Sept, 2015

To All Athletic Trainers and the Students at Loveland High School

Keith Kitchens

DeLee & Drez's

Orthopaedic Sports Medicine

PRINCIPLES AND PRACTICE

FOURTH EDITION

DELEE & DREZ'S

Orthopaedic Sports Medicine

PRINCIPLES AND PRACTICE

FOURTH EDITION

VOLUME II

MARK D. MILLER, MD
S. Ward Casscells Professor of Orthopaedic Surgery
Head, Division of Sports Medicine
University of Virginia
Charlottesville, Virginia
Adjunctive Clinical Professor and Team Physician
James Madison University
Harrisonburg, Virginia

STEPHEN R. THOMPSON, MD, MED, FRCSC
Orthopaedic Staff Surgeon
Department of Orthopaedics
Eastern Maine Medical Center
Bangor, Maine

ELSEVIER
SAUNDERS

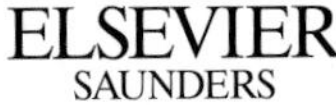

ELSEVIER
SAUNDERS

1600 John F. Kennedy Blvd.
Ste 1800
Philadelphia, PA 19103-2899

DELEE & DREZ'S ORTHOPAEDIC SPORTS MEDICINE: PRINCIPLES AND PRACTICE, FOURTH EDITION ISBN: 978-1-4557-4376-6

Notices

Knowledge and best practice in this field are constantly changing. As new research and experience broaden our understanding, changes in research methods, professional practices, or medical treatment may become necessary.

Practitioners and researchers must always rely on their own experience and knowledge in evaluating and using any information, methods, compounds, or experiments described herein. In using such information or methods they should be mindful of their own safety and the safety of others, including parties for whom they have a professional responsibility.

With respect to any drug or pharmaceutical products identified, readers are advised to check the most current information provided (i) on procedures featured or (ii) by the manufacturer of each product to be administered, to verify the recommended dose or formula, the method and duration of administration, and contraindications. It is the responsibility of practitioners, relying on their own experience and knowledge of their patients, to make diagnoses, to determine dosages and the best treatment for each individual patient, and to take all appropriate safety precautions.

To the fullest extent of the law, neither the Publisher nor the authors, contributors, or editors, assume any liability for any injury and/or damage to persons or property as a matter of products liability, negligence or otherwise, or from any use or operation of any methods, products, instructions, or ideas contained in the material herein.

ISBN: 978-1-4557-4376-6

Senior Content Strategist: Don Scholz
Senior Content Development Specialist: Joan Ryan
Publishing Services Manager: Patricia Tannian
Project Manager: Carrie Stetz
Design Direction: Ellen Zanolle

Printed in China

Last digit is the print number: 9 8 7 6 5 4 3 2 1

To my brilliant and beautiful wife, Ann,
for putting up with all my projects.

To my four children, all athletes in their own right.

And, to athletes everywhere and at every level—
being an athlete is like being a senator or a general—
once an athlete, always an athlete!

MARK D. MILLER

For Harper Finn: you are too young to read this now,
and you may choose never to read this later,
but it is nonetheless still for you.

And for Shannon: you have my unending gratitude
for letting me devote time to these things.

STEPHEN R. THOMPSON

Section Editors

Cy Frank, MD
Professor, Department of Surgery
Faculty of Medicine
University of Calgary
Calgary, Alberta, Canada
Basic Principles

Dilaawar J. Mistry, MD
Primary Care Team Physician, Colorado Rockies (Grand Junction)
Team Physician, USA Swimming
Western Orthopedics and Sports Medicine
Grand Junction, Colorado
Medical

Jeff G. Konin, PT, PhD
Professor and Chair, Physical Therapy Department
University of Rhode Island
Kingston, Rhode Island
Rehabilitation and Injury Prevention

Craig Bottoni, MD
Chief, Sports Medicine
Orthopaedic Surgery Service
Tripler Army Medical Center
Honolulu, Hawaii
Shoulder

Lance M. Brunton, MD
Clinical Assistant Professor
Department of Orthopaedic Surgery
University of Pittsburgh Medical Center
Pittsburgh, Pennsylvania;
Excela Health Orthopedics and Sports Medicine
Latrobe, Pennsylvania
Elbow, Wrist, and Hand

Victor Manuel Ilizaliturri Sánchez Jr., MD
Department Chief
Professor of Hip and Knee Surgery
National Institute of Rehabilitation
Mexico City, Mexico
Pelvis, Hip, and Thigh

F. Winston Gwathmey Jr., MD
Assistant Professor of Orthopaedic Surgery
University of Virginia School of Medicine
Charlottesville, Virginia
Pelvis, Hip, and Thigh

David R. McAllister, MD
Chief, Sports Medicine Service
Professor and Vice Chair
Department of Orthopaedic Surgery
David Geffen School of Medicine at UCLA
Los Angeles, California
Knee

Anish R. Kadakia, MD
Editor in Chief
Journal of Orthopedic Surgery and Research
Associate Professor of Orthopedic Surgery
Northwestern Memorial Hospital
Northwestern University Feinberg School of Medicine
Chicago, Illinois
Leg, Ankle, and Foot

William C. Lauerman, MD[†]
Professor of Orthopaedic Surgery
Chief, Division of Spine Surgery
Department of Orthopaedic Surgery
Georgetown University Hospital
Washington, DC
Spine and Head

Matthew Milewski, MD
Elite Sports Medicine
Connecticut Children's Medical Center
Farmington, Connecticut
Pediatric Sports Medicine

[†]Deceased.

Preface

Congratulations! You have the most up-to-date and comprehensive treatise on sports medicine in the world in your hands. *DeLee & Drez's Sports Medicine: Principles and Practice* has long been considered the most trusted source in the field, and this edition is the best yet. We have completely reorganized this textbook from the ground up; we completely revised the presentation of material and then invited only the best authors to contribute, regardless of who wrote previous chapters. We also took on the challenge of the figures and revised or replaced every piece of art. Finally, we developed a logical template for the structure of the chapters and insisted on its use—even to the point of returning chapters or re-assigning them to make sure that you, the reader, could find accurate and current information quickly and easily.

Important new information on concussion, hip and groin injuries (including an extensive expansion of the hip arthroscopy sections), medical management of the athlete, head and facial injuries, and the para-athlete highlight some of the most important features of this wonderfully put together fourth edition.

Like all comprehensive textbooks, this product is the result of the combined efforts of a dedicated team of authors, section editors, and publisher support. All of the section editors did a superb job, but special recognition must be given to Drs. Winston Gwathmey, Dave McCallister, Matt Milewski, Lance Brunton, Danny Mistry, Jeff Konin, and Anish Kadakia. We are deeply saddened that we cannot personally thank Dr. William Lauerman, who passed away suddenly before publication. He dutifully and meticulously edited the spine section. Instead, we dedicate this edition to his memory. He was a wonderful and dedicated surgeon, educator, investigator, and writer. Our edition was made all that much better with his involvement, and we will sorely miss him.

We would be remiss if we didn't give a special "shout out" to the master surgeons themselves, Drs. Jesse DeLee and David Drez. This textbook was their vision, and they were the architects; we are just the construction crew. Thank you for trusting us to help keep your knowledge of sports medicine on the cutting edge. We look forward to having you put it to use in the care of athletes of all ages and abilities.

Go Team!

Mark D. Miller

Stephen R. Thompson

Contributors

Kathleen C. Abalos
Resident, Internal Medicine
Beth Israel Deaconess Medical Center
Boston, Massachusetts

Alexander M. Aboka, MD, MPH
Orthopaedic Surgeon
Sports Medicine & Arthroscopy Specialist
Virginia Orthopaedic & Spine Specialists
Hampton Roads, Virginia

Jeffrey S. Abrams, MD
Clinical Professor
School of Graduate Medicine
Seton Hall University
South Orange, New Jersey;
Attending Surgeon
Department of Orthopaedic Surgery
University Medical Center of Princeton at Plainsboro
Princeton, New Jersey

Scott M. Adams, MD
Orthopaedic Surgeon
Sports Medicine
Orthopaedic Associates of Central Maryland
Baltimore, Maryland

Mohd Al Ateeq Al Dosari, MD
Director
Bone & Joint Institute
Head
Orthopedic Surgery
Hamad Medical Corporation
Doha, Qatar

Mauro Alini, PhD
Vice Director and Head
Musculoskeletal Regeneration Program
AO Research Institute
Davos, Switzerland

Ma'ad F. Al-Saati, MD
Consultant Orthopaedic Surgeon
Sports Medicine
Vice President
Saati Medical Center
Riyadh, Saudi Arabia

Peter E. Amato Jr., MD
Instructor of Anesthesiology
University of Virginia Health System
Charlottesville, Virginia

Annunziato Amendola, MD
Professor and Director
University of Iowa Sports Medicine Center
Department of Orthopaedics and Rehabilitation Faculty
University of Iowa Hospitals and Clinics
Iowa City, Iowa

Lindsay Andras, MD
Assistant Professor of Orthopaedic Surgery
Keck School of Medicine
University of Southern California
Children's Hospital Los Angeles
Los Angeles, California

James R. Andrews, MD
Medical Director
The Andrews Institute
Gulf Breeze, Florida;
Medical Director
The American Sports Medicine Institute
Birmingham, Alabama

Thomas Andriacchi, MD
Professor
Department of Mechanical Engineering and Department of Orthopedic Surgery
Palo Veterans Administration
Stanford University
Redwood City, California

Robert A. Arciero, MD
Professor and Chief
Sports Medicine Division
Department of Orthopaedic Surgery
University of Connecticut Health Center
Farmington, Connecticut

Kevin Asem, MD
Assistant Professor
Department of Family Medicine
Fowler Kennedy Sport Medicine Clinic
Western University
London, Ontario, Canada

Chad A. Asplund, MD
Medical Director
Sports Medicine and Student Health Services
Associate Professor, Family Medicine
Team Physician, Augusta Greenjackets
Georgia Regents University
Augusta, Georgia

Robert E. Atkinson, MD
Associate Professor
University of Hawaii Division of Orthopedic Surgery
John A. Burns School of Medicine
Honolulu, Hawaii

Luke S. Austin, MD
Assistant Professor of Orthopaedics
Rothman Institute
Egg Harbor Township, New Jersey

Bernard R. Bach Jr., MD
The Claude Lambert-Susan Thomsen Professor of Orthopedic Surgery
Director, Division of Sports Medicine
Director, Sports Medicine Fellowship Program
Rush University Medical Center
Chicago, Illinois

Aaron L. Baggish, MD
Cardiovascular Performance Program
Massachusetts General Hospital
Team Cardiologist, Boston Bruins and New England Patriots
Team Cardiologist, Harvard University
Boston, Massachusetts

Roald Bahr, MD, PhD
Professor of Sports Medicine
Department of Sports Medicine
Norwegian School of Sport Sciences
Chair, Oslo Sports Trauma Research
Oslo, Norway

Caroline Baratz
University of California–San Diego
San Diego, California

Mark E. Baratz, MD
Vice Chairman
Department of Orthopaedic Surgery
Allegheny General Hospital
Pittsburgh, Pennsylvania

Jeffrey T. Barth, PhD
Professor, Department of Psychiatry and Neurobehavioral Sciences
Director, Brain Injury and Sports Concussion Institute
University of Virginia School of Medicine
Charlottesville, Virginia

Robert W. Battle, MD
Team Cardiologist
Associate Professor of Medicine and Pediatrics
Department of Cardiology
University of Virginia
Charlottesville, Virginia

Frank Berkowitz, MD
Associate Professor of Radiology
Georgetown University School of Medicine
Chief of Neuroradiology
Georgetown University Hospital
Washington, DC

Thomas M. Best, MD, PhD
Professor and Pomerene Endowed Chair
Director, Division of Sports Medicine
Department of Family Medicine
Professor of Biomedical Engineering and Bioinformatics
The Ohio State University
Columbus, Ohio

Bruce Beynnon, PhD
McClure Professor of Musculoskeletal Research
Director of Research
Department of Orthopaedics and Rehabilitation
University of Vermont College of Medicine
McClure Musculoskeletal Research Center
Burlington, Vermont

Rishi Bhatnagar, MD
Precision Orthopaedics and Sports Medicine
Laurel, Maryland

Randy Bird, MS, RD
Director of Sports Nutrition
University of Virginia
Charlottesville, Virginia

Patrick M. Birmingham, MD
Sports Medicine & Orthopaedic Surgery
Northshore University Health System
Chicago, Illinois

Debdut Biswas, MD
Orthopaedic Surgery Resident
Section of Hand and Elbow Surgery
Department of Orthopaedic Surgery
Rush University Medical Center
Chicago, Illinois

Melanie Bonin, MD
Assistant Professor
Department of Family Medicine
Fowler Kennedy Sport Medicine Clinic
Western University
London, Ontario, Canada

Itamar B. Botser, MD
Clinical Fellow
Orthopaedic Sports Medicine
Stanford University
Redwood City, California

Margaret K. Boushell, MS
Biomaterials and Interface Tissue Engineering Laboratory
Department of Biomedical Engineering
Columbia University
New York, New York

Katherine Boyer, PhD
Assistant Professor
Department of Kinesiology
University of Massachusetts–Amherst
Amherst, Massachusetts

James P. Bradley, MD
Clinical Professor of Orthopaedic Surgery
University of Pittsburgh Medical Center
Pittsburgh, Pennsylvania

Jonathan T. Bravman, MD
Assistant Professor
Director of Sports Medicine Research
CU Sports Medicine
Division of Sports Medicine and Shoulder Surgery
University of Colorado
Denver, Colorado

Stephen F. Brockmeier, MD
Assistant Professor
Department of Orthopaedic Surgery
University of Virginia
Charlottesville, Virginia

Adam G. Brooks, MD
San Francisco Orthopaedic Residency Program
St. Mary's Medical Center
San Francisco, California

Donna K. Broshek, PhD
Associate Professor
Department of Psychiatry and Neurobehavioral Sciences
Associate Director
Brain Injury and Sports Concussion Institute
University of Virginia School of Medicine
Charlottesville, Virginia

Jefferey Brunelli, MD
Orthopedics and Sports Medicine
Liberty Orthopedics & Sports Medicine
Hinesville, Georgia

Lance M. Brunton, MD
Clinical Assistant Professor
Department of Orthopaedic Surgery
University of Pittsburgh Medical Center
Pittsburgh, Pennsylvania;
Excela Health Orthopedics & Sports Medicine
Latrobe, Pennsylvania

Brian Busconi, MD
Associate Professor of Orthopedics
Chief of Sports Medicine and Arthroscopy
University of Massachusetts Medical Center
Worcester, Massachusetts

Charles A. Bush-Joseph, MD
Professor, Department of Orthopaedic Surgery
Rush University Medical Center
Managing Member, Midwest Orthopaedics at Rush
Chicago, Illinois

Glenn Buterbaugh, MD
Clinical Associate Professor and President
Western PA Surgery Center
Clinical Associate Professor
University of Pittsburgh
Pittsburgh, Pennsylvania

David L. Butler, MD
Professor Emeritus
Tissue Engineering and Biomechanics Laboratories
University of Cincinnati, Ohio

J.W. Thomas Byrd, MD
Nashville Sports Medicine Foundation
Nashville, Tennessee

E. Lyle Cain Jr., MD
American Sports Medicine Institute
Andrews Sports Medicine and Orthopaedic Center
Birmingham, Alabama

John Campbell, MD
Orthopaedic Faculty
Institute for Foot and Ankle Reconstruction
Baltimore, Maryland

Kevin Caperton, MD
Orthopedics and Sports Medicine
Georgetown Orthopedics
Georgetown, Texas

Erik Carlson, MD
Chief Resident
Department of Orthopaedics and Rehabilitation
Yale University School of Medicine
New Haven, Connecticut

Rebecca Cerrato, MD
Orthopaedic Faculty
Institute for Foot and Ankle Reconstruction
Baltimore, Maryland

Jas Chahal, MD
Assistant Professor
Department of Surgery
Division of Orthopaedics
Toronto Western Hospital and Women's College Hospital
University of Toronto
Toronto, Ontario, Canada

Peter N. Chalmers, MD
Orthopaedic Resident
Orthopaedic Surgery
Rush University Medical Center
Chicago, Illinois

Aakash Chauhan, MD, MBA
Department of Orthopaedics
Allegheny General Hospital
Pittsburgh, Pennsylvania

A. Bobby Chhabra, MD
Lillian T. Pratt Distinguished Professor and Chair
Department of Orthopaedic Surgery
Professor of Plastic Surgery
Co-Director
UVA Hand Center
University of Virginia Health System
Charlottesville, Virginia

Eric Chicas, DPT
Physical Therapist
Memorial Hermann Ironman Sports Medicine Institute
Houston, Texas

John Jared Christophel, MD, MPH
Assistant Professor
Department of Otolaryngology–Head & Neck Surgery
University of Virginia
Charlottesville, Virginia

Philip J. Chuang, MS
Biomaterials and Interface Tissue Engineering Laboratory
Department of Biomedical Engineering
Columbia University
New York, New York

Mario Ciocca, MD
Director of Sports Medicine
Assistant Professor of Internal Medicine and Orthopaedics
Department of Internal Medicine/Orthopaedics
University of North Carolina
Chapel Hill, North Carolina

John P. Clement, MD, PhD
Musculoskeletal Radiologist
South Texas Radiology Group
San Antonio, Texas

Brian J. Cole, MD, MBA
Professor
Department of Orthopaedics
Department of Anatomy and Cell Biology
Section Head
Cartilage Restoration Center
Rush University Medical Center
Chicago, Illinois

Andrew J. Cosgarea, MD
Professor of Orthopaedic Surgery
Department of Orthopaedic Surgery
Director of Sports Medicine
Johns Hopkins University
Baltimore, Maryland

Juan Eugenio Cosme, MD
Radiologist
Professor of the Fellowship
Magnetic Resonance Unit
Instituto Nacional de la Nutrición Salvador Zubiran
Medica Sur Hospital
Mexico City, Mexico

Jeffrey Cunningham, MD
General Surgery
UPMC Mercy
Pittsburgh, Pennsylvania

Ralph J. Curtis, MD
Clinical Professor
Orthopaedic Surgery
University of Texas Health Science Center
Sports Medicine Associates of San Antonio
San Antonio, Texas

Shannon David, PhD
Professor of Orthopaedic Surgery
University of Southern California
Chief of Orthopaedic Surgery
Children's Hospital Los Angeles
Los Angeles, California

Thomas M. DeBerardino, MD
Associate Professor
Department of Orthopaedic Surgery
University of Connecticut Health Center
Orthopaedic Team Physician
University of Connecticut
Farmington, Connecticut

Richard E. Debski, PhD
Associate Professor
Orthopaedic Robotics Laboratory
Departments of Bioengineering and Orthopaedic Surgery
University of Pittsburgh, Pennsylvania

Marc M. DeHart, MD
Clinical Assistant Professor
Department of Orthopaedic Surgery and Rehabilitation
University of Texas Medical Branch
Galveston, Texas;
Clinical Assistant Professor
Department of Surgery
Texas A&M Health Science Center College of Medicine
Round Rock, Texas

Jeffrey M. DeLong, BS
Medical University of South Carolina
Charleston, South Carolina

Arthur Jason De Luigi, DO
Program Director
Sports Medicine Fellowship
Director, Sports Medicine
MedStar National Rehabilitation Hospital
Washington Hospital Center
Georgetown University Hospital
Associate Professor of Clinical Rehabilitation Medicine
Georgetown University School of Medicine
Washington, DC

Marco Demange, MD
Sports Medicine and Shoulder Surgery
Hospital for Special Surgery
New York, New York

John J. Densmore, MD, PhD
Associate Professor of Clinical Medicine
Division of Hematology/Oncology
University of Virginia
Charlottesville, Virginia

Ashvin K. Dewan, MD
House Staff
Orthopaedic Surgery
Johns Hopkins School of Medicine
Baltimore, Maryland

Seth D. Dodds, MD
Associate Professor
Hand and Upper Extremity Surgery
Department of Orthopaedics and Rehabilitation
Yale University School of Medicine
New Haven, Connecticut

Benjamin G. Domb, MD
Clinical Assistant Director
Loyola University Stritch School of Medicine
Medical Director
American Hip Institute
Hinsdale Orthopedics
Chicago, Illinois

William F. Donaldson III, MD
Professor and Chief of Spine Service
Department of Orthopaedic Surgery
University of Pittsburgh Medical Center
Pittsburgh, Pennsylvania

Jeffrey R. Dugas, MD
Andrews Sports Medicine and Orthopedic Center
Head Team Physician
Troy University
Fellowship Director
American Sports Medicine Institute
Birmingham, Alabama

Kostas J. Economopoulos, MD
Attending Orthopaedic Surgeon
The Orthopedic Clinic Association
Phoenix, Arizona

Marsha Eifert-Mangine, MD
Associate Professor
Health Sciences
College of Mount St. Joseph
Cincinnati, Ohio

Christoph Erggelet, MD, PhD
Professor of Orthopaedic Surgery
University of Freiburg Medical Center
Freiburg, Germany

Brandon J. Erickson, MD
Resident Physician
Rush University Medical Center
Chicago, Illinois

Fatih Ertem, MSc
Department of Biomechanics
Dokuz Eylul University Health Science Institute
Inciralti, Izmir, Turkey;
Visiting Graduate Researcher
Department of Orthopaedics and Rehabilitation
McClure Musculoskeletal Research Center
Burlington, Vermont

Mark S Eskander, MD
Spine Surgery
Christiana Spine Center
Newark, Delaware

Norman Espinosa, MD
Head of Foot and Ankle Surgery
Department of Orthopaedics
University of Zurich
Zurich, Switzerland

Jesse L. Even, MD
Sports Medicine
Arlington Orthopedic Associates
Arlington, Texas

Yale Fillingham, MD
Department of Orthopaedic Surgery
Rush University Medical Center
Chicago, Illinois

Lisa Fischer, BScPT, MD
Assistant Professor
Departments of Family Medicine and Kinesiology
Director, Primary Care Sports Medicine
Fowler Kennedy Sports Medicine Clinic
Western University
London, Ontario, Canada

Rachel M. Frank, MD
Department of Orthopaedic Surgery
Rush University Medical Center
Chicago, Illinois

Heather Freeman, PT, DHS
Physical Therapist
Assistant Research Coordinator
Shelbourne Knee Center
Indianapolis, Indiana

Jason R. Freeman, PhD
Associate Professor
Department of Psychiatry and Neurobehavioral Sciences
Associate Director
Brain Injury and Sports Concussion Institute
University of Virginia School of Medicine
Charlottesville, Virginia

Raffaele Garofalo, MD
Shoulder Service
F. Miulli Hospital
Acquaviva delle fonti-BA, Italy

William E. Garrett Jr., MD, PhD
Professor of Sports Medicine
Department of Orthopaedics
Duke University
Durham, North Carolina

R. Glenn Gaston, MD
Hand and Upper Extremity Surgeon
OrthoCarolina;
Chief of Hand Surgery
Department of Orthopedics
Carolinas Medical Center
Charlotte, North Carolina

Andrew G. Geeslin, MD
Orthopaedic Surgery Resident
Department of Orthopaedic Surgery
Western Michigan University School of Medicine
Kalamazoo, Michigan

William B. Geissler, MD
Professor and Chief
Division of Hand and Upper Extremity Surgery
University of Mississippi Health Care
Jackson, Mississippi

J. Robert Giffin, MD
Associate Professor
Department of Surgery
Western University
London, Ontario, Canada

Thomas A. Gill, MS
John A. Burns School of Medicine
University of Hawaii
Honolulu, Hawaii

Pau Golanó, MD
Professor of Human Anatomy
Laboratory of Arthroscopic and Surgical Anatomy
Human Anatomy and Embryology Unit
Department of Pathology and Experimental Therapeutics
University of Barcelona, Spain;
Department of Orthopaedic Surgery
University of Pittsburgh School of Medicine
Pittsburgh, Pennsylvania

Jorge Gómez, MD
Associate Professor
Adolescent Medicine & Sports Medicine
Baylor College of Medicine;
Assistant Team Physician
University of Houston
Houston, Texas

Andreas H. Gomoll, MD
Assistant Professor of Orthopaedic Surgery
Harvard Medical School
Department of Orthopaedic Surgery
Brigham and Women's Hospital
Boston, Massachusetts

Howard P. Goodkin, MD, PhD
The Shure Professor of Pediatric Neurology
Director
Division of Pediatric Neurology
Departments of Neurology and Pediatrics
University of Virginia
Charlottesville, Virginia

David Goodwin, MD
Resident Physician
Department of Orthopaedics
Georgetown University Hospital
Washington, DC

Thomas J. Graham, MD
Chief Innovation Officer
Justice Family Chair in Medical Innovations
Vice Chair
Department of Orthopaedic Surgery
Cleveland Clinic Innovations
Cleveland, Ohio

Phillip Gribble, PhD
Professor of Kinesiology
University of Toledo
Toledo, Ohio

Michael J. Griesser, MD
Orthopedic Surgeon
Performance Orthopaedics and Sports Medicine
Clinton Memorial Hospital
Wilmington, Ohio

Justin W. Griffin, MD
Resident Physician
Department of Orthopaedic Surgery
University of Virginia
Charlottesville, Virginia

Letha Griffin, MD, PhD
Peachtree Orthopaedic Clinic
Team Physician
Georgia State University
Atlanta, Georgia

Andrew J. Grove, MD
Primary Care/Sports Medicine Physician
Marquette University Medical Clinic
Team Physician
Department of Intercollegiate Athletics
Marquette University
Milwaukee, Wisconsin

Carlos A. Guanche, MD
Teaching Faculty
Southern California Orthopedic Institute
Van Nuys, California;
Adjunct Clinical Professor
University of Southern California
Los Angeles, California

James J. Guerra, MD
Clinical Associate Professor
Florida Gulf Coast University
Estero, Florida;
Attending Physician
Collier Sports Medicine and Orthopedic Center
Naples, Florida

Mark G. Hamming, MD
Orthopaedic Surgeon
Illinois Bone and Joint Institute
Lake Shore Orthopaedics
Lake Forest, Illinois

Daniel M. Hampton, MD
Greater Metropolitan Orthopaedic Institute
Alexandria, Virginia

Bryan T. Hanypsiak, MD
Voluntary Clinical Attending Physician
Mount Sinai Medical Center
New York, New York;
Director of Medical Education
Arthrex
Naples, Florida

Talal Hariri, DPT
Physical Therapist
Memorial Hermann Ironman Sports Medicine Institute
Houston, Texas

Joshua D. Harris, MD
Assistant Professor
Houston Methodist Hospital
Center for Orthopaedics and Sports Medicine
Houston, Texas

Jennifer A. Hart, MPAS, PA-C
Physician Assistant
Department of Orthopaedic Surgery
University of Virginia
Charlottesville, Virginia

Andrew Haskell, MD
Fellowship Co-Director and Department Co-Chair
Department of Orthopaedics
Palo Alto Medical Foundation
Palo Alto, California;
Assistant Clinical Professor
Department of Orthopaedic Surgery
University of California–San Francisco
San Francisco, California

Munif Hatem, MD
Hip Preservation Center
Baylor University Medical Center
Dallas, Texas

Bryan D. Haughom, MD
Resident Physician
Rush University Medical Center
Chicago, Illinois

Michael R. Hausman, MD
Professor of Orthopedic Surgery
Vice-Chairman
Department of Orthopedics
Mount Sinai Medical Center
New York, New York

Daniel Herman, MD, PhD
Assistant Professor
Divisions of PM&R, Sports Medicine, and Research
Department of Orthopaedics and Rehabilitation
University of Florida
Gainesville, Florida

C. Joel Hess, MD
Resident Physician
Physical Medicine and Rehabilitation
University of Virginia
Charlottesville, Virginia

Carolyn M. Hettrich, MD, MPH
Assistant Professor
Department of Orthopaedic Surgery and Rehabilitation
University of Iowa Sports Medicine Center
Iowa City, Iowa

MaCalus Hogan, MD
Assistant Professor
Division of Foot and Ankle Surgery
Assistant Residency Program Director
Department of Orthopaedic Surgery
University of Pittsburgh School of Medicine
University of Pittsburgh Medical Center
Pittsburgh, Pennsylvania

Christopher Hogrefe, MD
Clinical Assistant Professor
Emergency Medicine and Primary Care Sports Medicine
University of Iowa Hospitals and Clinics
Iowa City, Iowa

Catherine Hui, MD
Clinical Lecturer
Department of Surgery
Division of Orthopaedic Surgery
Glen Sather Sports Medicine Clinic
University of Alberta
Edmonton, Alberta, Canada

Waqas M. Hussain, MD
Sports Orthopaedic Fellow
Department of Orthopaedic Surgery
The Cleveland Clinic Foundation
Garfield Heights, Ohio

Victor Manuel Ilizaliturri Sánchez Jr., MD
Department Chief
Professor of Hip and Knee Surgery
National Institute of Rehabilitation
Mexico City, Mexico

John V. Ingari, MD
Chairman
Division of Orthopaedic Surgery
Fellowship Director
York Hospital Hand Fellowship
York Hospital
York, Pennsylvania

Todd A. Irwin, MD
Assistant Professor
Department of Orthopaedic Surgery
University of Michigan
Ann Arbor, Michigan

Nicolas V. Jaumard, MD
Postdoctoral Fellow
Department of Neurosurgery
Department of Bioengineering
University of Pennsylvania
Philadelphia, Pennsylvania

Tatiana Jevremovic, MD
Assistant Professor
Department of Family Medicine
Primary Care Physician
Fowler Kennedy Sport Medicine Clinic
Western University
London, Ontario, Canada

Darren L. Johnson, MD
Chairman
Department of Orthopaedic Surgery
University of Kentucky
Lexington, Kentucky

Don Johnson, MD
Director
Sports Medicine Clinic
Carleton University;
Assistant Professor of Orthopaedic Surgery
Department of Orthopaedics
University of Ottawa
Ottawa, Ontario, Canada

Jared S. Johnson, MD
The Steadman Clinic
Vail, Colorado

Ron M. Johnson, MPT
Facility Director
Excel Sports Therapy
Shiner, Texas

Grant L. Jones, MD
Associate Professor
Department of Orthopaedic Surgery
The Ohio State University
Columbus, Ohio

Anish R. Kadakia, MD
Editor in Chief
Journal of Orthopaedic Surgery and Research
Associate Professor of Orthopaedic Surgery
Northwestern Memorial Hospital
Northwestern University Feinberg School of Medicine
Chicago, Illinois

S. Babak Kalantar, MD
Assistant Professor of Spinal Surgery
Department of Orthopaedics
Georgetown University Hospital
Washington, DC

Kambiz Kalantari, MD
Associate Professor of Medicine
Division of Nephrology
University of Virginia Health System
Charlottesville, Virginia

Thomas W. Kaminski, PhD
Professor of Kinesiology & Applied Physiology
Professor & Director of Athletic Training Education
Department of Kinesiology & Applied Physiology
University of Delaware
Newark, Delaware

Christopher A. Keen, MD
Citrus Orthopaedic Joint and Bone Institute
Lecanto, Florida

Bryan T. Kelly, MD
Associate Professor of Orthopaedic Surgery
Weill Cornell Medical College
Associate Attending Orthopaedic Surgeon
New York—Presbyterian Hospital
Associate Attending Orthopaedic Surgeon
Hospital for Special Surgery
New York, New York

Susan E. Kirk, MD
Associate Professor of Medicine and Obstetrics and Gynecology
University of Virginia
Charlottesville, Virginia

Donald T. Kirkendall, PhD, ELS
Center for Learning Healthcare
Duke Clinical Research Institute
Durham, North Carolina

Mininder S. Kocher, MD, MPH
Professor of Orthopaedic Surgery
Harvard Medical School
Associate Director
Division of Sports Medicine
Children's Hospital Boston
Boston, Massachusetts

Sumant G. Krishnan, MD
The Shoulder Center
Baylor University Medical Center
Dallas, Texas

Marshall A. Kuremsky, MD
Triangle Orthopaedic Associates
Raleigh, North Carolina

Shawn M. Kutnik, MD
Hand and Upper Extremity Surgery
Premier Care Orthopedics
St. Louis, Missouri

Jessica Kynyk, MD
Assistant Professor of Internal Medicine
Department of Pulmonary, Allergy, Critical Care, and Sleep Medicine
Wexner Medical Center at Ohio State University
Columbus, Ohio

Robert F. LaPrade, MD, PhD
Chief Medical Research Officer
Deputy Director, Sports Medicine Fellowship Program
Director, International Scholar Program
Steadman Philippon Research Institute
The Steadman Clinic
Vail, Colorado

Christopher M. Larson, MD
Minnesota Orthopedic Sports Medicine Institute at Twin Cities Orthopedics
Edina, Minnesota

William C. Lauerman, MD†
Professor of Orthopaedic Surgery
Chief, Division of Spine Surgery
Department of Orthopaedic Surgery
Georgetown University Hospital
Washington, DC

Peter Lawrence, MD
Division of Vascular Surgery
David Geffen School of Medicine at UCLA
Los Angeles, California

Nicholas LeCursi, CO
Senior Orthotist
Orthotics and Prosthetics
University of Michigan
Ann Arbor, Michigan;
Lecturer/Clinical Director
Orthotics & Prosthetics
Department of Health Promotion and Human Performance
Eastern Michigan University
Ypsilanti, Michigan

William N. Levine, MD
Vice Chairman and Professor
Chief, Shoulder Service
Co-director, Center for Shoulder, Elbow, and Sports Medicine
Department of Orthopaedic Surgery
New York Presbyterian–Columbia University Medical Center
New York, New York

Thomas R. Lewis, MD
Assistant Professor
Department of Orthopaedic Surgery
University of Oklahoma College of Medicine
Oklahoma City, Oklahoma

Richard L. Lieber, PhD
Professor and Vice Chair
Department of Orthopaedic Surgery
University of California and VA Medical Centers
La Jolla, California

Kenneth Lindell, MD
Chief of Musculoskeletal Imaging
Department of Radiology
Tripler Army Medical Center
Honolulu, Hawaii

Thomas N. Lindenfeld, MD
Associate Director
Cincinnati Sports Medicine and Orthopaedic Center
Cincinnati, Ohio

Robert B. Litchfield, MD
Medical Director
Fowler Kennedy Sport Medicine Clinic
Associate Professor
University of Western Ontario
London, Ontario, Canada

Carlos A. Lopez, MD
St. Joseph's Health Centre
Toronto, Ontario, Canada

Gary M. Lourie, MD
Chief
Division of Hand Surgery
Atlanta Medical Center
The Hand and Upper Extremity Center of Georgia
Atlanta, Georgia

Walter R. Lowe, MD
Edward T. Smith Professor and Chairman
Department of Orthopedic Surgery
University of Texas Medical School
Houston, Texas

Helen H. Lu, PhD
Associate Professor of Biomedical Engineering
Associate Professor of Dental and Craniofacial Engineering
Columbia University
New York, New York

Richard Ma, MD
Sports Medicine and Shoulder Surgery
Hospital for Special Surgery
New York, New York

Travis G. Maak, MD
Assistant Professor of Orthopaedic Surgery
University of Utah
Salt Lake City, Utah

John MacKnight, MD
Professor of Internal Medicine and Orthopaedic Surgery
Medical Director for Sports Medicine
Primary Care Team Physician
University of Virginia
Charlottesville, Virginia

Henning Madry, MD
Professor of Experimental Orthopaedics and Osteoarthritis Research
Head, Center of Experimental Orthopaedics
Saarland University
Homburg, Germany

†Deceased.

Suzanne Maher, PhD
Associate Scientist
Hospital for Special Surgery
New York, New York

Francesc Malagelada, MD
Surgical Research Fellow and Orthopaedic Surgeon
South West London Elective Orthopaedic Centre
Epsom, Surrey, United Kingdom

Robert Mangine, MEd, PT
Assistant Professor of Physical Therapy
College of Mount St. Joseph;
Adjunct Assistant Professor
Department of Orthopaedics
Clinical Instructor of Rehabilitation
Sports Medicine Fellowship Training Program
University of Cincinnati;
National Director of Clinical Research and Education
NovaCare Rehabilitation
Cincinnati, Ohio

Michael A. Marchetti, MD
Clinical Research Fellow
Dermatology Service
Department of Medicine
Memorial Sloan-Kettering Cancer Center
New York, New York

Britt Marcussen, MD
Associate Professor of Family Medicine and Primary Care Sports Medicine
University of Iowa Hospitals and Clinics
Iowa City, Iowa

Hal David Martin, DO
Hip Preservation Center
Baylor University Medical Center
Dallas, Texas

Lyndon Mason, MB BCh
Foot and Ankle Fellow
Aintree University Hospital
Liverpool, United Kingdom

Elizabeth G. Matzkin, MD
Assistant Professor
Department of Orthopaedic Surgery
Harvard Medical School
Chief of Women's Sports Medicine
Department of Orthopedics
Brigham and Women's Hospital
Boston, Massachusetts

Augustus D. Mazzocca, MD
Director
New England Musculoskeletal Institute
Professor and Chairman
Department of Orthopaedic Surgery
University of Connecticut Health Center
Farmington, Connecticut

David R. McAllister, MD
Chief, Sports Medicine Service
Professor and Vice Chair
Department of Orthopaedic Surgery
David Geffen School of Medicine at UCLA
Los Angeles, California

Joseph C. McCarthy, MD
Vice Chairman
Department of Orthopedic Surgery
Massachusetts General Hospital
Boston, Massachusetts

Eric C. McCarty, MD
Chief, Sports Medicine & Shoulder Surgery
Associate Professor, Department of Orthopaedics
University of Colorado School of Medicine
Denver, Colorado;
Director, Sports Medicine
Department of Athletics
Associate Adjunct Professor
Department of Integrative Physiology
University of Colorado
Boulder, Colorado

Robert G. McCormack, MD
Associate Professor
Department of Orthopedic Surgery
University of British Columbia
Vancouver, British Columbia, Canada

Kelly R. McCormick, MD
Hope Orthopedics of Oregon
Salem, Oregon

Brett W. McCoy, MD
Sports Orthopaedic Fellow
Department of Orthopaedic Surgery
The Cleveland Clinic Foundation
Cleveland, Ohio

Sean McMillan, DO
Chief of Orthopedics
Director of Orthopedic Sports Medicine and Arthroscopy
Department of Orthopedics
Lourdes Medical Associates & Lourdes Medical Center at Burlington
Burlington, New Jersey

Kenneth R. Means Jr., MD
Attending Physician
Curtis National Hand Center at Union Memorial Hospital
Baltimore, Maryland

Matthew D. Milewski, MD
Elite Sports Medicine
Connecticut Children's Medical Center
Farmington, Connecticut

Wanda Millard, MD
Associate Professor
Department of Medicine
Division of Emergency Medicine
Fowler Kennedy Sport Medicine Clinic
Western University
London, Ontario, Canada

Mark D. Miller, MD
S. Ward Casscells Professor of Orthopaedic Surgery
Head, Division of Sports Medicine
University of Virginia
Charlottesville, Virginia;
Adjunct Clinical Professor and Team Physician
James Madison University
Harrisonburg, Virginia

R. Matthew Miller, MS
Orthopaedic Robotics Laboratory
Departments of Bioengineering and Orthopaedic Surgery
University of Pittsburgh, Pennsylvania

Dilaawar J. Mistry, MD
Primary Care Team Physician, Colorado Rockies (Grand Junction)
Team Physician, USA Swimming
Western Orthopedics and Sports Medicine
Grand Junction, Colorado

Todd Moen, MD
W.B. Carrell Memorial Clinic
Dallas, Texas

Peter J. Moley, MD
Assistant Professor of Clinical Rehabilitation Medicine
Weill Cornell Medical College
Assistant Attending Physiatrist
Hospital for Special Surgery
New York, New York

Andrew Molloy, MBChB, MRCS
Consultant Orthopaedic Surgeon
Trauma and Orthopaedics
University Hospital Aintree;
Consultant Orthopaedic Surgeon
BMI Sefton Hospital
Liverpool, United Kingdom

Timothy S. Mologne, MD
Sports Medicine Center
Appleton, Wisconsin

Michael Montano, MD
Sports Medicine Center
University of Massachusetts Memorial Medical Center
Worcester, Massachusetts

Scott R. Montgomery, MD
Orthopaedic Surgery Resident
Department of Orthopaedic Surgery
University of California–Los Angeles
Los Angeles, California

Claude T. Moorman III, MD
Professor and Vice Chair
Department of Orthopaedic Surgery
Director of Sports Medicine
Duke University Medical Center
Durham, North Carolina

Nathan M. Nair, MD, MPH
Assistant Professor
Department of Neurosurgery
Georgetown University Hospital
Washington, DC

Norimasa Nakamura, MD, PhD
Professor
Institute for Medical Science in Sports
Osaka Health Science University
Osaka, Japan

Nima Nassiri, BS
Division of Vascular Surgery
David Geffen School of Medicine at UCLA
Los Angeles, California

Rebecca J. Nesbitt, BS
Graduate Student Researcher
Tissue Engineering and Biomechanical Laboratories
University of Cincinnati, Ohio

Jared A. Niska, MD
Resident Surgeon
Department of Orthopaedic Surgery
David Geffen School of Medicine at UCLA
Los Angeles, California

Carl W. Nissen, MD
Elite Sports Medicine
Connecticut Children's Medical Center
Professor
Department of Orthopaedics
University of Connecticut
Farmington, Connecticut

Shelley M. Oliver, MD
Northern Colorado Orthopedic Associates
Fort Collins, Colorado

Anell Olivos Meza, MD
Fellow, Articular Surgery
National Institute of Rehabilitation
Mexico City, Mexico

James Onate, PhD
Associate Professor
School of Health & Rehabilitation Sciences
The Ohio State University
Columbus, Ohio

Scott I. Otallah, MD
Department of Neurology
University of Virginia
Charlottesville, Virginia

Brett D. Owens, MD, LTC MC USA
Chief, Orthopaedic Surgery
Keller Army Hospital
West Point, New York

Corey A. Pacek, MD
Orthopaedic Hand and Upper Extremity Surgeon
Tri Rivers Surgical Associates
Pittsburgh, Pennsylvania

Russ Paine, PT
Director of Rehabilitation and Research
Memorial Hermann Ironman Sports Medicine Institute
Houston, Texas

Ian James Palmer, PhD
Baylor University Medical Center
Hip Preservation Center
Dallas, Texas

Richard D. Parker, MD
Chairman
Department of Orthopaedic Surgery
The Cleveland Clinic Foundation
Cleveland, Ohio

Jonathan P. Parsons, MD
Associate Professor of Internal Medicine
Pulmonary, Allergy, Critical Care, and Sleep Medicine
Wexner Medical Center at Ohio State University
Columbus, Ohio

Anthony Perera, MBChB, PGDip Med Law
Consultant Orthopaedic Foot and Ankle Surgeon
University Hospital of Wales
Spire Cardiff Hospital
Cardiff, United Kingdom;
London Foot and Ankle Centre
Cromwell Hospital
London, United Kingdom

Leanne Peters, MD
Adjunct Professor
Department of Family Medicine
Primary Care Physician
Sports Medicine
Western University
London, Ontario, Canada

Ninoska Peterson, PhD
Community Faculty
Department of Psychiatry and Behavioral Sciences
Eastern Virginia Medical School
Norfolk, Virginia

William A. Petri Jr., MD, PhD
Chief
Division of Infectious Disease and International Health
University of Virginia Health System;
Wade Hampton Frost Professor of Epidemiology
University of Virginia
Charlottesville, Virginia

Frank A. Petrigliano, MD
Assistant Professor
Department of Orthopaedic Surgery
David Geffen School of Medicine at UCLA
Los Angeles, California

Rory J. Petteys, MD
Senior Resident
Department of Neurosurgery
Georgetown University Hospital
Washington, DC

Robert Pivec, MD
Associate
Rubin Institute for Advanced Orthopedics
Center for Joint Preservation and Replacement
Sinai Hospital of Baltimore
Baltimore, Maryland

Matthew A. Posner, MD, MAJ MC USA
Orthopaedic Surgeon
Blanchfield Army Community Hospital
Fort Campbell, Kentucky

Teodor T. Postolache, MD
Director, Mood and Anxiety Program
Department of Psychiatry
University of Maryland School of Medicine
Baltimore, Maryland

Tricia K. Prokop, PT, MS
Department of Physical Therapy
Division of Sports Medicine
Connecticut Children's Medical Center
Hartford, Connecticut;
Part-Time Faculty
University of Hartford
West Hartford, Connecticut

Matthew T. Provencher, MD
Chief
Sports Medicine Service
Department of Orthopaedic Surgery
Massachusetts General Hospital
Boston, Massachusetts

Jason A. Ramsey, MD
The Center for Orthopedic Surgery
Lubbock, Texas

John Redmond, MD
Chicago Comprehensive Hip Fellow
American Hip Institute
Chicago, Illinois

David R. Richardson, MD
Program Director
Orthopaedic Surgery
University of Tennessee Campbell Clinic
Memphis, Tennessee

Christopher J. Roach, MD, LTC MC USA
Orthopaedic Surgeon
Brooke Army Medical Center
San Antonio, Texas

Elliot P. Robinson, MD
Resident Physician
Department of Orthopaedics
Carolinas Medical Center
Charlotte, North Carolina

Scott A. Rodeo, MD
Professor of Orthopaedic Surgery
Weill Medical College of Cornell University
New York, New York

Anthony A. Romeo, MD
Section Head
Shoulder and Elbow Surgery
Professor
Department of Orthopaedic Surgery
Rush University Medical Center
Chicago, Illinois

Melvin P. Rosenwasser, MD
Carroll Professor of Surgery of the Hand
Department of Orthopaedic Surgery
Attending Orthopaedic Surgeon
New York Presbyterian Hospital/Columbia University Medical Center;
Director, Trauma Training Center
Director, Hand Fellowship
Department of Orthopaedic Surgery
Columbia University
New York, New York

Mitchell H. Rosner, MD
Professor of Medicine
Chairman
Department of Medicine
Division of Nephrology
University of Virginia Health System
Charlottesville, Virginia

Heidi C. Rossetti, PhD
Assistant Professor
Department of Psychiatry
UT Southwestern Medical Center
Dallas, Texas

Glen H. Rudolph, MD
The Marshfield Clinic
Rice Lake Center
Rice Lake, Wisconsin

Matthew Russo, MD
Resident Physician
Department of Orthopaedic Surgery
Georgetown University Hospital
Washington, DC

Marc Safran, MD
Professor of Orthopedic Surgery
Associate Director
Department of Sports Medicine
Stanford University
Redwood City, California

Mark Sakr, DO
Carolina Family Practice & Sports Medicine
Adjunct Instructor of Family Medicine
University of North Carolina
Chapel Hill, North Carolina

Timothy G. Sanders, MD
Medical Director
NationalRad
Deerfield Beach, Florida

Prasad J. Sawardeker, MD
Shoulder, Elbow, and Hand Surgeon
Department of Orthopaedic Surgery
Essentia Health
Fargo, North Dakota

Anousheh Sayah, MD
Assistant Professor of Radiology
Georgetown University School of Medicine
Georgetown University Hospital
Washington, DC

Michael Schaer, MD
Sports Medicine and Shoulder Surgery
Hospital for Special Surgery
New York, New York

Laura Scordino, MD
Resident Physician
Department of Orthopaedic Surgery
University of Connecticut
Farmington, Connecticut

David Selvan, MBChB
Speciality Registrar
University Hospital Aintree
Liverpool, United Kingdom

Jason T. Shearn, PhD
Associate Professor
Tissue Engineering and Biomechanics Laboratories
Biomedical Engineering Program
University of Cincinnati
Cincinnati, Ohio

K. Donald Shelbourne, MD
Orthopaedic Surgeon
Shelbourne Knee Center
Indianapolis, Indiana

Ashley Matthews Shilling, MD
Associate Professor of Anesthesiology
University of Virginia Medical Center
Charlottesville, Virginia

Adam Shimer, MD
Assistant Professor
Orthopaedic Surgery
University of Virginia
Charlottesville, Virginia

David L. Skaggs, MD, MMM
Professor of Orthopaedic Surgery
University of Southern California–Los Angeles
Chief of Orthopaedic Surgery
Children's Hospital Los Angeles
Los Angeles, California

Frederick S. Song, MD
Attending Surgeon
Department of Orthopaedic Surgery
University Medical Center of Princeton at Plainsboro
Princeton, New Jersey

Kurt Spindler, MD
Kenneth D. Schermerhorn Professor
Vice Chairman
Orthopaedics & Orthopaedic PCC
Head Team Physician
Vanderbilt Athletics
Vanderbilt University
Nashville, Tennessee

Alison Spouge, MD
Associate Professor
Schulich School of Medicine & Dentistry
Western University;
Staff Radiologist and Head
Department of Medical Imaging
University Hospital
London Health Sciences Centre
London, Ontario, Canada

Chad Starkey, PhD
Professor
Division of Athletic Training
College of Health Sciences and Professions
Ohio University
Athens, Ohio

Siobhan Statuta, MD
Assistant Professor
Family Medicine and Physical Medicine & Rehabilitation
University of Virginia Health System
Charlottesville, Virginia

John W. Stiller, MD
Chief Physician and Neurologist
Maryland State Athletic Commission
Baltimore, Maryland;
Director
Neurology Service
St. Elizabeth's Hospital
Washington, DC

J. Andy Sullivan, MD
Clinical Professor of Pediatric Orthopaedics
University of Oklahoma College of Medicine
Oklahoma City, Oklahoma

Stephan J. Sweet, MD, MPH
Orthopaedic Surgeon
Department of Orthopaedic Surgery
Southern California Permanente Medical Group
Woodland Hills, California

Peter P. Syré, MD
Neurosurgical Resident
Department of Neurosurgery
Department of Bioengineering
University of Pennsylvania
Philadelphia, Pennsylvania

Thomas Kyle Tabor, MD
Adjunct Professor
Department of Family Medicine
Fowler Kennedy Sport Medicine Clinic
London, Ontario, Canada

Eric W. Tan, MD
Chief Resident
Department of Orthopaedic Surgery
Johns Hopkins University
Baltimore, Maryland

Peter Tang, MD, MPH
Director
Hand, Upper Extremity, & Microvascular Fellowship
Allegheny General Hospital
Pittsburgh, Pennsylvania

Dean C. Taylor, MD
Professor of Orthopaedic Surgery
Director
Duke Sports Medicine Fellowship
Duke University
Durham, North Carolina

Kenneth F. Taylor, MD
Associate Professor and Chief
Division of Hand Surgery
Department of Orthopaedic Surgery and Rehabilitation
Penn State
Milton S. Hershey Medical Center
Hershey, Pennsylvania

Sam G. Tejwani, MD
Department of Orthopaedic Surgery
Division of Sports Medicine
Southern California Permanente Medical Group
Fontana, California

Raj Telhan, MD
Chief Resident
Physical Medicine and Rehabilitation
Hospital for Special Surgery
Memorial Sloan-Kettering Cancer Center
Columbia University Medical Center
Cornell University Medical Center
New York, New York

Stephen R. Thompson, MD, MEd
Orthopaedic Staff Surgeon
Department of Orthopaedics
Eastern Maine Medical Center
Bangor, Maine

Fotios P. Tjoumakaris, MD
Assistant Professor of Orthopaedics
Jefferson Medical College
Rothman Institute Orthopaedics
Egg Harbor Township, New Jersey

John M. Tokish, MD, Colonel, USAF MC
Director, Orthopedic Surgery Residency Program
Tripler Army Medical Center
Honolulu, Hawaii

Rachel Triche, MD
Santa Monica Orthopaedic and Sports Medicine Group
Santa Monica, California

Narayana Varhabhatla, MD
Assistant Professor of Anesthesiology
University of Virginia Medical Center
Charlottesville, Virginia

Aaron J. Vaughan, MD
MAHEC Family Physician
Sports Medicine Director
Asheville, North Carolina

Jordi Vega, MD
Orthopaedic Surgeon
Etzelclinic
Pfäffikon, Schwyz, Switzerland

Avaleen Vopicka, MD
Adjunct Professor
Fowler Kennedy Sport Medicine Clinic
Western University
London, Ontario, Canada

Stephen C. Weber, MD
Sacramento Knee and Sports Medicine
Sacramento, California

William M. Weiss, MD
Orthopedic Sports Medicine
Reconstruction & Arthroscopy Fellow
Plano Orthopedics & Sports Medicine
OrthoTexas
Plano, Texas

William C. Welch, MD
Professor and Vice-Chairman
Department of Neurosurgery
Department of Bioengineering
University of Pennsylvania
Philadelphia, Pennsylvania

Benjamin Williams, PhD
Neuropsychology Fellow
Resident in Psychology
Department of Psychiatry and Neurobehavioral Sciences
University of Virginia School of Medicine
Charlottesville, Virginia

Barbara Wilson, MD
Associate Professor of Dermatology
University of Virginia
Charlottesville, Virginia

Brian F. Wilson, MD
Department of Orthopaedic Surgery
University of Kentucky
Lexington, Kentucky

Beth A. Winkelstein, PhD
Professor of Neurosurgery and Bioengineering
Department of Neurosurgery
Department of Bioengineering
University of Pennsylvania
Philadelphia, Pennsylvania

Jennifer Moriatis Wolf, MD
Associate Professor
Department of Orthopaedic Surgery
University of Connecticut Health Center
Farmington, Connecticut

Valerie M. Wolfe, MD
Fellow
Department of Orthopaedic Surgery
New York Presbyterian Hospital
Columbia University
New York, New York

Robert W. Wysocki, MD
Assistant Professor
Section of Hand and Elbow Surgery
Department of Orthopaedic Surgery
Rush University Medical Center
Chicago, Illinois

Yi-Meng Yen, MD, PhD
Assistant Professor
Department of Orthopaedic Surgery
Children's Hospital Boston
Boston, Massachusetts

Hassaan Yousufi, BS
Mood and Anxiety Program
Department of Psychiatry
University of Maryland School of Medicine
Baltimore, Maryland

Tracy Zaslow, MD
Medical Director
Sports Medicine and Concussion Program
Children's Orthopaedic Center at Children's Hospital Los Angeles
President, Los Angeles Pediatric Society
Team Physician, Los Angeles Galaxy
Los Angeles, California

Xinzhi Zhang, MS
Biomaterials and Interface Tissue Engineering Laboratory
Department of Biomedical Engineering
Columbia University
New York, New York

Mary L. Zupanc, MD
Professor
Department of Neurology and Pediatrics
Division Chief, Pediatric Neurology
Director, Pediatric Comprehensive Epilepsy Program
University of California–Irvine
Children's Hospital of Orange County
Orange, California

Contents

VOLUME I

SECTION 1 *Basic Principles*

SECTION 2 *Medical*

SECTION 3 *Rehabilitation and Injury Prevention*

SECTION 4 *Shoulder*

SECTION 5 *Elbow, Wrist, and Hand*

VOLUME II

SECTION 6 *Pelvis, Hip, and Thigh*

SECTION 7 *Knee*

SECTION 8 *Leg, Ankle, and Foot*

SECTION 6

Pelvis, Hip, and Thigh

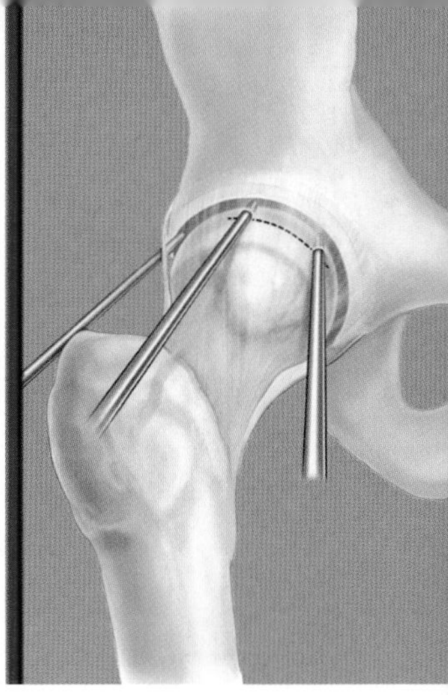

79

Hip Anatomy and Biomechanics

MARC SAFRAN • ITAMAR B. BOTSER

The hip joint (*coxa* in Latin) is the articulation connecting the pelvis and the femur. It is an encapsulated synovial joint with a ball and socket architecture in which the femoral head is the ball and the acetabulum is the socket. Although its structure may seem simple, it is actually very complicated with more than 20 muscles spanning the joint and a three-dimensional (3D) bony morphology that may vary widely among subjects. The acetabulum may be described as retroverted or anteverted, shallow or deep, and with high or low inclination of the weight-bearing surface. The femoral head may be overcovered by the acetabulum or undercovered, and the offset of the femoral head neck junction may be reduced or normal. The proximal femur may have a short or long neck, a high or low femoral neck-shaft angle, and be retroverted or anteverted. To further complicate matters, the head is not a completely round sphere; the socket is horseshoe shaped and the center of the femoral head moves relative to the socket, and as such it is not a true ball-in-socket joint.

The main function of the hip is to support the weight of the body in both static (e.g., standing) and dynamic (e.g., walking or running) situations. To address the biomechanical principles involved in the function of the human hip, it is essential to understand the anatomy of the proximal femur and pelvis, as well as the muscles, ligaments, and bony structures, which all contribute to the equilibrium of forces needed for controlled hip joint motion.

Prenatal Hip Joint Development

Knowledge regarding hip joint development is beneficial to the understanding of hip joint anatomy and biomechanics. Limb formation begins by the fourth week of the embryonic life. By the sixth week primitive chondroblasts accumulate at the proximal, center, and distal ends of the cellular femur template, forming chondrification centers, and a club-shaped cartilage model of the future femur arises from those centers. At the same time a shallow acetabulum begins to form proximal to the femoral head by the future ilium, ischium, and pubis precursor cells. Later, the chondrification process of these bones continues until fusion occurs. By the seventh week of development, the cartilage models of both the femur and the acetabulum are complete. By the eight week, the capsule, the acetabular labrum, the ligamentum teres, and the transverse ligament can be identified microscopically, and 3 weeks later they can be identified macroscopically.[1] At 16 weeks, the ossification of the femur is complete up to the lesser trochanter, and primary ossification centers have appeared in the three pelvic bones; however, ossification centers of the acetabulum do not appear until adolescence. Through the twentieth week of gestation, the differentiation of the hip joint ends and the process shifts to growth and maturation.[2]

Bony Anatomy

Acetabulum

Development

The acetabulum has two components: the triradiate cartilage in the center (Fig. 79-1) and the acetabular cartilage complex, which is formed by fusion of the ilium, ischium, and pubis.[2,3] The triradiate cartilage forms the nonarticular medial wall of the acetabulum, and its growth is crucial for acetabular height and depth. The acetabular cartilage complex, which is composed mainly of hyaline cartilage, forms the cup-shaped articular portion of the acetabulum.[2] Around the age of 8 to 9 years, secondary ossification centers appear at the acetabular rim (os acetabuli). In 1922, Perna identified three distinct os acetabuli—anterior, posterior, and superior.[4-6] Those ossification centers have an important role in the development of the acetabular rim and its depth.[3] In most cases, the superior os acetabulum fuses by adulthood; however, occasionally its fusion is delayed, and radiographically it may mimic a fracture of the acetabular rim. Normal acetabular development depends heavily on the interaction with the spherical femoral head as a template about which it forms.[2] Complete absence of the proximal femur yields an absent acetabulum.[7]

Acetabular Version

The normal acetabulum is angled 15 to 20 degrees anteriorly, or anteverted.[8] The acetabular version can be estimated by the appearance of the anterior and posterior acetabular walls on a straight (not tilted) anteroposterior pelvis radiograph, whereas computed tomography (CT) can be used to measure the acetabular version.[8,9] The anteverted acetabulum allows for hip flexion that is greater than hip extension. A retroverted acetabulum occurs when the acetabulum is angled less than 15 degrees anteriorly. The acetabulum may have a relative retroversion (still anteverted, but less than 15 degrees) or be truly retroverted, angled posteriorly. Additionally, cranial retroversion may be present, in which the anterior acetabular wall crosses over the posterior wall only

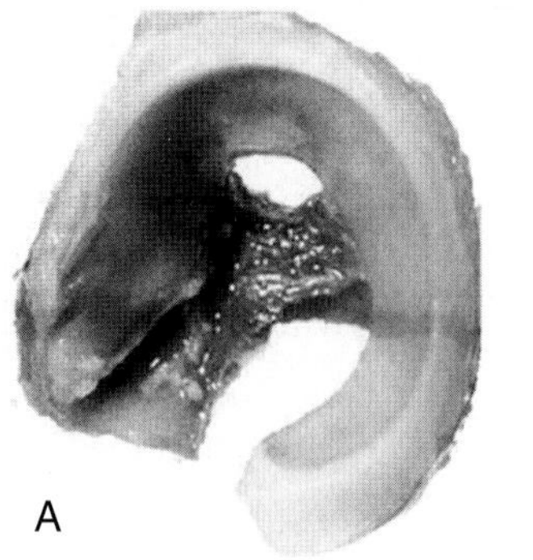

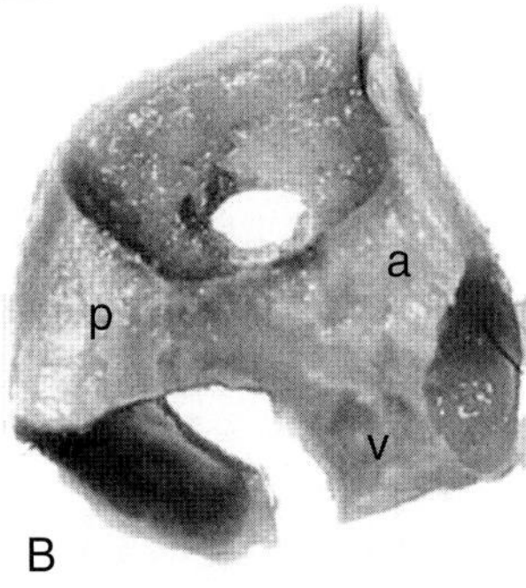

FIGURE 79-1 Triradiate cartilage. Lateral view (**A**) and medial view (**B**) of the normal acetabular cartilage complex of a 1-day-old infant. The ilium, ischium, and pubis have been removed with a curette. The lateral view shows the cup-shaped acetabulum, and the medial view shows the three flanges of the triradiate cartilage. The anterior flange (*a*) is located between the ilium and pubis and is slanted superiorly; the posterior flange (*p*) is horizontal and located between the ilium and ischium; and the vertical flange (*v*) is located between the pubis and ischium. *(Modified from Ponseti IV: Growth and development of the acetabulum in the normal child: anatomical, histological, and roentgenographic studies.* J Bone Joint Surg Am *60[5]:576, 1978.)*

superiorly (demonstrating a positive "cross-over sign" on radiographs).

Acetabulum Depth

On a cadaveric study of 154 hips, the mean values for the acetabular depth and diameter were 29.49 ± 4.2 mm and 54.29 ± 3.8 mm, respectively. The maximum and minimum measurements of acetabular diameter were 65.5 mm and 44.8 mm, respectively, and acetabular depth ranged from 38.6 to 22.6 mm, respectively.[10]

Another reported measure of acetabular depth can be determined from axial magnetic resonance or CT views of the hip joint as the distance between the center of the femoral head and the line connecting the anterior acetabular rim to the posterior acetabular rim. The value is positive if the center of the femoral neck is lateral to the line connecting the acetabular rim and negative if medial to it.[11] Murtha et al.[12] have studied the acetabular anatomy using 3D surface models of the normal hemipelvis derived from volumetric CT data on 42 patients. For the 22 female subjects, the mean acetabular depth was 0.79 mm (0.56 to 1.04), and for the 20 male subjects it was 0.85 mm (0.65 to 0.99).

Zeng et al.[13] studied acetabular morphologic differences between genders in a Chinese population; they measured the acetabular width as the inferior distance between the superolateral and lowermost points of the acetabulum and the acetabular depth as the perpendicular distance between the top and bottom of the acetabulum on an anteroposterior tomogram. Both width and depth were significantly smaller in women than in men, but the difference was not significant when adjusted for body height.

The acetabular depth can be also quantified radiographically on an anteroposterior pelvis view by the center edge angle (of Wiberg). The center edge angle is formed by a line drawn from the center of the femoral head to the outer edge of the acetabular roof and a vertical line drawn from the center of the femoral head directly superior.[6,14] Although currently somewhat a matter of controversy, the normal values of the center edge angle are between 25 and 35 degrees. A center edge angle of 20 to 25 degrees is often considered "borderline dysplasia," whereas the upper limits of the center edge angle may be reported as up to 40 degrees.

A deep acetabulum (profunda or protrusio) may result in pincer-type impingement, whereas on the other end of the spectrum, the acetabulum may not be deep enough. Failure of the secondary ossification centers to develop the acetabular rim and depth results in a shallow socket, also known as hip dysplasia.[3,14-16]

Proximal Femur

Development

At birth the ossification of the femoral shaft reaches the greater trochanter and the femoral neck. A few months later, two ossification centers appear, one in the center of the femoral head and one in the greater trochanter. Three growth plates are defined: longitudinal (between the femoral head and the neck), trochanteric (between the femoral neck and the greater trochanter), and the femoral neck isthmus.[2] These growth plates are essential for the growth and shape of the proximal femur.

The pressure exerted on the femoral head by the acetabulum is necessary to result in a spherical femoral head. Overall, the development of both the proximal femur and the acetabulum are related to correct development and positioning of each other.

Blood Supply

The main artery of the lower limb is the femoral artery, which is a continuation of the external iliac artery distal to the ilioinguinal ligament. The profunda femoris is a large lateral branch of the femoral artery that appears about 3.5 cm below the inguinal ligament. Branches from the profunda include the lateral circumflex, the medial circumflex, perforating arteries to the femur, muscular branches, and the descending genicular artery.[17]

The proximal femur is supplied by three main blood sources: (1) the nutrient artery of the shaft that arises from the perforating arteries; (2) the retinacular vessels of the capsule that arise from the circumflex arteries; and (3) the foveal artery of the ligamentum teres.

The nutrient artery enters the midshaft of the femur and may be single or double; its superior branch runs in the medullary cavity and anastomoses with the retinacular vessels in the metaphysis.[18] In adults over 13 years, the nutrient artery has been found to cross the epiphyseal plate from the metaphysis to the epiphysis.[18]

The retinacular vessels penetrate the capsule near its distal attachment and are the main blood supply to the femoral epiphysis and femoral head at all ages.[18-20] The three main groups of retinacular vessels—superior, inferior, and anterior—are all intracapsular and covered with a synovial membrane, sometimes in a mesenteric-like fold of synovial membrane. The anterior retinacular vessels are the smallest of the three, branching from the lateral femoral circumflex artery, and are less consistent. Overall, the lateral femoral circumflex artery contributes little to the vascularity of the femoral head.[19] The superior and inferior retinacular vessels arise from the deep branch medial femoral circumflex artery and run along the upper and lower borders of the femoral neck.[19] The medial circumflex femoral artery supplies blood to the neck of the femur and femoral head. It arises from the medial and posterior aspects of the profunda femoris artery and winds around the medial side of the femur, passing first between the iliopsoas and pectineus muscles and then between the obturator externus and adductor brevis. These two groups are fairly large and consistent between specimens. The superior group, which runs in the lateral retinacular fold, is larger, supplies the weight-bearing part of the femoral head, and may be the sole blood supply to the epiphysis.[18] Anastomoses of the deep branch of the medial femoral circumflex artery with other arteries have been described; a significant and consistent anastomosis with a branch of the inferior gluteal artery is found along the piriformis, and in some cases the inferior gluteal artery was found to be the main blood supply of the hip.[19,20]

The foveal artery, running within the ligamentum teres, is formed by the acetabular branches of the obturator or the medial circumflex or from both, and often its contribution to the femoral head blood supply is minute.[17,18] In some cases it was found to be anastomosing with the epiphyseal arteries, whereas in other cases it was found to supply only the area of insertion of the ligamentum teres to the fovea.[18] A recent study found no significant vascular contribution by the foveal artery.[20]

Femoral Neck Version

The femoral neck version is the angle between the femoral neck and the axis that crosses the distal femoral condyles; this angle can be measured through CT or magnetic resonance imaging (MRI) that includes both the knee and the hip.[21] Normally the proximal femur is anteverted. Femoral anteversion is greatest at birth and decreases with growth. Normal average anteversion ranges between 35 and 45 degrees at the time of birth, is 31 degrees at the age of 1 year, and decreases to 15.4 degrees by skeletal maturity (16 years of age).[2,8,22] Clinically, increased femoral anteversion can be seen as an "in-toed" appearance of the lower limb in a standing person, or squinting patellae, where the patellae point toward the midline.[8]

Neck Shaft Angle

The neck shaft angle is the angle measured between the axis of the femoral neck and the femoral shaft. This angle can be measured on plain anteroposterior pelvis radiographs, but internal or external rotation of the hip may increase the measured angle. Similar to the version angle, the neck shaft angle is highest at birth and declines with growth. The normal neck shaft angle is approximately 136 degrees at 1 year of age and decreases to 127 degrees by age 18 years.[2]

Femoral Head-Neck Junction

Normally the femoral head-neck junction is waist-shaped, with the femoral neck narrower than its head. The head-neck junction morphology can be quantified by the anterior offset or the alpha angle.[23-27] The offset is the difference between the anterior contour of the head and femoral neck on axial MRI or CT scans. On axial radiographs (cross-table or Dunn view), it is defined as the distance between the widest diameter of the femoral head and the most prominent part of the femoral neck.[28] The offset can be measured as the ratio between the femoral head and neck radii or as an absolute distance, which is normally measured as around 10 mm.[26,28]

The alpha angle was described by Notzli et al.[27] in 2002 as a measurement on axial MRI. The alpha angle is a simple method to quantify the concavity at femoral head-neck junction, and it was shown to correlate with anterior hip impingement. The alpha angle is composed of a line that connects the center of the femoral neck at its narrowest diameter to the center of the femoral head. The second line that composes the alpha angle is from the center of the femoral head to a point where the femoral head loses its sphericity, and thus where femoral head exceeds the normal radius of the femoral head. The alpha angle can also be measured on plain radiographs and was found to correlate well with the MRI values.[29-31] In general, normal alpha angle perimeters have fluctuated since the original report, being less than 50 or 55 degrees.

Internal Bony Architecture of the Femoral Neck

The first description of the bony trabecular orientation in the femoral neck is attributed to Ward in *Human Anatomy,* which was published in London in 1838; in 1961 it was cited by Garden,[32] who likened the trabecular structure within the femoral neck to that of a lamp bracket. Many other analogies of the trabecular pattern to other 3D weight-bearing subjects such as cranes are common as well.[33] Because the proximal femur is exposed to tensile and compressive forces during weight bearing, those forces lead to functional internal bony architecture of the femoral neck trabeculae lines as stated by Wolff's law of bone remodeling.[34] These trabeculae consist of a primary compressive group, which arises from the medial subtrochanteric cortex and ascends superiorly into the weight-bearing femoral head, and a primary tensile group, which spans from the foveal area of the femoral head, through the superior femoral neck, and into the lateral subtrochanteric cortex (Fig. 79-2).[35] Secondary compressive, secondary tensile, and a greater trochanteric group complete the pattern of trabecular orientation.[35] The calcar femorale was precisely defined anatomically by Merkle in 1874 as a dense plate of bone extending laterally from the posteromedial femoral cortex to the posterior aspect of the greater trochanter.[33,35,36] This bone spur is thickest medially and gradually thins as it extends laterally.[33,35,36] However, although defined anatomically as a cancellous bone spur, the term "calcar" is frequently (and some say mistakenly) used to describe the medial

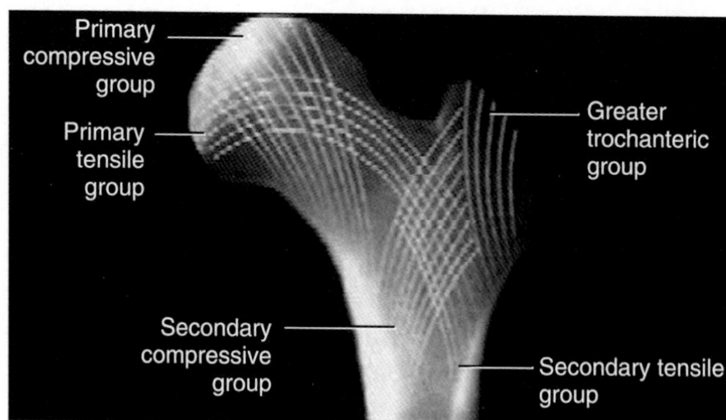

FIGURE 79-2 Trabecular pattern. An anteroposterior radiograph of the hip illustrating the primary and secondary compressive and tensile trabecular bone groups. A greater trochanteric group completes the pattern of trabecular orientation. *(From Hughes PE, Hsu JC, Matava MJ: Hip anatomy and biomechanics in the athlete.* Sports Med Arthrosc Rev *10[2]:103–114, 2002.)*

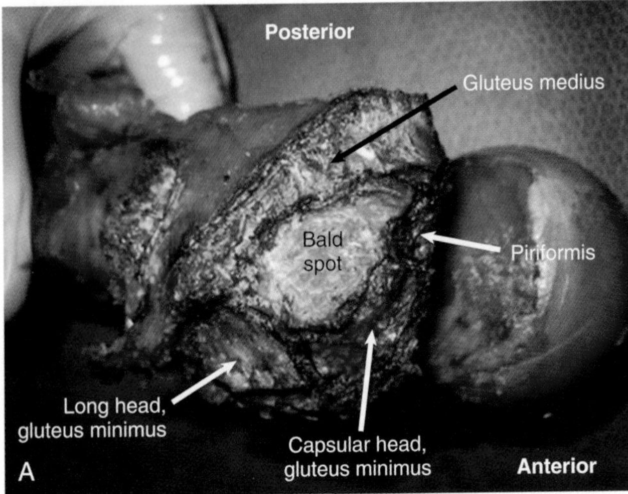

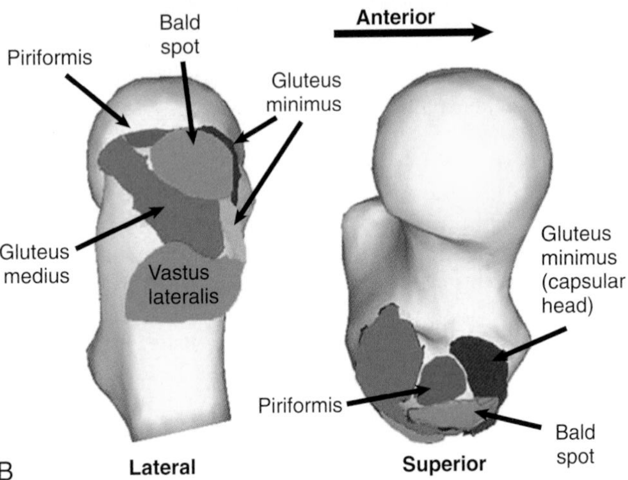

FIGURE 79-3 The bald spot is bordered posteriorly by the gluteus medius, anteriorly by the two heads of the gluteus minimus, and superiorly and medially by the piriformis. Examples of (**A**) a gross specimen and (**B**) the bone morphing model after navigated determination of tendon footprints are shown. *(From Gardner MJ, Robertson WJ, Boraiah S, et al: Anatomy of the greater trochanteric "bald spot": a potential portal for abductor sparing femoral nailing?* Clin Orthop Relat Res *466[9]:2196–2200, 2008.)*

cortical bone of the femoral neck, which is the thickest cortex of the femur bone and the strongest bone in the hip.[36] The medial cortex is also known as Adam's arch.[37]

Greater Trochanter

The greater trochanter can be divided into four different facets—anterior, lateral, posterior, and superoposterior.[38] Those facets are the insertions of the abductor complex; the gluteus medius muscle attaches to the superoposterior and lateral facets, and the gluteus minimus muscle attaches to the anterior facet.[38] A bald spot was described on the lateral facet of the greater trochanter, devoid of tendon insertion, and bordered anteriorly and distally by the gluteus minimus, posteriorly by the gluteus medius, and proximally by the piriformis tendon (Fig. 79-3).[39] Blood supply to the greater trochanteric area arises from the trochanteric branch of the medial femoral circumflex artery.[19]

Lesser Trochanter

The lesser trochanter is a pyramidal process that projects from the lower and posterior part of the base femoral neck. Medially it is in continuation with the lower border of the femoral neck, laterally with the intertrochanteric crest, and inferiorly with the linea aspera. The lesser trochanter is the insertion point of the iliopsoas muscle. The lesser trochanter varies in size in different subjects: its height is approximately 1.2 cm, and its width can range between 2 and 4.5 cm.[40]

Intraarticular Structures

Acetabular Labrum

The acetabular labrum is a horseshoe-shaped structure attached to the acetabular rim. Inferiorly the labrum joins the transverse ligament to bridge the acetabular notch, forming a complete circle.[41] It is triangular in its cross-sectional shape, with its base attached to the acetabulum and its apex forming a free edge (Fig. 79-4).[42] Petersen et al.[43] looked at the labrum under light microscopy and found that the majority of the collagen fibers have a circumferential orientation. The capsular side of the labrum is composed of dense connective tissue mainly consisting of collagen types I and III, whereas the articular side is composed of fibrocartilage.[43] At the articular side, the labrum is often separated from the articular cartilage by a physiologic cleft that is seen more frequently posteriorly, whereas anteriorly this cleft is usually absent and the transition between the labrum and articular cartilage is smooth.[43]

Seldes et al.[42] also studied the labrum histologically and found it to be widest in its inferior half and thickest at its superior half. On average, the acetabular labral size ranges from 4 to 8 mm. The average labral width as reported by Seldes et al.[42] ranged from 3.8 mm posterosuperiorly to 6.4 mm posteroinferiorly. However, the labral width may vary according to the forces that act on it. It appears that the labral size may be inversely proportional to the depth of the bony

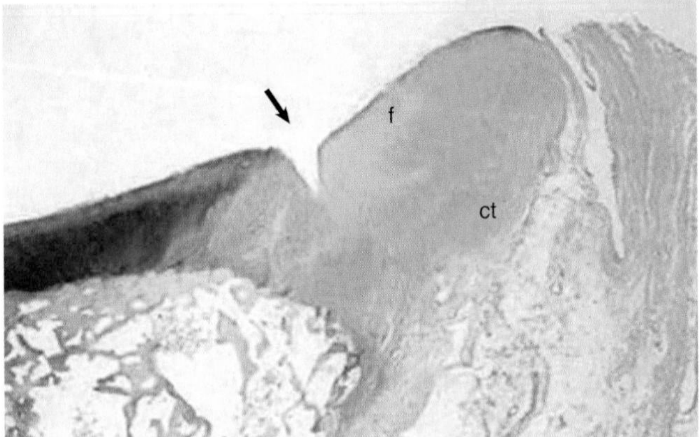

FIGURE 79-4 Histology of the labrum. Cross-sectional histology of the labrum: The labrum is separated from the articular cartilage by a physiological cleft (*arrow*) and is composed of two different tissues, fibrocartilage (*f*) on the articular side and connective tissue (*ct*) on the capsular side. This physiological cleft is seen more often in the posterior labrum. *(From Petersen W, Petersen F, Tillmann B: Structure and vascularization of the acetabular labrum with regard to the pathogenesis and healing of labral lesions.* Arch Orthop Trauma Surg *123[6]:283–288, 2003.)*

acetabular socket contribution to femoral head coverage. Thus the labrum may be small, with a width of less than 3 mm in coxa profunda, or it may be large/hypertrophic, with a width of up to 14 mm in a dysplastic hip.

Inferiorly, the labrum appears to be continuous with the transverse acetabular ligament over the cotyloid notch; however, a distinction is seen between the labrum and the transverse ligament. A bony acetabular tongue exists within the labrum with the labrum firmly attached to it with a well-defined tidemark. Histologically, the acetabular labrum merges with the articular hyaline cartilage of the joint surface of the acetabulum through a transition zone of 1 to 2 mm, particularly anteriorly.

The labrum is continuous with the articular cartilage of the acetabulum; however, differences exist in the transition between the anterior and posterior transition zones. The anterior labral-chondral transition is sharp and abrupt with minimal interdigitation of fibers, whereas the posterior labral-chondral transition is smooth and gradual. This appearance is due to differences in the orientation of collagen fibers of the labrum; the anterior fibers are parallel to the labral-chondral junction, whereas the posterior fibers are oriented perpendicularly.[44]

Blood Supply

The main vascular supply of the labrum arises from radial vessels on its capsular side embedded in a loose connective tissue between the labrum and the capsule (Fig. 79-5).[43,45,46] These vessels seem to supply only the outer third of the labrum.[43] Kalhor et al.[45] used a silicon injection technique to show a periacetabular vascular ring supplying the labrum, originating from the superior and inferior gluteal vessels, the medial and lateral femoral circumflex arteries, and the intrapelvic vascular system.

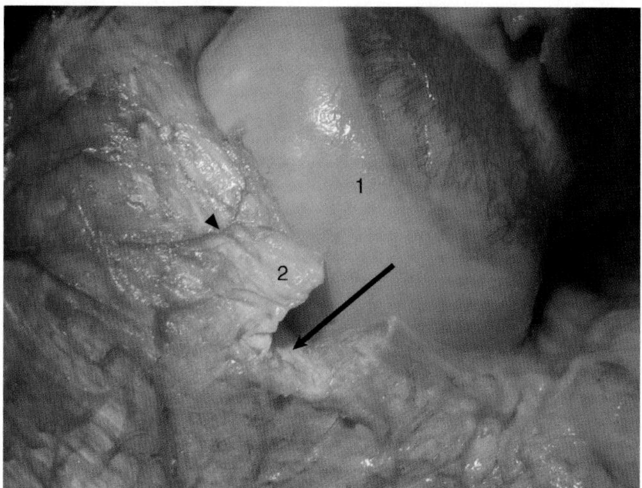

FIGURE 79-5 Vascular supply of the labrum. The posterior aspect of a right hip after resection of a segment of the labrum. The arrow points to the osseolabral junction and shows the absence of visible vessels traversing this boundary. The radial vessels on the labrum can be seen embedded in a layer of loose connective tissue. *1,* Femoral head; *2,* labrum. The arrowhead points to a radial vessel on the labrum that can be seen embedded in a layer of loose connective tissue.[58] *(From Kalhor M, Horowitz K, Beck M, et al: Vascular supply to the acetabular labrum.* J Bone Joint Surg Am *92[15]:2570–2575, 2010.)*

The acetabular bony rim that is embedded in the base of the labrum is another source of blood supply to the labrum. McCarthy et al.,[47] in an immunohistochemical study, showed abundant vessels within the bony acetabulum that reach the junction with the labrum. Seldes et al.[42] identified a group of three to four vessels located in the substance of the labrum that travels circumferentially around the labrum at its attachment site on the outer surface of the bony acetabular extension.

Innervation

The labrum has been shown to be richly populated by many neurologic structures. Kim and Azuma[48] found sensory nerves and organs such as Vater-Pacini, Golgi-Mazzoni, Ruffini, and Krause corpuscles within the acetabular labrum. Most of these sensory nerve end organs (86%) are in the articular side of the labrum. The corpuscles observed are receptors of pressure, deep sensation, and temperature sense. In addition, no differences in number or type of nerves and organs were found based on the age of the specimens, but more unmyelinated nerve endings, which function to sense pain, were identified in the superior and anterior quarters of the labrum.[48] Additionally, Gerhardt et al.[49] found that the anterior zone of the labrum contained the highest concentration of mechanoreceptors and sensory fibers, specifically Ruffini corpuscles. Thus the labrum may function to provide proprioceptive input, and a damaged labrum may be a source of hip pain.

Biomechanical Properties

The labrum deepens the acetabulum and acts as a suction seal, adding stability to the joint and protecting the articular cartilage. Seldes et al.[42] have shown that the labrum increases the acetabular surface area and volume by 22% and 33%, respectively.[50] Furthermore, the labrum creates a seal that opposes the flow of synovial fluid in and out of the central compartment. Safran et al.[51] have shown that the labrum has strain at rest, which increases and decreases in different locations of the labrum as the hip is taken through range of motion. According to biomechanical studies, with an intact labrum, the acetabular and femoral cartilage surfaces do not come into direct contact with each other because of a film of fluid contained by the labrum. Ferguson et al.[52] have found that hydrostatic fluid pressure within the intraarticular space was greater within the labrum than without, which may enhance joint lubrication, whereas labrum resection resulted in faster cartilage consolidation. Song et al.[53] also found that the acetabular labrum plays a role in maintaining a low-friction environment, possibly by sealing the joint from fluid exudation, because both complete and focal labral debridement resulted in increased joint friction, a condition that is thought to be detrimental to articular cartilage and leads to osteoarthritis. The sealing function of the labrum also helps maintain the negative intraarticular pressure that occurs in all joints. This negative intraarticular pressure helps resist distraction of the femoral head from the socket; this function is called the "suction effect" and is thought to improve the stability of the joint.[54]

Ligamentum Teres

The ligamentum teres, otherwise known as the round ligament of the femur, is a triangular double-band ligament with a length of 30 to 35 mm that attaches the femoral head to the acetabulum.[55-57] Medially, it is attached to either side of the acetabular notch by two bands that originate from the acetabular transverse ligament and the pubic and ischial margins. Laterally, its apex extends to the anterosuperior portion of the femoral head, merging with the fovea capitis femoris.

The ligament is composed of thick, well-organized, parallel, and slightly undulating or wavy fibers of collagen bundles that are composed of collagen types I, III, and V.[55-57] Embryonically, the ligamentum teres is defined around 8 weeks of intrauterine life as the joint space expands and is seen to attach to the medial border of the acetabular fossa, separating from the transverse acetabular ligament.

Blood Supply

An anterior branch of the posterior division of the obturator artery provides the blood supply to the ligamentum teres (Fig. 79-6). Vascular canals extend from the fovea capitis of the femoral head to supply the epiphysis of the femoral head; however, these arteries are not patent in a third of the population. These vessels do not anastomose with the distal arterial terminals in the femoral head until around age 15 years, when ossification of the head is nearly complete.[58]

Biomechanical Properties

The biomechanical role of the ligamentum teres has been debated in the medical literature since the nineteenth century, with proposed functions including that of a stabilizer, a fluid and force distributor in the acetabulum, and an embryonic remnant with no specific role in adults.[59-61] The ligamentum teres has also been previously described as a possible transmitter of somatosensory signals that act to help the hip avoid painful and excessive ranges of motion.[62] More recently, the ligamentum teres in the hip has been thought to provide functions comparable with the anterior cruciate ligament in the knee; with similar tensile strength, it has been proposed to provide some degree of stability in the hip, resisting dislocation and microinstability.[63] However, many other studies report that the ligamentum teres plays little role in the stability of the hip joint and suggest it is possibly a mere embryonic remnant.[56,64]

The ligamentum teres has been found to be taut in flexion, adduction, and external rotation,[55,56,63] and thus it may play a role in stability of the hip joint in those positions. In a recent study, Domb et al.[65] have found that the arthroscopic presence of ligamentum teres tears was associated with acetabular bony morphology and age. Ligamentum teres tears were less frequent in hips with a high lateral coverage index (center edge angle minus acetabular inclination) and also less frequent in patients younger than 30 years.

Innervation

Two histologic studies have found type IVa free nerve endings in the ligamentum teres, which are nociceptors and mechanoreceptors.[62,66] Leunig et al.[62] suggested that in addition to its mechanical and structural functions, the ligamentum teres may be involved in transmitting specific somatosensory afferent signals to the spinal and cerebral regulatory systems. Hence the ligamentum teres may be part of an integral reflex system involved in joint protection, acting as a rein to avoid excessive motion that may be potentially harmful to the joint.[62] Alternatively, Gerhardt et al.[49] identified a paucity of neural fibers in the ligamentum and did not find any sensory nerve fibers within it.

Although the function of the ligamentum teres has yet to be determined, its role as a source of hip pain after a full or a partial tear has been more clearly elucidated.[55,56,67-76]

Articular Cartilage

The articular cartilage of the hip, both on the acetabular side and the femoral side, has been shown to be highly

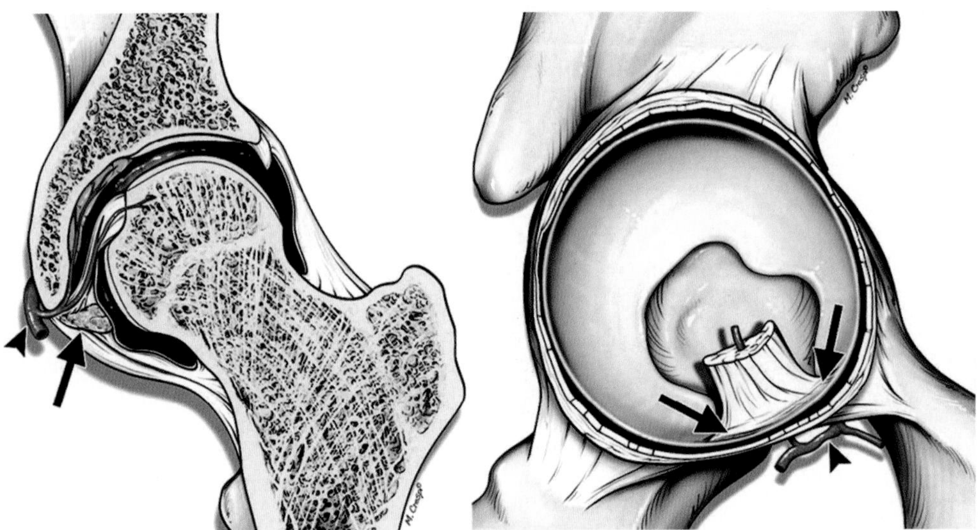

FIGURE 79-6 Ligamentum teres. Diagrams show the normal anatomy of the ligamentum teres. The ligamentum teres has a broad origin that blends with the entire transverse ligament of the acetabulum (*arrows*) and is attached to the ischial and pubic sides of the acetabular notch by two bands. It inserts into the fovea capitis femoris, and its arterial supply is provided by the anterior branch of the posterior division of the obturator artery (*arrowhead*). Vascular canals extend a short distance from the fovea capitis into the femoral head. *(From Cerezal L, Kassarjian A, Canga A, et al: Anatomy, biomechanics, imaging, and management of ligamentum teres injuries.* Radiographics *30[6]:1637–1651, 2010.)*

inhomogeneous in thickness distribution. Von Eisenhart et al.[77] studied the cartilage thickness and pressure on eight fresh cadaveric hip specimens during the phases of gait cycle. Maximum cartilage thickness was found ventrosuperiorly in the acetabulum and in the femoral head. The location of maximum thickness corresponded with the ventrosuperior location of maximum pressure recorded during the walking cycle; the maximal thickness ranged from 2.6 to 4.3 mm in the acetabulum (average, 3.3 mm) and from 2.4 to 5.3 mm in the femoral head (average, 3.5 mm). In general, cartilage thickness decreased with age. No statistical difference was found between the values for maximum thickness on both surfaces, although the mean thickness of the femoral cartilage (1.5 to 2.0 mm, with an average of 1.7 mm) was higher ($P < .01$) than that of the acetabulum (1.1 to 1.7 mm, with an average of 1.4 mm).

Hip Joint Capsule

The hip capsule is made up of internal fibers (within the joint) and external fibers (outside or away from the joint). The external fibers run longitudinally and comprise the iliofemoral ligament, ISFL, and pubofemoral ligament. The inner fibers comprise the zona orbicularis, which forms a collar around the femoral neck.[78,79] The capsule inserts on the bony acetabulum proximal to and distinct from the labrum, forming a recess between the two that ranges between 6.6 and 7.9 mm from the anteroinferior and posteroinferior quadrants, respectively.[42] From its acetabular attachment, the capsule extends to surround the femoral head and neck in a spiral fashion and is attached anteriorly to the intertrochanteric line, superiorly to the base of the femoral neck, superomedially to the intertrochanteric crest, and inferiorly to the femoral neck near the lesser trochanter.[78,80] One theory regarding the spiral architecture of the capsule is that it originated as humans began to walk upright. As humans transitioned from quadruped to biped, the hips were brought into relative extension, thus causing the capsular fibers to twist into a spiral pattern.[81-83] In normal stance, if the upper body is leaned slightly posteriorly, stability is provided primarily by the static restraints of the anterior capsule (mainly the iliofemoral ligament). If the anterior capsule is damaged or lax, maintaining the upright position may be difficult because the anterior muscle strength is not as powerful as the posterior muscle strength.

Capsular Ligaments

Iliofemoral Ligament

The iliofemoral ligament (ILFL), also known as the *Y ligament of Bigelow*, is shaped like an inverted "Y" and distally splits into two distinct arms, medial and lateral (Fig. 79-7). The single proximal insertion abuts the anterior inferior iliac spine, wrapping around the base like a crescent, and extends within a few millimeters of the acetabular rim along the anterior and anterolateral acetabulum. Distally, the ILFL lateral arm crosses the joint obliquely and inserts on the anterior prominence of the greater trochanteric crest, just superior to the origin of the intertrochanteric line, with an elongated oval-shaped footprint. The medial arm passes almost vertically inferior and inserts on a subtle angulated prominence of the anterior-inferior femur, at the level of the lesser trochanter, with a circular-shaped footprint. The individual arms of the ILFL diverge 57 mm (range, 50 to 64 mm) distal to the most superior aspect of the proximal attachment footprint; the medial and lateral insertional footprints are a few millimeters apart on intertrochanteric line.[80] The ILFL restricts external rotation in both flexion and extension and internal rotation in flexion.[84]

Pubofemoral Ligament

The pubofemoral ligament (PFL) originates on the iliopectineal eminence of the superior pubic ramus with a triangle-shaped insertional footprint (Fig. 79-7). The most inferomedial aspect of the insertional footprint extends to within a few millimeters of the acetabular rim. The PFL crosses inferoposteriorly under the medial arm of the ILFL and wraps around the femoral head like a sling or hammock, proximal to the zona orbicularis. The PFL terminates abruptly by blending with the proximal ischiofemoral ligament (ISFL), near the acetabular rim, beneath the inferior aspect of the femoral neck (Figure 79-7, *B*); the PFL lacks a bony femoral attachment.[80] The PFL blends anteriorly with the medial ILFL. The PFL controls external rotation in extension.[84]

Ischiofemoral Ligament

The ISFL resembles a large asymmetric triangle with a long tapered apex and consists of a single band (see Fig. 79-7). The proximal insertional footprint on the ischial acetabular margin is shaped like a broad triangle, beginning near the root of the ischial ramus and extending to within a few millimeters of the acetabular rim. The ISFL spirals superolaterally to insert at the base of the greater trochanter at the femoral neck-trochanteric junction, slightly anterior to the femoral neck axis; the distal ISFL footprint does not have a consistent shape.[80] The ISFL was noted to be the most significant restrictor of internal rotation both in internal and external rotation.[84]

Zona Orbicularis

The zona orbicularis is a thickening of the capsule, just distal to the femoral head-neck junction, that runs around the femoral neck, perpendicular to the axis of the femoral neck. The zona orbicularis has leashlike fibers organized in a spiral configuration; together with the anterior capsular ligaments, they tighten in a "screw home" mechanism during terminal extension and external rotation, further stabilizing the joint.[79,85] Additionally, the zona orbicularis may limit distraction of the femoral head from the acetabulum.[79]

Capsule Innervation

Sensory innervation of the hip capsule for proprioception and nociception has been studied extensively in the modern literature.[86-92] The capsule is generally thought to receive its innervation from branches of the obturator, femoral, sciatic, and superior gluteal nerves, the nerve to quadratus femoris, and possibly from the accessory obturator nerve. The complexity of the hip joint innervation results in a nonhomogenic pattern of pain referred from the hip joint, with hip pathology causing pain in the groin, all around the thigh, in the buttock, below the knee, and even in the foot.[93]

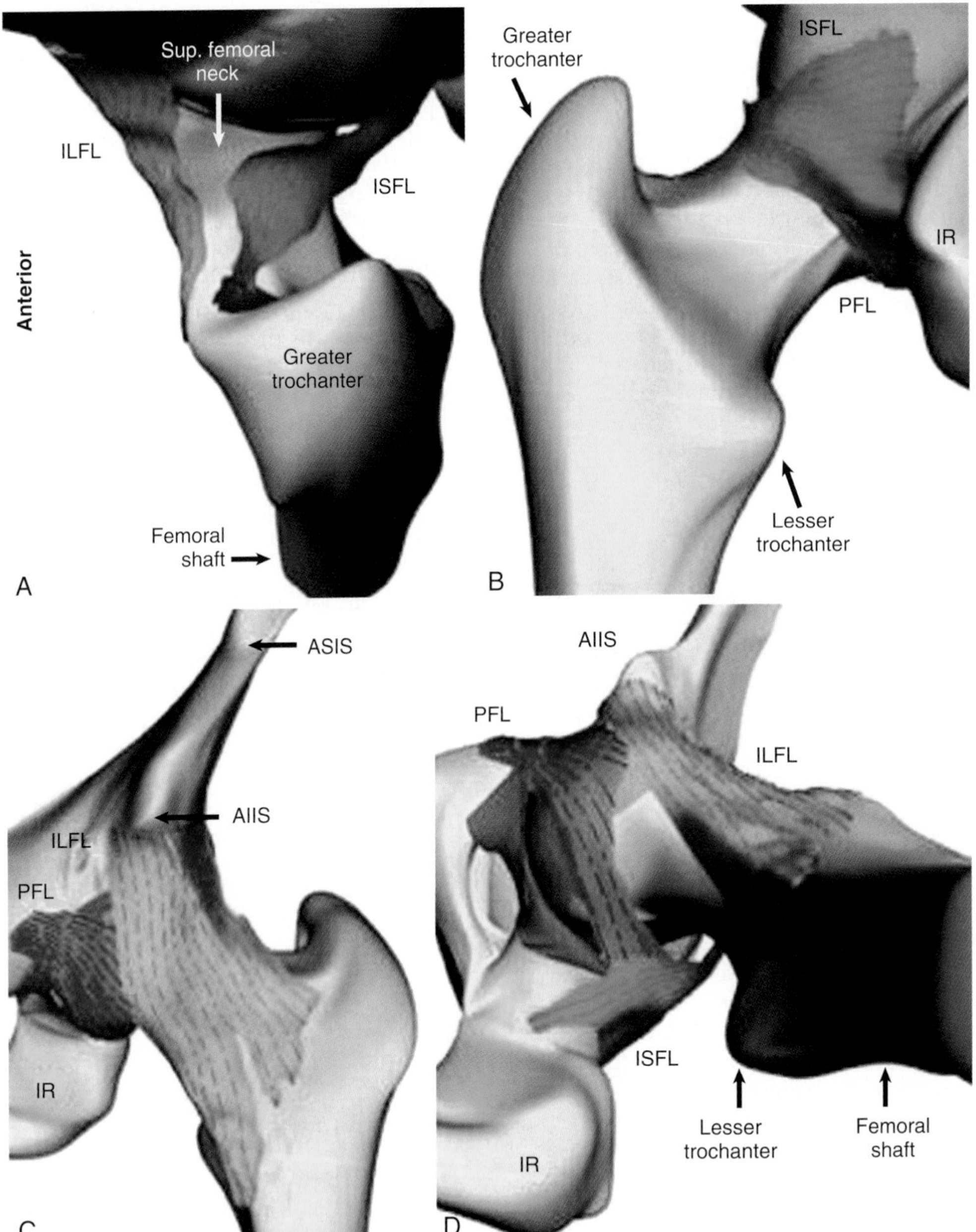

FIGURE 79-7 Ligamentous relationships of the hip capsule. **A,** A computer model demonstrating the relationship of the distal lateral iliofemoral ligament (*ILFL*) and the distal ischiofemoral ligament (*ISFL*), viewed from a superior position looking down the femoral shaft. **B,** A computer model showing the posterior blend of the pubofemoral ligament (*PFL*) and the ISFL. **C,** A computer model showing the anterior blend of the PFL and the ILFL. **D,** The relationships of all three ligaments as viewed from an inferior position looking upward at the inferior aspect of the femoral head. (*AIIS,* Anterior inferior ischial spine; *ASIS,* anterior superior ischial spine; *IR,* ischial ramus.)

Birnbaum et al.[86] examined 11 formalin-mounted human hips and described a separation between the anterior innervation of the capsule (obturator and femoral nerve) and its posterior innervation (sciatic nerve, superior gluteal nerve, and the nerve to the quadratus femoris).

Recently, Kampa et al.[89] dissected 20 formalin-fixed human hips to further explore the innervation of the capsule and to define its pattern more accurately. They chose to illustrate the capsular innervation arrangement by depicting the capsule as the face of a clock. The reference point from which measurements were taken was the inferior acetabular notch to depict the 6- o'clock position. Therefore the position between 12 and 6 o'clock represented the anterior aspect of the capsule and the position between 6 and 12 o'clock represented the posterior position. Their findings, discussed later in this chapter, were consistent with previous reports and demonstrate a richly innervated structure, innervated by five to seven nerves and a variable number of their branches (direct or muscular).[86-90]

Femoral Nerve

The femoral nerve is formed by the L2 to L4 nerve roots in the lumbar plexus. It courses along the iliacus muscle and alongside the psoas, descends under the inguinal ligament, innervates the anterior thigh musculature, and provides cutaneous innervation to the lower leg through its terminal branch of the saphenous nerve. The femoral nerve travels with (and lateral to) the femoral artery and vein. The capsular branches of the femoral nerve, which travel along the anterior margin of the capsule, pierce the capsule either medially or laterally over an arc of 75 degrees between the half-past 2- and 5-o'clock positions.[89]

Obturator Nerve

The obturator nerve roots from L2 to L4 descend through the fibers of the psoas major and emerge from the medial border and later enter the thigh through the obturator canal. The capsular branches of the obturator nerve travel along the anteroinferior margin of the capsule, entering the capsule primarily medially over an arc of 105 degrees between 3 o'clock and half past 6 o'clock, with an equal contribution from both the anterior and posterior branches.[60] The obturator nerve also provides innervation to the knee joint.

Accessory Obturator Nerve

In the past the accessory obturator nerve has been described as being present in between 10% and 30% of people.[87,88,90,92] However, Birnbaum et al.[86] did not find it at all in 11 specimens, and Kampa et al.[89] found it in only 1 of 20 hips (5%), where it crossed the anteroinferior margin of the capsule and entered it medially over an arc of 15 degrees between half past 5 and 6 o'clock.

Superior Gluteal Nerve

Originating at the sacral plexus from the L4 to S1 sacral nerves, the superior gluteal nerve leaves the pelvis through the greater sciatic foramen above the piriformis, accompanied by the superior gluteal artery and the superior gluteal vein. Kampa et al.[89] found that the superior gluteal nerve branches to the capsule are small and have a leash of vessels; they cross the superior and posterolateral aspects of the capsule and enter it medially or more commonly laterally over an arc of 75 degrees between half past 10 and 1 o'clock.[89]

Inferior Gluteal Nerve

The inferior gluteal nerve, a branch of the sacral plexus, leaves the pelvis through the lower part of the greater sciatic foramen, below the piriformis, and terminates by innervating the gluteus maximus. Kampa et al.[89] have found a contribution to capsular innervation from the inferior gluteal nerve in only two specimens (10%), and noted that the nerve entered the capsule laterally at 8 o'clock.

Sciatic Nerve

The sciatic nerve is formed by the joining of the L4 to S3 roots. The nerve courses laterally through the pelvis, exits at the greater sciatic foramen, and travels distally deep to the piriformis and superficially to the short external rotators. The nerve divides along the course of the posterior thigh into the common peroneal trunk and the tibial trunk. The common peroneal trunk lies more laterally. The area of the capsule supplied by the sciatic nerve overlaps with that of the superior gluteal nerve, with its branches traveling along the posterior margin of the capsule and entering the capsule mainly medially but also laterally over an arc of 90 degrees between 9 and 12 o'clock.[89]

Nerve to Quadratus Femoris

The nerve to the quadratus femoris is a sacral plexus nerve that arises from L4 to S1 and leaves the pelvis through the greater sciatic foramen. Its branches to the capsule supply the quadratus femoris posteroinferiorly and enter it predominantly medially and occasionally laterally over an arc of 105 degrees between half past 6 and 10 o'clock.[89]

Safe Zone of the Capsule

Kampa et al.[89] found that anterosuperiorly, between 1 o'clock and half past 2 o'clock, no nerves enter the capsule. This internervous plane, which is poorly innervated, was named the "safe zone" of the capsule (Fig. 79-8).

Capsule Vascularization

Kalhor et al.[94] have studied the vascularization of the hip capsule using intraarterial injection of colored silicon in 20 hips. In all specimens, contributions to the hip capsule vasculature arose from the medial femoral circumflex artery, lateral femoral circumflex artery, superior gluteal artery, and inferior gluteal artery. The circumflex arteries supplied the anterior capsule, whereas the posterior capsule was supplied by the gluteal arteries, augmented by contributions from the circumflex arteries (Fig. 79-9).

Muscles Around the Hip Joint

More than 20 muscles cross the hip joint (Table 79-1). They can be grouped according to their main function and innervation. The hip abductors and internal rotators (gluteus medius, gluteus minimus, and tensor fascia lata) are innervated by the superior gluteal nerve; the hip flexors (iliopsoas, rectus femoris, sartorius, and pectineus) are innervated by the femoral nerve; the hip adductors (adductor magnus, adductor longus, adductor brevis, and gracilis) are innervated by the obturator nerve; and the muscles of the hip extensors have mostly unique nerves that are named after the muscle they innervate.

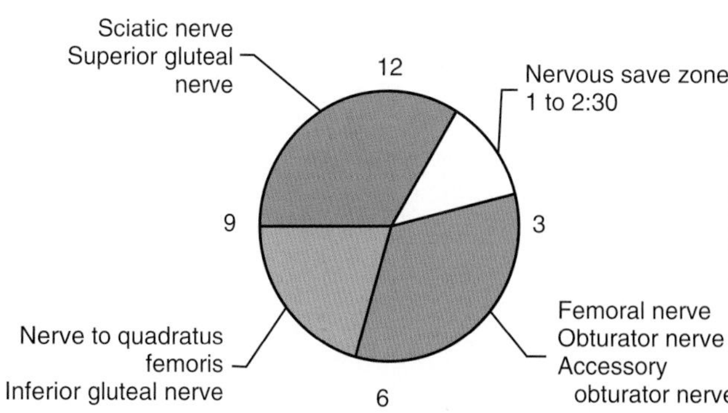

FIGURE 79-8 The capsule as the face of a clock. The pie chart demonstrates the different zones of innervation of the capsular and the internervous safe zone anterosuperiorly. *(From Kampa RJ, Prasthofer A, Lawrence-Watt DJ, et al: The internervous safe zone for incision of the capsule of the hip: a cadaver study.* J Bone Joint Surg Br *89-B[7]:971–976, 2007.)*

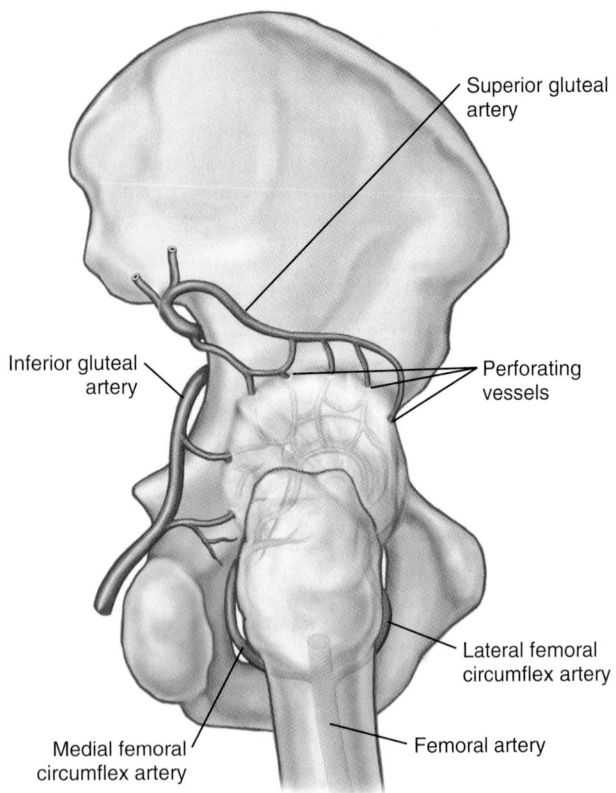

FIGURE 79-9 The hip from the posterior view, demonstrating the periacetabular vascular ring and anastomoses between distal and proximal vessels. *1,* Superior gluteal artery; *2,* inferior gluteal artery; *3,* medial femoral circumflex artery; *4,* lateral femoral circumflex artery; *5,* perforating vessels (cut surface). *(From Kalhor M, Beck M, Huff TW, et al: Capsular and pericapsular contributions to acetabular and femoral head perfusion.* J Bone Joint Surg Am *91[2]:409–418, 2009.)*

Abductors and Internal Rotators

The gluteus medius, gluteus minimus, and tensor fascia lata are abductors and internal rotators of the hip joint; all are innervated by the superior gluteal nerve, which originates from the sacral plexus (Table 79-1).

Gluteus Medius

The proximal attachment of the gluteus medius is at the anterior-superior iliac spine, along the outer edge of the iliac crest to the posterior-superior iliac spine.[95-97] The line of attachment is approximately 1-cm broad and limited to the iliac crest.[96] Robertson et al.[97] found that the gluteus medius tendon inserts into the greater trochanter by way of two distinct attachment sites, the superoposterior facet and the lateral facet. However, Gottschalk et al.[96] define the tendon attachment to be at the anterosuperior portion of the greater trochanter and not at its lateral aspect.

The muscle belly of the gluteus medius is composed of three distinct parts—anterior, middle, and posterior—and all three create a curved and fan-shaped muscle that tapers down to a flat tendon.[96-98] The muscle fibers of the posterior part are parallel to the femoral neck, whereas the anterior part fibers are nearly vertical.[96] Each one of the three parts of the gluteus medius is innervated by a separate branch of the superior gluteal nerve and has a different biomechanical function. The posterior part is thought to stabilize the femoral head in the acetabulum, together with the gluteus minimus. The middle is thought to initiate hip abduction. The anterior portion has two functions: its vertical fibers aid in abduction and its anterior fibers internally rotate the hip to allow pelvic rotation and swing-through of the contralateral lower limb.[96,97]

Gluteus Minimus

The gluteus minimus muscle attaches proximally on the iliac wing from the anterior inferior iliac spine to the posterior inferior iliac spine, along the middle gluteal line. Its distal attachment is on the anterior facet of the greater trochanter.[96,97] The fibers of this muscle tend to be horizontally orientated and run parallel to the neck of the femur.[96] The gluteus minimus is also innervated by the superior gluteal nerve. Both the gluteus medius and minimus have additional bursae deep to their respective tendons in the peritrochanteric area.

Tensor Fascia Lata

The tensor fascia lata arises from the anterior superior iliac spine and the outer lip of the anterior iliac crest and inserts distally between the two layers of the iliotibial band of the fascia lata. It is innervated by the superior gluteal nerve.

Flexors

Iliopsoas

The iliopsoas muscle is the main flexor of the hip joint, and in addition it acts as an external rotator. It is formed by two muscles, the iliacus and the psoas major, and is innervated by the femoral nerve. The iliacus muscle originates from the medial side of the iliac wing, whereas the psoas major arises from the transverse processes of the lumbar vertebrae, the intervertebral disks and adjacent vertebral margins of T12 to L5, and the tendinous arches.[99] Distally the iliopsoas attaches to the lesser trochanter in a unique muscle-tendon attachment where there is a direct muscular attachment in addition to the tendinous attachment. At the level of the joint the muscle/tendon ratio is around 50%.[100,101] As the iliopsoas travels distally, a greater percentage of the structure's area is tendon. The tendon passes anterior to the iliopectineal eminence and the anterior capsuloligamentous structures of the hip joint, with the iliopsoas bursa lying in between. The iliopsoas is also one of the dynamic stabilizers of the hip joint; its role as a stabilizer is more prominent in cases of inherent hip instability.[85,102]

Pectineus

The pectineus is a flat quadrangular muscle originating from the pectineal line on the superior ramus pubis and inserting to the femur distal to the lesser trochanter into the pectineal line of the femur. Its main functions are flexion and adduction of the hip. It is innervated mainly by the femoral nerve and sometimes has additional innervation from the obturator nerve.

Rectus Femoris

The rectus femoris is the only one of the four quadriceps muscles that crosses the hip joint. It is innervated by the

TABLE 79-1

MUSCLES AROUND THE HIP JOINT SORTED BY FUNCTION

Muscle	Origin	Insertion	Innervation	Spinal Level	Additional Function	Notes
Hip Abductors and Internal Rotators						
Gluteus medius	Ilium (between posterior-anterior gluteal lines)	Greater trochanter	Superior gluteal	L4–S1		
Gluteus minimus	Ilium (between anterior/inferior gluteal lines)	Greater trochanter	Superior gluteal	L4–S1		
Tensor fasciae latae	Anterior iliac crest	Iliotibial band (Gerdy's tubercle)	Superior gluteal	L4–S1		
Hip Flexors						
Iliopsoas	Iliac fossa (iliacus) transverse process L1-L5 (psoas)	Lesser trochanter	Femoral	L2–4	External rotation	Strongest hip flexor
Pectineus	Pectineal line of pubis bone	Pectineal line of femur	Femoral	L2–4	Adduction	
Rectus femoris	AIIS (straight head) anterior acetabular rim (reflected head)	Patella	Femoral	L2–4		Biarthrodial muscle
Sartorius	ASIS	Proximal medial tibia	Femoral	L2–4	External rotation	Biarthrodial muscle
Hip External Rotators						
Gluteus maximus	Ilium along crest posterior to posterior gluteal line	Iliotibial band/posterior femur	Inferior gluteal	L5–S2	Extension	
Piriformis	Anterior sacrum, through sciatic notch	Proximal greater trochanter (piriformis fossa)	Piriformis	S1–S2		
Obturator externus	Ischiopubic rami and external surface of the obturator membrane	Medial greater trochanter	Obturator (posterior branch)	L2–4	Adduction	
Obturator internus	Ischiopubic rami/obturator membrane	Medial greater trochanter	Obturator internus	L5–S2		
Superior gemellus	Ischial spine	Medial greater trochanter	Obturator internus	L5–S2		
Inferior gemellus	Ischial tuberosity	Medial greater trochanter	Quadratus femoris	L4–S1		
Quadratus femoris	Ischial tuberosity	Quadrate line of femur	Quadratus femoris	L4–S1		
Hip Extensors						
Gluteus maximus	Ilium along crest posterior to posterior gluteal line	Iliotibial band/posterior femur	Inferior gluteal	L5–S2	External rotation	
Long head of biceps femoris	Medial ischial tuberosity	Fibular head/lateral tibia	Tibial	L5–S2		Biarthrodial muscle, also flex the knee
Semitendinosus	Distal medial ischial tuberosity	Anterior tibial crest	Tibial	L5–S2		Biarthrodial muscle, also flex the knee
Semimembranosus	Proximal lateral ischial tuberosity	Posterior/medial tibia, posterior capsule, medial meniscus, popliteus, popliteal ligament	Tibial	L5–S2		Biarthrodial muscle, also flex the knee
Hip Adductors						
Adductor magnus	Inferior pubic ramus/ischial tuberosity	Linea aspera/adductor tubercle	Obturator (posterior branch) sciatic (tibial)	L2–4	Flexion, external rotation, extension	
Adductor brevis	Inferior pubic ramus	Linea aspera/pectineal line	Obturator (posterior branch)	L2–4	Flexion, external rotation	
Adductor longus	Anterior pubic ramus	Linea aspera	Obturator (anterior branch)	L2–4	Flexion, internal rotation	
Gracilis	Inferior symphysis/pubic arch	Proximal medial tibia	Obturator (anterior branch)	L2–4	Flexion, internal rotation	Biarthrodial muscle, also flex the knee

AIIS, Anterior inferior ischial spine; *ASIS,* anterior superior ischial spine.

femoral nerve and originates by two tendons: the anterior or straight head, from the anterior inferior iliac spine, and the posterior or reflected head, from a groove above the rim of the acetabulum. It is a biarthrodial muscle and inserts distally to the tibial tubercle with the patella within the combined quadriceps tendon.

Sartorius

The sartorius is the longest muscle in the body. It originates from the anterior superior iliac spine and inserts to the anteromedial surface of the upper tibia in the pes anserinus. The sartorius is innervated by the femoral nerve; it is a biarthrodial muscle that functions as a hip flexor and external rotator and also as a knee extensor.

Iliocapsularis

The iliocapsularis muscle is a little-known muscle that once was thought to be part of the iliopsoas muscle. It lies in the anterior aspect of the hip joint, originating from the inferior part of the anterior-inferior iliac spine and the anterior capsule, spanning directly on the anterior capsule and inserting distal to the lesser trochanter.[103] It is believed to play an important role in stabilizing dysplastic hips and was shown to be hypertrophic in that condition.[104]

Extensors

Hip extension is achieved by a synchronous activation of the gluteus maximus and the hamstring muscle complex.

Hamstrings

The hamstrings are a two-joint muscle complex crossing both the hip and the knee. The proximal hamstring complex is composed of the semimembranosus, the semitendinosus, and the long heads of the biceps femoris; they cross over the posterior hip joint and are innervated by the tibial nerve. The semitendinosus and the long head of the biceps have a common tendon attaching on the medial side of the ischial tuberosity, whereas the semimembranosus attaches laterally via a smaller footprint (Fig. 79-10).[105]

The short head of the biceps femoris is also part of the hamstring complex; however, it does not cross the hip joint. It attaches to the posterior aspect of the femur—the linea aspera—and is innervated by the common peroneal nerve and thus does not affect the hip joint motions directly.

Gluteus Maximus

The gluteus maximus is the largest of the three gluteal muscles. It is a wide and flat muscle that is responsible for hip extension and external rotation and is innervated by the inferior gluteal nerve. It has a wide origin proximally on the outer side of the ilium, the lumbar fascia, the sacrum, and the sacrotuberous ligament. Its fibers are directed obliquely in the lateral-inferior direction; distally it inserts to the gluteal tuberosity on the femur and the iliotibial band.

External Rotators

External rotation of the hip is performed by the gluteus maximus and the short external rotators, all of which originate from the posterior side of the pelvic ring.

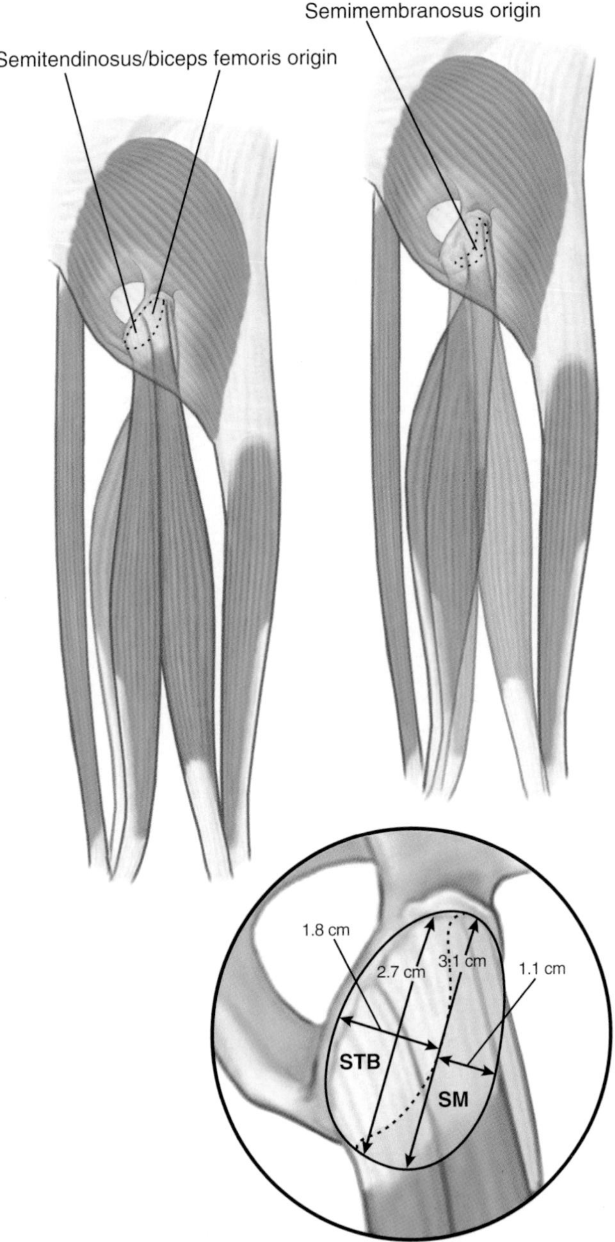

FIGURE 79-10 Posterior, right-sided views showing that the origin of the common tendon of the semitendinosus/biceps femoris (*STB*) is oval and measures 2.7 ± 0.5 cm from proximal to distal and 1.8 ± 0.2 cm from medial to lateral and that the semimembranosus (*SM*) origin is crescent shaped and measures 3.1 ± 0.3 cm from proximal to distal and 1.1 ± 0.5 cm from medial to lateral. The semimembranosus originates lateral to the common tendon of the semitendinosus/biceps femoris. *(From Miller SL, Gill J, Webb GR: The proximal origin of the hamstrings and surrounding anatomy encountered during repair: a cadaveric study.* J Bone Joint Surg Am *89[1]:44–48, 2007.)*

Short External Rotators

The short external rotators muscles include the piriformis, obturator externus, obturator internus, superior gemellus, inferior gemellus, and quadratus femoris. All the short external rotators are innervated by unique nerves named after the muscle they innervate. The piriformis is the superior muscle of the short rotators, originating from the anterior side of the sacrum, going posteriorly through the sciatic notch and inserting to the piriformis fossa on the proximal greater trochanter. The obturator internus, originating from the internal side of the obturator membrane and the posterior bony margins of obturator foramen, goes in between the superior and inferior gemelli, with all three of them joining together to form the conjoined tendon that inserts into the medial side of the greater trochanter. The obturator externus originates from the ischiopubic rami and external surface of the obturator membrane and inserts to the posteromedial surface of the greater trochanter. The quadratus femoris is the inferior muscle of the short rotators; it originates from the ischial tuberosity and inserts to the quadrate line of the femur.

Adductors

Adduction motion of the hip is performed by the adductor magnus, adductor brevis, adductor longus, and gracilis, all of which are innervated by the obturator nerve. The pectineus muscles also aid in adduction, and they are innervated by the femoral nerve. All the adductors originate in and around the pubic bone: the pectineus at the superior ramus pubis; the adductor longus at the anterior surface of the body of pubis, just lateral to the pubic symphysis; the adductor brevis at the anterior surface of inferior pubic ramus, inferior to origin of adductor longus; and the gracilis at the inferior margin of pubic symphysis. All adductors but the gracilis insert at the medioposterior side of the femur and the linea aspera, whereas the gracilis inserts at the medial surface of the proximal tibial shaft, just posterior to the sartorius (see Table 79-1).

The adductor magnus is composed of two parts: adductor and hamstring. The adductor part originates from the inferior pubic ramus and has relatively short horizontal fibers that insert onto the rough line leading from the greater trochanter to the linea aspera, medial to the gluteus maximus. This part is innervated by the posterior branch of the obturator nerve. The hamstring component originates from the ischial tuberosity and inserts at the adductor tubercle on the medial condyle of the distal femur. This hamstring part of the adductor magnus is innervated by the tibial nerve.

Bursae Around the Hip Joint

Trochanteric Bursae

The bursae in the greater trochanteric region, often referred as the *trochanteric bursa,* is a complex of several bursae that are intimately associated with the greater trochanter and the gluteal tendons. The three major bursae are the subgluteus maximus, the subgluteus medius, and the gluteofemoral bursae. The gluteus minimus bursa is a minor bursa located cephalad and ventral to the greater trochanter.[106] Dunn et al.[107] found a subgluteus-maximus bursa in 13 of 14 patients undergoing primary hip surgery. This bursa exists directly superficial to the common attachment of the gluteus medius, minimus, and vastus lateralis muscles onto the greater trochanter. It was termed the *deep bursa* or *dominant deep bursa* and *secondary deep bursa* if more than one was present. In five specimens, two bursae were present and could be separated easily through a fascial plane. The size of the deep bursae ranged from 1.5 to 4.7 cm long and 1.7 to 5.1 cm wide. In about half of the specimens, a smaller bursa was located on the deep surface of the gluteus maximus muscle and was termed the *superficial bursa*. In all specimens an additional deep bursa was located more distally, the gluteofemoral bursa, which was seen between the gluteus maximus and vastus lateralis muscles where the gluteus maximus muscle fibers insert onto the femur. In two specimens, branches of the inferior gluteal nerve (L5 to S2) were seen entering subgluteus-maximus bursae and the surrounding tissues.

Woodley et al.[108] also studied the bursae around the greater trochanter region in 18 embalmed human hips with use of macrodissection and histologic techniques. They demonstrated that multiple bursae are associated with the greater trochanter and are arranged in three distinct layers as determined by the planes of the gluteal tendons. Bursae in each layer differ with respect to morphology and location, although the centers of all bursae are positioned inferior to the apex of the greater trochanter. The mean number of bursae per hip was six, with a minimum of four and a maximum of nine bursae being found in any one specimen.

Iliopsoas Bursa

The iliopsoas bursa lies in between the anterior capsule of the hip joint and the iliopsoas tendon. This bursa has been described as the largest bursa in the body, measuring up to 7 cm long and 4 cm wide.[109,110] The portion of the anterior hip capsule between the iliofemoral and PFLs adjacent to the iliopsoas bursa is thin, with a communication between the hip joint and the bursa present in 14% to 25% of cadavers.[103,111-113]

General Hip Kinematics/Biomechanics

The hip joint is a ball and socket joint, with the acetabulum being the socket and the femoral head the ball. As with all ball and socket joints, it has six degrees of freedom: three planes of motion (flexion-extension, abduction-adduction, and internal-external rotation) and three planes of translations (anteroposterior, medial-lateral, and proximal-distal). Recent research has shown that the center of the femoral head moves relative to the acetabulum.[114,115] The joint motions are limited both by the bony anatomy and the soft tissues that surround the joint, mainly the hip capsule and ligaments.

Hip Motions

Hip range of motion may be affected by the bony morphology or ligamentous and muscle laxity. In general, a dysplastic acetabulum allows greater range of motion than a profunda acetabulum. However, hypermobility of a well-covered femoral head may be achieved by ligamentous and muscle laxity. In the standard hip, the range of motion is greatest in the sagittal plane; however, because many biarthrodial muscles (see Table 79-1) cross both the hip and the knee, the hip motion is also affected by the knee position. Hip flexion is around 120 to 140 degrees with the knee flexed actively and passively, and 90 degrees with the knee fully extended. Active hip extension is 10 to 20 degrees, and passive extension is as much as 30 degrees. Normal hip abduction is at least 50 degrees and adduction is 30 degrees (limited by the opposite extremity and the tensor fascia lata). Internal and external rotation of the flexed hip may range up to 70 and 90 degrees, respectively. Internal rotation is limited by the short external rotator muscles (obturator internus and externus, superior and inferior gemelli, quadratus femoris, and piriformis) and the ISFL. External rotation is limited by the lateral band of the ILFL, the PFL, the internal rotator muscles, and the degree of femoral neck anteversion.[35]

Hip Stability

Overall, the hip is considered a stable joint because of its bony architecture.[85,116-118] However, soft tissue has been shown to play a major role in the stability of the joint throughout a physiologic and supraphysiologic range of motion.[81,85,116-119] Biomechanical studies have suggested that the hip capsule works together with other static soft tissue stabilizers such as the acetabular labrum and transverse acetabular ligament.[81,85,116-119] In addition, dynamic stabilizers such as the iliopsoas, iliocapsularis, rectus femoris, and abductor complex also contribute to the overall maintenance of proper joint kinematics and force-coupled compression that enhance hip joint stability.[81,85,102,104] Nonetheless, the femoral head has been shown to move up to 3 mm relative to the acetabulum in intact cadaveric studies in which the hip is taken through the extremes of motion; average translation was 3.3 ± 2.8 mm medial-lateral, 1.4 ± 1.8 mm anteroposterior, and 0.3 ± 1.5 mm proximal-distal; these translations increased as more soft tissue was removed, except medial-lateral displacement.[115] In another study, ballet dancers with normal bony morphology were shown to have 1 to 6 mm of femoral head translation relative to the acetabulum when routine dancing motions were analyzed using optical tracker and 3D MRI.[114]

Gait Cycle

The gait cycle consists of two main phases: stance, while the foot is touching the ground, and swing, while the foot is in the air. In walking, the stance phase is longer and consists of about 60% of the gait cycle; thus, there is a double-support phase in which both feet are on the ground for approximately 20% of the total gait cycle. The double-support phase defines walking and occurs at the beginning and ending of each stance phase. When running, the stance phase is shorter than 50% of the gait cycle, and thus a float phase occurs in which both legs are in the air and at no time are both feet on the ground at the same time.[120-122] As the velocity of running increases, the stance phase shortens, and it has been reported to be 22% of the cycle in sprinting.[120]

The main motion of the hip during walking and running is in the sagittal plane—flexion and extension. During the stance phase the hip extends, adducts, and internally rotates, whereas during the swing phase the hip flexes, abducts, and externally rotates.[35,121,123] During normal walking the hip flexes to about 30 degrees and extends to around 10 degrees.[35,123] Flexion increases with running by approximately 20 degrees and another 10 to 15 degrees with sprinting.[120] Extension of the hip was found to differ slightly with running and was even reported to decrease with sprinting.[120,124] Anterior pelvic tilt is also a normal motion during both walking and running, and peak anterior pelvic tilt was found to have a significant positive correlation with peak hip extension.[124]

Another difference between running and walking is that during walking a wider base is found between the feet. In running the base narrows so that foot strike is more on the center line of progression. Hip adduction is 5 to 10 degrees in walking and 15 to 20 degrees during running.[35,123]

In general, the muscles around the hip joint work in conjunction with each other. Using electromyography, different activation patterns during walking and running beside the amplitude were shown.[125] Hip flexors are active mainly during the swing phase, and extensors are active during the stance phase. The gluteus maximus and the hamstrings also function at the same time to help decelerate the swinging thigh.[120,125] Hip adductor muscles are active throughout the running cycle, whereas in walking they are active only from the swing phase to the middle of the stance phase.[121] The gluteus medius and tensor fascia lata help stabilize the pelvis; during running they are active during the swing and early stance phases, whereas in walking they are active mainly during the stance phase.[125]

Forces Around the Hip Joint

The hip joint is complicated biomechanically and is difficult to study, because measuring the forces directly in a live person would require surgical intervention and implantation of transducers. Nonetheless, many methods have been used to investigate the forces throughout the hip joint: (1) simplification of the macro forces around the hip joint, also known as multibody dynamics; (2) measurement of forces in vivo in an implanted hip prosthesis; (3) in silico (computational simulation) micromechanics, also known as finite element analysis; (4) cadaveric studies; and (5) dynamic imaging studies with live volunteers.

Multibody Dynamics

A simple diagram of the forces around the hip joint during single leg stance is the most common use of multibody dynamics (Fig. 79-11).[123] The parameters in the equation are

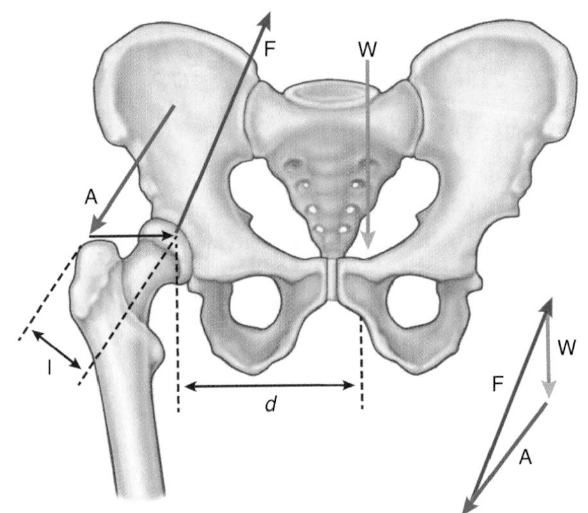

FIGURE 79-11 Forces acting on the hip joint during single-leg stance under conditions of equilibrium. Gravitational force (*W*), abductor muscle force (*A*), hip joint reaction force (*F*), abductor muscle moment arm (*l*), and force of gravity moment arm (*d*).

body weight (W) minus one leg weight (W – 1/6W), the abductors muscles force (A), the joint reaction force according to Newton's first law of motion (F), the moment arm from the center of gravity to the center of the hip joint (d), and the abductor muscle moment arm (l). The calculation takes into account that when standing on one leg the pelvis is in equilibrium, and thus the abductors muscles force (A) multiplied by the abductor muscle moment arm (l) is equal to the body weight (W) minus one leg (1/6W) multiplied by moment arm from the center of gravity to the center of the hip joint (d) or $A \times l = (W - 1/6W) \times d$. The joint reaction force (F) according to Newton's first law of motion is the force resulting in response to the weight and the abductors' muscle contraction. In general, when standing on one leg, the center of gravity shifts away from the stance leg, forcing the abductors to work harder, and as a result, increasing the joint force to 2.7 times the body weight with walking (see Fig. 79-11).[123]

In Vivo Studies

Bergmann et al.[126,127] have studied hip contact forces based on gait patterns during daily activities using instrumented implants, that is, implant pressure transducers into total hip prosthesis components. This method allows direct measurement of all the forces acting on the prosthetic hip joint. The measured forces were found to change with different gait activities: approximately 80% to 100% of body weight during two-legged stance, 250% during one-legged stance, 300% during slow walking, 350% to 400% with quick walking, up to 500% during jogging, to a maximum of more than 800% during stumbling.[127] The fact that the force during two-legged stance was not one half of the body weight is attributed to the persistent muscle forces acting on the hips.[123]

In Silico Studies

Finite element analysis methodology can simulate complex geometries and complex loads when all of the elements are reassembled during the solution process. This solution enables a simulation of static and dynamic situations. Typically, finite element analysis mesh geometries of musculoskeletal tissues are generated from CT and MRI data, whereas material properties are usually extrapolated from in vitro measurements.[128] This methodology has been used to calculate the forces throughout the femoral neck regarding stress fractures or pressure distribution within the hip joint. Russell et al.[129] used finite element analysis to calculate the contact force distribution throughout the acetabulum during the gait cycle phases from the resultant contact force applied during gait stance phase kinematics. Maximal load of twice the body weight was calculated within the joint during the midstance phase (Fig. 79-12).

In Vitro Studies

Cadaveric biomechanics studies have been used for many years to measure forces and motion in and around the hip joint. The main limitation of this method is the lack of muscle force and body weight, which need to be created artificially. Day et al.[130] have shown an increase of up to five times normal pressure in areas with thin fibrocartilage, mainly at the zenith of the acetabulum. Konrath et al.[131] measured the distribution of contact area and pressure between the acetabulum and the femoral head before and after cutting the acetabular labrum and transverse ligament. Simulating a single-limb stance, a peripheral distribution of load was seen in the intact acetabula. This pattern was altered only minimally after removal of the transverse acetabular ligament or the labrum, or both. Conversely, Ferguson et al.[132] checked the sealing effect of the acetabular labrum in vitro; a decrease in the intraarticular fluid pressure after labral resection was found, indicating the imperative sealing effect of the labrum. Song et al.[53] measured the resistance to rotation, which reflects articular cartilage friction, in five cadaveric hips joints during half, one, two, and three times body weight cyclic loading in the intact hip and after focal and complete labrectomy. Resistance to rotation was significantly increased after focal labrectomy at one to three times body weight loading and after complete labrectomy at all load levels.

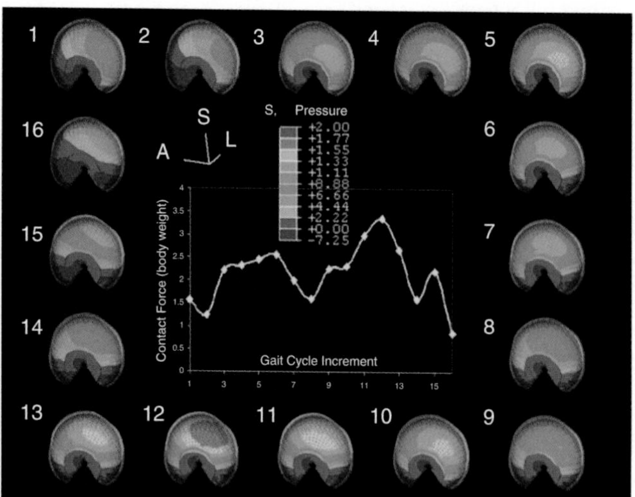

FIGURE 79-12 Acetabular loads. Applied loads and normal hip contact contours. Finite element control hip contact pressure contours at each gait cycle increment developed from the resultant contact force (*inset*) applied during gait stance phase kinematics. Maximal load of twice the body weight within the joint was found during the midstance phase. *(From Russell ME, Shivanna KH, Grosland NM, et al: Cartilage contact pressure elevations in dysplastic hips: a chronic overload model.* J Orthop Surg Res *1:6, 2006.)*

Dynamic Imaging Studies

Studies on live subjects have the potential to be the most accurate method to perform dynamic biomechanics studies. One option to perform those studies is to use an optical tracking system while the subjects perform different movements; the results are applied to a 3D model, which is based on the subject's MRI or CT images. Charbonnier et al.[114] used an optical tracking device with a combination of 3D MRI to study the hip motions of 11 pairs of female ballet dancers with no morphologic abnormalities. Based on their results, four dancing movements seemed to be potentially harmful for the hip joint, inducing significant stress in the hip joint, with high frequency of impingement and femoroacetabular translations ranging from 0.93 to 6.35 mm. For almost all movements, the computed zones of impingement were mainly located in the superior or posterosuperior quadrant of the acetabulum.

Hip-Spine Relationship

The hip and spine are closely related. Reduced range of motion in the hip may result in overuse of the lumbar spine,

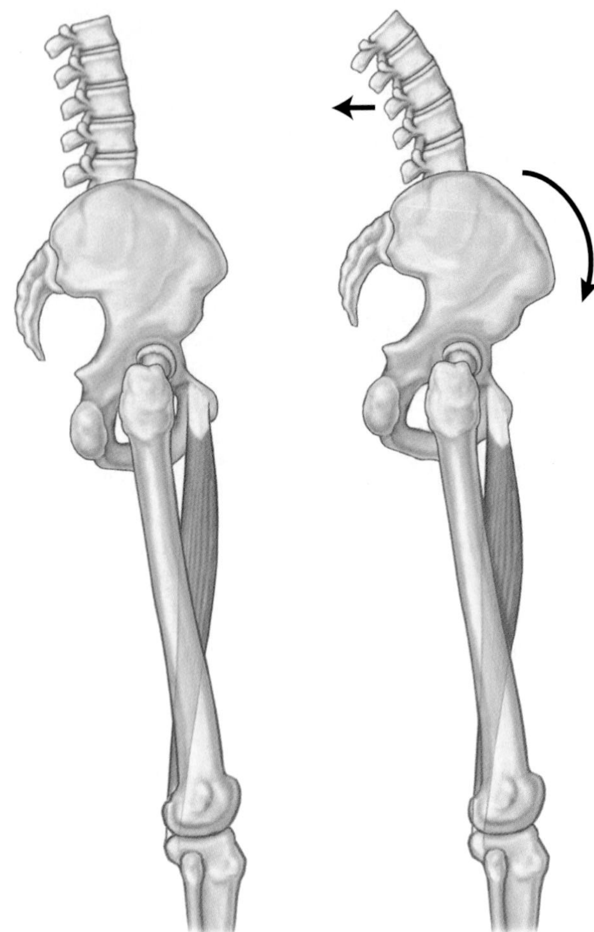

FIGURE 79-13 Hip/spine balance. Flexion deformity of the hip rotates the pelvis forward and hyperextends the lumbar spine.

and vice versa (Fig. 79-13). Esola et al.[133] have examined the role of the low back and the hip in forward bending in subjects with and without a history of back pain. Mean total forward bending for all subjects was 111 degrees—41.6 degrees from the lumbar spine and 69.4 degrees from the hips. The lumbar spine had a greater contribution to early forward bending, the lumbar spine and hips contributed almost equally to middle forward bending, and the hips had a greater contribution to late forward bending. Patients with a history of back pain tended to move more at their lumbar spine during early forward bending and had a significantly lower lumbar/hip flexion ratio during middle forward bending. Additionally, hip disorders can cause back pain secondarily by creating an abnormal sagittal balance and irregular gait that places further strain on the spine.[134,135]

Summary

Over the years the hip joint has been the subject of many anatomic and biomechanical studies. The anatomy of the hip joint seems simple on the basic level. However, more detailed inspection reveals that the hip joint is quite complex in anatomy, and particularly biomechanics. The hip appears to be a ball-and-socket joint, but it functions more like a gimbal joint. Although plenty of biomechanical studies exist, more advanced study of hip biomechanics is needed. The current chapter aimed to review the most updated studies in those areas, giving fundamental tools for understanding of the different hip joint pathologies.

For a complete list of references, go to expertconsult.com.

Suggested Readings

Citation: Safran MRLN, Zaffagnini S, Signorelli C, et al: In vitro analysis of periarticular soft tissues constraining effect on hip kinematics and joint stability. *Knee Surg Sports Traumatol Arthrosc* 21:1655–1663, 2012.

Level: III

Summary: This article pertains to an in vitro cadaveric study on the stability of the hip joint. The study showed that with hip motion, the femoral head is translating relatively to the acetabulum in all three planes. This translation increased with removal of the soft tissue around the joint, confirming its importance to hip stability.

Citation: Lee MC, Eberson CP: Growth and development of the child's hip. *Orthop Clin North Am* 37(2):119–132, 2006.

Level: III

Summary: This review regards the growth and development of the hip, beginning with prenatal cellular development. The authors discuss the ossification centers and blood supply of the femur and acetabulum.

Citation: Stops A, Wilcox R, Jin Z: Computational modeling of the natural hip: A review of finite element and multibody simulations. *Comput Methods Biomech Biomed Engin* 15(9):963–979, 2011.

Level: III

Summary: This article provides a review on finite element and multibody simulations of the hip. The former provide knowledge on contact pressures and the effects of musculoskeletal geometries, in particular cartilage and bone shapes, whereas the latter deal with the influence of gait patterns and muscle attachment locations on force magnitudes.

Citation: Franz JR, Paylo KW, Dicharry J, et al: Changes in the coordination of hip and pelvis kinematics with mode of locomotion. *Gait Posture* 29(3):494–498, 2009.

Level: III

Summary: This article summarizes a biomechanical/kinematic study on 73 healthy adult runners who were running on a treadmill. The influence of pick hip extension during walking and running on pelvic tilt and lumbar lordosis is explored.

Citation: Ferguson SJ, Bryant JT, Ganz R, et al: An in vitro investigation of the acetabular labral seal in hip joint mechanics. *J Biomech* 36(2):171–178, 2003.

Level: III

Summary: This article reviews a biomechanical study on the acetabular labrum and is one of the most-cited articles on the subject. It is shown that hydrostatic fluid pressurization within the intraarticular space is greater with the labrum than without it, which may enhance joint lubrication. It also is shown that cartilage consolidation is quicker without the labrum than with it, because the labrum adds an extra resistance to the flow path for interstitial fluid expression.

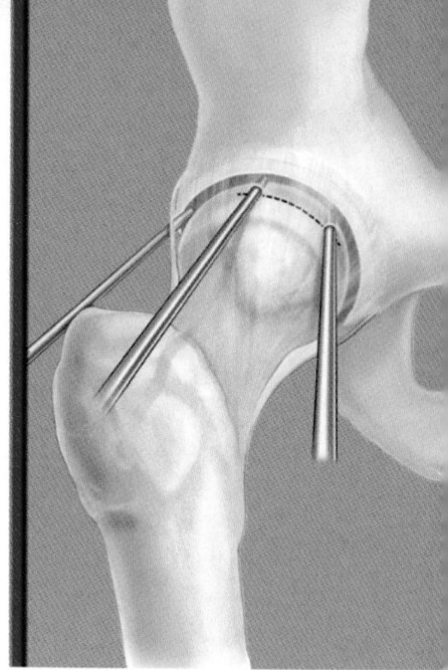

80

Hip Diagnosis and Decision Making

ADAM G. BROOKS • JOHN REDMOND • BENJAMIN G. DOMB

Overview of Pathologies

A solid understanding of the differential diagnosis for hip pathology is necessary before collecting a history and performing a physical examination. This background allows the clinician to tease out important elements in the history to narrow the differential and provide a focus for the physical examination. An overview of hip pathology is presented in the following sections (Box 80-1).

Soft Tissue Injuries

Inflammation and pain originating from the trochanteric, ischial, iliopsoas, and iliopectineal bursae are common. Movement at bone and soft tissue interfaces leads to repetitive friction and inflammation in these areas. Trochanteric bursitis is very common. Patients describe lateral thigh pain that can be reproduced with palpation on examination. Ischial bursitis typically presents with pain upon sitting and can be reproduced by palpation over the ischial tuberosity. The iliopsoas bursa lies between the iliopsoas muscle and pelvic brim.[1] Patients typically present with inguinal pain that is reproducible with provocative maneuvers such as the Thomas test. The iliopectineal bursa is adjacent to the iliopsoas bursa but lies over the iliopectineal eminence. Symptoms are similar to those of iliopsoas bursitis, although iliopectineal bursitis can be seen in conjunction with a snapping iliopsoas muscle over the iliopectineal eminence.[2]

Snapping hip syndrome, also referred to as *coxa saltans,* causes an audible or palpable "snap" with hip range of motion (ROM). The etiology of a snapping hip is classified as external, internal, or intraarticular.[3] An external snapping hip is caused by the iliotibial band gliding over the greater trochanter. An internal snapping hip is attributed to shifting of the iliopsoas tendon from medial to lateral over the femoral head, or iliopectineal eminence, during hip flexion and extension. An intraarticular snapping hip is related to labral tears, loose bodies, or osteochondral injuries.

Contusions involving the hip, thigh, and pelvis are frequently encountered in athletes and occur after low-energy trauma. An iliac crest contusion, or "hip pointer," results from a direct blow to the iliac crest, and an overlying hematoma often develops. Quadriceps contusions typically involve a direct blow to the anterior thigh, which can result in hematoma formation and difficulty ambulating. A direct blow to the inner thigh may result in a groin contusion. Myositis ossificans often occurs after a contusion and hematoma.[4] The hematoma organizes and calcifies, which can lead to pain and stiffness. Myositis ossificans can also be seen in the absence of trauma.

Muscle strains and ligamentous injuries in the area of the hip can be quite debilitating. Strains typically involve tearing at the musculotendinous junction and often occur during an eccentric contraction.[5] Strains are classified by the affected muscle groups, including adductor, iliopsoas, external oblique, hamstring, and quadriceps. With significant force during athletics, or in the setting of trauma, the strong sacroiliac ligaments can be sprained. Pain typically originates in the lower back and radiates into the buttock or groin.

Hernias involve the extrusion of abdominal contents through a defect in the abdominal wall. A delay in diagnosis is common because hernias can mimic other conditions that cause groin pain with activity. Three hernias can present as hip or pelvic pain: inguinal, femoral, and sports hernias. Inguinal hernias involve the protrusion of abdominal contents through the deep inguinal ring or medial to the deep inguinal ring. Femoral hernias occur when a hernia sac protrudes through the femoral sheath to enter the anterior thigh. The sports hernia is an increasingly recognized condition causing groin pain in athletes. The pathophysiology is incompletely understood, but it appears to involve weakness or tearing of the posterior inguinal wall. No true protrusion of abdominal contents occurs, but patients experience chronic groin pain that is often difficult to diagnose.[6]

Bone Injuries

Trauma during sporting events can result in fractures of the pelvis and femur. Pelvic ring injuries, acetabular fractures, femoral head and neck fractures, peritrochanteric fractures, and femoral shaft fractures lead to the acute onset of pain and difficulty with mobilization. Prompt recognition and treatment of the bony injury and soft tissue trauma is critical. Hip dislocations also occur when significant force disrupts the soft tissue restraints of the hip joint.[7] Hip dislocations are typically posterior, which leads to the patient having a shortened, internally rotated, and abducted hip. Less commonly, the dislocation will be anterior, which presents as an externally rotated and abducted hip. Expeditious recognition and reduction may be essential to prevent avascular necrosis.

Stress fractures of the pelvis and femur occur in the setting of repetitive submaximal loading of bone. Pain that is

BOX 80-1 Overview of Hip Pathology

Soft Tissue Injuries
- Bursitis
  - Trochanteric
  - Ischial
  - Iliopsoas
  - Iliopectineal
- Snapping hip syndrome
- Contusions
  - Iliac crest
  - Quadriceps
  - Groin
- Myositis ossificans
- Strains
  - Adductor
  - Iliopsoas
  - External oblique
  - Hamstring
  - Quadriceps
- Sacroiliac sprain
- Hernias
  - Inguinal
  - Femoral
  - Sports (athletic pubalgia)

Bone Injuries
- Traumatic fractures
- Dislocation
- Stress fractures
  - Pelvic
  - Sacral
  - Femoral neck
- Osteitis pubis
- Osteonecrosis

Degenerative Joint Disease

Nerve Entrapment Injuries
- Sciatic
- Obturator
- Pudendal
- Ilioinguinal
- Femoral
- Lateral femoral cutaneous

Intraarticular Pathology
- Labral tears
- Femoral acetabular impingement
- Loose bodies
- Chondral injuries
- Ruptured ligamentum teres

Infection

Pediatric Conditions
- Avulsion fracture
- SCFE
- Legg-Calvé-Perthes disease

SCFE, Slipped capital femoral epiphysis.

aggravated by activity and subsides with rest is the hallmark feature of a stress fracture. Pelvic rami and sacral stress fractures are seen in athletes who participate in high-impact activities such as running and jogging. The pain is typically in the groin, buttock, or thigh when the ramus is involved and in the low back when the sacrum is the source.[8] Femoral neck stress fractures typically present with activity-related groin pain. The location of the stress fracture is critical to determining treatment. Tension-sided femoral neck stress fractures along the superior lateral neck require surgical treatment to prevent nonunion, avascular necrosis, or fracture displacement. Compression-sided femoral neck stress fractures occur along the inferior medial neck and are often amenable to nonoperative treatment.[9]

Inflammation of the pubic symphysis is termed "osteitis pubis." Overuse of hip adductors and the gracilis may lead to this condition.[10] The pain is typically insidious in onset and midline over the symphysis.

Osteonecrosis, or avascular necrosis, of the femoral head is a cause of hip pain in young adults. Many conditions have been associated with osteonecrosis; however, the majority are related to corticosteroid use, trauma, alcohol abuse, and coagulopathy.[11] No cause is identified in 10% to 20% of cases, and this type of necrosis is termed "idiopathic avascular necrosis." Patients typically present with pain in the groin or buttock and often walk with a limp. Bilateral avascular necrosis has been found in 40% to 80% of patients.[11-13] Early identification may allow treatment that can prevent femoral head collapse and the need for arthroplasty.

Degenerative Joint Disease

Degenerative joint disease (DJD) results from the loss of cartilage in the hip joint and leads to progressive pain and stiffness. Although the process may be idiopathic, we now recognize that structural abnormalities of the hip are frequently associated with DJD.[14] The diagnosis is usually confirmed by observing joint space narrowing on plain radiographs. Patients typically present with the insidious onset of hip pain that worsens with activity.

Nerve Entrapment Injuries

Nerve entrapment surrounding the hip can involve the sciatic, obturator, pudendal, ilioinguinal, femoral, and lateral femoral cutaneous nerve. Diagnosing and treating these conditions can be difficult and frustrating for the patient and clinician. The pain often has a burning quality and is confined to a nerve root distribution. Electromyographic and nerve conduction studies are helpful in confirming the diagnosis and ruling out a lumbar radiculopathy. Sciatic nerve entrapment often presents with pain radiating down the buttock and posterior thigh. In some cases, this pain may be related to piriformis syndrome.[15] Obturator nerve entrapment causes pain in the medial thigh that can radiate toward the knee.[16] Prolonged compression during activities such as cycling can cause pudendal nerve entrapment.[17] Numbness and pain in the perineum and shaft of the penis are typical. Ilioinguinal nerve entrapment is a cause of inguinal pain that often radiates into the groin. Pain over the anterior thigh can be caused by femoral nerve entrapment, and when severe, it may cause quadriceps weakness and difficulty with gait.[18] Lateral femoral cutaneous nerve entrapment, or *meralgia paresthetica*, causes anterolateral thigh pain and numbness that extends toward the lateral knee.[19]

Intraarticular Pathology

Our understanding of intraarticular pathology has significantly expanded during the past few decades. Structural abnormalities of the hip joint seen in persons with dysplasia and femoroacetabular impingement often lead to injury of the labrum and chondral surface. Hip dysplasia, or developmental dysplasia of the hip, results in a broad spectrum of disease. The underlying abnormality is inadequate coverage of the femoral head, which in severe forms can cause hip dislocations in children. Often the degree of undercoverage is mild and leads to pathology during adulthood because of the concentration of forces on a shallow acetabulum.[20] Femoroacetabular impingement is caused by abnormalities of the femur and acetabulum that lead to abnormal contact within the hip joint.[21] Deformity on the femoral side is termed *cam impingement* and is due to an out-of-round femoral head. Deformity on the acetabular side is termed *pincer impingement* and occurs when the acetabulum is too deep. Frequently both abnormalities exist in the same hip joint, and this condition is termed *combined impingement*. The iliopsoas muscle can also cause direct anterior impingement.[22] Patients with intraarticular pathology typically present with groin or buttock pain. Scrutinizing hip radiographs will often help the clinician identify morphologic abnormalities of the hip that may lead to intraarticular pathology.[14] Multiple other sources of intraarticular pathology have also been described, such as ruptured ligamentum teres, loose bodies, and synovial disease.

Infection

Septic arthritis of the hip should always be considered in a patient who presents with the acute onset of pain. The patient is often febrile and lacks a history of trauma. Physical examination reveals pain with attempted passive ROM. Inflammatory markers are typically elevated. Prompt recognition and treatment are necessary to prevent long-term complications.[23]

Pediatric Hip Conditions

Skeletally immature patients often present with hip conditions that differ from the hip conditions of adults. Open physes and apophyses are areas of weakness and are frequently injured. When muscles are overloaded in children, failure can occur at the origin of the muscle, particularly when an apophysis is present.[24] This scenario causes an avulsion fracture at the muscle origin, which differs from the pathology seen in adults, who most frequently experience a fracture at the musculotendinous junction. Avulsion fractures occur at the anterior superior iliac spine, anterior inferior iliac spine, ischial tuberosity, and lesser trochanter when the sartorius, rectus femoris, hamstrings, and iliopsoas muscles, respectively, are overloaded.

Slipped capital femoral epiphysis (SCFE) is a disorder of the proximal femoral physis. The proximal femoral physis fails, leading to anterior superior displacement of the femur relative to the epiphysis.[25] This condition typically involves patients 11 to 14 years of age and often affects obese children. Displacement at the physis can frequently be identified with a frog-leg lateral radiograph. When SCFE is identified, surgical treatment is typically indicated.

Legg-Calvé-Perthes disease is a childhood disorder that leads to ischemic necrosis of the growing femoral head.[26] The process typically affects patients 5 to 8 years of age and predominantly involves boys. Parents notice that the child is limping, and the patient often has mild pain. Radiographs often identify abnormalities in the femoral epiphysis.

History

Evaluation of the hip should begin with a thorough history, including several standard components. The goal of the history should be to (1) rule out any alarming sources of hip pathology, including cancer, infection, or systemic disease; (2) begin to differentiate true hip pain from back pain, which can often be confused[27]; and (3) narrow the differential diagnosis to perform a focused physical examination. The clinician should ascertain the patient's age and profession, the chief complaint, the presence or absence of trauma, and any treatment modalities the patient may already have attempted to use. These modalities often include nonsteroidal antiinflammatory medications, assistive devices, interaction with other physicians, or physical therapy.[28] If the patient has experienced a recent trauma, a detailed history of that trauma should be elicited. A history of acute onset or trauma is a better prognostic indicator than an insidious onset of symptoms.[29] A detailed pain history includes the location, intensity, quality, onset, duration, alleviating factors, aggravating factors, and associated factors (Fig. 80-1). The clinician also should inquire about the presence of mechanical symptoms such as popping, locking, clicking, subjective instability, pain that is worse with activity, or pain that is worse with twisting maneuvers. Pain or catching during flexion and axial loading activities (e.g., rising from a seated position, walking up or down stairs, or entering and exiting a vehicle) also implies mechanical hip pain.[30] Patients also report pain with sexual intercourse or difficulty putting on shoes or socks because of rotational force and complex hip movements.[31]

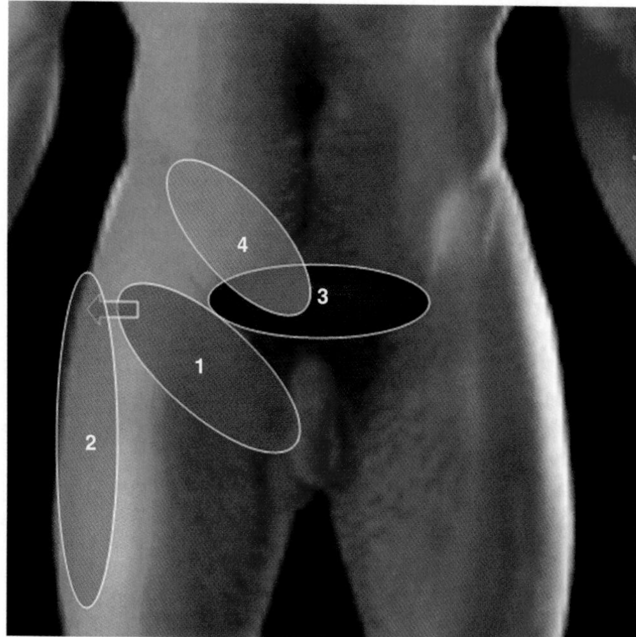

FIGURE 80-1 The location of pain can aid in diagnosis. *1,* Intraarticular pain can be caused by osteoarthritis or labral pathology. *2,* Lateral hip pain can be caused by trochanteric bursitis or abductor contracture. *3,* Symphyseal pain can be caused by osteitis pubis. *4,* Abdominal pain can be caused by athletic hernias.

The remainder of the standard history should not be overlooked. A medical and surgical history may uncover recent or remote illness including malignancy, an immune-compromised state, tuberculosis or other infection, trauma, previous hip dislocation, deep venous thrombosis, or hernia. A family history of cancer, systemic inflammatory arthritis, hip instability, or DJD is also useful. A social history detailing abuse of tobacco, alcohol, or illicit drugs is also important and may increase the index of suspicion for osteonecrosis of the femoral head or malignancy. Obtaining a sexual history as part of the social history can help evaluate the patient's risk of a sexually transmitted infection, which can cause septic arthritis. Pain with menses also should be noted. The social history should include a review of the patient's activities of daily living, work activities, hobbies, athletic activities, and impairments to these activities that are a result of the chief complaint.

BOX 80-2 Information Obtained from Patient History

Character and location of pain
Mechanism of injury (be specific if possible)
Duration of symptoms
Activity-related pain (e.g., does it subside with rest?)
Pain related to bowel or bladder activity or ingestion of food
Pain related to menses
Treatment history (injections, physical therapy, other physician evaluations)

Participation in running, soccer, ballet, hockey, golf, tennis, martial arts, or rugby is specifically associated with hip pathology.[32-34] A review of systems including recent fever, chills, malaise, night sweats, or unintended weight loss may raise red flags as well.[35] The clinician should remember that genitourinary, gastrointestinal, neurologic, or vascular pathology can also masquerade as hip pain.

When eliciting the history, the clinician should ask the patient what he or she believes is causing the pain. The patient's expectations of the encounter should be addressed, and he or she should be given a specific opportunity to ask questions or raise concerns. Additionally, the patient may provide or recall more pertinent history during the physical examination, and thus the clinician must listen attentively at all times (Box 80-2).

Physical Examination

The physical examination of the hip consists of several steps, including inspection, symptom localization, measurements, ROM, and special maneuvers.

Inspection

Several important pieces of information can be obtained simply by observing the patient. Stance and gait inspection are essential components of the physical examination. The patient's stance should be inspected for a slightly flexed position of the hip or knee, which may be indicative of hip pathology. The patient's stance should also be inspected for gross atrophy, spinal malalignment, or pelvic obliquity. While sitting, the patient should be observed for slouching to the unaffected side to avoid excessive flexion. The gait should be observed in multiple planes and for six to eight strides in the frontal and sagittal plane.[36]

The patient may present with one of several different gait abnormalities, including an antalgic gait, a pelvic wink, Trendelenburg's gait, excessive pelvic internal or external rotation, or true or false leg length discrepancies.[28] The antalgic gait involves a limp to decrease the time of stance phase on the affected side and limit weight bearing through the affected hip. An antalgic gait indicates pain in the hip, pelvis, or lower back. A pelvic wink is greater than 40 degrees of rotation in the axial plane toward the affected hip during terminal extension and signifies a hip flexion contracture in the setting of lumbar lordosis or forward-stooping posture. Trendelenburg's gait, also known as an abductor lurch, involves a lurching of the trunk toward the side of the affected hip. Abductors normally stabilize the pelvis when the contralateral leg is raised. If the abductor muscles or the nerves supplying those muscles are injured or not functioning, the patient will lurch to the ipsilateral side to prevent pelvic sagging. A Trendelenburg sign can be elicited by having the patient raise the contralateral leg. A pelvic sag of more than 2 cm on the ipsilateral side is a positive Trendelenburg sign, indicating abductor pathology. Internal or external rotation should be noted both during gait and once again in the sitting position, which stabilizes the pelvis. Decreased internal rotation is a sign of internal hip pathology.[37] Excessive internal rotation with decreased external rotation indicates increased femoral anteversion.[38] A short leg limp during gait may indicate a true or false leg length discrepancy, or the limp may be secondary to iliotibial (IT) band pathology. Children with leg length discrepancy may present with a circumduction gait or a vaulting gait to clear the long leg.[39]

Snapping or clicking noises should be noted as the patient walks. These noises can indicate iliopsoas, IT band, or intraarticular pathology. Lateral snapping is more likely with IT band pathology and generally is easily visualized.[40] Audible snapping is more likely a result of iliopsoas tendon pathology.

Symptom Localization

Numerous techniques can help localize symptoms. A simple tool involves asking the patient to localize his or her pain by using a single finger. This technique can narrow the differential. Additionally, examination of this location can be reserved for the end of the examination, thus enhancing the patient's trust by not causing pain at the beginning of the examination. This pain location in conjunction with Hilton's law can help distinguish the cause of pain in the hip region. Hilton's law states that "the same trunks of nerves whose branches supply the groups of muscles moving a joint furnish also a distribution of nerves to the skin over the insertion of the same muscles, and the interior of the joint receives its nerves from the same source."[41] This law helps explain why muscle spasms and superficial pain accompany hip pathology. The L3 nerve predominantly innervates the hip joint, and thus pain down the entire L3 dermatome (the anterior and medial thigh crossing laterally to the knee) can accompany hip pain. This pain can be confused with compression of the lateral femoral cutaneous nerve, also known as meralgia paresthetica, which will cause pain or neuralgia in the L2 or L3 dermatome.[42-45]

Another useful observation is the C sign. The C sign occurs when a patient cups his or her hand above the greater trochanter when describing hip pain. The hand forms a "C" and is placed on the lateral hip, which may lead the clinician to mistakenly consider lateral hip pathology such as IT band or trochanteric bursitis (Fig. 80-2). However, this sign is most characteristic of deep interior hip pain.[31,46] When a C sign is observed, the clinician should ensure that the examination and subsequent testing include a complete evaluation for intraarticular hip pain.

Palpation can also assist in localization of symptoms in the hip, although not as much as in other joints. The clinician must be familiar with the superficial and deep anatomy of the hip region for palpation to be of assistance. Initial palpation of the abdomen to check for fascial hernias or masses is important to rule out gastrointestinal or genitourinary sources of pain. Palpation of the lumbar spine, sacroiliac joint, ischium, iliac crest, greater trochanter, trochanteric bursa,

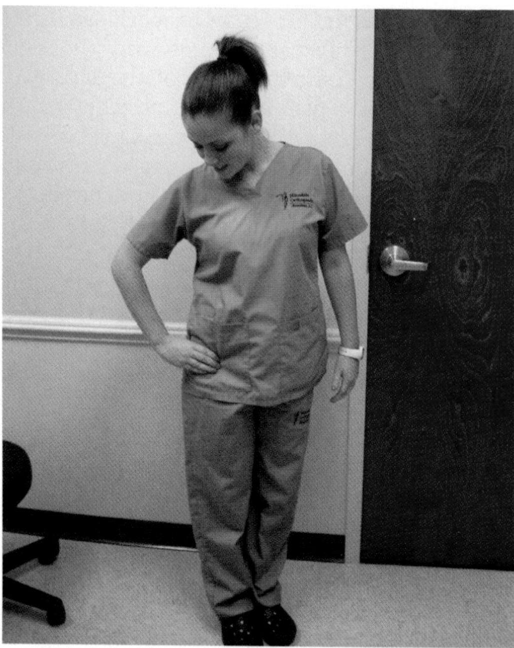

FIGURE 80-2 The C sign. Cupping the thumb and the index finger around the lateral thigh indicates deep hip pathology.

various muscle bellies, the adductor tubercle, and the pubic symphysis can help distinguish the location of pain (Fig. 80-3). Pubic symphysis pain can indicate fracture, calcification, or osteitis pubis. The clinician can also palpate the femoral nerve. A positive Tinel sign indicates a neurologic cause of pain. Identification of bursitis on examination is often extremely helpful in narrowing the differential and can be followed up with an injection of a local anesthetic to confirm the diagnosis. The addition of a steroid to the injection is often therapeutic as well.

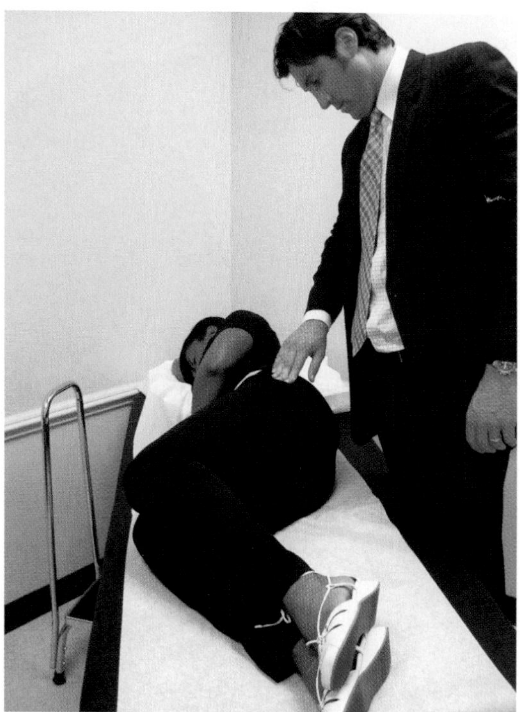

FIGURE 80-3 Greater trochanter palpation. Pain with palpation of the greater trochanter can indicate trochanteric bursitis or gluteus medius pathology.

A distal neurovascular examination should also be completed, including palpation of the dorsalis pedis and posterior tibial arteries, an assessment of capillary refill, and lymphatic return. A thorough motor and sensory examination can often be helpful in differentiating hip from lumbar pain. Strength testing of the iliopsoas, quadriceps, extensor hallicus longus, tibialis anterior, and gastrocnemius provides an assessment of the L2-S1 nerve roots. Any asymmetric weakness compared with the contralateral side may indicate a radicular component to the pain, and this finding should prompt further investigation into lumbar spine or peripheral nerve pathology. A thorough sensory examination will often help confirm radicular or peripheral nerve problems. When assessing numbness, the examiner should differentiate a radicular (L2-S1) pattern from a peripheral nerve pattern (femoral, peroneal) to provide a focus for additional testing. Intraarticular hip pain should not cause sensory disturbances or weakness in the foot. In the setting of injury, muscle testing also can be helpful. If the clinician believes that a specific muscle group has been affected, then resisted contraction can reproduce the patient's symptoms. Specifically, leg abductors (superior gluteal nerve L4-S1), leg adductors (obturator nerve L2-L4), knee extensors and hip flexors (femoral nerve L2-L4), hip extensors (inferior gluteal nerve L5-S2), and knee flexors and lower leg muscles (sciatic L4-S3) should be tested. The strength of patients with intraarticular pathology is often limited by pain, and the clinician should be aware that weakness in the iliopsoas or abductors may be a result of pain instead of being neurogenic. Diagnostic injections of the hip joint or epidural spinal injections can be helpful in differentiating hip and lumbar pathology.[47]

Both active ROM, passive ROM, and resisted ROM may reproduce hip pain. ROM examination can help differentiate muscle strains from intraarticular pathology. In general, passive ROM may reproduce hip pain but not pain from a muscle strain. A strain of the hip flexors can be detected with the active hip flexion but not passive hip flexion.

Measurements and ROM

Several measurements are important during the hip evaluation. Ipsilateral measurements from the shoulder of the iliac crest or from the anterior superior iliac spine to the medial malleolus can detect a true leg length discrepancy. Degenerative changes and collapsed avascular necrosis frequently cause a leg length discrepancy. Preoperative templating and the physical examination are the keys to successfully restoring leg length at the time of reconstruction.

The measurement of thigh circumference can detect muscle atrophy from chronic conditions. It is important to choose the same level of the thigh for circumference measurements. For example, 10 cm above the patella is a typical location for this measurement. The contralateral side must be measured for comparison, and this measurement can be taken at subsequent visits to gauge response to treatment.

Hip ROM must be accurately and reproducibly measured during the physical examination of the hip (Table 80-1). ROM can indicate the extent of hip pathology and the response to treatment. Hip flexion is best tested in the supine position,

TABLE 80-1

AVERAGE HIP RANGE OF MOTION

Motion	Degrees
Flexion	115
Abduction	50
Adduction	30
Internal rotation	45
External rotation	45

and the normal range is up to 120 degrees.[48] Hip extension is best tested in the prone position, and the normal range is up to 15 degrees. Internal and external rotation should be tested with the hip flexed at 90 degrees, which is best accomplished in the seated position to stabilize the pelvis. Normal internal rotation is up to 45 degrees, and normal external rotation is up to 50 degrees.[48] Arthritis, effusion, SCFE, or muscle contractures can cause a decrease in internal rotation.[38,49] Abduction and adduction should be measured with reference to the shaft of the femur at the midline of the pelvis. Normal abduction is 45 degrees, and normal adduction is up to 30 degrees.[48] An abductor contracture may decrease adduction ROM.[48] Differences between the normal and affected side can help detect hip pathology.[37] In patients with DJD, hip ROM is often globally decreased, with pain at the extremes of motion. Patients with dysplasia have shallow acetabuli and anterior superior undercoverage, which allows increased internal rotation with the hip flexed. Patients with femoroacetabular impingement (FAI) typically lack internal rotation in a flexed position because of the abnormal contact between the femoral head and neck with the acetabulum. After acetabular rim trimming and femoral osteoplasty, intraoperative ROM can be tested. Typically, as the impingement is relieved, the patient will gain internal rotation with the hip flexed.

Special Maneuvers

Supine

The straight-leg raise (SLR) is a test to assess lumber nerve root pathology. With the knee held in extension and the contralateral pelvis stabilized, the clinician passively raises the leg. When the patient feels pain, the hip should be extended 10 degrees and the foot dorsiflexed to elicit radicular symptoms. Pain from 0 to 30 degrees suggests a compressed nerve root, pain from 30 to 60 degrees may suggest sacroiliac disease, and pain after 60 degrees suggests sacroiliac disease.[50,51] The pain should be similar to the patient's chief complaint rather than generalized stiffness. Stretching of the hamstrings should not be confused with a positive SLR test.

An SLR against resistance, also known as an active SLR, can indicate hip pain. Again in the supine position, the patient flexes at the hip with the knee extended, but the clinician resists the flexion, thus generating force across the hip joint. Pain with the active SLR indicates hip pain.

The log roll test is the most specific test for intraarticular hip disease. The femur is gently rotated both internally and externally without motion of the pelvis or undue pressure on the surrounding muscles (Fig. 80-4). Pain is specific but not sensitive for hip pathology. The heel strike and Stinchfield tests can be useful accompaniments to the log roll test. Striking the heel with the fist causes an axial load through the hip and can recreate hip pain. The Stinchfield test involves gradually increasing resisted flexion of the hip, with pain indicating either joint pain or iliopsoas pathology.[38] Plain radiographs or magnetic resonance imaging (MRI) will often confirm physical examination findings for intraarticular pain. If the history and physical examination findings are confusing, a diagnostic injection of local anesthetic in the hip joint can be helpful in ruling out extraarticular pain.

The anterior impingement test involves forced flexion, adduction, and internal rotation (Fig. 80-5). This test is the most sensitive maneuver to detect subtle hip pathology, including femoroacetabular impingement. Because this maneuver may be uncomfortable in a normal hip, a comparison to the unaffected side is extremely important. This position of the hip loads the anterior superior aspect of the hip joint by bringing the femoral head and neck into contact with the anterosuperior acetabulum. When this test is positive, the clinician should scrutinize the patient's radiographs for signs of FAI or DJD. If no degenerative changes are observed, further workup with an MRI arthrogram may be helpful to further evaluate the hip joint. A positive anterior impingement test may also guide decision making intraoperatively by leading the surgeon to treat anterior pathology identified during arthroscopy.

The posterior impingement test is performed with the hip in extension and the leg flexed off the end of the examination table. The hip is then externally rotated to bring the femoral head and neck into the posterior acetabulum (Fig. 80-6). A positive test can be a sign of posterior labral pathology, excessive acetabular anteversion, or degenerative changes. Again,

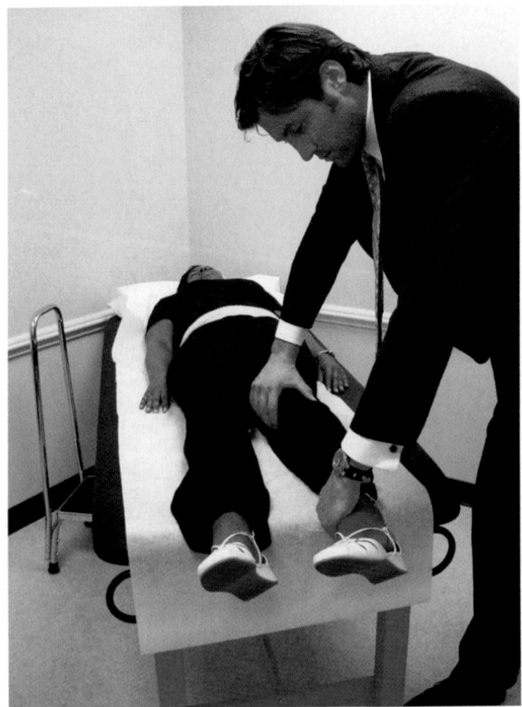

FIGURE 80-4 The log roll test. In the supine position with the hip and knee in a neutral position, pain with rotation at the hip is specific for intraarticular pathology.

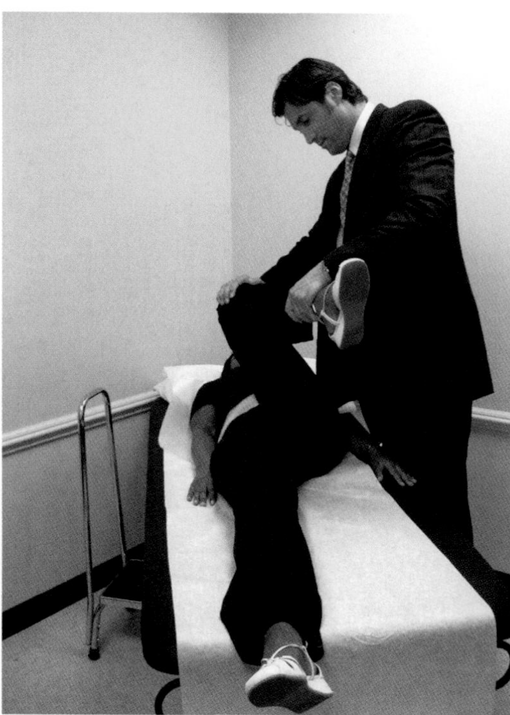

FIGURE 80-5 The anterior impingement test. In the supine position, pain with flexion, adduction, and internal rotation is the most sensitive test for intraarticular pathology.

this test can assist the surgeon preoperatively and intraoperatively by indicating when to address a posterior lesion.

The Patrick test, also known as the flexion, abduction, and external rotation (FABER) test, can stress the sacroiliac joint or imply lateral impingement or iliopsoas pathology. A figure-of-four is made in the supine position by placing the ipsilateral ankle over the contralateral knee. The ipsilateral knee is then pressed down. Posterior pain indicates sacroiliac joint disease, lateral pain indicates lateral impingement, and groin pain indicates iliopsoas pathology.[38]

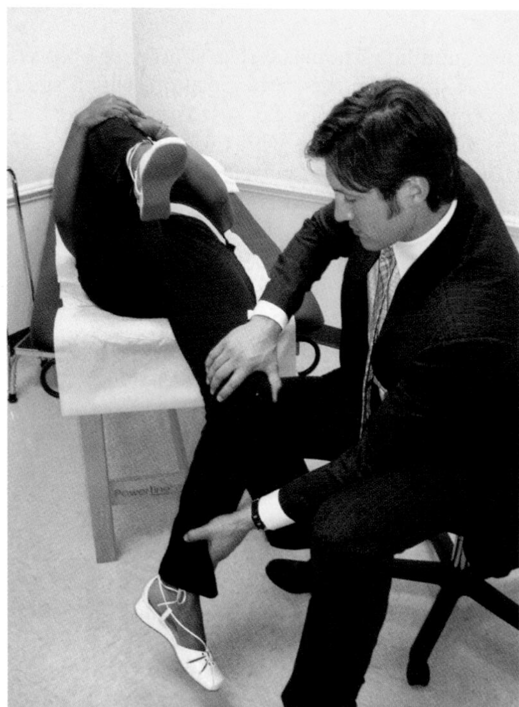

FIGURE 80-6 The posterior impingement test. In the supine position, pain with extension and external rotation indicates posterior impingement.

The McCarthy test involves bringing both hips in to full flexion in the supine position and then extending the affected hip in external rotation and internal rotation. Reproduction of the original pain during this arc of motion constitutes a positive McCarthy test and indicates labral pathology.[52-56]

The Scour test can help detect irregularities along the femoral head or acetabulum. The clinician flexes the hip and knee while pointing the knee to the shoulder. While taking the hip through its arc of motion, any bumps or catches should be noted. The presence of bumps or catches indicates a positive test and is suggestive of FAI.

The Thomas test determines the presence and degree of a flexion contracture (iliopsoas contracture) of the hip. The patient should flex the unaffected hip and draw the knee to the chest while lowering the affected leg to the table. A positive Thomas test occurs when the patient cannot lower the affected extremity to the table. Any popping or clicking during the Thomas test may indicate a labral tear.[35]

The Dial test of the hip can help detect hip capsular laxity. In the supine position, the patient's hip and knee are extended. The clinician places a hand on the femur and a hand on the tibia and internally rotates the entire lower extremity at the hip joint. The lower extremity is then released and allowed to externally rotate. External rotation less than 45 degrees with a firm end point constitutes a negative Dial test. Passive external rotation beyond 45 degrees constitutes a positive Dial test and is indicative of hip capsular laxity.[36]

Lateral

Several examinations may be performed to help evaluate the hip in the lateral position. Flexing and extending the hip while moving the abductor mechanism across the hip can recreate visual IT band snapping. However, the clinician should remember that the patient can often better reproduce a snapping IT band.

Abductor testing can be performed from the lateral position. Hip abduction against gravity or resistance may reveal weakness or pain (Fig. 80-7). When weakness is discovered, the cause may be neurologic or muscular. If neurologic weakness is suggested, an electromyogram can be a useful test for differentiating lumbar radiculopathy from superior gluteal nerve pathology. Painful weakness may suggest gluteus medius tendinopathy, trochanteric bursitis, or a trochanteric fracture. Further imaging with plain radiographs or MRI can be helpful in this setting.

Impingement testing with the flexion, adduction, and internal rotation maneuver can also be accomplished in the lateral position. While standing behind the patient, the clinician places one hand under the knee for support and the other hand on the hip joint with the index finger anterior and the thumb pointing posterior. If flexion, adduction, and internal rotation cause discomfort, the test is positive.

Ober testing comprises three parts: extension, neutral, and flexion. The extension test may detect an IT band contracture, the neutral test may detect a gluteus medius contracture, and the flexion test may detect a gluteus maximus contracture. The extension Ober test consists of flexing the knee, extending the hip, abducting the hip, and then releasing the hip. A delay in return to adduction indicates IT band pathology. The neutral Ober test consists of flexing the knee with the hip in the neutral position, abducting the hip, and then releasing the hip. A delay in return to adduction indicates gluteus medius pathology. The flexion Ober test consists of rotating the torso so that the patient's shoulders are flat on the table with the legs still in the lateral position, flexing the hip, extending the knee, abducting the hip, and then releasing the hip. A delay in return to adduction indicates gluteus maximus pathology.[57]

Finally, the abduction–extension–external rotation test can be conducted in the lateral position. The clinician extends the knee, abducts the leg 30 degrees, and flexes the hip 10 degrees (Fig. 80-8). Pain may be elicited by placing pressure on the greater trochanter while bringing the hip from 10 degrees flexion to full extension. Pain during this maneuver is suggestive of ligamentum teres injury or anterior capsular instability.[34] This test can reproduce femoral head subluxation in patients with developmental dysplasia of the hip.[20] Testing for general ligamentous laxity is a good complement to the abduction–extension–external rotation examination when instability is suspected. Laxity can be tested by bringing the patient's thumb to the anterior forearm. The ability to complete this task suggests laxity. Hyperextension of the knee and elbow beyond 5 degrees also suggests hyperlaxity of the ligaments.[34]

Prone

The modified Thomas test and Ely test can differentiate between iliopsoas contracture and rectus femoris contracture.

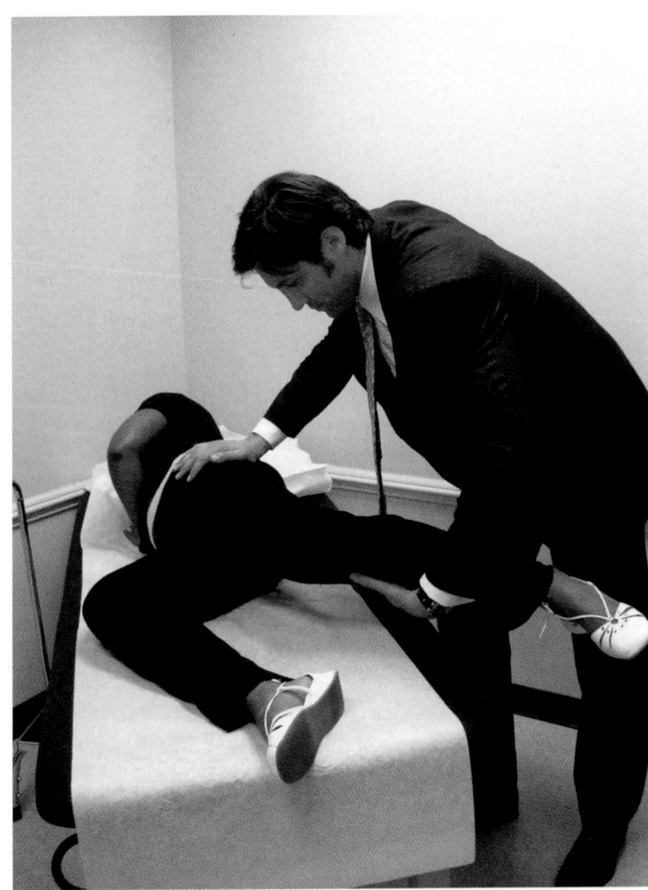

FIGURE 80-8 Abduction–extension–external rotation. Pain with this maneuver indicates anterior hip instability or ligamentum teres pathology.

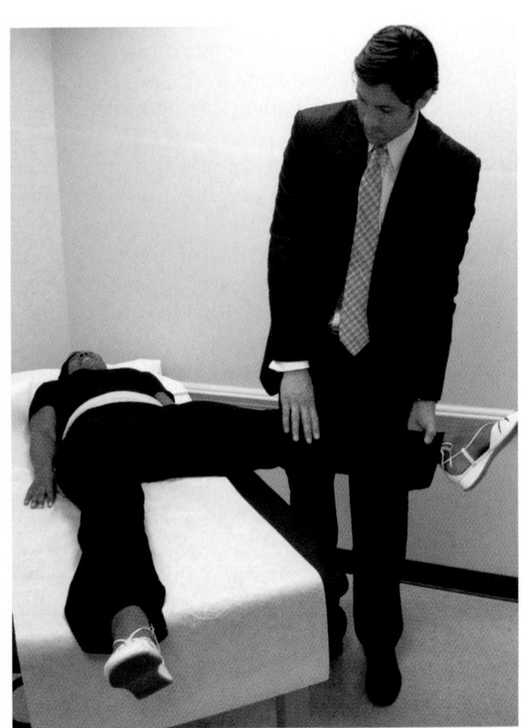

FIGURE 80-7 Resisted abduction. Pain with resisted abduction can indicate greater trochanter pathology or lateral impingement.

A positive modified Thomas test is simply an observation of the pelvis rising up in the prone position, which suggests an iliopsoas contracture.[48] The Ely test is performed by flexing the knee as far as possible with the patient prone. Upward motion of the buttocks and pelvis indicates a positive Ely test, which suggests a rectus femoris contracture because the rectus femoris crosses both the hip and knee joints.[34]

The femoral nerve stretch test should also be conducted in this position by flexing the knee. Nerve type pain with this maneuver indicates femoral nerve pathology instead of hip joint pathology.

Conclusion

A thoughtful, systematic approach to the hip joint is necessary for the diagnosis and treatment of hip pathology. Because hip, back, and knee pain can easily be confused for one another, a consistent and careful history and physical examination are crucial to avoid misdiagnosis.[37] The physical examination maneuvers previously described should allow the clinician to narrow the differential diagnosis and help determine whether the patient's pain is intraarticular or extraarticular. These distinctions are important given recent advances in imaging and treatment options for the hip.

For a complete list of references, go to expertconsult.com.

Selected Readings

Citation: Devin CJ, et al: Hip-spine syndrome. *J Am Acad Orthop Surg* 20(7):434–442, 2012.
Level of Evidence: V
Summary: This article discusses the difficulty in differentiating hip and spine pathology. Keys in the history, physical examination, diagnostic tests, and differential and a treatment algorithm are discussed.
Citation: Flynn JM, Widmann RF: The limping child: evaluation and diagnosis. *J Am Acad Orthop Surg* 9(2):89–98, 2001.
Level of Evidence: V
Summary: This article provides a framework for evaluating a child with a painful hip. The history, physical examination, and additional studies are outlined.
Citation: Parvizi J, Leunig M, Ganz R: Femoroacetabular impingement. *J Am Acad Orthop Surg* 15(9):561–570, 2007.
Level of Evidence: V
Summary: In this review article on femoroacetabular impingement, the pathophysiology, history, physical examination, and treatment are discussed.
Citation: Sanchez-Sotelo J, et al: Surgical treatment of developmental dysplasia of the hip in adults: I. Nonarthroplasty options. *J Am Acad Orthop Surg* 10(5):321–333, 2002.
Level of Evidence: V
Summary: In this review article on hip dysplasia in the adult patient, the pathophysiology, history, physical examination, and nonarthroplasty treatment options are discussed.
Citation: Domb BG, Brooks AG, Byrd JW: Clinical examination of the hip. *J Sports Rehab* 18:3–23, 2009.
Level of Evidence: V
Summary: This article provides a brief overview of the history, physical examination, and relevant imaging related to the athletic patient with hip pathology.

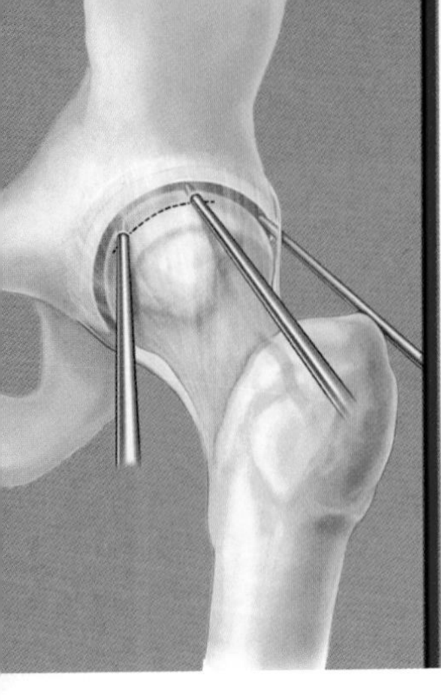

81

Hip Imaging

BRIAN BUSCONI • MICHAEL MONTANO •
SEAN McMILLAN • JUAN EUGENIO COSME

A multitude of structural hip disorders can occur in athletes with hip pain. Although the history and physical examination play a critical role in determining the diagnosis, it is also important to have a systematic approach to help diagnose these disorders radiographically. This chapter describes the key imaging studies used when examining a skeletally mature patient with a pathologic hip, as well as a systematic approach to interpretation of these studies.

Radiographic Techniques

Traditionally, the lateral hip radiograph demonstrates details of the femoral neck and helps identify cam impingement pathology, whereas the anteroposterior (AP) view demonstrates the acetabular version. Several radiographic views are important for proper evaluation of the hip. Among these, the most commonly referenced include the AP view of the pelvis (AP pelvic view),[1,2] a cross-table lateral view,[3] a 45-degree or 90-degree Dunn view,[4,5] a frog-leg lateral view,[6] and a false-profile view.[7] All views are technique dependent, and each demonstrates a different anatomic perspective of the hip joint. Descriptions of each view are provided in the following sections.

Standing Anteroposterior Pelvic View

A proper AP view should be taken with the patient standing. The x-ray tube–to-film distance should be approximately 120 cm, and the x-ray tube should be aimed perpendicular to the film. Both lower extremities should be internally rotated by 15 degrees to account for normal anatomic anteversion, and this position helps maximize the view of the femoral neck. The crosshairs of the beam should be centered on a point half the distance between the superior border of the pubic symphysis and on a line drawn connecting the anterior superior iliac spine.[8] The coccyx should be centered in line with the pubic symphysis. The radiographic teardrops, iliac wings, and obturator foramina should be symmetrical in appearance.[9] A 1- to 3-cm gap should be seen between the apex of the coccyx and the superior border of the pubic symphysis for proper pelvic inclination.[10] A standing rather than a supine AP radiograph is obtained because acetabular roof obliquity, center edge angle, and minimum joint space width may vary between weight-bearing and supine positions.[11]

The standing AP radiograph assesses (1) functional leg length inequalities; (2) neck shaft angle (NSA); (3) femoral neck trabecular patterns; (4) lateral and anterior center edge angles; (5) acetabular inclination; (6) joint space width; (7) lateralization; (8) head sphericity; (9) acetabular cup depth; and (10) anterior and posterior wall orientation (Figs. 81-1 and 81-2).[9]

Cross-Table Lateral View

For the cross-table lateral view radiograph, the patient should be supine on the x-ray table. The contralateral hip and knee should be flexed out of the way of the x-ray beam (typically >75 degrees). The hip of interest should be rotated internally 15 degrees to help accentuate the anterolateral surface of the femoral head-neck junction (Fig. 81-3). The x-ray beam should be parallel to the table and oriented at a 45-degree angle to the limb of interest with the crosshairs aimed at the center of the femoral head.[8]

45-Degree or 90-Degree Dunn View

The Dunn view is commonly used for assessment of femoral head sphericity in patients believed to have cam-type femoroacetabular impingement (FAI). It was originally described as a technique to measure femoral neck anteversion in children.

The 90-degree Dunn view assesses the patient with 90-degree hip flexion, whereas the 45-degree Dunn view ("modified Dunn view") assesses the patient with 45 degrees of hip flexion (Fig. 81-4). For both views, the film cassette is placed beneath the pelvis and the tube is centered over the upper border of the pubic symphysis. Each leg should be abducted 15 to 20 degrees from the midline, and the pelvis and tibia should be parallel to the long axis of the body (neutral rotation).[4] The crosshairs of the beam should be directed at a point midway between the anterior superior iliac spine (ASIS) and the pubic symphysis, and the tube-to-film distance should be approximately 40 inches in a line directed perpendicular to the table.[8]

Frog-Leg Lateral View

To obtain the frog-leg lateral view, the patient should be positioned supine on the x-ray table with the hip of interest abducted 45 degrees, the ipsilateral knee flexed 30 to 40 degrees, and the ipsilateral heel resting against the contralateral knee (Fig. 81-5). The cassette is positioned so that the top of the film rests at the ASIS. The crosshairs of the beam are directed at a point midway between the ASIS and the

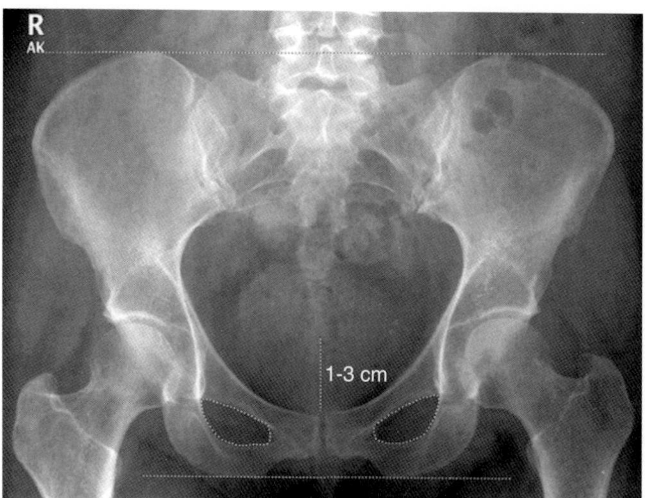

FIGURE 81-1 The standing anteroposterior radiograph is obtained with the feet in neutral rotation and shoulder width apart. The coccyx should be centered in line with the pubic symphysis, and the iliac wings, obturator foramina, and radiographic teardrops should be symmetrical in appearance. If pelvic inclination is appropriate, a 1- to 3-cm gap should be seen between the superior border of the pubic symphysis and the tip of the coccyx. *(From Martin HD: Clinical examination and imaging of the hip. In Thomas Byrd JW, Guanche CA, editors:* AANA Advanced Arthroscopy: The Hip, *Philadelphia, 2010, Elsevier.)*

pubic symphysis, with an x-ray tube–to-film distance of approximately 40 inches.[8]

This view permits assessment of another view of medial and lateral joint space width, femoral head sphericity, congruency, head-neck offset, alpha angle, and bone morphology.[9]

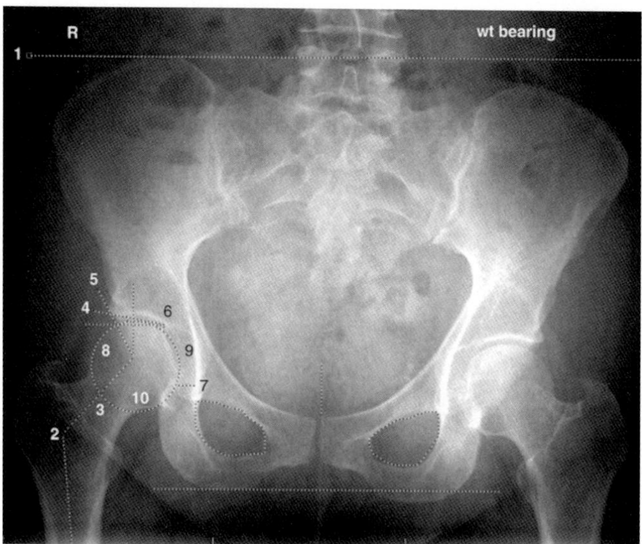

FIGURE 81-2 The standing anteroposterior radiograph assesses the following characteristics: *1,* functional leg length inequalities; *2,* neck shaft angle; *3,* femoral neck trabecular patterns; *4,* acetabular inclination; *5,* lateral center edge angles; *7,* lateralization; *8,* head sphericity; *9,* acetabular cup depth; and *10,* anterior and posterior wall orientation. *(From Martin HD: Clinical examination and imaging of the hip. In Thomas Byrd JW, Guanche CA, editors:* AANA Advanced Arthroscopy: The Hip, *Philadelphia, 2010, Elsevier.)*

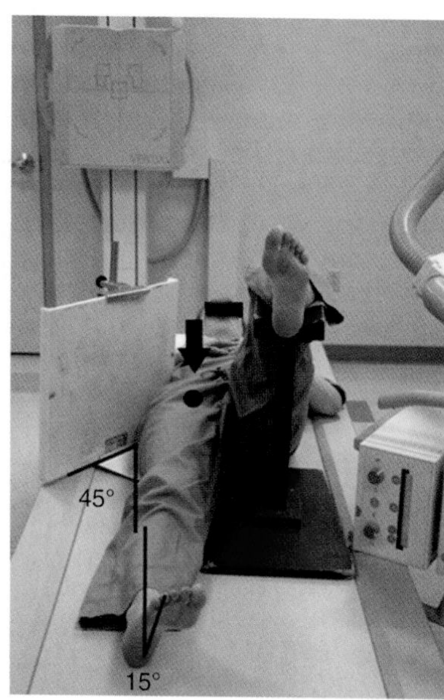

FIGURE 81-3 The positioning for a cross-table lateral radiograph with the limb in 15 degrees of internal rotation. The black arrow points to the center of the femoral head (*black dot*), the target for the crosshairs of the x-ray beam. *(From Clohisy JC, Carlisle JC, Beaulé PE, et al: A systematic approach to the plain radiographic evaluation of the young adult hip.* J Bone Joint Surg Am *90[suppl 4]:47–66, 2008.)*

False-Profile View

The false-profile view is helpful for evaluation of the anterior acetabular coverage of the femoral head. The view is obtained with the patient standing, the affected hip against the cassette, and the pelvis rotated 65 degrees from the plane of the cassette (Fig. 81-6). The beam is centered on the femoral head and perpendicular to the cassette. The tube-to-film distance should be approximately 40 inches.[8]

Interpretation of Plain Radiographic Images

Interpretation of both the false-profile and AP pelvic views generally helps to characterize the acetabular morphology, whereas the other views better describe the proximal femoral anatomy. By combining all views, we should be able to define the following parameters for each patient: leg length inequalities, NSA, femoral neck trabecular patterns, lateral and anterior center edge angles, acetabular inclination, joint space width, lateralization, head sphericity, acetabular cup depth, and anterior and posterior wall orientation.

Functional Leg Lengths

Functional leg lengths may be assessed on an AP pelvis radiograph by constructing a line horizontally off the superiormost portion of the iliac crest. Ideally this line should be symmetrical to the contralateral hemipelvis. A discrepancy greater than 2.0 cm corresponds with a functional leg length discrepancy and can have an adverse effect on the kinematic function of the hip.[12]

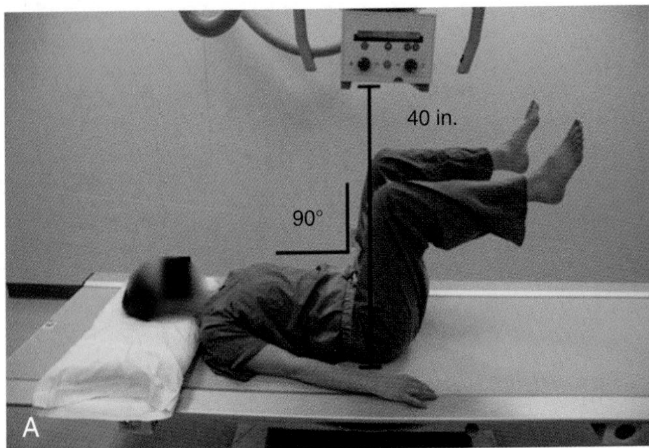

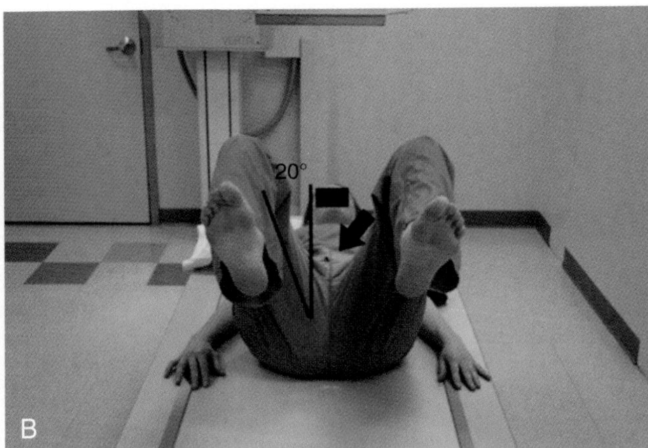

FIGURE 81-4 Positioning for a 90-degree Dunn view with the hips flexed and abducted 20 degrees. The black arrow (**B**) points to the crosshairs, centered at a point midway between the pubic symphysis and the anterior superior iliac spine. *(From Clohisy JC, Carlisle JC, Beaulé PE, et al: A systematic approach to the plain radiographic evaluation of the young adult hip.* J Bone Joint Surg Am *90[suppl 4]:47–66, 2008.)*

Neck Shaft Angle

The NSA is defined by the angle formed by the longitudinal axes of the femoral neck and the proximal femoral diaphyseal axis.[13] One line is drawn down the anatomic axis of the femoral neck, and the other is drawn down the anatomic axis of the femur. The angle formed represents the NSA. This angle is normally between 125 and 140 degrees. An angle less than 125 degrees is classified as coxa varus. An angle greater than 140 degrees corresponds to coxa valgus. The NSA dictates the load transfer from the femur to the acetabulum.[9]

Trabecular Pattern

The trabecular pattern is influenced directly by the NSA and reflects the compressive and tensile forces within the femoral neck. For cases of coxa varus, tensile trabeculae are more prominent. For cases of coxa valgus, compressive trabeculae are more prominent.[14]

Lateral Center Edge Angles

The lateral center edge angles can be used to assess the superolateral coverage of the femoral head by the acetabulum.[15] The

FIGURE 81-5 The positioning for a frog-leg lateral view with the hip abducted 45 degrees and the crosshairs centered at a point midway between the anterior superior iliac spine (*black dot*) and the pubic symphysis (*black line*). *(From Clohisy JC, Carlisle JC, Beaulé PE, et al: A systematic approach to the plain radiographic evaluation of the young adult hip.* J Bone Joint Surg Am *90[suppl 4]:47–66, 2008.)*

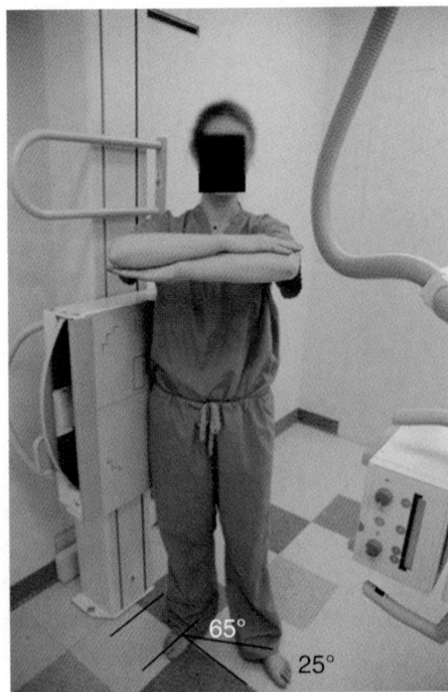

FIGURE 81-6 The false-profile view of the right hip is obtained with the pelvis rotated 65 degrees in relationship to the Bucky wall stand, with the foot on the affected side parallel to the radiographic cassette (shown in the *black lines*). *(From Clohisy JC, Carlisle JC, Beaulé PE, et al: A systematic approach to the plain radiographic evaluation of the young adult hip.* J Bone Joint Surg Am *90[suppl 4]:47–66, 2008.)*

lateral center edge angle is calculated by measuring the angle between two lines: (1) a line through the center of the femoral head, perpendicular to the transverse axis of the pelvis, and (2) a line through the center of the femoral head, passing through the most superolateral point of the sclerotic weight-bearing zone of the acetabulum.[8] Normal values range from 22 to 42 degrees in adults, although values less than 26 degrees may indicate inadequate coverage of the femoral head.[12]

Anterior Center Edge Angles

The anterior center edge angles are created through use of the false-profile view. This angle assesses the anterior coverage of the femoral head. It is calculated by measuring the angle between the vertical line through the center of the femoral head and a line connecting the center of the femoral head and the most anterior point of the acetabular sourcil.[16] Values of less than 20 degrees can be indicative of structural instability.[8]

Acetabular Inclination

Also known as the Tonnis angle, acetabular inclination is best appreciated on the AP view. It is formed by drawing a horizontal line and a tangent from the lowest point of the sclerotic zone of the acetabular roof to the lateral edge of the acetabulum. Three classifications are used for acetabular inclination[8,17]:

1. Normal = Tonnis angle of 0 to 10 degrees
2. Increased = Tonnis angle greater than 10 degrees, subject to structural instability (increased inclination)
3. Decreased = Tonnis angle less than 0 degrees, subject to pincer-type femoroacetabular impingement (decreased inclination)

Joint Space Width

Joint space width is described as the shortest distance between the surface of the femoral head and the acetabulum. Joint space width is examined using the standing AP radiograph because the effects of position influence the joint space observed.[18] Evidence of joint space narrowing can be classified using the Tonnis grade for osteoarthritis.[13]

Hip Center Position

For hip center position, the distance between the medial aspect of the femoral head and the ilioischial line is measured. If the distance is greater than 10 mm, then the hip is classified as lateralized. The distance of 10 mm should serve as a general reference point, and film magnification and patient body habitus must be taken into account and may influence this measurement.

Head Sphericity

Assessment of head sphericity should be performed with both the AP and frog-leg lateral views because a patient may have an apparently spherical head on one view and not on the other. The femoral head is classified as spherical if the epiphysis does not extend beyond the margin of reference circle by more than 2 mm, and it is classified as aspherical if it extends beyond this 2-mm margin.[19,20] The margin of reference is known as a Mose template (concentric circles).[21]

Acetabular Cup Depth

The acetabular cup depth is a relationship between the floor of the fossa acetabula and the femoral head relative to the ilioischial line. If the floor of the fossa acetabula touches or is medial to the ilioischial line or the posterior wall extends lateral to the center of axis of rotation, the hip is classified as coxa profunda.[9] If the medial aspect of the femoral head is medial to the ilioischial line, the head is classified as protrusion.[15] Additionally, the inner acetabular wall thickness, medial wall shape, and inferior cup orientation should be recognized.[9]

Acetabular Version

Normally, the acetabulum is anteverted by approximately 20 degrees. Acetabular version can be defined as either being retroverted or anteverted by identifying the presence or absence of a crossover sign on the AP view.[1] The acetabulum is considered to be anteverted if the line of the anterior aspect of the rim does not cross the line of the posterior aspect of the rim before reaching the lateral aspect of the sourcil, and it is considered to be retroverted if the line of the anterior aspect of the rim does cross the line of the posterior aspect of the rim before reaching the lateral edge of the sourcil.[8] It is important to note that true acetabular retroversion is associated with a deficient posterior wall,[1] whereas a hip with a crossover sign but no posterior wall deficiency refers to anterior overcoverage—cranial acetabular retroversion or anterior focal acetabular retroversion.[8,22]

Head-Neck Offset

Head-neck offset can be evaluated from the frog-leg lateral radiograph and is classified on the basis of the gross appearance of the relationship between the radius curvatures of the anterior aspect of the femoral head with the posterior aspect of the head-neck junction.[19] If the anterior and posterior concavities of the head-neck junction are symmetrical, then the head-neck offset is classified as symmetrical. If the anterior concavity has a radius of curvature greater than that at the posterior aspect of the head-neck junction, it is classified as having a moderate decrease in head-neck offset.[9] If the anterior aspect has a convexity, as opposed to a concavity, the head-neck junction is classified as having a prominence (cam-type FAI).[19]

Alpha Angle

The alpha angle is classically described for use with axial magnetic resonance imaging (MRI) scans; however, its use may be extrapolated to lateral radiographs. The angle is formed between a line connecting the center of the femoral head to the anatomic axis of the femoral neck and a second line running from the center of the femoral head to the prominence of the head-neck junction where the head sphericity ends. The angle between these two lines is known as the *alpha angle*. Values of more than 42 degrees are suggestive of head-neck offset deformity.[8]

Computed Tomography Evaluation of the Hip

Computed tomography (CT) is an ideal modality for characterization of the osseous structures in the area of the hip. Three-dimensional (3D) multiplanar reformatted CT images have been used to assess hip pathology. Although the CT images and the 3D reformatted images that they create are an excellent noninvasive method of demonstrating osseous morphology, the disadvantages of this technique are the utilization of ionizing radiation in the young patient population and the fact that CT does not allow direct visualization of intraarticular structures.[23] As a result, the workup of a painful hip should progress to MRI evaluation, which is discussed in the following section.

Magnetic Resonance Evaluation of the Hip

Although conventional and 3D CT scanning of the hip has been described for assessment of acetabular version and FAI, magnetic resonance arthrography (MRA) of the hip has gained popular acceptance for the diagnosis of these conditions. Compared with conventional MRI, magnetic resonance (MR) arthrograms can more readily identify intraarticular abnormalities such as cartilage defects, loose bodies, and labral tears.[24,25] The purpose of this section is to help the reader identify some of the most common pathologies within the hip joint with the use of MRA, including acetabular labral tears, FAI, hip sprains and dislocations, and stress fractures.

Labral Conditions

Labral pathology can often be stratified by patient age. In young patients, pathology is more likely to be caused by a traumatic mechanism, ranging from an acute twist injury of the hip during sport all the way to a hip dislocation. For middle-aged patients (<50 years), the mechanism is often FAI. More senior patients often experience degenerative tears associated with osteoarthritis.

Labral Variant

The acetabular labrum is a fibrocartilaginous rim that deepens the socket of the hip joint, although its role in hip stability remains unclear.[26] It encompasses approximately three fourths of the circumference of the acetabulum and is absent along its inferior aspect. It is here where the transverse acetabular ligament extends from the anterior to the posterior aspect of this inferior acetabular fossa.

Several clinically insignificant labral variations have been described in asymptomatic patients. The posterior inferior sublabral sulcus should not be misinterpreted as a posterior labral tear on axial images.[27] Additionally, an anterosuperior cleft may be seen as a normal variant in the presence of a normal lateral acetabular labrum. On anterior coronal or sagittal images, this cleft is seen as a partial undercutting of the labrum on a single image.[28] A transverse ligament labral junction sulcus is a normal sulcus found between the transverse ligament and the labrum either anteriorly or posteriorly. Finally, the perilabral sulcus resembles the normal space between the acetabular labrum and the capsule on coronal images (Figs. 81-7 and 81-8).

The shape of the labrum also varies among subjects. It most commonly has a triangular appearance (70% to 80%), although it may also be round, flat, irregular, or even absent (1% to 14%) in asymptomatic people.[28] An enlarged or hypertrophic labrum may occur in patients with mild developmental dysplasia of the hip (Fig. 81-9).

An area located above the anterosuperior margin of the acetabular fossa on the coronal view may appear deficient in articular cartilage. It is often stellate or creaselike in appearance (Fig. 81-10). This variant is normal and should not be confused with an osteochondral lesion.

Occasionally, contrast material may demonstrate tubelike intraosseous tracking within the posterior margin of the acetabular fossa (Fig. 81-11). This tracking is a common artifact that is posited to represent dilation of the nutrient foramina

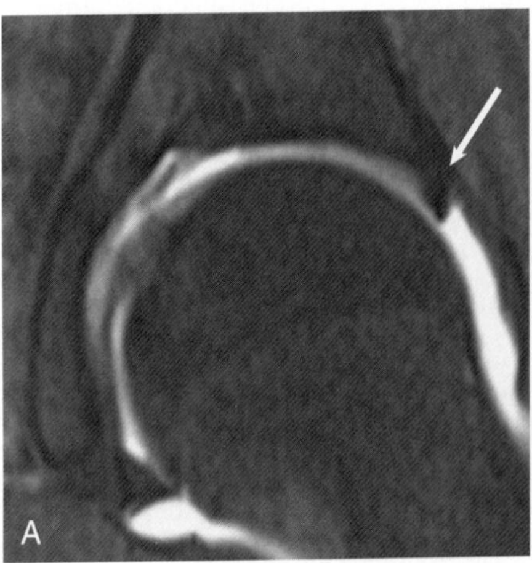

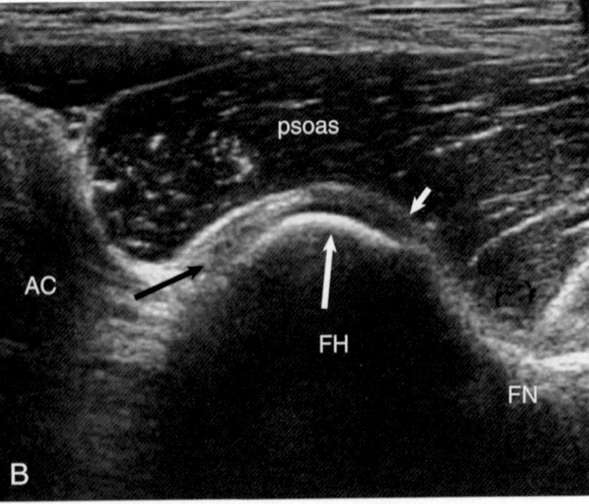

FIGURE 81-7 **A,** A coronal fat-saturated T1-weighted image shows a triangular-shaped superior labrum (*arrow*). **B,** An oblique sagittal ultrasound image shows the anterior labrum (*black arrow*), femoral head (*FH*), cortex (*large white arrow*), anterior joint capsule (*small white arrow*), femoral neck (*FN*), iliopsoas muscle (*psoas*), and acetabulum (*AC*). *(From Patel K, et al: Radiology. In Busconi BD, Miller MD, editors:* Clinics in Sports Medicine: Sport-Related Injuries of the Hip, *Philadelphia, 2011, Elsevier.)*

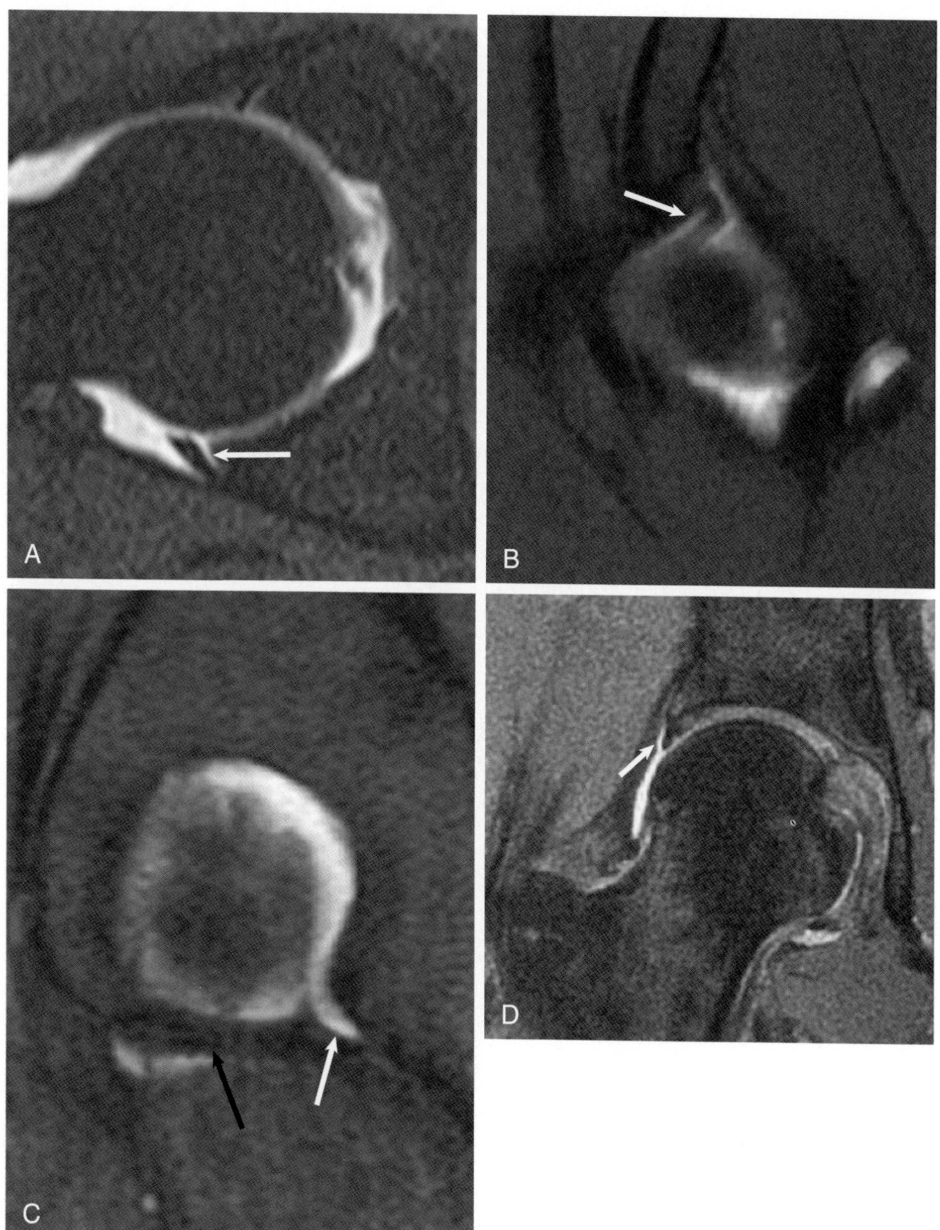

FIGURE 81-8 **A,** The posterior inferior sublabral sulcus or groove (*arrow*) does not extend completely underneath the labrum. **B,** The anterosuperior cleft (*arrow*) partially undercuts the labrum on a single coronal image, which does not extend completely through the labrum. **C,** A normal transverse ligament labral sulcus (*white arrow*) and transverse acetabular ligament (*black arrow*), which extends from the anterior to the posterior aspect at the inferior acetabular fossa. **D,** The perilabral sulcus (*arrow*), a normal space between the capsule, lateral acetabular rim, and labrum. *(From Patel K, et al: Radiology. In Busconi BD, Miller MD, editors:* Clinics in Sports Medicine: Sport-Related Injuries of the Hip*, Philadelphia, 2011, Elsevier.)*

along the anterior and posterior margin of the acetabular fossa.[29]

Finally, another entity often viewed on the MR arthrogram with unknown clinical significance is the pectinofoveal fold (Fig. 81-12). This fold may resemble a hip plica and can have various appearances and attachment sites.[30]

Labrum Tear

MRA appears to be superior to conventional MRI for the diagnosis of acetabular labral tears.[31] Criteria for tears on an MRA include contrast material extending into the labrum or acetabular/labral interface, blunted appearance, and displacement/detachment from the underlying bone.[32] It is important to distinguish normal variants (described previously) from true pathologic entities. With all this in mind, it is important to consider the sensitivity and specificity of MRA for the diagnosis of labral tears. Studies comparing MRA with surgical findings have shown a range of sensitivity from 60% to 100%[33] and a specificity from 44% to 100%.[34] These studies demonstrate that a negative scan does not fully rule out a labral tear and that hip arthroscopy remains the gold standard.[35]

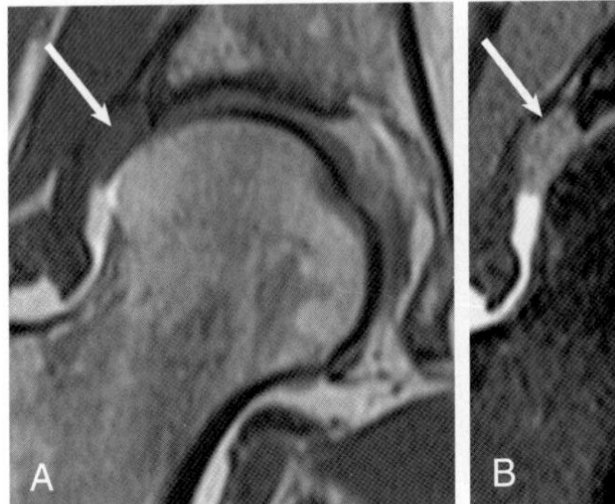

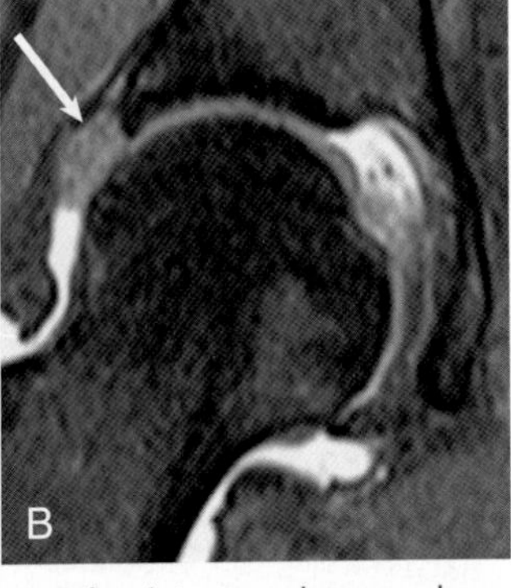

FIGURE 81-9 **A,** A coronal T1-weighted image shows a large hypertrophic superior labrum (*arrow*). **B,** A coronal proton density fat-saturated image shows increased signal intensity of hypertrophic labrum (*arrow*), suggesting intralabral degeneration. *(From Patel K, et al: Radiology. In Busconi BD, Miller MD, editors:* Clinics in Sports Medicine: Sport-Related Injuries of the Hip, *Philadelphia, 2011, Elsevier.)*

Most labral tears occur in the anterior superior labrum or posterior superior (which is more common in the younger population) and run along the base of the labrum or along the long axis (longitudinal tear).[28] The diagnosis of a labral tear is established when gadolinium is seen traversing or undercutting the labrum.

Labrum tears are frequently associated with developmental dysplasia, FAI, Legg-Calvé-Perthes disease, slipped capital femoral epiphysis, and degenerative hip disease. Traumatic tears may occur along the inner free margin with a radial flap, the most common type, or they may be unstable and displaced longitudinal tears (Fig. 81-13).[28] Overall, the frequency of tears by location is as follows from most to least: anterosuperior, posterosuperior, anteroinferior, and posteroinferior.[36]

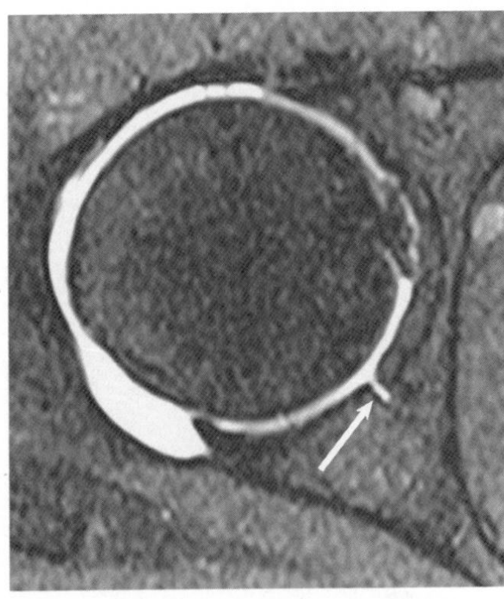

FIGURE 81-11 An axial fat-saturated T1-weighted image shows tubular acetabular intraosseous contrast tracking (*arrow*) along the posterior margin of the acetabular fossa, which likely represents dilatation of the nutrient foramina. *(From Patel K, et al: Radiology. In Busconi BD, Miller MD, editors:* Clinics in Sports Medicine: Sport-Related Injuries of the Hip, *Philadelphia, 2011, Elsevier.)*

Femoroacetabular Impingement

FAI occurs when morphologic abnormalities result in abnormal contact between the femoral neck/head and the acetabular margin, causing tearing of the labrum and avulsion of the underlying cartilage region, continued deterioration, and eventual onset of arthritis.[37] It is a major cause of early osteoarthritis of the hip, especially in young and active patients.[16] Ganz et al.[16] described two distinct types of FAI based on the pattern of chondral and labral lesions observed during surgical dislocation of the hip: cam impingement and pincer impingement.

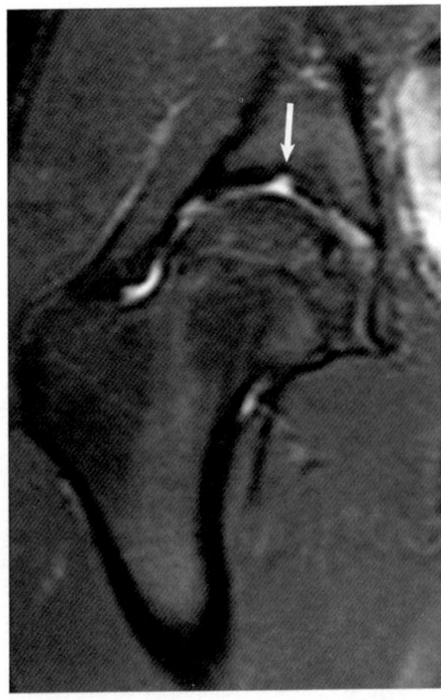

FIGURE 81-10 The stellate crease (*arrow*) represents a bare area deficient in hyaline cartilage and not degeneration. *(From Patel K, et al: Radiology. In Busconi BD, Miller MD, editors:* Clinics in Sports Medicine: Sport-Related Injuries of the Hip, *Philadelphia, 2011, Elsevier.)*

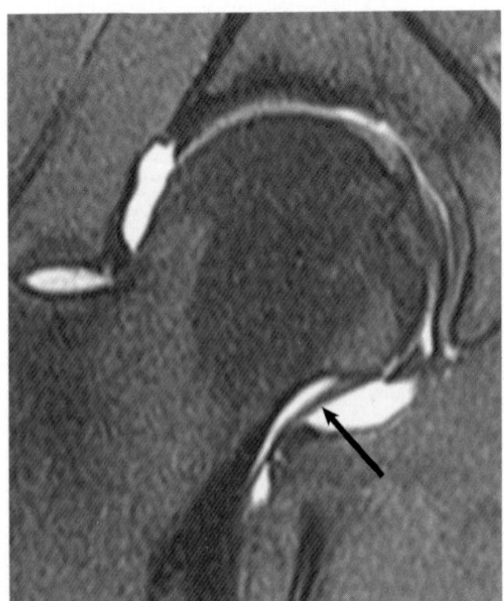

FIGURE 81-12 A coronal fat-saturated T1-weighted image shows the pectinofoveal fold (*arrow*) arising from the medial aspect of the femoral neck, extending inferiorly to attach on the proximal femur. The relationship of this fold to internal impingement is not known. *(From Patel K, et al: Radiology. In Busconi BD, Miller MD, editors:* Clinics in Sports Medicine: Sport-Related Injuries of the Hip, *Philadelphia, 2011, Elsevier.)*

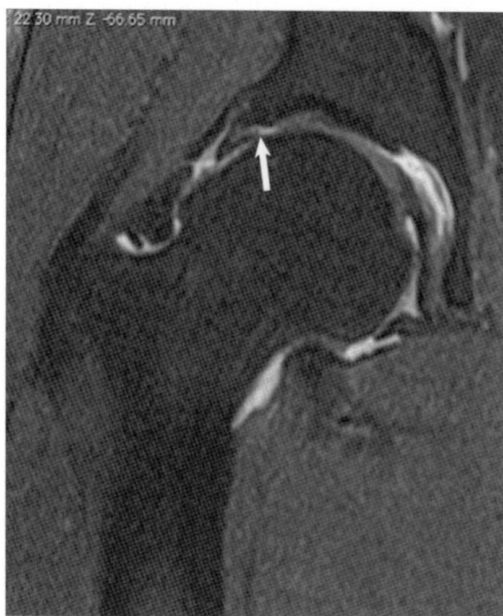

FIGURE 81-13 A coronal fat-saturated T1-weighted image shows a longitudinal cleavage tear (*arrow*) of the hypertrophic anterior superior labrum. *(From Patel K, et al: Radiology. In Busconi BD, Miller MD, editors:* Clinics in Sports Medicine: Sport-Related Injuries of the Hip, *Philadelphia, 2011, Elsevier.)*

Cam impingement is more common in young active males. The mechanism is related to an abnormally shaped femoral head (nonspherical) that gets jammed into the acetabulum during normal motion and especially during flexion. Downstream effects of this mechanism include tearing of the labrum from this abnormally prominent femoral neck being jammed into the acetabulum. The labral tear may extend to involve the acetabular cartilage and cause separation from the subchondral bone. The labral and chondral lesion is often observed in the anterosuperior area of the acetabulum.[38] The following triad of MRA findings has been described in patients with cam-type FAI: an abnormal alpha angle, an anterior/superior acetabular cartilage lesion, and an anterior/superior labral tear (Fig. 81-14).[39]

Pincer-type impingement is the acetabular cause and is more common in middle-aged and older women who engage in athletic activities. Abnormal contact occurs between the acetabular rim and the femoral neck. The femoral head in this situation may be normal, and the abutment is mostly a result of overcoverage of the femoral head in conditions such as coxa profunda[40] or acetabular retroversion.[1] The first structure to fail through this mechanism is usually the acetabular labrum, which often appears small but normally progresses to downstream degenerative changes in the labrum, intrasubstance ganglion formation, or ossification of the rim,[37] which may lead to further deepening of the acetabulum and worsening of the overcoverage. In persons with pincer-type impingement, the cartilage lesions are often seen along the posterior aspect of the acetabulum as a result of the countercoup type of injury because the femur abnormally touches the acetabular rim and the associated labral degeneration and tears are most commonly found in the anterosuperior labrum (Fig. 81-15).[28]

Most patients (86%) have a combination of both forms of impingement, which is called *mixed pincer and cam impingement;* only a minority (14%) have the pure FAI form of either cam or pincer impingement.[15]

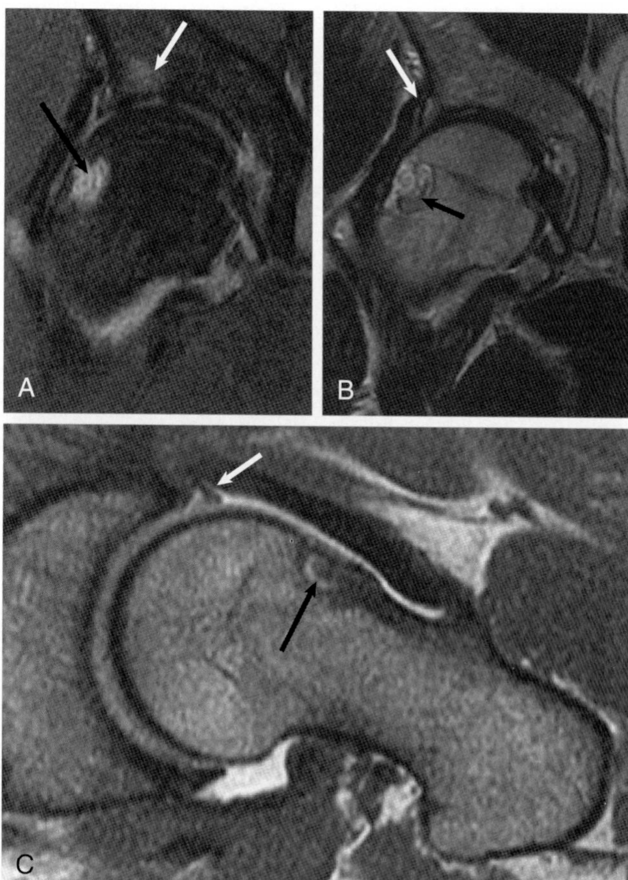

FIGURE 81-14 **A,** A coronal T1-weighted fat-saturated image shows anterior acetabular cartilage loss, subchondral edema (*white arrow*), an osseous bump, and fibrocystic changes of the femoral head (*black arrow*). **B,** A coronal T1-weighted image shows absent labrum (*black arrow*) and an acetabular bone spur (*white arrow*). **C,** An oblique axial T1-weighted image shows a displaced anterior labrum tear (*white arrow*), an osseous bump, and fibrocystic changes of the femoral neck. *(From Patel K, et al: Radiology. In Busconi BD, Miller MD, editors:* Clinics in Sports Medicine: Sport-Related Injuries of the Hip, *Philadelphia, 2011, Elsevier.)*

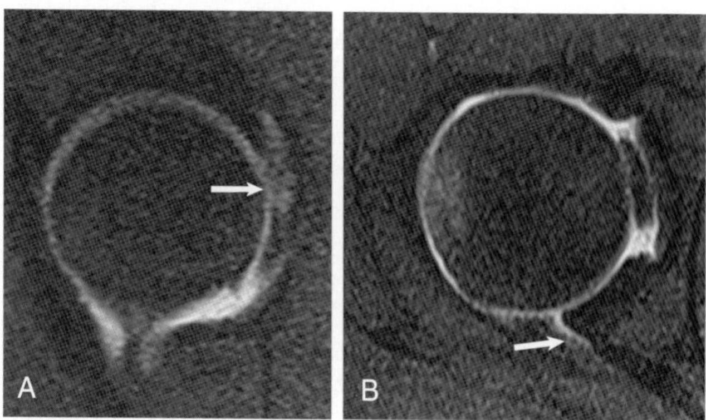

FIGURE 81-15 Sagittal (**A**) and axial (**B**) T1-weighted fat-saturated images show a posterior labrum tear (*arrows*). *(From Patel K, et al: Radiology. In Busconi BD, Miller MD, editors:* Clinics in Sports Medicine: Sport-Related Injuries of the Hip, *Philadelphia, 2011, Elsevier.)*

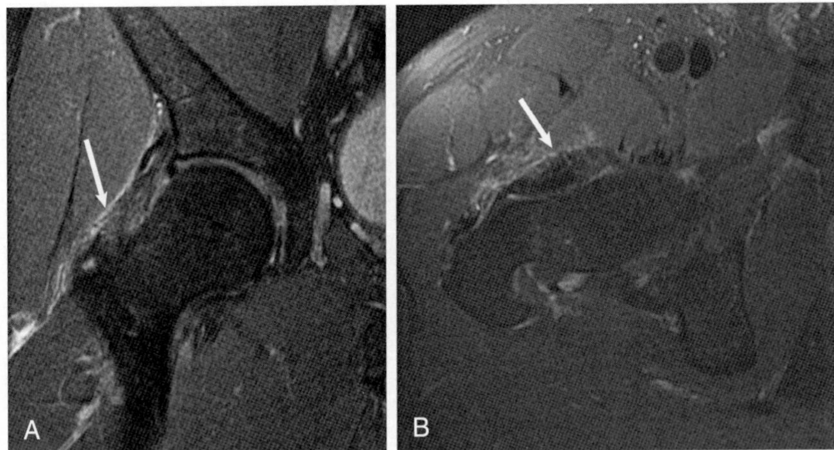

FIGURE 81-16 Proton density, fat-saturated T1-weighted coronal (**A**) and axial (**B**) images show pericapsular edema and a partial-thickness iliofemoral ligament tear (*arrows*) after a right hip sprain. *(From Patel K, et al: Radiology. In Busconi BD, Miller MD, editors:* Clinics in Sports Medicine: Sport-Related Injuries of the Hip*, Philadelphia, 2011, Elsevier.)*

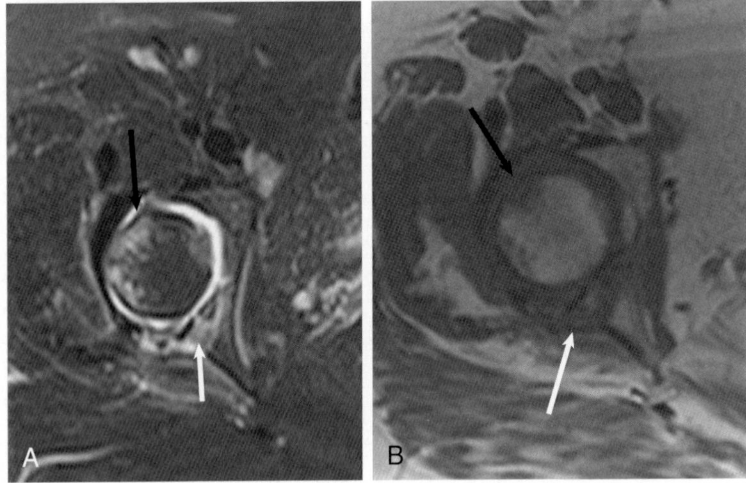

FIGURE 81-17 An axial short-tau inversion recovery image (**A**) and an axial T1-weighted image (**B**) show a posterior acetabular rim fracture (*white arrows*) and compression injury of anterior femoral head (*black arrows*). *(From Patel K, et al: Radiology. In Busconi BD, Miller MD, editors:* Clinics in Sports Medicine: Sport-Related Injuries of the Hip*, Philadelphia, 2011, Elsevier.)*

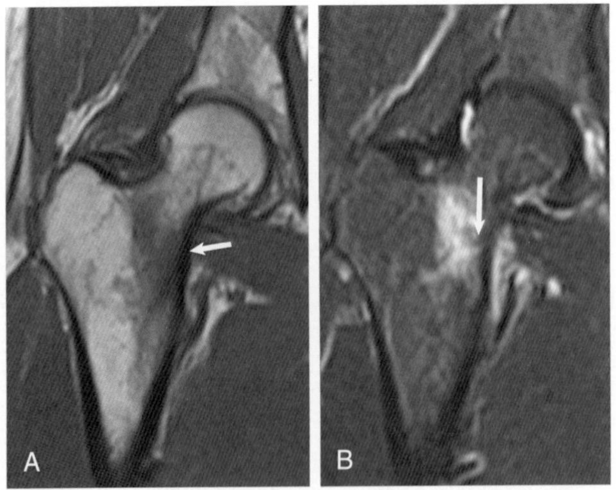

FIGURE 81-18 **A,** A coronal T1-weighted image shows medial femoral neck cortical thickening and edema (*arrow*). **B,** A coronal short-tau inversion recovery–weighted image shows an incomplete fracture line (*arrow*). *(From Patel K, et al: Radiology. In Busconi BD, Miller MD, editors:* Clinics in Sports Medicine: Sport-Related Injuries of the Hip*, Philadelphia, 2011, Elsevier.)*

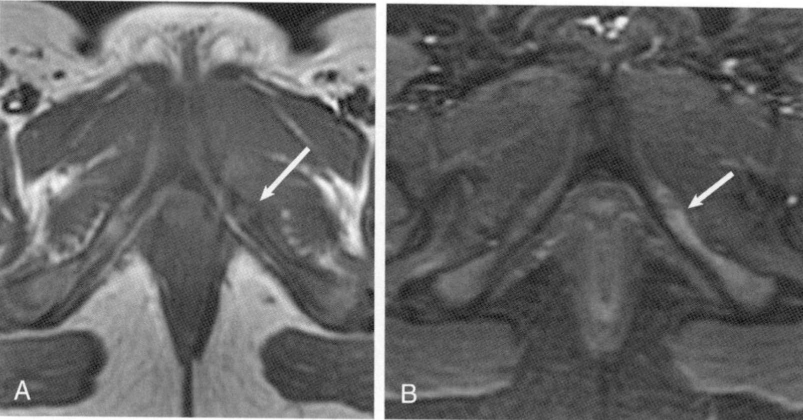

FIGURE 81-19 A T1-weighted image (**A**) and short-tau inversion recovery–weighted image (**B**) show a left inferior pubic ramus stress fracture. *(From Patel K, et al: Radiology. In Busconi BD, Miller MD, editors:* Clinics in Sports Medicine: Sport-Related Injuries of the Hip, *Philadelphia, 2011, Elsevier.)*

Hip Sprain and Dislocation

Hip sprain is an injury that occurs often in athletes, especially football players, when they fall onto a flexed and adducted hip. Radiographs often appear normal or may show a small posterior acetabular rim fracture. MRI may demonstrate pericapsular soft tissue edema and traumatic disruption of the iliofemoral ligament near its femoral attachment.[28]

Dislocation of the femoral head may occur during episodes of severe trauma. Hip dislocations represent approximately 5% of all dislocations and most frequently occur posteriorly (80% to 85%). This dislocation may result from a dashboard injury in which the flexed knee strikes the dashboard during a head-on automobile collision.[41] Radiographs typically demonstrate posterior acetabular rim fractures (Fig. 81-16). The MRI may show accompanying shear or compression fractures on the anterior and inferior portions of the femoral head (Fig. 81-17).[28]

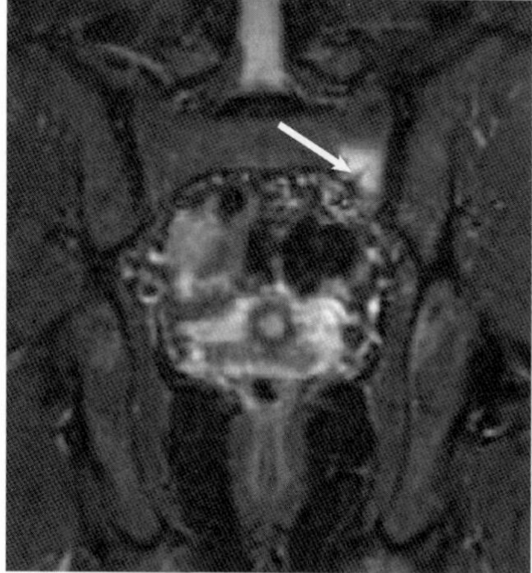

FIGURE 81-20 A coronal short-tau inversion recovery–weighted image shows an incomplete stress fracture of the left sacral ala (arrow). *(From Patel K, et al: Radiology. In Busconi BD, Miller MD, editors:* Clinics in Sports Medicine: Sport-Related Injuries of the Hip, *Philadelphia, 2011, Elsevier.)*

Stress Injuries

Stress fractures, including both fatigue and insufficiency fractures, are common injuries and may account for as many as 10% of all injuries seen in sports medicine clinics.[42] Wolff[43] describes bone as a dynamic tissue in which normal stresses stimulate remodeling, allowing adaptation to a changing mechanical environment. Bone remodeling is stimulated by fatigue damage, and fatigue damage occurs in the form of microfracture.[44]

Fatigue fractures are more common in runners who have recently started a new and intensive physical activity or who have recently changed their training regimen.[45] The femoral neck is typically involved, and the other most common pelvic bones involved are the pubic rami and sacrum.[46]

Radiographs are the usual initial imaging modality because of their wide availability and low cost; however, they are notoriously insensitive for finding stress fractures and have a sensitivity approaching 0% for stress fractures of the posterior pelvis and sacrum.[46,47] Bone scintigraphy is more sensitive for stress injuries or fracture, and abnormal findings of a bone scan may be seen as early as 6 to 72 hours after the injury occurred.[28] However, these scans are not specific for stress fractures, and increased uptake may be seen with infection, a tumor, or an early stage of avascular necrosis.[28] MRI is reported to be as sensitive as scintigraphy for stress fractures, approaching 100%; however, it is much more specific as well, given its higher level of soft tissue and bone marrow contrast (Figs. 81-18, 81-19, and 81-20).[46]

For a complete list of references, go to expertconsult.com.

Suggested Readings

Citation: Clohisy JC, et al: A systematic approach to the plain radiographic evaluation of the young adult hip. *J Bone Joint Surg Am* 90A(suppl 4):47–66, 2008.

Level of Evidence: V

Summary: This article describes a systematic algorithm for evaluating the young patient with hip pain. The techniques for obtaining proper radiographs are also discussed, and many supporting illustrations are provided.

Citation: Martin HD: Clinical examination and imaging of the hip. In Byrd TJ, editor: *AANA Advanced Arthroscopy: The Hip*, Philadelphia, 2010, Elsevier.

Level of Evidence: V

Summary: This chapter presents a broad overview of physical examination techniques for younger patients with hip pain.

Citation: Parvizi J, et al: Femoroacetabular impingement. *J Am Acad Ortho Surg* 15(9):561–570, 2007.
Level of Evidence: V
Summary: This article describes the mechanism of femoroacetabular impingement (FAI) and helps the reader properly diagnose it through radiographic, clinical, and physical examination techniques. It also presents a good overview of surgical versus nonsurgical treatments for FAI.

Citation: Patel K, et al: Radiology. In Miller M, editor: *Clinics in Sports Medicine: Sport-Related Injuries of the Hip*, Philadelphia, 2011, Elsevier.
Level of Evidence: V
Summary: This chapter delves into magnetic resonance imaging analysis of the patient with hip pain. It includes several illustrations depicting common pathologic conditions within the hip.

Citation: Smith T, et al: The diagnostic accuracy of acetabular labral tears using magnetic resonance imaging and magnetic resonance arthrography: A meta-analysis. *Eur Radiol* 21(4):863–874, 2011.
Level of Evidence: IV
Summary: This article compares the diagnosis of labral tears through magnetic resonance imaging (MRI) and magnetic resonance arthrography (MRA) imaging and concludes that MRA appears to be superior to conventional MRI. It also describes the five etiologic causes of labral tears and physical examination techniques that can help the practitioner better diagnose these tears.

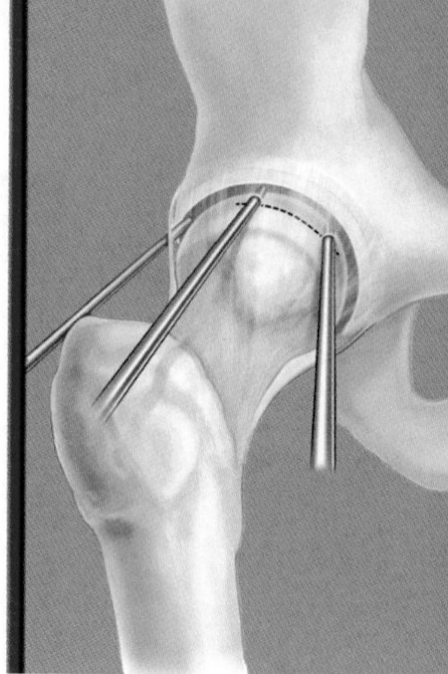

82

Hip Arthroscopy

VÍCTOR MANUEL ILIZALITURRI SÁNCHEZ JR • ANELL OLIVOS MEZA

History

Arthroscopic techniques have revolutionized surgery, and hip arthroscopy in particular has greatly advanced knowledge of the normal and pathologic hip.[1] Compared with other joints, however, arthroscopy of the hip has faced obstacles in application. The essential factor underlying the relatively slow development of hip arthroscopy is the anatomic constraint inherent in the hip joint. A thick, muscular, soft tissue envelope overlies the hip, and a thick fibrous capsule encompasses the joint. The femoral head is deeply recessed circumferentially into the acetabulum, limiting access to intraarticular structures. In the first account of hip arthroscopy in cadavers in 1931, Burman[2] acknowledged these challenges, writing, "it is manifestly impossible to insert a needle between the head of the femur and the acetabulum." The first clinical application, reported in 1939 by Takagi,[3] was for cases of Charcot disease, tuberculosis, and septic arthritis.

Whereas development of arthroscopic procedures for the knee and subsequently the shoulder progressed quickly in the later part of the twentieth century, hip arthroscopy lagged because of the technical demands and lack of indications. In the late 1980s, however, bolstered by improved recognition of intraarticular hip pathology and advances in technique such as the routine utilization of traction, hip arthroscopy emerged as a key component of the armamentarium for the diagnosis and treatment of hip disorders, as popularized by authors such as Glick, Byrd, and McCarty in North America and Villar in England. Increased utilization of hip arthroscopy contributed to a more comprehensive understanding of conditions that affect the hip joint. Many common hip conditions that were previously unrecognized and left untreated, such as femoroacetabular impingement (FAI) and structural instability, were elucidated by hip arthroscopy.[4,5] The indications and technology have continued to expand during the past two decades through the contributions of surgeons such as Byrd, Philippon, Sampson, and Ilizaliturri.[6-8]

With ever-expanding indications, improvements in technique, and innovative arthroscopic instrumentation, hip arthroscopy has become more standardized and reproducible.[1] The procedure has quickly grown from a diagnostic instrument to a powerful tool to treat hip pathology.

Indications and Purpose of the Treatment

The minimally invasive nature of hip arthroscopy is attractive to patients, surgeons, and the medical providers involved in patients' recovery and rehabilitation.[9,10] Open hip surgery requires a comparatively large incision and dissection, and the morbidity associated with the exposure may slow recovery. Use of the arthroscopic technique allows improved visualization of the labrum, articular cartilage of the femoral head, and acetabulum, as well the fovea, ligamentum teres, hip capsule, and adjacent synovia. Surgical tools developed specifically for hip arthroscopy can be used to provide the diagnosis and treatment of conditions involving the aforementioned structures.

Currently, the primary indications for hip arthroscopy include symptomatic labral tears (Fig. 82-1), focal symptomatic chondral lesions, loose bodies, ligamentum teres lesions, and capsular laxity.[11] A better understanding of the pathologic mechanism underlying FAI has expanded the role of arthroscopy in the treatment of this condition as well.[12] Arthroscopic treatment of pigmented villonodular synovitis and synovial chondromatosis has been reported. Other potential roles for hip arthroscopy include avascular necrosis and hip instability.[12] Arthroscopic and endoscopic access to structures in the area of the hip has also been introduced, and gluteus medius/minimus, iliotibial, and iliopsoas pathology may be addressed, as well as some nerve entrapment conditions.[10,13,14]

Like any surgical intervention, preoperative planning and careful patient selection is mandatory and should be considered the most important element in successful arthroscopy of the hip.[1,15] The suspected diagnosis based on the history and physical examination should be confirmed by imaging. Magnetic resonance imaging (MRI) has proved useful for intraarticular disorders, although it has limitations. In the case of labral pathology, a magnetic resonance arthrogram (MRA) is the best imaging study (Fig. 82-2). Computed tomography (CT) and three-dimensional reconstruction may help the surgeon understand bony deformities.[16]

The hip arthroscopist needs to be familiar with the anatomy in the area of the hip, as well as the normal arthroscopic anatomy and its variations. Hip arthroscopy is associated with a steep learning curve, and training in hip arthroscopy

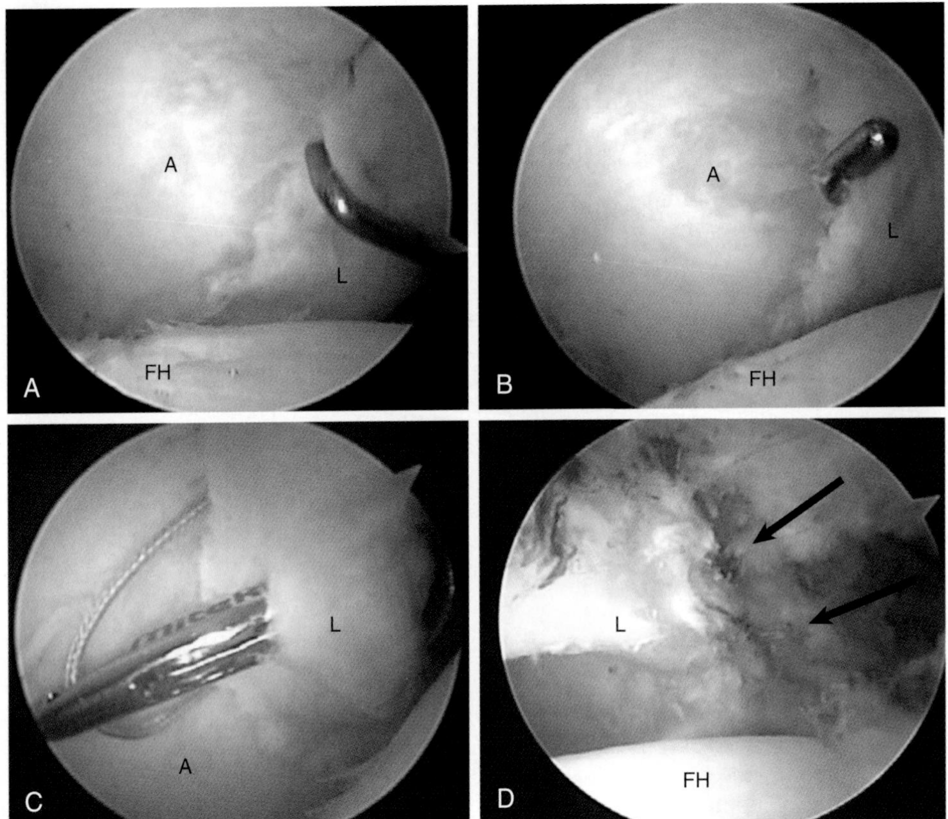

FIGURE 82-1 Arthroscopic sequence of a labral repair in a right hip. **A,** A hook probe is used to demonstrate a detachment of the anterior lateral labral (*L*); the acetabulum (*A*) is at the center of the photograph and the femoral head (*FH*) is at the bottom. **B,** The hook probe is positioned between the labral tear (*L*) and the anterior acetabulum (*A*). The FH is at the bottom. **C,** A suture anchor has been implanted on the anterior acetabular rim (*A*); in this figure, one limb of the suture is in the process of being passed through the labral (*L*) tissue. **D,** After completion of the labral repair, the black arrows point to the knots on the capsular side of the labrum (*L*); the FH is at the bottom.

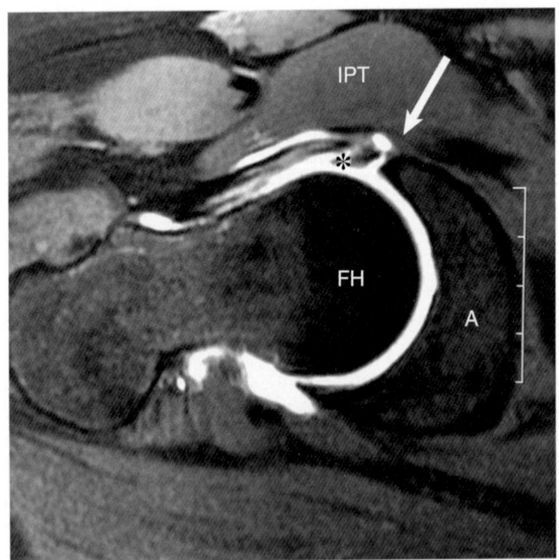

FIGURE 82-2 A magnetic resonance image of a right hip. Note the relation of the iliopsoas tendon with the anterior (*IPT*) aspect of the hip joint. The relation between the femoral head (*FH*) and the acetabulum (*A*) is normal. The arrow notes a labral tear and a paralabral cyst (note the contrast between the anterior acetabular rim and the labrum [*asterisk*]).

before performing one's first case is mandatory to avoid complications.[17] Training opportunities range from courses, cadaver laboratories, and symposiums to a formal dedicated fellowship.

Operative Room Setup and Positioning

Patient positioning is the first step to success in hip arthroscopy. Two positions have been described for hip arthroscopy: supine and lateral.[18] We prefer the lateral position with use of regional anesthesia, image intensifier control, and traction. Other physicians perform the procedure with the patient in the supine position.[1,19,20] Patient positioning and the site of arthroscopic portals differ among authors. Regardless of the position used, the positioning technique must be exact and reproducible. Poor patient positioning will result in inadequate distraction, with poor access to the central compartment or inadequate hip mobilization, limiting access to the hip periphery.[21] The setup must provide the capability of applying and releasing traction throughout the case.[18] Dynamic assessment of hip motion may help the surgeon in evaluating the clearance of hip mobility.[1,18]

Lateral Position

Glick[22] introduced the lateral position for hip arthroscopy. The patient is positioned in the lateral decubitus position on

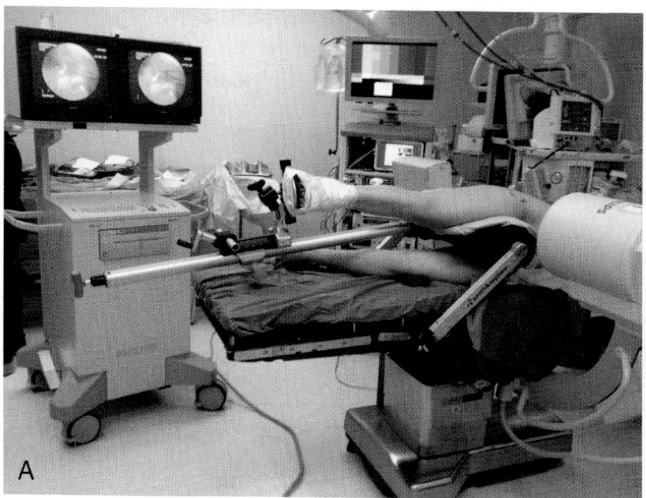
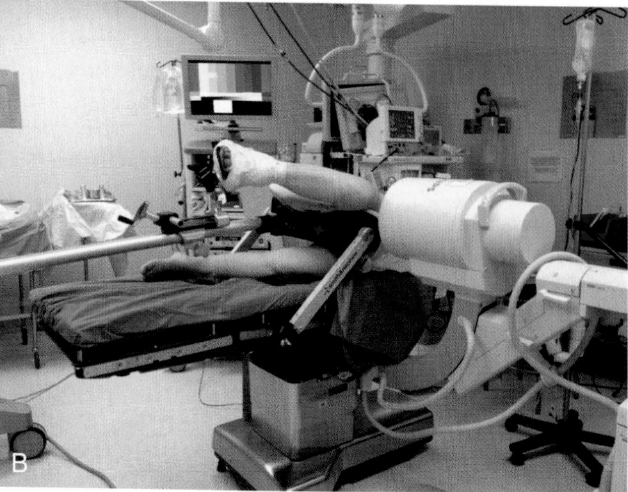

FIGURE 82-3 **A,** Patient positioning for hip arthroscopy in the lateral decubitus position. The hip is in traction, and the perineal post rests on the medial side of the groin and is elevated to provide a lateral vector for a traction force; the right foot is well padded and fixed to the traction device of the distractor. The image intensifier is positioned horizontally under the table to provide an anterior and posterior view of the right hip and to prevent the arch from obstructing the surgical area. **B,** To access the peripheral compartment, traction has been released and the hip is in flexion.

the operating table with the operative side upward (Fig. 82-3). Only the foot of the operative side is fixed to the traction device, and pelvic tilt is avoided by means of the patient's body weight. The opposite leg rests freely on the operating table with knee and hip flexion between 10 and 20 degrees. The operative hip is positioned in neutral abduction and flexion of 20 degrees to relax the anterior hip capsule. Flexion of more than 20 degrees does not improve distraction of the hip joint and increases the possibility of injury to the sciatic nerve. Neutral rotation is preferred while establishing arthroscopic portals to maximize the distance between the posterior edge of the greater trochanter and the sciatic nerve.

When the lateral position is used, the perineal post has extra padding, is oversized (with an outer diameter of 10 to 12 cm), has a horizontal orientation, and is positioned in the groin of the operative leg, which is not the case when the supine position is used. Elevation of the post provides lateralization of the force, and as a result, the traction direction is more in line with the femoral neck. Before traction is applied, the patient's genitalia should be inspected to verify that it is not being compressed. After a successful traction test is completed, the hip is taken through range of motion. Flexion of at least 40 degrees is important to adequately relax the anterior hip capsule and permit access the hip periphery. Flexion of at least 90 degrees along with internal and/or external rotation, as well as abduction and/or adduction, may be necessary to ensure complete decompression of impinging deformities. It is important to perform this test before draping because the operating room staff who have not undergone scrubbing will manipulate the table accessories, and they must be familiar with the manipulation of the traction device. In our experience a dedicated lateral hip distractor is preferred by the operating room staff because it is easier to manipulate under the drapes.

The surgeon stands in front of the patient to have better access to the anterior aspect of the hip (most of the pathology in the hip joint is anterior). The surgeon's assistant stands at the back side of the patient to facilitate participation in the procedure.[1,13] We believe that the arthroscopy tower should be positioned across from the surgeon on the back side of the patient. Placing the tower proximally toward the patient's head affords a direct view for the surgical assistant. An arthroscopy suite with multiple monitors would provide the assistant with an even better view.

Intraoperative fluoroscopy with a C-arm should be used for identification of the anatomic references to localize portal positions. The C-arm is covered by sterile drapes and is positioned horizontally under the operating table to provide an anteroposterior (AP) fluoroscopic view of the hip. In larger patients, the arch of the C-arm may not be big enough to reach the area of the hip joint from under the table, in which case it can be positioned over the table, focusing on the area of the hip joint with the arch tilted over the patient's head. The C-arm may be moved proximally toward the head when not in use. A lateral view is achieved by moving the hip joint rather than the C-arm. The screen of the image intensifier is also positioned at the back side of the patient adjacent to the feet to provide a direct unobstructed view to the surgeon and assistant. The scrub nurse with all the arthroscopic instrumentation is on the same side of the surgeon toward the feet of the patient.

Special operating table accessories are required to position a patient in the lateral decubitus position for hip arthroscopy on a fracture table. These accessories often are unavailable, which has made the supine approach more popular. More recently, dedicated distractors for hip arthroscopy in the lateral approach have been developed (McCarthy Type Distractor, Inomed, Boston, MA, and Smith & Nephew Lateral Distractor, Smith & Nephew Endoscopy, Andover, MA). These dedicated distractors may help make the lateral position more accessible to surgeons, especially in the surgery center setup.

Supine Position

Thomas Byrd developed supine positioning for hip arthroscopy. He describes the merits of supine positioning as follows:

it is the simplest and fastest positioning method; the orientation of the joint is familiar to the orthopaedic surgeon; it provides reliable access for all standard portals; it easily accommodates repositioning for arthroscopy of the peripheral compartment; and it permits other procedures to be performed, such as iliopsoas bursoscopy.[23] An important advantage of the supine approach is a reduced risk of intraabdominal fluid extravasation, which has been reported only in the lateral position.[24,25] Philippon has described the modified supine position in which the hip is in slight internal rotation (15 degrees), with 10-degree flexion, neutral abduction, and 10 degrees of lateral tilt.[26]

For supine hip arthroscopy, the patient is positioned on the operating table with both feet fixed to avoid pelvic tilt when traction is applied to the operative side. The surgeon, assistant, and scrub nurse work from the side of the operative hip, and the arthroscopy tower is positioned across the patient from the surgeon, with the fluoroscopy monitor at the foot. An oversized perineal post with extra padding (with an outer diameter of 12 cm) is vertically attached and positioned against the medial thigh of the operative leg, providing a lateralizing vector to the traction force.[1,23] The resulting direction of the traction is not in line with the femoral shaft but instead is more parallel to the femoral neck. The operative hip joint is positioned in extension, abduction (25 degrees), and neutral rotation during portal placement for proper orientation. The setup should allow easy rotation of the foot for intraoperative visualization of the femoral head.[23] The contralateral leg is abducted in the traction apparatus to neutralize the force on the pelvis. The C-arm is brought in between the legs in a vertical position over the operative side to provide an AP image of the hip. Slight traction is applied first to the contralateral extremity to stabilize the torso and pelvis on the table. After the pelvis is stabilized, traction is applied to the surgical leg, and adequate distraction of the joint line is confirmed by fluoroscopy.

Traction

Access to the hip joint for arthroscopy is provided by traction. The fundamental advantage of traction is opening of the joint line to allow entrance of the instruments (Fig. 82-4). Traction affords a thorough exploration of the central compartment with reduced risk of iatrogenic chondral or labral damage. The main disadvantages of traction include stretching of soft tissue structures such as the lateral femoral cutaneous nerve, compression of perineal structures against the post, and pressure on the foot.[1,12] In a patient who has not been anesthetized, forces of up to 900 N may be necessary to open the joint 10 mm (see Fig. 82-4, *B*).[27] This traction may be reduced to 300 N with inducement of proper anesthesia and muscle relaxation.[28] According to Byrd[22] and Glick,[23] necessary traction force to obtain appropriate visualization may approach 80 lb (25 to 30 kg). Special traction devices are available for both supine and lateral approaches.[12,29]

A traction test is always performed before preparing and draping the patient to confirm effective separation of the femoral head from the acetabulum at the image intensifier. This separation should be at least 10 mm. When separation does not occur, the foot fixation should be verified, because a poorly secured foot is the most common cause of ineffective traction. The foot must be well padded to avoid compression injuries. Different options are available for foot fixation to the traction device. A "ski boot" design was introduced by McCarthy and is very effective in providing foot fixation to the traction device. Most fracture tables have "booties" that fix the foot with use of Velcro straps or belt buckles.

Preparing and Draping

After the traction test is performed, the hip is brought back to the starting position without traction and the surgical area is prepared for surgery. When applying sterile drapes, we first start by covering both ends of the C-arm using sterile bags.[1] Waterproof adhesive sterile drapes are then placed in a standard fashion. The surgeon should be careful not to cover portal sites with the drapes. The medial drape should be slightly medial to the anterior superior iliac spine, the posterior drape should be behind the posterior edge of the greater trochanter, the superior drape should be above the level of the anterior superior iliac spine, and the distal drape should be at least 10 to 15 cm below the tip of the greater

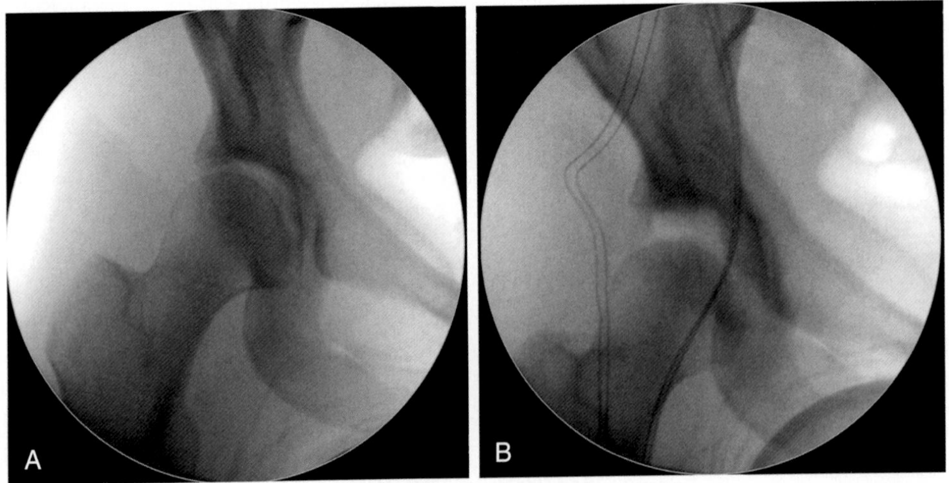

FIGURE 82-4 Fluoroscopic image of a right hip. **A,** Traction has not been applied to the hip. **B,** After traction is applied, separation is observed between the acetabulum and the femoral head (a 10-mm space between the acetabular margin and the superior aspect of the femoral head is recommended).

trochanter.[18] After drapes are in position, sterile gauze is placed over the area where the portals will be established, and an adhesive transparent surgical drape is placed over the surgical area (including the gauze). This seal will prevent fluid from leaking under the drapes to the patient when the procedure starts.[1]

After cables and tubes for arthroscopy are ready, traction is applied (traction starting time should be recorded to monitor its duration). With the traction established, the gauze is removed from the surgical area with the adhesive drape that covers it and landmarks are identified and marked on the skin with a skin marker (we prefer to mark the skin after traction is applied to avoid migration of the marks).[1]

Hip Arthroscopy Equipment and Instrumentation

Use of a set of dedicated hip arthroscopy instruments is mandatory when attempting arthroscopic access to the hip joint. The use of standard arthroscopy equipment for access to the hip joint will increase the possibility of iatrogenic damage to structures inside and around the hip joint.[26]

An arthroscopy tower should contain the monitor, digital camera, high-flow/low-pressure arthroscopy pump, shaver and radiofrequency control console, and an image processing system. Specially designed extra-long arthroscopic instruments are used, which include a long spinal needle and a specially designed flexible guide wire to reach the depth of the hip joint. We use a specially designed hip arthroscopy instrument set (Hip Access System, Smith & Nephew) that is based on a slotted cannula and is designed to be used in combination with standard length 4.0-mm arthroscopes of 30 and 70 degrees. The scissors and graspers used for hip arthroscopy also should be longer than conventional ones.[1] Although most patients can be treated using standard-length shaving tips and burrs, use of extra-long instruments is recommended. Curved instruments are needed to accommodate the spherical anatomy of the hip. Flexible radiofrequency devices are also very helpful. Cannulated instruments are the workhorse of hip arthroscopy and are included in every commercially available hip arthroscopy instrument set.[1] Standard cannulas may limit access of curved devices, and thus slotted cannulas may be used for these devices.

Irrigation should be always assisted by a fluid pump to provide clear visualization without the need for excessive pressure. Because of the possibility of intraabdominal extravasation of fluid, the amount of fluid and the intraarticular pressure must be monitored. We recommend a low pressure (50 to 60 mm Hg) and high flow pump.[1,30]

Landmarks and Topographic Anatomy of the Hip Joint

Surface landmarks around the hip joint and their relationship to anatomic structures are the road map of hip arthroscopy. Understanding portal placement in relation to these landmarks and the anatomic structures around the portal path in every anatomic layer is paramount in performing safe and successful hip arthroscopy.

The most important and apparent surface landmarks are the greater trochanter and the anterior superior iliac spine

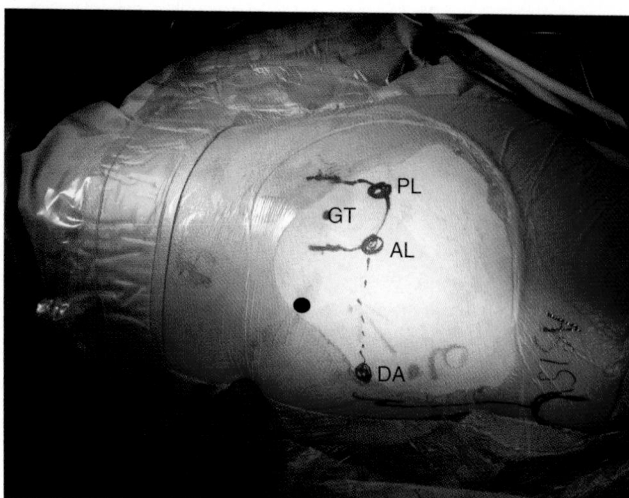

FIGURE 82-5 The position of arthroscopic portals in a right hip. The patient's head is to the right and the front is to the bottom (i.e., the patient is in the lateral decubitus position). The anterior superior iliac spine (*ASIS*) and the greater trochanter (*GT*) have been outlined on the skin. The site of the anterolateral portal (*AL*) is at the superior anterior corner of the GT. The site of the posterolateral portal (*PL*) is at the posterior superior corner of the GT. The direct anterior portal (*DA*) is at the intersection of a vertical line coming down from the ASIS and a horizontal line directed anteriorly from the tip of the GT. The black circle indicates the location of the mid anterior portal, which can substitute for the DA or be used as an accessory portal.

(Fig. 82-5). These landmarks should always be marked before the surgery is started.

Byrd et al.[31] performed a cadaveric anatomic study and described the relation of the classic central compartment portals, skin landmarks, and the anatomic structures around the hip joint. The sciatic nerve lies about 1.5 cm posterior to the posterior aspect of the greater trochanter. The femoral neurovascular bundle lies medial to the vertical line coming down from the anterior superior iliac spine. Two or three branches of the lateral femoral cutaneous nerve traverse the anterior hip and are at most risk of injury when anterior portals are established.

An image intensifier is used for all cases, and surface landmarks are verified with fluoroscopy, which is important to ensure precise portal placement and minimize the risk of iatrogenic damage. Once displacement of the joint line of at least 10 mm is achieved with traction, the first portal (in our practice, the anterolateral portal) can be placed.

Portals

Most hip arthroscopies can be performed through a visualization portal and working portal, although some surgeons use additional portals as needed depending on the pathology.[1] Three standard portals are described for hip arthroscopy: anterolateral, anterior, and posterolateral.[1,23] Several accessory portals are also used.

Anterolateral

The anterolateral portal is also known as the anterior peritrochanteric portal because of its location at the anterosuperior corner of the greater trochanter. The anterolateral portal is considered the easiest and safest portal to establish because it is located most centrally in the "safe zone," and for this reason, we establish it first. This portal penetrates the gluteus medius before entering the lateral aspect of the capsule. Entrance into the hip is monitored closely with fluoroscopy to minimize iatrogenic chondral injury or penetration of the labrum. The superior gluteal nerve travels an average of 4.4 to 5 cm superior to this portal.[1,32]

Anterior

The anterior portal site is established at the intersection of a vertical line extending distally from the anterior superior iliac spine and a horizontal line extending medially from the greater trochanter (Fig. 82-6). The trajectory of this portal from the skin into the hip is approximately 45 degrees cephalic and 30 degrees toward the midline. Branches of the lateral femoral cutaneous nerve (LFCN) are at risk when the anterior portal is established. The portal courses through the sartorius and rectus muscles en route to the hip joint.[1,32] Some surgeons prefer to position the direct anterior portal 1 cm lateral to vertical line from the anterior superior iliac spine to avoid penetrating the rectus femoris tendon and limit risk of injury to branches of the LFCN. This portal is typically created under arthroscopic visualization to ensure appropriate position within the joint (Fig. 82-7).

Posterolateral

The posterolateral portal is located at posterosuperior corner of the greater trochanter and is also known as the posterior peritrochanteric portal. The posterolateral portal penetrates both the gluteus medius and minimus before entering the lateral capsule at its posterior margin. Its route is superior and anterior to the piriformis tendon. This portal lies closest to the sciatic nerve at the level of the capsule with an average distance of 2.9 to 3 cm. Approximately 4.4 cm separates the posterolateral portal from the superior gluteal nerve.[1,32]

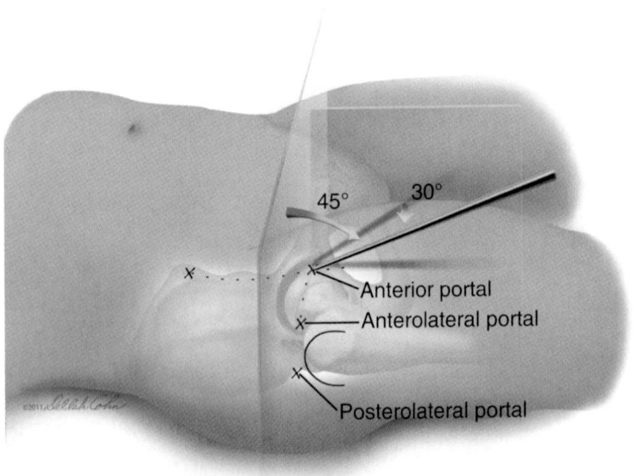

FIGURE 82-6 The anterior portal is located at the intersection of a line extending distally from the anterior superior iliac spine and medially from the anterolateral portal. *(Courtesy Dr. Thomas Byrd.)*

Accessory Portals

To accommodate some central compartment instrumentation and to access the hip periphery, variations of the original portals and other accessory portals have been introduced. Robertson and Kelly[32] described the anatomic relationships of eight different skin incisions (including the traditional anterolateral, posterolateral, and direct anterior portal) with 11 different portal trajectories that have been used for hip arthroscopy and the peritrochanteric space by different authors, using a study design similar to that of the study by Byrd (Fig. 82-8).[31]

Surgical Technique

Atraumatic technique is essential when performing hip arthroscopy, and every step should be performed with caution. A systematic approach for the complete visualization of the joint is the key for an accurate diagnosis and treatment of hip pathology. Doffman and Boyer[32a] divided the hip joint in two compartments, central and peripheral, divided by the labrum. In this regard, a complete arthroscopic inspection of the hip can be achieved with use of a combined procedure. The central hip compartment can be scoped only by distraction of the joint; the periphery of the hip can be seen without traction.[12]

For most indications, hip arthroscopy is started within the central compartment with the assistance of traction. As previously stated, the anterolateral portal is typically the initial portal established because of its relatively safe location. However, because this portal is established with use of fluoroscopy and without direct intraarticular visualization, intraarticular structures such as the labrum and chondral surfaces are at risk. To establish this portal, fluoroscopy is used to carefully navigate a spinal needle into the hip joint between the separated acetabulum and femoral head (Fig. 82-9). To minimize risk of iatrogenic damage to the labrum, the needle should be introduced as close as possible to the femoral head, away from the free margin of the lateral labrum, with the tip of the needle pointing away from the femoral head. After feeling the needle penetrate the thick hip capsule, the joint may be distended with approximately 40 cm^3 of saline solution, and the intracapsular position of the needle is confirmed by backflow of fluid. The position of the spinal needle with use of fluoroscopy before and after fluid distention should be noted. As the joint space expands, the needle should move distally with the femoral head. If it remains fixed to the acetabular rim, the surgeon should suspect that the needle is piercing the labrum and reposition it closer to the femoral head to avoid further damage to the labrum. A blunt-ended guide wire may be introduced to palpate the medial wall of the acetabulum to verify the intraarticular position. Nitinol guide wires are preferred because they are more flexible than standard Kirschner wires and are more tolerant to bending before kinking and breaking.

Once the portal position is satisfactory, the spinal needle is removed, leaving the guide wire in the joint. A skin incision is performed around the guide wire to allow passage of cannulated instruments. A sharp cannulated trocar is used to penetrate only the joint capsule, followed by a blunt cannulated trocar, to avoid damage to the articular cartilage. Our preference is to use a cannulated switching stick mounted on

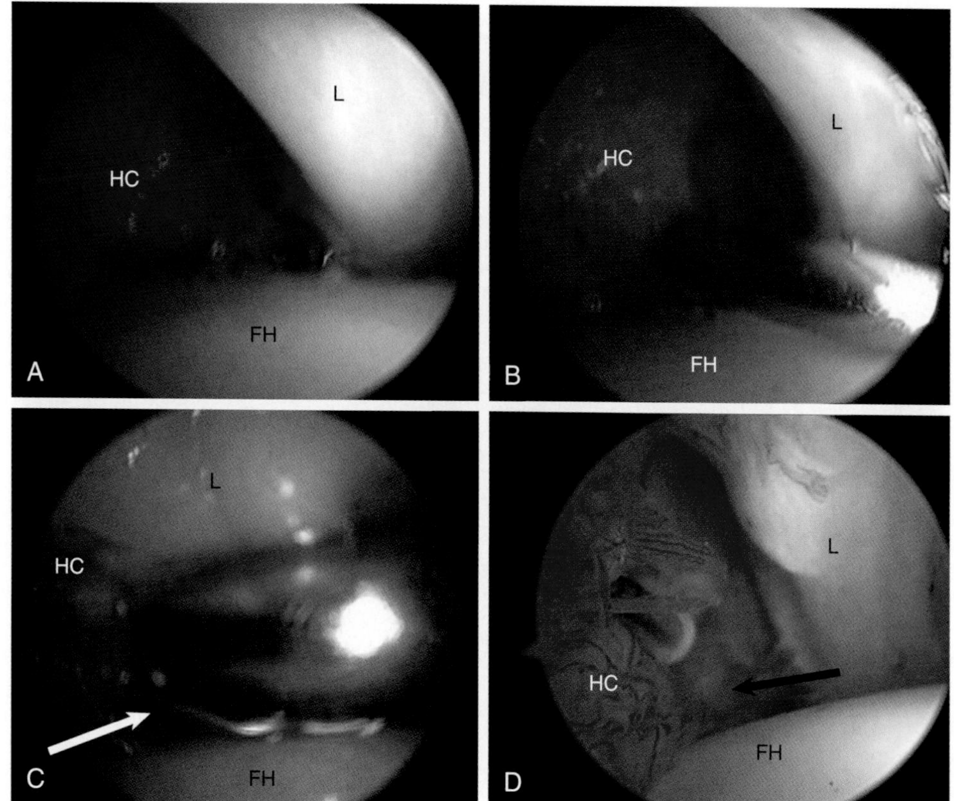

FIGURE 82-7 Arthroscopic sequence of establishments of the direct anterior portal under arthroscopic vision (left hip). **A,** This photograph demonstrates the anterior labrum (*L*), the femoral head (*FH*), and a triangle space between them limited by the field of view by the scope. The area within this triangle is the anterior hip capsule (*HC*). The join does not contain any fluid. **B,** The free margin of the anterior labrum (*L*) is at the top; the FH is at the bottom. A spinal needle is observed as it pierces the anterior HC. The joint does not contain any fluid. **C,** The labrum (*L*) is at the top, and the FH is at the bottom. A direct anterior portal has been established with a switching stick. The white arrow points to a slotted cannula as it is introduced around the switching stick. The joint does not contain any fluid. **D,** The anterior labrum (*L*) is at the top; the FH is in the bottom. A radiofrequency hook probe is used to create a capsulotomy (*black arrow*) of the anterior HC.

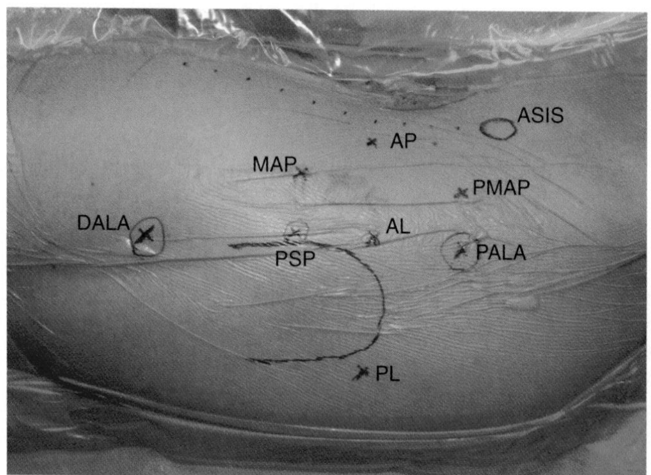

FIGURE 82-8 Arthroscopic portals for a left hip. Standard portals include the anterior portal (*AP*), anterolateral portal (*AL*), and posterolateral portal (*PL*). Accessory portals include the mid anterior portal (*MAP*), proximal mid anterior portal (*PMAP*), the proximal and distal anterolateral portals (*PALA* and *DALA*), and the peritrochanteric space portal (*PSP*). *ASIS,* Anterior superior iliac spine. *(From Robertson WJ, Kelly BT: The safe zone for hip arthroscopy: a cadaveric assessment of central, peripheral, and lateral compartment portal placement.* Arthroscopy *24:1019–1026, 2008.)*

a special handle, which uses the nitinol guide wire as a monorail to follow it into the hip joint. Once the switching stick is in its intraarticular position, the handle is removed, and the standard arthroscopy cannula is introduced over the guide wire. A 70-degree 4-mm arthroscope is positioned in the arthroscopy cannula after the switching stick is removed.

The other portals are established under direct arthroscopic vision. Most surgeons establish the direct anterior portal or one of its variants. A spinal needle is introduced at the site of the direct anterior portal and triangulated to the tip of the arthroscope inside the hip joint. The needle should be observed entering the joint at the anterior safety triangle limited superiorly by the free margin of the anterolateral labrum, inferiorly by the femoral head, and laterally by the limit of the arthroscopic field of view. The stylus is removed from the needle and a nitinol guide wire is introduced. The needle is removed and the guide wire is used as a monorail to introduce cannulated instruments to establish a working portal.

Two techniques are used with the working portal—a modular cannula system or a slotted cannula system. In the modular system, a cannulated obturator is used to introduce modular cannulas into the hip joint. The cannulated obturator and modular cannula assembly are introduced into the portal using the nitinol guide wire. Modular cannulas are

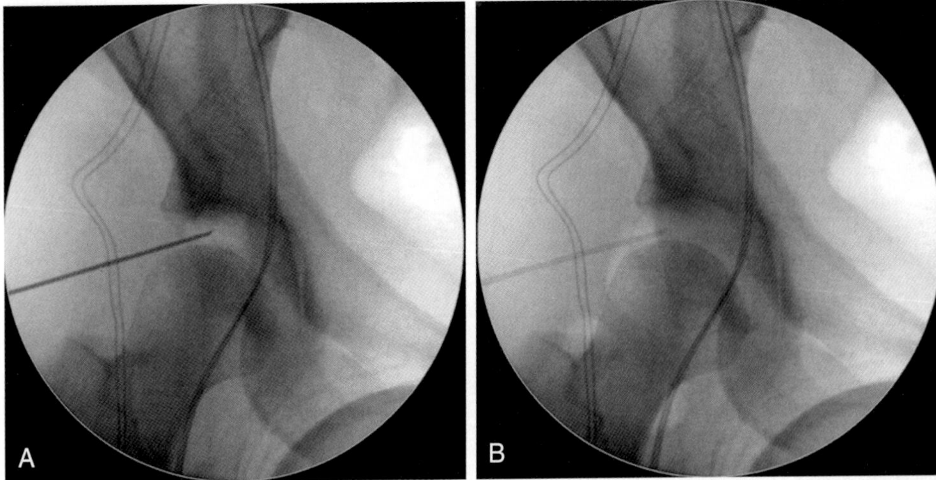

FIGURE 82-9 Fluoroscopic image of a right hip. **A,** A spinal needle is introduced at the site of the anterolateral portal and navigated into the joint with use of fluoroscopy. Note that the needle is closer to the femoral head to maximize the distance to the free margin of the labrum and prevent labral penetration. The blunt side of the beveled needle is toward the head to prevent damage to the femoral head cartilage. **B,** The stylus to the needle is removed and water is used to distend the joint. As the space between the acetabulum and femoral head increases, the needle stays closer to the femoral head, indicating that it is not incarcerated by the labrum.

available in different diameters and have a proximal attachment for a modular fluid management bridge that serves to lock the arthroscope inside the cannula, thus working as and arthroscopy cannulas and also as a working cannula. The system is based on the philosophy of positioning different cannulas in each portal; the arthroscope can then be interchanged between these cannulas to access different parts of the joint as needed, allowing the free cannulas to serve as working cannulas. With the slotted cannula system, a switching stick is typically positioned over the nitinol guide wire into the joint and the slotted cannula is slid around the switching stick to enter the hip joint (Fig. 82-10). With the slotted cannula inside the hip joint, the switching stick is exchanged for an arthroscopic instrument and the slotted cannula is removed. After the selected instrument has been used, it serves as a guide to reinsert the slotted cannula, preparing the portal for the introduction of a different instrument or for portal exchange. Portal exchange with a slotted cannula is slightly more complicated than it is with a closed cannula system; a switching stick is introduced into the joint with use of the slotted cannula, which is removed to be reinserted around the arthroscopy cannula (where the scope is positioned) and confirmed inside the joint with the arthroscope. The cannula/arthroscope assembly is removed from the slotted cannula, leaving the later in position inside the portal. The arthroscope is removed from the arthroscopy cannula and is introduced at the other portal over the switching stick. The switching stick is removed and the arthroscope is positioned inside the arthroscopy cannula.

When working portals are established with use of either the modular cannula or the slotted cannula method, instruments are brought into the joint under direct arthroscopic vision to prevent iatrogenic damage.

Once the portals are established, a hip capsulotomy is typically performed to increase instrument mobility within the joint. The capsulotomy is typically performed with use of a banana arthroscopic knife. Other instruments such as radiofrequency devices of different shapes may also be used to perform the capsulotomy. An effective technique for a capsulotomy is to connect the anterolateral and direct anterior

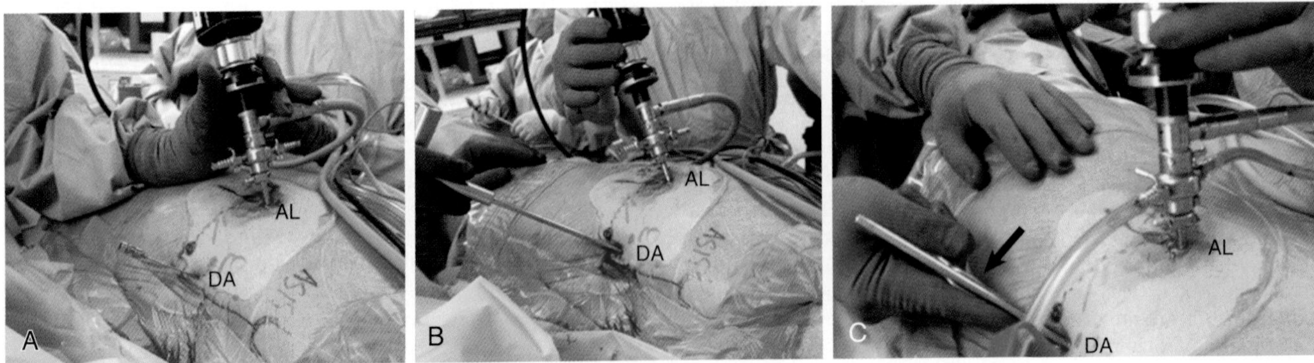

FIGURE 82-10 The sequence of portal establishment using a cannulated technique (in a right hip in the lateral decubitus position). The arthroscope is in the anterolateral portal (*AL*). **A,** A spinal needle is introduced through the direct anterior portal (*DA*) and triangulated toward the tip of the arthroscope under direct arthroscopic control. **B,** After a nitinol wire is placed through the spinal needle, a cannulated switching stick is passed over the wire. **C,** A slotted cannula (*black arrow*) is used to establish the working portal.

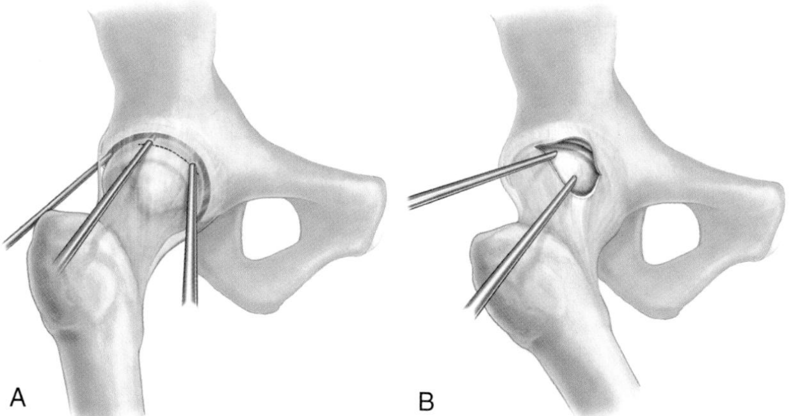

FIGURE 82-11 **A,** An arthroscopic knife or electrocautery is used to connect the direct anterior and anterolateral portals. **B,** Dividing the capsule between the two portals facilitates navigation and instrumentation within the hip joint. *(Courtesy Dr. Thomas Byrd.)*

portals inside the hip joint, because this technique will produce a capsulotomy that is parallel to the anterior acetabular rim (Fig. 82-11). With this exposure it is very easy to identify the free margin and the capsular side of the labrum, providing access to the labral insertion on the acetabular rim. Visualization can be improved by combining the technique with a limited capsulectomy. With the area exposed, the surgeon may proceed to remodel the pincer deformity and treat labral pathology.

Access to the hip periphery is better without traction and with hip flexion to relax the anterior hip capsule. A number of accessory portals have been described to access the hip periphery; they can be established with the aid of fluoroscopy and using the cannulated instruments with the same technique as described for the central compartment.

Intraarticular Orientation

Central Compartment

As previously mentioned, a systematic initial inspection of the join is imperative. The surgeon should avoid spending considerable time on obvious aspects of the pathology and instead focus on detecting and addressing coexistent lesions. Whereas the central acetabulum and the periphery of the femoral head may be viewed with a 30-degree arthroscope, a 70-degree arthroscope is needed to thoroughly evaluate the periphery of the acetabulum, the labrum, the articular capsule, and the superior pole of the femoral head. Two methods have been described to systematically document anatomy and pathology within the central compartment, the clock face method and the geographic zone method.[1]

Clock Face Method

Given the circular orientation of the acetabulum, using a clock face to document arthroscopic findings has been widely accepted. In this method, an imaginary analog clock is applied to the acetabulum, and a description of the geographic situation of lesions of the acetabulum or the labrum is expressed in times on the clock face. For orientation, the 6-o'clock position is directed inferiorly from the opening (center) of the acetabular fossa to the obturator foramen. The 12-o'clock position is directly opposite the 6-o'clock position and generally marks the superolateral aspect of the acetabulum.

This clock-face method is easy to understand and is familiar to surgeons with experience in shoulder arthroscopy. However, a few disadvantages are encountered with use of this method. The clock-face method can only be applied to the acetabulum. In addition, based on how a surgeon documents findings, the clock-face positions for the anterior and posterior aspects of the acetabulum may change for the right and left hip. In a right hip, the anterior acetabulum is between 1 and 5 o'clock, and in a left hip, the anterior acetabulum is between 7 and 11 o'clock. When reporting findings for an operative report, this situation must be specified. Some surgeons invert the clock face artificially to have the anterior acetabulum between 1 and 5 o'clock regardless of laterality. However, clock-face orientation is not standardized and may generate confusion when data are presented to other surgeons.

The precise definition of the 12- and 6-'clock positions may also create issues with reproducible documentation with the clock face. Pelvic inclination, as well as acetabular version and inclination, may affect the arthroscopic perception of the 12-o'clock position. Additionally, the location of the 12-o'clock position may be altered during arthroscopy with rim shaving for pincer lesions.

Geographic Zone Method

The geographic zone method, recently developed through consensus of a group of hip arthroscopy experts, facilitates accurate documentation of intraarticular lesions of the acetabulum and the femoral head (Fig. 82-12).[32] With this method, the acetabular fossa is the main landmark for zone subdivision of both the acetabulum and the femoral head. Two imaginary vertical lines are positioned in the acetabulum at the anterior and posterior limits of the acetabular fossa, dividing the acetabulum into three parts. An imaginary horizontal line is positioned in alignment with the most superior aspect of the acetabular fossa, dividing the acetabulum in a superior and inferior half. The result is a subdivision of the acetabulum in six different zones. The anterior-inferior zone is assigned number 1, and then progressive numbers are assigned to the zones that surround the acetabular fossa so that number 5 is given to the posterior inferior zone. Finally, number 6 is

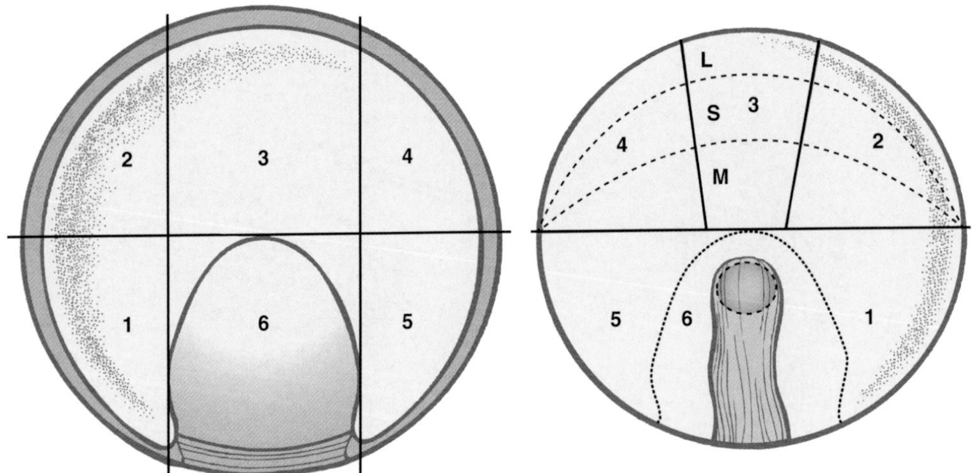

FIGURE 82-12 The geographic zone method of documenting acetabular and femoral head pathology. On the acetabulum, the acetabular fossa is used as the main landmark. Two vertical lines on either side of the fossa divide the acetabulum into thirds, and a horizontal line at the superior aspect of the fossa creates six zones. On the femoral head, the ligamentum teres is used as the primary landmark, and like the acetabulum, two vertical lines on either side of the ligamentum teres divide the femoral head into thirds. A horizontal line at the top of the ligamentum teres creates six zones. Zones 2, 3, and 4 make up the main weight-bearing portion of the femoral head and are further subdivided into medial (*M*), superior (*S*), and lateral (*L*) zones. The femoral head zones correspond to the acetabular zones. *(From Ilizaliturri VM Jr, Byrd JW, Sampson TG, et al: A geographic zone method to describe intra-articular pathology in hip arthroscopy: cadaveric study and preliminary report.* Arthroscopy *24:534–539, 2008.)*

assigned to the acetabular fossa. The process is the same for a right or left acetabulum. Each of the zones from 1 to 5 includes the corresponding acetabular cartilage and rim (including the labrum).

On the femoral head, the area that corresponds to the acetabular fossa is positioned around the ligamentum teres. Imaginary lines are then placed around the projection of the fossa on the femoral head following the same pattern as the acetabulum, which divides the femoral head in 6 different zones. As in the acetabulum zone, 1 is assigned to the anteroinferior subdivision and progressive numbers are assigned to the zones around the projection of the acetabular fossa so that zone 5 is the posterior inferior zone. The number 6 is assigned to the zone that contains ligamentum teres. On the femoral head, zones 2, 3, and 4 (which correspond to the superior half of the head) are assigned subdivisions: medial, superior, and lateral.

Contraindications

Contraindications for hip arthroscopy include medical contraindications, advanced osteoarthritis, avascular necrosis with collapse, an ankylosed joint, arthrofibrosis and capsular contractions, ulcerous or skin-infected injuries adjacent to the area of the portals, significant heterotopic ossification, morbid obesity, or any other condition that prohibits entry into the hip joint.[1,12]

Complications

Complications during hip arthroscopy are uncommon (Table 82-1). In a study of 1054 patients, Clarke and Villar reported a complication rate of 1.4%.[32b] These findings are similar to the review by Byrd[34] of 1491 cases performed by different experienced surgeons in which the complication rate was 1.34%. Sampson[25] reported a 6.4% complication rate in a study of 530 patients. The nature and rate of complications change as the surgeon gains experience, and generally with improved efficiency and technique, complications can be limited (Box 82-1).

BOX 82-1 Recommendations to Minimize Hip Arthroscopy Complications

Traction and Perineal Post

- Magnitude of traction force should be limited to 22.7 kg (50 lb)
- Traction should be limited to <2 hours
- For prolonged cases, traction should be intermittent
- The perineal post diameter should be at least 9 cm and adequately padded
- An adequate foot fixation device should be used

Scope Injuries

- Adequate distraction of the joint is required (10 mm)
- Joint distention should be performed with 20 to 40 mL of saline solution
- Rim osteophytes and capsulotomy should be resected (in cases of cam-type impingement)
- A cannula should be used for instrument or portal exchange
- The length of instrumentation should be at least 16 cm
- Special equipment for hip arthroscopy should be used

Fluid Extravasation

- Inflow fluid pressure should be low (40-50 mm Hg)
- Surgery time should be reduced
- Psoas endoscopic release should be performed last
- The abdomen should be examined periodically

Heterotopic Ossification

- The joint should be washed out at the end of the surgery

TABLE 82-1

HIP ARTHROSCOPY COMPLICATIONS

Type of Complication	Technical Error
Neurovascular Traction Injuries	
Transient palsy of the sciatic nerve	Excess flexion of the hip
Neurapraxia of the pudendal nerve	Magnitude of the intraoperative traction
Transient dysesthesia of the pudendal nerve	Prolonged traction
Transient palsy of the femoral nerve	Traction and excessive extension of the hip
Hematoma and edema of the labia majora	Inadequate padding of the perineal post
Pressure necrosis of the scrotum (1 case)	Inadequate padding of the perineal post
Vaginal tear (1 case)	Inadequate padding of the perineal post
Trochanteric bursitis (1 case)	Excessive distraction
Avascular necrosis of the femoral head (2 cases)	Prolonged traction
Portal Placement	
Periportal hematoma (0.3%)	Inadequate placement of portals
Pseudoaneurysm (rupture of the inferior gluteal artery)	Incorrect placement of the accessory PLP
Sciatic nerve injuries	Incorrect placement of the posterior portal
Lateral femoral cutaneous nerve injuries	Incorrect placement of the anterolateral portal
Iatrogenic	
Chondral damage (1%-18%)	Scope and instrumentation direct trauma
Labral lesion (18%-20%)	Incorrect establishment of the initial portal
Intraarticular instrument breakages (0.3%-0.4%)	Incorrect manipulation of the tools
Lateral cutaneous nerve damage	Inadequate introduction of the instruments
Skin irritation	Instruments passed in and out numerous times
Retroperitoneal extravasation of the fluid	Longer operative time and outflow pump pressure
Fluid extravasation into the thigh	Iliopsoas tendon release
Anchor placement complications	Malplacement or intraarticular penetration
Other Complications	
Heterotopic ossification (1.6%-6%)	
Joint instability (4 cases)	
Adhesions (79%-92% of revisions)	
Femoral neck fractures (4 cases)	
Deep venous thrombosis (3.7%)	
Hypothermia (2.7%)	
Portal infection (0.001%)	
Pulmonary embolism (1 case)	
Septic arthritis	

PLP, Posterolateral portal.

Complications that occur as a result of traction are observed in 0.5% to 6.4% of cases.[33,35-37] The surgeon must be vigilant regarding the magnitude and duration of traction, and ensuring safe traction is critical to avoiding traction-related complications. Traction-type injuries are usually associated with prolonged procedures or application of excessive force that causes transient nerve palsies.[8,37,38] In a series of 106 cases in which a fracture table was used for femoral fracture intramedullary nailing, Brumback et al.[39] noted that traction forces greater than 50 kg were safe only when applied for short periods. Large distraction forces applied for long periods were associated with a higher risk of nerve palsy.

To minimize the amount of time that traction is applied, Griffin and Villar[36] have proposed a "trial of traction." This trial involves applying traction temporarily to set the adequate distraction space, releasing traction while preparing the skin and draping, and then reapplying the traction when the procedure starts. Similar to tourniquet-associated ischemia time, traction time should be closely monitored and kept to less than 2 hours. Traction should be released when it is not necessary for visualization, such as during arthroscopy of the peripheral compartment. A tensiometer is a helpful tool for monitoring adequate and safe joint distraction.[23] If more time is necessary, the traction should be released and reinitiated after a rest period of at least 15 minutes.[40]

The perineal post usually causes complications attributed to compression, with the pudendal nerve and perineal structures being at risk. Glick[22] has demonstrated that a well-padded post with an outer diameter of at least 12 cm significantly decreases the risk of compressive neuropathy in the perineum. The top of the foot should also be well padded to decrease trauma to the skin and underlying structures.

Iatrogenic nerve injury is possible with portal placement. Direct injury to branches of the LFCN may be caused during placement of the anterior portal.[1] The portal should be established with a superficial skin incision and blunt dissection to protect direct injury to branches of the LFCN. Most of these injuries are transient, although persistent numbness in the anterolateral thigh is possible. The superior gluteal nerve and sciatic nerve are potentially at risk with establishment of the anterolateral and posterolateral portals, respectively.

Although underreported, direct injury from the arthroscope may occur during hip arthroscopy. In the series by Sampson,[25] significant arthroscope-associated injury was considered to be less than 1%. Labral injury may occur with portal establishment, and the anterosuperior labrum is at risk with the initial portal. Careful observation of the relationship between the spinal needle and the femoral head during insufflation of the joint may help avoid piercing the labrum with the initial portal.[23] If the needle stays with the acetabulum when the femoral head is pushed away by the fluid, placement of the needle through the labrum should be suspected, and the needle should be redirected. Papavasiliou and Bardakos[41] recommend additional caution when accessing dysplastic hips to avoid damage to the hypertrophic labrum in these patients.

Chondral lesions occur in as many as 18% of cases and usually affect the femoral head. Adequate distraction and joint distention are central to avoiding chondral injury. The femoral head should be separated at least 10 mm from the acetabulum to gain access to the central compartment. If sufficient separation is not possible, the periphery should be accessed first.[40,41] In treatment of cam-type impingement, a resection of rim osteophytes along with ample capsulotomies may facilitate femoral head–acetabular separation and access to the central compartment. Additionally, hip-specific arthroscopic instrumentation should be used to decrease the risk of iatrogenic chondral injury. Monllau et al.[18] observed that the appropriate length of the instruments should be at least 16 cm and emphasized that cannulated equipment should be used.

Incomplete decompression of the femoroacetabular impingement (FAI) deformity is underreported and is possibly more frequent with the arthroscopic technique. Although incomplete reshaping has not been presented as a major complication in the literature, it has been the most frequent indication for revision hip arthroscopy. Philippon and Schenker[43] reported that incomplete reshaping was the primary indication in 92% of patients who underwent revision arthroscopy. In another series by Heyworth et al.,[44] repeat arthroscopic reshaping was the reason for revision arthroscopy in 79% of cases.

Obtaining preoperative images to understand the deformity is essential. Three-dimensional CT and MRA with radial cuts are powerful tools that help delineate the shape of the deformity. During arthroscopy, adequate exposure of the deformity on the acetabular and femoral side is mandatory. This exposure can be improved by capsulotomy and sometimes capsulectomy in difficult cases. Fluoroscopy is used to assist in navigating the depth of the resection and the extent of the lateral decompression on the femoral neck. A complete lateral decompression is important to avoid impingement in high degrees of motion.[40] The crossover sign can be used to plan the distal limit of resection of the anterior acetabular rim during arthroscopy. Philippon and Schenker[43] observed that during rim trimming, 1.5 mm of resection corresponds to 1 degree of acetabular coverage. A center-edge angle less than 20 degrees is a contraindication for rim trimming to prevent hip instability.[43] The pincer deformity is usually exposed using an anterior hip capsulectomy parallel to the anterior acetabular rim. If the labrum can be detached for rim trimming and reattached in the remodeled rim, it should be carefully preserved and retracted while rim remodeling is performed.[40]

Avascular necrosis of the femoral head may occur after arthroscopic treatment of FAI if the femoral circumflex vessels are damaged, and these vessels are most at risk when cam reshaping is performed. If posterior or lateral rim trimming is performed, the blood supply may also be jeopardized by a far-posterior capsulotomy. The most lateral aspect of the cam deformity is closer to the critical area where the blood supply enters the hip. A constant and reliable landmark to identify the hip blood supply arthroscopically is the lateral synovial fold. The branches of the medial femoral circumflex artery are behind this landmark.[21] The lateral synovial fold can be identified arthroscopically with a 30-degree arthroscope as viewed from the anterior portal or an anterior accessory portal. No capsular or bony resection can be performed posterior to the lateral synovial fold. Sampson[25] reported one case of avascular necrosis in a series of 1000 consecutive hip arthroscopies 7 months after a partial labral resection and debridement for osteoarthritis without treatment of FAI deformities.

Femoral neck fracture in the arthroscopic treatment of cam-type impingement is a concern. The field of arthroscopy is limited because the femoral head-neck junction cannot be completely visualized. A complete exploration with a scope in different positions is necessary to understand the shape and size of the deformity. The medial, lateral, superior, and inferior limits of the deformity should be identified before starting the first bone cut. In a cadaveric study, Mardones et al.[45] concluded that resection of up to 30% of the anterolateral quadrant of the femoral head-neck junction did not alter the load-bearing capacity of the proximal femur. However, a 30% resection decreased the amount of energy required to produce a fracture by 20%. These investigators recommended 30% as the largest amount of bone resection.[45] When removing a cam-type deformity, the resection is usually carried out to the depth of the normal neck profile, which is typically 15% of the bone volume. Sampson[25] reported one femoral neck fracture after arthroscopic reshaping of a cam deformity in a series of 120 cases.

Hip instability may occur after hip arthroscopy, especially when an anterior hip capsulotomy or capsulectomy is performed. Theoretically, the iatrogenic injury to the iliofemoral ligament may produce an unstable hip; however, this phenomenon has not been reported in the literature. Excessive bone resection from the anterior acetabular rim may result in anterior hip dislocation. A careful study of the preoperative radiographs and evaluation of the center-edge angle is mandatory before bone resection from the acetabular rim. No bone resection can be performed in cases that have center-edge angles of 20 degrees or less as measured in the anteroposterior pelvis radiograph.[40]

Fluid extravasation is a potentially dangerous complication of hip arthroscopy. Prolonged surgery time, use of high-pressure irrigation equipment, and use of normal saline solution as irrigation are factors related to this complication. Intraabdominal fluid extravasation is also associated with arthroscopy postacetabular fracture, as well as periarticular endoscopy (iliopsoas bursa or peritrochanteric space).[41] The fluid can migrate into the retroperitoneal space through the iliopsoas sheath.[41] Femoral nerve palsy has been reported as a result of fluid extravasation into the thigh. The suggestive symptoms are abdominal distention, subcutaneous edema of the thigh, and hypothermia. Byrd and Chern[46] have recommended performing the operation in an expeditious fashion, and if difficulties are encountered and extravasation becomes a problem, it is better to terminate the procedure. A high-flow management system is recommended, allowing adequate flow without excessive pressure. Waiting several weeks after acetabular fractures to perform hip arthroscopy is advisable.[40]

The incidence of hypothermia below 35°C in patients undergoing hip arthroscopy has being reported by Parodi et al.,[47] with a rate of 2.7%. They found that prolonged surgery time, low mass index, low blood pressure during the procedure, and low-temperature arthroscopic irrigation fluid are the factors that contribute to the development of hypothermia.[47]

Deep venous thrombosis is uncommon after hip arthroscopy. Bushnell et al.[48] reported 0% incidence in more than 5500 cases of hip arthroscopy but suggested that prophylaxis should be established based on the patient's risk factors, including advanced age, personal family history of venous thrombosis or pulmonary embolism, obesity, and tobacco use.

For a complete list of references, go to expertconsult.com.

Suggested Readings

Citation: Ilizaliturri VM Jr, Byrd JW, Sampson TG, et al: A geographic zone method to describe intra-articular pathology in hip arthroscopy: cadaveric study and preliminary report. *Arthroscopy* 24:534–539, 2008.
Level of Evidence: I (testing of previously developed diagnostic criteria in series of consecutive patients)
Summary: This article reports on the development of an alternative method to divide the acetabulum and femoral head based on anatomic landmarks to facilitate reporting of intraarticular injuries.

Citation: Robertson W, Kelly BT: The safe zone for hip arthroscopy: A cadaveric assessment of central, peripheral, and lateral compartment portal placement. *Arthroscopy* 24:1019–1026, 2008.
Level of Evidence: IV (case series)
Summary: In this article, it is reported that all arthroscopic portals can be safely inserted; however, the greatest risk still comes from the proximity of the anterior portal to the lateral femoral cutaneous nerve.

Citation: Kelly BT, Williams RJ, Philippon MJ: Hip arthroscopy: Current indications, treatment options, and management issues. *Am J Sports Med* 31:1020–1037, 2003.
Level of Evidence: V (expert opinion)
Summary: In this article the most common clinical and radiographic methods to detect early hip joint disease are discussed and the indications and surgical techniques of hip arthroscopy are described.

Citation: Mei-Dan O, McConkey MO, Brick M: Catastrophic failure of hip arthroscopy due to iatrogenic instability: Can partial division of the ligamentum teres and iliofemoral ligament cause subluxation? *Arthroscopy* 28:440–445, 2012.
Level of Evidence: IV (case report)
Summary: This article provides a description of a case of rapid clinical and radiographic deterioration after hip arthroscopy as a result of femoral head subluxation, despite minimal disruption of the static stabilizers.

Citation: McCormick F, Kleweno CP, Kim YJ, et al: Vascular safe zones in hip arthroscopy. *Am J Sports Med* 39:64S–71S, 2011.
Level of Evidence: IV (case series)
Summary: In this article, vascular safe zones are identified using anatomic and intracapsular landmarks to reduce the risk of damage during hip arthroscopic surgery.

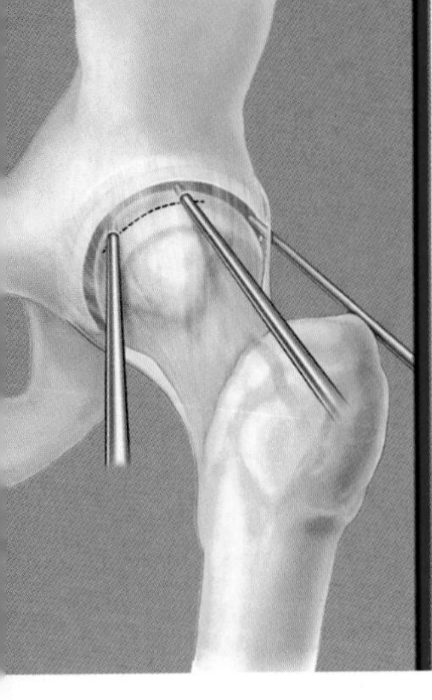

83

Athletic Pubalgia

CHRISTOPHER M. LARSON • PATRICK M. BIRMINGHAM • SHELLEY M. OLIVER

Athletic pubalgia or "sports hernia" is an umbrella term describing several anatomic injury patterns. Correctly diagnosing and treating this entity can be challenging.[1,2] A number of different terms, including "sports hernia," "Gilmore's groin," osteitis pubis, "slap-shot gut," "sportsman's hernia," and adductor or rectus strain have been used to describe a wide variety of pathologies in the area of the groin.[2-5] However, recognition is growing that groin injuries in athletes comprise a complex set of injuries to the musculature of the abdominal wall, the adductors, the hip joint, the pubic symphysis, and the sacroiliac joint that can be a source of significant disability.[3,4,6,7]

Anatomy

The complexity of the anatomy of the hip joint, pelvis, pubic symphysis, and the associated abdominal wall necessitates careful evaluation to accurately diagnose the source of an athlete's pain. The pubic symphysis is a nonsynovial amphiarthroidal joint.[8] Static stability of the joint is provided by the disk and four ligaments. The arcuate or inferior ligament has attachments to the inferior articular disk, the inferior attachment of the rectus abdominis, and the adductor and gracilis aponeurosis. The superior ligament spans the space between the pubic tubercles. The anterior ligament blends with fibers of the external oblique and rectus abdominis superficially. The deep portion of the anterior ligament attaches to the intraarticular disk. The posterior ligament is poorly developed. The pubic symphysis acts as the fulcrum for forces generated at the anterior pelvis. It represents the common attachment of the confluence of the rectus abdominis fascial sheath with the fascial sheath of the adductor longus, which merge anterior to the pubis to form a common sheath.[8-10] The abdominal wall has a layered structure. From superficial to deep, the structures of the abdominal wall are skin, fascia, external oblique fascia and muscle, internal oblique fascia and muscle, transversus abdominis muscle and fascia, and the transversalis fascia. The posterior fascia is deficient in the lower third of the rectus. Fibers from the rectus, conjoint tendon (the fusion of the internal oblique and transversus abdominis fascia), and external oblique merge to form the pubic aponeurosis, which is confluent with the adductor and gracilis origin. The conjoint tendon inserts anterior to the rectus abdominis on the pubis (Fig. 83-1).[11]

Given the clinical identification of an association between athletic pubalgia and femoroacetabular impingement (FAI)[7,9] and the recognition that loss of internal rotation of the hip is related to the development of groin pain and osteitis pubis,[12] Birmingham et al.[13] performed a cadaveric study looking at the effect of FAI on rotation at the pubic symphysis. At higher torque values, motion through the symphysis was much greater in cadavers with simulated cam morphology than in the native hip state. This finding supports the previous hypothesis that the altered rotational profile seen in the setting of FAI contributes to altered mechanics at the pubic symphysis.

One other possible source of pain has been theorized to be the result of entrapment of the genital branches of the ilioinguinal or genitofemoral nerves.[14] The symphysis itself is innervated by branches of the pudendal and genitofemoral nerves.[8] Some other reports have suggested that the iliohypogastric or obturator nerves could be involved.[15,16]

Historical Background

Groin injuries have been discussed within the medical literature as early as 1932, when Spinelli[17] reported on pubic pain in fencers. Gilmore[18] recognized a "severe musculotendinous injury of the groin" in 1980 in three professional soccer players. He identified a triad of pathology including injuries to the external oblique aponeurosis and conjoint tendon, avulsion of the conjoint tendon from the pubic tubercle, and dehiscence of the conjoint tendon from the inguinal ligament,[3] and later reported a 97% rate of return to sport after surgical repair.

In 1993, Hackney[19] first used the term "sports hernia" to describe a syndrome of groin pain in athletes for whom nonsurgical management had failed. At surgery, he identified weakening of the transversalis fascia with separation of that fascia from the conjoint tendon, dilation of the inguinal ring, and one case of a small direct hernia. He treated all patients with a surgical repair of the posterior inguinal wall and obtained an 87% return to sport rate in 15 athletes. Irshad et al.[20] described "hockey groin syndrome" in 22 National Hockey League players in 2001. These investigators found tearing of the external oblique aponeurosis and entrapment of the ilioinguinal nerve. Meyers et al.[2] have proposed that use of the term "athletic pubalgia"[4] is more appropriate than the more commonly used "sports hernia" for the constellation of injuries to the abdominal wall, hip flexors, adductors, and pubic symphysis presenting with pubic area or inguinal pain. They proposed that the primary pathology in athletic pubalgia is an imbalance between the strong adductors and the relatively weak abdominal muscles. Meyers et al.[21] describe 17

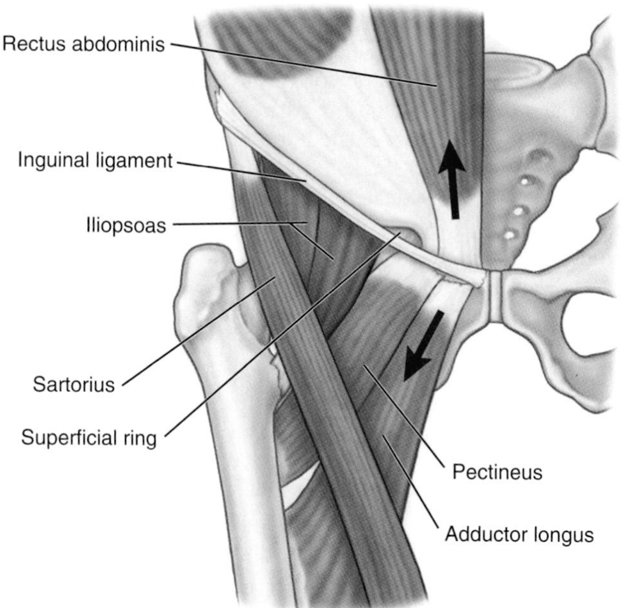

FIGURE 83-1 Injury to the abdominal wall at the fascial attachments of the rectus and adductors onto the pubis is implicated in athletic pubalgia.

different variants of athletic pubalgia, the most common of which are multiple tears or detachment of the anterior and anterolateral fibers of the rectus abdominis from the pubis and combined injuries to the rectus and adductors.[21]

As the understanding of intraarticular hip pathology has improved, the coexistence of labral pathology and femoroacetabular impingement with athletic pubalgia has increasingly been recognized.[7,9] Larson et al.[7] reported surgical treatment in a subset of athletes with coexistent femoroacetabular impingement and athletic pubalgia. Failure to treat both pathologies resulted in a low return to sport rate (25% if athletic pubalgia was addressed in isolation and 50% if the intraarticular hip pathology was addressed in isolation). This study resulted in the development of a surgical protocol to address both etiologies at the same surgery when athletes present with both symptomatic athletic pubalgia and intraarticular hip disorders (FAI). Using this approach, they achieved an 85% to 93% return to sport rate.[7]

When addressing the athlete with groin pain, it is important to carefully investigate other potential sources of the athlete's pain. Careful screening must be conducted for intraarticular hip pathology and associated hip pathomorphology if symptoms are present and are limiting. Additionally, it is important to be aware of the broader differential diagnosis of groin pain. Disorders of the gastrointestinal, genitourinary, or gynecological systems must also be considered, with several authors identifying tumors, Crohn disease, and other pathologies in the evaluation of the athlete with groin pain.[2,22]

History

Groin injuries are particularly common among persons who participate in sports requiring repetitive twisting, pivoting, and cutting motions, as well as activity requiring frequent acceleration and deceleration. Hockey, soccer, ice hockey, and rugby players have a particularly high incidence, with a lower incidence reported in American football, basketball, and baseball players.[3,20,23] Meyers et al.[21] noted that in the 1980s, fewer than 1% of their patients with athletic pubalgia were female. During the past two decades, however, that situation has changed dramatically, and female patients now represent 15% of patients presenting with athletic pubalgia.

Athletes may report insidious onset of groin pain or less commonly have a more acute presentation. Although some variability exists in the location and characteristic of symptoms, Meyers et al.[6] found that all of their athletes reported lower abdominal pain with exertion, whereas 92% had minimal to no pain at rest. Forty-three percent had bilateral symptoms and 67% had adductor pain after the onset of lower abdominal pain. Pain may also radiate to the rectus, perineum, or testicular region.[7] Exacerbation typically occurs during activities involving kicking, acceleration, and pivoting.[6,23] Abdominal crunches or sit-ups, coughing, or sneezing may also reproduce symptoms. Osteitis pubis presents in a similar fashion with pubic pain that may radiate to the adductors and is typically exacerbated by weight bearing.[19] Intraarticular hip pathology typically presents with deep groin pain that may radiate to the anterior thigh and lateral hip. Considerable overlap exists between intraarticular hip and athletic pubalgia/sports hernia symptom presentation, which increases the complexity in making an accurate diagnosis on the basis of symptoms alone.

Physical Examination

Assessment for athletic pubalgia/sports hernia should begin with palpation of the pubic symphysis, the insertion of the rectus abdominis, the adductor origin, the external and internal obliques, the transverses abdominis, the pectineus, the gracilis, and the inguinal ring for areas of tenderness. Pain can be precipitated via simulated coughing, resisted sit-ups (46%; Fig. 83-2), and hip adduction or the Valsalva maneuver.[6] A hernia is not detectable upon palpation; however, tenderness is usually present around the conjoint tendon, pubic tubercle (22%), adductor longus (36%), superficial inguinal ring, or posterior inguinal canal.[6,24,25]

Examination findings for osteitis pubis frequently overlap with athletic pubalgia and include tenderness of the pubic symphysis (67%), adductor origin tenderness (59%), pain with the adductor squeeze test (96%),[5] and apprehension throughout hip range of motion.[26] More severe cases may present with a typical "waddling" gait pattern.[27]

Diagnostic Injections

As previously indicated, the symptoms of femoroacetabular impingement, athletic pubalgia, osteitis pubis, and adductor strain can present with overlapping symptomatology and physical examination findings. An intraarticular injection of local anesthetic into the hip followed by physical examination or by having the athlete perform activities that typically provoke their pain can be useful. Pain that resolves with this injection can be assumed to be related to intraarticular hip pathology and treated accordingly.[7] Persistent pain in the lower abdominal and proximal adductor regions after intraarticular injections are consistent with coexistent athletic pubalgia. Similarly, injection of the pubic symphysis may be

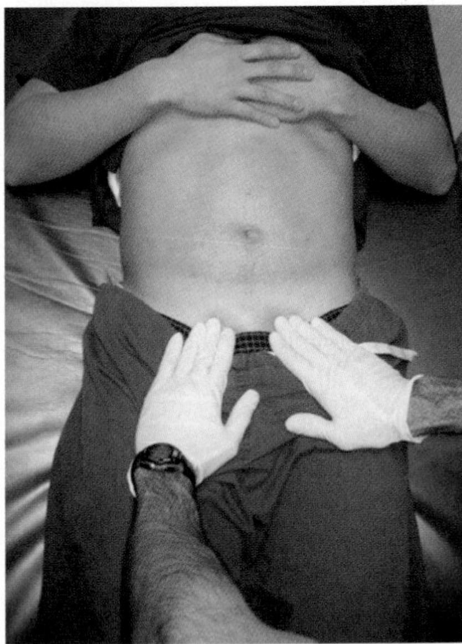

FIGURE 83-2 Pubic and/or groin pain with resisted sit-ups is associated with athletic pubalgia. *(Reprinted with permission from Minnich JM, Hanks JB, Muschaweck U, et al: Sports hernia: diagnosis and treatment highlighting a minimal repair surgical technique.* Am J Sports Med *39[6]:1341–1349, 2011.)*

useful for confirming the diagnosis of osteitis pubis. Radiocontrast dye can be used for the symphyseal injection, and extravasation of this dye up the rectus abdominis tract or down the adductor tract may indicate athletic pubalgia. Adductor pathology can be ruled in or out with an injection of anesthetic to the adductor cleft. Additionally, if psoas disorders are suspected, a diagnostic psoas bursal injection with anesthetic can be carried out as well. If impingement is suspected from the anterior inferior iliac spine, a subspine injection can be performed.

Imaging

Radiographic Analysis

Plain radiographs are vital in the initial evaluation of the athlete with hip or groin pain. A number of pathologies including osteitis pubis, avulsion fractures, stress fractures, apophysitis, osteoarthritis, and femoroacetabular impingement/dysplasia may be identified on radiographs. It is essential to obtain good quality, properly oriented images according to an established imaging protocol.[28]

The anteroposterior (AP) view (Fig. 83-3) may be used to evaluate the pubic symphysis for evidence of osteitis pubis, including sclerosis, fragmentation, and cyst formation within the pubic ramus, as well as symphyseal widening. When evaluating for FAI, femoral head neck deformities and acetabular depth and version are assessed. In the adolescent athlete, the AP view can be useful to identify apophyseal injuries. Additionally, stress fractures of the femoral neck and pubic rami and sacroiliitis may be identified.[11]

Stability of the pubic symphysis can be determined on single leg stance AP views. Symphyseal widening greater than 7 mm or vertical translation greater than 2 mm on a single leg stance view suggests instability of the pubic symphysis.[26]

Magnetic Resonance Imaging

Magnetic resonance (MR) arthrography has been used for the assessment of intraarticular hip pathology. More recently, noncontrast MR has been evaluated and found to be sensitive for intraarticular pathology, including articular cartilage injury and labral pathology. Ideally, coronal oblique and axial oblique sequences through the rectus insertion and pubic symphysis should be obtained in addition to standard sagittal, coronal, and axial sequences. Magnetic resonance imaging (MRI) is 68% sensitive and 100% specific for rectus abdominis pathology when compared with findings at surgery and 86% sensitive and 89% specific for adductor pathology. It is 100% sensitive for osteitis pubis.[29] Nonarthrogram studies may be preferred for in-season athletes to avoid the potential for irritation as a result of intraarticular contrast administration.

The MRI should be evaluated in a systematic fashion. The pubic bones should be evaluated for edema, subchondral sclerosis, and cysts suggestive of osteitis pubis (Fig. 83-4).[10,30] Evaluation of the tendinous insertions around the pubic symphysis should then be performed (Fig. 83-5). Frequent findings include fluid signal within the rectus abdominis or adductor origin, thickening of either structure, peritendinous fluid, or partial or complete disruption of either tendon. Most commonly, a confluent fluid signal is present that extends from the anterior-inferior insertion of the rectus abdominis into the adductor origin, with a corresponding fluid signal in the pubis.[29]

Decision-Making Principles

Treatment decisions are based on the degree of limitations and the ability to participate in the athlete's respective sport, duration of symptoms, pathology identified on physical examination and imaging, response to prior treatment modalities, and where the athlete is with respect to his or her training, sport season, and upcoming athletic events. Conservative management should be attempted prior to surgical intervention. The

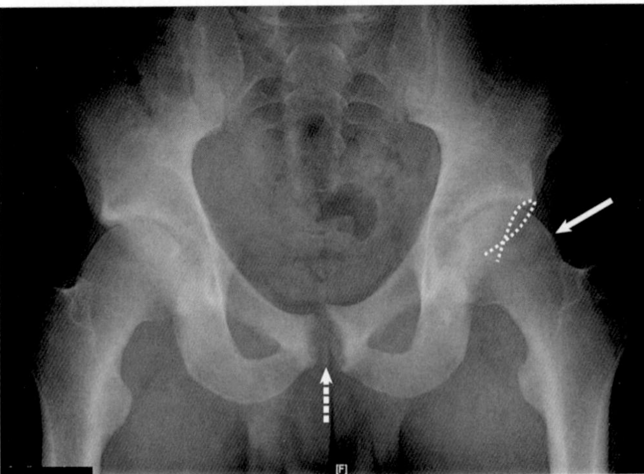

FIGURE 83-3 A well-aligned anteroposterior pelvis radiograph; note that the coccyx is centered over the pubic symphysis and a centimeter proximal. This radiograph reveals findings consistent with osteitis pubis (*dashed arrow*), including erosion, irregularity, and cyst formation. Additionally, a positive cross-over sign is noted, suggesting pincer impingement and a large cam lesion on the femoral neck (*solid arrow*).

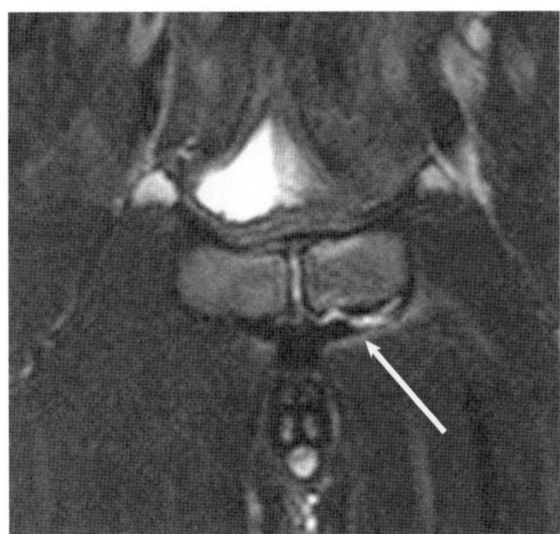

FIGURE 83-4 An oblique axial fat suppression T2-weighted magnetic resonance imaging scan of the pubic symphysis. Disruption of the left rectus aponeurosis is noted as it inserts on the anterior aspect of the superior pubic ramus (*tip of arrow*).

common locations of pain are the groin (FAI, athletic pubalgia, or adductor), lower abdomen or pubic symphysis (athletic pubalgia or adductor longus), posterior hip (FAI, proximal hamstring, low back, sacroiliac joint, or sciatic nerve entrapment disorders), or lateral thigh/hip (iliotibial band or gluteus medius/minimus). If no treatment has been provided, then rest, use of nonsteroidal antiinflammatory drugs (NSAIDs), physical therapy, and injections in select situations should be initiated. If the athlete continues to be symptomatic after 6 to 12 weeks of nonsurgical treatment, surgery might be considered. The timing of the surgery depends on the degree of disability and the point in the season. If the athlete's season is underway, an attempt can be made to delay surgery until the season is completed if the athlete is productive and functional. Surgery can then be performed at the end of the season if the athlete remains symptomatic. If the athlete is not able to compete at a reasonable level, then in-season or season-ending surgery can be considered. If the athlete has a combined pathology such as FAI and athletic pubalgia, these conditions can be surgically addressed at the same setting to minimize postoperative rehabilitation time and total time lost from participation. However, no evidence has indicated that carrying out these procedures separately or in a staged manner has any negative impact on outcome.[7]

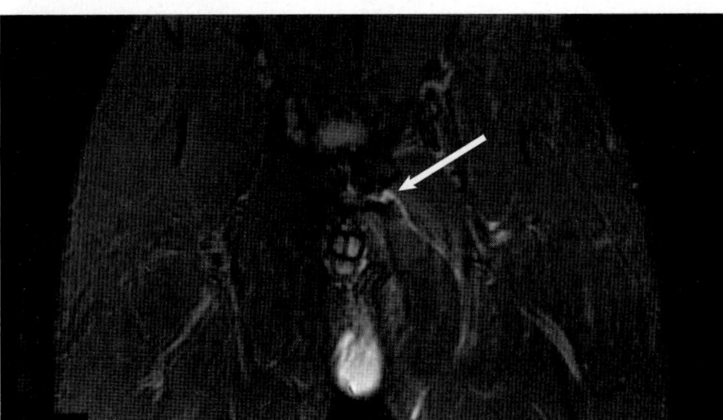

FIGURE 83-5 Coronal fat-suppression T2-weighted imaging of the pelvis demonstrating injury to the left adductor longus at its origin on the anterior-inferior aspect of the superior pubic ramus. Fluid signal is coursing linearly distally through the proximal muscle fibers (*tip of arrow*).

Treatment Options

Adductor Strain

Muscle imbalance between the abductors and adductors appears to contribute to injury. Tyler et al.[31] found that professional hockey players were 17 times more likely to sustain an adductor strain if their adductor strength was less than 80% of their abductor strength. In a follow-up study, they were able to demonstrate a clinically and statistically significant decrease in adductor strains in the same population with institution of a preventative adductor strengthening program.[32]

Nonoperative Management

Treatment starts with a brief period of rest, judicious use of ice and NSAIDs, and institution of a core and contralateral lower extremity strengthening program. Once the athlete is able to perform a pain-free concentric contraction of the adductor against resistance, the program can be progressed to core strengthening and adductor-specific exercises. It has been suggested that the athlete can progress to sport-specific training when the adductor strength is 75% of the ipsilateral abductor and passive range of motion is normal.[32,33]

One randomized clinical trial is available that presents 8- to 12-year follow-up data after nonoperative management of adductor-related groin pain.[34] The initial study randomly assigned 59 athletes to either a passive rehabilitation protocol consisting of modalities and stretching or an active rehabilitation protocol emphasizing strengthening of the core, abductors, and adductors.[34] In the initial study period, 23 of 29 patients treated with 8 to 12 weeks of active therapy had returned to sport by 4 months after initiating treatment.[33] In the passive therapy group, only 4 of 30 patients had returned to sport at the 4-month mark. At 8 to 12 years after treatment, 50% of the active rehabilitation group had no adductor pain with activity, no groin pain during or after activity, and were active in athletic activity at or one level below their previous level of athletic activity in the same sport. Only 22% of the passive therapy group met the same criteria.

The literature includes one case report of injection of a complete tear of the adductor longus with platelet rich plasma, with return to competitive soccer without surgery.[35] However, evidence for platelet rich plasma injections in the area of the hip and pelvis is lacking.

Operative Management

Surgical treatment of proximal adductor pain is indicated when 3 to 6 months of conservative management has failed to improve symptoms. Akermark and Johansson[35] published a case series of 16 competitive athletes with long-standing (mean, 18 months) and recurrent groin pain localized on physical examination to the adductor origin. Conservative management with rest, stretching, NSAIDs, and corticosteroid injections had failed for all of the athletes. Surgical treatment involved open tenotomy 1 cm from the adductor origin. All patients experienced improvement and were able to resume sporting activities at some level. Ten of 16 patients were pain free. The leg treated with surgery was weaker in adduction torque in all patients after full recovery.

Atkinson et al.[36] reported on 48 athletes who underwent 68 percutaneous adductor tenotomies for adductor strain. All patients were significantly restricted in their chosen sport before surgery, and 54% were able to return to full participation in their sport at a mean of 18.5 weeks.[37] Schlegel et al.[38] reported on 19 professional football players who sustained spontaneous rupture of the adductor longus. Twelve of 19 had groin or abdominal pain that preceded acute rupture. Of the 19 athletes identified, 14 were treated conservatively and nine underwent surgical repair with suture anchors. The nonoperative group returned to play at an average of 6 weeks after injury with no noted strength deficits. The group that

AUTHORS' PREFERRED TREATMENT

Adductor Strain

We prefer to perform a fractional lengthening or recession of the adductor longus through a 2-cm incision (Fig. 83-6). The adductor tendon is released 4 to 5 cm distal to its origin, leaving the underlying muscle intact (Fig. 83-7). This procedure may have less potential for longer term adductor weakness. In the setting of significant degenerative tearing and tendinosis proximally, however, a proximal release near the origin is performed.

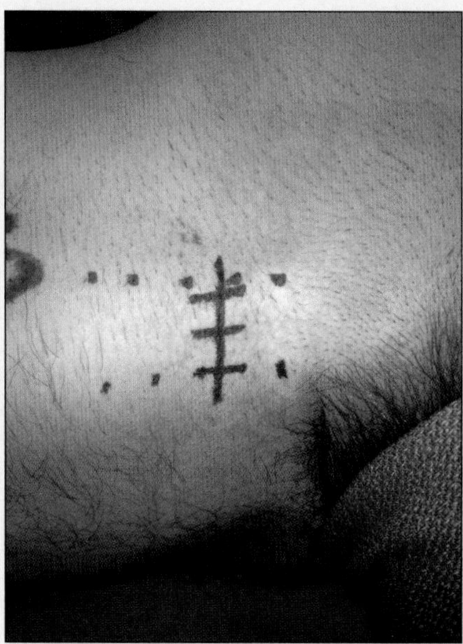

FIGURE 83-6 Skin markings for the 2-cm incision used for open adductor tenotomy. Note the dotted lines marking the borders of the adductor tendon and the location of the incision 4 to 5 cm distal to the origin.

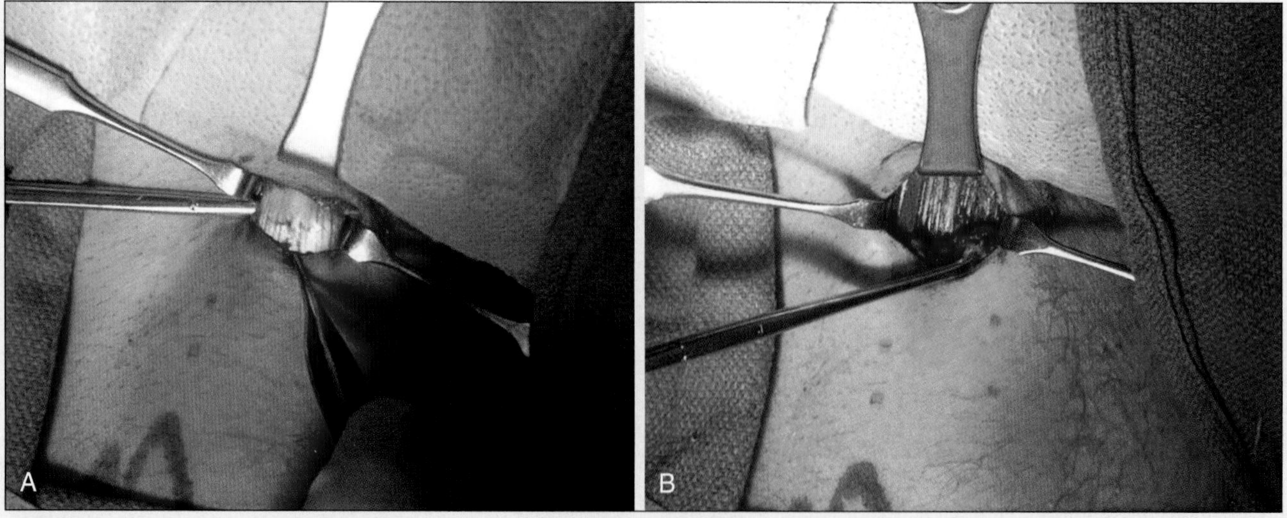

FIGURE 83-7 **A,** The exposed adductor longus tendon. **B,** The underlying adductor muscle belly after release of the tendinous portion.

underwent surgery returned to play at an average of 12 weeks after injury, and 20% experienced wound complications. Given that minimal functional deficits occur after spontaneous rupture of the adductor at its origin, controlled release in the context of a surgical procedure might similarly have few long-term functional consequences.

Athletic Pubalgia/Sports Hernia

Nonoperative Management

Generally, a brief period of rest is indicated for persons with athletic pubalgia/sports hernia. Physical therapy should emphasize core strengthening and identification and treatment of weakness and restricted motion in the musculature of the hip and pelvis. Ice and NSAIDs can be helpful for managing pain. During this period of rehabilitation, it is advisable to avoid heavy weight lifting, deep hip flexion, low repetition exercises, squats, lunges, and clean exercises.

Operative Management

A variety of surgical procedures have been described for the treatment of athletic pubalgia. Gilmore first described "Gilmore's groin" as a cause of chronic groin pain in athletes in 1980.[10] His repair involves plication of the transversalis fascia, reapproximation of the conjoint tendon to the inguinal ligament, and approximation of the external oblique aponeurosis. With use of this technique, the reported return to sport rate is 96% to 97% within 10 to 12 weeks.[18,39] Hackney[19] published his technique in 1993. He presented a series of 15 patients with an average duration of groin pain for 20 months prior to surgical intervention. Upon surgical exploration, weakness of the transversalis fascia with separation from the conjoint tendon and dilatation of the internal inguinal ring was identified. A direct repair was performed with the goal of reconstituting the internal inguinal ring, plication of the transversalis fascia, and apposition of the conjoint tendon to the internal inguinal ring.[19] Postoperatively, swimming and cycling were allowed at 3 weeks, running at 4 to 5 weeks, and sport-specific exercise at 6 weeks. Eighty-seven percent of the athletes were able to resume full participation in sporting activities.

Meyers et al.[6] have published extensively on the treatment of athletic pubalgia with use of a "pelvic floor repair." This procedure involves an open surgical approach with reattachment of the anteroinferior rectus abdominis to the pubis and a variation of an adductor release. In 276 athletes evaluated for groin pain, 157 had clinical symptoms and examination findings consistent with athletic pubalgia and underwent primary pelvic floor repair. Imaging and intraoperative findings were somewhat variable and included unilateral or bilateral tearing or scarring of the rectus, tearing of the external oblique aponeurosis, and scarring of the adductor origin. Postoperatively, 152 athletes were able to return to their preinjury level of competition. Evaluation of the results of their procedure over 20 years showed that 95.3% of athletes were able to return to sports by 3 months after surgery. Meyers et al.[21] reported that athletes who underwent surgery more recently were following either a 3- or 6-week return to sport protocol, after which the majority of athletes were able to return to full participation.

Using a laparoscopic approach, Genitsaris et al.[39] identified 131 athletes with groin pain for whom 2 to 8 months of physical therapy had failed to resolve symptoms. All of these patients underwent bilateral mesh repairs, with the mesh extending from the pubis to the anterior superior iliac spine bilaterally. The peritoneum was closed over the mesh. All patients were able to return to full sporting activities 2 to 3 weeks after surgery.[39]

Kluin et al.[40] identified 14 athletes with groin pain that persisted despite 3 months of conservative management. During laparoscopic exploration, nine occult inguinal hernias, four occult femoral hernias, and three preperitoneal lipomas were identified along with other pathology. The athletes were treated with laparoscopic mesh repair, and 13 of 14 athletes were able to return to sport by 3 months. Ingoldby[41] compared traditional open and laparoscopic results in 28 athletes; 14 open procedures and 14 laparoscopic procedures were performed. Full training was resumed at an average of 5 weeks after the open procedures and 3 weeks after the laparoscopic procedures.[41]

Muschaweck and Berger[42] developed a "minimal repair" technique in 2003 (Fig. 83-8). They identified patients with

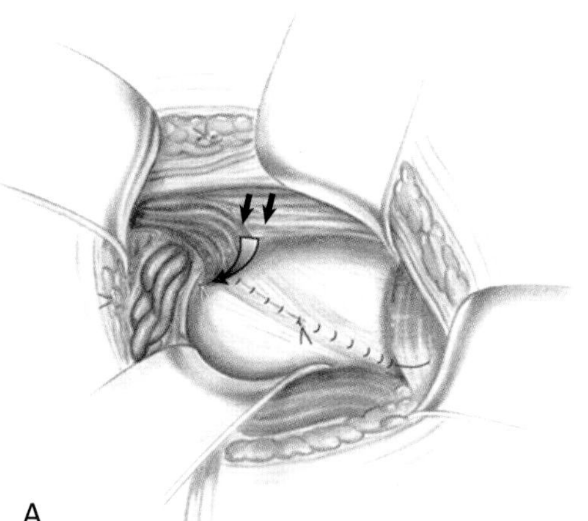

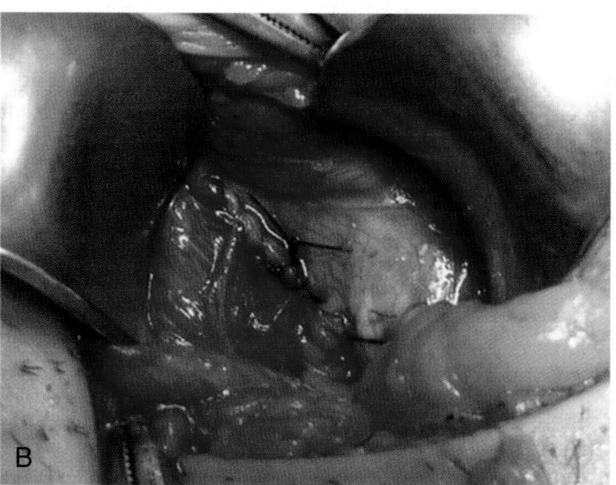

FIGURE 83-8 Illustration (**A**) and intraoperative picture (**B**) of a tension-free repair of the defect in the posterior wall of the inguinal canal. *(From Minnich JM, Hanks JB, Muschaweck U, et al: Sports hernia: diagnosis and treatment highlighting a minimal repair surgical technique.* Am J Sports Med *39[6]:1341–1349, 2011.)*

"sportsmen's groin" on the basis of a clinical history of groin pain radiating to the inner thigh, pubis, testicles, or scrotum, examination findings of tenderness on palpation of the internal inguinal ring, and an ultrasound confirming bulging of the posterior inguinal wall with the Valsalva maneuver. Their "minimal repair" involves decompression of the genital branch of the genitofemoral nerve with a tension-free suture repair of any defect in the posterior wall of the inguinal canal. Return to sport generally occurred by day 14. A total of 132 procedures were performed in 128 patients, including 89 high-level athletes. At 28 days after surgery, 83.7% of the athletes were fully competitive in their sport. No long-term follow-up was provided.

Paajanen et al.[43] performed a prospective randomized controlled trial comparing nonoperative management with laparoscopic sports hernia repair. All athletes reported 3 to 6 months of symptoms prior to enrollment in the study. The subjects were either professional or high-level recreational athletes. The group randomly assigned to nonoperative management underwent a period of rest followed by physical therapy and local injections of corticosteroids, and they used oral NSAIDs for a total of 8 weeks. At 1 month, 20% of athletes had returned to sport, and at 3 months, 27% had returned to sport. At 6 months, 7 of 30 had elected to switch to the operative arm of the study. At 1 year, 15 had returned to sport and 14 reported complete relief of pain. Operative management consisted of a laparoscopic procedure with insertion of a preperitoneal mesh repair. Adductor tenotomy was performed in six patients who had adductor tenderness preoperatively; 67% had returned to sport at 1 month postoperatively, and 90% had returned at 3 months. Twenty-nine of 30 athletes had returned to full participation and were pain free 1 year after surgery. Pain scores and patient satisfaction scores were better in the operative group at all points up to a year out from surgery.[43]

AUTHORS' PREFERRED TREATMENT

Athletic Pubalgia/Sports Hernia

We refer patients with suspected sports hernia/athletic pubalgia to an experienced general surgeon with an interest in sports hip injuries. Ideally, the treatment performed should address the pathology that is present, which can include oblique and transverses abdominis injury and tears, rectus abdominis and adductor aponeurosis disruptions, and proximal adductor–related injury and pathology. Little evidence exists to suggest that primary repairs, mesh reinforcement, minimal incision, laparoscopic repairs, or broad pelvic floor repairs have a distinct advantage.

Osteitis Pubis

Nonoperative Management

Options for nonoperative management of osteitis include rest, use of therapeutic modalities, oral NSAIDs and corticosteroid injections, and rehabilitation that focuses on strengthening of the core and pelvic musculature. Currently all available studies of nonoperative management of osteitis pubis provide level IV evidence.[44]

In a prospective cohort study, Verrall et al.[12] identified 27 professional Australian-rules football players with chronic groin injuries diagnosed on the basis of history and a physical examination. MRI showed that these athletes had findings consistent with osteitis pubis. Treatment consisted of non–weight bearing for 12 weeks. Swimming and upper body lifting activities were allowed initially. Cycling was allowed at 3 weeks, along with a core/pelvic strengthening program as long as this activity did not provoke pain. Stair stepping was initiated at 6 weeks, followed by a graduated running program at 12 weeks. With this protocol, 89% were able to return to sport by 1 year after initiation of treatment. By the second season, 100% of the athletes had returned and 81% did not have symptoms.[12]

Rodriguez et al.[45] identified 44 professional soccer players with osteitis pubis on the basis of history, physical examination, radiographic findings that included irregularity of the pubic symphysis and rami, and a bone scan demonstrating increased uptake in the pubic rami. Thirty-five athletes underwent a conservative rehabilitation protocol that included multiple therapeutic modalities (electrical stimulation or ultrasound, ice massage, and infrared laser) for the first 14 days in conjunction with high-dose NSAIDs. Subsequently, the athletes followed a gradual activity progression including stretching, strengthening of the adductors, abductors, and abdominal muscles, running progression, plyometrics, and kicking progression. Athletes with mild symptoms returned to sport an average of 3.8 weeks after initiation of treatment. Athletes with moderate symptoms returned to sport 6.7 weeks after the initiation of treatment. No long-term follow-up was available.

Some level IV evidence in the literature supports the use of additional modalities, including injection of corticosteroids into the pubic symphysis. O'Connell et al.[46] found that 14 of 16 in-season athletes were able to return to sport within 48 hours of symphyseal injection of corticosteroid with significant pain relief. However, at 6 months only 5 of 16 athletes were pain free, and four patients required an additional period of rest before returning to full activity.[46]

Holt et al.[47] presented a case control study of 12 athletes at the University of Wisconsin who presented with physical examination and radiographic findings consistent with osteitis pubis. In the initial arm, nine athletes underwent 4 months of conservative management consisting of rest, NSAIDs, stretching, and gradual return to sport-specific activities. After this protocol failed to resolve symptoms, eight athletes underwent symphyseal injection of corticosteroids. Seven of eight athletes were able to return to sport after one to three injections and an additional period of rest ranging from 4 to 24 weeks. In the second arm, three athletes with osteitis pubis were identified; they underwent 7 to 10 days of conservative management, and after failure of early treatment, they received an injection. All three athletes were able to return to sport within 2 weeks and remained symptom free at 1 year after injection. The authors advocated early consideration of corticosteroid injection after diagnosis of osteitis pubis because it may allow early return to sport and sustained symptom relief.

Operative Treatment

Operative treatment of osteitis pubis is generally considered a salvage technique and is used most frequently in the scenario of demonstrable instability on radiographic studies or failure of several months of conservative management. Techniques described in the literature include curettage of the symphysis,[48] wedge resection,[49] mesh reinforcement of the symphysis, and arthrodesis of the symphysis with bone graft and compression plating.[25]

Wedge resection of the pubic symphysis was first described in 1961 by Schnute[50] in a case series. He reported that use of the wedge resection resulted in significant clinical improvement in patients who were severely limited by pain. Grace et al.[49] reported on 10 patients who underwent wedge resection an average of 32 months after the onset of symptoms. Three patients experienced chronic pain and one required fusion of the sacroiliac joints for posterior instability that developed as a result of the wedge resection. Moore et al.[51] reported the cases of two additional patients who experienced sacroiliac instability after wedge resection. No study has been published that documents the use of this procedure in high-level athletes, and given the relatively high risk of developing late posterior instability, this technique should be used cautiously in the athletic population.

Williams et al.[25] described fusion of the pubic symphysis with compression plating and bone grafting as a viable treatment option for chronic osteitis pubis. They treated seven rugby players with chronic groin pain who were diagnosed as having osteitis pubis on the basis of physical examination and radiographic findings. Surgical treatment involved excision of the articular surface of the pubis, cancellous bone grafting, and application of a compression plate. One athlete also underwent mesh repair by Gilmore after injuries to the external oblique aponeurosis and conjoint tendon were identified. The athletes returned to sport approximately 6 months after surgery. All seven athletes were able to return to sport, and at an average of 52 months after surgery, all were pain free.

In the largest published study of operative treatment of osteitis pubis in athletes, Radic and Annear[48] treated 23 patients with curettage of the pubic symphysis. Surgical treatment involved curettage of the articular surface until all articular cartilage was removed and bleeding bone was encountered. No stabilization of the joint was performed. Initially 70% were able to return to their previous level of activity at an average of 5.6 months after surgery. However, with longer follow-up, 39% remained asymptomatic and 26% had experienced a one-time recurrence of their symptoms that resolved with rest. Thirty percent of their cohort were never able to resume their preinjury level of activity and did not consider the surgical procedure to have been worthwhile.

Mesh reinforcement of the pubic symphysis was described in 2005 by Paajanen et al.[52,53] They identified 16 athletes with a clinical history suggestive of osteitis pubis and MRI demonstrating pubic bone marrow edema and a positive bone scan. Eight patients with more severe symptoms, for whom 6 months of conservative management had failed to relieve symptoms, elected to undergo surgical intervention that involved laparoscopic placement of mesh behind the pubis that was held in place with titanium tacks. Two athletes underwent concomitant adductor or gracilis release. Seven of 8 patients treated with surgery returned to sport at an average of 2 months postoperatively. At an average of 2.7 years after surgery, all surgically treated patients were competing at their preinjury level. The authors also reported on eight patients with more mild symptoms who were treated nonoperatively. Four of eight conservatively managed patients were able to return to their preinjury level of activity after 1 to 1.5 years of conservative management, and four were competing with some pain at one level below their preinjury level.[53] The authors believed that surgical management with mesh repair allowed their cohort to return to sport more quickly with better resolution of pain compared with conservative management.

The literature includes one report of treatment of osteitis pubis with an endoscopic decompression of the pubic symphysis in a chronic case that occurred in association with FAI.[55] The FAI was also treated arthroscopically at the same setting, and the patient experienced improvement, with resolution of the presenting waddling gait pattern.

Meyers et al.[6] initially excluded athletes with osteitis pubis from surgical treatment of athletic pubalgia. However, as clinical experience increased, they called back prior patients who had been diagnosed with osteitis pubis, treated them with the same surgical repair as their series of patients with athletic pubalgia, and noted a similar outcome as in the patients with athletic pubalgia.[21] This finding reinforces the hypothesis that athletic pubalgia and osteitis pubis represent a spectrum of injuries caused by abnormal forces in the area of the pubic symphysis.

AUTHORS' PREFERRED TREATMENT

It is our experience that mild symphyseal instability can be the result of disruption of the central pivot or rectus abdominis adductor aponeurosis. A repair of the central pivot appears to stabilize the pubic symphysis in this situation. For greater degrees of instability or in recalcitrant cases despite a pelvic floor repair, more aggressive surgical stabilization with open reduction internal fixation and fusion may be warranted. However, we have not encountered the need for fusion in our practice. In the absence of athletic pubalgia or sports hernia, an open or endoscopic decompression may be warranted, but further outcomes are necessary to better define the results after these procedures in an athletic population.

Complications

Athletic Pubalgia

The most common postoperative complaint is minor bruising or edema involving the abdomen, thighs, genitals, and perineum. Postoperative hematoma requiring a repeat operation occurred in 0.3% of patients, and the wound infection rate was 0.4%. Nerve dysesthesia of the ilioinguinal, genitofemoral, anterior, or lateral femoral cutaneous nerve distribution occurred in 0.3% of patients. Penile vein thrombosis occurred in 0.1% of patients, but all cases resolved.[21] The potential for postoperative scar tissue and subsequent neural dysesthesias also exists. The most common reason for a repeat operation was development of similar symptoms on the contralateral side. The second most common was for adductor release not carried out at the first surgery.[21] Another common reason for continued disability after surgical treatment results from failure to identify associated intraarticular hip pathology (i.e., FAI).[7,21]

Osteitis Pubis

Complications associated with curettage of the symphysis for osteitis pubis include hemospermia and intermittent scrotal swelling.[27]

Adductor Tenotomy

For proximal adductor procedures, the potential exists for spermatic cord injury if dissection is carried medial to the gracilis origin on the pubis.[55]

Future Considerations

The understanding of diagnosis and treatment of athletic pubalgia is constantly expanding. Although formerly it was thought to be an isolated pathology, evidence now suggests otherwise. As our understanding evolves, an approach with a greater focus on the targeting of pathology is emerging. Based on the evidence supporting a link between athletic pubalgia and FAI in athletes presenting with groin or pelvic pain, both FAI and athletic pubalgia should be considered. One important question is whether all athletes presenting with symptoms consistent with both intraarticular hip pathology and athletic pubalgia/sports hernia require treatment of both entities initially. This scenario is challenging because a transition point probably exists at which addressing FAI alone is inadequate because permanent injury has occurred to the anterior pelvic musculature, leading to athletic pubalgia. At this time we have no clear-cut indicators with regard to when the athletic pubalgia symptoms/pathology are beyond a point that healing can occur with restoration of hip range of motion after FAI corrective procedures. When timing is an issue, both might be best treated at the same setting.

More sensitive imaging modalities would be helpful to determine the exact location of subtle anatomic injuries for athletic pubalgia and FAI. Determination of the exact location would provide some conformity with respect to which athletic pubalgia surgical approach would be best indicated for a particular patient, because several variants are available. If future studies focused on the variable anatomic pathology and specific approaches used for treatment of these entities, we might develop a better understanding with respect to the optimal pathology-specific approaches to use for this challenging patient population.

For a complete list of references, go to expertconsult.com.

Suggested Readings

Citation: Birmingham PM, Kelly BT, Jacobs R, et al: The effect of dynamic femoroacetabular impingement on pubic symphysis motion: A cadaveric study. *Am J Sports Med* 40(5):1113–1118, 2012.
Level of Evidence: Controlled cadaveric laboratory study
Summary: In this cadaveric study, the investigators examined motion through the pubic symphysis in the native state and with a simulated cam lesion. The authors found that rotation was increased through the symphysis in the presence of dynamic femoroacetabular impingement caused by a cam lesion and hypothesized that this pathologic motion could contribute to the development of athletic pubalgia.

Citation: Larson CM, Pierce BR, Giveans MR: Treatment of athletes with symptomatic intra-articular hip pathology and athletic pubalgia/sports hernia: A case series. *Arthroscopy* 27(6):768–775, 2011.
Level of Evidence: IV (therapeutic case series)
Summary: In a retrospective review, the authors identified 31 athletes (37 hips) who presented with symptoms consistent with both femoroacetabular impingement and athletic pubalgia. Treating either entity in isolation resulted in a low return to sport rate (25% in athletes treated for athletic pubalgia alone and 50% in athletes treated for femoroacetabular impingement alone), which led the authors to treat both entities in a staged or concurrent fashion with an 85% to 93% rate of return to sports.

Citation: Meyers WC, McKechnie A, Philippon MJ, et al: Experience with "sports hernia" spanning two decades. *Ann Surg* 248(4):656–665, 2008.
Level of Evidence: IV (retrospective review)
Summary: The authors presented their experience with 8490 patients who were diagnosed with a sports hernia, 5218 of whom underwent surgical treatment. The investigators noted an increase in the percentage of patients who opted for surgical treatment and a changing patient demographic during the past 20 years.

Citation: Zoga AC, Kavanagh EC, Omar IM, et al: Athletic pubalgia and the "sports hernia": MR imaging findings. *Radiology* 247(3):797–807, 2008.
Level of Evidence: IV (retrospective review)
Summary: The authors retrospectively reviewed the magnetic resonance imaging (MRI) scans of 141 patients with symptoms of athletic pubalgia to determine the sensitivity and specificity of imaging findings when compared with the standards of surgical or physical examination findings. MRI was 68% sensitive and 100% specific for injuries to the rectus abdominis and 86% sensitive and 89% specific for adductor tendon injuries.

Citation: Holmich P, Nyvold P, Larsen K: Continuing significant effect of physical training as treatment for overuse injury: 8- to 12-year outcome of a randomized clinical trial. *Am J Sports Med* 39(11):2447–2451, 2011.
Level of Evidence: I (randomized controlled trial, 80% long-term follow-up)
Summary: In the initial randomized controlled trial, the authors compared an active physical therapy program that emphasized core stability and eccentric strengthening with a passive therapy program in the treatment of adductor-related groin pain in athletes. At long-term follow-up, the active therapy group demonstrated sustained improvement in outcome scores when compared with the passive therapy group.

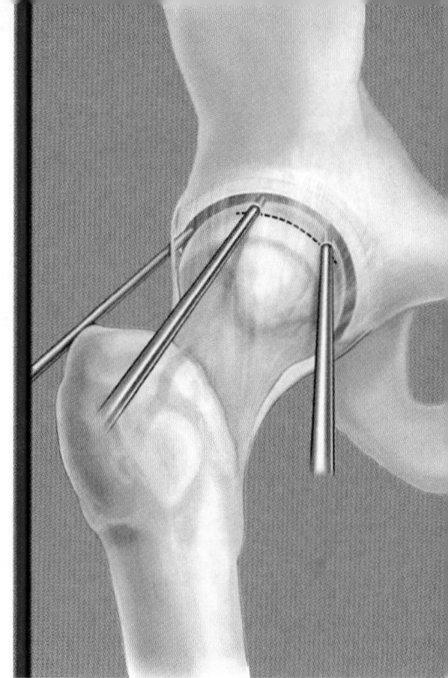

84

Femoroacetabular Impingement in Athletes

J. W. THOMAS BYRD

The implication that abnormal hip structure leads to secondary joint damage has been variously described for almost 100 years.[1,2] However, the concept of femoroacetabular impingement (FAI) as a cause of osteoarthritis is credited to Professor Reinhold Ganz and his colleagues from Bern, Switzerland.[3] Early-onset osteoarthritis among adults in their fourth and fifth decades is often attributed to this process. It is now recognized that FAI can cause serious joint damage among young athletes, even in their second and third decades. As athletes push their bodies beyond physiologic limits, breakdown occurs. Among these athletes with impingement, the threshold for breakdown is much lower and occurs with loads and activities that are tolerated by their counterparts with normal joint structure. Thus severe joint damage is often encountered in these athletes who, if they were less active, would only start to present with findings of osteoarthritis at a later age. FAI refers to the process by which a misshapen hip joint secondarily leads to breakdown of the intraarticular structures causing pain and associated dysfunction, followed by the premature development of osteoarthritis. Three types of FAI have been identified: a pincer type, a cam type, and combined impingement.

Pincer impingement is caused by an excessive prominence of the anterolateral rim of the acetabulum. This condition can occur simply from overgrowth of the anterior edge or as a result of retroversion of the acetabulum, which is a condition in which the face of the acetabulum tilts slightly backward instead of being in its normal forward position. Sometimes a separate piece of bone is found along the anterolateral rim, which is referred to as an *os acetabulum*. With hip flexion, the prominent rim of the acetabulum crushes the labrum against the femoral neck (Fig. 84-1). This cyclical submaximal repetitive microtrauma leads to breakdown and failure of the acetabular labrum. Secondarily, over time, a variable amount of articular failure within the adjacent acetabulum occurs. Pincer impingement occurs just about equally in males and females and more commonly starts to cause symptoms in middle age.[4]

Cam impingement refers to the cam effect caused by a nonspherical femoral head rotating inside the acetabulum. This condition has long been recognized as a sequela of a slipped capital femoral epiphysis in which posterior displacement of capitis leaves a prominence of the anterior neck, resulting in severely limited internal rotation of the hip. Operations performed to excise this bony prominence have been referred to as a *cheilectomy*.[5] However, more subtle forms of an aspherical femoral head are much more common and have only more recently been recognized as a cause of problems. This "pistol-grip" deformity is seen in association with early-onset osteoarthritis in adults.[6] It may be due to premature eccentric closure of the capital physis in adolescence, resulting in the nonspherical shape of the femoral head. It has been postulated that intense physical activity at a young age may somehow precipitate this partial physeal arrest and cause the cam lesion. This concept has not yet been substantiated. Thus although cam impingement is clearly a causative factor in joint damage among athletic persons, it is not clear whether athletic activity caused the impingement. With flexion, the nonspherical portion of the head rotates into the acetabulum, creating a shear force on the anterolateral edge of the acetabular articular surface (Fig. 84-2). With repetitive motion, this force eventually results in articular delamination and failure of the acetabular cartilage. Persons with this condition have preferential articular pathology and relative labral preservation. Over time the labrum eventually starts to fail, but only after the process is advanced on the articular surface. Cam impingement has approximately a 3:1 predilection for males and often presents with problems in young adulthood.[7]

Combinations of pincer and cam impingement can occur. The demographics are intermediate between pincer and cam forms. One pattern or the other may predominate, or athletes may have an equal contribution from both, which may have some influence on the optimal method of treatment.

Impingement (or FAI) has gained much attention in the past few years. In the past, this pathologic process simply went undiagnosed. Athletes often experienced poorly explained groin pain that remained an ill-defined, unsolved problem, eventually ending their competitive careers. With growing recognition and treatment, many athletes have been able to resume competitive activities and thus have created more awareness of this disorder. It is important not to neglect findings of impingement, but it is also important not to overtreat all abnormal radiographic findings. We have much to learn about why some athletes with impingement-shaped hips continue to function at high levels for years without experiencing secondary joint damage.

History

The onset of symptoms associated with FAI in athletes is variable, but the damage results from the cumulative effect of

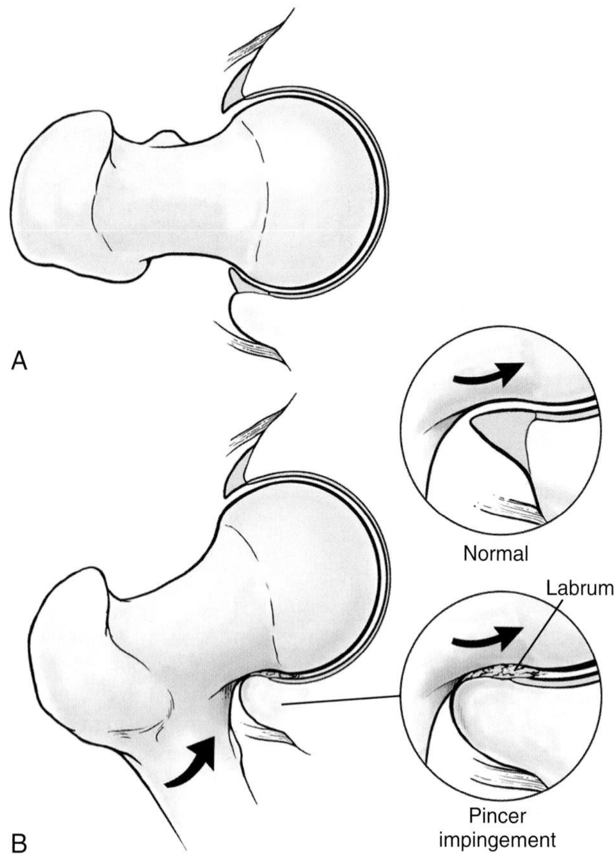

FIGURE 84-1 **A,** Bony overcoverage of the anterior labrum sets the stage for pincer impingement. **B,** With hip flexion, the anterior labrum gets crushed by the pincer lesion against the neck of the femur. Secondary articular failure occurs over time. In normal circumstances, clearance is adequate for the labrum during hip flexion. *(Courtesy J.W. Thomas Byrd, MD.)*

cyclical abnormal wear associated with the altered joint structure. The onset may be gradual, but athletes often recount an acute precipitating episode or event, prior to which they were relatively asymptomatic. However, on close questioning, the athlete frequently recalls prior nonspecific symptoms of a groin strain. Also, many athletes who experience pathologic impingement recount that, in their early years, they were never as flexible as other teammates. Although they may demonstrate specific examples of loss of flexibility, it is rarely a functional problem for them. Diminished range of motion is better compensated in the hip than in other joints by increased pelvic and lumbosacral motion. These compensatory pathomechanics create other problems that commonly coexist with FAI such as athletic pubalgia, trochanteric or iliopsoas bursitis, and/or sacroiliac pain.

Hip joint disorders often go undetected for a protracted period. In one study of athletes, 60% were treated for an average of 7 months before it was recognized that the joint could be the source of symptoms.[8] As the athlete attempts to compensate for the damaged joint, he or she may experience symptoms associated with secondary disorders created by compensating for the hip. For example, chronic gluteal discomfort may be present, or lateral pain from trochanteric bursitis and abductor irritability may be experienced. On examination, these secondary findings may be more evident and obscure the underlying element of primary hip dysfunction.

Hip joint symptoms typically emanate from the anterior groin and may radiate to the medial thigh.[9] Athletes often demonstrate the C sign when describing deep interior hip pain (Fig. 84-3); that is, the hand is cupped above the greater trochanter with the fingers gripping into the anterior groin. Mechanical symptoms associated with intraarticular pathology are typically characterized by intermittent sharp stabbing pain or catching. These symptoms are often precipitated by turning, twisting, pivoting, or lateral movement. Maximal flexion is uncomfortable and extension of the flexed hip against resistance, such as rising from a squatted or seated position, may elicit pain. With chronic degeneration, the symptoms may become more constant with activities and less intermittent.

Physical Examination

Physical examination usually elicits evidence of hip joint irritability.[9] However, keep in mind that, as an examiner, you may not create the level of forces across the joint that an athlete can generate with physical activities that precipitate symptoms.

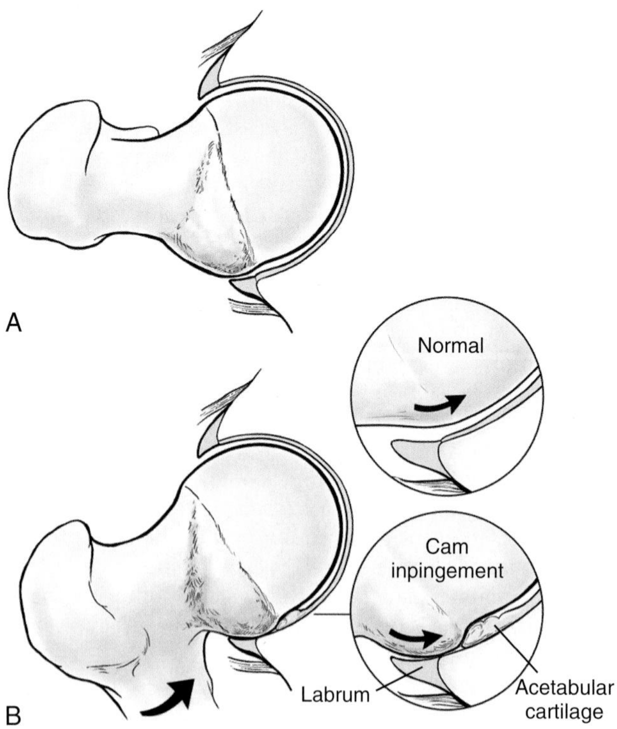

FIGURE 84-2 **A,** The cam lesion is characterized by the bony prominence centered on the anterolateral femoral head-neck junction. **B,** Cam impingement occurs with hip flexion as the nonspherical portion of the femoral head (cam lesion) glides under the labrum, engaging the edge of the articular cartilage and resulting in progressive delamination. Initially the labrum is relatively preserved, but secondary failure occurs over time. *(Courtesy J.W. Thomas Byrd, MD.)*

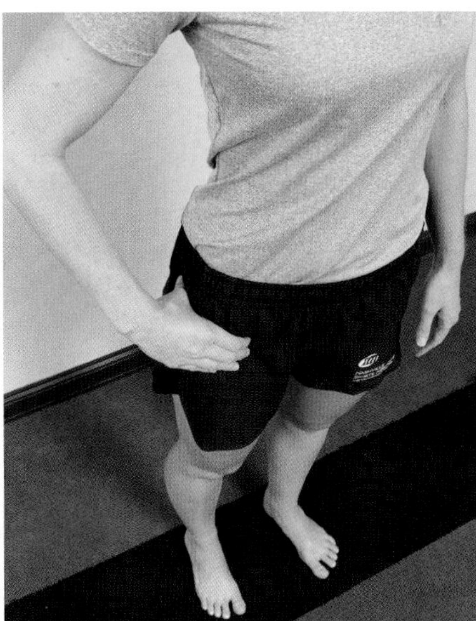

FIGURE 84-3 The C sign. This term reflects the shape of the hand when a patient describes deep interior hip pain. The hand is cupped above the greater trochanter with the thumb posterior and the fingers gripping deep into the anterior groin. *(Courtesy J.W. Thomas Byrd, MD.)*

The trademark feature of FAI is diminished internal rotation caused by the altered bony architecture of the joint. However, much variation is found in the normative data on hip range of motion. Also, although only one hip may be symptomatic, the altered structure is usually present in both hips, and there may not be much asymmetry in motion when comparing the symptomatic with the asymptomatic side. Be aware that many athletes may demonstrate reduced internal rotation and still not have pathologic impingement. Also, pathologic impingement may occasionally be observed in athletes with normal or even increased internal rotation.

The log roll test, although not sensitive, is the most specific test for hip joint pathology independent of its etiology (Fig. 84-4). Rolling the leg back and forth rotates only the femoral head in relation to the acetabulum and the capsule, without stressing any of the surrounding structures. Forced flexion, adduction, and internal rotation is called the *impingement test* in reference to eliciting symptoms associated with impingement (Fig. 84-5). However, virtually any person with an irritable hip, regardless of the etiology, will be uncomfortable with this maneuver. Thus although it is quite sensitive, it is not necessarily specific for impingement. This maneuver may normally be a little uncomfortable, and thus the symptomatic side must be compared with the asymptomatic side. Most important is whether this maneuver recreates the characteristic type of pain that the athlete experiences with activities. Less frequently, posterior impingement may be encountered and is assessed by external rotation of the extended hip (Fig. 84-6).

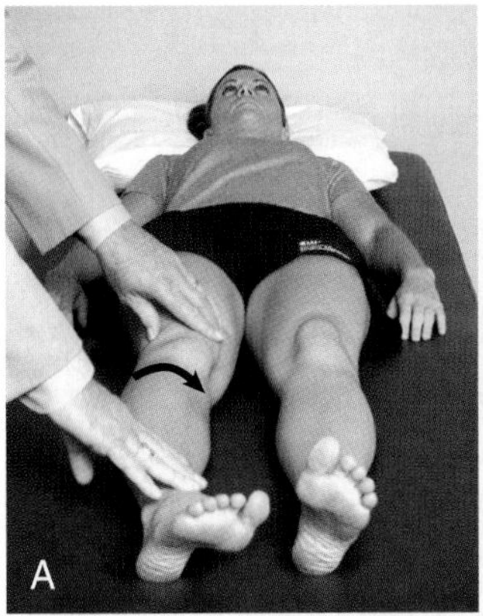

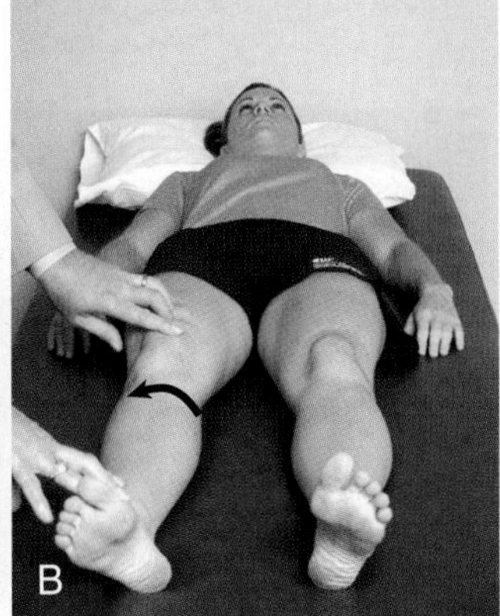

FIGURE 84-4 The log roll test is the single most specific test for hip pathology. With the patient supine, gently rolling the thigh internally (**A**) and externally (**B**) moves the articular surface of the femoral head in relation to the acetabulum but does not stress any of the surrounding extraarticular structures. *(Courtesy J.W. Thomas Byrd, MD.)*

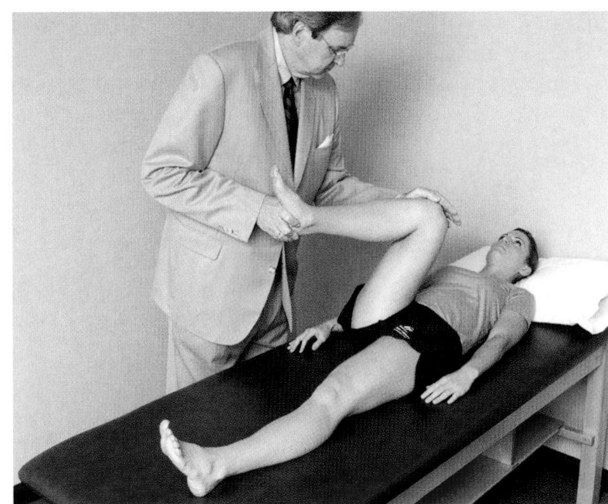

FIGURE 84-5 The impingement test is performed by provoking pain with flexion, adduction, and internal rotation of the symptomatic hip. *(Courtesy J.W. Thomas Byrd, MD.)*

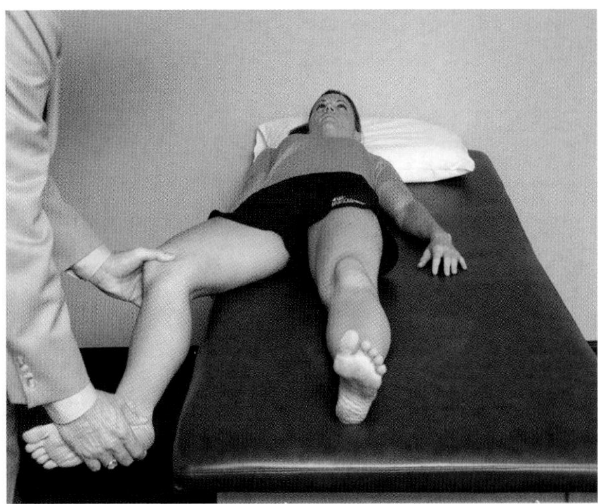

FIGURE 84-6 Supine, the patient is positioned close to the edge of the table so the hip can be extended along with maximal external rotation, which can elicit symptoms of painful posterior impingement. However, anterior translation of the femoral head in this position may also evoke symptoms of anterior instability or possibly elicit pain by entrapping an anterior labral tear. Thus the maneuver may be positive for various forms of hip joint pathology. *(Courtesy J.W. Thomas Byrd, MD.)*

These conditions often have a chronic component, even at the time of initial evaluation, and thus secondary findings may be present as a result of compensatory mechanisms. Lateral pain may be present from trochanteric bursitis, and posterior tenderness within the gluteal muscles may be present from overfiring in an attempt to splint the joint. These secondary features may be more easily recognized on examination and can obscure the underlying primary joint pathology.

The anterior groin and lower abdominal and adductor area must be carefully palpated to localize tenderness suggestive of athletic pubalgia.[10] This tenderness can mimic or coexist with FAI. Tenderness with resisted sit-ups and hip flexion or adduction should raise an index of suspicion for athletic pubalgia. Pain with passive flexion and internal rotation is more indicative of an intraarticular source.

Snapping of the iliopsoas tendon is assessed by bringing the hip from a flexed, abducted, externally rotated position into extension with internal rotation. Alternatively, the athlete may better demonstrate the audible clunk when taking the hip from a flexed to an extended position. The snapping can be a source of symptoms and warrant treatment, or it may just be an incidental finding. Because it is usually noticeable to the athlete, it is important to assess its contribution to the individual's symptoms when determining the appropriate treatment algorithm.

Diagnostic Intraarticular Injection

The athlete's history and examination are the most powerful clinical assessment tools. Beyond that, a diagnostic intraarticular injection with an anesthetic provides the greatest clinical relevance with regard to the presence of hip pathology as a cause of symptoms and disability. Historically, this injection has been performed under fluoroscopic guidance, commonly in association with gadolinium arthrography for magnetic resonance imaging (MRI).[16] The proficiency with which clinicians perform fluoroscopic-guided intraarticular injections can be variable and, if the test causes pain, it may be difficult to reliably assess the response to the anesthetic. Also, anecdotal observations by experienced clinicians have suggested that when the test is performed in conjunction with gadolinium, use of the contrast material may negate the expected response to the anesthetic, resulting in a false-negative interpretation.

More recently, office-based ultrasound injection of the hip has gained some popularity.[11] With training, it is simple to perform and is much easier on the athlete than alternate methods. It is also much more convenient because it can be performed during the course of a normal office visit (Fig. 84-7).[12]

Examining the athlete before and after the injection can provide valuable information. However, most important is the athlete's subjective sense of pain relief. Sometimes symptoms are provoked only by vigorous activities and cannot be elicited simply by an examiner. Thus it can often be helpful to inject anesthetic into the joint and send the athlete to therapy or a training room to perform activities that would normally precipitate symptoms. For this purpose, it is preferable to use a long-acting anesthetic so the athlete can more reliably assess the level of pain relief that may be too brief with a short-acting anesthetic.

When the history and examination findings are clearly indicative of a joint problem, diagnostic injections are not necessary. However, sometimes the clinical presentation may not be entirely clear or other factors may be contributing to the generation of pain. The response to the injection aids the clinician but, more importantly, may help educate the athlete about which portion of the symptoms is emanating from the joint. This information is important because treatment of the hip may ultimately only be successful at treating part of the symptoms.

Imaging

Radiographs

If an athlete has symptoms troublesome enough to warrant management beyond a couple of training room treatments, then radiographs should be obtained. Radiographs should include a well-centered anteroposterior pelvis view and a lateral view of the affected hip.[13] These views are important for assessing impingement, as well as evaluating joint space preservation and other acute or chronic bony changes. Overcoverage of the anterior acetabulum, characteristic of pincer impingement, is evaluated by the presence of a crossover sign

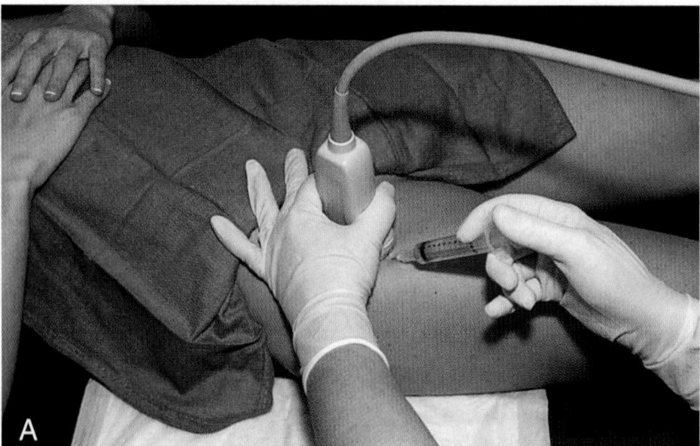

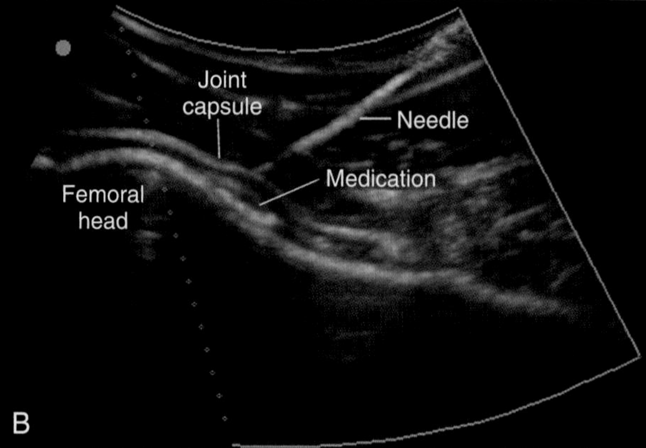

FIGURE 84-7 **A,** The transducer is held over the femoral head-neck junction in long axis and slightly oblique. The injection is performed in plane with the transducer, allowing visualization of the needle throughout its course of advancement to the capsule. **B,** The medication can be visualized entering the joint capsule. *(Courtesy J.W. Thomas Byrd, MD.)*

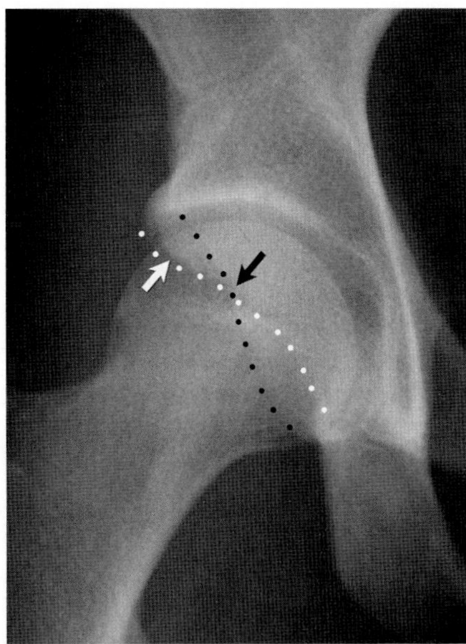

FIGURE 84-8 An anteroposterior view of the right hip. The anterior (*white dots*) and posterior (*black dots*) rims of the acetabulum are marked. The superior portion of the anterior rim lies lateral to the posterior rim (*white arrow*), indicating overcoverage of the acetabulum. Anteriorly, it assumes a more normal medial position, creating the crossover sign (*black arrow*) as a positive indicator of pincer impingement. *(Courtesy J.W. Thomas Byrd, MD.)*

(Fig. 84-8). Overcoverage can be due to acetabular retroversion, indicated by the posterior wall sign (Fig. 84-9) and the prominent ischial spine sign (Fig. 84-10). Global overcoverage may be associated with acetabular profunda (Fig. 84-11) and protrusio (Fig. 84-12), which are commonly accompanied by an excessive center-edge angle. The presence of an os acetabulum can also be evaluated (Fig. 84-13). The etiology and the significance of an os acetabulum are variable, ranging from an unfused apophysis, a traction phenomenon from pull of the rectus femoris origin, or a rim fracture as a result of cam impingement.

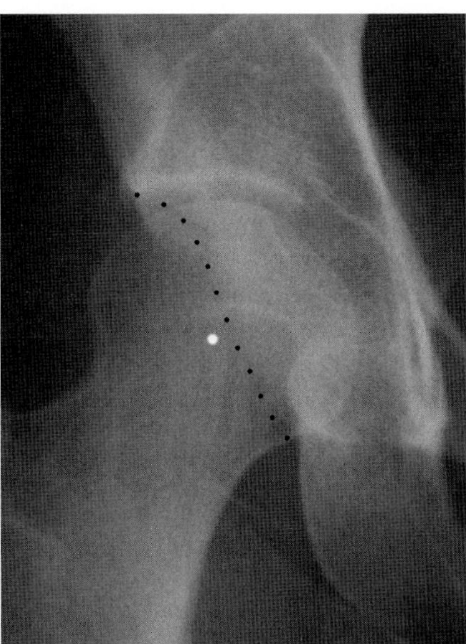

FIGURE 84-9 Anteroposterior view of the right hip. Acetabular retroversion as a cause of pincer impingement is indicated by a shallow posterior wall in which the posterior rim of the acetabulum (*black dots*) lies medial to the center of rotation of the femoral head (*white dot*). *(Courtesy J.W. Thomas Byrd, MD.)*

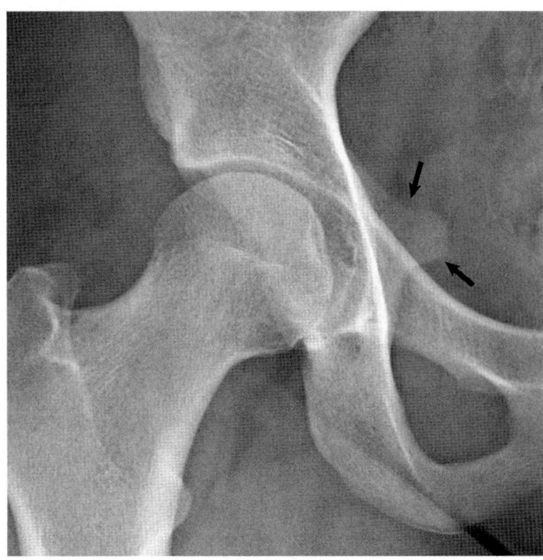

FIGURE 84-10 This ischial spine is normally hidden behind the acetabulum. Acetabular retroversion is significantly correlated with prominence of the ischial spine (*arrows*) extending inside the pelvis. *(Courtesy J.W. Thomas Byrd, MD.)*

The sphericity of the femoral head is assessed on both the anteroposterior and lateral views (Fig. 84-14). Some controversy exists regarding the optimal lateral radiograph. One study showed that the 40-degree Dunn view most predictably demonstrates the cam lesion.[14] However, because of the variable shape and location of the lesion, no radiograph is consistently reliable. A frog lateral view is easy to obtain in a reproducible fashion and has demonstrated efficacy in

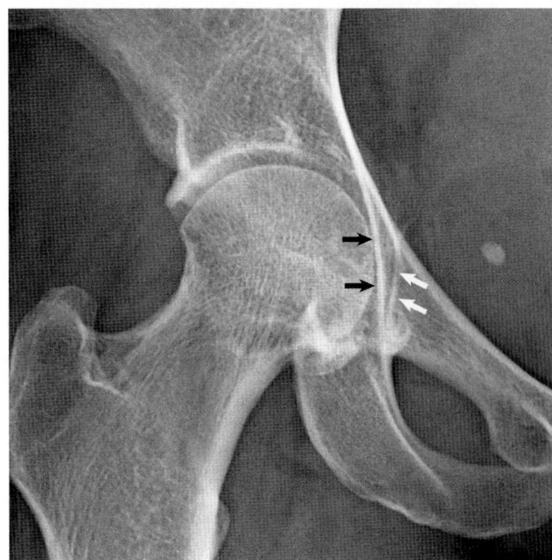

FIGURE 84-11 Coxa profunda exists when the floor of the acetabular fossa (*white arrows*) touches or is medial to the ischiofemoral line (*black arrows*). *(Courtesy J.W. Thomas Byrd, MD.)*

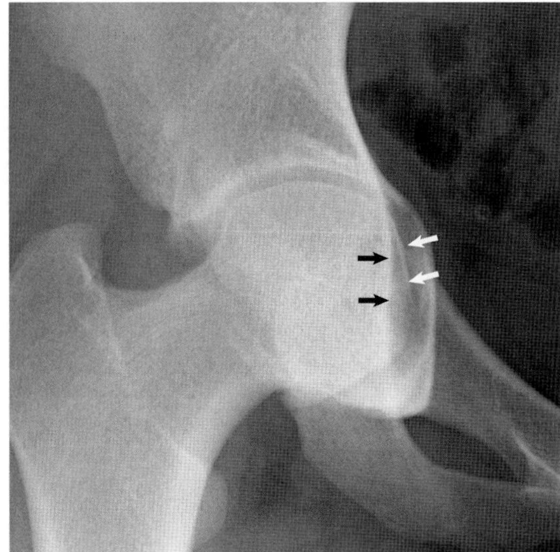

FIGURE 84-12 Acetabular protrusio is defined when the medial aspect of the femoral head (*white arrows*) is medial to the ischiofemoral line (*black arrows*). *(Courtesy J.W. Thomas Byrd, MD.)*

assessing the cam lesion. Whatever lateral radiograph is chosen, the clinician must be cognizant that it can underinterpret the extent of a cam lesion. A herniation pit may be present in the region of the anterolateral femoral head-neck junction (Fig. 84-15). This pit has been reported with 30% prevalence in pathologic cases of FAI but is sometimes observed in asymptomatic persons.[15] Repetitive compression of the cam lesion against the surface of the acetabulum results in cystic erosion into the subcortical femoral surface. This cystic structure can become large and difficult to distinguish from a benign neoplasm. However, the characteristic location usually supports its identity as a simple herniation pit.

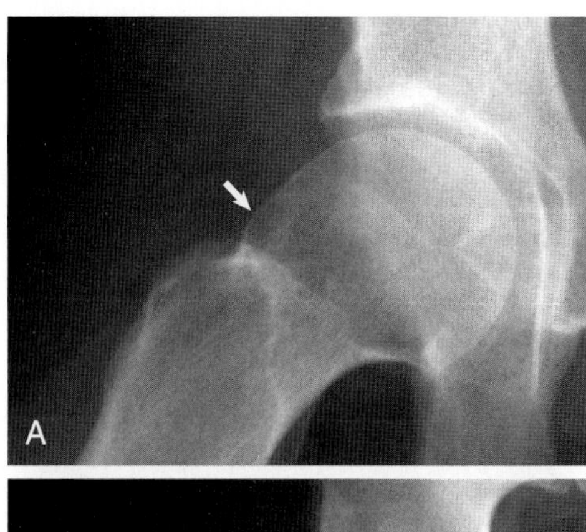

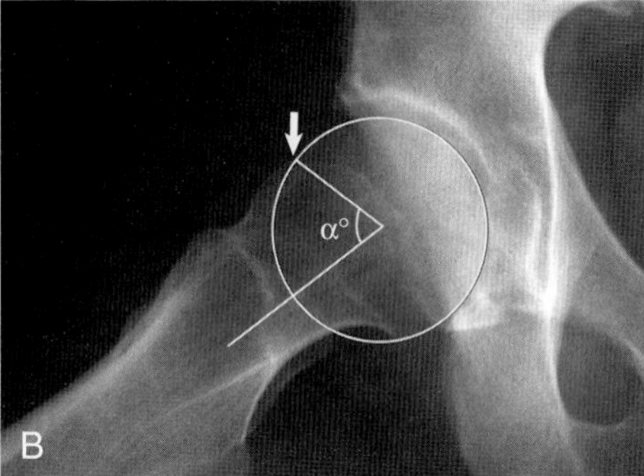

FIGURE 84-14 A frog lateral view of the right hip. **A,** The cam lesion (*arrow*) is evident as the convex abnormality at the head-neck junction where normally a concave slope of the femoral neck is present. **B,** The alpha angle is used to quantitate the severity of the cam lesion. A circle is placed over the femoral head. The alpha angle is formed by a line along the axis of the femoral neck (1) and a line (2) from the center of the femoral head to the point where the head diverges outside the circle (*arrow*). An alpha angle >50 degrees is associated with femoroacetabular impingement. *(Courtesy J.W. Thomas Byrd, MD.)*

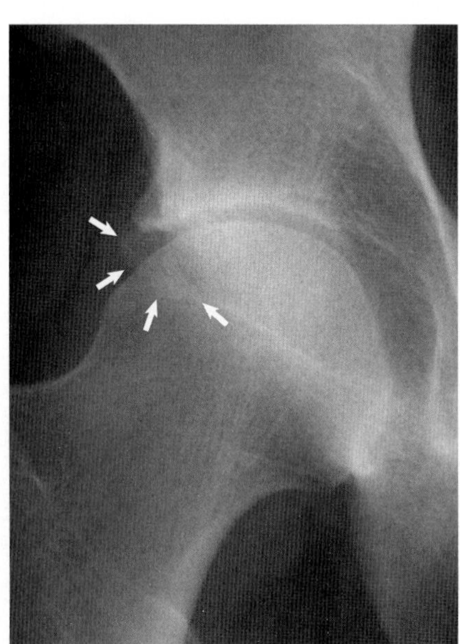

FIGURE 84-13 An anteroposterior radiograph of a right hip. An os acetabulum (*arrows*) is present and, although the etiology is variable, it is often associated with femoroacetabular impingement. *(Courtesy J.W. Thomas Byrd, MD.)*

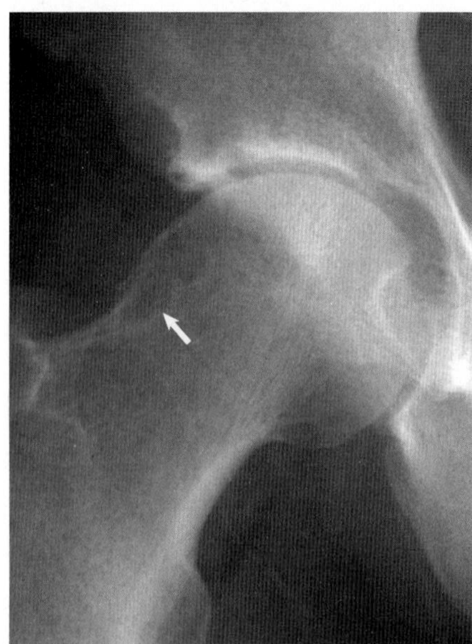

FIGURE 84-15 An anteroposterior radiograph of a right hip. A herniation pit is present (*arrow*), which is often associated with cam impingement. *(Courtesy J.W. Thomas Byrd, MD.)*

Several caveats must be considered regarding radiographic interpretation of FAI. Indexes of pincer impingement are assessed on a supine pelvis radiograph, and it is uncertain how this view can be extrapolated to the orientation of the pelvis when standing. Dynamic positioning of the pelvis is influenced by numerous other factors, such as lumbar lordosis or kyphosis. The shape of cam lesions is variable, and the epicenter may be more anterior or lateral. Thus radiographs represent a poor two-dimensional image of the lesion's three-dimensional anatomy.

Magnetic Resonance Imaging

MRI scans have different degrees of effectiveness. Low-resolution images provided by open scanners and small magnets are ineffectual at demonstrating most hip joint pathology. High-resolution small field-of-view images necessitate at least a 1.5-Tesla magnet with surface coils.[16] The thick, noncompliant capsule does not allow for much fluid accumulation in the joint, and thus any amount of effusion in a symptomatic hip is significant indirect evidence of joint pathology. The sensitivity of conventional MRI to detect labral pathology is much improved, but the ability to detect articular damage, which is usually present in association with FAI, is variable and often poor. In general, if labral pathology is evident, one must assume that some amount of associated articular damage probably exists. Increased signal on T2-weighted images in the anterior acetabulum, which is indicative of subchondral edema, must be carefully evaluated. Sometimes this increased signal is incorrectly interpreted as a stress fracture of the anterior inferior iliac spine but is more likely indicative of a subchondral stress reaction in the anterior acetabulum as a result of failure of the subjacent articular surface. Thus subchondral edema of the anterior acetabulum should be taken as a worrisome warning sign of significant associated articular pathology (Fig. 84-16).

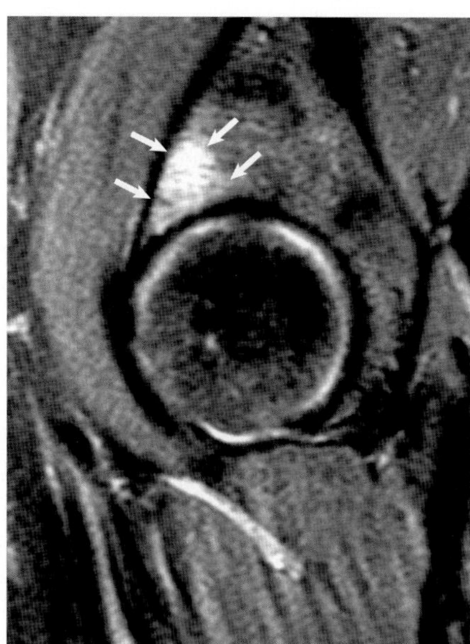

FIGURE 84-16 A sagittal T2-weighted magnetic resonance image of a right hip. Subchondral edema of the acetabulum (*arrows*) is present as an indicator of subjacent articular failure seen in association with cam impingement. *(Courtesy J.W. Thomas Byrd, MD.)*

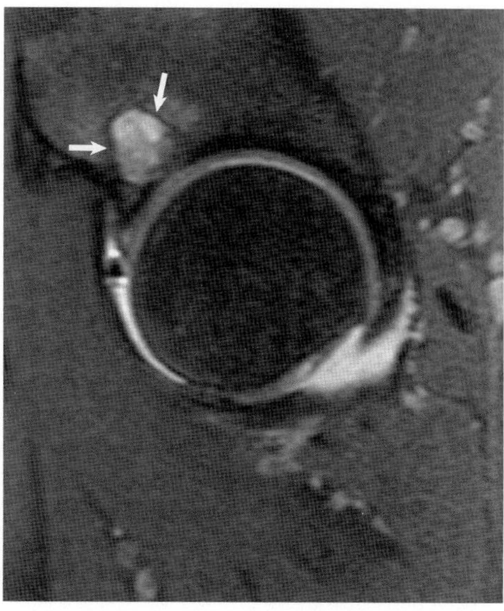

FIGURE 84-17 A sagittal T2-weighted MRI image of a right hip demonstrates a subchondral cyst (*arrows*) indicative of associated articular damage. *(Courtesy J.W. Thomas Byrd, MD.)*

Increased activity within the area of a herniation pit may be associated with active disease as a result of cam impingement. This area of involvement can be sizable, and the differential diagnosis may include osteoid osteoma and other benign tumors, which are considerably less likely. Other generally reliable indirect indicators of joint pathology are a paralabral cyst, which is pathognomonic of associated labral pathology, and subchondral cysts, which usually indicate associated articular damage (Fig. 84-17). Currently much work is underway to develop more cartilage-sensitive sequencing, including delayed gadolinium-enhanced MRI of cartilage (dGEMRIC) studies.[17]

Gadolinium Arthrography with MRI

MRI enhanced with intraarticular contrast (magnetic resonance arthrography; MRA) demonstrates greater sensitivity at detecting intraarticular pathology than other imaging methods.[16] It is better than other imaging methods at detecting labral lesions but is still not completely reliable with regard to the assessment of associated articular problems. A labral cleft, characterized by a normal separation between the labrum and the rim of the acetabulum, may be evident as contrast material separating these two structures. This cleft should not be interpreted as a tear and is distinguished by its smooth margins and lack of interdigitation within the substance of the labral tissue that would be present with a tear (Fig. 84-18). Because posterior labral tears are uncommon, in most cases, separation of the posterior labrum can be assumed to be a normal cleft.

The clinician must interpret how the imaging findings correlate with the athlete's clinical presentation. In this respect, a most useful aspect of MRA is the concomitant injection of long-acting anesthetic along with the contrast material. Whether the athlete experiences a temporary period of pain relief is usually more relevant than interpretation of the images. For example, the study may not fully define the joint damage responsible for the athlete's symptoms, but it can be

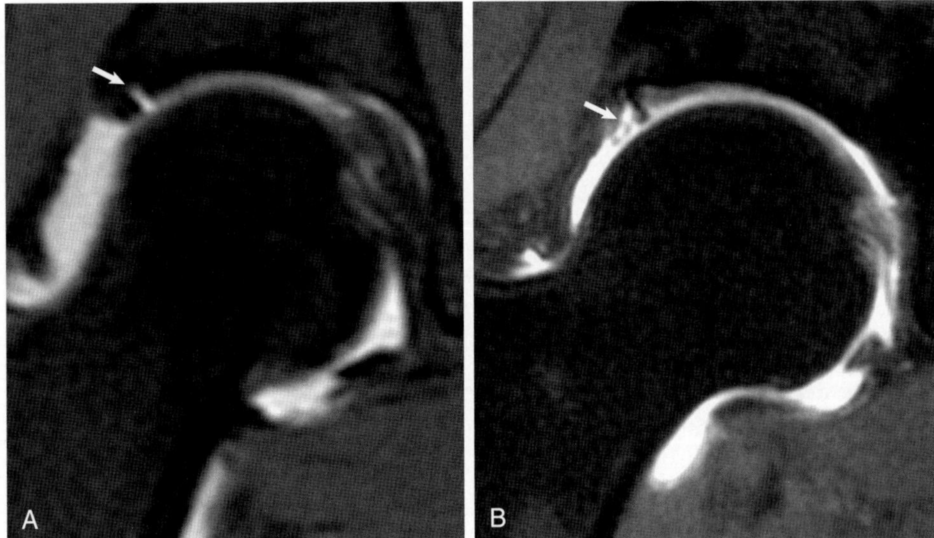

FIGURE 84-18 **A,** A coronal magnetic resonance arthrography (MRA) image of a right hip demonstrates contrast material separating the lateral acetabulum from the labrum (*arrow*). Although a labral detachment cannot be ruled out, the smooth margins suggest a normal labral cleft. **B,** A coronal MRA image of a right hip demonstrates contrast interdigitating within the substance of the lateral labrum (*arrow*), which is indicative of true labral pathology. *(Courtesy J.W. Thomas Byrd, MD.)*

indirectly substantiated by the response to the injection. Conversely, imaging abnormalities may be present but not responsible for the athlete's symptoms. If the injection does not provide some pain relief, the clinician must look closely for other causes. The validity of this response is dependent on two factors. First, the athlete must predictably be able to perform activities to generate pain prior to the injection. Second, the athlete must perform these activities after the injection to accurately assess the response. Usually the athlete needs to go to a training room or therapy department to simulate functional pain-provoking activities.

MRA has disadvantages compared with conventional MRI. The contrast material eliminates the opportunity to assess whether an effusion is present. In addition, postcontrast imaging sequences may less clearly detect subchondral signal changes present within the bone. An optimal protocol would include a select series of both pre- and postcontrast images.

Computed Tomography

Computed tomography (CT) is much better at showing bone architecture and structure than MRI and MRA, which often cannot distinguish an os acetabulum and have difficulty defining the amount of joint space narrowing. For some cases, CT provides information that complements these other studies. However, quantitating cam lesions is difficult with all planar two-dimensional images, whether from MRI or CT. Unless the image happens to bisect the variable apex or epicenter of the cam lesion, it often underestimates its magnitude. CT with three-dimensional reconstructions provides the clearest image of the cam lesion and its structure. These images are especially helpful in arthroscopic management. They aid the arthroscopic surgeon in understanding the exact shape of the abnormal bone that must then be fully exposed and resected. These images are not necessary with traditional open techniques for correcting impingement because of the luxury of the exposure provided by the extensile approach.

Treatment

Prevention

Currently no formal prevention programs exist for FAI. When an athlete experiences symptoms from intraarticular pathology, the causal relationship of the underlying impingement and the importance of its correction are well understood. However, some athletes have abnormally shaped hips (impingement *morphology*) that do not necessarily develop secondary joint damage (impingement *pathology*). Thus the value or efficacy of preventative programs is uncertain until good demographic data are available to understand the risk of impingement morphology causing impingement pathology. Nonetheless, a sense of awareness is important.

Pilot programs are being developed to assess proper screening. Evaluation for reduced internal rotation as a predictor of underlying impingement would be easy, and radiographs might be appropriate for persons deemed at risk. It is difficult to recommend substantial alterations for an athlete who is asymptomatic, but screening may provide early warning regarding any future symptoms and can be incorporated into methods of conservative treatment.

Conservative Treatment

Conservative treatment begins with an emphasis on early recognition. Pain in an athlete with FAI should be taken as a worrisome warning sign of progressive damage within the joint. It is important to be aware that many athletes demonstrate high pain tolerance, sometimes to the point of a true insensitivity to pain, and thus the damage to the joint can be severe, even in persons who continue to function at a high level. Thus although it may not be appropriate to intercede in someone who is asymptomatic, it should not be a matter of simply waiting to see how severe the symptoms may become. If the symptoms are stable, a trial of conservative management is certainly reasonable.

The mainstay of treatment is identifying and modifying offending activities that precipitate symptoms. Efforts are made to optimize mobility of the joint, but these efforts are only modestly effective because motion is limited by the bony architecture, which cannot be corrected by manual techniques. Decompensatory disorders are the secondary problems that develop as an athlete struggles to compensate for the chronic limitations imposed by the impingement. Assessing and optimizing core strength are important because these actions can help the athlete compensate more effectively.

Squats, which have long been a mainstay of most weight training programs, are especially deleterious to a hip at risk. A normal joint may tolerate squats well, but in a person with impingement, they can cause or perpetuate problems. Few sporting activities necessitate squats as a functional training tool, and thus they can often be eliminated completely. Squats can at least be modified, limiting hip flexion to 45 degrees and thus protecting the joint from the forces encountered with greater amounts of flexion.

Surgical Treatment

Open Surgical Dislocation

Surgical correction of FAI was first described with the open dislocation technique.[3] This method is still preferred for persons with severe deformities when periacetabular or proximal femoral osteotomy is required.

Mini Open Procedure with Concomitant Arthroscopy

The mini open technique was popularized to avoid problems associated with the trochanteric osteotomy used with conventional surgical dislocation.[18] The intraarticular pathology is addressed arthroscopically, and the cam lesion is corrected through the limited open anterior exposure. The mini open procedure is a popular transitional method for surgeons experienced in the open technique as they integrate the use of arthroscopy into their practice and is often abandoned as the surgeons become more proficient with the arthroscope to address all aspects of the joint pathology.

Arthroscopic Technique

Arthroscopic management of FAI begins with arthroscopy of the central compartment. The patient is positioned supine and traction is applied. Three standard portals are created to provide optimal access for surveying and accessing intraarticular pathology.[19-21]

Pincer impingement has three arthroscopic parameters. First is the presence of anterior labral pathology that must be present to have pathologic pincer impingement. Second, positioning of the anterior portal may be difficult despite adequate distraction because of the bony prominence of the anterolateral acetabulum. Third is the presence of bone overhanging the labrum, whereas normally there would just be a capsular reflection when pincer impingement is not present.

In general, labral preservation is preferred.[22,23] Sometimes the bony lesion can be exposed on the capsular side of the labrum and recontoured without compromising the structural integrity of the labrum. More often, when the labrum is failing as a result of pincer impingement but maintains reasonable quality tissue, it can be mobilized to correct the pincer lesion and then refixed (Fig. 84-19). The labrum is sharply dissected from the overlying bone to expose the pincer lesion. The acetabulum is then recontoured with a high-speed burr, taking care to preserve the mobilized labrum. It is then refixed with suture anchors. Anchor placement usually requires a more distal entry site to ensure that it diverges from the joint, avoiding perforation of the articular surface.

Sometimes, by middle age, if the extent of labral degeneration is extensive, it may be appropriately managed with simple debridement. Debridement of the deteriorated portion exposes the abnormal overhanging bone, which is recontoured to eliminate the pincer lesion (Fig. 84-20). The labral damage may not be salvaged, but recontouring the acetabulum opens the joint and may substantially improve mobility and symptoms.

Management of cam impingement also begins with arthroscopy of the central compartment, with assessment for articular failure of the anterolateral acetabulum characteristic of pathologic cam impingement (Fig. 84-21). The intraarticular damage is addressed and attention is then turned to the cam lesion via the peripheral compartment.

A capsular window is created by connecting the anterior and anterolateral portals. While maintaining these two portals just outside the joint, the traction is released and the hip is slightly flexed, which brings the cam lesion within the peripheral compartment into view. Further capsular dissection fully exposes the abnormal bone, and a proximal anterolateral portal aids in providing complete access. After fully defining the lesion, its overlying fibrous and fibrocartilaginous tissue is removed. The bone is then reshaped, recreating the normal concave relationship at the junction of the articular surface and eliminating the cam lesion (Fig. 84-22). The lateral retinacular vessels are identified and preserved.

Postoperative Rehabilitation

The recovery strategy depends on the extent of pathology that is encountered at the time of arthroscopy and what is done to address it. For simple labral debridement and recontouring of the acetabular rim, the athlete is allowed to bear weight as tolerated, with an emphasis on range of motion and joint stabilization. If the labrum is refixed, precautions are necessary to protect the repair site during the early healing phase. These precautions include protected weight bearing and avoiding extremes of flexion and external rotation for the first 4 weeks.

Reshaping of the femoral head-neck junction necessitates some precautions. Fracture of the femoral neck is an unlikely but potentially serious complication. The athlete is allowed to bear weight fully, but crutches are used to avoid awkward twisting movements during the first 4 weeks. Once full motor control has been regained, the joint is adequately protected for light activities. Full bony remodeling takes 3 months, during which time some precautions are necessary to avoid high impact or torsional forces. If microfracture is performed, the athlete must maintain a strict protected weight-bearing status for 2 months to optimize the early maturation of the fibrocartilaginous healing response. During this time, gentle range of motion is emphasized to stimulate the healing process.

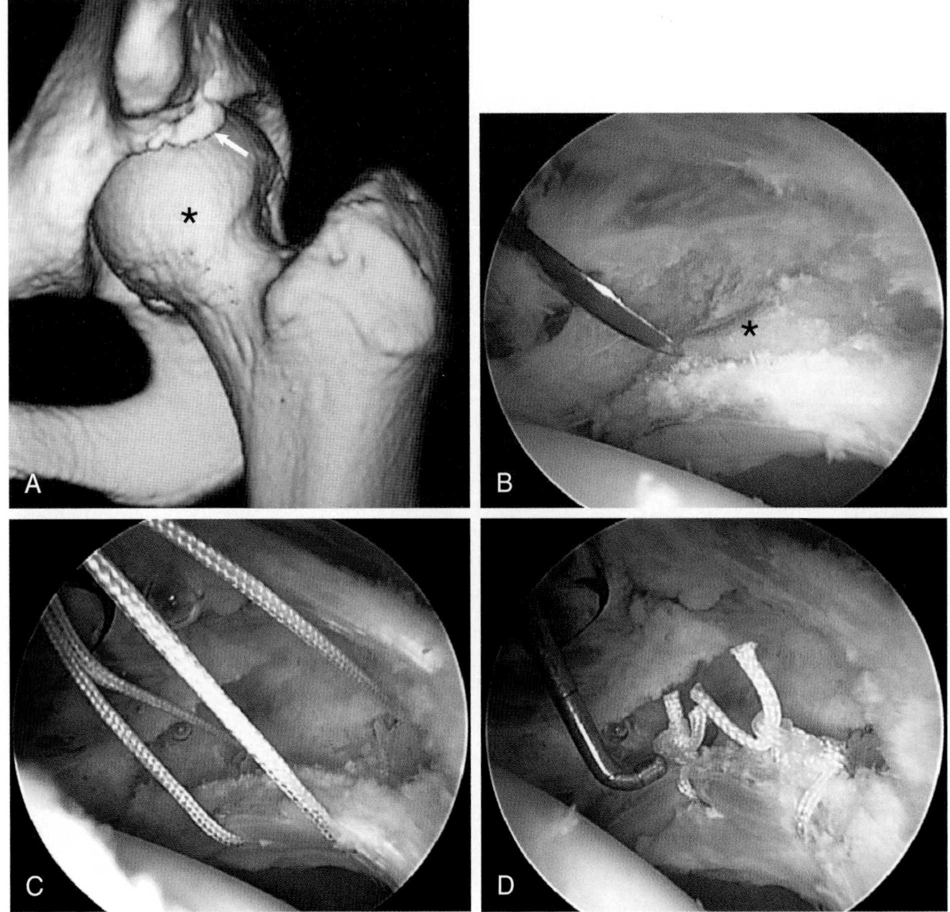

FIGURE 84-19 A 15-year-old female gymnast with pain and reduced internal rotation of the left hip. **A,** A three-dimensional computed tomography scan shows a pincer lesion with accompanying os acetabulum (*arrow*) and a cam lesion (*asterisk*). **B,** When viewed from the anterolateral portal, the pincer lesion and os acetabulum (*asterisk*) are exposed, with the labrum being sharply released with an arthroscopic knife. **C,** The acetabular fragment has been removed and the rim trimmed with anchors placed to repair the labrum. **D,** The labrum has been refixed. *(Courtesy J.W. Thomas Byrd, MD.)*

At 3 months, specific precautions are lifted and functional progression is allowed. The speed with which the athlete advances is variable and may require another 1 to 3 months for full return to sport. Thus athletes are generally advised that return to sports after surgical correction of FAI can take 4 to 6 months.

Results

In 2011, my colleague and I published findings regarding the largest series ever reported of athletes undergoing surgical correction for FAI; our study included 200 consecutive athletes treated with an arthroscopic technique, with a minimum of 1-year follow-up.[24] The median preoperative modified Harris hip score was 72, which improved to 96 after surgery. Ninety-five percent of professional athletes and 85% of intercollegiate athletes were able to return to their previous level of competition. Overall these results were very favorable, but the discrepancy between professional and intercollegiate athletes reflects the finding that more than just the procedure is involved in an athlete's ability to return to sport. Motivation of the athlete and counseling regarding future problems are just two of numerous potential confounding variables. Five transient neurapraxias were encountered, all of which resolved, and one minor case of heterotopic ossification occurred. One athlete (0.5%) underwent conversion to a total hip arthroplasty, and four athletes (2%) underwent a second arthroscopic procedure.

Philippon et al.[25] provided the first report on arthroscopic management of FAI among athletes. Their study included 45 professional athletes with an average follow-up of 1.6 years. Forty-two (93%) were able to resume their sport, although that number declined to 35 (78%) during the follow-up period. In a subsequent publication regarding correction of FAI in 28 professional hockey players, Philippon et al.[26] reported that all the athletes were able to return to hockey activities, although two required repeat surgery.[26] These investigators also reported early outcomes on arthroscopic treatment of FAI in adolescents, with 35-point improvement (according to a modified Harris hip score) among 16 athletes younger than 16 years.[27]

Bizzini et al.[28] published the first study of open surgical dislocation for the treatment of FAI in athletes, reporting on five professional hockey players, three (60%) of whom were able to resume their previous level of competition. Subsequently, Naal et al.[29] reported on 26 professional athletes

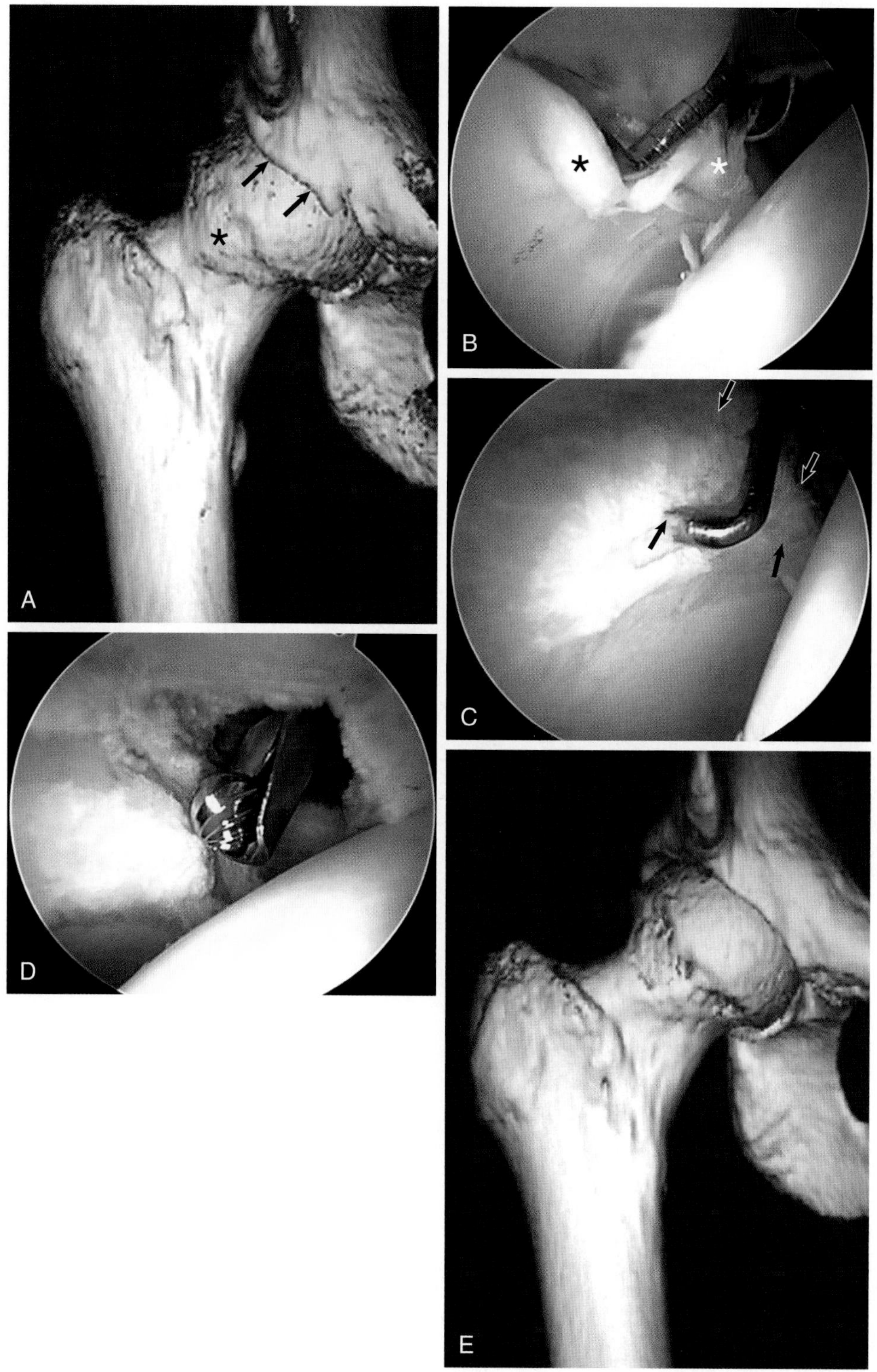

FIGURE 84-20 A 38-year-old woman with progressive pain and loss of motion of the right hip. **A,** A three-dimensional (3D) computed tomography (CT) scan illustrates pincer impingement (*arrows*), as well as a kissing lesion characterized by osteophyte formation on the femoral head (*asterisk*). **B,** As viewed anteriorly from the anterolateral portal, maceration of the anterior labrum (*white asterisk*) and some associated articular delamination (*black asterisk*) are observed. **C,** Debridement of the degenerate labrum exposes the pincer lesion (*arrows*). **D,** The pincer lesion is recontoured with a burr. **E,** A postoperative 3D CT scan demonstrates the extent of bony recontouring of the acetabulum and the femoral head. *(Courtesy J.W. Thomas Byrd, MD.)*

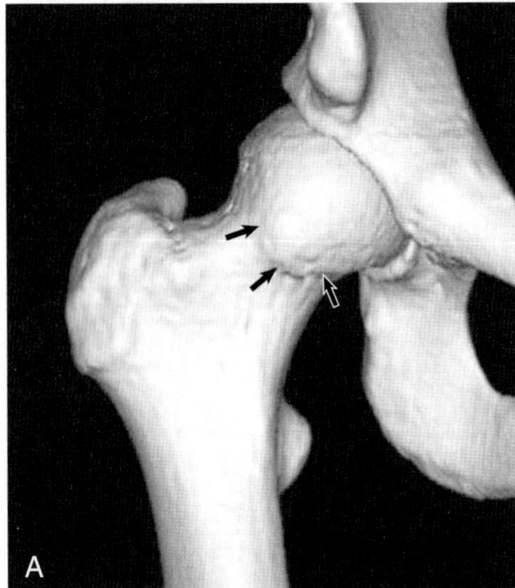

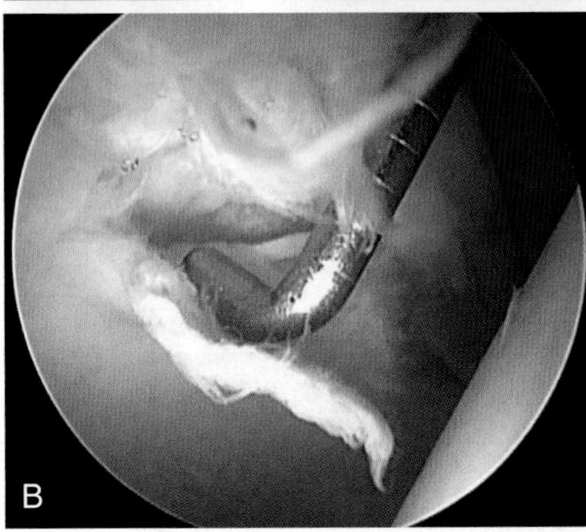

FIGURE 84-21 A 20-year-old hockey player with a 4-year history of right hip pain. **A,** A three-dimensional computed tomography scan defines the cam lesion (*arrows*). **B,** As viewed from the anterolateral portal, the probe introduced anteriorly displaces an area of articular delamination from the anterolateral acetabulum characteristic of the peel-back phenomenon created when the bony lesion shears the articular surface during hip flexion. *(Courtesy J.W. Thomas Byrd, MD.)*

treated with surgical dislocation. Four athletes were excluded from their results because of advanced osteoarthritis. Among the remaining 22 subjects, 21 (95%) returned to sport, although that number diminished to 88% by 2-year follow-up. The investigators reported no complications, but one athlete underwent repeat surgery and six required removal of trochanteric screws. Overall, 18 subjects (82%) were satisfied with the procedure and would do it again. Among these professional athletes, the fact that some returned to their sport despite not being satisfied with the procedure again reflects that other variables, such as motivation, may influence the ability to return to sport.

The literature includes one study on the use of the mini anterior approach for correcting FAI in athletes by Cohen et al.[30] These investigators did not use adjuvant arthroscopy and relied on manual traction to inspect the central compartment. They reported on 47 hips in 44 athletes, among whom 55% returned to sport. A 20% incidence of neurapraxia of the lateral femoral cutaneous nerve and one femoral nerve palsy were reported, all of which eventually resolved.

Numerous other studies have now been published regarding arthroscopic management of FAI. Nho et al.[31] reported on a group of 47 high school, collegiate, and professional athletes with a minimum 1-year follow-up. Fourteen (30%) were lost to follow-up. Among the remaining subjects, 79% returned to sport, and no complications were mentioned. Fabricant et al.[32] examined the arthroscopic correction of FAI in adolescents 19 years of age or younger. These investigators reported on 21 athletes (27 hips) with a 21-point improvement (according to a modified Harris hip score). No complications occurred, but details on return to sport were not provided.

Larson et al.[33] have also examined the relationship between treatment of hip joint problems and concomitant athletic pubalgia. Upon studying 37 athletes (37 hips), they found that the best outcomes occurred when both the hip joint problem and athletic pubalgia were surgically corrected, regardless of whether this correction was performed as a combined or staged procedure. These investigators reported that 89% of the subjects who underwent correction of both problems returned to sport.

Complications

Major potential complications of FAI surgery include osteonecrosis of the femoral head, femoral neck fracture, inadequate osteochondroplasty, heterotopic ossification limiting hip range of motion, trochanteric nonunion, failure of labral refixation, postoperative hip instability, intraabdominal fluid extravasation, and deep infection.[34,35] Other complications include superficial infections, transient neurapraxias, clinically insignificant heterotopic ossification, symptomatic hardware, and bursitis.

The types and rates of complication are dependent upon the treatment technique used. Rates of major complications range from 0 to 20% with open dislocation, 0 to 17% with the mini open technique, and 0 to 5% with arthroscopic treatment.[35] Open dislocation has the associated morbidity inherent with the larger exposure and trochanteric osteotomy. A longer period of protected weight bearing may be required to protect the trochanteric fixation, and stiffness, trochanteric nonunion, symptomatic hardware, and trochanteric bursitis may occur.[36-38] Mini open femoroacetabular osteochondroplasty involves an anterior approach to the hip and risks injury to the lateral femoral cutaneous nerve.[39] Inadequate decompression of the impinging lesions and failure of labral refixation are also possible with this technique.[40]

In a study of 1054 hip arthroscopies, Clarke et al.[41] report an overall complication rate of 1.4%. Nonetheless, although the literature supports the relative safety of hip arthroscopy, the procedure should be performed only by surgeons with experience in the technique to avoid potential complications.[35] Arthroscopic treatment for FAI adds the element of traction, as well as the associated risks. Pudendal, sciatic, and lateral femoral cutaneous nerve palsies have been reported but spontaneously resolve in most cases.[7,42] Injury to perineal structures, heterotopic ossification, and inadequate osteochondroplasty are also possible risks of arthroscopic treatment.[22,42] Although rare, intraabdominal fluid extravasation, a potentially life-threatening condition, has been reported with hip arthroscopy.[43]

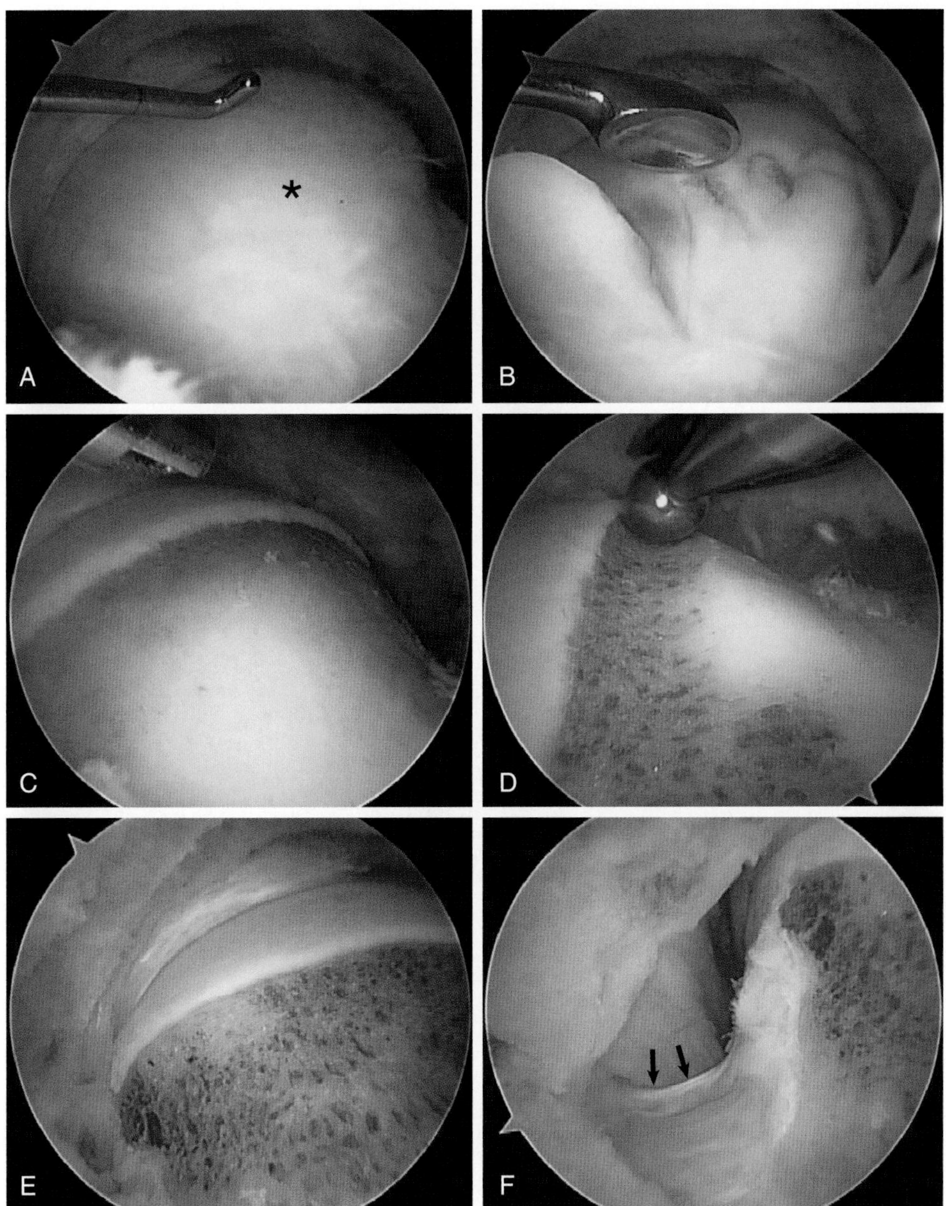

FIGURE 84-22 Views from the periphery. **A,** The cam lesion is identified covered in fibrocartilage (*asterisk*). **B,** An arthroscopic curette is used to denude the abnormal bone. **C,** The area to be excised has been fully exposed. The soft tissue preparation aids in precisely defining the margins to be excised. **D,** Bony resection is begun at the articular margin. **E,** The completed recontouring is surveyed. **F,** As viewed laterally on the base of the neck, the lateral retinacular vessels are identified (*arrows*) and preserved during the recontouring. *(Courtesy J.W. Thomas Byrd, MD.)*

Conclusions

Substantial strides have been made in understanding the role of hip joint pathology as a source of dysfunction and disability among athletes. Historically, most of these disorders were not recognized and not treated, leading athletes to relinquish their competitive careers. FAI is a common cause of joint damage among athletes. Recognition of this entity and the development of surgical techniques to address it have allowed many athletes to resume their athletic careers. However, surgical intervention can never restore a truly normal joint, and thus emphasis is placed on earlier recognition for the purpose of injury prevention. With careful assessment, the clinician can accurately assess hip problems, including joint damage and other associated disorders that may coexist or mimic joint pathology. Many athletes may demonstrate imaging findings of FAI and require little more than close observation. However, in the presence of progressively worsening symptoms, a proactive surgical approach is the preferred strategy.

For a complete list of references, go to expertconsult.com.

Suggested Readings

Citation: Ganz R, Parvizi J, Beck M, et al: Femoroacetabular impingement: A cause for osteoarthritis of the hip. *Clin Orthop Relat Res* 417:112–120, 2003.
Level of Evidence: II
Summary: In this landmark article, femoroacetabular impingement as a cause of secondary joint damage and early-age–onset osteoarthritis is described.

Citation: Byrd JWT: Femoroacetabular impingement in athletes, part I: Cause and assessment. *Sports Health* 2(4):321–333, 2010.
Level of Evidence: IV
Summary: In part I of this article, the presentation and evaluation of athletes with femoroacetabular impingement are detailed.
Citation: Byrd JWT: Femoroacetabular impingement in athletes, part II: Treatment and outcomes. *Sports Health* 2(5):403–409, 2010.
Level of Evidence: IV
Summary: In part II of this article, the treatment options for femoroacetabular impingement are detailed, including conservative measures, open, mini open, and arthroscopic strategies, and results are provided.
Citation: Krych AJ, Thompson M, Knutson Z, et al: Arthroscopic labral repair versus selective labral debridement in female patients with femoroacetabular impingement: A prospective randomized study. *Arthroscopy* 29(1):46–53, 2013.
Level of Evidence: I
Summary: In this level I, prospective, randomized study, superior results of labral refixation compared with debridement are reported.
Citation: Bedi A, Kelly BT: Femoroacetabular impingement. *J Bone Joint Surg Am* 95A(1):82–92, 2013.
Level of Evidence: III
Summary: In this review article, treatment strategies for femoroacetabular impingement are detailed.

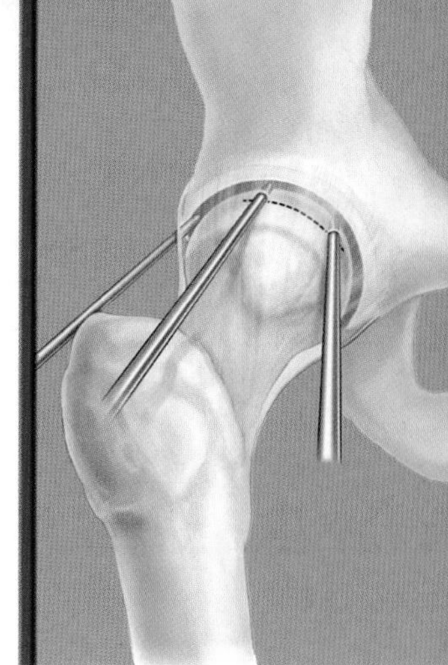

85

Hip and Pelvis Overuse Syndromes

RAJ TELHAN • BRYAN T. KELLY • PETER J. MOLEY

The hip is the specialized structure connecting the hemipelvis to the femur. The interaction of the femoral head, neck, and trochanters to the acetabulum and pelvis involves a complex array of tissue. Abnormalities of the bony morphology or soft tissues can lead to overload. It has been proposed that 5% to 6% of sports injuries of the hip occur at the hip and pelvis.[1] Overuse is the most prevalent etiologic cause of such injuries. Certain activities can lead to a "conflict" between the acetabulum and femur, resulting in injury.[2] In the absence of direct impact of tissue, endurance sports can result in a hip overuse injury as a result of a mismatch between the active and recovery phases of training.[3-5] Regardless of the sport or activity, classification by level of involvement—osteochondral, inert soft tissue, contractile muscle, or neural—is helpful in establishing a diagnosis and treatment plan. The chapter outlines hip overuse injuries using the previously described schema.

This chapter also provides a framework to evaluate and treat overuse injuries of the hip. To organize and provide a framework for this chapter, a layered approach characterized by the senior author (B.T.K.) is used. The layered understanding of potential etiologic contributors to hip pain is useful (Table 85-1). The first layer, the osteochondral layer, which comprises the bone architecture of the hip and pelvis, determines many of the kinetic/kinematic forces that contribute to hip overuse injury. Surrounding the osteochondral layer is the inert layer—primarily the labrum and the hip joint capsule. Biomechanical forces act on the labrum and capsule, which are susceptible to mechanical impingement and failure under asymmetric biomechanical forces. The next layer is the contractile or dynamic layer, including the muscles that cross the hip joint. The contractile layer is best organized by region: anterior, lateral, posterior, and medial. Lastly, the neural layer must be considered when developing a differential of pain relating to overuse of the hip.

Initial Evaluation

A thorough history, physical examination, and knowledge of hip anatomy and function are fundamental to making an accurate diagnosis. The differential diagnosis of hip and groin pain in athletes is broad and determined by factors such as age and activity type.[5-7] Before establishing a musculoskeletal diagnosis, causes of referred hip pain must be considered. These causes may include intraabdominal disorders, genitourinary abnormalities, or gynecological abnormalities. Lumbar spine pathology also may cause hip or pelvis pain. Extraarticular versus intraarticular pathology can be accurately distinguished with a meticulous history, physical examination, and workup. Stress fractures in women of relevant age should prompt assessment for amenorrhea, eating disorders, and osteoporosis.

Evaluation of gait, biomechanics, and alignment should be performed in addition to focal evaluation of the area of injury. Complete examination of the hip should include inspection, palpation, range of motion testing, strength testing, sensory examination, neurovascular examination, and special tests, with comparison between the injured and uninjured limb. Braly et al.[8] presented an 11-point physical evaluation tool including systematic evaluation in the standing, seated, supine, lateral, and prone positions.[9]

Osteochondral Layer

Femoroacetabular Impingement

Irregularities of the femoroacetabular articulation are a possible source of hip pain in athletes.[10] Morphologic femoroacetabular abnormalities can cause labral and chondral damage.[11,12] Most patients with labral tears also have bony abnormalities such as hip dysplasia and femoroacetabular impingement (FAI).[10] In patients with FAI, morphopathology of the femur or acetabulum damages the chondrolabral structures during normal joint motion.[13] The most common type of morphopathology is the mixed cam and pincer lesion, which occurs along the anterior femoral neck and the anterior-superior acetabular rim.[13,14] The accepted mechanism of flexion and internal rotation produces abutment and impingement of the labrum and cartilage. Such repetitive microtrauma results in joint degeneration.[14]

Biomechanically, cam lesions result from a decrease in femoral head-neck offset, resulting in additional bone overgrowth. Cam lesions are most commonly seen on the anterior and anterosuperior aspect of the femoral neck and are seen in people with FAI.[14] Pincer impingement is bony change in the acetabulum itself and is observed in 42% of people with FAI. Structured pincer lesions manifest as either a deep acetabulum or retroverted acetabulum, which leads to an apparent deeper anterior acetabular wall.[13] FAI can result in pathology including primary labral tears, chondropathy, and hip osteoarthritis when the hip joint is placed into a position of impingement in a repetitive fashion during sporting activities.

TABLE 85-1
LAYERS OF THE HIP

Layer	Description
Osteochondral	Bony structure of hip and pelvis/ femoroacetabular articulation
Inert	Static stabilizing structures including the hip capsule, ligaments, and labrum
Contractile/dynamic	Muscles that cross the hip joint
Neural	Sensory and motor nerves in the hip region

No gold standard exists for diagnosing FAI, and not all persons with FAI experience hip pathology. Signs associated with FAI include reduced hip internal rotation with hip flexion and a positive flexion, adduction, and internal rotation (FADIR). Positive FADIR testing is common in persons with FAI and may warrant radiographic examination. Therapeutic intervention involves decreasing frequency and duration of positional impingement. Flexion, internal rotation, and adduction should be limited.[13]

Stress Fracture

Femoral Neck Stress Fractures

The mechanical loading and arthrokinematics of femoroacetabular morphology interact with gravity to produce injury. Together, bony architecture and the muscles in the hip and pelvis play a role in the development of stress injuries. The muscles in the hip and pelvis are important in balancing torque forces such as those at the femoral neck. If the muscles become fatigued with activity and, particularly in areas of baseline weakness, the ability of the muscles to absorb gravitational forces is lost, these forces are transmitted to a greater degree to the bone. Additionally, these forces can be transmitted asymmetrically through the hip joint, resulting in a stress injury in the setting of morphologic abnormality.[15]

A compression-side femoral neck stress fracture is defined as sclerosis or localization of injury to the compression side of the femoral neck on the basis of imaging studies, with subdivisions based on the presence of a fatigue line (Fig. 85-1). The three subtypes consist of no fatigue line, a fatigue line greater than 50%, and a fatigue line less than 50% of the femoral neck. Stage 1 is characterized by normal radiographs and abnormal uptake on a bone scan, or magnetic resonance imaging (MRI) signal intensity on T2-weighted or short tau inversion recovery images. Stage 2 is notable for endosteal or periosteal callous without overt fracture, and stage 3 is notable for evidence of a cortical crack without displacement.[15] In tension-side fractures, a callus or disruption of the cortical surface on the tension side (superior) of the femoral neck is observed. In the case of tension-side stress fractures, surgical management is required to stabilize the fracture to avoid the complications of a femoral neck fracture.

Pelvic and Sacral Stress Fractures

A pelvic stress fracture is defined by damage to the inferior pubic rami, likely from shear force between the medial adductor muscle group and the lateral hamstring attachment, causing repetitive overload and increasing the likelihood of a stress fracture. Sacral stress fractures are rare and occur as a result of vertical force transmission through the spinal column to the sacrum and ilium.[16,17] Sacral stress fractures occur unilaterally, primarily at the sacral ala (Fig. 85-2).

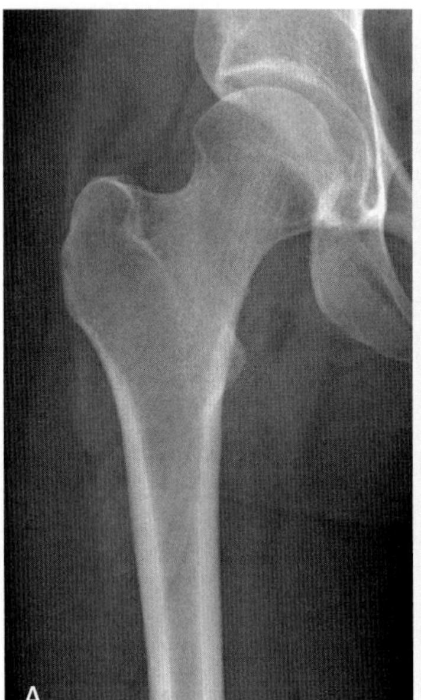

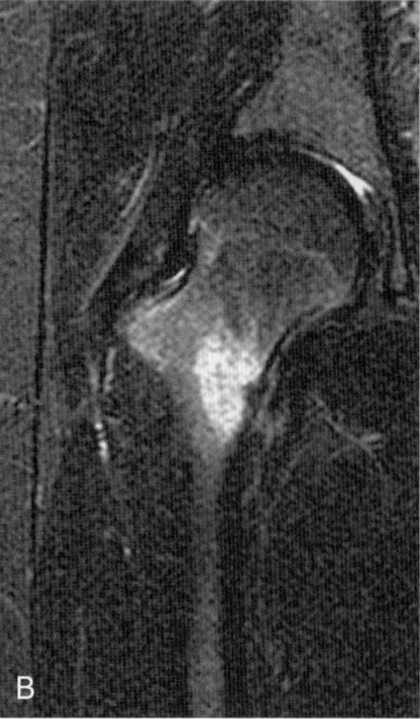

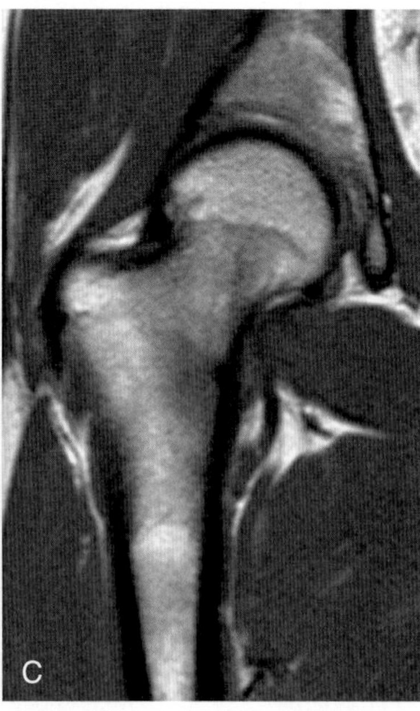

FIGURE 85-1 **A,** An anteroposterior radiograph in a runner with hip pain. **B,** A coronal T2-weighted magnetic resonance imaging (MRI) scan with fat saturation demonstrates increased signal within the medial femoral neck, which is of concern for edema associated with a stress fracture. **C,** A coronal T1-weighted MRI scan shows a small, focal, low signal intensity region along the medial femoral neck, confirming a stress fracture. *(From Pearce DH: Skeletal assessment of fractures of the proximal femur. In Waddell J, editor:* Fractures of the proximal femur: improving outcomes, *Philadelphia, 2010, Elsevier.)*

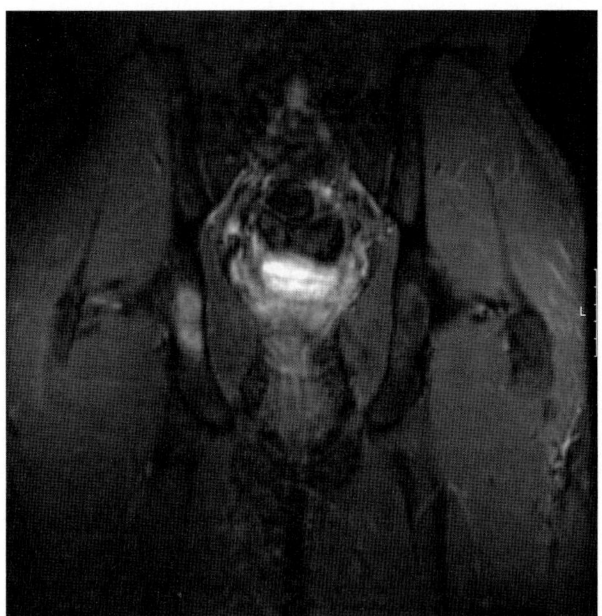

FIGURE 85-2 A T2-weighted coronal magnetic resonance image of the pelvis demonstrates increased fluid signal in the right ischium consistent with bony edema from a stress reaction.

Inert Layer

Acetabular Labral Tears

Acetabular labral tears are common causes of hip pain in athletes.[10,18,19] Functionally, the labrum deepens the acetabulum, contributing to the hip dynamic stability by maintaining femoral head contact within the acetabulum.[18,20,21] Negative intraarticular pressure of the joint is maintained by the acetabular labrum. Causes of acetabular labral tears are multifactorial. They are associated with tearing as a result of direct trauma, Legg-Calvé-Perthes disease, osteoarthritis, classic hip dysplasia, microinstability, and FAI.[18,20,21] Wenger et al.[21] reported that 87% of 31 patients with labral tears were found to have at least one structural abnormality, including retroverted acetabulum, abnormal femoral head-neck offset, and coxa valga. Repetitive microtrauma is also a potential mechanism of injury in these patients.

Plain radiographs are useful in localizing structural bony abnormalities but not soft tissue injury.[22,23] As many as two thirds of labral tears occur in the anterosuperior labrum,[18] possibly because of poor vascular supply and exposure to higher forces or stresses[24] as a result of anterosuperior impingement in FAI.[12] Repetitive twisting, hyperextension, hyperflexion, hyperabduction, and/or frequent external rotation of the hip may result in labral tears.[20,25]

The mechanism of injury for labral tears is repetitive high impact within the joint, resulting in anteromedial groin pain and limited hip range of motion.

In summary, labral tears are commonly seen as a result of overuse injuries. FAI and developmental hip dysplasia increase the risk of labral tears.[26] Conservative management should always precede surgical intervention. Improving hip joint neuromotor control should be a goal in physical therapy by activating deep stabilizing muscles. Gait retraining should aim to reduce excessive hip extension and loading of anterior hip structures.[20]

Structural risk factors for labral tears include static overload, dynamic impingement, and dynamic instability. Static overload includes lateral or anterior undercoverage, femoral anteversion, or femoral valgus. Dynamic impingement would include FAI, femoral retroversion, and femoral varus. Finally, dynamic instability can occur when functional range is greater than the morphologic constraints. An example would be posterior subluxation from an anterior cam, levering the hip in excessive flexion.[27]

Contractile Layer

Hip pain from overuse is often linked to muscle imbalances, with muscle strains tending to be the most common type of injuries. Muscles that cross two joints and fast-twitch type 2 fibers are most often involved, especially during activities requiring eccentric contraction.[3,28,29] When injury does occur, it is commonly at the myotendinous junction where biomechanical shear forces are most focal.[28] Ultrasound can be used to assess tendon degradation and muscle tear.[30] MRI can provide high-resolution multiplanar visualization of the tissues involved.[3,29] Classification of muscle strain based on MRI findings is possible as follows: first degree (stretch injury), second degree (partial tear), and third degree (complete rupture).[29] Modifiable risk factors include muscle imbalance between agonists and antagonists, fatigue, lack of flexibility, and poor trunk coordination. Overuse can involve the anterior, lateral, medial, and/or posterior hip musculature.

Anterior Hip

Iliopsoas Tendonitis/Bursitis

The iliopsoas is the main flexor of the hip joint. From its origin off the anterior bodies and transverse processes of the lumbar vertebrae, the muscle courses across the pelvic brim to its insertion on the lesser trochanter of the femur.[31] The most common causes for iliopsoas tendonitis/bursitis are rheumatoid arthritis, acute trauma, and overuse.[31] The iliopsoas bursa is the largest bursa in the hip, positioned between iliopsoas and the pelvic brim. Iliopsoas bursitis is most common in young female athletes[29] who may present with a combination of anterior hip pain and a palpable audible snap (Fig. 85-3).[1,32,33]

It is postulated that repetitive hip flexion and extension is the primary biomechanical mode of injury, which is often seen in high-risk sports such as rowing and running. In rowers, excessive hip flexion during the stroke can irritate the iliopsoas bursa via internal snapping of the hip.[34] Paluska[35] has highlighted the role of sprinting and hill climbing in causing friction of the iliopsoas tendon on the iliopectineal eminence, anterior femoral head, and anterior hip capsules, effectively causing iliopsoas bursitis. Additional evidence is now available that implicates the iliopsoas in hip impingement.[36] Patient presentation includes a positive FADIR test, painful resisted hip flexion, and tenderness over the iliopsoas on palpation. Radiographic findings show normal head-neck offset, but a labral tear is seen on imaging and intraoperatively.

Coxa Saltans Syndrome (Snapping Hip)

Snapping hip syndrome—coxa saltans—is characterized by an audible snap or catch of the hip.[1,29,37] External coxa saltans

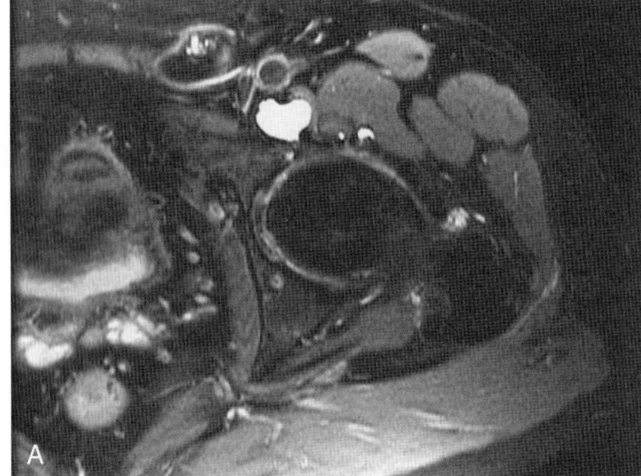

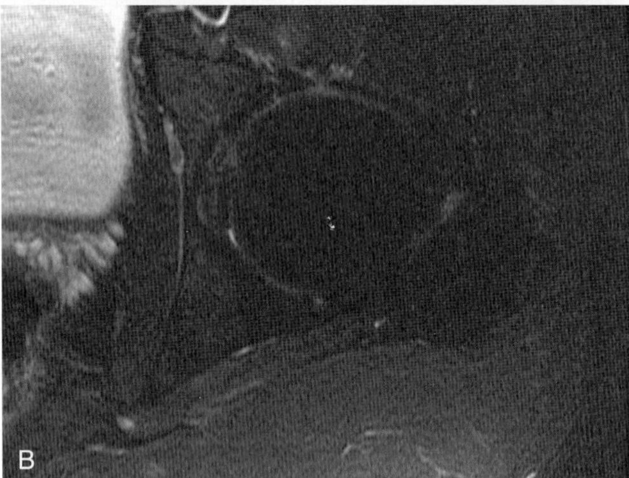

FIGURE 85-3 **A,** A T2-weighted axial magnetic resonance image (MRI) of the hip demonstrates high signal adjacent the iliopsoas tendon, representing bursitis. Iliopsoas bursitis can accompany snapping hip. **B,** A T2-weighted axial MRI of the hip shows edema in the area of the iliopsoas tendon consistent with tendinitis. *(From Byrd JT, Guanche C, editors:* AANA advanced arthroscopy: the hip, *Philadelphia, 2010, Elsevier.)*

defines lateral symptoms, and internal coxa saltans describes medial symptoms. Mechanistically, snapping of the iliopsoas over the iliopectineal eminence, anterior femoral head, or anterior hip results in audible internal snapping. Other mechanical hypotheses for internal snapping include accessory iliopsoas tendinous slips, stenosing tenosynovitis of the iliopsoas insertion, iliopsoas tendon snapping over a bony ridge at its insertion at the lesser trochanter, snapping of the iliofemoral ligament over the anterior femoral head, and subluxation of the long head of the biceps femoris at the ischium (snapping bottom).[1,37] More recent ultrasound investigation has demonstrated snapping over the iliacus muscle.[32] Persons at risk include those who perform movements with high flexion angles (associated with internal and external rotation) or repetitive hip flexion maneuvers.[1,37]

The snapping of the iliotibial band across the greater trochanter results in visible external (lateral) snapping.[38] Mechanistically, the iliotibial band glides over the trochanter when moving from extension to flexion,[29] as in biking and running.[1] External snapping hip is more common than internal snapping hip. Palpable snapping of these tendons during examination confirms diagnosis. Although the utility of imaging is limited, dynamic ultrasound analysis has been suggested to be useful in differentiating the diagnosis.[1,37] Repetitive snapping in both cases may lead to iliopsoas bursitis or tendonitis.

Rectus Femoris Injury/Overuse

The rectus femoris (straight and reflected head) and the sartorius are also hip flexors. Strains in these muscles generally occur at the myotendinous junction (Fig. 85-4, *A*). In addition, muscles that cross two joints are at higher risk for strains.[3] Both have also been implicated in apophyseal avulsion injuries in skeletally immature patients.[38,39] Although this issue predominantly affects adolescents, a case report demonstrated a proximal avulsion in two National Football League kickers,[40] soon followed by a larger National Football League

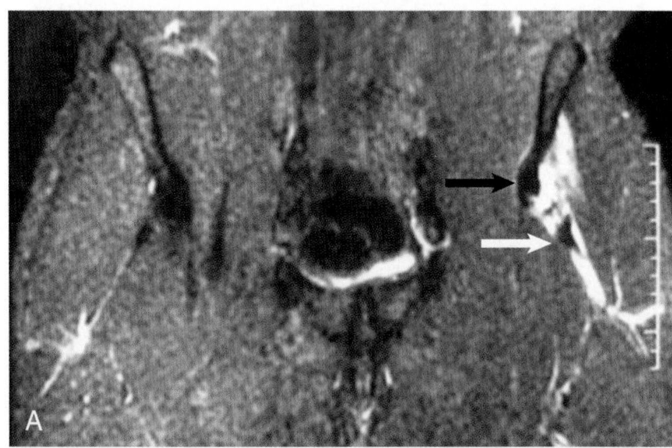

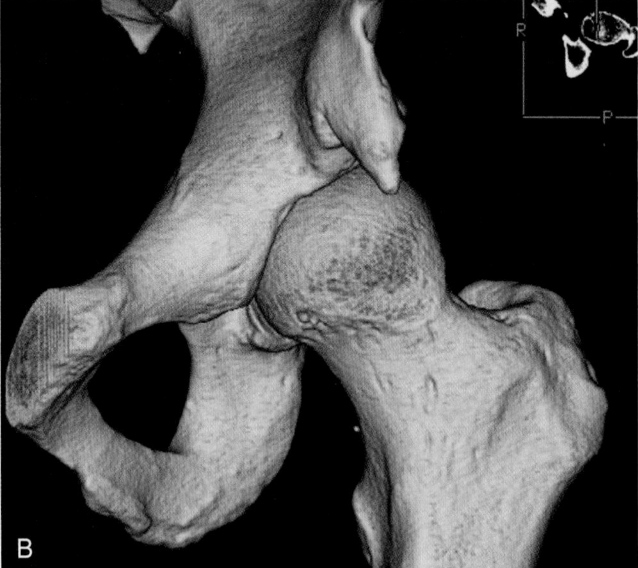

FIGURE 85-4 **A,** A fat-suppressed magnetic resonance image of the left hip demonstrates a rectus avulsion injury (*white arrow*) from the anterior inferior iliac spine (AIIS; *black arrow*). **B,** A computed tomography reconstruction of the left hip demonstrates a healed avulsion of the AIIS. This bony prominence superior to the hip may cause subspine impingement as the hip is brought into flexion. *(**A,** From Bedi A, Dolan M, Leunig M, et al: Static and dynamic mechanical causes of hip pain.* Arthroscopy *27[2]:235–251, 2011.)*

survey.[41] Investigators surmise that these injuries occur in kickers who go from a hip-extended/knee-flexed starting point to a hip-flexed/knee-extended position. These injuries can be managed conservatively. One complication has been extraarticular impingement, specifically subspine impingement in patients with rectus femoris avulsions.[42,43] Subspine impingement is characterized by pain in straight flexion, causing the inferior portion of the femoral neck to abut the overhanging anterior inferior iliac spine (Fig. 85-4, *B*).

Lateral Hip

Hip Abductor Overuse

Muscle imbalance and overuse of the hip abductors is a major cause of hip abductor injury (Fig. 85-5). The wider female pelvis has been postulated to increase the likelihood of injury in women.[30] Morphologic abnormalities such as hip dysplasia can cause biomechanical overload of the abductor group.[44]

In terms of muscle imbalances, weak gluteus medius in the presence of a normal tensor fascia lata may lead to overuse.[44] Clinically, patients have hip and gluteal pain that is worse with periods of prolonged sitting and side lying.[44] Objective findings may include pain on palpation of the gluteal muscles over the insertion of the greater trochanter and Trendelenburg gait. Abnormalities in the kinetic chain can result in progressive low back pain and lumbar facet arthropathy, that is, greater trochanteric pain syndrome (GTPS).[44]

Greater Trochanteric Pain Syndrome

Four distinct muscles implicated in GTPS either attach to or cross over the greater trochanter: They are the gluteus maximus and tensor fascia lata with their connection to the iliotibial band (ITB). The gluteus medius and gluteus minimus attach directly to the trochanter.[30] Three bursae are present between the muscle layers—the subgluteus maximus bursa, the subgluteus medius bursa, and the gluteus minimus bursa—with the deep subgluteus maximus bursa being more commonly irritated[30] in classic trochanteric bursitis. The greater trochanteric bursa lies between the tensor fascia lata and the gluteus medius and the greater trochanter of the femur. Overuse of the hip abductor, facet arthropathy in the lumbar spine, and snapping hip are all associated with GTPS.[29]

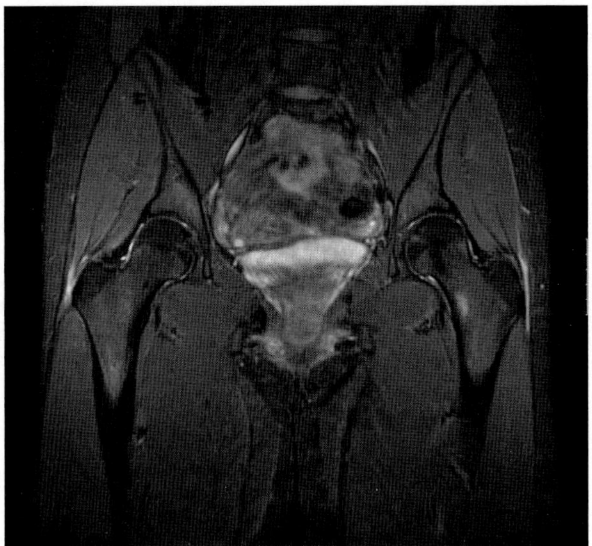

FIGURE 85-5 A T2-weighted coronal magnetic resonance image of the pelvis demonstrates increased signal in the insertion of the right gluteus medius onto the greater trochanter and partial tearing of the tendon.

Up to one quarter of the general population may experience GTPS.[30] Clinical presentation includes tenderness to palpation along the greater trochanter and increased pain with FABER testing and lying on one's side. Factors contributing to hip overuse in athletes include imbalance of hip abductor strength and tension on the ITB in cyclists with high-riding seats.[45]

Iliotibial Band Syndrome

The connective tissues of the gluteus maximus and tensor fascia lata run together to form the ITB. From its origin on the iliac crest, it runs down the lateral aspect of the thigh and inserts on Gerdy's tibial tubercle. ITB syndrome is diagnosed on the basis of clinical evaluation, not imaging. Mechanically, ITB dysfunction occurs as a result of friction microtrauma from the lateral femoral condyle, leading to inflammation and pain on the lateral aspect of knee at 30 degrees of knee flexion.[46-49] Greater hip adduction and knee internal rotation movements lead to greater ITB tensile strain.[50]

Biomechanical variables linked to ITB syndrome include leg length discrepancy, forefoot varus, rearfoot eversion, hip abductor weakness, hip abductor or ITB tightness, and increased Q angles.[46,47,49] Overuse in athletic training contributes to ITB syndrome.

ITB syndrome is the most common cause of lateral knee pain in runners.[46] Biomechanical evaluation reveals that the injury occurs during the deceleration phase or early stance phase of the gait cycle in runners.[49] Clinical symptoms include greater pain with activity, including running and stair descent. Management includes activity modification and biomechanical gait/running form corrections.

Medial Hip

Adductor Tendinopathies and Tears

Adductor muscle group damage is most likely to occur during moments of fast acceleration and sudden directional change.[51,52] Clinical presentation may include medial thigh or groin pain with tenderness to palpation along the pubic ramus. Resisted isometric hip adduction may also cause pain,[53] but it can also be seen in patients with osteitis pubis. It is important to differentiate adductor magnus injury from hamstring injury by understanding the mechanism of injury. For example, in swimmers, hip adductor overuse injury results from repetitive forceful adduction.[52]

Athletic Pubalgia

Athletic pubalgia describes debilitating abdominal and inguinal exertional pain that can progress to include hip adductor pain.[54-56] Clinically, symptoms are generated upon resisted hip adduction and abdominal contraction. A suggested mechanical hypothesis is that the pain results from a complex injury to the flexion and adduction apparatus of the low abdomen and hip.[54,55] Hammoud et al.[54] review the characteristics of the so-called *pubic joint,* which is comprised of the right and left pubic symphyses and their combined musculotendinous attachments. It is suggested that the uneven distribution of extreme force around this apparatus generates a constellation of abdominal and pelvic pain.[56,57]

Mechanically, restriction of terminal flexion and external rotation has been hypothesized to result in secondary abnormal motion of the hemipelvis, resulting in injury to the posterior inguinal wall, rectus abdominis, and adductor musculature that is linked with sports hernia.[54-56]

In terms of epidemiology, the most common types of hip injuries include muscle strain, contusion, and intraarticular injury and sprain.[54,58] It is hypothesized that these injuries are part of a linked triad that occurs as a constellation associated with FAI and can exacerbate muscle injury of the pelvis, including athletic pubalgia, in athletes.[54]

The best treatment consists of stretching, postural/balance exercises, and flexibility training. Initial treatment should include a standard protocol of rest, ice, physical therapy, and range of motion exercises. More interventional procedures include corticosteroid injection to the adductor enthesis and, in cases of refractory pain, surgery for proximal hamstring and iliopsoas tendonitis.[54,58,59]

The goal of surgical repair (which is up to 95% effective) is to relieve tension on the pubic symphysis by performing selective epimysiotomy or detachment of structures that attach there to create tensile force.[54-56]

Posterior Hip

Hamstring Tendinopathy

The hamstrings are the most commonly strained muscles of the hip, in the following order of injury: biceps femoris, semimembranosus, and semitendinosus.[3,29,51] The mechanism of injury is most often sudden eccentric contraction (especially at the long head of the biceps) during running.[51,60] During dance and kicking sports, extreme stretch during hip flexion with the knee extended can result in injury to the proximal tendon, which has been associated with tears, worse outcomes, and longer recovery.[51] Clinical presentation often includes sudden-onset posterior thigh pain, weak knee flexion and hip extension, reduced range of motion at the hip, and tenderness to palpation over the ischial tuberosity.[51,61] In cases of partial or complete tear, an audible snap, local bruising, and a local palpable defect may be present. Proximity to the site of the hamstring origin is correlated with increased recovery time.[60]

During workup, avulsion must be ruled out in athletes with sudden-onset high-acuity hamstring pain with use of radiography, computed tomography, or MRI. Generally, treatment will entail progressive strengthening followed by ultrasound-guided injections of a corticosteroid and a local anesthetic, which can help reduce pain in the short term for patients who fail to respond to conservative therapy. Surgical intervention may be necessary for cases of complete avulsion because hip power generation can be reduced, which can limit future sporting performance. Recurrence of hamstring injuries is highly likely.[62]

Ischial Tuberosity Bursitis

The ischiogluteal bursa is positioned between the hamstring tendons and the ischial tuberosity. Irritation of the bursa often occurs as a result of prolonged sitting[29] and has been seen in rowers, cyclists, and runners as a result of compression and overuse injury to the hamstring tendon origin.[63] Inadequate bike saddle fit can cause friction on the ischial bursae.[64] Athletes will present with buttock pain that may irradiate down the posterior thigh if the sciatic nerve gets irritated with the bursa inflammation.[29] Ischiogluteal bursitis is difficult to differentiate from hamstring tendinopathy, but hamstring tendinitis is far more common than ischiotibial bursitis.

Neural Layer

Hip pain can result from referred neural pain. Posterior thigh and hamstring pain may be a result of lumbar spine pathology, including discogenic pain, facet arthropathy, and nerve root impingement that causes dermatomal distribution pain that overlaps with the hip, pelvis, and groin. Accordingly, a complete neurologic examination assessing for underlying focal strength deficits, reflex changes, and a change in sensorium is essential.

Nerve Entrapments

Neuroanatomically, the tibial branch of the sciatic nerve supplies most of the hamstring muscle group. Injury to the nerve, including at the level of the nerve root and lumbosacral plexus, can cause referred pain. Mechanisms of injury include compression and direct trauma through sports-related injury. Compression of the sciatic nerve can be caused as it courses through the piriformis and the hip external rotators.[65,66]

Meralgia paresthetica refers to lateral femoral cutaneous nerve injury, causing anterior thigh pain from this purely sensory nerve. Injury is most commonly noted as a result of blunt compressive forces in proximity to the ASIS, resulting in entrapment and/or irritation. Rugby has been implicated, as well as activities requiring repeated hip flexion and extension.[67] Treatment of choice is nonsurgical conservative management including rest and use of nonsteroidal antiinflammatory drugs until symptoms have resolved.

Fascial entrapment of the obturator nerve within the adductor compartment is also common and can present as exercise-induced groin pain.[68] The usual presentation of obturator nerve entrapment is a deep ache in the region of the adductor origin. Physical examination assists in diagnosis, especially when the patient exercises at a level that generates typical pain. It is recommended that the patient be examined immediately after exercise that induces pain. One should check for weakness in resisted adduction and numbness over the distal medial thigh for confirmation of the diagnosis. The mainstay of treatment is surgical fascial release, with conservative measures yielding limited improvement.[68]

Ilioinguinal nerve impingement, genitofemoral nerve impingement, lateral cutaneous nerve impingement, and pudendal nerve entrapment can also be a source of groin pain. Labat et al.[69] describes the following criteria for the diagnosis of pudendal nerve entrapment: (1) pain in the region innervated by the pudendal nerve (i.e., from anus to clitoris/penis; (2) pain that does not awake the patient at night; (3) pain that is not associated with objective sensory impairment; and (4) pain that is relieved by diagnostic pudendal nerve block.

Most nerve impingements resolve spontaneously and do not necessitate surgical intervention. Corticosteroid injection around certain nerves (e.g., the lateral femoral cutaneous nerve) may relieve pain symptoms. In refractory cases of entrapment, surgical myofascial release is necessary.

Treatment Options

For all of the aforementioned musculotendinous pathologic processes, proper treatment rests upon accurate diagnosis. With proper treatment, safe return to play and guidance regarding minimization of future overuse injury is possible. The mainstay of treatment is conservative therapy as a first-line intervention for the vast majority of hip injuries related to overuse.[3] The customized combination of rest, ice, pain control, and physical therapy is the foundation of any effective recovery plan. Additionally, neuromuscular reeducation and biomechanical retraining to counteract muscle fatigue, imbalance, and training errors is essential. Training regimens must also be carefully crafted to prevent sudden or drastic increases in workload. As previously mentioned, the best treatment plan is one that is customized to the patient's sport-specific or activity-specific injury. Loucks[70] has written about the importance of evaluating diet and energy expenditure to ensure proper nutritional support for bone and muscle healing/repair. Interdisciplinary treatment managed by physicians, physical therapists, and trainers is highly recommended.

Rehabilitation/Physical Therapy

The layered understanding of potential etiologic contributors—osteochondral, static, contractile, and neural—to hip pain is useful in crafting a comprehensive rehabilitation regimen. Important variables to consider include functional interaction between underlying bony architecture, surrounding muscular structures, pelvic stability, intraarticular pathology, and neural overlay.[71] Treatment goals include pain reduction, restoration of motion, improvement of strength and flexibility, and return to sport. In the acute phase, treatment should include rest, ice, compression, and elevation. If the patient has an antalgic gait, weight unloading may be considered via crutches.[71]

Strengthening exercises of the hip musculature and abdominal core are useful.[71-73] Ekstrom et al.[74] found that specific exercises, such as the bridge, unilateral bridge, prone bridge on elbows and toes, and quadruped arm/lower extremity lift, had increased muscle signal activation during electromyography for endurance training and stabilization of trunk and hips. Initially, static (isometric) strengthening may be initiated, and then the patient may progress to dynamic (isokinetic) strengthening.[73]

As pain-free strength and range of motion improves, the exercises can progress from passive to active training regimens that emphasize eccentric resistance.[3,51,71,73] Sport-specific training should only be initiated once full pain-free range of motion is achieved.

Prognosis for resolution with conservative management is excellent in the absence of an underlying fracture.[35] Intraarticular degeneration may be treated nonoperatively at first, but if conservative measures fail to address fixed biomechanical or structural defects, interventional procedures should be considered.

Therapeutic Injections

The role of corticosteroid injection is reduction of pain and inflammation in acute injuries that are severe enough to inhibit function as a result of tendonitis or bursitis. Such injections may be performed with use of ultrasound or fluoroscopic guidance. When data regarding improvement of pain were analyzed, significant gains were found with injection of corticosteroid and local anesthetic at the site of the greater trochanteric bursa.[30,75,76] Similar injections have been suggested to relieve pain resulting from greater trochanteric syndrome associated with external coax saltans.[29,30] Injections should always be combined with other modalities and physical therapy, a combination that has been found to be most effective in treating the symptoms.[77]

Training and Activity Modifications

Cardiovascular warm-up should be followed by dynamic stretching that incorporates sport-specific movements prior to competitions or training.[71] Static stretching should be performed at the end of the athletic activity. Finally, we have found that activity modification is one of the most useful means of decreasing pain and facilitating the athlete's return to sport.

For a complete list of references, go to expertconsult.com.

Suggested Readings

Citation: Feeley BT, Powell JW, Muller MS, et al: Hip injuries and labral tears in the national football league. *Am J Sports Med* 36(11):2187–2195, 2008.
Level of Evidence: IV
Summary: This descriptive epidemiology study in National Football League players found 738 hip-related injuries out of a total of 23,806 total injuries reported. The most common hip injuries sustained by these elite athletes are reviewed.

Citation: Bedi A, Dolan M, Leunig M, et al: Static and dynamic mechanical causes of hip pain. *Arthroscopy* 27(2):235–251, 2011.
Level of Evidence: V
Summary: This literature review includes descriptions of dynamic and static factors associated with mechanical hip pain, the combinations of dynamic and static stresses that are commonly identified in hip pain, and common patterns of compensatory injury in patients with femoroacetabular impingement.

Citation: Shin A, Gillingham B: Fatigue fractures of the femoral neck in athletes. *J Am Acad Orthop Surg* 5(6):293–302, 1997.
Level of Evidence: V
Summary: In this review article the demographics, pathophysiology, diagnosis, and management of stress fractures of the femoral neck are detailed.

Citation: Overdeck KH, Palmer WE: Imaging of hip and groin injuries in athletes. *Semin Musculoskelet Radiol* 8(1):41–55, 2004.
Level of Evidence: V
Summary: In this article several pathologic conditions of the hip and groin in both recreational and professional athletes are reviewed, with an emphasis on magnetic resonance imaging as the modality of choice in the diagnosis of these injuries.

Citation: Tyler TF, Slattery AA: Rehabilitation of the hip following sports injury. *Clin Sports Med* 29(1):107–126, 2010.
Level of Evidence: V
Summary: In this article the approach to the athlete with hip pain is reviewed, emphasizing the biomechanics and forces across the hip joint. The principles of rehabilitation after hip injury are outlined.

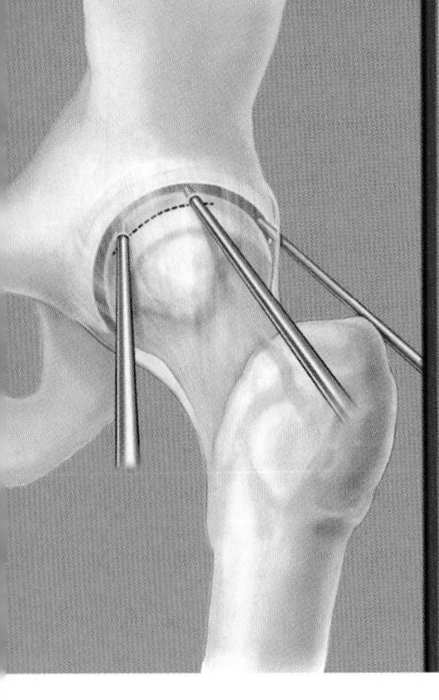

86

Snapping Hip Syndrome

VÍCTOR MANUEL ILIZALITURRI SÁNCHEZ JR • ANELL OLIVOS MEZA

The snapping hip, also known as *coxa saltans* or *dancer's hip,* is defined as an audible or palpable clicking that usually is accompanied by pain during movement of the hip joint.[1-8] Initially this phenomenon was classified in two main categories, intraarticular and extraarticular. More recently, use of the term "intraarticular snapping hip" has been discontinued because of increasing knowledge of intraarticular hip pathology. Currently snapping hip is divided into internal and external cases, based on whether the snap occurs on the medial or lateral aspect of the thigh, respectively.[1,5,6,8-11]

Snapping hip was described in the literature in the first third of the last century. This pathology was usually attributed to the iliotibial band until Nunziata and Blumenfeld[12] proposed an alternate etiology—slippage of the psoas tendon over the iliopectineal eminence. During the past 20 years, several reports have attempted to clarify the pathoanatomic features, assessment, and treatment of these hip disorders. Schaberg et al.[13] distinguished "external" from "internal" etiologies, and the term "coxa saltans" was later introduced as a general description encompassing all different types.[14] Occasionally we encounter a patient with painful clicking or popping symptoms without identifiable intraarticular pathology or lesions of the iliopsoas tendon or iliotibial band, known as idiopathic etiologies.[10]

Internal snapping hip is an unusual but potentially debilitating disorder produced by the iliopsoas tendon slipping over underlying bony prominences.[2,9,10,14] It was first recognized and described in 1951 by Nunziata and Blumenfeld in Argentina. The question of whether the iliopsoas tendon snaps over the anterior brim, femoral head, or lesser trochanter is debated.[2,3,12] Gruen et al.[2] and Spina[5] have reported that the tight iliopsoas tendon is tethered over the pelvic brim and contributes to the anterior hip and pelvic pain. The snap may be painful and can relate to exercise or sports activity.[15] Snapping of the iliopsoas tendon can be difficult to differentiate from intraarticular pathology because the symptoms may mimic a mechanical intraarticular process and both emanate from deep in the anterior groin (immediately adjacent to the joint).[14]

Snapping of the iliotibial band, or external coxa saltans, is a more evident phenomenon, initially described by Binnie[16] in 1913. Potential causes include snapping of the proximal hamstring tendon over the ischial tuberosity, or more commonly, snapping of the iliotibial band, fascia lata, gluteus maximus, or a combination of the aforementioned over the greater trochanter.[5,9,10,17] Although iliotibial snapping may occur after trauma, symptomatic cases are usually associated with repetitive activities, especially sports.[14] Other possible causes have been reported as iatrogenic processes after surgical procedures that leave the greater trochanter more prominent or in a lateral displacement position after hip arthroplasty, especially when a longer neck is used and a higher offset is created.[6,14]

Epidemiology

Internal snapping hip occurs in between 5% to 10% of the population, and a significant number of painless cases may be incidental.[14] Iliopsoas tendon snapping may be present as a bilateral disease with progressive unilateral or bilateral pain. Sometimes the patient has a history of trauma, and in some cases it is possible that the asymptomatic snapping was not recognized until it became painful.[14] Patients involved in certain activities, such as ballet, may be at risk for the development of this pathology as an insidious overuse phenomenon.

The frequency of snapping hip syndrome has been reported in up to 90% of elite ballet dancers and with bilateral involvement in 80%. The clinician must be careful to differentiate whether snapping hip is the true cause of groin pain and whether the problem is solely intraarticular, extraarticular, or both.[3]

Pathophysiology

The internal snapping phenomenon occurs as the iliopsoas tendon subluxes from lateral to medial, which typically occurs as the hip moves from flexion, abduction, and external rotation to extension and internal rotation.[16] The structure responsible for transiently impeding the translation of the iliopsoas, thus creating the snapping phenomenon, is a source of continuous controversy. The most popular theories are that the tendon snaps back and forth across the anterior aspect of the femoral head or the capsule or over the pectineal eminence. Other authors believe that an exostosis of the lesser trochanter can be the cause of the snapping.[14]

The external coxa saltans is frequently produced by a band formed by posterior thickening of the iliotibial band and anterior thickening of the gluteus maximus fibers. In hip extension, this band lies posterior to the greater trochanter but snaps over the greater trochanter with flexion.[14] In more severe cases, the phenomenon also may be reproduced with hip rotation. Tightness of the iliotibial band may be an exacerbating feature.[14] The iliotibial band is a long, nonelastic collagen structure that crosses both the hip and knee joints on the lateral thigh. The complex origin and insertion of this structure allows it to be taut during all motions of the hip. Any increase in this tension combined with repetitive motion can result in increased friction over the greater trochanter that may produce irritation and inflammation of the trochanteric bursa, as well as chronic degenerative changes such as fibrosis.[5]

Various biomechanical causes have been proposed to act as predisposing anatomic factors to increase tension, including femoral retroversion or anteversion, internal tibial torsion, excessive foot pronation, and ipsilateral long leg.[5,6] Another anatomic issue to consider is the wide insertion of the gluteus maximus muscle into the iliotibial tract. The broad coverage and wide area of action of this structure may be responsible for residual snapping, even after surgical release.[6] A case of snapping hip as a result of fibrosis of the band muscle attributed to repeated intramuscular injections has also been reported.[17]

Diagnosis

Clinical Presentation

Patients with internal snapping hip syndrome have chronic symptoms that begin with mildly painful snapping that grows in frequency and intensity over a period of months to years.[2] When this phenomenon is asymptomatic, no treatment is required.[3] Persons with a symptomatic internal snapping hip characteristically describe a painful clicking sensation emanating from deep within the anterior groin. Sometimes the pain may also be found at the ipsilateral flank. Patients can commonly pinpoint the area of pain on the groin and often volunteer to demonstrate the snapping.[15] Surgical treatment is indicated only for symptomatic cases that do not improve with conservative measures.[3]

Most external snapping hips are asymptomatic; however, repetitive motion in sports such as running, dancing, and rowing may also incite inflammation, pain, and disability.[6] The patient will describe a snapping or subluxation type sensation on the lateral aspect of the hip. The iliotibial snapping can be detected with the patient lying on his or her side and then passively flexing and extending the hip. In some cases the snapping phenomenon may be visible under the skin, and in other cases it may be palpated over the area of the greater trochanter by placing the fully extended palm over the area.[6]

A different form of external snapping hip is also described by some patients as the ability to "dislocate the hip," which is often demonstrated by rotating the affected hip while tilting the pelvis in the standing position. The voluntary "dislocators" are more frequently painless and should only be treated with stretching exercises of the iliotibial band.

Physical Examination

Examination of patients with internal snapping hip reveals medial groin pain centered at or just below the pelvic brim.[2] Physical examination of the internal snapping hip is performed with the patient in the supine position. The affected hip is flexed more than 90 degrees and extended to the neutral position (Fig. 86-1). This maneuver will reproduce the

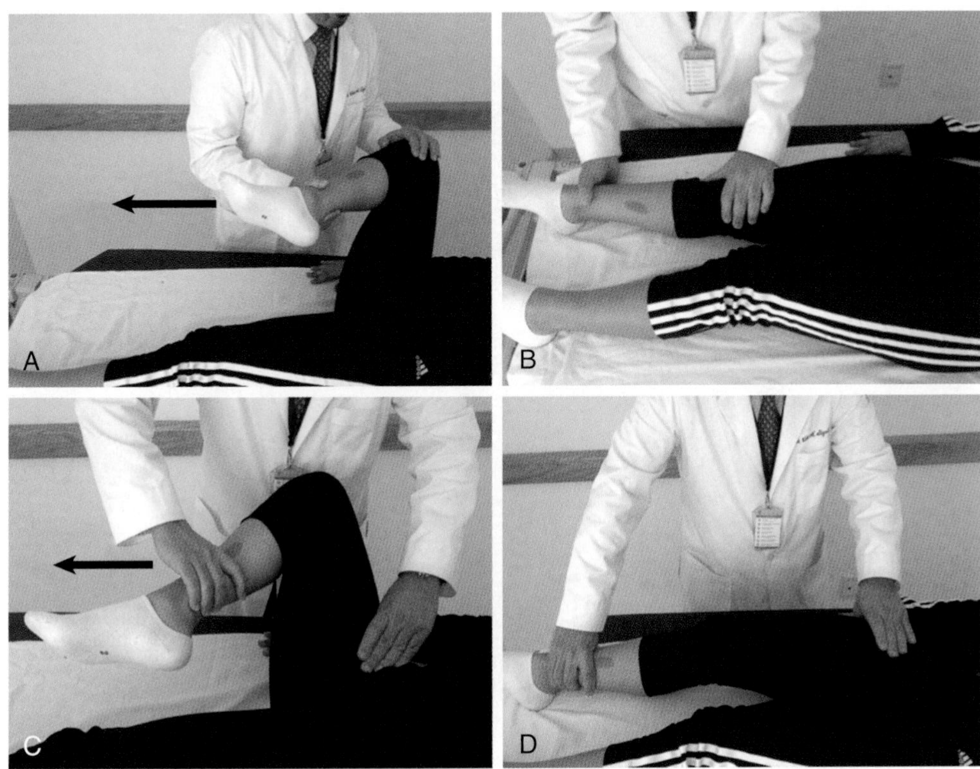

FIGURE 86-1 Physical examination of internal snapping hip syndrome in a right hip. **A** and **B,** The hip is flexed more than 90 degrees, abducted, and externally rotated as it is brought to extension with neutral rotation and abduction. The snapping phenomenon may be reproduced in the front of the groin. The snapping is frequently audible, or the patient may tell the examiner that the snapping occurs. **C** and **D,** The same examination maneuver described in **A** and **B** is reproduced, with the examiner's hand positioned in the front of the joint to detect the snapping phenomenon.

snapping phenomenon at the front of the groin. The snapping phenomenon usually cannot be observed through the skin but often produces an audible snap. Upon palpation, the snapping phenomenon is felt by placing the hand over the affected groin. The examiner can frequently reproduce the painful snapping by abduction and external rotation in flexion and by adduction and internal rotation while extending. Painful snapping with this maneuver is key to the diagnosis.[2] Occasionally the patient can reproduce the snapping phenomenon when walking as the hip goes into extension during the late stance phase of gait. When the snapping is symptomatic, the patient always has an apprehension response when it occurs. Other related findings are the presence of a C sign, a positive log roll test, or a positive impingement; however, those findings are more often associated with intraarticular hip pathology. More than 50% of patients with internal snapping hip have concomitant intraarticular hip pathology.[18]

Symptomatic external snapping hip syndrome is always accompanied with pain in the greater trochanteric region (Fig. 86-2). The pain is a result of greater trochanteric bursitis, inflammation of the iliotibial band itself, or abductor tendon pathology. A positive Ober test may also be found at physical examination (Fig. 86-3). The Trendelenburg gait may be seen in a person with an associated abductor muscle tear or weakness. A pathologic gait may not be present initially but will develop with fatigue of the abductor complex, which can be elicited with a Trendelenburg test (Fig. 86-4). This test consists of asking the patient to perform a single leg stand over periods of 10 seconds with a 10-second increment in each period; if abductor pathology is present, the sign becomes positive within 20 seconds.[18] The test is carried out comparatively.

Imaging

Plain radiographs usually appear normal, although in some cases a femoroacetabular impingement deformity may be documented. Iliopsoas bursography is useful and may document the snapping phenomenon dynamically when combined with fluoroscopy.[15] The main disadvantage of this technique is that it is dependent on the ability of the technician to reproduce the snapping during hip motion within the range of view of the C arm. Ultrasound is becoming increasingly useful as a dynamic noninvasive study that may document pathologic changes with the iliopsoas tendon and bursa, as well as the snapping phenomenon. With use of dynamic ultrasound, slippage of the tendon over bony prominences while the hip is extended may be demonstrated.[15,19] Iliopsoas ultrasonography also depends on the ability and experience of the examiner. More recently, ultrasonography has also been

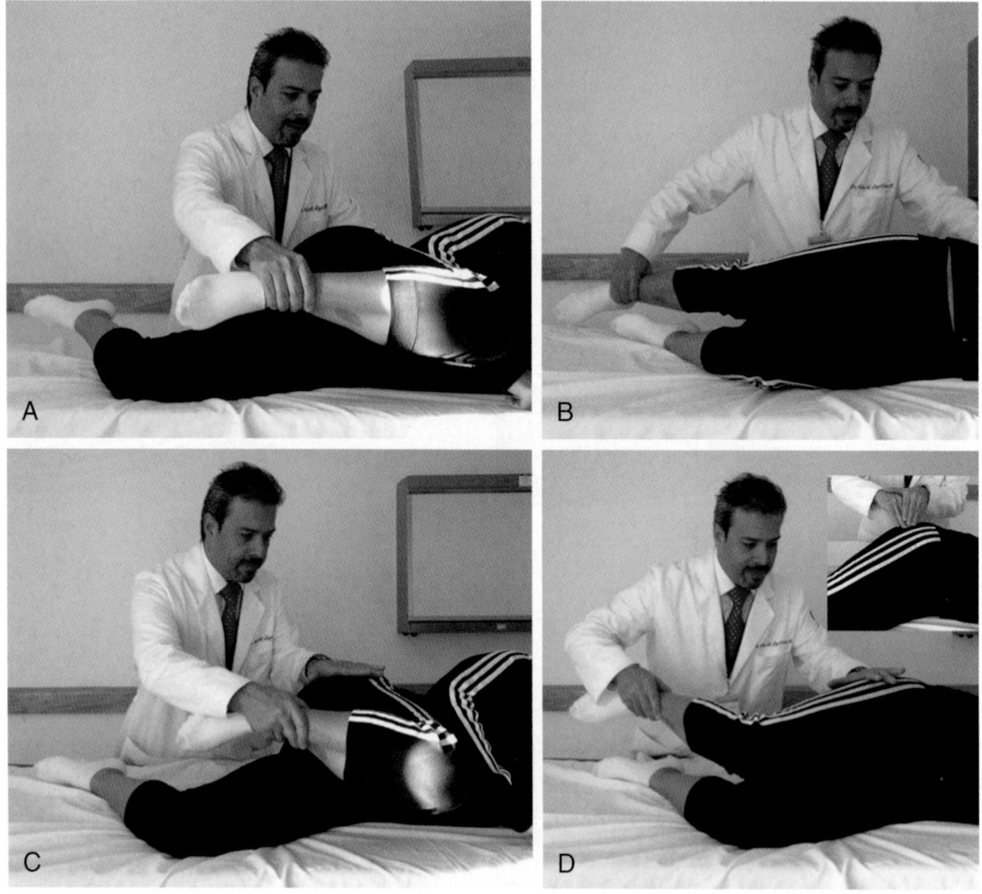

FIGURE 86-2 Physical examination of an external snapping hip syndrome. **A** and **B,** With the patient in the lateral decubitus position, the hip and knee are cycled through flexion and extension, which will reproduce the snapping phenomenon on the greater trochanteric area. The snapping may be observed through the skin, or the patient refers to it as it occurs. **C** and **D,** The examiner may palpate the snapping with the extended palm over the greater trochanteric area. **D,** *Upper right,* A tender spot is frequently found posterior to the greater trochanter.

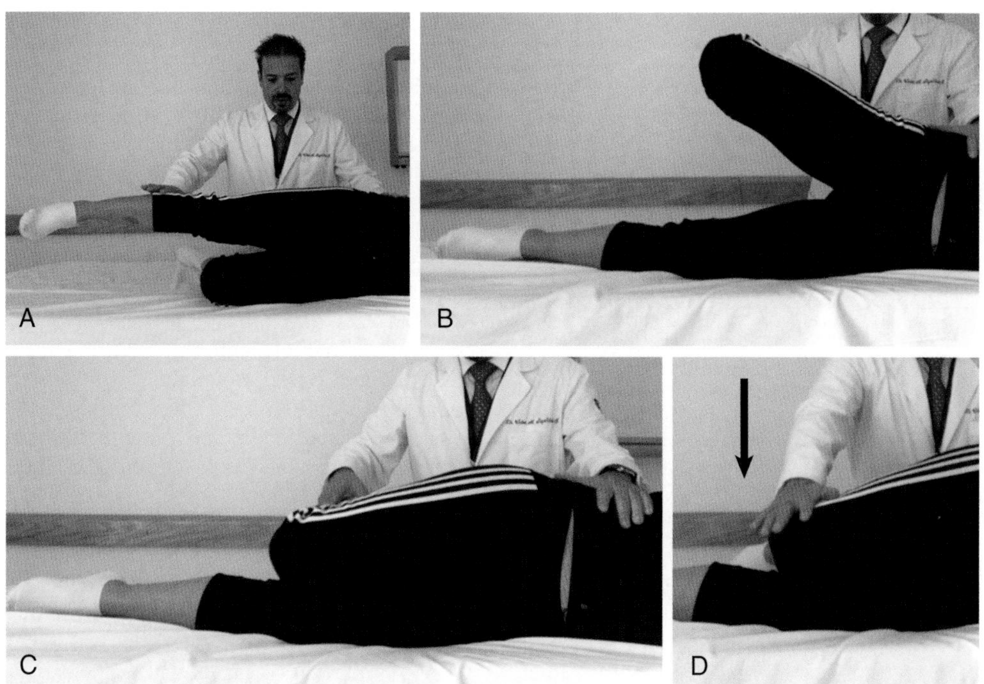

FIGURE 86-3 In this sequence, a lateral leg raise and the Ober test are presented. **A,** In the lateral decubitus position, the patient is asked to perform an active straight lateral leg raise. The examiner may then evaluate muscle strength by asking the patient to perform a lateral leg raise against force. **B,** With the patient in active hip abduction, the knee is flexed. **C,** The patient is asked to release active abduction. For a negative test, the knee should fold on the opposite knee (for a positive test, the hip remains abducted). **D,** If the test is positive, a spring effect may be found by pushing downward on the knee.

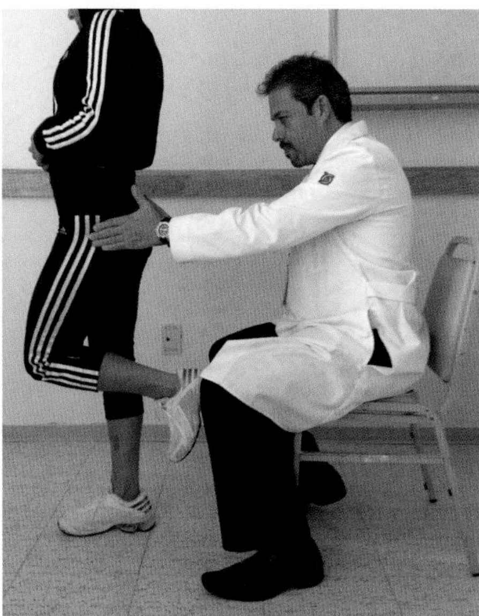

FIGURE 86-4 The Trendelenburg test. The examiner is seated behind the patient and puts his or her hands on both greater trochanteric areas; the patient is then asked to perform a single leg stand, and the examiner observes pelvic tilt. With a positive test the pelvis tilts toward the side of the elevated limb. A variation is to perform a fatigue Trendelenburg test by performing this test over a period of 10, 20, and 30 seconds. The test is always compared with the opposite side.

used to describe new mechanisms of iliopsoas snapping, such as the bifid iliopsoas tendon or snapping of the iliopsoas over the iliacus muscle and snapping of the iliopsoas tendon over paralabral cysts. Conventional magnetic resonance imaging can show tendonitis of the psoas or bursitis in some cases.[15] Magnetic resonance arthrography, however, is the preferred diagnostic study to evaluate persons who have a painful hip with internal snapping, because almost half of the patients with internal snapping hip syndrome have associated intraarticular hip pathology (Fig. 86-5). Magnetic resonance arthrography can show intraarticular pathology in addition to changes related to the iliopsoas tendon and bursa.[15]

Anteroposterior pelvis radiographs should always be performed to identify bony abnormalities, calcifications, or other pathology. Dynamic ultrasonography may document the snapping phenomenon and can also detect associated pathology such as tendonitis, bursitis or muscle tears, and iliopsoas bursitis.[6,14,19,20] Ultrasound can be useful to measure tendon thickness and bursa size. Magnetic resonance imaging is complementary. Axial T1-weighted images best demonstrate thickening of the iliotibial tract or the focal thickening of the anterior edge of the gluteus muscle, and with these images it also is possible to identify secondary atrophy of the remainder of the gluteus maximum muscle.[20]

Treatment

Nonoperative

Treatment of internal hip snapping is initially nonoperative and includes rest, stretching exercises, and use of oral antiinflammatory medications.[5] Steroid injections of the iliopsoas

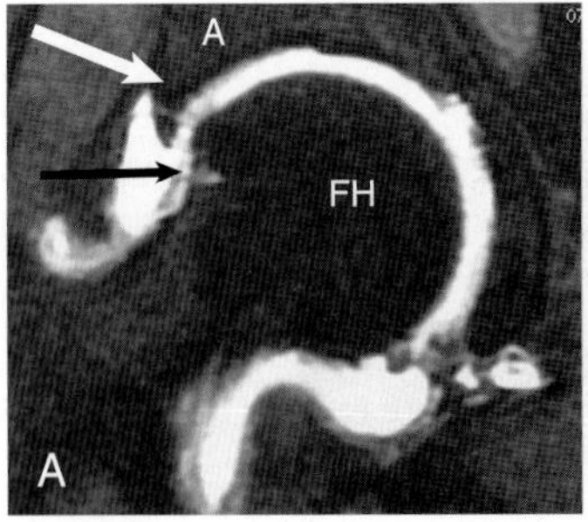

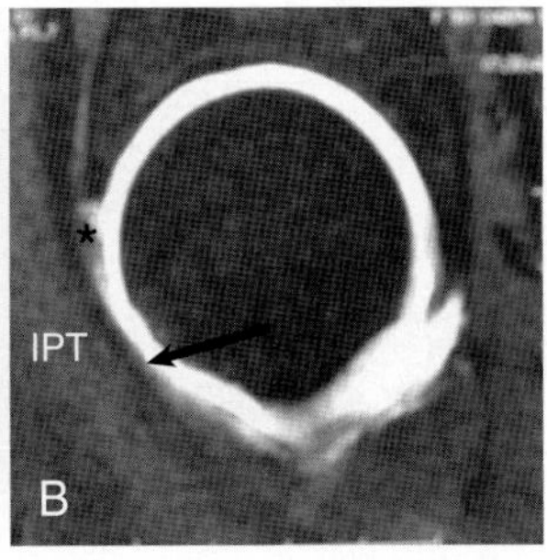

FIGURE 86-5 Magnetic resonance arthrogram of a right hip with PINCER impingement as a result of coxa profunda and an internal snapping hip. **A,** The white arrow indicates the acetabular (*A*) over coverage. The black arrow indicates an area of notching of the femoral head (*FH*) neck junction. **B,** In this sagittal image, the relationship between the iliopsoas tendon (*IPT*) and anterior capsule (*black arrow*) is demonstrated. The labrum (*asterisk*) is also in very close relationship with the anterior hip capsule and the IPT. Note that contrast is observed between the rim and the labrum, which corresponds to a tear.

bursa have also been used to treat this problem, with studies demonstrating relief of up to 3 months in 80% of the patients who received an injection.[9,10] In a series of 30 patients reported by Gruen et al.,[2] 19 patients (63%) improved with a 3-month period of stretching of the hip internal and external rotators and eccentric strengthening of the hip flexor and extensors.

In most cases of external snapping hip, nonoperative treatment should be attempted initially.[5] The patient should be educated about which offending activities to avoid, and most patients with symptoms improve with activity modification, stretching, and nonsteroidal antiinflammatory therapy. Formal physical therapy and corticosteroid infiltration of the greater trochanter bursa may also be helpful. Surgery should be considered for persons who do not respond to conservative treatment.

Operative Treatment: Internal Snapping Hip

Surgical treatment of internal snapping hip is reserved for symptomatic patients who do not improve after undergoing conservative treatment.[5] Surgical approaches include open and endoscopic procedures that involve either a release of the iliopsoas tendon or a lengthening of the muscle-tendon unit (MTU).[9]

Evaluation of the surgical anatomy of the iliopsoas tendon is important when performing a release. The level of the release will determine the volume of the tendon that is cut and the resulting volume of the muscle fibers that are not released. In a cross-sectional anatomic study of the iliopsoas tendon, Blomberg et al.[21] reported the average diameter and percentage of tendon and muscle at different levels. Using 20 embalmed cadavers, they measured the diameter of the MTU of the iliopsoas at the level of the labrum and the hip periphery and its insertion on the lesser trochanter. At each one of the described levels, they looked at the percentage of tendon and muscle. They reported that the average circumference of the iliopsoas MTU at the level of the labrum, the hip periphery, and the lesser trochanter was 68.3, 58, and 45.7 mm in diameter, respectively.[21] The MTU consisted of 40% tendon and 60% muscle at the level of the labrum, 53% tendon and 47% muscle at the level of the hip periphery, and 60% tendon and 40% muscle at the level of the lesser trochanter insertion (Fig. 86-6). Based on this information, a more proximal release will leave more muscle tissue intact and have less of an affect on the overall volume of the MTU. In theory, this approach may produce less functional compromise but also could be related to more frequency of recurrence of the snapping phenomenon after release.

Open Procedures for Iliopsoas Tendon

Surgical treatment for internal snapping hip was first described by Nunziata and Blumenfeld.[12] In this report, the authors performed lengthening of the iliopsoas tendon in two of three patients and found that the patients who underwent surgery had decreased pain and snapping of their hips. Schaberg et al.[13] reviewed eight patients with a snapping hip, six of whom had a lengthening procedure in which the tendon was partially divided near its insertion on the lesser trochanter through a modified anterior approach. These investigators found that two patients had a bony ridge on the anteromedial aspect of the lesser trochanter that was believed to contribute to the symptomatic snapping hip. The exostosis was removed. At a range of 1 to 8 months after surgery, five of the six patients were reported to be asymptomatic. Jacobson and Allen[22] reported a population of 14 patients treated by the partial division of the iliopsoas tendon below the pelvic brim near the lesser trochanter. Six of the patients had recurrence of the snapping, three patients reported weakness in hip

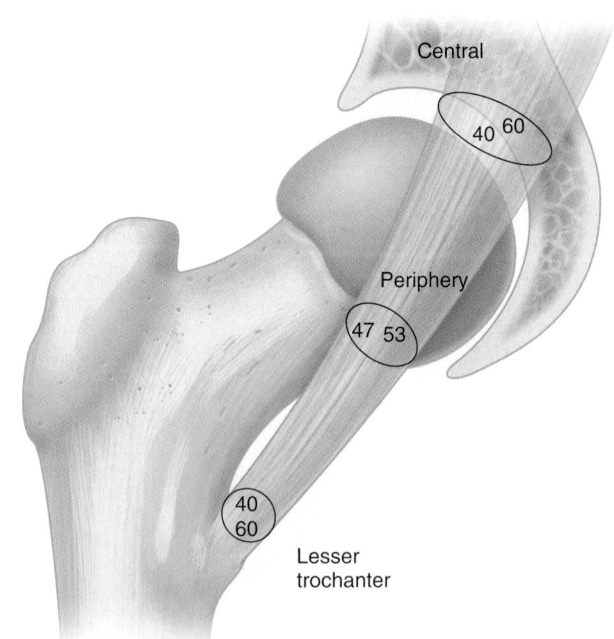

FIGURE 86-6 A schematic representation of the locations for iliopsoas tendon release. In all the techniques presented, only the tendinous portion of the iliopsoas is released. The central compartment release cuts 40% of the muscle tendon unit (MTU), the periphery release cuts 47% of the MTU, and the lesser trochanter iliopsoas tendon release cuts the 60% of the MTU.

flexion, and two required an additional operation.[22] The most common complication reported in this study was periincisional loss of sensation. Taylor and Clarke[23] reported 14 patients with snapping hip treated with partial iliopsoas tendon release below the pelvic brim, close to the insertion of the tendon on the lesser trochanter. Although all patients reported improvement of pain, two of the patients had postoperative weakness in the flexion of the hip above 90 degrees, and six patients continued to have snapping symptoms after surgery. Gruen et al.[2] described the fractional lengthening of the iliopsoas tendon in 11 subjects with no recurrence of snapping in any patient, and the pain relief achieved was the same as that reported by other authors. All of their procedures were performed with an ilioinguinal approach involving more proximal release of the iliopsoas tendon within the substance of the muscle, which allows a fractional lengthening to be performed directly over the pelvic brim. Proximal release of the tendon may protect the patient from flexion weakness by avoiding damage to the distal insertion of the tendon on the lesser trochanter.[2,7]

Endoscopic Release of the Iliopsoas Tendon

The traditional surgical techniques described for the treatment of painful hips due to snapping of the iliopsoas tendon have been open procedures. However, problems reported with these surgical approaches include morbidity from the approach, recurrent snapping tendon, persistent hip pain, and sensory nerve injuries caused by the surgical incision.[2,18] Endoscopic release of the iliopsoas tendon procedure avoids complications of open surgery and provides long-term relief from a painful internal snapping hip.[3,11]

Endoscopically, the iliopsoas tendon can be released at two different levels—at the insertion of the tendon on the lesser trochanter, or at the level of the hip joint through an anterior hip capsulotomy (the so-called *transcapsular technique*).[3,18] The release at the iliopsoas insertion can be performed from the central compartment or from the hip periphery. Either of these techniques may be performed in the supine or lateral decubitus position.[15]

At the level of the labrum, the iliopsoas tendon makes up about 40% of the MTU.[10] Some authors recommend performing the tenotomy at this level as opposed to at the lesser trochanter because the latter would be equivalent to the release of the entire iliopsoas muscle belly–tendon complex.[10] However, the clinical results and the frequency of complications for both techniques are not clear in the literature. Ilizaliturri et al.[3] found no statistical difference in the postoperative WOMAC scores between the insertion tendon release and transcapsular technique, and no complications were seen in a study of 19 patients.

Transcapsular Iliopsoas Tendon Release

Central Compartment Release

Iliopsoas tendon release from the central compartment is performed with the hip joint in traction.[18] The anterolateral portal is used as the viewing portal through which the anterior capsule is visualized with a 70-degree arthroscope. From the direct anterior portal, a radiofrequency hook probe or an arthroscopic banana knife is introduced to create an anterior hip capsulotomy (Fig. 86-7) relative to the 2- and 3-o'clock position of the labrum in a right hip or geographic zone 1. Fibers of the iliopsoas tendon are visualized through the capsulotomy. The tendon is further exposed using a mechanical shaver. A radiofrequency hook probe is used to release the tendon in a retrograde fashion, leaving the iliacus muscle intact.

Release from the Hip Periphery

Iliopsoas tendon release from the hip periphery is performed without traction.[18] A 70- or 30-degree arthroscope is positioned into the peripheral compartment anterior and inferior to the femoral neck through the anterolateral portal (Fig. 86-8). The medial synovial fold serves as the best landmark to identify the inferior aspect of the head and neck (at the 6-o'clock position). The proximal origin of the medial synovial fold at the inferior head-neck junction is visualized. The field of view is rotated to the anterior hip capsule. The mid anterior portal is used to introduce instruments into the peripheral compartment. A capsulotomy is performed between the zona orbicularis and the labrum, directly above the medial synovial fold, which exposes the iliopsoas tendon fibers. In some cases a natural communication between the anterior hip capsule and the iliopsoas bursa is already present at this level. The tendon is further exposed using a mechanical shaver, and the iliopsoas tendon is released in a retrograde fashion using a radiofrequency hook probe. The iliacus muscle is left intact behind the released iliopsoas tendon.

Iliopsoas Bursa Release

Using an accessory portal, a spinal needle is introduced into the iliopsoas immediately proximal to the lesser trochanter (Fig. 86-9). The anterior aspect of the proximal femur may be palpated to navigate the needle in the sagittal plane, and an image intensifier is used to navigate the needle in the coronal plane. With the needle in position directly proximal to the lesser trochanter, a guide wire is introduced and the cannulated hip arthroscopy instruments are used to establish a viewing portal. A 30-degree arthroscope is introduced, and the fibers of the iliopsoas tendon at its insertion on the lesser trochanter are identified. A second accessory portal is established, triangulating a spinal needle to the tip of the arthroscope. Once the needle is observed inside the iliopsoas bursa, a guide wire and cannulated hip arthroscopy instruments are used to establish a working portal. The iliopsoas tendon is further exposed with use of a mechanical shaver and released in a retrograde fashion with use of a radiofrequency hook probe.

Operative Treatment: External Snapping Hip

The objective of the surgical treatment of external snapping hip is to relax the iliotibial band over the greater trochanter to eliminate the snapping phenomenon. Different techniques have been described in the literature with variable results, and no evidence indicates that any one procedure is more beneficial than others.[5,14] Open iliotibial band release or lengthening has been the traditional surgical option to treat external snapping hip syndrome. Traditional surgical techniques include Z-plasty, diagonal osteotomy of the trochanter, anchoring of the iliotibial tract to the trochanter, cruciate incision with sutured flaps to the tract, resection of the posterior half of the tract at the gluteus maximus insertion, and ellipsoid resection

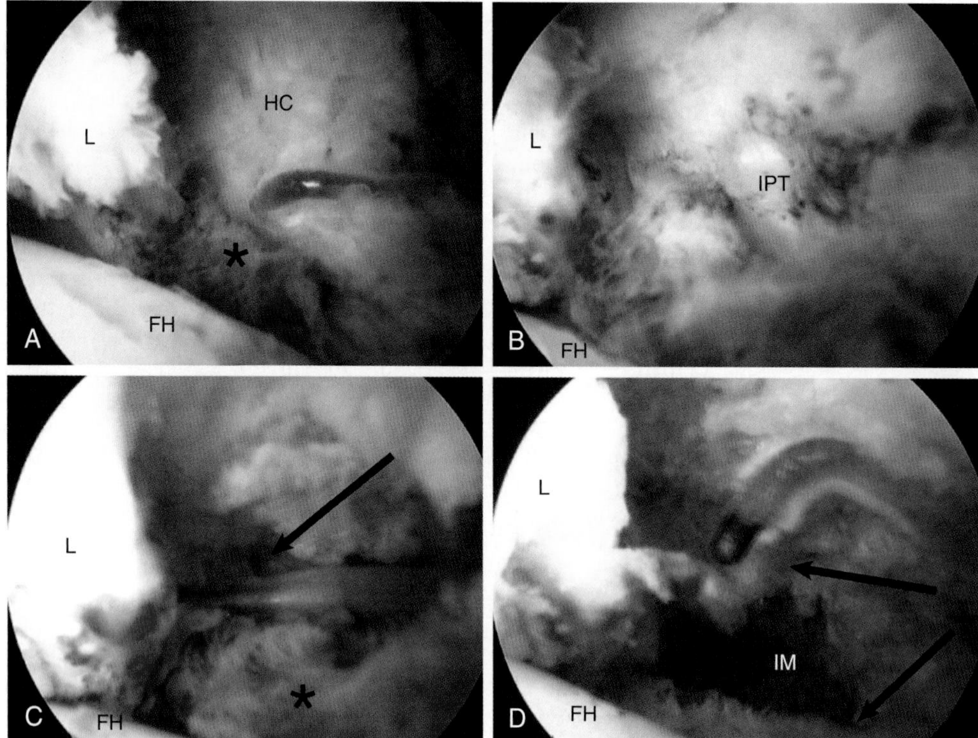

FIGURE 86-7 Arthroscopic sequence of a central compartment of iliopsoas tendon (*IPT*) release. **A,** The femoral head (*FH*) is to the bottom and the labrum (*L*) is to the left; a radiofrequency hook probe is used to perform an anterior cut on the hip capsule (*HC*) to expose the IPT. Note the severe inflammation of the hip capsule (*asterisk*). **B,** The FH is to the bottom and the L is to the left. The IPT is observed through the anterior hip capsulotomy. **C,** A radiofrequency hook probe is used to cut the IPT (*black arrow*) in a retrograde fashion. The FH is at the bottom and the L is at the left. **D,** The black arrows indicate the stumps of the IPT; the iliacus muscle (*IM*) is observed intact behind the stumps. The FH is at the bottom and the L is at the left.

of the tract over the trochanter.[5,6] Recent advances in minimal invasive surgery have led to significant evolution in the endoscopic treatment of external snapping hip syndrome.

Endoscopic Release of the Iliotibial Band

Outside-in Technique

The endoscopic outside-in technique for the iliotibial band has shown to be effective and reproducible, and results are compared with those of open procedures in the short term.[18] For this surgical procedure, our preference is to perform the endoscopic release in lateral position, similar to the setup for a total hip arthroplasty. Surgical drapes must allow free range of motion of the lower extremity to permit reproduction of the snapping phenomenon during surgery. No traction is necessary to access the greater trochanteric bursa and the iliotibial band. The greater trochanter is the main landmark for portal placement and is marked on the skin with use of a skin marker.

We use two portals: proximal trochanteric and distal trochanteric. The area of snapping should be between both portals to ensure iliotibial band release and will include the area that generates the problem. The skin area of snapping is marked and the space under the iliotibial band is infiltrated with 40 to 50 mL of saline solution. Next the inferior trochanteric portal is established with use of a standard arthroscopic cannula directed proximally to the site of the superior trochanteric portal. The blunt obturator is used to develop a working space above the iliotibial band. The site of the proximal trochanteric portal is identified endoscopically by inserting a needle at the portal landmark. The skin incision is made and a shaver is introduced to dissect subcutaneous tissue from the iliotibial band situated between the portals. The pump pressure should be kept low while working on the subcutaneous space to avoid complications with the skin, and hemostasis is important to allow clear visualization of the iliotibial band.

Once the iliotibial band is well visualized, a radiofrequency hook probe is introduced from the proximal trochanteric portal, and a 4- to 6-cm vertical retrograde cut is performed on the iliotibial band starting at the level of the inferior trochanteric portal (Fig. 86-10). The pump pressure can be increased after the vertical cut on the iliotibial band is complete. A transverse anterior cut of 2 cm in length is performed starting at the middle of the vertical cut. The resulting superior and inferior anterior flaps are resected with use of a shaver, developing a triangular defect on the anterior iliotibial band that will provide access to the posterior iliotibial band. Next a transverse posterior cut is started at the same level of the transverse anterior cut. This release is the most important and should be carried out until the snapping phenomenon is solved. Finally, the superior and inferior posterior flaps are resected, which results in a diamond-shaped defect on the iliotibial band (Fig. 86-11). The greater trochanter will rotate freely within the defect without snapping. The greater trochanteric bursa should be removed through the defect on the iliotibial band, and the abductor tendons should be inspected for tears.[18]

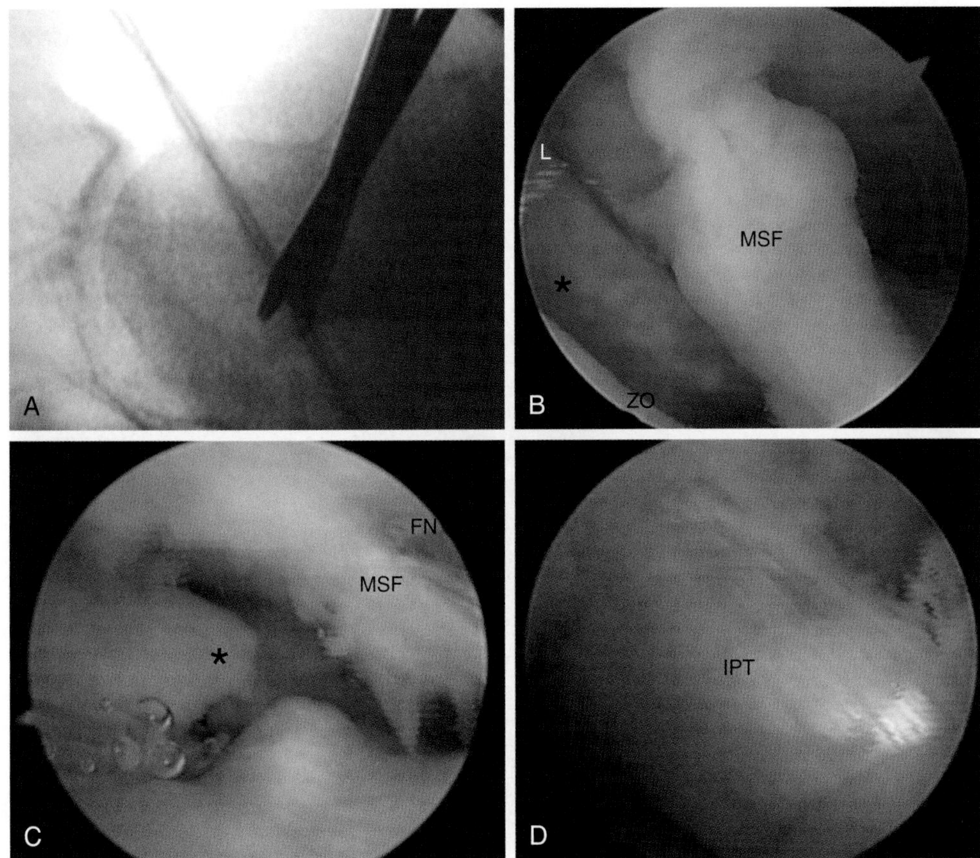

FIGURE 86-8 Peripheral release of the iliopsoas tendon (*IPT*). **A,** A fluoroscopy image demonstrates the position of an arthroscope and switching stick located anterior and medial to the femoral head (FH) inside the hip periphery. **B,** A corresponding arthroscopic photograph that shows the anatomy of the aforementioned area. The medial synovial fold (*MSF*) is at the center, the femoral neck (*FN*) is to the right, and the anterior inferior labrum (AL) is to the left. The anterior inferior zone orbicularis (ZO) is to the bottom. To access the IPT, a capsulotomy is performed between the AL and the ZO (*asterisk*). **C,** The MSF and FN are to the right. A capsulotomy is performed (*asterisk*) using a radiofrequency hook probe. **D,** The IPT is exposed through the capsulotomy.

Inside-out Technique

In the inside-out endoscopic technique, the release is performed from the peritrochanteric space deep to the iliotibial band.[24] Three portals are recommended: anterior, distal posterior, and proximal posterior. The anterior portal is placed 1 cm lateral to the anterior superior iliac spine within the interval between the tensor fascia lata and sartorius. This portal offers the best access into the peritrochanteric space. Once the portal is localized, a cannula is directed into the peritrochanteric space with the leg in full extension and held in 0 degrees of adduction and 10 to 15 degrees of internal

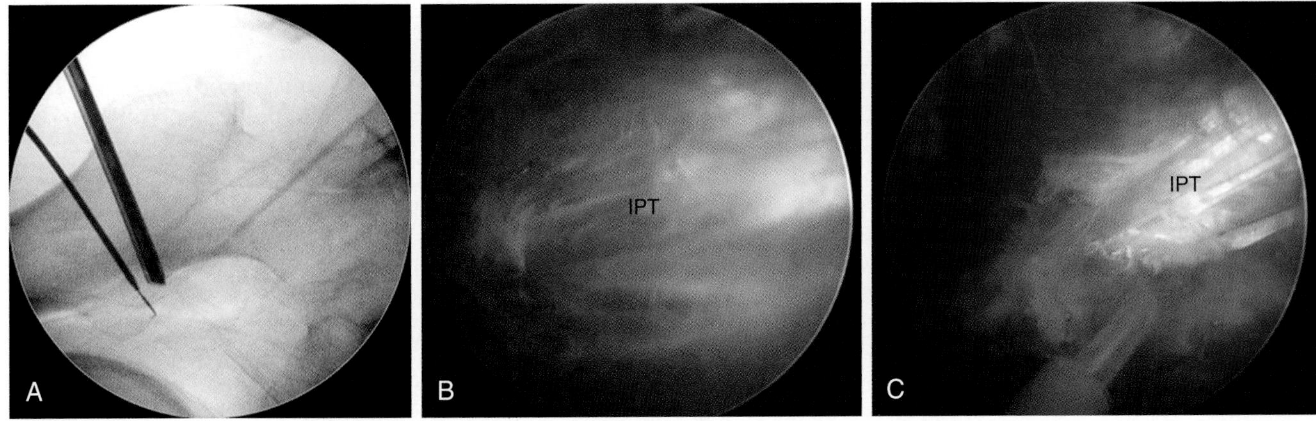

FIGURE 86-9 Release of the iliopsoas tendon (*IPT*) at the lesser trochanter. **A,** A fluoroscopic image of a right hip; note the arthroscope and the radiofrequency hook probe in position proximal to the lesser trochanter. **B,** A corresponding endoscopic photograph of the IPT. **C,** The IPT release with a radiofrequency hook probe.

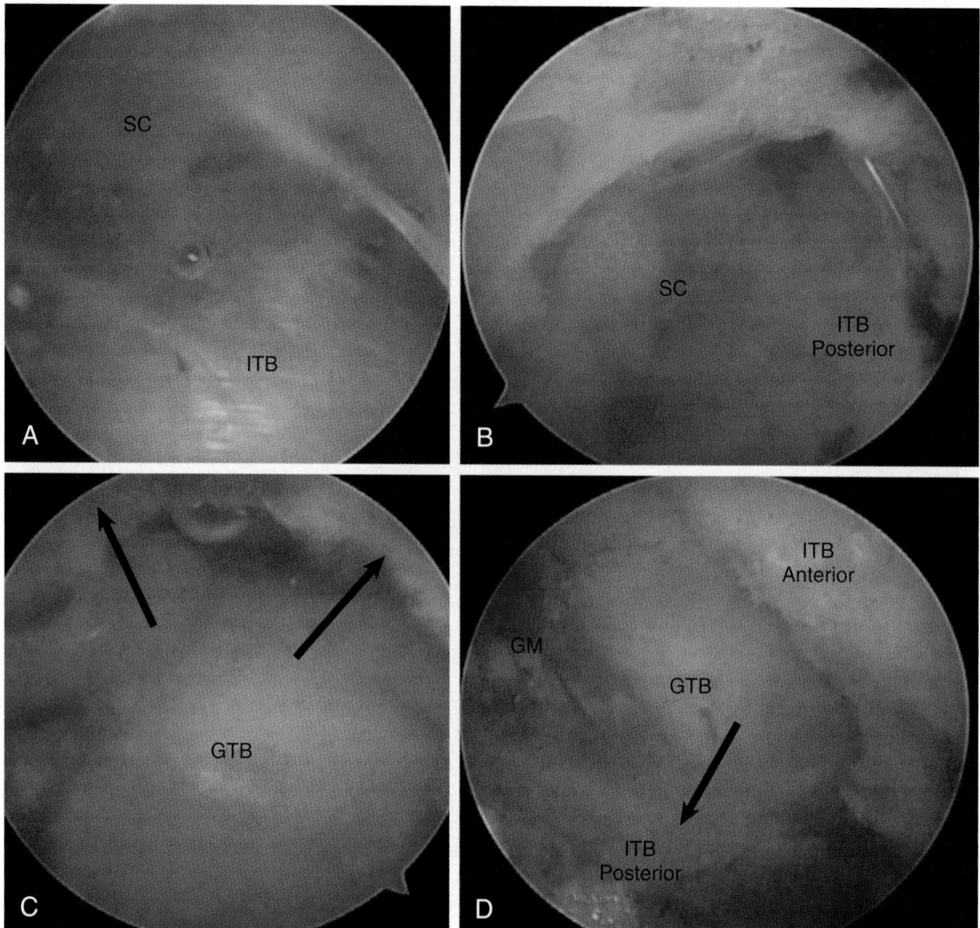

FIGURE 86-10 An endoscopic sequence demonstrating iliotibial band (*ITB*) release in a right hip. **A,** The endoscopic view of the subcutaneous space at the region of the greater trochanter; the subcutaneous (SC) tissue is observed to the left and the ITB is clearly exposed at the bottom of the photograph. A radiofrequency probe is used for hemostasis. **B,** The ITB is released vertically from distal to proximal. **C,** After the vertical and the anterior horizontal cuts are completed, the flaps are resected and the anterior half of the diamond release is obtained. The arrows point to the margins of the resected flaps. The greater trochanteric bursa (*GTB*) is observed through the defect of the ITB. **D,** The *black arrow* points to the side of the posterior horizontal release of the ITB. Note the insertion of the gluteus maximus (*GM*) on the posterior ITB. The greater trochanteric bursa is observed through the defect.

rotation.[24,25] The cannula is directed posteriorly and swept back and forth within the trochanteric bursa between the iliotibial band and the greater trochanter. With appropriate portal placement, a clear space beneath the iliotibial band can easily be established. Fluoroscopy may be helpful to confirm the cannula position.[19] A 70-degree arthroscope is introduced by the anterior portal and oriented distally. The initial view includes the insertion of the gluteus maximus into the posterior border of the iliotibial band. The distal posterior portal is established next between the tip of the greater trochanter and the vastus tubercle along the posterior one third of the greater trochanteric midline followed by proximal posterior portal placement proximal to the tip of the greater trochanter in line with the distal posterior portal. Proper portal placement is the key in the appropriate understanding of the peritrochanteric space. Inspection should proceed in a counterclockwise fashion starting distally and posterior at the gluteus maximus insertion and then proceeding proximally and anterior toward the vastus lateralis. The arthroscope should be turned toward the iliotibial band. The release should be performed along the posterolateral portion of the greater trochanter, beginning at the vastus tubercle insertion and extending to the tip of the greater trochanter in a z-type release of 1 cm anterior, 3 cm distal, and 1 cm posterior.[24,26]

Complications

Surgical treatment of internal and external hip snapping is associated with minimal complications. Complications related to open treatment are typically from the morbidity of the approach. Persistence or recurrence of the snapping phenomenon, which can be considered failure of the treatment, may occur with incomplete or insufficient release. Flexion or abduction weakness may be seen with excessive release and/or injury to surrounding muscles in internal or external snapping hip, respectively. Heterotopic ossification may result from iatrogenic injury to the muscles around the hip[18]; it is more commonly encountered with iliopsoas release at the level of the lesser trochanter, and prophylaxis with indomethacin or another antiinflammatory agent may help reduce risk. In the surgical treatment of external snapping hip, the sciatic nerve traverses in close proximity to the posterior

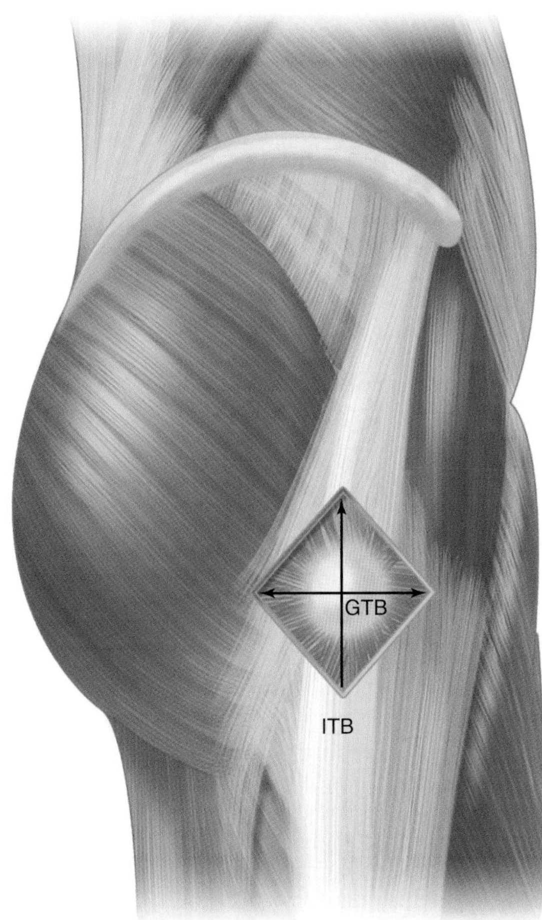

FIGURE 86-11 A schematic demonstration of the release technique of the iliotibial band (*ITB*) endoscopically. The vertical arrow shows the direction of the first cut; the second and third cuts are demonstrated by the horizontal arrows. By resection of the resulting flaps, a diamond shape defect is obtained of the ITB and the greater trochanteric bursa (*GTB*) is observed through the defect.

margin of the greater trochanter and should be protected when surgery of the peritrochanteric space is performed. More studies and follow-up are needed to identify and describe possible complications.

Discussion

The objective of this chapter is to present the general aspects of the snapping hip. Painless snapping is common and usually does not require treatment beyond stretching and activity modification. Initial treatment for the painful snapping phenomenon should be conservative with rest, stretching exercises, and use of oral antiinflammatory medications. Therapy and injections are also options. Surgical procedures are indicated for refractory cases, with a trend toward endoscopic release rather than use of a traditional open technique. A thorough understanding of the anatomy around the hip is required for the effective and safe treatment of the snapping hip.

For a complete list of references, go to expertconsult.com.

Suggested Readings

Citation: Ilizaliturri VM, Chaidez C, Villegas P, et al: Prospective randomized study of 2 different techniques for endoscopic iliopsoas tendon release in the treatment of internal snapping hip syndrome. *Arthroscopy* 25(2):159–163, 2009.

Level of Evidence: I (randomized controlled trial)

Summary: The authors evaluated short-term results of two different techniques of endoscopic iliopsoas tendon release for the treatment of internal snapping hip syndrome. They found no clinical difference in the results of the iliopsoas tendon release at the level of the lesser trochanter or at the level of the hip joint.

Citation: Ilizaliturri VM, Martínez-Escalante FA, Chaidez PA, et al: Endoscopic iliotibial band release for external snapping hip syndrome. *Arthroscopy* 22(5):505–510, 2006.

Level of Evidence: IV (therapeutic case series)

Summary: This prospective study describes an endoscopic iliotibial band release for the treatment of external snapping hip syndrome. Ten of 11 patients had good results, with an average 2-year follow-up. One patient had a nonpainful recurrence of snapping hip. The results are comparable with those reported for open procedures.

Citation: Blomberg JR, Zellner BS, Keene JS: Cross-sectional analysis of iliopsoas-muscle-tendon units at the sites of arthroscopic tenotomies. *Am J Sports Med* 39(1):58S–63S, 2011.

Level of Evidence: Controlled cadaveric laboratory study

Summary: In this very interesting cadaveric study, the authors describe the average circumference and percentage of muscle and tendon of the iliopsoas muscle-tendon unit (MTU) at the three levels where the arthroscopic tenotomies are usually performed. The authors found a clinical relevance of releasing the iliopsoas tendon at the level of the lesser trochanter, preserving 40% of the MTU.

Citation: Wettstein M, Jung J, Dienst M: Arthroscopic psoas tenotomy. *Arthroscopy* 22(8):907e1–907e4, 2006.

Level of Evidence: IV (therapeutic case series)

Summary: The arthroscopic release of the psoas tendon through the anterior capsule is described. The authors described the application of this technique in nine patients with no complications, and hip flexion strength was restored to normal within 3 months.

Citation: Sun Choi Y, Moon Lee S, Yong Song B, et al: Dynamic sonography of external snapping hip syndrome. *J Ultrasound Med* 7:753–758, 2002.

Level of Evidence IV (diagnosis case series)

Summary: The authors describe a series of seven cases of painful external snapping hip evaluated by dynamic sonography. They analyzed real-time images and found sudden abnormal displacement of the iliotibial band or gluteus maximus muscle overlying the greater trochanter during the hip motion.

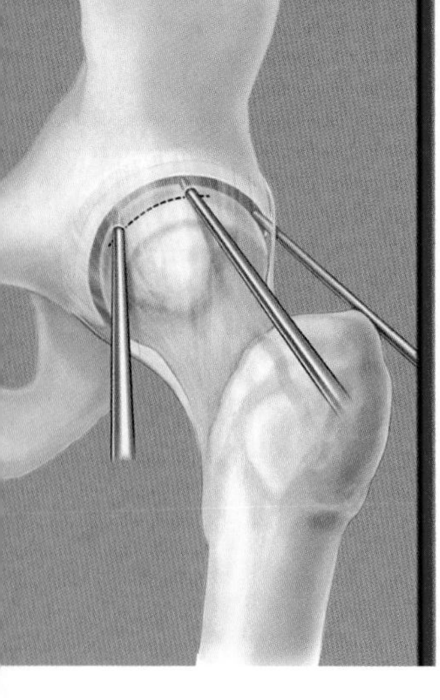

87

Hip and Thigh Contusions and Strains

SEAN McMILLAN • BRIAN BUSCONI • MICHAEL MONTANO

The muscles that surround the hip are vulnerable to injury from direct impact (contusion) or forceful contraction of a stretched muscle (strain). This chapter will cover contusions and strains around the hip joint. Hamstring injuries is covered in Chapter 88.

Contusions

Contusions are the most common injury to the hip, thigh, and pelvis. Collisions with other athletes or falls to the ground are the most common cause of contusions. Contusions can be superficial and limited to the subcutaneous tissue, or they can be deep and involve the bone, muscle, and ligaments. When associated with muscle involvement, contusions can result in slow bleeding with significant hematoma formation. Depending on the depth of the contusion and the extent of the injury, symptoms may occur immediately or after a 24- to 48-hour delay. Often, particularly with superficial contusions, treatment is of short duration and is based on the patient's symptoms. Patients generally have a rapid return to play. With the diagnosis of a deep contusion, however, the treatment period may be extended. Aside from icing, treatment should be delayed 48 hours to ensure that all bleeding has stopped. After 48 hours, treatment with antiinflammatory drugs, heat, massage, and physical therapy is implemented. Rehabilitation should be aimed at maintaining flexibility and muscle mass. Range of motion (ROM) should be monitored because patients are prone to the development of myositis ossificans after sustaining deep contusions involving the muscle.

Iliac Crest Contusion

Iliac crest contusion, commonly known as a hip pointer, is an anterior pelvic contusion that commonly affects athletes involved in contact sports. These contusions result from either a direct fall onto the iliac crest or from a direct blow, as seen in football or hockey.[1,2]

History

The athlete will almost immediately note pain over the iliac crest and/or greater trochanter after a fall or collision. He or she will note an inability to ambulate without a limp and pain with side-to-side or attempted crossover movements.[3]

Physical Examination

Examination of the injured athlete will reveal an antalgic gait, pain with palpation of the pelvic brim, bruising, and swelling. Active ROM of the hip will be decreased. Strength testing will demonstrate a marked decrease in any or all of the following muscle groups, depending on the location of the contusion: hip flexors; sartorius and rectus femoris; the internal and external obliques; the tensor fascia lata; the gluteus medius; the latissimus dorsi; and the paraspinal muscles.[3,4]

Imaging

Diagnosis of a hip pointer is made primarily on the basis of the history and physical examination. Radiographs are used only to rule out further injury, such as a fracture. Adolescent athletes are susceptible to avulsion fractures and may require a radiograph should an avulsion injury be suspected. Rarely, magnetic resonance imaging (MRI) or ultrasound are needed; however, some investigators have advocated their role in the evaluation of hematoma formation in an effort to quantify return to play.[3]

Treatment Options

Nonoperative treatment with protection rest, ice, compression, and elevation (PRICE) is central to treatment of hip pointers. Crutches may be used for the first few days. Ice, rest, and compression should be instituted for the first 48 hours to decrease the risk of hematoma formation. Antiinflammatory agents also may be used during the first 5 to 7 days. Beginning on day 3, the athlete may begin painless ROM activities. Some investigators have advocated delivery of a cortisone injection to the affected area to decrease pain and swelling; however, the risks of such injections must be weighed. Physical therapy may be initiated once a painless

AUTHORS' PREFERRED TECHNIQUE

Iliac Crest Contusion

Our preferred technique is to initiate PRICE and use of crutches for the initial 24 hours. A repeat physical examination in the office should be undertaken within 3 to 4 days of the injury. Provided an avulsion fracture is not suspected, ROM exercises and gentle stretches are begun. A localized cortisone injection is considered for athletes who are not progressing as rapidly as anticipated. In those instances, activities are ceased for 48 to 72 hours, and rehabilitation is then resumed in earnest. Return to play is expected in 2 to 4 weeks once the athlete has completed strength testing and sport-specific drills.

ROM has been established. Therapy should include stretches, sport-specific massage, and strengthening. Surgery is rarely indicated for hip pointer injuries; however, concomitant injuries such as sports hernias must be ruled out.[5]

Return to Play

Return to play is anticipated 2 to 4 weeks after the time of injury. Sport-specific drills and strength testing of the affected limb must be completed prior to resumption of competitive activities. Upon returning to activities, appropriate padding should be worn to prevent reinjury.[3,6]

Results

The treatment of hip pointers has yielded excellent results. Almost all athletes are able to return to their previous level of competition and performance once the injury has sufficiently healed.[3,4,7]

Complications

Complications after hip pointers are rare. The complications most commonly seen include hematoma formation, cutaneous nerve injury, or myositis ossificans. Missed fractures or avulsions injuries are rare complications.[3,5,7]

Quadriceps Contusion

The quadriceps consists of the rectus femoris and the vastus musculature (medialis, lateralis, and intermedius; Fig. 87-1). Quadriceps contusions are the result of a direct blow or trauma to the thigh. They typically occur in the anterior or lateral compartment and are most commonly associated with football, soccer, rugby, or high-speed traumas. The pathophysiology associated with quadriceps contusions involves microtrauma to the muscle fibers with resultant swelling and edema. More significant contusions can also result in hemorrhage formation, myositis ossificans, or even tears.

Jackson and Feagin[8] established a classification system based on knee flexion. They describe the muscle contusion as mild, moderate, or severe. Forty-eight hours after injury, mild contusions are able to flex greater than 90 degrees; moderate contusions, from 45 to 90 degrees; and severe contusions, less than 45 degrees (Table 87-1). This classification helps guide counseling and treatment, and resolution occurs on days 6.5, 56, and 72, respectively. No corresponding MRI classification system has been developed. Persons with injuries classified as moderate to severe contusions were significantly more likely to experience myositis ossificans than were persons with mild contusions.[8,9]

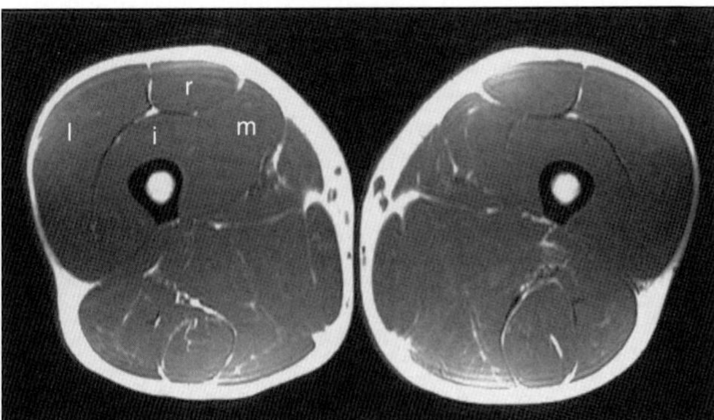

FIGURE 87-1 Cross-sectional anatomy of the thigh on a T1-weighted axial magnetic resonance image. The quadriceps is composed of the rectus femoris (*r*), vastus lateralis (*l*), vastus medialis (*m*), and vastus intermedius (*i*).

TABLE 87-1

CLASSIFICATION OF QUADRICEPS CONTUSIONS

Grade	Range of Motion
Mild	>90 degrees
Moderate	45-90 degrees
Severe	<45 degrees

History

Typically the patient will present on the field with a chief complaint of pain, lack of movement, or explosiveness and an antalgic gait. Twenty-four to 48 hours later, the patient may note similar or amplified symptoms, with noticeable limitations of knee ROM, thigh pain, loss of function, and swelling.[9] As previously stated, the mechanism of injury is usually a helmet or a severe kick to the thigh.

Physical Examination

Physical examination begins by evaluating the gait of the patient as he or she walks. Typically an antalgic gait is noted in persons with a moderate to severe contusion. A localized physical examination will note a tender, swollen, and oftentimes ecchymotic thigh in the area corresponding to the blunt trauma that was sustained. The thigh should be compared with the contralateral side as well. Palpation of the affected thigh may yield a palpable defect found in persons with severe contusions, indicating a partial or complete tear. In addition, a firm thigh compared with the contralateral side has been associated with longer recovery times.[10] However, the most important component of the physical examination is the ROM of the knee, because this component correlates with the severity of the injury and the anticipated return to activity.[9,10] Rarely, symptoms of an anterior thigh compartment syndrome can be identified on the basis of the physical examination.[10]

Imaging

Plain radiographs may be taken in the initial setting to rule out fracture; however, they typically have a low yield if a thorough history and physical examination are conducted. However, radiographs may have a more substantial role 2 to 4 weeks after injury if a firm mass is palpated to evaluate for developing myositis ossificans.[11,12]

MRI and ultrasound also may be used to evaluate the extent of the muscular edema and hemorrhage; however, no level I studies have shown that imaging evaluations will accurately correlate with the severity of the contusion or predict return a play better than the Jackson and Feagin knee flexion classification.[8,10,13,14]

Treatment Options

Nonoperative Treatment

The treatment of quadriceps contusions is usually managed in a nonoperative or conservative fashion (Table 87-2).

TABLE 87-2

CLINICAL GRADING SYSTEM FOR STRAINS

Grade	Muscle Tearing	Strength Loss	Pain	Physical Examination: Muscle Defect
I	Minor	Minimal/none	Mild	Absent
II	Moderate	Moderate/severe	Moderate/severe	Possible palpable defect
IIIA	Severe	Severe	Severe	Frequent palpable defect (complete rupture of musculotendinous unit)
IIIB	Severe	Severe	Severe	Frequent palpable defect (avulsion fracture at the tendon's origin or insertion)

Depending on the severity of the injury, some athletes may be able to continue their activity and present after competition or training for evaluation. Based on military studies, knee immobilization with the knee flexed to 120 degrees for the initial 24 hours is recommended.[15] Severe contusions may benefit from flexion immobilization for up to 48 hours.[9,15] This immobilizations can be achieved with either a hinged knee brace with locking capabilities, a compressive elastic wrap, or an anteriorly placed splint. Ice and compression should also be initiated in the first 24 to 48 hours, followed by elevation (the PRICE protocol). After the initial period of flexion, active, pain-free ROM exercises should be initiated. For severe contusions, crutches may be used until quadriceps control has returned. In these cases, physical therapy may be warranted, as well as the use of electrical stimulation. Ryan et al.[9] demonstrated a shortened recovery time for the moderate and severe groups from 56 to 19 days and from 72 to 21 days, respectively, via utilization of the aforementioned protocol. After return to pain-free motion, patients are allowed to return to noncontact sport-specific training. Return to contact sports is allowed after the thigh firmness has resolved and the muscle is not tender to palpation. If the patient is involved in a contact sport, a thigh pad with a ring should be recommended to minimize recurrence (Fig. 87-2).[9,15]

Nonsteroidal antiinflammatory drugs (NSAIDs) are used initially to decrease pain and swelling, but long-term use is discouraged. However, for persons with severe contusions or contusions with firm masses that do not dissipate in the initial 7 to 10 days, NSAIDs may be used to prevent heterotopic bone formation or myositis ossificans. Although randomized controlled studies have not been performed to examine the effectiveness of NSAIDs in the treatment of myositis ossificans, their presumed effectiveness is based on animal studies and reports of their usage in patients who have had a total hip replacement.[15-17]

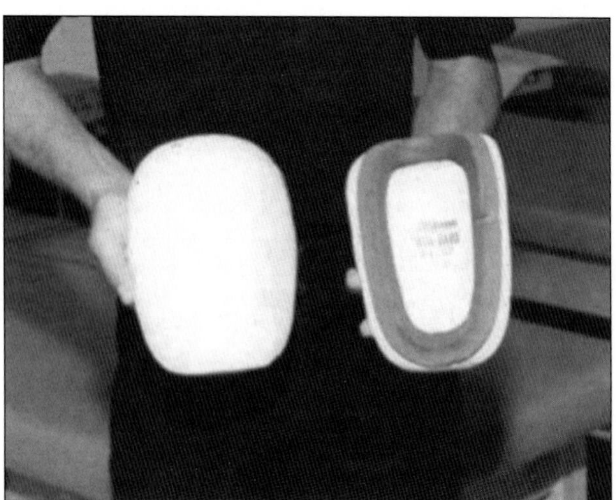

FIGURE 87-2 A thigh pad with a ring.

Operative Treatment

Operative treatment of quadriceps contusions is primarily reserved for persons with compartment syndromes.[18-20] Aspiration or surgical decompression of a thigh hematoma has been reported; however, no literature is available to support the effectiveness of these treatments.[18] Aspiration of knee effusions associated with severe contusions may decrease painful ROM, but support of this treatment is anecdotal. Other surgical considerations are reserved for partial or complete quadriceps tears or avulsion off the patella. Operative treatment of myositis ossificans should be reserved for patients with symptomatic loss of motion, pain, and strength once bone maturation has been demonstrated on a three-phase bone scan. Such treatment usually is performed 12 to 24 months after the time of injury.[21-23]

Postoperatively, compressive dressings, ice, rest, elevation, and standard surgical site care should be instituted. Again, early ROM is critical to increase healing and decrease the risk of heterotopic bone formation.

Decision-Making Principles

The ROM classification system by Jackson and Feagin[8] currently serves as the gold standard for the treatment and prognosis of thigh contusions. As a rule, nonoperative treatment should be pursued when possible, provided compartment syndrome has not been identified. The aforementioned military studies have demonstrated the quickest return to activity with immediate flexion of the affected knee to 120 degrees during the initial 24 to 48 hours from the time of injury. Subsequent early range of active ROM should follow to prevent heterotopic bone formation and to increase rates of return to play.[9,11] Heterotopic bone formation should be managed with the previously outlined contusion rehabilitation protocol and may be monitored with triple-phase bone scans to evaluate for skeletal maturity. Surgical intervention should only be considered for myositis ossificans if loss of strength and ROM has not resolved during the ensuing months. Bony maturation must be identified prior to excision to prevent local recurrence.[23-25]

AUTHORS' PREFERRED TECHNIQUE

Quadriceps Contusion

Timely evaluation of the patient should be undertaken to assess the severity of the contusion and to rule out more severe sequelae such as compartment syndrome. Ice, knee flexion, and a gentle compressive wrap are instituted if assessment takes place on the field. For patients with moderate to severe contusions, we prefer to institute immediate knee flexion to 120 degrees with a locked, hinged knee brace. Use of ice and a compressive wrap or sleeve is also instituted with rest. The patient is reevaluated within 24 to 48 hours by one of us or a therapist, and active ROM of the knee is begun, with a greater than 120-degree return to ROM desired as soon as possible. Electrical stimulation is added as warranted. If no contraindication exists, NSAIDs are begun at prescription-strength dosage for 5 to 7 days around the clock. However, they are discontinued if the patient cannot tolerate them. Noncontact training is permitted once quadriceps control and painless full ROM has returned, which is typically seen in 10 to 14 days. Full contact is permitted at the 3- to 4-week mark provided no further setbacks occur and if a thigh pad is worn. For patients who demonstrate worsening symptoms at the 14- to 21-day mark, radiographs are repeated and return to sporting activities is tabled.

Return to Play

A mild contusion may be managed symptomatically with ROM exercises and NSAIDs, thus allowing the athlete to continue to competition or training. Noncontact training is permitted once quadriceps control and painless full ROM has returned, which is typically seen in 10 to 14 days. Full contact is permitted at the 3- to 4-week mark provided no further setbacks occur and if a thigh pad is worn. The patient should be seen and cleared by a physician, and dedicated strength testing may be warranted to ensure the patient's safety.[8-10]

Results

A review of the literature on management and outcomes after thigh contusions is mostly based on case studies or anecdotal evidence, with some exceptions. Nonetheless, most reports note good to excellent results, with almost all athletes retuning to play. Ryan et al.[9] demonstrated a shortened recovery time for the moderate and severe groups from 56 to 19 days and from 72 to 21 days, respectively, with utilization of immediate flexion of the knee to 120 degrees, followed by early ROM exercises. These findings were echoed by Aronen et al.[15]

Complications

Myositis ossificans and the sequelae of thigh compartment syndromes are two significant complications associated with quadriceps contusions. In their military studies, Ryan et al.[9] identified the greatest risk factors for myositis ossificans: knee flexion less than 120 degrees, sustaining the injury while playing football, having a previous quadriceps injury, experiencing a delay in treatment greater than 3 days, and having an ipsilateral knee effusion. Myositis ossificans is generally associated with a severe contusion and has a reported occurrence rate of 9% to 14%.[26-28]

Thigh compartment syndrome is rare, and treatment of this condition remains controversial. Most authors advocate emergent fasciotomies, but some reports in the literature advocate nonsurgical intervention, even when compartment pressure standards are met for a diagnosis of compartment syndrome.[18-20,29] The rationale for this proposal is derived from Robinson et al.[29] and others, who note that in cases of sports-related thigh compartment syndromes with pressures greater than 55 mm Hg, no adverse sequelae were identified at 1 year with a return to preinjury strength and ROM.[29] Standard compartment syndrome measurement should be taken, and identification is made on the basis of one of the following criteria: compartment pressures of 30 mm Hg, 45 mm Hg, or less than 30 mm Hg from diastolic pressure, as identified in different studies.[30-32]

Future Considerations

Future consideration should be given to the pursuit of level I and II studies on the management of quadriceps contusions. Additionally, exploration of the nonoperative management of thigh compartment syndrome is also warranted.

Groin Contusions

Groin contusions involve the adductor musculature and usually occur from a direct blow to the inner thigh. They are often seen in soccer players and cyclists (Fig. 87-3). Aside from standard contusion treatment of ice, antiinflammatory drugs, physical therapy, and gradual return to play, the treating clinician should be aware of the possibility that vascular complications may develop, such as phlebitis and thrombosis. Ultrasound is a useful noninvasive method of diagnosing vascular complications.

Myositis Ossificans

Myositis ossificans is heterotopic ossification in an area of muscle, soft tissue, or disrupted periosteum (Fig. 87-4). Although this disease process can occur without a history of trauma, athletes can usually describe a sentinel event that causes a hematoma formation. The hematoma organizes, and calcium deposits are formed by the body. In a process that is not entirely understood, osteoblasts invade the formed

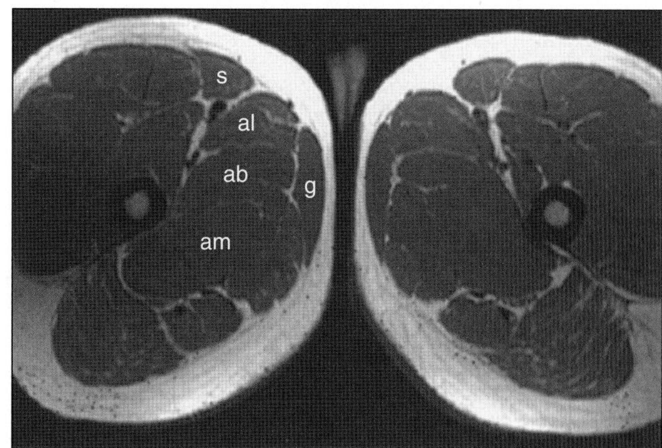

FIGURE 87-3 Cross-sectional anatomy of the thigh on a T1-weighted axial magnetic resonance image. The musculature of the medial thigh includes the adductor longus (*al*); adductor brevis (*ab*); adductor magnus (*am*); gracilis (*g*); and sartorius (*s*).

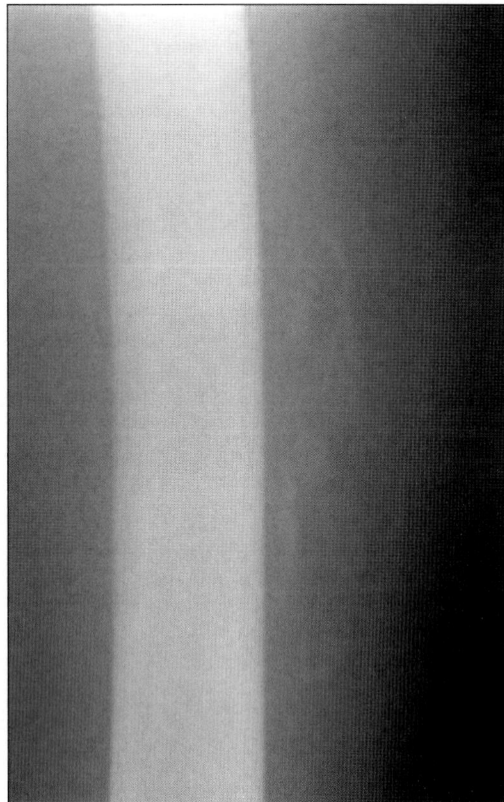

FIGURE 87-4 Myositis ossificans of the quadriceps.

hematoma and begin to make bony spicules.[33] This process tends to occur near joints and at tendon origins, but it can occur anywhere along the course of a muscle. The process can start as soon as 1 week after injury and can be detected on plain films a minimum of 3 weeks after injury. Patients present with a rapid enlargement within the soft tissues, decreased range of motion, and significant pain 1 to 2 weeks after injury. The patient has swelling and warmth at the site, as well as an increased erythrocyte sedimentation rate and serum alkaline phosphatase level.[23] Any treatment modalities implemented should not promote hematoma formation. Massage and manipulation should be avoided. Therapy should consist of active stretching and strengthening. Passive ROM should be delayed for at least 3 to 6 months.[34] For patients with refractory loss of ROM, surgery should be considered. Surgery, if warranted, should be delayed for at least 9 to 12 months to allow the lesion to mature. A bone scan can help ascertain the maturity of the lesion. Despite surgical removal, patients and clinicians should be aware that the lesion may recur.

Strains

Muscle strains are among the most common athletic injuries, representing 30% to 50% of all injuries.[23,35,36] Most strains occur at the myotendinous junction in fast-twitch type 2 muscle fibers of biarticular muscles undergoing an eccentric contraction. Although most strains occur at this interface, muscle strains can occur anywhere along the length of the muscle.[37,38] While following up on a professional soccer team, Volpi and colleagues[39] noted that 32% of strains involved the quadriceps, 28% involved the hamstring, 19% involved the adductor, and 12% involved the gastrocnemius.

Classification

The clinical classification system depends on the severity of the muscle injury: mild, moderate, or severe (see Table 87-2). Mild (grade I) sprains involve tearing of a few muscle fibers with mild pain and minimal loss of strength. Moderate (grade II) sprains involve increased tearing of muscle fibers with some strength loss. Severe (grade III) sprains include tearing of the entire muscle with complete loss of strength.[40,41] More commonly in adolescents and a small subset of adults, the tendons of origin or insertion may be avulsed and are classified as grade IIIB.

Quadriceps Strains

The only biarticular muscle in the quadriceps is the rectus femoris, but all muscles receive innervation from the femoral nerve. The indirect head of the rectus femoris gives rise to a central tendon in the proximal thigh, allowing strains to occur proximal to the musculotendinous junction. The primary function of these muscles is knee extension.[15]

Quadriceps strain typically affects the rectus femoris. These strains can occur proximally or distally. The quadriceps is commonly affected for several reasons; it crosses two joints, has a high percentage of type II fibers, and has a complex musculotendinous architecture. Sudden forceful eccentric muscle contraction of the quadriceps is required during hip extension and knee flexion and can lead to increased forces across the muscle-tendon interface, resulting in strains.[35,42-44]

History

Athletes with a quadriceps strain typically are found in sports that require cutting, jumping, or kicking, such as soccer, rugby, football, and basketball. A thorough history will tend to reveal the onset of anterior thigh pain either during the maximal extension phase of the thigh, after a sudden change in direction, or during deceleration after a forceful kick.[45] Oftentimes patients will have an antalgic gait, loss of knee flexion, or an anterior thigh mass.[42,46-49] Most commonly, quadriceps strains occur distally at the musculotendinous junction; however, they also can occur proximally or centrally.[48] Pain may be reported immediately after the injury has occurred, but often the athlete may be able to continue playing through a practice or game, with the onset of symptoms occurring after a cooling-down period.[40,43,50]

Physical Examination

Initially, physical examination is best carried out with the patient lying supine and concludes with a prone examination. With the patient prone, a thorough palpation of the muscle should be undertaken to assess for tenderness, swelling, masses, or defects. Ecchymosis may occur 24 hours or more after the onset of injury, after which ROM of the knee and hip should be performed and compared with the contralateral side. Next, evaluation of knee extension should be undertaken with the hip flexed to 90 degrees and then with the hip in extension. Weakness identified in hip flexion indicates injury to the rectus, whereas weakness seen in hip extension points toward a vastus injury. It should be noted that rectus injuries have a slower recovery time than do those that occur in the vastus.[21,51] Once the supine examination is complete, the patient is positioned prone and strength is retested, which

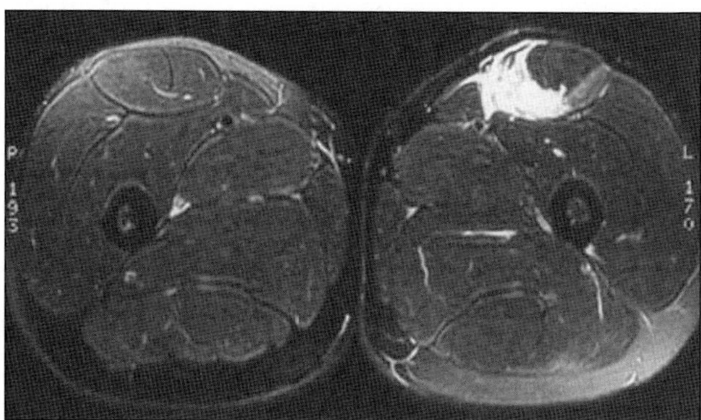

FIGURE 87-5 A T2-weighted axial magnetic resonance image of the thighs showing increased fluid in the rectus femoris indicative of a quadriceps strain.

can help isolate the quadriceps for motion and strength evaluation. For moderate to severe strains, pain is usually felt with resisted knee extension.

Imaging

Imaging in quadriceps strains is typically used more as an adjunct than for diagnosis. Radiographs, ultrasound, and MRI may all be used and can provide information regarding the length of recovery. Radiographs are routinely normal; however, in the young athlete they can be particularly important in identifying avulsion fractures or stress fractures. Ultrasound and MRI are most beneficial in predicting recovery time. Finlay and Friedman[67] reported that ultrasound is a highly sensitive and specific method for evaluating acute quadriceps injuries. The use of dynamic ultrasound with the knee in flexion and extension can allow differentiation between hematoma and muscle tears; however, ultrasound is highly operator-dependent. MRI is still considered to be the gold standard for quadriceps evaluation (Fig. 87-5).[52-54] However, its use in the initial evaluation phase is usually restricted to high-level or professional athletes to better predict a return to play. For recreational athletes, MRI is indicated if the symptoms do not improve after 2 to 3 weeks of rehabilitation or for evaluation of chronic (>8 weeks) strains.[37] Cross et al.[50] reported that MRI can estimate the size of the quadriceps strain and predict the duration of rehabilitation. Furthermore, involvement of the central tendon signifies a significantly longer rehabilitation interval.[50]

Treatment Options

Most quadriceps strains can be managed nonoperatively (Table 87-3). In the acute phase, the treatment of quadriceps strains begins with the standard PRICE protocol in an effort to decrease swelling and hematoma formation. Severe strains may require a short period of crutch use. Passive, pain-free stretching should also be initiated in the first 24 to 48 hours.[21,51] At the 3- to 5-day mark, the active rehabilitation phase may begin. First, isometric exercises and increasing movement within pain-free arc of motion are begun. Eccentric contraction of the quadriceps should be avoided. As strength and ROM continue to improve, the patient is transitioned to isotonic training with increasing resistance as tolerated.[21] When improving strength, isokinetic exercises should focus on low resistance and high speeds. A progressive running and kicking program should then be initiated, starting with a slow jog and

TABLE 87-3

TREATMENT PROTOCOL FOR A QUADRICEPS STRAIN

Phase	Activity
I	RICE, NSAIDs
II	Isometric exercises
III	Isotonic exercises
IV	Isokinetic exercises
V	Running, plyometrics, jumping exercises
VI	Sport-specific training

NSAIDs, Nonsteroidal antiinflammatory drugs; *RICE,* rest, ice, compression, and elevation.

advancing to sprinting. When sprinting is tolerated, kicking may be started with a light ball over short distances, advancing to a normal-weight ball over longer distances.[50] Finally, sport-specific training should begin. The patient may return to play after completion of this training but should continue to work on a quadriceps rehabilitation program involving stretching, isokinetic strengthening, and conditioning.

Surgical intervention is reserved for total or near-total muscle tears, persistent pain with nonoperative treatment, reattachment of avulsion fractures, and large hematoma evacuation. Time until return to play after rectus reattachment surgery was noted to be 9 months in one report (Fig. 87-6).[21,45,55]

Decision-Making Principles

Nonoperative treatment should be pursued whenever possible for quadriceps strains. There are very few indications for surgical intervention. Moreover, controversy exists regarding the value of surgical decompression of large hematomas, as well as the need for operative intervention for rectus avulsion injuries. Complete muscle tears, true fractures associated with quadriceps strains, or symptomatic mature myositis ossificans appear to be the only criteria for surgical intervention. However, recalcitrant nonoperative treatment of severe quadriceps strains may also warrant surgical intervention based on some published reports.[45]

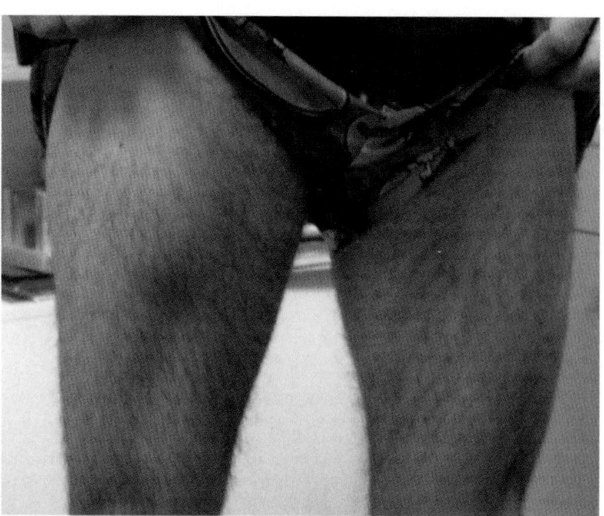

FIGURE 87-6 Quadriceps rupture with retraction.

AUTHORS' PREFERRED TECHNIQUE

Quadriceps Strains

We prefer to use nonsurgical management. In initial 24 to 72 hours, PRICE, NSAIDs, and gentle ROM are begun. If sufficient progress is noted, the rehabilitation protocol is then begun at day 3 to 5, with a focus on pain-free motion. If at any point a setback is experienced, the protocol is backed down. Antiinflammatory modalities are also instituted by the trainer or physical therapist, along with ultrasound and electrical stimulation for moderate to severe strains. Operative intervention is only considered for avulsion fractures that are symptomatic for 12 months or more. Gentle passive ROM is begun 7 to 10 days after the surgery, with an emphasis on avoiding eccentric muscle contractions. Once patients can tolerate this gentle passive ROM, they may begin the aforementioned rehabilitation protocol.

Return to Play

A review of the literature by Orchard et al.[51] noted a lack of consensus for safe return to play after muscle strains. Despite this finding, certain criteria that appear in the literature seem to lower the risk of reinjury after a quadriceps strain. Range of motion of the knee should be equal to the contralateral leg. Isokinetic quadriceps strength should fall within 15% of the contralateral side. Ideally, completion of a sport-specific program should be completed, including observed straight-ahead sprinting and figure-eight cutting sprints. Most patients are able to return to play within 2 to 3 weeks while wearing a compressive thigh wrap and continuing a dedicated stretching and strengthening program.

Results

Good to excellent results have been reported with use of the phased treatment protocol for quadriceps strain. In recent articles it has been advocated that higher level athletes should resume play earlier, with the understanding that the risk of reinjury is higher. Stratification of the risk of reinjury can be aided by imaging, such as ultrasound or MRI, to quantify the severity of the initial injury.[51] Based on imaging, injuries involving greater than 15% of the rectus cross-sectional area have demonstrated a longer recovery phase (14.6 days vs. 8.9 days). Strains greater than 13 cm in length also resulted in a doubling of recovery time. The contrast enhancement around the central tendon, the so-called acute bulls-eye lesion, also revealed a significantly worse prognosis (26.8 days vs. 9.2 days) (Fig. 87-7).[38,42] Although many investigators have recommended surgical treatment for proximal avulsion fractures, Hsu and coworkers[55] treated two National Football League kickers with a nonoperative treatment regimen and noted that both patients were able to return to full practice after 3 to 12 weeks.

Limited data exist for surgical outcomes for quadriceps strains, with the majority of the information being case reports. Straw et al.[45] reported a full return of strength and return to competition after repairing a chronic proximal rectus avulsion in a semiprofessional soccer player. Similar reports exist in the literature, noting a return to previous activity level with nearly symmetrical strength in athletes treated surgically for chronic rectus weakness.[55]

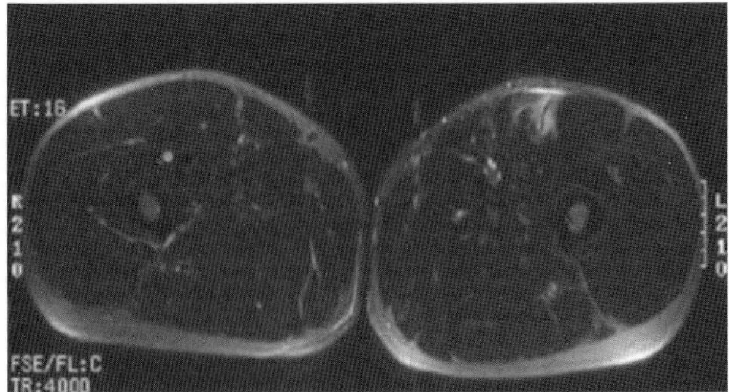

FIGURE 87-7 An acute bulls-eye lesion.

Complications

Complications associated with quadriceps strains include myositis ossificans, reinjury, residual weakness, and compartment syndrome. Risk stratification for reinjury is only used as a guide, further emphasizing the need for dedicated return to play criteria and a thorough warm-up and stretching program. Residual weakness that persists for more than 12 months should warrant evaluation of surgical intervention. Myositis ossificans has previously been discussed in the contusion section, and urgent intervention in the initial 24 to 72 hours for severe strains is warranted.

Future Considerations

The future of quadriceps strains lies in identifying more rapid improved return-to-play criteria while limiting reinjury risk. Some persons have advocated removing the athlete from competition completely until all symptoms have resolved. However, some investigators are advocating a return to play even before the full return-to-play criteria have been met. Anecdotally, it is the physician's charge to protect the athlete and limit short- and long-term risk.

Adductor Strains

Adductor strains, which are the most common groin injuries in athletes, occur as a result of a forced push-off or side-to-side motion.[56,57] These injuries are seen more often in athletes who play soccer, hockey, rugby, martial arts, and football. Their reported incidence ranges from 13% to 43%.[58-61] Adductor strains commonly are the result of a forceful abduction of the thigh during an intentional adduction movement. The musculotendinous junction of the adductor longus is most commonly involved.[57,62] Inflexibility, previous injury, and strength imbalance between adductors and abductors have been implicated as risk factors for adductor strains.

Adductor strains can be graded from I to III. Mild (grade I) strains result in pain with minimal strength loss, moderate (grade II) strains result in strength loss and pain, and severe (grade III) strains result in complete functional and motor loss.

History

The athlete will typically present with a chief complaint of acute groin pain, tenderness, and swelling. The mechanism may be a sudden change in direction, or the athlete may note that he or she was attempting a forceful kick that was met with opposite resistance, such as an opposing player blocking the kick. Pain will be noted to be worse with side-to-side movement. Often the patient has a history of an adductor injury. A review of the literature suggests the need for a thorough history and examination, because groin pain in 27% to 90% of athletes has more than one cause.[63,64] A differential of groin pain includes osteitis pubis, athletic pubalgia, hernias, and stress fractures.

Physical Examination

Patients with moderate to severe injuries may display an antalgic gait, and in rare instances they may not be able to bear weight on the affected limb. A complete palpatory examination of the medial groin should be performed to look for tenderness, swelling, ecchymosis, and defects. ROM and strength should also be assessed. Medial groin pain is accentuated with resisted hip adduction. In addition, the pubic rami and inferior abdominal wall should be inspected to rule out other causes of pain.

Adductor strains must be differentiated from other sources of groin pain. Tenderness to palpation at the pubis may result from osteitis pubis, athletic pubalgia, or muscular origin avulsion injury. Osteitis pubis results in tenderness over the pubic tubercle or inguinal ring and often can be differentiated because symptoms exacerbate with sit-ups.[65,66] Persons with athletic pubalgia may have tenderness over the pubic tubercle, and this tenderness can be reproduced with resisted sit-ups or the Valsalva maneuver. An inguinal hernia examination should also be performed.

Imaging

Plain radiographs with the patient standing on one leg are the initial imaging modality of choice. These radiographs are acquired less for diagnosis of adductor strains and more to rule out other pathology, such as avulsion fractures or osteitis pubis. A bone scan, MRI, and ultrasound have also been used to varying degrees. An MRI is not routinely ordered and is only used as a guide in estimating the length of recovery. Much like with other strains of the thigh, involvement of greater than 50% of the cross-sectional area, tissue fluid collection, and deep muscle tears are predictive of a slower return to sport.[35] Ultrasound has been used to evaluate the musculotendinous junction and to aid in the differentiation of a strain from other conditions, including hernia.[67]

Treatment Options

Nonoperative

Adductor strains are managed similar to quadriceps and hamstring strains. The majority of these injuries are treated nonsurgically. PRICE, NSAIDs, and a progressive rehabilitation program are initiated. Typically persons with grade I strains do not seek medical attention; however, if they do seek treatment, a 3- to 7-day course of progressive ROM and strengthening is recommended. Sport-specific drills should be performed and observed prior to clearance. For persons with more severe strains, early stretching sometimes has been noted to aggravate the injury. A gentle progression through isometric, isotonic, and isokinetic exercises should be initiated, and the patient should be noted to be pain-free before advancing to sport-specific drills. Upper body and core exercises may begin in phase II. Swimming and use of a stationary bike and elliptical machine may begin in phase III. Sports-specific drills may begin once the patient has ROM and adductor strength that is 75% of ipsilateral abductors. Emphasis should be placed on reinjury prevention via a focused stretching and strengthening program designed to create an adduction-to-abduction strength ratio of 0.8 or higher.[68] Corticosteroid injections and platelet-rich plasma injections have yet to yield sufficient data to be considered front-line treatment options.

Operative

Surgical intervention is rarely required for adductor strains. Strains recalcitrant to conservative care with persistent pain and weakness may require tenotomy versus repair. The literature for surgical intervention is predominately based on case reports. Persons with complete avulsions who have had persistent symptoms for 6 months or longer may be treated with repair. For incomplete tears that are symptomatic, tenotomy may be best indicated.[57,69]

Decision-Making Principles

Nonoperative treatment is the overwhelming option of choice for adductor strains. Although a high reinjury rate applies, surgical intervention is very rarely warranted and has had mixed results. Proper education of the athlete and the trainer as to the rehabilitation course and future prevention is the key to a successful outcome. Surgical intervention is only considered for complete avulsions that hinder return to play for 6 months or more or for chronic partial tears that may require tenotomy after a similar amount of time.

AUTHORS' PREFERRED TECHNIQUE

Adductor Strains

We prefer nonsurgical management, with an emphasis on normalizing abductor-adductor strength imbalance while rehabilitating the athlete. The athlete is initially treated with the standard PRICE protocol and a 5- to 7-day course of NSAIDs. Beginning on day 3, passive ROM and gentle isometric exercises are begun. Eccentric loading is avoided in phase I. Advancement to phase II is permitted once the athlete can adduct against gravity without pain. Phase II consists of isotonic exercises under supervision. Stationary biking and swimming are permitted, as is core and upper body training. Stretching, which is typically avoided in phase I, is permitted to the level of discomfort without pain. Attention to abductor-adductor strengthening is begun. Progression to phase III occurs once the patient demonstrates pain-free strength against submaximal abduction-adduction resistance. In phase III, isokinetic training is incorporated, followed by sport-specific drills. A dedicated warm-up and stretching program should be instituted to focus on reinjury awareness for the athlete. Return to play is permitted once single-leg strength is demonstrated to be equal to the contralateral side in all planes and the adduction-to-abduction strength ratio is greater than 80%.

Return to Play

Return to competition is permitted once pain-free sport-specific movements can be performed with adductor strength within 20% of the contralateral side. Although most patients return to play in 2 to 3 weeks, severe cases may take 8 to 12 weeks. Dedicated warm-up stretching should be emphasized, as should in-season strengthening. Return to play prior to pain-free sport-specific training has been associated with chronic adductor strains.[68] Reinjury education and prevention is warranted as well. Return to play after tenotomy for chronic adductor pain ranges from 8 to 12 weeks.

Results

Return to play rates after surgical tenotomy for chronic adductor strains have been demonstrated to range from 60% to 90%. Concomitant injuries, such as sports hernias and subsequent repair, have been shown to affect outcome.[70,71] Adductor strains treated with a dedicated rehabilitation program and injury prevention awareness have demonstrated excellent results. Tyler et al.[72] reported a greater than fourfold reduction in adductor strains in the National Hockey League after institution of a dedicated adductor strengthening and stretching program. Holmich et al.[73] noted that active therapy in persons with chronic adductor strains provided better results than those seen in patients treated with passive therapy programs.[73]

Complications

The most common complication of adductor strains is reinjury. Seward et al.[74] and Tyler and associates[72] report recurrence rates of 32% and 44%, respectively. The highest risk factor for adductor strain is an adductor-to-abductor strength of 80% or less.[68] Other complications include myositis ossificans, compartment syndrome, calcific tendinitis, and chronic groin pain.

Future Considerations

Preemptive injury prevention training and identification may be a future consideration for athletes participating in high-risk sports. In addition, evaluation of platelet-rich plasma and other nonsurgical modalities for chronic adductor strains may be warranted because of mixed data on return to competition after tenotomy.

For a complete list of references, go to expertconsult.com.

Suggested Readings

Citation: Ryan JB, Hopkinson WJ, Wheeler JH, et al: Quadriceps contusions. West Point update. *Am J Sports Med* 19(3):299–304, 1991.
Level of Evidence: II
Summary: In this article, the authors provided defining data for appropriate management of quadriceps contusion that altered previous standards of care. Current treatment regimens are predicated on the findings presented in this article.

Citation: Beiner JM, Jokl P: Muscle contusion injury and myositis ossificans traumatica. *Clin Orthop Relat Res* 403S:S110–S119, 2002.
Level of Evidence: II
Summary: In this article, the authors provide analysis of the etiology, treatment, and outcomes of myositis ossificans.

Citation: Orchard J, Best TM, Verrall GM: Return to play following muscle strains. *Clin J Sport Med* 15(6):436–441, 2005.
Level of Evidence: III
Summary: Consensus regarding return-to-play guidelines has been lacking in the literature. This article provides treatment parameters and offers a perspective on earlier return to competition.

Citation: Beiner JM, Jokl P: Muscle contusion injury and myositis ossificans traumatica. *Clin Orthop Relat Res* 403S:S110–S119, 2002.
Level of Evidence: III
Summary: The authors provide a comprehensive review of hamstring injuries, treatments, and outcomes. Gaps within the hamstring injury literature are also identified.

Citation: Lovell G: The diagnosis of chronic groin pain in athletes: A review of 189 cases. *Aust J Sci Med Sport* 27(3):76–79, 1995.
Level of Evidence: III
Summary: The author provides a systematic review that evaluates the effectiveness of exercise therapy for groin pain in athletes and the treatment of this disorder.

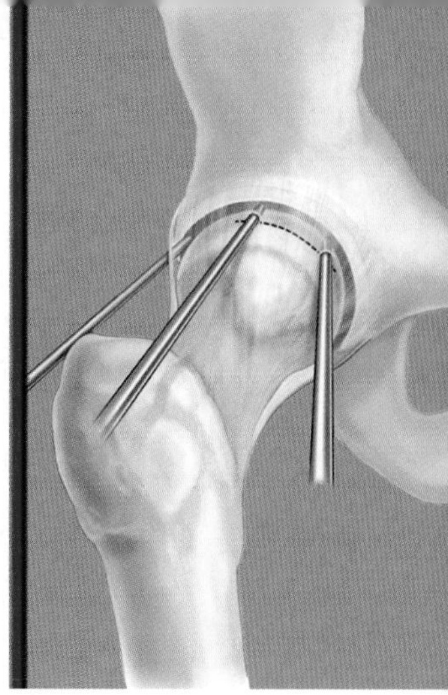

88

Hamstring Injuries

CARLOS A. GUANCHE

Hamstring injuries are common in athletic populations and can affect athletes at all levels of competition.[1-4] Several studies have shown that the rates of muscle strain in high school football (12% to 24%) and collegiate football (18.9% to 22.2%) are fairly high.[5-9] In one study, the National Football League surveillance system identified 1716 hamstring strains among all players, with a range of 132 to 210 injuries per year,[10] which accounts for an overall injury rate of 0.77 per 1000 athlete-exposures and a reinjury rate of 16.5%. One literature review identified previous hamstring injury as the greatest risk factor for reinjury.[11] The injured muscle may have an altered compliance or deformation pattern, predisposing it to less tissue motion or higher muscle strain. Age was also found to be an independent risk factor for hamstring injury. Although some studies suggest that contact activities are the cause of hamstring injuries, most studies have shown that more than 90% of injuries occur without contact, with the classic injury being sustained by a water skier who gets pulled up by the boat.[5,12]

The thigh contains a large cross-sectional area of muscles with three main muscle groups: hamstrings, quadriceps, and adductors. The hamstring complex consists of the biceps femoris, semitendinosus, and semimembranosus. The semitendinosus, semimembranosus, and long head of the biceps are biarticular and are innervated by the tibial portion of the sciatic nerve. The short head of the biceps is monarticular and is innervated by the common peroneal nerve. These muscles work together to extend the hip, flex the knee, and externally rotate the hip and knee.[12] The myotendinous junctions of the hamstrings have significant overlap.

The proximal hamstring complex has a strong bony attachment on the ischial tuberosity (Fig. 88-1). Their footprint on the ischium is composed of the semitendinosus and the long head of biceps femoris beginning as a common proximal tendon and footprint, and there is a distinct semimembranosus footprint.[13] The semimembranosus footprint is medial (and anterior) to the crescent-shaped footprint of the common insertion of the semitendinosus and long head of the biceps femoris (see Fig. 88-1).

Biomechanically, the hamstrings are subjected to high tensile load given their extensive eccentric role. During initial swing, the knee and hip are flexing, which requires simultaneous eccentric and concentric activity of the hamstrings. During the last portion of swing, the hamstrings continue to play a dual role of controlling knee extension while extending the hip. The hamstrings work synergistically with the gluteal muscles to stabilize, decelerate, and propel the hip. During the propulsion phase, the medial hamstrings assist in decelerating hip external rotation, which maintains the gluteus maximus at an ideal length to act as an accelerator (along with the hamstrings) of the femur in the sagittal plane. The hamstrings, along with the rectus abdominis, also are decelerators of pelvic anterior tilt throughout stance. Given these functional relationships, it is conceivable that hamstring strain or rupture has its source in the inhibition and weakness of its closest synergists, the gluteal and abdominal muscles.[14]

Hamstring injuries occur on a continuum that can range from musculotendinous strains to avulsion injuries.[1,2] A strain is a partial or complete disruption of the musculotendinous unit.[1,4] A complete tear or avulsion, in contrast, is a discontinuity of the unit. In one study, 12.3% of 170 cases of hamstring injuries were tendon tears; the majority (90.5%) were muscle belly injuries.[15] Most hamstring strains do not require surgical intervention and resolve with a variety of modalities and rest. The most important point in evaluating these patients is to differentiate the complete or partial tears from the muscle strain subgroup, because patients with complete or partial tears can experience more substantial disabilities.

History

The history of an acute injury usually involves a traumatic event with forced hip flexion and the knee in extension, as is classically observed in waterskiing.[2,16-18] However, the injury can result from a wide variety of sporting activities that require rapid acceleration and deceleration.[2,19,20]

Proximal hamstring injuries can be categorized as complete tendinous avulsions, partial tendinous avulsions, apophyseal avulsions, and degenerative (tendinosis) avulsions.[19] Degenerative tears of the hamstring origin are more insidious in onset and are commonly seen as an overuse injury in middle- and long-distance runners. The mechanism of injury in these patients is presumably repetitive irritation of the medial aspect of the hamstring tendon (typically along the lateral aspect of the tuberosity, where the bursa resides), ultimately causing an attritional tear of the tendon.

Commonly, athletes with proximal hamstring tendon tears typically describe a popping or tearing sensation with associated pain and bruising over the posterior hip.[21,22] They may also have weakness with active knee flexion, a sensation of instability, or difficulty controlling their

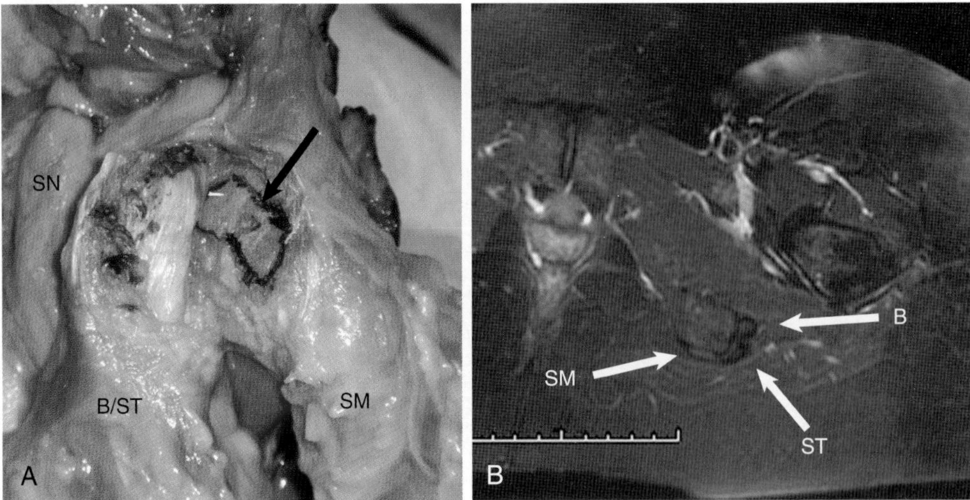

FIGURE 88-1 Normal anatomy of the hamstring origin. **A,** The posterior view of a cadaveric dissection of the ischium in a left hip. The arrow is pointing to the origin of the biceps and semitendinosus (*B/ST*) muscles, which have been elevated and retracted laterally. **B,** An axial T2-weighted magnetic resonance image depicting the anatomy of the hamstring origin in a left hip. *B,* Biceps origin; *SN,* sciatic nerve; *SM,* origin of semimembranosus.

legs.[20,22-25] Occasionally, patients who present with either acute or chronic tears may report a pins-and-needles sensation in sciatic nerve distribution, much like sciatica.[20,22,24,26] This sensation may be due to acute compression of a hematoma in the proximity of the sciatic nerve or chronic scarring and tethering of the tendon to the nerve.

Symptoms of ischial bursitis include buttock or hip pain and localized tenderness overlying the ischial tuberosity. Additional symptoms of chronic ischial bursitis may include tingling into the buttock that spreads down the leg, presumably from local inflammation and swelling in the area of the sciatic nerve.[26] The symptoms usually worsen while sitting. Clinically, the persons most affected tend to sit with the painful buttock elevated off their seat.

Physical Examination

The examination is typically performed with the patient in the prone position. Maintaining the knee in a slightly flexed position will limit muscle spasms and make the examination more comfortable for persons with acute ruptures. Inspection and palpation of the posterior thigh may reveal muscle spasm. Ecchymosis may only be observed if the fascial covering is also disrupted. Palpation of the entire posterior thigh is very important to localize the injury. Persons with acute injuries typically have focal tenderness and swelling. However, with delayed presentation, patients are more likely to have diffuse swelling and tenderness. Persons with low-grade strains typically have limited swelling and tenderness, whereas in persons with a more severe strain, a palpable defect may be appreciated.

An examination technique has been described in which the patient is positioned prone and asked to actively apply tension to his or her hamstring tendon.[21] The degree of tension is then compared with the passive tendon tension while sitting. Decreased tension compared with the normal side suggests a proximal tendon rupture. In a cohort of 25 patients with complete tears, the examiner was able to identify all patients with tendon tears (100% sensitivity); however, specificity was not measured because the examination was not applied to healthy subjects.

The most critical aspect of the examination is to have a high degree of suspicion for a tear. In less acute situations in which the tear is several days old, it is possible that even a large defect may not be palpable clinically as a result of the overlying hematoma. It is especially critical to assess these patients with imaging studies to delineate the type of tear that is present.

Imaging

If a high level of suspicion exists for a proximal hamstring injury, both routine and advanced imaging is performed. Plain radiographs of the pelvis and a lateral radiograph of the affected hip are obtained to rule out any apophyseal avulsions, particularly to the ischial tuberosity in adolescent athletes (Fig. 88-2). If a fracture is identified, a computed tomography scan may assist in assessing the displacement and fracture configuration for surgical planning.

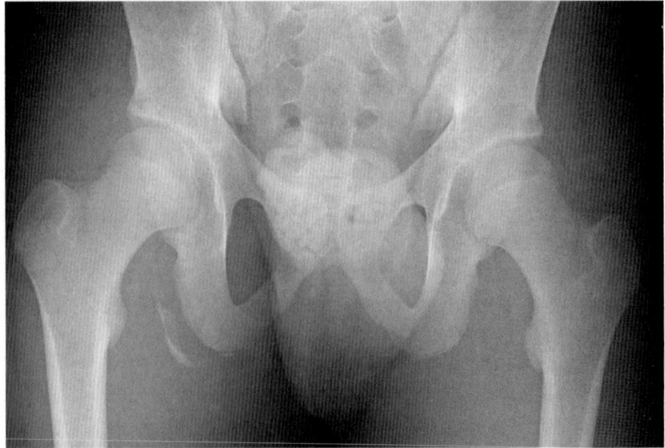

FIGURE 88-2 An anteroposterior radiograph of the pelvis showing a bony avulsion of the right ischial tuberosity.

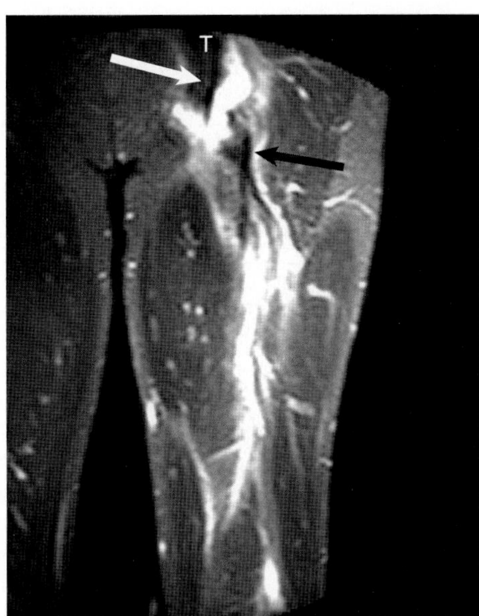

FIGURE 88-3 A coronal T2-weighted magnetic resonance image of a complete three-tendon rupture of the proximal hamstring. The black arrow points to the common avulsed tendon. The white arrow identifies the tuberosity (*T*).

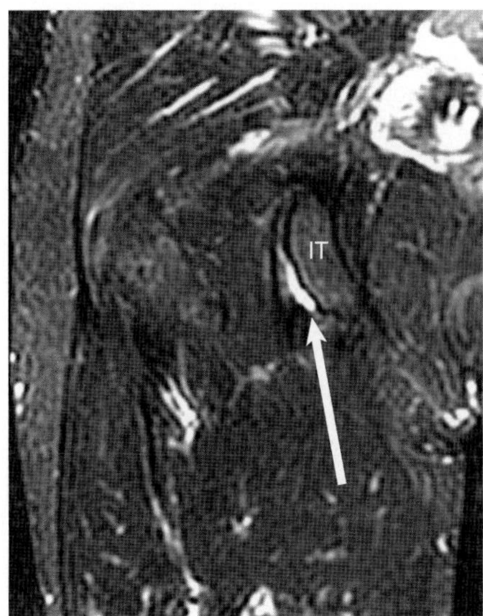

FIGURE 88-4 A coronal T2-weighted magnetic resonance image of a right hip showing the sickle sign (*arrow*), which indicates fluid within the ischial bursa. *IT,* Ischial tuberosity.

More commonly, no fractures are identified and magnetic resonance imaging (MRI) is used to assess the proximal hamstring insertion on the ischial tuberosity. A number of different combinations of injury can thus occur at this tendon insertion. A complete rupture of all three tendons is common and most easily identified on an MRI scan, with accurate measurement of the amount of retraction possible (Fig. 88-3).[23] All three MRI planes (coronal, sagittal, and axial) should be used to define the tear pattern. A commonly associated finding with an acute complete hamstring avulsion is a large posterior thigh hematoma.

Partial hamstring origin tears are somewhat more difficult to diagnose, particularly in the case of two-tendon tears, which commonly have an associated musculotendinous junction injury to the third "intact" tendon. Unfortunately, retraction of the two tendons more than 2 cm typically renders the intact tendon functionally impaired and is clinically comparable to a complete rupture. Despite this diagnostic difficulty, MRI is very helpful in distinguishing complete versus partial tears. As such, one or two tendon injuries can be identified, and this distinction often determines a patient's need for surgical repair. In addition, partial insertional tears without any significant retraction can be seen on MRI as a "sickle sign" (Fig. 88-4). These tears are typically partial avulsion of the common biceps and semitendinosus origin.

Another imaging modality that can be used in the assessment of proximal hamstring injuries is ultrasound. Although ultrasound can be extremely user specific, it can also be highly accurate to evaluate partial tears and insertional tendinosis.[27] Its potential for bedside use as a dynamic test may lead to the detection of more subtle injuries, particularly in the athletic population. Currently, however, ultrasound is still less sensitive than MRI, and it does not supplant this modality. In one study, 170 cases of hamstring muscle strains were evaluated with MRI and ultrasound.[15] In 21 patients with complete tears, 100% of the tears were identified with MRI, whereas 58% were identified with ultrasound. With use of ultrasound, large hematomas can produce mixed echogenic patterns, which can make visualization of retracted tendons difficult (Fig. 88-5).

Decision-Making Principles

Whether the surgical procedure is performed with an open approach or endoscopically, the indications are the same. The only certain indication for the open procedure is a large retracted tear with chronic atrophy as noted on MRI imaging. In these cases, the procedure would more than likely require extensive mobilization and probably the use of a graft for reconstruction of the avulsed segment, which must be performed in an open fashion at this time. The first indication for surgery is an acute hamstring avulsion in an active patient with greater than 2 cm of retraction. Some patients have a clinically evident partial hamstring avulsion involving the biceps/semitendinosus tendon, with refractory ischial pain

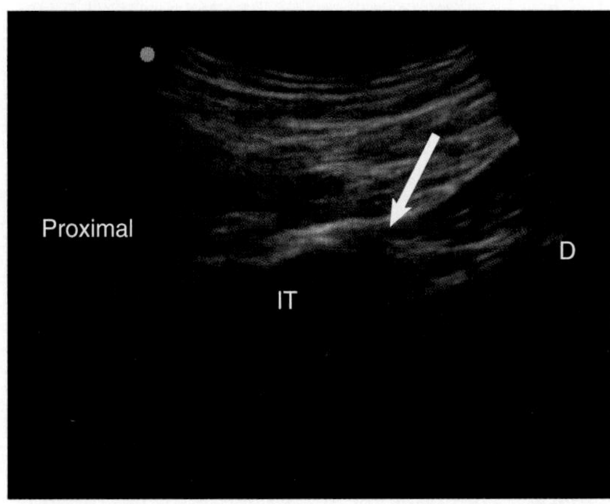

FIGURE 88-5 Ultrasound image of left hamstring origin (*arrow*). *D,* Distal; *IT,* ischial tuberosity.

and the inability to return to high-level sports. Finally, patients are also candidates for surgical intervention when they have a history of refractory ischial bursitis and no discernable tear and conservative treatment has failed, including at least 6 weeks of physical therapy and two ultrasound-guided ischial injections.

Treatment

Nonoperative

Nonoperative treatment of proximal hamstring injuries is most commonly recommended in the setting of low-grade partial tears and insertional tendinosis. Initial treatment consists of active rest, use of oral nonsteroidal antiinflammatory medications, and a physical therapy program, which consists of a gentle hamstring stretching and strengthening program. As the initial symptoms resolve, core, hip, and quadriceps exercises can be added in association with a more aggressive hamstring injury prevention program.[28] Full return to sports and activities is allowed when the patient is asymptomatic.[11] If progress does not occur with this program, an ultrasound-guided corticosteroid injection may be used and has been shown to provide initial relief in up to 50% of patients at 1 month.[27] Patients who experience failure of nonoperative treatment of partial tears may benefit from surgical debridement and repair, similar to patients with other commonly seen partial tendon tears (i.e., the patella, quadriceps, and biceps). As will be described, newer and less invasive endoscopic techniques are perfectly suited for this problem.

Nonoperative treatment of complete ruptures of the proximal hamstring is less frequently recommended because surgical repair has resulted in the successful return of patients to a high level of function.[16,18,21,22,26,29-31] One study identified a group of water skiers with hamstring avulsion injuries that initially were treated nonoperatively. Persistent cramping or pulling with vigorous activity was experienced by 83% of the patients.[18] Seven patients returned to sports activities but at a lower level, and five patients were only able to perform limited activities. Upon Cybex testing, these patients had a hamstring and quadriceps deficit of 61% and 23%, respectively. Two patients ultimately underwent delayed surgical repairs.

Surgical Treatment

Endoscopic

To date, no reports of endoscopic management of these injuries have been published. After gaining experience in the open management of these injuries, I have developed an endoscopic technique that allows a safe approach to the area of damage in most tears, including acute disruptions. It is expected that the benefits of a more direct approach—without elevating the gluteus maximus and with the use of endoscopic magnification to protect the sciatic nerve—will improve the management of these injuries and reduce the morbidities associated with the open approach.

The patient is placed in the prone position after induction of anesthesia, with all prominences and neurovascular structures protected. The table is flat (as opposed to the slightly flexed position of the table in the open repair procedure) to help maintain the space between the gluteal musculature and the ischium. The posterior aspect of the hip is then sterilized, ensuring that the leg and thigh are free so that the leg and hip can be repositioned intraoperatively (Fig. 88-6).

Two portals are then created, 2 cm medial and 2 cm lateral to the palpable ischial tuberosity (Fig. 88-7). The lateral portal is established first by using blunt dissection with a switching stick, as the gluteus maximus muscle is penetrated and the submuscular plane is created. The switching stick serves to palpate the prominence of the tuberosity and identify the medial and lateral borders of the ischium. The medial portal is then established, taking care to palpate the medial aspect of the ischium. A 30-degree arthroscope is then inserted in the lateral portal and an electrocautery device is placed in the medial portal. The space between the ischium and the gluteus muscle is then developed, taking care to stay along the central and medial portions of the ischium to avoid any damage to

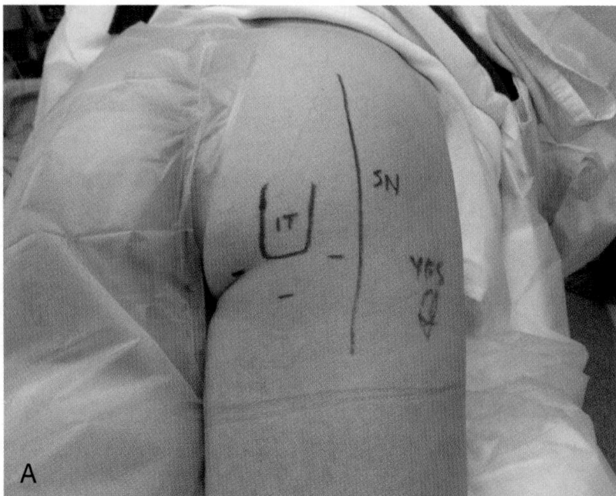

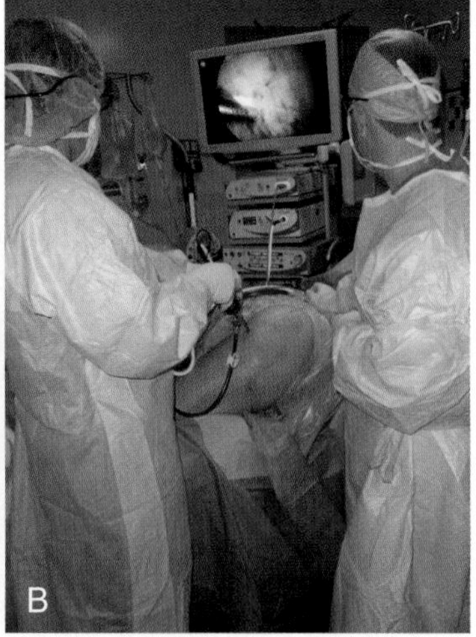

FIGURE 88-6 Positioning of the patient. **A,** In the prone position with the leg draped free. The view is of a right hip, with the patient in the prone position. Note that the table is flat with no flexion. **B,** The surgeon and assistant are positioned on the same side. The arthroscopic equipment is positioned on the contralateral side.

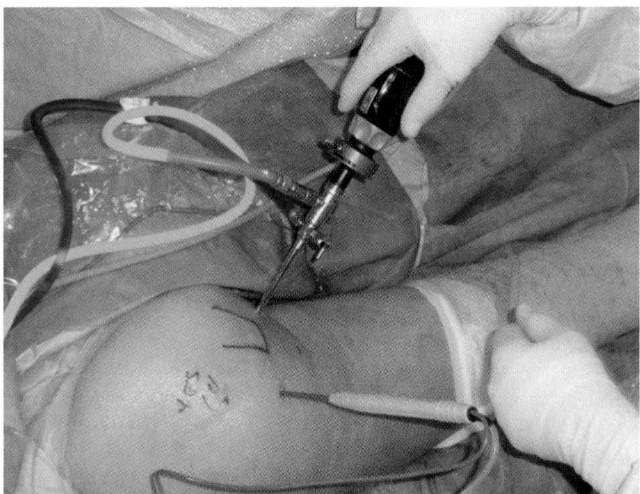

FIGURE 88-7 Portals for the endoscopic approach. Note that the arthroscope is in the medial portal and the empty portal is the distal portal. The ablator is in the lateral portal.

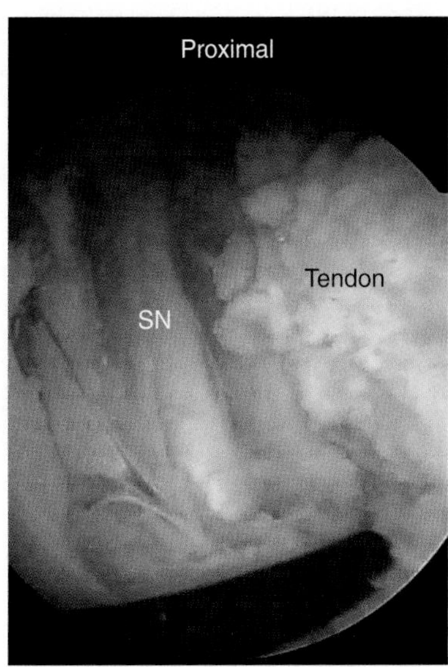

FIGURE 88-9 Exposure of the sciatic nerve (*SN*) in a patient with a history of a hamstring avulsion about 2 months earlier. Note the significant scar bands over the SN prior to exposure.

the sciatic nerve. The lateral aspect is then exposed with the use of a switching stick as a soft tissue dissector. With the lateral aspect identified, the dissection continues anteriorly and laterally toward the known area of the sciatic nerve (Fig. 88-8). Very careful and methodical release of any soft tissue bands is then undertaken in a proximal to distal direction to mobilize the nerve and protect it throughout the exposure and ultimate repair of the hamstring tendon. In cases of acute disruptions in which some scarring is taking place, significant bands are often encountered (Fig. 88-9).

Once the nerve has been identified and protected, attention is directed once again to the area of the tendinous avulsion. The tip of the ischium is identified through palpation with the instruments. The tendinous origin is then inspected to identify any obvious tearing (Fig. 88-10). With acute tears the area is obvious and the tendon is often retracted distally. In these cases, a large hematoma occasionally is present and must be evacuated. It is especially important to protect the sciatic nerve during this portion of the procedure, because it is sometimes obscured by the hematoma.

Once the area of pathology is identified (in persons with incomplete tears), an endoscopic knife can be used to longitudinally split the tendon along its fibers (Fig. 88-11). This area often can be identified through palpation, because softening typically is present over the area of the detachment, making the tissue ballotable against the ischium. The hamstring is then undermined and the partial tearing is debrided with an oscillating shaver. The lateral wall of the ischium is cleared of devitalized tissue and a bleeding bed is established in preparation for the tendon repair. The inferior ischium and the ischial bursa can also be resected and cleared of inflamed tissues as the lateral ischial tissue is mobilized. By retracting the anterior tissues, the bursa can be entered and debrided (see Fig. 88-11).

An inferior portal may then be created approximately 4 cm distal to the tip of the ischium and equidistant from the medial and lateral portals. This portal is used for insertion of suture anchors, as well as suture management. A variety of

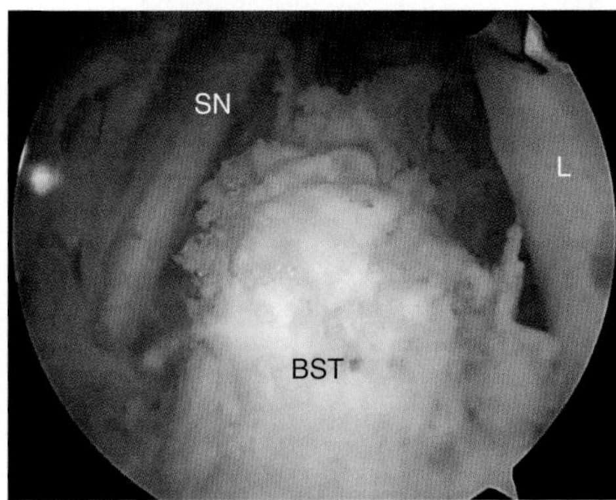

FIGURE 88-8 Normal arthroscopic anatomy exposure in a left hip as viewed from the lateral portal. Note the tool entering from the medial portal. *SN,* Sciatic nerve; *BST,* common biceps/semitendinosus; *L,* lateral ischium.

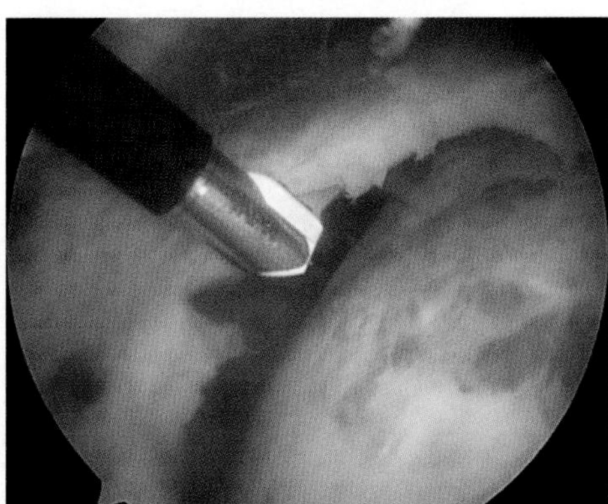

FIGURE 88-10 The distal end of the ischium cleared of soft tissue. The view is from the medial portal and shows all of the avulsed area of ischium. The visualized device is elevating the remaining sheath tissue from the lateral portal.

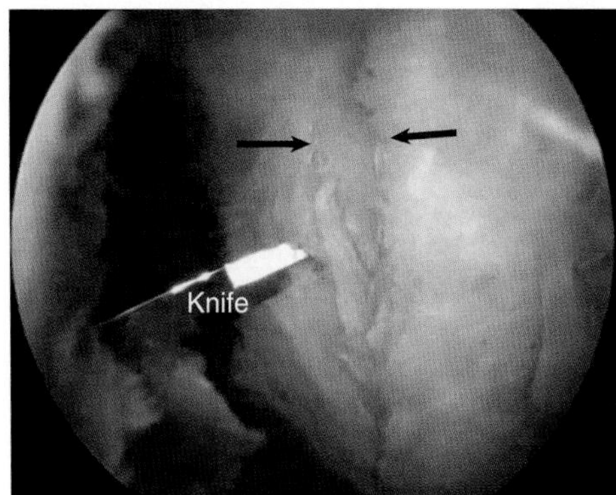

FIGURE 88-11 The incision of a tendon to explore an area of tearing and ischial bursa exposes detached lateral hamstring complex. Note the arrows showing the area of separation after the incision.

suture-passing devices can then be used for the repair. The principles are essentially the same as those used in arthroscopic rotator cuff repair. Once all of the sutures are passed through the tissue of the avulsed hamstring, the sutures are tied and a solid repair of the tendon is completed. In general, one suture anchor is used per centimeter of detachment (Fig. 88-12). Alternatively, a more proximal portal can also be established to mobilize a retracted tendon in patients with acute disruptions.

Postoperatively, the patient is fitted with a hinged knee brace that is fixed at 90 degrees of flexion for 4 weeks to limit not only weight bearing but also to restrict excursion of the hamstring tendons and protect the repair. At 4 weeks, the knee is gradually extended by about 30 degrees per week to allow full weight bearing by 6 to 8 weeks while maintaining the use of crutches. Physical therapy is instituted at this point, with the initial phase focused on hip and knee range of motion. Hamstring strengthening is begun at 10 to 12 weeks, predicated on full range of motion and a painless gait. Full, unrestricted activity is allowed at approximately 4 to 6 months.

Open

The indications for surgical treatment of proximal hamstring ruptures include all acute complete three-tendon tears and two-tendon tears with retraction of 2 cm or more.[30] Acute surgical repair initially is not indicated for patients with a one-tendon or two-tendon tear with less than 2 cm of retraction; they are treated surgically if nonoperative treatment is not successful. In addition, less active patients or patients who are unable to comply with the postoperative rehabilitation protocol should be managed nonoperatively. Patients with complete or partial tears for whom conservative management fails may be candidates for delayed repair.

The patient is placed prone with all bony prominences well padded and the trunk in slight flexion. A transverse incision in the gluteal crease inferior to the ischial tuberosity is used.[17,19,30,31] The sciatic nerve is only dissected free in cases of chronic injury with scarring or preoperative sciatic nerve symptoms. Once the ruptured tendon is visualized, freed from scar tissue, and debrided, it is tagged for repair. The ischial tuberosity is identified, cleared of devitalized tissue, and decorticated to provide for optimal healing. The conjoined hamstring tendons are repaired together to bone suture

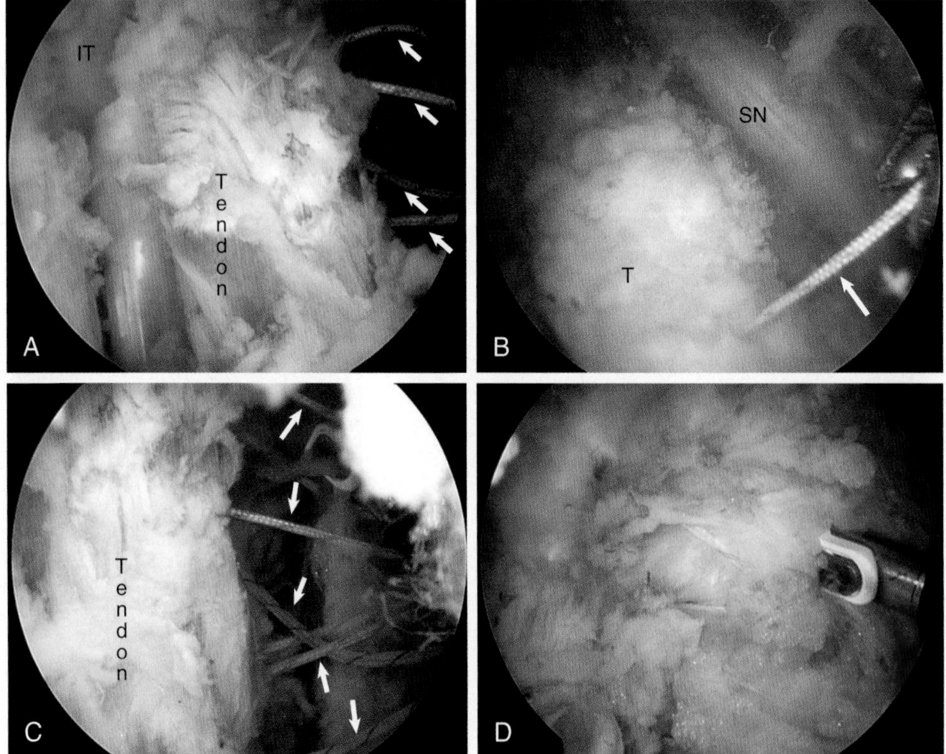

FIGURE 88-12 Repair of a tendinous avulsion. **A,** The prepared surface with sutures in place (*arrows*). **B,** The suture in place (*arrow*). Note the proximity of the sciatic nerve (*SN*) to the repair. **C,** Final mattress sutures in place in the substance of the tendon (*arrows*). **D,** Final tendon repair with closure of the defect. Multiple crossing sutures are seen. *IT,* Ischial tuberosity; *T,* tendon.

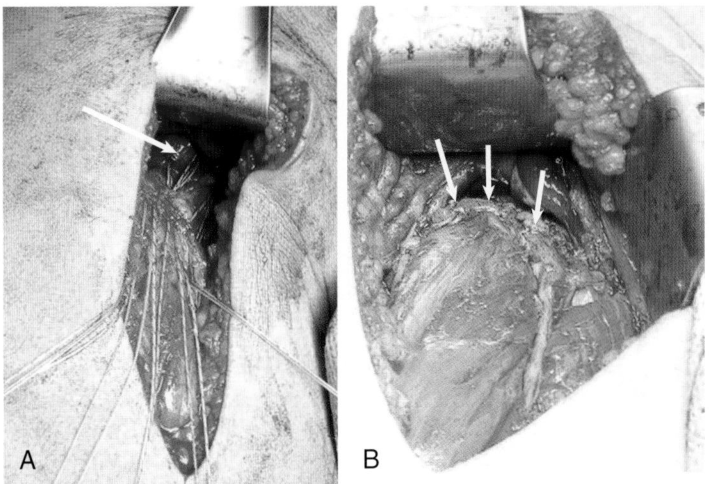

FIGURE 88-13 Open repair of the proximal hamstring on the ischial tuberosity *(arrow)*. **A,** The view is of a longitudinal incision in the left hip. Multiple sutures are in place with the ischial tuberosity visualized in the wound. **B,** Final repair of the hamstring, with multiple suture points visualized *(arrows)*.

anchors. Sutures are passed through the tendon using horizontal mattress sutures placed from inferior to superior and are tied down from superior to inferior with the knee flexed to at least 30 degrees. The tendon should be placed on the lateral aspect of the ischial tuberosity and should lay down flat to allow optimal bony healing, as well as to prevent prominence (Fig. 88-13).

Results

In one study of 52 patients in which the open technique was used for both acute[32] and chronic[11] repairs, a 96% satisfaction rate was found with use of subjective validated outcome scales and at an average of 27 months follow-up.[33] Lower Extremity Functional Scale results indicated that acute repairs had statistically significant greater outcomes than did chronic repairs ($P = .023$). Thirty-five patients (67%) reported that they could participate in strenuous activities at their latest follow-up.

Another study of eight patients with a similar suture anchor repair revealed postoperative Cybex testing at 88% of peak torque, with the ratio of hamstring-to-quadriceps strength being 0.55, which was not significantly different from the other side.[23] An analysis of 10 athletes with acute complete hamstring tendon tears revealed that the average peak torque was 82% and the hamstring-to-quadriceps strength ratio was 0.56.[24] Nine of 10 patients returned to their previous level of professional sports activities. Three patients had acute sciatic nerve symptoms that were successfully treated with hematoma evacuation and neurolysis.

Most studies evaluating late surgical repairs have been in patients with chronic tears for complaints of pain while sitting, hamstring weakness, and sciatic nerve symptoms due to scarring, also known as hamstring syndrome.[21,31,34] These chronic tear repairs yield less consistent results, and the potential exists of scarring of the hamstring-avulsed tissue to the sciatic nerve. These repairs could require concomitant dissection of the nerve from the avulsed tendons, followed by sciatic neurolysis, and may be an indication for endoscopic neurolysis with either open or endoscopic repair, depending on the comfort level of the surgeon and the exposure obtained. As a result of the inferior results, most surgeons experienced in proximal hamstring repair recommend early reattachment compared with delayed repair.[35] In the study by Sarimo et al.,[22] 41 athletes underwent either acute or chronic surgical repair. The authors found that the odds ratio of having a moderate or poor result was 29-fold with a delay of surgical repair of greater than 3 months.[22] In a few patients who have early surgery, decreased activity, pain, weakness, neuralgia, and difficulty walking may still occur, which is attributed to immobilization and possibly injuries to branches of the sciatic nerve. The surgical outcome may be confounded by one of several issues: retracted tendons can be difficult to repair anatomically, denervated muscles can have attenuated tissue quality and be prone to repeated rupture, and retracted tendons can be adherent down with the nerves, predisposing the nerves to potential injury with neurolysis.

For patients with chronic ruptures who undergo repair, an allograft may be necessary for reattachment to the ischial tuberosity.[35] The literature includes few results with regard to this procedure; however, Folsom and Larson[32] reported on five patients who required Achilles tendon allograft reconstruction for repair of a chronic rupture. They found that reconstruction of chronic ruptures with an Achilles allograft appeared to restore function and strength at a level comparable with acute repairs.

For patients with high-grade partial insertional tears who fail to respond to nonoperative treatment, surgical repair is performed. The surgical approach is the same as previously described. Once the tendon is exposed, it is incised and released from the tuberosity with use of an elevator. It is then repaired using the same technique for complete tears with suture anchors. Treatment of partial tears has been reported by Lempainen et al.,[37] with high levels of satisfaction in 47 athletes.

Chronic proximal hamstring tendinopathy has also traditionally been included in the generic term *hamstring syndrome*. In this specific injury, the tendon is traumatized from repetitive overuse injury. Theoretically, the tendon undergoes repetitive stretch and mechanical overload and is unable to fully heal. The sciatic nerve can undergo similar types of stress, leading to scarring, adhesion, and impingement from the thickened tendon. In the cohort in the study by Lempainen et al.,[37] surgical treatment was performed with tenotomy of the thickened semimembranosus tendon and tenodesis to the biceps femoris; 89% of the patients had good to excellent results. A few patients with poor outcomes had persistent adhesions or regenerated semimembranosus tendons that recreated impingement.

As with the endoscopic repairs, the repair is protected with a hinged knee brace that is typically fixed at 90 degrees for the first 4 weeks. With this more invasive approach, patients take aspirin for 4 weeks after surgery for deep vein thrombosis prophylaxis.

The endoscopic approach has been developed during the past 18 months and used in a group of 15 patients. All patients underwent the surgery as described with no need to abandon the procedure because of failure to visualize any of the structures. All of the patients underwent suture anchor fixation with no anchor complications to date. Two patients initially reported numbness over the posterior thigh with resolution of their symptoms by 6 weeks after surgery. No wound complications or sciatic nerve dysfunction occurred. One patient (who had preoperative refractory ischial bursitis) has had a subsequent guided injection as a result of recurrent ischial pain.

Rehabilitation

Assuming that hamstring strain or rupture has its source in the inhibition and weakness of its closest synergists, the gluteal and abdominal muscles, it is important to focus on both groups in the rehabilitation of these injuries, whether they are treated surgically or not. Because the gluteal muscles work in conjunction with the hamstrings to extend the hip, when the agonists (gluteal muscles) for hip extension are weak, an increased relative effort of the hamstrings is required to control trunk and hip flexion during the loading phase of running.[38] In one prospective evaluation, 24 athletes were rehabilitated in one of two protocols: either an isolated hamstring stretching and progressive strengthening protocol or a progressive agility and trunk stabilization protocol.[39] At both short (2 weeks) and long (1 year) follow-up, the authors found a significantly higher reinjury rate in athletes treated with the isolated hamstring rehabilitation protocol (54.5% vs. 0% and 70% vs. 7.7%, respectively). This finding suggests that good strong neuromuscular control of the lumbopelvic region allows the lower extremity muscle to function at high velocity while maintaining a protected range of motion for hamstring muscles.

Using the synergistic concept as the premise for the rehabilitation program, the patient ambulates on crutches with non–weight bearing for the first 2 to 4 weeks, depending on the quality of tension on the repair. Weight bearing is advanced to full weight bearing by 4 weeks with continued use of crutches until 6 weeks, as the knee brace is extended by about 15 degrees per week. The brace is removed between 6 and 8 weeks after surgery. Passive hip range of motion is begun with a therapist at 2 weeks and active hip flexion is started at 4 weeks. Isotonic strengthening (at 6 weeks), isokinetic strengthening (at 8 weeks), and aqua therapy are initiated with progression of core pelvic and closed-chain exercises. Dry land training and sport-specific training are initiated at 12 weeks, with return to full sports participation between 5 to 8 months after surgery.

Complications

Potential complications associated with proximal hamstring ruptures prior to surgical treatment are related to the mechanism of injury. The complications can be early or delayed. The early complications most commonly involve a neurapraxia injury to the sciatic nerve as a result of a stretch injury. Depending on the mechanism and force of the injury, the sciatic nerve can be damaged, leading to burning symptoms radiating down the leg and weakness of the foot. During the initial examination it is critical to determine if the sciatic nerve is functioning appropriately to document and ensure that no iatrogenic injury is present at the time of surgery. Fortunately, neurapraxia injury most commonly resolves over time, despite being troubling to the patient initially. Delayed complications of nonoperative treatment of proximal hamstring ruptures have been described by Puranen and Orava.[34] These complications include knee flexion and hip extension weakness, difficulty sitting, hamstring deformity, and the potential development of symptoms similar to those of hamstring syndrome as the tendons scar down to the sciatic nerve. Hamstring syndrome consists of local posterior buttock pain and discomfort over the ischial tuberosity. In addition, the pain may worsen with stretching and during exercise (e.g., sprinting, hurdling, and kicking).

Surgical repair of proximal hamstring ruptures also has its inherent risks. Superficial and deep wound infections can occur, as with other surgeries; however, the location of the incision can potentially increase this risk because of the proximity of the incision to the perineum. Additionally, the three main nervous structures at risk of iatrogenic injury are the posterior femoral cutaneous, inferior gluteal, and sciatic nerves. The posterior femoral cutaneous nerve exits the sacral plexus and enters the pelvis through the greater sciatic foramen, below the piriformis muscle. It then descends beneath the gluteus maximus with the inferior gluteal artery and runs down the back of the thigh beneath the fascia lata and over the long head of the biceps femoris to the back of the knee.[37,40] It provides sensation to the skin of the posterior surface of the thigh and leg, as well as to the skin of the perineum. It can be injured during the surgical approach for repair if it is not protected. The inferior gluteal nerve is the major innervation of the gluteus maximus, which is the principal extensor of the thigh. This nerve can be injured with aggressive retraction of the gluteus during the surgical approach.[40]

The sciatic nerve is the longest and widest single nerve in the human body and provides innervation of the skin of the leg, as well as the muscles of the posterior compartment of the thigh; it also provides the motor function of the calf and foot. The nerve is in close proximity to the ischial tuberosity as it runs along the lateral aspect.[40] It may be injured from retraction during exposure of the tuberosity for repair.[22,26]

Other potential complications associated with proximal hamstring repair include repeat rupture, weakness, and sitting pain. According to the reports on hamstring repair, repeat ruptures are rare. In the cohort in the study by Sarimo et al.,[22] failure of surgical repair was found in 3 of 41 patients. Upon a repeat operation, anatomic repair of the injury could not be achieved. The authors believed that the deteriorated tendon quality can be a result of delays in surgical treatment, fatty degeneration, and muscle denervation from nerve injury.[22]

Several studies have tested postoperative hamstring strength after repair. Recently, Carmichael et al.[26] found that mean postoperative isotonic strength was 84% compared with the contralateral side; however, other studies have shown a return of strength ranging from 60% to 90% after repair.[19,23,29,31]

A concern unique to the endoscopic approach is that of fluid extravasation into the pelvis as a result of the fluid used in the distension of the potential space around the hamstring tendon. Every effort should be made to regularly check the abdomen for any evidence of abdominal distension. Likewise, any unusual blood pressure decreases that may be due to fluid compression from retroperitoneal extravasation need to be kept in mind. In general, an attempt should be made to maintain the fluid inflow pressures as low as is feasible for good visualization, and an attempt should be made to keep track of fluid ingress and egress volumes to ensure that extravasation is avoided.

One of the most important aspects in the treatment of proximal hamstring ruptures is early recognition and early treatment. Early recognition of the injury allows for early repair of the acute injury, which is substantially easier to perform immediately after the injury occurs (within 4 weeks). Later recognition and delayed surgery lead to a more difficult repair that ultimately may result in increased surgical complications and poorer patient outcomes. Patients who undergo repairs of acute injuries have had better outcomes in the literature compared with patients who undergo repairs of chronic injuries.[21,22]

The surgical approach for hamstring repair may be slightly intimidating for surgeons because it is not a common area for surgical treatment and is infrequently encountered during our orthopaedic training. Although this surgical area may be unfamiliar, the anatomy should be well known, in particular the areas of concern, including the sciatic nerve. It is recommended that a first-time repair be performed in the acute setting in a fairly slender patient to provide an easier approach to the ischial tuberosity.

In summary, recognition of proximal hamstring ruptures allows early treatment with surgical repair. With proper treatment, good functional results can be achieved.

Future Considerations

Few clinical studies have been conducted to test hamstring strength in patients who have undergone nonoperative treatment of acute ruptures to assist in determining a range of strength deficit if the tendon is not repaired.[21] As a result, when discussing the options of repair or conservative treatment with patients after a diagnosis of a complete proximal hamstring rupture, it is difficult to provide patients with a percentage of weakness expected if the repair is not performed. As previously mentioned with regard to distal biceps ruptures, future studies may accurately document associated weakness either prior to repair or in patients with chronic ruptures.

In addition, further development and refinement of the endoscopic technique is necessary, because presently it is clearly in its earliest phases. The extent to which this technique can be used in all tears remains to be seen. The technique definitely allows a more thorough assessment of the entire constellation of findings, including sciatic nerve involvement. Further studies are necessary to document the outcomes of the technique and compare it with the traditional open procedures.

For a complete list of references, go to expertconsult.com.

Suggested Readings

Citation: Elliott MC, Zarins B, Powell JW, et al: Hamstring muscle strains in professional football players: A 10-year review. *Am J Sports Med* 39:843–850, 2011.

Level of Evidence: IV

Summary: The authors of this article provide a summary of the types of strains and ruptures seen in the professional athlete.

Citation: Miller SL, Gill J, Webb GR: The proximal origin of the hamstrings and surrounding anatomy encountered during repair. A cadaveric study. *J Bone Joint Surg Am* 89(A):44–48, 2007.

Level of Evidence: Anatomic study

Summary: The authors of this article provide a review of the pertinent surgical anatomy that delineates the appropriate anatomic areas to understand in approaching the area.

Citation: Blasier RL, Morawa LG: Complete rupture of the hamstring origin from a water skiing injury. *Am J Sports Med* 18:435–437, 1990.

Level of Evidence: V (case report)

Summary: This article is one of the original articles in which the most common mechanism of acute ruptures is described.

Citation: Sarimo J, Lempainen L, Mattila K, et al: Complete proximal hamstring avulsions: A series of 41 patients with operative treatment. *Am J Sports Med* 36:1110–1115, 2008.

Level of Evidence: IV

Summary: This articles includes the largest series published, with a good summary of the mechanisms, treatment, and outcomes of the open procedure.

Citation: Folsom GJ, Larson CM: Surgical treatment of acute versus chronic complete proximal hamstring ruptures: Results of a new allograft technique for chronic reconstructions. *Am J Sports Med* 36:104–109, 2008.

Level of Evidence: II

Summary: In this article the surgical technique and indications for reconstruction of the hamstring in chronic rupture cases are described.

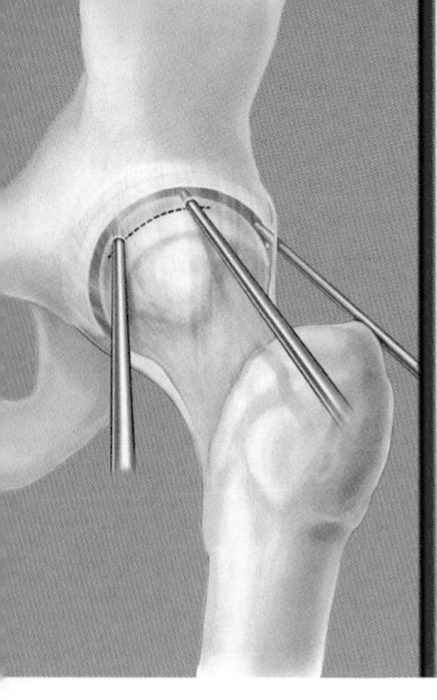

89

Nerve Entrapment Lesions of the Hip and Thigh

HAL DAVID MARTIN • IAN JAMES PALMER • MUNIF HATEM

Neurologic hip and thigh pain can present a challenging diagnostic situation. A structured and comprehensive physical examination is essential for a correct diagnosis.[1] The assessment should incorporate the four layers of the hip: osseous, capsulolabral, musculotendinous, and neurovascular. The neurovascular layer is influenced by the other layers, including the fifth layer, the kinematic chain. To effectively treat hip and thigh nerve entrapments, diagnostic strategies require the interpretation of abnormal anatomy and biomechanics of each layer. Isolated treatments of single layers may not provide a complete solution, leading to frustration for both the patient and physician.

This chapter presents a short review covering general nerve and entrapment characteristics and describes specific nerve entrapments from posterior to anterior.

General Characteristics

Peripheral nerve fibers are arranged in widely variable numbers into bundles (fascicles) (Fig. 89-1). Each fascicle is surrounded by the perineurium, a multilayered epithelial sheath.[2] The space among the perineurium/fascicles is filled by connective tissue, including vessels. Finally, the nerve is surrounded by the epineurium, a thicker, highly vascular areolar tissue that provides a cushion for the nerves. Although the endoneurium offers little mechanical support, the perineurium is dense, providing strength in tension and maintaining the pressurized blood-nerve barrier. The fascicular pattern is continually modified along the length of peripheral nerves with an interchange of nervous fibers among different fascicles.[3] Vascular considerations for peripheral nerves should not only include the inflow but also the outflow, because varicosities can cause dilations within the nerve.[4] Another important consideration is that the vascular supply for hip and thigh nerves is different from that of the upper body (Fig. 89-2).[5] Peripheral nerves possess the ability to glide and stretch, accommodating normal joint biomechanics. The nerve is susceptible to mechanical compression or especially stretch injury[5a] as it courses around musculotendinous, osseous, and ligamentous structures.

Peripheral nerve entrapment syndromes comprise nerve dysfunction because of localized interference of microvascular function and structural changes in the nerve or adjacent tissues. Acute and chronic nerve compression increases vascular permeability with edema formation and, consequently, impairment of axonal transport.[6] Diabetes mellitus and other metabolic and unknown factors can increase the susceptibility to compression injuries or influence the treatment outcome.

General symptoms include a burning or lancinating pain to the area supplied by the nerve. Physical examination may reveal evidence of impaired sensory perception of the nerve and pain relief with an anesthetic injection to the site where pain occurs. However, vague and poorly localized symptoms can produce complex clinical presentations. Furthermore, peripheral nerve entrapments can occur at more than one point in the same nerve fiber or coexist with lumbosacral root compression. This concept has been developed in the upper limb and termed *double crush syndrome*.[7]

Magnetic resonance is the most useful imaging method for evaluating peripheral nerve entrapment. The findings include direct and indirect signs of nerve injury.[8] In fluid-sensitive images, hyperintensity that is focal or similar to that of adjacent vessels is more likely to be significant.[8] Abnormalities in nerve size or fascicular pattern or blurring of the perineural fat tissue are suggestive of neural injury, although these features are difficult to note in small-diameter nerves.[8] The main indirect sign of nerve entrapment injury is muscular denervation edema.[9] Ultrasonography is an important method of guiding nerve blocks and has been increasingly used for nerve evaluation, because it offers the advantages of dynamic evaluation and Doppler assessment of nerves and vessels.

Electrodiagnostic studies for lower extremity nerve entrapments are more complex than for the upper limb.[10] Obesity, edema, and age can affect the acquisition of sensory nerve action potentials in the lower limb, mainly in the proximally located nerves. Moreover, asymptomatic (usually elderly) patients often display neurogenic changes in electrodiagnostic studies.[10] These features may be problematic for the differential diagnosis between lumbosacral and peripheral entrapment.[10] However, electrodiagnostic assessment can be useful when it is associated with an adequate physical examination and nerve block.

The following conservative measures can control symptoms in most patients: oral and topical analgesic agents; steroidal and nonsteroidal antiinflammatory drugs; neuromodulation drugs, including tricyclic antidepressants, gabapentin, and pregabalin; physiotherapy; transcutaneous electric nerve stimulation; cryoablation; and nerve blocks.

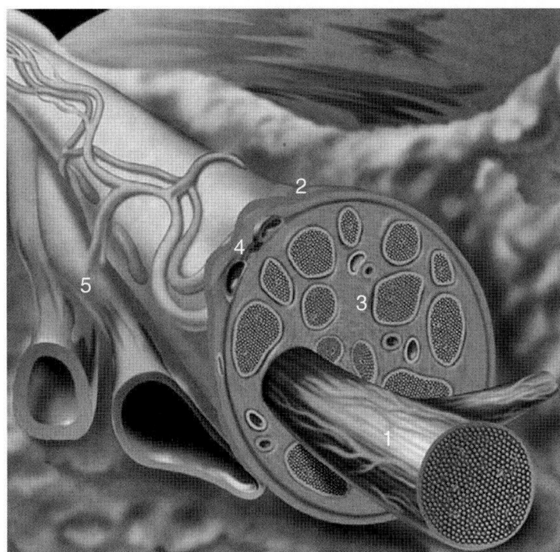

FIGURE 89-1 Organization of a peripheral nerve. *1,* Nerve fascicle with endoneurium and evolved by perineurium. *2,* Epineural sheath enveloping the bundle of fascicles. *3,* Connective tissue among the fascicles. *4,* Epineural blood vessels. *5,* Neighboring vasculature. *(From Enneking FK, Chan V, Greger J, et al: Lower-extremity peripheral nerve blockade: essentials of our current understanding.* Reg Anesth Pain Med *30[1]:4–35, 2005.)*

Entrapments of the Posterior Nerves

Deep Gluteal Syndrome/Sciatic Nerve Entrapment

In recent years, the identification of a number of etiologies of sciatic nerve entrapment has given rise to the term *deep gluteal syndrome* (DGS).[11] Entrapment of the sciatic nerve is characterized by nondiscogenic, extrapelvic nerve compression presenting with symptoms of pain and dysesthesias in the buttock area, hip, or posterior thigh and/or as radicular pain.

Anatomy

The deep gluteal space is anterior and beneath the gluteus maximus and posterior to the posterior border of the femoral neck, the linea aspera (lateral), the sacrotuberous and falciform fascia (medial), the inferior margin of the sciatic notch (superior), and the hamstring origin (inferior) (Fig. 89-3). The sciatic nerve, formed by L4-S3 sacral roots, courses distally through the deep gluteal space anterior to the piriformis muscle and posterior to the obturator/gemelli complex and quadratus femoris. Variations exist concerning the relationship between the piriformis muscle and sciatic nerve. Six categories have been described[12] and are important for the surgeon to recognize; however, the anomaly itself may not be the etiology of DGS symptoms. The prevalence of piriformis/sciatic nerve anomalies is 16% to 17% (Fig. 89-4).[13]

Etiology

The piriformis muscle and tendon is the most common source of extrapelvic sciatic nerve impingement. In many cases, a thick tendon can hide under the belly of the piriformis overlying the nerve. Hypertrophy of the piriformis muscle has been attributed to sciatic nerve entrapment[14]; however, Benson and Schutzer[15] found that only 2 of 14 patients had larger piriformis muscles on the symptomatic side, and seven appeared smaller than on the unaffected side. Atypical fibrovascular scar bands and greater trochanteric bursae hypertrophy have been reported in many cases of sciatic nerve entrapment.[16] The obturator internus/gemelli complex can also be a source of sciatica-like pain. The sciatic nerve exits the sciatic notch anterior to the piriformis and posterior to the superior gemelli/obturator internus, which can cause a scissor effect between the two muscles, resulting in entrapment. Distally at the ischium, the insertion of the hamstring tendon (especially the semimembranosis) can be thickened as a result of trauma or hamstring avulsion and subsequently decrease the ischiofemoral space, which may involve the sciatic nerve. Other sources of sciatic nerve entrapment include malunion of the ischium or healed avulsions, acetabular fracture, posthip reconstruction, tumor, vascular abnormalities, and gluteus maximus (scarring and subluxation from a prior iliotibial band release). The greater trochanter can cause sciatic nerve

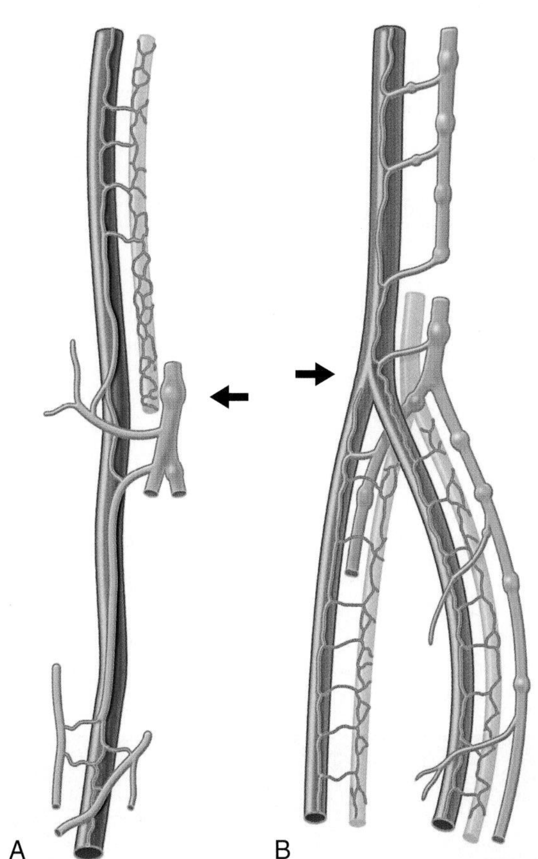

FIGURE 89-2 From proximal to distal, the dominant venous drainage of the median and sciatic nerves. The arrows designate the level of the elbow and knee. **A,** The median nerve is to the plexus around the brachial artery and via muscular veins in the arm. In the forearm, the dominant venous drainage is provided by the median vein. **B,** The sciatic nerve is via the perforators of the profunda system in the thigh and directly to the popliteal vein at the knee. In the leg, the anterior and posterior tibial nerves drain predominantly to the plexus around their accompanying arteries, as well as to muscular veins. *(Modified from Del Piñal F, Taylor GI: The venous drainage of nerves; anatomical study and clinical implications.* Br J Plast Surg *43[5]:511–520, 1990.)*

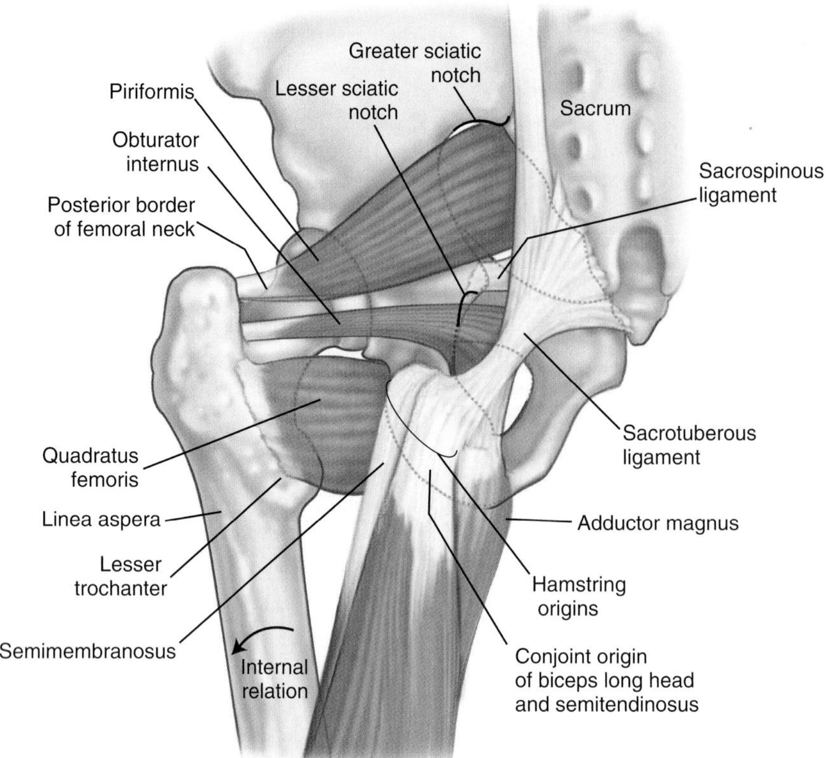

FIGURE 89-3 The deep gluteal space. *(Modified from Thomas Byrd JW, editor:* Operative hip arthroscopy, *ed 3, New York, 2012, Springer.)*

compression in deep flexion, abduction, and external rotation. Intrapelvic pathologies must be considered, including gynecologic conditions (Fig. 89-5) and vascular entrapment of sacral neural roots.[17] Varicosities associated with incompetent veins along the sciatic nerve have been also reported to be a source of sciatic nerve symptoms.[4]

Diagnosis

Potential sources of entrapment involve each layer, and thus a comprehensive physical examination, a detailed history, and standardized radiographic interpretation are paramount in evaluating hip pain.[1,16,18] In all cases of suspected sciatic nerve entrapment, the spine must first be ruled out as the cause of symptoms. Clinical presentation often includes a history of trauma and symptoms of pain while sitting (i.e., the inability to sit for more than 30 minutes), radicular pain of the lower back or hip, and paresthesias of the affected leg.[15,16] Some patients may present with the neurologic symptoms of abnormal reflexes or motor weakness. Symptoms related to nerves other than the sciatic nerve may be observed, such as weakness of the gluteus medius and minimus muscles (superior gluteal nerve), weakness of the gluteus maximus (inferior gluteal nerve), perineal sensory loss (pudendal nerve), or loss of posterior thigh sensation (posterior femoral cutaneous nerve). Patients with intrapelvic sciatic nerve endometriosis present with symptom variations related to menses.

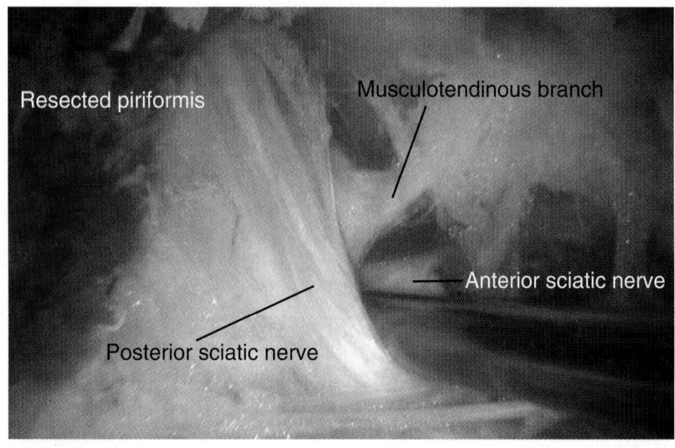

FIGURE 89-4 The ancillary musculotendinous branch through the sciatic nerve.

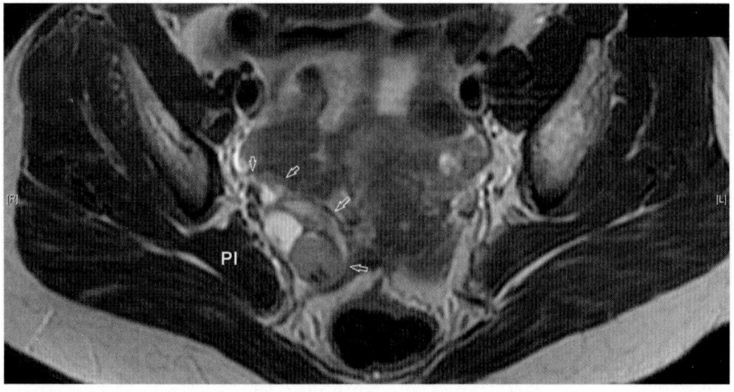

FIGURE 89-5 Magnetic resonance image of the pelvis demonstrating an ovarian cyst on the right side (*arrows*). The sacral plexus and gluteal vessels are located between the piriformis muscle (*PI*) and the ovarian cyst.

The physical examination of patients with possible sciatic nerve entrapment is based on three tests: palpation; the seated piriformis stretch test; and the active piriformis test. In a recent study, the combination of the seated piriformis stretch test with the piriformis active test had a sensitivity of 91% and specificity of 80% for the endoscopic finding of sciatic nerve entrapment.[18a] The seated piriformis stretch test (Fig. 89-6, *A*) is a flexion and adduction with internal rotation test performed with the patient in the seated position.[1] The examiner extends the knee (engaging the sciatic nerve) and passively moves the flexed hip into adduction with internal rotation while palpating 1 cm lateral to the ischium (with the middle finger) and proximally at the sciatic notch (with the index finger). A positive test is the recreation of the posterior pain at the level of the piriformis or external rotators. An active piriformis test is performed by having the patient push the heel down into the table and abduct and externally rotate the leg against resistance while the examiner monitors the piriformis (Fig. 89-6, *B*).

Guided injection tests are important in supporting the diagnosis of DGS when the piriformis is involved. Complementary diagnostic studies include electromyography and nerve conduction studies, which can be beneficial in the diagnosis of DGS. Piriformis entrapment of the sciatic nerve is often indicated by H-reflex disturbances of the tibial and/or perineal nerves. This study is performed dynamically with the knee in extension and the hip in adduction with internal rotation and compared side to side.

DGS is characterized by lateral and superior pain at the level of the external rotators or piriformis muscle along the sciatic tract. Four main differential diagnoses should be considered with use of the ischial tuberosity as a reference[19]: (1) ischiofemoral impingement (pain lateral to the ischium); (2) ischial tunnel syndrome (pain lateral to the ischium); (3) hamstring issues (pain at the ischium); and (4) pudendal nerve entrapment (pain medial to the ischium).

Nonoperative Treatment

Nonoperative treatment for DGS begins with a conservative approach addressing the suspected site of entrapment. Treatment of entrapment from a hypertrophied, contracted, or inflamed muscle (e.g., the piriformis, quadratus femoris, obturator internus, or superior/inferior gemellus) begins with rest, use of antiinflammatory drugs and muscle relaxants, and physical therapy. The physical therapy program should include stretching maneuvers aimed at the external rotators. The piriformis stretch involves placing the leg in flexion, adduction, and internal rotation (Fig. 89-7). Patients with cam impingement, anterior pincer impingement, or acetabular retroversion may not be able to stretch adequately into this position and should be evaluated and treated primarily for femoroacetabular impingement because most cases will resolve with appropriate surgical intervention. Imaging-guided injections of anesthetics and corticosteroids can provide pain relief in patients who do not respond to physical therapy. A trial of three injections has been recommended before opting for more aggressive treatment, with evaluation on a case-by-case basis. Most cases of DGS/sciatic nerve entrapment will respond to conservative nonoperative measures.

Operative Treatment

Options for operative treatment include open and endoscopic techniques. The open transgluteal approach has been described to effectively perform piriformis muscle resection and neuroplasty of the sciatic and posterior femoral cutaneous nerves.[14] A number of case studies have reported success with an open approach, and the largest case series have reported good to excellent outcomes in 75% to 100% of the procedures.[14,15] Additionally, release of the hamstrings and neurolysis of the sciatic nerve at the hamstring origin have been performed, with achievement of satisfactory results with significant pain relief and increased hamstring strength.[20]

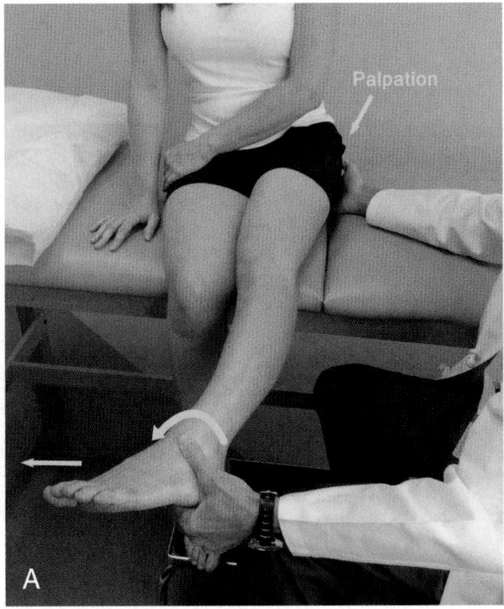

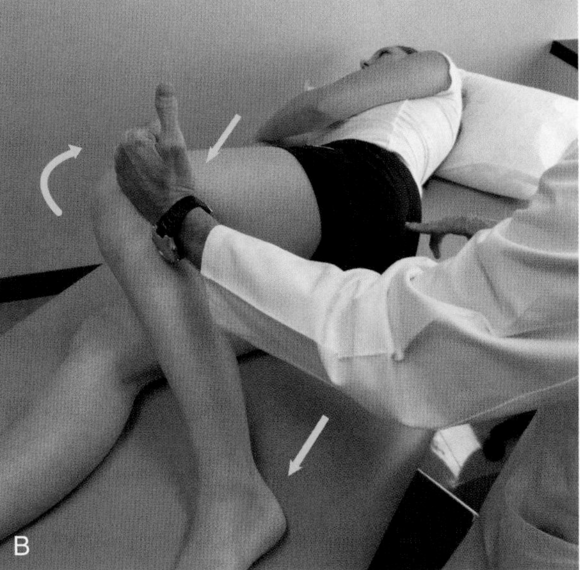

FIGURE 89-6 The seated piriformis stretch test and active piriformis test. **A,** The patient is in the seated position with knee extension. The examiner passively moves the flexed hip into adduction with internal rotation while palpating 1 cm lateral to the ischium (with the middle finger) and proximally at the piriformis (with the index finger). **B,** With the patient in the lateral position, the examiner palpates the piriformis. The patient drives the heel into the examining table, thus initiating external hip rotation while actively abducting and externally rotating against resistance.

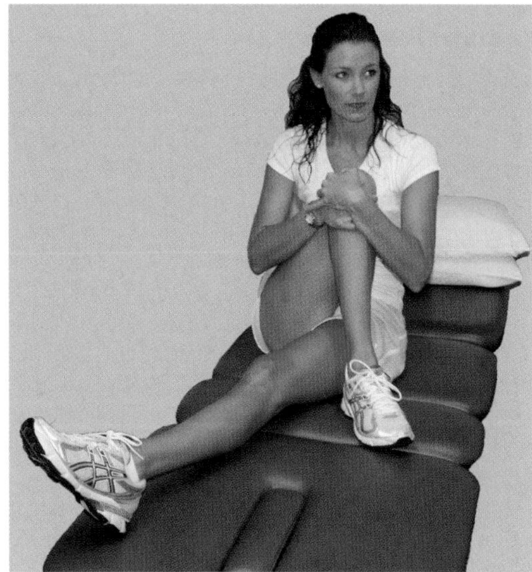

FIGURE 89-7 Piriformis stretch. In a seated position, the patient brings the knee into the chest and across midline and pulls the knee to the opposite shoulder.

Endoscopy is an effective and minimally invasive approach to the treatment of DGS. Dezawa et al.[21] first reported on six cases of endoscopic piriformis muscle release. We described an endoscopic technique for sciatic nerve decompression in the supine position with use of an orthopaedic table.[16] In this technique, a 70-degree-long scope and adjustable/lengthening cannulas are used through three portals: anterolateral, posterolateral, and auxiliary posterolateral (Fig. 89-8). We reported on a case series of 35 patients treated with endoscopic sciatic nerve decompression with a 12-month follow-up.[16] The average duration of symptoms was 3.7 years with an average preoperative verbal analog pain score of 7, which decreased to 2.4 after surgery. The preoperative modified Harris Hip Score was 54.4, and this score increased to 78 postoperatively. Twenty-one patients reported preoperative use of narcotics for pain; two continued to take narcotics after surgery (for reasons unrelated to the initial complaint). Eighty-three percent of patients had no postoperative sciatic pain while sitting (i.e., the inability to sit for >30 minutes).[16] Among 200 cases, complications continue to be extremely low; however, poor outcomes are related to femoral retroversion and previous abdominal surgery. It is very important to assess acetabular and femoral version, which have an effect on sciatic nerve biomechanics.[22] In cases of sciatic nerve compression by the greater trochanter (with deep flexion and external rotation) or ischium, greater trochanteric osteoplasty or osteotomy may be a consideration. Complications have involved a hematoma brought on by early postoperative use of nonsteroidal antiinflammatory drugs with excessive postoperative activity. Concomitant pudendal nerve and sciatic nerve complaints are often resolved; however, in two cases the pudendal complaints worsened. Knowledge of proper rehabilitation is important for successful outcomes. By understanding the anatomy and biomechanics and applying clinical tests and diagnostic strategies, adequate treatment of all four layers can be obtained as a part of a comprehensive plan of treatment.

Pudendal Nerve Entrapment

The pudendal nerve arises from S2-S4 ventral rami and exits the pelvis through the greater sciatic foramen and below the

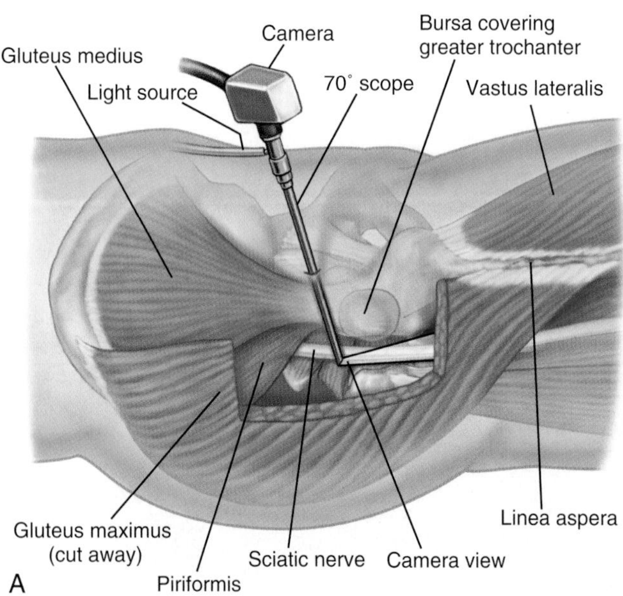

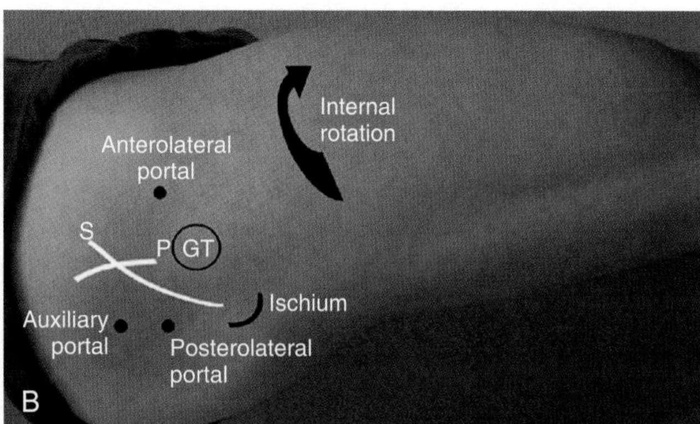

FIGURE 89-8 Peritrochanteric space (PTS) and portal placement. **A,** The PTS and anatomic landmarks with orientation of the arthroscope and light source. The scope is introduced into the PTS and turned around to introduce the auxiliary portal. **B,** The anterolateral portal placement is 1 cm anterior and 1 cm superior to the greater trochanter (*GT*). The posterolateral portal placement is 3 cm posterior to the greater trochanter and in line with the anterolateral portal. The auxiliary portal is positioned 3 cm posterior and 3 cm superior to the greater trochanter. The course of the sciatic nerve (*S*) and piriformis (*P*) are depicted in relation to the greater trochanter and ischium. *(**A,** From Martin H: Diagnostic arthroscopy. In Kelly BT, Philippon MJ, editors:* Arthroscopic techniques of the hip: a visual guide, *Thorofare, NJ, 2009, Slack. **B,** From Martin HD, Shears SA, Johnson JC, et al: The endoscopic treatment of sciatic nerve entrapment/deep gluteal syndrome.* Arthroscopy *27:172–181, 2011.)*

piriformis muscle. It crosses the sacrospinous ligament close to its insertion to the ischial spine or passes over the ischial spine. The pudendal nerve then enters the Alcock (pudendal) canal formed by the obturator fascia and sacrotuberous ligament (Fig. 89-9). In the posterior part of the Alcock canal, the pudendal nerve gives rise to the inferior rectal nerve, the perineal nerve, and the dorsal nerves of the penis or clitoris.[23]

Pudendal nerve entrapment can occur in different places from its origin until terminal branches.[24] Cycling, endometriosis, previous pelvic surgery, and vascular abnormalities have been described as possible etiologies of pudendal nerve entrapment.[25] Antolak et al.[26] have suggested that aberrant development and subsequent malpositioning of the ischial spine found in men with pudendal nerve entrapment could be associated with athletic injuries during their youth.

The diagnosis of pudendal neuralgia has been primarily clinical and empirical[27]; however, progress in clinical nerve imaging and injection techniques are aiding in the differential diagnosis of pudendal nerve entrapment.[24] In 2008, Labat et al.[27] described the Nantes criteria with five essential diagnostic criteria: (1) pain in the anatomic territory of the pudendal nerve; (2) pain that is worsened by sitting (relief is achieved when sitting on a toilet seat); (3) the pain does not wake the patient at night, (4) pain with no objective sensory impairment; and (5) the pain is relieved by a diagnostic pudendal nerve block. Also defined in the report are complementary diagnostic criteria, exclusion criteria, and associated signs, not excluding the diagnosis.[27] The physical examination and injections are useful for preliminarily sorting patients into different points of entrapment categories: type I, sciatic notch tenderness only; type II, midischial tenderness; type IIIa, obturator internus muscle tenderness only; type IIIb, obturator and piriformis muscle tenderness; and type IV, no palpable tenderness.[24]

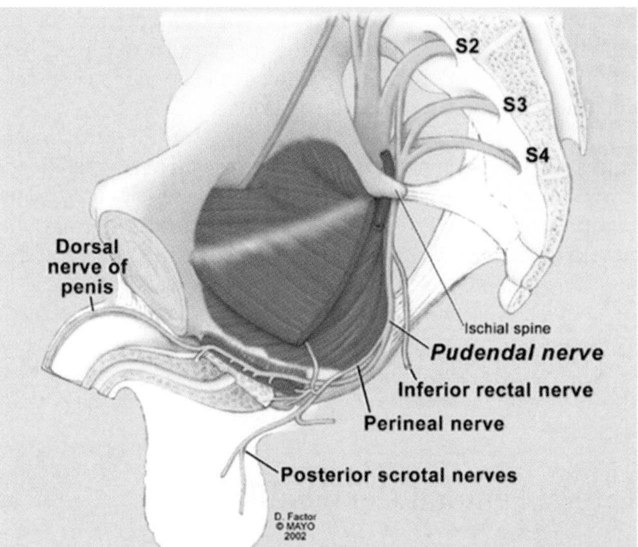

FIGURE 89-9 Pudendal nerve course and branches. *(From Hough DM, Wittenberg KH, Pawlina W, et al: Chronic perineal pain caused by pudendal nerve entrapment: anatomy and CT-guided perineural injection technique.* AJR Am J Roentgenol *181[2]:561–567, 2003.)*

Conservative treatment includes use of pain medications, physical therapy of the pelvic floor muscles, and guided anesthetic nerve blocks, including steroids. Surgical decompression may be considered when nonsurgical treatments have failed and is traditionally performed through transgluteal open approaches. One published randomized controlled trial compared 16 patients who were surgically treated with 16 who were conservatively treated. At 12 months, 71% of the surgery group improved compared with 13% of the nonsurgery group.[28] In contrast to extrapelvic approaches, a laparoscopic intrapelvic decompression technique has been described in a case series including 18 patients; 15 patients (83%) had significant pain relief, with a mean follow-up of 21 months.[25]

Superior and Inferior Gluteal Nerves

The superior gluteal nerve arises from L4, L5, and S1 ventral rami.[23] The inferior gluteal nerve arises from L5, S1, and S2 ventral rami.[23] Both nerves access the deep gluteal space through the greater sciatic foramen, passing above (superior gluteal nerve) and below (inferior gluteal nerve) the piriformis.

The gluteal nerves are at risk of being damaged in lateral or posterior surgical approaches to the hip or via percutaneous iliosacral screws, gluteal injections, bone calluses related to fracture, and prominent osteophytes. Sacroiliac inflammatory and infectious processes can cause gluteal nerve neuropathy because of the anatomic proximity.

Limp or gait pattern changes can be noted in patients with dysfunction of gluteal nerves. Weakness of the abductor musculature and a positive Trendelenburg test are also found in persons with superior gluteal nerve neuropathies. Superior or inferior nerve entrapment usually does not cause obvious gait abnormalities.

Conservative treatment is usually indicated in cases of gluteal nerve neuropathy. Surgical excision of bone or screw compression should be considered in some cases. In cases of severe abductor dysfunction with good gluteus maximus function, gluteus maximus flap transfer is an option. Limiting proximal extension of the gluteal medius incision to 3 cm cranial to the greater trochanter is indicated to avoid superior gluteal nerve damage in lateral hip approaches. In posterior approaches, gluteus maximus splitting of more than 5 cm from the greater trochanter should be avoided to protect the inferior gluteal nerve.[28a]

Entrapments of the Anterior Nerves

Obturator Nerve

The obturator nerve arises in the lumbar plexus from the merging of the posterior divisions of the L2-L4 ventral rami.[23] After its intrapelvic trajectory, the obturator nerve crosses the 3-cm–long obturator canal at the upper part of the obturator foramen, entering the thigh and dividing into anterior and posterior branches. The obturator externus and adductor brevis muscles separate these two neural divisions (Fig. 89-10).[23]

The obturator nerve is most often damaged by direct damage or stretching associated with trauma, pelvic surgery, or hip surgery. Entrapment of the obturator nerve can be

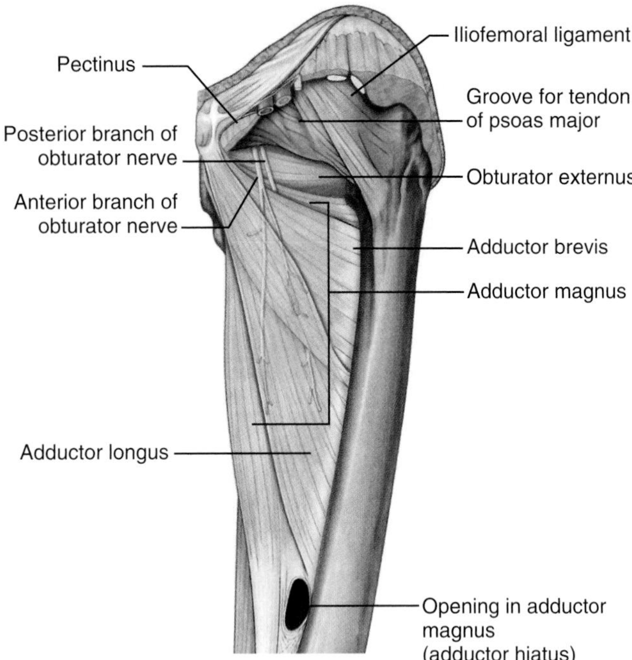

FIGURE 89-10 The obturator nerve and its anterior and posterior divisions, separated by the adductor brevis muscle. *(From Standring S, editor:* Gray's anatomy: the anatomical basis of clinical practice, *ed 40, London, 2008, Elsevier.)*

associated with the following etiologies: hernia and pelvic floor repair using synthetic mesh or tape; herniation at the obturator canal; tumor; bursae or periarticular cysts; endometriosis; and bone cement used for a total hip arthroplasty. Athletes can also experience obturator nerve entrapment at a thick fascia overlying the short adductor muscle.[29]

Sensory and motor complaints can be seen in patients with entrapment of the obturator nerve. The patient presents with paresthesias, sensory loss, and pain in the medial thigh extending medially from the hip to the knee.[30] Movements of abduction and extension increase the symptoms by stretching the obturator nerve. Athletes present a characteristic clinical pattern of exercise-induced medial thigh pain commencing in the region of the adductor muscle origin and radiating distally along the medial thigh,[29] and this condition should be differentiated from isolated adductor tendinitis. The hip adductors on the affected side are weak, and in severe cases the gait can assume an abductor pattern. The gracilis and obturator externus muscle functions are compensated by muscles supplied by other nerves.

Treatment of the obturator nerve entrapment includes pain medications, nerve blocks, and rehabilitation aiming at adductor muscle reinforcement. Rigaud et al.[31] reported good results with laparoscopic neurolysis and freeing of the obturator nerve in 13 patients; 8 patients presented with synthetic mesh or tape related to the entrapment. Kitagawa et al.[32] also reported good results in five surgeries for obturator nerve entrapment caused by tumor or gynecologic surgery. Bradshaw et al.[29] reported good results in 32 cases of obturator nerve decompression in athletes and suggested that obturator neuropathy is a form of focal nerve entrapment by fascial or vascular structures or both, but in some cases the condition may have an inflammatory or fibrotic basis.[29]

Femoral Nerve

The femoral nerve is formed in the lumbar plexus by the anterior divisions of the L2-L4 ventral rami. It descends through the psoas major muscle, emerging laterally from this muscle at the pelvis.[23] After coursing in the pelvis, it passes posterior to the inguinal ligament and is separated from the femoral artery and vein by the iliopectineal fascia. In the thigh, the femoral nerve divides into several motor and sensory branches.

Entrapment of the femoral nerve is more frequent within the iliacus compartment and at the level of the inguinal ligament.[8] Hematomas resulting from trauma, surgery, or anticoagulant therapy can cause a subacute compartment syndrome with progressive edema, swelling, and ischemia of the iliacus compartment. Urologic, gynecologic, orthopaedic, vascular, and hernia repair surgical procedures are a known cause of femoral intraoperative injury. Surgeries performed through lithotomy positioning have an increased risk for femoral nerve entrapment. Hip flexion contractures greater than 30 degrees can cause intrapelvic femoral nerve entrapment by the iliopsoas tendon. Tumors and giant iliopsoas bursa are other causes of femoral nerve compression in the pelvis or proximal thigh. Some infectious pathologies, as well as primary iliopsoas pyomyositis, are described as causing femoral nerve symptoms with a subacute clinical presentation. The saphenous nerve may be compressed by fibrous bands or branches of the femoral vessels as it leaves the adductor canal or more proximally[33]; however, this nerve and the infrapatellar branches are more often damaged as a consequence of vascular and orthopaedic surgical procedures.

The main clinical feature of patients with femoral nerve entrapment is quadriceps muscle weakness,[34] although numbness and paresthesias may be noted in the anterior thigh and areas supplied by the saphenous nerve. Patients with proximal nerve injury often present with iliopsoas muscle weakness. However, the proximal psoas muscle is also directly innervated by the L2 and L3 nerve roots and may function without femoral nerve innervation. Severe femoral nerve lesions produce wasting of the quadriceps muscle and absence of the patellar tendon reflex, causing the inability to step up when climbing stairs and forcing the patient to keep the knee hyperextended when walking on level ground.[30]

Femoral nerve entrapment is usually treated with conservative methods, including pain management medications, nerve blocks, and rehabilitation. In cases of hematoma compression, surgical or percutaneous drainage may be necessary. Femoral nerve neurolysis, sutures, or grafting techniques can be used in some cases of iatrogenic, traumatic, or neoplastic injuries. Kuntzer et al.[34] described the features of femoral nerve neuropathies in 32 patients (most as a result of hip surgery): functional improvement was seen in two thirds of patients within 2 years of onset, but no later than this time.

Lateral Femoral Cutaneous Nerve

The lateral femoral cutaneous nerve (LFCN) supplies the anterior and lateral thigh skin as far as the knee. It arises from the L2 and L3 ventral rami (Table 89-1) and emerges from the lateral border of psoas major.[23] After crossing the iliacus muscle, it usually accesses the thigh within 2 cm medial to

TABLE 89-1

SUMMARY OF FUNCTION OF THE LATERAL FEMORAL CUTANEOUS, ILIOINGUINAL, ILIOHYPOGASTRIC, AND GENITOFEMORAL NERVES

Nerve	Motor Innervation	Sensory Innervation
Lateral femoral cutaneous nerve	None	Parietal peritoneum in the iliac fossa Anterior and lateral thigh until knee
Ilioinguinal	Transversus abdominis and internal oblique	Transversus abdominis and internal oblique muscles Proximal medial skin of the thigh Root of the penis and upper scrotum skin, males Mons pubis and adjacent labia majora skin, females
Iliohypogastric		
Lateral cutaneous branch	None	Posterolateral gluteal
Anterior branch	Transversus abdominis and internal oblique	Transversus abdominis, internal and external oblique muscles Suprapubic skin
Genitofemoral		
Genital branch	Cremaster muscle	Skin of scrotum in males or mons pubis and labia majora in females
Femoral branch	None	Anteromedial skin of the thigh

the anterior superior iliac spine and under the inguinal ligament,[35] although variations in this pattern occur frequently.

Sensory symptoms in the LFCN innervation territory are known as meralgia paresthetica[36] and can be caused by nerve entrapment. The point of irritation is usually where the LFCN perforates or crosses the inguinal ligament, lying at an acute angle in hip extension.[36] Most cases are idiopathic, although hip arthroscopy, pelvic surgeries, trauma, and direct compression are possible etiologies. The LFCN is at risk of injury during laparoscopic inguinal hernia repair.[37] Obesity, pregnancy, or entities raising abdominal pressure are considered risk factors. The suggested mechanism is an increased demand on the inguinal ligament and consequent traction on the nerve.[38] External compression is associated with LFCN entrapment, mainly with use of tight trousers[38] or prone positioning for spine surgery.

The LFCN is an exclusively sensory nerve, and its neuropathy is manifested by a tingling, stinging, or burning sensation in the anterior lateral thigh, often associated with numbness and hypersensitivity to touch. Ecker and Woltman[38] reported bilateral disease in 22% of the patients but stated that the symptoms usually begin unilaterally in these patients. Symptom exacerbation is found with extension of the hip, prolonged standing,[38] and nerve palpation at the point where the nerve crosses the inguinal ligament or distal to the anterior inferior iliac spine. The symptoms are commonly mild and resolve spontaneously, but they may also be severe and cause limitation in daily activities. Anesthetic block at the point of Tinel's reproduction is used to confirm the diagnosis.

Conservative treatment is successful in approximately 90% of patients[39] and includes use of analgesic agents, topical antiinflammatory drugs, and nerve anesthetic/steroid blocks, weight loss in obese patients, and avoiding sources of external compression, such as tightly fitting clothes and belts. In patients with persistent and disabling symptoms, surgical treatment with neurolysis or neurectomy should be considered.[40] Compared with neurolysis, neurectomy is more effective in relieving pain and has a lower rate of symptom recurrence.[39,40] The numbness resulting from resection usually does not disturb the patient.[40] Neurectomy is also indicated when neurolysis has failed to resolve the symptoms.

Ilioinguinal and Iliohypogastric Nerves

The ilioinguinal and iliohypogastric nerves usually originate from L1 ventral rami and run within the retroperitoneum before its trajectory through the abdominal wall muscles (Fig. 89-11). Next, the ilioinguinal nerve passes in the inguinal canal and emerges with the spermatic cord from the

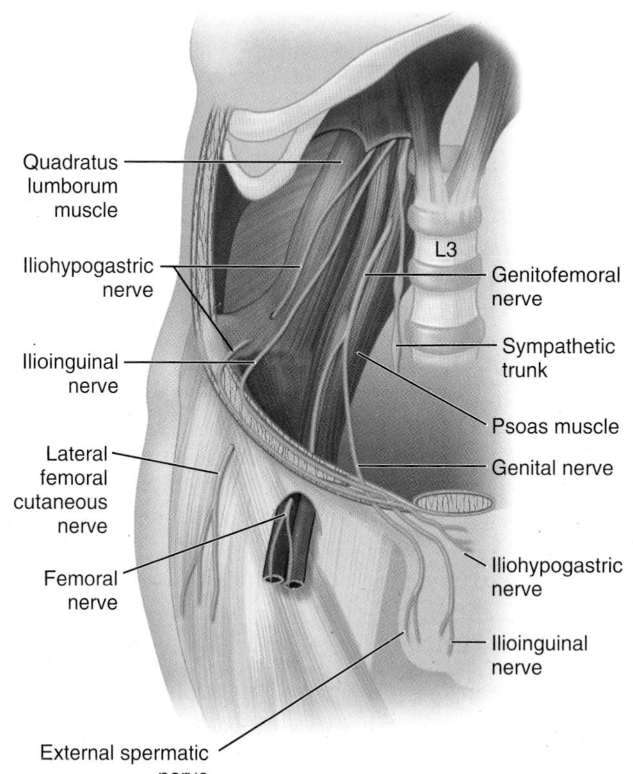

FIGURE 89-11 Courses of the genitofemoral, ilioinguinal, iliohypogastric, and genitofemoral nerves. *(Modified from Starling JR, Harms BA: Diagnosis and treatment of genitofemoral and ilioinguinal neuralgia.* World J Surg *13[5]:586–591, 1989.)*

superficial inguinal ring, whereas the iliohypogastric nerve ends in the suprapubic skin (see Table 89-1).[23] These nerves often have communication with dermatome overlapping.

Entrapment of the ilioinguinal or iliohypogastric nerve is consequent to previous abdominal surgeries such as hernia repair, urologic and gynecologic procedures, and different surgeries performed through Pfannenstiel or other incisions in the lower abdomen. Stark found a 1.1% incidence of ilioinguinal nerve entrapment in 893 patients who underwent hernia repairs, with a greater incidence associated with laparoscopic repair compared with open surgery.[37] Shin observed that ilioinguinal and iliohypogastric nerve entrapment as a consequence of laparoscopic surgery is associated with suture entrapment during fascial closure.[41] Trauma can also cause entrapment of these nerves.[42] Kopell et al.[43] suggested that the mechanical irritation of the nerve from the musculofascial edges in the inguinal region could cause ilioinguinal and iliohypogastric neuropathy symptoms. Akita noted that the ilioinguinal nerve and the genital branch of the genitofemoral nerve may be most affected in persons with a sports hernia, and entrapment of a branch may be a reasonable explanation for the cause of chronic groin pain.[42]

A history of lower abdominal surgery usually suggests the diagnosis of ilioinguinal or iliohypogastric compression. Stabbing or cutting pain in the neural territory is the main symptom and can be elicited by stretching movements.[44] The pain may begin just after surgery but may also start months or years later, possibly as a result of the development of fibrosis or a neuroma.[44] Sensory loss, allodynia, and a positive Tinel sign at the emergence from the oblique internus can be found.[45] Pain relief with an anesthetic block at the site of nerve emergence is important to make the diagnosis and exclude differential diagnoses. Madura et al.[46] suggests an "arch and twist" maneuver to stretch the affected nerves. This maneuver should be followed by a nerve block, which produces temporary relief. Differentiating ilioinguinal from genitofemoral nerve entrapment can be difficult, with the main consideration being a possible communication between these nerves and resultant overlap of sensory innervation.

Medical treatment including tricyclic antidepressants, anticonvulsive drugs, transcutaneous electric nerve stimulation, acupuncture, and repeated nerve blocks can be tried. Results of surgical decompression of the ilioinguinal nerve have not been good.[43,46] Some authors have described significant pain relief in patients who have undergone ilioinguinal nerve resection,[45,47] and a recent randomized controlled trial concluded that nerve resection was superior to medical treatment.[44] Laparoscopic resection can also be performed. Neurectomy of the ilioinguinal nerve during inguinal hernia repair has been demonstrated to decrease the incidence of postoperative neuralgia.[48]

Genitofemoral Nerve

The genitofemoral nerve originates from the L1 and L2 ventral rami (see Fig. 89-11). It divides into genital and femoral branches above the inguinal ligament or close to its origin in the lumbar plexus. The genital branch crosses the external iliac artery and accesses the inguinal canal via the deep inguinal ring. The femoral branch pierces the femoral sheath and fascia lata, emerging in the anterosuperior part of the femoral triangle.[23]

Entrapment of the genitofemoral nerve is associated with inguinal herniorrhaphy, appendectomy, and other surgical procedures in the pelvis and lower abdomen. When studying nerve irritation after inguinal hernia repair, Stark et al.[37] reported that the genitofemoral nerve was affected at a frequency of 2% compared with 1.1% for each ilioinguinal nerve and the lateral femoral cutaneous nerve.

Chronic pain and paresthesias in the distribution of the genitofemoral nerve characterize the entrapment. Walking and hip hyperextension typically intensify the symptoms. As in ilioinguinal and iliohypogastric nerve entrapment, the "arch and twist" maneuver is used to stretch the entrapped nerve.[46] Harms et al.[49] state the importance in differentiating genitofemoral from ilioinguinal nerve entrapment in patients with persistent pain and paresthesias in the inguinal region after surgery. To define the source of the symptoms, they recommend an ilioinguinal nerve block and, depending on result, a paravertebral block of L1 and L2. Communication between the ilioinguinal and genitofemoral nerves occurs in around 13% of persons,[42] and therefore discriminating ilioinguinal from genitofemoral nerve entrapment can be difficult.

The symptoms are usually temporary and controlled by conservative treatment, including analgesic agents, antiinflammatory drugs, neuropathic pain medications, transcutaneous electric nerve stimulation, and anesthetic/steroid blocks. In cases of entrapment resulting from herniorrhaphy, the patients are usually pain free after 6 weeks.[37] Removal of clips may be necessary. In cases in which the symptoms were not controlled by the previously cited measures, open or laparoscopic resection of the genitofemoral nerve over the psoas muscle should be considered. Identification of the nerve anatomy during mesh placement and a reduction in the number of clips can help prevent nerve entrapment as a result of herniorrhaphy.[37]

Conclusion

A structured physical examination that incorporates the four layers of the hip (the osseous, capsulolabral, musculotendinous, and neurovascular layers) is essential for a differential diagnosis in patients with hip pain.[1] The four-layer approach will help avoid frustration for both the patient and physician. The neurovascular layer can present a challenging diagnostic condition, and an appreciation for each layer, including the fifth layer, the kinematic chain, is necessary. The osseous contribution must be understood in all three planes because it affects nerve biomechanics in motion. Use of a comprehensive approach will develop a detailed understanding of neurologic hip pain. To treat pathologic conditions of hip and thigh nerves, a complete treatment plan should address all layers of the hip.

For a complete list of references, go to expertconsult.com.

Suggested Readings

Citation: Martin H: Clinical Examination and Imaging of the Hip. In Byrd J, Guanche C, editors: *AANA Advanced Arthroscopy: The Hip*, Philadelphia, 2010, Elsevier.
Level of Evidence: V
Summary: The author details a comprehensive approach for the physical examination of the hip, including a four-layer assessment. It is important to consider osseous, capsular labral, and musculotendinous influences on the neurovascular layer and consequently nerve entrapment pathologies.

Citation: Martin HD, Hatem MA, Champlin K, et al: The endoscopic treatment of sciatic nerve entrapment/deep gluteal syndrome. *Arthroscopy* 27:172–181, 2011.

Level of Evidence: V

Summary: The authors provide a useful review of the surgical treatment of sciatic nerve entrapment. An updated review of the differential diagnoses for posterior hip pain and sciatic entrapment is included in the article.

Citation: Smoll NR: Variations of the piriformis and sciatic nerve with clinical consequence: A review. *Clin Anat* 23:8–17, 2010.

Level of Evidence: Anatomic review

Summary: The authors provide a systematic review and metaanalysis of the prevalence of piriformis and sciatic nerve anomalies in humans using previously published literature. After pooling the results of 18 studies and 6062 cadavers, the prevalence of the anomaly in cadavers was 16.9%. Anomalies of the piriformis and sciatic nerve occur frequently, and awareness of these anomalies is necessary to correctly diagnose sciatic nerve pain.

Citation: Labat JJ, Riant T, Robert R, et al: Diagnostic criteria for pudendal neuralgia by pudendal nerve entrapment (Nantes criteria). *Neurourol Urodyn* 27:306–310, 2008.

Level of Evidence: V

Summary: The authors reported diagnostic criteria and the clinical characteristics of pudendal nerve entrapment. The diagnosis of pudendal neuralgia by pudendal nerve entrapment syndrome is essentially clinical, and five diagnostic criteria are described.

Citation: Robert R, Labat JJ, Bensignor M, et al: Decompression and transposition of the pudendal nerve in pudendal neuralgia: A randomized controlled trial and long-term evaluation. *Eur Urol* 47:403–408, 2005.

Level of Evidence: I

Summary: A randomized controlled trial was performed to compare decompression of the pudendal nerve with nonsurgical treatment. Each group was composed of 16 patients, and at 12 months, improvement was seen in 71.4% of the surgery group compared with 13.3% of the nonsurgery group. Decompression of the pudendal nerve is an effective treatment for cases of pudendal nerve entrapment that have been unresponsive to conservative treatment.

Citation: Hahn L: Treatment of ilioinguinal nerve entrapment—a randomized controlled trial. *Acta Obstet Gynecol Scand* 90:955–960, 2011.

Level of Evidence: I

Summary: Nineteen patients were randomly allocated to surgical transection or nonsurgical treatment of ilioinguinal nerve entrapment. Improvements were found in the group randomly allocated to surgery. Nine of 10 women discontinued the medical arm of treatment because of adverse effects and/or lack of effect. After being shifted over to the surgery group, similar improvements were noted. The positive results found here indicate that surgery is superior to medical treatment in persons with ilioinguinal nerve entrapment of unknown cause, as well as after previous surgery.

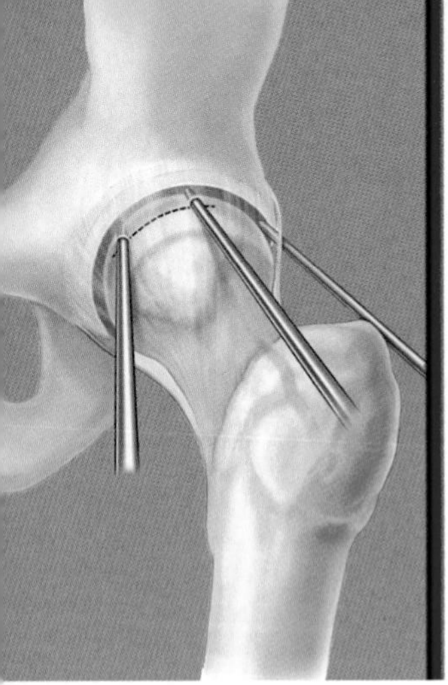

90

Hip Arthritis (Including Osteotomy and Total Hip Arthroplasty)

JOSEPH C. McCARTHY • SEAN McMILLAN • BRIAN BUSCONI • ROBERT PIVEC

Osteoarthritis is a progressive degenerative joint disease caused by primary or secondary factors (Table 90-1).[1,2] Whereas primary osteoarthritis is believed to be caused by an interplay of genetic and environmental factors that eventually lead to late joint degeneration in older persons (i.e., persons generally older than 60 years), secondary osteoarthritis is frequently found in a much younger patient population. Although some pathophysiologic overlap occurs between primary and secondary osteoarthritis, the latter is commonly observed as a consequence of a structural abnormality of the hip joint that causes indirect cartilage damage or a known deficiency in normal cellular function that directly affects hyaline cartilage.[3] Conditions that lead to indirect cartilage damage occur as a result of the development of morphologic abnormalities in the femur or acetabulum that cause labral damage and mechanical overload of the articular cartilage and ultimately induce a chronic degenerative process involving the cartilage, subchondral bone, and synovium, which leads to the characteristic findings seen in osteoarthritis.[4-6]

Epidemiologic studies have estimated that the incidence of osteoarthritis in the United States for patients younger than 50 years is 21 per 100,000 population.[7] The etiology is multifactorial, but anatomic abnormalities, metabolic diseases, and environmental factors have all been implicated.[8,9] Several of these mechanisms represent modifiable risk factors; in several studies and joint registry reports it has been observed that young patients who are overweight or who participate in high-impact athletic activities, particularly professional athletes, have an increased risk for the development of osteoarthritis.[3,10-12]

Treating patients with osteoarthritis who are younger than 50 years may be challenging.[13,14] Although implant survivorship has markedly increased with the advent of modern cementless stem and cup designs, large-diameter femoral heads, and newer generations of highly cross-linked polyethylene that have improved wear properties, many young patients may still require revisions at some point in their lifetime.[13] Although alternative bearing surfaces such as ceramic-on-ceramic or metal-on-metal bearings have been evaluated as a potential replacement for traditional metal-on-polyethylene bearings because of their better wear properties, they have been found to have drawbacks.[15,16] Concerns regarding implant fracture or chipping with ceramic bearings and early failure from adverse tissue reactions to metallic wear debris have restricted their use.[17-20]

With an increased understanding of the etiology and pathologic processes that occur in persons with primary and secondary osteoarthritis, there has been a trend toward increased emphasis on activity modification and joint-preserving procedures that attempt to delay the need for total hip arthroplasty (THA). However, despite efforts to save the patient's native joint, many of these patients will still require a THA at some point in their lives.[21] Consequently, it is important to properly educate this younger subset of patients on the limitations of hip arthroplasty because they are likely to demand greater motion and partake in more physical activity than the traditional THA population.

Various treatment options for young patients with hip arthritis are discussed in this chapter, with a focus on surgical treatment options such as hip arthroscopy, osteotomy, and THA. The complications observed in these patients and their postoperative management are also discussed, with particular attention to a return to previous athletic activities.

History

Hip arthritis in the young patient may present a diagnostic challenge, but the correct diagnosis of the specific condition is imperative to achieve a successful clinical outcome. The surgeon should first elicit a complete history, including family information, and exclude other conditions that may lead to referred hip pain. These conditions may include lumbar spinal involvement, sacroiliac joint involvement, greater trochanteric bursitis, tendinitis, athletic pubalgia, or an inguinal hernia (Box 90-1).[22,23] The surgeon should also carefully consider potential nonarthritic causes of hip pain that may include labral tears, loose bodies due to synovial chondromatosis, synovitis, and, rarely, sepsis.[23]

Patients with arthritis commonly report a history of vague, dull pain that localizes to the groin and has a gradual onset. The pain is exacerbated by activity and is usually associated with stiffness and, less commonly, buckling. Usually patients relate an antecedent event such as a minor trauma or a misstep while playing sports to which they attribute their pain. Unlike conditions that may mimic hip arthritis, patients with true osteoarthritis classically present with pain after activity and stiffness after a period of rest such as prolonged sitting or sleeping. When asked to localize their pain, they may demonstrate the classic C sign, which helps distinguish arthritis from other more common causes of pain such as bursitis. The

TABLE 90-1

ETIOLOGY OF HIP OSTEOARTHRITIS

Type	Etiology
Primary	Idiopathic Genetic factors Environmental factors (e.g., weight and activity level)
Secondary	
Direct causes	Rheumatoid arthritis Septic arthritis Posttraumatic arthritis Rapidly progressive osteoarthritis
Indirect causes	Developmental dysplasia of the hip Femoroacetabular impingement Slipped capital femoral epiphysis Legg-Calvé-Perthes disease Osteonecrosis

patient may also report a family history of "early arthritis" that may be indicative of an underlying anatomic abnormality or rheumatologic disease.

Symptoms of catching, locking, or clicking are more indicative of labral pathology or loose bodies than arthritis, although both of these conditions can be considered secondary risk factors for arthritis.[24] A history of pain along the lateral aspect of the hip is likely due to greater trochanteric bursitis, whereas lumbar or gluteal pain may be indicative of a peripheral neuropathy. Although rare, the presence of vascular pathology such as a delayed presentation of a pseudoaneurysm may also be a cause of hip pain.[25] This condition is more commonly seen in patients after a major trauma or prior pelvic surgical procedures, and it can be distinguished from arthritis by the acute onset of groin pain that is usually associated with a pulsatile mass and, in extreme cases, hemodynamic compromise.[26]

The surgeon should be careful to rule out the possibility of athletic pubalgia (sportsman's hernia), which is a condition caused by dilation of the superficial inguinal ring.[27] In a recent study by Hammoud et al.,[28] 32% of patients treated for femoroacetabular impingement (FAI) had previously undergone surgery for athletic pubalgia and had not experienced symptom resolution. These patients frequently present with reports of hip pain with physical activity and stiffness after prolonged rest, and their condition can be difficult to distinguish from the early presentation of arthritis. The presence of classic findings seen on magnetic resonance imaging (MRI) helps distinguish this condition from other causes of hip pain.[29]

Many patients who present with hip pain will have a benign, self-limited course in which the symptoms disappear with time. Thus examining the temporal relationships between the onset of pain or stiffness, the location of the pain, and any response to a prior course of nonoperative therapy is often the best way to differentiate arthritis from other potential causes of hip pain.

BOX 90-1 Etiologies that May Mimic Hip/Groin Pain

- Greater trochanteric bursitis
- Iliotibial band tendonitis
- Athletic pubalgia (sportsman's hernia)
- Inguinal hernia
- Femoral hernia
- Lumbar pathology
- Sacroiliac joint arthritis
- Pelvic arterial pseudoaneurysm
- Tumor

Physical Examination

Through physical examination of a young patient with hip pain, the clinician should aim to arrive at a definitive diagnosis while ruling out other potential sources for hip pain that require different treatment approaches (see Box 90-1). The examination should always begin with a complete visual inspection of the involved extremity, with particular attention given to any marked anatomic abnormalities, abnormal gait, and the presence of any discoloration, masses, or scars on the skin.

True joint pain should be distinguished from referred back pain by having the patient perform a passive straight leg raising test to provoke radicular symptoms and comparing the results with pain elicited with active hip flexion against resistance. Patients who have true hip pain will note pain or yield to resisted active hip flexion but will have no radicular symptoms with passive hip flexion.[30]

Assessment of the patient's range of motion includes hip flexion, extension, and internal and external rotation. Patients with FAI will present with loss of internal rotation, whereas patients with arthritis due to other causes lose external rotation. Pain is frequently observed at the extremes of range of motion, although in some patients stiffness compared with the contralateral limb may be the only physical finding. In advanced stages of osteoarthritis, range of motion is restricted globally.[31]

FAI can be diagnosed by the presence of a positive impingement sign that reproduces the patient's pain.[32] Two different tests may be used, the anterior and posterior impingement tests, both of which are performed with the patient supine (Fig. 90-1, *A* and *B*). In the anterior impingement test, the hip is passively flexed to 90 degrees and internally rotated, which causes anterior impingement between the femoral neck and labrum, eliciting the pain. Similarly, the posterior impingement test is the reverse, where the hip is passively extended and externally rotated. However, the presence of an impingement sign is a nonspecific finding. Other conditions that can elicit a positive impingement sign may include iliopsoas bursitis, displaced labral tears, and a tight anterior capsule.[33]

In equivocal cases, fluoroscopically guided intraarticular injections may help distinguish hip pain from other sources of referred pain.[34] When combined with corticosteroid injections, they can be both diagnostic and therapeutic. Patients should be instructed to record their pain with physical activity.[34] Injections are an attractive option that allow patients to continue with physical therapy while helping to diagnose the source of the hip pain before obtaining advanced imaging studies.

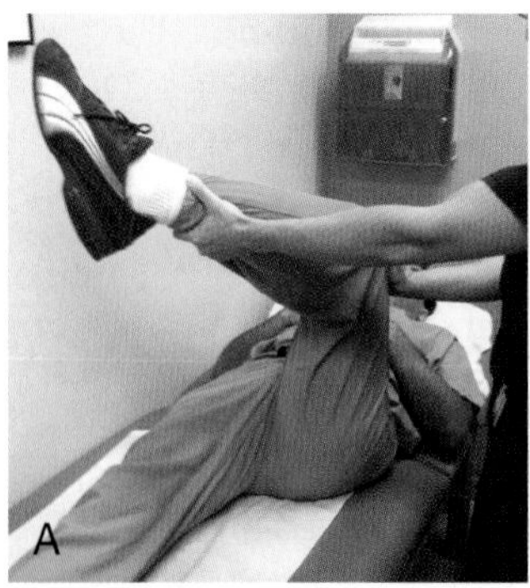
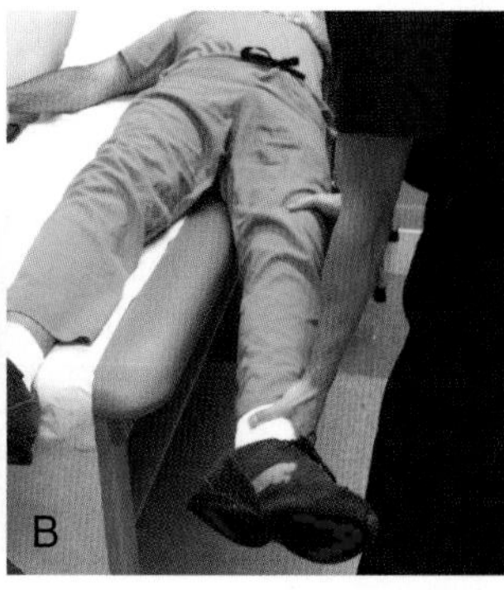

FIGURE 90-1 Femoroacetabular impingement can be diagnosed clinically with use of the anterior and posterior impingement tests. A positive impingement sign occurs when the maneuver reproduces the patient's pain. **A,** The anterior impingement test is performed with the patient supine; the hip is passively flexed to 90 degrees and internally rotated to cause anterior impingement. **B,** The posterior impingement is best performed with the patient supine and the affected hip off the side of the examination table. The patient's hip is passively extended and externally rotated to cause posterior impingement.

Imaging

Even when a thorough history and physical examination have been performed, a definitive diagnosis often is reached only after evaluation of radiographic studies. Standard radiographs include an anteroposterior view of the pelvis and a frog-leg lateral view of the affected hip (Fig. 90-2, *A* and *B*). Both the affected hip and the contralateral hip should be evaluated. In patients with early evidence of arthritis, subtle indications of early degeneration can lead to a diagnosis without the need for advanced imaging studies.[35]

Classic radiographic findings include joint space narrowing, osteophytes, cysts, and subchondral sclerosis. In a subset of patients who have a condition known as rapidly progressive osteoarthritis, rapid joint space narrowing occurs, which is defined as more than 2 mm per year of joint space loss.[36] In severe forms of this disease, massive femoral head osteolysis may occur within 1 year of symptom onset.[36,37]

TABLE 90-2

TYPES OF CAM AND PINCER LESIONS

Type of Lesion	Plain Radiographic Findings
Cam	Aspherical head Pistol grip deformity (lateral contour deformity) Coxa brevis Prior slipped capitol femoral epiphysis
Pincer	Coxa profunda Protrusio Acetabular retroversion Ossified labrum

For patients with signs of impingement, the surgeon should evaluate the sphericity of the femoral head and the morphology of the acetabulum for signs of a cam or pincer lesion (Table 90-2).[38-40] However, it should be noted that many patients with aspherical heads are completely asymptomatic throughout their lifetimes. The acetabulum should be evaluated for pincer lesions, retroversion, or a shallow acetabular index, which may help guide future surgical treatment options. The crossover sign is a clear indication of acetabular retroversion and posterior impingement. The surgeon should note the presence of inferior and notch osteophytes, which, although often more subtle than other indications, are signs of an early presentation of osteoarthritis. Notch osteophytes in particular place increased sheer pressures on the femoral head and may contribute to early degeneration. In severe cases, labral calcification (os acetabuli) can also be observed on plain radiographs late in the disease course.

Determination of the α angle on either a lateral plain radiograph or oblique MRI section can help stratify patients and determine the risk of progression of cam lesion disease. The α angle is defined as the angle between a line from the center of the femoral head through the femoral neck and a line from the center of the femoral head to the head-neck junction (Fig. 90-3). Notzli et al.[41] noted that patients who

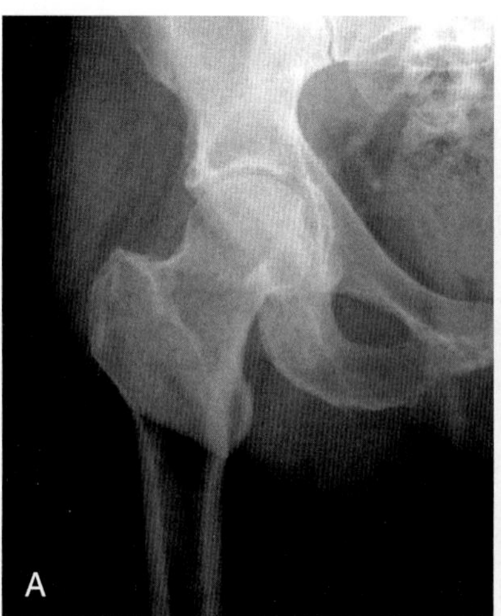
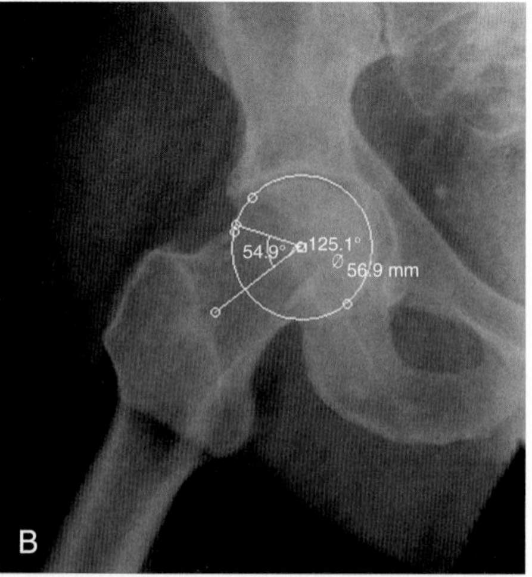

FIGURE 90-2 Anteroposterior (**A**) and frog-leg lateral (**B**) radiographs of the right hip in a 32-year-old patient with insidious onset of right groin pain. Evaluation of the lateral radiographs demonstrates an α angle of 55 degrees.

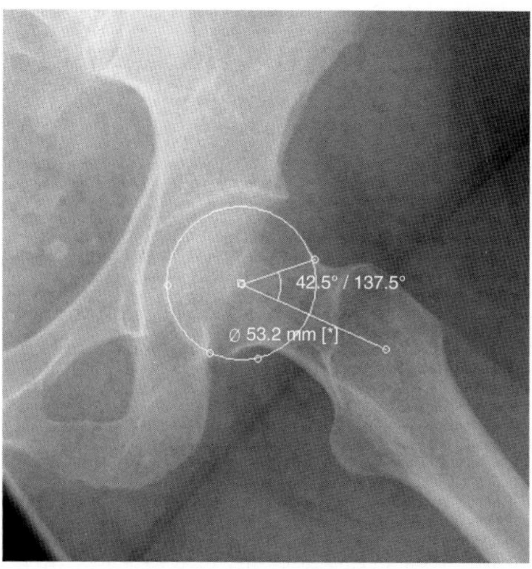

FIGURE 90-3 A frog-leg lateral radiograph of the left hip in a 36-year-old woman demonstrating a normal α angle. The α angle is determined by measuring the angle between a line drawn from the center of the femoral head through the midpoint of the femoral neck and a second line from the center of the femoral head to the head-neck junction. An α angle greater than 55 degrees has been considered to be radiographic evidence of cam impingement.

have an α angle greater than 55 degrees are considered to have radiographic evidence of impingement. The sensitivity and specificity of plain radiographic measurement of the α angle has been reported as 91% and 88%, respectively.[42]

Furthermore, normal plain radiographs do not exclude the early presentation of arthritis. In equivocal cases, an MRI of the hip can be obtained to determine the cause of hip pain and rule out other causes such as labral tears, osteonecrosis, or tumors. An early sign of arthritis on MRI is articular cartilage delamination, although it may be difficult to visualize. In patients with labral pathology, an MRI scan is the most sensitive and specific study available; however, noncontrast studies may be limited in their ability to visualize chondral lesions. Gadolinium arthrogram MRI scans have been demonstrated to have 92% sensitivity for identifying labral tears.[43] Coronal, sagittal, and axial (oblique) scans should be obtained to completely visualize the entire labrum, particularly the anterior labrum, where most pathology is observed.

Decision-Making Principles

The goal of treating young patients with hip arthritis is to preserve the native joint and delay the need for THA as long as possible. This process begins with the correct diagnosis of the patient's underlying pathology and timely treatment with the appropriate techniques. Surgeons should be comfortable performing the necessary intervention and should not hesitate to refer the patient to a specialist center if they are not familiar with the appropriate treatment options.

Patients with normal plain radiographs and an equivocal physical examination that is suggestive of an early presentation of arthritis should first undergo a course of nonoperative therapy with analgesics, activity modification, and injections. However, in the setting of clear abnormalities, early surgical intervention is likely to have greater long-term benefits than continued nonoperative treatments. Particularly in patients with FAI or acetabular abnormalities, no amount of nonoperative therapy will reverse the underlying mechanical causes that are the source of the patient's disability. In this situation, the surgeon should attempt early joint salvage rather than waiting and increasing the likelihood that earlier THA will be required.

In late-stage disease with evidence of osteoarthritis on plain radiographs and clear patient symptomatology, it is best to proceed immediately to THA. Worse postoperative clinical outcomes have been observed when surgery is delayed. A recent study by Vergara et al.[44] demonstrated significantly lower postoperative clinical scores in patients who waited 6 months rather than only 3 months for THA.

Any concomitant conditions that may have a negative effect on postoperative rehabilitation or outcomes also should be assessed prior to any surgical intervention. Several studies have demonstrated poor outcomes for patients who are depressed or have other sources of pain, such as lumbar stenosis.[45,46] If necessary, the patient should be referred to a psychiatrist or specialist to resolve, to the extent possible, any outstanding comorbidities prior to surgery.

Economic considerations are also important when caring for young patients with arthritis because these patients are still in the productive part of their lives. Because of employment demands, young patients may not be able to engage in physical therapy, and a prolonged time away from work may represent a substantial economic burden.[47] It has been estimated that for young patients with severe osteoarthritis, the annual cost of lost productivity may be as high as $17,000, and continued nonoperative therapy may be twice as expensive as THA when all costs are considered.[48]

Patient education regarding expected outcomes with surgical intervention is paramount in the mature athlete with osteoarthritis, particularly when managing expectations after hip arthroscopy. Recent literature has suggested a role for arthroscopy in the face of mild to moderate osteoarthritis in the mature adult (younger than 55 years).[49] However, preoperative education and postoperative management are necessary to optimize patient satisfaction.

Arthroscopy of the hip is a minimally invasive procedure that can be performed for patients with varying degrees of osteoarthritis who have not responded to conservative measures and may not yet be a candidate for a THA. In patients with osteoarthritis, hip arthroplasty may be used to remove loose bodies and perform joint lavage, labral repairs or debridement, synovectomy, femoral osteoplasty, or acetabuloplasty.[50]

Cartilage lesions often are dormant on plain radiographs or poorly visualized on magnetic resonance arthrography. The Outerbridge grading classification of chondral lesions is not specific for osteoarthritis.[51] Conversely, the Tönnis classification represents radiographic changes.[52] Arthroscopic evaluation of these lesions can better lend itself to both current and future expectations, which is particularly true in lesions that may not have declared themselves radiographically. Although uniformity of hip osteoarthritis may not be present, a universal theme across the literature is that the outcomes are poorer in patients with more advanced osteoarthritis. Sampson[53] attempted to classify osteochondral lesions of the femoral head and acetabulum to better predict outcomes (Boxes 90-2 and 90-3). In this classification, poorer outcomes were noted

BOX 90-2 Femoral Head Cartilage Lesions

SAMPSON CLASSIFICATION OF FEMORAL HEAD CARTILAGE LESIONS

Intact Head Substrate Bone with Chondral Damage (No Avascular Necrosis)

HC 0 5 No damage
HC 0T 5 Uniform thinning
HC 1 5 Softening
HC 2 5 Fibrillation
HC 3 5 Exposed bone
HC 4 5 Any delamination

Special Class

HTD 5 Traumatic defect (size in mm)
HDZ 5 Demarcation zone from femoroacetabular impingement

HC, Femoral head cartilage; *HDZ,* demarcation zone for femoroacetabular impingement; *HTD,* femoral head traumatic defect; *T,* thinning.

with higher grade lesions. More aggressive intervention is recommended as well in these higher grade lesions in an effort to maximize outcomes and stave off further surgical intervention. Furthermore, the nature of the osteochondral defect must be understood. Most lesions may be classified as either substance loss of the articular cartilage (partial or full thickness) or delamination. Sampson[53] again noted that with an intact labrocartilage junction, the cartilage may be repaired with the labrum back to bone as a flap. When the junction is torn the labrum may be repaired, although the cartilage may need to be excised.[53]

Recent literature has suggested a role for arthroscopy in the face of mild to moderate osteoarthritis in mature adults who are younger than 55 years. Haviv and O'Donnell[49] retrospectively reported on 564 patients who underwent hip arthroscopy. They noted that over a 7-year period, 16% of all participants eventually required THA. These investigators concluded that the time from the first arthroscopy to a hip replacement was found to be longer in patients younger than 55 years and in those who were diagnosed as being in a milder osteoarthritic stage. The patients who underwent osteoplasties also had a lower incidence of needing a THA.[49]

McCarthy et al.[50] performed a 10-year retrospective study in which 106 hip arthroscopies were analyzed. On the basis of their findings, lower Harris hip scores and older age were predictive of poorer outcomes. No difference in outcome was observed with regard to gender; however, it was found that older age had a 3.6 times higher likelihood of leading to subsequent THA. In addition, chondral defects of either the femoral head or acetabulum were 20 to 60 times more likely to lead to a THA; however, it was noted that patients with Outerbridge scores of 0 to 2 were less likely to need a replacement.[50] These findings, which corroborated those of the multivariate 10-year analysis by Byrd and Jones,[54] suggested that patients older than 40 years with any grade 3 or 4 chondral lesions had a 90% chance of progressing to a THA.

Appropriate patient counseling of the risks and benefits and expected outcomes after hip arthroscopy will almost certainly lead to higher patient satisfaction. Appropriate postsurgical rehabilitation must be emphasized to offload pressures across the hip joint. Additionally, activity modifications based on intraoperative findings may lead to longevity of the procedure and pain relief. An example of this modification includes switching from running to swimming or elliptical training. Although hip arthroscopy may be an effective treatment for mechanical symptoms or for symptomatic osteoarthritis, it must be emphasized to the patient that it is unlikely to significantly halt the progression of the condition in patients with higher grades of disease. Hip arthroscopy in this setting should be viewed as a palliative and delaying intervention rather than a curative measure. During the decision-making process, appropriate patient selection and expectation management should guide the surgeon through the treatment algorithm.

Treatment Options

Nonoperative

Nonoperative treatment options include use of medication and physical therapy. Patients should always be instructed to attempt lifestyle modifications such as weight loss, light aerobic physical activity, and avoidance of activities that exacerbate their symptoms. In the case of nonprofessional athletes, it may be reasonable to recommend that they switch from high-level sports to recreational activities. Patients who wish to remain active should be encouraged to partake in low-impact sports such as swimming, cycling, or walking that do not result in repetitive demands for hip movement at the extremes of range of motion seen in high-impact sports such as football, soccer, or gymnastics.

Symptomatic treatment can be achieved through the use of nonnarcotic analgesics and nonsteroidal antiinflammatory drugs (NSAIDs). Because of the risks involved with chronic NSAID administration, it is recommended that acetaminophen be prescribed as a first-line analgesic. In a metaanalysis, Wegman et al.[55] observed that acetaminophen is just as effective as NSAIDs while having fewer adverse effects. If this regimen does not alleviate symptoms, the physician may consider prescribing antiinflammatory agents, but low doses

BOX 90-3 Acetabular Cartilage Lesions

SAMPSON CLASSIFICATION OF ACETABULAR ARTICULAR CARTILAGE LESIONS

AC 0 5 No damage
AC 1 5 Softening no wave sign
AC 1w 5 Softening with wave sign intact labrocartilage junction
AC 1wTj 5 Softening with wave sign and torn labrocartilage junction
AC 1wD 5 Softening with wave sign and intact labrocartilage junction with delamination
AC 1wTjD 5 Softening with wave sign and torn labrocartilage junction with delamination
AC 2 5 Fibrillation
AC 2Tj 5 Fibrillation with torn labrocartilage junction
AC 3 5 Exposed bone small area <1 cm^2
AC 4 5 Exposed bone large area >1 cm^2

A, Acetabulum; *C,* cartilage defects; *D,* with delamination; *Tj,* torn labrocartilage junction; *w,* with wave sign.

should be used along with a gastroprotective agent, especially in patients with a history of gastric ulcers or upper gastrointestinal bleeding. In patients who do not tolerate nonselective NSAIDs, selective cyclooxygenase-2 inhibitors may be used. Narcotic pain medications should be avoided when possible and if necessary should only be used as a bridge until definitive surgical treatment has been provided. Worse postoperative clinical outcomes for total joint arthroplasty are seen in patients who take opioid medications on a long-term basis before surgery.[56]

Corticosteroid injections can also be used as an adjunct[57] and were demonstrated to be efficacious for up to 3 months in a recent study by Robinson et al.[58] The authors noted that a prednisone dose-equivalent of 80 mg was necessary to demonstrate efficacy at 3 months and that lower doses have variable efficacy and duration.[58] Hip injections are technically more demanding than knee injections and present a potential risk for damage to neurovascular structures in the anterior compartment. Intraarticular injections should not be attempted without fluoroscopic guidance.[34]

Operative

Arthroscopy

As a consequence of our increased understanding of lesions that are a potential precursor to osteoarthritis, along with the refinement of arthroscopic instrumentation and surgical technique, hip arthroscopy has become a mainstay of early joint-preservation efforts. Hip arthroscopy is ideal for the removal of loose or foreign bodies, the repair of labral damage, and the treatment of small chondral lesions, FAI, and synovial chondromatosis.[59]

In the setting of FAI, arthroscopy is an ideal option to resolve any size mismatch between the femoral head and acetabulum that is causing mechanical overload of the articular cartilage, while enabling concurrent labral repair. Although this procedure can be performed with use of an open or mini open technique, arthroscopy requires less tissue dissection, which leads to shorter hospital stays, fewer complications, and faster recovery periods when compared with open debridement.[60]

Arthroscopy requires distraction of the hip to reach the central compartment, whereas the peripheral compartment can be examined without distraction. Most of the resistance to distraction is caused by negative hydrostatic pressure within the hip joint, and the remainder is caused by the ligamentous structures and dynamic resistance from the surrounding musculature.[61] To reduce the required distraction force, patients should be anesthetized and the muscles completely relaxed. Negative hydrostatic pressure can be reduced via injection of sterile saline solution prior to distraction. Although the necessary distraction force is highly variable, in most patients, adequate visualization of the central compartment can be obtained with 50 lb of distraction force.[62]

The patient may be positioned in a supine or lateral decubitus position according to the preference of the surgeon. Benefits of the lateral decubitus position include ease of instrument insertion as a result of less overlying soft tissue laterally, having the greater trochanter as a readily palpable fixed landmark, and being able to access both anterior and posterior structures via the paratrochanteric portals.[61]

The choice of entry portal depends on the location of hip pathology, but the anterolateral portals (supine) or anterior paratrochanteric portals (lateral decubitus) are most commonly used because most hip pathology is present anteriorly.[61] Other portals that can be used are the proximal and posterior paratrochanteric portals and the posterior portal. The surgeon should be familiar with the surrounding anatomy and the neurovascular structures that are at risk. The lateral femoral cutaneous nerve is at risk with use of the anterior portal and the sciatic nerve is at risk with use of the posterior portal. If the posterior portal is to be used, it is recommended that a small incision be used initially to identify the posterior capsule and sciatic nerve, thus preventing injury. Insertion of the trocar too deeply through the anterior portals, although less common, risks damage to the femoral neurovascular bundle.

Osteotomy

Pelvic and femoral osteotomies are other joint-preserving treatment options that are ideal in the setting of symptomatic developmental dysplasia of the hip or other structural abnormalities that lead to a decreased joint contact area or impingement. The majority of the pathology is observed on the acetabular side, although a small subset of patients may have a femoral deformity that is amenable to osteotomy. It is imperative to ensure that potential osteotomy candidates have viable articular cartilage. Otherwise, the resultant procedure may improve the mechanical properties within the joint but will have no effect on the patient's symptoms or long-term survival of the joint.[63,64]

A pelvic osteotomy is necessary to reorient the acetabulum in cases of a shallow acetabular index to obtain increased femoral head coverage (thereby decreasing the load per unit area and contact stress) or to correct a pincer lesion. Several different procedures have been described in the literature during the past 50 years, including innominate (single, double, or triple) and periacetabular osteotomies. Single innominate osteotomies may lead to lateralization of the hip joint, which was addressed by the development of the triple innominate osteotomy. Although triple osteotomies lead to improved acetabular coverage with less joint lateralization, they may result in nonunions, particularly in the anterior pelvic ring, which may require a second procedure. The risk for nonunions in the superior public ramus is of particular concern with external rotation of the osteotomy fragment to achieve better head coverage. This complication can be avoided by medialization of the fragment or by bone grafting.[65]

The periacetabular osteotomy was developed as an alternative to innominate osteotomies. It offers the advantage of maintaining the continuity of the pelvic ring and obviates the need for postoperative traction or immobilization. However, necrosis of the acetabular fragment is a risk because of disruption of the normal blood supply, which in the immediate postoperative period is provided primarily by the hip capsule.[66]

Femoral osteotomies are less commonly used and are limited to patients with a deformity localized to the proximal femur. A varus osteotomy may lead to inequality of leg length and in rare cases can lead to instability and decreased strength because of laxity of the secondary stabilizers of the hip joint. This problem can be corrected by advancement of the greater trochanter. Similarly, a valgus osteotomy may lead to the opposite complication with increased leg length, hip tightness, and, in rare cases, sciatic neuropathy. Rotational osteotomies have also been described that may be used to treat small osteonecrotic lesions in the weight-bearing portion of the femoral head. As with all osteotomies, femoral nonunion is a risk.[67,68]

The osteotomy is a challenging joint-preserving treatment option that should only be attempted by experienced surgeons who have received training in the procedure.

Total Hip Arthroplasty

THA is often the only option for patients who have not responded to nonoperative therapy or joint-preserving procedures. Although arthroplasty provides excellent pain relief and return to function, concerns exist regarding implant durability and survivorship in younger, more active patients. Furthermore, the presence of abnormal anatomy as a consequence of the patient's underlying disease or as a result of prior surgical procedures adds a further layer of complexity regarding implant choice, positioning, and the surgical approach.[13]

As mentioned previously, joint salvage is the goal; however, in the presence of worsening symptoms, the patient and surgeon should not delay THA. Unnecessary waiting or prolonged nonoperative treatment courses place an increased economic burden on the patient and decrease the likelihood that they will be able to achieve a similar level of postoperative function had surgery not been delayed.[44,48]

Cementless fixation of the femoral and acetabular component has become the standard procedure in the United States. Cementless fixation offers the benefit of biologic fixation at the bone-implant interface, which has the potential to remodel over time. The use of proximally porous coated stems offers the advantage of proximally loading the femur, which may lead to less thigh pain and proximal stress shielding. Excellent long-term survivorship has been observed with these stem designs. Another option is resurfacing arthroplasty or use of short neck-preserving stems. These bone-preserving options may facilitate future revisions by maintaining proximal bone stock and allowing use of a metaphyseal rather than a diaphyseal engaging stem during a future revision, if necessary.

The choice of surgical approach is based on the surgeon's preference and experience, as well as the presence of prior surgical scars. The anterior or anterolateral approach both provide excellent exposure while avoiding disruption of the posterior soft tissues. Dislocation rates of less than 1% have been reported with these approaches even in the absence of any hip precautions.[13] Dislocation or instability can be further avoided with the use of large-diameter femoral heads or dual-mobility bearings.[13]

The choice of bearing selection is an important consideration. Factors that need to be assessed include durability and wear, the maximal femoral head size that can be used with the system, and the risk for complications. The complications that have been reported in the literature with metal-on-metal and ceramic-on-ceramic bearings have led to decreased usage of these bearing surfaces in the United States.[69]

Although ceramic bearings display excellent wear properties (5 μm/year linear wear), problems with chipping and squeaking of ceramic bearings have been well reported in the literature. However, these problems appear to have been largely solved with newer generation ceramics. The incidence of squeaking is less than 2.5% in recent studies, and a chipping rate of less than 0.005% has been observed in hip simulators.[70] One potential drawback of ceramic bearings is that they may require the use of small femoral heads. This factor is particularly relevant in women who have small dysplastic acetabuli, which necessitates the use of small cups that cannot accept femoral heads measuring 36 mm or larger.

Adverse tissue reactions and higher levels of failure of stemmed metal-on-metal total hip arthroplasties compared with metal-on-polyethylene bearings have been well documented in national joint registry data.[20] Although these alternative bearing surfaces were originally developed to address dislocation rates seen with polyethylene bearings that used small-diameter femoral heads, recent advances in component and polyethylene design have obviated the need for metal-on-metal articulations to gain the benefits of a large-diameter femoral head.

Modern metal-on-polyethylene bearings utilizing highly cross-linked polyethylene have excellent wear that has been reported to be 58% to 74% lower than that of conventional polyethylene.[71] Use of this material has allowed the use of thinner polyethylene liners (3.9 mm) and 36-mm femoral heads even in patients with small acetabular cups. A recent study by Sayeed et al.[72] demonstrated very low wear and no acetabular rim fractures, wear through, or early failures of a 3.9-mm polyethylene liner at 2-year follow-up. Another option is to use a dual mobility bearing that has demonstrated excellent clinical results and low dislocation rates in Europe and has recently been introduced in the United States. Dislocation rates with this bearing system have been reported to be less than 1% in a recent systematic review.[73]

Postoperative Management

Postoperative management of the young patient with arthritis of the hip differs based on the surgical treatment. In all cases the goal is to promote early range of motion and ambulation when possible. Patients should be enrolled in formal physical therapy and be educated about lifestyle modifications.

Timing of return to sports and activities is a frequent concern after these procedures. Several studies have addressed the return of patients to preinjury activity levels.[74,75] A systematic review by Alradwan et al.[74] demonstrated that 92% of athletes treated for FAI returned to their preinjury sport, with 88% continuing to play at the same level of competition. Tippett[75] reported on a patient who returned to competitive singles tennis 1 year after undergoing a periacetabular osteotomy; the patient participated in a structured physical therapy regimen that included gradual reintroduction to high-impact physical activity.

No guidelines for activity after a THA have been validated. Although patients can run short distances if necessary, most surgeons discourage repetitive, high-impact activities such as running, which may decrease the durability of the implant. Patients should be advised to engage in low-impact closed-chain exercises instead. However, many of these guidelines were based on early data that observed a correlation between activity levels and implant failure. It is unclear whether these same precautions apply to modern stem design and modern highly cross-linked polyethylene.[76] Recent studies have demonstrated that most patients return to lower-impact activities on their own after undergoing a THA. Schmidutz et al.[77]

AUTHORS' PREFERRED TECHNIQUE

Hip Arthritis

Young patients with significant anterior groin and thigh pain are often faced with a decision regarding continued nonsurgical treatment or surgical intervention such as arthroscopy, osteotomy, and THA. These decisions are very difficult and require extensive clinical evaluation and discussion with the patient and, when necessary, with the patient's family. In general, patients who may be a candidate for osteotomy tend to be younger, often younger than 20 or 25 years. In addition, they have a structural deformity of the acetabulum and/or femur that is correctable and sufficient joint space cartilage thickness to allow ongoing function. This group of patients is select and limited. This procedure should be performed by an experienced osteotomy surgeon. More commonly, the decision in a middle-aged patient is between hip arthroscopy and THA.

It is our belief that hip arthroscopy may be of value to a patient with some arthritic changes with the following caveats. First, patients must have 2 mm or more of joint space between the femoral head and acetabulum. Second, they must have a functional range of motion for day-to-day activities, as well as their exercise hobbies. Third, their symptoms should be predominantly mechanical—that is, catching, buckling, locking, and/or giving way. Fourth, they must have reasonable expectations for adherence to the operative treatment program and their postoperative function. In addition, use of an intraarticular joint injection has generally improved their hip symptoms significantly. Finally, they are cognizant of the limitations of arthroscopy and the fact that the procedure does not eliminate the possibility of a THA at some time later in life.

For patients who are candidates for arthroscopy, the procedure allows repair of a labral tear, elimination of loose bodies, resection of hypertrophic and impinging synovium, and treatment of chondral lesions through debridement of chondral picking. It is also possible to perform bumpectomies or osteophyte resection to reduce any bony impingement that may be present.

It is our preference to perform this operation in the lateral decubitus position with use of superior trochanteric portals along with an anterolateral portal. This approach allows access not only to the central compartment but also to the peripheral compartment to address the aforementioned issues. Postoperatively, patients use crutches during the first week or two depending on the extent of the procedure and their intraoperative pathology, which is discussed with them.

For patients for whom a THA is more applicable, again, making the decision to undergo this procedure can be daunting. It is our preference to consider a total hip replacement when the patient's joint space is less than 2 mm, the patient has significant decreased range of motion, or a hip flexion contracture is present. In contrast, for patients with unrealistic expectations, ongoing nonsurgical treatment should be considered. A THA also allows correction of congenital or developmental abnormalities such as dysplasia, leg length inequality, or significant femoral distortions and excessive anteversion that cannot be accomplished with arthroscopy. In addition, a THA can improve the patient's range of motion, whereas arthroscopy generally will not significantly improve range of motion.

We prefer to perform the THA procedure with the patient in the lateral decubitus position with use of a posterolateral approach. The abductor tendons are completely preserved. The short external rotators and capsule are incised but repaired at the end of the procedure. Complete exposure of the joint is critically important to facilitate optimal component position and correction of the patient's preoperative deformity. The goal is to optimize the patient's impingement-free range of motion and reproduce joint kinematics. We prefer to use cementless components on both the acetabulum and the femur, generally with a tapered stem and an ingrowth acetabular component, with use of screws when necessary. Regarding bearing surfaces, we do not use metal-on-metal bearings or femoral heads larger than 36 mm because both have had adverse clinical sequelae. For younger patients, a ceramic femoral head of 36 mm or less in diameter is generally used, along with a highly cross-linked polyethylene liner. The impingement-free range of motion is then tested intraoperatively and the capsule and soft tissues are repaired during closure. After surgery, a postoperative program that is explained later in this chapter is well detailed.

analyzed 76 persons who underwent short-stem arthroplasties at a mean 2.7-year follow-up and noted increased frequency of sports activities but a shift from high- to low-impact sports.

Patients who undergo total hip resurfacing arthroplasty have traditionally been released to participate in high-impact activities more frequently than other patients. However, sustaining a femoral neck fracture is a risk during these activities, and it is unclear at what time patients can be safely released from postoperative activity restrictions. Bedigrew et al.[78] compared 90 patients (96 hips) who underwent either resurfacing or THA and noted increased bone mineral density in the resurfacing group that peaked at 6 months. The authors concluded that it was safe to release patients for participation in high-impact activities at 6 months without an increased risk for fracture.[78]

Results

Overall, joint-preserving surgery that is performed early in the disease course has demonstrated excellent clinical outcomes and the ability to substantially delay the need for THA. When THA is required, patients demonstrate excellent mid- to long-term survivorship when modern stem designs and liners are used.

In a study of 111 hips treated with arthroscopy for pain or catching, McCarthy et al.[50] demonstrated survivorship of the native hip in 63% of patients at a mean 13-year follow-up. When patients were further substratified according to Outerbridge grade, Kaplan-Meier survivorship at 10 years with arthroplasty as a clinical end point was 80% for both the acetabulum and femur in persons with low-grade lesions (Outerbridge grade 0 to II), whereas survivorship decreased

TABLE 90-3

NATIVE HIP JOINT SURVIVORSHIP AFTER A PERIACETABULAR OSTEOTOMY

Study	Follow-up (yr)	Survivorship (%)
Burke et al. (2012)	5	94
Matheney et al. (2009)	9	76
Troelsen et al. (2009)	9	82
Matta et al. (1999)	4	89
Murphy et al. (1999)	5	96

to 22% and 12% for the acetabulum and femur, respectively, for persons with high-grade lesions (Outerbridge grade III/IV). In a patient who is 40 years or younger, these findings represent a 10% probability of requiring THA within 10 years if a low-grade lesion is present compared with a 99% probability if a high-grade lesion is present.[50] Similar results were reported by Ng et al.,[79] who performed a systematic review of the literature and demonstrated that overall up to 30% of patients will require THA, with patients who had Outerbridge grade III or IV chondral lesions having worse clinical outcomes.

Osteotomies have also demonstrated successful outcomes similar to the outcomes reported for hip arthroscopy (Table 90-3). Troelsen et al.[80] reported a 82% survivorship with THA as an end point in 116 osteotomies at a mean follow-up of 9 years. Risk factors that predisposed patients to conversion included severe dysplasia, decreased acetabular anteversion, and os acetabuli.[81] Nearly identical results were reported by Matheney et al.,[81] who demonstrated 76% survivorship at a mean of 9 years in 135 hips. When assessing for predictors of failure, the authors observed a 95% probability of requiring arthroplasty if severe dysplasia was present preoperatively and the patient was older than 35 years.[81]

THA demonstrates high implant survivorship at 5- to 10-year follow-up (Table 90-4). The rate of implant survivorship for modern ceramic-on-ceramic and metal-on-polyethylene bearings is greater than 98% at mid- to long-term follow-up, and in several studies that report more than 10-year follow-up, a greater than 95% rate of implant survivorship is maintained.[82,83] Studies of young patients who underwent THA with conventional polyethylene bearings showed that implant survivorship was markedly lower at long-term follow-up. Several of these studies reported a 54% to 68% rate of implant survivorship at 13- to 15-year follow-up.[84,85] Overall, clinical outcomes and implant survivorship rates are excellent with modern implants at 10-year follow-up. However, further study is required to confirm whether this rate of survivorship is maintained at a follow-up of 15 years or longer.

Complications

Complications after hip arthroscopy are rare, with a reported rate of 4% in a recent metaanalysis by Kowalczuk et al.[86]

TABLE 90-4

TOTAL HIP ARTHROPLASTY IMPLANT SURVIVORSHIP

Study	Bearing Type	Hips	Mean Age at Surgery (yr)	Follow-up (yr)	Survivorship (%)
Kim et al. (2012)	CoC	127	<30	15	99.2
Byun et al. (2012)	CoC	56	<30	6	100
Finkbone et al. (2012)	CoC	24	16	5.5	96
Kamath et al. (2012)	CoC	21	18	4	95
Hwang et al. (2012)	MoM (stemmed)	78	<50	12	98.7
Faldini et al. (2011)	MoP	34	47	12	100
Kim et al. (2011)	CoP	73	45	8.5	100
Girard et al. (2010)	MoM (stemmed)	47	25	11	94.5
Almeida et al. (2010)	MoP	75	38	10	88
Clohisy et al. (2010)	MoP	102	<25	4	98
Liang et al. (2010)	MoP	81	<50	6	95
Kang et al. (2010)	MoP	45	<45	12	89
Kim et al. (2010)	CoC	93	<45	10	100
Jialiang et al. (2010)	MoP	67	<50	6	100
Baek and Kim (2008)	CoC	71	39	7	100
Wangan et al. (2008)	MoP	49	<30	13	51
Nizard et al. (2008)	CoC	132	23	15	72
Ha et al. (2007)	CoC	74	37	6	100
Mont et al. (2006)	MoP	104	38	2	97
Archibeck et al. (2006)	MoP	100	39	9	87
Yoo et al. (2006)	CoC	72	30	5	100
McAuley et al. (2004)	MoP	256	<40	15	54
Pignatti et al. (2003)	CoC	123	32	5	96
Bessette et al. (2003)	MoP	16	16	13.5	68

CoC, Ceramic-on-ceramic; *CoP,* ceramic-on-polyethylene; *MoM,* metal-on-metal; *MoP,* metal-on-polyethylene.

Common complications include damage to the cartilage, surrounding soft tissues, or neurovascular structures (particularly with errant portal placement) and traction neuropathy as a result of prolonged distraction.[87] In most cases sciatic or pudendal neuropathy resolves within 3 months, but patients should be informed of this risk. Some male patients may experience weak erections but should be informed that this condition is usually self-limiting. Ankle fractures and other quite rare complications after distraction have also been reported in the literature.[88] Many complications can be avoided by careful portal placement, the use of well-padded, laterally placed perineal posts with a diameter greater than 9 cm, and intermittent distraction release.[87]

Complications associated with periacetabular osteotomies include neurovascular damage, pelvic nonunion, and necrosis of the osteotomy fragment. A substantial learning curve is associated with this procedure, and higher complication rates are observed for surgeons who have not mastered the technique. A study by Davey and Santore demonstrated a decrease in major complications from 17% to 2.9% after the second 35 cases performed by a single surgeon compared with the first 35 cases. The most common complications the authors observed were intraoperative bleeding and sciatic nerve neuropraxia.[89] Similar results were reported by Thawrani et al.,[90] who observed a 3.6% major complication rate in 83 osteotomies, of which one was an intraoperative hemorrhage requiring embolization, with two cases involving postoperative osteonecrosis. The authors also noted a 22% minor complication rate that included nonunion of the superior pubic ramus osteotomy that required no further intervention in five hips and transient lateral femoral cutaneous nerve palsy in four hips.[90]

Complications after THA in young patients are similar to those observed in the standard THA population. Aseptic loosening of the acetabular component is a common cause of revision, whereas the femoral component often remains well fixed. Dislocation was rarely seen even with the use of 22-mm femoral heads. Kim et al.[91] reported only one dislocation in 118 cementless total hips at a mean follow-up of 10 years but did note thigh pain in 10% of patients. In all cases the thigh pain was transitory.[91] In patients with ceramic-on-ceramic bearings, component chipping or fracture is rare. Ha et al.[92] noted no failure of ceramic components in a series of 78 hips at 5-year follow-up, whereas Yoo et al.[93] noted only one ceramic fracture that occurred after a motor vehicle accident. Other complications were also reported by Clohisy and colleagues[94] in a recent study of 88 patients (102 hips) who had a mean age of 20 years. The authors noted major complications that required a return to the operating room in 9% of the cases. These complications included four dislocations (three of which were revised), two peroneal nerve palsies, one periprosthetic fracture, and one femoral artery intimal tear.[94]

Future Considerations

Advances in our knowledge of the pathophysiologic processes that lead to joint degeneration will likely lead to the development of more joint-preserving treatment options. Although THA demonstrates excellent results, it is questionable whether the majority of young patients who undergo this procedure will be able to remain revision-free at 20 or even 30 years. The combination of increased life expectancy and expanded surgical indication for the treatment of hip disease will drive the development of diagnostic imaging and surgical techniques that identify and treat hip arthritis and its precursor lesions early in the disease process before the degenerative pathway has begun.

For a complete list of references, go to expertconsult.com.

Suggested Readings

Citation: Samora JB, Ng VY, Ellis TJ: Femoroacetabular impingement: A common cause of hip pain in young adults. *Clin J Sport Med* 21(1):51–56, 2011.

Level of Evidence: V

Summary: In this article the authors provide a current review of diagnostic, nonoperative, and operative treatment strategies for hip pain in young adults.

Citation: Polkowski GG, Callaghan JJ, Mont MA, et al: Total hip arthroplasty in the very young patient. *J Am Acad Orthop Surg* 20(8):487–497, 2012.

Level of Evidence: V

Summary: This article summarizes current treatment considerations for persons younger than 30 years who are in need of total hip arthroplasty. The information within this article is helpful in guiding treatment options in young patients for whom all other forms of nonarthroplasty management have failed.

Citation: De Kam DC, Busch VJ, Veth RP, et al: Total hip arthroplasties in young patients under 50 years: Limited evidence for current trends. A descriptive literature review. *Hip Int* 21(5):518–525, 2011.

Level of Evidence: V

Summary: The controversial topic of total hip arthroplasty is explored and evaluations of current trends are summarized to provide an effective treatment algorithm.

Citation: Litwin DE, Sneider EB, McEnaney PM, et al: Athletic pubalgia (sports hernia). *Clin Sports Med* 30(2):417–434, 2011.

Level of Evidence: V

Summary: This brief chapter provides a concise and comprehensive review of diagnosis, treatment, and outcomes for athletic pubalgia by some of the field's pioneers.

Citation: McCarthy JC, Jarrett BT, Ojeifo O, et al: What factors influence long-term survivorship after hip arthroscopy? *Clin Orthop Relat Res* 469(2):362–371, 2011.

Level of Evidence: V

Summary: With hip arthroscopy indications rapidly evolving, this article helps better define patient selection and factors that will guide outcomes in patients who undergo hip arthroscopy.

Citation: Matsuda DK, Carlisle JC, Arthurs SC, et al: Comparative systematic review of the open dislocation, mini-open, and arthroscopic surgeries for femoroacetabular impingement. *Arthroscopy* 27(2):252–269, 2011.

Level of Evidence: IV

Summary: In this article, three different techniques for the treatment of bony lesions related to femoral-acetabular impingement are identified and reviewed.

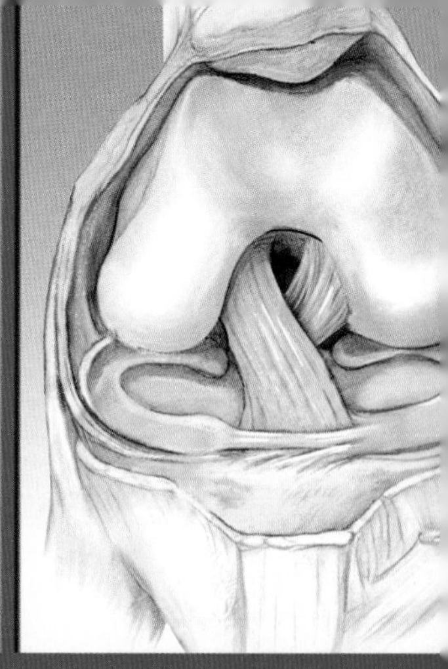

SECTION 7

Knee

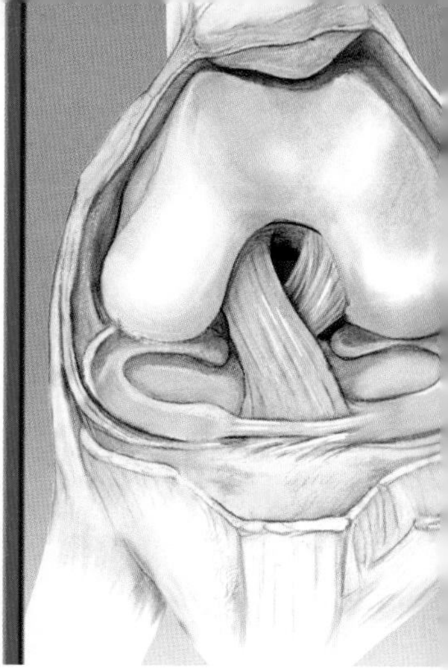

91

Knee Anatomy and Biomechanics of the Knee

FRANCESC MALAGELADA • JORDI VEGA • PAU GOLANÓ • BRUCE BEYNNON • FATIH ERTEM

Knee Anatomy

Francesc Malagelada • Jordi Vega • Pau Golanó

The knee is the largest joint in the human body and one of the most complex from a functional point of view. It is also one of the most often injured joints because of its anatomic characteristics, the interrelation of its structural components, and the significant external forces that act on it. For this reason, any orthopaedic surgeon or sports medicine physician who is presented with a patient with a knee problem must have a broad knowledge of the knee's anatomy, both superficial and deep.

The first objective of this chapter is to describe the anatomy of the knee, with the goal of helping the reader more easily comprehend the content presented in the following chapters.

Superficial Anatomy

An understanding of the superficial anatomy is essential to explore the knee in a correct manner (Fig. 91-1).

When the knee is viewed from the anterior aspect, the presence of the patella is highlighted. It is located in the center of the joint, and on its anterior face, the entire perimeter of the patella can be palpated. The motion of the patella from lateral to medial and from proximal to distal can functionally vary based on the position of the knee and the contraction of the quadriceps femoris muscle. The more extended the knee and the more relaxed the quadriceps femoris muscle, the more mobile the patella will be, whereas as the knee flexes, the patella follows the femoral trochlear groove (patellar surface) and becomes more immobile. On the other hand, the normal superficial appearance of the patella can be altered by inflammatory processes that affect the prepatellar bursa, which can cause the typical morphologic appearance of the anterior knee to disappear.

On the superior border of the patella the tendon of the quadriceps femoris muscle can be palpated, and on either side, the vastus medialis and lateralis, components of the same muscle, can be palpated. At the level of the apex of the patella, and directed distally, the patellar tendon can be identified as it descends to the tibial tuberosity, which is easily visible and palpable. This tuberosity continues distally with the anterior border of the tibia. Lateral to this anterior border, the muscle masses of the anterior compartment of the leg can be palpated, specifically the tibialis anterior muscle, and lateral and proximal to this tuberosity the anterior tubercle or Gerdy's tubercle can be palpated, which constitutes the point of insertion for the iliotibial tract. Medial to the tubercle, palpation can lead to recognition of the insertion, on the medial aspect of the tibia, of the tendons of the sartorius, gracilis, and semitendinosus muscles, also known as the pes anserinus tendons. The most superficial structure corresponds to the sartorius muscle, and deep to this muscle, the tendons of the gracilis and semitendinosus muscles can be appreciated. At the upper limit of the pes anserinus, the cordlike tendon of the gracilis muscle can be palpated, which is located about 2 cm distal to the tibial tubercle. This understanding will prove useful during anterior cruciate ligament (ACL) reconstruction with use of autograft tendons from the pes anserinus (hamstring tendons).

Approximately two fingerbreadths proximal to the tibial tubercle, and on either side of the patellar tendon, the femoral condyles, medial and lateral, and the proximal region of the tibia or the tibial condyles can be palpated. The femoral and tibial condyles can be palpated most easily with the knee in 90 degrees of flexion. In this position, the space delineated between the femoral and tibial condyles forms a triangle on either side of the patellar tendon. This triangle, which by palpation corresponds to a soft spot, is where the anteromedial and anterolateral arthroscopic portals can be positioned. On the other hand, in cases of articular effusion, which is frequently associated with intraarticular pathology of the knee, the appearance of this triangular space can be more difficult to appreciate.

In the lateral region of the knee, distal to the lateral condyle of the tibia, the prominence of the fibular head can be observed. With the knee flexed to 90 degrees, and with varus articular force, one may palpate, and occasionally visualize, a cordlike structure that runs from the fibular head to the lateral condyle of the femur. This structure corresponds to the lateral

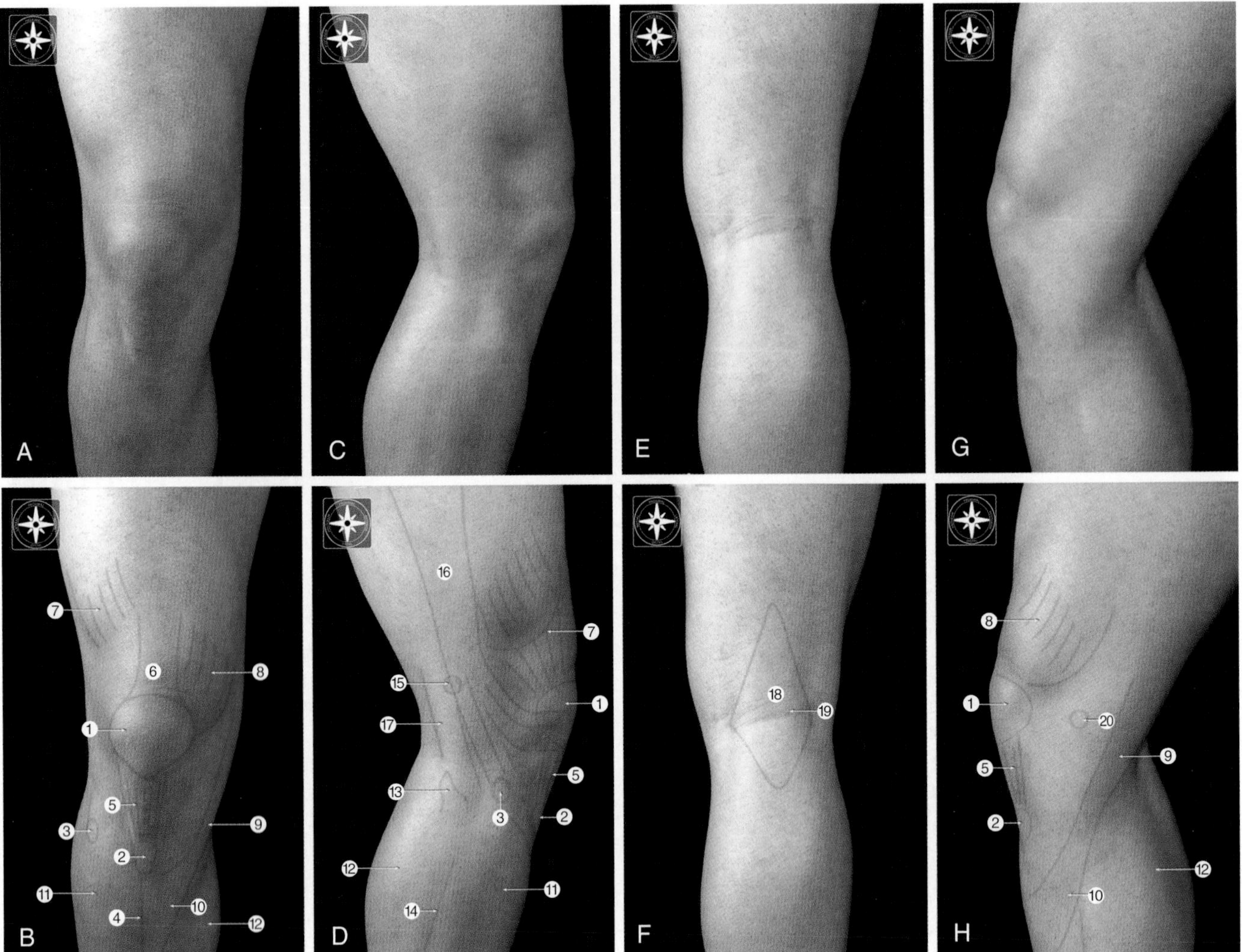

FIGURE 91-1 Surface anatomy. **A** and **B,** Anterior view. **C** and **D,** Lateral view. **E** and **F,** Posterior view. **G** and **H,** Medial view. *1,* Patella. *2,* Tibial tuberosity. *3,* Anterior tubercle or Gerdy's tubercle. *4,* Anterior border of the tibia. *5,* Patellar tendon. *6,* Quadriceps tendon. *7,* Vastus lateralis. *8,* Vastus medialis. *9,* Pes anserinus tendons. *10,* Pes anserinus area in the medial face of the tibia. *11,* Muscles of the anterior compartment of the leg. *12,* Muscles of the posterior compartment of the leg. *13,* Head of the fibula. *14,* Shaft of the fibula. *15,* Lateral epicondyle. *16,* Iliotibial tract. *17,* Biceps femoris muscle. *18,* Popliteal fossa. *19,* Flexion crease of the knee. *20,* Medial epicondyle. *(Copyright Pau Golanó.)*

collateral ligament (LCL). At the same level, but in the medial region, the medial collateral ligament (MCL) can be found, but because it is a flat structure, it is not possible to see or palpate it.

In the posterior region, osseous structures cannot be observed because they are covered with muscular structures. From a posterior view, with the knee in extension, a space that forms a rhombus can be appreciated; this space is called the popliteal fossa. This view is more easily defined when the patient actively flexes the knee. The popliteal fossa is traversed, in its medial zone, by a horizontal line that corresponds to the flexion crease of the knee. The edges of this rhombus correspond to the margins or limits of different muscle groups and the center of the popliteal fossa.

The inferior borders of the popliteal fossa correspond to the medial and lateral head of the gastrocnemius muscle, which are divergent at their origin but converge distally to reunite with the soleus muscle to form the calcaneal or Achilles tendon. The superomedial border corresponds to the tendons of the semitendinosus superficially and the semimembranosus deeply at their musculotendinous junction. With the knee flexed, these tendons are more easily appreciable, and they can even be pinched between one's fingers. In persons in whom the pes anserinus tendons have been used as an autograft for ACL reconstruction, this border may disappear or may appear altered. Finally, the superolateral border corresponds to the tendon of the biceps femoris, on its path to its insertion on the fibular head. At this level, one can begin to appreciate the thick iliotibial tract.

In the popliteal fossa, one can palpate diverse neurovascular structures: the tibial nerve, the common peroneal nerve, and the popliteal artery. The tibial nerve is encountered in the medial region of the popliteal fossa and can be recognized as a thick cordlike structure. One technique to highlight the nerve during exploration consists of placing the patient in the lateral decubitus position with the hip flexed to 90 degrees. In this position, one maintains the patient's knee slightly flexed with the ankle in dorsiflexion. Using the index finger, the hand can be passed from the inferior portion of the knee toward an anterior position and the nerve palpated. The common peroneal nerve can be localized in the lateral region of this fossa. With the knee in flexion, by sliding the index finger laterally, one may palpate a cordlike structure that is much smaller than that of the tibial nerve. The popliteal artery can be localized medial to the tibial nerve and is easily recognizable by palpation of its pulse.

Osseous Anatomy

The knee contains three osseous components, the femur, the tibia, and the patella (Fig. 91-2). These three structures form the tibiofemoral and the patellofemoral articulations, which together comprise the knee joint. In the lateral region of the knee, a third articulation is encountered, the proximal tibiofibular joint, which does not truly participate in the flexion-extension movement of the knee but is involved in the lateral stability of the knee via the insertion of the LCL and the biceps femoris tendon onto the fibular head.[1]

Femur

The distal region of the femur is formed by the two condyles, one medial and one lateral. A prominence named the *lateral epicondyle* is located on the lateral condyle, and the LCL inserts onto this prominence. At the level of the medial condyle is the adductor tubercle, and anterior and distal to this tubercle lies the medial epicondyle, the origin of the MCL.

Both femoral condyles, which are united at the anterior level by the femoral trochlear groove (patellar surface), are separated at the posterior level by a great notch, the intercondylar notch. The femoral trochlear groove permits the patella to slide during the movements of knee flexion and extension. The

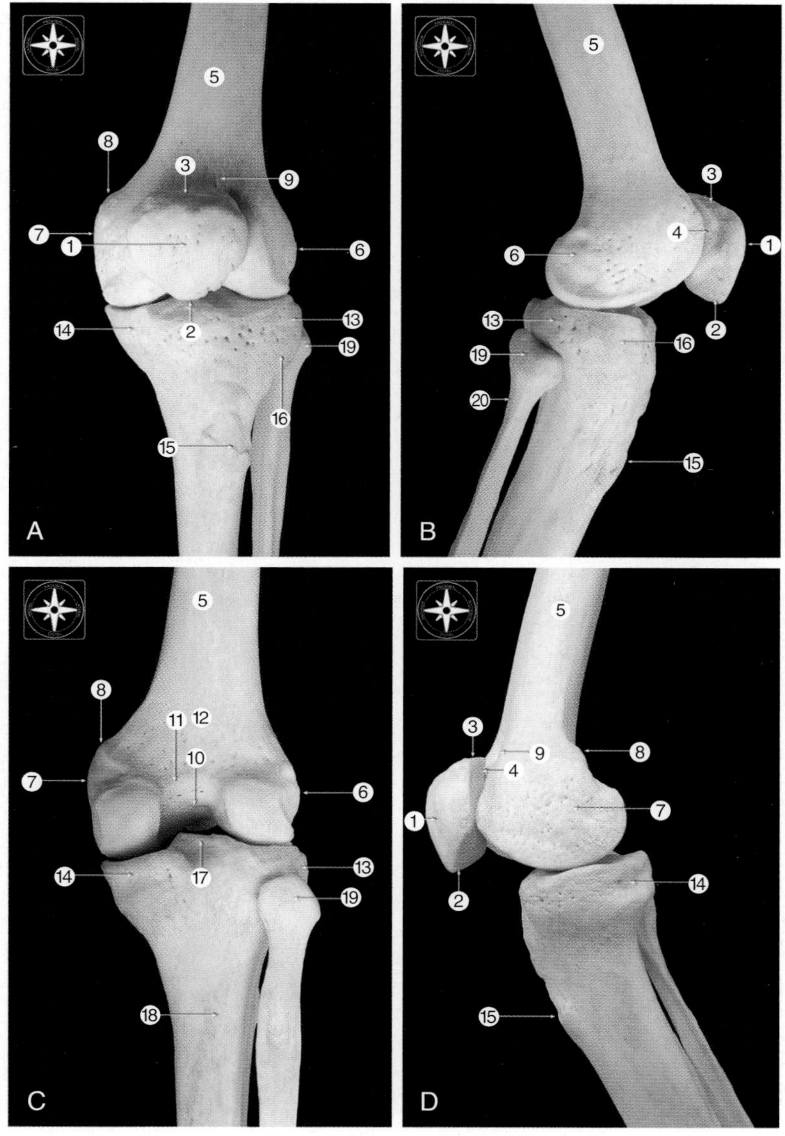

FIGURE 91-2 Bony anatomy. **A,** Anterior view. **B,** Lateral view. **C,** Posterior view. **D,** Medial view. Patella: *1,* Anterior surface. *2,* Apex. *3,* Base. *4,* Articular surface. Femur: *5,* Shaft. *6,* Lateral condyle and lateral epicondyle. *7,* Medial condyle and medial epicondyle. *8,* Adductor tubercle. *9,* Supratrochlear fossa. *10,* Intercondylar notch. *11,* Posterolateral rim of the intercondylar notch. *12,* Popliteal surface. Tibia: *13,* Lateral condyle. *14,* Medial condyle. *15,* Tibial tuberosity. *16,* Anterior tubercle or Gerdy's tubercle. *17,* Intercondylar eminence. *18,* Soleal line. Fibula: *19,* Head and apex. *20,* Neck. *(Copyright Pau Golanó.)*

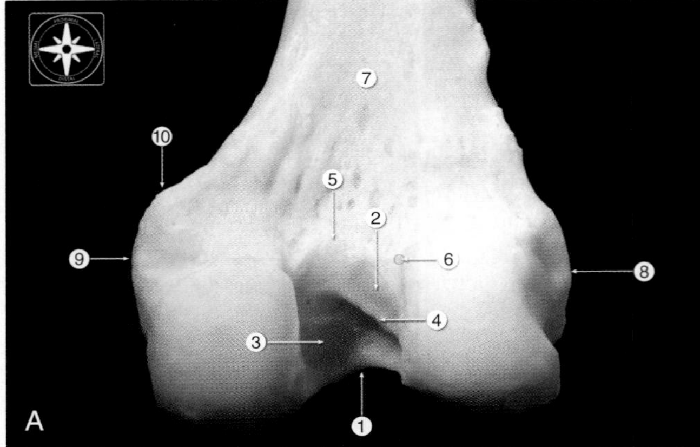

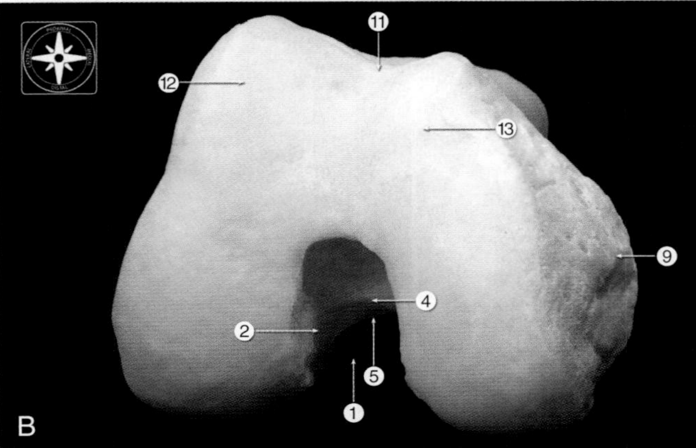

FIGURE 91-3 Intercondylar notch morphology. **A,** Posterior view of the distal epiphysis of the femur (knee in extension). **B,** Distal view of the distal epiphysis of the femur (knee at 90 degrees of flexion). *1,* Intercondylar notch. *2,* Femoral footprint of anterior cruciate ligament. *3,* Femoral footprint of posterior cruciate ligament. *4,* Lateral intercondylar ridge or resident's ridge. *5,* Posterolateral rim of the intercondylar notch. *6,* Over the top. *7,* Popliteal surface. *8,* Lateral condyle and lateral epicondyle. *9,* Medial condyle and medial epicondyle. *10,* Adductor tubercle. *11,* Femoral trochlear groove (patellar surface). *12,* Lateral slope of the patellar surface. *13,* Medial slope of the patellar surface. *(Copyright Pau Golanó.)*

intercondylar notch is the point of proximal insertion of the ACL and the posterior cruciate ligament (PCL). A wide zone on the medial wall of the notch constitutes the origin of the PCL, whereas the lateral wall has a flattened area that represents the proximal origin of the ACL. This area includes discrete bony prominences that are used as landmarks for the reconstructive surgery of the ACL. The prominences that are referenced for the correct positioning of the osseous tunnels are the lateral intercondylar ridge and the lateral bifurcate ridge.[2-4] The lateral bifurcate ridge is located perpendicular to the lateral intercondylar ridge, and in their posterior margin, an imaginary "T" is formed between them. The lateral intercondylar ridge is considered the anterior limit of the ACL and the lateral bifurcate ridge represents the separation of the two bundles (anteromedial and posterolateral) of the ACL.[4] Because of the confusion of the lateral intercondylar ridge with the posterolateral rim of the intercondylar notch during localization of the femoral tunnel for anterior ligamentoplasty, this prominence is now popularly called *resident's ridge* (Fig. 91-3).[5-7]

Tibia

The proximal epiphysis of the tibia forms two flattened surfaces, named the tibial plateaus or condyles. The medial tibial surface is larger and its shape is almost flat, whereas the lateral surface is more narrow and convex. Both present posterior declination of approximately 10 degrees with respect to the tibial diaphysis. At the posterior level, the lateral tibial condyle presents a flat and oval articulation with the fibula. In its most posterior zone, the medial tibial condyle presents a deep transverse groove for the insertion of the semimembranosus muscle (reflected tendon) and another medially for the insertion of the MCL.

The central region, located between the tibial plateaus, is occupied by the intercondylar eminences with the medial and lateral spines (medial and lateral intercondylar tubercle). Anterior and posterior to these eminences one can find the anterior and posterior intercondylar areas, respectively, which offer insertion for the cruciate ligaments and menisci.

The tibial tuberosity protrudes on the anterior face of the tibia, which corresponds to the insertion of the patellar tendon. Approximately 2 to 3 cm lateral to this tuberosity, the anterior tubercle or Gerdy's tubercle is encountered, which constitutes the point of insertion for the iliotibial tract.

Patella

The patella is the largest sesamoid bone in the human body. It has a triangular shape, and we can highlight three edges, two surfaces, and one apex. The anterior surface is separated from the skin by the prepatellar bursa. The posterior or articular surface is divided by a central ridge into a medial articular surface and a larger lateral surface that occupies approximately two thirds of the patella (Fig. 91-4).

The superior edge (base) of the patella is the location of insertion for the fibers of the tendon of the quadriceps femoris, principally the rectus femoris, vastus lateralis, and vastus intermedius. Most of the fibers of the vastus medialis insert

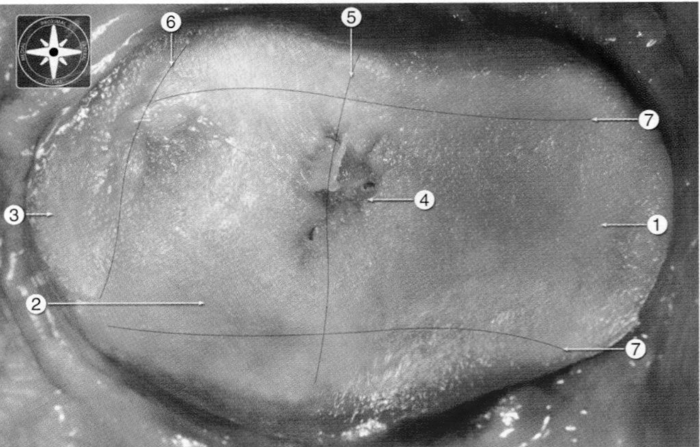

FIGURE 91-4 Posterior (intraarticular) view of the patella. *1,* Lateral facet. *2,* Medial facet. *3,* Odd facet. This facet comes in contact with the femur only when the knee approaches full flexion. *4,* Articular cartilage lesion (grade III-IV Outerbridge classification). *5,* Central ridge, which corresponds to the femoral trochlear groove (patellar surface). *6,* Vertical ridge. *7,* Horizontal ridges. *(Copyright Pau Golanó.)*

on the medial edge; only a small portion insert along the superior edge. The fibers of the quadriceps femoris tendon envelop the anterior surface of the patella and merge at the level of the patellar vertex with the patellar tendon or ligament (Fig. 91-5).

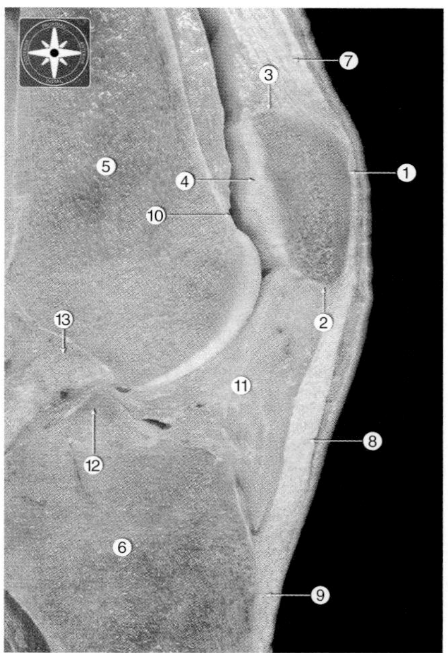

FIGURE 91-5 Sagittal section of the knee joint. *1,* Anterior surface of patella. *2,* Apex of patella. *3,* Base of patella. *4,* Posterior or articular surface of patella. *5,* Femur. *6,* Tibia. *7,* Quadriceps tendon. *8,* Patellar tendon. *9,* Tibial tuberosity. *10,* Supratrochlear fossa. *11,* Infrapatellar fat pad (Hoffa's fat pad). *12,* Tibial insertion of anterior cruciate ligament. *13,* Femoral insertion of posterior cruciate ligament. *(Copyright Pau Golanó.)*

Muscular Anatomy

The muscles that act on the knee joint may be divided schematically and with regard to their location into four groups (Fig. 91-6): anterior, posterior, medial, and lateral. In some anatomy texts these muscle groups are referred to as *dynamic elements* of the knee, but instead of following that discussion in this chapter, we only refer to them with regard to their origin and insertion and provide some anatomic detail that may prove useful to the reader.

Anterior

The anterior group is formed by the quadriceps femoris muscle, which is the primary extensor of the knee joint. It is formed in turn by four muscular components, the rectus femoris (which also functions as a hip flexor), vastus intermedius, vastus lateralis, and vastus medialis. The insertion of this muscle at the level of the base of the patella has been described previously in the osseous anatomy section.

Posterior

In the posterior region of the knee and in its most proximal zone, three muscles belonging to the posterior muscle compartment of the thigh may be observed: the semimembranosus and semitendinosus (more superficial) muscles on the

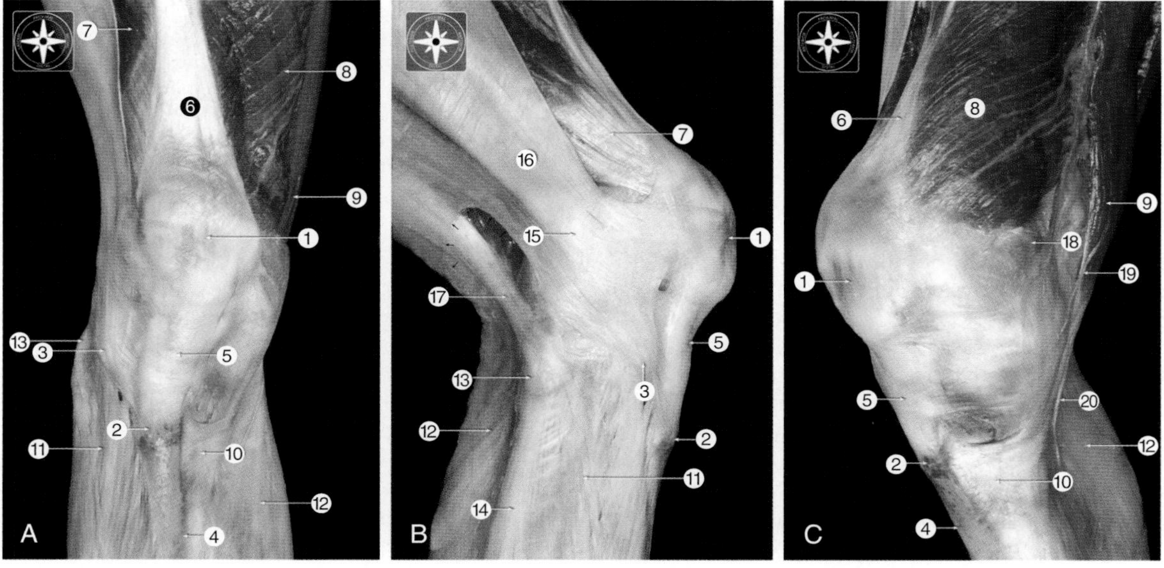

FIGURE 91-6 Muscular anatomy. **A,** Anterior view. **B,** Lateral view. **C,** Medial view. *1,* Patella. *2,* Tibial tuberosity. *3,* Anterior tubercle or Gerdy's tubercle. *4,* Anterior border of the tibia. *5,* Patellar tendon. *6,* Quadriceps tendon. *7,* Vastus lateralis. *8,* Vastus medialis. *9,* Sartorius muscle. *10,* Pes anserinus area in the medial surface of the tibia. *11,* Muscles of the anterior compartment of the leg. *12,* Muscles of the posterior compartment of the leg. *13,* Head of the fibula. *14,* Shaft of the fibula (peroneus longus muscle). *15,* Lateral epicondyle. *16,* Iliotibial tract. *17,* Biceps femoris muscle (femoral fascia opened). *18,* Medial epicondyle. *19,* Infrapatellar branch (cut) of the saphenous nerve. *20,* Saphenous nerve (cut). *(Copyright Pau Golanó.)*

medial side and the biceps femoris muscle on the lateral side, all of which act as knee flexors. In the distal zone the popliteus muscle and the gastrocnemius muscle, muscles of the posterior compartment of the leg, deep and superficial, respectively, also have a flexor function.

The semimembranosus is one of the hamstring muscles. The distal semimembranosus tendinous insertions are important structures that contribute to the stability of the posterior medial corner of the knee.[8] The semimembranosus inserts at the posterior level of the knee joint through five tendinous expansions: the anterior or tibial expansion (the reflected expansion), the direct expansion, the inferior or popliteal expansion, the capsular expansion, and the oblique popliteal ligament. The anterior expansion extends anteriorly, passing under the posterior oblique ligament, and inserts in the medial aspect of the proximal tibia under the MCL. The direct expansion also has an anterior course, deep to the anterior arm, and attaches in the posterior medial aspect of the tibia. The inferior expansion extends more distally than the anterior and the direct expansions. It passes under the distal tibial segments of the posterior oblique ligament and the MCL, inserting just above the tibial attachment of the MCL. The capsular expansion is adjacent to the posterior oblique ligament. The oblique popliteal ligament is a thin, broad lateral extension of the semimembranosus tendon that covers and blends with the posterior medial capsule and extends beyond the midline of the joint to intertwine its fibers with the arcuate ligament from the lateral posterior aspect of the knee (Fig. 91-7).[8,9]

The popliteus muscle originates on the posterior aspect of the tibia and inserts on the lateral femoral epicondyle. Because of its multiple attachments to other posterior and posterolateral structures, the popliteus muscle is an important structure that provides dorsolateral stability, stabilizes the lateral meniscus, and balances the neutral tibial rotation.[10,11] This muscle possesses a tendon of some 2.5 cm in length that runs across a hiatus located in the segment medial and posterior to the lateral meniscus, making its visualization possible during arthroscopic exploration of the knee.

The gastrocnemius muscle comes from the lateral and medial femoral condyles through two heads of origin. Together with the soleus and plantaris muscles, they form the superficial posterior compartment of the leg.

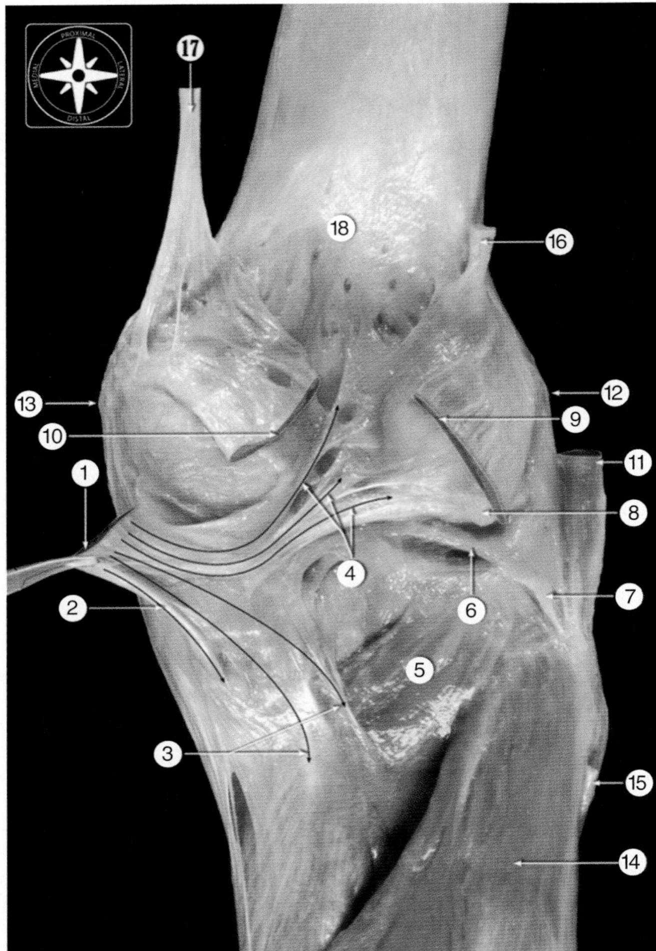

FIGURE 91-7 Posterior view of the capsular structures of the knee joint. *1,* Semimembranosus tendon (cut). *2,* Direct expansion. *3,* Inferior or popliteal expansion. *4,* Oblique popliteal ligament. *5,* Popliteus muscle. *6,* Popliteus capsular extension. *7,* Fabellofibular ligament. *8,* Os fabella. *9,* Lateral head of gastrocnemius muscle (cut). *10,* Medial head of gastrocnemius muscle (cut). *11,* Biceps femoris tendon (cut). *12,* Lateral epicondyle. *13,* Medial epicondyle. *14,* Fibular origin of the soleus muscle. *15,* Common peroneal nerve (cut). *16,* Lateral intermuscular septum insertion (cut). *17,* Adductor magnus tendon insertion (cut). *18,* Popliteal surface. *(Copyright Pau Golanó.)*

Medial

The medial musculature of the knee includes two muscles, the sartorius muscle of the anterior compartment of the thigh and the gracilis muscle of the medial or adductor compartment of the thigh. These muscles act at the level of the knee as flexors and internal rotators of the leg. Their insertion on the medial region of the tibia is characteristic and, together with the insertion of the semitendinosus muscle, is known as the *pes anserinus* (see Fig. 91-6, *C,* and Fig. 91-8). Knowledge of the anatomy and position of these tendons at the level of the pes anserinus is fundamental to correctly harvest autografts during reconstruction of the ACL or PCL.[12]

The pes anserinus insertion is, on average, 19 mm (range, 10-25 mm) distal and 22.5 mm (range, 13-30 mm) medial to the apex of the tibial tubercle, with an average width of 20 mm (range, 15-34 mm).[12] The sartorius inserts more anterior and superficially than the gracilis and the semitendinosus and forms an aponeurotic fascia. On the superior margin of this fascia is a thickened band that can be confused with the tendon of the gracilis, which is immediately distal. This confusion at the moment of obtaining the graft would result in a tendon of smaller length and attached to a muscle belly. Posteriorly, and deep to the sartorius, lies the tendon of the gracilis at the proximal level and the tendon of the semitendinosus muscle at the distal level.[13] These last two tendons can be used for ACL reconstruction procedures. Both tendons (semitendinosus and gracilis) have tendinous expansions directed toward the fascia of the medial head of the gastrocnemius muscle[13] that need to be sectioned for correct harvesting of both tendons. If these expansions are not carefully freed from the tendons, the tendon stripper can inadvertedly transect the main tendon, leaving the surgeon with a shortened graft (Fig. 91-8).[12,14]

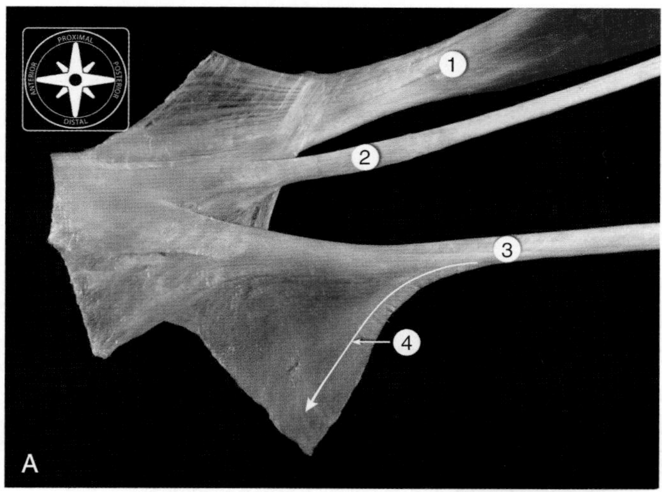

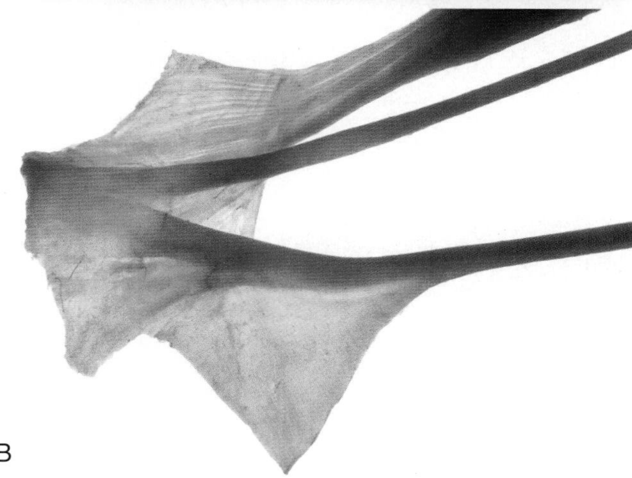

FIGURE 91-8 Pes anserinus anatomy. Deep view. **A,** Anatomical dissection. **B,** Anatomical dissection by transillumination. *1,* Sartorius tendon (superficial layer). *2,* Gracilis tendon. *3,* Semitendinosus tendon. *4,* Semitendinosus tendinous expansions directed toward the fascia of the medial head of the gastrocnemius muscle. *(Copyright Pau Golanó.)*

Lateral

The tendon of the biceps femoris muscle is the only tendon located at the lateral side of the knee. Its insertion is formed by three bands, one that is directed to the lateral part of the fibular head, another to the lateral condyle of the tibia, where it merges with the iliotibial tract, and finally a third one that comprises the deep fascia of the lateral part of the leg, where it coincides with the joint capsule of the knee. This muscle is a flexor at the level of the knee and an external rotator for the leg.

Bursae

The knee has a system of bursae that is the most extensive and complex in the human body. Twelve bursae are described. However, based on their clinical importance, only the prepatellar, superficial infrapatellar, anserine, and gastrocnemius bursae are described.

The prepatellar bursa is located in the anterior region of the knee, at the subcutaneous level, anterior to the inferior half of the patella and to the superior half of the patellar tendon. Inflammation of this bursa is known as *housemaid's knee*.

The superficial infrapatellar bursa is also located in the anterior aspect of the knee and similarly in the subcutaneous plane, above the distal limit of the patellar tendon and the tibial tuberosity.

The anserine bursa is in the medial aspect of the knee. This bursa is located three fingerbreadths below the medial joint line and between the medial surface of the tibia, the MCL, and the tendons of the pes anserinus at the level of their insertion.

Two bursae are found in the posterior area, located deep between the heads of the medial and lateral gastrocnemius and the posterior joint capsule. The lateral subtendinous gastrocnemius bursa rarely communicates with the knee joint, but the medial bursa does so commonly. In certain occasions, the medial subtendinous gastrocnemius bursa may enlarge and create a space known as a *Baker* or *popliteal cyst*.[15]

Ligaments

Medial Collateral Ligament

The MCL, with a more or less triangular shape, is an intrinsic ligament that is intimately related to the medial meniscus and joint capsule, forming the medial meniscoligamentous complex. This ligament has two layers, one deep and the other superficial. The fibers of the deep layer extend from the medial femoral condyle to the medial tibial condyle. The fibers of the superficial layer extend like a fan from the medial epicondyle to the medial tibial condyle, posteriorly to the insertion of the pes anserinus, approximately 10 cm distal to the medial joint line. It then merges with the posterior joint capsule, where they form a strong capsular reinforcement known as the posterior oblique ligament (Fig. 91-9).[9,13]

Lateral Collateral Ligament

The LCL, a cordlike band, is considered an extrinsic capsular ligament between 5.5 and 7.1 cm in length[1] that extends from the lateral femoral condyle to the fibular head (Fig. 91-10). At the proximal level the ligament is closely related to the joint capsule, which is separated by fat, through which run the lateral inferior articular artery and veins at the level of the joint line. Its distal insertion is augmented by the iliotibial tract.[1,16,17]

Joint Capsule and Synovial Membrane

The knee has the most extensive joint cavity and synovial membrane of the human organism. The capsule extends from the patella and the patellar tendon anteriorly to the medial, lateral, and posterior expansions. Proximally it inserts on the femur, some three to four fingerbreadths above the patella, and distally it presents a circular insertion over the tibial ridge, except at the point where the popliteus tendon penetrates the joint traversing to its hiatus.

The capsule is constituted of a fibrous membrane with a number of areas of thickening that act as reinforcement and are considered intrinsic ligaments (especially the medial and

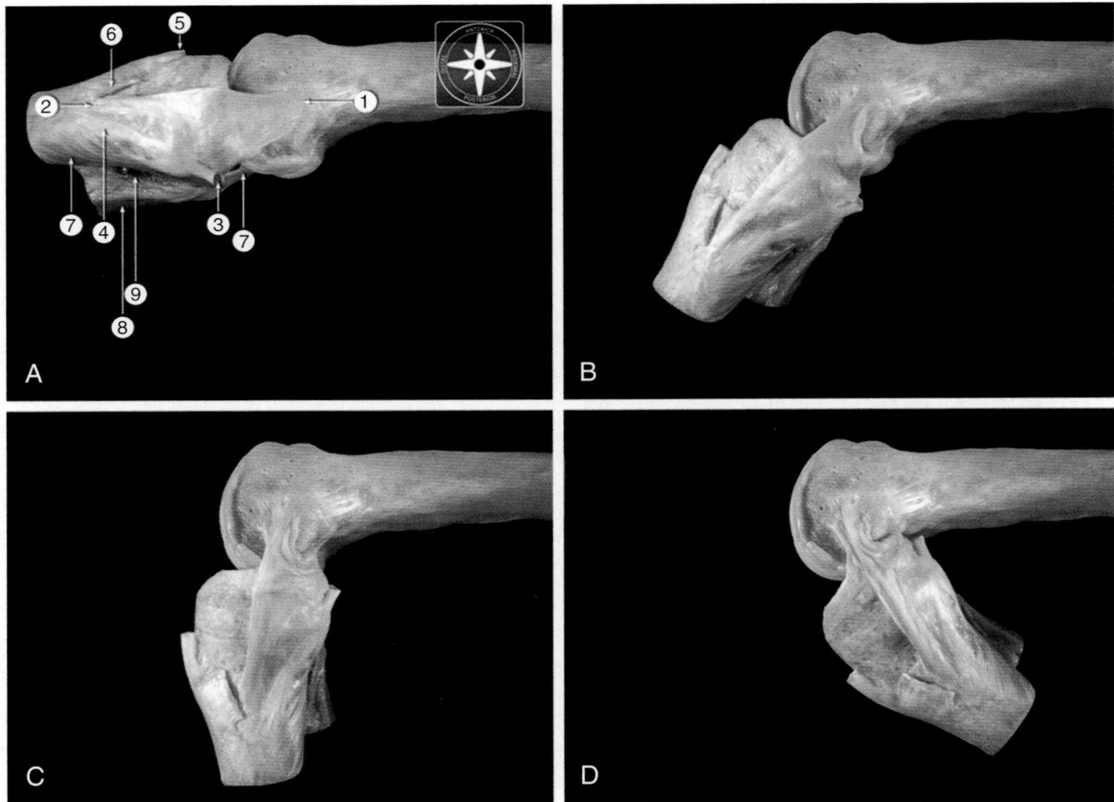

FIGURE 91-9 Osteoarticular anatomic dissection of the medial collateral ligament during the range of motion of the knee joint (**A,** extension to **D,** maximal flexion). *1,* Medial epicondyle. *2,* Tibial insertion of medial collateral ligament. *3,* Semimembranosus tendon (cut). *4,* Inferior or popliteal expansion of the semimembranosus tendon. *5,* Patellar tendon (cut). *6,* Pes anserinus (cut). *7,* Popliteus muscle. *8,* Soleus muscle (cut). *9,* Neurovascular bundle (popliteal artery, veins and tibial nerve). *(Copyright Pau Golanó.)*

lateral patellofemoral ligaments). The capsule is reinforced posteriorly by the oblique popliteal ligament, an expansion of the semimembranosus that extends from medial and distal to proximal and lateral. The arcuate complex is found in the posterolateral corner.[11] These two structures contribute to the posterior stability of the knee. The popliteal oblique ligament is found in the floor of the popliteal fossa, the space for the popliteal artery and vein, and more superficially for the tibial nerve.

The synovial membrane not only covers the internal walls of the capsule but also surrounds the cruciate ligaments, the popliteus tendon, the coronal recesses situated beneath the menisci, and the infrapatellar fat pad (the Hoffa fat pad), situated behind the patellar tendon. The synovial folds are quite numerous, especially at the level of the suprapatellar pouch. Plicae are synovial folds and are considered vestigial synovial septae that were never reabsorbed during the developmental process of the knee. The three most frequent plicae or synovial folds are the infrapatellar (ligamentum mucosum), suprapatellar, and medial patellar plicae.[18-20]

The infrapatellar plica or ligamentum mucosum is encountered most frequently and is considered a normal structure in the knee joint (Fig. 91-11).[21] The medial patellar plica is the one that most frequently becomes symptomatic.[19]

The posterior synovial cavity communicates with the medial subtendinous bursa of the gastrocnemius muscle and can participate in the generation of a popliteal or Baker cyst.[15]

Menisci

The menisci, medial and lateral, are two half-moon–shaped fibrocartilage structures that cover the peripheral portion of the medial and lateral tibial condyles (Fig. 91-12). In section, they are triangular with a peripheral base. Their superior surface is slightly concave, whereas the inferior is flat, adapting to the articular surface of the femoral and tibial condyles, respectively. Each meniscus is differentiated into three parts, the center or meniscal body and the meniscal ends or anterior and posterior horns. The horns insert into the anterior and posterior intercondylar area. They are also inserted into the tibial condylar ridge through their capsular union or coronary ligament. In 50% to 90% of knees, the anterior horns are connected by a dense fibrous band named the anterior transverse ligament, anterior intermeniscal ligament, or anterior transverse geniculate ligament.[22-24] Both menisci slide with flexion and extension of the knee. The degree of this movement is larger for the lateral meniscus, with 9 mm, compared with 3 mm for the medial meniscus.[25,26]

Medial Meniscus

The medial meniscus possesses a semilunar or “C” shape. Because of its strong insertions at the level of the body and posterior horn, this meniscus is less mobile than the lateral and is exposed to a greater risk of injury. Anteriorly the

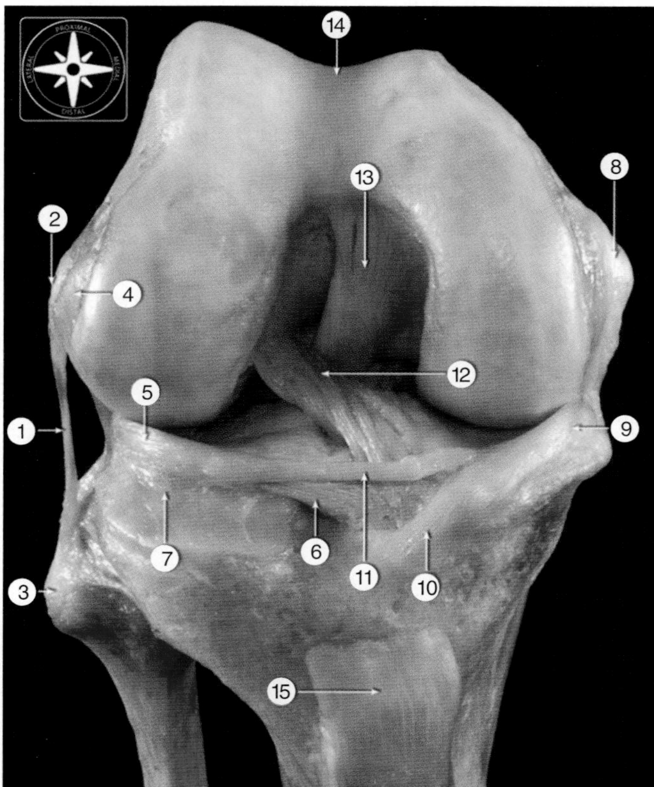

FIGURE 91-10 Anterior view of the osteoarticular dissection of the knee joint. *1,* Lateral collateral ligament. *2,* Lateral epicondyle. *3,* Head of the fibula. *4,* Popliteus tendon insertion. *5,* Lateral meniscus. *6,* Anterior horn of the lateral meniscus. *7,* Coronary ligament (meniscotibial capsule). *8,* Medial epicondyle. *9,* Medial meniscus. *10,* Anterior horn of the medial meniscus. *11,* Anterior transverse ligament, anterior intermeniscal ligament, or anterior transverse geniculate ligament. *12,* Anterior cruciate ligament. *13,* Posterior cruciate ligament. *14,* Femoral trochlear groove (patellar surface). *15,* Patellar tendon (cut). *(Copyright Pau Golanó.)*

meniscus does not have a connection to the capsular tissue or fat pad. Whereas in its medial portion it is firmly inserted into the deep capsular ligament, in its posterior body the meniscus is firmly fixed by the oblique popliteal ligament to blend with the joint capsule.

Lateral Meniscus

The lateral meniscus is almost circular, with an "O" shape. Because of the poor union of the meniscus to the margin of the lateral tibial condyle and the absence of insertion in the zone where the popliteus tendon courses, the meniscus possesses a mobility that relatively protects it from injury. In 69% to 74% of knees, a dense fibrous band can be observed arising from the posterior meniscal horn and running upward and posteriorly to the PCL; it inserts on the medial femoral condyle, known as the posterior meniscofemoral ligament or the ligament of Wrisberg (Fig. 91-13).[27-30] In approximately 50% to 74% of knees, another fibrous band can be observed arising from the posterior horn and passing upward and in front of the PCL, also terminating on the medial femoral

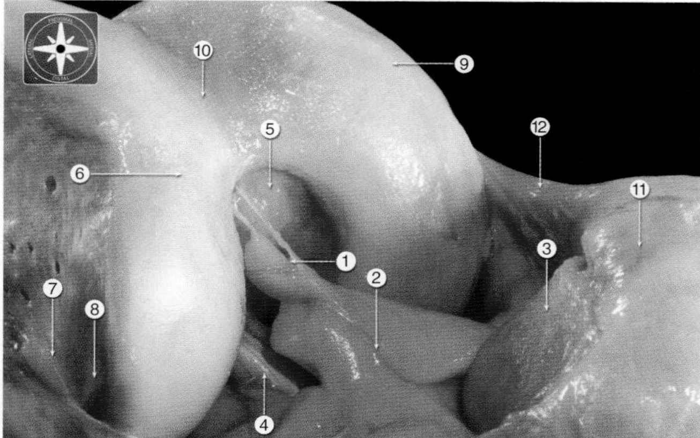

FIGURE 91-11 Anatomic dissection of the anterior region of the knee joint showing the morphology and relationship of the infrapatellar plica or ligamentum mucosum. *1,* Infrapatellar plica. *2,* Infrapatellar fat pad (Hoffa's fat pad). *3,* Posterior surface or articular surface of patella. *4,* Anterior cruciate ligament. *5,* Femoral insertion of posterior cruciate ligament covered by a synovial fat pad. *6,* Lateral slope of the patellar surface. *7,* Epicondyle insertion of lateral collateral ligament. *8,* Popliteus tendon insertion. *9,* Medial slope of the patellar surface. *10,* Femoral trochlear groove. *11,* Deep surface of quadriceps tendon. *12,* Joint capsule. *(Copyright Pau Golanó.)*

condyle; it is named the anterior meniscofemoral ligament or the ligament of Humphry.[27,29-31] Approximately 4% of people have both ligaments in the same knee.[32]

The most common congenital abnormality of the meniscus is a discoid meniscus with a frequency of 1.5% to 4.6% for the lateral[33] and 0.3% for the medial.[34]

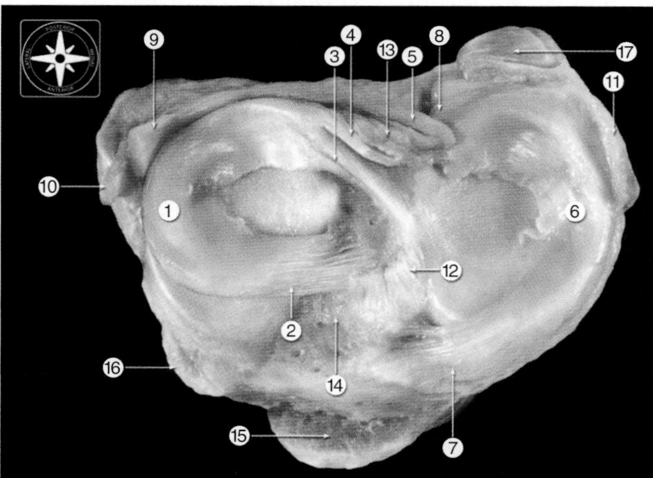

FIGURE 91-12 Osteoarticular dissection showing the morphology and relationship of the proximal epiphysis of the tibia in a superior view. *1,* Lateral meniscus. *2,* Anterior horn of the lateral meniscus. *3,* Posterior horn of the lateral meniscus. *4,* Anterior meniscofemoral ligament. *5,* Posterior meniscofemoral ligament. *6,* Medial meniscus. *7,* Anterior horn of the medial meniscus. *8,* Posterior horn of the medial meniscus. *9,* Popliteus tendon (cut). *10,* Lateral collateral ligament (cut). *11,* Medial collateral ligament (cut). *12,* Tibial footprint of the anterior cruciate ligament. *13,* Posterior cruciate ligament (cut). *14,* Anterior intercondylar area. *15,* Patellar tendon (cut). *16,* Iliotibial tract insertion in the anterior tubercle or Gerdy's tubercle (cut). *17,* Semimembranosus tendon (cut). *(Copyright Pau Golanó.)*

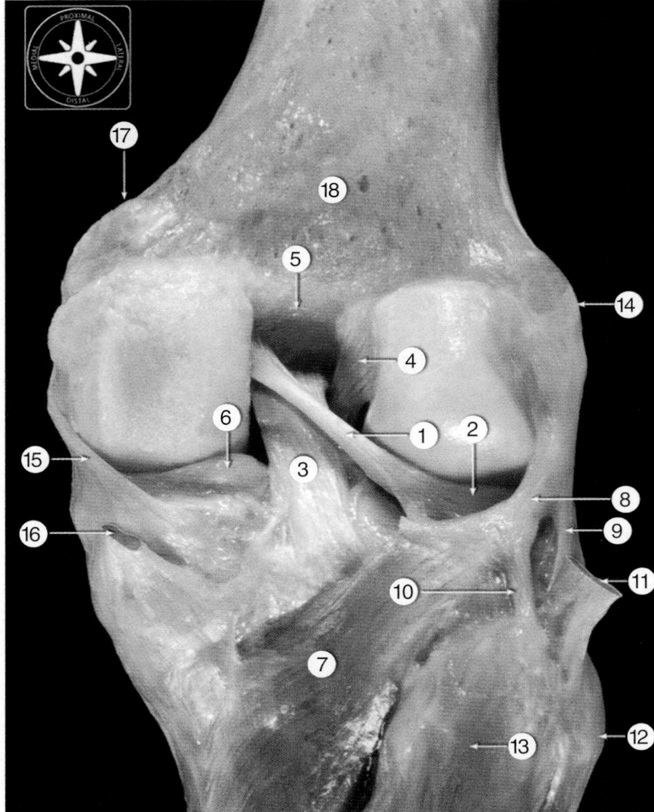

FIGURE 91-13 Osteoarticular dissection showing the posterior structures of the knee joint after removing the joint capsule. *1,* Posterior meniscofemoral ligament or the ligament of Wrisberg. *2,* Lateral meniscus. *3,* Posterior cruciate ligament. *4,* Femoral insertion of the anterior cruciate ligament. *5,* Intercondylar notch. *6,* Medial meniscus. *7,* Popliteus muscle. *8,* Popliteus tendon. *9,* Lateral collateral ligament. *10,* Popliteus capsular extension. *11,* Biceps femoris tendon (cut). *12,* Head of the fibula. *13,* Soleus fibular insertion muscle. *14,* Lateral epicondyle. *15,* Medial collateral ligament. *16,* Semimembranosus tendon (cut). *17,* Adductor tubercle. *18,* Popliteal surface. *(Copyright Pau Golanó.)*

Because many functions of the meniscus have been described, its resection can cause mechanical alterations that can lead to degenerative articular changes.[35] For this reason, avoidance of complete meniscal resection is advised.

Cruciate Ligaments

The ACL is thinner and longer than the PCL. They are both located near the center of the joint, slightly nearer to the posterior than to the anterior wall.

Anterior Cruciate Ligament

The ACL inserts in the anterior intercondylar area of the tibia and is directed, in a spiral fashion, to its attachment on the lateral wall of the femoral intercondylar notch. The native ligament can be broadly divided into two fascicles or bundles, the anteromedial (AM) and the posterolateral (PL). This terminology was chosen according to their insertion on the tibia. The fibers of the AM bundle insert on the most AM part of the tibia and originate on the most proximal part of its femoral insertion, whereas the PL bundle inserts on the most PL part of the tibia and originates on the most distal portion of the femoral insertion (Fig. 91-14). Both bundles contribute in a different way to the rotational and anteroposterior stability of the knee (Fig. 91-15).[36] The AM bundle is tight in flexion, whereas the PL tightens in extension. For this reason, some authors have reported on reconstructing the ACL using two bundles with two separate tunnels in the femur and another two in the tibia.[37,38]

Posterior Cruciate Ligament

The PCL inserts in the posterior intercondylar area of the tibia and is directed to its attachment on the medial wall of the femoral intercondylar notch. As with the ACL, the presence

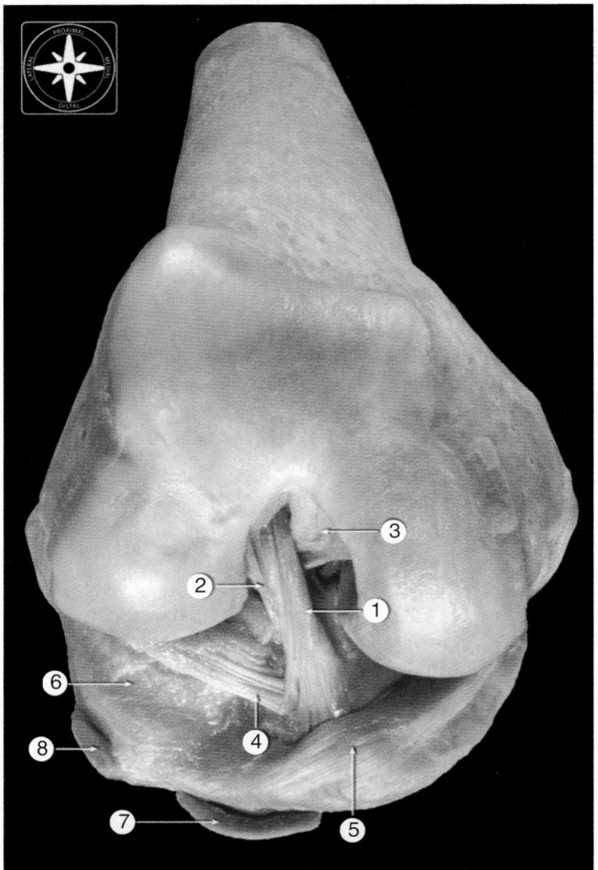

FIGURE 91-14 Osteoarticular dissection showing the anterior cruciate ligament. Superior view with the knee in maximal flexion. *1,* Anterior cruciate ligament (anteromedial bundle). *2,* Anterior cruciate ligament (posterolateral bundle). *3,* Femoral insertion of the posterior cruciate ligament. *4,* Anterior horn of the lateral meniscus. *5,* Anterior horn of the medial meniscus. *6,* Coronary ligament (meniscotibial capsule). *7,* Patellar tendon (cut). *8,* Iliotibial tract insertion in the anterior tubercle or Gerdy's tubercle (cut). *(Copyright Pau Golanó.)*

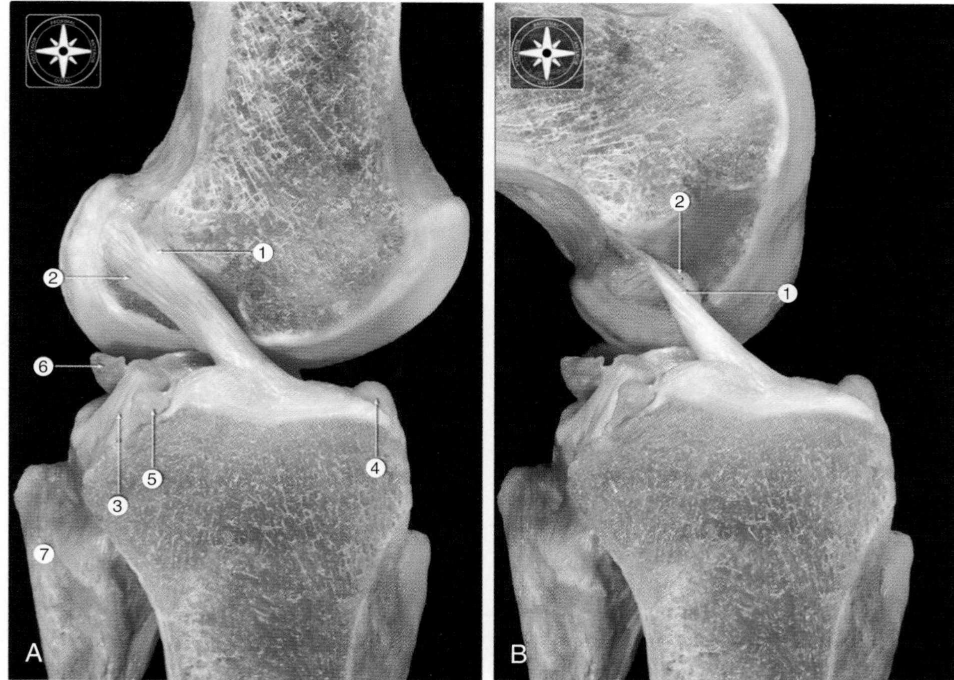

FIGURE 91-15 Sagittal section of the knee joint showing the different tension patterns of fascicles of the anterior cruciate ligament. The medial femoral condyle was cut off through the intercondylar notch for better visualization of the anterior cruciate ligament and its femoral attachment. **A,** Knee in extension. **B,** Knee at 90 degrees of flexion. *1,* Anteromedial bundle. *2,* Posterolateral bundle. *3,* Posterior cruciate ligament (cut). *4,* Anterior horn of the medial meniscus (cut). *5,* Posterior horn of the medial meniscus (cut). *6,* Posterior meniscofemoral ligament. *7,* Head of the fibula. *(Copyright Pau Golanó.)*

of two different bundles has been described, the anterolateral (AL) and the posteromedial (PM). In complete extension, the PM bundle of the ligament encounters more tension than the AL bundle, whereas during flexion, the PM fibers relax and the AL fibers are taut.

Neurovascular Anatomy

Vascularization

The knee is vascularized by an extensive arterial plexus, superficial and deep, formed by seven arterial branches: five articular or genicular arteries, which are branches of the popliteal artery; the descending articular artery, a branch of the femoral artery; and the recurrent anterior artery, a branch of the anterior tibial artery.[39]

The superficial plexus forms a vascular circle around the patella.[40] The deep plexus is located between the inferior margin of the femur and the superior margin of the tibia. Of all the arteries that form the plexus, three require special attention for their contribution to the cruciate ligaments and the menisci: the lateral inferior genicular artery, the medial inferior genicular artery, and the middle genicular artery.

The blood supply of the menisci predominantly originates from the inferior medial and lateral genicular arteries.[41] Their branches give off the parameniscal capillary plexus located on the peripheral ridge of the meniscus around its insertion on the posterior capsule. At the lateral side, the proximity of the articular genicular to the meniscal insertion to the capsule makes it susceptible to injury during lateral meniscal resection. On the medial side, the genicular artery lies some two fingerbreadths below the joint line and passes through a tunnel formed by the tibia and the MCL.

The vascularity of the cruciate ligaments is provided by the middle genicular artery and by a few branches of the inferior medial and lateral genicular arteries.[42-44] Although the medial genicular artery offers additional branches to the distal femoral epiphysis and to the proximal tibial epiphysis, the osseoligamentous junction of the cruciate ligaments does not significantly contribute to ligament vascularity. Although the ACL is capable of offering a vascular response after injury, spontaneous repair does not occur.[45]

Innervation

From a clinical point of view, it is worth mentioning the common peroneal nerve and the infrapatellar branch of the saphenous nerve.

- The common peroneal nerve is the terminal branch of the lateral sciatic nerve. It runs parallel and posterior to the tendon of the biceps femoris muscle in the posterolateral region of the knee until it reaches the fibular head.
- The infrapatellar branch of the saphenous nerve, a branch arising from the femoral nerve, runs through the medial and infrapatellar area of the knee, innervating the skin of the anteromedial aspect of the knee. It can be

injured when a medial knee incision is performed to obtain the gracilis and semitendinosus tendons, which are used for cruciate ligament reconstruction, MCL repair, or medial meniscus repair. Injury to this nerve can generate an anesthetic zone over the medial, anterior, and distal leg.[12,46-48]

Acknowledgment

We thank Dr. C. Jan Gilmore, Department of Orthopaedic Surgery, Sports Medicine, Presbyterian Hospital, Albuquerque, NM, for his expert translation of the anatomy section of this chapter.

Biomechanics of the Knee

Bruce Beynnon • Fatih Ertem

The knee joint is the largest and most complex joint in the human body. The joint capsule and ligaments, which provide structural stability to the knee, are particularly vulnerable to injury by large moments that can be created through the forces acting along the long lever arms of the lower limb, and thus it is not surprising that the knee is one of the most frequently injured joints. An injury to the knee, such as disruption of the ACL, can result in an extensive disability because this injury may alter normal knee biomechanics and therefore locomotion. Knowledge of knee biomechanics provides an essential framework for understanding the consequences of injury and joint disorders; it aids in the intelligent planning of surgical procedures, serves as the basis for developing objective rehabilitation programs, and describes the effects of different types of orthoses on the knee joint.

The knee joint is composed of three independent articulations, one between the patella and femur and the remaining two between the lateral and medial tibial and femoral condyles. The patellofemoral articulation consists of the patella, which has a multifaceted dorsal surface that articulates with the femoral trochlear groove. The tibiofemoral articulations consist of femoral condyles with saddle-shaped tibial condyles and interposing menisci. The posterior aspects of the femoral condyles are spherical in profile, whereas the anterior aspects of the femoral condyles are more elliptical. Thus, in extension, the flat portions of the femoral condyles are in contact with the tibia, and in flexion, the spherical portions of the femoral condyles are in contact with the tibia.

To the untrained observer, the knee joint may appear to function as a simple pinned hinge (ginglymus), with flexion-extension rotation the only apparent motion between the femur and tibia. However, the motion characteristics of the knee joint are complex, requiring a full 6 degrees of freedom (three translations and three rotations) to completely describe the coupled, or simultaneous, joint motions (Fig. 91-16). An example of coupled motion is demonstrated with flexion rotation of the knee from the extended position. With this rotation, there is a coupled posterior movement of the femoral contact regions on the tibial surface in the sagittal plane and an internal rotation of the tibia relative to the femur in the transverse plane. By use of the Eulerian-based coordinate system described by Hefzy and Grood,[49] the translations and rotations can be described in anatomically referenced directions (see Fig. 91-16). Although many different types of coordinate systems have been used to describe three-dimensional knee motion, this system is appealing because it allows joint rotation to be expressed in terms familiar to the clinician. Grood and Noyes[50] have applied the three-dimensional coordinate system to the interpretation of various clinical examination techniques and have developed a "bumper model" of the knee joint. This model is useful in describing the soft tissue restraints to anteroposterior translation and internal-external rotation of the knee joint. In addition, the model can be applied to demonstrate the types of tibiofemoral subluxations that may result when different soft tissue structures are disrupted. Application of this approach may aid in the examination of injuries to the knee ligaments and capsular structures.

This section assumes a working knowledge of the biomechanical terms essential to the description of knee function. For an introduction to basic knee biomechanics, the reader is encouraged to review the work of Mow and Hayes,[51] along with the definition of biomechanical terms as they apply to the knee presented by Noyes and coworkers.[52] A review of experimental studies of the tibiofemoral and the patellofemoral joints with associated contact morphometry studies is presented in this section.

Description of Biomechanical Techniques

The American Society of Biomechanics has defined the term *biomechanics* as the study of the structure and function of biologic systems using the methods of mechanics. Specifically for the knee joint, this process involves modeling and experimental investigation techniques. Perhaps the most commonly described knee model is the crossed four-bar linkage called the *cruciate linkage*.[49,51,53-56] This approach has been used to study the interaction of the cruciate ligaments with the tibiofemoral joint (Fig. 91-17). The model consists of two crossed rods representing the cruciate ligaments and two connecting bars representing the tibial and femoral attachments of these ligaments. This approach has been used to describe the shape of both the tibial and femoral condyles, the path of the instantaneous center of knee joint rotation, and the posterior migration of the tibiofemoral contact point that occurs with knee flexion. The four-bar approach is based on rigid interconnecting cruciate linkages that are not allowed to elongate. Because the cruciate ligaments elongate and twist during normal joint articulation,[57-59] this technique may be inadequate for

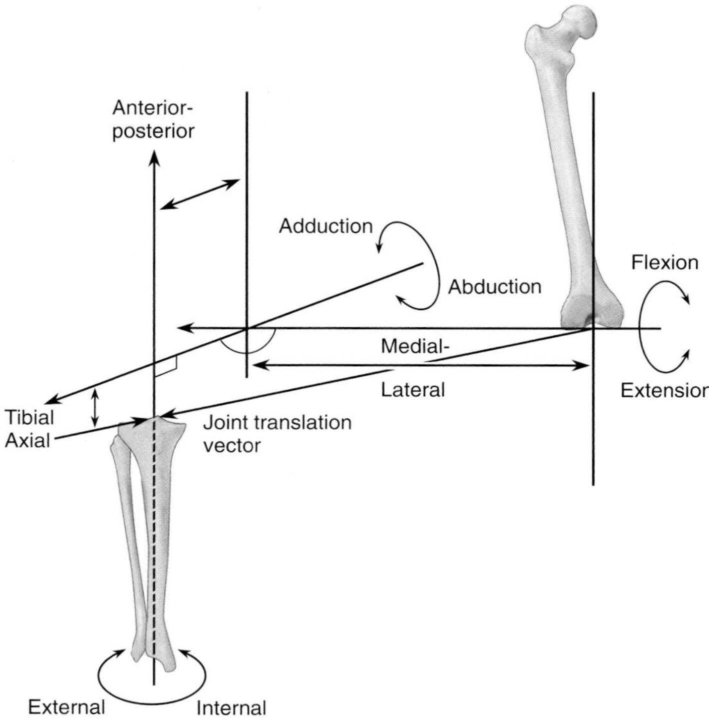

FIGURE 91-16 Coordinate system for knee joint rotations and translations. Flexion-extension rotation is about the fixed femoral axis. Internal-external rotation is about a fixed tibial axis. Abduction-adduction is about an axis that is perpendicular to the femoral and tibial axes. The joint translations occur along each of the three coordinate axes. *(From Hefzy MS, Grood ES: Review of knee models.* Appl Mech Rev *41:1–13, 1988.)*

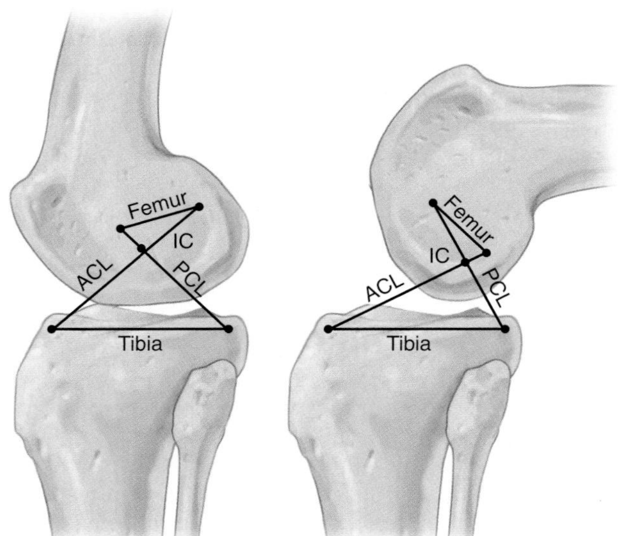

FIGURE 91-17 The four-bar cruciate linkage model. The model includes two crossed bars, which represent the anterior and posterior cruciate ligaments (*ACL, PCL*). The remaining two bars represent the tibial and femoral attachments of the ligaments. *IC,* Instantaneous center of joint rotation. *(From Hefzy MS, Grood ES: Review of knee models.* Appl Mech Rev *41:1–13, 1988.)*

modeling the detailed interaction of the cruciate ligaments with the tibiofemoral joint.

Churchill and associates[60] described the knee in passive and active flexion, respectively, in three dimensions with use of a compound-hinge model. Flexion is described about the transepicondylar axis, and internal-external rotation is described about an axis parallel to the longitudinal axis of the tibia (Fig. 91-18). The model accounts for three-dimensional kinematics while allowing the axes to remain fixed in bone. Previous models use the concept of an instantaneous center of rotation, which accounts for femoral rollback by using a different center of rotation with each flexion angle.[61-63]

Coughlin and coworkers[64] characterized the 6 degrees of freedom of the tibiofemoral joint in terms of two rotations about the femoral epicondylar (FE) axis and an axis parallel to the anatomic tibial axis. The FE axis is defined as the line passing through the spherical centers of the medial and lateral condyles. In the midsagittal plane, the patella follows a circular arc with a constant radius of curvature. These axes remain nearly perpendicular, with the patella tracking along a circular arc that can be described relative to the FE axis during flexion from 0 to 90 degrees. The authors suggest this model has clinical application in identifying the FE axis intraoperatively.[64]

Tibiofemoral Joint Biomechanics

Force Measurement of Ligaments

Measurement of ligament or tendon force continues to be one of the biggest challenges in orthopaedic biomechanics. To

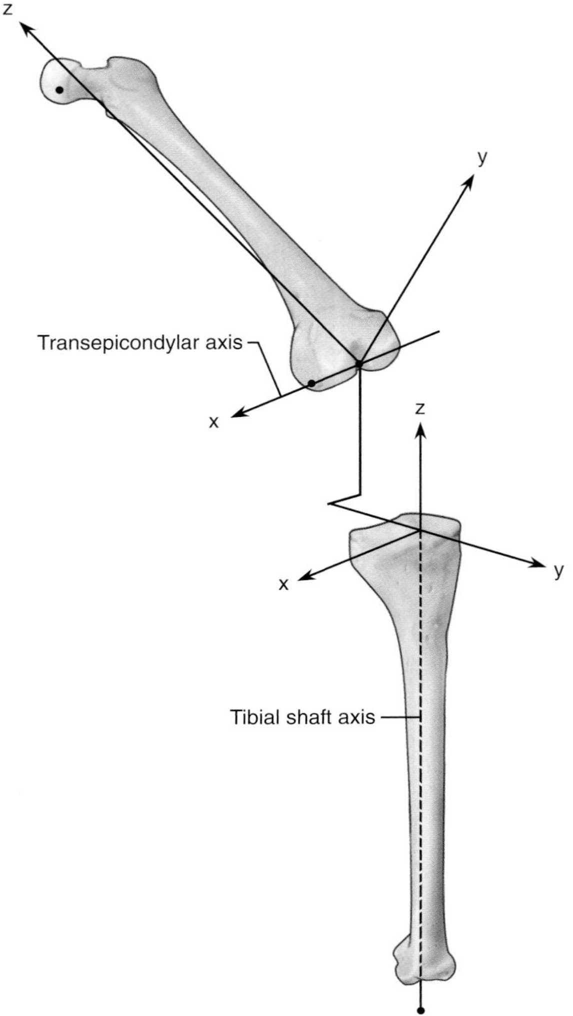

FIGURE 91-18 The compound-hinge model describes the three-dimensional kinematics of the knee using two axes: the transepicondylar axis and an axis parallel to the longitudinal axis of the tibia.

meet this challenge, Salmons[65] introduced the buckle transducer. The buckle transducer is a structure containing a beam over which the ligament is looped to create bending of the buckle frame. The beam is attached separately, and therefore transverse cutting of the ligament is not required. Lengthwise incisions are required, however, disrupting many ligament fibers and altering the normal function of the ligament by dissociating one group of fiber bundles from another.[66-68] Salmons[65] and other investigators[69-71] have applied this technique to various knee ligaments. This approach is limited to in vitro applications in which a knee ligament is instrumented with the transducer and then the knee joint is loaded, and the output from the buckle transducer is then directly recorded. After the tissue is tested in situ, it is dissected free from one of its bony attachments so that a known load can be applied to the tissue-buckle system and a calibration of the gauge–soft tissue system can be made. With use of this approach, the load can be determined for the tissue in situ.

Markolf and colleagues[72-75] have presented a direct approach to the measurement of ACL and PCL force in cadaveric knees. This technique involves isolating the tibial attachment of the cruciate ligament by creating a bone plug with a coring cutter and attaching a load sensor to the external portion of the bone plug. This approach facilitates the measurement of resultant cruciate ligament force. For example, the authors have used this approach to demonstrate that passive flexion-extension motion of the knee from 10 degrees to full flexion does not load the ACL, whereas loading of the quadriceps musculature (simulating active extension of the lower limb against gravity) developed ACL loading between the limits of 0 and 45 degrees. In later studies using human cadaver knees, Markolf and coworkers[76] demonstrated that hamstring loading has a greater effect on cruciate force than does quadriceps loading. PCL force increases significantly with hamstring loading beyond 30 degrees of flexion.

Although direct force measurements of the cruciate ligaments are desirable, the current state-of-the-art force transducers allow the associated errors to fall within relatively large error bounds. Fleming and colleagues[77] reported mean errors ranging from 20% to 29% for the arthroscopically implantable force probe (AIFP), if it is calibrated after implantation. They noted that similar limitations have been reported for other force transducers that operate on the same principle, although the errors associated with other arthroscopic force transducers have not been reported. In addition, Fleming and colleagues[78] determined that the output of AIFPs is specimen dependent. When the force transducer was removed and reimplanted into the same location, the results were not repeatable, with errors ranging from 4% to 109%. Upon reimplantation into another location in the same ACL, the percentage errors ranged from 2% to 203%. These findings highlight a need for a more repeatable transducer that yields relative measurements of ACL stress in vivo. Because stress is directly related to strain, several investigators have chosen to measure strain in the ligaments. Beynnon and Fleming and coworkers[79,80] have shown that the accuracy associated with strain measurements in the ACL is on the order of 0.2% and 0.1% with use of the Hall-effect strain transducer and the differential variable reluctance transducer (DVRT), respectively.

Strain Measurement of Ligaments

Several investigators have measured ligament displacement, enabling the calculation of strain pattern, to understand the effect of knee joint position and muscle activity on ligament biomechanics.[81-86] Most of this work has been carried out in vitro, and the results are conflicting.

Edwards,[83] Kennedy,[84] Brown,[82] Berns,[87] Hull,[88] and their associates used mercury-filled strain gauges to measure the length of ligaments at various angles of knee flexion. Henning and colleagues[89] have constructed a device to measure displacement in the ACL in vivo.

Butler and associates[90] and Woo and colleagues[91] have developed optical techniques for mapping surface strains in various tissues. Butler and coworkers[90,92] used high-speed cameras to record the movements of surface markers and measured both midsubstance and insertion-site deformations of soft tissues. These techniques are ideal methods for monitoring surface strains, particularly during high-rate tests, but they are not useful for out-of-plane movements or for ligaments such as the cruciate ligaments that cannot be directly viewed. They also suffer from the theoretical disadvantage that the tissue of interest has to be exposed and therefore is not in a physiologic state.

Other investigators have calculated strain by measurement of the change of ligament attachment length under various applied joint loadings. For example, Wang and colleagues[86] measured the three-dimensional coordinates of pins stuck in a cadaveric joint at the palpated origin and insertion points of the major knee ligaments. They recorded the relationship between torque and angular rotation of the femur relative to the tibia. After excision of certain ligaments, the tests were repeated to determine the contribution of these elements to torsional restraint. In the most extensive and elegant studies, Sidles and associates[93] used a three-dimensional digitizer to compute ligament length patterns. In a slightly different approach, Trent and colleagues[94] used pins embedded in the ligament attachments and measured the displacement of one pin relative to the other. In addition, in this study they located the instant centers of transverse joint rotation. Warren and coworkers[95] also used pins placed at ligament origins but measured displacements with a radiographic technique.

The pins or other markers used as locators of ligament origin generally estimate average ligament strain. This technique may produce confusing results because of both the difficulty in choosing the center of a ligament insertion and the changes in strain from place to place within a ligament. For example, Covey and colleagues[96] demonstrated that the fiber anatomy across the PCL leads to differences in strain measurement among four geographically distinct areas of the ligament.

Previous work at the University of Vermont has focused on the measurement of ACL displacement in vitro by use of the Hall-effect strain transducer and, more recently, a DVRT, which allow calculation of strain.[81,85,97,98] This technique has been applied to the measurement of ACL strain in vivo.[57,58,80,97,99-101]

Ligament Biomechanics

The primary functions of the knee ligaments are to stabilize the knee, control normal kinematics, and prevent abnormal displacements and rotations that may damage articular surfaces. Ligaments are the most important static stabilizers and are primarily composed of type I collagen, the constituent that provides resistance to a tensile load developed along the length of the ligament; collagen fibers and their orientation within the tissue are responsible for the primary biomechanical behavior of these structures. The fibers of the large distinct ligaments are almost all arranged in parallel bundles, making them ideal for withstanding tensile loads, whereas capsular structures have a less consistent orientation, making them more compliant and not as strong in resisting axial loading. The fibers within ligaments do not act uniformly across a ligament during loading, however; using excursion filaments implanted in four distinct fiber regions of the PCL, Covey and associates[96] demonstrated the differential behavior of the fiber regions.

The ligament insertion sites are designed to reduce the chance of failure by distributing the stresses at the bone-ligament interface in a gradual fashion. This goal is accomplished by the passing of the collagen fibers from the ligament into the bone through four distinct zones: (1) ligament substance, (2) fibrocartilaginous matrix, (3) mineralized fibrocartilage, and (4) bone itself.[102] Despite the transitions, Noyes and colleagues[103] demonstrated that some strain concentration occurs near the ligamentous insertion sites. The knee ligaments can best control motion of the bones relative to each other if the motion takes place along the direction of the ligament fibers. For example, when the knee is loaded in valgus, the medial collateral ligament develops a tensile stress in combination with a compressive force across the lateral compartment of the knee, and a resistance to medial joint opening is provided. Acting alone, ligaments cannot restrain the relative rotation associated with applied torques because the ligament would simply rotate about its bony insertion sites. A second force, usually developed through cartilage-to-cartilage compression, is required. For example, as the knee is loaded with an internal torque, a transverse rotation causes the femoral condyles to ride up the tibial spines (Fig. 91-19). This combination creates a compressive force across the tibiofemoral contact regions and an oppositely directed tensile force along the cruciate and collateral ligaments. This example may help demonstrate the mechanism by which the ACL interacts with tibiofemoral articular compression to resist an applied internal rotation to the knee joint.

The ability of a ligament to resist applied tensile loading may best be described through examination of the load-elongation curve produced during tensile failure testing of an ACL (Fig. 91-20). As a tensile load is applied, the ligament elongates; the slope of the measured load-displacement

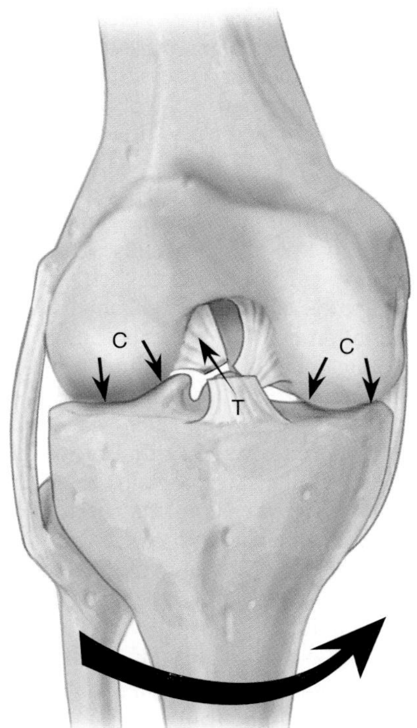

FIGURE 91-19 Internal rotation of the tibia relative to the femur. The internal rotation causes the femoral condyles to ride up on the tibial spine, producing tension in the cruciate ligaments and a compressive force across the articular surfaces. *C,* Compressive force produced between the tibiofemoral articular surfaces; *T,* Tensile load developed along the anterior cruciate ligament.

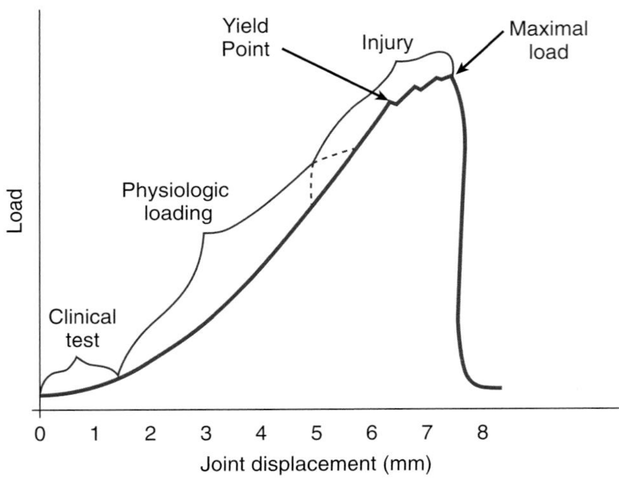

FIGURE 91-20 Load-elongation curve for the tensile failure of the anterior cruciate ligament. *(From Cabaud HB: Biomechanics of the anterior cruciate ligament.* Clin Orthop *172:26, 1988.)*

relationship represents the stiffness of the ligament. The steeper the slope of this curve, the stiffer the ligament. In the unloaded state, the ligament fibers are under minimal tension, and the collagen fibers have a wavy pattern. As a tensile load is applied, the wavy pattern begins to straighten. Initially, little load is required to elongate the ligament, which is characterized by the relatively flat "toe" region of the curve. The change from the toe to the linear portion of the curve represents the change in stiffness that an examiner perceives during a clinical laxity examination when a ligament's end point is reached. As the tensile load continues to increase, all the collagen fibers are straightened, and the curve becomes nearly linear. This region of the curve characterizes the elastic deformation of the ligament until the yield point is reached. At this point, there is a sudden loss in the ability of the ligament to transmit load because some fibers within the ligament fail. If loading continues, a maximal or ultimate failure load is reached, and a sudden drop in load is recorded when many or all fibers fail, representing total failure of the ligament. The area under the load-deformation curve represents the amount of energy absorbed by a ligament during failure testing. Noyes and associates demonstrated that the characteristics of the ACL's load-displacement curve are dramatically affected by variables such as age,[104] strain rate,[105] and duration of immobilization (disuse).[106] Young adults have a yield point that can be as much as three times greater than that of an older person.[104] In addition, Chandrashekar and coworkers[107] revealed sex-based differences in the material properties of the ACL. The female ACL withstood 8.3% lower strain at failure when evaluated in a tensile failure test, 14.3% lower stress, and 22.5% lower modulus of elasticity. Recent studies have revealed gender-based differences in joint laxity; Hsu and associates[108] found that the application of simultaneous tibial and valgus torque revealed 25% lower torsional joint stiffness in female knees as well as rotary joint laxity 30% higher than that for male knees.[108]

Most orthopaedic surgeons who operatively restore the function of the ACL perform an intraarticular reconstruction with autograft material.[109] Noyes and associates[103] characterized the relative strength of the various ligament replacement materials, demonstrating that a 14-mm wide bone–patella tendon–bone preparation was 168% as strong as the normal ACL, with the strength of all other autogenous replacements being less in comparison with the normal ACL. Woo and coworkers[110] have demonstrated that the normal tensile strength of the ACL may be as high as 2500 N rather than the original 1725 N standard presented by Noyes and associates.[103] This finding has led some surgeons to use combinations of autogenous graft material in an effort to increase the strength of the ACL replacement. Butler[111] used the primate model to demonstrate that maintaining a vascular supply to an ACL graft produces no material property differences in comparison with a similar free graft 1 year after implantation.

Papannagari and associates[112] demonstrated that bone–patellar tendon–bone autograft reconstruction does not restore normal knee kinematics under physiologic loading conditions. Three months after surgery, subjects displayed an additional 2.9-mm anterior translation of the tibia relative to the femur at full extension and 2.2-mm anterior translation at 15 degrees of flexion compared with the contralateral knee under weight-bearing conditions. Tashman and colleagues[113] developed a three-dimensional system to accurately assess dynamic joint motion, revealing abnormal kinematics in ACL-reconstructed knees during weight-bearing motion. A combination of radiographic targets inserted into bone to eliminate skin artifact for biplane imaging (radiographic stereophotogrammetric analysis) and subject-specific bone modeling revealed an additional 4-degree external rotation and 3-degree adduction in the tibiofemoral joint of the ACL-reconstructed knee compared with the contralateral normal limb during dynamic weight-bearing motion.[113]

Zantop and coworkers[114] assessed the role of the anteromedial bundle (AMB) and posterolateral bundle (PLB) of the ACL in tibial translation and rotary laxity. AMB transection significantly increased anterior tibial translation at 60 and 90 degrees, whereas isolated PLB transection resulted in increased tibial translation at 30 degrees of flexion in addition to increased combined internal-external rotation in response to internal-external rotary load. From these results, the investigators concluded that ACL reconstruction should include both bundles to restore normal translational and rotational kinematics. Mae and colleagues[115] examined the force sharing of anteromedial and posterolateral grafts in "anatomic" two-bundle reconstruction in response to 134-N anterior tibial loading. They observed that this reconstruction technique yielded grafts that shared force similarly to the two bundles of the normal ACL.[115]

Function of the Cruciate Ligaments in Controlling Joint Biomechanics

The concept of primary and secondary knee stabilizers was introduced by Butler and colleagues,[116] who demonstrated that the ACL is a primary restraint to anterior translation of the tibia relative to the femur, providing an average restraint of 87.2% to the applied load at 30 degrees. With the knee at 90 degrees, this restraint was 85.1%. After ACL transection, the remaining intact ligamentous structures provided little restraint to anterior subluxation, leading Butler to describe the function of the remaining soft tissues as secondary restraints to this particular motion. The remaining ligament and capsular structures each contributed less than 3% to the total restraining force resulting from an applied anterior shear load. Butler and colleagues[116] demonstrated that the PCL is the primary restraint to posterior translation of the tibia relative to the femur, providing 94% of the restraining force at 90 and 30 degrees of knee flexion. None of the remaining ligamentous and capsular secondary structures contributed more than 2% of the total restraining force to an applied posterior shear load. Markolf and colleagues[117] compared posterior tibial translation after isolated transection of the PLB of the PCL and found small increases in laxity after transection at 0 and 10 degrees of flexion. Sectioning of the PLB had no significant effect at higher flexion up to 90 degrees. Force measurements of the anterolateral bundle remained unchanged with posteromedial bundle sectioning, leading the authors to conclude that the anterolateral bundle was the primary restraint to posterior tibial translation.

Fukubayashi and associates[118] investigated the coupled behavior between anteroposterior shear loading and internal-external tibiofemoral rotation in human cadavers. They showed that interaction of the ACL with tibiofemoral geometry produces an internal tibial rotation with anterior-directed shear load applied across the tibiofemoral joint, whereas the PCL produces an external tibial rotation with applied posterior shear loading. The magnitude of tibial rotation, coupled with applied anteroposterior shear loading, decreased after transection of either cruciate ligament.

Gollehon and coworkers[119] investigated the role of the cruciate ligaments, LCL, and deep complex (arcuate ligament and popliteus tendon) in joint stability. This investigation showed that the PCL was the principal structure resisting posterior translation of the tibia relative to the femur. Isolated transection of the PCL did not affect varus or external rotation of the knee. Transection of the PCL, LCL, and deep complex was then performed to investigate the effects of a combined injury. This transection created a significant increase in varus rotation, posterior translation, and external rotation at all angles of knee flexion, suggesting that subjects with such a combined injury may have a functionally impaired joint. Combined sectioning of the ACL and the posterolateral structures produced a significant increase in internal-external rotation of the tibia, indicating that patients with this combined injury may also have compromised knee function.[119]

Similar methods were used by Markolf and coworkers, and their coupled-motion results are in agreement with those of Gollehon and colleagues. Markolf et al.[120] also measured force in the cruciate ligaments and found that the cruciate ligaments become load-bearing structures with the application of varus rotation after transection of the LCL and deep complex.[120] The same group measured force in the ACL and the PCL in the intact cadaveric knee under combined loading conditions.[75,121] They found that force in the ACL increases most in response to anterior directed forces applied to the tibia combined with internal tibial torque when the knee is near full extension. Force in the ACL was also increased when anterior tibial force was combined with a valgus moment at knee flexion angles greater than 10 degrees. The combination of posterior tibial force, varus moment, and internal torque produced the greatest forces in the PCL. In addition, they reported that the forces in the ACL were higher than the forces in the PCL in forced hyperflexion.[73,74,120] More recently, Withrow and coworkers[122] confirmed the results of Markolf and colleagues regarding the effect of valgus loading on the ACL. Peak strain in the anteromedial aspect of the ACL increased 30% with the addition of valgus loading in combination with impulsive compression loading, leading the authors to suggest that minimizing valgus loading, or abduction, during impulsive compression may reduce ACL strain.

Grood and associates[123] investigated the role of the PCL and posterolateral structures (LCL, arcuate ligament, and popliteus tendon) in the control of knee joint biomechanics. Isolated sectioning of the PCL revealed that the amount of posterior tibial translation, measured relative to the femur, was twice as much at 90 degrees compared with that at 30 degrees of knee flexion. This amount of translation occurred without abnormal axial tibial rotation and varus-valgus rotation. The concurrent increase in posterior laxity with flexion of the knee was attributed to slackening of the posterior portion of the joint capsule, which provides a secondary restraint to posterior translation. The authors concluded that clinical examination of the PCL should be performed at 90 degrees of flexion, because at this degree the secondary restraints are less effective in blocking posterior tibial translation.[123] At this knee angle the clinician can gain a full appreciation of the PCL contribution to joint laxity. Removal of the posterolateral complex while leaving the PCL intact produced an increase in both external tibial rotation and varus rotation. The increase in external rotation was greatest at 30 degrees of flexion, at which point it was two times larger compared with that measured at 90 degrees. This finding demonstrated that the posterolateral complex provides the primary restraint to external rotation with the knee at 30 degrees. Therefore the authors recommend clinical examination of the posterolateral complex with the external rotation examination while the knee is between 20 and 40 degrees of flexion.[123] A significant increase in external tibial rotation with the knee flexed to 90 degrees required transection of both the PCL and the posterolateral complex. This finding suggests that in a clinical examination demonstrating a significant increase in external tibial rotation with the knee at 90 degrees of flexion, deficiencies in both the PCL and posterolateral complex may exist.

Several investigators have measured ACL displacement patterns, enabling calculation of strain pattern, to understand the effect of knee joint position and muscle activity on ligament biomechanics.[68,81,84,87,93,95,124] Most of this work has been carried out in vitro, and the results are conflicting. The results of in vitro studies do not capture the effects of muscle activity or the effects of body weight, soft tissues, and secondary stabilizers in the knee.

In vivo studies have used magnetic resonance imaging and three-dimensional computer modeling techniques to observe morphologic changes in ligaments, such as elongation, rotation, and twist.[59,125] Li and coworkers[125] demonstrated the elongation and rotation that the ACL undergoes during weight-bearing flexion. The ACL length decreased by 10% at 90 degrees flexion compared with full extension. At 30 degrees of flexion, the ACL exhibited a 20-degree internal rotation. At lower flexion angles, the ACL oriented 60 degrees vertically and 10 degrees laterally, leading the authors to suggest that the ACL may have a greater role in weight-bearing activities at lower flexion angles. Li and associates[59] used the same technique to demonstrate the reciprocal behavior of the ACL and PCL in vivo during weight-bearing flexion. The AMB of the ACL displayed a relatively constant length from full extension to 90 degrees of flexion, whereas the PLB shortened. Both bundles of the PCL elongated during flexion, leading the authors to highlight the reciprocal behavior of the ACL and PCL under weight-bearing flexion, rather than that of the two bands of the ACL.[59]

Beynnon and Fleming and colleagues[57,58,97,99,126] have measured the in vivo strain biomechanics of the ACL in humans. This work involved arthroscopic implantation of the Hall-effect strain transducer or the DVRT into the AMB of the ACL after the routine surgical procedure was complete. These subjects had normal ACLs and consented to have their surgery performed with use of local anesthesia, allowing them full control of the lower limb musculature. The objective of these studies was to provide invaluable data for the clinical management of patients with ACL ruptures.

It was revealed that anterior shear loads of 150 N applied at 30 degrees of flexion (the Lachman test) produced more strain within the normal AMB than did shear testing at 90 degrees (the anterior drawer test).[58,126] It was possible to predict AMB strain from anterior tibial translation at 30 degrees of flexion but not at 90 degrees of flexion.[126] These in vivo results[58] are in agreement with previously published studies that used either instrumented knee laxity testing or clinical impressions to assess the behavior of the ACL under clinical examination conditions and to confirm that the Lachman test is the clinical examination of choice to evaluate the integrity of the ACL.[127-132]

The in vivo study revealed that no significant change in ACL strain occurred during isometric quadriceps contraction when the knee was maintained at a flexion angle of 90 degrees.[58] At this flexion angle, the ACL remained unstrained as quadriceps activity increased. Isometric quadriceps strengthening should therefore be safe in the ACL-injured or reconstructed knee if the flexion angle is maintained at 60 and 90 degrees. At 15 and 30 degrees of knee flexion, isometric quadriceps activity produces a large increase in AMB strain and should be carefully controlled, especially during the early stages of rehabilitation after reconstruction in which soft tissue fixation may be tenuous.[58,133] The in vivo ACL strain study[58] indicated that the knee flexion angle at which isometric quadriceps activity produced an increase in ACL strain and may become unsafe for the injured or reconstructed ACL was somewhere between 45 and 50 degrees. The model predictions presented by Nisell and coworkers[134] suggest that isometric quadriceps extension efforts at knee angles between 60 and 0 degrees may become unsafe for a newly reconstructed ACL, whereas this activity would be safe for a PCL reconstruction. Isometric quadriceps extension with the knee positioned between 60 degrees and full flexion may be unsafe for a PCL reconstruction, whereas this activity would be safe for an ACL reconstruction.

Fleming and coworkers[135] used in vivo strain measurement to demonstrate that the gastrocnemius muscle acts as an antagonist to the ACL. Gastrocnemius contraction produced greater strain on the ACL at 5 and 15 degrees of flexion than at 30 and 45 degrees. The authors proposed that development of rehabilitation programs should take into account knee flexor torque supported by the gastrocnemius when it is desirable to minimize strain on the healing ACL graft.[135]

In vivo strain measurement within the ACL when a seated subject performed an isotonic quadriceps contraction (active range of motion [AROM]) consistently revealed ACL strain between 10 and 48 degrees and an unstrained region between 48 and 110 degrees of flexion.[58] AROM rehabilitation programs may now be prescribed with these two flexion angle regions adapted to the clinician's requirements. In the unstrained region, quadriceps activity associated with AROM did not produce significantly different ACL strain values in comparison with the same knee motion without contraction of the leg musculature (flexion-extension motion of the subject's knee performed by an investigator and termed *passive range of motion* [PROM]).[58] This finding suggests that AROM between the limits of 50 and 100 degrees may be performed safely immediately after ACL reconstruction. The AROM activity may then move to flexion angles nearer full extension when the ACL graft and fixation will tolerate greater levels of strain.[58] The maximal AROM strain values were greater (ranging between 4.1% and 1.5%) than the maximal PROM strain values.[58] Application of a 10-lb boot to a subject's foot during the AROM activity increased the ACL strain values compared with the same activity without a weighted boot.

ACL strain was also evaluated during open and closed kinetic chain exercises and revealed no significant differences between the two exercises evaluated.[97] This finding suggests that the specific closed kinetic chain exercise evaluated (squatting with and without resistance) is not necessarily "safer" than the open kinetic chain exercise tested (active flexion-extension). The results conflict with the results of some cadaveric studies, which conclude that closed kinetic chain activities are safer for the ACL than open kinetic chain activities.[72,136] In a separate study, our group reported strains of the same magnitude (about 2.7%) during stair climbing.[100] In addition, we investigated strain in the ACL during steady-state cycling and found the mean peak strain to be half of that experienced during closed kinetic chain exercises (squatting) or open kinetic chain exercises (active flexion-extension).[101] The results imply that cycling may be a safe method of rehabilitating the knee musculature without damaging a healing ACL.

Fleming and coworkers[137] evaluated strain in the ACL during flexor-extensor exercises against resistance torque with and without a compressive load applied at the foot. Application of compressive load did not reduce the peak strain measurement of the ACL. However, ACL strain did not increase with an increase in resistance while the compressive load was applied.[134] The same group later demonstrated that one-legged closed kinetic chain exercises did not produce more strain on the ACL than two-legged exercises.[138] Peak ACL strain values at 30, 50, and 70 degrees of flexion were similar during four exercises: single-leg step-up and step-down, lunge, and one-legged sit-to-stand. The strain values were greatest at 30 degrees of flexion across all exercises. These results led the investigators to suggest that closed kinetic chain exercises can be used with increased resistance to rehabilitate muscles without placing additional strain on the healing ACL graft.[137,138]

Our findings illustrate that both muscle activity and knee position determine ACL strain at rest and with joint motion.[58] A ranked comparison of the different activities evaluated in subjects with normal ACLs, ordered from high to low risk on the basis of peak strain values, has been used to develop rehabilitation programs after ACL reconstruction.[139]

In vivo strain measurement within the ACL for PROM between 110 degrees and full extension revealed that the ACL is strained as the joint is brought into extension, and measurement remains at or below the zero strain level between the limits of 11.5 and 110 degrees of flexion when distal leg support loading is used.[58] Therefore continuous passive motion of the knee within these limits should be safe for the reconstructed ACL immediately after surgery when the leg is supported throughout flexion-extension motion without applied varus or valgus loading, internal or external torques, or anterior shear forces. However, the limits of near extension (0 to 10 degrees) can cause small magnitudes of strain (1% or less).[58] We believe this should not be viewed as a constraint to bracing a patient's knee in the fully extended position (0 degrees) or to the use of continuous passive motion during a rehabilitation program.

The cruciate ligaments serve several functions as passive stabilizers of the knee. The cruciate ligaments guide the knee joint through normal biomechanics, as demonstrated by the four-bar linkage model. The anterior and posterior cruciate ligaments are the primary restraints to corresponding anterior and posterior translation of the tibia relative to the femur and have a reciprocal relationship during weight-bearing flexion. The coupled internal and external tibial rotation that occurs with corresponding anterior and posterior shear loading is controlled in part by the cruciate ligaments and should be considered a significant aspect of the clinical examination. In addition, the cruciate ligaments act as secondary restraints to varus-valgus motion of the knee joint.

Medial and Lateral Collateral Ligaments and Their Function in Controlling Joint Biomechanics

Warren and associates[95] assessed the restraining action of the MCL complex in human cadaver specimens. They demonstrated that sectioning of the superficial long fibers of the MCL complex produced a significant increase in valgus rotation of the tibiofemoral joint in experiments performed at 0 and 45 degrees of knee flexion. Sectioning the posterior oblique or deep medial portions of the MCL complex had no significant effect on increasing valgus knee angulation.

Grood and colleagues[140] also investigated the medial ligament complex and presented results that support the findings of the Warren group.[95] More recently, Ellis and associates[141] demonstrated in cadaveric knees that ACL deficiency led to an increase in MCL insertion site and contact forces during anterior tibial loading and had no effect during valgus loading, indicating that the ACL does not play a role in valgus restraint. These results led the investigators to suggest that increased valgus laxity during clinical examination of an ACL-deficient knee would indicate MCL compromise.[141]

Grood and coworkers[140] demonstrated that the long superficial portion of the MCL complex provided 57% of the valgus restraint at 5 degrees, which increased to 78% at 25 degrees of flexion. The variable restraint behavior with valgus loading was attributed to the restraint provided by the posterior medial capsule, which decreased as the knee was moved from an extended into a flexed position. Haimes et al.[142] studied intact and MCL-deficient cadaveric knees and found that a coupled external rotation is associated with abduction in an MCL-deficient knee at extension, 15 degrees of flexion, and 30 degrees of flexion. In contrast, the intact knees studied had a coupled internal rotation associated with abduction. This finding—that is, the presence of a coupled external rotation as opposed to a coupled internal rotation—may be used in physical examination for diagnosis of isolated MCL injuries.

Grood and coworkers[140] investigated the LCL complex. They demonstrated that in response to varus stress, this complex limits lateral opening of the joint. In response to varus loading, the LCL was found to provide 55% of the total restraint at 5 degrees and 69% at 25 degrees of knee flexion. An increase in the contribution of the LCL to the total varus restraint resulted as the knee was brought from an extended to a flexed position. This change was attributed to a decrease in resistive support provided by the posterior portion of the lateral capsule as the knee was flexed. With the knee joint in full extension, the investigators demonstrated that the secondary restraints (including the cruciate ligaments and the posterior portion of the joint capsule) block opening of the knee joint after the collateral ligaments have been cut.[143] Simulating the forces applied by the dynamic stabilizers (the iliotibial tract and biceps muscles) revealed their important contribution to varus stability of the knee in vivo.[140] The contribution of the dynamic stabilizers to overall laxity of the knee is difficult to assess because the actual muscle force magnitudes for a specific activity are unknown. In a later investigation, Gollehon and associates[119] studied the contribution of the LCL and deep ligament complex (popliteus tendon and arcuate ligament) to joint laxity. They demonstrated that the LCL and deep ligament complex function together as the principal structures resisting varus and external rotation of the tibia.[119] Höher and colleagues[144] conducted a cadaver study and concluded that the LCL and popliteus carry most of the force in PCL-deficient knees under a posterior load at high flexion angles. Further, they loaded the popliteus in tension to simulate muscle activation and found that the force in the popliteus complex was significantly greater than the force in the LCL at all flexion angles tested (0 to 90 degrees) in both intact cadaveric knees and PCL-deficient knees.

Meniscal Biomechanics

Function of the Meniscus in Load Transmission

Meniscal injury is thought to be the most common injury sustained by athletes.[145] The menisci were originally thought to be vestigial structures that served no significant function for the tibiofemoral joint.[146] The meniscus was thought to be an expendable structure; this perspective prompted many orthopaedists to treat meniscal tears by completely removing the meniscus.[147-151] As recently as 1971, Smillie[151] recommended complete removal of the meniscus even if the posterior horn was the only structure suspected of being damaged at the time of anterior arthrotomy. Conversely, as early as 1948, Fairbank[152] had suggested the load-transmission function of the meniscus and postulated that a complete meniscectomy frequently resulted in tibiofemoral joint space narrowing, flattening of the femoral condyles, and osteophyte formation. In long-term follow-up studies performed in the late 1960s and 1970s, several investigators confirmed Fairbank's observations, reporting a high incidence of unsatisfactory results after a complete meniscectomy was performed.[153-155] It was not until the mid-1970s that several biomechanical studies confirmed the clinical observations by measuring the load-transmission function of the meniscus.[143,156-163] These investigations predicted that between 30% and 99% of the load transmitted across the tibiofemoral joint passes through the menisci during weight-bearing activities.

Maquet and colleagues[158] used a contrast injection radiography technique to measure contact area in human cadaver specimens subjected to a physiologic compressive load. This study revealed a posterior translation of the medial and lateral contact areas as the knee was brought from an extended to a flexed position along with a decrease in contact surface area with knee flexion. The contact area also decreased significantly with meniscectomy, leading Maquet and colleagues to postulate that the menisci transmitted a significant proportion of tibiofemoral compressive load.

Seedhom and Hargreaves[159,160] reported that 70% to 99% of the tibiofemoral compressive load is transmitted through the normal menisci and that all of the load is transmitted through the posterior horns of the menisci with joint flexion past 75 degrees. These investigators also revealed that partial removal of the meniscus decreased the compressive stress transmission of the joint to a lesser extent compared with removal of the entire structure, provided that the circumferential continuity of the meniscus was maintained. More recently, Zielinska and Donahue[164] used a three-dimensional finite element model to quantify changes in contact pressure in response to varying degrees of medial meniscectomy. The maximal contact pressure and contact area were linearly correlated with the proportion of the meniscus removed. The investigators revealed that removal of 60% of the medial meniscus increases the contact pressure on the remaining meniscus by 65% and by 55% on the medial tibial plateau.[164]

Krause and coworkers[157] reported an increase in stress across the knee joint of about three times in the canine model and two and one-half times in human cadaver knees after removal of both menisci. The investigators also measured the circumferential displacement of the medial meniscus with an applied axial compressive load, demonstrating the presence of "hoop," or tangential stress, acting at the outside fibers of the meniscus. This observation led Johnson and Pope[165] to demonstrate how the meniscus absorbs energy by undergoing circumferential elongation as a load is developed across the knee joint. As the joint compresses, fibers elongate. Thus the meniscus absorbs energy and reduces the impulsive shock loading that would otherwise be developed across the articular cartilage and subchondral bone.

Ahmed and Burke[166] directly measured the tibiofemoral pressure distribution using a microindentation transducer. They demonstrated that the medial and lateral menisci transmit at least 50% of the compressive load imposed on the tibiofemoral joint in the flexion range between 0 and 90 degrees. Removal of the medial meniscus caused a reduction in the contact area that ranged between 50% and 70%, with the latter reduction occurring at greater axial load. Because articular contact stress is inversely proportional to contact area, a 50% decrease in the contact area would cause a twofold increase in contact stress.

Allen and colleagues[167] determined the resultant load acting on the meniscus in human cadaver knees using an instrumented testing system. They found that the application of a 134-N anterior tibial load on an ACL-deficient knee significantly increases the resultant force acting on the medial meniscus compared with an intact knee at all flexion angles tested (0, 15, 30, 60, and 90 degrees). On the basis of the results, they suggest that ACL reconstruction contributes to the goal of preserving meniscal integrity.

These biomechanical investigations provide a basis for the concept of partial meniscectomy, which has been made possible with the technology provided by modern arthroscopic surgery. There can be no doubt that partial meniscectomy provides better results compared with total excision of that structure.[168]

Function of the Meniscus in Joint Stability

The menisci have been shown to provide increased geometric conformity to the tibiofemoral joint (thereby optimizing contact stress) and to share efficiently in the transmission of the tibiofemoral compressive load. Johnson and associates[154] and Tapper and Hoover[155] have performed postoperative clinical examinations in patients undergoing meniscectomy. Both studies revealed an increased varus-valgus and anteroposterior laxity in 10% to 25% of these patients, leading the investigators to conclude that the menisci provide some ability to stabilize the knee joint in connection with knee ligaments and bony geometry. The clinical follow-up study presented by the authors suggested a relationship between an increase in joint laxity after complete meniscectomy and sequelae of marginal spur formation and even degenerative changes.[154]

Bylski-Austrow and coworkers[169] subjected human cadaver knees to physiologic loads at three flexion angles and measured displacements of the menisci radiographically. The tibias were either loaded in the anteroposterior direction with 100 to 150 N or torqued to 10 to 15 Nm. In all cases, a 1000-N compressive load was applied to the tibiofemoral joint. Internal rotation caused the lateral meniscus to move 3 to 7 mm farther posteriorly than the medial meniscus moved anteriorly. Similarly, external rotation caused the medial meniscus to move posteriorly and the lateral meniscus to move a greater distance anteriorly. In all cases, the menisci "stayed with the femur" as the tibia was moved. The authors suggest that increased or decreased meniscal displacement, caused by ligament injury, meniscal repair, or meniscal replacement, might increase the risk for meniscal injury.

Shefelbine and associates[170] performed an in vivo study of human knees using magnetic resonance imaging to demonstrate that meniscal translation was not affected by ACL deficiency, but bone kinematics were altered. With a 125-N compressive load applied at the foot, the femur in ACL-deficient knees translated, on average, 4.3 mm further anteriorly from 0 to 45 degrees flexion than observed in the healthy knees. At full extension, the contact area centroid was shifted posteriorly relative to the tibia in the ACL-deficient knee. Translation of the medial meniscus did not differ between ACL-deficient and normal knees, leading the authors to suggest that altered bone kinematics subsequent to ACL injury, coupled with lack of compensation in meniscal translation, may increase the risk for secondary meniscal injury. Von Eisenhart-Rothe and colleagues[171] revealed similar findings: magnetic resonance imaging revealed posterior translation of the medial femoral condyle relative to the tibia in

ACL-deficient knees during isometric contraction of flexor and extensor muscles. Meniscal translation was the same across healthy and ACL-deficient knees.

Allen and colleagues[167] conducted a study to measure anteroposterior translation in intact cadaveric knees, ACL-deficient knees, and ACL-deficient knees that underwent a medial meniscectomy. Their findings agreed with those of Hsieh and Walker[172]: the anteroposterior laxity of the intact knee was significantly different from the anteroposterior laxity of both groups of ACL-deficient knees. Further, they found that the coupled internal rotation associated with the anterior tibial load was less for both groups of ACL-deficient knees than for the intact knees. In both loading scenarios, the ACL-deficient knee that underwent a meniscectomy was the most lax, followed by the ACL-deficient knee, indicating that both the ACL and the meniscus are important in preventing anteroposterior laxity in the knee.

Beynnon and associates[173] conducted in vivo testing to assess tibial movement relative to the femur during transition from non–weight-bearing to weight-bearing subsequent to ACL injury. Knees with ACL insufficiency demonstrated an average anterior tibial translation of 3.4 mm compared with 0.8 mm observed in the healthy, contralateral knee. The authors hypothesized that further translation is prevented by the posterior horn of the medial meniscus, which would experience greater strain during transition to weight-bearing after ACL injury.[173]

Hollis and colleagues[174] conducted testing similar to that performed by Allen and coworkers[167] in nine human cadaver knees. They loaded the tibia from 0 to 38 N in the anteroposterior direction while applying a 200-N axial force along the axis of the tibia and measured meniscal strains in cadaveric knees with intact ACLs, sectioned ACLs, and reconstructed ACLs. Their results showed that meniscal strains increase after the ACL has been sectioned. After ACL reconstruction, however, the meniscal strains return to levels observed in the ACL-intact state, suggesting that ACL reconstruction reduces the likelihood of meniscal damage. Conversely, Pearsall and Hollis[175] evaluated lateral and medial meniscal strain using DVRT strain gauges in eight cadaveric knees with intact PCLs, sectioned PCLs, and reconstructed PCLs. Strain in both menisci increased at 60 and 90 degrees of flexion in knees with sectioned PCLs. Similar to the results of Hollis and associates,[174] PCL reconstruction reduced meniscal strain to PCL-intact levels.[175]

Markolf and colleagues[74] evaluated the effect of meniscectomy on anteroposterior, varus-valgus, and rotary knee laxity in human cadavers with an instrumented laxity-testing device. They observed that bicompartmental removal of the menisci increased anteroposterior joint laxity between 45 and 90 degrees of knee flexion, whereas only a minor increase in laxity occurred in the rotary and varus-valgus planes. In a later study, these researchers demonstrated that although bicompartmental meniscectomy made the unloaded knee looser, in the knees with a developed tibiofemoral compressive load, laxity measurements were little affected.[136] Bargar et al.[69] used the instrumented laxity-testing device to evaluate anteroposterior load-displacement and varus-valgus torque-rotation responses of a subject's knee joint in vivo. They demonstrated that medial meniscectomy alone does not create a measurable increase in varus-valgus laxity, whereas a trend of increased anteroposterior laxity was observed. A significant increase in anteroposterior laxity was observed in subjects with a combined medial meniscectomy and torn ACL.[69]

Levy and associates[176] used human cadavers to investigate the effects of isolated medial meniscectomy and to study the effects of medial meniscectomy in the ACL-deficient knee. They demonstrated that an isolated medial meniscectomy did not produce a significant change in the anteroposterior load-displacement response of the knee. This finding is corroborated by the previous works presented by Hsieh and Walker[172] and Bargar and associates.[69] In the ACL-deficient knee without a compressive joint load, Levy and coworkers[176] demonstrated that resection of the meniscus caused a significant increase in the anterior displacement of the tibia relative to the femur at 30, 60, and 90 degrees of knee flexion. This observation led these researchers to suggest that in the ACL-deficient knee, the posterior horn of the meniscus acts as a wedge between the tibiofemoral articular surfaces, resisting anterior excursion of the tibia relative to the femur. In a later study, this observation was confirmed by Sullivan and colleagues.[177] In this work, the medial ligament structures in an ACL-deficient knee with an intact meniscus were sectioned, revealing an increase in anterior tibial displacement relative to the femur in comparison with the knee in which only the ACL was cut. In the ACL-deficient knee with an intact medial ligament complex, the mechanism of anterior tibial restraint was demonstrated to be the wedging apart of tibiofemoral articular surfaces by the meniscus—a distraction resisted by the intact medial ligament complex and capsular structures—and the development of a tibiofemoral compressive load.[177] The authors hypothesized that this may be one of the mechanisms that produces posterior horn tears of the menisci in an ACL-deficient knee.[177]

Tienen and coworkers[178] demonstrated the relative immobility of the posterior horn of the medial meniscus with use of cadaveric knees. In the absence of tibial torque, the anterior horn moved further posteriorly and laterally than did the posterior horn during flexion. Application of external torque revealed constrained posterior horn displacement during the first 30 degrees of flexion. Watanabe and associates[179] demonstrated that anterior tibial translation increases after two-thirds and complete resection of the posterior horn of the medial meniscus. Additionally, applied varus torque increased external tibial rotation by 2.2 and 6.7 degrees after two-thirds and complete resection of the posterior horn, respectively.[179]

In a later study, Levy and coworkers[180] investigated the effect of lateral meniscectomy on the motion of the human knee joint without compressive joint loading. They determined that isolated lateral meniscectomy did not produce a significant change in the anteroposterior load-displacement behavior of the knee. In addition, these investigators revealed that the lateral meniscus does not act as a restraint to anterior translation of the tibia relative to the femur, leading the researchers to suggest that this structure may not behave like the medial meniscus in providing an effective posterior wedge to anterior translation.[180] It is important that the results of these investigations of the meniscus be applied to events that occur without a compressive joint load, such as the swing phase of gait, and not to activities that include compressive joint loading.

The menisci have also been thought to assist with joint lubrication, provide resistance to extreme joint flexion or extension, and aid in the damping of impulsive loads transmitted across the tibiofemoral joint. These functions are difficult to characterize biomechanically or to describe with clinical impressions.

Patellofemoral Joint Biomechanics

A study of patellofemoral joint biomechanics is necessary to understand the pathologic processes, develop rational treatment regimens, and understand the effects that various rehabilitation programs have on this joint. For example, an abnormally high compressive patellofemoral joint reaction (PFJR) force produces abnormally high stress across the articular cartilage and is thought to be one of the initiating factors of alterations in articular cartilage metabolism, chondromalacia, and subsequent osteoarthritis.[181-184] In addition, morphometric abnormalities in the trochlear groove or the dorsal articular surface of the patella in combination with high lateral forces at the patellofemoral articulation have been thought to cause lateral subluxation or dislocation of the patella.[184-187]

Patellofemoral Contact Area

In the normal knee, the patellofemoral contact area is optimally designed to respond to the increase in PFJR load developed with knee flexion through a corresponding increase in contact area. This mechanism helps distribute the contact force while minimizing patellofemoral contact stress.

Goodfellow and colleagues[188] used the dye method to measure patellofemoral contact area in human cadaver knees subjected to simulated weight-bearing conditions. Area measurements were made at 20, 45, 90, and 135 degrees of knee flexion and are presented in Figure 91-21. Movement of the knee from full extension to 90 degrees revealed that the contact area on the dorsal aspect of the patella moves in a continuous zone from the inferior to the superior pole of the patella. Continued flexion of the knee to 135 degrees developed two separate contact regions, one on the “odd medial facet” and the other on the lateral aspect of the patella (see Fig. 91-21). Singerman and colleagues[189,190] calculated the center of pressure from a 6-degrees-of-freedom patellar transducer in human cadaver knees and reported that the center of pressure translates superiorly and medially as the knee is flexed to 90 degrees. At flexion angles greater than 85 degrees, the results were somewhat variable, but the center of pressure always moved inferiorly with extension.[189] Huberti and Hayes[191] used pressure-sensitive film to measure the increase of patellofemoral contact area that occurs concurrently with knee flexion (Fig. 91-22). At a flexion angle of 10 degrees, contact between the dorsal surface of the patella and the trochlea is initiated. The length of the patellar tendon controls when patellar-trochlear contact occurs. In patients in whom the patellar tendon is too long, patella alta may be present, and flexion of the knee greater than 10 degrees may be required to seat the patella adequately in the trochlear groove. Von Eisenhart-Rothe and colleagues[192] used an open magnetic resonance system coupled with three-dimensional image postprocessing to evaluate kinematics and contact areas in the knee compartment in vivo. Patella tilt decreases during flexion from 30 to 90 degrees, coupled with an increase in lateral patellar shift. The femur rotates externally and translates posteriorly relative to the tibia in the same flexion range. These movements result in a significant increase in contact area.[192]

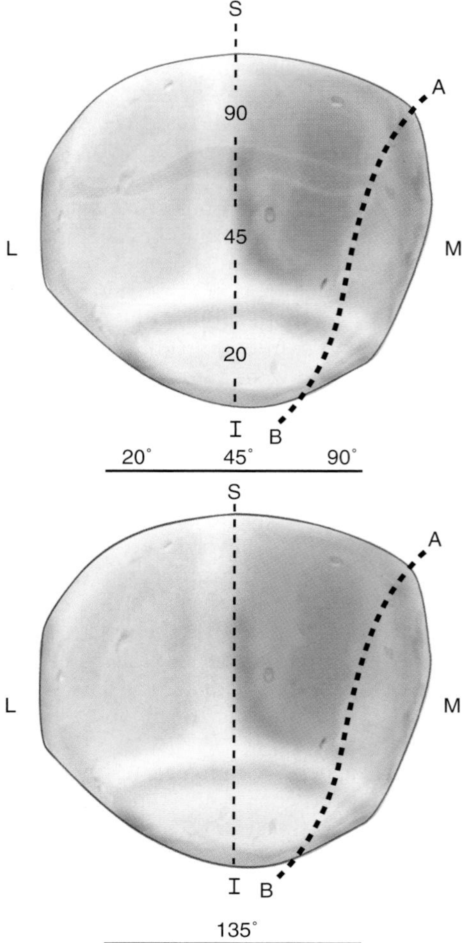

FIGURE 91-21 Patellofemoral contact regions at different knee flexion angles. *I,* Inferior; *L,* lateral; *M,* medial; *S,* superior. *(From Goodfellow J, Hungerford DS, Zindel M: Patellofemoral joint mechanics and pathology.* J Bone Joint Surg Br *58:287–290, 1976.)*

With knee movement between extension and 90 degrees, the patella was found to be the only component of the extensor mechanism that contacts the femur, holding the quadriceps tendon away from the femur. With knee motion between 90 and 135 degrees, the quadriceps tendon contacts the femur.[193] Once the quadriceps tendon contacts the femur, the compressive PFJR force is divided between contact of the broad band of the quadriceps tendon with the femur and patellofemoral contact.

The interaction between the patellofemoral contact area and PFJR force can be demonstrated with the squatting activity. During this activity, as knee flexion increases, the PFJR force initially increases, whereas the patellofemoral contact area available for distributing the contact force also increases, effectively distributing the articular contact stress. Besier and colleagues[194] demonstrated that patellofemoral contact area increased on average by 24% during weight-bearing knee flexion in both female and male subjects. The opposite situation may occur with knee extension during weight-training programs that apply a weight to the distal aspect of the tibia with the athlete in a seated position. For this activity, the patellofemoral contact area decreases as the PFJR force

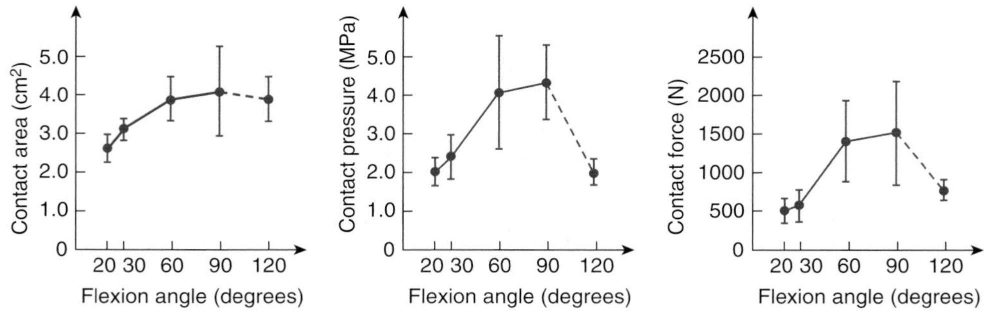

FIGURE 91-22 Experimental measurement of patellofemoral contact made in human cadaver specimens for the squatting activity with a normal Q angle. Values between 90 and 120 degrees have been extrapolated. *Left,* Contact area; *middle,* contact pressure; *right,* contact force. *(From Huberti HH, Hayes WC: Patellofemoral contact pressures: the influence of Q-angle and tibiofemoral contact.* J Bone Joint Surg Am *66A:715–724, 1984.)*

increases; therefore the PFJR stress may become high even if light weights are applied to the distal aspect of the tibia. This example may help explain why isotonic or isokinetic exercises through a full range of motion are not advised in the treatment of patellofemoral pain syndromes. Quadriceps exercises extending the knee only through the last 15 to 20 degrees of extension are more likely to be tolerated, as demonstrated by the decrease in PFJR force in Figure 91-22.

Patellofemoral Force Transmission

The patella transmits force from the quadriceps muscle group to the patellar tendon while developing a large PFJR force. This mechanism serves to stabilize the knee against gravity when the joint is in a flexed position and assists in the forward propulsion of the body as the knee is extended during gait. Therefore the loads developed along the patellar tendon and the PFJR force are a function of both quadriceps force and knee flexion angle. A sagittal plane analysis can be used to demonstrate this concept. This analysis applies statics to describe the forces and moments required to maintain the knee joint in equilibrium. For example, with use of this technique, the quadriceps force (F_{Quads}), the PFJR force, and the patellar tendon force (F_{PT}) may be related at chosen knee flexion angles. Figure 91-23 is a simplified sagittal plane static representation of the relation between the PFJR and the quadriceps muscle forces. The mass of the upper body (W), assumed to act at the hip joint, is supported by the F_{Quads} developed by the quadriceps muscle groups. The vertical line below the center of mass at the subject's hip joint represents the force vector due to upper body weight, which falls well behind the flexion axis of the knee. The distance from the center of mass force vector to the flexion axis of the knee is defined as the moment arm (c). The moment arm is relatively small with the knee near extension. Therefore the support mechanism provided by the F_{Quads} and the developed PFJR are relatively small. In the right portion of Figure 91-23, the knee is in a position of greater flexion with an associated increase in the moment arm (c′). To maintain the knee in static equilibrium, the new force (F_{Quads}) generated by the quadriceps must increase significantly. As a result of the increased quadriceps force, the PFJR must also be larger. This model may help explain the mechanism by which both PFJR and F_{Quads} increase during squatting activities.

In the earlier force analysis studies, the patella-trochlea articulation was represented as a frictionless pulley.[181,185,195-201]

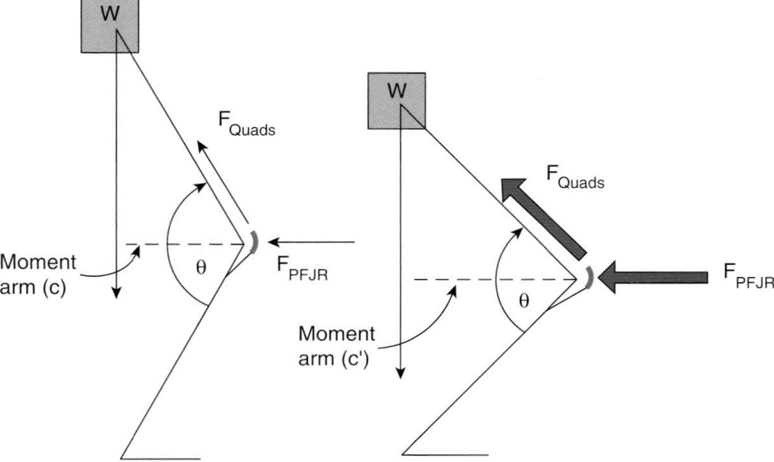

FIGURE 91-23 Static model of the patellofemoral joint reaction force (F_{PFJR}) at two positions of knee flexion. With the knee in the flexed position (*right*), the values of F_{Quads} and F_{PFJR} are large, supporting the weight (*W*) of the upper body acting through a large moment arm (*c′*). The F_{Quads} and F_{PFJR} values are much less with the knee in a more extended position (*left*), in which the moment arm (*c*) is smaller.

This assumption was justified on the basis of the low coefficient of friction between the patellofemoral articular surfaces. With this approach, the forces developed by the quadriceps muscle group were assumed to be equal to the force developed along the patellar tendon throughout the full range of knee motion, with the direction of the PFJR force defined as the bisector of the angle between the quadriceps and the patellar tendon force vectors. Using the mechanics principle of static equilibrium, and with the assumption that the patella-trochlea articulation behaves like a frictionless pulley, Reilly and Martens[200] predicted a compressive PFJR force of 0.5 times body weight for level walking. For ascending and descending stairs, the PFJR was estimated to reach 3.3 times body weight.[200] Analysis of the squatting activity revealed that a maximal PFJR of 2.9 times body weight occurred at 90 degrees of flexion.[200] Active extension of the lower leg with a 9-kg boot while the femur was orientated in a horizontal position produced a peak PFJR at 36 degrees of flexion.[200] Maquet[202,203] questioned the frictionless pulley assumption and demonstrated with a lateral vector diagram of the patellofemoral articulation that the forces in the quadriceps mechanism and patellar tendon can differ and can also vary as a function of knee flexion angle. Several investigators have confirmed Maquet's findings.[204-209]

In later work performed by Huberti,[204] Van Eijden,[209] Buff,[207] Ahmed,[205] Singerman,[189] and their coworkers, the combined tibia, femur, and patella were evaluated with use of both experimental and theoretical techniques. Because the force values F_{PT} and F_{Quads} are unequal, these researchers have chosen to report results by calculating the ratio between the two force values (F_{PT}/F_{Quads}) at selected knee flexion angles. Huberti's group simulated the squatting activity in human cadaver specimens while measuring F_{Quads} with a tensile load cell and the F_{PT} with a buckle transducer.[204] They demonstrated that for knee flexion between 0 and 45 degrees, the F_{PT} developed was greater than F_{Quads} (Fig. 91-24). With continued knee flexion to 120 degrees, the F_{PT} was consistently less in comparison with F_{Quads}. The authors suggested that not only does the patella function as a pulley that changes the magnitude and direction of forces in the quadriceps and patellar tendon, but the patella also has two distinct mechanical functions.[204] In the first and more classically described function, the anteroposterior thickness of the patella can be attributed to increasing the effective moment arm of the quadriceps muscles and patellar ligament, whereas in the second function, the patella acts as a lever (Fig. 91-25). Therefore the parameters that define the proximal and distal lever arms of the patella have a direct effect on the balance of forces in the quadriceps and patellar tendon. The researchers reasoned that the parameters were the length of the patella, the location of the patellofemoral contact area, and the angle between the quadriceps tendon and patellar tendon.[204] In a parallel experimental investigation of the squatting activity, Huberti and Hayes[191] estimated that the compressive PFJR force reached a maximal value of 6.5 times body weight. With knee flexion to 120 degrees, tendofemoral contact supported one third of the compressive PFJR force.[188]

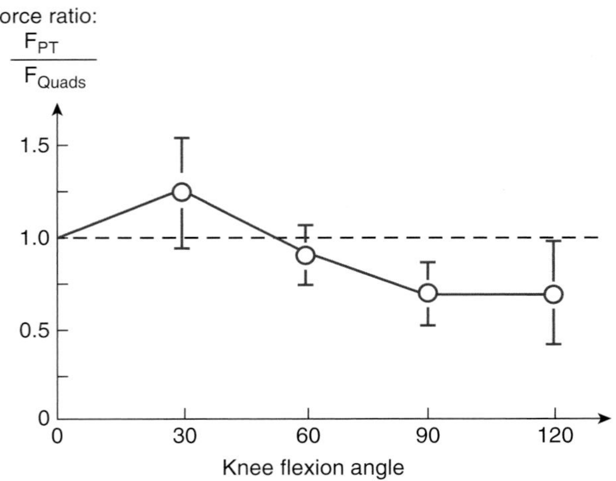

FIGURE 91-24 The predicted force ratio F_{PT}/F_{Quads} for the knee positioned between 0 and 120 degrees of flexion. Between 0 degrees and 45 degrees, the force developed in the patellar tendon is greater than that developed by the quadriceps musculature, whereas from 45 to 120 degrees, the patellar tendon force is less. *(From Huberti HH, Hayes WC, Stone JL, et al: Force ratios in the quadriceps and the ligamentous patellae.* J Orthop Res *2:49, 1984.)*

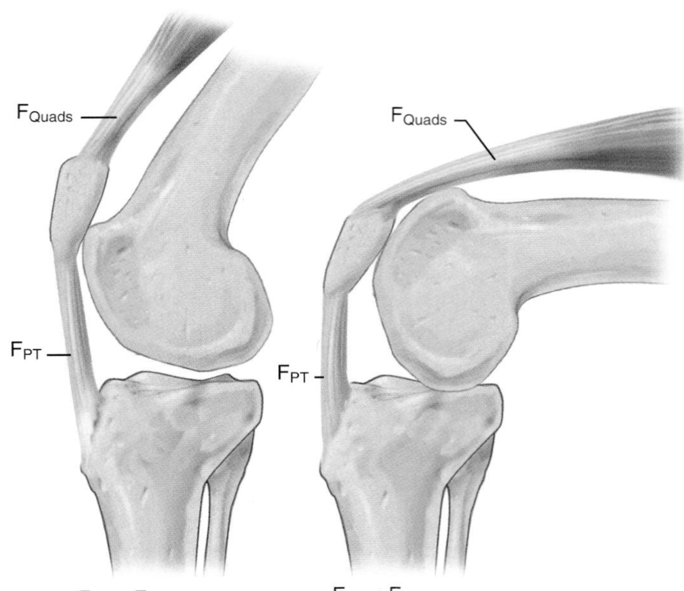

FIGURE 91-25 The mechanical function of the patella as a lever and as a spacer to increase the patellar tendon moment arm. *Left,* With the knee near the extended position, the levering action of the patellar mechanism produces greater force values in the patellar tendon (F_{PT}) in comparison with those developed by quadriceps contraction (F_{Quads}). *Right,* With the knee in the flexed position, the levering action of the patella is decreased, and the force values developed in the patellar tendon are less than those developed by the quadriceps. *(From Huberti HH, Hayes WC, Stone JL, et al: Force ratios in the quadriceps tendon and ligamentous patellae.* J Orthop Res *2:49, 1984.)*

Van Eijden and associates[209] developed a mathematical model of the patellofemoral articulation and verified model predictions with experimental findings. Predictions of the F_{PT}/F_{Quads} ratio were similar to the experimental findings presented by Huberti,[204] Ahmed,[205] Buff,[207] and their coworkers. Van Eijden's group demonstrated that the PFJR is about 50% of the quadriceps force at full extension and increases to 100%

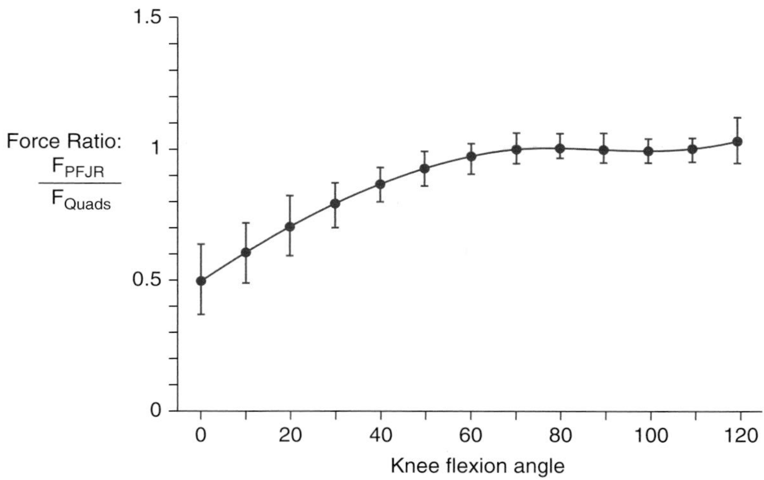

FIGURE 91-26 The predicted force ratio patellofemoral joint reaction force/quadriceps force (F_{PFJR}/F_{Quads}) for the knee positioned between 0 and 120 degrees of flexion. Between 0 and 70 degrees, F_{PFJR} is less than that developed by quadriceps contraction, whereas from 70 to 120 degrees, F_{PFJR} is equal to F_{Quads}. *(From van Eijden TM, Kouwenhoven E, Verburg J, et al: A mathematical model of the patellofemoral joint.* J Biomechan *19:219–288, 1986.)*

of the quadriceps force with the knee positioned between 70 and 120 degrees of flexion (Fig. 91-26).[209]

These studies have important implications for knee rehabilitation programs that are designed to minimize patellar tendon forces, as in patellar tendinitis. In these programs, application of the large isokinetic or isometric knee moments with the knee in positions between extension and 45 degrees should be avoided. In this flexion range, quadriceps activity actually produces forces of greater magnitude in the patellar tendon. This finding has been demonstrated by the work of Huberti and colleagues,[204] who showed that the F_{PT}/F_{Quads} ratio is greater than 1.0 for knee positions between extension and 45 degrees (see Fig. 91-24). It may be advisable to restrict rehabilitation programs for patellar tendinitis to flexion angles between 45 and 120 degrees, in which the F_{PT}/F_{Quads} ratio is less than 1.0. This constraint prevents an amplification of F_{PT}. This restriction would not apply to normal gait, in which the bending moments and therefore F_{Quads} are not high. Because of the changing relationship between developed F_{Quads} and resulting F_{PT} as the knee courses from extension through full flexion, the effectiveness of the quadriceps in developing an extension moment becomes substantially smaller at larger knee flexion angles, which also prevents the amplification of F_{PT}.

These studies also have important implications in the rehabilitation and surgical treatment of patellofemoral pain syndromes. Rehabilitation programs designed to minimize the PFJR but not the F_{Quads} should avoid large isokinetic, isotonic, or isometric moments with the knee positioned between 60 and 120 degrees of flexion. In this range, the predicted PFJR force is equal to the F_{Quads} (see Fig. 91-26).[209] With the requirement of minimizing the PFJR force, it may be advisable to restrict knee rehabilitation to range between the limits of extension, when the PFJR is about 50% of the F_{Quads}, and 40 degrees, when the PFJR is 90% of the F_{Quads}.[209] Maquet[183] has investigated the surgical treatment of patellofemoral pain, demonstrating that by increasing the extensor moment arm by a 2-cm elevation of the tibial tubercle, a 50% reduction in the PFJR force occurred when the knee is flexed to 45 degrees. Ferguson and associates[210] investigated the effect of anterior displacement of the tibial tubercle on patellofemoral contact stress. In this study, the patella-trochlea interfaces of human cadaver specimens were instrumented with miniature force sensors to monitor the patellofemoral contact stress. They revealed that anterior displacement of the tibial tubercle decreased the patellofemoral contact stress between 0 and 90 degrees of flexion.[210] The largest decrease in contact stress was achieved with a 12.5-mm elevation of the tubercle; further elevation produced only a minimal decrease in contact stress.[210] This finding demonstrates the importance of the anteroposterior position of the patellar tendon and its role in controlling the extensor moment arm. In addition, the proximal-distal location of the patellofemoral contact point is critical to the function of the patella as a lever (as explained earlier).

In the frontal plane, the axis of the F_{Quads} forms an angle with the patellar tendon. This angle has been defined as the Q angle and is measured as the intersection of the center line of the patellar tendon and the line from the center of the patella to the anterior superior iliac spine.[208] The normal Q angle is reported to range between 10 and 15 degrees with the knee in full extension.[212,213] With knee flexion, the Q angle decreases because a coupled internal rotation of the tibia occurs relative to the femur.[185] Contraction of the quadriceps creates a bowstring effect that displaces the patella in a lateral direction, producing a contact force against the lateral margin of the femoral trochlear groove. Abnormal tracking of the patella, which allows lateral subluxation of only a few millimeters, markedly decreases the contact area, greatly increasing the local stress (force per unit area) (Fig. 91-27).

This mechanism may contribute to patellofemoral pain and degeneration of the patellar articular cartilage (chondromalacia). Other anatomic conditions can also contribute to abnormal patellar tracking. These conditions include hypoplasia of the trochlear groove, abnormal patellar articular configuration, underdevelopment of the vastus medialis, transverse plane rotational malalignment of the proximal tibia relative to the distal femur, and an abnormally high Q angle. Huberti

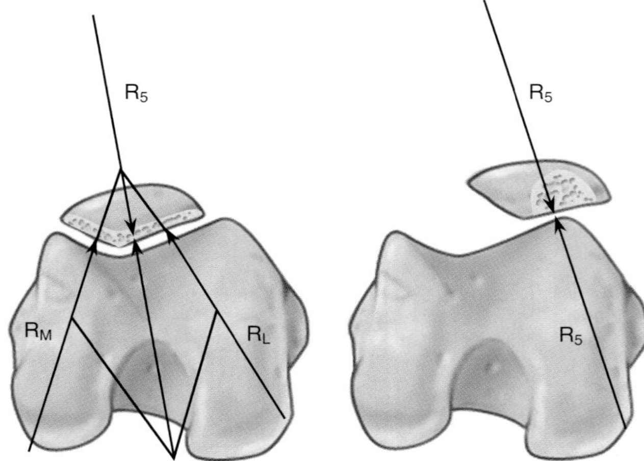

FIGURE 91-27 Patellofemoral joint reaction forces for the normal knee (*left*). The joint reaction force (R_5) is resisted by the lateral (R_L) and medial (R_M) components. In the knee with a lateralized patella (*right*), the joint reaction force is resisted by the lateral component only (R_5). *(From Maquet P: Mechanics and osteoarthritis of the patellofemoral joint.* Clin Orthop *144:70, 979.)*

and Hayes[191] studied the effect of different Q angles by simulating the squatting activity in human cadaver specimens while measuring patellofemoral contact pressure with pressure-sensitive film. They demonstrated that either an increase or a decrease in Q angle developed an increased peak patellofemoral pressure and the associated unpredictable patterns of cartilage loading. Cox[214] has presented a retrospective study of the Roux-Elmslie-Trillat procedure for realignment of the knee extensor mechanism and prevention of recurrent subluxation of the patella. An evaluation of 116 patients observed for at least 1 year demonstrated that this procedure is a satisfactory method for the prevention of lateral subluxation, with recurrence in only 7% of the cases. Careful attention to the medial transfer of the tibial tuberosity without a posterior displacement was emphasized as the key to successful long-term results.[214] Procedures resulting in some posterior transfer of the tibial tuberosity, such as that described by Hauser, decrease the patellar tendon moment arm and consequently increase the patellofemoral contact stress. Fulkerson and Hungerford[215] have reviewed the clinical and radiological outcomes of the Hauser procedure and have presented evidence of progressive knee joint degeneration.

For a complete list of references, go to expertconsult.com.

Suggested Readings

Citation: Farrow LD, Chen MR, Cooperman DR, et al: Morphology of the femoral intercondylar notch. *J Bone Joint Surg Am* 89A(10):2150–2155, 2007.

Level of Evidence: V

Summary: In this study the morphologic features of the femoral intercondylar notch are described. The posterolateral rim of the intercondylar notch is not well defined. Accurate placement of commercial femoral tunnel aiming guides may be difficult.

Citation: Warren LF, Marshall JL: The supporting structures and layers on the medial side of the knee: An anatomical analysis. *J Bone Joint Surg Am* 61A:56–62, 1979.

Level of Evidence: V

Summary: In this study the anatomic structures in the medial side of the knee are described. This study is one of the most important works describing the medial side of the knee. Only minor variations in the overall anatomic pattern are found.

Citation: LaPrade RF, Morgan PM, Wentorf FA, et al: The anatomy of the posterior aspect of the knee. An anatomic study. *J Bone Joint Surg Am* 89A:758–764, 2007.

Level of Evidence: V

Summary: In this study an anatomic detailed description of the posterior aspect of the knee is provided.

Citation: LaPrade RF, Engebretsen AH, Ly TV, et al: The anatomy of the medial part of the knee. *J Bone Joint Surg Am* 89A:2000–2010, 2007.

Level of Evidence: V

Summary: In this study an anatomic description of the medial aspect of the knee is provided.

Citation: Beynnon BD, Fleming BC: Anterior cruciate ligament strain in vivo: A review of previous work. *J Biomech* 31:519–525, 1998.

Level of Evidence: IV

Summary: The strain behavior of the anterior cruciate ligament (ACL) has been measured by arthroscopic implantation of the differential variable reluctance transducer while subjects are experiencing local anesthesia. Movement of the knee from a flexed to an extended position, either passively or through contraction of the leg muscles, produces an increase in ACL strain values. Isolated contraction of the dominant quadriceps with the knee between 50 degrees and extension creates substantial increases in strain. In contrast, isolated contraction of the hamstrings at any knee position does not increase ACL strain. With the knee unweighted, the protective strain shielding effect of a functional knee brace decreases as the magnitude of anterior shear load applied to the tibia increases. The approach used in this study is novel in that it can be used to measure an important portion of the ACL's strain distribution while clinically relevant loads are applied to the knee, subjects perform rehabilitation exercises, or in the presence of different orthoses such as functional knee braces.

Citation: Beynnon BD, Fleming BC, Labovitch R: Chronic anterior-cruciate ligament deficiency is associated with increased anterior translation of the tibia during the transition from non-weightbearing to weightbearing. *J Orthop Res* 20:332–337, 2002.

Level of Evidence: III

Summary: Translation of the tibia relative to the femur was measured while a group of subjects with normal knees and a group with anterior cruciate ligament (ACL) tears underwent transition from non–weight-bearing to weight-bearing stance. A fourfold increase in anterior translation of the tibia for the knees with ACL tears compared with the contralateral side is a concern because it is substantially greater than the 95% confidence limits of the side-to-side differences in anteroposterior knee laxity measured from subjects with normal knees. This observation could explain, at least in part, one of the mechanisms that initiates damage to the meniscus and articular cartilage in subjects who have sustained an ACL tear.

Citation: Beynnon BD, Johnson RJ, Naud S, et al: Accelerated versus nonaccelerated rehabilitation after anterior cruciate ligament reconstruction: A prospective, double-blind investigation evaluating knee joint laxity using roentgen stereophotogrammetric analysis. *Am J Sports Med* 39(12):2536–2548, 2011.

Level of Evidence: I

Summary: Rehabilitation with the accelerated and nonaccelerated programs administered in this study produced the same increase in the envelope of knee laxity. Most of the increase in the envelope of knee laxity occurred during healing when exercises were advanced and activity level increased. Patients in both programs had the same clinical assessment, functional performance, proprioception, and thigh muscle strength, which returned to normal levels after healing was complete. For participants in both treatment programs, the Knee Injury and Osteoarthritis Outcome Score assessment of quality of life did not return to preinjury levels.

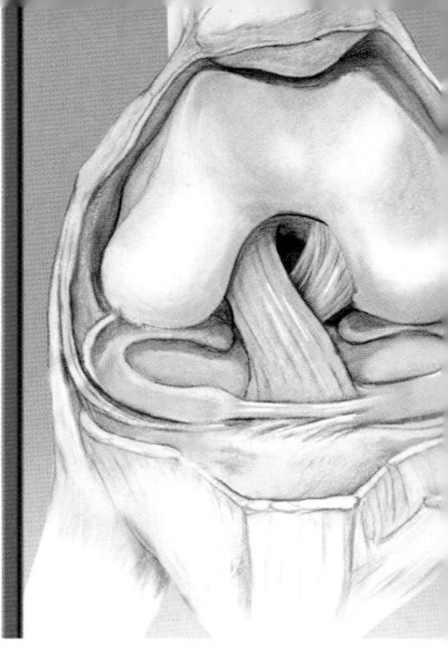

92

Knee Diagnosis and Decision Making

PETER N. CHALMERS • JAS CHAHAL • BERNARD R. BACH JR

For the experienced practitioner, the history and physical examination remains the most efficient, sensitive, specific, accurate, and cost-effective method of establishing a diagnosis in patients with knee-related complaints. Several investigators have demonstrated that the history and physical examination have equivalent sensitivity and specificity to magnetic resonance imaging (MRI) for a variety of intraarticular pathologies, with an overall accuracy of 93%.[1,2] When taking a systematic approach to patients with knee-related concerns, assessing each structure in question sequentially for possible injury is critical.[2] Developing an intuitive and comprehensive approach to the physical examination requires a detailed understanding of knee anatomy, in particular the relation of the surface skin to the underlying structures, to be able to relate tenderness to pathology. A complete description of the relevant anatomy is described in Chapter 91. In-depth knowledge of knee pathology can be helpful so that the history and examination can be dynamically tailored; pertinent clinical conditions are described in Chapters 95-108.

History

Eliciting the history starts with the chief or primary complaint that leads the patient to present for an evaluation. We endeavor to record this complaint in the patient's own words, because they provide the first clues regarding the patient's reason for the office visit. Asking an open-ended question such as, "What brings you to the office today?" is very helpful. Giving patients the opportunity to "tell their story" also allows them to develop a more significant and meaningful relationship with their physician.

Once the patient has completed his or her initial response, the surgeon can return to the beginning of the story as necessary to fill in gaps and collect more details. In particular, the examiner must determine the duration of the complaint and the date of onset. Important details often can be gathered from the patient's recollection of the inciting event or trauma, should one exist. If the injury occurred during an athletic endeavor, the examiner should obtain a full account of the event, including whether this incident was a contact or noncontact injury and if it occurred during practice or during a competition. These details may provide the first clues as to the underlying pathology. For instance, a valgus stress suggests an injury to the medial collateral ligament (MCL), whereas a high-energy trauma such as a motorcycle accident may suggest a knee dislocation or multiligamentous injury. In comparison, noncontact ACL injuries usually occur in the context of stopping quickly, cutting sharply, and landing and changing direction with the foot planted. The mechanism of ACL injury in skiers is different—when skiers injure the ACL, they are moving out of control with the knee bent or extended. The uphill arm is back, the body is off balance, the hips are lower than the knees, and the weight is placed on the inside edge of the downhill ski. This mechanism of injury has been referred to as the "phantom foot" mechanism.[3] Recollection of an auditory pop or a tearing sensation may be present. Up to 66% of patients with an ACL injury describe such a sensation.[4,5] Swelling immediately after the event may also occur. Indeed, a hemarthrosis develops in most persons with ACL injuries within 3 hours of the initial tear (Table 92-1).

If no specific event can be recalled, the patient should be asked if he or she has had a recent change in activity, which might suggest overuse. Commonly patients may have changed training techniques (e.g., increased frequency, increased distances, or a change in terrain or surfaces). A recent increase in running may suggest a stress fracture or patellofemoral syndrome. Acute changes from inactivity to activity may lead deconditioned patients to subject their knees to nonphysiologic kinetics as a result of loss of neuromuscular control.

The major symptoms on which to focus for a patient presenting with knee-related concerns include (1) pain, (2) instability, (3) mechanical symptoms, (4) stiffness, and (5) swelling. The patient should be asked about the continued presence of pain and any change in character or severity of the pain. Use of visual analog scales can be helpful. Pain ratings based on a 0 to 10 scale can be used. It is helpful to hear whether the pain is constant, is only related to activities, or occurs after activity. Pain related to stair climbing or prolonged sitting suggests a patellofemoral etiology, whereas pain with twisting or rotating activities (e.g., rolling over in bed or getting out of a car) is suggestive of meniscal pathology.

Subjective instability should be explored, with attention paid to determining the frequency and inciting events or activities surrounding each instability event. For example, patients with an ACL tear often state that they experience instability with pivoting, twisting, or cutting activities. They may also describe a sensation of movement with their knees that they often explain by placing two fists together and moving one with respect to the other in what has been called the *two-fist sign*. In contrast, instability that is experienced linearly, as in walking on level ground or on stairs, is often associated with quadriceps weakness and deconditioning.

TABLE 92-1

POTENTIAL ETIOLOGIES FOR A HEMARTHROSIS OF THE KNEE

Traumatic	Atraumatic
Anterior cruciate ligament tear	Pigmented villonodular synovitis
Posterior cruciate ligament injury	Hemangioma
Chondral fracture	Hemophilia
Patellar dislocation	Sickle cell anemia
Meniscal tear	Charcot arthropathy
Intraarticular fracture	Pharmacologic coagulopathy
Tear in the deep portion of the joint capsule	Thrombocytopenia

Side-to-side instability on level ground may suggest valgus or varus laxity, whereas instability when descending a ramp may also be experienced by patients with damage to the posterolateral corner (PLC).

The patient should be asked about any evaluation or treatment he or she received at the time of the injury or subsequent to the injury. It may also be helpful to know if weight-bearing restrictions were recommended. Knowledge of previous immobilization is also helpful, particularly if the patient has residual loss of range of motion. For any patient with a prior surgical intervention, the operative report and arthroscopy images can provide valuable information. Finally, the physician should ask which, if any, of these treatments have benefited the patient. These questions help guide the surgeon in creating a treatment plan that avoids replication of prior failed treatments.

Once the history surrounding the present complaint is fully understood, the physician should collect general medical, surgical, and social histories. For athletes, a more complete understanding of their athletic history should be sought, including their current and past level of play, the number of hours per week that they play, and their skill level, potential, and athletic goals. These factors all play a role in surgical decision making.[6] In particular, in the patient with an ACL tear who plans to return to category I hard cutting or pivoting sports such as basketball, football, rugby, volleyball, or mogul/black diamond skiing, the risk for reinjury with nonoperative treatment of an ACL tear is high.[6] The surgeon should also obtain an occupational history, because a patient who is reliant upon the injured extremity for his or her livelihood likely requires a more aggressive treatment regimen.

A review of systems should always be collected as well. A particular focus should be placed on pain and swelling in other joints, eye disease, back pain, pain with urination, and skin disorders, all of which may hint at a diagnosis of an inflammatory arthropathy. Similarly, a history of fevers, night sweats, or drainage may lead the physician to suspect infection. A history of atraumatic knee pain with an associated mass with primarily nocturnal or constant pain may lead the physician to a neoplastic diagnosis. Pain out of proportion, hypersensitivity, and color and/or temperature changes to the knee should lead the physician to suspect a complex regional pain syndrome.

Finally, the physician must discuss goals and expectations with the patient. Expectations frequently need to be tempered. In athletes and former athletes presenting with a knee injury, it behooves the surgeon to come to a better understanding of whether the athlete would like to return to play or simply desires a painless knee for activities of daily living. The patient is most likely to achieve a successful result if he or she understands the goals of the treatment program for the presumed diagnosis.

Physical Examination

Physical examination of the knee requires an in-depth understanding of the anatomic structures and the function of these structures, because each provocative test seeks to isolate the function of each structure. We often view the examination as a multistep process: (1) inspection, (2) palpation, (3) range of motion and strength testing, (4) patellar testing, (5) meniscal testing, (6) ligamentous stability testing, (7) gait assessment, (8) evaluation of muscle weakness and imbalance (e.g., hamstring tightness, quadriceps tightness, or core weakness), and (9) assessment of the back, hip, and feet. We start by examining the noninjured extremity, which may provide important information regarding baseline abnormalities and also helps to relax the patient.

Inspection

A great deal of information can be gained from inspection of the patient before taking a history or performing a focused physical examination (Box 92-1). If possible, patients should be observed as they enter the examination room or at some other time when they do not know they are being observed.[7] Once the patient is in the examination room, the physician can gain insight into the patient's general mobility by observing him or her transfer from a chair to the examination table.

The periarticular skin should be carefully inspected for (1) any surgical scars, which may affect future surgical planning; (2) erythema, which should be demarcated with a skin-marking pen if it is believed to reflect an underlying cellulitis; (3) ecchymoses, which reflect subcutaneous hemorrhage that may signal a capsular injury (Fig. 92-1); and (4) abrasions, which may provide a clue to the direction of the primary trauma. In particular, an anterior tibial abrasion is classically associated with a posterior cruciate ligament (PCL) injury because of the posteriorly directed force on the anterior tibia at the time of injury (Fig. 92-2). Attention should be directed to the presence or absence of effusion, any localized swelling, and muscle tone within the periarticular muscles, in particular the quadriceps and vastus medialis obliquus. The examiner should examine a patient with a suspected dislocation for the presence of any abnormal skin furrows or dimpling, which

BOX 92-1 Diagnosis by Visualization

Atrophy
Effusion
Ecchymosis
Malalignment
Gait abnormalities
Extensor mechanism disruption

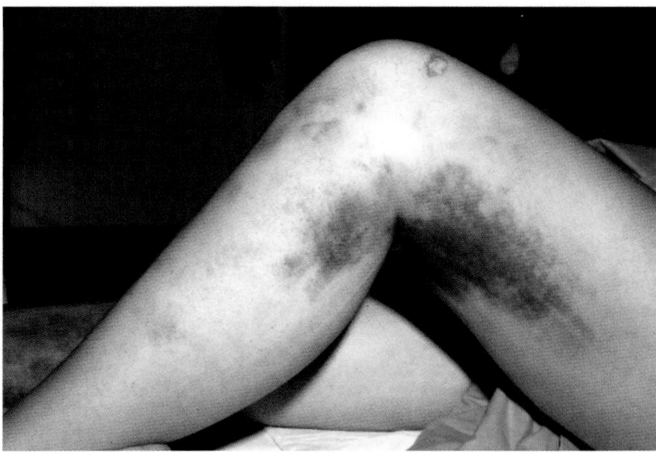

FIGURE 92-1 Ecchymoses reflect a subcutaneous hemorrhage and may signal a capsular injury. These posterolateral hemorrhages raise suspicion for a posterolateral corner ligamentous injury.

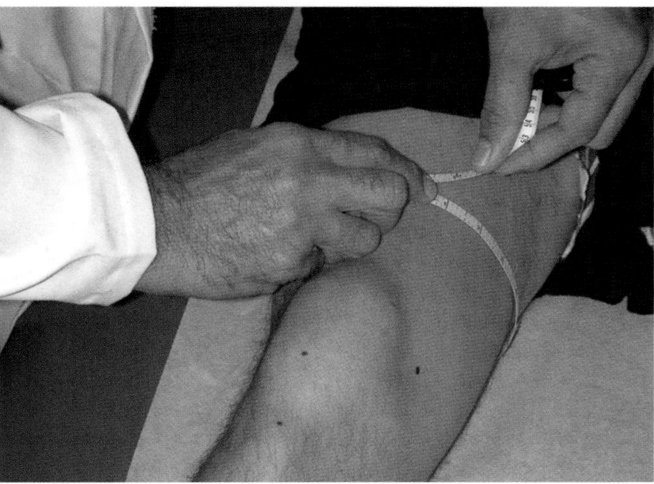

FIGURE 92-3 Thigh circumference, which the examiner should always measure at the same distance proximal to the superior patellar pole, is a sensitive measure of quadriceps atrophy.

could signal buttonholing of the condyles through the capsule and the need for open reduction.[8,9] Although general inspection may reveal atrophy, the most sensitive measurement of atrophy is a comparison of thigh circumference with the contralateral knee (Fig. 92-3). This measurement can be used as a marker for the rehabilitation process after surgery. General inspection may reveal stigmata of other general medical conditions, such as signs of venous stasis, ulcerations, or prior amputations as a result of diabetic neuropathy or vascular insufficiency, as well as signs of chronic infections or abscesses. Predrawn knee schematics may be helpful for recording findings from visual inspection. Alternatively, obtaining a photograph at the time of presentation can be invaluable for comparison at a later date. Photographs can be entered into the electronic medical record. Serial examinations can be crucial for the determination of progression, especially in the acutely injured patient.

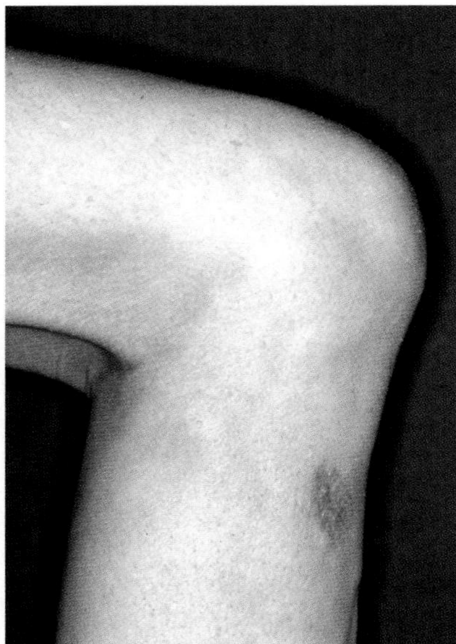

FIGURE 92-2 An anterior tibial abrasion is shown with associated posterior subluxation of the tibia, suggesting a posterior cruciate ligament injury.

Patients should remove their shoes so that the entire limb can be inspected. Overall limb alignment should be visually estimated within the coronal, sagittal, and axial planes. Any deformity should be fully inspected visually and radiographically. Specific attention should be directed to malrotation.[10] With the patient supine, the examiner should also visually inspect the height level of the patella for alta or baja. The physician may also want to measure limb length. Although the most accurate method for limb length measurement is the placement of sized standing blocks under the short leg until the pelvis is level, a rapid, rough estimation can be gained with a glance at the relative heights of the medial malleoli in the supine patient. The physician can also estimate the Q angle visually and measure it with a goniometer, although this measurement can be affected by a variety of other deformities. Deformities within the foot should also be observed. For instance, pes planus may be a contributing factor to genu valgum or may be a sign of generalized ligamentous laxity. Core strength can also be observed by asking patients to stand on one leg. An inability to maintain a level pelvis indicates weakness of the core trunk stabilizers that can indirectly contribute to patellofemoral symptoms.

The patient's gait should be observed. Although gait is a complex process requiring normal function of the foot, ankle, knee, hip, and lumbosacral spine, some gait abnormalities can also be referred to the knee. One should observe for varus and valgus thrusts, an antalgic gait with shortening of the stance phase for the affected limb, and the foot progression angle. Patients with ACL deficiency may exhibit a quadriceps avoidance gait, possibly to prevent excess anterior tibial translation.[11]

Palpation

It should be noted that many patients in the acute postinjury phase have generalized inflammation with diffuse tenderness that tends to be nondiagnostic; as a result, the patient may need to return at a later date for a repeat examination.

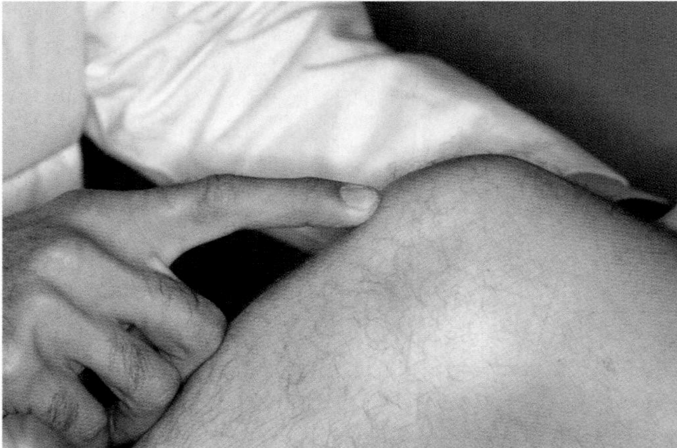

FIGURE 92-4 Tenderness at the inferior pole of the patella suggests patellar tendonitis.

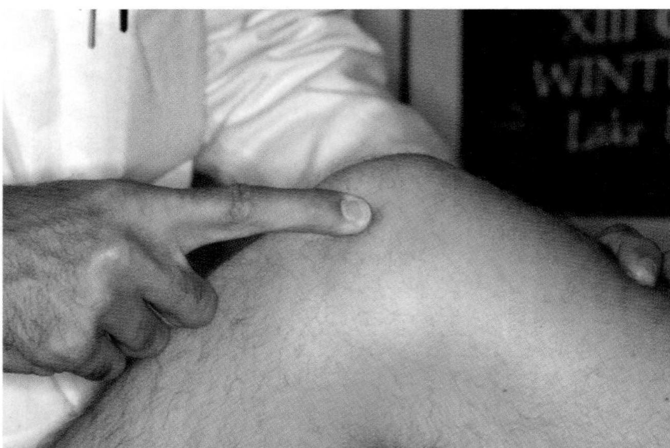

FIGURE 92-6 A tender palpable band, which may snap back and forth over the medial femoral condyle, suggests medial plica syndrome.

The knee should be palpated for the presence or absence of an effusion. The examiner can milk fluid down from the suprapatellar bursa while holding the patella between the thumb and forefinger of the contralateral hand to assess for the ability to ballot the patella. Alternatively, the examiner can feel for swelling at the soft spots medial and lateral to the patellar tendon, where the capsule is fairly subcutaneous. The other area where the surgeon may be able to palpate synovial fluid is in a Baker cyst, which is most commonly posteromedial between the semimembranosus and the medial head of the gastrocnemius.

The quadriceps tendon and its patellar insertion can be palpated both for tenderness associated with quadriceps tendonitis and a gap associated with a quadriceps tendon tear. The patella should be palpated for prepatellar tenderness or fullness that may be a sign of prepatellar bursitis. The patellar tendon and its patellar origin should be palpated for tenderness associated with patellar tendonitis (Fig. 92-4), as well as for a gap associated with a patellar tendon tear. The tibial tubercle should be palpated (Fig. 92-5) for bony tenderness, which may be associated with Osgood-Schlatter syndrome.

On the medial side of the knee, the entire course of the medial collateral ligament should be palpated for tenderness. The femoral and patellar attachments of the medial patellofemoral ligament should be evaluated for a palpable gap or tenderness. The medial tibial plateau should be palpated for tenderness because it might be associated with an acute fracture or stress fracture. The region just anteromedial to the patella should be assessed for a palpable tender band from plica syndrome (Fig. 92-6). The distal insertion of the sartorius, semitendinosus, and gracilis tendons should be palpated for pes anserine bursitis. The posteromedial joint line should also be palpated for a possible meniscal tear. Whereas anteromedial (Fig. 92-7) and medial joint line tenderness is often associated with plica syndrome or hypertrophic fat pad syndrome, displaced bucket hand meniscal tears characteristically have more tenderness anterior than the classic posteromedial location associated with most meniscal tears.

Similarly, the surgeon must also palpate the lateral structures. The lateral collateral ligament is best identified with the knee in the "figure of four" position, where varus stress makes the ligament taut and more easily palpable. The other structures of the PLC, such as the popliteus tendon and the popliteofibular ligament, can be more difficult to assess with

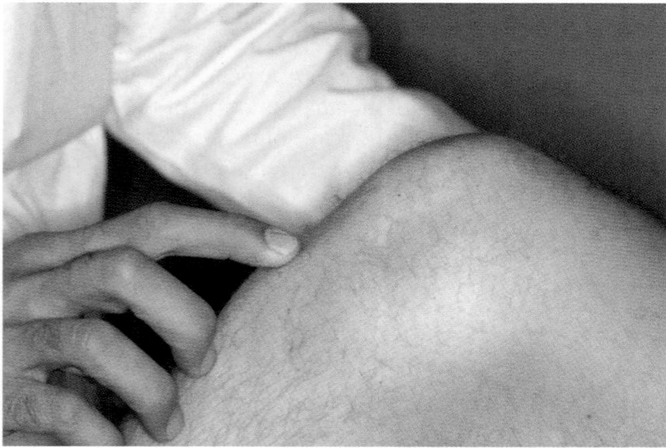

FIGURE 92-5 Tenderness to palpation at the tibial tubercle suggests Osgood-Schlatter syndrome, fracture of the tibial tubercle, or possibly insertional patellar tendonitis.

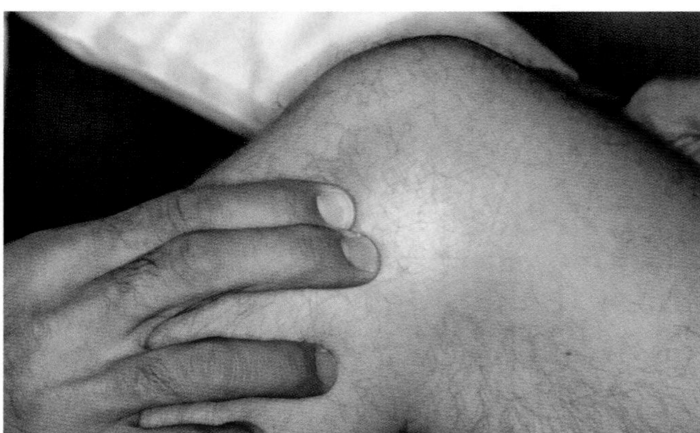

FIGURE 92-7 Palpation for tenderness at the anterior medial joint line.

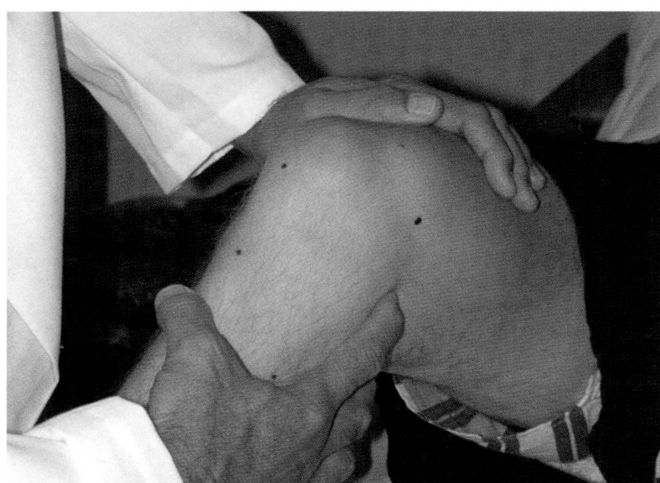

FIGURE 92-8 Palpation for tenderness at the posterior lateral joint line.

palpation. The biceps tendon is most easily assessed as a cord at the posterolateral surface of the fibular head. Just anterior to the biceps tendon is the iliotibial band, which can be palpated as it passes over the lateral femoral condyle and at its tibial attachment at Gerdy's tubercle. The fibular head should also be assessed. The lateral tibial plateau should be palpated for tenderness, which might be associated with an acute fracture or stress fracture. The posterolateral joint line (Fig. 92-8) is palpated for a possible meniscal tear. As on the medial side, anterolateral joint line tenderness can be associated with hypertrophic fat pad syndrome or a displaced bucket handle tear. Just distal to the fibular head, the examiner can commonly palpate the common peroneal nerve. In patients with suspected pathology of the peroneal nerve, the examiner should attempt to elicit a Tinel sign. Pain associated with common peroneal neuritis may be referred to the anterolateral proximal tibial region.

Range of Motion and Strength Testing

Range of motion is a fairly sensitive predictor of intraarticular pathology and is critical for knee function. Normal knee range of motion has been described as 0 to 120 degrees,[7,12] although the range of motion actively used for gait is 10 to 120 degrees.[13] However, considerable variation exists. At terminal extension many persons have up to 5 degrees of hyperextension, which, in combination with range from 0 to 10 degrees of flexion, may be useful for the "screw home" mechanism of internal rotation that tensions the cruciate ligaments and "locks" the knee at full extension. Many persons have additional passive flexion beyond their active range; in men this is commonly 140 degrees and in women it is 143 degrees, although in societies where kneeling is common, such as in Japan, India, and the Middle East, passive flexion to 165 degrees is common.[12] One hundred twenty-five degrees of flexion are necessary to squat, whereas 110 degrees of flexion is required to descend stairs in normal fashion. The loss of as little as 10 degrees of flexion will affect running speed. The loss of as little as 5 degrees of extension can cause a limp with increased quadriceps activation during gait and resultant quadriceps strain and fatigue, as well as patellofemoral pain. Differences between passive and active range of motion should be noted. A loss of both is considered a "contracture" and implies a block to motion, whereas a loss of active range of motion with preserved passive range of motion is considered a "lag" and implies a muscle tightness or imbalance.

Several methods may be used to test range of motion. A goniometer can be placed on the lateral side of the knee with the proximal end pointed toward the greater trochanter and the distal end pointed toward the lateral malleolus. This method has high inter- and intraobserver reliability.[14] A more sensitive indicator of full extension and flexion is the measurement of the heel-height difference with the patient placed in the prone position (Fig. 92-9). Similarly, the heel-buttock distance can be measured in full flexion in the supine position. One centimeter correlates with approximately 1 degree.[13]

Range of motion testing should also be performed on the ankle and hip joints and lumbar spine. We also commonly test for generalized ligamentous laxity, specifically by examining for elbow recurvatum, hyperextension at the metacarpophalangeal joint, the ability to abduct the thumb to meet the forearm, and excess external rotation of the humerus in adduction, all of which may signal a connective tissue abnormality. It should be noted that some confusion exists in the literature regarding the terms *laxity* and *instability*. *Laxity* is a term used to describe a finding on physical examination, whereas *instability* is a term used to describe a patient's subjective experience of this same entity. It is possible for a person to have generalized ligamentous laxity with no instability, and vice versa.

Several other structures can be assessed during range of motion testing. For instance, if the patient reports lateral knee pain with a palpable snap, the examiner can flex the knee, internally rotate, and then extend the knee to elicit snapping of the biceps tendon over a prominent fibula head (Fig. 92-10).[15] This observation may not be detected with external or neutral tibial rotation. It is important to consider this entity because it can mimic an unstable lateral meniscal tear. More commonly, the patient should be assessed for hamstring

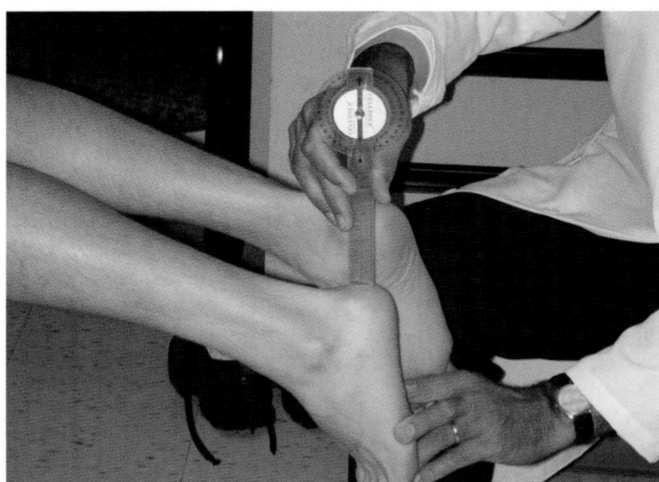

FIGURE 92-9 The most sensitive way to measure extension deficit is to measure the heel-height distance difference with the patient in the prone position. A 1-cm difference roughly correlates with a 1-degree difference.

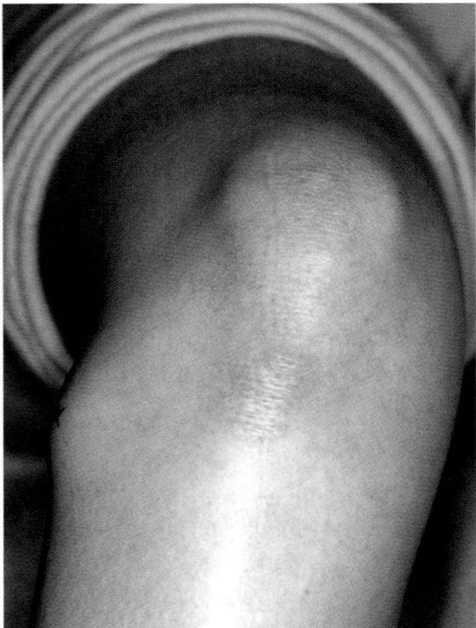

FIGURE 92-10 Observation may reveal prominence of the fibular head, which may predispose to snapping of the biceps tendon with flexion/extension.

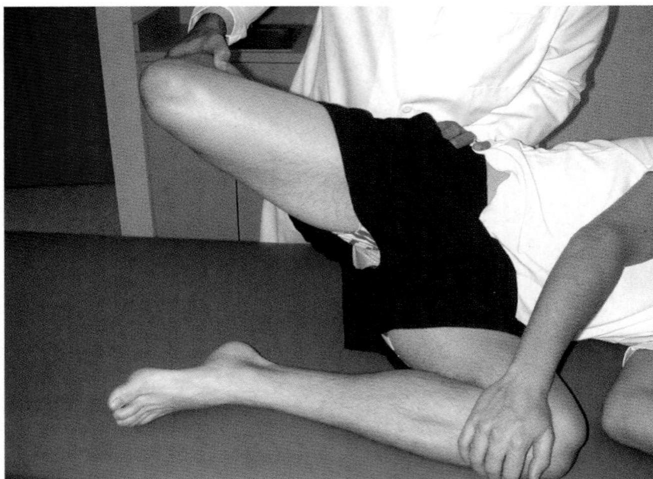

FIGURE 92-11 To test for contracture of the iliotibial band, the examiner can use the Ober test, in which the patient is placed in the lateral decubitus position and the knee is flexed to 90 degrees while the hip is abducted to 40 degrees and fully extended and an attempt is then made to adduct the hip. An inability to adduct past midline signifies tightness within the iliotibial band.

tightness in the supine position with the examiner attempting to flex the hip with the knee extended. We grade hamstring flexibility in degrees from the examination table. In this same position, the patient should be assessed for the ability to perform a straight leg raise. The examiner may also wish to assess for iliotibial band tightness using the Ober test. In this test, the patient is placed in the lateral decubitus position with both hips and knees flexed to 90 degrees so as not to flatten the lumbar spine. Concomitantly, the affected leg is abducted to 40 degrees and fully extended, and an attempt is then made to adduct the hip. An inability to adduct past midline signifies an iliotibial band contracture (Fig. 92-11).

Range of motion testing is also an excellent time to assess muscular strength, including hip abduction, knee flexion and extension, ankle flexion and extension, foot eversion and inversion, and extension of the hallux. In a patient with demonstrable weakness, one must determine whether neuromuscular inhibition due to pain may be contributory. While testing distal strength, one should assess distal sensory function in the sural nerve at the lateral border of the foot, the saphenous nerve at the medial ankle, the superficial peroneal nerve over the dorsum of the foot, the deep peroneal nerve at the dorsal first web space, and the tibial nerve over the plantar surface of the foot. Patients with previous longitudinal anterior knee incisions should be assessed for residual numbness in the distribution of the infrapatellar branch of the saphenous nerve; any numbness would be lateral to any incision because the nerve runs from medial to lateral. Whereas testing sensation to light touch is commonly sufficient for examination of the knee in the setting of a sports physician's office, testing with a 5.08 Semmes-Weinstein monofilament is the most sensitive method of testing for a sensory deficit in this region of the body and the preferred method in patients with suspected diabetic neuropathy.

The vascular status of the limb can be assessed with palpation of pulses at the posterior tibial artery at the posteromedial ankle, the dorsalis pedis artery over the proximal dorsal foot, and the popliteal artery at the posterior knee. Patients without palpable pulses require assessment with a Doppler device. This portion of the examination is crucial in the acute assessment of any patient with trauma to the knee, particularly patients with suspected or confirmed knee dislocations. These patients may require additional assessment with an ankle-brachial index, and any patient with an ankle-brachial index score of less than 0.8 requires further investigation with an angiogram or magnetic resonance angiogram.[16]

Patella

To assess the retinaculum and peripatellar capsular structures, the examiner can assess patella mobility with the knee in extension before it engages with the trochlea (Fig. 92-12). In anxious patients, the examiner may wish to repeat this portion

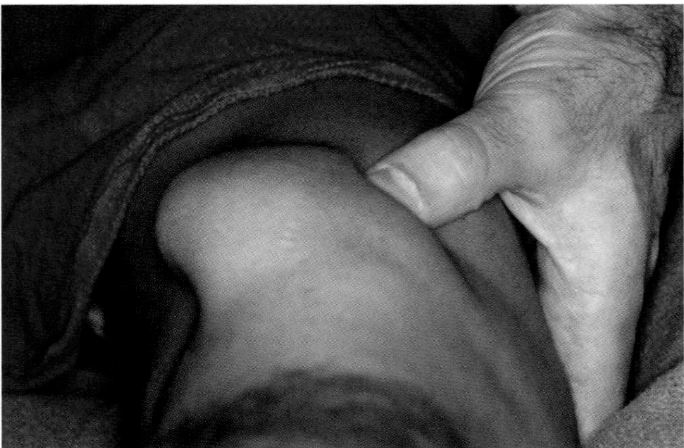

FIGURE 92-12 Patellar mobility can be assessed in full extension to assess fibrosis within the retinaculum, capsule, and other peripatellar tissues.

of the examination with the patient in the prone position, which relaxes the quadriceps.[10] The knee can then be flexed to 30 degrees when the patella has fully engaged into the trochlea where the retinaculum is tightened. At this position, patellar tilt can be assessed and palpated by attempting to lift the lateral patella from the lateral trochlea. Furthermore, the examiner should palpate the lateral edge of the patella and determine if static lateral translation of the patella is present in relation to the lateral femoral condyle and whether this translation is correctable. The lateral edge of the patella can be palpated to determine if it overhangs the lateral femoral sulcus; if anatomically positioned, both structures are palpable. The apprehension sign can be elicited by pressing laterally on the medial border of the patella (Fig. 92-13). In a patient who has undergone a previous lateral release, a medially directed positive apprehension sign indicates an overzealous lateral retinacular release with subsequent medial instability. The examiner should also assess how far the patella can be translated laterally, which is then graded into quadrants. As a rule of thumb, the examiner should not be able to displace the patella more than half of its width laterally. The knee can then be taken through a flexion/extension cycle with the examiner's hand on the patella to feel for crepitus (Fig. 92-14), as well as any dynamic maltracking (Fig. 92-15). While observing patellar movement during range of motion, one should determine whether the patella subluxes in extension or in flexion. Specifically, the examiner should note the presence or absence of a "J sign" as the patella translates laterally out of the trochlea in terminal extension. Finally, with the knee in 60 to 90 degrees of flexion, the examiner can press with one hand on the patella and stabilize the ankle with the other hand while asking the patient to attempt to actively straighten his or her knee. If this maneuver elicits pain, the examiner should suspect patellofemoral pathology.[10] The degree of flexion of the knee at the time of the pain may signal chondral injury more proximally versus distally within the groove. However, even in healthy patients, synovium can become entrapped between the patella and the trochlea and cause pain with compression against the patella.

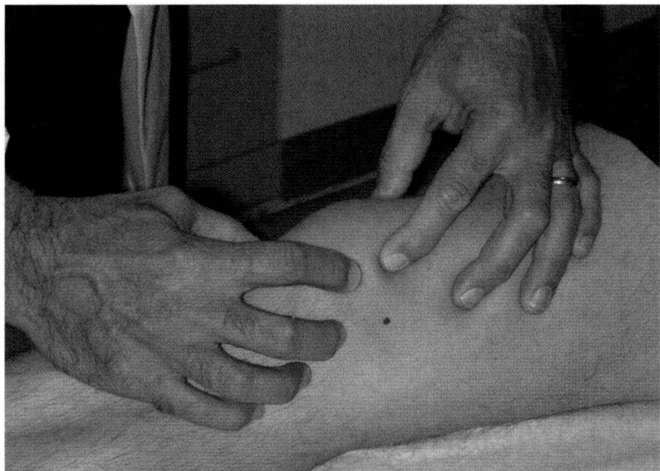

FIGURE 92-13 Patellar apprehension, a sign of instability, is present if pressure laterally on the medial border of the patella causes pain or patient concern for impending dislocation or subluxation.

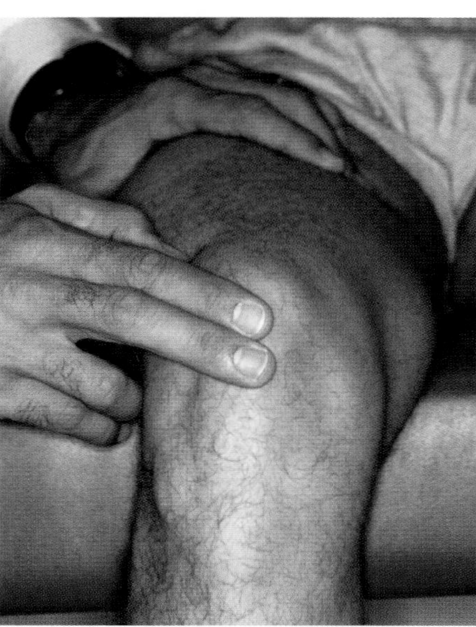

FIGURE 92-14 Palpation of the patella during flexion/extension cycles allows the examiner to assess for crepitus and maltracking.

The Q angle should be observed with the knee between 70 and 90 degrees of flexion. External rotation of the tibia may create a dynamic Q angle, which in some patients may exceed 45 degrees. In a patient with a long-standing distal extensor mechanism reconstruction (e.g., Hauser procedure), the Q angle may be negative, with resultant posteriorization of the patellar force vectors. Arthroscopic assessment consequently will demonstrate severe medial patellofemoral arthritis as a result of this slingshot effect.

Meniscus

A variety of meniscal examination maneuvers have been described. In a recent metaanalysis of numerous previously published studies examining the sensitivity, specificity, and accuracy of the various physical examination tests for meniscal pathology, joint line tenderness was found to be the most

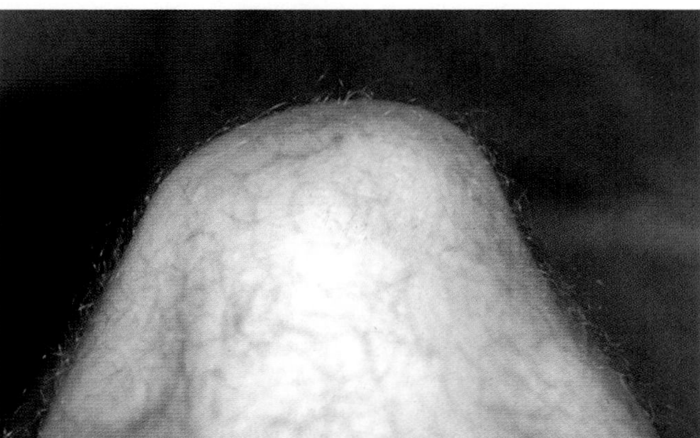

FIGURE 92-15 Lateral patellar maltracking.

sensitive test overall, whereas the McMurray test is the most specific.[17] Joint line tenderness can be elicited with palpation as a sign of a meniscal tear, commonly posterior to the midaxial line in the sagittal plane, although a displaced bucket handle tear is more tender anteromedially or anterolaterally at the anterior apex of the "bucket."

The most commonly used provocative meniscal test is the McMurray test, which is performed with the patient supine. To test the medial meniscus, the knee is flexed and brought into a varus stress and externally rotated and then slowly extended while palpating the medial joint for a mechanical click and asking the patient for any sensation of pain (Fig. 92-16). To test the lateral side, the aforementioned maneuver is performed with a valgus stress.[18] The senior author has not found the position of tibial rotation to be particularly sensitive; instead, we assess for pain referred to the affected compartment with hyperflexing, rotating, and extension maneuvers. The Apley test is performed with the patient in the prone position. The knee is brought into 90 degrees of flexion and then internally and externally rotated while applying an axial load (Fig. 92-17). A positive test occurs with the reproduction of pain or a catching or locking sensation. In addition, the test can be repeated in distraction across the joint, with continued pain and symptomatology signaling an articular cartilage lesion instead of a meniscal tear.[19] The Thessaly test is performed with the patient's own weight causing the compression. In this test, the patient stands on the affected leg, supported with his or her outstretched hands by the examiner and flexes the affected knee to 5 degrees while internally and externally rotating three times. The test is repeated in 20 degrees of flexion. In the original description of this test, the accuracy was 94% for medial meniscal tears and 96% for lateral meniscal tears, with all other tests having lesser accuracy—78% to 84% for the McMurray tests, 75% to 82% for the Apley test, and 81% to 89% for joint line tenderness.[20]

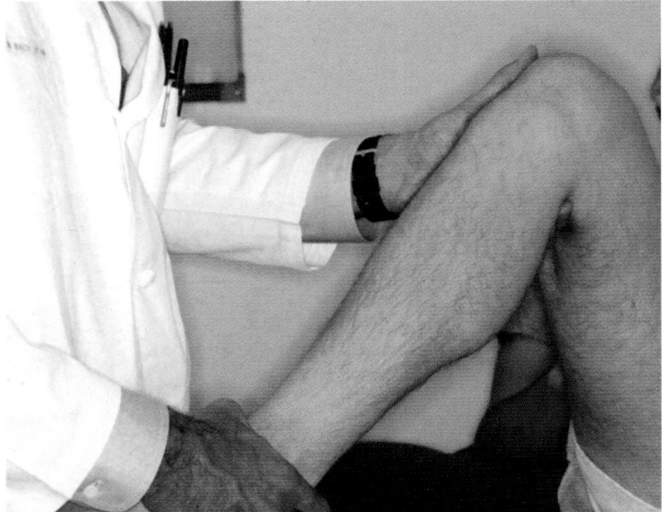

FIGURE 92-16 The McMurray meniscal test involves flexion, external rotation, and either varus or valgus stress with either medial or lateral joint line palpation for tears within the medial and lateral menisci, respectively.

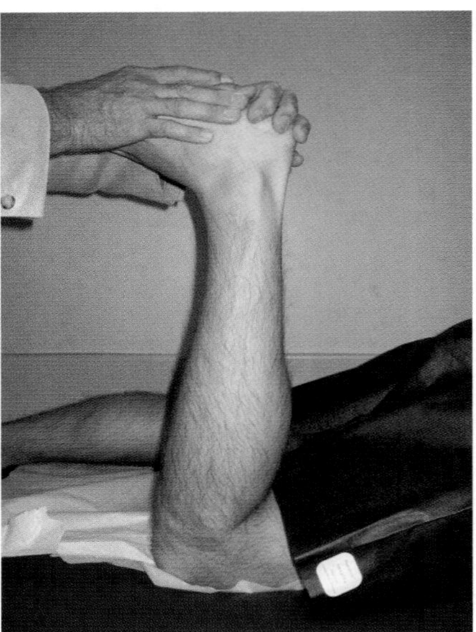

FIGURE 92-17 The Apley meniscal test involves prone positioning, flexion of the knee to 90 degrees, axial compression, and then internal and external rotatory movements.

Ligamentous Stability

Ligamentous stability testing in the knee is among the most difficult to learn aspects of the physical examination and also one of the most important portions of the examination.[21,22] A variety of tests have been described for testing the ACL. The anterior drawer test is historically the oldest test but is the least sensitive. With this test, one attempts to anteriorly translate the tibia with the knee flexed to 90 degrees with the ankle stabilized. Generally, this test is only positive with loss of not only the ACL but also the secondary restraints to anterior tibial translation such as the posterior horn of the medial meniscus (e.g., meniscal resection or an unstable peripheral meniscal tear). If the anterior drawer test is more positive than the Lachman test, one should suspect a PCL injury because the tibia is in a posterior resting position and is being translated to its neutral position. Increased anteromedial rotation of the tibia while flexed at 90 degrees is suggestive of a posteromedial corner injury.

The Lachman test is the most sensitive test for determining an ACL injury. The examiner attempts to anteriorly translate the tibia with the knee at 30 degrees of flexion (Fig. 92-18).[23,24] We perform this test with one hand stabilizing the distal femur and the other hand gripping the distal tibia such that a thumb is placed on the joint line and can palpate the translation of the tibia relative to the femur. This distance is then used to grade the test; grade 1 has 0 to 5 mm of translation, grade 2 has 5 to 10 mm of translation, and grade 3 has greater than 10 mm of translation (Fig. 92-19).[25] When compared with the opposite knee, the examiner should also assess for the true presence of a "soft" or "firm" end point. The sensitivity of the Lachman test is 94% to 98% in a patient who is awake.[26]

The most definitive test for assessing the functional integrity of the ACL is the pivot shift test, which characterizes the subluxation-reduction phenomenon of ACL deficiency. The goal of ACL reconstruction surgery is to eliminate the pivot shift regardless of the preoperative grade. Unfortunately,

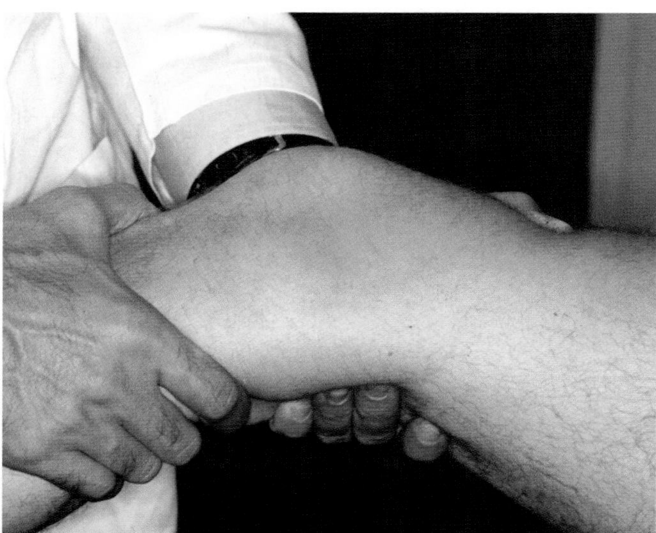

FIGURE 92-18 Lachman testing, which is similar to anterior drawer testing but performed at 30 degrees of flexion.

eliciting a positive pivot shift in the office can be difficult because patients are often apprehensive and guarding their knee. Furthermore, once a physician has elicited this sensation, subsequent efforts are usually met with patient guarding. In the office, we prefer to note that the patient is guarding on pivot shift maneuvers rather than stating that the test is negative. It is of interest that after reconstruction, if the ACL is functionally stable, the patient will allow the physician to perform multiple pivot shift attempts without apprehension. The pivot shift phenomenon is a complex combination of subluxation, rotation, and reduction motions. It is most easily conceptualized as a subluxation of the tibia in extension and a reduction with knee flexion. The pivot shift, as described by Galway (the Hughston "jerk test") and Noyes ("flexion rotation drawer"), as well as the Losee test, the Slocum test, and the Bach-Warren test, are all subtle modifications of this phenomenon.[27] An excellent overview of the various described maneuvers has been presented by Lane et al.[27] It is critical to

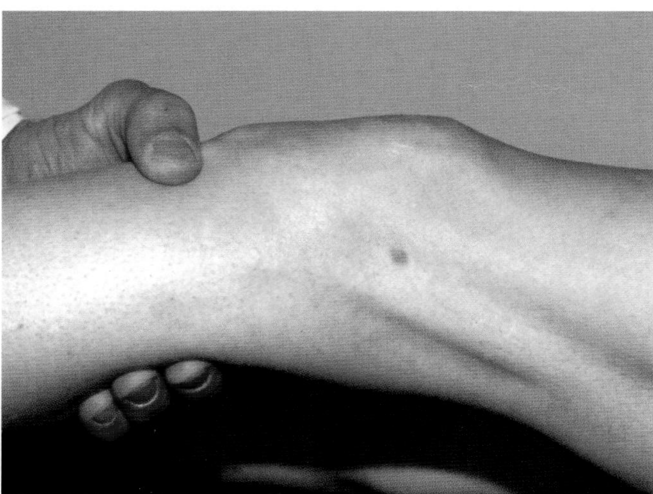

FIGURE 92-19 A positive Lachman test with anterior subluxation of the tibia.

recognize that axial load and valgus force can have an impact on the grade of the pivot shift phenomenon. Incarcerated ACL stumps, displaced meniscal fragments, meniscal deficiency, associated ligamentous patholaxity (e.g., MCL), knee stiffness, arthritis, the position of the thigh when tested (abduction vs. adduction), and tibial rotation (external vs. internal rotation) can affect the pivot shift phenomenon. Perfecting this examination is an art form that takes years to master. It is easily inadequately performed, interpreted improperly, or sadly, not performed as part of an examination with the patient anesthetized prior to arthroscopic evaluation. We have encountered many patients who have been informed that they have a partial ACL tear (as determined by MRI, physical examination, and/or arthroscopy) but who are found to have an obvious pivot shift phenomenon upon careful examination.

To perform the pivot shift maneuver, the physician exerts a valgus and internal rotation moment on the tibia with the knee extended and then slowly flexes the knee (Fig. 92-20). A positive result is a subluxing sensation at roughly 20 to 30 degrees of flexion.[28] The biomechanical explanation for this maneuver is that in the ACL-deficient knee the tibia subluxes anteriorly at full extension. Valgus stress traps the lateral condyle in this subluxed position. With increasing flexion, the periarticular soft tissues exert an increasing ligamentotaxis effect, pulling the tibia posteriorly. Eventually this force causes the posterior lip of the tibia to be pulled posteriorly over the convex femoral condyle, reducing the knee with a palpable clunk.[29] One modification of this test is the "pivot jerk" maneuver in which the knee is brought from flexion to extension with a similar valgus and internal rotation force, with the clunk experienced as the reduced tibia subluxes anteriorly.[7]

Several grading scales have been proposed for the pivot shift test. In the most commonly used scale, grade I is a gliding sensation without a palpable clunk, grade II is a palpable and sometimes audible clunk or jump, and grade III is

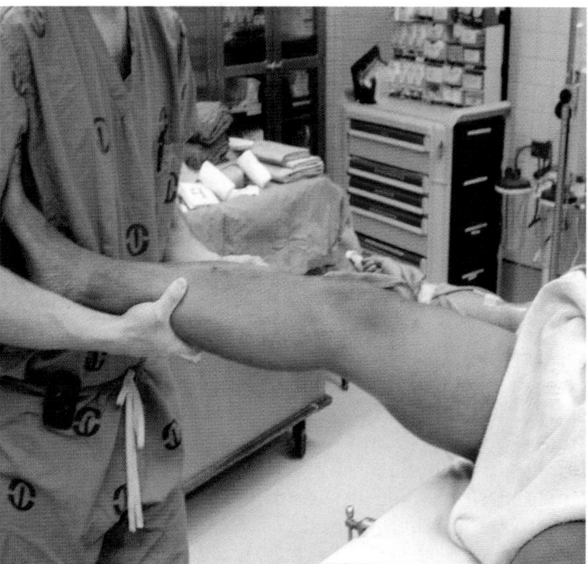

FIGURE 92-20 Pivot shift testing, shown preoperatively after administration of an anesthetic. In this examination maneuver, the examiner applies an external rotation and valgus stress to the fully extended knee and then slowly flexes, feeling for a reduction "clunk" at 20 to 30 degrees of flexion.

a locked knee. Transient locking is usually observed with associated meniscal deficiency. In 1987, Jakob and colleagues[29a] proposed an alternate grading scale in which a grade I pivot is "trace," that is, only elicited with the patient anesthetized; a grade II pivot is positive in internal rotation and neutral; and a grade III pivot is positive in external rotation and less obviously so in internal rotation. Conversely, Bach and colleagues[30] noted improved sensitivity of the pivot shift test with hip abduction and tibial external rotation, an effect believed to be due to the tenodesis effect of the iliotibial band. The iliotibial band is one of several structures that can affect the ability of the ACL-deficient knee to pivot; with an MCL injury, valgus stress no longer causes a compressive force across the lateral compartment, and a flexion contracture of bucket handle meniscal tear prevents making full extension. Conversely, several injuries can accentuate the pivot further; injury to the PLC increases the examiner's ability to externally rotate the tibia and thus increase the pivot. A prior medial meniscectomy can also result in increased anterior tibial translation and an increased pivot shift.

Unfortunately, the pivot shift maneuver is subject to poor interobserver reliability because of the vast variation in force applied by the examiner during the maneuver.[29] In addition, because of patient anxiety and guarding, these rotatory instability tests may be difficult to elicit. Any patient scheduled to have a surgical knee intervention should undergo repeat ligamentous testing once general anesthesia has been induced. Sensitivity of the pivot shift maneuver without use of an anesthetic has been described to be as low as 32% to 40%, rising to 97% to 100% with use of an anesthetic.[27] The senior author can recall only a single patient in 26 years who, when examined after inducement of anesthesia, had a negative pivot shift despite complete ACL disruption. Authors of other studies have described sensitivities as high as 89% with the pivot shift maneuver.[31] Almost all studies have described specificities for the anterior drawer, Lachman, and pivot shift tests in excess of 95%.[31]

The most important examination for PCL diagnosis is the posterior drawer test. The knee is flexed to 90 degrees and a posteriorly directed force is placed on the tibia while the examiner feels and observes for posterior translation. Similar to the anterior drawer and Lachman tests, this test is commonly graded I for 0- to 5-mm translation, II for 5- to 10-mm translation, and III for 10- to 15-mm translation compared with the opposite knee (Fig. 92-21).[1] Differentiating between grades has important prognostic significance.[22,32,33] A grade III injury may only be possible with concomitant injury to the PLC, capsule, and/or MCL and should cause the examiner to examine closely for such a combined injury.[21,34] In the quadriceps activation modification, the knee is brought to 70 degrees of knee flexion and the patient is asked to actively extend at the knee while the ankle is stabilized, while the examiner watches for anterior tibial translation, which signifies an abnormally posterior resting tibial position. The anterior medial tibial plateau normally has an anterior step-off relative to the medial femoral condyle. In a knee with a PCL injury, this step-off is reduced. In a grade III PCL injury, the tibia may be flush with the femoral condyle (Fig. 92-22).[22] The posterior drawer test is the most sensitive and specific test for PCL injury, although in combination, these clinical examination tests have an accuracy of 96%, a sensitivity of 90%, and a specificity of 99%.[35]

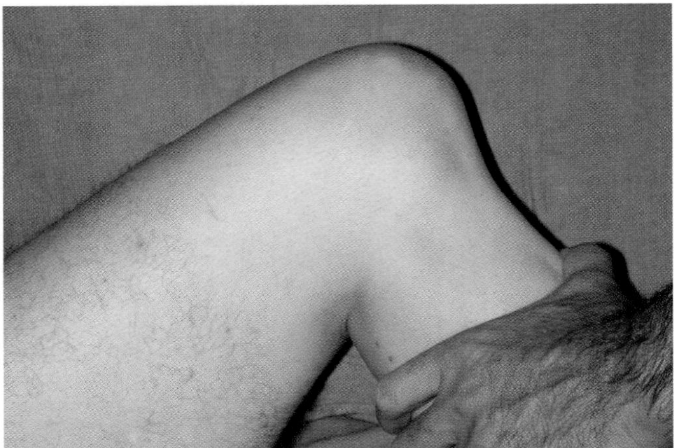

FIGURE 92-21 A positive posterior drawer test demonstrates posterior subluxation of the tibia relative to the femur.

Testing of the MCL starts with palpation, as previously described, with which the examiner may be able to specify whether injury occurs at the proximal or distal end of the ligament.[36] This differentiation may have prognostic clinical significance because proximal MCL injuries have been demonstrated to have a slower recovery of full range of motion than distal MCL injuries.[37] The integrity of the MCL can be tested clinically with the patient in the supine position and the ankle cradled between the torso and the elbow while the examiner's hand on the lateral side of the knee exerts a valgus stress and the hand on the medial side of the knee rests with fingers at the joint line to measure the tibiofemoral separation. Similar to tests for the ACL and PCL, this test is commonly graded I for 0- to 5-mm separation, II for 6- to 10-mm separation, and III for greater than 10-mm separation.[25,38] This test should be performed at both full extension and 30 degrees of flexion (Fig. 92-23). Although an isolated MCL injury will cause valgus laxity at 30 degrees, no laxity is observed at full extension without injury to the secondary restraints such as the cruciate ligaments, posterior capsule, or posterior oblique ligament.[38,39] These tests must be interpreted in combination to determine the degree of injury (which, it should be noted, is separate from the grade of the valgus stress test), with first-degree injuries exhibiting tenderness without instability;

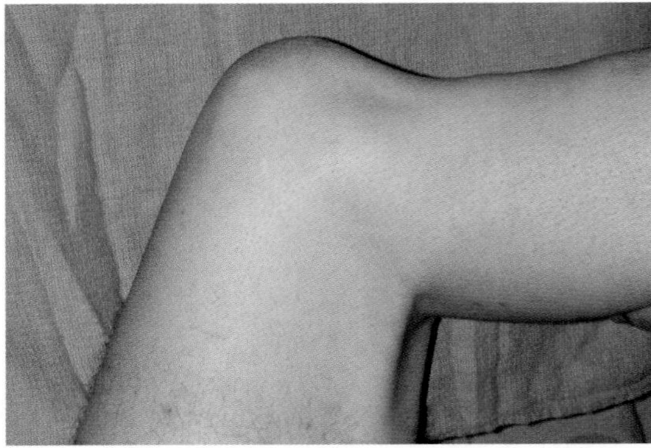

FIGURE 92-22 The posterior sag test is similar to the posterior drawer test but allows gravity to provide the subluxation force. This tibia demonstrates posterior subluxation.

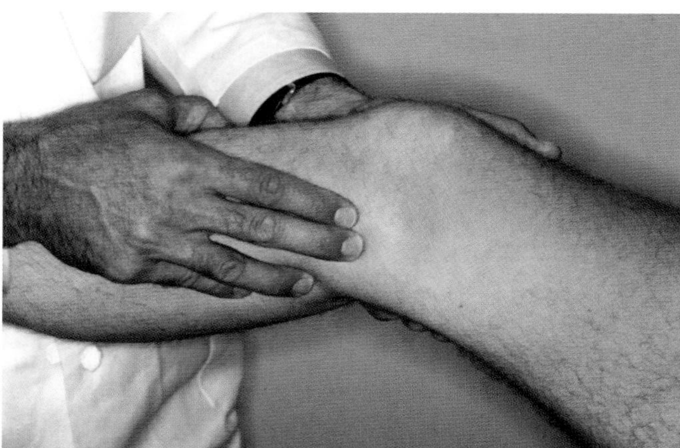

FIGURE 92-23 Valgus stress testing performed at 30 degrees of flexion to assess the medial collateral ligament. Note the examiner's fingers on the medial joint line to assess tibiofemoral separation.

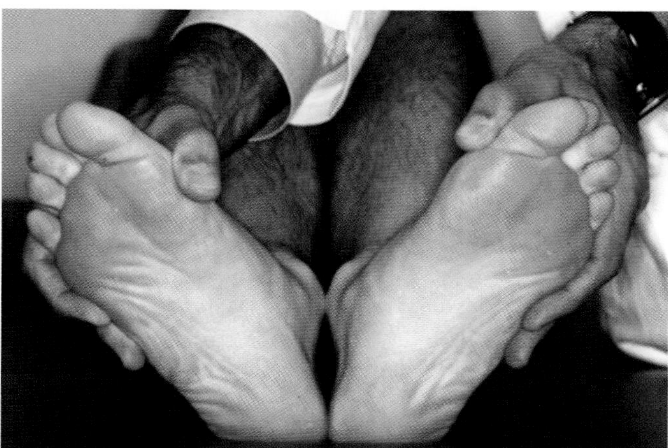

FIGURE 92-25 Dial testing performed with the patient supine at 30 degrees of flexion. The side-to-side difference in the angle between the foot and the axis of the tibia denotes degree of laxity of the posterolateral corner.

second-degree injuries exhibiting laxity to valgus stress but with a firm end point; and third-degree injuries exhibiting laxity to valgus stress with no end point.[36,38]

We commonly conclude with testing of the structures of the PLC. Similar to the medial side, the examiner can examine for tibiofemoral separation with varus stress at both full extension and 30 degrees of flexion (Fig. 92-24), the latter of which tests the lateral collateral ligament. Also similarly, this test is commonly graded I for a 0- to 5-mm opening, II for a 5- to 10-mm opening, and III for a 10- to 15-mm opening.[25] Similar to valgus stress testing, a positive result at 30 degrees suggests an injury to the lateral structures, whereas a positive result at 0 degrees suggests concomitant injury to the secondary stabilizers in addition to the lateral collateral ligament, cruciate ligaments, and posterior capsule.[39] However, to fully test the remainder of the structures, the physician must also perform rotatory testing. The most commonly used rotatory test is the dial test, in which the physician attempts to maximally externally rotate both tibia at both 30 and 90 degrees of flexion (Fig. 92-25). Side-to-side testing is crucial, and a side-to-side-difference of less than 10 degrees is considered a mild injury, whereas 10 to 20 degrees is considered moderate and greater than 20 degrees is considered severe. Generally, an abnormality at 30 degrees of knee flexion is considered to be an isolated PLC injury, whereas abnormality noted at both 30 and 90 degrees requires injury to both the PLC and PCL.[40] Of note, a complete MCL injury may also allow excess external rotation (because of anteromedial rotation of the tibia).[38,41] The dial test can also be performed in the supine or seated position, again with the examiner assessing for asymmetric thigh-foot angles.

Several additional rotatory tests have been described, many of which describe overlapping functions of the PLC and PCL.[42] For instance, in the recurvatum test, the examiner holds the knee extended by the hallux in the supine and relaxed patient and observes for asymmetric and excess recurvatum and external rotation (Fig. 92-26).[43] Similarly, with the patient at 90 degrees of flexion and the ankle stabilized, the

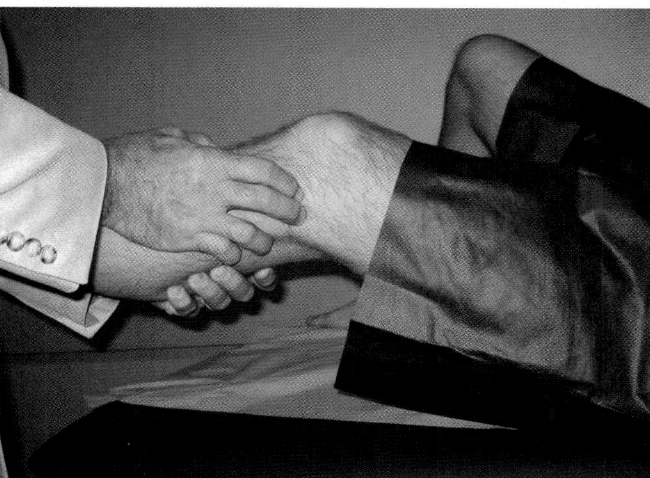

FIGURE 92-24 Varus stress testing performed at 30 degrees of flexion. Again, note the position of the examiner's fingers on the lateral joint line.

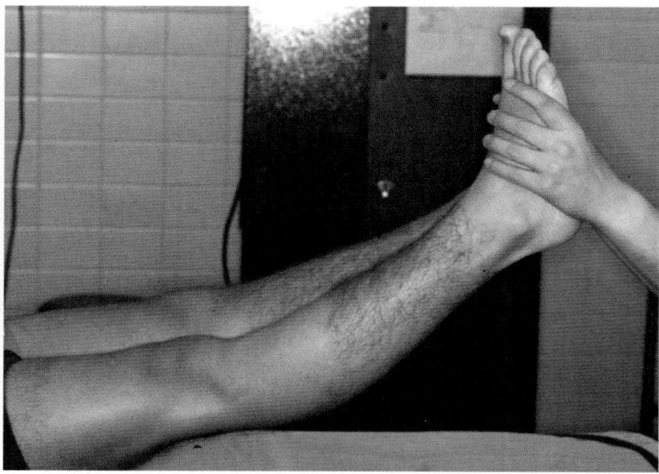

FIGURE 92-26 External recurvatum testing performed preoperatively after administration of an anesthetic.

examiner can test the ability of the tibia to abnormally spin posterolaterally (also described as the external rotation drawer test), a finding most likely to be positive with both PCL and PLC injuries. In addition, a reverse pivot shift maneuver has been described in which the knee is held flexed and a valgus and external rotation stress is placed as the knee is extended, feeling for a reduction "clunk" at 30 to 40 degrees of flexion. In this maneuver, the tibia begins in a posteriorly subluxed position and is forced to reduce anteriorly with increasing extension.[35] Although this test is most likely to be positive with both PLC and PCL injuries, it can also be positive with isolated injuries to either ligamentous structure. These tests have varying sensitivity; the posterolateral external rotation spin test has a sensitivity of 76%, and the external rotation recurvatum test has a sensitivity of 73%.[44]

It should be noted that although these tests are not highly specific to any single structure within the PLC, the examiner may be able to gather some idea of which structures are injured based on the physical findings. Category A injuries have increased external rotation with injury to the popliteofibular ligament and popliteus tendon. Category B injuries have increased external rotation and opening to varus stress of 5 mm at 30 degrees of flexion with injury to the category A structures, as well as attenuation of the lateral collateral ligament. Category C injuries have increased external rotation and opening of 10 mm at varus stress at 30 degrees with injury to the category A structures, as well as tears of the lateral collateral ligament, lateral capsule, and possibly the cruciate ligaments.[8] LaPrade and Terry[44] found that a positive reverse pivot was associated with injuries to the lateral collateral ligament, popliteus, and mid third lateral capsular ligaments, whereas a positive spin test was associated with lateral collateral ligament and lateral gastrocnemius injuries and a positive varus stress test was associated with injury to the posterior arcuate ligament. Patients with these injuries must be closely examined for injuries to the peroneal nerve as well.

Synthesis and Decision Making

A busy office setting often requires one to perform an efficient and focused physical examination. Although experience remains the most valuable tool that will inform which questions to ask and which examination maneuvers to perform in a given patient, we have attempted to synthesize the information provided in this chapter into useful algorithms (Figs. 92-27 and 92-28) that can guide physicians with respect to performing a focused examination and efficiently reaching a clinical diagnosis.

After obtaining a history and performing a physical examination, the practitioner must form a working differential

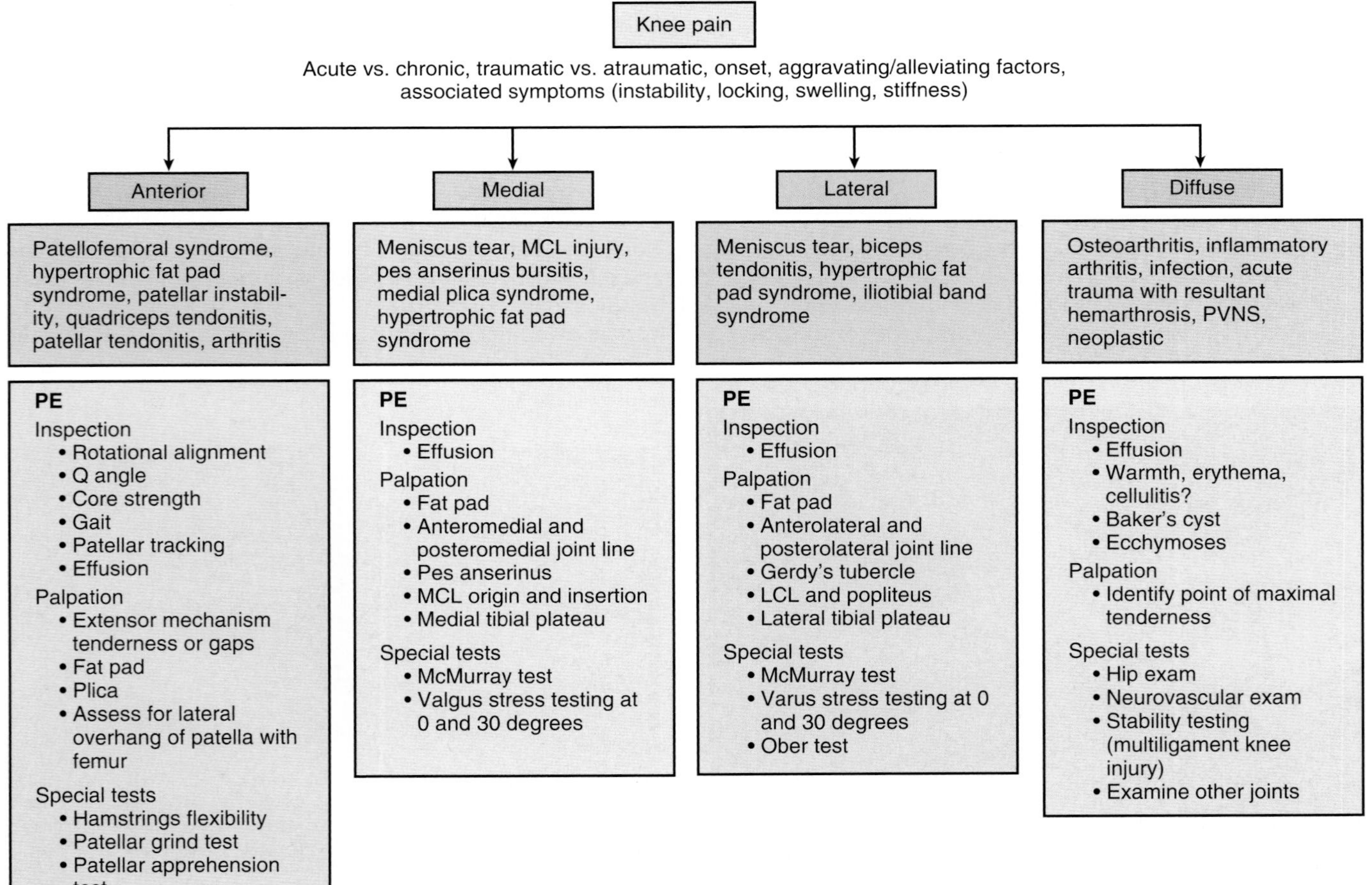

FIGURE 92-27 Algorithm for the evaluation of knee pain. *LCL,* Lateral collateral ligament; *MCL,* medial collateral ligament; *PE,* physical examination; *PVNS,* pigmented villonodular synovitis.

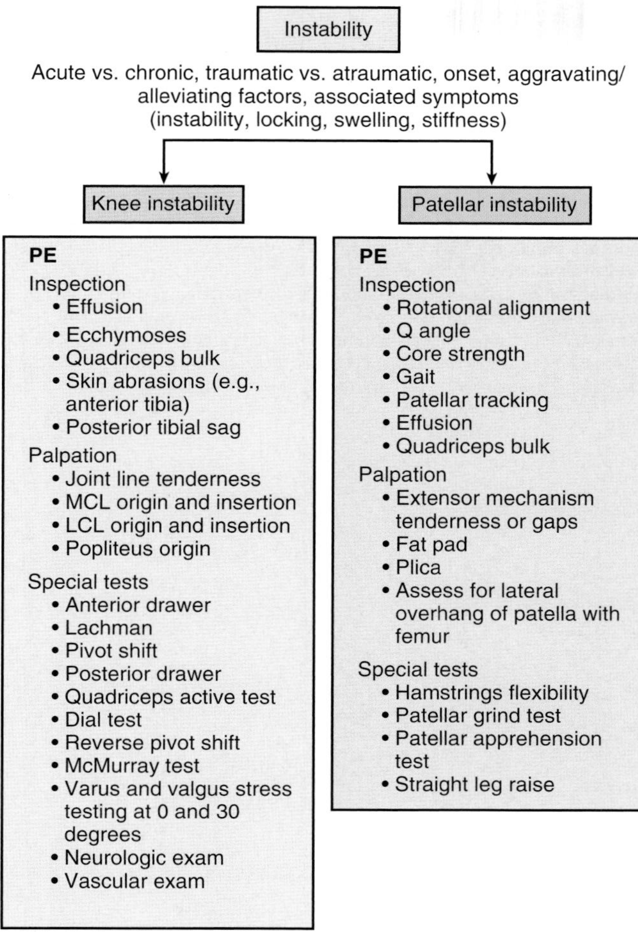

FIGURE 92-28 Algorithm for the evaluation of knee instability. *LCL,* Lateral collateral ligament; *MCL,* medial collateral ligament; *PE,* physical examination.

diagnosis that is to be followed initially with plain radiographs. We suggest that all new patients undergo standing bilateral anteroposterior, 30-degree flexion posteroanterior, lateral, and sunrise views of the knees. In the setting of varus or valgus malalignment, 3-ft standing anteroposterior views are also recommended to evaluate the mechanical axis. When ligamentous, meniscal, and/or cartilaginous pathologic features are suspected, we routinely order MRI scans to help elucidate and confirm the diagnosis. Finally, in the setting of patellar instability, a computed tomography scan can be obtained to assess the distance between the tibial tuberosity and the deepest point of trochlear groove on superimposed axial images. Computed tomography can also be helpful in the setting of revision ligamentous surgery to assess for tunnel osteolysis. More detailed information regarding cross-sectional imaging tests can be found in Chapter 93.

Although most sports-related knee conditions are initially treated with a trial of nonoperative treatment consisting of physical therapy, medications, and bracing, certain conditions require early surgical intervention. These conditions include displaced bucket handle meniscus tears (isolated or in the setting of a concomitant ligamentous injury), irreducible knee dislocations, multiligament knee injuries with associated vascular injury, acute PCL osseous avulsions, acute displaced osteochondral injuries, patellar dislocations with a loose osteochondral fragment causing mechanical symptoms, extensor mechanism tear, and intraarticular sepsis. The decision to proceed with immediate surgical care can only be made with an accurate diagnosis that once again is dependent on a systematic and focused history and physical examination.

The physiologic age of the knee is also an important factor to consider in the decision-making process. A patient in his or her fifties may have a healthy knee with no degenerative changes, whereas another person in his or thirties may present with a knee with posttraumatic arthritis. We believe that the chronologic age of the patient should not necessarily influence who is offered surgical reconstruction. Other factors to consider when deciding between forms of treatment include a patient's activity level, occupation, off-season timelines, and, as previously outlined, his or her expectations and goals.

Although an individualized treatment plan should be tailored according to the aforementioned patient factors, certain findings from the history and clinical examination can be used to guide treatment as well. For example, patients with acute ACL tears who have an effusion and quadriceps inhibition should not undergo surgical reconstruction until range of motion and quadriceps function have been optimized. Associated injuries must also be taken into account. A patient with an ACL injury who has a coexisting bucket handle meniscal tear will be treated more emergently than a patient with an isolated ACL tear. A patient's mechanical axis alignment can also influence decision making regarding the knee. Significant varus or valgus malalignment may require corrective osteotomies in the setting of ipsilateral compartmental pathology, as in the case of cartilage regenerative or reparative procedures, meniscus transplantation, or early unicompartmental osteoarthritis. One of the most challenging patients is the person who has degenerative joint disease and meniscal pathology noted on MRI. The history of a short duration of symptoms (<3 months) and mechanical symptoms are the two best prognosticators that the patient will benefit from an arthroscopic partial meniscectomy.

Conclusion

Although they are difficult to master given the complexity of the underlying anatomy, history and physical examination remain the most safe, cost-effective, and accurate methods of arriving at a diagnosis in a patient with knee-related complaints. We encourage practitioners to develop a systematic approach when evaluating patients, which is important not only to efficiently arrive at a diagnosis but also to prevent missing conditions that require emergent intervention or associated injuries that can affect treatment decision making and prognosis.

For a complete list of references, go to expertconsult.com.

Suggested Readings

Citation: Karachalios T, Hantes M, Zibis AH, et al: Diagnostic accuracy of a new clinical test (the Thessaly test) for early detection of meniscal tears. *J Bone Joint Surg Am* 87(5):955–962, 2005.
Level of Evidence: I (diagnostic)
Summary: This large prospective review of several physical examination tests for meniscal injury demonstrates excellent diagnostic accuracy for the Thessaly test and for joint line tenderness.

Citation: Kocher MS, Steadman JR, Briggs KK, et al: Relationships between objective assessment of ligament stability and subjective assessment of symptoms and function after anterior cruciate ligament reconstruction. *Am J Sports Med* 32(3):629–634, 2004.
Level of Evidence: II (diagnostic)
Summary: The retrospective correlation between postoperative physical examination findings and clinical outcome after anterior cruciate ligament reconstruction demonstrates a significant association between the pivot shift examination and a variety of functional outcomes, without a similar relationship between instrumented laxity or the Lachman test.

Citation: Lane CG, Warren R, Pearle AD: The pivot shift. *J Am Acad Orthop Surg* 16(12):679–688, 2008.
Level of Evidence: Not applicable
Summary: This article provides an excellent recent summary of the biomechanics, anatomic features, modifications, mitigating and aggravating factors, and clinical evidence surrounding the pivot shift maneuver.

Citation: LaPrade RF, Terry GC: Injuries to the posterolateral aspect of the knee. Association of anatomic injury patterns with clinical instability. *Am J Sports Med* 25(4):433–438, 1997.
Level of Evidence: I (diagnostic)
Summary: This large prospective examination of the correlation between a variety of physical examination maneuvers is designed to assay the structures of the posterolateral corner and the intraoperative pathologic findings.

Citation: Rubinstein RA, Shelbourne KD, McCarroll JR, et al: The accuracy of the clinical examination in the setting of posterior cruciate ligament injuries. *Am J Sports Med* 22(4):550–557, 1994.
Level of Evidence: I (diagnostic)
Summary: This prospective, randomized, controlled examination of a variety of examination maneuvers in patients with isolated posterior cruciate ligament tears, isolated anterior crucial ligament knees, and normal knees demonstrates that the posterior drawer test is the most sensitive and specific test for isolated injuries to the posterior cruciate ligament.

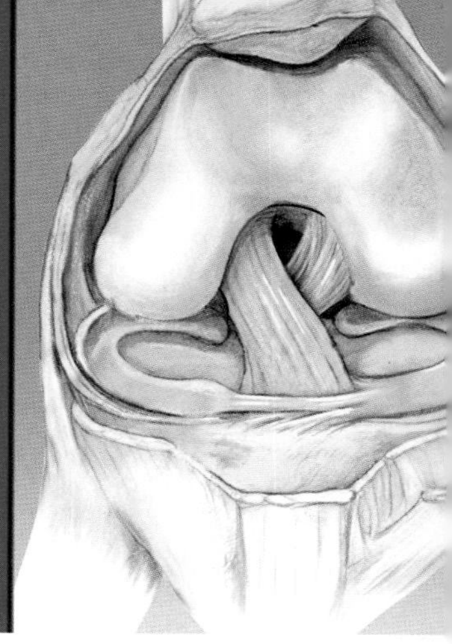

93

Imaging of the Knee

TIMOTHY SANDERS

Radiographs

Radiographs are often the initial imaging study performed for a patient presenting with knee pain, swelling, or decreased range of motion. Radiographs can also aid in the evaluation of numerous other clinical presentations, including suspected arthritis, osteonecrosis, instability, malalignment, patellofemoral tracking abnormalities, and postoperative pain. Radiographs are usually the initial imaging study performed to assess a suspected bone lesion (e.g., a tumor or infection) and to evaluate fracture healing or hardware complications. Standard imaging protocols vary depending on the clinical presentation but often include an anteroposterior, lateral, and tunnel view of the affected knee. Other supplemental views may be added depending on the clinical presentation (Table 93-1).

Radiographs are best suited for depicting abnormalities of the osseous structures such as fractures, dislocations, or bone lesions. Most athletic knee injuries, however, involve soft tissue structures rather than the bones, and the presence of subtle and seemingly insignificant osseous abnormalities can sometimes indicate the presence of a more serious soft tissue injury (Table 93-2). A thorough evaluation of the soft tissues should include a search for soft tissue swelling, loss of normal fat planes, soft tissue calcification (e.g., intraarticular body and vascular calcification), and joint effusion (including a fat-fluid level).

Computed Tomography

The most current generation of multidetector computed tomography (CT) scanners are capable of providing high-resolution images in all imaging planes and are superb for evaluating the extent and location of intraarticular fractures in the area of the knee. CT imaging can accurately depict the extent and location of articular surface incongruity, particularly as it pertains to the tibial plateau. It is also an excellent method of assessing fracture healing, including evaluation of malunion or nonunion, which is a common complication of fractures in the region of the tibial shaft and the area of the knee. CT imaging is the modality of choice in the evaluation of bone loss and tunnel position after anterior cruciate ligament (ACL) reconstruction. CT imaging can also accurately depict the matrix of a bone lesion, demonstrating osteoid, cartilage, or fibrous matrix to aid in diagnosing focal bone lesions. The administration of intraarticular contrast followed by CT imaging through the knee (CT arthrography) is an accurate means of assessing for internal derangement in patients who have a contraindication to magnetic resonance imaging (MRI).

Ultrasound

Ultrasound has limited usefulness with regard to evaluation of the knee. Although a few studies have been performed to assess the accuracy of detecting meniscal pathology with use of ultrasound, it has been shown that only the most peripheral portions of the meniscus can be assessed with ultrasound and that MRI is far more accurate for detection of meniscal tears and other internal derangement of the knee such as the cruciate ligament injury. Ultrasound can accurately assess the status of the collateral ligaments, as well as the quadriceps and patellar tendons, in cases of suspected injury. Ultrasound can also be a useful tool when a targeted evaluation of one of these structures is required. However, ultrasound is not generally accepted as a standard imaging technique for providing a global survey of the knee. The most common use of ultrasound of the knee is to assess for the presence of a Baker cyst and for directing aspiration of a cyst. Ultrasound is also an excellent means of assessing the large vessels of the knee and calf for the presence of arterial disease or deep venous thrombosis.

Magnetic Resonance Imaging

MRI is well accepted as the primary noninvasive imaging modality for global assessment of the knee and accurately depicts abnormalities of the ligaments, tendons, menisci, articular cartilage, and bones. It has a high negative predictive value with regard to the knee. Imaging protocols vary widely depending on the available equipment and the preferences of the imager. However, it is generally accepted that high-field strength magnets provide the highest quality images. Advancements in low-field strength system technology during the past few years have resulted in significant improvements in the overall image quality on the low field systems that are commonly used in the evaluation of the musculoskeletal system.

Use of a dedicated surface coil is mandatory to provide high-quality images regardless of the field strength of the magnetic resonance (MR) system. Images are performed in the sagittal, axial, and coronal imaging planes. The T2-weighted

TABLE 93-1

SUPPLEMENTAL RADIOGRAPHIC VIEWS OF THE KNEE

View	Clinical Concern
Standing anteroposterior	Alignment/joint space narrowing/arthritis
Axial (Merchant view)	Patellofemoral joint
Cross-table lateral	Joint effusion often accompanies internal derangement Fat-fluid level indicates intracapsular fracture
Oblique views	Identification of subtle fractures
Stress views	Ligamentous injury

images are often referred to as the *pathology images* and best depict injuries of the muscles, tendons, ligaments, and bone. Fat-saturation techniques are commonly applied to the T2-weighted sequences to improve conspicuity of the fluid, which is particularly helpful in the detection of bone marrow abnormalities such as bone contusions. T1-weighted and proton density images have the highest signal-to-noise ratio and are often described as the *anatomy images*. These images are best suited for detecting meniscal pathology and for depicting the anatomy of the knee.

MR arthrography (MRA) can be performed with either direct injection of gadolinium into the joint (direct MRA) or after injection of intravenous gadolinium (indirect MRA). MRA has been shown to more accurately assess the postoperative meniscus for persistent or recurrent tears compared with conventional MRI. It can also be helpful in the detection of intraarticular bodies and in the grading of osteochondral lesions. Studies have shown that direct and indirect MRA are equivalent in the evaluation of the postoperative meniscus except during the first postoperative year after meniscal repair, when indirect MRA can result in enhancement of the granulation tissue at the site of repair and mimic a recurrent tear, resulting in a false-positive study. Compared with direct MRA, indirect MRA has the advantage of being less invasive and does not necessarily require the presence of an on-site physician for administration of the contrast medium.

TABLE 93-2

SUBTLE RADIOGRAPHIC SIGNS ASSOCIATED WITH INTERNAL DERANGEMENT

Radiographic Sign	Associated Abnormality
Effusion	Internal derangement (nonspecific)
Fat-fluid level	Intracapsular fracture
Segond fracture	Anterior cruciate ligament tear
Deep lateral femoral sulcus	Anterior cruciate ligament tear
Arcuate sign (avulsion fracture fibular head)	Posterolateral corner injury
Avulsion fracture medial patellar facet	Transient patellar dislocation

Menisci

The presence of meniscal pathology is the most common reason for knee arthroscopy, and MRI is well accepted as an accurate, noninvasive, preoperative screening method for meniscal evaluation. The reported accuracy of MRI ranges between 92% and 95% for detection of meniscal tears, and it has been shown that the experience of the person who reads the images is an important factor with regard to overall accuracy. A thorough knowledge of the normal meniscal MR appearance and primary and secondary MRI signs of meniscal tear, along with an understanding of the common pitfalls and common sources of diagnostic error, are mandatory for achieving the highest level of accuracy with regard to the detection of meniscal pathology.

Normal MRI Appearance

The menisci are composed of fibrocartilage and therefore appear dark on all MR pulse sequences. The normal meniscus can demonstrate intrasubstance signal, but signal extending to the superior or inferior articular surfaces of the meniscus is usually indicative of pathology. Intrameniscal signal in a child or adolescent usually represents normal meniscal vascularity, whereas in an adult it most commonly indicates the presence of myxoid degeneration or meniscal contusion.

The sagittal and coronal low echo time pulse sequences (T1 and proton density) are the primary sequences used to detect meniscal pathology, and these images provide the highest sensitivity with regard to the detection of meniscal tears. The axial imaging plane can be complementary, particularly in the detection of a radial tear or a medial meniscal root injury. The T2-weighted images lack sensitivity with regard to detecting meniscal tears but provide increased specificity when compared with T1/proton density imaging.

Direct MRI Signs of Meniscal Tear

- Unequivocal surfacing signal seen on two contiguous images in the same imaging plane or in different imaging planes is nearly diagnostic of a meniscal tear (Fig. 93-1).

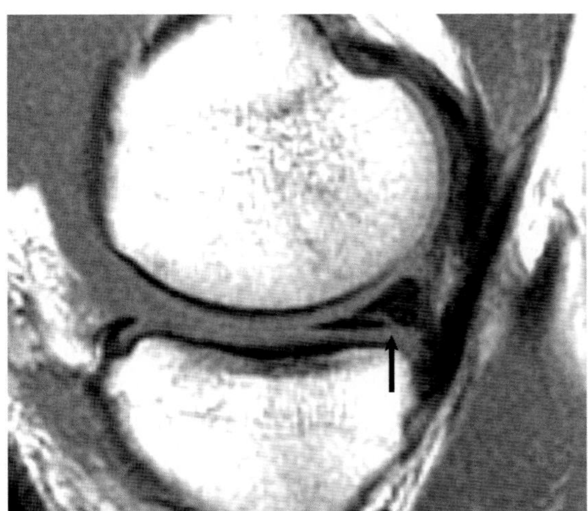

FIGURE 93-1 A meniscal tear. Unequivocal surfacing signal (*arrow*) extending to the articular surface of the meniscus is a direct magnetic resonance imaging sign of a meniscal tear.

The presence of surfacing signal on only a single image has no more than a 50% chance of representing a tear.

- Abnormal meniscal morphology in the absence of prior meniscal surgery, including missing or displaced meniscal tissue, is also diagnostic of a tear.
  - A double posterior cruciate ligament (PCL) sign (Fig. 93-2) results from a displaced bucket handle fragment of the medial meniscus located within the intercondylar notch just anterior to the PCL.
- Meniscocapsular separation is a sign of a meniscal tear.
- The presence of intrameniscal fluid signal on T2-weighted imaging is strongly indicative of a tear even in the absence of a surfacing signal.

Indirect MRI Signs of Meniscal Tear

Although most meniscal tears are easily identified with use of direct MRI signs, occasionally equivocal findings make detection of a meniscal tear difficult. In these instances, the presence of secondary or indirect signs can increase the confidence level of detecting a tear. Indirect imaging signs in and of themselves are not diagnostic of a meniscal tear but add significance to the presence of equivocal MR findings.

- The presence of a parameniscal cyst is usually associated with a horizontal or complex tear of the adjacent meniscus. A parameniscal cyst appears as a lobulated fluid-signal intensity mass on T2-weighted images and is usually located in direct contact with the adjacent meniscus (Fig. 93-3). Other cystic lesions about the knee, such as a pericruciate ganglion or fluid-filled bursae or ganglia, can mimic a parameniscal cyst on MRI.
- The presence of focal subchondral marrow edema underlying the meniscus or pericapsular soft tissue edema in cases of nonspecific findings is often seen in association with meniscal tears.
- Greater than 3 mm of extrusion of the meniscus along the medial joint line is often associated with a radial tear or meniscal root injury of the affected meniscus.

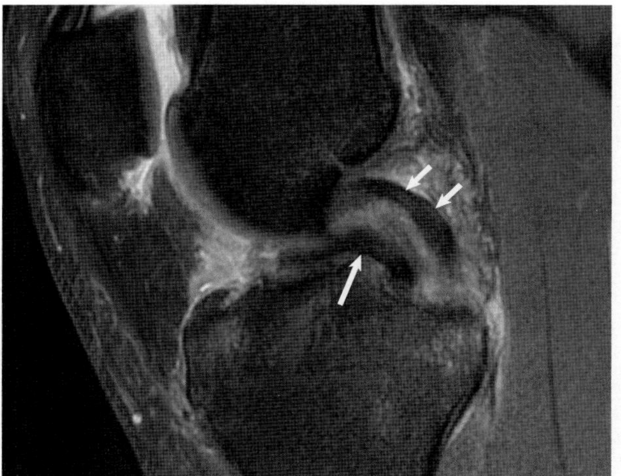

FIGURE 93-2 Double posterior cruciate ligament (PCL) sign. A displaced bucket handle fragment (*long arrow*) of the medial meniscus is located within the intercondylar notch just anterior to the PCL (*short arrows*). This appearance has been termed the "double PCL" sign and indicates a bucket handle tear of the medial meniscus.

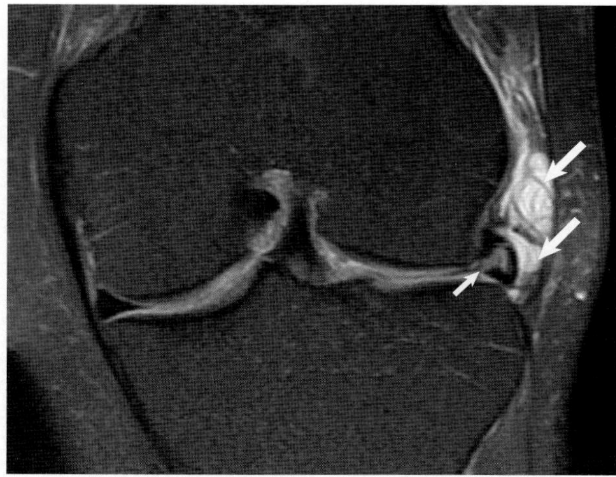

FIGURE 93-3 A parameniscal cyst. A complex fluid signal–intensity mass located in direct contact with the meniscus represents a parameniscal cyst (*large arrows*). The *small arrow* points to the associated meniscal tear of the lateral meniscus.

Pitfalls and Sources of Diagnostic Error with Regard to Detection of Meniscal Pathology

Although the overall accuracy of MRI in detecting meniscal tears is often quoted as being between 92% and 95%, to achieve this level of accuracy, the person reading the images must have a thorough knowledge and understanding of the common pitfalls and sources of diagnostic errors. These sources of errors can be broadly grouped into four categories:

- **MR artifact:** One of the most common sources of diagnostic error is the presence of patient motion artifact, which can result in an artifactual surfacing signal (Fig. 93-4). Great care should be taken when attempting to diagnose a meniscal tear in the presence of a patient motion artifact. Repeat imaging without patient motion is necessary to confirm the presence of true surfacing signal.
- **Normal anatomic structures located in close anatomic position to the meniscus:** The presence of an anatomic structure in close proximity to the meniscus can occasionally mimic grade III surfacing signal. The most common sources of errors include:
  - **Anterior transverse meniscal ligament** mimicking a tear of the anterior horn lateral meniscus (Fig. 93-5)
  - **Meniscofemoral ligament** mimicking a tear of the posterior horn lateral meniscus (Fig. 93-6)
  - **Popliteus tendon sheath** mimicking a tear of the posterior horn lateral meniscus
- **Miscellaneous conditions of the meniscus**
  - **Discoid meniscus** (Fig. 93-7) indicates a congenitally enlarged meniscus, involves the lateral meniscus in more than 90% of cases, and is associated with an increased incidence of both medial and lateral meniscal tears.
  - **Meniscal ossicles** represent an intrameniscal ossification, which most often occurs in the posterior horn of the medial meniscus near the meniscal root and demonstrates MR signal characteristics similar to

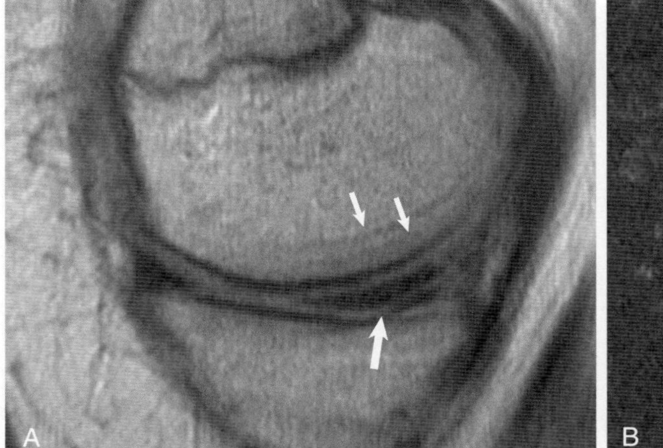

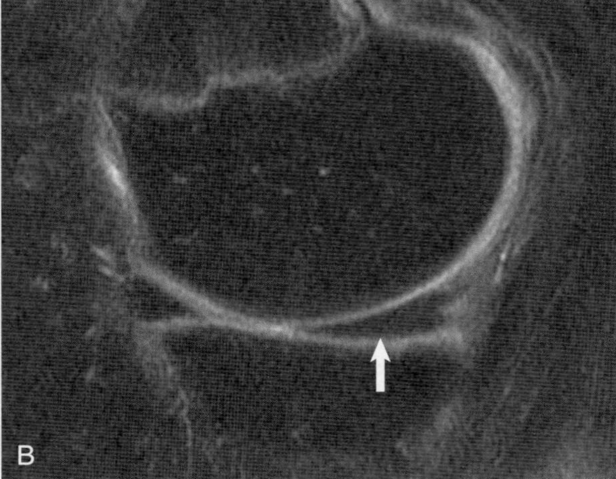

FIGURE 93-4 A motion artifact simulating a meniscal tear. The presence of patient motion on the image (**A**) results in a blurred image with repeating lines (*small arrows*) projected across the anatomy. One of these lines crosses the meniscus and simulates a tear (*large arrow*), resulting in a potential false-positive scan. The second image (**B**) obtained just moments later in the same patient who is lying still reveals a normal meniscus (*arrow*) with no evidence of a tear.

bone (increased T1-weighted signal) within the substance of the meniscus.

- **Postoperative meniscus**
  - The normal postoperative meniscus may demonstrate abnormal morphology or a persistent surfacing T1 signal. However, the presence of a surfacing fluid signal (seen on T2-weighted imaging), a displaced meniscal fragment, or a meniscal abnormality remote from the site of previous meniscal surgery are signs of persistent or recurrent meniscal tears.
  - Having knowledge of prior meniscal surgery is critical to avoid this pitfall. MRI scans often contain clues that indicate prior arthroscopic surgery, such as linear arthrofibrosis in Hoffa's fat pad that correlates with the arthroscopic surgical tract.
  - Postoperative changes that can mimic a tear include a persistent surfacing signal on low echo time sequences, abnormal meniscal morphology, or missing meniscal tissue.

Anterior Cruciate Ligament

The ACL is composed of two separate bundles, the anteromedial and posterolateral bundles, so named for their tibial attachments. The ligament originates along the intercondylar notch portion of the lateral femoral condyle and inserts distally on the tibia near the anterior tibial spine.

High-quality MRI is considered approximately 95% accurate in the detection of an acute ACL tear (similar to that of physical examination) and is slightly less accurate in the detection of chronic ACL disruption. The role of MRI is to confirm the clinical suspicion of ACL injury and to differentiate a partial-thickness tear from a full-thickness tear. MRI can also delineate the location of a tear (proximal, midsubstance,

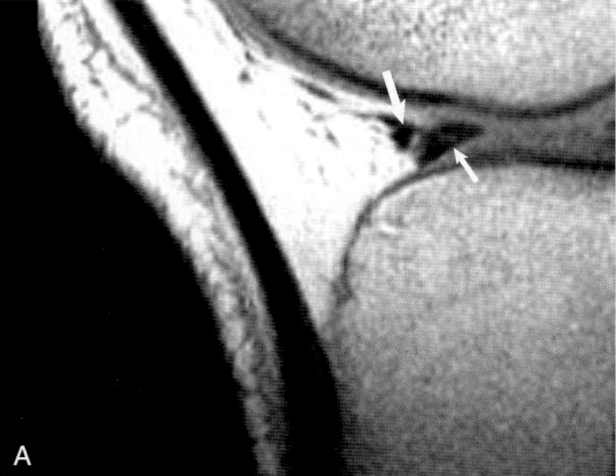

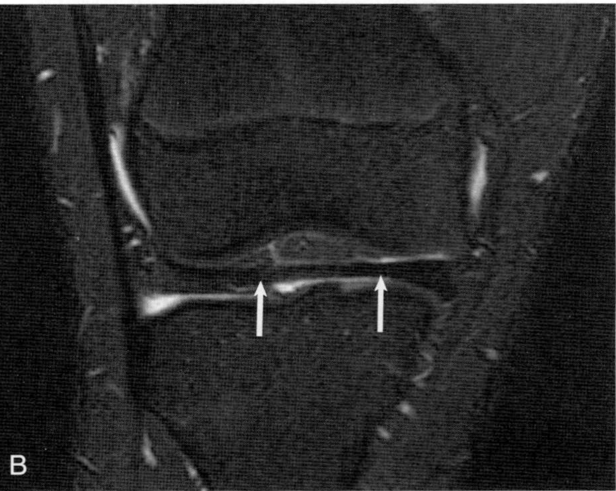

FIGURE 93-5 An anterior transverse meniscal ligament simulating a meniscal tear. A sagittal image through the anterior aspect of the knee (**A**) demonstrates a gap between the anterior transverse meniscal ligament (*large arrow*) and the adjacent anterior horn of the lateral meniscus (*small arrow*), which can simulate surfacing signal and potentially mimic a meniscal tear. A coronal image through the anterior aspect of the knee (**B**) shows the anterior transverse meniscal ligament (*arrows*).

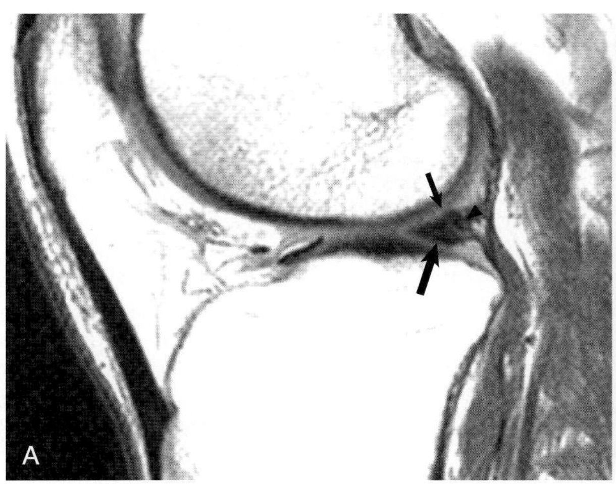

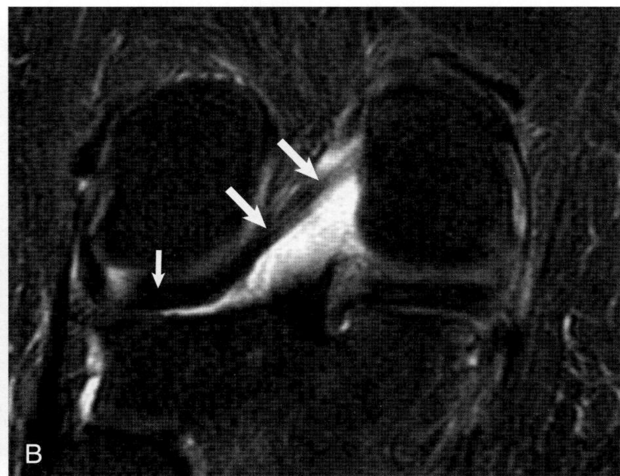

FIGURE 93-6 A meniscofemoral ligament simulating a meniscal tear. A sagittal image through the posterolateral aspect of the knee (**A**) shows the attachment of the meniscofemoral ligament (*arrowhead*) to the posterior horn lateral meniscus (*large arrow*). The linear signal (*small arrow*) between the two structures can mimic a tear of the lateral meniscus. A coronal image through the posterior aspect of the knee (**B**) shows the course of the meniscofemoral ligament (*large arrows*) as it extends from the inner aspect of the medial femoral condyle to attach to the posterior horn of the lateral meniscus (*small arrow*).

or distal) and detect the presence of an osseous avulsion injury. In addition, MRI plays an important role in the detection of associated meniscal, cartilage, and concomitant ligament injury.

Normal MRI Appearance of the Anterior Cruciate Ligament

Sagittal T2-weighted images provide the primary evaluation of the ACL (Fig. 93-8), with coronal and axial T2-weighted images being complementary. The axial images are particularly useful in the evaluation of the proximal attachment of the ACL. The two bundles are closely opposed proximally but fan out distally with broadening of the ligament distally with interspersed fibro-fatty tissue that results in intermediate signal striations within the substance of the ACL fibers distally. The striated appearance of the distal ACL should not be misinterpreted as an ACL injury. The ACL fibers should appear continuous, and on the sagittal images, the ACL should parallel but not touch the roof of the intercondylar notch.

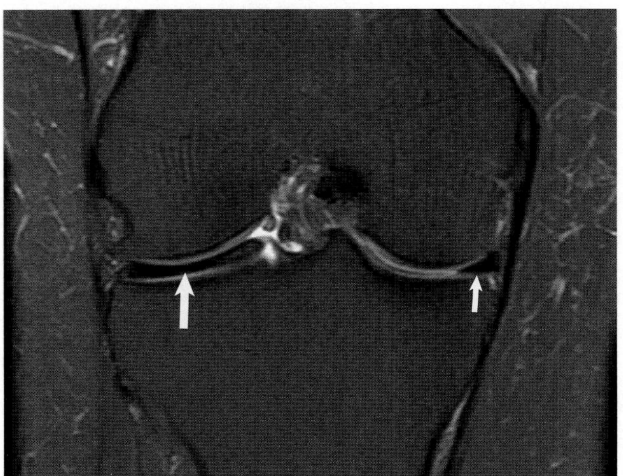

FIGURE 93-7 A large lateral discoid meniscus (*large arrow*). Note the size of the normal medial meniscus (*small arrow*).

Direct Signs of Anterior Cruciate Ligament Tear

The presence of any of the following findings indicates an ACL injury.

- Complete disruption or discontinuity of the ACL fibers (Fig. 93-9)
- An edematous-appearing mass in the expected location of the ACL fibers

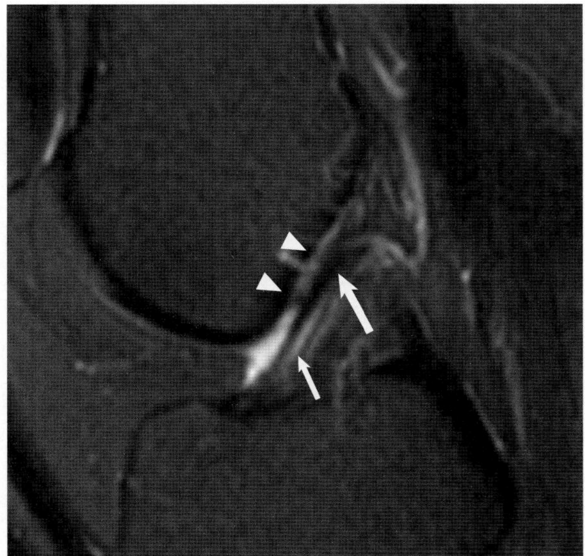

FIGURE 93-8 The normal magnetic resonance imaging appearance of the anterior cruciate ligament (ACL) in the sagittal imaging plane. The ACL fibers (*large arrow*) appear taut and parallel the roof of the intercondylar notch (*arrowheads*). Notice that the normal distal ACL (*small arrow*) demonstrates a striated appearance that represents fibro-fatty tissue located between the two bundles of the ACL. This appearance should not be mistaken for ACL injury.

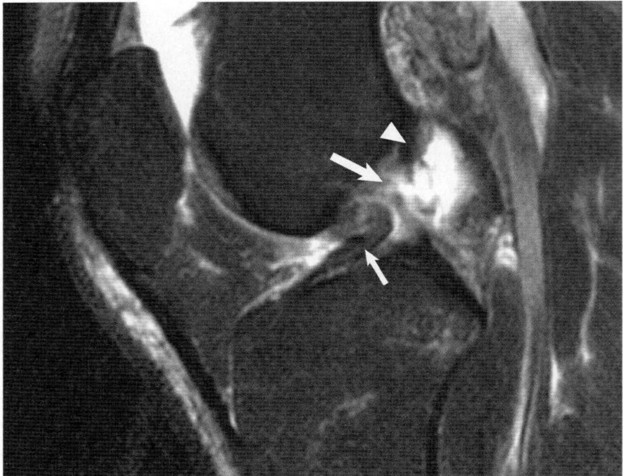

FIGURE 93-9 Complete disruption of the anterior cruciate ligament (ACL). A fluid-filled gap (*large arrow*) is located between the proximal ACL fibers (*arrowhead*) and the distal fibers (*small arrow*) that are displaced inferiorly within the intercondylar notch.

- The "empty notch" sign: fluid signal is seen at the expected proximal attachment site (best depicted on axial T2-weighted images)
- Avulsion fracture at the distal attachment site (most commonly occurs in adolescents and young adults)
- Posterior or inferior drooping of the ACL fibers
- Partial-thickness tear: edema/fluid signal within the substance of the ligament but with some definite intact fibers or single bundle disruption with an intact second bundle
- Chronic disruption: nonvisualization of the ACL fibers in all imaging planes

Indirect Signs Associated with an Anterior Cruciate Ligament Tear

Secondary imaging signs include numerous osseous abnormalities that occur at the time of injury and are usually most prominent in the setting of an acute ACL injury, becoming less obvious over time. The presence of an indirect sign of ACL injury is a strong indicator of ACL injury and should prompt a thorough search for direct signs confirming the presence of an ACL injury:

- Pivot shift bone contusion pattern: lateral femoral condyle and posterolateral tibia (Fig. 93-10)
- The presence of marrow edema within the posteromedial tibia in the setting of an ACL tear, which has a very high association with an accompanying medial meniscal tear
- The deep lateral femoral sulcus sign measuring greater than 1.5 mm in depth with irregularity of the cortex in the region of the lateral femoral sulcus (often seen in conjunction with a pivot shift bone contusion pattern)
- A Segond fracture (an avulsion fracture of the lateral tibial cortex associated with lateral capsule avulsion)
- The anterior drawer sign, buckling of the PCL, and acute hemarthrosis are less specific findings that are often seen in association with an ACL injury

Pitfalls and Sources of Diagnostic Error with Regard to Detection of Anterior Cruciate Ligament Tears

- Poor image quality and patient motion artifact are two sources of common diagnostic error.
- A small cortical fracture fragment at the distal attachment site of the ACL can easily be overlooked, especially on T2-weighted images. T1-weighted images without fat saturation are best for depicting a small cortical avulsion fracture fragment at the distal attachment site of the ACL.
- Myxoid degeneration of the ACL (Fig. 93-11) is a degenerative process of the ACL often seen in conjunction with pericruciate or intracruciate ganglion formation and can mimic an ACL injury. The appearance of ACL myxoid degeneration has been described as a "celery stalk" appearance with thickening and splaying of the fibers with intermediate signal within the fibers, but no discontinuity of the fibers and the absence of indirect imaging signs of an ACL injury. Myxoid degeneration of the ACL is often seen in association with a posterior horn medial meniscal root avulsion injury.

Posterior Cruciate Ligament

The PCL arises along the inner aspect of the medial femoral condyle and inserts distally onto the posterior slanted portion of the tibia. The PCL has three separate components that are named for their femoral attachments followed by their tibial attachment site: an anterolateral bundle, followed by the smaller posteromedial bundle, and finally the meniscofemoral ligaments of Humphrey and Wrisberg. The PCL is less commonly injured than the ACL, and injury is often partial thickness in nature.

Normal MRI Appearance of the Posterior Cruciate Ligament

The PCL (Fig. 93-12) is best evaluated using T2-weighted sagittal images; axial and coronal images are complementary

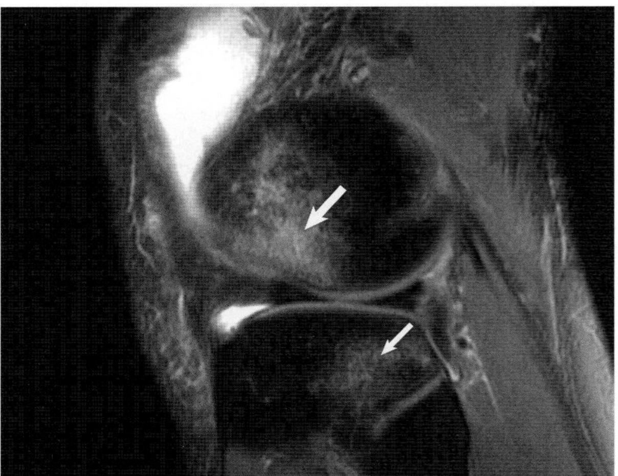

FIGURE 93-10 A pivot shift bone contusion pattern. Bone contusions within the midportion of the lateral femoral condyle (*large arrow*) and the posterior aspect of the lateral tibial plateau (*small arrow*) indicate a recent pivot shift injury and have a high association with an anterior cruciate ligament tear. Note the large associated joint effusion.

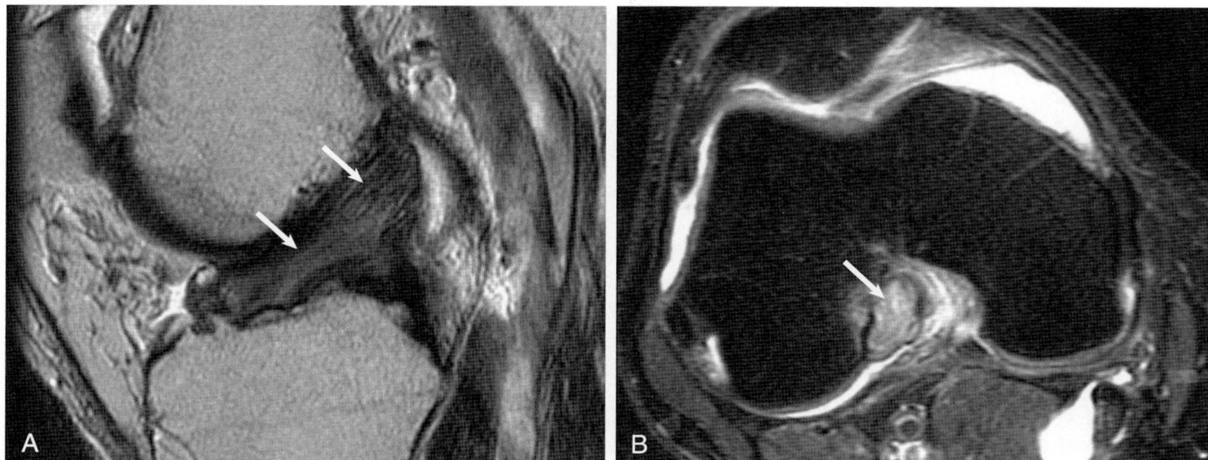

FIGURE 93-11 Myxoid degeneration of the anterior cruciate ligament (ACL). A sagittal image (**A**) reveals thickening and splaying of the ACL fibers (*arrows*) typical of myxoid degeneration. An axial image (**B**) also reveals thickening and splaying of the ACL fibers (*arrow*). The fibers are intact, and this appearance should not be mistaken for an ACL tear/injury.

but rarely necessary to establish the diagnosis of a PCL injury. The PCL is roughly twice the thickness of the ACL and typically demonstrates uniformly low signal throughout. MRI of the knee is routinely performed with the knee in full extension. As a result, the PCL is lax and is seen as a curved or arcuate-appearing bandlike structure that extends from the inner aspect of the medial femoral condyle to the posterior slanted portion of the tibia. The meniscofemoral ligaments are best depicted on the sagittal and coronal images seen extending from the inner aspect of the medial femoral condyle and inserting onto the posterior horn of the lateral meniscus.

Direct Signs of Posterior Cruciate Ligament Injury

Most PCL injuries are partial thickness in nature and appear on MRI as edema within the substance of the ligament or fluid signal, extending partially through the substance of the ligament, most often involving the posteromedial bundle.

Full-thickness tears are less common and appear as complete disruption or discontinuity of the fibers (with the fluid signal on T2 images completely traversing the fibers of the PCL), most often in the midsubstance of the ligament (Fig. 93-13). Avulsion fractures can occur at the tibial attachment site. These fracture fragments are often large with varying degrees of fracture fragment displacement. MRI demonstrates discontinuity of the cortex with cortical step-off and associated marrow edema. An avulsion fracture can rarely occur at the femoral attachment site and is referred to as a *peel-off injury*, best depicted on T1-weighted images.

Chronic injury may present as complete absence of PCL fibers on MRI, or occasionally in the setting of a chronic PCL

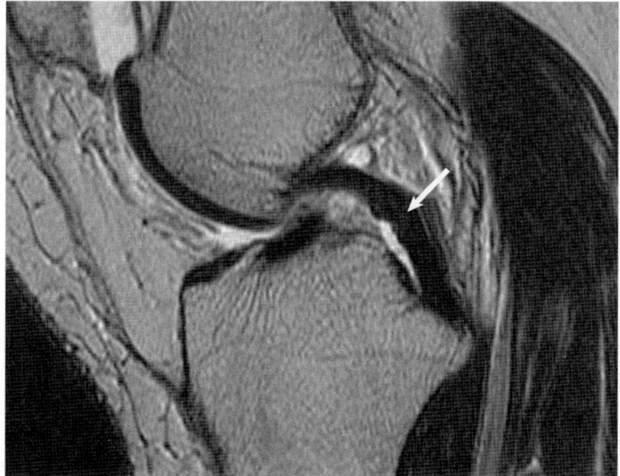

FIGURE 93-12 The normal magnetic resonance imaging (MRI) appearance of the posterior cruciate ligament (PCL). The PCL (*arrow*) is roughly twice the thickness of the anterior cruciate ligament and appears as a curvilinear low–signal-intensity structure on sagittal MRI.

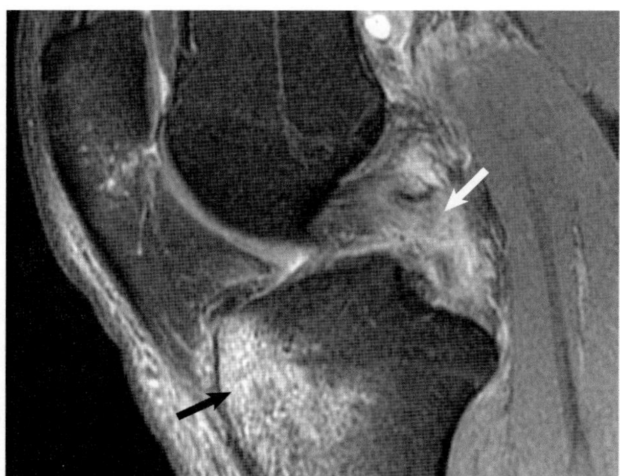

FIGURE 93-13 A complete tear of the posterior cruciate ligament (PCL). Complete discontinuity of the PCL fibers is seen (*white arrow*). A bone contusion (*black arrow*) of the anterior proximal tibia is referred to as the "dashboard" bone contusion pattern, which is commonly associated with PCL injury.

injury, the edema and fluid signal associated with the acute injury resolves and the torn PCL fibers will attach to an adjacent structure through scarring, giving the appearance of an intact PCL in the setting of a clinically incompetent ligament.

Indirect Signs of a Posterior Cruciate Ligament Injury

As with ACL injuries, the secondary signs of a PCL injury are typically bone abnormalities that result from contusions that occur at the time of injury.

- The most common secondary finding of PCL injury is the "dashboard" bone contusion pattern (Fig. 93-13) that is located within the anterior aspect of the proximal tibia and occurs as a result of the flexed knee striking against an object such as the dashboard during an motor vehicle accident or against the ground at the time of a fall. The dashboard contusion pattern has a high association with PCL injury.
- Less common and less specific secondary findings associated with PCL injury include a "kissing" contusion pattern of a hyperextension mechanism of injury, a fibular head avulsion fracture associated with conjoined tendon avulsion, and the medial Segond fracture resulting from an avulsion of the medial capsular structures.

Pitfalls and Sources of Diagnostic Error with Regard to Detection of Posterior Cruciate Ligament Tears

Small cortical avulsion fractures at the proximal attachment site of the PCL can be difficult to detect on MRI and are often associated with only minimal marrow edema. The T1-weighted images are usually best for detecting small avulsion fracture fragments. Myxoid degeneration and pericruciate ganglion formation of the PCL can mimic PCL sprain or partial-thickness injury. Myxoid degeneration typically appears as slightly increased T2-signal with mild thickening of the ligament but lacks fluid signal within the substance of the ligament. Secondary signs such as the dashboard contusion pattern are absent in the setting of myxoid degeneration but are often present with PCL injury.

Medial Collateral Ligament

The medial collateral ligament (MCL) complex has been divided into three anatomic layers. The most superficial layer includes the deep fascia along the medial aspect of the knee. The second layer is composed of the superficial fibers of the MCL. The third layer is composed of the medial joint line capsule and includes the deep fibers of the MCL.

Normal MRI Appearance of the Medial Collateral Ligament

The MCL is best evaluated on coronal T2-weighted images with a fat saturation technique that increases the conspicuity of adjacent soft tissue edema. The MCL is a bandlike structure that appears dark on T2-weighted images and has a proximal femoral attachment on the adductor tubercle. The fibers extend in a vertical fashion and attach distally to the tibia approximately 5 cm below the joint line. The MCL measures approximately 8 to 10 cm in length and 1.5 cm in anteroposterior dimension.

Direct MRI Signs of Medial Collateral Ligament Injury

A three-point MRI grading system is used to describe the extent of an MCL injury. The location of an MCL injury should be described as proximal or distal.

- Grade I (sprain): Edema (seen as an increased T2 signal) is noted superficially or within the substance of the MCL, often with thickening of the fibers (Fig. 93-14, *A*)
- Grade II (partial-thickness tear): A partial-thickness tear or discontinuity of the superficial fibers of the MCL, often with retraction of the superficial fibers; the deep fibers remain intact (Fig. 93-14, *B*)
- Grade III (full-thickness tear): A complete tear is seen as a disruption of the superficial and deep fibers of the MCL, often with retraction of the torn fibers and adjacent soft tissue edema (Fig. 93-14, *C*)

Old or chronic MCL injuries are often depicted on MRI as persistent thickening of the MCL fibers but lack the acute findings of soft tissue edema. *Pellegrini-Stieda* refers to heterotopic bone formation within the substance of the MCL that is often associated with an old injury and is best depicted on radiographs of the knee.

Indirect MRI Signs of Medial Collateral Ligament Injury

The most common indirect sign of MCL injury is a bone contusion located along the peripheral aspect of the lateral femoral condyle resulting from a direct contact injury to the lateral aspect of the knee associated with a valgus mechanism of injury, such as occurs during a "clipping" mechanism of injury often seen in American football (see Fig. 93-14, *C*).

Pitfalls and Sources of Diagnostic Error with Regard to Detection of Medial Collateral Ligament Tears

Soft tissue edema deep to the MCL is most often reactive in nature and associated with an intraarticular process such as internal derangement and should not be misinterpreted as an injury of the MCL. Edema isolated to the region of the adductor tubercle may be associated with injury to the medial patellofemoral ligament and associated with a previous patellar dislocation rather than an MCL injury.

Lateral Collateral Ligament Complex/ Posterolateral Corner Structures

The iliotibial band that is the distal extension of the iliotibial track represents the most anterior structure on the lateral side of the knee and inserts distally onto the tibia at the level of Gerdy's tubercle. The lateral collateral ligament complex/ posterolateral corner (PLC) is composed of a group of superficial structures that include the lateral head gastrocnemius muscle and tendon, fibular collateral ligament, biceps femoris tendon, and conjoined tendon. Deep structures include the popliteus muscle and tendon, arcuate and popliteofibular ligament, and finally the posterior capsule.

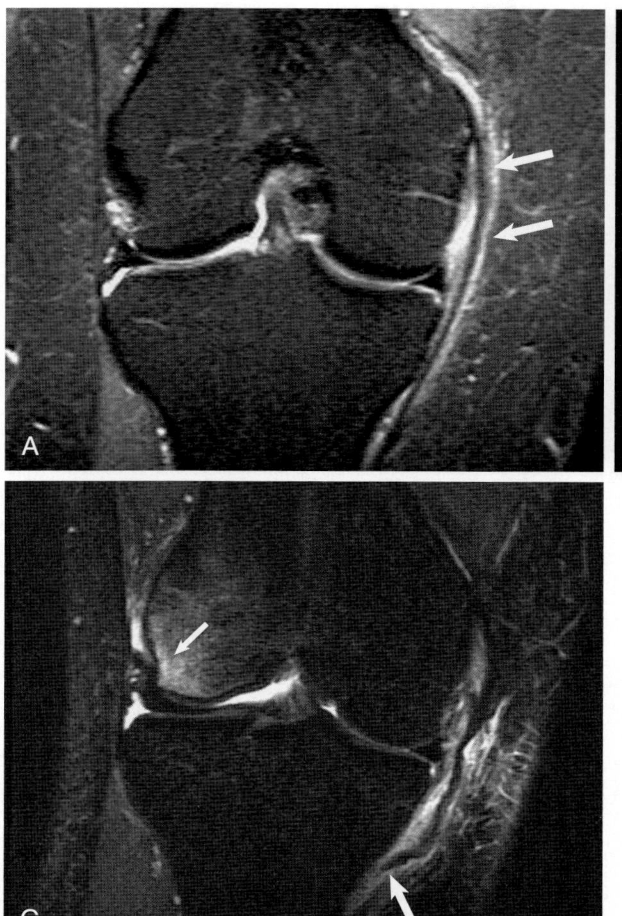

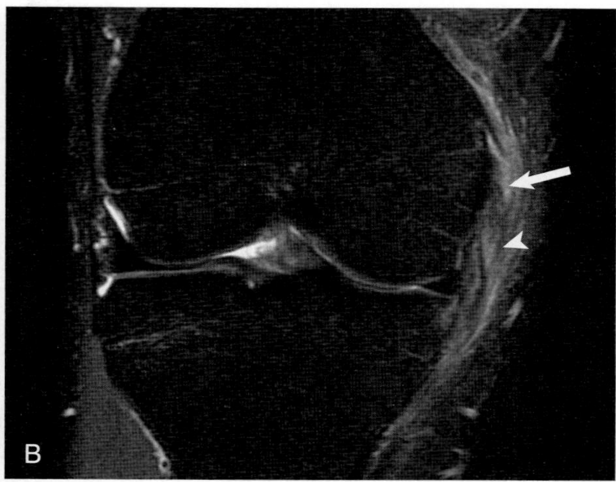

FIGURE 93-14 The magnetic resonance imaging grading system of medial collateral ligament (MCL) injuries. **A,** Grade I injury shows soft tissue edema (*arrows*) superficial to MCL fibers, which appear intact. **B,** Grade II injury shows thickening and edema of the MCL fibers (*arrows*), indicating partial-thickness tearing of the fibers. **C,** A grade III injury of the MCL at its distal attachment site shows a complete disruption, with retraction of the torn fibers (*arrow*). A bone contusion (*arrowhead*) within the lateral femoral condyle indicates a recent injury resulting from direct trauma to the lateral aspect of the knee.

Normal MRI Appearance of the Lateral Collateral Ligament Complex

The iliotibial band is a long, thin, bandlike, low–signal-intensity structure that extends along the anterolateral aspect of the knee just superficial to the lateral femoral condyle and inserts distally onto Gerdy's tubercle. The anatomy of the PLC is complex, and an accurate assessment with MRI requires a separate evaluation of each anatomic structure using all three imaging planes. PLC injury is often accompanied by soft tissue edema located along the posterolateral aspect of the knee. The presence of edema along the posterolateral aspect of the knee mandates assessment of the PLC structures. T2-weighted images with fat saturation in all three planes are required to detect the extent of injury.

Direct Signs of Lateral Collateral Ligament/ Posterolateral Corner Structure Injury

Iliotibial band friction syndrome is best depicted on coronal T2-weighted MRI. Soft tissue edema is seen deep to the iliotibial band and superficial to the lateral femoral condyle (Fig. 93-15). In severe or chronic cases, thickening of the iliotibial band or subcortical marrow edema of the lateral femoral condyle may occur. A tear of the iliotibial band appears as complete disruption of the structure or as an avulsion fracture of Gerdy's tubercle.

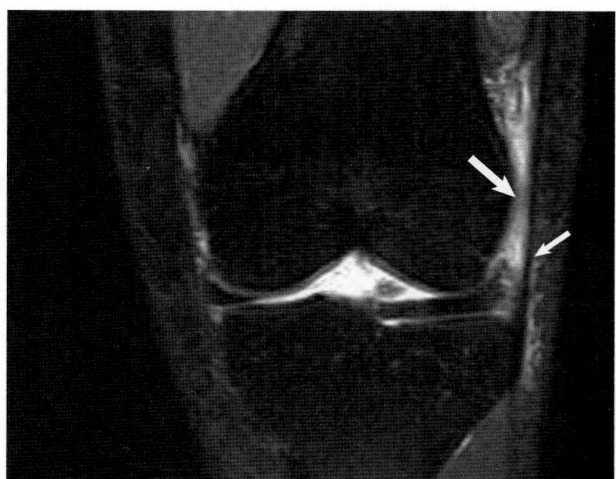

FIGURE 93-15 Iliotibial band syndrome. Soft tissue edema (*large arrow*) is noted deep to the iliotibial band (*small arrow*), indicative of iliotibial band syndrome.

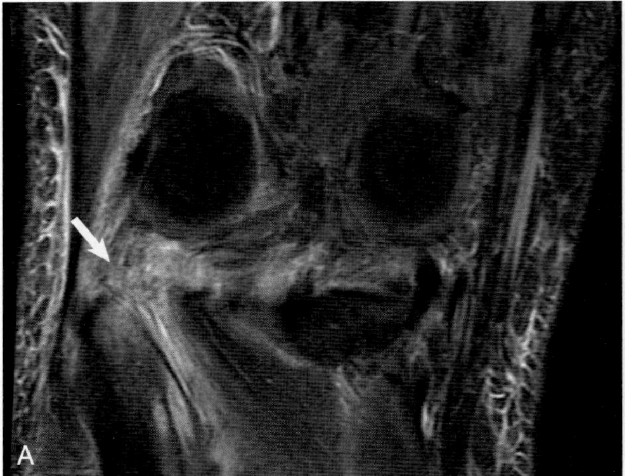

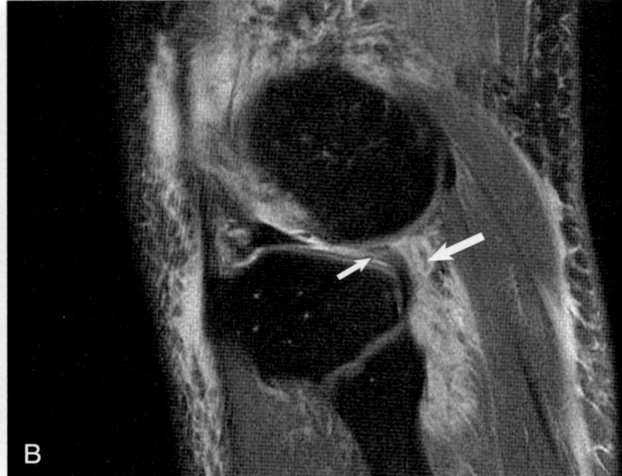

FIGURE 93-16 Posterolateral corner injury. A coronal T2-weighted image (**A**) shows extensive soft tissue edema (*arrow*) along the posterolateral aspect of the knee. A sagittal T2-weighted image (**B**) shows a high-grade tear of the posterolateral corner structures (*large arrow*) with a tear (*small arrow*) of the posterior horn of the lateral meniscus.

Injury of the PLC structures is graded similar to an MCL injury, with each anatomic structure evaluated and graded separately (Fig. 93-16) as follows: grade I = sprain, grade II = partial-thickness tear, and grade III = full-thickness tear.

Indirect Signs of Lateral Collateral Ligament/Posterolateral Corner Structure Injury

Diffuse soft tissue edema located along the posterolateral aspect of the knee can be associated with an ACL injury. The presence of soft tissue edema requires a thorough evaluation of each separate anatomic structure.

Pitfalls and Sources of Diagnostic Error with Regard to Detection of Iliotibial Band/Posterolateral Corner Injury

The most common source of error with regard to diagnosing iliotibial friction band syndrome is to misinterpret the presence of joint fluid as soft tissue edema deep to the iliotibial band. Axial T2-weighted images can help differentiate joint fluid from soft tissue edema deep to the iliotibial band.

In the presence of a massive complete disruption of the PLC, it is rarely challenging to make the appropriate diagnosis on MRI. Partial-thickness injury or a subtle high-grade injury such as avulsion of the popliteofibular ligament from the fibular head can be clinically important, and detection requires a systematic evaluation of each anatomic structure using all three imaging planes.

Extensor Mechanism

The extensor mechanism is a complex anatomic region of the knee. The patella, which tracks within the trochlear groove portion of the distal femur, is the largest sesamoid in the body. The medial and lateral patellar retinaculum act to stabilize the patella within the trochlear groove. Finally, the suprapatellar and infrapatellar fat pads and the adjacent bursae act to cushion and protect the other structures of the extensor mechanism. Several pathologic processes can affect this anatomic region of the knee, including patellar instability and tracking abnormalities, quadriceps and patellar injuries, and inflammatory changes of the fat pads and bursae.

Normal MRI Appearance of the Extensor Mechanism

The quadriceps tendon is a multislip tendon that arises out of the distal quadriceps musculature and inserts onto the superior pole of the patella. Although the tendon appears dark on MR pulse sequences, it contains longitudinally oriented intermediate signal intensity striations or streaks that represent fibro-fatty tissue situated between the various strands of the multislip tendon. The patellar tendon arises along the inferior pole of the patella and inserts onto the anterior tibial tubercle. It demonstrates homogeneously low signal and lacks the internal striations that are seen within the quadriceps tendon. On MRI, the medial soft tissue restraints of the patella appear as thin bandlike structures arising along the medial aspect of the patella. The medial soft tissue restraints are composed of the medial retinaculum, the medial patellotibial ligament, which extends from the inferior pole of the patella to insert on the tibia, and the medial patellofemoral ligament, which extends from the superior pole of the patella to attach on the adductor tubercle of the distal femur. The fat pads demonstrate fat signal intensity on all MR pulse sequences and in the absence of disease should be free of edema and inflammatory changes.

Sagittal T2-weighted images are the primary means of evaluating the patellar and quadriceps tendons, the articular surface of the trochlear groove, and the bursae and fat pads. Axial images serve a complementary role with regard to evaluating each of these structures and serve as the primary means of evaluating the articular surface of the patella and the patellar reticulum.

Direct MRI Signs of Extensor Mechanism Injury

Injuries of the quadriceps and patellar tendons include tendinosis, partial-thickness tears, and full-thickness tears. In the acute setting, tendinosis appears as thickening and an intermediate signal within the substance of the tendon. A partial-thickness tear appears as fluid signal extending partially through the involved structure (Fig. 93-17), whereas an acute full-thickness tear appears as complete discontinuity of the tendon with retraction of the tendon ends and a fluid-filled gap (Fig. 93-18). In the setting of chronic tendinosis, soft

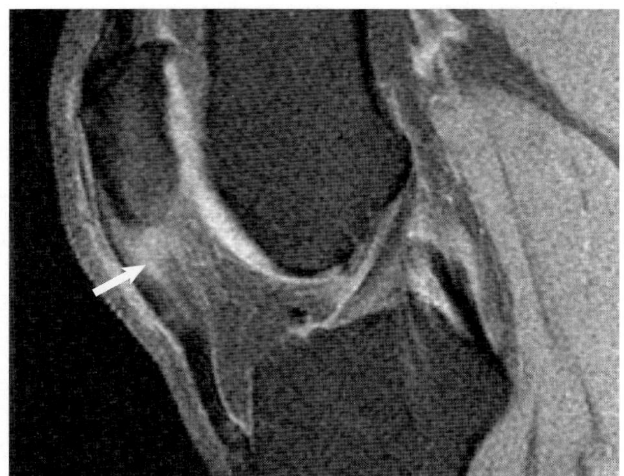

FIGURE 93-17 A partial-thickness tear of the patellar tendon. Thickening and edema of the proximal patellar tendon is present, with a linear area of bright T2-weighted signal indicating a partial-thickness longitudinal tear (*arrow*).

tissue calcification may appear within the substance of the involved tendon. Edema within Hoffa's fat pad may indicate a primary abnormality of the fat pad or may represent reactive changes associated with adjacent pathology.

Indirect MRI Signs of Extensor Mechanism Injury

Soft tissue edema and swelling is often noted adjacent to an area of patellar or quadriceps tendon abnormality. These changes may occur within the prepatellar soft tissues, in the underlying fat pad, or within an adjacent bursa. Patella baja can occur with a quadriceps tendon tear, whereas patella alta is often seen in association with a tear of the patellar tendon.

Pitfalls and Sources of Diagnostic Error with Regard to Detection of an Extensor Mechanism Injury

- Subtle increased T1 signal abnormality is often noted at the proximal attachment of the patellar tendon and in the absence of an abnormal T2 signal is considered a normal finding and should not be considered a sign of patellar tendinosis.
- The intrasubstance linear striations within the distal 3 to 4 cm of the quadriceps tendon are considered a normal MR appearance representing the multislip appearance of the tendon. Tendinosis presents as thickening and ill-defined increased signal within the tendon.
- Thickening of the distal insertion of the patellar tendon associated with enlargement or fragmentation of the tibial tubercle can represent an asymptomatic finding associated with a previous case of Osgood-Schlatter disease. An acute process of the distal patellar tendon attachment usually is accompanied by adjacent soft tissue swelling, marrow edema, and pain.

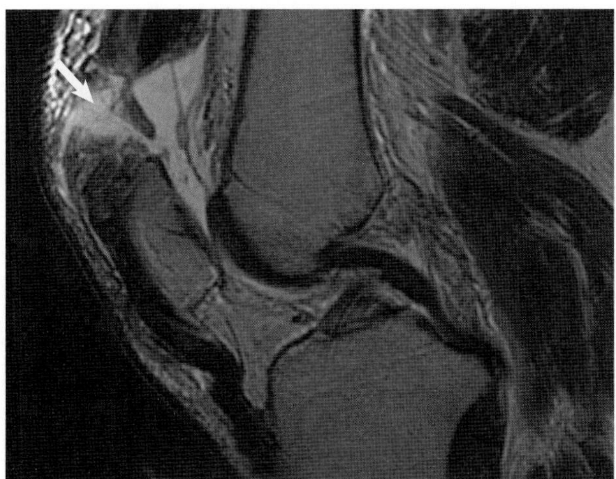

FIGURE 93-18 A complete tear of the quadriceps tendon. Complete discontinuity of the quadriceps tendon is seen with a fluid-filled gap (*arrow*) indicating a full-thickness tear.

Patella

MRI After Transient Dislocation of the Patella

Transient dislocation of the patella usually occurs in young athletes as a result of a twisting injury. If the patella spontaneously reduces after transient dislocation, the patient may not realize the true nature of the injury.

Direct MRI Signs of Recent Transient Dislocation of the Patella

- Bone contusion of the lateral femoral condyle and lower pole medial patellar facet occurs as a result of the patella impacting the lateral femoral condyle at the time of dislocation (Fig. 93-19).
- Osteochondral injuries can occur in the region of the lower pole of the patella or along the peripheral margin of the lateral femoral condyle. Chondral injuries can range from low-grade fissuring and fraying to full-thickness osteochondral lesions with detached and displaced osteochondral fragments (see Fig. 93-19).

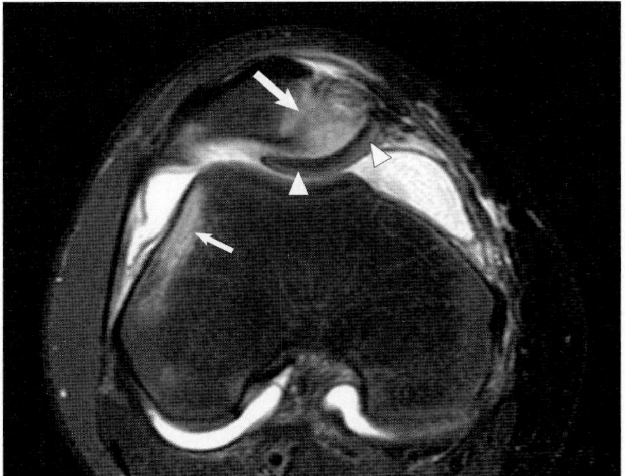

FIGURE 93-19 A previous transient patellar dislocation. A bone contusion of the anterior peripheral aspect of the lateral femoral condyle (*small arrow*) and of the lower pole of the medial patellar facet (*large arrow*) is present, indicating a recent transient dislocation of the patella. A large detached and displaced osteochondral fragment (*arrowheads*) is also present within the anterior aspect of the knee.

- Injury to the soft tissue restraints of the patella can include injury of the medial patellar retinaculum and the medial patellofemoral ligament. On MRI, the medial patellofemoral ligament appears as a bandlike structure that extends from the superior pole of the patella to the adductor tubercle and sits just deep to the vastus medialis obliquus muscle; it is best evaluated with T2-weighted axial images. Injuries are graded as grade I sprain, grade II partial-thickness tear, and grade III complete tear. Injury usually occurs at the femoral attachment site but can also occur at the patellar attachment site.

Indirect Signs of Recent Transient Dislocation of the Patella

- Large joint hemarthrosis or lipohemarthrosis in the presence of an osteochondral fracture of the patella
- Loose bodies in the setting of the typical bone contusion pattern

Osseous Structures and Articular Surfaces

Normal MRI Appearance of Articular Cartilage

Articular cartilage demonstrates intermediate signal intensity on T2-weighted and proton density imaging. The underlying cortex of bone appears as a dark low–signal-intensity line, and the cartilage is easily differentiated from fluid in the joint, which appears bright on T2-weighted and proton density imaging. Numerous cartilage-specific MR pulse sequences have been developed; however, T2-weighted and proton density with fat saturation are by far the most common pulse sequences used in everyday practice to evaluate the articular surfaces. MRI accuracy ranges between 90% and 94% in the detection of arthroscopically visible cartilage lesions of the knee.

It is essential to use all three imaging planes to adequately assess all of the articular surfaces of the knee. The patellar articular cartilage is best evaluated on axial and sagittal images, whereas the tibial plateau and femoral condyle articular surfaces are best seen on coronal and sagittal images. The trochlear groove articular cartilage is best evaluated using the sagittal images.

Direct MRI Signs of Articular Cartilage Abnormalities

Several MR grading systems have been proposed for describing chondral abnormalities. A commonly used system is a four-point variation of the Outerbridge classification system.

- Grade 0: Normal articular cartilage
- Grade I: Chondral signal change in the absence of morphologic abnormalities, thought to represent chondral softening; MRI correlates poorly with grade I softening of the articular cartilage found at arthroscopy
- Grade II: Chondral surface irregularity, fissuring, and fraying that extends up to 50% through the thickness of the cartilage (Fig. 93-20)
- Grade III: Deep chondral fissuring and fraying extending greater than 50% through the thickness of the articular cartilage
- Grade IV: Full-thickness chondral loss with exposed underlying bone, often associated with subchondral signal abnormalities such as edema, sclerosis, and subchondral cysts

In addition to this grading system, other modifiers such as "chondral fissuring," "fraying," "flap tear," or "delamination injuries" are often used to further describe chondral lesions.

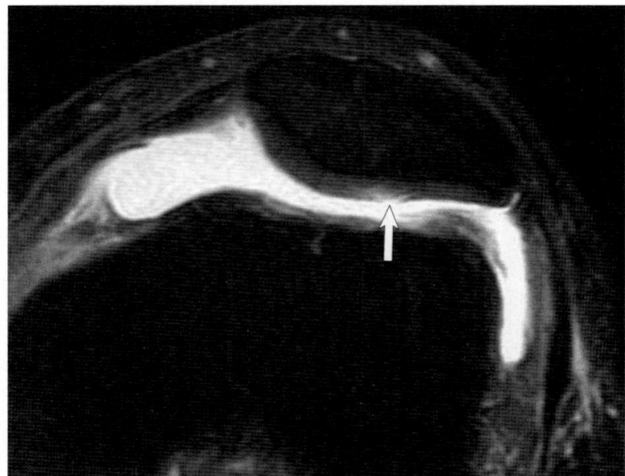

FIGURE 93-20 Chondromalacia patella. A focal area of grade II chondromalacia of the patella is seen with partial-thickness fissuring and fraying (*arrow*) of the articular cartilage of the lateral patellar facet.

Osteochondritis dissecans (OCD) refers to a focal isolated osteochondral lesion in the absence of other chondral abnormalities. The juvenile form refers to an OCD lesion that occurs in the presence of open growth plates and has a better prognosis than the adult form of OCD, which occurs after closure of the growth plates. The MR grading system of osteochondritis dissecans is as follows:

- Grade I: Focal subchondral marrow edema with intact overlying cortex and articular cartilage
- Grade II: A partially detached osteochondral fragment with fluid signal partially undermining the lesion
- Grade III: A completely detached but nondisplaced osteochondral fragment with fluid signal completely undermining the osteochondral fragment (Fig. 93-21)
- Grade IV: A detached and displaced osteochondral fragment

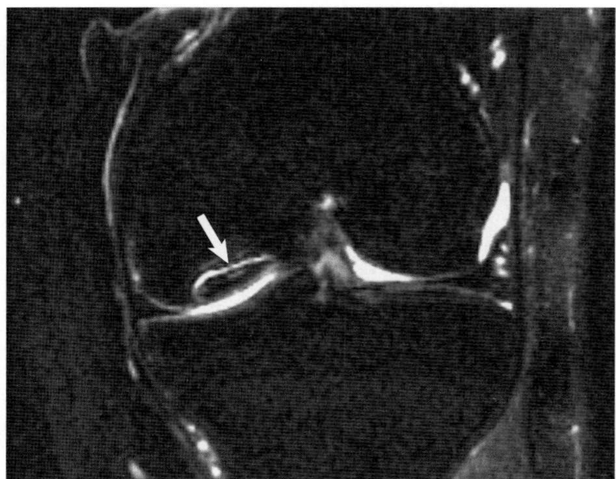

FIGURE 93-21 An osteochondritis dissecans lesion of the medial femoral condyle. Fluid signal (*arrow*) is nearly completely surrounding an osteochondral fragment of the medial femoral condyle, indicating a grade III lesion.

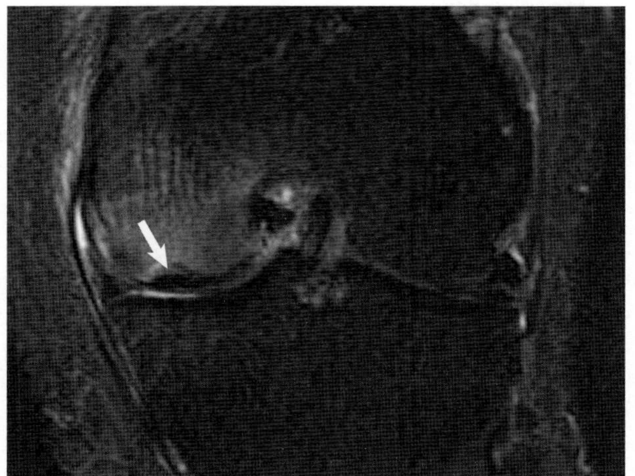

FIGURE 93-22 Spontaneous osteonecrosis of the knee medial femoral condyle. A low–signal-intensity line is noted within the subchondral region of the medial femoral condyle, representing a subchondral fatigue fracture *(arrow)*, which often is referred to as spontaneous osteonecrosis of the knee. Adjacent subchondral reactive marrow edema is present.

Spontaneous Osteonecrosis of the Knee

Spontaneous osteonecrosis is currently thought to represent a subchondral fatigue fracture that can involve any articular surface of the knee but is most often seen involving the medial femoral condyle (Fig. 93-22). It typically occurs in patients older than 50 years and is most often associated with meniscal tears or occurs after a partial meniscectomy. It likely results from abnormal stresses on the bone associated with altered weight-bearing after changes in meniscal morphology. MRI most often demonstrates a subchondral line that parallels the articular surface of the bone with diffuse adjacent reactive subchondral marrow edema. The subchondral fracture may heal without further sequelae or may progress to cortical collapse and fragmentation, leading to rapid onset of focal osteoarthritis.

MR Imaging of the Osseous Structures

Bone marrow is composed largely of fat and hematopoietic cells. The fat cells are the predominant cell type within the marrow of adults. As a result, the signal within the bone marrow should largely follow that of fat, revealing a bright T1-weighted signal and a low signal on T2-weighted images with fat saturation. Hematopoietic cells demonstrate an intermediate T1-weighted signal, which is typically brighter than adjacent muscle. A T1-weighted signal that is lower in signal intensity than adjacent muscle is suspicious for an abnormal marrow process such as bone contusion, infection, avascular necrosis, or tumor. The cortex of bone appears dark on all pulse sequences.

Fractures

Fractures are seen on MRI as a low–signal-intensity line with associated cortical discontinuity. In the acute setting, bone marrow edema/contusion is often seen adjacent to the fracture. MRI is an excellent means of detecting a radiographically occult fracture and is helpful in determining the extent of articular surface involvement and step-off.

Bone Contusion Patterns Associated with Soft Tissue Injury

Bone contusions can occur at the time of knee injury and typically result from either direct trauma to the bone or from compressive forces of two bones having an impact on one another. Bone contusions appear as a low signal on T1-weighted images or as a bright signal on T2-weighted images. Five specific bone contusion patterns have been described in the area of the knee, and these bone contusions have been referred to as the "footprint" left behind at the time of injury. Identification of a specific bone contusion pattern indicates the mechanism of injury and in turn can be used to accurately predict the type of soft tissue injury that is likely to be present.

- Pivot shift injury: Bone contusions on the lateral femoral condyle and posterior tibia; associated with ACL injury (see Figure 93-10)
- Dashboard injury: Bone contusion on the anterior aspect of the proximal tibia; associated with PCL injury (see Figure 93-13)
- Hyperextension injury: Kissing contusions of the anterior tibia and the adjacent anterior femur; associated with ACL and or PCL injury and posterior capsular injury
- Clipping injury: Bone contusions of the lateral femoral condyle; associated with MCL injury (see Fig. 93-14, *C*)
- Lateral patellar dislocation: Bone contusions on the anterior peripheral lateral femoral condyle and medical patellar facet, osteochondral lesions of the patella and lateral femoral condyle, as well as injury of the medial patellofemoral ligament (see Fig. 93-19)

Stress Fracture

Stress fractures typically appear on MRI as an ill-defined low–signal-intensity line that extends perpendicular to the primary trabecular pattern of the involved bone. In the acute setting, adjacent marrow edema is usually present (Fig. 93-23). Stress

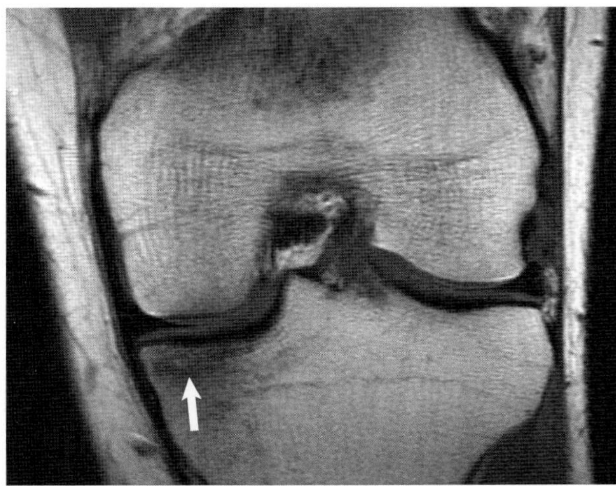

FIGURE 93-23 A stress fracture of the medial tibial metaphyseal region. An ill-defined low–signal-intensity line *(arrow)* is present within the medial tibial metaphyseal region, with surrounding marrow edema representing a stress fracture. The overlying cortex and articular cartilage is intact.

fractures are typically incomplete and nondisplaced, but if the offending stress continues, the fracture can progress to a complete fracture. In the area of the knee, stress fractures most commonly occur in the tibial metaphysis but can also occur in the distal femur and along the lower pole of the patella.

Suggested Reading

Citation: Sanders TG: Imaging of the knee. In Morrison WB, Sanders TG, editors: *Problem Solving in Musculoskeletal Imaging*, Philadelphia, 2008, Elsevier.
Level of Evidence: V
Summary: In this chapter a systematic approach to the evaluation of magnetic resonance imaging of the knee is described, including the magnetic resonance appearance of normal anatomic structures, normal variants, and the primary and secondary findings of specific injuries of the knee.
Citation: Anderson MW: MR imaging of the meniscus. *Radiol Clin North Am* 40:1081–1094, 2002.
Level of Evidence: V
Summary: In this article the normal magnetic resonance (MR) appearance of the menisci is described, with a review of the MR appearance of various meniscal injuries and the common pitfalls for detecting meniscal pathology.
Citation: Mosher TJ: MRI of osteochondral injuries of the knee and ankle in the athlete. *Clin Sports Med* 25:843–866, 2006.
Level of Evidence: V
Summary: In this article the normal magnetic resonance (MR) appearance of articular cartilage is described, with a review of the various MR classifications for cartilage injury and postoperative imaging of knee cartilage.
Citation: Hayes CW, Coggins CA: Sports-related injuries of the knee: An approach to MRI interpretation. *Clin Sports Med* 25:659–679, 2006.
Level of Evidence: V
Summary: An overview of an approach to interpreting magnetic resonance imaging of the knee is provided in this article.
Citation: Sanders TG, Medynski MA, Feller JF, et al: Bone contusion patterns of the knee at MR imaging: Footprint of the mechanism of injury. *RadioGraphics* 20:S135–S151, 2000.
Level of Evidence: V
Summary: In this article the authors describe various bone contusion patterns of the knee, relate these bone contusion patterns to a specific mechanism of injury, and describe the typical soft tissue injury patterns associated with the various mechanism of injury.
Citation: White LW, Miniaci A: Cruciate and posterolateral corner injuries in the athlete: Clinical and magnetic resonance imaging features. *Semin Musculoskelet Radiol* 8:111–131, 2004.
Level of Evidence: V
Summary: In this article, the magnetic resonance imaging features of posterolateral corner injuries are described.
Citation: Sanders TG, Miller MD: A systematic approach to magnetic resonance imaging interpretation of sports medicine injuries of the shoulder. *Am J Sports Med* 33:1088–1105, 2005.
Level of Evidence: V
Summary: In this article the authors provide a nice review of an approach to interpreting magnetic resonance imaging of the knee.

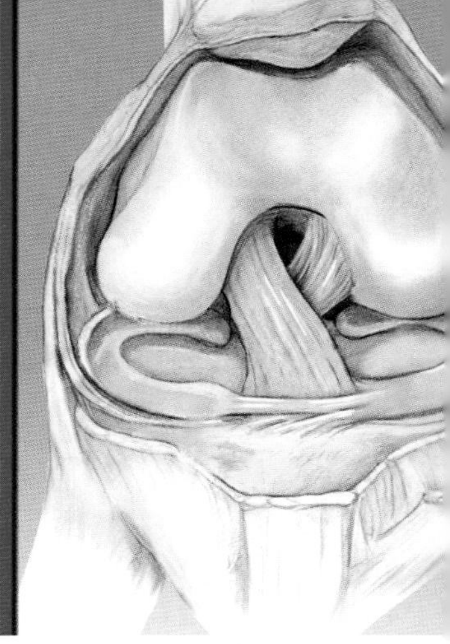

94

Basics of Knee Arthroscopy

JUSTIN W. GRIFFIN • JENNIFER A. HART •
STEPHEN R. THOMPSON • MARK D. MILLER

Few areas in orthopaedic surgery have grown as rapidly as knee arthroscopy. Arthroscopy often can be performed more quickly and with increased accuracy, lower complication rates, decreased hospitalization time, and shorter recovery periods compared with many more open operative techniques. The effective use of arthroscopy is based on the understanding of the benefits and indications for arthroscopy, as well as its limitations.

The knee was the first joint to be examined arthroscopically, and many of the fundamental principles of arthroscopy were developed for the knee.[1] The first knee arthroscopy was performed in Europe and was advanced significantly by Japanese surgeons (Takagi and Watanabe).[1] Applications continue to expand, and the future scope of arthroscopic applications is limited only by the imagination of the arthroscopist.

Preoperative Evaluation

Indications for knee arthroscopy continue to expand at a rapid rate. Each patient's unique anatomy must be considered before initiating arthroscopy. Systematic evaluation of the entire knee includes a thorough physical examination and history. Additional studies including radiographs and advanced imaging should be reviewed, and proper documentation must be performed.[2] Preoperative consultation with appropriate medical specialties and an anesthesiologist help reduce perioperative complications.[3] Postoperative prophylaxis for deep vein thrombosis (DVT) should be considered in at-risk patients. Local, regional, and general anesthetic considerations should be reviewed with the patient and the anesthesia team.

Indications

Arthroscopy has diverse application in various forms of knee disease. Diagnostic arthroscopy helps confirm suspected knee injuries.[4] An arthroscopic synovectomy can be useful for synovial biopsies to aid in the diagnosis of rheumatologic disorders, to remove diseased synovium and loose bodies, and to resect synovial folds or plicae. Arthroscopic treatment of septic arthritis of the knee has increased in frequency. Treatment of meniscal disease is perhaps the most common application of arthroscopy. Meniscal tears and repairs account for about half of knee injuries that require surgery. Osteochondral lesions commonly are addressed arthroscopically. Microfracture, autologous chondrocyte implantation, and osteochondral plug transfers are also performed arthroscopically.

Injuries to the cruciate ligaments can be diagnosed easily with arthroscopy and subsequently treated. Arthroscopic-assisted reconstruction of these ligaments is one of the most common orthopaedic procedures today.[5] Other procedures that sometimes are aided with arthroscopy include tibial plateau fracture reduction, reduction and fixation of tibial eminence fractures, loose body removal, anterior fat pad debridement, and lateral release for patellar malalignment.[3]

Contraindications for knee arthroscopy must be considered as well. One such consideration includes local skin infections over the portal sites. Additionally, alternative treatments should be considered for patients who have too high a risk for surgery and those who are not expected to be compliant with postoperative rehabilitation.[6]

Positioning

Two different forms of positioning are commonly used for knee arthroscopy. The patient can be positioned supine on the operating table, and a lateral post can be used for countertraction. Alternatively, the operative leg can be positioned in a commercially available leg holder (Fig. 94-1). The operative leg is allowed to hang freely over the end of the operating table, and the opposite leg is positioned in a well-padded leg holder, taking care not to compress the peroneal nerve.

Portal Placement

Landmarks, including the inferior pole of the patella and the joint line, are marked. Portal incisions are typically vertical, 1 cm in length, and made with a No. 11 blade while the knee is flexed.[4] A spinal needle can be used for localization of the anteromedial portal (Fig. 94-2). Portal placement is key to successful knee arthroscopy. Standard arthroscopic portals for knee arthroscopy have traditionally included a superomedial or superolateral portal for fluid inflow and outflow and inferomedial and inferolateral portals positioned just above the joint line on both sides of the patellar tendon for arthroscopy and instrumentation (Fig. 94-3).[7] Typically the inferolateral portal is used for arthroscopic visualization and the inferomedial

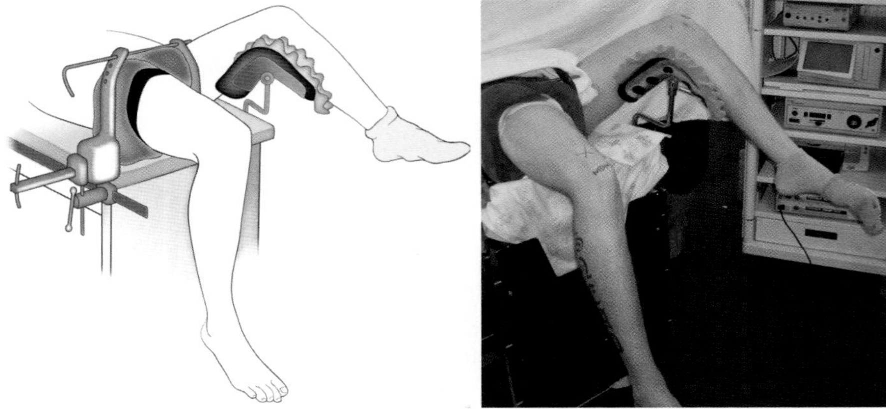

FIGURE 94-1 The patient is positioned supine with use of a leg holder on the lateral post. *(From Miller MD, Chhabra AB, Safran MR:* Primer of arthroscopy, *Philadelphia, 2010, Elsevier.)*

portal is used for instrumentation, although alternating instrumentation between the medial and lateral portal is often necessary to reach certain structures (Fig. 94-4). Newer arthroscopic fluid control systems have now made the use of superior outflow portals optional. The use of a far proximal superior portal can still be helpful for visualization of patellar tracking (see Fig. 94-3).

Accessory portals for the knee include the posteromedial, posterolateral, far medial and lateral, and proximal superomedial portals. The posteromedial portal is often helpful for visualizing the posterior cruciate ligament and the posterior horn of the medial meniscus (Fig. 94-5).[8] The posterolateral portal, located just posterior to the lateral collateral ligament between the iliotibial band and the biceps tendon, sometimes is helpful, but extreme care should be taken to ensure that the portal is anterior to the biceps tendon to avoid injury to the peroneal nerve (Fig. 94-6). An accessory medial portal has been developed for obtaining access to the appropriate angle for anatomic femoral tunnel placement in ACL surgery.[9] Other portals include the midpatellar portal, far medial and lateral portals (which are sometimes helpful for instrument placement in hard-to-reach areas), and the proximal superomedial portal, located 4 cm proximal to and in line with the medial edge of the patella (for assessment of patellar tracking).

Diagnostic Arthroscopy

As with any joint, systematic examination of the knee is appropriate. Before positioning the patient, a complete examination is conducted after induction of anesthesia to assess instability in all planes. An arthroscopic cannula is placed in the superomedial or superolateral portal for inflow and outflow (although the use of these superior portals is now optional with many of the new pump systems), and the obturator and sheath are introduced into the inferolateral portal after incision with the knee flexed at 60 to 90 degrees, angled toward the notch. As the knee is brought into extension, the obturator and sheath are advanced into the suprapatellar pouch and the obturator is replaced by a camera for visualization. The anteromedial portal can be made at the outset of the case or created under visualization with the spinal needle (see Fig. 94-2). Although many examination sequences are possible, it is important to visualize the suprapatellar pouch, patellofemoral joint (Fig. 94-7), medial and lateral gutters, medial and lateral compartments (meniscus and articular cartilage), and intercondylar notch (cruciate ligaments) in all patients.[4] Surgeons differ with regard to fat pad excision for visualization and therapeutic purposes.

The patellofemoral joint is inspected and articulation is examined, including the patella facets and trochlea.

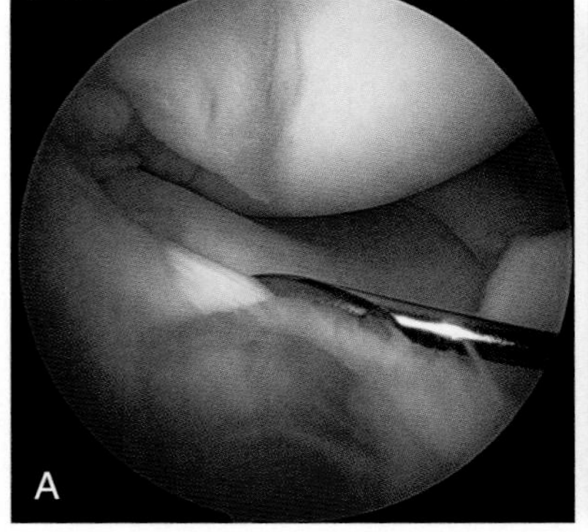

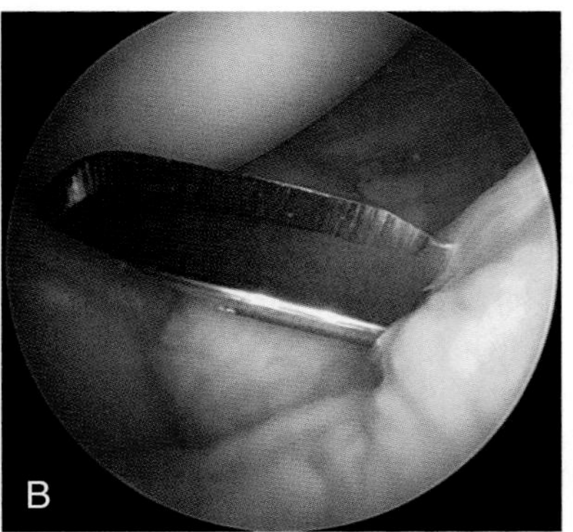

FIGURE 94-2 Anteromedial portal localization. **A,** The arthroscope is turned toward the anteromedial capsule. A spinal needle is inserted and positioned until it is just above the meniscus and its trajectory is satisfactory for intraarticular work. **B,** The spinal needle is carefully removed and a No. 15 or No. 11 blade is inserted blade-side up.

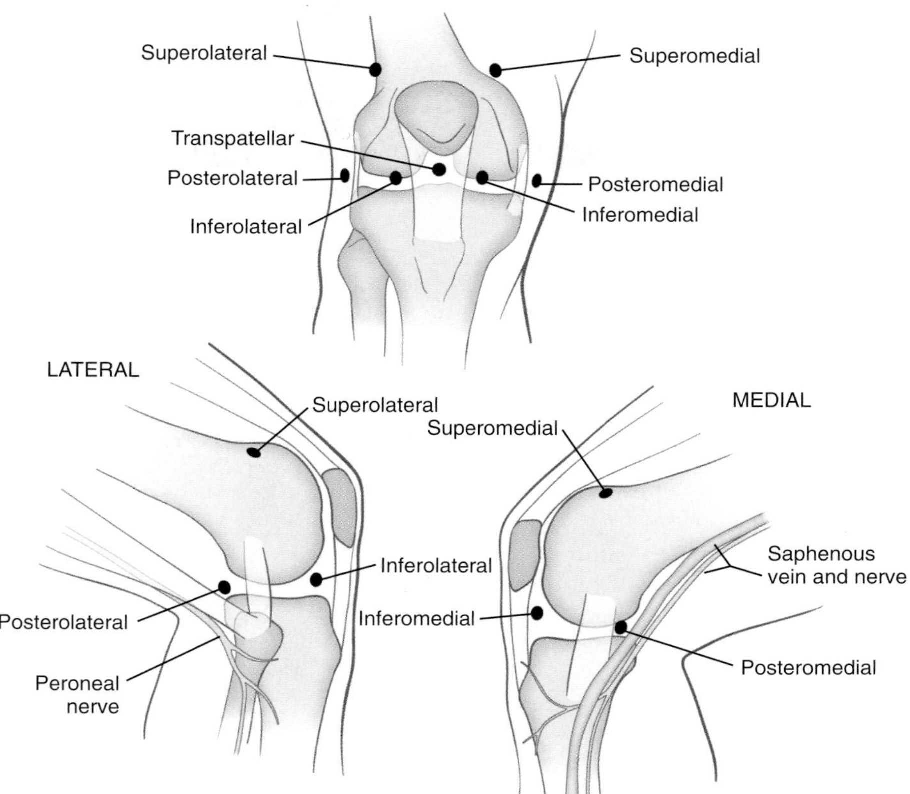

FIGURE 94-3 Portal placement for knee arthroscopy. *(From Miller MD, Chhabra AB, Safran MR:* Primer of arthroscopy, *Philadelphia, 2010, Elsevier.)*

Engagement should be full at 40 degrees. The gutters are examined for loose bodies. The knee is flexed and the scope is brought down into the intercondylar notch. The ACL is inspected by directing the scope to view it laterally and by probing the ligament (Fig. 94-8). The ACL is composed of the two separate bundles that are often not distinct but can occasionally be recognized. The posterior cruciate ligament is also evaluated, although often only the femoral side is examined, with the remainder hidden by the ACL.[10] The medial compartment is then visualized with valgus stress and extension using an assistant or with the surgeon resting the ankle on his or her hip. The foot can be externally rotated to improve access. The meniscus and articular surfaces are examined. Once all lesions are characterized, the lateral compartment is visualized in the same fashion in the figure-of-four position.

Accessory viewing portals are established as necessary if other areas need to be evaluated. A posteromedial portal can be helpful whenever medial meniscus pathology is suspected but is unable to be identified from the anterior portals. This portal is established by introducing the arthroscopic cannula into the back of the knee by directing it from anterior to posterior on the notch side of the medial femoral condyle. Care must be taken to avoid the saphenous nerve and vein. A spinal needle is used to establish the position of the portal. Next, a small incision is made in the skin only, followed by spreading with a blunt instrument down to the capsule. Once the arthroscope is in the posterior aspect of the knee, the posterior horn of the medial meniscus can be visualized. Use of a 70-degree scope may be helpful. After a complete evaluation of the joint is performed, all surgical pathology is addressed accordingly.

Instrumentation

A 30-degree arthroscope is most commonly used, although a 70-degree scope may be helpful in the posterior corners.[8] An arthroscopic probe can be used and provides a sense of touch to the arthroscopist. Instruments angled upward, including biters, are best for the medial compartment, whereas straight instruments often work best in the lateral compartment. Arthroscopic shavers are available in both large and small sizes and should be chosen on the basis of the dimensions of the compartment.[5]

Postoperative Care

Upon completion of the procedure, the fluid is evacuated from the joint and the instruments are removed. Typically, nonabsorbable monofilament is used to closed the portals and is removed 10 to 14 days after surgery. In some centers, portals are routinely left open, because it is believed that open portals permit easier fluid extravasation and reduce postoperative swelling and pain.[11] A local anesthetic can be injected at the end of the surgery into the skin only. Although the weight-bearing status may differ depending on the surgery performed, most patients require crutches for some period of

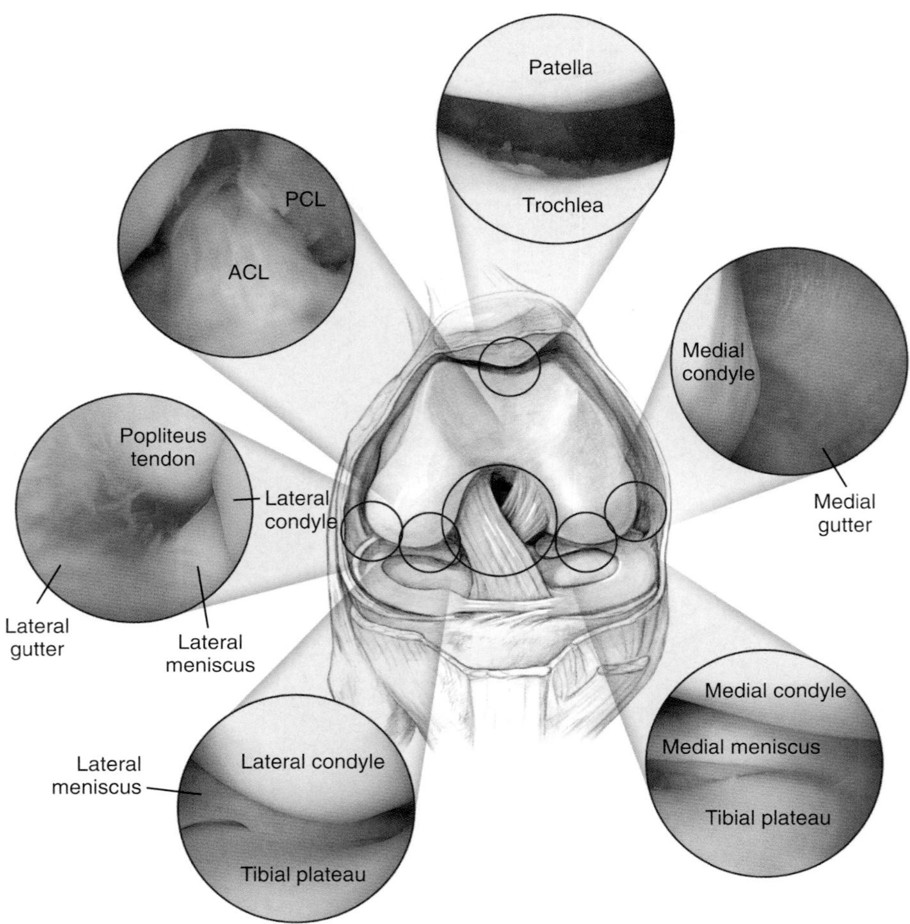

FIGURE 94-4 Visualization during diagnostic arthroscopy. *ACL,* Anterior cruciate ligament; *PCL,* posterior cruciate ligament. *(From Miller MD, Chhabra AB, Safran MR:* Primer of arthroscopy, *Philadelphia, 2010, Elsevier.)*

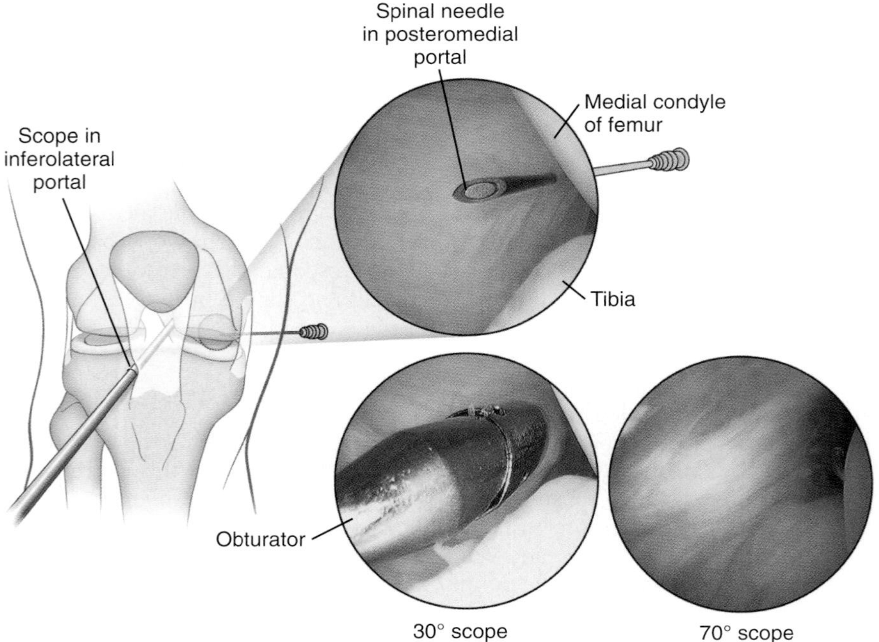

FIGURE 94-5 View of the intercondylar notch from the posteromedial portal. *(From Miller MD, Chhabra AB, Safran MR:* Primer of arthroscopy, *Philadelphia, 2010, Elsevier.)*

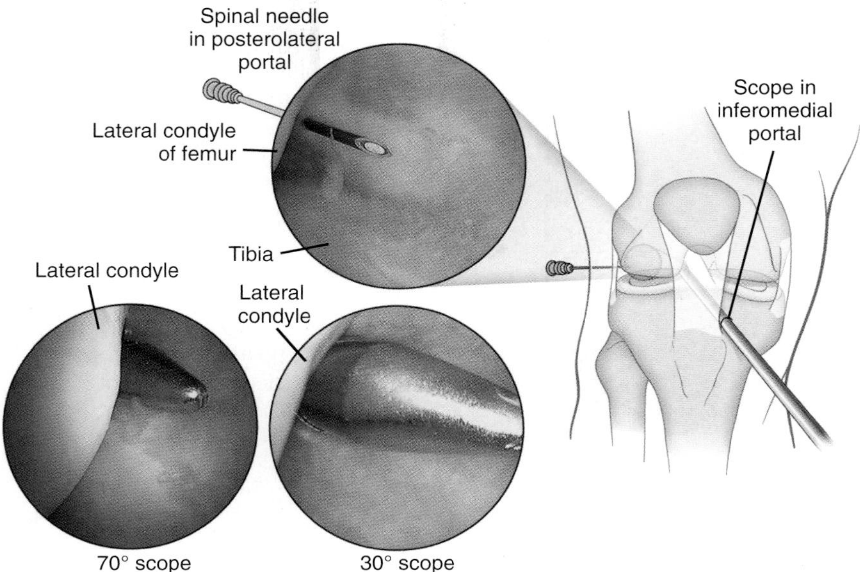

FIGURE 94-6 View of the intercondylar notch from the posterolateral portal. *(From Miller MD, Chhabra AB, Safran MR:* Primer of arthroscopy, *Philadelphia, 2010, Saunders.)*

time. Postoperative pain medicines are typically prescribed for a short period for most patients undergoing knee arthroscopy.

Complications

Postoperative complications can include infection, arthrofibrosis, nerve and vessel injury, iatrogenic cartilage injury, compartment syndrome, collateral ligament injury, and DVT or pulmonary embolism.[6,12] Perhaps the most common complication is inadvertent damage to the intraarticular structures.[12] This risk is inversely proportional to the surgeon's experience and the care with which the surgeon performs the procedure. Proper portal placement, use of a gentle technique, and attention to detail are crucial. The exact prevalence and long-term sequelae of iatrogenic cartilage lesions are unknown, but studies involving second-look arthroscopy and animal models have shown that this is a true risk and that the lesions do not tend to fill with time. Nerve or vessel injury can result from improper placement of the portals.[7] For this reason, a thorough knowledge of local anatomy is necessary before performing arthroscopy.

Tourniquet paresis can be reduced with use of a wide cuff and by limiting tourniquet time whenever possible.

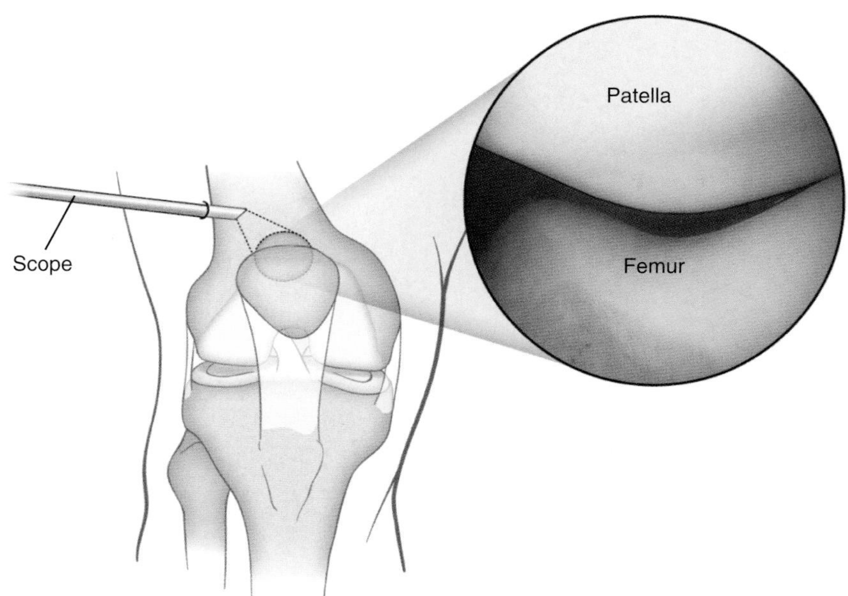

FIGURE 94-7 Visualization of the patellofemoral joint. *(From Miller MD, Chhabra AB, Safran MR:* Primer of arthroscopy, *Philadelphia, 2010, Elsevier.)*

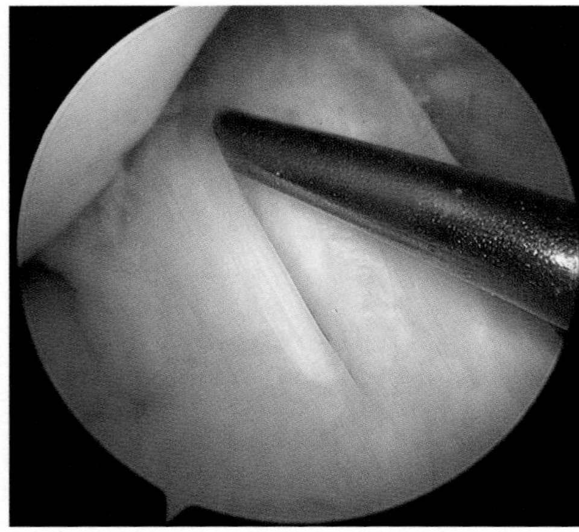

FIGURE 94-8 Arthroscopic appearance of the two bundles of the anterior cruciate ligament. *(From Miller MD, Chhabra AB, Safran MR:* Primer of arthroscopy, *Philadelphia, 2010, Elsevier.)*

Positioning devices (e.g., leg holders) can have a tourniquet effect, even when the tourniquet is not inflated. Fluid extravasation has been reported, although the incidence of this complication can be reduced with careful placement of inflow cannulas and proper use of inflow pumps. Synovial fistula formation is a rare complication of arthroscopy and is usually remedied by 7 to 10 days of immobilization and, occasionally, delayed closure. Infection is an extremely rare complication of arthroscopy with less than a 1% occurrence rate and is usually the result of a break in sterile technique. High-dose antibiotics and arthroscopic irrigation and debridement may be indicated in severe cases. Hemarthrosis can occur as well, although it can be avoided with meticulous technique and care after procedures such as a lateral release.[5]

Arthrofibrosis is unusual after knee arthroscopy, although it can occur with procedures such as ACL reconstruction and multiligamentous knee reconstructions. Attainment of full motion preoperatively and early motion postoperatively are key to avoiding such an outcome.

An unusual but potentially life-threatening complication of knee arthroscopy is the development of a postoperative DVT or pulmonary embolism. Although the risk for these events is low, careful screening of risk factors must be performed to identify patients who require routine prophylaxis.[3,6] These risk factors include immobilization, increased body mass index, personal or family history of clotting disorder, and advancing age.

Summary

Knee arthroscopy is effective in treating a number of intraarticular knee pathologies. Proper evaluation and management is key to successful patient outcomes. Results vary based on the underlying etiology, but they do appear to help patients in the symptomatic management of intraarticular disorders.

For a complete list of references, go to expertconsult.com.

Suggested Readings

Citation: Hoogeslag RA, Brouwer RW, van Raay JJ: The value of tourniquet use for visibility during arthroscopy of the knee: A double-blind, randomized controlled trial. *Arthroscopy* 26(9 Suppl):S67–S72, 2010.
Level of Evidence: I
Summary: In this randomized controlled trial, significantly improved visibility during routine knee arthroscopy was demonstrated with use of a tourniquet.
Citation: Jameson SS, Dowen D, James P, et al: The burden of arthroscopy of the knee: A contemporary analysis of data from the English NHS. *J Bone Joint Surg Br* 93B(10):1327–1333, 2011.
Level of Evidence: II
Summary: In this article a prospective, large-volume registry analysis of knee arthroscopies occurring in the United Kingdom National Health Service is provided. The overall rate of complications was less than 1%.
Citation: Sikand M, Murtaza A, Desai VV: Healing of arthroscopic portals: A randomised trial comparing three methods of portal closure. *Acta Orthop Belg* 72(5):583–586, 2006.
Level of Evidence: II
Summary: In this article a prospective randomized controlled trial comparing suture closure of arthroscopy portals with Steri-Strip application or no closure whatsoever is described. Swelling was significantly lower in the two groups without suture closure. Patient satisfaction with regard to final scar appearance was higher in the two groups without suture closure.

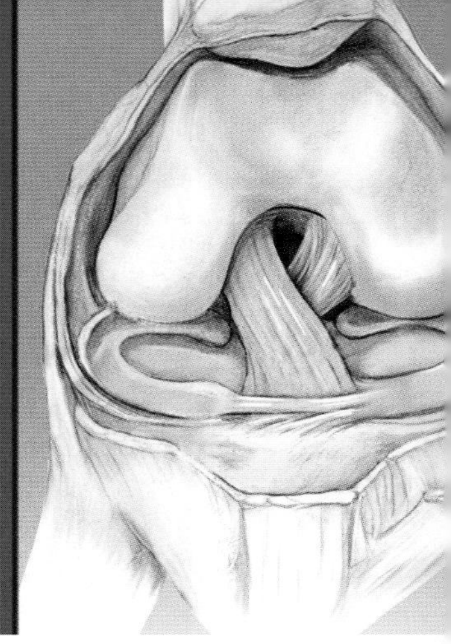

95

Arthroscopic Synovectomy of the Knee

BRYAN D. HAUGHOM • BRANDON J. ERICKSON • CHARLES A. BUSH-JOSEPH

The synovial lining is a specialized mesenchymal tissue that is integral to the normal functioning of a joint. Synovial disorders can involve varying amounts of the synovium. Rheumatoid arthritis shows total joint involvement, whereas on the other end of the spectrum, plica syndrome is caused by an isolated synovial lesion.

Volkman performed the first synovectomy in 1855 for tuberculous synovitis. Although the indications and technique have changed over time, the procedure is still performed, and the objective of removing the diseased synovium remains the same.[1] Compared with open procedures, arthroscopic techniques have enabled surgeons to perform a synovectomy without a large arthrotomy, decreasing the risk of postoperative arthrofibrosis. Arthroscopy also serves as an effective technique to remove synovium in the posterior compartment and allows viewing of synovial lesions that may be missed with open procedures. Arthroscopic synovectomy can be used in the surgical treatment of rheumatoid arthritis, pigmented villonodular synovitis, hemophilic synovitis, plicae, synovial hemangioma, synovial osteochondromatosis, and degenerative synovitis.

As with all orthopaedic conditions, a complete workup including a thorough history and physical examination and complete imaging analysis is needed to evaluate these patients. Additionally, a trial of medical management should be performed before initiation of surgical treatment. Surgical treatment consists of arthroscopically removing varying amounts of synovium, the amount of which is based on the underlying disease process.

Clinical Evaluation

History

A complete history is important in the evaluation of patients with synovial disorders. The presence of other affected joints, the length of time symptoms have been experienced, exacerbating symptoms, and the amount of disability experienced by the patient on a daily basis are important pieces of information. Patients with rheumatoid arthritis may have more systemic complaints, including morning stiffness and other affected joints, particularly the small joints of the hands and feet. Pigmented villonodular synovitis (PVNS) is typically a monoarticular process that affects adults in the third or fourth decade of life. Symptoms are mechanical in nature and may be similar to those seen in patients with meniscal tears.[2] Clinically patients have the insidious onset of localized warmth, swelling, and stiffness with occasional locking and a palpable mass. Plica syndrome is a finding in patients with anteromedial knee pain. Patients experience tightness, snapping, giving way, and pain with repetitive activities. Clinically it is difficult to distinguish plica syndrome from other causes of knee pain such as meniscal tears, patellar tendinitis, or patellofemoral pain syndrome.

Physical Examination and Laboratory Tests

A full rheumatologic workup should be completed for patients with systemic diseases, and appropriate laboratory tests should be up to date. Patients with hemophilia require a consultation with a hematologist. If surgical treatment is to be pursued, it is essential to have a well–thought-out plan for perioperative management of clotting factors.

Other joints may be affected in patients with rheumatic or autoimmune disorders, and these joints should be evaluated. Patients with rheumatoid arthritis often have a flexion contracture and quadriceps atrophy in the knee region.[3] The skin should be examined and previous incisions and subcutaneous nodules should be evaluated. The knee should be examined to determine overall alignment, range of motion, the presence of an effusion, warmth, tenderness, crepitus, strength, meniscal integrity, and stability. Collateral ligament instability or bony malalignment suggests more severe articular loss, and patients with these conditions are poor candidates for a synovectomy.

The physical examination for PVNS is often nonspecific. An effusion is associated with diffuse involvement. Palpation of the joint may show warmth and tenderness. Aspiration of the joint fluid may show a dark-brown fluid that is a result of recurrent bleeding into the joint. Cytologic studies of the aspirate may show hemosiderin pigment and multinucleated foreign body giant cells, but often the findings of these studies are normal.[4] Ligamentous instability is uncommon in persons with PVNS.

Plica syndrome begins insidiously. Tenderness over the medial parapatellar region is common. A plica may sometimes be directly palpated and rolled under the finger, recreating the patient's symptoms. If the medial border of the patella is palpated while pushing the patella medially with one hand and the other hand produces a valgus stress with external rotation

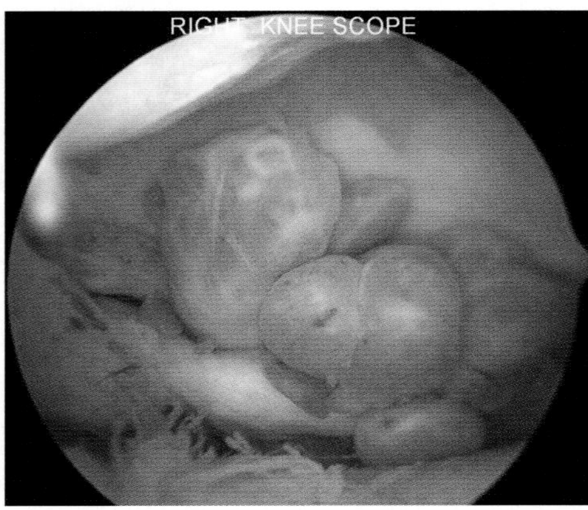

FIGURE 95-1 Arthroscopic appearance of localized pigmented villonodular synovitis.

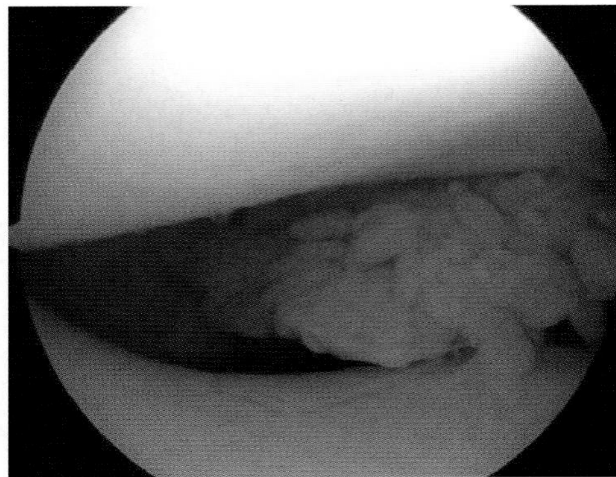

FIGURE 95-3 The patellofemoral joint of a left knee in a 39-year-old patient with rheumatoid arthritis. Despite conservative treatment, the patient experienced a flexion contracture with uncontrolled swelling and elected to undergo arthroscopic synovectomy.

of the tibia, pain may be elicited, suggesting plica syndrome.[5] An effusion is not typically present in persons with plica syndrome.

Imaging

In patients with rheumatoid arthritis, cervical spine flexion and extension views should be obtained in preoperative patients to rule out cervical instability. Radiographs of the knee should be obtained. Patients with rheumatoid arthritis may have periarticular erosions and osteopenia. Radiographs in patients with PVNS can show erosive, cystic, and sclerotic lesions of the articular surface. If enough synovium that contains hemosiderin is present, soft tissue masses may be seen, but often the findings of the films are normal with well-maintained joint spaces. Magnetic resonance imaging is considered to be the most diagnostic study for PVNS. It may show nodular intraarticular masses of low signal intensity on T1- and T2-weighted images and also allows evaluation of the location and extent of disease.

Treatment

In disorders associated with a localized lesion, such as a localized PVNS (Figs. 95-1 and 95-2) or plica, arthroscopic intervention can remove the pathology in its entirety. Persons with diffuse conditions such as rheumatoid arthritis (Figs. 95-3 through 95-6) or hemophilia can undergo surgery to decrease the severity of disease symptoms once conservative measures have been exhausted. Recently, medical management of rheumatoid arthritis has improved significantly. The goals of medical treatment include reducing the number of painful and swollen joints, suppressing the acute phase response, decreasing the rheumatoid factor titer, and slowing radiographic progression of the disease. A patient with rheumatoid arthritis and minimal degenerative changes on radiographs would be a candidate for arthroscopic synovectomy after failure of approximately 6 months of medical management. Medical management should consist of a combination of disease-modifying antirheumatic drugs, nonsteroidal antiinflammatory drugs, an appropriate physical therapy regimen, activity modification, and intraarticular steroid injections (in general, no more than three steroid injections should be administered in one joint in a given year).[6] Significant joint space narrowing or mechanical malalignment is a relative contraindication to synovectomy for inflammatory synovial knee disorders.

Hemophilic synovitis can also be associated with significant joint destruction and has shown favorable improvement in symptoms with synovectomy.[7-9] Radiosynovectomy is indicated as the first procedure in persons with hemophilic

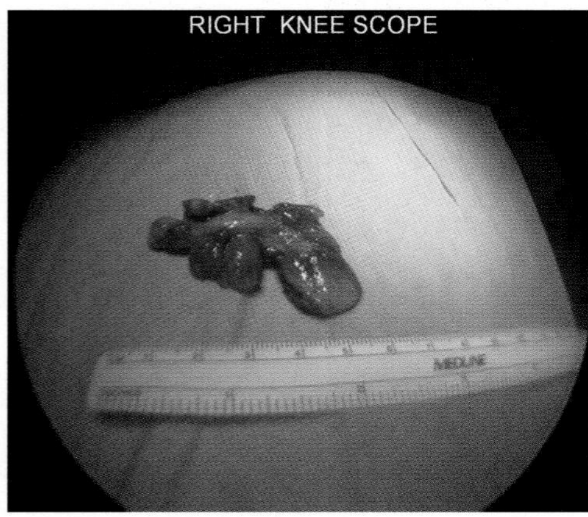

FIGURE 95-2 Gross view of the localized pigmented villonodular synovitis specimen from Figure 95-1.

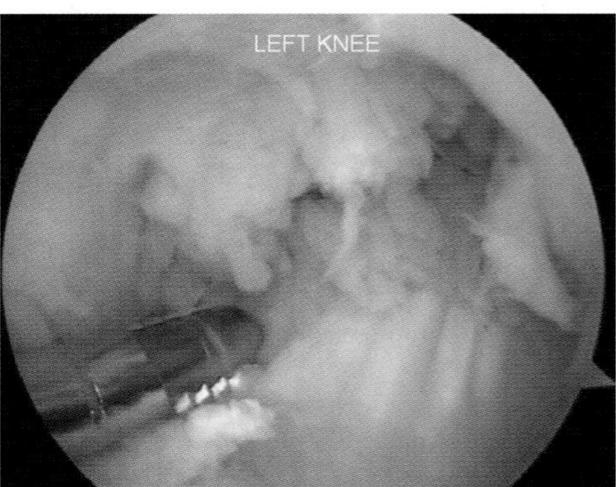

FIGURE 95-4 The arthroscopic view of the notch before debridement in the left knee of the patient in Figure 95-3.

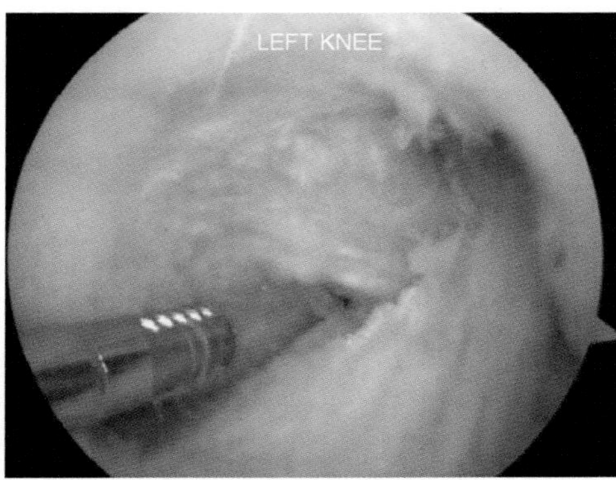

FIGURE 95-5 The arthroscopic view of the notch after debridement in the same patient shown in Figure 95-3.

synovitis, with satisfactory results in 80% of patients.[10] No more than three radiosynovectomies can be performed per year. If the three radiosynovectomy procedures fail to relieve symptoms, an arthroscopic synovectomy is indicated.[10] Although joint deterioration is not preventable, a synovectomy can reduce recurrent hemarthrosis and maintain range of motion. A hemophilic synovectomy requires an inpatient stay for coordinated management of clotting factors with the patient's hematologist.

Surgical Technique

Because arthroscopic synovectomy requires the use of multiple portals to access all spaces in the knee joint, good preoperative planning and patient setup is essential for a successful operation. Because a synovectomy can be a long procedure, induction of general anesthesia is recommended, and use of a Foley catheter should be considered. An epidural can be used if required for medical reasons and may also help with postoperative pain relief.

Examination After Inducement of Anesthesia

Both knees are examined for an assessment of the range of motion, ligamentous stability, patellar mobility, patellar tracking, and the presence of an effusion.

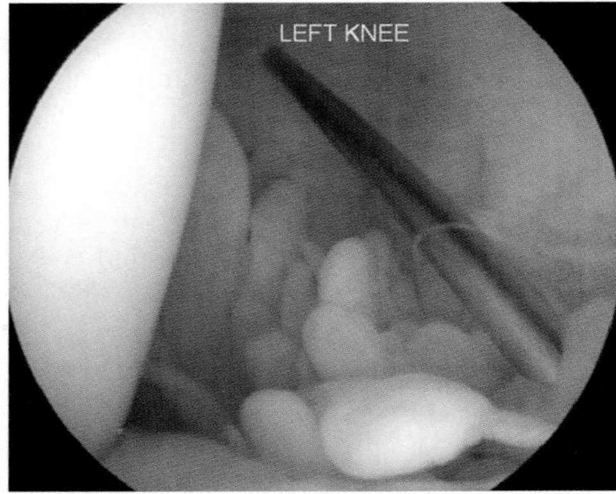

FIGURE 95-6 The arthroscopic view of the posteromedial compartment of the patient shown in Figure 95-1. The spinal needle is used to localize the ideal portal location.

Positioning

The patient is placed supine on the operating room table. The well leg is appropriately padded and secured in a well leg holder after placement of a compressive stocking and sequential compression device. A leg holder is not used on the operative leg because it may interfere with use of the superomedial and superolateral portals. The foot of the operating table is dropped and the mid portion of the table is flexed to avoid hip hyperextension. A well-padded thigh tourniquet is placed high on the operative leg.

Surgical Steps

Anterior Compartments

After standard prepping and draping is performed, the extremity is exsanguinated and the tourniquet is inflated to between 250 and 300 mm Hg. The tissue obtained from the synovectomy should be collected and sent for pathologic evaluation. The anterior aspect of the knee is addressed first. A superomedial outflow portal is created and the outflow cannula is placed here. Standard inferolateral and inferomedial portals are created. The arthroscope is placed in the inferolateral portal, and an initial diagnostic arthroscopy is performed. The synovectomy then proceeds with use of an arthroscopic shaver. While viewing from the inferolateral portal with the knee in extension, the shaver is used in the superolateral and inferomedial portals to remove all synovial tissue but avoiding injury to surrounding muscle, tendon, and fascia (Table 95-1).

Posterior Compartments

The anterior compartment should now be finished, and attention is turned to the posterior compartments, beginning with the posteromedial compartment. Typically the posterior compartments can be visualized with a 30-degree scope; however, a 70-degree scope can be used if difficulty is encountered. The arthroscope must first be placed in the posterior compartment. The blunt-tipped trocar is placed in the arthroscopic sheath and inserted into the inferolateral portal. The trocar is directed toward the medial femoral condyle, and when it is contacted, the trocar is carefully advanced posteriorly through the interval between the medial femoral condyle and the posterior cruciate ligament, raising the hand with insertion to match the slope of the tibia. If this maneuver proves difficult, a central and vertically oriented patellar tendon portal may provide easier access to the posterior compartment. The arthroscope is inserted, and the posterior portion of the medial femoral condyle and the posterior horn of the medial meniscus should be visible (Fig. 95-7). While looking medially, a spinal needle is inserted anterior to the medial head of the gastrocnemius into the posteromedial compartment. The needle is used to ensure that all areas in the posterior knee that are in need of synovectomy can easily be reached. Once the ideal portal location has been determined, a longitudinal incision is made in the skin. A hemostat is used to bluntly dissect and then penetrate the capsule, and a cannula is placed. The shaver is placed through the cannula, and the synovium in the posteromedial compartment is resected.

The posterolateral compartment is accessed in a manner similar to the posteromedial compartment. A blunt-tipped trocar is placed in the arthroscopic cannula in the inferomedial portal between the lateral femoral condyle and the

TABLE 95-1

STEPS FOR PERFORMING AN ARTHROSCOPIC SYNOVECTOMY OF THE KNEE

Step	Area of Synovial Resection	Camera Portal/Leg Position	Instrument Portal
1	A. Suprapatellar pouch B. Lateral gutter	Inferolateral/extension	Superolateral
2	A. Begin medial gutter B. Medial aspect suprapatellar pouch C. Intercondylar notch	Inferolateral/extension	Inferomedial
3	A. Finish medial gutter B. Medial suprapatellar pouch	Inferolateral/flexion	Superomedial
4	A. Retropatellar space B. Inferolateral gutter	Superolateral/extension	Inferolateral
5	A. Retropatellar space B. Inferomedial gutter	Superolateral/extension	Inferomedial
6	A. Posteromedial compartment	Inferolateral/flexion	Posteromedial
7	A. Posterolateral compartment	Inferomedial/flexion	Posterolateral

anterior cruciate ligament. The hand is gently raised and advanced posteriorly, taking care not to violate the posterior capsule, which could put the neurovascular structures at risk. The arthroscope replaces the trocar, and the posterior lateral femoral condyle and the posterior horn of the lateral meniscus are viewed. Again, a spinal needle is used to make a posterolateral portal under direct visualization. Placing the needle in the soft spot, anterior to the biceps femoris muscle and posterior to the iliotibial band, helps protect the common peroneal nerve. The needle should be inserted posterior to the fibular collateral ligament and anterior to the lateral head of the gastrocnemius. Once it is determined that the spinal needle is placed so that all areas that require synovectomy can be reached, the skin is incised and a hemostat is used to dissect to the posterior capsule. The capsule is then punctured under direct visualization and a cannula is placed. The shaver is placed through the cannula, and the posterolateral compartment synovectomy is performed.

After the synovectomy is complete, the tourniquet is deflated and an electrocautery device is used to achieve hemostasis. It is common to use a suction drain for 24 hours to help minimize hemarthrosis. Ice, elevation, and a light compressive dressing are used to minimize swelling, and early motion is encouraged.

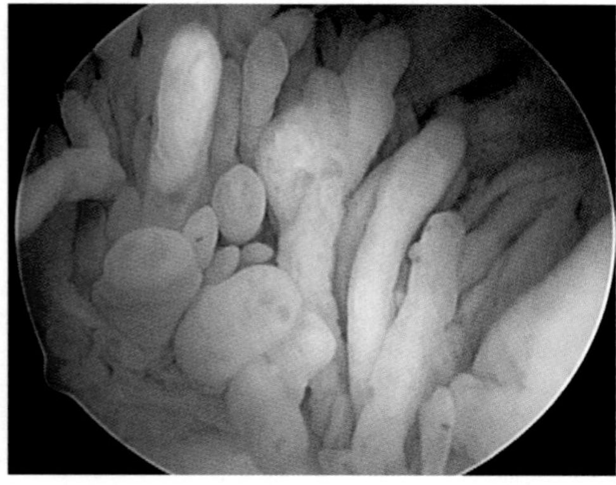

FIGURE 95-7 The arthroscopic appearance of the synovium in a patient with diffuse pigmented villonodular synovitis.

Postoperative Management

The patient can bear weight as tolerated after surgery. Physical therapy is begun on postoperative day 1 after drain removal and concentrates on closed chain exercises. The most immediate goals are regaining knee extension and quadriceps function. A continuous passive motion machine can be used for the first few days after surgery.

Complications

After synovectomy, a recurrent hemarthrosis may occur. The fluid can often be aspirated with a large-bore needle, but an arthroscopic washout may be needed. Joint stiffness and loss of extension may occur after a synovectomy. Performing aggressive and early range of motion exercises, using extension boards, and dynamic bracing may help with these symptoms. A septic joint or neurovascular injury can also occur. With use of careful technique, these complications can be minimized.

Results

Goetz et al.[11] evaluated 32 knees at 14-year follow-up after combined arthroscopic and radiation synovectomy for rheumatoid arthritis. These investigators concluded that combined arthroscopic and radiation synovectomy led to a stable improvement of knee function for a minimum of 5 years, but repeat surgery was frequent, with 56% of patients having another operation by 10 years.[11] If total knee arthroplasty was considered the end point, the joint survival rate was 88.5% at 5 years, 53.9% at 10 years, and 39.6% at 14 years.[11] Carl et al.[12] studied 11 patients with rheumatoid arthritis who were undergoing a synovectomy. These investigators found that a synovectomy led to an overall reduction of acute inflammatory infiltrates by 82.1% and of chronic inflammatory infiltrates by 62.5%.[12]

Although few follow-up data are available regarding synovectomy in patients with hemophilia in general, Verma et al.[13] suggest that the primary predictor of outcome in hemophiliacs is the degree of intraarticular preexisting degenerative changes. In more severe cases, the results of arthroscopic synovectomy are less predictable, and total joint arthroplasty should be considered.

Rhee et al.[14] performed a retrospective study to determine the long-term results of arthroscopic treatment of localized PVNS. Follow-up was 112 months for 11 patients. The authors concluded that excision of localized PVNS can improve symptoms and that patients can return to preoperative activity levels.[14] Sharma and Cheng[15] reported a recurrence-free survival of 62% at 2 years and 48% at 5 years in patients treated for diffuse and localized PVNS with arthroscopic synovectomy. Although synovectomy can prevent recurrence of PVNS, it appears that the joint may still progress to secondary osteoarthritis.

Summary

Arthroscopic synovectomy is a procedure that is the treatment of choice for a number of synovial disorders. The procedure requires thoughtful preparation and extensive preoperative workup. Results vary based on the underlying etiology, but the procedure does appear to help patients with the symptomatic management of synovial disorders.

For a complete list of references, go to expertconsult.com.

Selected Readings

Citation: Goetz M, et al: Combined arthroscopic and radiation synovectomy of the knee joint in rheumatoid arthritis: 14-year follow-up. *Arthroscopy* 27(1):52–59, 2011.
Level of Evidence: IV (therapeutic case series)
Summary: The authors evaluated the outcome of 32 knees treated with combined arthroscopic and radiation synovectomy of the knee joint in early cases of rheumatoid arthritis in terms of knee function and the need for repeat surgical intervention. At an average of 14 years of follow-up, with any repeat surgical intervention as the end point, the survival rate was 32%, challenging the long-term benefit of the procedure.

Citation: Carl HD, et al: Site-specific intraoperative efficacy of arthroscopic knee joint synovectomy in rheumatoid arthritis. *Arthroscopy* 21(10):1209–1218, 2005.
Level of Evidence: III
Summary: The authors assessed site-specific intraoperative reduction of inflammatory infiltrates achieved with arthroscopic knee synovectomy in patients with rheumatoid arthritis using preoperative and postoperative synovial tissue samples. They concluded that arthroscopic synovectomy reduces acute and chronic inflammatory infiltrates in patients with rheumatoid arthritis. However, this reduction appears to depend on the anatomic region of the joint.

Citation: Sharma V, Cheng EY: Outcomes after excision of pigmented villonodular synovitis of the knee. *Clin Orthop Relat Res* 467(11):2852–2858, 2009.
Level of Evidence: IV (therapeutic study)
Summary: The authors retrospectively determined recurrence-free survival (RFS) after excision, RFS after salvage surgery for relapse, and factors associated with relapse in 49 patients with pigmented villonodular synovitis. These investigators found that diffuse disease and arthroscopic synovectomy were associated with relapse and that recurrence was frequent after synovectomy.

Citation: Kim TK, et al: Neurovascular complications of knee arthroscopy. *Am J Sports Med* 30:619–629, 2002.
Level of Evidence: IV (review article)
Summary: The authors summarize causes and frequencies of complications related to arthroscopic procedures, including anterior and posterior compartment synovectomy. Complication management and medicolegal implications are reviewed.

Citation: Rhee PC, et al: Arthroscopic treatment of localized pigmented villonodular synovitis: Long-term functional results. *Am J Orthop* 39(9):E90–E94, 2010.
Level of Evidence: IV (therapeutic case series)
Summary: The authors review outcomes of patients undergoing arthroscopic resections of localized pigmented villonodular synovitis lesions. Complications and recurrence rates are presented.

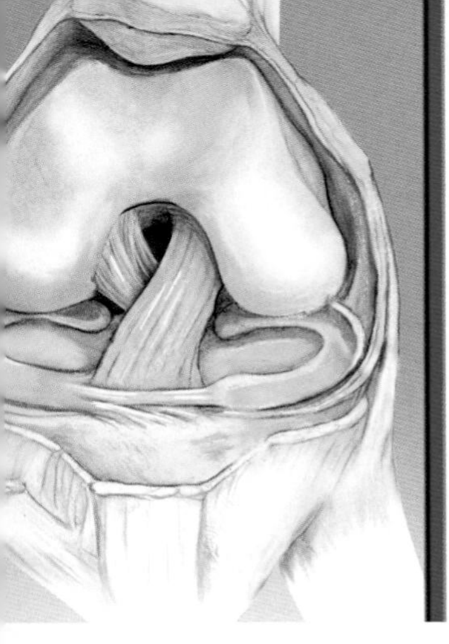

96

Meniscal Injuries

TRAVIS G. MAAK • SCOTT A. RODEO

History of the Meniscus

One of the earliest descriptions of the menisci was recorded by Bland-Sutton in 1897. At that time, the menisci were thought to be vestigial tissue and were depicted as "the functionless remnants of intra-articular leg muscles."[1] Further advances in our understanding of the menisci have demonstrated that the menisci provide mechanical support and secondary stabilization, localized pressure distribution and load sharing, lubrication, and proprioception to the knee joint.[2,3]

In 1936, King[4,5] initially documented meniscal healing at the meniscosynovial junction in a canine model. He also documented minimal healing with intrasubstance tears. Significant articular chondral degeneration was documented in the setting of partial or complete meniscectomy. These data suggested that the available vascular supply may serve a crucial role in meniscal healing and that the menisci may have a role in chondroprotection.[4,5]

Fairbank substantiated this chondroprotective role in 1948 using radiographic evaluation of patients after a total meniscectomy. This study documented specific radiographic "Fairbank changes," including formation of an anteroposterior ridge extending from the femoral condylar margin, marginal flattening of the femoral articular surface, and joint space narrowing. These radiographic findings were identified as early as 5 months after a complete meniscectomy and demonstrated time-dependent progression. These observations led to the conclusion that the menisci may have a function during weight bearing and that a complete meniscectomy may contribute to intraarticular degenerative changes. This awareness, in conjunction with further substantiating data,[6-8] increased the focus on meniscal preservation through limited partial meniscectomy, meniscal repair, biologic stimulation procedures, and an advanced algorithm to guide the effective use of these treatment options.

Meniscus Anatomy and Structure

The menisci are fibrocartilaginous structures that are semilunar in shape and wedge-shaped in cross-section. Two menisci (medial and lateral) exist between the femoral and tibial articulation. The femoral articulating meniscal surface is concave, whereas the tibial articulating surface is convex. These surfaces conform to the convex and concave opposing chondral surfaces, respectively. The conforming articulation provides perfect congruency between the femoral condyle, meniscus, and tibial plateau, which establishes the foundation for the biomechanical function of the menisci.

The medial and lateral menisci are significantly different in shape largely because of the structural differences between the medial and lateral femoral condyles and tibial plateau (Fig. 96-1). Both the macroscopic and microscopic anatomy of the menisci determine its function. The medial and lateral menisci are two C-shaped fibrocartilaginous structures attached anteriorly and posteriorly to the tibial plateau. The medial meniscus is longer in the anteroposterior direction compared with the lateral meniscus. The anterior horn of the medial meniscus is smaller in sagittal cross-section compared with the posterior horn. The anterior and posterior horns of the lateral meniscus, on the other hand, are similar in size. Approximately 50% of the medial tibial plateau is covered by the medial meniscus, compared with 59% coverage of the lateral tibial plateau by the lateral meniscus.[9]

Anchoring of the menisci occurs through insertional fibers and ligament attachments. Insertional fibers anchor both menisci to the subchondral bone at their anterior and posterior horns. The intermeniscal ligament also directly attaches the anterior horns of both menisci in most patients. The medial meniscus is continuous with the deep fibers of the medial collateral ligament and medial joint capsule, rendering it less mobile than the lateral meniscus. Nevertheless, the posterior horn of the medial meniscus remains mobile up to 5 mm to accommodate femoral rollback.[2,10] The lateral meniscus, on the other hand, has significantly fewer capsular and ligamentous attachments and thus is more mobile. Normal lateral meniscal excursion has been documented up to 11 mm and may partially explain the reduced incidence of lateral meniscal injuries.[10] The intraarticular portion of the popliteus tendon can be identified at the popliteal hiatus located between the posterolateral border of the lateral meniscus and the posterior knee capsule. This area of potential hypermobility is stabilized by the superior and inferior popliteomeniscal fasciculi that secure the posterolateral meniscus to the popliteus and posterior joint capsule (Fig. 96-2).[11] Fascicular injury can produce lateral meniscus hypermobility and may require meniscocapsular repair to reestablish meniscal stability.

In addition to the fasciculi, additional lateral meniscal stability may be achieved through accessory meniscofemoral ligaments in up to 66% of patients. Two accessory ligaments are frequently encountered: the ligament of Humphrey and the ligament of Wrisberg. Although uncommon, a Wrisberg ligament variant may also exist in the setting of a discoid

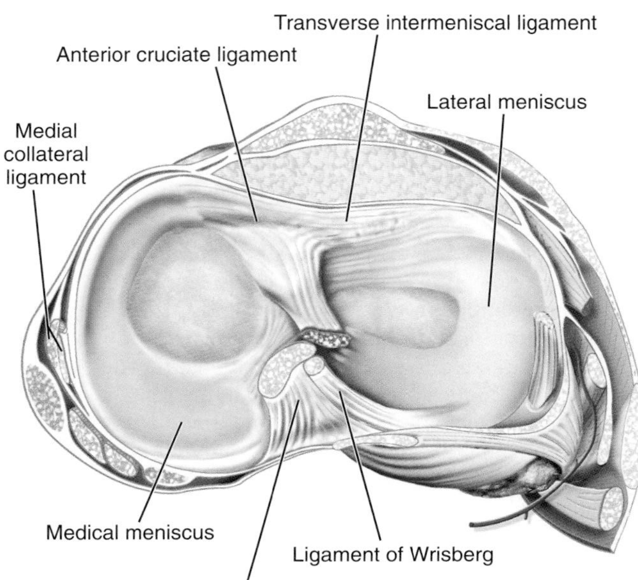

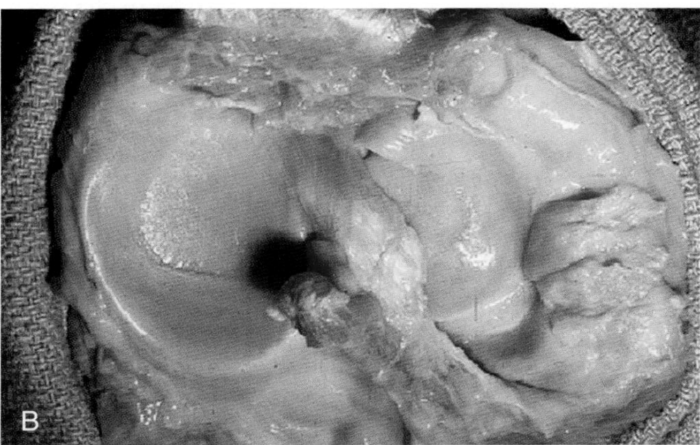

FIGURE 96-1 Superior schematic (**A**) and cadaveric dissection (**B**) views of meniscal axial anatomy demonstrate the structural differences and specific attachment sites of the anterior and posterior horns of the medial and lateral meniscus. *(Modified from Pagnani MJ, Warren RF, Arnoczky SP, et al: Anatomy of the knee. In Nicholas JA, Hershman EB, editors:* The lower extremity and spine in sports medicine, *ed 2, St Louis, 1995, Mosby.)*

lateral meniscus, in which there is deficiency of the meniscocapsular attachments, with only a stout Wrisberg ligament stabilizing the posterior horn (see Figs. 96-1 and 96-2). The ligament of Humphrey extends from the medial femoral condyle to the posterior horn of the lateral meniscus and courses anterior to the posterior cruciate ligament (PCL). The ligament of Wrisberg and Wrisberg's variant have similar attachments but course posterior to the PCL.

Histologically, dense fibrocartilage is composed of collagen fibers that are arranged circumferentially (to disperse compressive loads or "hoop stresses") with some radial fibers as well (to resist longitudinal tearing). At the surface, collagen fibers are arranged randomly to disperse shear stress associated with flexion and extension of the knee joint (Fig. 96-3).[2] Proteoglycan macromolecules hold and retain water, which is paramount to the compressive, shock-absorbing properties of

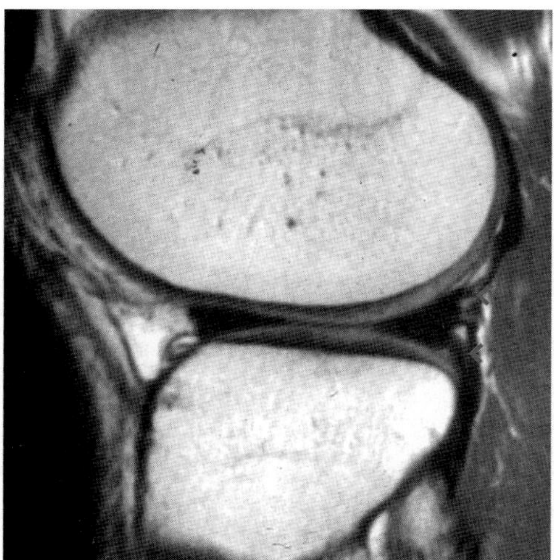

FIGURE 96-2 A sagittal magnetic resonance imaging scan demonstrating the anatomic relationship of the superior and inferior popliteomeniscal fasciculi of the lateral meniscus (*red arrowheads*).

the menisci and augments its ability to aid in lubrication of the knee joint.

The blood supply of the menisci originates at the periphery in the perimeniscal capillary plexus, which are tributaries of the medial and lateral geniculate arteries. Importantly, only the peripheral 25% to 30% of the meniscus is vascularized (Fig. 96-4).[12] The gradient attenuation in vascularity from the periphery to the central portion of the menisci is gradual, but the need for ease of clinical classification led to the designation of three vascular "zones." The outer third is known as the "red-red zone" because of its relatively high concentration of vascular channels. In this zone, bleeding at the site of injury promotes fibrovascular scar formation and migration of anabolic cells in response to cytokines released during the inflammatory response. As a result, tears in this zone have the highest healing potential. The middle vascular zone is termed

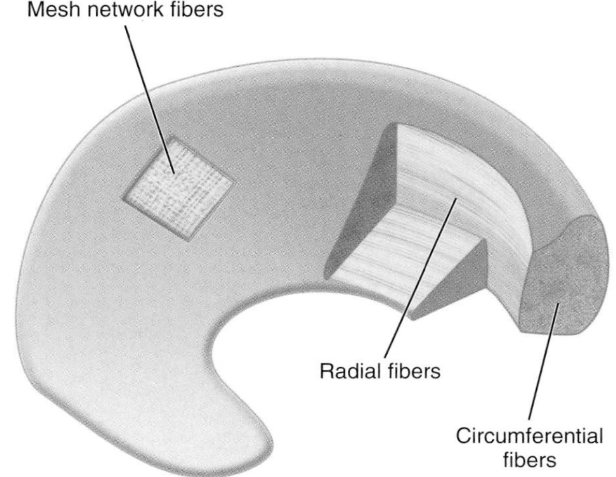

FIGURE 96-3 Meniscal microstructure. *(From Bullough PG, Munuera L, Murphy J, et al: The strength of the menisci of the knee as it relates to their fine structure.* J Bone Joint Surg Br *52B:564–567, 1970.)*

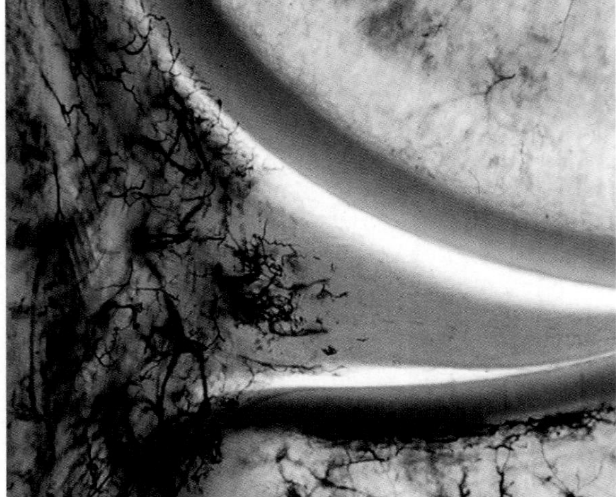

FIGURE 96-4 Adult meniscal microvasculature.

the *red-white zone*. This zone has intermediate vascularity, which leads to a less predictable result with regard to healing of meniscal tears. If a repair is attempted in this zone, ancillary techniques such as synovial abrasion, vascular access channels, and a fibrin clot may be used to increase local blood flow and maximize healing potential. The red-red and red-white zones combine to form the outer 4 mm of the meniscus.[13] The remainder of the meniscus is avascular in adults and is therefore called the *white-white zone*. Nutrition of this tissue is achieved solely from the synovial fluid via passive diffusion, which is aided by motion of the knee joint. Consequently, injury in the white-white zone of the meniscus does not stimulate a healing response, and the prognosis for healing after attempted repair is poor.

Meniscal neuroanatomy and vascular anatomy are extremely similar both in density and location. The periphery and anterior and posterior horns of the menisci have a significantly higher density of neural components compared with the central regions.[2,8] Both mechanical and sensory fibers have been identified in these locations and may contribute to pain and proprioception during knee range of motion. Dye et al.[14] substantiated these basic science data through clinical study with use of neurosensory meniscal mapping. This study documented significant neural activity at the meniscocapsular junction and meniscal periphery, compared with limited activity in the central region. These data suggest that mechanical loading of the peripheral meniscal rim and meniscocapsular junction may be responsible for most of the pain experienced after a meniscal injury.

Meniscus Biomechanics and Function

The medial and lateral menisci function to provide mechanical support and secondary stabilization, localized pressure distribution and load sharing, lubrication, and proprioception to the knee joint.[2,3] Mechanically, the menisci also transmit at least 50% to 75% of the axial load in knee extension and up to 85% with the knee in 90 degrees of flexion (Fig. 96-5).[15]

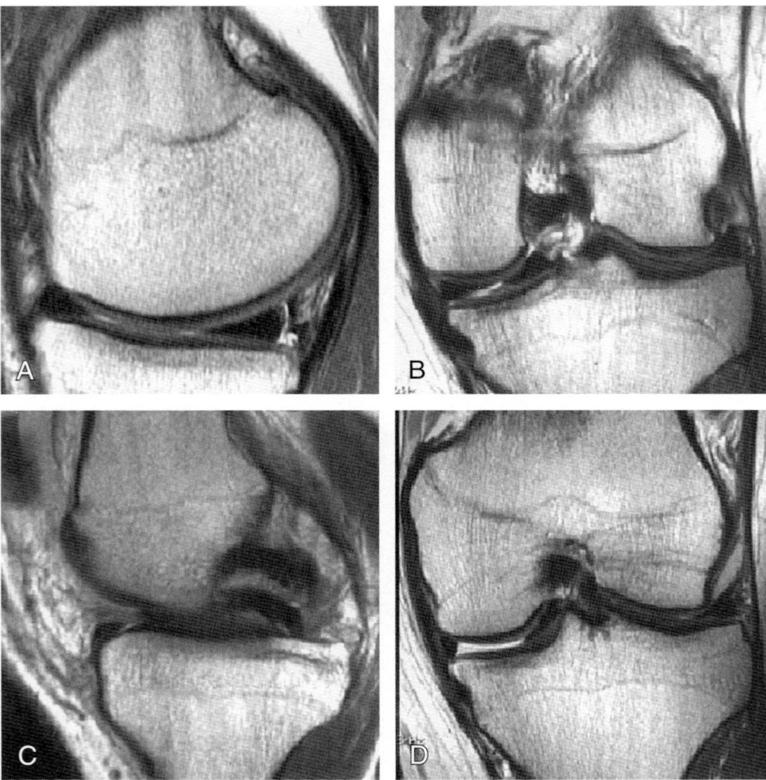

FIGURE 96-5 Magnetic resonance imaging of the medial and lateral menisci. **A,** A sagittal image demonstrates increased signal within the peripheral rim of the posterior horn of the medial meniscus, indicating a peripheral vertical meniscal tear. **B,** A coronal view demonstrates a complex medial meniscal tear. **C,** A double posterior cruciate ligament sign indicates a bucket handle meniscal tear displaced into the notch. **D,** A coronal view demonstrates an absent posterior horn due to a displaced bucket handle tear that can be visualized in the notch.

The femoral and tibial radii of curvature are significantly different and thus are poorly congruent at the point of articulation. The menisci provide the congruency necessary for both load transmission and knee stability. They decrease the peak contact stresses at the articular surface by 100% to 200%.[16-18] Removal of the menisci during partial or total meniscectomy results in increased point contact loading at the femorotibial articulation and significantly increased contract stresses focused in a small area. A recent biomechanical study by Lee et al.[19] highlighted this function by documenting increased contact stress with incrementally increasing meniscectomy in a dose-response fashion. Moreover, resection of 75% of the posterior horn can increase contact stresses similar to those present after a total meniscectomy.[16,19]

This process is particularly notable in the lateral compartment because of its specific anatomic differences. The femoral and tibial articulation is a convex-convex articulation that is buffered by the lateral meniscus, which covers up to 70% of the tibial surface area. This articulation is in direct contrast to the convex-concave femorotibial articulation in the medial compartment. For this reason, partial or complete removal of the lateral meniscus results in greater contact stresses and increased risk for progression of osteoarthrosis compared with the medial compartment.[17,20]

The menisci perform a crucial role in shock absorption in addition to contact stress distribution. The meniscal collagen ultrastructure is organized in a circumferential fashion with radial linking fibers, thereby allowing conversion of axial loads to horizontal “hoop” stresses. This shock absorption is also aided by the reduced meniscal cartilage stiffness, increased elasticity, and biphasic structure. Prior data have demonstrated that total meniscectomy results in a 20% decrease in shock absorption, and thus preservation of meniscal integrity is crucial to minimize chondral damage.[21]

The role of the meniscus as a secondary stabilizer of the knee has also been well documented. Bedi et al.[22] noted that transection of the anterior cruciate ligament (ACL) and meniscectomy resulted in nearly double the anterior tibial translation in both Lachman and pivot shift testing compared with that of the ACL alone, as measured with knee-specific computer navigation software. The secondary stabilizing effect is primarily due to the posterior horn of the medial meniscus in resisting anterior tibial translation as demonstrated during a Lachman maneuver.[22,23] Prior data have demonstrated that deficiency of the posterior horn of the medial meniscus in the setting of primary ACL reconstruction is associated with a higher risk of graft elongation and recurrent joint laxity.[24] In this setting, the posterior horn of the medial meniscus functions as a wedge buttress to inhibit anterior tibial translation. Prior data have documented a 58% increase in anterior tibial translation with medial meniscectomy in the flexed ACL-deficient knee.[25]

The biomechanical stabilizing effect of the lateral meniscus has also been well documented. Lateral meniscal deficiency may significantly reduce knee stability, specifically with tibial internal rotation (and subsequent pivot shift).[26] Musahl et al.[27] used computer-assisted navigation in a cadaveric model to document a significant 6-mm increase in anterior tibial translation after a lateral meniscectomy in ACL-deficient knees during the pivot shift but not Lachman maneuvers. These data demonstrate the importance of the lateral meniscus as a stabilizer during axial, rotatory loading of the knee.

Epidemiology

Acute and chronic tears of the menisci are very common orthopaedic injuries that affect patients of various ages and activity levels. Meniscal injury often causes pain and physical impairment, and clinical symptoms such as catching, locking, and decreased range of motion may frequently require surgical intervention for relief. The treatment for meniscal tears has evolved over the course of several decades with both technological and intellectual advances in orthopaedic surgery.

Since 1936, when total meniscectomy was the treatment of choice,[28] abundant research has led to the understanding that meniscal tissue should be retained whenever feasible.[29,30] For this reason, recent measures have attempted to preserve as much of the meniscus as possible. These measures have evolved from open total meniscectomy to open partial meniscectomy and finally to arthroscopic partial meniscectomy or repair. Meniscal injury was recently noted to be the most common musculoskeletal injury, occurring with a frequency of 23.8/100,000 per year.[31] The American Academy of Orthopedic Surgeons estimates that arthroscopy procedures of the knee total 636,000 cases per year in the United States as of 1999.[32] Within this cohort, arthroscopic treatment of meniscal injury is among the most common procedure performed, accounting for 10% to 20% of all surgeries at some centers.[33]

Improved understanding of the etiology, management, and outcomes for meniscal injury has been obtained from epidemiologic data regarding gender, age, activity level and type, and patient comorbidities.[7,34-40] Men are up to four times more likely than women to sustain a meniscal tear.[2,34] Cutting and pivoting sports requiring knee flexion at high activity levels generate the highest risk for meniscal injury, including basketball, soccer, gymnastics, wrestling, football, and skiing. Additionally, lateral meniscal tears are less common than medial meniscal tears for most of these activities and all age groups.[34,37-40]

Recent advances in radiology including magnetic resonance imaging (MRI) have significantly improved the diagnosis of meniscal injury. However, improved imaging has also increased the frequency of incidental meniscal pathology that does not necessarily correlate with clinical symptoms. Prior data have documented a 5.6% incidence of asymptomatic meniscal tears in a young patient population (mean age: 35 years).[41] Abnormal signal characteristics were also identified in the posterior horn of the medial meniscus in 24% of patients. These incidental findings significantly increase with age, with a 76% prevalence of meniscal tears in asymptomatic older patients (mean age, 65 years).[42]

Advanced imaging techniques have also aided in diagnosing meniscal pathology in the setting of concomitant ligament injury. Injury to the ACL has been associated with a significantly increased risk of lateral and medial meniscal tears due to the mechanism of acute ACL injury and secondary stabilizing effects in chronic ACL tears, respectively. Prior data have documented a 60% to 70% prevalence of meniscal tears in the setting of acute ACL injury.[43] Lateral meniscal tears more commonly occur as a result of the rotational and translational mechanism of injury.[43,44] Previous data in a young population with acute ACL ruptures documented a 57% and 36% prevalence of concomitant lateral and medial meniscal tears, respectively.[43] However, medial meniscal tears are more commonly identified in the setting of chronic ACL tears.

Meniscal Injury: Classification

Multiple types of tears have been described, including vertical (longitudinal or circumferential), radial, horizontal (transverse or cleavage), degenerative, and complex tears and horn detachment (Fig. 96-6). Vertical, oblique, and longitudinal patterns are most common in the younger population, whereas complex degenerative tears are more often seen in patients older than 40 years. Numerous authors have observed that tear type and configuration were predictive of outcome, with complex unstable tears (i.e., those with >3-mm displacement upon examination with an arthroscopic probe) faring worse than simple vertical-longitudinal tear types.[45,46]

Vertical (longitudinal or circumferential) meniscal tears are frequently due to a traumatic etiology such as an ACL tear. These tears are also termed *bucket handle tears* when they are large (>1 cm), displaced, and unstable. Bucket handle tears may frequently cause mechanical symptoms, including locking and the inability to fully extend the knee. They more frequently occur in the medial meniscus because of the limited motion afforded by the strong peripheral meniscocapsular attachments. Smaller, incomplete vertical tears more commonly occur and are frequently identified at the time of arthroscopy. These incomplete tears do not require intervention in the setting of concomitant ACL injury if they are determined to be stable when manually probed.[47,48]

Oblique (parrot beak or flap) tears commonly occur at the junction of the posterior and middle body of the meniscus. These unstable tears frequently cause mechanical symptoms including locking and catching during knee motion that may or may not produce pain. The associated pain has been hypothesized to be associated with irritation of the meniscocapsular junction and surrounding synovium. This tear type is not typically amenable to repair because it most commonly occurs in the white-white meniscal region. Excision of the unstable fragment is effective in addressing the mechanical symptoms.

Radial tears are oriented perpendicular to the circumferential fibers and are commonly identified in the lateral meniscus after an acute ACL rupture. Again, variability exists in the length of these tears, which range from small to large tears that extend from the white-white zone through to the periphery. A small radial tear involving less than 60% of the meniscus does not significantly influence compartment biomechanics, whereas a large radial tear that extends through more than 90% of the meniscus to the periphery results in a significant increase in peak compartment pressures.[49] Partial tears preserve the crucial peripheral circumferential fibers and thus the load distribution ability of the meniscus. This radial tear subtype can be debrided to a stable edge in most circumstances. Complete tears, on the other hand, result in complete circumferential fiber disruption, which not only compromises the function of the meniscus but also increases the biomechanical tendency for repair diastasis with axial load. Although diastasis significantly impairs healing, repair of this tear type should be attempted, because the only alternative treatment is effectively a near-total meniscectomy. Strict non–weight-bearing rehabilitation should be instituted after repair of complete radial tears to reduce the potential for tear diastasis.

Horizontal tears often develop from variable shear stress between the superior and inferior meniscal regions in the early stage of meniscal degeneration. This tear type is typically a degenerative tear and may be associated with meniscal cyst formation that may communicate with the periphery. These tears have been commonly identified on MRI; however, their presence is not necessarily linked to clinical symptoms.[50] Although some data suggest that cyst aspiration and suture repair of the horizontal tear may obviate the need for meniscectomy,[51] in our opinion, most horizontal tears, including associated flaps, can be treated with a partial meniscectomy.

Complex tears of the meniscus occur in a stellate pattern and propagate through multiple planes, although the horizontal cleavage plane is most common. These tears most commonly occur at the posterior root, are degenerative in nature, and should be treated with partial meniscectomy if surgical management is indicated.

A meniscal tear zone classification has been documented and divides each meniscus into three radial and four circumferential zones. This classification system permits improved clinical documentation and comparison of outcomes (Fig. 96-7).[52]

History

Meniscal tears can be either traumatic or degenerative. Degenerative tears have been closely associated with osteoarthritis. Acute tears are often related to trauma, most frequently as a result of a twisting motion. Early diagnosis and treatment of acute meniscal tears can significantly affect the short-term meniscal viability and subsequent long-term articular chondral protection. This treatment is particularly critical in a younger population given the high incidence of acute,

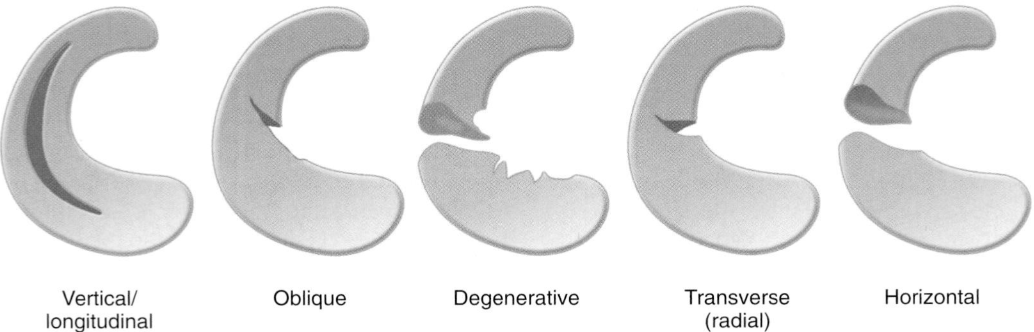

FIGURE 96-6 A descriptive classification of meniscal tears. *(Modified from Ciccotti MG, Shields CL, El Attrache NS: Meniscectomy. In Fu FH, Harner CD, Vince KG, editors:* Knee surgery*, Baltimore, 1994, Williams & Wilkins.)*

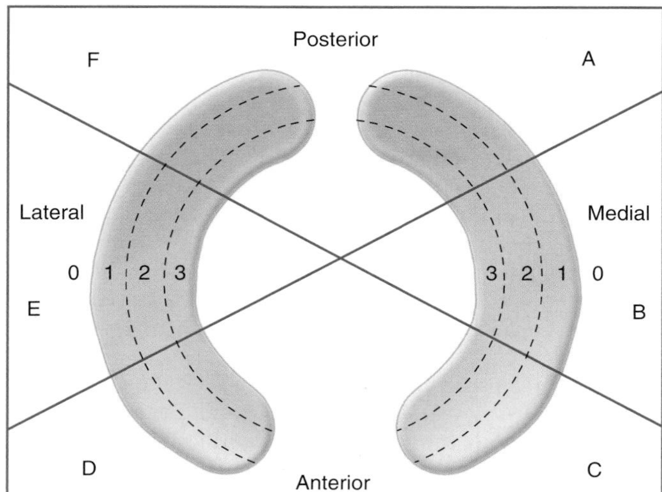

FIGURE 96-7 Classification of a meniscal tear according to the anatomic position and vascularity. *(Modified from Cooper DE, Arnoczky SP, Warren RF: Arthroscopic meniscal repair.* Clin Sports Med *9:589–607, 1990.)*

traumatic meniscal tears and the importance of joint preservation at an early age.

A carefully completed history, physical examination, and diagnostic imaging evaluation facilitates efficient and accurate diagnosis and guide appropriate treatment. The aforementioned epidemiology should aid in guiding the patient history with regard to age, mechanism of injury, activity level, concomitant pathology, and previous ipsilateral injury or surgery. Additionally, fundamental questions should also be asked, including the location and duration of symptoms, exacerbating activities, and alleviating mechanisms, including medication and activity modification.

Patients may or may not be able to recall a single traumatic event. These events typically include twisting or hyperflexion with or without a mild effusion that may be noticed the day after injury. Notably, this effusion is nonspecific for meniscal pathology. Pain is often localized to the joint line and is usually intermittent. Constant pain or pain at rest usually indicates separate or additional pathology, such as osteoarthritis. Mechanical symptoms may also herald an unstable flap or bucket handle meniscal tear; these symptoms include catching, locking, popping, pinching, or the feeling of having to move the knee through a specific range of motion to "reset" the joint. Clear evidence of locking due to an incarcerated torn meniscal fragment must be described as an inability to achieve full extension. Unlike traumatic tears, degenerative, chronic meniscal tears are atraumatic and are rarely associated with an acute effusion. Instead, patients may describe mild intermittent effusions, infrequent mechanical symptoms, and generalized joint-line pain. These tears more commonly affect an older, less active population and may exist with concomitant osteoarthrosis.

Physical Examination

Physical examination of the patient with a possible meniscus tear should include an evaluation of gait, standing alignment, range of motion and strength testing of the hip and knee, ligament stability testing, and a careful inspection and palpation of the knee with particular attention directed to the joint line. Additional specialized tests including the McMurray and Apley grind tests may also be included.[53-58] The contralateral extremity should also be examined for comparison because of the variability and patient-specific nature of these physical examination findings.

Physical examination may reveal an antalgic gait with varus or valgus alignment. This alignment may prove to be pertinent to the etiology and treatment of the meniscal tear. Displaced tears may present with a mechanical block to range of motion that is also associated with distinct pain at that end point. Pain with deep knee flexion is nonspecific but is common for posterior horn injuries. Cruciate and collateral ligament stability should then be evaluated. A visible knee effusion may also exist that can be exaggerated with "milking" or manipulation of the suprapatellar pouch to maximize the size of the effusion inferiorly. At this time, palpation for point tenderness should be performed with a focus on ligamentous and tendinous origins and insertions and the joint line. We prefer to perform the palpation component of the examination with the patient in a supine position with the hip externally rotated and the knee flexed to 90 degrees. Notably, palpable joint line tenderness has been repeatedly identified as the most sensitive and specific physical examination finding for meniscal pathology.[44,53,56,59] However, joint-line tenderness is significantly less accurate for identifying meniscal pathology in the setting of an ACL injury.[57]

Provocative maneuvers that cause meniscal fragment impingement between the femoral and tibial surfaces have also been described. The McMurray test is performed on the medial meniscus by flexing the knee, creating a varus stress by internally rotating the tibia, and bringing the knee into full extension. Reproducible pain with a palpable mechanical click or pop indicates a positive examination. Conversely, the lateral meniscus is tested with an applied valgus stress and external tibial rotation. Another commonly performed test is the Apley grind test, in which an axial load is created with concurrent internal and external rotation ("grind") with the patient positioned prone and the affected knee flexed to 90 degrees. A positive examination is defined as pain at the medial and/or lateral joint line. A new clinical test, termed the *Thessaly test,* has been used to increase the diagnostic accuracy of the physical examination for meniscal tears by dynamically reproducing the load transmission in the knee joint at 5 and 20 degrees of knee flexion. The Thessaly test is performed with the examiner holding the patient's outstretched hands while he or she performs a single leg stance flat-footed on the affected extremity and axially rotates three times with the knee in 5 degrees and then 20 degrees of flexion. A positive test is documented with the presence of medial or lateral joint-line pain and possible mechanical symptoms. When this test is performed in 20 degrees of flexion, a 94% and 96% accuracy has been documented for medial and lateral meniscal tears, respectively, with low false-positive and false-negative results.[58]

Imaging

Isolated meniscal pathology can be accurately diagnosed in more than 90% of patients with history and physical examination alone. Nevertheless, diagnostic imaging, including plain radiographs and MRI, is critical to confirm clinical suspicions, evaluate alignment, and identify concomitant pathology. Imaging is particularly useful when concomitant chondral or ligament pathology exists because the history and physical examination are far less accurate in this setting.

Plain radiographs should be the first-line radiographic study but are not sensitive or specific to meniscal pathology. Weight-bearing anteroposterior, lateral, and 45-degree flexed posteroanterior views should be obtained. A Merchant patellar view allows evaluation of patellofemoral pathology. Standing knee alignment can be assessed and correlated with meniscal pathology and, if a significant concern exists for abnormal alignment, a full-length, standing, long cassette, anteroposterior hip to ankle view of both lower extremities should be obtained. Degenerative joint disease may indicate a degenerative meniscal tear, but acute tears have no specific radiographic findings.

MRI is the ideal radiographic study for visualizing soft tissue pathology, including injury to the meniscus, capsule, ligaments, and articular cartilage. Arthrography was historically used prior to MRI to identify meniscal tears and may be considered in the setting of a contraindication to MRI. MRI is a noninvasive study that is performed without exposure to ionizing radiation and is able to image in multiple planes, thereby providing a three-dimensional depiction of soft tissue and osseous structures. Previous studies have documented a very high accuracy for MRI identification of meniscal abnormalities.[60,61]

We routinely obtain MRI imaging for evaluation of meniscal pathology using both fat-suppressed and diffusion-weighted fast spin-echo (cartilage sensitive) axial, coronal, and sagittal images (Fig. 96-8). Normal meniscal architecture is demonstrated by uniform low signal intensity on both fast spin-echo and fat-suppressed images. A high signal within the meniscal substance but not extending to the articular surface frequently exists as a result of intrasubstance degeneration. This signal may lead to an overinterpretation of a meniscal tear. Grading of the meniscal high signal can minimize this overinterpretation (see Fig. 96-8).[62] Grade I is characterized by a nonfocal intrasubstance high signal without articular extension. Grade II is a focal linear high-signal region without articular extension. Grade III is a focal linear high-signal region located at the free edge of the meniscus with superior or inferior articular extension. A grade III signal that is identified on two or more MRI images has 90% sensitivity for representing a true meniscal tear.[62] Nevertheless, careful evaluation of the surrounding structures, including the meniscofemoral and intermeniscal ligaments and popliteus tendon, should be conducted because they may mimic a meniscal tear.

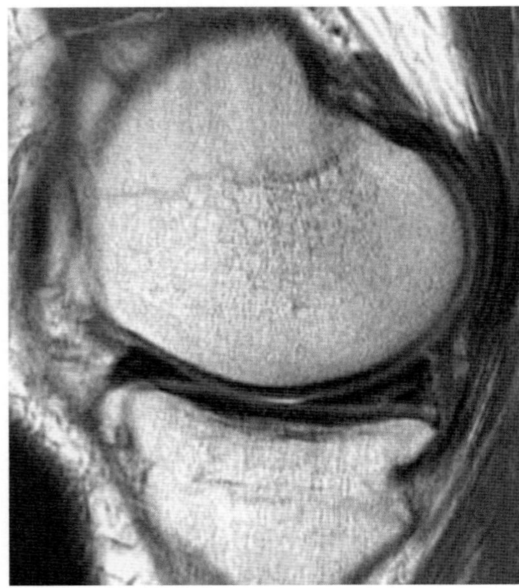

FIGURE 96-8 A sagittal fat-suppressed magnetic resonance imaging slice demonstrates a grade III linear signal communicating with joint space through the inferior surface of the meniscus.

Sagittal meniscal windows may aid in identifying acute, vertical meniscal tears and bucket handle tears, whereas coronal images are most helpful for identification of horizontal degenerative tears. Axial imaging may further confirm the existence of radial and flap tears. Bucket handle tears should be carefully evaluated at the intercondylar notch with the classic double PCL sign where the displaced meniscal tissue may be identified as a second low-signal line parallel and anterior to the PCL.

Despite the high sensitivity and noninvasive attributes of MRI, significant limitations exist, including higher cost and technical errors in both imaging technique and interpretation. Multiple studies have shown a high percentage of asymptomatic meniscal tears on MRI examination ranging from 36%[63] to 76%.[64] This percentage increases significantly with patient age.[65] Prior MRI data from asymptomatic patients older than 65 years documented a 67% prevalence of meniscal tears.[42] This prevalence increased to 86% in the setting of symptomatic osteoarthritis. For this reason, it is important to correlate MRI findings with the history and physical examination and, when indicated, findings on arthroscopy.

Treatment Options

Nonoperative Management

Nonoperative management of meniscal tears is not designed to facilitate healing of the tear but rather is directed at symptom management. Although prior data have documented spontaneous healing of stable, isolated peripheral meniscal tears, this outcome is a rare exception. Most unrepaired meniscal tears will not progress to healing,[66] and therefore nonoperative management must be directed at reducing symptoms in carefully selected patients. Our experience suggests that most symptomatic meniscal lesions in the absence of significant concomitant osteoarthrosis do not respond well to nonoperative management, especially in the setting of mechanical symptoms, despite some evidence that symptom resolution may occur with this approach.[66] However, nonoperative treatment is frequently used in the setting of associated medial or lateral compartment osteoarthrosis with concomitant meniscal tears and the absence of mechanical symptoms.

Nonoperative management should include rest, use of ice and nonsteroidal antiinflammatory medications, and activity modification for 6 to 12 weeks. Intraarticular injections of corticosteroids, analgesic medications such as lidocaine or bupivacaine, and viscosupplementation may also be used if concomitant osteoarthrosis is present. We do not suggest this methodology in the absence of osteoarthrosis, and it should be noted that corticosteroids may impair meniscal healing and that bupivacaine may lead to chondral damage.[67-69] It is important to note that nonoperative management of an unstable, repairable meniscal tear may also result in tear propagation, thereby producing an irreparable tear that must be excised.

Operative Management

Surgical Indications

The definitive treatment of meniscal tears involves either repair or excision of the pathologic tissue. Surgery is indicated in patients who have persistent mechanical symptoms and/or pain and have not responded to a course of nonoperative treatment. The indications for arthroscopy include (1) symptoms of meniscal injury that affect activities of daily living, work, and/or sports participation, such as instability, locking, effusion, and pain; (2) positive physical findings of joint-line tenderness, joint effusion, limitation of motion, and provocative signs, such as pain with squatting, a positive pinch test, or a positive McMurray test; (3) failure to respond to nonsurgical treatment, including activity modification, medication, and a rehabilitation program; and (4) ruling out other causes of knee pain identified by patient history, physical examination, plain radiographs, or other imaging studies.[70,71]

Timing of the injury and surgical management must also be considered. Acute tears have a higher rate of successful healing compared with chronic ones; it is understood that repairs of tears less than 8 weeks old heal more frequently compared with older tears.[72] Additionally, patients undergoing repairs of traumatic meniscal tears have better 6-year functional results than do persons with degenerative meniscal tears.[73,74] The majority of these studies, however, combine traumatic meniscal tear and concomitant injury. Stein et al.[75] recently compared long-term outcomes after arthroscopic meniscal repair versus partial meniscectomy for traumatic meniscal tears and documented no difference in function score. However, the meniscal repair group demonstrated a higher rate of return to preinjury and sporting activity levels. Additionally, only 40% of the meniscal repair group demonstrated osteoarthritic progression at 8-year follow-up compared with 81% of the partial meniscectomy group. For these reasons, a recent traumatic history should be considered a good prognostic factor for meniscal healing within the meniscal repair algorithm.

The influence of patient age on meniscal repair outcome has been well documented. Prior data have documented a reduced cellularity and healing response in patients older than 40 years.[76] Increased repeat tear rates have also been documented in patients older than 30 years,[77] although failure occurred later in older patients.[78] The association between increased age and worse outcome seems to be negated in the setting of avascular tears and meniscal tears with concomitant ACL rupture. No difference between younger patients and older patients (>40 years) has been found with regard to clinical success after meniscal repairs performed for tears with relative avascularity.[79,80] Kalliakmanis et al.[81] recently documented no difference in repair failure between older or younger patients younger than 35 years of age in the setting of a concomitant ACL tear. Although prognostic factors including avascular tears, concomitant ACL rupture, and continued ligamentous instability seem to play identical roles in younger patients,[82] the consequence of postmeniscectomy arthritis remains significantly greater.

From the aforementioned variables, one may synthesize surgical indications for meniscal repair that can predict healing prognosis. Contraindications for repair include older or sedentary patients or patients who are unable to perform the necessary postoperative rehabilitation. Additionally, isolated inner third white-white tears with a remaining rim greater than 6 mm should not be repaired. Borderline tears including middle third white-white tears should only be considered for repair if extension exists into the red-white or red-red region. Degenerative or stable longitudinal (<12 mm in length) tears should also not be repaired. Meniscal tears with a peripheral rim less than 4 mm should be considered for repair, because removal of this large tear will result in biomechanical alterations similar to a total meniscectomy.[83] Particular consideration should be given in this circumstance to patients younger than 40 years of age and those with active lifestyles. Meniscal repair is ideal in younger patients with acute traumatic tears. The adverse sequelae of meniscectomy are most marked after a lateral meniscectomy in young, active women, with some patients demonstrating a relatively rapid progression to lateral compartment arthrosis. Thus aggressive attempts should be made to repair the lateral meniscus in this setting.

Arthroscopy

Arthroscopy can be used both to confirm the diagnosis and to treat meniscal pathology. Careful evaluation of the meniscal tear configuration should aid in preoperative planning regarding potential meniscectomy, meniscal repair, or even transplantation. Nevertheless, a complete diagnostic arthroscopy with careful probing of all intraarticular structures remains the gold standard for diagnosis of meniscal injury and should be conducted to confirm the preoperative diagnosis and identify other potential intraarticular pathology.

Special Circumstances

Meniscal Root Tears

Diagnosis and treatment of a tear in the anterior or posterior root of the medial or lateral meniscus is extremely important because of the biomechanical role that these attachments play in meniscal stability. These tears often occur with concomitant ligamentous injury, including ACL ruptures and multiligamentous knee injury. Unstable posterior root tears of the lateral meniscus may be identified with high-energy acute ACL tears because of the translation and impaction of the posterolateral meniscus and the tibial plateau that occur during the traumatic pivot shift.[84]

Anterior or posterior root tears can be repaired through an arthroscopic approach. Bone tunnel and suture anchor repairs have been described with good success. Both techniques should include preparation of the anatomic insertion site with osseous abrasion to stimulate a vascular footprint. The first step of the bone tunnel repair requires passing nonabsorbable sutures through the anterior or posterior root tissue. An arthroscopic guide can then be used to facilitate the creation of a bone tunnel from the anterior tibial cortex to the meniscal root footprint. The nonabsorbable sutures should then be retrieved through the tunnel and secured at the anterior tibial aperture over a bone bridge or other preferred cortical fixation device. The suture anchor repair is performed by placing a suture anchor in the footprint of the meniscal root followed by passing the loaded sutures through the meniscal root and subsequent reduction and fixation. A posteromedial or posterolateral accessory portal is required to place the suture anchor in the correct position for posterior horn tears.

Lateral Meniscus Fascicular Tears

Tears of the fascicular attachments to the lateral meniscus represent a unique injury to the lateral meniscus. Stabilization of the lateral meniscus differs from the medial meniscus because of the intraarticular position of the popliteus tendon. For this reason, direct meniscocapsular attachment is not possible in this region. Two popliteomeniscal fasciculi that anchor the lateral meniscus to the popliteus tendon have been described.[11] Fascicular tears can produce an unstable posterolateral meniscus and mechanical symptoms. Repair of these anchoring fasciculi can be achieved using an inside-out or all-inside repair because of the vascular nature of these peripheral attachments. Incarceration of the popliteal tendon should be avoided during suture placement.

Meniscal Cysts

Meniscal cysts may also be identified in conjunction with an adjacent meniscal tear. Meniscal tears may lead to the formation of meniscal cysts, likely because of a one-way valve mechanism that allows extravasation and capture of synovial fluid. This mechanism is particularly prevalent with horizontal cleavage tears in the anterior meniscal region. Prior data have suggested that cysts are up to seven times more common in the lateral compartment, but recent MRI data have documented an equivalent prevalence.[85,86]

Treatment of both the cyst and the associated meniscal tears is important to effectively address the one-way valve mechanism by which the cyst likely occurred. Arthroscopic partial meniscectomy and debridement remove the one-way valve mechanism created by the opposing flaps and provide access to and decompression of the associated cyst. Intraarticular extravasation of the cyst fluid may be observed during the arthroscopic debridement and can serve as a confirmatory sign of effective management. Open cystectomy may also be performed in rare cases with no associated meniscal pathology or an unusually large fluid collection. Both surgical techniques have been associated with good outcomes.[87-90] Ultrasound-guided aspiration of the cyst is rarely a definitive treatment, because the fluid in the cyst may reaccumulate.

Discoid Meniscus and Meniscal Variants

Young[91] first identified the discoid meniscus during a cadaveric dissection in 1889. This variant likely occurs as a congenital anatomic variant but has been previously thought to occur because of abnormal embryologic apoptosis of the central meniscus during development. The prevalence of the discoid meniscus variant is approximately 5% but may be increased in the Asian population.[92-98] Both medial and lateral discoid menisci have been described, but the lateral side is much more common.[94,96,99] Bilateral discoid menisci may also occur in up to 20% of cases.

Three main lateral discoid meniscal variants exist according the classification system described by Watanabe et al.[100] This system was developed from arthroscopic observations of the lateral meniscus and its tibial attachments (Fig. 96-9). Type I describes a discoid variant that fully covers the lateral tibial plateau and has intact peripheral attachments. This type is the most common of the three variants. Type II is an incomplete variant that also has intact peripheral attachments but does not fully cover the tibial plateau. Type III, or the Wrisberg ligament type, is lacking the normal posterior meniscal attachments and is posteriorly anchored solely by the meniscofemoral ligament of Wrisberg. For this reason, this type has increased mobility of the posterior meniscal body and subsequent clinical instability. This instability has been termed *snapping-knee syndrome*. Fortunately, this unstable variant has a low prevalence of between 0 and 33%.[93,101-104] Notably, the posterior meniscal instability has been most commonly identified in younger patients with complete discoid morphology.[95] Absence of capsular attachments of the anterior aspect of a discoid meniscus with resultant instability of this portion of the meniscus has also been described.[105] Other classification systems also exist that attempt to provide a more specific description of the stability and structure and may prove more useful in guiding treatment.[106]

The majority of discoid menisci are incidentally identified and asymptomatic and thus do not require treatment; however, some discoid menisci require operative intervention because of symptomatic tears that occur from high intraarticular sheer

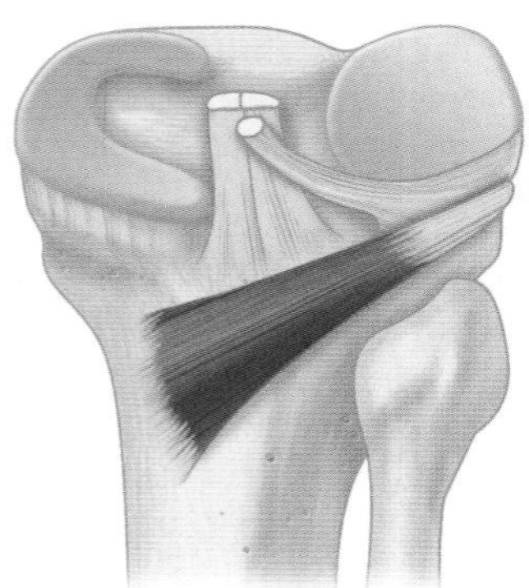
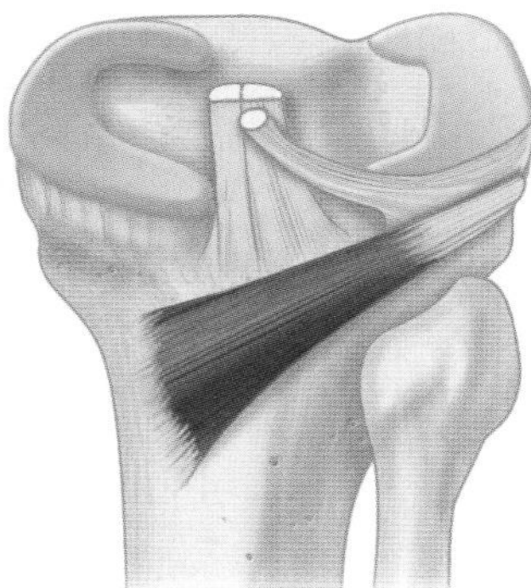
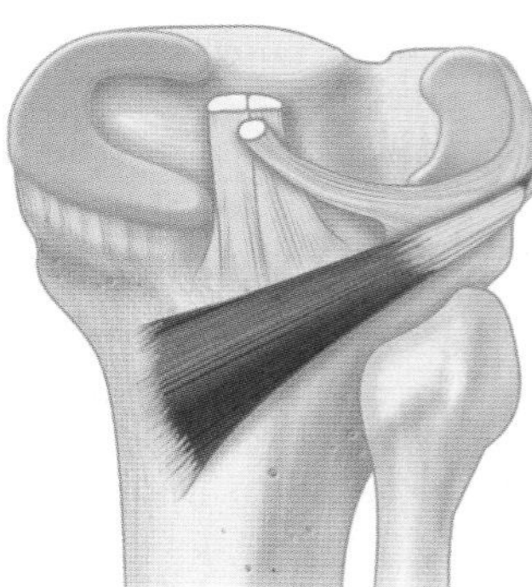

FIGURE 96-9 The Watanabe classification for discoid lateral menisci. *(From Kocher MS, Klingele K, Rassman SO: Meniscal disorders: Normal, discoid, and cysts.* Orthop Clin North Am *34:329–340, 2003.)*

stress. Common symptoms include mechanical snapping or clicking with type III discoid menisci or tears in previously stable type I or II variants. These mechanical symptoms may be associated with lateral joint-line pain and swelling. The patient may or may not be able to recall a specific traumatic event that was associated with the symptoms. Joint-line palpation may reveal focal tenderness at the location of the tear with or without a palpable click during motion. Diagnostic imaging should be performed, including plain radiographs, which can demonstrate lateral joint space widening and tibial plateau concavity, a flattened lateral femoral condyle, tibial spine hypoplasia, meniscal calcification, and concomitant lateral femoral condyle osteochondritis dissecans.[107,108] MRI evaluation should also be used to specifically evaluate the morphology of the meniscus and identify any tears. An absent "bow-tie" sign may be identified, demonstrating meniscal continuity between the anterior and posterior horns in three or more consecutive 5-mm coronal images (Fig. 96-10). Although this sign can be easily used to identify type I and II discoid variants, it is less effective for the type III variant. The type III variant can only be identified by the absence of small peripheral attachments because of the otherwise normal meniscal morphology.[107,109] Diagnostic arthroscopy should be used to confirm a clinical suspicion in this case.

Symptomatic type I and II variants should be treated with arthroscopic "saucerization" or partial meniscectomy with contouring to mimic normal meniscal morphology (see Fig. 96-9).[103,104,110-115] A motorized shaver or arthroscopic biter can be used to resect the abnormal central tissue and other associated torn or degenerative tissue. A peripheral 6- to 8-cm meniscal rim should be maintained and contoured to avoid potential repeat tearing. Careful technique should be used to avoid iatrogenic chondral injury, because the discoid meniscus is frequently associated with a tight, narrow joint space and thickened meniscus. The techniques previously described for partial meniscectomy should also be applied in this case. If a large meniscal tear that extends to the periphery or an unstable peripheral detachment is present, the surgeon should consider repair and stabilization according to the techniques described in the meniscal repair section.

The combination of saucerization and peripheral repair is particularly suited for treatment of a symptomatic, unstable type III discoid lateral meniscus. Careful evaluation of the stability of the peripheral rim should be performed to confirm an adequate repair and stabilization, because this variant can be significantly unstable. We suggest using an inside-out repair technique for these cases because of the young age and significant instability of this variant. Nevertheless, continued improvements in all-inside implants may increase the utility of the all-inside technique in this setting.

A total meniscectomy should be avoided, if possible, because of the clear association with early compartmental arthrosis.[116-120] Long-term data after a total meniscectomy have documented increased compartmental degeneration and arthrosis. Saucerization and repair, on the other hand, have been correlated with good to excellent early clinical and radiographic results.[103,104,111-114,121] Unfortunately, a total meniscectomy is required in some circumstances because of significant tissue degeneration or tearing without the possibility of repair. Patients in whom total meniscectomy is required should be observed carefully for early signs and symptoms of meniscal

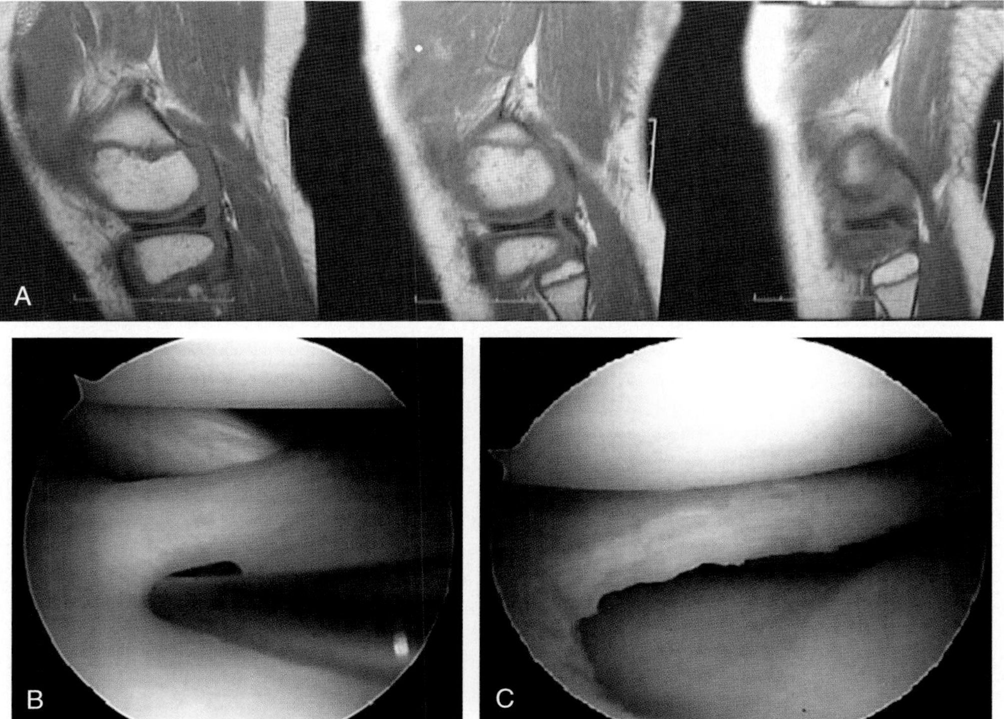

FIGURE 96-10 Discoid lateral meniscus. **A,** Diagnostic magnetic resonance imaging scans demonstrate absence of the classic "bow-tie" appearance of the lateral meniscus in three successive 5-mm cuts. **B,** The arthroscopic view of a complete discoid lateral meniscus. **C,** The arthroscopic view of a final saucerization procedure.

deficiency (i.e., early arthrosis) to optimize the potential for a future meniscal transplant when indicated.

Meniscal Allograft Transplantation

Although recent improvements in the understanding of meniscal biomechanics and pathology and advancement in surgical techniques have resulted in more focused attempts to preserve the meniscal integrity and structure, this goal is not possible in many cases. Severe cases may require total meniscectomy or segmental meniscal excision with subsequent chondral deterioration and osteoarthrosis. This degeneration can result in significant pain, activity limitation, and functional impairment. In these circumstances, a meniscal allograft transplant has been used as a surgical management option. Clinical and radiographic evaluation, surgical indications and techniques, and postoperative management for meniscal allograft transplantation are discussed later in this chapter.

Decision-Making Principles

We believe that the history and physical examination are the most important components for optimizing the management of a patient with meniscal pathology. The specific age, activity level, occupation, and sport-specific requirements must be carefully considered when developing an individualized treatment plan.

We routinely obtain an MRI for any patient with potential meniscal pathology. Noncontrast cartilage-specific MRI is used to carefully evaluate the menisci, ligaments, and articular cartilage. Although performing MRI routinely can be costly, we believe that the information provided is crucial for diagnosis and management. MRI can provide confirmation of a meniscal tear or identify mimicking pathology such as an articular chondral injury. Tailored nonoperative management or preoperative planning can be carefully constructed on the basis of these diagnostic imaging data. A concomitant articular chondral injury may also be identified and, when indicated, addressed at the time of surgery.

We believe that early diagnosis and management of a meniscal injury optimizes the biologic and clinical outcome. This early intervention is particularly important for younger patients. We perform most meniscal surgery procedures on an outpatient, ambulatory basis with use of a regional anesthetic. We typically use the anteromedial and anterolateral portals for most meniscal procedures but may create accessory posteromedial or posterolateral portals for improved visualization and instrumentation. We do not routinely use a superomedial or superolateral outflow portal because it is rarely required for visualization and can unnecessarily injure the quadriceps muscle.

In our institution, we use isolated trephination and synovial abrasion for partial-thickness tears and stable, vertical tears less than 10 mm in length. The remaining reparable tears undergo formal repair. Improvements in instrumentation have allowed a transition to an all-inside technique for most vertical posterior and midbody tears using the FasT-Fix suture system (Smith & Nephew, Andover, Massachusetts). Nevertheless, we continue to use the formal inside-out technique for a subset of patients, including those of a younger age and those who have large bucket-handle tears and unstable type III discoid variants. These techniques do not need to be used in isolation, and thus we frequently perform an all-inside repair for the posterior component of a tear followed by use of inside-out and outside-in techniques for anterior tear extension. We only consider repairing meniscal tears in the avascular zone in young patients who have a large fragment, particularly in the setting of concomitant ACL reconstruction.

Partial meniscectomy is reserved for irreparable tears, including radial, horizontal, oblique, and degenerative tear configurations. We carefully limit the meniscal resection to only that which is necessary to maintain a stable construct. Both ipsilateral and contralateral portals are used to maximize visualization and instrument access. A motorized shaver is used for final contouring of the meniscectomy. We prefer to use a curved shaver because the shaving edge can be easily mobilized with rotation and it provides excellent access to the posterior meniscal tissue.

The most important surgical decision regarding a meniscal injury is whether to excise or repair the lesion. This decision is directly dependent on the aforementioned vascular supply of the meniscal region in which the tear occurs—red-red, red-white, or white-white zones. Vertical tears are particularly amenable to repair if they occur at the meniscal periphery in the red-red zone. Repair of a centrally located red-white tear, on the other hand, is less successful because of the presence of vascular supply for only half of the meniscal substance. Nevertheless, meniscal repair may be considered in this region depending on the tear type. White-white tears, on the other hand, have an exceedingly low likelihood for successful repair, and thus a partial meniscectomy should be performed in this region.[52,122-127]

Surgical Techniques

Meniscectomy

Surgical meniscectomy should be performed after arthroscopic confirmation of an irreparable, unstable meniscal tear. The size of the tear should be carefully delineated using an arthroscopic probe to ensure that meniscal tissue is maximally preserved and all unstable fragments are removed. Fragments that can be displaced above or below the stable meniscal body or into the articular surface should be removed (Fig. 96-12).

Resection of meniscal tears can be performed efficiently using arthroscopic instruments including meniscal biters, punches, or motorized shavers. The position of the meniscal tear should be considered prior to instrument selection. Posterior horn tears of the medial meniscus may be easily viewed from the anterolateral portal, whereas an up-going punch can be placed through the anteromedial portal for resection. This arrangement should be reversed for posterior horn tears of the lateral meniscus, and a straight biter may prove more useful given the convexity of the lateral tibial surface. Care should be taken during meniscectomy to minimize iatrogenic chondral injury that can occur with intraarticular instrument introduction and movement within the joint. Positioning of the extremity can assist in minimizing this injury by increasing the space within each specific compartment. Applying a valgus force with concomitant flexion or extension can widen the medial compartment joint space. The "figure of four" position is used to provide a varus force to increase the lateral compartment joint space, again with concomitant flexion or extension as necessary. Lastly, other surgeons have used radiofrequency probes for meniscectomy and meniscal contouring[128,129]; however, we prefer not to use this technique because

AUTHORS' PREFERRED TECHNIQUE

Meniscal Repair

Careful preoperative surgical planning and setup will enable improved efficiency, intraoperative ease, and postoperative outcome. Most arthroscopic meniscal surgeries are ambulatory using a general, regional, or local anesthetic. The patient is positioned in the supine position with use of a thigh-level leg holder or lateral post to provide lateral resistance to allow application of valgus loading and improved medial compartment distraction. This method reduces medial compartment iatrogenic chondral injury and improves access and visualization of the posterior meniscus. However, excessive valgus loading can lead to iatrogenic injury of the medial collateral ligament and should be avoided if possible.

Standard surgical instrumentation includes an arthroscopic cannula system with inflow and outflow cannulae. A 30-degree arthroscope is sufficient for addressing most meniscal pathology, although a 70-degree arthroscope may be used if necessary. Excision instrumentation includes straight, up-going, and side-directed duckbill meniscal punches, as well as a motorized shaver to facilitate fragment excision and meniscal rim contouring. A curved 4.5-mm shaver is very helpful for posterior meniscectomy in the standard knee, and a curved 3.5-mm shaver may be used in a knee with particularly tight ligaments to minimize chondral damage.

Each arthroscopic procedure should include a systematic and repeatable diagnostic evaluation. This technique ensures that all pathology is effectively identified and addressed. Careful probing of the menisci aids in identifying tears that may be difficult to visualize. Peripheral vertical tears or meniscocapsular detachments may also be identified by meniscal hypermobility and subluxation. Undersurface horizontal cleavage tears may only be visualized by lifting the superior flap to view the inferior undersurface. The probe should also be used to discriminate between stable and unstable meniscal tears. Meticulous evaluation of the posterior rim and root should be completed, because injuries in this region are subtle. Posteromedial and posterolateral visualization can be accomplished by passing the arthroscope between the PCL and medial femoral condyle or ACL and lateral femoral condyle, respectively (Fig. 96-11). Alternatively, posteromedial and posterolateral portals can be established to improve visualization and instrumentation in these regions if necessary. Surgical familiarity with these techniques allows complete and effective diagnosis and management of all meniscal pathology.

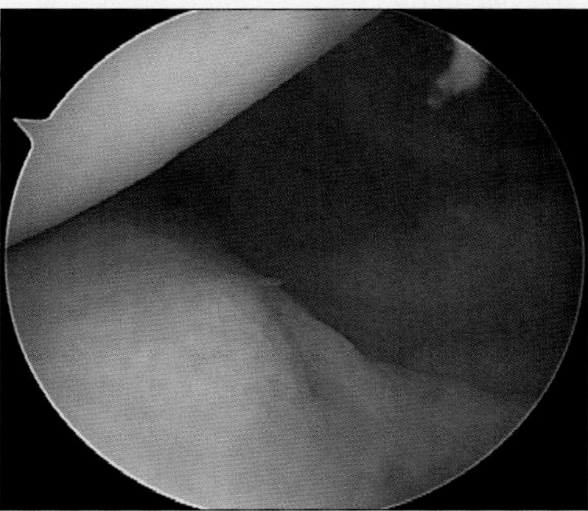

FIGURE 96-11 An arthroscopic view in the posterior compartment of the knee with visualization of the posterior horn of the medial meniscus and the meniscotibial attachments.

of the potential undesired meniscal and chondral damage that may occur as a result of thermal injury.

Meniscal Repair: The Basics

The first reported meniscal repair was performed in an open fashion in 1885.[130] This procedure was infrequently used until the importance of the meniscus was appreciated within the past 30 years. Recent advances in arthroscopic techniques have replaced open meniscal repair and include inside-out, outside-in, and all-inside arthroscopic repairs. Careful arthroscopic evaluation of the tear should be performed, including probing to identify the location, configuration, and

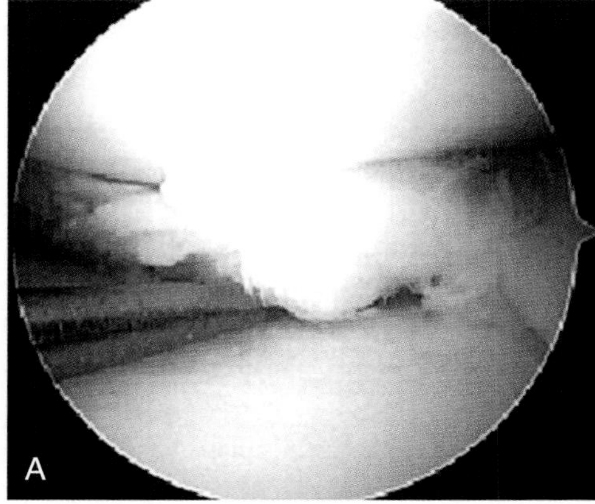

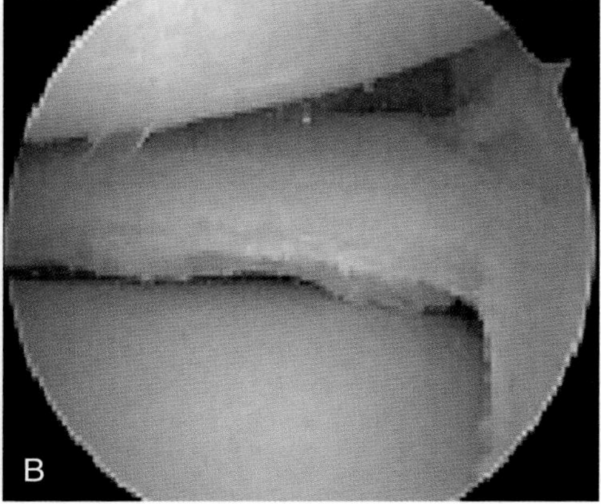

FIGURE 96-12 A complex meniscal tear with an unstable, inverted flap. **A,** The flap is reduced with an arthroscopic probe. **B,** The appearance after a partial meniscectomy. Meniscal tissue should be preserved when possible, and resection should be limited to only unstable parts of the meniscus. Careful contouring of the remaining meniscus may minimize the risk of a repeat tear.

extent of the meniscal tear. These factors, in combination with the patient history, should then be considered in determining the potential for meniscal healing. The synovial fringe and healing bed should be stimulated on both sides of the tear using a combination of meniscal rasps and a small, 3.5-mm shaver. This technique should maximize the vascular response and subsequent healing potential. All frayed edges of the meniscal tear should be removed to minimize mechanical prominences surrounding the repair. After the site has been adequately prepared, the tear can be repaired using crossing sutures or appropriate implants. Vertical mattress sutures provide optimal biomechanical strength because of the capture of longitudinally oriented collagen fibers and should be used whenever possible.[131-133]

Meniscal Repair: Inside-out

The inside-out technique was initially described in 1986 by Scott et al.[134] as a minimally invasive substitute for open meniscal repair. Double-limbed sutures are passed using arthroscopic assistance through the meniscus and capsule and are then retrieved through a small, extracapsular counter incision. Meticulous positioning of the incision and instrumentation is crucial for the inside-out repair. The neurovascular structures including the peroneal and saphenous nerves and popliteal artery should be protected throughout the procedure because injury to these structures may occur during surgical dissection and suture placement, especially during repair of posterior horn meniscal tears. Meniscal tears that occur in the anteriormost location are difficult to repair with use of this technique because placement of the arthroscopic guide is limited by the posteriorly directed angle.

The inside-out repair is best performed with the patient in the supine position and the operative knee flexed to 90 degrees for access to the lateral compartment and just slight flexion for the medial compartment. This position optimizes visualization while providing access to the posterior aspect of the knee. This access is required for the counter incision and suture retrieval. We use a lateral post that is placed in an elevated position to allow buttressing of the lateral thigh. A footrest may also be used to provide hands-free extremity positioning. After confirmation of the tear location and size, the arthroscope should be placed in the ipsilateral anterior portal. The arthroscopic needle guide is then placed in the contralateral portal to ensure that the needles are not angled directly posterior. This position minimizes the risk of neurovascular injury and facilitates needle recovery through the counter incision. A variety of needle-guide cannulas are available, including single- and double-barreled, curved, and straight cannulas. Vertical mattress sutures are used whenever possible.

Careful placement of the posteromedial or posterolateral counter incision and exposure of the joint capsule are crucial for easy, safe suture passage and knot placement (Fig. 96-13). A 3- to 4-cm incision should be placed posterior to the mid axis, and it should be 2 to 3 cm distal and 1 cm proximal to the joint line. The medial dissection proceeds to the anterior margin of the sartorius fascia, which is longitudinally incised. Blunt dissection should then be used to define and posteriorly retract the sartorius, gracilis, and semitendinosus. Care to avoid injury to the saphenous nerve is necessary. The medial head of the gastrocnemius is then exposed and should be elevated from the underlying posteromedial capsule and retracted posteriorly. A Henning or popliteal retractor should be placed between the gastrocnemius and posteromedial capsule to protect the infrapatellar branch of the saphenous nerve posteriorly and facilitate suture retrieval.

Joint-line positioning of the incision is similar for the lateral counter incision. The dissection plane is between the iliotibial band and biceps femoris. The posterior margin of the iliotibial band is incised longitudinally, and the interval between these structures is developed. Care should be taken to retract the biceps femoris posteriorly, thereby protecting the peroneal nerve that is located posterior to the biceps tendon. The lateral head of the gastrocnemius can then be visualized and should be posteriorly mobilized from the underlying posterolateral capsule. The aforementioned preferred retractor should then be placed in the interval between the gastrocnemius and capsule to protect the posterior neurovascular bundle and facilitate suture retrieval. Care needs to be taken to avoid injury to the lateral inferior geniculate artery.

The surgical ease of suture passage and retrieval for the inside-out approach directly depends on the intraarticular visualization and extraarticular capsular exposure (Fig. 96-14). Double-limbed 2-0 absorbable or nonabsorbable sutures attached to flexible long needles are used for repair. The surgeon should focus on guide cannula placement, arthroscopic visualization, and suture passage while an assistant retrieves the sutures through the counter incision. The guided needle can be used to pierce a single limb of the meniscal tear and then functions as a joystick to guide the optimal capsular placement. The needle should then be advanced through the capsule until it encounters the protecting posterior retractor and is then retrieved through the counter incision. The needle from the second limb of the suture can then be passed in a similar fashion to position and reduce the opposing meniscal tissue. This sequence should be repeated with suture spacing at approximately 3- to 5-mm increments until the entire tear is fully repaired. Ideally, sutures should be placed on the superior and inferior aspects of the meniscus to improve rigid meniscal fixation. After all sutures have been placed, the knee should be flexed to 15 to 20 degrees and the sutures can be directly tied to the extraarticular side of the capsule under direct visualization.

Although the basics of the inside-out meniscal repair are straightforward, a few surgical tips may improve efficiency and avoid complications. First and foremost, careful positioning of the counter incision and retractor placement significantly minimizes the risk of neurovascular injury and difficulty with suture retrieval. If the needle is not easily visualized during passage and the posterior retractor is not encountered, the surgeon should reposition the retractor. Frequently, the incision and subsequent retractor placement is too proximal and the retractor should be replaced into a distal, inferior position. Initial tear reduction also may be difficult and can be aided by placement of the first suture pair into the middle of the tear along the superior flap of the meniscus, which facilitates accurate reduction of most tears.

Meniscal Repair: Outside-in

Rodeo and Warren[135,136] described the outside-in technique in an attempt to minimize the incidence of neurovascular injury that was associated with the inside-out repair. Repair of tears of the anterior third of the meniscus and anterior meniscal allograft fixation are also more easily performed with use of

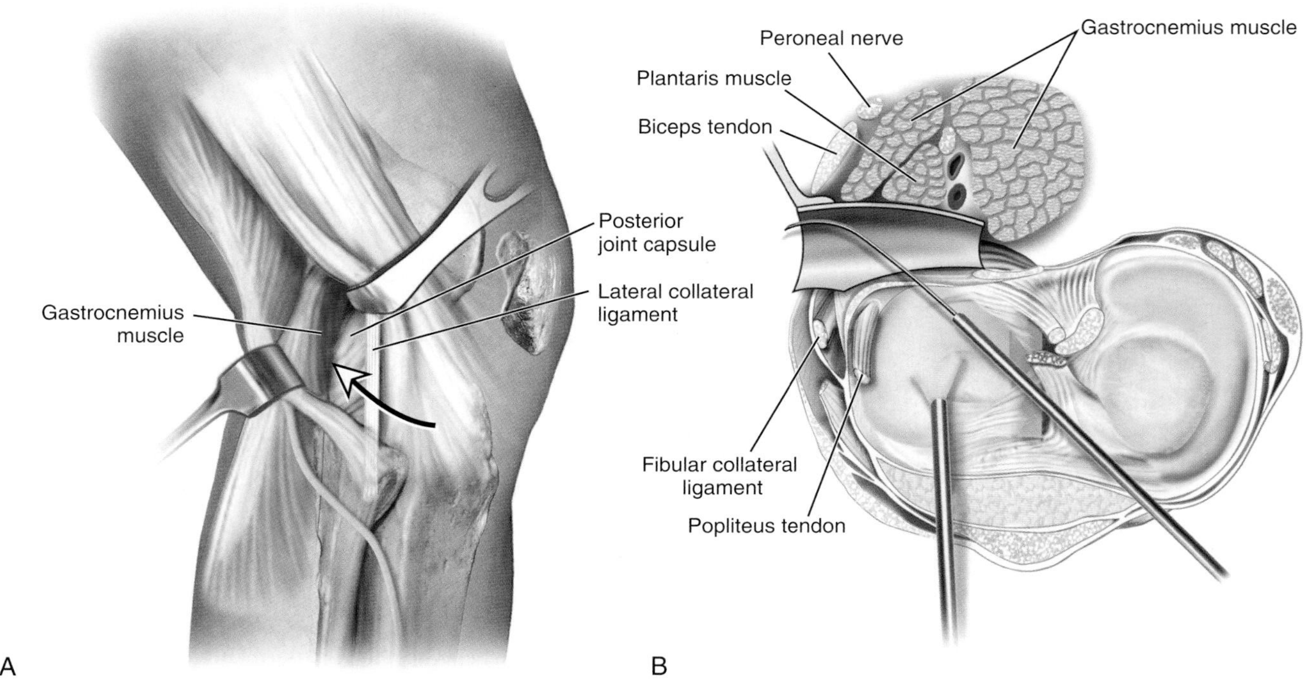

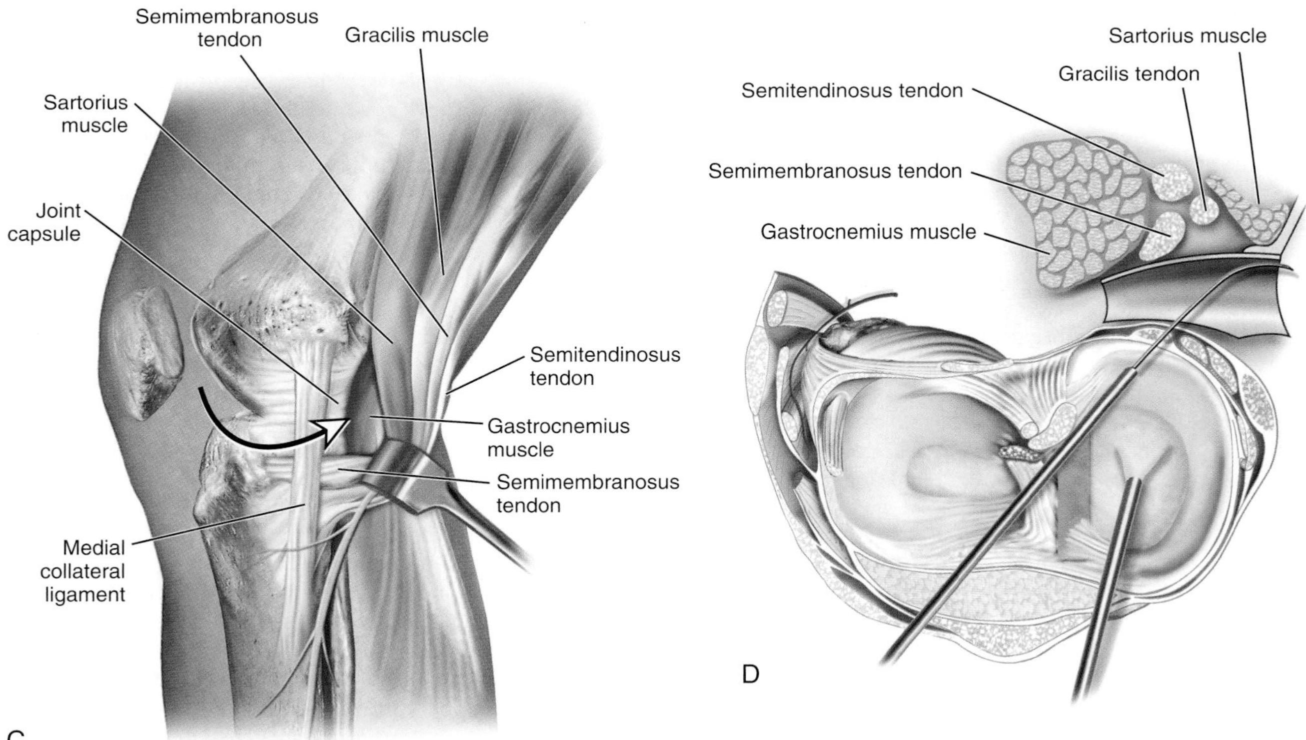

FIGURE 96-13 A schematic representation of the inside-out lateral (**A** and **B**) and medial (**C** and **D**) meniscal repair with the counter incision and subsequent surgical exposure. *(Modified from Noyes FR, Barber-Westin SD, Rankin M: Meniscal transplantation in symptomatic patients less than fifty years old.* J Bone Joint Surg Am *87:149–165, 2005.)*

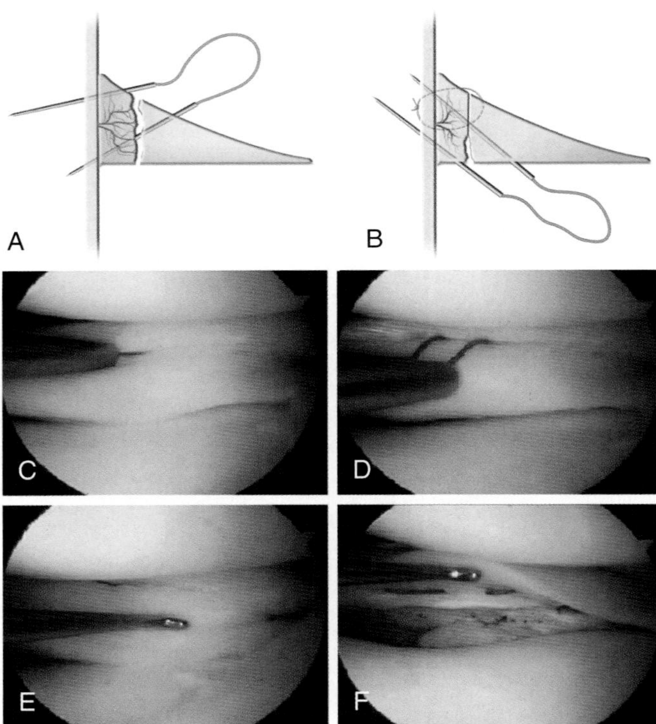

FIGURE 96-14 Inside-out meniscal repair. A schematic representation of vertical mattress suture placement into the superior (**A**) and inferior (**B**) surfaces. **C** to **F,** Arthroscopic images demonstrate the needle guide, suture placement, and final construct. *(From Rubman MH, Noyes FR, Barber-Westin SD: Arthroscopic repair of meniscal tears that extend into the avascular zone: a review of 198 single and complex tears.* Am J Sports Med *26:87–95, 1998.)*

this technique. This technique can also be used to produce any desired suture configuration allowed by spinal needle insertion, and thus difficult meniscal tears including radial and flap tears may be more easily and successfully addressed in this manner.[125] However, the outside-in technique can prove difficult for repairs of the posterior third of either meniscus because of the close proximity of the neurovascular structures.

The outside-in surgical technique uses an 18-gauge spinal needle as a guide for suture passage and retrieval with an arthroscopic grasper under direct arthroscopic visualization. The spinal needle is introduced percutaneously and is advanced through the meniscus on each side of the tear. The needle should exit through the central aspect of the desired superior or inferior meniscal leaf. An arthroscopic probe or grasper can be used for meniscal positioning prior to needle puncture to optimize final suture fixation and repair position. These instruments can also provide counter pressure during passage of the needle. A second spinal needle is placed in a similar fashion at the desired position. After needle placement, one 0-0 or 2-0 polydioxanone (PDS) suture is passed through each spinal needle and retrieved with a grasping device through the contralateral portal. Early techniques used mulberry knots that were tied on each end of the sutures to reduce the meniscal tear with tension placed against the meniscus at the knot-meniscal interface (Fig. 96-15). A small incision was then used to retrieve the extracapsular suture ends, which are then tied over the capsule. We prefer to use a modified technique in which the initial sutures are used as shuttle sutures to pass a single PDS or nonabsorbable braided suture in an inside-out direction. These sutures are then tied over the capsule in a similar fashion. This modification eliminates the necessity for mulberry knots and also offers the possibility of placing spanning sutures across the meniscal tear. This technique is particularly useful during placement of horizontal mattress sutures to approximate a displaced radial tear. The outside-in technique has been used to effectively repair anterior meniscal tears with excellent results in up to 90% of patients.[135,136]

Meniscal Repair: All-Inside

Early techniques for all-inside meniscal repairs used shuttling devices and arthroscopic knot tying to complete the meniscal repair. These techniques were technically challenging and required posterior accessory portals for posterior horn repairs. In many circumstances, this technique was more challenging than the aforementioned options.

Recent technical advances and improved implants have attempted to reduce the incidence of complications associated with early implants and the aforementioned technical challenges. Additionally, newer implants aimed to improve the strength and healing rates of the meniscal repair. Currently used devices include the RapidLoc (Mitek, Westwood, Massachusetts), FasT-Fix, and Meniscal Cinch (Arthrex, Naples, Florida). The RapidLoc is designed as a hybrid device that incorporates an intraarticular poly-L-lactide acid or PDS “top hat” that is anchored with connecting 2-0 Ethibond suture to an extracapsular poly-L-lactide acid “backstop.” This anchor is deployed with use of an implant-specific introducer followed by suture tensioning of the top hat at the intraarticular meniscal surface. Prior data have documented early successful outcomes with this technique.[137-139] However, the rigid intraarticular component of this device has been linked to chondral injury due to a mechanism similar to the rigid fixation devices.[140,141]

Unlike the RapidLoc, the FasT-Fix and Meniscal Cinch do not use a rigid intraarticular component and thus reduce the potential chondral injury that may occur at the interface between the device and the articular cartilage (Fig. 96-16). Instead, the FasT-Fix and Meniscal Cinch consist of two anchors constructed of polyetheretherketone polymer that are connected with a pretied 0-0 Ethibond or 2-0 FiberWire suture bridge, respectively. These anchors are sequentially deployed through the meniscus and capsule with use of an implant-specific introducer and deployment mechanism. The introduction sheath is designed to protect the chondral surface during needle positioning. This sheath is retracted or removed. The device is then automatically deployed after penetration of the meniscus and capsule with the needle-pledget construct. This sequence is repeated to deploy the second anchor followed by removal of the introducer and the use of a knot-pusher and cutter to secure the knot and remove the excess suture material. The knot-pusher should be used to advance the pretied knot until appropriate tension is applied to the suture before cutting the suture at the meniscal edge.

The all-inside suture-based implants that do not use intraarticular rigid components have several advantages over their rigid counterparts. The most notable advantage is the low risk of chondral injury that may occur at the interface between the implant and articular cartilage. Additionally, improved instrumentation, including the introducer sheath

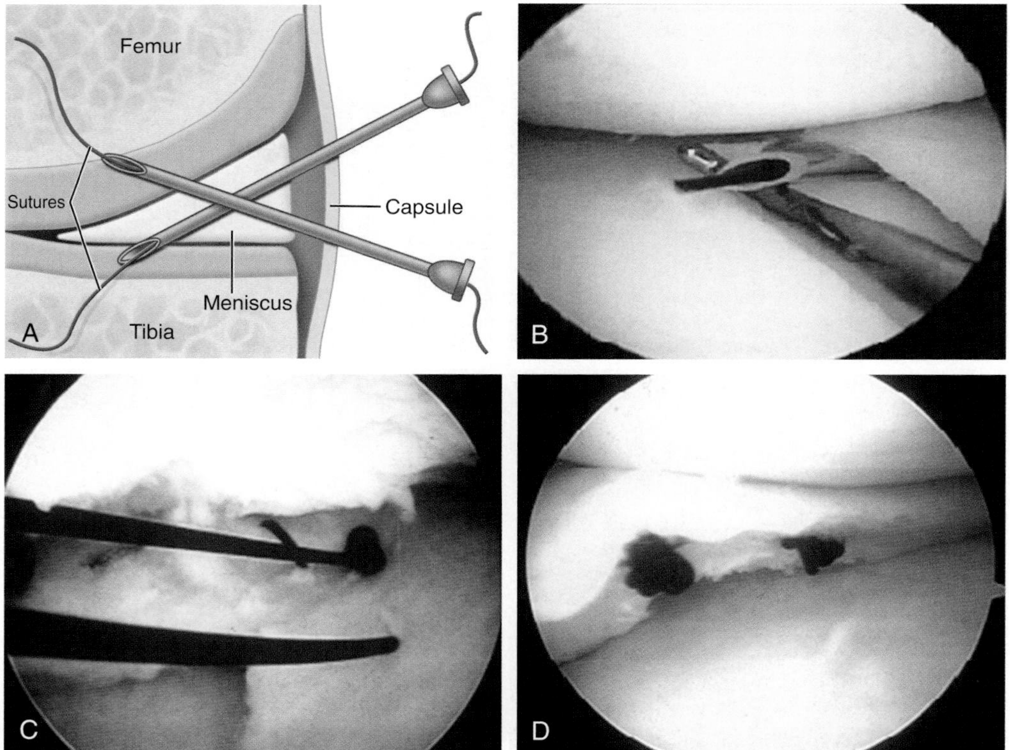

FIGURE 96-15 Outside-in meniscal repair. **A,** A schematic representation of spinal needle and suture placement through the superior or inferior meniscus. **B,** An arthroscopic view demonstrates spinal needle placement through the inferior meniscal margin and polydioxanone suture introduction. **C,** Suture shuttled through the working portal. **D,** The final construct using intraarticular mulberry knots.

and dual anchor constructs, minimizes iatrogenic injury and permits multiple suture orientations, including vertical, oblique, and horizontal mattress sutures. Superior and inferior meniscal leaf placement is also possible. Previous biomechanical data have demonstrated that the FasT-Fix construct has strength equivalent to inside-out vertical mattress sutures and superior to other all-inside constructs.[142-146] Additionally, early clinical outcomes have demonstrated excellent results with this method.[147,148]

Biologic Stimulation

Despite the many technical and implant-related advances, meniscal healing continues to rely on the biologic healing response that occurs after repair. For this reason, extensive research has been directed toward stimulating and maximizing this biologic meniscal healing response. Some of these methods include trephination, synovial abrasion, fibrin clot augmentation, and meniscal scaffolds. In fact, isolated synovial abrasion and trephination without direct repair has been used to successfully facilitate healing of small, stable, and incomplete tears.[123,126,127]

Trephination is designed to theoretically introduce vascular access channels into an avascular region of the meniscus to aid in stimulating a proliferation of fibrovascular tissue into the repair site. This technique is performed arthroscopically by repeatedly passing a spinal needle or small trephine in an outside-in fashion through the desired meniscal tissue. The resultant channels should theoretically allow neovascularization and tissue ingrowth. Although trephination can be easily performed in an arthroscopic fashion, there exists some risk of permanent disruption and fragmentation of the meniscal tissue during this process. This risk directly increases with the caliber of the horizontal channels.

Synovial abrasion is also easily accomplished with the use of a motorized shaver or arthroscopic rasp. This technique is also designed to stimulate a fibrovascular pannus that should creep from the synovial periphery into the tear site and aid in a reparative response. The shaver or rasp is used under direct arthroscopic visualization to abrade the synovial tissue adjacent to the desired repair site to stimulate visible bleeding and subsequent repair.[149]

Fibrin clot augmentation was initially described in an animal model by Arnoczky et al.[122] This technique was designed to introduce an exogenous fibrin clot into the tear site to serve as a reparative scaffold and to provide a chemotactic and mitogenic stimulus. The surgical technique requires drawing blood from a peripheral vein followed by hemoagitation to produce a semisolid clot. The clot is introduced directly between the flaps of the meniscal tear with the goal of facilitating a local proliferation of fibrovascular tissue to aid in the healing process. Prior data have documented improved healing of meniscal tears with tenuous vascularity when they were treated with fibrin clot augmentation.[124,125]

Postoperative Management

We divide our postoperative rehabilitation after meniscal repair into three distinct phases. This protocol is designed to maximize early healing and limit the healing time required

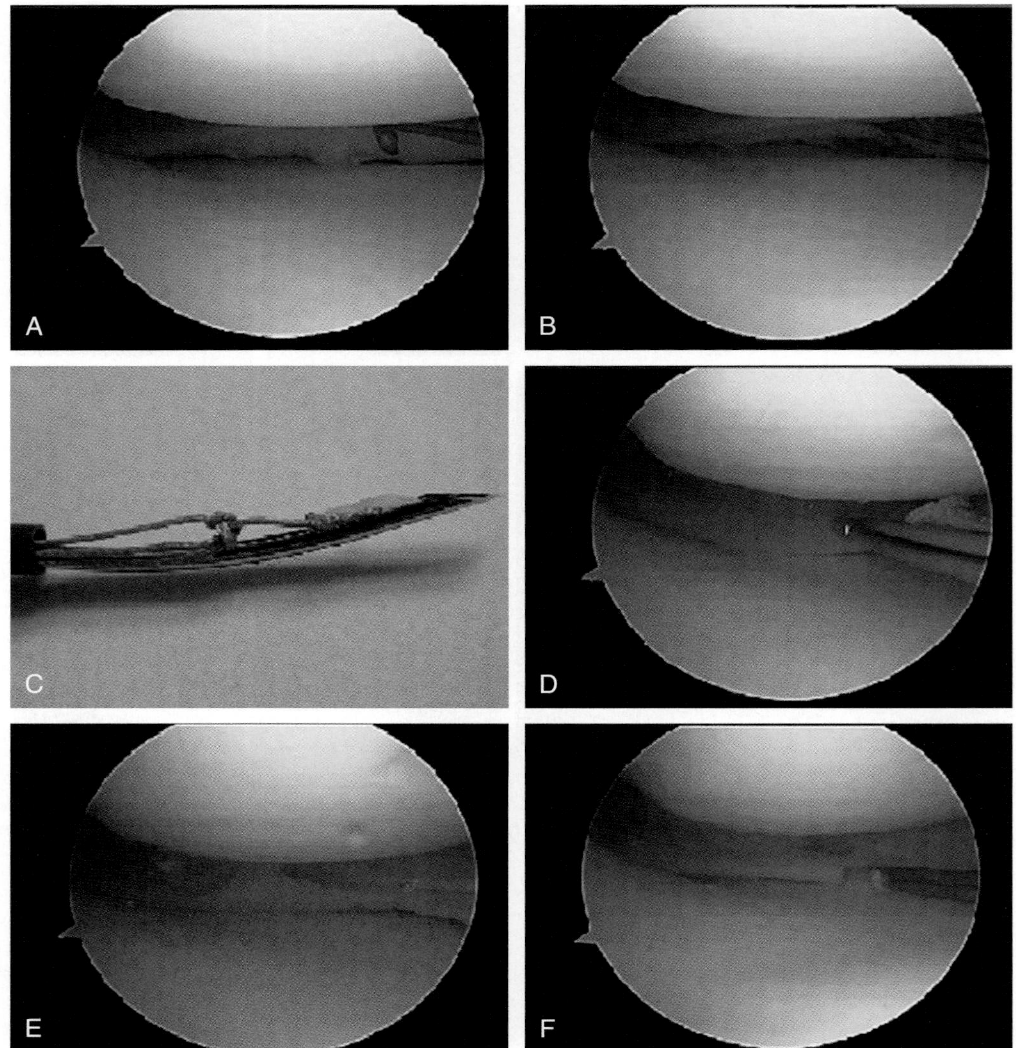

FIGURE 96-16 All-inside meniscal repair. Arthroscopic views demonstrate identification and delineation of a vertical tear, red-white zone, and medial meniscus (**A** and **B**), a FasT-Fix device (**C**), the initial trajectory for placement of the first anchor of the device (**D**), the appearance after placement of the second anchor and initial knot tensioning (**E**), and the final suture construct (**F**).

prior to return to sports. These protocols are carefully individualized with regard to the tear configuration and location, repair type, concomitant procedures, and patient activity. Immediate range of motion is initiated in the recovery room for all patients and continues throughout the rehabilitation program. We may limit knee flexion to 90 degrees for the first 4 weeks after repair of radial or complex tears. Progressive weight bearing is allowed, beginning with toe-touch ambulation. Early weight bearing with the knee in full extension is encouraged after repair of vertical or bucke thandle tears because it provides a compressive load across the repair site that may facilitate healing. Weight bearing after repair of radial and complex tears, on the other hand, may create a distraction force at the repair and thus is more restricted. We allow toe-touch ambulation for the first 4 to 6 weeks followed by progressive ambulation in persons who have undergone these tenuous repair types.

Phase 1 of our rehabilitation protocol is initiated in the recovery room and continues for approximately 6 weeks after surgery. Notably, progression through these phases depends primarily on patient recovery and ability, whereas the time-specific guidelines function solely as rough estimates. Immediate passive and active-assisted range of motion is initiated in the recovery room with a motion goal of full extension to 90 degrees of flexion prior to progression to phase 2. We may restrict flexion to 90 degrees in the setting of posterior horn repairs in an attempt to minimize the shear and distraction forces that occur at the posterior meniscocapsular junction during deep flexion. Weight bearing is allowed in the aforementioned fashion according to repair type. A nonantalgic gait is required prior to discontinuation of assisted ambulation. We also immediately initiate quadriceps strengthening with straight leg raises and isometric exercises to minimize postoperative quadriceps atrophy.

Phase 2 typically occurs during weeks 6 to 14 and is focused on progressing range of motion to achieve a normal arc and initiating muscle strengthening and proprioception. Strengthening exercises should be delayed until a full, normal range of motion is obtained. Postoperative bracing is discontinued during phase 2 when functional quadriceps control is demonstrated. We frequently use pool and bicycle therapy during this phase to facilitate a return to functional activities while improving range of motion and strength.

Phase 3 typically occurs during weeks 14 to 22 and is designed to facilitate strengthening and initiate functional sports-specific activities. Running begins early in this phase, followed by agility and sport-specific exercises. Isokinetic and plyometric training are introduced, with deep flexion and pivoting activities incorporated in the later stages of this phase.

Return to Play

Successful return to play occurs after completion of phase 3 of our rehabilitation protocol. Although no data exist regarding strict return-to-play criteria, we have identified some tests that have proven useful. Full range of motion, absence of mechanical symptoms, and strength greater than 80% of the strength of the contralateral extremity are required prior to return to play. We also use the single-leg hop and crossover hop tests because they both require significant proprioception and ipsilateral strength. For this reason, patients may return to play if they can demonstrate less than a 15% deficit during these strenuous tests. Most patients are able to return to sporting activities at approximately 6 months, but this time frame is dependent on the patient's progress.

Results

Long-term data are plentiful regarding the impact of surgical and demographic variables on the end result of removal of meniscal tissue.[71] A great deal of data have supported the hypothesis that increased meniscal resection predicts worse radiographic and functional long-term status.[150-154] Obesity[155,156] and advanced age[157,158] have been shown to be further predictive of even poorer functional and clinical results after resection of meniscal tissue. Data regarding medial versus lateral arthroscopic partial meniscectomy are mixed. Although in vitro computer modeling postulates that lateral partial meniscectomy may lead to more degenerative changes when compared with medial partial meniscectomy,[159] in vivo studies have shown no significant clinical differences.[157] Short- and medium-term analyses of outcomes regarding gender differences at 8.5 to 14.5 years after surgery demonstrate no difference in surgical outcome between men and women.[153,160,161] Nevertheless, 15- to 22-year follow-up data indicate that symptoms and functional limitations are worse in women who have undergone meniscectomy compared with men,[158] and osteoarthritis tends to develop more frequently in women.[155] Radiographic osteoarthritis is accelerated in patients with malalignment, because an even greater amount of stress is placed on the affected compartment.[160] Therefore meniscal tissue is salvaged through meniscal repair whenever possible, and a substantial body of research has identified predictors of improved prognosis after meniscal repair.

Meniscal repair has been associated with excellent outcomes and is considered preferable to meniscectomy in the setting of a meniscal tear with increased healing potential, such as those in the red-red or red-white vascular zone. Long-term success has been documented with use of an inside-out meniscal repair technique. Success rates up to 92% have been reported with complete resolution of symptoms and an 80% return to previous activity.[134] Second-look arthroscopy demonstrated complete healing in 61.8% and incomplete, stable healing in 16.9% of patients. Healing rates were notably increased after repairs of narrow (<2 mm) peripheral (>2 mm) tears or associated concomitant ACL reconstruction. Other series have substantiated these results.[162,163]

Meniscal vasculature and the specific vascular zones also play an important role in healing after repair. Prior outcome data regarding repair of meniscal tears in the central avascular zone demonstrated an 80% rate of complete resolution of symptoms at a mean of 42 months after surgery.[79] However, second-look arthroscopic evaluation demonstrated complete healing in only 25% of tears and incomplete healing in 38% of tears. Noyes and Barber-Westin[164] have suggested that improved healing rates may be accomplished in the avascular zone in a subset of patients younger than 20 years. This study documented a 75% rate of clinical success in 71 meniscal repairs. These indications were then extended to patients older than 40 years who had meniscal tears that also extended into the avascular zone. An 87% successful clinical outcome was observed as measured by absence of symptoms at a mean 33-month follow-up.[80] Nevertheless, the excellent clinical outcomes that have been reported after repair of avascular meniscal tears may not correlate with complete meniscal healing. Fortunately, these healing rates significantly increase with repair of tears in the vascular zones with similarly good clinical outcomes. Theoretically, the risk of a repeat meniscal tear may be higher in the setting of incomplete healing, and thus we favor the use of partial meniscectomy in all but a limited subset of patients with avascular tears, including young, active persons with tear extension from the vascular zone into the avascular zone.

Complications

Complications after meniscal repair include chondral injury, implant failure, postoperative joint-line irritation, nerve injury, arthrofibrosis, effusion, infection, deep venous thrombosis, and pulmonary embolus.[165,166] When all these complications are included, they occur in approximately 2.5% of knee arthroscopies and 1.2% of meniscal surgeries.[167] Bleeding or pseudoaneurysms may occur after meniscal surgery but are primarily associated with posterior horn resection and not meniscal repair.[168,169] The incidence of infection after knee arthroscopy is less than 0.1%, with increased risk in patients who have longer surgeries, undergo multiple procedures, have had prior surgery, and are given corticosteroids intraoperatively. Although deep venous thrombosis (DVT) has been documented in up to 18% of knee arthroscopies, fatal pulmonary embolism remains an extremely rare event. Nevertheless, risk factors for DVT include obesity, advanced age (>40 years), a history of DVT, tobacco use, and oral contraceptive use. We frequently prescribe enteric-coated aspirin for many patients during the perioperative period in an attempt to minimize this risk.

Nerve injury has also been documented with meniscal repair techniques. Medial meniscal repair has been associated with injury to the saphenous nerve, producing transient neurapraxia, but permanent injury has only been identified in 0.4% to 1% of documented cases.[167,170,171] Peroneal nerve injury is a rare but devastating injury that may occur during lateral meniscal repair. A carefully dissected posterolateral safety incision with proper retractor placement significantly reduces this risk.[172] The most commonly encountered complications were saphenous neuropathy and arthrofibrosis. A 13% and 19% risk was documented for lateral and medial repairs, respectively.

Meniscal Allograft Transplantation

Clinical Evaluation

A complete patient history, physical examination, and radiographic assessment are crucial for evaluation of the patient when considering meniscus transplantation. Thorough evaluation is particularly important in this setting, because patient selection can be difficult given the complexity of the associated pathology. A detailed description of the patient's symptoms should be obtained. Reports of instability with increased joint line tenderness localized to the involved compartment are common. Intermittent swelling may also be present, specifically with an increased level of activity. Emphasis should be placed on reports of increasing pain in a particular compartment, because this pain may be associated with increased compartment loading and chondral damage.

The patient history can serve to guide a focused physical examination. Limb alignment and gait should be evaluated, because malalignment may require concomitant surgical correction in the setting of a meniscal transplant. Range of motion should be evaluated, and restricted motion should be carefully documented, because meniscal transplantation should not be performed if motion is restricted. Ligamentous instability and signs of chondral damage should also be identified. A painless effusion may be a sign of early chondral damage. Concomitant, unrecognized ligamentous laxity can increase the chance of meniscal allograft transplant failure and thus should be recognized and addressed prior to or during meniscal transplantation. Joint-line tenderness is commonly identified and may be localized to the meniscal-deficient compartment. Pain during palpation of the medial or lateral femoral condyles can also suggest compartment overload and chondral damage.

Careful imaging evaluation should be performed after the history and physical examination. Several modalities are available, including plain radiographs, MRI, triple-phase bone scan, and three-dimensional gait analysis. Initial evaluation with routine plain radiographs should include weight-bearing anteroposterior extension views of both knees, a weight-bearing 45-degree flexion posteroanterior or tunnel view, a 45-degree flexion non–weight-bearing lateral view, and axial (Merchant) views of both patellofemoral joints. The tunnel view allows improved assessment of posterior tibiofemoral chondral damage.[173] Additionally, a standing full-length lower extremity anteroposterior radiograph of both limbs should be obtained to evaluate limb alignment.

MRI should be obtained to evaluate the status of the menisci, ligaments, cartilage, and subchondral bone (Fig. 96-17). Additional cartilage-specific MRI sequences including three-dimensional fat suppression, proton density, and two-dimensional fast spin-echo can be used to fully assess patellofemoral and tibiofemoral hyaline cartilage and subchondral bone.[174] Cartilage signal intensity and morphology should be noted. Increased signal within the chondral layer, chondral fissuring, and subchondral sclerosis or edema may be identified and are suggestive of chondral damage. Increased uptake on a bone scan may suggest compartment overload and impending chondral damage, thus increasing the importance of attempting to restore the compartment load-sharing through meniscal allograft transplantation. Malalignment should be considered during preoperative planning, because correction of malalignment with a high tibial osteotomy or distal femoral osteotomy may be required with or without a meniscal transplant. The patient's response to a trial in an unloader brace provides helpful information about relative compartment overload.

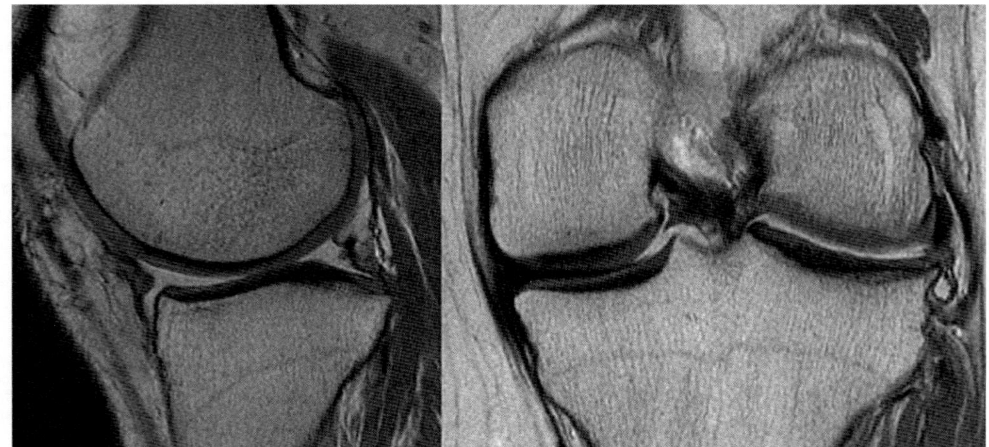

FIGURE 96-17 Preoperative sagittal and coronal magnetic resonance imaging (MRI) slices demonstrate meniscal deficiency after a total lateral meniscectomy. Preoperative MRI evaluation should be obtained to facilitate surgical planning by quantifying the meniscal remnant and evaluating the chondral surfaces.

Surgical Indications

Meniscal allograft transplantation (MAT) is primarily indicated for young, nonobese patients with stable, well-aligned knees and minimal to no arthritis. The most commonly associated symptom is pain in the affected compartment due to compartment overload. Although age is not a contraindication for meniscus transplantation, it is not commonly recommended in patients older than 50 years because of concomitant degenerative changes. Skeletal maturity should also be confirmed to minimize the risk of intraoperative physeal injury. Obesity is also a relative contraindication for MAT because it creates a suboptimal mechanical environment for the allograft and increases the risk of early failure. Knee instability also places abnormal stresses on the meniscus and can be a cause of early failure, and thus it must be identified and addressed prior to or during MAT. Early lateral meniscus transplantation may be considered in young female patients after a subtotal lateral meniscectomy, because these patients often experience relatively rapid progression of lateral compartment degenerative changes.

Significant controversy exists regarding the acceptable degree of degenerative changes in the setting of MAT. The most common contraindication to MAT is the presence of osteoarthritis with grade III to IV Fairbank changes. However, many surgeons believe that MAT may be contraindicated in the setting of Outerbridge grade I or II cartilage changes. Nevertheless, focal areas of grade III or IV degeneration might not preclude a positive outcome, especially if they can be addressed with a concomitant cartilage restoration procedure. Knee arthrosis due to lower extremity malalignment is also a contraindication to MAT. In young patients without arthritis, angular malalignment may need to be addressed, and the surgeon should have a low threshold to perform a concurrent osteotomy during MAT to optimize the mechanical environment of the knee and reduce the risk of meniscus allograft failure.

Most surgeons now agree that meniscal transplant has a minimal role in knees in which moderate to severe degenerative joint disease has already developed, because the likelihood of symptom improvement in this mechanical environment is quite low. In addition, meniscal transplants are contraindicated in patients with active inflammatory arthropathies or any history of an infectious, immunologic, or metabolic condition affecting the knee given the high risk for potential complications and early graft failure.

Basic Science, Allograft Procurement, Processing, and Sizing

Meniscal allograft selection for MAT requires consideration of graft procurement, processing, storage, and sizing and timing for donor matching and implantation. Although the specifics of these basic science and procurement variables must be considered, they are beyond the scope of this chapter. Many studies have outlined these specifics and should be reviewed preoperatively.[175-179] Preoperative allograft sizing specifics should also be carefully reviewed and optimized.[180]

Surgical Technique

Diagnostic arthroscopy should be performed prior to MAT in cases of revision ACL reconstruction. Radiographic and clinical findings should be visually confirmed and chondral surfaces should be inspected to rule out advanced arthrosis. This inspection is particularly important if the index and revision surgeons differ.

After diagnostic arthroscopy, the residual meniscal tissue in the desired transplant compartment should be debrided until punctate bleeding is encountered within 1 to 2 mm of the peripheral rim. Preservation of meniscal vasculature is an important factor in meniscal repair or transplantation. The osseous insertions of the anterior and posterior horns should also be identified for anatomic transplant tunnel or slot placement. A sub-PCL medial femoral condylar notchplasty or sub-ACL lateral femoral condylar notchplasty may then be performed to provide increased visualization of the posterior horn insertion. This notchplasty also allows improved passage of the bone plug or keyhole bridge. An open posteromedial or posterolateral approach should also be used in preparation for inside-out meniscal capsular suturing.

The manner of preparation of the meniscal allograft depends directly on the fixation method that is used by the revising surgeon. This method should be determined during preoperative planning. Excess soft tissue should be removed from the plateau, leaving only meniscal tissue and bone. The anterior and posterior horns should then be identified and marked with a sterile marker to ensure anatomic placement and minimize confusion. The hemiplateau can then be machined for either bone plug or keyhole fixation. Sutures are placed through the bone plugs to aid in graft placement and fixation (Fig. 96-18). A traction suture should also be placed at the junction of the middle and posterior third of the meniscus. This suture serves to facilitate meniscal orientation and reduction during placement. Fixation of the soft tissue meniscal body can be performed after the initial osseous fixation.

Postoperative rehabilitation after meniscal transplantation begins with knee range of motion limited to 90 degrees of flexion. Flexion angles great than 90 degrees increase loads to the posterior meniscal horn and should be avoided for the first 4 postoperative weeks. Focus should be placed on obtaining full extension and preserving quadriceps function with braced straight leg raises and quadriceps isometric contraction in extension. Toe-touch weight bearing is maintained with a double-upright hinged knee brace for 4 weeks followed by incremental progression to full weight bearing by 6 weeks. Progressive range of motion is allowed after 4 weeks with continued bracing. Strengthening should begin at approximately 6 to 8 weeks as range of motion gradually improves. The brace is discontinued at approximately 4 to 6 weeks. An unloader brace is sometimes used once the patient has resumed full weight bearing (from week 6 to week 12) to continue to protect the meniscus. Light jogging is allowed at 4 to 6 months based on restoration of appropriate strength, endurance, coordination, and balance. Return to high-impact activities is generally not recommended after meniscus transplantation but may be considered at 6 to 8 months after transplantation depending on the patient's goals and desires and after careful discussion regarding the risk to the transplanted meniscus.

We view MAT as an interim approach to joint preservation, with the recognition that further surgery may be required in the future. This procedure is used in young, active, symptomatic patients with an absent meniscus and evidence of

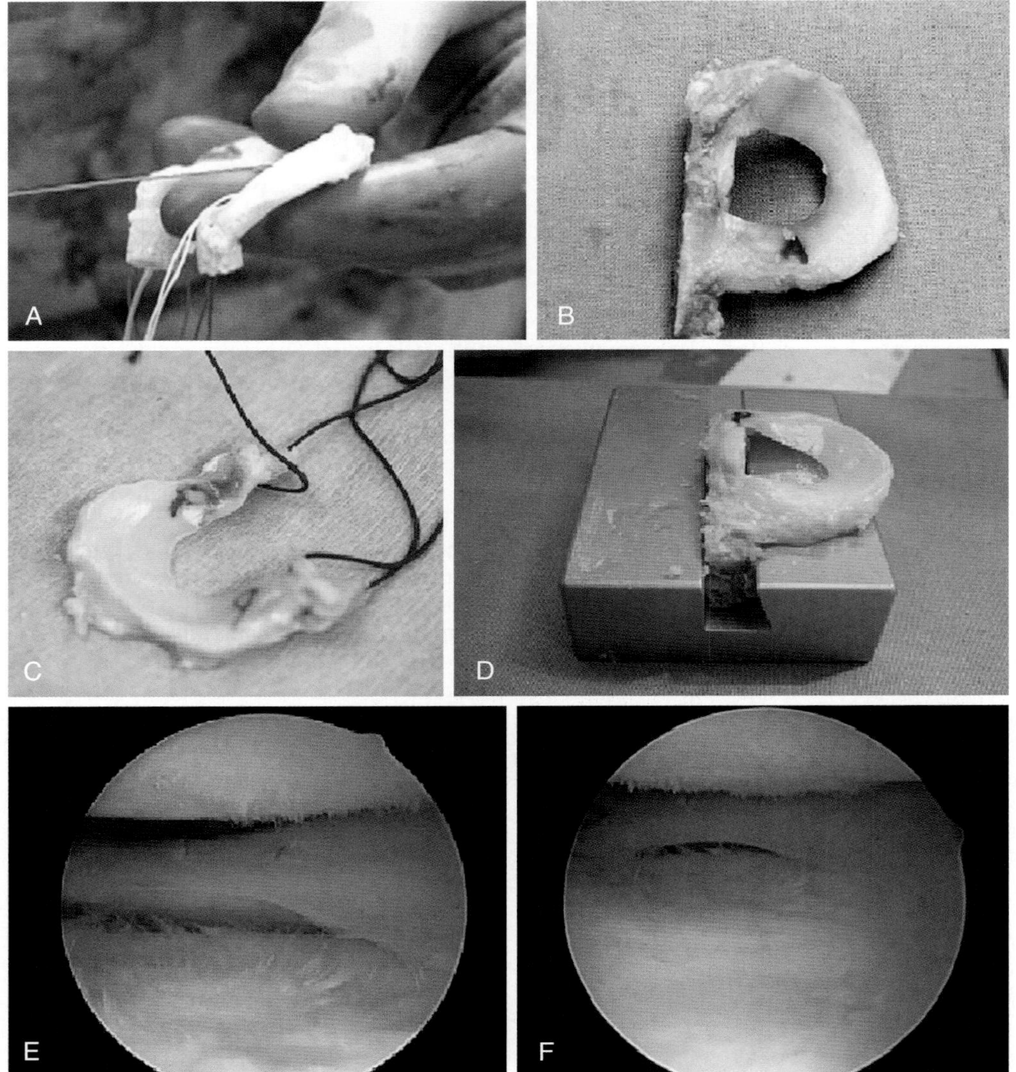

FIGURE 96-18 Medial (**A** and **C**) and lateral (**B** and **D**) meniscal allografts. Cylindrical bone-plug (**C**) or keyhole-slot (**D**) techniques may be used for graft fixation. Slot preparation should ensure that the bone is broader on its inferior surface (demonstrated in **D**). **E** and **F**, Second-look arthroscopic views of a lateral meniscal allograft.

compartmental overload. We believe that this alternative is preferable to progression of compartmental arthrosis in this patient population despite the risk of complications and failure.

Future Considerations

This chapter has outlined many areas in which improvements in basic science and operative management should occur. Implant improvements have allowed use of the all-inside technique with excellent results, but research continues to produce new, improved implants and techniques. Two principal areas of improvement were also identified, including avascular meniscal tears and younger patients with significant meniscal tissue deficiency. Current research and development efforts are aimed at addressing these two areas. Cellular and acellular meniscal repair and regeneration techniques have been developed with some available preliminary data. These techniques are designed to stimulate and maximize repair healing or function as a scaffold for new meniscal tissue regeneration. The tissue engineering and regenerative medicine field has proven crucial for the latter goal. It is our hope that the combination of innovative repair methods, biologic stimulation, and scaffold-based regeneration will provide improved, sustainable outcomes in the near future.

Current basic science and tissue engineering research and development may prove fundamental to the future treatment of avascular meniscal repair. Previous attempts at biologic modulation of meniscal healing include the use of an autologous fibrin clot to stimulate a fibrocartilaginous matrix. Recent cellular-based modalities aimed at stimulating or augmenting the repair have been attempted, including platelet-rich plasma, concentrated stem cells obtained from bone marrow aspirate, application of growth factors, chondrocytes, mesenchymal stem cells, and meniscal scaffolds.[181,182]

Management of young patients with significant meniscal tissue deficiency is particularly difficult, because this scenario requires the theoretical regeneration of new tissue. Novel tissue engineering research has produced synthetic meniscal scaffolds that can be contoured to a specific defect and impregnated with autologous cellular components such as bone marrow aspirate. These scaffolds have included collagen-based and polyurethane acellular implants,[183-188] a hydrogel meniscus constructed from polyvinyl pyrrolidine and cross-linked polyvinyl alcohol,[189] and small intestinal submucosa scaffolds.[190] Limited data exist regarding the efficacy of these modalities, but preliminary results appear promising.[191,192] A recent systematic review of the available preclinical and clinical trials supported the application of meniscal scaffolds and documented excellent safety and good preliminary results.[191] Current indications for these clinical trials include (1) young patients, (2) significant meniscal tissue deficiency with an intact anterior and posterior horn and peripheral rim, (3) ligamentous stability, and (4) no malalignment. These clinical trials include only acellular scaffolds, whereas recent preclinical trials have advanced to scaffolds augmented with cells and/or growth factors. It is likely that cellular augmentation of acellular scaffolds will facilitate improved tissue ingrowth and regeneration. Although significant obstacles remain regarding the ideal regenerative meniscal scaffold, we believe that tissue engineering and regenerative medicine may represent the future for treatment of meniscal injuries.

Critical Points

The roles of the menisci in force transmission and chondral protection within the knee have been well documented. Knowledge of the gross and microscopic meniscal anatomy, biomechanical function, and role in articular congruity and shock absorption is important for diagnosis and treatment. The range of repairable meniscal tears is expanding because of recent augmentation techniques and improved understanding of meniscal healing. Clinical and radiographic identification of repairable meniscal tears is crucial to healing success and improved outcomes. Careful consideration should be given to the factors that may contribute to or inhibit meniscal healing, including tear location, tear type, tear etiology, concomitant injury, and patient profile. Treatment of all identified repairable meniscal tears should be carefully managed to maximize the healing potential after repair. Focus should be placed on optimizing the biologic environment and mechanical stability of the repaired meniscus to maximize healing. Careful observation should be performed after a total meniscectomy in the young patient to identify potential candidates for MAT, because the outcomes may be optimized if this procedure is performed prior to compartment degeneration. Finally, the outcomes of meniscal repair and transplantation should be reported to aid the current understanding of meniscal healing and improve this crucial process.

For a complete list of references, go to expertconsult.com.

Suggested Readings

Citation: Arnoczky SP, Warren RF: Microvasculature of the human meniscus. *Am J Sports Med* 10(2):90–95, 1982.
Level of Evidence: V (cadaveric study)
Summary: In this study 20 cadaver specimens were histologically evaluated regarding the meniscal microvascular blood supply. These data demonstrated the presence of a perimeniscal capillary plexus that supplied the peripheral 10% to 25% of the menisci.

Citation: Burks RT, Metcalf MH, Metcalf RW: Fifteen-year follow-up of arthroscopic partial meniscectomy. *Arthroscopy* 13:673–679, 1997.
Level of Evidence: IV (case series)
Summary: This study is a large cohort retrospective case series with 14.7-year follow-up of 146 patients after a partial meniscectomy. The data demonstrated an 88% rate of good to excellent results in knees with stable ligaments and suggested that valgus alignment was protective after a partial medial meniscectomy.

Citation: Dienst M, Greis PE, Ellis BJ, et al: Effect of lateral meniscal allograft sizing on contact mechanics of the lateral tibial plateau: An experimental study in human cadaveric knee joints. *Am J Sports Med* 35(1):34–42, 2007.
Level of Evidence V (cadaveric study)
Summary: In this study the effect of allograft sizing on the contact mechanics of the lateral tibial plateau was evaluated. Oversized allografts resulted in increased contact forces compared with undersized allografts, and 10% size variability above or below normal was demonstrated to have mechanics similar to those of intact knees.

Citation: Lee SL, Aadalen KJ, Malaviya P, et al: Tibiofemoral contact mechanics after serial medial meniscectomies in the human cadaveric knee. *Am J Sports Med* 34(8):1334–1344, 2006.
Level of Evidence: V (cadaveric study)
Summary: In this study 12 cadaveric knees were evaluated after serial medial meniscectomies. Incrementally increased contact pressures were documented after each meniscectomy, with the greatest effect demonstrated after removal of the posterior and peripheral zones.

Citation: Rubman MH, Noyes FR, Barber-Westin SD: Arthroscopic repair of meniscal tears that extend into the avascular zone: A review of 198 single and complex tears. *Am J Sports Med* 26(1):87–95, 1998.
Level of Evidence: IV (retrospective case series)
Summary: In this study 198 meniscal tears were evaluated at a mean 42 months after repair of a major central avascular segment with partial extension into the vascular zone. Eighty percent of tears were asymptomatic and 20% required revision meniscectomy. Ninety-one repairs were evaluated arthroscopically and demonstrated a 63% rate of partial or full healing.

Citation: Shoemaker SC, Markolf KL: The role of the meniscus in the anterior-posterior stability of the loaded anterior cruciate-deficient knee: Effects of partial versus total excision. *J Bone Joint Surg Am* 68:71–79, 1986.
Level of Evidence: V (cadaveric study)
Summary: In this study the anteroposterior biomechanical effect of the menisci on the ACL-deficient knee was evaluated. A 10% increase in anteroposterior laxity was demonstrated after total medial meniscectomy, with an additional 10% increase after subsequent removal of the lateral meniscus.

Citation: Tenuta JJ, Arciero RA: Arthroscopic evaluation of meniscal repairs: Factors that effect healing. *Am J Sports Med* 22(6):797–802, 1994.
Level of Evidence: IV (case series)
Summary: In this study 54 meniscal repairs were arthroscopically evaluated at a mean of 11 months after repair in an attempt to identify factors that affect healing. Notably, patients with simultaneous meniscal repair and ACL reconstruction had a significantly higher healing rate (84%), whereas patients with an intact meniscal rim width greater than 4 mm had a 0% healing rate.

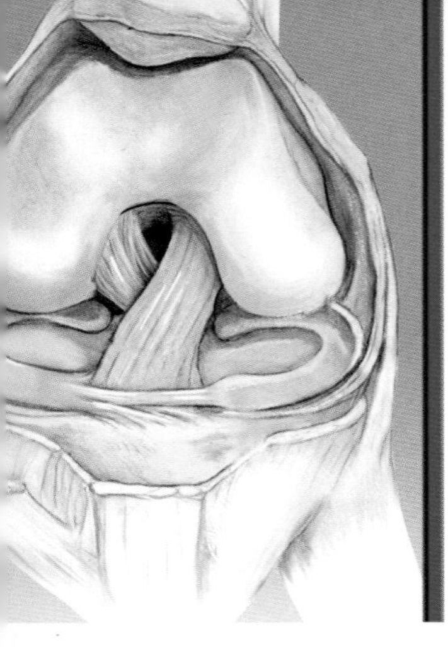

97

Articular Cartilage Lesion

ANDREAS H. GOMOLL • BRIAN J. COLE

Cartilage repair remains one of the fastest evolving areas within the field of orthopaedic surgery. Indications continue to be refined and new techniques emerge yearly, with more than 10 new implant technologies in mid- to late-stage clinical trials at this time.

In this chapter we provide a concise overview of current techniques for cartilage repair, present new developments in this evolving area, and subsequently discuss our preferred techniques in more detail.

Damage to the articular cartilage comprises a spectrum of disease ranging from single, focal chondral defects to diffuse osteoarthritis, the latter of which is not discussed in this review. Left untreated, articular cartilage defects have no spontaneous repair potential, and therefore various techniques have evolved to stimulate defect repair or overtly replace damaged cartilage and bone.

Conventional marrow-stimulation techniques, such as abrasion arthroplasty, drilling, or microfracture, attempt to fill the defect with a fibrocartilaginous scar produced by marrow-derived pluripotent stem cells. This tissue, however, is of lesser biologic and mechanical quality than hyaline cartilage and is therefore inadequate to treat larger defects. Tissue engineering technologies, such as autologous chondrocyte implantation (ACI) or matrix autologous chondrocyte implantation (MACI), achieve a tissue that more closely approximates the original hyaline cartilage, but they are expensive and more invasive, at least in their present form.

Relevant Anatomy and Biomechanics

Partial-thickness chondral lesions do not penetrate the subchondral bone and are therefore avascular, do not heal, and may enlarge over time. Full-thickness defects, especially with injury to the underlying vascular bone, have the potential to fill with a fibrocartilaginous scar formed by cells invading from the marrow cavity. The resulting tissue, however, is predominantly composed of type I collagen, resulting in inferior mechanical properties compared with type II collagen-rich hyaline cartilage.

Long implicated in the subsequent development of osteoarthritis, focal chondral defects result from various etiologies. Patients are approximately evenly divided in reporting a traumatic versus an insidious onset of symptoms; athletic activities are the most common inciting event associated with the diagnosis of chondral lesions.[1] Traumatic events and developmental etiologies such as osteochondritis dissecans (OCD) predominate in younger age groups. For example, traumatic hemarthroses in young athletes with knee injuries are associated with chondral defects in up to 10% of cases.[2] Patellar dislocation is strongly associated with damage to the articular surface, with chondral defects of the patella seen in up to 95% of patients[3]; the incidence of OCD is estimated at 30 to 60 cases per 100,000 people.[4] Several large studies have found high-grade chondral lesions (Outerbridge grade III and IV) in 5% to 11% of younger patients (i.e., younger than 40 years), and up to 60% in older age groups.[1,5,6] The most common locations for these defects are the medial femoral condyle (up to 32%) and the patella,[5,6] and most are detected incidentally during meniscectomy or anterior cruciate ligament (ACL) reconstruction.[1,7] Notably, despite this relatively high incidence, many of these defects are incidental in nature and asymptomatic.

Upon careful evaluation, a large percentage of chondral defects are found to be associated with structural abnormalities, such as malalignment, patellar instability, and insufficiency of the ligamentous and meniscal structures. The disappointing early results of cartilage repair have been explained by the failure to diagnose and correct these associated bony and ligamentous abnormalities. For example, in early studies of patellar defects treated with ACI alone, good and excellent results were found in only one third of patients.[8] Later studies, however, identified patellar maltracking as an important associated abnormality, and performance of a corrective osteotomy concurrently with cartilage repair led to good or excellent results in 70% to 80% of patients.[9-11] These reports emphasize the importance of a thorough patient evaluation to correctly identify and treat all associated abnormalities to ensure the long-term success of chondral repair.

Varus or valgus malalignment of the lower extremity results in compartment overload and is associated with degeneration of the articular surface. Coventry's early work with osteotomies popularized this technique for the treatment of osteoarthritis with comparatively large correction angles.[12] The population treated for chondral defects today, however, is predominantly athletic and does not tolerate large degrees of overcorrection. When performed concurrently with cartilage repair, osteotomy around the knee should restore the mechanical axis to neutral alignment, with the goal of decreasing abnormal pressures to normal rather than unloading the respective compartment through overcorrection. Even in patients with early joint space narrowing, overcorrection of the mechanical axis should be limited to 2 degrees or less.

Ligamentous insufficiency, most commonly of the ACL, increases shear forces in the knee joint and predisposes the joint to further injury and thus contributes to chondral damage. Any patient undergoing cartilage repair should therefore be carefully evaluated for instability, which can be corrected in a staged or concomitant fashion.

Meniscal insufficiency, such as after a subtotal meniscectomy, increases contact stresses by up to 300% in the respective compartment and is associated with the development of osteoarthritis.[13] In carefully selected patients with meniscal insufficiency, meniscal allograft transplantation can provide pain relief and improved function. The ideal candidate for allograft transplantation has a history of prior total or subtotal meniscectomy with refractory, activity-related pain localized to the involved compartment. After meniscal allograft transplantation, good to excellent results are achieved in nearly 85% of cases, and patients demonstrate a measurable decrease in pain and increase in activity level.[14]

Classification

Earlier classification schemes were mainly descriptive in nature and have largely been abandoned. Newer systems have evolved to classify chondral defects based on size and depth to establish a universal language among clinicians and researchers and to ideally provide a correlation of lesion grade with clinical outcome. Currently, the most commonly used arthroscopic classifications are the Outerbridge[15] and International Cartilage Repair Society systems (Table 97-1, Fig. 97-1).[16] The International Cartilage Repair Society has also published a grading system for arthroscopic evaluation after prior cartilage repair procedures (see Table 97-1).

TABLE 97-1

CLASSIFICATION SYSTEMS FOR CARTILAGE DEFECTS

	DESCRIPTION	
Lesion Grade	**Outerbridge Classification**	**ICRS Classification (with Subclassifications)**
0	Normal cartilage	Normal cartilage
1	Cartilage with softening and swelling	A. Softening or fibrillations B. Superficial fissuring
2	Partial-thickness defect with fissures on the surface that do not reach subchondral bone or exceed 1.5 cm in diameter	Less than one-half cartilage depth
3	Fissuring to the level of subchondral bone in an area with a diameter >1.5 cm	More than one-half cartilage depth, and A. Not to the calcified layer B. To the calcified layer C. To the subchondral bone D. Blisters
4	Exposed subchondral bone	Osteochondral lesion violating the subchondral plate

ICRS, International Cartilage Repair Society.

History

Patients often present with a history of knee injury or prior surgical procedures such as meniscectomy or ACL reconstruction. They report activity-related knee pain and swelling, especially with impact activities such as running. The pain often localizes to the affected compartment and occasionally synovitis develops, resulting in diffuse pain. Larger defects can be associated with mechanical symptoms, profound crepitus, popping, and giving-way.

Physical Examination

Depending on the acuity of symptoms, typical physical examination findings include an antalgic gait, soft tissue swelling, joint effusion, quadriceps atrophy, tenderness with palpation of the joint line and femoral condyle, and occasionally mild varus/valgus laxity due to loss of cartilage and/or meniscal substance. With the exception of very advanced cases, or in large lesions with loose bodies, motion is generally preserved. It is important to evaluate limb alignment and ligamentous stability, because any deficiencies should be treated in either staged or concomitant procedures.

Imaging

Radiographic evaluation should include a standard weight-bearing anteroposterior view in extension, a posteroanterior view in 45 degrees of flexion (Rosenberg view), a flexion lateral view, and an axial view of the patellofemoral joint (Merchant or skyline view). Double-stance, weight-bearing, long-leg radiographs are obtained to quantify lower extremity alignment to determine if a corrective osteotomy is required.

Computed tomography (CT) scans are used infrequently unless the lesion also affects the subchondral bone, such as in persons with OCD, traumatic osteochondral defects, or failed prior marrow stimulation techniques. Here, CT, especially when combined with arthrography, can be very helpful to more precisely delineate the exact dimensions of the defect and assess bone healing (Fig. 97-2).

Magnetic resonance imaging (MRI) assessment of the articular surface has received increased attention because of newly developed protocols for cartilage-specific high-resolution imaging and contrast enhancement with intravenous and intraarticular gadolinium. Delayed gadolinium-enhanced MRI of cartilage is an imaging protocol that provides an assessment of the glycosaminoglycan content of cartilage (Fig. 97-3).[17] It represents a useful tool for noninvasive follow-up evaluation after cartilage repair techniques such as ACI. The recent discovery of gadolinium-associated nephrogenic systemic fibrosis[18] has raised concerns about the use of contrast MRI; however, this disease predominately appears to affect patients with renal insufficiency. Additional noncontrast techniques are being developed, including T2-weighted mapping and T1-rho that allow indirect evaluation of the biochemical composition of cartilage, such as the glycosaminoglycan and collagen content.[19] Although arthroscopy remains the gold

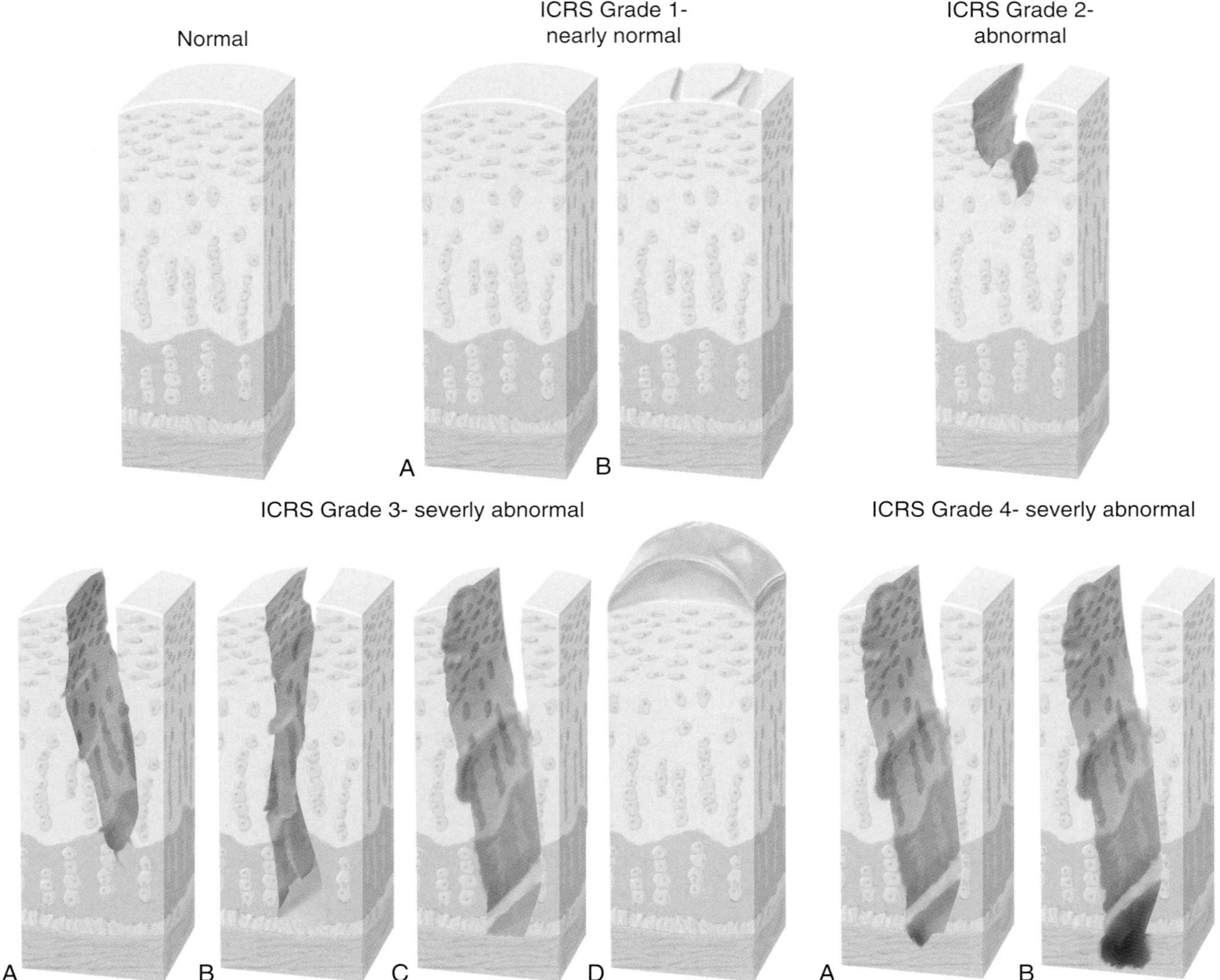

FIGURE 97-1 International Cartilage Repair Society classification of chondral defects. Please refer to Table 97-1 for further explanation of grades. *ICRS,* International Cartilage Repair Society.

standard for assessing articular injury, sensitivities and specificities approaching 90% have been reported with MRI protocols using a 1.5-Tesla magnet.[20-23] However, the choice of correct sequences is more important than magnet strength (Fig. 97-4). Furthermore, MRI provides additional information on the ligamentous and meniscal structures, which, if compromised, would require staged or concomitant treatment. Several scoring systems have been developed to characterize the structural outcomes after cartilage repair, such as the MOCART system.[24] At this time, however, no clinical correlation has been demonstrated between MRI and clinical outcomes.

Another application for both CT and MRI is in the evaluation of patellofemoral cartilage lesions because these lesions allow calculation of the tibial tubercle-to-trochlear groove distance, a measure of the lateral translation of the tibial tubercle in relation to the trochlear groove. This parameter is considered more objective than the clinical evaluation of the quadriceps (Q) angle and is important when considering a tibial tubercle osteotomy or anteromedialization. A normal range is less than 15 mm, whereas patients with patellar instability typically demonstrate a tibial tubercle to trochlear groove distance greater than 20 mm.

Decision-Making Principles

Indications for Cartilage Repair

Many cartilage defects seen on imaging or arthroscopy are asymptomatic, and thus careful assessment of alternative sources of pain is necessary. Conservative treatment with physical therapy should be continued for at least 3 to 6 months in conjunction with activity modification and weight normalization unless a young patient has a large defect that can be expected to deteriorate over time. Injection therapy, although not indicated in these young patients, might be considered in older patients who are within a few years of age eligibility for joint replacement surgery.

Surgical intervention is indicated for a full-thickness (grade 3 or 4) cartilage defect and after adequate nonoperative

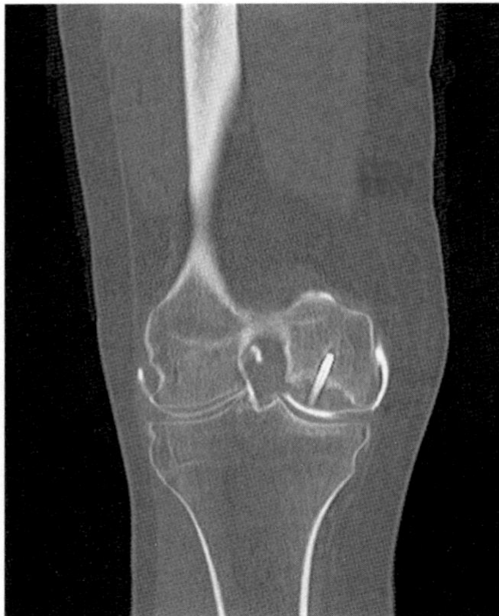

FIGURE 97-2 A computed tomography arthrogram demonstrating an osteochondritis dissecans lesion in the medial femoral condyle. The defect has previously been treated with arthroscopic fixation with use of multiple screws.

management has failed to provide acceptable pain relief. A thorough discussion of the details of this complex surgery and recovery is a necessary part of the informed consent process.

Contraindications

Smoking,[25] obesity (body mass index >35),[26] inflammatory conditions, or uncorrected articular comorbidities such as malalignment, meniscal deficiency, and ligamentous laxity are contraindications to cartilage repair. Advanced degenerative changes (>50% joint space narrowing) are considered a contraindication to cartilage repair in all but very young patients who have intolerable symptoms and no other options.

Treatment Algorithm

Treatment strategies for cartilage repair are based primarily on defect location and size. The two most common locations for cartilage defects are on the (medial) femoral condyle and the patellofemoral joint.[5] The tibiofemoral and patellofemoral compartments behave quite differently and require different treatment approaches.[27,28]

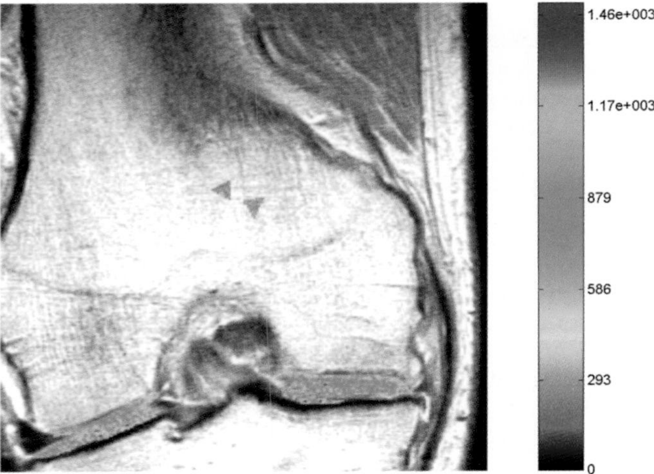

FIGURE 97-3 Color-coded delayed gadolinium-enhanced magnetic resonance imaging of cartilage allows assessment of the glycosaminoglycan content of a defect after cartilage repair, here after autologous chondrocyte implantation. *(Courtesy Dr. Tom Minas.)*

Treatment Choice Based on Defect Location

Treatment decisions in the tibiofemoral compartment are based on defect size. Knutsen et al.[29] conducted a randomized controlled trial (RCT) of microfracture versus ACI and reported similar overall clinical results. However, larger defects (>4 cm^2) treated with microfracture did significantly worse, whereas ACI outcomes were not correlated with size. The authors therefore recommended that larger defects should be considered for ACI. Basad et al.[30] investigated this issue further with an RCT of ACI and microfracture, specifically for defects larger than the threshold found in Knutsen's trial (4 cm^2), and reported significantly better results with ACI. Another recent RCT demonstrated significantly better histologic and functional outcomes after ACI when compared with microfracture for defects that were not yet chronic (<3 years).[31-33]

Other studies have reported that the microfracture technique should be limited to smaller lesions, for which this technique, as well as osteochondral autograft transfer (OAT), produce good and excellent results in 60% to 80% of patients.[26,34-41]

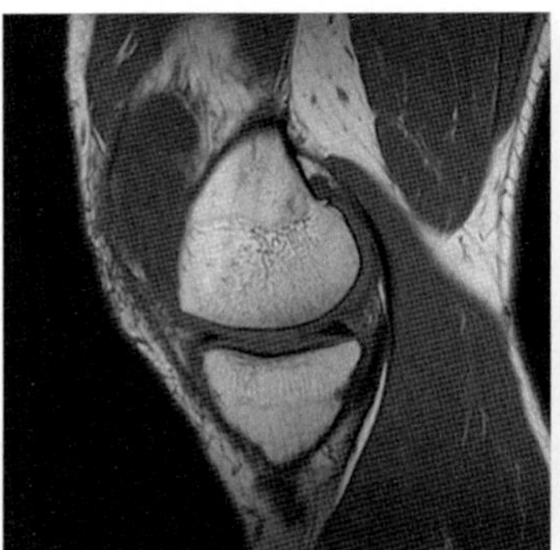
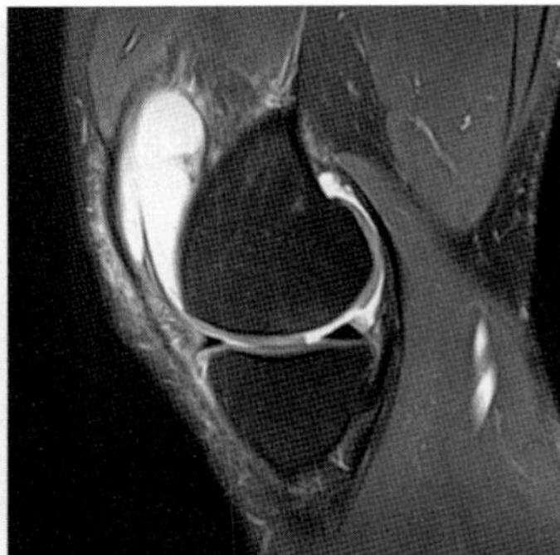
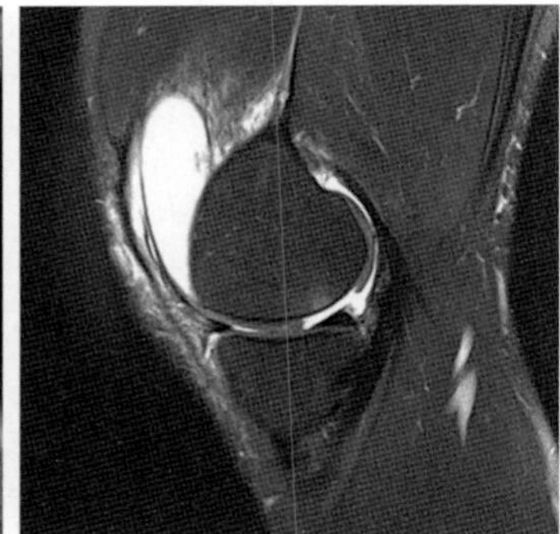

FIGURE 97-4 Sagittal magnetic resonance images showing the same focal chondral defect in the medial femoral condyle, using different pulse sequences (*left,* T1-weighted; *middle,* proton density, fat suppressed; *right,* T2-weighted, fat suppressed).

The decision to use microfracture versus OAT is based on several factors, including the surgeon's familiarity with the techniques, patient demand, and associated bone loss. The incidence and magnitude of OAT harvest site morbidity are controversial but are generally considered to be approximately 5%.[42] An athletic population has shown better return to play with OAT when compared with microfracture (93% vs. 52%, respectively).[37] Therefore OAT is recommended for smaller lesions, lesions in athletes who place a high demand on their knees, and for patients with associated bone loss, whereas microfracture is suited for medium-size defects with little or no bone loss in patients who place a lower demand on their knees.

Both ACI and osteochondral allograft transplantation have produced good and excellent results in more than 70% of patients presenting with larger defects, but no randomized trials have been conducted to compare the two procedures.[8,28,43-51] Surgeon and patient preference, as well as graft availability, are key factors guiding the treatment decision. Furthermore, associated bone loss or bone abnormalities (e.g., cysts, sclerosis, and edema) influence the decision; bone loss of 8 to 10 mm or more severe bony abnormalities can be treated with ACI but would require bone grafting in a staged or concurrent fashion (sandwich ACI),[52] whereas osteochondral allografting presents a single-stage treatment option.

The patellofemoral (PF) compartment is a challenging location, and all interventions, including partial replacements, do worse here when compared with the femoral condyles. The aggressive correction of patellar maltracking is crucial for success.

Although microfracture, OAT, and osteochondral allograft procedures have generally good outcomes in the femoral condyles, on the basis of limited studies and expert opinion, consensus is growing that they should be used cautiously in the PF compartment. Kreuz et al.[27] found only transient improvement for 18 to 36 months after microfracture in the PF compartment. The use of OAT in the PF compartment has shown varying results. Hangody and Fules[38] reported results only slightly worse than in the femoral condyle, whereas Bentley and colleagues[28] reported universal failure of OAT in the patella. Jamali et al.[53] investigated the use of osteochondral allografts in the PF compartment and reported 60% good and excellent results. Recent studies of ACI report successful outcomes in more than 80% of patients.[9-11,54] Therefore even though use of ACI in the patella is an off-label indication, it has emerged as the cartilage repair option of choice in the PF compartment.

Osteochondritis Dissecans Lesions

Symptomatic osteochondral defects, such as OCD or fresh osteochondral fractures after patellar dislocation, should be repaired whenever possible. One exception is the adolescent with open growth plates, for whom nonoperative treatment of stable OCD lesions can be successful.

Debridement alone without subsequent repair can provide good short-term pain relief but should only be considered in specific circumstances, such as when athletes are in the midst of their playing season, when defects are very small, and when patients are unable or unwilling to follow the rehabilitation associated with repair. In long-term follow-up studies, high rates of osteoarthritis were found as early as 9 years after fragment removal, especially in lesions larger than 2 cm^2.[55-57] Repair for OCD defects with OAT revealed better outcomes than did repair with microfracture at 4 years in a randomized trial (83% vs. 63%, respectively).[58] ACI is associated with greater than 80% success in younger patients,[59,60] and osteochondral allograft transplantation is successful in approximately 70%.[46]

Patient Age and Defect Chronicity

The most age-dependent procedure appears to be microfracture, with patients older than 35 years demonstrating worse outcomes.[29,37,40,61] Although older patients generally do less well than younger patients, this age dependency is less pronounced for other procedures, such as OAT, ACI, and osteochondral allograft transplantation.[62]

Chronic defects demonstrate worse outcomes, whereas repairs of acute injuries tend to demonstrate better results.[26,33]

Treatment Options

Prior to the development of modern bioengineering technology, orthopaedists were restricted to procedures that aim to palliate the effects of chondral lesions or attempt to stimulate a healing response initiated from the subchondral bone, resulting in the formation of a fibrocartilaginous repair tissue. Simple arthroscopic lavage and debridement of arthritic joints has been used since the 1940s[63] in an effort to reduce symptoms resulting from loose bodies and cartilage flaps. Although lavage alone has not been found to be effective, in combination with debridement, it can result in adequate pain reduction in slightly more than half of patients.[64,65] The goal of debridement of chondral defects is to remove any loose flaps of articular cartilage and create a defect shouldered by a stable rim of intact cartilage leading to reduced mechanical stresses in the defect bed. Currently, its use is limited to the treatment of small, incidental lesions found during arthroscopy or for larger and usually more diffuse arthritic lesions associated with mechanical symptoms in an attempt to delay the need for more invasive procedures such as total joint replacement.

Marrow stimulation techniques (MSTs), such as drilling, abrasion arthroplasty, and microfracture, attempt to induce a reparative response. This response is achieved by perforation of the subchondral bone after radical debridement of damaged cartilage and removal of the tide mark "calcified" zone, which has been found to enhance the volume and integration of repair tissue.[66] The currently favored technique is microfracture, in which an awl is used to perform multiple perforations in the subchondral plate. However, recent studies have demonstrated that subchondral drilling with a drill bit (rather than smooth Kirschner wire) results in the formation of better repair tissue and better reconstitution of the subchondral bone.[67-69] Perforation of the subchondral bone results in the extravasation of blood and marrow elements with formation of a blood clot in the defect. Over time, this blood clot, and the primitive mesenchymal cells contained within, differentiate into fibrocartilaginous repair tissue that fills the defect. Unlike hyaline cartilage, fibrocartilage largely consists of type I collagen and exhibits inferior wear characteristics. Postoperatively, MSTs require extended periods of relative non–weight bearing for 6 or more weeks, as well as the use of continuous passive motion (CPM) for up to 6 hours per day to enhance maturation of the repair tissue. Even though MSTs result in reparative tissue with inferior wear characteristics, treatment of smaller defects (<4 cm^2) results in good outcomes in 60% to 70% of patients.[26] However, especially with larger defects or those located in the PF compartment, symptoms tend to worsen again after 18 to 24 months.[27]

Osteochondral Autograft Transfer

OAT brings mature autologous cartilage from a lesser weight-bearing area of the knee into the defect, using instrumentation such as OATS (Arthrex, Naples, FL), COR (Mitek, Raynham, MA), or mosaicplasty (Smith & Nephew, Andover, MA) to address medium-size defects (1 to 4 cm^2). In this technique, multiple small osteochondral cylinders are harvested from lesser weight-bearing areas of the same knee joint, mostly from the lateral or medial aspects of the trochlea, the sulcus terminalis, or the intercondylar notch. Traditionally the lateral trochlea was the preferred harvest site, but studies have demonstrated lesser PF loading in the medial trochlea, which might therefore be a more advantageous harvest site.[70] The chondral defect is prepared with a punch to create a recipient hole that matches the graft cylinders, which are then press-fitted into the defect. Commonly, multiple cylinders must be transferred to fill larger defects. Osteochondral autografting is limited by the amount of cartilage that can be harvested without substantially violating the weight-bearing articular surface.[70] The main advantage lies in its autogeneity, thus avoiding the risk of disease transmission, providing immediate graft availability through harvesting of the patient's own tissue, and resulting in a decreased cost of this single-stage procedure. Furthermore, because of the transfer of mature cartilage with primary bone-to-bone healing, return to play is generally faster than for procedures that require graft maturation, such as marrow stimulation and ACI.

Autologous Chondrocyte Implantation

ACI introduces chondrogenic cells into the defect area, resulting in the formation of a repair tissue that more closely resembles the collagen type-II rich hyaline cartilage. The original technique of ACI was developed more than 15 years ago[8] and has been used in the United States to treat more than 10,000 patients since its approval by the Food and Drug Administration (FDA) in 1997. Second- and third-generation techniques that involve the use of collagen matrices to replace the periosteal patch cover or as a preseeded carrier are available in Europe, with more than 5-year follow-up results. These techniques offer the benefit of a less-invasive surgical approach through arthroscopic application and have demonstrated excellent results without the periosteum-related problems seen in conventional ACI, but they have not yet been approved by the FDA.[71]

ACI is indicated for the treatment of medium- to large-size chondral defects with either no osseous deficits or shallow associated osseous deficits. ACI has been approved by the FDA for application in the femoral condyle (medial, lateral, and trochlea) after failure of an MST, but it has also been used to treat patellar defects in an off-label fashion. Originally reported in 1994 for the treatment of chondral defects in the knee,[8] it has more recently been applied to other joints such as the shoulder[72] and ankle,[73] although such use is off-label.

ACI in its current form is a two-stage procedure in which a cartilage biopsy of approximately 200 to 300 mg is harvested during an initial arthroscopic procedure, most commonly from the intercondylar notch or the trochlear margin. The tissue contains approximately 200,000 to 300,000 chondrocytes, which are released by enzymatic digestion of the surrounding matrix and expanded in a monolayer culture for several weeks followed by staged reimplantation through an arthrotomy. Although the ideal cell density for reimplantation is controversial, in current practice, reimplantation of approximately 12 million cells is recommended for an average size lesion of 4 to 6 cm^2. The postoperative rehabilitation is similar to that of marrow-stimulating techniques, utilizing protected weight bearing for 6 to 8 weeks and CPM for up to 6 weeks. Return to impact and pivoting activities is considered after 9 to 12 months.

Particulated Juvenile Cartilage Allograft

Rather than transplanting osteochondral cylinders, the particulated juvenile cartilage allograft technique (DeNovo NT; Zimmer, Warsaw, IN) uses only articular cartilage allografts. The cartilage is retrieved from juvenile donors, because the density and metabolic activity of chondrocytes is substantially higher in this age group. The tissue is minced into cubes with a side length of 1 mm, promoting chondrocyte migration out of the extracellular matrix.[74] The chondrocytes then attach to the subchondral plate of the defect and produce new matrix, slowly filling the defect with repair tissue in a process comparable with other cell-based therapies.[75] At this point, few clinical outcomes data have been published, because the graft is regulated as minimally manipulated allograft tissue, and therefore it did not require the same extensive FDA-mandated studies necessary for other products in the United States.

Preserved Osteochondral Allograft

The preserved osteochondral allograft (Chondrofix; Zimmer) was recently developed to address major logistical issues in the use of fresh osteochondral grafts, namely limited availability and a short window to schedule surgery once a suitable graft has been found. Although frozen grafts offer similar benefits, the freezing process causes substantial damage not only to the chondrocytes but also to the extracellular matrix itself, causing decreased survival of frozen grafts. The proprietary processing protocol used to treat the preserved osteochondral allograft cylinders removes cells, lipids, and potential pathogens, allowing off-the-shelf storage at room temperature. Given that grafts are provided preshaped in various diameters (7, 9, 11, and 15 mm) and a length of 10 mm, there is no need for size, side, or compartment-specific matching, which has greatly improved graft availability. Depending on diameter, the grafts can be implanted either arthroscopically or through a mini arthrotomy. The technique is closely related to OAT but avoids the need for graft harvest with its associated issues of donor site morbidity, mismatch in donor/recipient site cartilage thickness, and the technical difficulty of harvesting a perpendicular graft.

The implant is regulated as minimally manipulated human allograft tissue and therefore no clinical outcome data were generated during the approval process. Therefore, until the clinical outcomes have been established, the procedure should be viewed as an investigational second-line treatment option.

Osteochondral Allograft Transplantation

More than 750,000 musculoskeletal allografts were transplanted in 1999, mainly for the treatment of bone defects and reconstruction of the ACL. More recently, the treatment of chondral defects with fresh osteochondral allografts has garnered significant attention because of its potential to restore and resurface even extensive areas of damaged cartilage and bone. Unfortunately, the supply of osteochondral allograft tissue remains limited because of issues related to the donor pool and aseptic processing. However, improved preservation techniques have been developed that allow storage times of up to 4 weeks with acceptable compromise in chondrocyte viability with grafts stored at 4°C.

Osteochondral allograft transplantation is used predominantly in the treatment of large and deep osteochondral lesions resulting from osteochondritis dissecans, osteonecrosis, and traumatic osteochondral fractures, but it can also be used to treat peripherally uncontained cartilage and bone defects. Furthermore, osteochondral allografting presents a viable salvage option after failure of other cartilage resurfacing procedures. When it is used for the treatment of cartilage or shallow osteochondral lesions, a thin subchondral bone graft (5 to 7 mm) results in the most rapid integration and best chance of success, because the mechanism of bulk allograft failure historically has been through creeping substitution and collapse of the transplanted osseous bed rather than failure of the articular cartilage itself.

The main advantages compared with OAT are the ability to closely match the curvature and thickness of the recipient cartilage by harvesting the graft from a corresponding location in the donor condyle, the ability to transplant large grafts, and the avoidance of donor site morbidity. These techniques require relatively atraumatic seating of the osteochondral plugs; multiple studies have demonstrated deleterious effects of excessive forces during the insertion, such as using a mallet to seat the plug all the way flush with the surrounding articular surface.[76-78]

The main concern with fresh allograft transplantation is the small risk of disease transmission, which is estimated at 1 in 1.6 million for the transmission of human immunodeficiency virus.[79] Since the advent of strict donor screening criteria in combination with polymerase chain reaction testing for human immunodeficiency virus and hepatitis, no cases of viral disease transmission have been identified.

Postoperative Management

The rehabilitation protocol after cell-based therapy such as microfracture, particulated cartilage allograft, and ACI is divided into three phases, based on the slow maturation of the repair tissue, which at the same time must be protected from overloading and stimulated to encourage tissue maturation. The three phases of the healing process are the proliferative (fill) phase, the transitional (integration) phase, and the remodeling (hardening) phase, each of which can accommodate increasing amounts of load. During the initial proliferative phase, protection of the graft is paramount, and the patient is limited to touch-down weight bearing for 6 weeks. During this phase, patients also use a CPM machine for 6 to 8 hours per day to reduce the likelihood of adhesions and aid in maturation of the transplant. Depending on the location and the size of the graft, different limitations of motion can be used. Traditionally, PF defects were advanced more slowly than defects on the femoral condyles, frequently limiting flexion to less than 40 to 60 degrees. Although acceptable for arthroscopic marrow stimulation techniques, the open approaches necessary for ACI raise the risk for arthrofibrosis. Therefore many centers have switched to more aggressive rehabilitation protocols that involve increasing range of motion on the CPM machine to 90 degrees of flexion over the course of the first 2 weeks.

The initial period is followed by the transitional stage in which patients advance to full weight bearing over the course of several weeks. Additional exercises are prescribed based on the specific location and type of the defect; for example, open-chain exercises should be avoided altogether in persons with PF grafts. During the final remodeling phase that begins approximately 3 months after transplantation, the joint is increasingly loaded with strengthening and impact-loading activities. A full return to high-impact and pivoting activities should be delayed for at least 9 to 12 months until near-complete graft maturation has been achieved. Complete maturation is not expected until 12 to 24 months, depending on the size and location of the graft.

Rehabilitation after OAT and allograft transplantation is comparatively unsophisticated, consisting of an initial period of protected weight bearing to allow for primary bone-to-bone healing, generally for 6 weeks. Thereafter, activities can be advanced more quickly, and return to play is mainly limited by residual swelling and strength deficits. High-impact activities such as longer distance running should be avoided for the first year after allograft transplantation, with hopes of reducing the risk of graft collapse during the phase of early creeping substitution.

Return to Play

Most cartilage repair procedures require extensive postoperative rehabilitation and delayed return to athletic activities. As a general rule, the involved extremity should be relatively pain free and without residual stiffness, swelling, or muscle atrophy before a return to play can be considered. More important than following these general guidelines, however, is that cartilage repair requires a protracted healing period that frequently extends long after aforementioned criteria have been met. The need for this protracted healing period is not apparent to outside observation by the patients, who therefore have to be frequently reminded of their restrictions. Return to play is individualized based on the specific procedure and sport; participation in high-impact and pivoting activities such as basketball and soccer is delayed for 9 to 12 months, whereas impact-free activities such as stationary biking can be considered as early as 8 to 12 weeks after surgery.

Results

Commonly used outcome measures include functional scores, such as the Lysholm, Tegner activity, Knee Injury and Osteoarthritis Outcome, and International Knee Documentation Committee rating systems, as well as health surveys including the Short Form-12 or Short Form-36. Other measures include subjective parameters such as patient satisfaction and

Text continued on p. 1146

AUTHORS' PREFERRED METHOD

Articular Cartilage Lesion

We have developed a comprehensive treatment algorithm based on defect size and location that takes into consideration the patient's activity and demand level (Fig. 97-5).[80] In the following sections, we discuss four commonly used techniques and their application in our clinical practice.

Marrow Stimulation

Marrow stimulation is most commonly performed as an all-arthroscopic procedure, and the setup and patient positioning is the same as that for routine knee arthroscopy. In very posterior defects, the patient should be positioned so that knee hyperflexion can be achieved.

Approach and Defect Preparation

After routine diagnostic arthroscopy to evaluate the cartilage defect (Fig. 97-6, *A*), loose chondral flaps are first debrided with the shaver; a curette is then used to achieve stable vertical shoulders and remove the layer of calcified cartilage (Fig. 97-6, *B*).

Marrow Stimulation

After thorough debridement, multiple holes are created in the subchondral bone with a microfracture awl or small drill bit (Fig. 97-6, *C*). In an effort to remain perpendicular to the chondral surface, it may be necessary to rotate the articular surface in line with the awl or create accessory portals. It is important to preserve the integrity of the subchondral bone, which can be violated if holes are not spaced wide enough and thus connect or become confluent. Ideally, the holes should be spaced approximately 3 to 4 mm apart, resulting in 3 to 4 holes per cm^2. Stability of the transition zone between surrounding cartilage and regenerate fibrocartilage can be improved by placing holes directly adjacent to the defect shoulders. After completion of the microfracture, pump pressure is lowered and bleeding should be observed from all holes.

Closure

Arthroscopy portals are closed with interrupted sutures. The patient should be counseled that occasionally joint aspiration may become necessary because of persistent bleeding from the treated defect.

Osteochondral Autograft Transplantation

Osteochondral autograft transplantation can be performed through either an arthroscopic or open approach

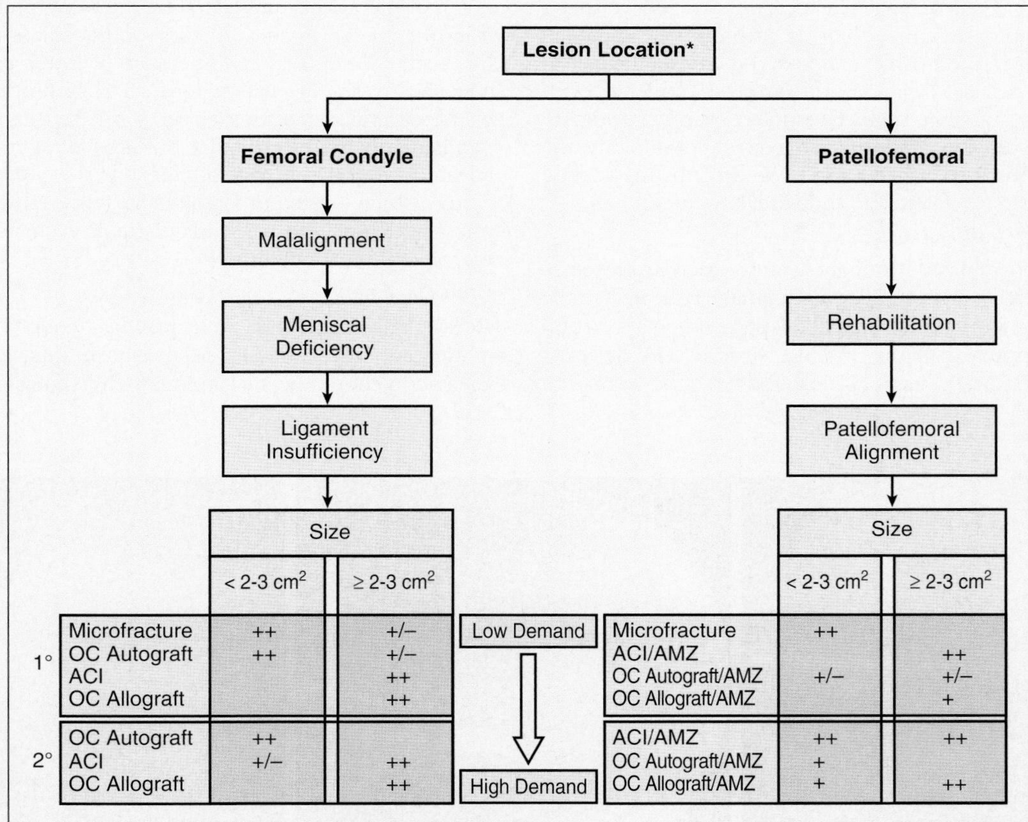

FIGURE 97-5 A treatment algorithm for isolated femoral and patellofemoral focal chondral lesions. For condylar lesions, comorbidities of ligament instability, meniscal deficiency, and malalignment must be assessed and corrected if needed. For trochlear and patellar lesions, patellofemoral alignment must be evaluated to select the proper degree of anteromedialization. *ACI,* Autologous chondrocyte implantation; *AMZ,* anteromedialization tibial tubercle osteotomy; *OC,* osteochondral. *Assumes minimal bone loss. Note: AMZ is often performed for lateral and central patellofemoral lesions and is of questionable benefit for medially located patellofemoral lesions. *(Modified from Alford JW, Cole BJ: Cartilage restoration, part 2: Techniques, outcomes, and future directions.* Am J Sports Med *33[3]:443–460, 2005.)*

Continued

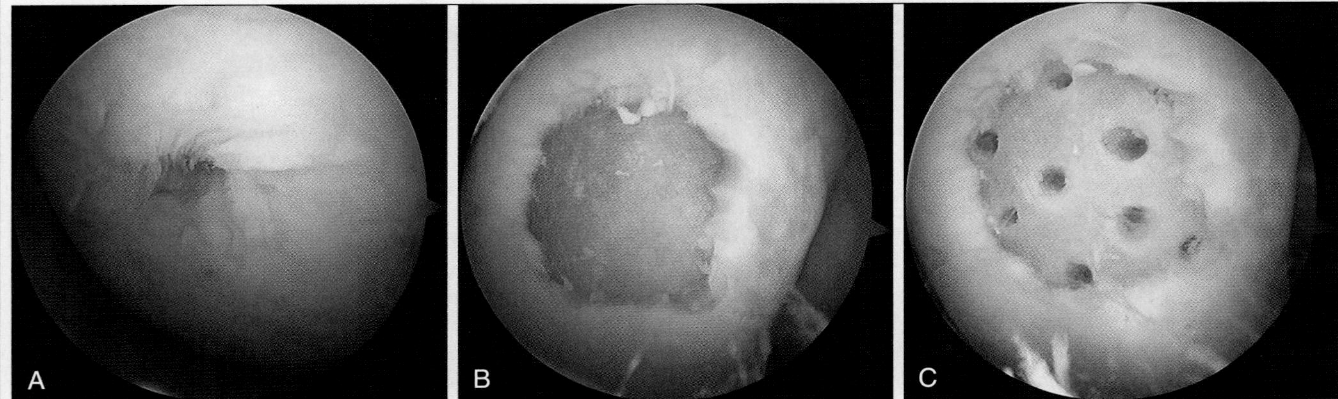

FIGURE 97-6 **A,** An arthroscopic image showing a full-thickness chondral defect on the femoral condyle. **B,** The cartilage defect after preparation of vertical shoulders of stable cartilage and removal of the layer of calcified cartilage with a ring curette. **C,** Multiple pick holes have been created with the microfracture awl, starting close to the periphery, but being mindful not to create holes that become confluent.

(Fig. 97-7, *A*), based on the exact defect size and location and the surgeon's preference.

We frequently assess the defect arthroscopically, followed by harvesting of the autograft from the trochlear ridge through a small 1.5- to 2-cm parapatellar incision. We believe that a mini open approach rather than an arthroscopic approach allows a more reproducible graft harvest perpendicular to the articular surface, which is the greatest challenge with osteochondral autograft transplantation. Several proprietary systems are available, and the surgeon should follow the guidelines of the system being used. We describe the general technique without reference to individual systems.

Approach and Graft Harvest

The lesion is evaluated through routine knee arthroscopy. Needle localization with an 18-gauge spinal needle aids in the creation of accessory portals that allow perpendicular orientation of the approach to the articular surface. The defect is evaluated and sized, using sizing rods or the probe to determine the size and number of plugs required to cover the defect. An accessory portal is created after needle localization, or, more frequently, we recommend a small 1.5- to 2-cm incision. Common donor locations include the intercondylar notch or the medial and lateral trochlea. We prefer to harvest from the medial trochlea or close to the sulcus terminalis in the lateral femoral condyle because of lower patellofemoral contact stresses in that region.[70] The appropriate, slightly oversized graft harvesting chisel is selected and placed perpendicularly to the articular surface. With a mallet, it is advanced to a depth of approximately 8 to 10 mm; the harvester is then twisted or toggled and retrieved with the graft. The graft length and perpendicularity is evaluated to create a corresponding recipient slot.

Graft Placement

Occasionally, a central, transpatellar tendon approach is required for perpendicular placement. In this case, the patellar tendon should be split in line with its fibers and repaired

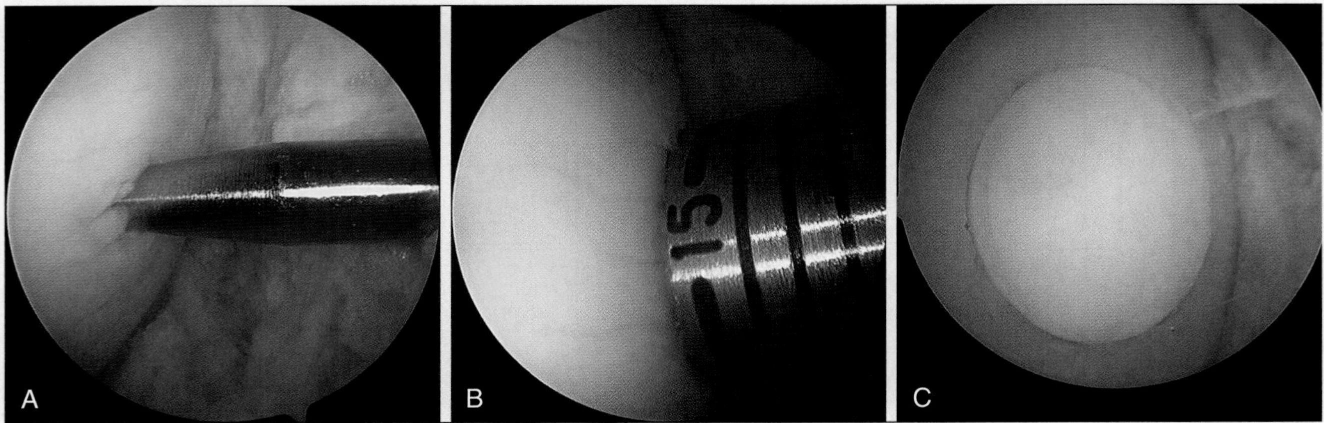

FIGURE 97-7 **A,** A previously microfractured defect on the femoral condyle had developed a subchondral cyst with persistent pain. The microfracture awl here is used to locate the cyst. **B,** The recipient slot is created with the harvesting tube. **C,** An osteochondral cylinder has been transferred from the lateral trochlea to the recipient site and seated with an oversized tamp.

at the end of the procedure. An appropriately sized tube is selected and a recipient hole of the appropriate depth is created. This procedure is best performed with use of a tourniquet to improve visualization. The depth of the recipient site is measured to ensure that the defect is approximately 1 mm deeper than the length of the graft. The graft is then advanced within the harvesting tube so that the end is just visible (Fig. 97-7, *B*). The harvester is introduced into the joint and oriented perpendicularly to the articular surface, and the graft is slowly advanced into the recipient site. Subsequently the harvester is removed and the graft is fully seated and made flush by gentle pressure with an oversized tamp. It is preferable to slightly recess the graft rather than leaving it proud (Fig. 97-7, *C*). This process is repeated until the required number of osteochondral plugs has been placed. The donor site can be left untreated or filled with synthetic graft.

Closure

The arthroscopic portals are closed with interrupted sutures. A mini arthrotomy should be closed in layers, including the joint capsule and retinaculum.

Autologous Chondrocyte Implantation

After arthroscopic cartilage biopsy and culture, a process that usually takes approximately 6 weeks, the cell suspension is shipped to the surgical facility. The patient is positioned supine on a standard operating table with a tourniquet on the thigh. Especially in very posterior lesions of the femoral condyle, a leg-positioning device is helpful to stabilize the knee in hyperflexion. If periosteum is to be used, the drapes should allow access to the level of the mid tibia for patch harvesting.

Approach

For single lesions of the femoral condyles, a parapatellar arthrotomy is used. Adequate exposure is critical, and it may become necessary to sublux the patella (Fig. 97-8, *A*) or mobilize the meniscus by incising the coronary ligament and releasing the anterior root and intermeniscal ligament, with subsequent repair at the end of the procedure. Correct placement of the retractors is crucial, especially in limited incisions. A bent Hohmann or Z retractor placed into the intercondylar notch is helpful to displace the patella to the contralateral side. A Z retractor or rake retractor is helpful to control the peripheral soft tissues. For multiple defects, a standard medial parapatellar arthrotomy is performed with lateral subluxation or dislocation of the patella.

Defect Preparation

Meticulous preparation of the lesion is critical for the success of the procedure. The defect must be cleaned of all degenerated tissue to achieve a stable rim of healthy cartilage with vertical shoulders. This preparation is performed by first outlining the defect with a scalpel incision down to the subchondral plate, taking as much of the surrounding cartilage as necessary to remove all unstable or undermined areas. However, if this procedure would transform a contained into an uncontained lesion, it is advisable to leave a small rim of degenerated cartilage to sew to rather than using bone tunnels or suture anchors. The defect is then thoroughly debrided with small ring or conventional curettes (Fig. 97-8, *B*) while maintaining an intact subchondral plate to minimize bleeding, which would result in migration of a mixed stem cell population from the marrow cavity into the chondral defect. If the subchondral plate is sclerotic, such as with chronic defects, partially healed OCD lesions, or after prior microfracture, we prefer to carefully thin out the sclerotic bone with a fine burr and cold irrigation. Minor bleeding from the subchondral bone is controlled with thrombin, fibrin glue, or rarely, a needle-tipped electrocautery device in the cutting mode. Once the defect is prepared, it is templated using glove paper. If periosteum is to be used, the template should be oversized by approximately 2 mm in both length and width to allow for

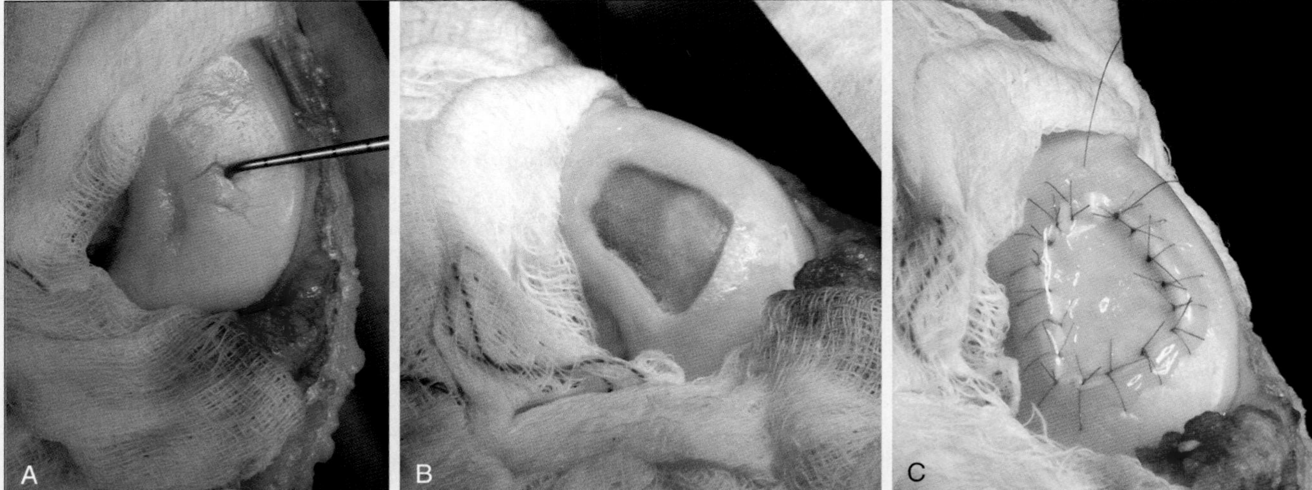

FIGURE 97-8 **A,** A chondral defect on the weight-bearing femoral condyle is being probed. The patient had sustained direct impact trauma to this area 2 years ago. The probed cartilage was found to be extremely soft and fissured. **B,** All degenerated cartilage has been removed and the layer of calcified cartilage has been debrided carefully so as not to injure the subchondral plate. **C,** A collagen patch has been sutured in place, and the suture line has been waterproofed with fibrin glue.

Continued

shrinkage of the periosteum. More commonly, an artificial membrane consisting of a bilayer type I/III collagen matrix is used. However, the use of collagen membranes for ACI is an off-label indication in the United States and must be discussed with the patient.

Periosteal Harvest

The most accessible site for procurement of the periosteal patch is the proximal medial tibia distal to the pes anserine to avoid the fibrous extensions of the sartorius fascia. Either the arthrotomy is extended distally or a second incision is made located centrally over the anteromedial surface of the proximal tibia starting 3 to 5 cm inferior to the pes anserine insertion. The subcutaneous fat is incised superficially, and further dissection with Metzenbaum scissors will expose the tibial periosteum. The template is used to outline the periosteum, which is incised using a fresh No. 15 blade and mobilized with a small, sharp periosteal elevator. The patch should be very gently removed from its bony bed to avoid tearing; the periosteum is pulled upward with a nontoothed microforceps as it is gently removed from the tibia with a gentle pushing motion of the periosteal elevator. After the patch has been harvested, it should be spread out on a moist sponge to avoid desiccation and shrinkage. If a tourniquet has been used, it can be deflated at this point for the remainder of the procedure.

Patch Fixation

The periosteal patch is retrieved from the back table and placed over the defect, with the cambium layer facing the defect. The periosteum is gently unfolded and stretched with a nontoothed forceps; a collagen patch is usually cut dry, then moistened with saline solution. An obviously oversized patch can be trimmed back carefully at this time, preserving a small rim of 1 to 2 mm. Suturing is performed with 6-0 Vicryl on a P-1 cutting needle immersed in mineral oil or glycerin for better handling. The sutures are placed through the patch and then through the articular cartilage, exiting approximately 3 mm away from the defect edge, everting the edge slightly to provide a better seal against the defect wall. The knots are tied on the patch side to remain below the level of the adjacent cartilage. Interrupted sutures are initially placed on each side of the patch (at 3, 6, 9 and 12 o'clock), adjusting the tension of the patch after each suture and trimming the patch as needed to obtain appropriate tension that is neither too loose, thus allowing the patch to sag into the defect, nor so tight that it would cut out of the sutures. Thereafter, additional sutures are placed in between to circumferentially close the gaps. An opening wide enough to accept an Angiocath is left in the most superior aspect of the patch to inject the chondrocytes (Fig. 97-8, *C*). If any concerns exist about water tightness of the suture line, testing can be performed by slowly injecting saline solution into the covered defect with a tuberculin syringe and plastic 18-gauge Angiocath. Any leakage should be addressed with additional sutures or fibrin glue as needed. Lastly, the saline solution is reaspirated to prepare the defect for implantation.

Chondrocyte Implantation

The cells are now resuspended and sterilely aspirated from the transport tubes with a tuberculin syringe through an 18-gauge or larger needle because smaller gauge needles can damage the cells. The needle is then removed and replaced with a flexible, plastic 18-gauge 2-inch Angiocath. The Angiocath is introduced into the defect through the residual opening of the periosteal patch. As the Angiocath is slowly withdrawn, cells are injected until the defect is filled with fluid. One or two additional sutures and fibrin glue are then used to close the injection site.

Wound Closure

We minimize the use of intraarticular drains to avoid damage to the graft. When drains are used, they should be used without suction and with care to position the tubing away from the defect. The wound is closed in layers, and a soft dressing is applied to the knee.

Particulated Juvenile Cartilage Allograft

The defect is approached through a standard arthrotomy, chosen on the basis of the defect location (Fig. 97-9, *A*). The cartilage defect is then debrided according to the microfracture/ACI technique: creation of vertical shoulders of stable cartilage and removal of all degenerated tissue, as well as the layer of calcified cartilage. The allograft tissue is then placed into the defect, using at least 1 vial per 2.5 cm^2 (Fig. 97-9, *B*). Fibrin glue is added to secure the graft in place (Fig. 97-9, *C*). Alternatively, an aluminum foil mold of the defect can be created, and the tissue and fibrin glue can be mixed on the back table. The finished implant is then placed into the defect with additional fibrin glue for fixation. In larger defects, or when stability and containment are of concern, the graft can be covered with a collagen membrane that is sutured to the surrounding cartilage (use of the collagen membrane is off-label, because none is approved for cartilage repair in the United States).

Preserved Osteochondral Allograft

Overall, the same technique is used with a preserved osteochondral allograft as with OAT. It can be performed either arthroscopically or with a (mini) open procedure. Placement of the allograft cylinders involves impaction of a hollow coring tube to the implant depth (10 mm), followed by removal of the bone that is contained within by a reamer (Fig. 97-10, *A*). The implant is then introduced into the recipient site and seated flush to the surrounding cartilage with an oversized tamp (Fig. 97-10, *B*).

Osteochondral Allograft Transplantation

Osteochondral allograft transplantation is performed through an arthrotomy sized to be consistent with the location and extent of the lesion. The patient is positioned supine on a standard operating room table. A leg-positioning device can be helpful for very posterior lesions that require hyperflexion of the knee. The most commonly used technique is the press-fit plug or mega-OATS technique, which is discussed here. Several proprietary systems have been developed to facilitate graft sizing and preparation.

Approach

Most commonly, an anterior midline incision is made from the proximal pole of the patella to the tibial tubercle, but medial or lateral paramedian incisions can be used as well. A medial or lateral peripatellar capsulotomy is performed from the superior pole of the patellar to the tibial tubercle. Recently, more limited incisions such as the subvastus or mid vastus

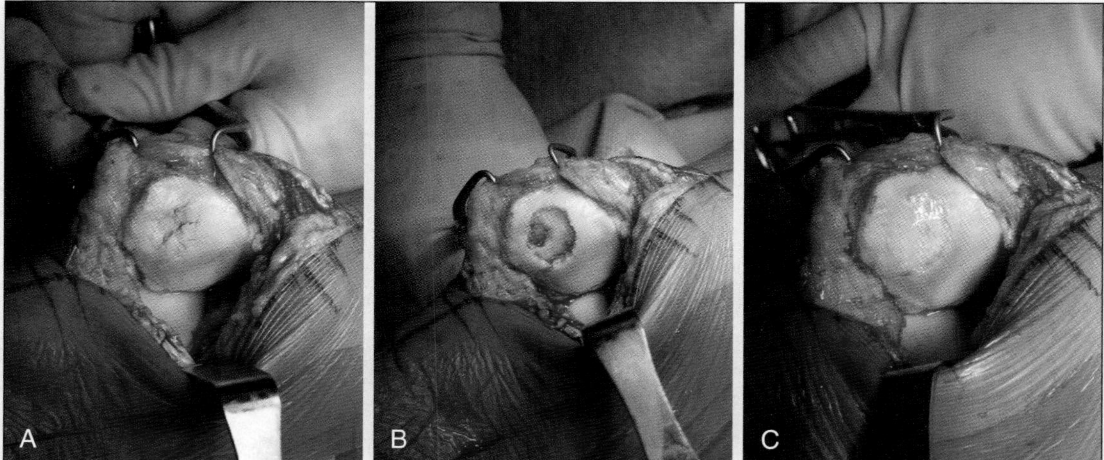

FIGURE 97-9 **A,** A large chondral defect of the patella after prior failed osteochondral autograft transfer (OAT). **B,** The defect has been debrided back to a stable rim. The abnormal bone in the area of prior OAT is clearly visible. **C,** The defect after placement of particulated cartilage allograft and fibrin glue fixation.

approaches have gained popularity, and we believe that these approaches allow for accelerated postoperative quadriceps rehabilitation. The patella is retracted with either a Z retractor or bent Hohman retractor placed into the notch. We have found it helpful to release the fat pad and dissect the anterior meniscal horn from the capsule to provide better exposure, especially with small incisions.

Defect Preparation

Once the lesion is exposed, the abnormal cartilage is identified (Fig. 97-11, *A*). It is of utmost importance to reconstruct the normal geometry of the articular surface with the donor graft. A cannulated cylindrical sizing guide is placed over the defect to determine the optimal plug diameter, and a guide pin is drilled perpendicularly to the articular surface through the sizing guide. A 6- to 8-mm deep recipient socket is created with a cannulated reamer (Fig. 97-11, *B* and *C*), and the exact depth of the defect is measured in all four quadrants. Multiple drill holes are created in the floor of the defect to improve blood supply. If subchondral cysts are present, autologous bone grafting of the cavities should be performed rather than reaming deeper so that the amount of transplanted allograft bone can be minimized.

Graft Preparation

The appropriate donor site is then identified on the allograft condyle (Fig. 97-11, *D*), which is secured in the workstation, and a mark is made at the 12-o'clock position to aid in orientation. A bushing of the appropriate diameter is selected and oriented perpendicularly to the articular surface. Using the coring reamer, an osteochondral cylinder is harvested. After extracting the graft from the reamer, the

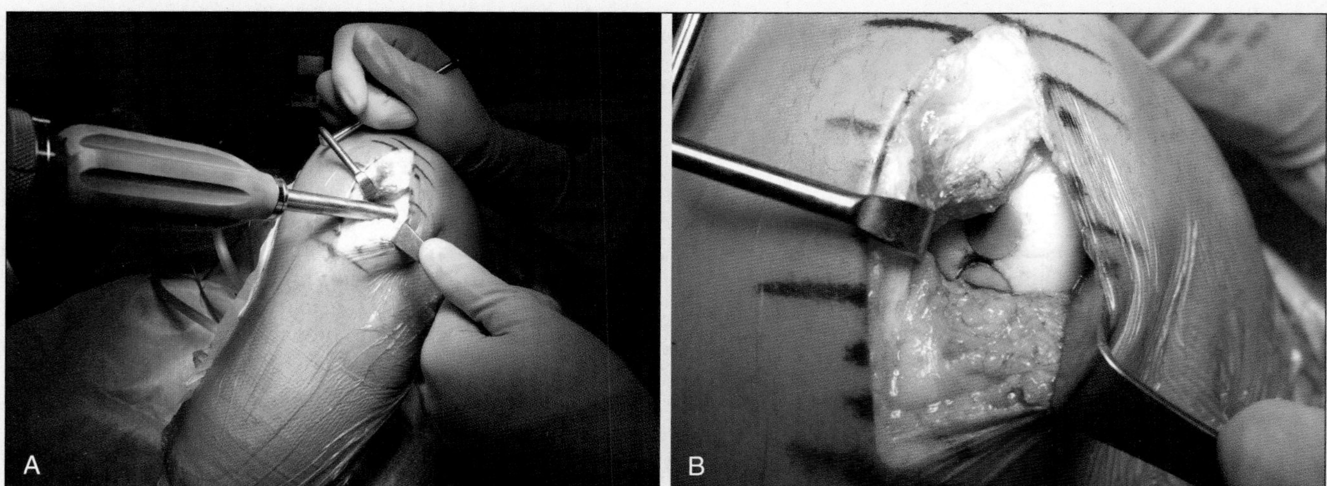

FIGURE 97-10 **A,** Creating the recipient slot with a reamer. **B,** Two preserved osteochondral allograft plugs seated flush to the articular surface for treatment of an oblong chondral defect in the femoral condyle.

Continued

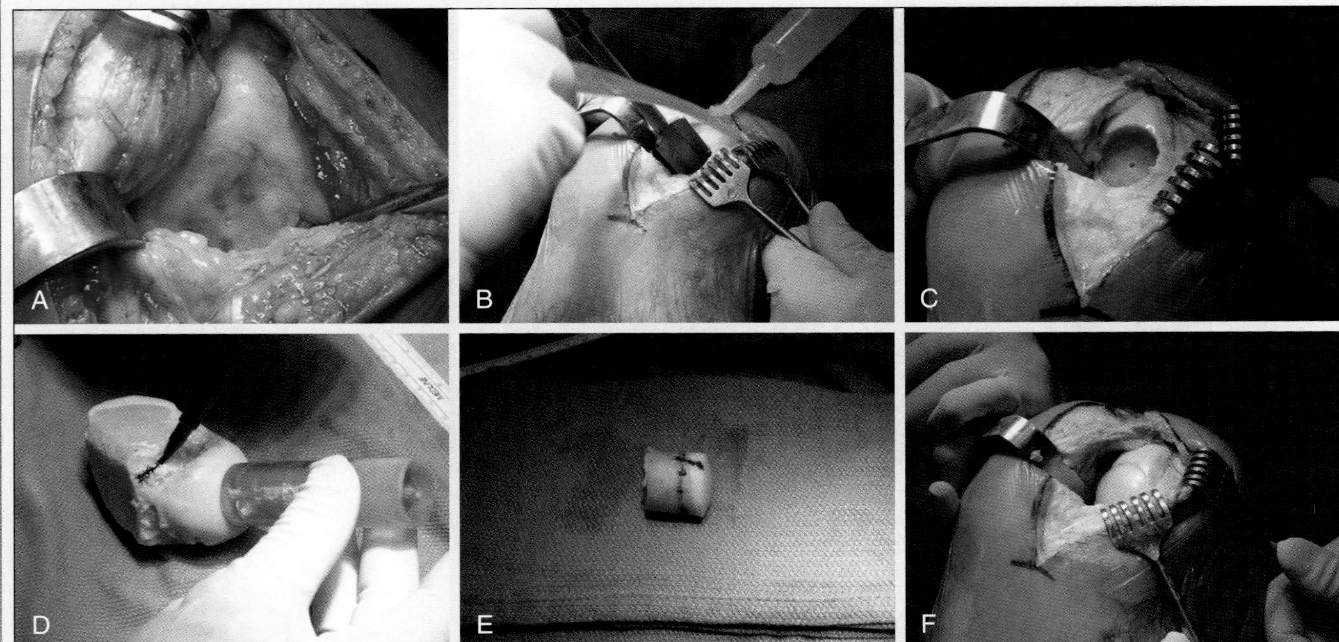

FIGURE 97-11 **A,** A large chondral defect of the weight-bearing femoral condyle is exposed through a limited, peripatellar approach. **B,** A guide pin has been introduced perpendicularly into the defect and is being overdrilled with an appropriately sized reamer. **C,** The prepared defect after reaming to a depth of approximately 6 to 8 mm. **D,** Selecting the appropriate harvest site on the fresh allograft hemicondyle. **E,** The allograft cylinder prior to trimming to the appropriate depth, which has been marked out for each quadrant. **F,** The transplant has been introduced into the recipient site. Press-fit fixation is usually sufficient but can be augmented with resorbable pins.

four quadrants of the graft are marked (Fig. 97-11, *E*) and trimmed down to match the depths previously recorded from the recipient site. It is helpful to slightly bevel the edges of the graft to facilitate insertion and avoid excessive impaction pressures.

Graft Insertion

The recipient site is now prepared for insertion with a calibrated dilator and the graft is press-fit with manual pressure and ranging of the knee, without the use of impaction forces (Fig. 97-11, *F*). It is preferable to slightly recess the graft rather than leaving it proud. Absorbable pins or screws may be used for supplemental fixation if concerns about stability exist.

Closure

Standard layered closure is performed after repair of the capsulotomy. Drains can be used if necessary.

objective ones such as range of motion, swelling, quadriceps atrophy, radiographic joint space narrowing, and others.

Microfracture

Marrow stimulation techniques result in a fibrocartilaginous repair tissue with inferior wear characteristics. However, several studies evaluating the efficacy of treatment have demonstrated good outcomes in 60% to 80% of patients, provided strict indications are followed: smaller defects (<2 to 4 cm^2) on the femoral condyles (not the PF joint!) in younger patients (<40 years) with relatively short chronicity (<3 years).[26,27,36,41,61]

Osteochondral Autograft Transfer

Patients treated with OAT experienced good to excellent results in approximately 91% of condylar lesions, 86% of tibial defects, and 74% of trochlear lesions; 5% of patients experienced donor site morbidity with PF pain.[38,42] The treatment of patellar defects remains controversial, with some groups reporting almost universal failure in this location.[28,81] An RCT compared the outcomes of OAT with those after microfracture, demonstrating higher functional scores (96% vs. 52%, respectively), better rates of return to play (93% vs. 52%, respectively), and better macroscopic appearance during second-look arthroscopy (84% vs. 57%, respectively) for OAT.[37]

Autologous Chondrocyte Implantation

Several long-term studies have reported good to excellent results in 70% to 80% of patients after ACI for the treatment of chondral lesions in the knee.[10,35,81-87] Although the outcomes of ACI for the treatment of large lesions (>4 cm^2) exceed those of other forms of treatment, such as debridement,[88] microfracture,[29,84] and OAT,[28,81] smaller lesions demonstrate comparable short- and mid-term clinical outcomes regardless of the specific cartilage repair technique used. Several studies have investigated size-specific outcomes with ACI and microfracture; Knutsen et al.[29] reported that overall no significant clinical differences were found between groups. However, when outcomes were stratified by size, lesions larger than 4 cm^2 did poorly with microfracture, whereas ACI demonstrated no correlation with size; the authors therefore recommended cell-based therapy for larger defects.[29] A recent 5-year follow-up study of medium-sized lesions (average defect size, 2.5 cm^2) demonstrated significantly better functional outcomes for ACI in patients who had symptoms for less than 3 years. No difference was observed between the (overall inferior) outcomes in chronic defects.[33] Basad et al.[84] specifically investigated outcomes in larger defects, only enrolling patients with defects larger than 4 cm^2, for whom they demonstrated significantly better results with membrane-induced ACI.

Inferior results are seen with ACI in patients who smoke or are obese, as well as patients who had previously been treated with marrow stimulation or have persistent severe subchondral edema.[25,89-91]

Although the treatment of patellar defects is considered an off-label indication, its use has demonstrated convincing outcomes provided that patellar maltracking issues are adequately addressed, most commonly through tibial tubercle osteotomy.[10,11,86,92]

Periosteal patch hypertrophy resulting in mechanical symptoms such as clicking and popping occurs in up to 15% to 20% of patients, typically 7 to 9 months after the procedure.[93] Therefore many surgeons have abandoned the use of periosteum in favor of type I/III bilayer collagen membranes, thus decreasing the intervention rate for hypertrophy by approximately 80% without compromising clinical outcomes.[71,94,95]

Particulated Juvenile Cartilage Allograft

Limited clinical data exist for particulated juvenile cartilage allografts, with its use described in the knee and ankle in several case reports and small cohorts.[75,96,97]

Preserved Osteochondral Allograft

No clinical studies of the use of preserved osteochondral allografts have been published to date. A registry trial is currently under way, with patients prospectively followed up with use of clinical and MRI techniques.

Osteochondral Allograft Transplantation

After osteochondral allograft transplantation, good to excellent results are generally achieved in nearly 85% to 90% of cases at 5- to 10-year follow-up.[49] The treatment of osteonecrosis and PF defects, as well as the use of bipolar grafts in the tibiofemoral compartments, is associated with lowered graft survival of approximately 70% to 80%.[98-100]

Complications

General complications inherent to knee surgery are infection, thrombosis, and arthrofibrosis, which are more common with open than with arthroscopic procedures. Nerve damage after knee surgery usually takes the form of injury to the infrapatellar branch of the saphenous nerve, resulting in a numb area over the lateral aspect of the knee. Rarely, nerve damage can result from direct injury to the peroneal nerve or indirect, tourniquet-related injury to the sciatic and tibial nerves. Specific risks associated with individual procedures are graft detachment or delamination after ACI and subchondral collapse or nonunion after osteochondral allograft transplantation, which generally are addressed by revision cartilage repair.

Future Considerations

Future Developments

Matrices were introduced to improve on a number of perceived shortcomings of the first-generation ACI (ACI-P, for periosteal cover). These techniques are also performed as staged procedures, with an initial arthroscopic cartilage biopsy followed by cellular expansion and reimplantation. The second-generation technique (ACI-C, for collagen cover) replaces the periosteal patch with a collagen matrix, commonly a two-layered, type I/III porcine collagen or other synthetic construct. This modification was successful in virtually eliminating patch hypertrophy[94] and obviates the need to harvest the periosteal patch, thus decreasing surgical time and morbidity associated with a wider exposure. For third-generation ACI, or MACI (Genzyme/Sanofi BioSurgery, Cambridge, MA), the chondrocytes are seeded onto a type I/III porcine-derived collagen carrier matrix after initial expansion in culture. During implantation, the matrix is sized to match the defect and placed through either a mini open approach or arthroscopically with fibrin glue fixation. The use of a preseeded matrix also addresses disadvantages of the ACI procedure that are associated with implantation of a cell suspension such as the risk of cell leakage from the defect and the potentially uneven cell distribution within the defect. European studies investigating MACI have shown clinical results comparable with the ACI-P and ACI-C techniques.[43] However, as with ACI, MACI is limited by relatively slow cell growth and differentiation, which precludes early aggressive rehabilitation. MACI is currently not available in the United States. However, a large randomized trial in Europe of MACI versus microfracture was recently concluded, and the data will be submitted to the FDA soon for U.S. approval.

Multiple other technologies are currently undergoing clinical evaluation, generally combining autologous chondrocytes with various membranes that can be implanted in a minimally invasive manner without the need for suturing. Because most of these technologies are minor variations of the previously discussed MACI technology, only two technologies that are substantially different are briefly discussed here.

An autologous chondrocyte graft treated in the laboratory for 6 weeks with pressure perfusion is presently undergoing phase III clinical trials in the United States (NeoCart; Histogenics Inc., Northampton, MA) for the treatment of small lesions (2 to 3 cm^2). The chondrocytes are harvested arthroscopically in an initial staging procedure. The cells are then grown to confluence in 2 to 3 days, seeded on a type I bovine collagen membrane, and placed in a fluid chamber that pressure cycles nutrients through the matrix until near-mature tissue is produced. During reimplantation, the tissue is cut to fit the templated defect and secured to the subchondral bone with a proprietary glue.

Allogenic tissue-engineered cartilage grafts derived from chondrocytes of adolescent donors younger than 12 years are currently being investigated in a phase III trial in the United States (DeNovo ET; ISTO Technologies, St. Louis, MO). The chondrocytes are grown in a matrix-free culture and implanted with fibrin glue.

The successful application of biologic matrices as carrier devices for autologous chondrocytes has led several groups to investigate the use of such matrices in conjunction with MSTs. A collagen matrix is placed into a chondral defect after microfracture to stabilize the resultant blood clot and allow cell adherence. In comparison with ACI and MACI, no initial harvest procedure is needed to obtain a cartilage biopsy. Most importantly, the decision to perform this type of chondral repair can be made intraoperatively because the acellular carrier matrix has an extended shelf life and is not patient-specific. Early work with this technique in a sheep model demonstrated results worse than microfracture alone[101]; however, several clinical studies have shown more promising outcomes.[102] Future research to modify these matrices with growth factors to enhance cell adherence and differentiation holds promise to improve the results of this technology.

Another technique currently in phase III clinical trials uses a resorbable scaffold that is seeded with particulated autologous cartilage in the operating room just prior to implantation (cartilage autograft implantation system; DePuy, Raynham, MA). A cartilage biopsy is harvested from the patient's knee, minced, and then fixated on a resorbable polymer matrix with fibrin glue. The resultant construct is then reimplanted during the same setting using resorbable staples. In vitro studies have demonstrated the viability of chondrocytes and the outgrowth of matrix after the mincing process.[74] A phase I/II clinical study demonstrated promising short-term outcomes.[103]

Synthetic Osteochondral Implants

Synthetic osteochondral implants appear to be a promising alternative to treat small defects without the potential donor site morbidity associated with OAT. Several implants are under investigation. Although some implants are in clinical application outside the United States, none has been approved by the FDA for cartilage repair. Generally, most implants are based on a collagen scaffold that is treated with various forms of calcium, either hydroxy apatite or calcium phosphate. Early studies have demonstrated promising short-term results.[104]

Synthetic polylactic/polyglycolic calcium sulfate plugs (TruFit, Smith & Nephew, Andover, MA) have been approved by the FDA to back-fill donor sites in an attempt to decrease morbidity after OAT. Although animal models had demonstrated promising results,[105] a recent clinical study with CT follow-up of 9 patients demonstrated subchondral cyst formation in all cases.[106] Currently, this plug technology has not been approved by the FDA to treat chondral defects.

Stem Cells

Mesenchymal stem cells (MSCs) have the ability to differentiate into many diverse cell lineages, including chondrocytes. Initially identified in bone marrow aspirates, MSCs have also been isolated from adipose tissue, skin, umbilical cord, and peripheral blood. MSCs are autogenous, can be obtained through simple in-office biopsy of muscle or fatty tissue, and expand more than 500-fold with a potential cell yield in the billions.[107] Studies are under way to seed the expanded cells onto a suitable carrier matrix and then expose them to a combination of environmental factors, such as hypoxia and hydrostatic pressure, and biochemical agents, such as growth factors, to commit the cells to the chondrogenic pathway[108] prior to surgical implantation. Comparatively few clinical trials have investigated the application of stem cells for cartilage repair, including a U.S. trial, in which allogeneic stem cells in a hyaluronic carrier were injected into the knee joint, and a Korean trial that used umbilical cord blood–derived stem cells to surgically treat cartilage defects.

For a complete list of references, go to expertconsult.com.

Suggested Readings

Citation: Gudas R, Gudaite A, Pocius A, et al: Ten-year follow-up of a prospective, randomized clinical study of mosaic osteochondral autologous transplantation versus microfracture for the treatment of osteochondral defects in the knee joint of athletes. *Am J Sports Med* 40(11):2499–2508, 2012.

Level of Evidence: I

Summary: This prospective randomized trial of microfracture (MFx) versus mosaicplasty (osteochondral autograft transfer; OAT) demonstrates significantly better outcomes for mosaicplasty in terms of failure rate (MFx, 38%; OAT, 14%), and International Cartilage Repair Society scores. Seventy-five percent of patients who underwent OAT, but only 37% of patients who underwent MFx, maintained their previous level of physical activity.

Citation: Basad E, Ishaque B, Bachmann G, et al: Matrix-induced autologous chondrocyte implantation versus microfracture in the treatment of cartilage defects of the knee: A 2-year randomised study. *Knee Surg Sports Traumatol Arthrosc* 18(4):519–527, 2010.

Level of Evidence: I

Summary: This prospective randomized trial of microfracture versus autologous chondrocyte implantation (ACI) specifically investigated defects larger than 4 cm^2, the classic indication for ACI. It demonstrated significantly better outcomes for ACI after 2 years according to the Lysholm, Tegner, and International Cartilage Repair Society scores.

Citation: Knutsen G, Engebretsen L, Ludvigsen TC, et al: Autologous chondrocyte implantation compared with microfracture in the knee. A randomized trial. *J Bone Joint Surg Am* 86A(3):455–464, 2004.

Level of Evidence: I

Summary: This prospective randomized trial of microfracture (MFx) versus autologous chondrocyte implantation (ACI) demonstrated no significant differences between groups overall. Defects larger than 4 cm^2 treated with MFx, however, demonstrated worse outcomes. The authors recommended use of ACI for the treatment of larger defects.

Citation: Saris DB, Vanlauwe J, Victor J, et al: Treatment of symptomatic cartilage defects of the knee: Characterized chondrocyte implantation results in better clinical outcome at 36 months in a randomized trial compared to microfracture. *Am J Sports Med* 37(Suppl 1):10S–19S, 2009.

Level of Evidence: I

Summary: This prospective randomized trial of microfracture (MFx) versus autologous chondrocyte implantation (ACI) demonstrated greater improvement in the Knee Injury and Osteoarthritis Outcome Score with ACI and worsening of subchondral bone changes with MFx.

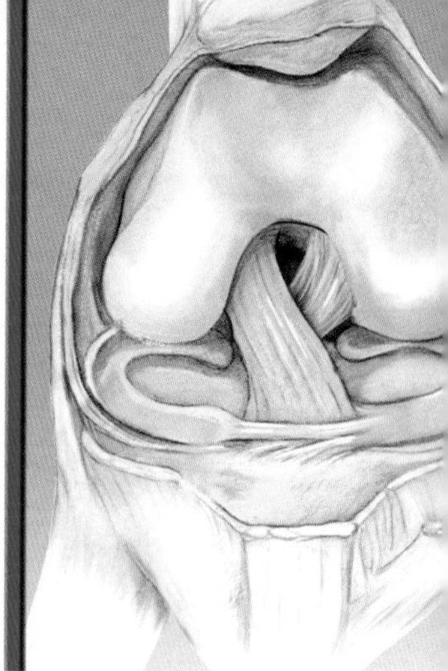

98

Anterior Cruciate Ligament Injuries (Including Revision)

JARED A. NISKA • FRANK A. PETRIGLIANO • DAVID R. McALLISTER

History

The surgical treatment of anterior cruciate ligament (ACL) injuries began in the early 1900s with attempted primary repair. Patients treated with primary repair had poor results, including recurrent instability, which led to the advent of ACL reconstruction in the 1970s. The MacIntosh and Ellison procedures, two of the original reconstruction techniques, used the iliotibial band for extraarticular stabilization of the knee. A high incidence of arthrofibrosis and overall poor clinical outcome[1] led to the development of an anatomic intraarticular reconstruction through an open approach in the 1980s. A variety of synthetic grafts, such as polypropylene and Gore-tex, were used in the early stages. Over time, these grafts stretched and fragmented, leading to high failure rates, sterile effusions, pain, and instability. Tendon autografts and allografts, including hamstrings (HS) and bone–patellar tendon–bone (BPTB), quickly became the standard of care.[1,2]

The development of arthroscopic instrumentation in the early 1990s facilitated transition to an arthroscopically assisted reconstruction. Initially, femoral and tibial tunnels were drilled independently through a two-incision technique and the grafts were fixed on the anterior tibia and lateral femur. However, in the early 1990s, a single-incision ACL reconstruction in which the femoral tunnel was drilled through the tibial tunnel became popular. In some instances, this approach resulted in a relatively vertical femoral tunnel. Recent biomechanical evidence has suggested that a femoral tunnel placed in the center of the native femoral footprint may convey a biomechanical advantage.[3,4] Consequently, there has been a heightened awareness of the native ACL anatomy and a renewed focus on techniques that result in more anatomic placement of the graft.

Anatomy and Biomechanics

The ACL originates on the tibial articular surface lateral and anterior to the medial intercondylar spine. Proximally, it courses posterior and lateral to insert on the posteromedial wall of the lateral femoral condyle.[5] Two functional bundles are present, the anteromedial (AM) and the posterolateral (PL), which are named for their tibial insertion sites (Fig. 98-1).[6,7] The ACL provides rotational stability and resists anterior tibial translation, varus stress, and valgus stress.[8]

The position of the AM and PL bundles varies with flexion and extension of the knee. In extension, the AM and PL bundles are parallel, but as the knee flexes, the bundles cross and the posterolateral bundle moves anteriorly. The PL bundle is tight in extension and the AM bundle is tight in flexion.[7,9] The femoral attachment of the ACL spans an area of 113 mm^2 and is circular in shape. The ACL attaches on the tibial side over an oval area, comprising approximately 136 mm^2.[10] ACL fibers do not pass anterior to the cruciate ridge (also referred to as the lateral intercondylar ridge), which runs proximal to distal on the lateral femoral condyle.[11]

Indirect comparison from various studies suggests that ACL strength decreases with age.[12] Under normal walking conditions, the ACL experiences forces of approximately 400 N, whereas passive knee motion produces only 100 N. High-level activities such as cutting, accelerating, and decelerating are estimated to produce forces up to 1700 N, which approaches the average maximal tensile strength of the ligament, 2160 ± 157 N.[13] Despite this narrow window, the ACL works in concert with other stabilizing structures in the knee to resist force and usually requires an abnormally high load to fail.[9,14] Many other structures in the knee can be injured in conjunction with an ACL rupture, including the menisci, collateral ligaments, articular cartilage, and joint capsule.[15-17]

Basic Science

Microanatomy

The ACL is composed of longitudinal collagen fibrils that range in diameter from 20 to 170 μm. The fibrils are composed primarily of type I collagen but also contain type III collagen.[18] They arrange to form a unit called the *subfascicular unit,* which is surrounded by a layer of connective tissue called the *endotendineum*. These units combine to form the fasciculus, which has an outer layer called the *epitendineum*. The fasciculus is ensheathed by the paratenon, forming the largest ligamentous unit. The microscopic architecture changes to a more fibrocartilaginous appearance near the bony attachments on the tibia and femur.[19,20]

The blood supply to the ACL comes from branches of the middle genicular artery and secondarily from branches of the inferior medial and lateral genicular arteries, as well as the infrapatellar fat pad and synovium. The proximal portion of

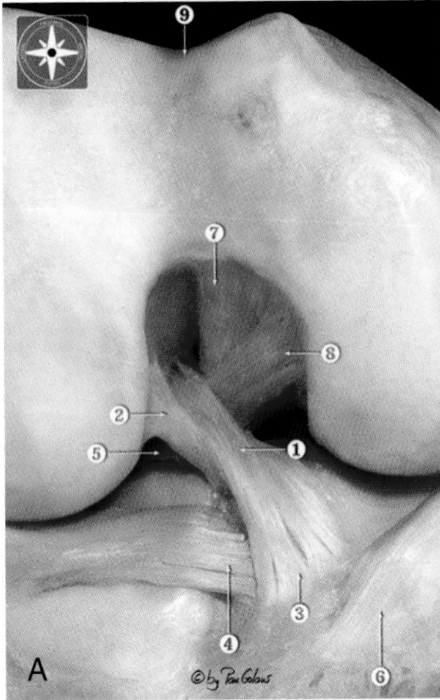

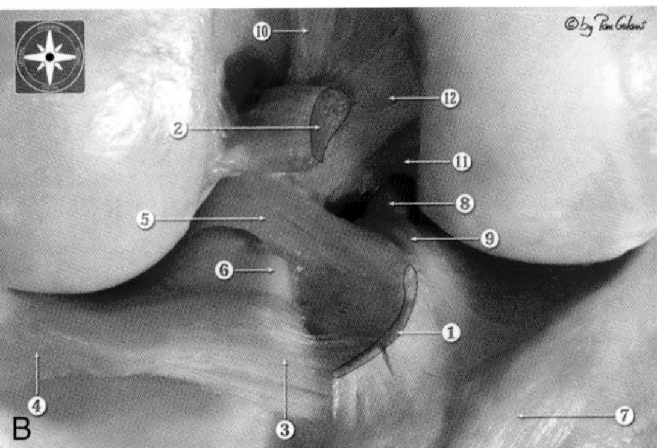

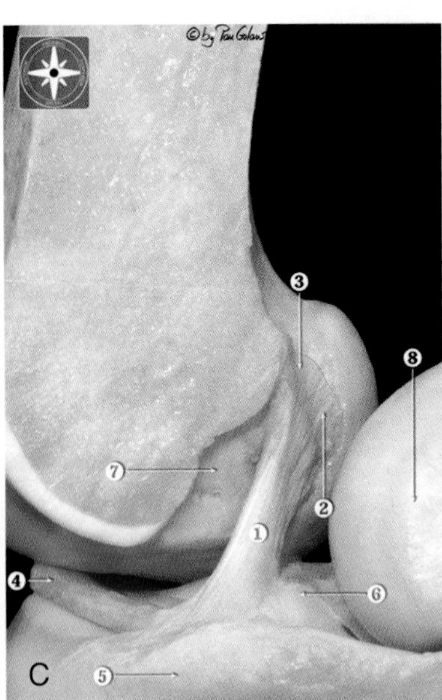

FIGURE 98-1 Functional bundles of anterior cruciate ligament (ACL) in a cadaveric specimen. **A,** The anterior view with the knee in 90 degrees of flexion. *1,* The anteromedial bundle of the ACL; *2,* the posterolateral bundle of the ACL; *3,* the tibial insertion of the ACL; *4,* the anterior horn of the lateral meniscus; *5,* the posterior horn of the lateral meniscus; *6,* the anterior horn of the medial meniscus; *7,* the femoral insertion of the posterior cruciate ligament; *8,* the anterior meniscofemoral ligament (Humphrey ligament); and *9,* the femoral trochlear groove. **B,** The anterior view of the intercondylar notch with the ACL midsubstance resected. *1,* The ACL tibial footprint; *2,* the ACL femoral stump; *3,* the anterior horn of the lateral meniscus; *4,* the body of the lateral meniscus; *5,* the posterior horn of the lateral meniscus; *6,* the lateral tibial spine; *7,* the anterior horn of the medial meniscus; *8,* the posterior horn of the medial meniscus; *9,* the medial tibial spine; *10,* the anterolateral bundle of the posterior cruciate ligament; *11,* the posteromedial bundle of the posterior cruciate ligament; and *12,* the anterior meniscofemoral ligament (Humphrey ligament). **C,** The sagittal view of the intercondylar notch and ACL. *1,* The ACL midsubstance; *2,* the anteromedial bundle of the ACL; *3,* the posterolateral bundle of the ACL; *4,* the body of the lateral meniscus; *5,* the anterior horn of the medial meniscus; *6,* the medial tibial spine; *7,* the medial wall of the lateral femoral condyle; and *8,* the medial femoral condyle. *(Copyright Pau Golanó.)*

the ACL has better vascularity, because the middle genicular artery gives rise to ligamentous branches proximally and courses distally along the dorsal aspect of the ACL. The largest ligamentous branch is the tibial intercondylar artery, which arises proximally and bifurcates distally at the tibial spine to supply the tibial condyles.[21,22]

Nerve fibers have been found in all regions of the ACL, primarily running parallel with the vasculature in a longitudinal manner, but also incorporating freely into the connective tissue. The appearance of the nerve fibers suggests a role in vasomotor control. However, the diameter of the nerve fibers in the connective tissue suggests a role in pain or reflex activity.[21] This role is supported by findings of altered proprioception in patients with capsuloligamentous injury and partial restoration of this function with ligamentous reconstruction.[23]

Biology of ACL Injury

The ACL is an intraarticular structure encased by a thin soft tissue envelope formed by the synovial lining. Rupture of the ligament usually causes disruption of this synovial lining and hematoma formation throughout the joint space with very little local reaction. Extraarticular ligaments, such as the medial collateral ligament (MCL), are contained within a robust soft tissue envelope. Injury to these ligaments causes formation of local hematoma and fibrinogen mesh that allows for invasion of inflammatory cells, resulting in healing with granulation tissue and eventually organized fibrous tissue.[24]

Biology of ACL Reconstruction

Epidemiology

ACL injuries comprise 40% to 50% of all ligamentous knee injuries, primarily as a result of sporting activity.[25] Injury to the ACL is most common in young athletes, especially female athletes in their adolescent years.[26] Sports in which athletes are particularly prone to ACL injury are skiing, soccer, basketball, and football. The majority of injuries are from noncontact mechanisms and often occur during landing. Some studies have shown that the maximum strain on the ACL occurs with the knee near extension and a valgus force applied with internal tibial rotation and anterior tibial translation.[27,28] Females have a higher risk of ACL injury, which is possibly due to gender differences in knee biomechanical forces during landing. Females have increased quadriceps to HS strength and land in a more erect posture, which creates a larger anterior shear force and a greater strain on the ACL.[29,30]

It is estimated that 200,000 ACL reconstructions are performed annually, with an 8% failure rate.[31] Failure can occur early or late, with early failure occurring within 6 months of reconstruction and late failure occurring after 6 months. Early failure is largely due to technical error in 22% to 79% of cases, with tunnel malposition being the primary culprit. Late failure is most commonly due to repeat trauma to the graft but can also be due to tunnel malposition, most commonly a vertical femoral tunnel.[31,32]

History (Clinical Presentation)

It is important to obtain a detailed patient history, including the injury mechanism and symptoms, as a first step to diagnosing an ACL injury. These injuries generally occur during a rotational movement or deceleration, and only one third of these injuries occur with direct contact. Most patients are unable to recall the exact mechanism of injury, but studies have shown that most acute hemarthroses and ACL injuries occur as a result of twisting injuries of the knee.[33] Many patients report a popping sensation; however, the correlation between a popping sensation and an ACL injury is fairly nonspecific.[34,35] A large proportion of patients with an ACL rupture experience immediate pain, swelling, and a feeling of instability. Most are unable to return to sport.

The most sensitive marker for an acute ACL injury is a severe effusion within 2 to 12 hours of the injury.[33,35,36] Injury to the ligament disrupts the blood supply and causes a large hemarthrosis that is a hallmark of an ACL injury. It must be noted, however, that hemarthrosis can be caused by injury to the menisci or posterior cruciate ligament (PCL) or by osteochondral fractures.[33] Moreover, lack of severe effusion should not exclude injury to the ACL.

Physical Examination

Physical examination is very important in diagnosing an ACL injury. Together with the patient history, the physical examination can often provide enough information for a definitive diagnosis. It is critically important to examine both the affected and unaffected knee to get a baseline measure for each patient. Examining the unaffected knee first calms the patient and helps him or her to relax, which is important when testing for ligamentous stability of the injured knee.

Examination of the acutely injured knee should begin with inspection. Patients who have significant knee injuries, such as an ACL rupture, usually present with a large effusion. The affected knee is often flexed to relieve the increased pressure in the joint caused by the hemarthrosis. If several days or weeks have passed since the injury occurred, the quadriceps may be atrophied compared with the contralateral leg.[37]

Palpation should be performed to evaluate for warmth, degree of effusion, crepitus, and local tenderness. Warmth and effusion indicate inflammation, which correlates with a large hemarthrosis in the setting of an ACL injury. A large majority of acutely injured knees have tenderness to palpation either medially, laterally, or on both sides.[35] Local swelling or tenderness over the lateral or medial aspects of the knee suggests injury to the MCL or lateral collateral ligament (LCL). Focal joint-line tenderness could indicate meniscal or chondral injury. Osteochondral injury may also present with crepitus on range of motion (ROM) testing of the knee.[37]

ROM is restricted in almost 90% of patients with acute ACL injury. Apprehension and guarding are common, and physical examination findings can be more revealing after aspiration or local intraarticular injection.[37] Although it is not commonly performed, aspiration can also provide clues to the diagnosis because a hemarthrosis suggests ligamentous injury, whereas the presence of fat globules suggests a bony injury. Both active and passive ROM should be tested to determine if there is injury to the extensor mechanism or mechanical block from a meniscal tear, loose body, or torn ACL that is obstructing motion.

Ligament Laxity

Although some studies have reported less than 30% sensitivity of the ligamentous examinations in patients with acute ACL injuries, a recent metaanalysis showed that the sensitivity and specificity of a combined ligamentous examination (anterior drawer, pivot shift, and Lachman testing) was 84% and 92%, respectively.[37] The Lachman test showed a sensitivity ranging from 60% to 100% (mean, 84%) and specificity of 100% in a single study. Anterior drawer testing is 9% to 93% sensitive (mean, 62%) for ACL injury, with specificity ranging from 23% to 100% (mean, 67%).[37] The anterior drawer and Lachman test address anteroposterior stability of the knee but not rotational stability. The pivot-shift test addresses rotational stability by combining a valgus stress on the knee with rotation and axial load during knee flexion. A positive test is marked by a palpable clunk produced by reduction of the subluxed lateral tibial plateau by the iliotibial band when moving from full extension into flexion. This test is 27% to 95% sensitive (mean, 38%) and is limited in patients who are awake because of guarding.[35,37] It is also important to test for varus and valgus stability of the knee to evaluate for injury to the LCL or MCL, which can also be injured in the setting of an ACL rupture.

In one study, arthroscopic examination in athletes with acute knee injuries and hemarthrosis who had no obvious clinical laxity on examination revealed surgical-type injuries in 90% of patients. Seventy-two percent had ACL tears, and two thirds of these patients had associated meniscal tears. Other injuries included isolated major meniscal injuries, osteochondral fractures, and injuries to the PCL.[36] Other studies have confirmed these findings, and the authors recommend arthroscopy in patients who experience tense effusion within 12 hours of injury.[33]

Arthrometers such as the KT-1000 and KT-2000 can be used as an adjunct to manual maneuvers such as the Lachman and anterior drawer tests, but they are not necessary to make the diagnosis of an ACL rupture. Thus they are most commonly used for research purposes.[13]

Imaging

Imaging studies including radiographs and magnetic resonance imaging (MRI) can help confirm the diagnosis of an ACL injury. Radiographic evidence of a lateral capsular avulsion of the proximal tibia (often referred to as a Segond fracture) is pathognomonic for an ACL injury.[38] Standard radiographs can help exclude associated injuries such as loose bodies, tibial eminence avulsion fractures in younger patients, degenerative changes, and acute fractures of the proximal tibia or distal femur.

MRI is the gold standard for diagnosing an ACL injury because it is both highly sensitive and specific in detecting ACL tears (Fig. 98-2).[39] The majority of ACL tears occur in the midsubstance of the ligament and are visualized on MRI

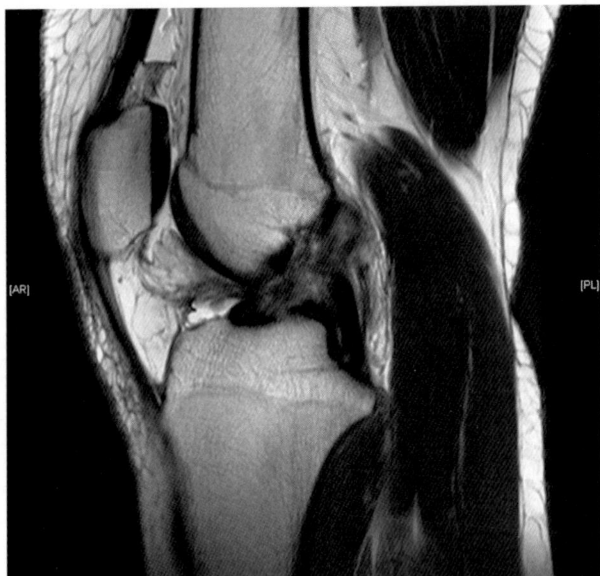

FIGURE 98-2 A sagittal magnetic resonance imaging scan of the anterior cruciate ligament showing complete rupture.

as increased signal intensity with discontinuity of the ligamentous fibers. Hemarthrosis is common, and the presence of a bone bruise is observed on MRI in 84% of patients with an ACL rupture, with the highest incidence on the lateral tibial plateau and lateral femoral condyle, at 73% and 68%, respectively. Secondary signs of ACL rupture may include buckling of the PCL and uncovering of the posterior horn of the lateral meniscus on sagittal MRI sequences due to anterior translation of the tibia relative to the femur. Additionally, the LCL, which is oblique in orientation and typically not visualized in its entirety, may be seen from its origin to insertion on a single coronal image. MRI is also useful for evaluating meniscal injury and osteochondral defects. In patients with ACL rupture, injury is observed to the medial meniscus in 51% of patients and to the lateral meniscus in 54% of patients, with injury to both menisci observed in 33% of patients. MCL injury is observed in 23% of patients with an ACL rupture.[40-42]

Decision-Making Principles

Operative Versus Nonoperative Treatment

The desired activity level of the patient must factor into the decision about whether to pursue nonoperative management of an ACL rupture or ACL reconstruction. The most common complaint of patients with a deficient ACL is recurrent instability and "giving way," and as a result, fewer than 20% of patients return to their preinjury activity level.[43] No large prospective trials have been conducted to demonstrate the natural history of ACL deficiency and the risk for further injury and osteoarthritis. However, it is accepted that high-level athletes with ACL deficiency have a significantly increased risk of symptomatic instability and meniscal injury without ACL reconstruction, which was demonstrated in a group of East German Olympic athletes who continued to compete after sustaining an ACL rupture. Thirty-five year follow-up after the injury revealed that 18 of the 19 athletes had undergone surgery for at least a partial meniscectomy, and 10 of 19 patients had severe osteoarthritis that was treated with a total knee arthroplasty.[44] Other studies have confirmed the increased incidence of meniscal tears with chronic ACL insufficiency,[45] which is thought to occur as a result of decreased rotational stability. Bray and Dandy[46] showed a significantly higher incidence of meniscal injury in patients who had positive results of a pivot-shift test after ACL reconstruction. Although ACL reconstruction may protect the meniscus, it does not completely guard against subsequent injury, nor does it prevent subsequent osteoarthritis.[47]

Age

A study of middle-aged patients who elected nonoperative treatment revealed that 83% had a satisfactory outcome despite a very high incidence of instability. Eighty-seven percent had little to no change on radiographs at 7-year mean follow-up.[48] However, at 4-year follow-up of patients treated conservatively, only 14% were able to return to unlimited athletic activity.[43] Five-year follow-up in athletic persons showed that 74% were unable to participate in twisting or turning activity and 69% had pain with strenuous activity. More importantly, at 11-year follow-up, 44% of patients had radiographic evidence of moderate to severe degenerative joint disease and moderate to severe disability.[49]

The success of ACL reconstruction is age independent, with 91% of patients older than 40 years reporting excellent or good results at 2-year follow-up, compared with 89% for patients younger than 40 years.[50] Nonoperative management with activity modification produces good to excellent results in 57% of patients older than 40 years.[50] Older patients often have more social and professional obligations that may prevent them from proceeding with ACL reconstruction and successfully completing a rehabilitation program, which highlights the importance of stratifying patients by activity level to determine the indication for ACL reconstruction. The use of an allograft instead of an autograft in the older population decreases morbidity and has been shown to produce comparable results.[51]

Gender

Female athletes are at a two- to eightfold greater risk for ACL injury compared with their male counterparts. Most studies have looked at high school and collegiate athletes in soccer, basketball, and volleyball. The majority of injuries occurred as a result of noncontact mechanisms, which led to investigation and speculation about gender differences that can account for this significant disparity.[52,53] Possible etiologies have centered on hormonal and neuromuscular differences, environmental conditions, and differences in anatomy, such as alignment or joint laxity.[29,53]

Anatomic differences that have been evaluated include Q angle, the size and shape of the intercondylar notch, the size of the ACL, material properties of the ACL, foot pronation, body mass index, and generalized ligament laxity. None of these differences alone places females at a greater risk of ACL injury. However, a study of West Point cadets produced a logistic regression model that could predict risk for noncontact ACL injury in 75% of cases, based on a narrow femoral notch, body mass index one standard deviation above the mean, and generalized joint laxity. Some studies have shown that hormonal changes during the menstrual cycle affect the material and mechanical properties of the ACL, which could make it more vulnerable to injury during specific phases of the cycle.[54] However, this effect has not been shown definitively and requires further investigation.[55]

Partial ACL Tears

Diagnosis of a partial ACL tear can be challenging and requires close evaluation of the history, physical examination, and MRI findings, although the gold standard for diagnosis is arthroscopy.[56] Partial tears comprise 10% to 28% of all ACL tears, and if left untreated, 42% will proceed to complete rupture. In addition, a large majority of patients with partial tears are unable to return to their preinjury activity level.[57] KT-2000 arthrometer testing in patients with partial tears has shown only minimal differences in anterior tibial translation.[58] Decision making regarding treatment of partial ACL tears should include evaluation of the patient's desired activity level, the degree of laxity, and symptomatic instability. Options for conservative management include rehabilitation, focusing on HS strengthening, activity modification, and brace wear during activity. Well-designed prospective clinical trials are needed to accurately compare treatment regimens for partial ACL injuries.

Associated Injuries

Rupture of the ACL is associated with injury to other structures in the knee, including the medial and lateral menisci, MCL and LCL, chondral surfaces, PL corner structures, and fracture of the distal femur and proximal tibia.[59] Many years ago, the phrase "unhappy triad" was coined by O'Donoghue to refer to the constellation of ACL rupture, MCL injury, and tearing of the medial meniscus.[15] Subsequent studies have shown that lateral meniscal tears are equally common with ACL rupture.[41] A review of meniscal injury in the setting of ACL rupture showed a predominance of lateral meniscal tears (56%) in persons with an acutely injured ACL and increased incidence of medial meniscal tears (70%) in persons with chronic ACL insufficiency. In addition, the authors found increased reparability with tears to the medial meniscus and increased likelihood of successful repair with concomitant ACL reconstruction. The likelihood of successful meniscal repair decreased with increased time from injury to surgery.[45] An additional study of pediatric and adolescent patients demonstrated an increased risk of medial meniscal tears with delay in ACL reconstruction.[60]

All associated injuries should be evaluated individually to form an overall management plan. Partial-thickness vertical tears posterior to the popliteus tendon that are stable at the time of ACL reconstruction may respond particularly well to nonoperative management.[61] Injury to the medial meniscus should be addressed aggressively, and it has been shown that repair of stable peripheral tears decreases the risk of postoperative pain and the need for subsequent partial meniscectomy.[62]

MCL injuries are common in the setting of ACL rupture, occurring in approximately 23% of cases.[41,63] It was previously thought that high-grade MCL injuries may need to be treated operatively in the setting of ACL rupture. However, recent data have shown that nonoperative bracing of MCL injuries after ACL reconstruction results in equivalent clinical outcome as tested by anterior tibial displacement, function, participation in sporting activities, strength, and one-leg–hop testing.[63,64] Another prospective randomized study found no difference between operative and nonoperative groups for treatment of grade III MCL injury combined with ACL rupture.[65] However, in some persons with severe combined ligamentous injuries, MCL repair may be indicated, although it is often not necessary.

Revision ACL

As the number of ACL reconstructions continues to increase, so does the total number of failures. These failures can typically be categorized as biologic, technical, or traumatic. The majority of failures in the past were due to technical errors, such as improper graft placement, inadequate notchplasty, inadequate graft fixation, improper graft tensioning, use of a graft with inadequate tensile strength, or failure to correct other causes of instability in the knee.[66,67] However, more recent data have shown that traumatic reinjury, which occurs in 32% of patients, is the primary mode of failure.[32] The technical approach to revision ACL reconstruction has been refined during the past 10 to 20 years; however, the results of revision surgery are worse than those for primary reconstruction.[68-70] The risk of chondral damage in the lateral compartment and patellofemoral space is increased with revision ACL reconstruction.[71] Moreover, risk of chondral lesions at revision reconstruction increases in the presence of a previous partial meniscectomy.[72] Patients must be counseled regarding the limitations of revision surgery and the potential for future failures.

Treatment Options

Nonoperative Options

Nonoperative management of ACL rupture can lead to recurrent instability and meniscal injury in athletes.[43,44] For this reason, ACL reconstruction is recommended in patients who are active and require the ability to cut or pivot during physical activity. Persons older than 40 years can do well with a conservative training program but should be advised that a return to their previous activity level is unlikely.[48] Patients should not make a decision regarding surgical management based on their age because studies have shown equivalent outcomes in patients younger and older than 40 years.[50] In a recent randomized controlled trial of young, active adults, early reconstruction versus rehabilitation with the option of delayed reconstruction was evaluated. Patients undergoing delayed reconstruction had outcomes similar to those receiving early reconstruction, and the majority of patients assigned to the rehabilitation group elected to continue with nonoperative management.[73]

Operative Options

ACL reconstruction is commonly recommended for young, active patients. The timing of when to reconstruct ACL injuries has been debated, but most studies have recommended delayed reconstruction. A few studies have shown an increased risk of arthrofibrosis with early reconstruction within the first month.[74-76] Another study showed that rehabilitation prior to the operation can decrease the risk of arthrofibrosis, suggesting that operative treatment should wait for 2 to 6 weeks when motion returns.[77] However, a metaanalysis of the current literature found no difference in clinical outcome between early reconstruction (performed within 3 weeks of the injury) and late reconstruction (performed more than 6 weeks after the injury).[78]

Loss of terminal extension is the primary difficulty encountered, and patient satisfaction is greatly influenced by stiffness and restricted ROM.[79] Patients who have an effusion, swelling, inflammation, and stiffness beyond 4 weeks after the injury was sustained, and who undergo ACL reconstruction, have an equal likelihood of experiencing arthrofibrosis, suggesting that it is the amount of effusion, stiffness, and inflammation present at the time of surgery that results in an increased risk of the development of arthrofibrosis.[74] Currently the only strong indications for immediate reconstruction are associated injury to the PL corner or a repairable meniscal injury.[77]

Preoperative loss of motion has a significant correlation with postoperative loss of motion. Sixty-seven percent of patients who have restricted ROM after surgery had limited ROM at the time of reconstruction.[75] More recent studies have shown that excellent clinical results can be obtained with acute reconstruction (within 2 to 17 days) if a postoperative rehabilitation protocol emphasizing early ROM and terminal knee extension is used.[80] We believe that the best approach is to allow time for the swelling to resolve and wait for the patient to regain good preoperative ROM prior to surgery.

Graft Selection

The keys to choosing an appropriate graft are that it exhibits properties similar to the native ACL, allows for secure fixation, incorporates into the bone tunnels, and limits donor site morbidity.[81] All tendon autografts (BPTB, quadruple HS, and quadriceps tendon) and BPTB allografts have greater tensile strength and stiffness compared with the native ACL.[69,82,83] Synthetic devices are no longer used in the United States because of an unacceptably high rate of complications, including failure and persistent effusion.[84] HS and BPTB autografts are popular, but the choice of graft should be discussed with the patient.

The first choice in decision making is allograft versus autograft. An autograft incorporates into bone earlier, matures more rapidly, and avoids the risk of a host immune reaction, as well as disease transmission. Conversely, the use of an allograft is associated with less morbidity and requires a shorter surgical time.[85,86] A metaanalysis of BPTB autografts versus allografts showed that patients treated with an autograft had a lower incidence of graft rupture and performed better on hop testing. However, when irradiated and chemically processed allografts were excluded from the analysis, no differences were found between autografts and allografts.[87] Patients who underwent allograft reconstruction more commonly reported a final International Knee Documentation Committee (IKDC) score of A (normal knee). However, if a good result was defined as an IKDC score of A or B, no difference existed between the groups.[88] Patients often prefer use of autografts rather than allografts because of a general aversion to allograft tissue. Physician recommendation also has a significant impact on graft selection, because more than two thirds of patients identified physician recommendation as the primary factor in their decision making.[89] Recent evidence suggests a higher failure rate of ACL allografts in young, active patients. A retrospective cohort study found that patients 25 years and younger undergoing ACL reconstruction had a 29.2% failure rate with allograft tissue compared with an 11.8% failure rate with BPTB autografts.[90] Another study showed that higher activity level after ACL reconstruction and allograft use for reconstruction were risk factors for ACL graft failure.[91]

Allografts sterilized with radiation or ethylene oxide are significantly weakened, but current techniques using cryopreservation maintain the biomechanical properties of the tendon allografts.[92,93] Disease transmission from tendon allografts has been reported, but the incidence is quite infrequent, occurring on average in less than one patient per year. Stringent guidelines have almost eliminated the risk of hepatitis C or human immunodeficiency virus, but theoretically a risk still exists. These risks are between 1 in 173,000 and 1 in 1 million for human immunodeficiency virus and approximately 1 in 421,000 for hepatitis C.[94] A few reports of bacterial infection from donor grafts have been reported in the past 10 years,[95] although a recent study specific for allograft ACL reconstruction found no increased risk of infection with allografts compared with autografts.[96]

BPTB and HS tissues are most commonly used for ACL reconstruction. A metaanalysis comparing BPTB and HS autografts showed lower rates of graft failure (4.9% vs. 1.9%) and less anterior laxity on arthrometer testing in the BPTB group. However, the use of the patellar tendon is not without complication, because a greater number of patients in that group reported anterior knee pain (17.4% vs. 11.5%) and required manipulation under anesthesia for lysis of adhesions (6.3% vs. 3.3%).[97] Additionally, the risk of patellar tendon rupture, patellar fracture, and quadriceps weakness is increased with a BPTB autograft. The primary morbidity associated with an HS autograft is pain from hardware prominence, which results in a higher rate of hardware removal (5.5% vs. 3.1%). HS autografts are also associated with HS weakness, but this weakness generally resolves within 1 year.[97,98] A systematic review of current literature found that no single graft source is clearly superior to others.[99] Another systematic review of outcomes using HS or BPTB autografts showed equivalent functional and clinical results but increased anterior knee pain and pain upon kneeling in the BPTB group.[100]

We prefer using autografts rather than allografts in most patients having an index procedure because of the lower failure rate with autografts and the slight risk of disease transmission with allografts. Our preferred choice for an autograft in patients who place a high demand on their knees is BPTB because of earlier incorporation of the bone plugs into the tibial and femoral tunnels and excellent clinical results. We reserve the use of allografts for patients who place a lower demand on their knees, in the revision setting, or in cases of specific patient preference.

Graft Harvest

Harvesting of each type of tendon provides unique technical challenges. Patellar tendon autografts require harvesting bone from the patella and tibial tubercle, which can increase the risk of fracture and damage the articular cartilage of the patella.[81] Many surgeons prefer repairing the paratenon to improve glide and prevent scarring to the overlying tissue.[101] HS harvest requires elevating the sartorius to access the semitendinosus and gracilis and can put the superficial branch of the saphenous nerve at risk. Amputating the tendon prematurely during the harvest is also a risk. The quadriceps tendon is another autograft option.[81]

Graft Tension and Fixation

Graft tension is influenced by the amount of force placed on the graft, as well as the amount of knee flexion and rotation. The graft needs enough tension to stabilize the knee, but too much tension can stretch the graft and lead to failure of the graft itself or failure of fixation. Cadaveric studies have evaluated knee stability under various amounts of tension and showed that 40 N to 60 N with the knee in full extension is ideal for HS and BPTB grafts.[102,103] Some authors recommend providing tension with the knee in full extension, whereas other authors argue that it is best to provide tension with the knee in 20 to 30 degrees of flexion.[104] It has also been suggested that grafts should be preconditioned prior to implantation to prevent creep. Evaluation of outcome is complicated because most surgeons provide tension manually and in various knee positions. Graft-tensioning boots are used by some surgeons because they eliminate the need for manual provision of tension and allow the surgeon to use both hands for tibial fixation. Further trials are required to provide more comprehensive data regarding provision of graft tension.

Graft fixation should be strong enough to withstand closed-chain exercises for at least 12 weeks until the bone or tendon is able to incorporate into the bone tunnels. Closed-chain exercises produce on average 200 N of force but can produce up to 500 N of force.[77] Poor fixation can cause the graft to slip or the fixation to fail altogether.[77] Interference screw fixation of patellar bone blocks has the highest stiffness and fixation strength, ranging from 423 N to 558 N.[105] Screw placement parallel to the bone block is optimal for maximum pull-out strength, whereas divergence greater than 30 degrees has increased risk of failure from pullout.[106] Screw diameter and length also influence fixation strength.[107,108] The use of tibial dilators has no effect on fixation strength, nor does the use of bioabsorbable instead of metallic screws.[109,110]

Many graft fixation devices are commercially available. Soft tissue grafts can be secured with use of interference screws, suture posts, screw and washer constructs, and staples on the tibial side. Similar fixation can be used on the femoral side in addition to cross-pins and buttons.[81] Cross-pins, screw and washer constructs, and buttons all provide indirect fixation, meaning the graft is suspended within the bony tunnel. All others provide direct fixation, which compresses the graft against the side of the bone tunnel. It should be noted that the clinical implications of most biomechanical fixation pull-out studies are limited because they were performed on porcine and bovine specimens at time zero.

Graft Healing

A successful ACL reconstruction relies on incorporation of the graft into the surrounding bone, as well as ligamentization and revascularization of the graft. Bone-to-bone healing is stronger and faster than soft tissue healing to bone. BPTB allografts and autografts heal in a process similar to fracture healing.[81] With soft tissue grafts, the tendon takes 12 weeks to incorporate into the surrounding bone through remodeling of a cellular and fibrous layer formed at the tendon-bone interface. At 12 weeks, collagen fibers form an attachment to bone that resembles Sharpey fibers.[111] At 12 months after ACL reconstruction, all histologic markers of ligamentization and revascularization, including fiber pattern, cellularity, and degree of metaplasia, resemble those of a native ACL. Vascularity and fiber pattern demonstrate no maturation after 6 months, suggesting that tendon autografts may be mature enough at 6 months to proceed with more aggressive rehabilitation and possible return to sport.[112]

Patellar tendon autografts incorporate faster than allografts and have stronger mechanical properties at 6 months. Allografts have a prolonged inflammatory response, decreased strength, and a slower rate of incorporation and tissue remodeling at the 6-month time point.[85]

Revision Options

Determining the cause of failure is the key to successful revision ACL reconstruction. The surgeon should discuss with the patient the expected outcome and the anticipated postoperative activity level. Planning for a revision ACL reconstruction should involve all the steps of a primary reconstruction, including evaluation for associated injuries. In addition, thought should be given to correcting any technical error from the primary surgery and graft selection for revision. The same graft options in primary ACL reconstruction exist for revision surgery, although reharvesting previously harvested graft tissue is not advised.

In one recent study, it was reported that only 54% of patients returned to their preinjury activity level after revision surgery.[113] Patellar tendon autografts and allografts used for revision ACL reconstruction have produced equivalent clinical results and ligamentous stability on arthrometer testing.[70] Overall, revision ACL reconstruction should be viewed largely as a salvage procedure, and patients should be aware that they may never return to their preinjury function and activity level.

Postoperative Management

Rehabilitation

Advancements in surgical technique and graft fixation have enabled patients to participate in early postoperative rehabilitation, focusing on ROM and progressing to patellar mobilization and strengthening. Patients can bear weight on the affected limb immediately. Early weight bearing and rehabilitation do not compromise ligamentous stability and result in a lower incidence of anterior knee pain compared with non–weight bearing.[118-120]

Bracing of the knee in full extension or even hyperextension during early stages of rehabilitation can help to achieve full extension 3 months after surgery, with no adverse effects to knee flexion or stability.[121] In addition, postoperative bracing can help limit swelling, hemarthrosis, pain, and wound drainage. Despite good short-term benefits, postoperative bracing has equivalent long-term clinical outcome,

Text continued on p. 1160

AUTHORS' PREFERRED TECHNIQUE

Primary ACL Reconstruction

A single-bundle ACL reconstruction uses one large graft that is fixed in place at the insertion site of the ACL on the tibia and femur (the so-called footprints of the ACL). If the insertion site is large enough, some surgeons attempt to recreate the AM and PL bundles as two distinct structures using two grafts in a procedure referred to as a *double-bundle* ACL reconstruction. This section presents a single-bundle ACL reconstruction.

Positioning and Setup

The patient is positioned supine on the operating table. After administration of an appropriate anesthetic, both the operative and uninvolved legs are examined, including ROM and anterior drawer, Lachman, and pivot-shift tests. Special attention is given to varus, valgus, and posterolateral instability because those structures are not assessed arthroscopically. A post is placed proximally and laterally against the thigh to allow for valgus stress on the knee and visualization of the medial compartment.

Graft Harvest

If examination of the anesthetized patient confirms the diagnosis of an ACL tear, we proceed directly to harvesting of the graft. We most commonly use a BPTB autograft. The incision is marked 1 cm medial to the inferior pole of the patella, extending longitudinally 1 cm medial to the tibial tubercle (Fig. 98-3). The skin is incised and sharp dissection is carried down through the skin and subcutaneous tissue to the level of the patellar tendon paratedon. The parateon is incised at the midline and separated from the underlying tendon with use of a scalpel. The knee is slightly flexed and a scalpel is used to harvest the central portion (usually 9 to 10 mm) of the patellar tendon. An oscillating saw is used to make the bone cut on the tibial side. Our goal is to make the tibial bone plug 20 to 25 mm in length and trapezoidal in shape, which is achieved by making a cut perpendicular to the surface of the bone medially and a lateral cut that is angled 20 degrees toward the medial cut. The distal cut is made last, and the bone plug is extracted by hand with use of a 0.5-inch curved osteotome (Fig. 98-4).

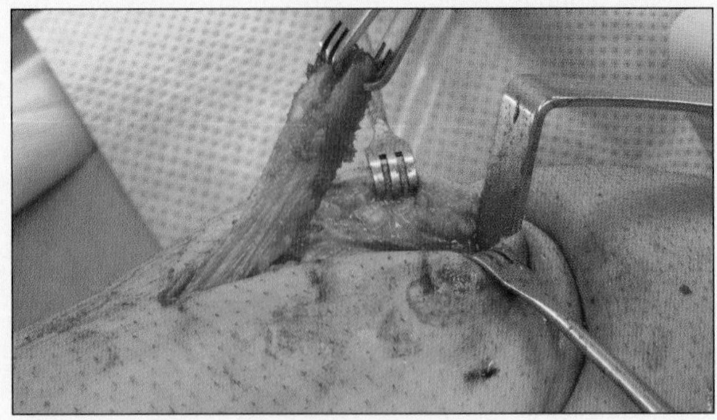

FIGURE 98-4 Harvesting of the patellar tendon.

The knee is then placed into extension with the inferior two thirds of the patella exposed. The patellar bone cut should be 20 to 25 mm in length and triangular in shape, which is achieved by making medial and lateral bone cuts angled 45 degrees from the bone surface with an oscillating saw. The cuts should be made to a depth of 10 to 12 mm and should meet, allowing for easy extraction.

Graft Preparation

The bone plugs are shaped to fit into a 10-mm tunnel, and any excess bone is reduced to morsels for bone grafting of the patellar defect (Fig. 98-5). Because loss of fixation is more likely in the tibial tunnel, the patellar bone plug (which has a denser architecture) is placed into the tibial tunnel to maximize purchase with the interference screw. Two perpendicular 2-mm drill holes are made at the distal one third of the patellar bone plug, and two drill holes are placed in the tibial bone plug. Heavy nonabsorbable suture is loaded onto a Keith needle and passed through each hole. The bone-tendon junction is marked with a sterile marker to allow for visualization during graft passage. The tendinous portion of the graft is measured with a sterile ruler.

Portal Placement and Diagnostic Arthroscopy

The AM, anterolateral, and superolateral arthroscopic portals are established. The suprapatellar pouch, patellofemoral joint,

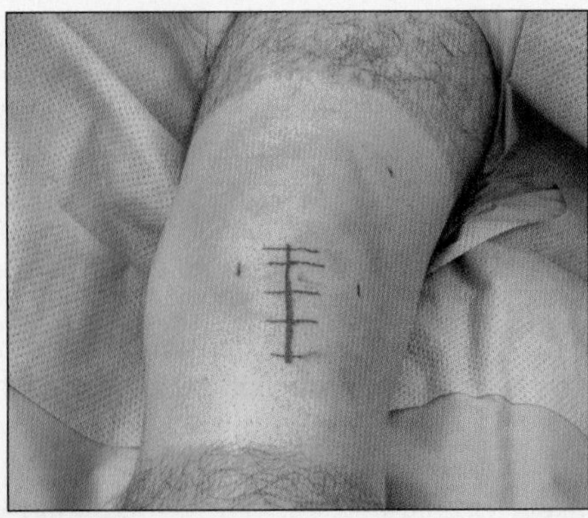

FIGURE 98-3 Superolateral, anteromedial, and anterolateral portal sites and the patellar tendon graft incision.

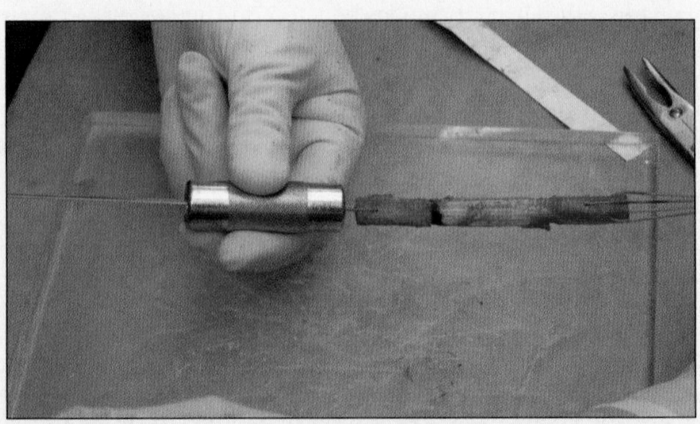

FIGURE 98-5 Sizing of the patellar tendon autograft.

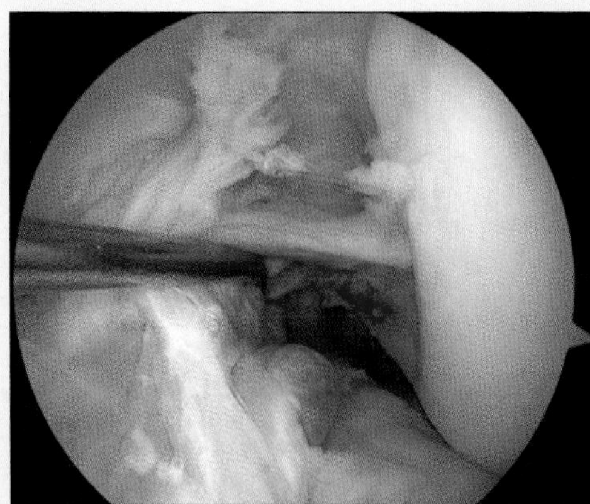

FIGURE 98-6 The arthroscopic view of a torn anterior cruciate ligament.

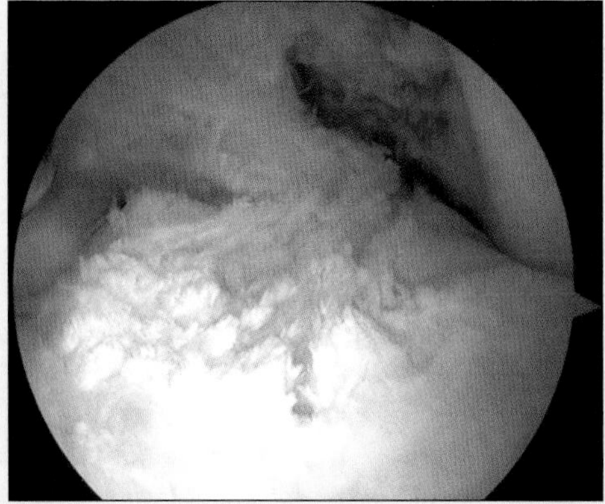

FIGURE 98-8 The tibial footprint of the anterior cruciate ligament (ACL). The insertion of the ACL remains as a guide for positioning of the tibial tunnel.

medial and lateral gutters, medial and lateral compartments, and femoral notch (Fig. 98-6) are evaluated for concomitant intraarticular pathology. Meniscal injuries in the poorly vascularized white zone are debrided. Meniscal tears in the red-red or red-white zones are repaired whenever possible using an inside-out or all-inside technique.

Tunnel Placement

The precise positions for both femoral and tibial tunnel placement remain a matter of debate. The definition of an "anatomic reconstruction" has not been consistently described, and accordingly, we avoid this nomenclature. However, the available literature suggests that (1) the graft should be placed in an oblique position to resist rotational laxity and (2) the femoral and tibial tunnels should be placed within the native footprint of the ACL to achieve this goal. We typically use a motorized shaver to debride the torn ACL down to the footprint on both the femur and tibia. A small portion of the footprint is left intact to permit identification of the native ACL origin and insertion. Enough tissue should be debrided from the lateral and superior aspects of the notch to allow for visualization of the over-the-top position (Fig. 98-7). A motorized burr is used to perform a notchplasty as needed to prevent impingement of the graft and to visualize the periosteum on the posterior aspect of the lateral condyle.

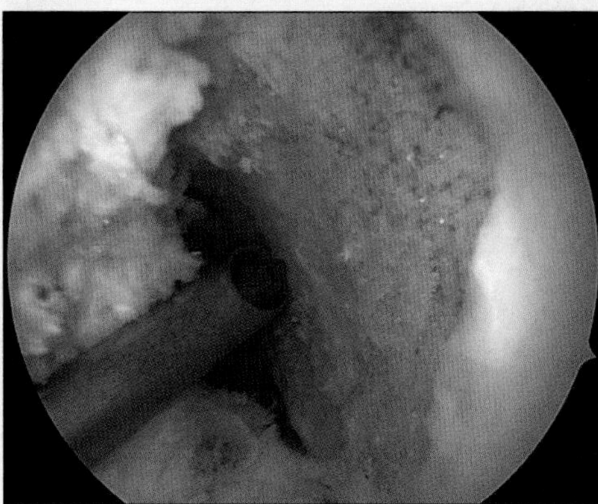

FIGURE 98-7 An anteromedial guide wire placed in the center of the femoral anterior cruciate ligament footprint.

The center of the femoral footprint is then marked with an awl or curette. This position is typically 6 to 7 mm anterior to the back wall. The position of this mark can be confirmed by switching the 30-degree scope to the AM portal. The angle on the tibial drill guide is set to N+7, in which N is the length (mm) of the tendinous portion of the graft.[114] The guide arm is oriented so the path of the guide pin points from the ACL footprint on the tibia to the footprint on the lateral condyle of the femur. The drill should penetrate the center of the tibial footprint, which is typically located in line with the posterior aspect of the anterior horn of the lateral meniscus (Fig. 98-8). The length of the tunnel is measured from the tibial drill guide and should be at least 2 mm longer than the soft tissue portion of the tendon graft based on the N+2 rule if using a BPTB graft.[115] If the proposed tunnel length is too short, it can be lengthened by increasing the angle on the guide. After the proper tibial tunnel length is confirmed, the guide wire is advanced and the tibial tunnel is created with use of a cannulated drill. A large curette is used to control the guide pin and protect the articular cartilage during drilling. The reamings are collected and used later for bone grafting of the patellar defect. A rasp is used to smooth out the surface of the tibial tunnel, and a shaver is used to remove soft tissue around the tibial tunnel entrance.

A Beath pin is placed through the tibial tunnel and directed toward the previously marked spot at the center of the femoral footprint. The pin is advanced through the femur and out the anterolateral thigh. This maneuver is referred to as the *transtibial technique* because the femoral tunnel is established through the tibial tunnel. A cannulated reamer is advanced to a depth of 10 mm and the posterior wall is visualized to confirm adequate positioning and bone tunnel integrity (Fig. 98-9). If the tunnel position is adequate, the tunnel is drilled to a depth of 30 mm.

In some cases, it is not possible to reach the appropriate position in the femoral notch via a transtibial approach. In these cases, the femoral tunnel can be drilled through the AM portal with a straight reamer or flexible reamer system. Commercially available flexible reamers permit reaming through

Continued

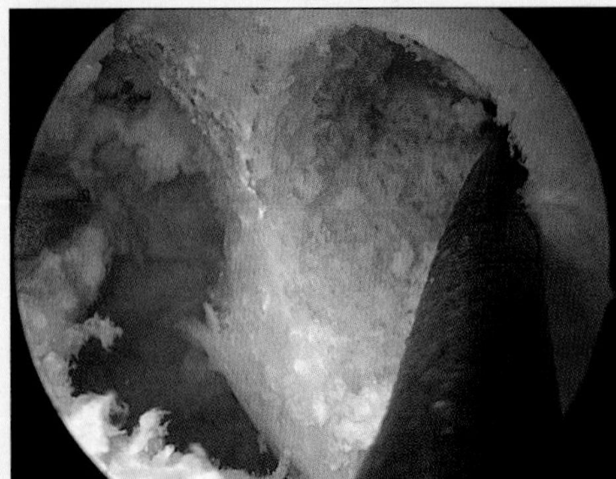

FIGURE 98-9 The intact back wall after flexible anteromedial reaming.

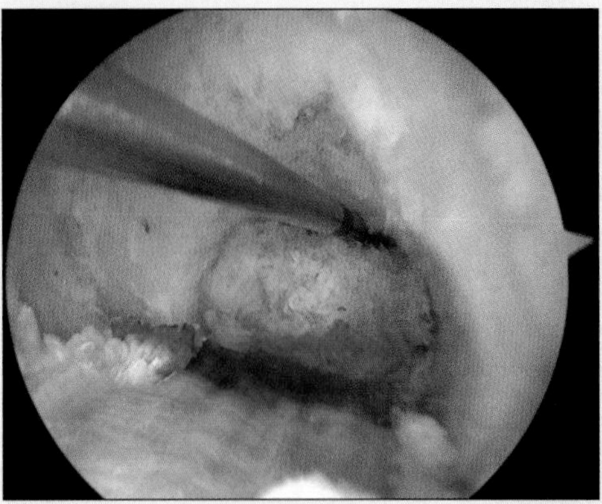

FIGURE 98-10 Tibial bone block docking in the femoral tunnel. A guide wire is placed for later interference screw fixation.

the AM portal with knee flexion of 100 to 110 degrees. When using a flexible reamer system, a flexible guide wire is introduced through the AM portal with a cannulated guide to position the guide wire in a superior and lateral position prior to advancing the wire into the femoral footprint and out the anterolateral thigh. A flexible 10-mm reamer is placed over the guide wire under direct visualization to avoid damaging the medial femoral condyle. Another approach to achieving the appropriate position of the femoral tunnel is to use a straight reamer introduced through an AM portal. In these cases, it is important to hyperflex the knee during femoral tunnel reaming to avoid creating a short tunnel or violating the back wall of the femoral tunnel. Finally, an outside-in or two-incision technique can be used to ream the femoral tunnel. In these instances, a femoral aiming guide is placed through a second incision over the anterolateral femur and reamed from outside-in.

Graft Placement and Fixation

If the femoral tunnel was made transtibially, the eyelet of the pin is loaded with the suture from the graft and the graft is gently pulled into the femoral and tibial tunnels. If the femoral tunnel was created via AM portal reaming, a suture is placed through the eyelet of the guide pin and the pin is passed through the femoral tunnel. A probe is used to retrieve the suture loop through the tibial tunnel. Suture on the tibial tubercle bone plug (intended for the femoral tunnel) is placed through the loop of suture and the graft is passed through the tunnels. When an AM reaming portal is used, the femoral bone plug is often shortened to 20 mm to facilitate passage of the graft through the acute angle between the tibial and femoral tunnels. The bone plug is then oriented in the femoral tunnel with the cancellous side facing anteriorly. The bone plug is left slightly proud on the articular surface to allow for placement of the interference screw guide wire. A guide wire is introduced through the AM portal and placed anteriorly between the graft and tunnel (Fig. 98-10). The graft is advanced so it is flush with the surrounding bone and a 7 × 20 mm or 25 mm cannulated metal interference screw is inserted over the guide wire (Fig. 98-11). The interference screw should be flush with the bone block, and care should be taken to avoid damaging the tendon with the threads of the screw. The knee should be ranged under visualization to evaluate for impingement of the graft on the femoral notch.

The knee is cycled 20 times with approximately 10 lb of tension with use of the sutures in the distal bone plug to create tension. The graft should tighten (shorten) over the terminal 30 degrees of each cycle. Tibial fixation is performed with the knee in 0 to 30 degrees of flexion. Grafts fixed closer to extension will avoid excessive tension on the graft in extension. A guide wire is placed between the bone plug and tunnel wall. Manual tension should be maintained while a 9 × 20 mm or 25 mm tibial interference screw is placed over the guide wire. We do not apply a posterior drawer force on the proximal tibia during fixation. The Lachman test is performed to ensure adequate fixation and elimination of anterior laxity.

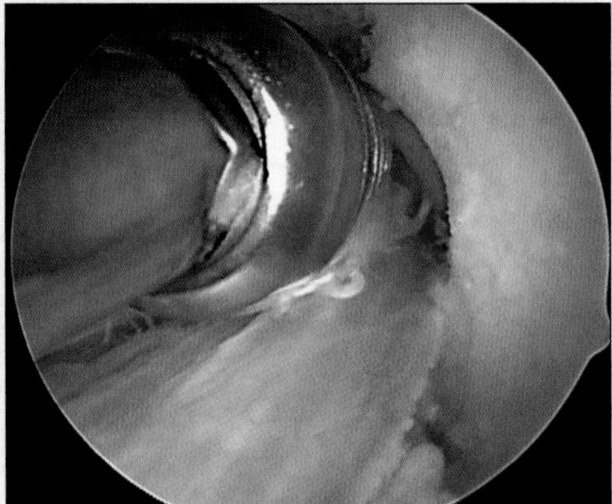

FIGURE 98-11 Femoral interference screw placement.

AUTHORS' PREFERRED TECHNIQUE

Revision ACL Reconstruction

Preoperative Planning

Formulating a detailed preoperative plan is the key to a successful revision ACL reconstruction. It is important to differentiate between symptoms of pain and stiffness versus true instability, including which activities cause a feeling of instability. History, physical examination, and radiographic findings should help to determine whether the failure is due to traumatic repeat rupture, technical error, or biologic failure. It is also important to identify concomitant injuries such as meniscal deficiency, chondral damage, malalignment, or other ligamentous injury so they can be incorporated into a comprehensive surgical plan. Previous operative reports and the patient's postoperative course, age, and activity level prior to the index procedure can be helpful in decision making. Arthroscopic photographs and implant records from the index surgery can help in determining the cause of failure and assist in planning for hardware removal if necessary. It is also helpful to know if the reconstruction was double or single bundle and if the femoral tunnel was drilled transtibially or through the AM portal.

Varus knee alignment and other knee pathology, such as MCL laxity, medial meniscal injury or deficiency, or PL laxity, can contribute to failure of ACL reconstruction.[116,117] We routinely obtain bilateral standing radiographs and a true lateral radiograph to evaluate tunnel positioning. Plain radiographs can provide information regarding assessment of tunnel placement, retained hardware, potential areas of graft impingement, patellofemoral pathology, and tunnel osteolysis (Fig. 98-12). If tunnel widening is present, a CT scan may be obtained to determine if bone grafting is necessary prior to reconstruction. MRI is obtained if concomitant injuries to other ligaments, the meniscus, or articular cartilage are a concern. We usually perform a one-stage revision operation. However, if a large bony defect is present, we initially perform a bone graft at the site of the defect and return 3 to 6 months later for revision ACL reconstruction.

Prior to surgery, the patient should be made aware that revision ACL reconstruction is a salvage procedure and has worse outcomes than primary ACL reconstruction.[31,32] In addition, it is important to discuss graft options and anticipated activity level after surgery. We recommend use of a contralateral BPTB autograft or an HS autograft in young, active patients. We recommend use of an allograft in patients who place a lower demand on their knees, in patients who have had multiple ligament reconstructions, and when availability of autograft tissue is limited.

Positioning and Setup

Our positioning of the patient for revision surgery is the same as for primary reconstruction. An examination after inducement of anesthesia is performed on both the operative and uninvolved leg.

Portal Placement

When performing revision surgery, we proceed directly to diagnostic arthroscopy. If the femoral tunnel was drilled through the tibial tunnel in the index procedure, we prefer to perform the revision through an AM portal. If the index procedure established the femoral tunnel through the AM portal, we attempt to perform the revision through a transtibial

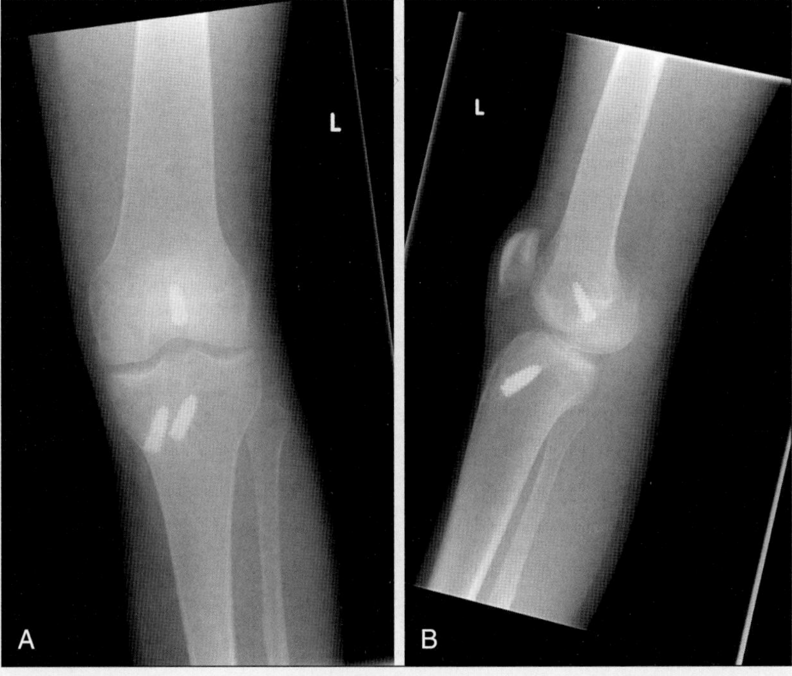

FIGURE 98-12 Radiographs of a failed anterior cruciate ligament reconstruction. **A,** Preoperative anteroposterior radiograph. **B,** Preoperative lateral radiograph. Note the anterior and vertical position of the femoral interference screw, indicating malpositioning of the femoral tunnel position.

Continued

tunnel. It should be noted that each revision ACL reconstruction is unique and that anatomic variations may require other approaches from time to time.

Tunnel Placement

After diagnostic arthroscopy, we identify the previously used femoral and tibial tunnels. If the fixation devices from the index surgery are not interfering with the new tunnels, we leave them in place. The goal is to create divergent revision tunnels that will have a bridge of bone separating the majority of old and new tunnels whenever possible (Fig. 98-13). In the case of a traumatic repeat rupture with adequate placement of the previously placed tunnels, we attempt to use the old tunnels. If retained hardware needs to be removed, it is extracted with use of instruments specific to the implant used in the index surgery. If implant-specific trays are not available, we have a commercially available ACL revision tray available at the time of surgery.

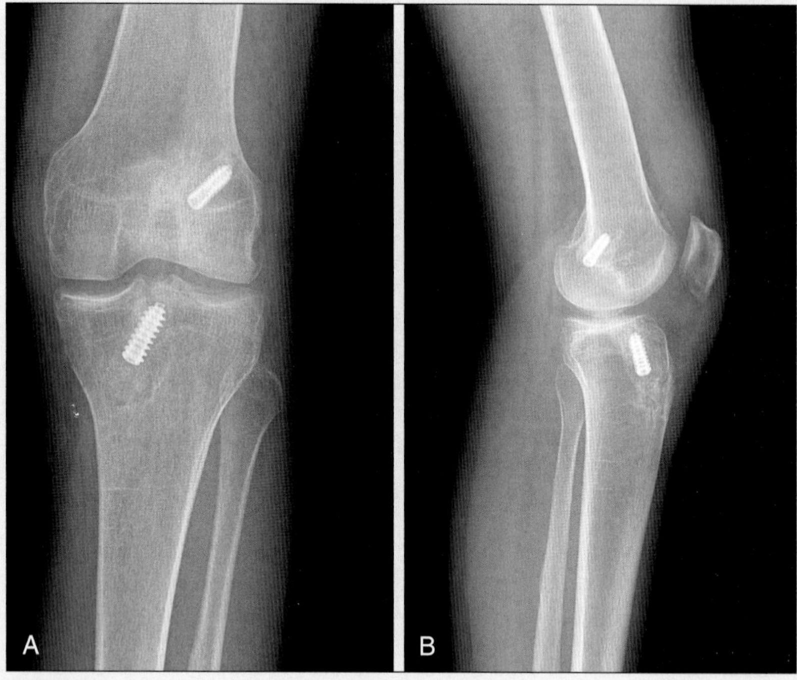

FIGURE 98-13 Radiographs after a revision anterior cruciate ligament procedure. **A,** Postoperative anteroposterior radiograph. **B,** Postoperative lateral radiograph.

ROM, ligamentous stability, activity, and function compared with patients without postoperative bracing.[122]

The goal during rehabilitation in the early postoperative period is to preserve full extension and work on gaining 10 degrees of flexion every day. A continuous passive motion machine can be used to supplement early active and passive ROM, although we do not routinely use this machine.

Muscle Training (Open and Closed Kinetic Chain)

Quadriceps strength correlates with functional stability of the knee postoperatively and has been the focus of many postoperative training programs.[123] However, biomechanical studies of quadriceps and HS contraction showed that HS contraction decreases strain on the ACL through a posterior force on the proximal tibia during knee flexion.[124] Analysis of forces during knee flexion showed that force of contraction between the quadriceps and HS is balanced at a flexion angle of 22 degrees. At flexion angles greater than 22 degrees, the quadriceps, HS, and gastrocnemius muscle groups work together to unload the ACL.[124]

Debate in postoperative rehabilitation protocols has focused on open versus closed kinetic chain exercises. In the early postoperative period, closed-chain exercises are thought to be safer than open-chain exercises. Closed kinetic chain exercises are performed with the foot fixed in place in constant contact with the ground. Examples of closed kinetic chain exercises are squats and the leg press, which require activation of multiple muscle groups for stabilization and also distribute ground reaction force to all lower limb joints (Fig. 98-14, *A*). During open kinetic chain exercises, such as leg extension, the limb is free to move and the joint reactive force is focused on the knee (Fig. 98-14, *B*). In a study by Kvist and Gillquist,[125] it was found that tibial translation is less in closed-chain exercises (between 10 and 40 degrees of knee flexion) but is greater at knee flexion greater than 70 degrees. These investigators also found that squats with the center of gravity behind the feet result in the least amount of tibial translation. A prospective randomized trial of patients participating in open versus closed kinetic chain exercises after ACL reconstruction showed superior results with closed-chain exercises. Subjects in the closed-chain group had greater knee stability, less patellofemoral pain, and greater overall satisfaction and return to activity. Ninety-five percent of patients in both groups regained full ROM.[126] Closed-chain exercises result in greater muscle activation than open-chain exercises.[125]

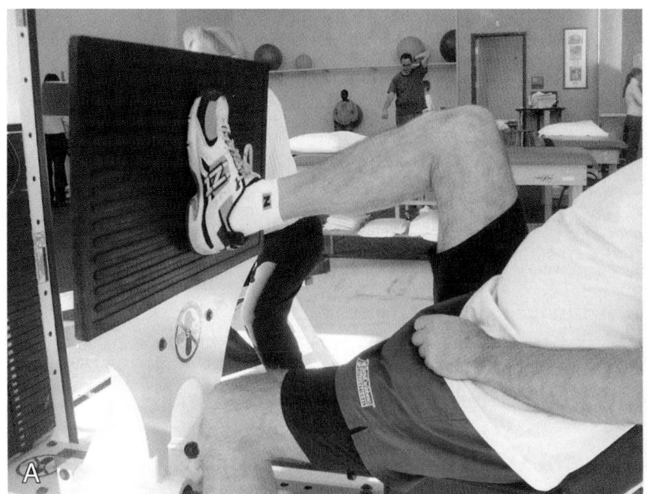

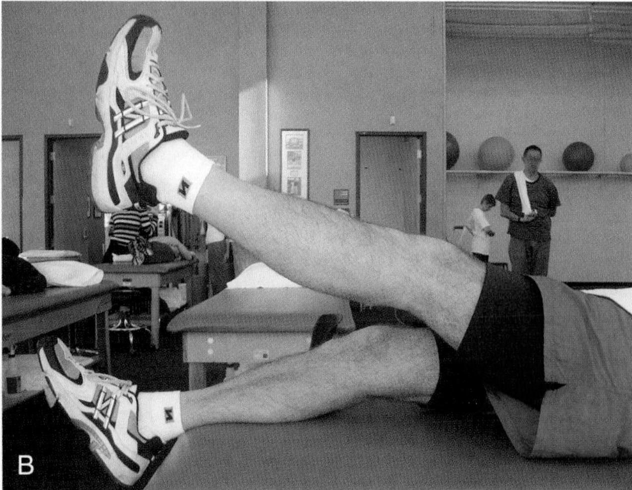

FIGURE 98-14 Closed-chain (**A**) and open-chain (**B**) kinetic exercises after anterior cruciate ligament reconstruction.

Other reviews of current literature suggest that a combination of open and closed kinetic chain exercises should be considered, especially in patients who require strengthening of the quadriceps muscle. Proponents of integrating open-chain exercises argue that the exercises can be modified to minimize strain on the ACL and decrease stress on the patellofemoral joint.[127] Functional outcomes are similar in patients participating in open versus closed kinetic chain exercises in the first 2 to 6 weeks after surgery.[128] However, patients who participate in open kinetic chain exercises plus closed kinetic chain exercises starting 6 weeks after surgery increase their quadriceps torque and return to sports 2 months earlier compared with patients who performed closed-chain exercises alone.[129] Thus the body of literature seems to suggest that it is important to begin rehabilitation using closed-chain exercises and progress to a combination of open- and closed-chain exercises at some point.

Electrical Stimulation, Biofeedback, and Proprioception

The use of electrical stimulation in the rehabilitation protocol is controversial because it has not produced consistent results. However, all studies have shown that it is safe, and when combined with volitional exercises, it can result in a more normal gait pattern and stronger quadriceps muscle activity.[130] A recent review of eight randomized controlled trials found that neuromuscular electrical stimulation may be more effective than exercise alone in restoring quadriceps strength after ACL reconstruction. The effect on functional performance was inconclusive, and overall analysis was complicated by inconsistencies in electrical stimulation protocols.[131]

Muscle strength depends on neural signaling, motor unit activation, and muscle contraction. Although electrical stimulation addresses muscle contraction, it does not require initiation of the movement or a sustained effort by the patient to maintain muscle contraction. Electromyographic biofeedback has been used to help patients monitor the quality of muscle contraction during a voluntary contraction. This modality is more effective than electrical stimulation in restoring peak torque in the quadriceps extensor mechanism after ACL reconstruction.[132]

The importance of proprioception has been described by several studies that have examined the neural anatomy of the ACL and how disruption of the sensory system can lead to decreased functional stability. Johansson and colleagues[133] showed that the ACL has a sensory system and mechanoreceptors that detect stretching at moderate loads, which signals to modify muscular stiffness around the knee. Knee proprioception is impaired for 6 to 12 months after ACL reconstruction, and improved proprioception correlates well with improved functional outcome and patient satisfaction after surgery.[134,135] These findings suggest that restoring mechanical stability alone is insufficient for optimizing functional outcome. Because proprioception does not return for up to 1 year after reconstruction, patients should incorporate proprioception training exercises throughout the rehabilitation process.

Functional Training

Rehabilitation programs have advanced in the past 10 years to incorporate proprioception and neuromuscular control. A greater focus is now placed on joint repositioning, closed kinetic chain exercises, single-leg stance, cone stepping, and lateral lunge drills, which provide a neurologic stimulus that allows the patient to regain dynamic stability.[136] In addition to restoring basic proprioception, it is important to emphasize neuromuscular control when the dynamic stabilizers are fatigued, especially in athletes, who require endurance and muscle stabilization at the end of exercise. Low-resistance exercises such as stair climbing, cycling, use of an elliptical machine, and slide boards are safe repetitive activities that can be used at the end of a training session to encourage dynamic stabilization.[136] A systematic review of neuromuscular training activities in female athletes has provided positive results, showing that plyometric power, biomechanics, technique, strength, balance, and core stability training can reduce the rate of ACL injury through improved neuromuscular control.[137]

Techniques to Limit Pain and Swelling

Cryotherapy has been used to lower the temperature of the knee joint and surrounding tissue, which can provide pain relief and shorten the recovery period after ACL reconstruction. Improved pain relief allows for more aggressive early rehabilitation, which is thought to result in better long-term results.[138] However, a metaanalysis of all studies on cryotherapy showed that it is effective for pain control but does not influence long-term outcome.[139] Standard measures such as compression and elevation also work to limit swelling and provide analgesia. For more severe pain, narcotic medications are prescribed.

Rehabilitation Protocol

Our patients who undergo primary and revision ACL reconstruction are allowed to bear weight on the surgical extremity with crutches after surgery with a hinged knee brace locked in extension. Physical therapy begins immediately, with initial emphasis on ROM and progressing to patellar mobilization and strengthening. Use of the brace is discontinued 1 to 2 weeks after surgery. Stationary cycling begins when the patient is out of the brace. Associated meniscal injuries that were repaired at the time of ACL reconstruction do not change the rehabilitation program. Studies have shown that no difference exists in the failure rate of meniscal repair in patients who underwent ACL reconstruction and immediate postoperative rehabilitation compared with the published rate for meniscal repair alone.[140,141]

Return to Play

No standard or objective criteria are currently available to determine when a patient is ready to return to competitive sport or unrestricted activity after ACL reconstruction. Functional testing provides an inaccurate marker for risk of injury because tests are performed under nonfatigued conditions.[142] Patients evaluated at a mean of 11 months after ACL reconstruction exhibit normal single-leg hop symmetry when they are nonfatigued, but 68% exhibit abnormal hop testing when they are fatigued.[142] Dynamic testing under weight-bearing conditions is also more accurate for testing of knee stability. Thus it may be important to incorporate weight bearing and fatigue testing into the postoperative rehabilitation program before clearing patients for return to full activity.[142,143]

Participating in a functional sports agility program when knee ROM reaches 0 to 120 degrees and quadriceps muscle strength is 60% that of the contralateral leg does not affect graft stability and is thought to be safe. Patients can participate in a rehabilitation program as early as 4 weeks and at a mean of 5.1 weeks[120] and return to sport 5 to 9 months after surgery. Patients are required to demonstrate ligamentous stability and no knee effusion on clinical examination before proceeding with full activity.[144] In general, if ROM and strength have returned, we allow patients to begin running in a straight line at 3 months after surgery and return to full sport at 8 to 9 months after surgery.

Results (Level I and Level II Evidence)

Good overall results have been achieved with ACL reconstruction using BPTB and HS grafts. Patient satisfaction rates are greater than 90%, and 95% of patients report normal to near-normal knee function at long-term follow-up.[145] Return to sport at the same level or higher is reported to be between 70% to 90%.[146,147]

Graft Type

Current level I evidence from randomized controlled trials shows no overall difference in outcome between BPTB and quadrupled HS grafts in postoperative laxity, clinical outcome, return to sport, one-leg–hop test, ROM, anterior knee sensory deficit, patellofemoral crepitus, osteoarthritis, or thigh muscle circumference.[98] A systematic review of patients after ACL reconstruction found greater anterior knee pain and kneeling pain in the BPTB group but equivalent patient-recorded outcomes and clinical assessments in both groups.[98,100]

Single Versus Double Bundle

It is currently unclear if the native ACL bundles function independently of one another. Double-bundle reconstruction has been advocated by some authors because it more closely mimics the normal anatomy of the ACL. However, clinical studies of conventional anatomic single-bundle and anatomic double-bundle ACL reconstruction have shown mixed results. Some studies have shown increased rotatory laxity on pivot-shift examination after single-bundle reconstruction but no difference in clinical outcome, return to sports, or functionality between the single-bundle and double-bundle groups.[98] Other studies have shown no difference in anterior laxity or rotatory stability in patients treated with double-bundle versus single-bundle reconstruction.[148,149] Most studies have failed to show a difference in clinical outcome as measured by Lysholm scores, IKDC scores, or other outcome measures.[98,149-151] Therefore further randomized studies are required to show superiority of the double-bundle repair.

Complications

The most severe complications of ACL reconstruction are infection and graft failure. Fortunately, infection occurs in less than 0.9% of patients.[152] The graft failure rate is around 5% and is generally due to improper tunnel placement, traumatic repeat rupture, or failure to diagnose concurrent injury to other structures in the knee.[152] Loss of ROM is the most common complication[121] and can be minimized by regaining full ROM prior to surgery and being diligent with postoperative rehabilitation under supervision. Patellar fracture and patellar tendon rupture can occur with BPTB autograft reconstruction but are rare occurrences. Between 20% and 42% of patients report anterior knee pain with BPTB reconstruction; however, the pain improves with time and usually does not prevent high-level athletic activity.[98] Injury to the saphenous nerve is a concern with harvesting of the HS and can result in decreased sensation but is rarely a concern in the long term.[153] Osteoarthritis develops in many patients who rupture their ACL, but evidence is lacking to show that ACL reconstruction protects patients from the development of osteoarthritis.

Tunnel widening is a known radiographic complication of ACL reconstruction. Two separate studies of patients who underwent ACL reconstruction with HS versus BPTB showed a significant increase in tibial and femoral tunnel diameters in the HS group, although the two groups had similar clinical outcomes.[154]

Future Considerations

Soft tissue grafts have a slower rate of healing and incorporate into the bone tunnel at a later time point than do bone grafts (BPTB). Many techniques for accelerating the healing process have been explored, including the use of growth factors, mesenchymal stem cells (MSCs), and periosteum augmentation. Platelet-derived growth factor and transforming growth factor β-1 have shown some promise in increasing the density of collagen fibrils.[155,156] Bone morphogenic protein-2 has been used to accelerate bone growth around the graft.[157] Periosteum has been used to enhance soft tissue and bone-graft incorporation into the surrounding bone tunnel. A prospective clinical trial using HS autograft enveloped with autologous periosteum found decreased femoral tunnel widening after reconstruction.[158] Animal studies using MSCs demonstrated healing that more closely resembled ligamentous insertion. Moreover, knees treated with MSC had higher failure loads and greater stiffness compared with control subjects.[159]

Attempts have also been made to create ligaments in vitro through tissue engineering. However, further efforts are required to make this process a reality. A recent study by Vavken and colleagues demonstrated comparable biomechanical results with bioenhanced ACL repair using a collagen-platelet composite compared with ACL reconstruction in a large animal model.[160] However, this technique is still under investigation and has not been introduced into clinical practice.

For a complete list of references, go to expertconsult.com.

Suggested Readings

Citation: Beynnon BD, Johnson RJ, Abate JA, et al: Treatment of anterior cruciate ligament injuries, part 1. *Am J Sports Med* 33(10):1579–1602, 2005.

Level of Evidence: III (retrospective cohort)

Summary: The authors of this article provide a review of the current knowledge regarding anterior cruciate ligament (ACL) injuries, focusing on biomechanics of the ACL, prevalence of injury and risk factors, natural history of ACL-deficient knees, associated injuries, indications for treatment, and management.

Citation: Beynnon BD, Johnson RJ, Abate JA, et al: Treatment of anterior cruciate ligament injuries, part 2. *Am J Sports Med* 33(11):1751–1767, 2005.

Level of Evidence: III (retrospective cohort)

Summary: The authors of this article provide a review of the technical aspects of anterior cruciate ligament reconstruction, bone tunnel widening, graft healing, rehabilitation, and the effect of age, sex, and activity level on outcome.

Citation: Barrett AM, Craft JA, Replogle WH, et al: Anterior cruciate ligament graft failure: A comparison of graft type based on age and Tegner activity level. *Am J Sports Med* 39:2194–2198, 2011.

Level of Evidence: III (cohort study)

Summary: Bone–patellar tendon–bone autografts had a lower failure rate (11.8%) than did allografts (29.2%) or hamstring tendon autografts (25%) in patients 25 years and younger. Overall failure rate after anterior cruciate ligament reconstruction was higher in patients 25 years and younger (16.5% vs. 8.3%).

Citation: Markolf KL, Park S, Jackson SR, et al: Simulated pivot-shift testing with single and double-bundle anterior cruciate ligament reconstructions. *J Bone Joint Surg Am* 90A(8):1681–1689, 2008.

Level of Evidence: III (observational study)

Summary: Biomechanical testing after single-bundle and anatomic double-bundle anterior cruciate ligament reconstruction revealed that single-bundle reconstruction was sufficient in restoring intact knee kinematics as tested by a simulated pivot-shift event. Double-bundle reconstructions resulted in less tibial rotation and displacement, as well as higher graft forces than an intact knee. The clinical consequence of this difference is unknown.

Citation: McAllister DR, Joyce M, Mann B, et al: Allograft update: The current status of tissue regulation, procurement, processing, and sterilization. *Am J Sports Med* 35(12):2148–2158, 2007.

Level of Evidence: V (descriptive study, expert opinion)

Summary: Allografts are commonly used in knee surgeries, and most surgeons believe that sterilized allografts are safe. The Food and Drug Administration has created mandates for the processing of allogenic tissue, but the process of sterilization remains relatively unknown. This article describes the process of procuring and processing allograft tissue in the United States.

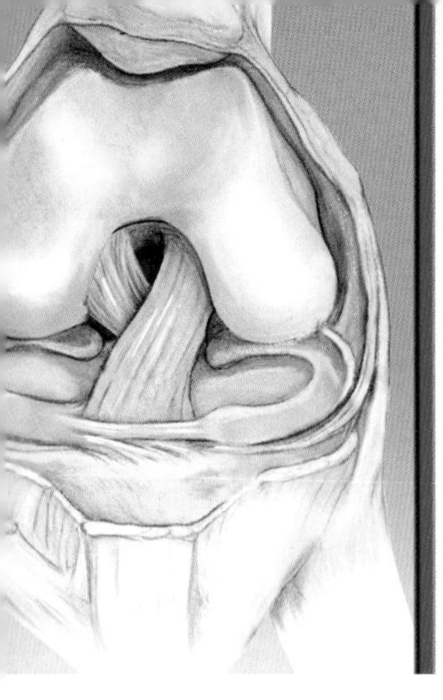

99

Posterior Cruciate Ligament Injuries

FRANK A. PETRIGLIANO • SCOTT R. MONTGOMERY • JARED S. JOHNSON • DAVID R. McALLISTER

The treatment of posterior cruciate ligament (PCL) injuries is a controversial topic in orthopaedic surgery. In contrast to anterior cruciate ligament (ACL) injuries, for which an abundance of basic science and clinical data is available, the PCL has only recently become a topic of intense investigation. PCL injuries are less common compared with ACL injuries, and thus studies on outcomes are underpowered, making it difficult to draw definitive conclusions regarding management. However, recent biomechanical and clinical data have highlighted the importance of the PCL in knee stability and function. Injury to the PCL, which acts as the primary restraint to posterior tibial translation, may lead to instability, pain, diminished function, and eventually arthrosis.

The purpose of this chapter is to discuss the evaluation, diagnosis, and management of PCL injuries and to present the relevant historic and recent literature on these topics. After a brief review of the pertinent components of the history, physical examination, and imaging modalities, we discuss important considerations in decision making and treatment options in patients with PCL injuries, as well as our preferred surgical technique and outcomes of surgical management of PCL injuries. Decision making in this patient population is largely dependent on the grade of PCL injury and the presence or absence of concomitant ligamentous injuries in the knee. We also focus on the latest evidence regarding transtibial versus the tibial inlay technique, single- versus double-bundle methods of reconstruction, and the outcomes of these various surgical treatment options.

History

The true incidence and prevalence of PCL injuries is unknown and difficult to estimate because many of these injuries, particularly prior to the introduction of magnetic resonance imaging (MRI), are not diagnosed.[1] The reported incidence of PCL injuries has differed depending on the population studied. The incidence is as low as 3% in the outpatient setting[2] and as high as 37% in the traumatic setting.[3] Traumatic injuries and sports-related injuries account for the majority of PCL injuries. A prospective analysis of patients presenting with acute hemarthrosis of the knee and diagnosed with a PCL injury demonstrated that 56.5% of patients were trauma victims, whereas 32.9% had a sports-related injury.[3] Yet isolated PCL injuries were infrequent in this cohort, with 96.5% being part of a multiligamentous injury. Similarly, in a retrospective cohort of 494 patients with PCL insufficiency, Schulz et al.[4] found traffic accidents (45%) and athletic injuries (40%) to be the most common causes of injury. Among specific sports, the incidence of PCL injury tends to be greater in those involving contact, such as football, soccer, and rugby. In the cohort reviewed by Schulz and colleagues,[4] skiing and soccer were the sports with the highest incidence of PCL injuries. Overall, the incidence of PCL injury has been estimated to be relatively low in athletes across a variety of sports.[5-8]

Important information can be obtained from the history of the patient presenting with acute knee pain or trauma. Any patient with knee pain and swelling with a high-energy mechanism of injury should be suspected of having a PCL injury, another capsuloligamentous injury, or both. Patients commonly report the inability to bear weight, instability, and decreased knee range of motion. In contrast to ACL injuries, which often result from a noncontact event, PCL injuries are typically due to external trauma. The classic "dashboard injury" pattern results from a posteriorly directed force on the anterior aspect of the proximal tibia with the knee in a flexed position. In patients with a higher energy mechanism of injury, it is possible that a knee dislocation occurred at the time of the injury even if the knee is reduced at the time of the evaluation.

In athletics, the typical mechanism of isolated PCL injury is a direct blow to the anterior tibia (Fig. 99-1, *A*) or a fall onto the knee with the foot plantar flexed. When the foot is in a position of dorsiflexion, the force is transmitted to the patella and distal femur, decreasing the risk of injury to the PCL (Fig. 99-2). Noncontact mechanisms of injury, although less common, have also been reported. Most commonly, this mechanism of injury occurs via forced hyperflexion of the knee (Fig. 99-1, *B*).[9] In a small cohort reported by Fowler and Messieh,[9] these injuries would often lead to incomplete tearing of the PCL with the posteromedial (PM) fibers intact. Knee hyperextension has also been described as a mechanism of injury, which is usually combined with a varus or valgus force that results in multiple ligament injury (Fig. 99-1, *C*). Isolated injuries may have more subtle presentations, with patients reporting stiffness, swelling, and pain located in the back of the knee or pain with deep knee flexion (squatting and kneeling). In contrast to acute ACL tears, a "pop" is usually not reported with isolated PCL injuries and athletes are often able to continue to play. Reports of anterior knee

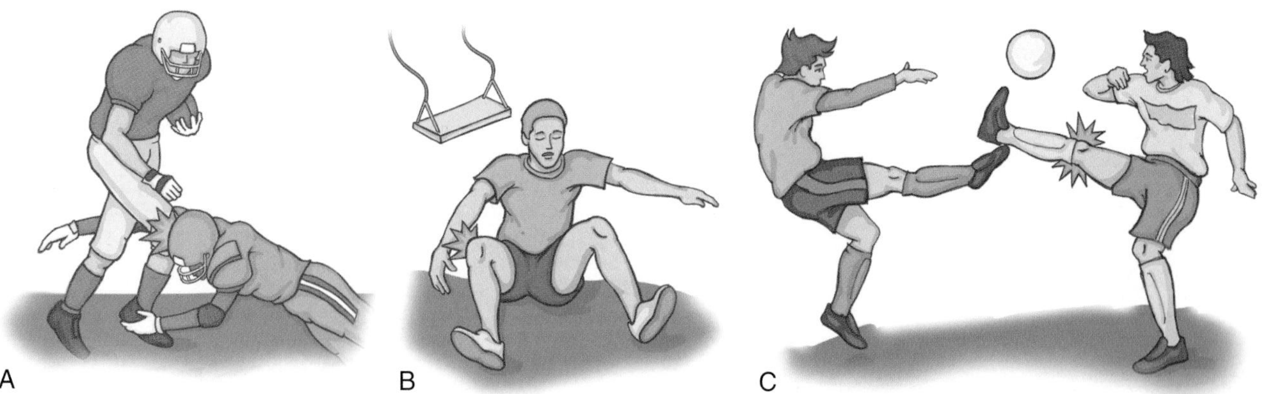

FIGURE 99-1 Posterior cruciate ligament injuries are most frequently the result of a blow to the front of the flexed knee.

pain, difficulty ascending stairs, and instability are common when patients present in the chronic phase of an isolated PCL injury.[10]

Physical Examination

Posterior Drawer Test

The posterior drawer test was described initially by Hughston et al.[11] in 1976 and later by Clancy et al.[12] in 1983 and is considered the most accurate clinical test to assess the integrity of the PCL, with a sensitivity of 90% and 99% specificity.[13,14] The results of this examination also guide treatment recommendations. A posteriorly directed force is placed on the proximal tibia with the patient lying supine and the knee flexed to 90 degrees. This test can be performed with the tibia in neutral, external, and internal rotation. It is important to remember that with a PCL injury, the tibia subluxes posteriorly. Thus it is important to first apply an anteriorly directed force to reduce the posterior subluxation before applying the posteriorly directed force (Fig. 99-3). In cases of isolated PCL tears, a decrease occurs in posterior tibial translation with internal tibial rotation.[15] The superficial medial collateral ligament (MCL) and posterior oblique ligament act as a secondary restraint with the tibia in internal rotation.[16] Translation is measured as the change in distance of step-off between the medial tibial plateau relative to the medial femoral condyle. It is critical to examine the contralateral knee, because the normal relationship between the medial tibial plateau and medial femoral condyle is variable, with the plateau normally resting on average 1 cm anterior to the condyle. Understanding this relationship is also critical in avoiding a false-positive anterior drawer test. The presence or lack of a firm end point should also be noted.

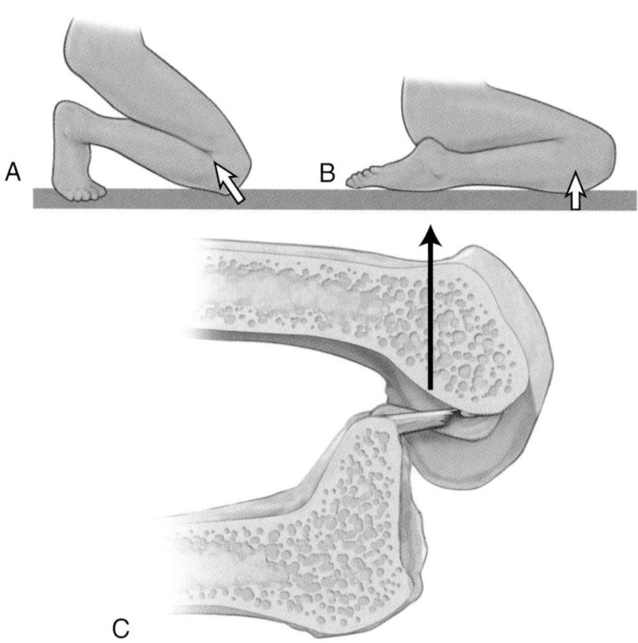

FIGURE 99-2 **A,** Falling on a flexed knee with the foot in a dorsiflexed position spares injury to the posterior cruciate ligament (PCL) by transmitting the force to the patellofemoral joint. **B,** Landing with the foot in a plantar flexed position injures the PCL because the posteriorly directed force is applied to the tibial tubercle. **C,** Hyperflexion of the knee without a direct blow is a common mechanism of PCL injury in athletes.

The amount of posterior translation observed during the posterior drawer test is used to grade the PCL injury. In grade I injuries, 0 to 5 mm of increased posterior translation is observed compared with the contralateral knee, but the anterior step-off of the plateau relative to the condyle is maintained. Grade II injuries are defined as those with 6 to 10 mm of posterior translation, which results in the plateau being flush with, but not posterior to, the medial femoral condyle. In both grade I and II injuries, the PCL is usually partially torn. With grade III injuries, posterior translation exceeds 10 mm and the medial tibial plateau displaces posterior to the medial femoral condyle during the posterior drawer test. This finding usually represents a complete tear of the PCL and could also represent a combined PCL and posterolateral corner (PLC) injury.

Posterior Sag Test (Godfrey Test) and Quadriceps Active Test

The posterior sag test may be positive in patients with complete PCL tears or partial tears. The patient lies supine with the hip and knee flexed to 90 degrees and the limb supported at the foot by the examiner. The anterior aspect of the proximal tibia is viewed from the side and compared with the uninjured, contralateral knee. Gravity displaces the tibia posterior to the femur in the case of a complete tear (Fig. 99-4).

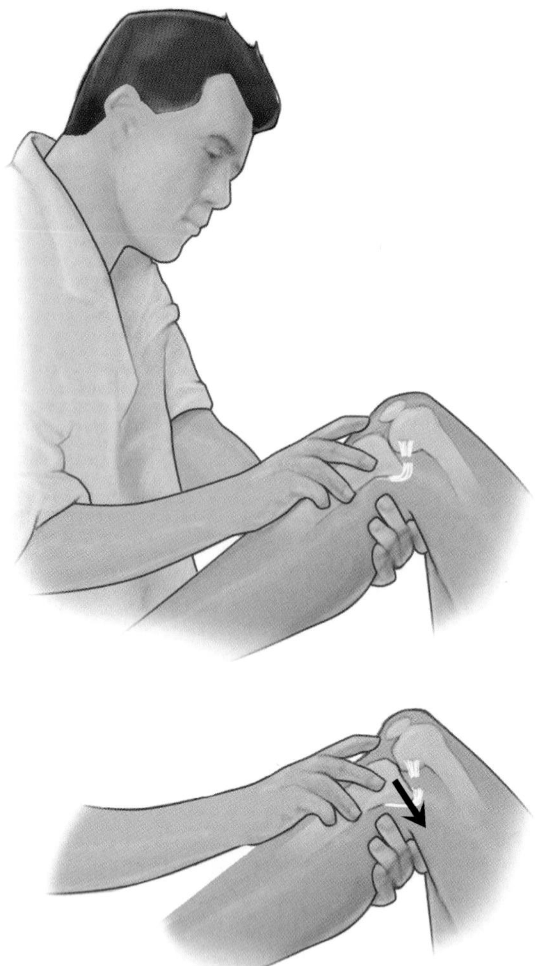

FIGURE 99-3 Assessing the tibial step-off before performing the posterior drawer examination. *(Modified from Miller MD, Harner CD, Koshiwaguchi S: Acute posterior cruciate ligament injuries. In Fu FH, Harner CD, Vince KG, editors:* Knee surgery, vol 1, *Baltimore, 1994, Williams & Wilkins.)*

The quadriceps active test can aid in the diagnosis of complete tears. With this test, the patient lies supine and the knee is placed at 90 degrees of flexion. While the examiner stabilizes the foot, the patient is asked to contract the quadriceps isometrically. In the presence of a complete tear of the PCL (grade III), the patient will achieve dynamic reduction of the posteriorly displaced tibia.

External Rotation of the Tibia (Dial Test)

The dial test is performed to evaluate for concomitant injuries to the PLC, which will affect decision making and treatment options because these patients are more likely to require surgery. The PLC cannot be accurately assessed in persons with grade III PCL injuries in which the tibia is subluxed posteriorly. The dial test is performed with the patient positioned prone or supine, while an external rotation force is applied to both feet with the knee positioned at 30 degrees and then 90 degrees of flexion. The degree of external tibial rotation is measured by comparing the medial border of the foot with the axis of the femur. It is essential to compare the results with the contralateral side because wide variability of external rotation is possible at these positions.[18,19] More than a 10-degree side-to-side difference is considered abnormal.[20] At all degrees of knee flexion, the popliteus complex portion of the PLC is the primary restraint to external rotation, but its effect is maximal at 30 degrees. An increase of 10 degrees or more of external rotation at 30 degrees of knee flexion, but not at 90 degrees, is considered diagnostic of an isolated PLC injury.[21] Increased external rotation at both 30 and 90 degrees of knee flexion suggests a combined PCL and PLC injury.

Reverse Pivot-Shift Test

The reverse pivot-shift test is also used to assess combined injuries and is performed with the patient supine. The knee is passively extended from 90 degrees of flexion with the foot externally rotated and a valgus force applied to the tibia. A positive result is observed when the posteriorly subluxed lateral tibial plateau is abruptly reduced by the iliotibial band at 20 to 30 degrees of flexion. A positive test typically indicates injury to the PCL and another capsuloligamentous structure, usually the PLC.[22]

Collateral Ligament Assessment

Varus and valgus stress tests are used to assess the lateral collateral ligament (LCL) portion of the PLC. The tests are performed with the knee in full extension and in 30 degrees of flexion. Although an isolated PCL injury does not significantly affect varus or valgus stability, increased varus opening at 30

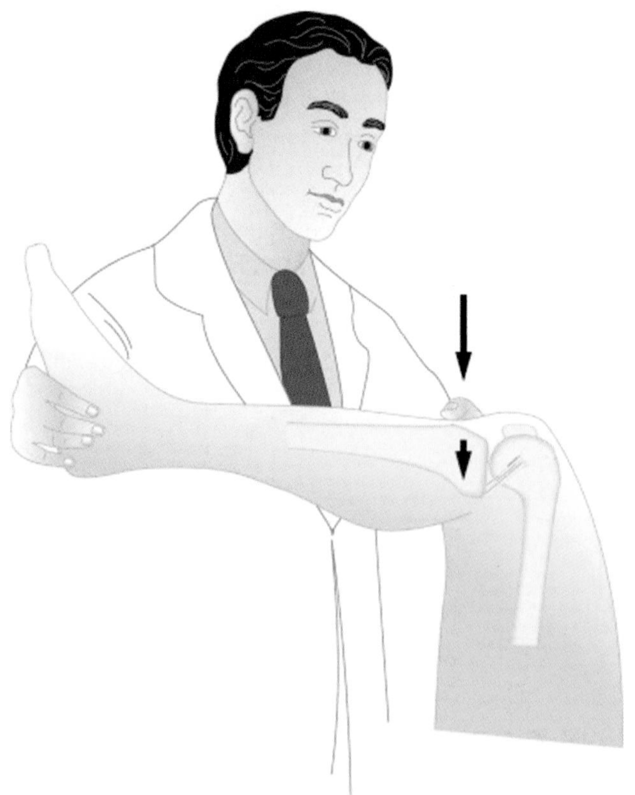

FIGURE 99-4 A positive Godfrey test. *(Modified from Miller MD, Harner CD, Koshiwaguchi S: Acute posterior cruciate ligament injuries. In Fu FH, Harner CD, Vince KG, editors:* Knee surgery, vol 1, *Baltimore, 1994, Williams & Wilkins.)*

degrees of knee flexion indicates an injury to the LCL and possibly the popliteus complex. If a significant degree of varus opening is noted at full extension, a combined injury of the PLC, PCL, and/or ACL is likely present.[24,25]

Gait and Limb Alignment

The evaluation of gait and limb alignment is particularly important for persons with chronic injury of the PCL or the PLC. In these patients, varus alignment, external rotation, and varus thrust may be observed. Compromised function of the stabilizers of the lateral knee can lead to excessive posterolateral rotation and varus opening (or thrust) in the stance phase of gait.

Imaging

Radiography

In the acute setting, plain radiographs of the knee should be performed, including bilateral standing anteroposterior, flexion posteroanterior 45 degrees with weight bearing, and Merchant patellar and lateral radiographs. These views are evaluated for posterior tibial subluxation, avulsion fractures, posterior tibial slope, and tibial plateau fractures. Tibial plateau fractures often indicate a high-energy injury with multiligament involvement. Bony avulsion fractures can be seen at the insertion of the PCL and at the fibular head, medial tibial plateau (medial Segond fracture), or the tibial tubercle.[26] Identification of bony avulsion injuries of the PCL, when recognized acutely, may be repaired primarily with superior results compared with late reconstruction.[26,27] Identification of tibial tubercle fractures is also critical. The unopposed pull of the hamstrings causes posterior tibial subluxation in this scenario, which can become fixed within a short time, requiring open reduction. Medial Segond fractures represent a medial capsular avulsion in PCL injuries that may be associated with a peripheral medial meniscus tear.[28,29] Lastly, hip-to-ankle cassette views are critical to evaluate overall lower extremity alignment, particularly varus, in chronic or revision cases.

Stress radiographs are not necessary to diagnose a PCL injury but may be helpful to differentiate between complete and partial PCL tears. However, these radiographs are most commonly used for research purposes. In a retrospective review of 21 patients with partial or complete PCL tears, Hewitt and colleagues[31] found that stress radiographs were more accurate than KT-1000 measurements in diagnosing PCL tears. With the knee flexed to 70 degrees and an 89-N weight suspended from the tibia at the level of the tibial tubercle, a lateral radiograph was taken. The mean translation of the medial tibial plateau was 12.2 mm in the presence of a complete tear compared with 5.2 mm seen with a partial tear as confirmed with diagnostic arthroscopy. The magnitude of posterior tibial translation during stress radiography has been correlated with the presence of combined ligament injury. In a cadaveric study by Sekiya et al.,[32] the authors demonstrated that greater than 10 mm of posterior tibial translation on stress radiography correlated with the presence of a PLC injury in addition to a complete disruption of the PCL. It should be noted that the accuracy of stress radiography may be decreased by patient guarding and partial reduction of the tibia with quadriceps activation; in addition, this infrequently performed examination is operator dependent. Stress radiographs can also be influenced by tibial rotation, and thus some authors have concluded that physical examination may be equally sensitive to stress radiographs in determining the presence and extent of a PCL tear.[33]

Magnetic Resonance Imaging

MRI has become the imaging modality of choice for confirming the presence of an acute PCL tear and to diagnose associated injuries with a sensitivity of up to 100%.[14,34,35] The location and physical characteristics of the tear can also be assessed with MRI and may have implications for prognosis and treatment.[36,37] MRI may be less sensitive in the diagnoses of chronic tears. The normal PCL appears dark on T1- and T2-weighted sequences and is curvilinear in appearance.[38] In contrast, chronic tears of the PCL can heal and assume the aforementioned curvilinear appearance; thus MRIs are much less sensitive for chronic PCL tears, and the appearance of a normal shape of the ligament should not be used as a criterion for a normal PCL.[39,40]

Lastly, MRI provides important information on the status of the menisci, articular cartilage, and other ligaments in the knee, because concomitant injuries affect treatment decision making and prognosis.[41] Bone bruises have been found in 83% of grade II and III PCL injuries on MRI, but in contrast to the bone bruise associated with ACL tears, the location is variable.[42] The utility of MRI for the diagnosis of associated injuries to the PLC has previously been evaluated. With use of thin-slice coronal oblique T1-weighted images through the entire fibular head, LaPrade and colleagues[43] were able to identify injury to the posterolateral structures with an accuracy of 68.8% to 94.4%, depending on the structure. Similarly, Theodorou et al.[44] found that MRI has an accuracy of 79% to 100% for the diagnoses of posterolateral injuries confirmed with arthroscopy.

Bone Scan

Although a bone scan is not frequently used, it can be useful in the evaluation and management of chronic PCL injuries. In particular, patients with these injuries are predisposed to early medial and patellofemoral compartment chondrosis.[12,45,46] In the setting of an isolated PCL-deficient knee with medial or patellofemoral compartment pain and normal radiographs, a bone scan to assess these compartments may be indicated. Increased uptake suggests that surgical intervention may be beneficial,[47] although this supposition has not been proven definitively.

Decision Making

Decision making in the treatment of PCL injuries is dependent on the natural history of the disease, with most treatment recommendations made on the basis of symptoms, activity level, grade of the injury, and associated injuries. As with any orthopaedic ailment, operative intervention should be chosen only if it results in superior outcomes compared with nonsurgical management. Controversy exists regarding PCL treatment because the extent to which posterior laxity causes symptoms or accelerates the development of degenerative joint disease (DJD) is unclear. Furthermore, it is unknown whether reconstruction sufficiently mitigates laxity to result in clinical improvement and slow the development of DJD. Reducing posterior laxity with reconstruction may improve long-term outcomes in patients with PCL injuries, and yet residual laxity is common even after reconstruction.[48,49] Some investigators propose that isolated PCL tears follow a benign course in the short term without reconstruction[1,9,47,50] but that diminishing results may be seen at later point.[51] To date, no study has demonstrated that PCL reconstruction can prevent the development of DJD.[52]

Controversy remains regarding indications for nonoperative versus operative management because few clinical studies have sufficient sample sizes and duration of follow-up to draw definitive conclusions. Additionally, a variety of PCL reconstructions are currently used, and the treatment of isolated PCL injuries is often reported in conjunction with combined injuries, such as PLC injuries, making outcome studies relatively heterogeneous. Currently most studies are retrospective in nature and use various outcome measurements, which make comparisons difficult. Until randomized prospective clinical trials are conducted, this debate will likely continue. The next section reviews the results of nonoperative management of PCL injuries and conclude the section with our decision-making rationale.

Nonoperative Treatment

Many studies have found favorable outcomes when isolated PCL injuries are treated conservatively. Parolie and Bergfeld[1] evaluated patient satisfaction in 25 persons with isolated PCL tears that had resulted from sporting injuries at a minimum of 2 years of follow-up. These investigators found that 68% of patients returned to their previous level of activity and 80% were satisfied with their knee function. They evaluated laxity and found no correlation with DJD. More recently, Shelbourne and Muthukaruppan[53] prospectively evaluated 215 conservatively treated patients with isolated PCL tears. Their study focused on patients with grade II laxity or less. These investigators found that subjective scores did not correlate with the degree of laxity and mean scores did not decrease with time from injury. They were unable to identify any risk factors that would predict which patients would have a decline in knee function over time. Patel et al.,[54] in another recent retrospective review of 57 patients with grade A or B PCL tears, a grading system proposed by MacGillivray and colleagues,[55] also found that functional scores did not correlate with the degree of PCL laxity. Lysholm knee scores were excellent in 40% and good in 52%. Patel et al.[54] found grade I medial compartment osteoarthritis (OA) in seven knees, grade II in three knees, and mild patellofemoral OA in four knees at an average of 6.8 years of follow-up. They concluded that most patients with acute, isolated PCL tears do well with nonoperative management at intermediate follow-up.

Other investigators have also found good initial clinical outcomes with nonoperative treatment but have found deterioration at extended follow-up. Boynton and Tietjens[51] observed 38 patients with isolated tears for a mean of 13.4 years. Of these patients, eight had subsequent meniscal injuries and surgery. Of the remaining 30 patients with normal menisci, 24 (81%) had occasional pain, 17 (56%) had occasional swelling, and a positive increase in articular cartilage degeneration was seen on radiographs over time. Fowler and Messieh[9] prospectively followed up 13 patients with acute isolated PCL tears that were confirmed by arthroscopy and treated with physiotherapy. All patients had a good subjective functional score according to the Houston criteria, but objective scores were good in only 3 patients and only fair in the other 10 patients.

Although relatively good results have been observed with nonoperative treatment, it should be noted that many of the patients in these series had grade II laxity or less and not all patients achieved a normal outcome, especially patients with grade III injuries. The benign course observed may be due to the integrity of the secondary restraints and various portions of the PCL complex remaining intact in persons with less serious injuries. Tibial slope may also affect the stability of the PCL deficient knee. In a cadaveric study, increasing the posterior tibial slope decreased the static posterior instability of the PCL/PLC-deficient knee, whereas decreasing the tibial slope increased posterior instability and the magnitude of the reverse pivot-shift test.[56]

Despite acceptable clinical results with nonoperative treatment, it is well understood that PCL deficiency alters knee kinematics and the distribution of load during activity. It has been shown that the PCL-deficient knee experiences increased contact pressures in the patellofemoral and medial compartments.[57,58] Logan et al.[57] evaluated the effect of PCL rupture on tibiofemoral motion during squatting with use of MRI. They concluded that PCL deficiency is similar to a medial meniscus resection and results in a "fixed" anterior subluxation of the medial femoral condyle (posterior subluxation of the medial tibial plateau). This subluxation changes the kinematics of the knee and may explain the increase in medial compartment OA seen in PCL-deficient knees. Currently more attention is being placed on additional injuries that are commonly associated with grade III tears that lead to greater instability and more severely altered biomechanics.

Although it is known that the kinematics of the knee are altered in the presence of a PCL injury, specific prognostic factors that predict outcome have proven elusive. In many studies the time from injury and objective instability have not correlated well with final outcome and radiographic changes. Surgical reconstruction is not recommended for isolated grade I injuries. Because many patients with isolated grade II posterior laxity only improve to grade I laxity with reconstruction, we agree with other authors that operative intervention in these patients may not offer improved outcome when compared with nonoperative treatment.[48,53] The treatment of acute isolated grade III PCL injuries is controversial. In these patients, some surgeons favor a more aggressive approach involving PCL reconstruction, whereas others recommend nonsurgical treatment. In cases with greater than 10 mm of abnormal posterior laxity, the clinician should remember to have a high index of suspicion for a combined ligamentous injury involving the PLC.

Level I evidence does not currently exist to support strong recommendations on the management of PCL injuries. However, based on the previously described data, we recommend nonoperative management for the treatment of acute and chronic isolated grade I and II PCL injuries (Figs. 99-5 and 99-6). Operative management is reserved for chronic isolated grade III PCL injuries with symptoms of pain or instability when an adequate course of conservative treatment has failed. In addition, surgical treatment is usually

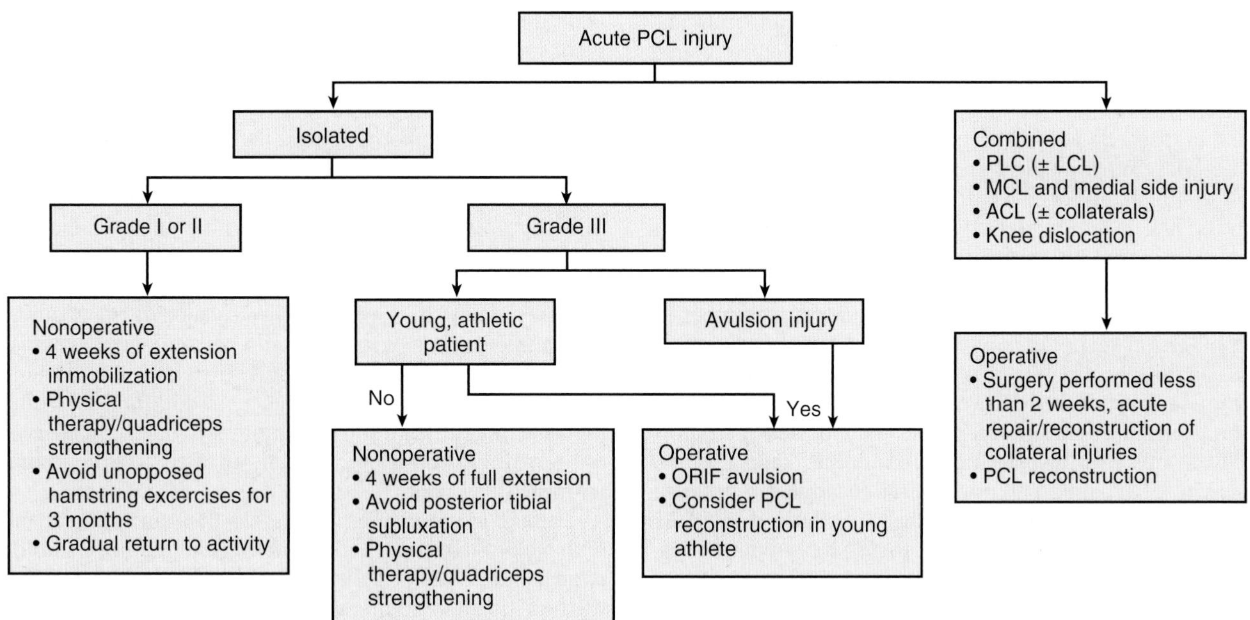

FIGURE 99-5 Treatment recommendations for acute injuries of the posterior cruciate ligament (PCL). *ACL,* Anterior cruciate ligament; *LCL,* lateral collateral ligament; *MCL,* medial collateral ligament; *ORIF,* open reduction, internal fixation.

recommended for acute and chronic combined ligamentous injuries. The treatment of acute grade III PCL tears is controversial, with some surgeons recommending PCL reconstruction and others recommending nonoperative treatment. Lastly, open reduction and internal fixation are recommended for acute avulsion fractures at the PCL tibial attachment site.

Treatment Options

Nonoperative Treatment

As discussed in the previous section, nonoperative treatment is recommended in patients with acute, isolated grade I or II PCL tears.[1,45] Nonoperative management is aimed at

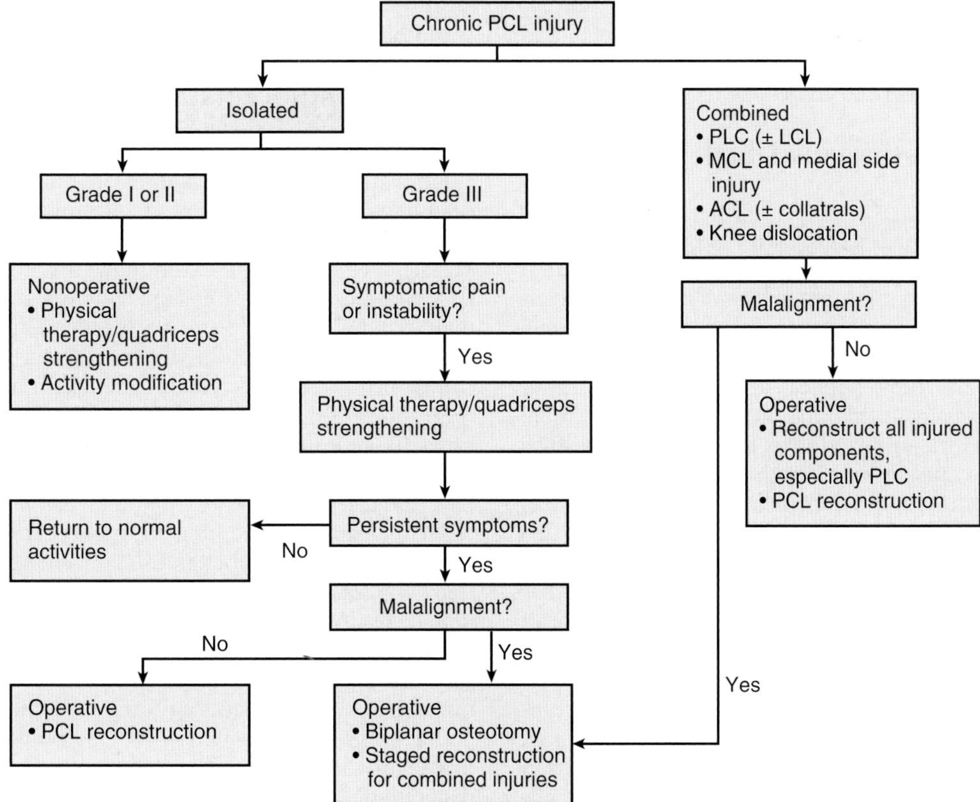

FIGURE 99-6 Treatment recommendations for chronic injuries of the posterior cruciate ligament (PCL). *ACL,* Anterior cruciate ligament; *LCL,* lateral collateral ligament; *MCL,* medial collateral ligament.

counteracting the forces of gravity and the hamstring muscles, which act to sublux the tibia posteriorly on the femur. Pierce and colleagues[60] have recently reviewed the literature on rehabilitation protocols for nonoperative and operative treatment of PCL injuries. Based on the finding of the reviewed studies, a three-phase rehabilitation protocol was recommended. We follow a similar protocol at our institution.

In the first 6 weeks after injury (phase I), rehabilitation is focused on partial weight bearing, hamstring and gastrocnemius stretching to reduce the posterior pull on the tibia, and quadriceps strengthening. In this initial phase, a number of immobilization techniques have been described to decrease stress on the healing ligament. These techniques include bracing the knee locked between 0 and 60 degrees of knee flexion,[61] use of a cylindrical leg cast with a posterior support to prevent posterior displacement of the tibia,[62] and use of a brace with a dynamic anterior drawer to apply an anterior force on the posterior proximal tibia.[63] In phase II, 6 to 12 weeks after injury, the focus is on progressive strengthening, reestablishment of full range of motion, and improving proprioception. In phase III, 13 to 18 weeks after the injury occurred, the patient is allowed to begin running and to perform sports-specific exercises, with return to sports allowed 4 to 6 months after the initial injury, assuming quadriceps strength is comparable to that of the contralateral leg.

Operative Treatment

A number of surgical techniques for PCL reconstruction can be considered. Current surgical treatment options include transtibial and tibial inlay reconstruction techniques with single- or double-bundle reconstruction and a variety of fixation methods. Several biomechanical and anatomic studies have been published recently investigating the benefits and pitfalls of these techniques. However, no consensus currently exists on the best method of PCL reconstruction.

Transtibial Tunnel Versus Tibial Inlay Techniques

The transtibial technique is a commonly used method of PCL reconstruction. In this technique, the tibial and femoral tunnels are drilled and the graft must make a sharp turn around the "killer turn" as it surfaces from the tibial tunnel and changes direction before entering the knee joint. This acute turn has been implicated as the cause of graft abrasion with subsequent thinning of the graft and eventual graft rupture or excessive laxity.[64] The residual posterior knee laxity observed clinically after traditional transtibial PCL reconstruction techniques may be related to this acute turn. To address the concern of graft attenuation resulting from this tunnel, the tibial inlay technique was developed and reported by Jakob and Ruegsegger,[65] as well as by Berg.[66] In this technique, direct fixation occurs at the tibial attachment site of the PCL, preventing an acute turn as the graft passes from the tibia to the femoral tunnel.

A number of cadaveric biomechanical studies have compared the transtibial and tibial inlay techniques. Although McAllister et al.[67] found no significant differences in mean knee laxities between the tibial tunnel and tibial inlay techniques at time zero, increased laxity was observed with this technique after cyclic loading. Bergfeld et al.[68] assessed anteroposterior laxity in cadaveric knees undergoing tunnel reconstruction or inlay reconstruction. Minimal differences in anteroposterior laxity were observed in the inlay group when compared with the tunnel group from 30 to 90 degrees of knee flexion and after repetitive loading at 90 degrees of knee flexion. However, evaluation of the grafts after testing demonstrated evidence of graft thinning and attenuation in the tunnel group but not in the inlay group. In a detailed cyclic loading analysis, Markolf and colleagues[69] also evaluated cadaver knees with tibial inlay and transtibial reconstruction. Ten of 31 grafts in the tunnel group failed at the acute angle before 2000 cycles of testing could be completed, whereas all 31 grafts that had been fixed to the tibia with use of the inlay method survived the testing intact. In addition, a significant increase in graft thinning and stretching out was observed in the remaining tunnel grafts that survived testing compared with the inlay grafts.

Thus in vitro analyses comparing the transtibial technique with tibial inlay suggest that although initial knee stability is equivalent, posterior laxity increases with cyclic loading with the transtibial technique when compared with the tibial inlay technique. Attempts have also been made to decrease the effects of the killer turn by reducing the sharp edge at the tibial tunnel exit, but this technique has only been attempted in an animal model.[70] Weimann and colleagues[70] found that rounding the sharp edge of the tibial tunnel decreased graft damage associated with the killer turn in a porcine model of PCL reconstruction. To date, retrospective studies comparing patients undergoing transtibial versus tibial inlay procedures[55,71] have not shown significant differences in subjective outcome or knee laxity measurements. Thus although the tibial inlay technique may have some biomechanical advantages when tested in a cadaveric model, these advantages have yet to be realized in the clinical setting.

Single-Bundle Versus Double-Bundle Reconstruction

Controversy also exists regarding the utility of single- versus double-bundle techniques of PCL reconstruction. The native PCL can be divided into an anterolateral (AL) and a PM bundle (Fig. 99-7). The AL bundle is tight in knee flexion and becomes lax in extension, whereas the PM bundle is tight in knee extension and becomes lax in flexion. The AL bundle is larger in cross-sectional area and thus is most commonly reconstructed in single-bundle procedures (Fig. 99-8). Double-bundle PCL reconstructions were proposed to more closely reproduce the anatomy and biomechanical properties of the intact PCL. Biomechanical studies have indicated that the two bundles demonstrate reciprocal tightening during knee range of motion and both are active in reducing posterior tibial translation and external tibial rotation, suggesting that both are required for normal knee kinematics.[72,73]

Single- versus double-bundle PCL reconstruction have been compared in several biomechanical studies, and some investigators have suggested improved biomechanics with double-bundle reconstruction.[74,75] Tsukada et al.[76] compared single anterolateral bundle reconstruction, single posteromedial bundle reconstruction, and double-bundle reconstruction in cadaveric human knees at different angles of knee flexion. The double-bundle reconstruction resisted posterior

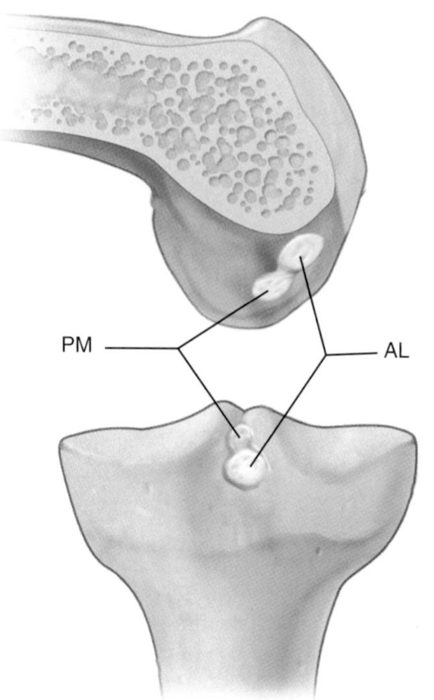

FIGURE 99-7 Femoral and tibial insertion sites of the posteromedial (PM) and anterolateral (AL) bundles of the posterior cruciate ligament.

tibial load better than the anterolateral single bundle at 0 and 30 degrees of knee flexion and better than the posteromedial single bundle at 30, 60, and 90 degrees of knee flexion under the posterior tibial load, leading the authors to conclude that double-bundle reconstruction reduces laxity in extension.

Additional studies have demonstrated potential drawbacks of double-bundle reconstruction, and some studies have been unable to demonstrate a benefit. Whiddon et al.[77] compared single- and double-bundle tibial inlay reconstruction in a cadaver model and found that the double-bundle technique improved rotational stability and posterior translation in knees with a concomitant PLC injury. However, no advantage was seen with a double-bundle reconstruction when compared with a single-bundle reconstruction with regard to posterior translation with the PLC intact. In addition, excessive rotational constraint was observed at 30 degrees. Wiley and colleagues[78] also observed that although posterior laxity was reduced compared with single-bundle reconstruction, overconstraint at 30 degrees of flexion was seen with double-bundle reconstruction. In a comparison of single-bundle AL reconstruction with double-bundle reconstruction in cadaver knees, Markolf and colleagues[79] found that the addition of a PM bundle reduced laxity from 0 to 30 degrees of flexion but at the expense of increased PCL graft forces. Bergfeld et al.[80] compared single- and double-bundle tibial inlay reconstruction in cadaveric knees using Achilles tendon

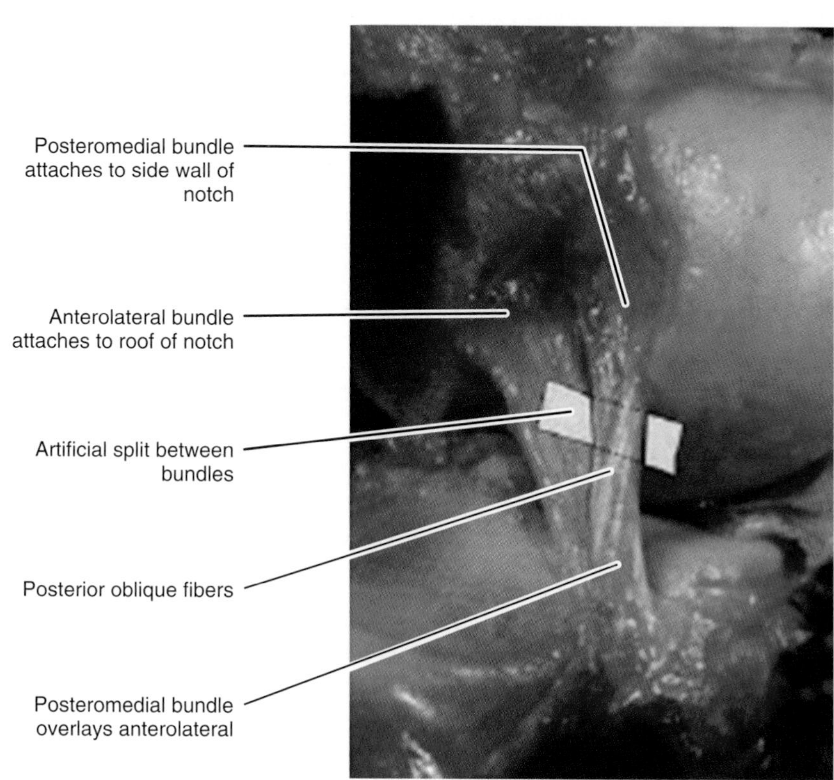

FIGURE 99-8 Posterolateral view of the left knee showing double-bundle architecture of the native posterior cruciate ligament. *(From Amis AA, Gupte CM, Bull AMJ, et al: Anatomy of the posterior cruciate ligament and the meniscofemoral ligaments.* Knee Surg Sports Traumatol Arthrosc *14[3]:257–263, 2006.)*

grafts. No differences in translation between the single- and double-bundle reconstruction were observed at any flexion angle.

A number of clinical studies have shown no significant differences in subjective and objective results between single- and double-bundle PCL graft reconstructions.[81-83] Based on the literature to date, we believe evidence is lacking to support the routine use of double-bundle reconstruction. However, this type of reconstruction remains a topic of interest and is undergoing continued investigation in the treatment of PCL injuries.

Graft Choice and Fixation

Graft choice and fixation techniques are also important considerations when discussing treatment options for surgery. Both autograft and allograft tissues have been used for PCL reconstruction. Bone–patellar tendon–bone, hamstring, and quadriceps tendons are common autograft sources. The Achilles tendon, as well as anterior and posterior tibial tendons, are frequently used allografts. Among autografts, bone–patellar tendon–bone grafts have the advantage of bone-to-bone healing in the bone tunnel. In comparison, the tendon portion of the quadriceps graft and both ends of hamstring grafts require tendon-to-bone healing in the bone tunnel, which may have inferior biomechanical properties.[84] Weakening of the quadriceps tendon, which acts synergistically with the PCL to prevent posterior tibial translation, is a concern with this graft option, as is the variable length of the tendinous portion.[85] Allograft tissue has the advantage of avoiding donor site morbidity, reducing operating time, and offering improved graft diameter with greater collagen tissue when Achilles and tibialis anterior tendons are used. Pitfalls of allografts include a small risk of disease transmission, cost, and availability. In a survey of orthopaedic surgeons, Dennis et al.[86] reported that allograft Achilles tendon was the most commonly used graft for acute (43%) and chronic (50%) PCL reconstructions. For the reasons previously discussed, we favor the use of Achilles tendon allografts for PCL reconstruction.

A number of biomechanical studies have investigated various graft fixation constructs used in PCL reconstruction. Most recently, Lim et al.[87] compared cross-pin fixation in a porcine model with bone blocks, interference screw fixation with bone blocks, cross-pin fixation of soft tissue with backup fixation, and interference screw fixation of soft tissue with backup fixation on the tibial side using Achilles allograft PCL reconstruction. Although cross-pin fixation with backup fixation had a higher maximum failure load and stiffness, tendon graft displacement was increased compared with bone-block fixation. Gupta and colleagues compared bioabsorbable to metallic screws for inlay fixation and found no difference in failure load or linear stiffness.[88] Markolf and colleagues[89] demonstrated the importance of bone-block position and orientation within the tibial tunnel; they found that positioning the bone–patellar tendon–bone graft flush with the posterior tunnel opening with the graft oriented so the bone block faced anteriorly in the tibial tunnel was the position with the best biomechanical properties. Margheritini et al.[90] found that combining distal and proximal tibial fixation resulted in significantly less posterior tibial translation and more closely restored intact PCL in situ forces at 90 degrees than did reconstruction with distal fixation.

High Tibial Osteotomy for Chronic PCL Injuries

A chronic isolated PCL injury results in posterior translation of the tibia and external rotation of the tibia in relation to the femur. These anatomic changes result in increased forces and subsequent development of OA in the medial and patellofemoral compartments.[91-93] Additionally, a chronic combined PCL and PLC injury can result in chronic posterolateral instability and varus malalignment associated with bony deformity, lateral soft tissue deficiency, and hyperextension and external rotation as a result of PLC deficiency (i.e., triple varus).[94] In cases of chronic PCL or combined PCL/PLC injury with resultant varus malalignment and posterior or posterolateral instability, soft tissue procedures alone may be insufficient, whereas performance of a high tibial osteotomy (HTO) prior to soft tissue reconstruction may improve outcomes by decreasing forces across the lateral supporting structures of the knee.

A medial opening wedge HTO can improve alignment and decrease instability by addressing both coronal and sagittal malalignment. In addition to correcting varus malalignment, a medial opening wedge osteotomy with the anteromedial gap equal or larger than the posterior medial gap increases the posterior tibial slope[95] and thus decreases the posterior resting position of the tibia.[96] In contrast, a lateral closing wedge osteotomy may decrease posterior tibial slope, consequently increasing the posterior resting position of the tibia,[97] and thus may not be appropriate in the knee with a PCL injury. Several investigators have demonstrated a concomitant increase in posterior tibial slope with opening wedge HTO.[98,95] Specifically, Noyes et al.[95] calculated that for each increase of 1 mm in the anterior gap, an increase of 2 degrees occurs in the posterior tibial slope. In the coronal plane, in the absence of medial compartment OA, the osteotomy should result in the mechanical axis crossing the center of the knee. If medial compartment joint space narrowing is present, some authors have recommended valgus hypercorrection with the mechanical axis crossing lateral to the center of the knee.[94]

Although satisfactory long-term outcomes have been observed in patients undergoing HTO for medial compartment OA,[99] studies reporting results of HTO specifically for chronic PCL deficiency or combined PCL/PLC insufficiency are limited and heterogeneous in patient population, duration of follow-up, and outcomes. In a case series of 17 HTOs for symptomatic hyperextension varus thrust that included four patients with isolated PCL injuries and seven with combined PCL and posterolateral ligament injuries, improved subjective activity scores were observed postoperatively at a mean follow-up of 56 months.[98] Similarly, Badhe and Forster[100] reported the results of HTO with or without ligament reconstruction in 14 patients with knee instability and varus alignment, including nine patients with PLC or combined PCL injury. The mean time from injury to HTO was 8.3 years. Although the mean Cincinnati Knee Score improved from a mean preoperative score of 53 to a mean postoperative score of 74, no patients were able to participate in competitive sports, and more than 30% had continued knee pain at follow-up. Thus although biomechanical studies suggest that HTO may improve alignment and stability in patients with chronic PCL insufficiency or combined PCL/PLC injury with varus malalignment and instability, data on outcomes in this patient population are currently minimal.

AUTHORS' PREFERRED TECHNIQUE

PCL Reconstruction

As discussed previously, many techniques have been described for PCL reconstruction. We prefer the tibial inlay method of reconstruction with an Achilles tendon allograft. The tibial inlay approach avoids the "killer turn" that may predispose the graft to stretch-out and failure. We also believe that the acute angle of the graft as it enters the notch in the transtibial technique can make tensioning more difficult. Some surgeons are concerned that the posterior approach to the tibia needed for the open inlay procedure, which may involve a change to the prone position, is more technically demanding. We believe that with experience these challenges are easily overcome and that this technique leads to better biomechanical stability.

Previous studies have demonstrated that the AL bundle is the most important component of the native PCL. The AL bundle has a higher cross-sectional area and is stronger than the PM bundle. Therefore the goal of a single-bundle reconstruction is to recreate the native AL bundle. However, it should be remembered that the footprint of the native PCL is much larger than the typical drill used to create the femoral tunnel, and thus the surgeon must choose which portion of the PCL to reconstruct. Clinical studies comparing single versus double-bundle reconstructions have not found any significant differences in patient outcome scores. Multiple options are available for graft tissue, and no study has conclusively demonstrated a superior graft. We use an Achilles tendon allograft for most of our PCL reconstructions. We prefer to use the Achilles tendon because of its size, strength, and versatility. For the aforementioned reasons, we prefer to use a single-bundle tibial inlay technique with use of an Achilles allograft for PCL reconstruction. This procedure is described in the following sections.

Graft Preparation

The soft tissue portion of the Achilles allograft is sized for a 10-mm bone tunnel. The bone plug is then fashioned into a trapezoidal shape 25 mm in length and 13 mm in width. The bone plug is predrilled and tapped for a 6.5-mm cancellous screw. The bone plug is drilled with a 4.5-mm drill from the cancellous to cortical surface to protect the soft tissue and is then tapped with a 6.5-mm tap. A 6.5-mm cancellous screw, approximately 35 mm in length, and a metal washer are then placed into the bone plug from the soft tissue/cortical surface to the cancellous surface. The screw is placed so that the tip is 5 mm past the cancellous surface to facilitate later tibial fixation. A running locking stitch is then placed along approximately 30 mm of tendon using a No. 2 braided polyester suture, which tabularizes the graft to aid in passage through the femoral tunnel.

Arthroscopy/Femoral Tunnel

For the arthroscopic portion of the case, the patient is laid supine on the operative table. We recommend that the patient be intubated to protect the airway during position changes. A complete examination is performed after inducement of anesthesia prior to placement of a tourniquet. It is very important to evaluate for both PCL and associated capsuloligamentous injuries at this time. A thigh tourniquet is then placed but not inflated. A routine diagnostic arthroscopy is performed, and any meniscal or chondral injuries are treated at this time. The ACL may appear lax because of posterior tibial subluxation and should tighten with an applied anterior drawer. The PCL is then examined, and often, the ligament is lax or stretched out rather than frankly torn (Fig. 99-9). Once incompetence of the PCL has been confirmed, the residual PCL tissue is removed with a shaver and hand-operated punches. If the ligaments of Humphry and Wrisberg are present, they are preserved if possible. The native footprint is preserved as a guide for femoral tunnel placement. Our goal of reconstruction is to restore the AL bundle of the PCL. The tunnel is placed in the distal and anterior portion of the native PCL footprint. A small medial incision is made through the skin and then through the medial retinaculum, which facilitates optimal drill guide placement with the tunnel oriented slightly posteriorly. The medial articular margin is used as a landmark for the guide. An outside-in arthroscopic guide is used to establish the tunnel position, and a femoral guide pin is placed. The femoral tunnel is created with a cannulated drill over the guide pin (Fig. 99-10). The drill size is determined by the size of the graft and is typically 10 mm in width. An

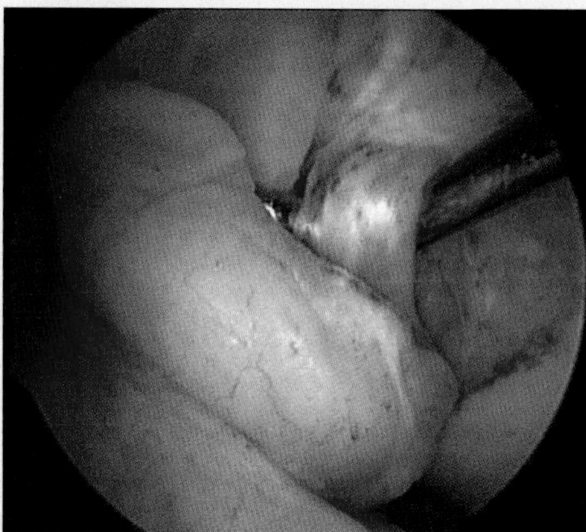

FIGURE 99-9 An arthroscopic view of a posterior cruciate ligament tear.

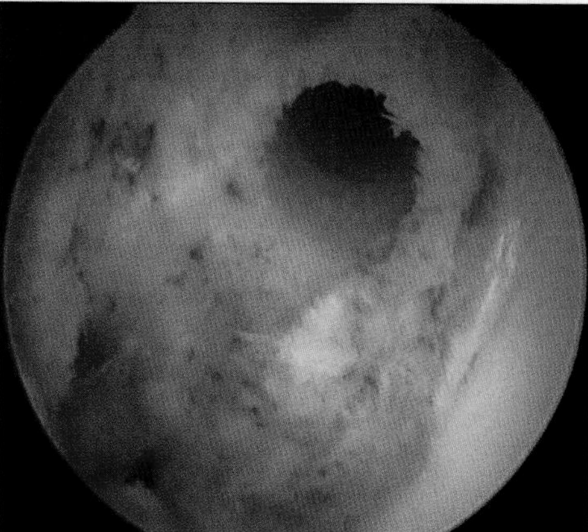

FIGURE 99-10 An arthroscopic view of the femoral tunnel created in the footprint of the native anterolateral bundle with a cannulated drill over a guide pin.

Continued

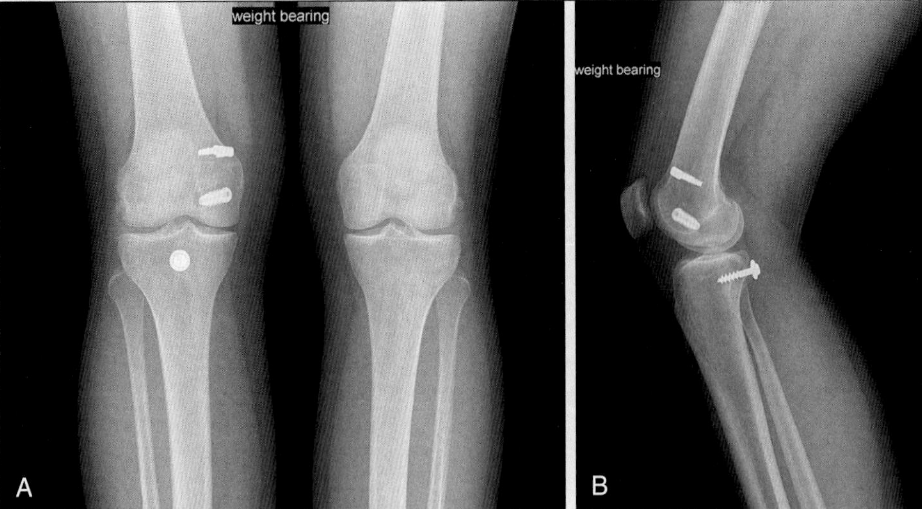

FIGURE 99-11 Anteroposterior and lateral radiographs of the knee after completion of single-bundle posterior cruciate ligament reconstruction.

18-gauge wire loop is passed through the femoral tunnel from the outside and positioned in the posterior notch to be retrieved later for graft passage.

Tibial Inlay

The patient is then rotated into the prone position in a sterile fashion in preparation for the tibial inlay portion of the case. The extremity is exsanguinated and a tourniquet is inflated. The posteromedial exposure to the tibia, as described by Burks,[101] is then performed. The skin incision is a gentle curve with a horizontal end at the medial popliteal crease and vertical limb overlying the medial aspect of the gastrocnemius. Dissection is carried down the investing fascial layer, which is incised over the medial head of the gastrocnemius. The medial sural cutaneous nerve can be at risk but typically perforates the fascia distal to the horizontal limb of the incision. The medial border of the medial gastrocnemius is identified. The interval between the medial gastrocnemius and semimembranosus tendon is developed. Blunt dissection is performed down to the joint capsule. The medial head of the gastrocnemius is then retracted laterally with a blunt-tipped retractor, which protects its motor branch and neurovascular structures. At this point the posterior proximal tibia and posterior femoral condyles are palpated and a vertical incision is made through the posterior capsule. The posterior notch and tibial attachment of the PCL should now be exposed and the tibial insertion site of the native PCL is prepared for placement of the graft. Typically two prominent processes are found on the medial and lateral borders of the PCL that can be palpated. The insertion site is resected using osteotomes, a rongeur, and/or a burr. A graft recipient site is created that will anatomically accommodate the previously prepared graft. The bone graft is then placed into the site and secured with a 6.5-mm cancellous screw and washer (Fig. 99-11). The sutures in the tendinous portion of the graft are shuttled through the femoral tunnel using the previously placed wire loop. After the sutures are passed, the capsule is repaired. The tourniquet is deflated and hemostasis is achieved. The wound is irrigated and closed in layers.

Graft Tensioning

After wound closure the patient is again returned to the supine position in a sterile fashion. The arthroscope is placed back into the knee and the graft is inspected, entering the femoral tunnel (Fig. 99-12). The knee is cycled several times, which allows the surgeon to evaluate range of motion and helps apply tension to the graft. Tension is applied to the graft in 70 to 90 degrees of flexion with an anterior drawer force placed on the proximal tibia. A 9 × 25 mm soft tissue interference screw is then used to fix the graft in the femoral tunnel. A staple is then placed over the soft tissue portion of the graft into the medial femoral condyle to augment fixation. The arthroscopic portals and the incision for the femoral tunnel are closed in the standard fashion.

Transtibial Technique and Double-Bundle Reconstruction

Alternatively, PCL reconstruction can be achieved via an arthroscopic transtibial technique. The patient is positioned supine. A detailed examination is performed after inducement of anesthesia followed by arthroscopic assessment of the knee

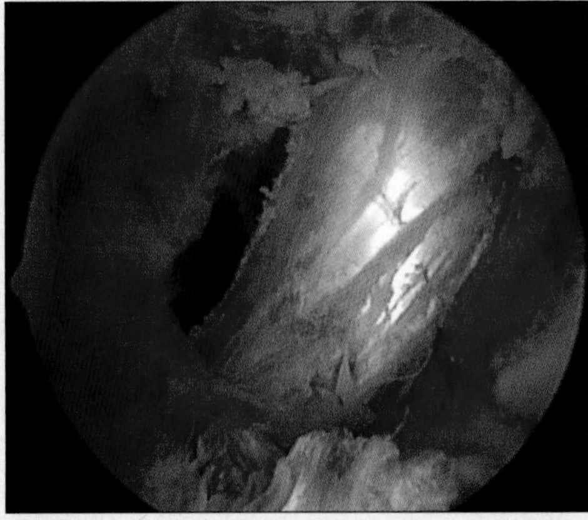

FIGURE 99-12 An arthroscopic view of a completed posterior cruciate ligament reconstruction.

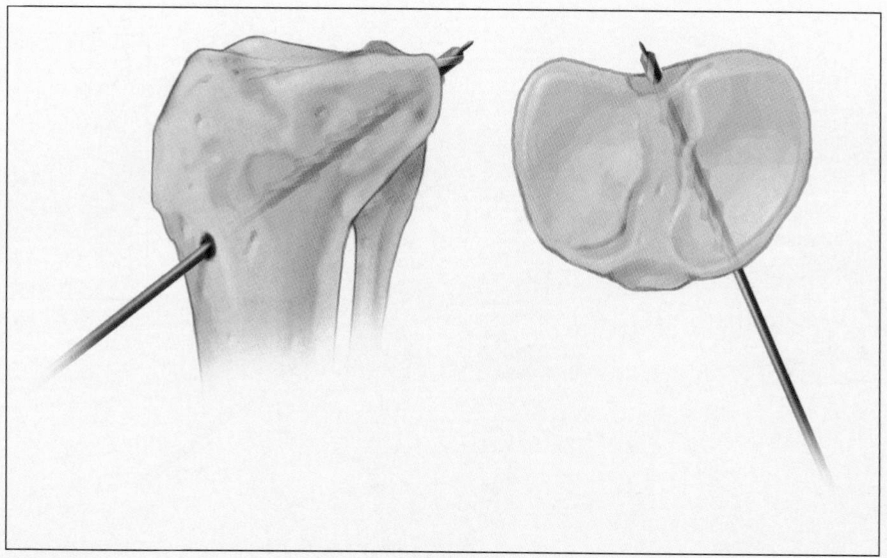

FIGURE 99-13 Posterior cruciate ligament tibial guide wire placement and drilling. *(Modified from Miller MD, Harner CD, Koshiwaguchi S: Acute posterior cruciate ligament injuries. In Fu FH, Harner CD, Vince KG, editors:* Knee surgery, vol 1, *Baltimore, 1994, Williams & Wilkins.)*

joint to confirm the extent of the injury and to assist with the repair or reconstructive procedure. The tibial footprint is prepared via an accessory anteromedial portal, and occasionally with use of a 70-degree arthroscope. A tibial tunnel is then created from the anteromedial tibia and directed posteriorly to the native PCL tibial attachment (Fig. 99-13). If a single-bundle procedure is performed, care is taken to place the single guide wire in the center of the tibial footprint via direct visualization and/or radiographic guidance with use of a guide. If a double-bundle reconstruction is performed, two guide wires are placed and confirmed radiographically, with the AL guide wire being more lateral and distal and the PM guide wire being more medial and proximal. The tunnel(s) is (are) reamed under power to the posterior cortex and then completed by hand with direct visualization.

After the tibial tunnels are completed, attention is focused on creating the femoral tunnels. The femoral insertion site anatomy is identified, and the appropriate tunnel position is marked for a single-bundle reconstruction or double-bundle reconstruction. The lateral portal is enlarged, and the knee is hyperflexed to drill the femoral tunnel(s) (Fig. 99-14, *A*). One or two grafts are used depending on whether a single-bundle or double-bundle reconstruction is being performed. These grafts are passed anterograde through the tibial tunnel (Fig. 99-15) and subsequently retrograde into the femur. The grafts are fixed on the femoral or tibial side and then tension is applied to the other side of the graft and it is fixed. Tension is applied to the AL bundle and it is fixed at 90 degrees of flexion, whereas tension is applied to the posteromedial bundle and it is fixed at 30 degrees of flexion.

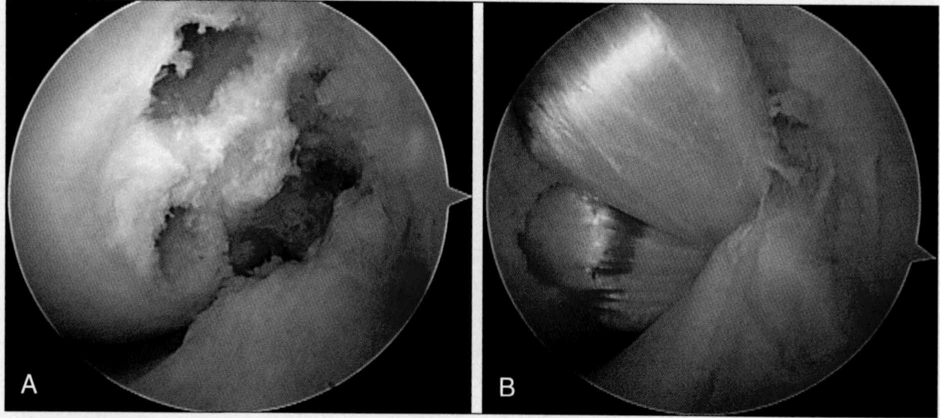

FIGURE 99-14 Positioning of femoral tunnels for double-bundle reconstruction. **A,** Femoral tunnel position for anterolateral and posteromedial bundles. Note that the anterolateral bundle is more anterior. **B,** Double-bundle reconstruction with tibialis anterior allografts.

Continued

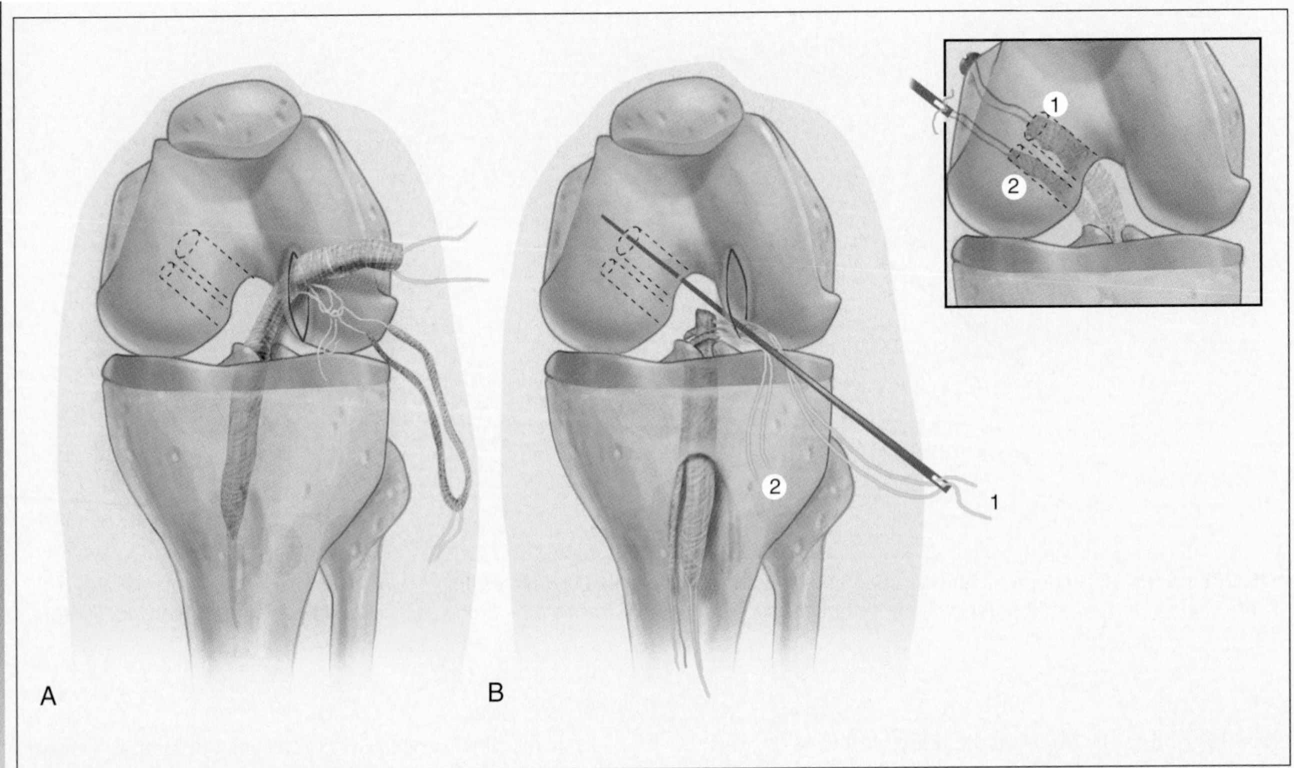

FIGURE 99-15 Graft placement. **A,** The graft for the anterolateral bundle (inset, *1*) and a second graft for the posteromedial bundle (inset, *2*) are passed in anterograde fashion through the tibial tunnel. **B,** The grafts are then fixed to corresponding femoral tunnels. *(Modified from Petrie RS, Harner CD: Double bundle posterior cruciate ligament reconstruction technique: University of Pittsburgh approach.* Op Tech Sports Med *7:118–126, 1999.)*

Postoperative Management

Although rehabilitation after ACL reconstruction has been investigated by numerous authors, postoperative management after PCL reconstruction has been studied less extensively. Because PCL reconstruction has not been as successful as ACL reconstruction in restoring objective stability, many surgeons recommend a more conservative postoperative course. No level I studies have been performed to compare different protocols, and in a recent review of the literature, Pierce et al.[60] found that currently no consensus exists regarding a set of optimal guidelines. In general, rehabilitation should focus on quadriceps strengthening and regaining range of motion while avoiding posterior tibial translation, which places stress on the graft. These goals are usually achieved by initial immobilization and avoidance of active hamstring forces, limited range of motion, and progressive weight bearing and strengthening based on the time from surgery and the patient's progress.

The aim of reconstruction and rehabilitation is to help the patient return to previous levels of function. The goal of most protocols is to achieve this goal around 9 months after surgery. Postoperative protocols use functional progression to determine the patient's advancement. Functional status is determined using a combination of subjective patient assessment and objective data. These data include joint stability, range of motion, effusion, proprioception deficits, muscle strength, and gait abnormalities. Careful monitoring of these factors during rehabilitation can help the surgeon identify and manage potential complications early during the postoperative course. It is important for the patient to understand that strict compliance with the postoperative protocol is critical to a good outcome.

Traditionally, PCL protocols are divided into specific phases, and advancement is based on time from surgery and patient progression. The nature of these phases varies among surgeons, but many similarities exist. The first phase usually emphasizes protecting the graft from stress, range of motion within limits, non–weight bearing, effusion prevention, and reactivation of the quadriceps. The next phase focuses on regaining full range of motion, advancement of weight bearing, and low-impact strengthening. The length and method of immobilization have varied among different studies. The initiation of range of motion exercises and degrees of motion allowed during the early phases also differs among studies. Progression through the subsequent phases depends on patient function. Factors that influence progression include strength, stability, endurance, and agility. Patients are allowed to return to play when they regain appropriate quadriceps strength and painless active range of motion, which, as previously stated, is usually at around 9 months after surgery.

To regain strength and proprioception, most protocols include open and closed kinetic chain exercises. For this

AUTHORS' PREFERRED TECHNIQUE

Postoperative Management

A. Acute Immediate Postoperative Phase (Early Protection Phase)
- Bracing: After surgery, the hinged brace is locked at zero
- Range of motion: passive range of motion (initiated after 2 to 3 weeks of immobilization in extension)—patient-assisted tibial lift into flexion (0 to 70 degrees) with passive knee flexion
- Exercises:
  - Quadriceps isometrics, straight leg raise—adduction, abduction proximal weight

B. Acute Phase (Maximal Protection Phase)
- Goals:
  - Minimize external forces to protect the graft
  - Prevention of quadriceps atrophy
  - Control postsurgical effusion
- Weight bearing: weight bearing as tolerated with an assistive device
- Range of motion: as tolerated to 90 degrees
- Exercises:
  - Continue isometric exercises and quadriceps strengthening
  - Closed kinetic chain mini-squat, shuttle, bike
  - Open kinetic chain knee extension (60 degrees to 0 degrees)
  - Proprioception training
  - Weight shifts
- Brace: Fit with a functional brace at 4 to 6 weeks after surgery

C. Progressive Range of Motion/Strengthening Phase
- Weight bearing: weight bearing as tolerated without an assistive device
- Range of motion: as tolerated to 125 degrees flexion
- Exercises:
  - Continue quadriceps strength training
  - Begin isotonic quadriceps strength exercises
  - Leg press (0 to 60 degrees)
  - Step-ups
  - Sport-cord progression program
  - Rowing, NordicTrack
  - Initiate closed kinetic chain terminal knee extension

D. Functional Activity Phase

Few scientific data are available to help determine the best method of rehabilitation as the patient transitions into functional stages, and thus progression at this level is determined by the patient's tolerance to exercise and level of function. The evaluation of power and endurance that have been used for ACL programs should theoretically measure total length, strength, and endurance and can be used for the PCL reconstructed knee. As previously stated, the anticipated return to previous activity after PCL reconstruction is anticipated to take approximately 9 months.

reason it is important that open and closed chain exercises be part of the PCL rehabilitation program. Open-chain knee flexion resulting from hamstring contraction causes significant posterior translational forces across the tibia and should be avoided during early phases of rehabilitation.[102] Open-chain knee extension can protect the graft by producing anteriorly directed shear forces across the tibia, and most investigators advocate that these forces be initiated early.[60,102] Closed kinetic chain exercises at low arcs of motion have also been shown to decrease posterior shear forces and are included in PCL rehabilitation. We use the following protocol.

Results of Operative Treatment

Isolated Posterior Cruciate Ligament Injuries

The results of isolated PCL reconstruction have been evaluated in many published studies. Although most patients demonstrate improvement, some patients report persistent knee symptoms and have residual laxity that may inhibit return to preinjury-level activities.[55,64,81,82,103-115] The main limitation of these studies is the low incidence of isolated PCL injury requiring reconstruction, which results in a small sample size. Many of these studies are also retrospective case series that differ in operative technique, outcome measurements, and postoperative treatment, making direct comparison between studies difficult. A summary of these studies can be found in Table 99-1.[105,113,114,116-123]

Hermans et al.[105] evaluated 25 patients who underwent isolated AL bundle PCL reconstructions at an average follow-up of 9.1 years. They used an arthroscopic transtibial, single-bundle approach with use of various graft types. The final International Knee Documentation Committee (IKDC), Lysholm, and functional Visual Analog Scale scores were significantly better than preoperative scores, but only 41% of patients had normal or near-normal clinical findings according to the IKDC guidelines. This finding was mostly attributed to residual laxity with a mean side-to-side difference of 4.7 mm by Telos stress radiographs at final follow-up. Preoperative symptomatic instability greater than 1 year and chondrosis at the time of surgery correlated with poorer subjective outcomes. These findings confirm that although isolated PCL reconstruction often results in improved functional outcome, many patients have residual laxity. Lahner et al.[114] prospectively followed up on 33 patients with chronic symptomatic PCL injuries who underwent isolated single-bundle transtibial reconstruction. These patients were followed up over 2 years, and during this time, their IKDC scores improved from 41.8 to 69.5, and 72.8% regained normal to near-normal knee function. In this study, nine patients (27.4%) showed no improvement in knee function postoperatively. Chen and Gao[113] evaluated a transtibial double-bundle reconstruction using a suture suspension technique at a minimum follow-up of 2 years. In their series of 19 patients, 78.9% regained normal knee function and 15.8% regained near-normal knee function. These rates are significantly higher than those reported in other studies and may be attributable to higher preoperative scores. The patients in this series had an average preoperative IKDC score of 65.6 and less posterior laxity compared with subjects in other studies.

TABLE 99-1

RESULTS OF ISOLATED POSTERIOR CRUCIATE LIGAMENT RECONSTRUCTION

Study	No. of Patients	Age (yr)	Follow-up (yr)	Chronicity/Grade	Graft Type	Surgical Technique
Lahner et al. (2012),[114] prospective	33	32.5	2	Chronic 13 grade II 20 grade III	Hamstring autograft	Transtibial, single bundle
Hermans et al. (2009),[105] retrospective	25	30.8	9.1	7 acute, 18 chronic, grade II or more	9 BPTB autograft 7 quadrupled hamstring autograft 8 double hamstring autograft	Transtibial, single bundle
Chen and Gao (2009)[113]	19	39	Minimum of 2	Unknown Average time 14 mo 15 grade II 4 grade III	8-strand hamstring autograft	Transtibial, double bundle
Chan et al. (2006),[116] prospective	20	29	3.3	Unknown Average time 4 mo All grade III	Quadrupled hamstring autograft	Transtibial
Sekiya et al. (2005),[117] retrospective	21	38	5.9	5 acute 16 chronic All grade III	Achilles allograft	Transtibial
Ahn et al. (2005),[118] retrospective	Group I: 18	30	2.9	All chronic 11 grade II 7 grade III	Hamstring autograft	Transtibial
	Group II: 18	31	2.3	10 grade II 8 grade III	Achilles allograft	Transtibial
Jung et al. (2004),[119] retrospective	12	29	4.3	Unknown Average time 5.4 mo Range 1-10 mo	Patellar tendon autograft	Tibial inlay
Wang et al. (2003),[120] retrospective	30	32	3.3	13 acute 17 chronic All grade III	Mixed	Transtibial
Deehan et al. (2003),[121] prospective	27	27	3.3	All chronic (16 patients 4-12 mo after injury, 11 patients >1 yr) Grade II and III injuries	Hamstring autograft	Transtibial
Chen et al. (2002),[122] retrospective	Group A (quad tendon): 22	29	2.5	All grade III 12 acute 10 chronic	Quadriceps tendon autograft	Transtibial
	Group B (hamstring tendon): 27	27	2.2	16 acute 11 chronic	Quadrupled hamstring autograft	
Mariani et al. (1997),[123] retrospective	24	26	2.2	All chronic	Patellar tendon autograft	Transtibial

A, Abnormal; *bio,* biologic; *BPTB,* bone–patellar tendon–bone; *IKDC,* International Knee Documentation Committee; *IS,* interference screw; *KT,* KT-1000 testing; *N,* normal; *NA,* not available; *NN,* near-normal; *OAK,* Orthopädische Arbeitsgruppe Knie; *SA,* severely abnormal.

Fixation	Subjective Outcome	Instrumented Laxity	Posterior Drawer	Miscellaneous
Tibia: bio IS + button Femur: FlippTack	IKDC: 69, 72.8% N/NN Tegner: 5.9	Telos radiograph: 5 mm	Grade I: 25 grade II: 8	Minor extension deficit 3-5 degrees in only 2 patients
Tibia: IS Femur: IS	IKDC: 65 Lysholm 75 Tegner 5.7	KT posterior drawer: 4.7 mm Side-side difference: 2.1 mm	Grade 0: 2 grade I: 15 grade II: 5	11 patients with residual positive quadriceps active test IKDC N to NN in only 41% Poorer results in chronic injuries
Suture suspension	Lysholm: 92.1 IKDC: 92.1, 78.9% N, 15.8% NN	KT posterior drawer: 9.4 preoperative to 1.0 postoperative Stress radiograph: 2.0	Grade 0: 17 Grade I: 1 Grade II: 1	Average preoperative IKDC score 65.6
Tibia: bio IS + screw and washer Femur: bio IS + washer	Lysholm: 93 Tegner: 6.3 IKDC: 85% N/NN	Average postoperative KT posterior drawer: 3.8 mm	Grade I: 16 grade II: 3 grade III: 1	18/20 showed no radiographic deterioration 3 patients had stiffness
Tibia: screw and washer Femur: metal IS	IKDC knee function: 57% N/NN, 43% A/SA IKDC activity level: 62% N/NN, 38% A/SA	KT posterior drawer: 4.5 mm KT side-side difference: 1.96 mm	IKDC acute/ subacute: 75% N/NN Chronic: 40% N/NN	Acute/subacute group had significantly better IKDC and KT-1000 than chronic group
Femur: IS and screw and washer	Lysholm: 90 IKDC: 16 N/NN, 2 A	Telos stress radiograph posterior displacement: 2.2 mm	NA	No difference in outcome between groups
Tibia: IS and screw and washer	Lysholm: 85 IKDC: 14 N/NN, 3 A, 1 SA	2.0 mm	NA	
Femur: IS Tibia: screw and washer	OAK score: 92.5; 7 excellent, 4 good IKDC: 11/11 were N/NN	Stress radiographs: 3.4 mm side-side difference; KT side-side difference, 1.8 mm	NA	
Femur: IS; tibia: screw and post	Lysholm: 92 (24 excellent/ good, 6 fair/poor) Tegner: 4.5	NA	Grade I: 16 grade II: 12 grade III: 3	Significant correlation between poor results and more chronic injuries
Femur: IS Tibia: IS	Lysholm: 94 IKDC: 25 N/NN, 2 A/SA	KT side-side difference <2 mm: 17 patients 3-4 mm, 6 patients	Grade 0/I: 23 grade II: 1	No correlation between time from injury to surgery and outcome
Tibia: suture and post Femur: metal IS	Lysholm: 90.63 IKDC: 18 N/NN, 4 A/SA	Average postoperative KT posterior drawer: 3.72 mm	NA	1 patient had stiffness 86% had normal radiographs
Tibia: screw and washer Femur: screw and washer	Lysholm: 91.44 IKDC: 22 N/NN, 5 A/SA	Average postoperative KT posterior drawer: 4.11 mm		1 patient had stiffness 92% had normal radiographs
Tibia and femur: metal IS	Lysholm: 94 Tegner: 5.4 IKDC: 19 N/NN, 5 A/SA	KT side-side differences: 6, 0-2 mm 13, 3.5 mm 3, 6-10 mm 2, >10 mm	NA	Significant correlation between poor results and more chronic injuries

Transtibial Versus Tibial Inlay

Several case series have compared the outcomes of transtibial and tibial inlay methods of PCL reconstruction. No significant difference in clinical outcome scores between the two techniques have been identified. The details of these studies are outlined in Table 99-2. MacGillivray et al.[55] evaluated 20 patients who underwent reconstruction of an isolated PCL injury. The mean follow-up was 5.7 years. Thirteen patients underwent transtibial reconstruction and seven underwent tibial inlay, all with a single-bundle graft. These investigators found that the posterior drawer improved in 57% of patients in the inlay group and in 38% in the transtibial group. No significant difference in Tegner, Lysholm, or American Academy of Orthopaedic Surgeons knee scores was found between the two groups. The investigators concluded that neither method predictably restores original laxity and that there was no difference in outcome scores.

Seon and Song[71] retrospectively reviewed 21 isolated transtibial and 22 tibial inlay reconstructions. They found a significant improvement in Lysholm knee scores in both groups but no intergroup differences. Postoperative Tegner scores were also improved in both groups. Final follow-up found normal or grade I laxity on posterior drawer in 19 patients in the transtibial group and in 20 patients in the inlay group. Mean side-to-side differences were also improved, with no significant difference between the two groups. The authors concluded that the transtibial and inlay techniques resulted in relatively good clinical and objective outcomes and are both satisfactory options for reconstruction. Kim et al.[108] compared three different PCL reconstruction techniques. Twenty-nine patients underwent single- or double-bundle arthroscopic tibial inlay reconstruction or transtibial single bundle reconstruction. These investigators found a significant difference in postoperative posterior tibial translation when the double-bundle tibial inlay group was compared with the single-bundle transtibial group, with less translation in the former. Although they noted a difference in translation, they found no significant difference in postoperative Lysholm scores or range of motion.

Single Versus Double Bundle

A number of in vivo studies have compared single-bundle and double-bundle PCL reconstructions. Yoon et al.[124] prospectively followed up 53 patients who underwent single- or double-bundle reconstruction. All reconstructions were performed with a transtibial approach using Achilles tendon allograft and had a minimum of 2-year follow-up. At final follow-up, patients were evaluated for range of motion and posterior stability using stress radiography and by subjective knee scoring. The authors found no significant difference in range of motion, Tegner activity scores, Lysholm scores, and IKDC evaluation. The only difference that could be identified was in posterior laxity. Both groups had improved stability postoperatively; however, the double-bundle group had less posterior translation with a difference of 1.4 mm, which was statistically significant. Although they did have less instability on objective testing, the patients' clinical outcomes as measured by subjective scoring were the same in both groups.

Several studies to date have shown no significant differences in subjective or objective results between single- and double-bundle PCL graft reconstructions. Wang et al.[120] prospectively compared single- and double-bundle PCL reconstruction using hamstring autograft. No significant differences were observed between the two groups with regard to functional score, ligament laxity, and radiographic changes of the knee. Hatayama and colleagues[83] were also unable to detect a difference in posterior tibial translation between patients treated with single- compared with double-bundle PCL reconstruction. Similarly, in a comparison of bone–patellar tendon–bone in one femoral tunnel compared with hamstring autograft in two tunnels, Houe and Jorgensen[82] found no difference in postoperative laxity or Lysholm and Tegner scores.

Complications

The complications of PCL reconstruction include the more common problems that occur with orthopaedic surgery, such as infection and stiffness. In addition, some complications are associated with the specific nature of the procedure. One of the most common problems after PCL reconstruction is persistent posterior laxity. Hermans et al.[105] found that 11 patients in a case series of 25 patients had a positive quadriceps active test after surgery. In addition, four patients required hardware removal because of soreness, and one patient required open capsular release for postoperative arthrofibrosis and decreased range of motion. The exact incidence of complication after PCL reconstruction is unknown.

Vascular injury during PCL reconstruction is rare but is a known complication. Nemani et al.[106] reported on a case involving a popliteal venotomy that occurred during PCL reconstruction in the setting of a previous popliteal artery bypass graft. In this case the patient had sustained a knee dislocation with vascular injury. During the PCL reconstruction, the popliteal vein was found to be adherent to the PCL remnant, and a venotomy was noted after debridement. The authors recommend caution in the setting of previous surgery because the relationship of the neurovascular structures can be altered. Although complications appear to be uncommon, the clinician should have a frank discussion with the patient preoperatively to discuss the potential risks associated with the procedure.

Future Considerations

The optimal treatment for the PCL-deficient knee remains unclear. Future studies will help to better define the indications for the different treatment options. These studies will attempt to overcome the limitations of prior investigations. A need exists for randomized and prospectively designed studies with controlled variables that will allow clinicians to draw definitive conclusions. The difficulties encountered in PCL study design have been discussed, but small sample size due to low incidence is probably one of the most significant. Multicenter trials will likely be required to achieve the necessary power to derive treatment recommendations. Conducting multicenter trials is difficult because of different surgical indications and methods of reconstruction that would need to be controlled. Future efforts should focus on overcoming these limitations and thus providing data that could help elucidate the best treatment recommendations for PCL injuries.

TABLE 99-2

RESULTS OF ISOLATED POSTERIOR CRUCIATE LIGAMENT RECONSTRUCTION: TRANSTIBIAL VERSUS INLAY

Study	No. of Patients	Age (yr)	Follow-up (yr)	Chronicity/ Grade	Graft Type	Surgical Technique	Fixation	Subjective Outcome	Instrumented Laxity*	Posterior Drawer	Miscellaneous
Kim et al. (2009),[108] retrospective	Group T (transtibial): 8	32.4	3.9	Average time to surgery, 9.4 mo; all grade III	Achilles allograft in all cases	Transtibial single bundle	Tibia: bio IS Femur: bio IS	Lysholm: 86.9	Telos side-to-side difference: 5.6 mm	NA	Significant difference in posterior translation between groups T and I2 No significant difference in Lysholm scores
	Group I1 (inlay): 11	31.9	I1: 3.0			AS inlay single bundle	Tibia: bio IS and washer Femur: bio IS	Lysholm: 79.7	4.7 mm		
	Group I2 (inlay): 10	33.6	I2: 2.5			AS inlay double bundle	Tibia: bio IS and washer Femur: bio IS	Lysholm: 84.3	3.6 mm		
Seon & Song (2006),[71] retrospective	Group A (transtibial): 21	29.1	2.6	All chronic; all grade II or greater	Hamstring autograft;	Transtibial	Tibia: bio IS Femur: anchor screw	Lysholm: 91.3 Tegner: 5.6	Telos side-side difference: 3.7 mm	19 normal/ grade I 2 grade II	No significant differences between groups
	Group B (tibial inlay): 22	29.4	3.0		Patellar tendon autograft	Tibial inlay	Tibia: screw and washer Femur: bio IS screw	Lysholm: 92.8 Tegner: 6.1	Telos side-side difference: 3.3 mm	20 normal/ grade I 2 grade II	
MacGillivray et al (2006),[55] retrospective	Group I (transtibial): 13	29	6.3	All chronic 5 grade II 8 grade III	Mixed	Transtibial	Tibia: IS Femur: IS	Lysholm: 81 Tegner: 6	KT posterior drawer: 5.9 mm	3 grade I 6 grade II 4 grade III	Neither method restored anteroposterior stability to the knee
	group II (tibial inlay): 7	31	4.8	3 grade II 4 grade III		Tibial inlay	Tibia: screw/ washer Femur: IS	Lysholm: 76 Tegner: 6	KT posterior drawer: 5.5 mm	3 grade I 3 grade II 1 grade III	

AS, Arthroscopic; *bio*, biologic; *IS*, interference screw; *KT*, KT-1000 testing; *NA*, not available.

For a complete list of references, go to expertconsult.com.

Suggested Readings

Citation: Markolf KL, Zemanovic JR, McAllister DR: Cyclic loading of posterior cruciate ligament replacements fixed with tibial tunnel and tibial inlay methods. *J Bone Joint Surg Am* 84A(4):518–524, 2002.

Level of Evidence: Biomechanical study

Summary: Markolf and colleagues performed a cadaveric study comparing posterior cruciate ligament reconstruction fixed with tibial tunnel and tibial inlay techniques. Knees were subjected to 2000 cycles of tensile force of 50 to 300 N. The authors found that the inlay technique resulted in less graft failure and graft thinning.

Citation: McAllister DR, Petrigliano FA: Diagnosis and treatment of posterior cruciate ligament injuries. *Curr Sports Med Rep* 6(5):293–299, 2007.

Level of Evidence: Review

Summary: McAllister and Petrigliano reviewed current concepts in the diagnosis and treatment of posterior cruciate ligament injuries.

Citation: Yoon KH, Bae DK, Song SJ, et al: A prospective randomized study comparing arthroscopic single-bundle and double-bundle posterior cruciate ligament reconstructions preserving remnant fibers. *Am J Sports Med* 39(3):474–480, 2011.

Level of Evidence: II

Summary: Yoon and colleagues compared single- and double-bundle posterior cruciate ligament reconstruction in a prospective, randomized study. Although a small benefit was observed with regard to posterior laxity in the double-bundle group, no difference was seen with subjective outcome measures.

Citation: Margheritini F, Mariani P: Diagnostic evaluation of posterior cruciate ligament injuries. *Knee Surg Sports Traumatol Arthrosc* 11(5):282–288, 2003.

Level of Evidence: Review

Summary: In this review by Margheritini and Mariani, a focus is placed on the principles of diagnostic evaluation of posterior cruciate ligaments.

Citation: Fanelli GC, Edson CJ: Posterior cruciate ligament injuries in trauma patients: Part II. *Arthroscopy* 11(5):526–529, 1995.

Level of Evidence: IV

Summary: Fanelli and Edson offer one of the few studies on the incidence of PCL injuries in trauma patients with acute hemarthrosis of the knee. More than 200 acute knee injuries with hemarthrosis were reviewed. PCL injuries occurred in 38% of acute knee injuries; 56.5% were trauma patients, and 32.9% were sports related.

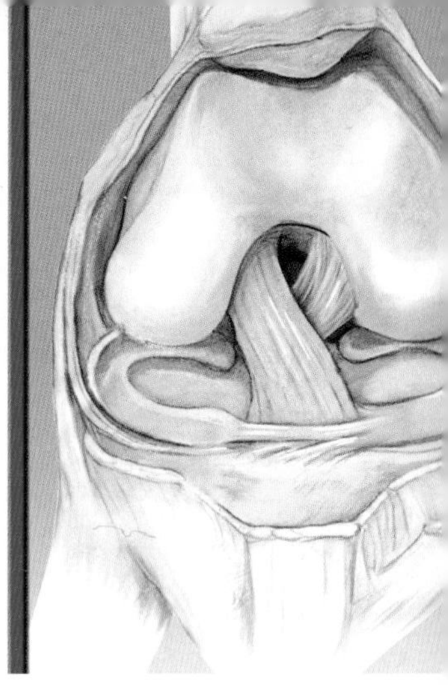

100

Medial Collateral Ligament and Posterior Medial Corner Injuries

BRIAN F. WILSON • DARREN L. JOHNSON

Medial ligament injuries of the knee are often assumed to be only medial collateral ligament (MCL) injuries. However, the medial ligament includes not only the MCL but also posteromedial structures that play a vital role in the stability of the knee. Recent work of LaPrade and colleagues[1,2] has demonstrated that the posterior oblique ligament (POL) is an important valgus and rotational stabilizer of the knee. The management of the MCL has evolved during the past 30 years. Most isolated MCL injuries are treated conservatively, with a rare role for surgical intervention. However, the treatment of MCL sprains with anterior cruciate ligament (ACL) injury (or any other concomitant ligamentous injury for that matter), along with the timing of ACL reconstruction, continue to be controversial. This chapter describes the anatomy of the medial knee (including the often forgotten posteromedial corner), evaluation of the knee, treatment of medial ligament injuries, and the role of rehabilitation.

History

The history will depend on whether the injury is witnessed by the physician on the sidelines or elicited from the patient in the clinic. Most of these injuries present in the office setting as potentially chronic conditions. A description of the mechanism of injury should be elicited in as much detail as possible. It is important to ascertain when the patient was hurt and how. Typically the injury is the result of a blow to the lateral aspect of the leg or lower thigh. The mechanism may be a result of a clipping injury in football or a noncontact injury from cutting, pivoting, or twisting. Skiers are prone to medial-side injuries, with 60% of skiing knee injuries affecting the MCL.[3,4] In addition, it is important to ask the patients about pain, onset of swelling, ability to ambulate, the sensation of a "pop," and the presence of a deformity necessitating a reduction, such as patellar dislocation or a more severe knee dislocation. In addition, a history of knee injuries or surgeries should be elicited because they can cloud an acute knee injury examination.

Physical Examination

Ideally, the examination of the knee should occur at the time of injury before the onset of muscle spasm. However, most of these injuries are examined in the office setting after some time has elapsed after the injury. A thorough knee examination includes observation of the patient's gait, documentation of the neurovascular status, palpation of the knee for tenderness, swelling, and ecchymosis, and assessment of stability. The physician should follow some basic principles: (1) assess the ligaments and muscles while the patient is as relaxed as possible, (2) perform the physical examination as gently as possible, and (3) examine the uninjured knee before assessing the injured knee.

The patient's gait should be observed as the patient walks into the room or at some point during the examination. Gait may be misleading, however, because patients with a complete MCL tear may walk with a barely perceptible limp. Hughston and colleagues[5,6] found that 50% of athletes with grade III injuries could walk into the office unassisted and reported that a complete disruption of the medial compartment can occur "without subsequent significant pain, effusion, or disability for walking." However, patients with an MCL tear may exhibit a vaulting-type gait in which the quadriceps is activated, allowing stabilization of the medial-sided structures during gait. This gait differs from that of a patient with an ACL or meniscus tear who may walk with a bent knee gait because of pain or an effusion. As with any orthopaedic injury, the neurovascular status of the limb should be assessed. Pedal pulses should be palpated and sensation should be assessed over the dorsum, plantar, and first web space of the foot. If a knee dislocation is a possibility, ankle brachial indices should be performed to evaluate for vascular injury. Compartments should be examined to rule out compartment syndrome. The ability to passive and actively dorsiflex and plantarflex the ankle and great toe should be assessed.

On the skin, the physician should look for edema, effusion, and ecchymosis to help localize the site of injury. It is important to differentiate between localized edema and an intraarticular effusion. Isolated MCL injuries usually have localized swelling. Hemarthrosis of the knee may indicate intraarticular pathology, such as an ACL or peripheral meniscal tear. Severe medial complex injuries with an ACL tear frequently show no evidence of effusion because the capsular rent is large enough to allow extravasation of fluid and blood. If hemarthrosis is present, the examiner should exclude other injuries such as a torn cruciate, patellar dislocation, an osteochondral fracture, and a peripheral meniscal tear. Along with assessment of swelling, palpation of the anatomic sites of attachment can provide clues to the diagnosis. The entire course of the MCL should be palpated from proximal to distal. Pain at the medial femoral epicondyle signifies injury at the femoral insertion of the MCL. With tibial-sided injuries, patients have pain along the proximal tibia around the pes anserine adjacent to the tibial tubercle. Mid-substance tears result in pain at the joint line, and such pain may also present with a medial meniscal injury, posing a diagnostic dilemma. Hughston and colleagues[5] showed that point tenderness can accurately identify the location of injury in 78% of cases, and localized edema can identify a tear in the medial meniscus 64% of the time. A valgus injury that disrupts the MCL may also result in lateral meniscus tears or osteochondral fracture to the lateral femoral condyle or lateral tibial plateau. Therefore a thorough examination of the lateral knee should also be performed.

Valgus stress testing at 30 degrees of knee flexion is still the gold standard for assessing isolated injury to the MCL. This test should be performed with the foot in external rotation because increased instability will be noted if the knee moves from internal to external rotation. To relax the hamstrings and quadriceps muscles, the thigh should rest on the examination table and the foreleg should move freely off the edge of the table at 30 degrees of flexion. The examiner then grasps the ankle and applies a valgus stress with the other hand resting on the medial side of the knee to assess the amount of opening and the quality of the end point compared with the uninjured side. The laxity of the MCL can be recorded based on a grading system or the amount of opening. According to the Noyes classification, 5 to 8 mm of medial opening signifies a significant collateral ligament injury with "impairment of the ligament's restraining effect."[7] The grading system has three grades: (1) stress examination produces little to no opening with pain along the line of the collateral ligament; (2) some opening to stress occurs but with a firm end point; and (3) significant opening of the joint occurs with no end point. After assessing the degree of opening, a repeat valgus stress should be performed with the examiner palpating the medial meniscus to assess if it subluxates in and out of the joint, indicative of injury to the meniscotibial ligament.[8]

In addition to valgus testing in flexion, opening of the medial joint should be assessed with the knee in full extension. The cruciate ligaments, POL, posteromedial capsule, and MCL all contribute to knee stability in full extension. Asymmetric joint opening compared with the contralateral side should alert the physician to the possibility of a combined MCL injury with a cruciate tear or posteromedial complex injury. If any increased laxity is observed in full extension compared with the uninvolved knee, it is unlikely that an isolated MCL injury is present; rather, it is likely that the patient has a concomitant injury to the posteromedial capsule and POL in addition to the MCL lesion. The ACL should be assessed with the Lachman test because the pivot shift is difficult to perform as a result of guarding and the loss of the pivot axis with medial instability. In addition, the posterior cruciate ligament and lateral ligamentous structures should be examined. Along with cruciate injury, patellar instability and tearing of the vastus medialis obliquus are associated with laxity in full extension. Hunter and colleagues[9] found 18 of 40 laterally displaceable patellae on stress radiographs in patients with medial-sided injuries and a 9% to 21% incidence of damage to the extensor mechanism with medial ligament injury. In addition to valgus testing at 30 and 0 degrees, the Slocum modified anterior drawer test and an anterior drawer test in external rotation should be performed to assess for medial-sided injuries (Table 100-1).

Imaging

Radiography, arthrography, magnetic resonance imaging (MRI), and arthroscopy can provide information regarding knee injuries. Radiography with anteroposterior, lateral, and sunrise views should be performed for both knees. These radiographs should be evaluated for occult fractures, the lateral capsular sign (Segond fracture), ligamentous avulsions, old Pellegrini-Stieda lesions (i.e., an old MCL injury) (Fig. 100-1), and loose bodies. In adolescent and pediatric patients, stress radiographs help differentiate between physeal and ligamentous injuries.

MRI without contrast is the imaging study of choice for evaluating MCL tears because it is less invasive than other studies and provides detail for lesions of the medial meniscus, superficial MCL, POL, posteromedial complex, and semimembranosus tendon (Fig. 100-2). In addition, MRI is beneficial in assessing injuries to anterior and posterior cruciate ligaments, the meniscus, and osteochondral structures. Loredo and associates[10] showed that intraarticular contrast may help highlight and better define the structures of the posteromedial complex but still concluded that the assessment of the posteromedial complex was difficult. They found that the posteromedial complex was best visualized on coronal and axial images. Indelicato and Linton[11] stated that MRI can provide advantages in four circumstances: (1) when the status of the ACL remains uncertain despite physical examination; (2) when the status of the meniscus is in question; (3) when surgical repair of the MCL is indicated and localization of the tear will help limit the exposure; and (4) when an unexplainable effusion occurs during rehabilitation. However, MRI does not always provide concrete diagnosis, and the clinical examination becomes the deciding factor. Examination after administration of an anesthetic is another tool the physician can use to assess the injury pattern in patients who present long after an injury has occurred or in patients for whom the office examination and MRI do not provide a diagnosis. Upon examination with use of an anesthetic, Norwood and coworkers[12] found that 18% of patients had anterolateral rotatory instability that was not suspected preoperatively. In addition to MRI, arthrograms can be used to evaluate meniscal disease and capsular tearing with extravasation of contrast material. Kimori and colleagues[13] found arthrography to be more useful than arthroscopy in diagnosing tears of the meniscotibial and meniscofemoral ligaments.

With the increased use of MRI, arthroscopy is used infrequently as a diagnostic tool. ACL and meniscal tears may be identified on MRI. Also, it is rare to find an intrasubstance medial meniscal tear in an isolated MCL rupture because meniscocapsular separation occurs, and thus the fulcrum to load the medial compartment and tear the medial meniscus is lost.

Decision-Making Principles

When considering treatment of the MCL, one must remember that most MCL injuries heal reliably with conservative management. For injuries that are chronic or involve the posterior oblique ligament or for concomitant ligamentous injuries, the debate continues regarding nonoperative versus surgical treatment. Other associated injuries or rotational instability resulting from a POL injury may require surgical treatment. Surgical

TABLE 100-1

METHODS FOR EXAMINING THE MEDIAL COLLATERAL LIGAMENT

Examination	Technique	Grading	Significance
Valgus stress at 0 and 30 degrees	Valgus force applied to tibia while stabilizing the femur; this should be done at 0 and 30 degrees of flexion and compared with the opposite leg	Grade I: 0- to 5-mm opening, firm end point Grade II: 5- to 10-mm opening, firm end point Grade III: 10- to 15-mm opening, soft end point	Opening at 30 degrees occurs from isolated MCL injuries; valgus stress at 0 degrees is associated with other ligament tears (anterior cruciate ligament, posterior collateral ligament, or posterior oblique ligament)
The Slocum modified anterior drawer test	Valgus force in 15 degrees of external rotation and 80 degrees of flexion	This test is positive if there is a noticeably increased prominence of the medial condyle compared with the other side	The disruption of the deep MCL allows the meniscus to move freely and allows the medial tibial plateau to rotate anteriorly, leading to an increased prominence of the medial tibial condyle
Anterior drawer test in external rotation	Anterior drawer test at 90 degrees of knee flexion with an external rotation applied to proximal tibia	This test is positive if a noticeably increased anterior translation of the medial condyle is present	A disruption of the MCL alone should not lead to an increased anteromedial translation; an increased anteromedial translation indicates an anteromedial rotatory instability that involves an injury of the posteromedial structures

MCL, Medial collateral ligament.

management of chronic laxity of the medial structures can be quite difficult, and therefore anatomic repair of the medial support structures in the acute setting is preferred when indicated. With most MCL injuries, clinical outcomes will be satisfactory after a period of immobilization and recovery of motion and strength, followed by progressive activities. In the small subset of patients with continued pain, instability, or impaired performance, surgical management must be considered.

A review of literature for nonoperative versus operative treatment of complete isolated MCL injuries does not delineate the site of injury. The site of injury may have a role in the functional recovery of patients who place a high demand on their knees. In our practice caring for Division I collegiate

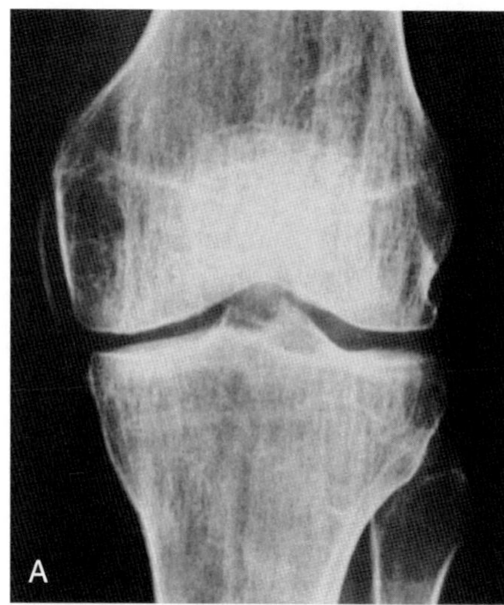

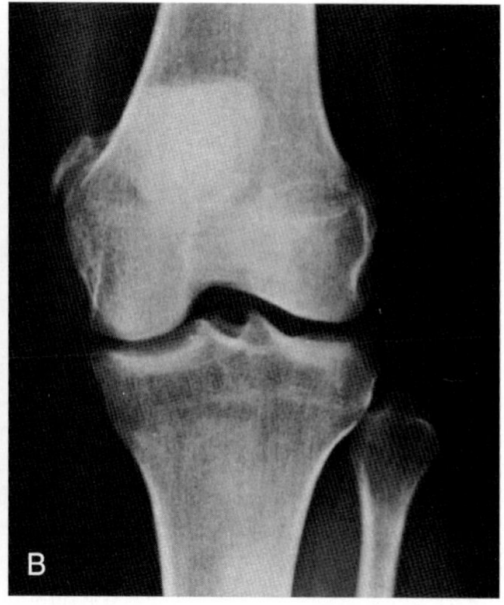

FIGURE 100-1 **A** and **B,** A Pellegrini-Stieda lesion. *(From Pavlov H: Radiology for the orthopedic surgeon.* Contemp Orthop *6:85, 1993.)*

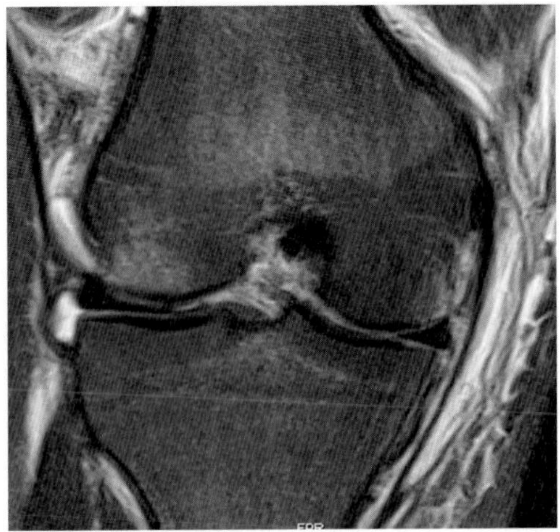

FIGURE 100-2 Magnetic resonance image showing a medial collateral ligament tear.

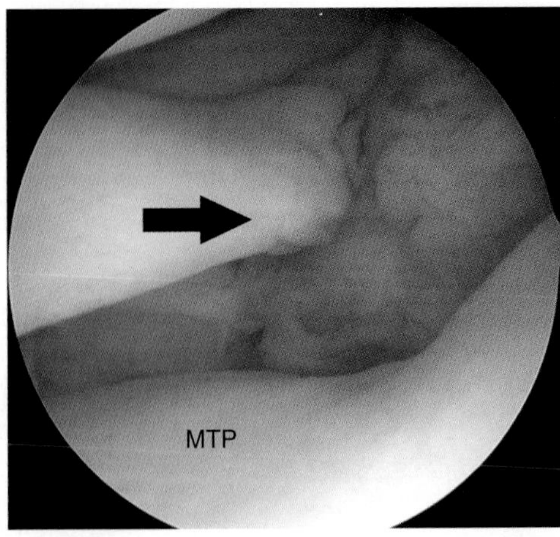

FIGURE 100-3 Arthroscopic image of the medial compartment of the knee. The *arrow* points to the posterior horn of the medial meniscus avulsion injury. *MTP,* Medial tibial plateau.

athletes, several complete injuries of the MCL off the tibial insertion failed to heal reliably with nonoperative treatment. After recovery, athletes may have varying amounts of valgus knee instability, preventing return to competitive sports and resulting in dysfunction in activities of daily living. Most MCL sprains should be treated nonoperatively. Complete avulsions of the superficial and deep MCL from the tibia with disruption of the meniscal coronary ligament have a poorer prognosis with nonoperative treatment and may be optimally managed with acute surgical repair for improved valgus stability of the knee.

Before proceeding with a treatment plan, it is essential to know the extent of injury. Initially we perform a thorough history and physical examination. With MCL injuries, we assess the grade of injury of the MCL and any associated ligamentous, meniscal, posteromedial corner, or patellar injuries. We obtain radiographs as a routine diagnostic tool to rule out fracture or any signs of chronic medial insufficiency (Pellegrini-Stieda lesion) and chronic ACL deficiency (the deep femoral notch sign, peaked tibial spines, or a cupula lesion). The use of MRI is dependent on the grade of the MCL lesion and associated injury. Isolated grade I or II injuries can be diagnosed with clinical examination and do not require MRI. However, in a grade I or II injury with an indeterminate cruciate examination and effusion, we order an MRI. We also obtain MRI for all grade III injuries because the site of involvement—tibia or femur—is important in our decision making, particularly the extent of injury to the POL and posteromedial capsule. With grade III laxity in full extension and complete involvement of the POL and capsule, avulsion of the posterior horn of the medial meniscus root may be seen (Fig. 100-3) and demands surgical intervention. In addition, most grade III lesions are associated with concomitant ligamentous injuries. Our treatment algorithm is outlined in Figure 100-4.

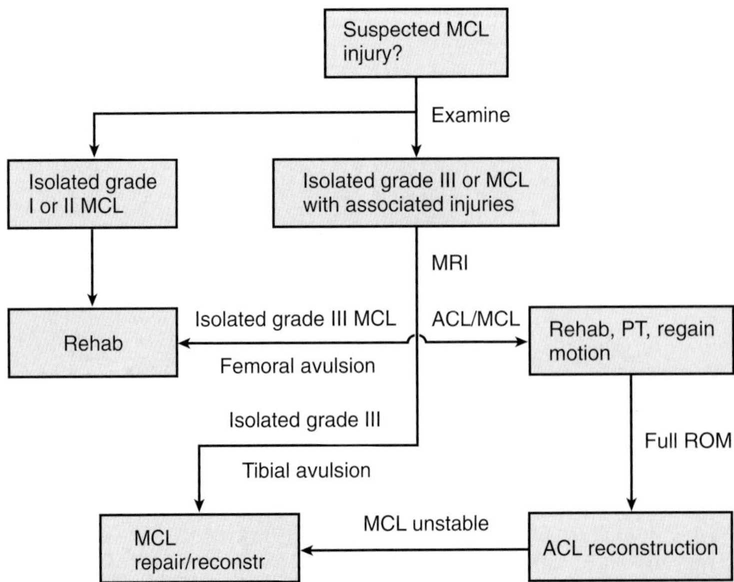

FIGURE 100-4 Algorithm for treatment of medial collateral ligament (MCL) injuries. *ACL,* Anterior cruciate ligament; *PT,* physical therapy; *ROM,* range of motion.

Management of grade III injuries is much more controversial. Even with physical examination and advanced imaging, it remains difficult to gauge the extent of damage to the POL and posteromedial capsule in combined injuries. The treatment of grade III MCL sprains has significantly evolved during the past 20 years. The general consensus has been to treat isolated grade III injuries conservatively. We believe that the treatment of grade III injury is dependent not only on the specific location of the MCL rupture but also the degree of laxity on physical examination, as well as the degree of the arthroscopic drive-through sign. The extent of injury and laxity of the injury to the POL and posterior capsule is instrumental in our decision making. Nonoperative management of these injuries may lead to a rotational instability in addition to valgus laxity, which is not well tolerated by athletes involved in pivoting sports. Grade III injuries not only involve complete disruption of its fibers but also are frequently associated with additional ligamentous injuries.

Treatment Options

Management of the MCL and medial-sided knee injuries can be divided into operative and nonoperative approaches. Numerous factors, including the timing, severity, location, and associated injuries such as an ACL tear need to be taken into account when formulating a treatment plan. The MCL has the greatest capacity to heal of any of the four major knee ligaments because of its anatomic and biologic properties.[14,15] As a result of multiple biomechanical, clinical, and functional studies, the trend has been toward a conservative, nonsurgical method for most MCL injuries.

Grade I and II isolated tears of the MCL generally respond well to nonoperative management. Partial tears are treated routinely with temporary immobilization and protected weight bearing with crutches. Once the swelling subsides, range of motion, resistive exercises, and progressive weight bearing are initiated. Nonsteroidal antiinflammatory drugs can be used to help with pain and swelling. Studies have shown no deleterious effect of nonsteroidal drugs on ligament healing.[16]

Management of grade III injuries remains much more controversial. Even with physical examination and advanced imaging, it remains difficult to gauge the extent of damage to the POL and posteromedial capsule in combined injuries. Nonoperative management of these injuries may lead to a rotational instability in addition to valgus laxity, which is not well tolerated by athletes involved in pivoting sports. Grade III injuries not only involve complete disruption of its fibers but also are frequently associated with additional ligamentous injuries. Recently, posteromedial corner injuries have been recognized as a separate entity from MCL injuries and may need to be addressed more aggressively because of rotational laxity and instability that can result from their injury.[1,2,17]

Anatomic medial knee reconstruction has been described recently in the literature.[2,18,19] For grade III injuries requiring surgery, the reconstruction techniques addressing the posterior oblique ligament offer improved clinical stability and restoration of knee mechanics.[1,20-23]

AUTHORS' PREFERRED TECHNIQUE

Medial Collateral Ligament Injury

We treat isolated grade I and II MCL injuries conservatively. In the first 48 hours, we encourage rest and use of ice, compression, and elevation to help reduce swelling. In addition, we have all patients use a hinged knee brace and provide crutches for protected weight bearing. If patients have significant pain and valgus laxity, initially we lock the brace in extension. Once the swelling subsides and pain is improved, we encourage aggressive range-of-motion exercises and straight leg raises with quadriceps exercises. Once the patient has regained full range of motion and ambulation without a limp, use of crutches and the brace can be discontinued. Stationary bicycle and progressive resistive exercises are instituted as tolerated. Once full range of motion and 80% strength of the opposite side have been achieved, closed-chain kinetic exercises and jogging are allowed. Once athletes have achieved 75% of the maximal running speed, sport-specific training is allowed. Return to sports is permitted after the patient has strength, agility, and proprioception equal to the other side. We recommend a functional brace for contact or high-risk sports.

Patients with grade I sprains usually return to sports in 10 to 14 days; because immobilization is temporary, these patients regain strength and motion quickly. However, return to play after grade II sprains is much more variable. With grade II sprains, the period of immobilization can be up to 3 weeks to allow the pain to dissipate. Therefore patients can lose more strength and motion with increased time of immobilization compared with patients with grade I sprains. Patients are allowed to return to play when they have equal strength of both knees and no pain is experienced with valgus stress.

The treatment of grade III MCL sprains has significantly evolved during the past 20 years. The general consensus has been to treat isolated grade III injuries conservatively. We believe that the treatment of grade III injury is dependent not only on the specific location of the MCL rupture but also the degree of laxity on physical examination, as well as the degree of the arthroscopic drive-through sign. The extent of injury and laxity of the injury to the POL and posterior capsule is instrumental in our decision making.

Diagnostic arthroscopy is performed initially to evaluate intraarticular injuries. The medial opening is assessed arthroscopically, termed the "medial drive-through" finding. This part of the examination is critical in that it indicates where the MCL injury is primarily based and where it will be necessary to operate and perform a repair. For femoral-sided MCL injuries, the medial meniscus remains reduced with the tibia upon valgus opening (i.e., a gap forms above the medial meniscus). On the other hand, tibial-sided MCL injuries demonstrate that the medial meniscus remains reduced with the femur on valgus opening (i.e., a gap forms between

Continued

medial meniscus and tibia, with the medial meniscus lifting off the tibia).

With valgus opening of the knee during arthroscopic examination, it may be observed whether the knee opens posteriorly to the medial meniscus, particularly as the knee is slowly extended with valgus load. If the capsule is exposed with this maneuver posteriorly, the patient has an injury of the POL and posterior medial capsule, which needs to be addressed at the time of surgical correction.

If the injury is acute, medial repair is attempted. For chronic injuries, the medial structures are repaired and reconstructed or augmented.

For acute repair, the origins and insertions of the deep and superficial MCL are evaluated. Typically the lesion is on the tibial side. Isolated femoral-sided lesions often heal reliably without surgical repair.

The surgical approach is a fairly easy one in that the incision is similar to a hamstring harvest incision, except the length of the incision is longer in the proximal direction. The surgical incision is longitudinal between the tibial tubercle and the medial aspect of the knee. This exposure is carried from the inferior margin of the superficial MCL and may be taken proximally to the femoral insertion if required. The sartorial fascia is incised to expose the MCL. The hamstrings are retracted for dissection deeper to the MCL insertion to the tibia.

The initial approach is made from the inferior aspect of the lesion by placing grasping tension sutures in the entire MCL structure. Careful dissection is performed while lifting it off the tibia with a scalpel or periosteal elevator, following its course superiorly and posteriorly. Following the MCL structures superior to the medial joint line and exposing the insertion of the deep MCL results in further dissection.

Repair of the deep MCL insertion is performed by placing multiple suture anchors from posterior to anterior along the tibial joint line; four anchors with double-loaded nonabsorbable sutures are typically used.

Sutures are then passed through the deep and superficial MCL structures and tied down to the tibia while maintaining tension on the grasping sutures placed at the start of dissection. Tying of sutures to the tibial insertion is performed at 30 degrees of flexion with a varus load applied to the knee. The tibial insertion of the superficial MCL is often secured to the tibia with a large fragment screw and spiked-washer construct distally with the grasping sutures.

Posteriorly to the repaired MCL structures, the POL and capsular tissue are reefed from multiple posterior to anterior directed sutures, typically figure-8 sutures or horizontal mattress sutures. The objective is to take the laxity and slack out of the medial POL, which helps tighten the rotational instability caused from the injury.

Chronic medial-sided injuries are also assessed initially with arthroscopy. As previously described, the liftoff test is performed in a valgus maneuver to the knee. If the medial meniscus lifts off the tibia with valgus stress to the knee, we approach reconstruction of the tibial side. If the medial meniscus stays to the tibia with valgus stress to the knee, it is a more femoral-based injury. Surgical exposure and approach is the same as stated previously in the acute repair.

For chronic MCL injury reconstructions, if postoperative stiffness is not a concern or if the patient has an isolated MCL injury, an autograft hamstring tendon is harvested in the same surgical incision. Otherwise, allograft tendon is used for reconstruction.

The deep MCL structures and capsule are repaired to the anatomic origin and insertion of the femur and tibia with suture anchors and double-loaded with nonabsorbable sutures, as described previously for the acute injury repair. The tissue is reefed to remove laxity and slack in the injured structures. Augmentation with the autograft or allograft is performed once this maneuver is complete.

To augment the repair, autograft semitendinosus hamstring is harvested with an open-ended tendon stripper, leaving the distal attachment intact to the tibia at the pes anserine. The muscle tissue is cleaned from the semitendinosus tendon proximally with a large periosteal elevator, and a nonabsorbable whipstitch suture is placed in the free end of the tendon. All accessory attachments of the semitendinosus distally are carefully freed. A Kirschner wire is inserted at the medial epicondyle. The tendon is looped over the wire and the isometry of the tendon is evaluated with the knee in flexion and extension. If the excursion is more than 2 mm, the wire is moved to a position of isometry. Once isometry is confirmed, a large fragment screw and spiked washer are placed provisionally in the femur without fully setting the head at that isometric position of the medial femoral epicondyle. A bone trough is made around the screw shank. The tendon is looped around the screw. The screw is then tightened to the femur with the knee in 30 degrees if flexion, and varus stress is applied to the knee.

A right-angled hemostat is used to create a window in the direct head semimembranosus tendon attachment of the femur posteriorly. The free end of the semitendinosus tendon autograft is then directed posterior and obliquely and pulled through this window, recreating the central arm of the POL. The autograft is sutured to the semimembranosus tendon with use of a nonabsorbable suture.

If an allograft tendon is used, the aforementioned technique is modified, with attachment of the tibial limb of the allograft augment secured to the tibial insertion of the superficial MCL with another large fragment screw and spiked-washer fixation.

For multiple ligamentous knee injuries, the ACL is reconstructed and the medial structures are addressed with the previously described techniques depending on the time from injury.

A case example is that of a 16-year-old high school football player who sustained a contact MCL and ACL injury that was treated operatively in a staged fashion (Figs. 100-5 to 100-7). After treatment, he was allowed full return to contact sports 1 year from injury. Although most femoral-sided tears can be treated successfully with conservative methods, complete tibial-sided avulsions of the deep and superficial MCL, although rare, often heal with residual laxity.[24] In athletes who participate in level I sports, we frequently favor operative repair of these tibial-sided complete avulsions that display retraction of the deep or superficial MCL on MRI (see Fig. 100-8). Figures 100-8 and 100-9

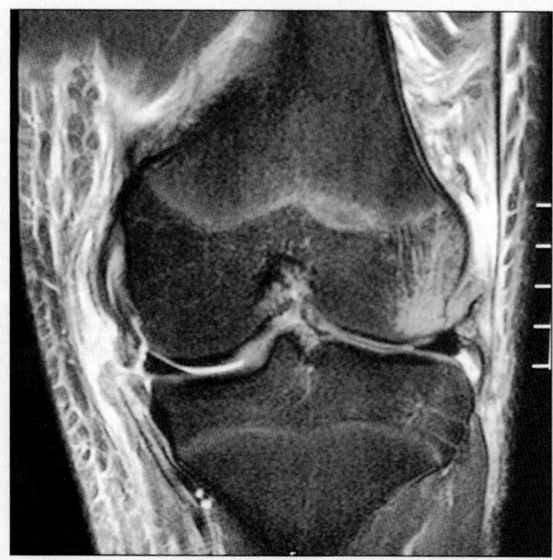

FIGURE 100-5 Coronal magnetic resonance image shows complete avulsion of the superficial and deep medial collateral ligament with an unattached medial meniscus.

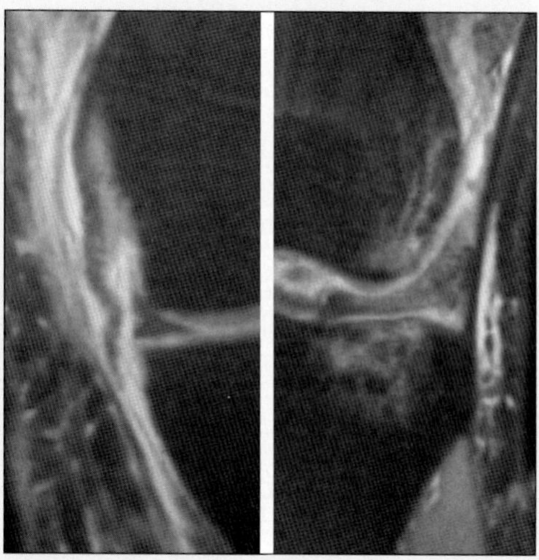

FIGURE 100-8 A coronal magnetic resonance image shows tibial-sided avulsion of the medial collateral ligament with retraction and a contrecoup bipolar bone bruise lesion laterally, which suggest a high-energy injury pattern.

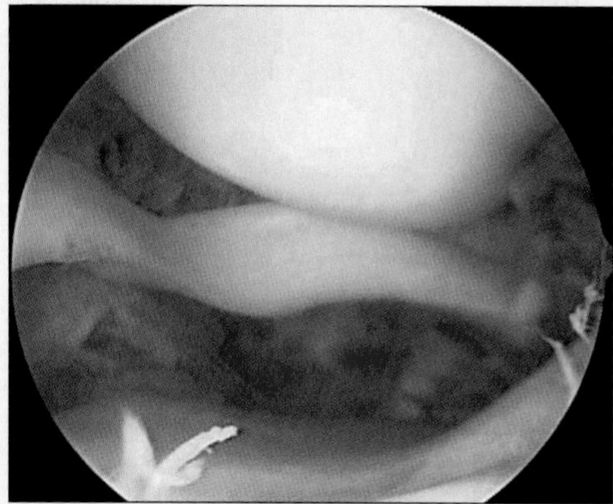

FIGURE 100-6 Arthroscopy confirms gross laxity of the medial compartment with complete disruption of medial support structures and a free-floating meniscus.

highlight a case example of a Division I football player with an isolated tibial-sided complete MCL avulsion with gross laxity and an impressive arthroscopic drive-through sign that was treated surgically.

Our rehabilitation protocol for grade III lesions is placement in a long-leg hinged knee brace locked in extension with weight bearing as tolerated on crutches for 2 weeks. After approximately 2 weeks we unlock the brace during weight bearing. In the first 4 weeks, our goal is to have the patient attain nearly full range of motion and normal gait pattern with full weight bearing in a hinged knee brace and begin quadriceps and hamstring strengthening.

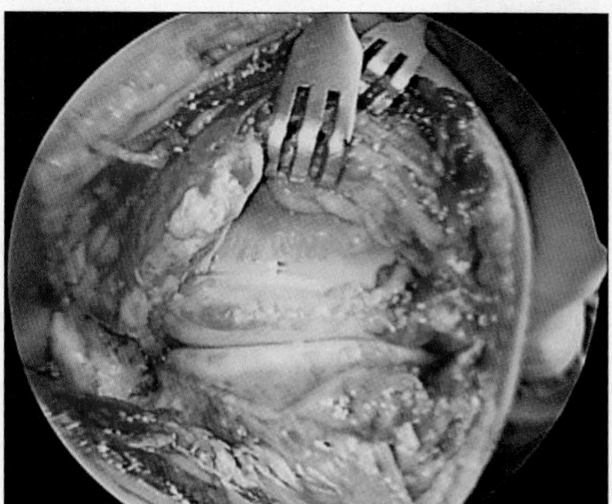

FIGURE 100-7 Open surgery confirms complete avulsion of the medial collateral ligament from the tibia with a free-floating, unattached medial meniscus between the articular cartilage of the medial femoral condyle and the tibial plateau.

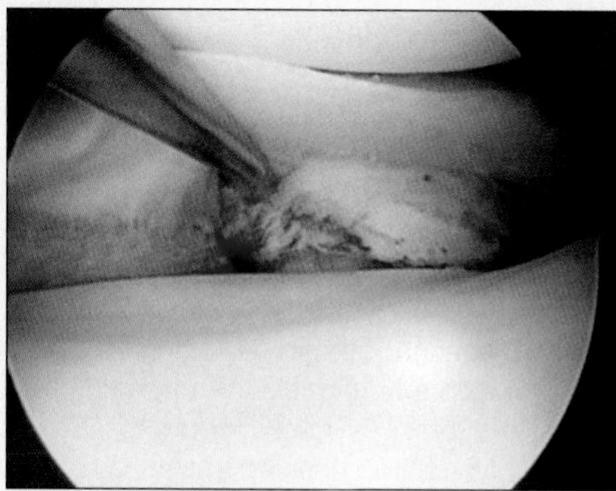

FIGURE 100-9 Arthroscopy confirms a drive-through sign with liftoff of the medial meniscus from the tibia requiring open repair of medial structures.

Continued

In contrast, patients who undergo a repair of the MCL follow a different protocol. Postoperatively, a hinged knee brace is locked from 30 to 90 degrees for 3 weeks, followed by unlimited motion. Weight bearing is limited for 3 weeks with crutches and then progressed to full weight by 4 to 6 weeks. Bracing is discontinued at 6 weeks and nonimpact conditioning is allowed, with running started by 3 months.

Chronic laxity of the medial support structures after nonoperative management is difficult to treat. A firefighter we treated after nonoperative management of his grade III medial lesion had chronic medial instability, which for him was a significant safety issue for performance of his duties as a firefighter. Figure 100-10 shows medial reconstruction of his POL and MCL using allograft tissue and performed anatomically as an isolated procedure for chronic medial stability.

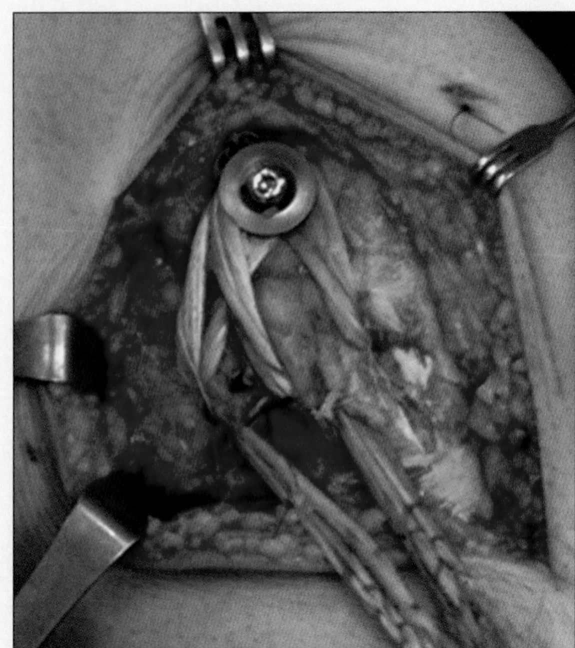

FIGURE 100-10 The medial side of the knee illustrating medial reconstruction of the medial collateral ligament and posterior oblique ligament using allograft tissue and performed anatomically.

Postoperative Management

The treatment of MCL injuries initially promotes nonoperative management, and thus rehabilitation is pivotal and is the primary modality for treatment. No one perfect rehabilitation protocol exists that will work for every athlete. Upon reviewing the literature, no apparent consensus exists regarding the most efficacious rehabilitation protocol, and protocols are usually based on surgeon preference and experience. Steadman,[25] Bergfeld,[26] O'Connor,[27] Cox,[28] and Wilk[29] have had excellent success with their individual protocols for treatment of MCL injuries. To effectively treat MCL injuries, the grade of the injury must be determined because the parameters of rehabilitation are based on the degree of injury. Table 100-2 shows the general principles for rehabilitation of MCL injuries.

Isolated grade I sprains are treated with rest, ice, compression, and elevation for the first couple of days to help reduce swelling. Patients are allowed weight bearing as tolerated with use of an assistive device if pain is experienced with walking. The only exception is patients with significant valgus deformity, because they will place more stress on the MCL, affecting healing. In these patients, it may be safer to allow partial weight bearing for a couple of weeks. With grade I MCL tears, immobilization in a brace is rarely required, and if patient compliance is of concern, a short leg hinged brace is used to control valgus and rotational stresses. Range of motion is begun immediately to prevent arthrofibrosis and stiffness. In addition, quadriceps strengthening and closed chain exercises are started. Once the patient regains full range of motion, resistive exercises are begun along with sport-specific drills.

Isolated grade II injuries are treated similarly to grade I injuries with rest, ice, elevation, and compression. Because grade II injuries involve a greater degree of damage to the ligament with increased valgus instability, a long-leg hinged brace is usually needed. Patients are allowed to progressively bear weight as tolerated in the brace; however, if the patient is having significant pain, the brace can be locked in extension until the pain subsides, usually in 1 week. Assistive devices are used until the patient has a nonantalgic gait. Active range-of-motion exercises are started immediately. During the early period, quadriceps strengthening is performed in a non–weight-bearing fashion with straight leg raises, quadriceps-setting exercises, and electrical stimulation. Once the patient

TABLE 100-2

PRINCIPLES FOR REHABILITATION OF THE MEDIAL COLLATERAL LIGAMENT

Phase	Goals	Criteria for Progression
Maximal protection phase	Early protected ROM Decrease effusion and pain Prevent quadriceps atrophy	No increase in instability No increase in swelling Minimal tenderness Passive ROM at least 10 to 100 degrees
Moderate protection phase	Full painless ROM Restore strength Ambulation without crutches	No instability No swelling or tenderness Full painless ROM
Minimal protection phase	Increase strength and power	

ROM, Range of motion.

has achieved full range of motion and functional strength, proprioceptive and agility drills can be initiated.

Isolated grade III injuries usually involve disruption of both the superficial and deep fibers. Therefore the rehabilitation process is slower, and a longer period of immobilization is required.

The treatment of grade III injuries can be divided into stages. In the first phase (for about 4 weeks), the patient should wear a brace locked in extension and progressively increase weight bearing to attain a normal gait pattern. Also, the patient needs to perform range-of-motion exercises with eccentric strengthening of the quadriceps and hamstrings. In phase II, which lasts 4 to 6 weeks, the patient continues to attain full range of motion, unlocks the brace, and achieves quadriceps and hamstring strengthening. After 6 weeks, the brace can be discontinued if the patient has a nonantalgic gait and has regained quadriceps strength for daily ambulation. Phase III starts after 6 weeks and includes squatting, light jogging with agility drills, and continued strengthening to return to sports.

After surgical repair of an isolated MCL, the brace is locked at 30 degrees and the patient is allowed to perform toe-touch weight bearing for 3 weeks. The patient is encouraged to continue range of motion from 30 to 90 degrees. The patient also continues strengthening of the quadriceps and hamstring while wearing a brace. After 3 weeks, the patient is allowed to progress to full weight bearing with full-time brace wear to continue to protect the repair. The brace can be worn unlocked to allow free range of motion, as well as valgus and rotational stability. From 3 to 6 weeks, the goal is to restore full range of motion along with continued strengthening with closed kinetic chain exercises. After 6 weeks, the patient continues to progressively increase activities with resistive and sport-specific exercises.

Combined injuries of the MCL and ACL require additional steps compared with the rehabilitation of isolated MCL tears. Upon reviewing the literature on ACL and MCL injuries, as stated previously, conservative treatment of MCL injuries followed by surgical reconstruction of the ACL is the favored management in most patients. Initially the protocol focuses on the severity of the MCL injury. For example, a grade I MCL injury with an ACL injury will proceed with the protocol presented earlier for grade I injuries. The patient will quickly regain range of motion and functional strength, and then the surgeon can proceed with reconstruction of the ACL. Conversely, the patient with a grade III injury with an ACL injury will take much longer because of the slower protocol for type III injuries. Regaining range of motion and functional strength training may take 8 to 10 weeks, and therefore it will take longer to proceed with ACL reconstruction with a type III injury. The ACL is reconstructed accompanied by conservative treatment of the MCL, following the rehabilitation protocol for an ACL reconstruction. After a combined ACL reconstruction and medial-sided repair, the knee is braced in full extension, and a standard ACL protocol is followed with protected weight bearing. In a combined ACL and MCL injury, it is important to remember that ACL rehabilitation takes precedence over medial-sided repair.

For return-to-play guidelines, see Box 100-1.

BOX 100-1 Return-to-Play Guidelines

Full range of motion
No instability
Muscle strength 85% of the contralateral side
Proprioception ability is satisfactory
No tenderness over the medial collateral ligament
No effusion
Quadriceps strength; torque/body weight
Use of a lateral knee brace (if necessary)

Results

Numerous authors have shown excellent results with nonoperative treatment of grade I and II MCL tears.[30-33] Ellsasser and associates[30] looked at 74 knees in professional football players and achieved a 98% success rate with a nonoperative protocol. They had strict inclusion criteria to ensure an isolated MCL injury was present: (1) up to grade II laxity with a firm end point in flexion, (2) no instability to valgus stress in extension, (3) no significant rotatory or anteroposterior subluxation, (4) no significant effusion, and (5) normal stress radiograph findings. In this series, patients were treated with crutches, no brace, and progressive weight bearing. Based on their experience, Ellsasser and associates concluded that by 1 week, patients should progress to full extension, have no effusion, and perceive decreased tenderness. The players returned to football in 3 to 8 weeks. The only failure occurred in a patient with an osteochondral fracture that was found at later follow-up.

Derscheid and Garrick[31] performed a prospective study that examines 51 grade I and grade II MCL injuries in college football players. They used a nonoperative rehabilitation protocol with a knee immobilizer initially. Players with a grade I injury returned to full participation at an average of 10.6 days, and players with a grade II injury returned at an average of 19.5 days. At long-term follow-up, these patients showed slight increases in medial instability. Injured knees had a higher incidence of reinjury than did control knees, but this finding was not statistically significant. Bassett and associates[32] and Hastings[33] studied the use of a cast brace in treating isolated MCL ruptures. In both studies, early return to athletics was found with the use of the cast brace. Nonoperative treatment varies from casting to functional bracing to no bracing, and good outcomes occur with all three forms of treatment.

Fetto and Marshall[34] found an 80% incidence of concomitant ligamentous injuries with a grade III MCL tear, with 95% of the associated injuries being an ACL tear. Early authors recommend primary repair for grade III injuries. O'Donoghue[35] stressed the importance of immediate repair of complete tears of the MCL. Hughston and Barrett[36] supported primary repair of all medial structures, including the superficial MCL and POL. They believed that repair and advancement of the POL was key to restoring medial stability. Their results were good to excellent in 77% to 94% of patients. Muller[37] reported 65% good and 31% excellent results in repair of isolated grade III MCL injuries. He repaired the superficial MCL avulsion with screws and washers and intrasubstance tears with a combination of approximation and tension-relieving sutures. Hughston and Barrett,[36] O'Donoghue,[35] Muller,[37] Collins,[38] Kannus,[24] and most recently LaPrade and Wijdicks[1,2] have written that surgical intervention is necessary for complete ruptures of the MCL.

Although good results have been demonstrated with surgical repair of the MCL, many studies have focused on the nonoperative management of grade III MCL injuries. Fetto and Marshall[34] were among the first to assess outcomes after nonoperative treatment of grade III MCL injuries. They studied 265 MCL injuries and found that patients with grade II injuries did much better than patients with grade III injuries (97% compared with 73%). Initially in their study, all patients with grade III injuries underwent operative intervention. However, some patients with grade III injuries did not have an operation because of skin lesions and infection. At follow-up, patients with operative treatment of isolated MCL ruptures had no improved outcome compared with the nonsurgical group. This incidental finding led the way for more prospective studies to investigate the role of nonoperative treatment in patients with isolated grade III MCL injuries.

Indelicato[39] prospectively compared operative and nonoperative treatment of isolated third-degree ruptures. All patients underwent examination with use of an anesthetic and arthroscopy to rule out any other pathology, such as ACL and meniscal tears. Indelicato[39] found objectively stable knees in 15 of 16 patients treated operatively and in 17 of 20 patients treated nonoperatively. Both groups followed a rigid rehabilitation protocol including casting at 30 degrees of flexion for 2 weeks and then 4 weeks longer in a cast brace with hinges that allowed motion from 30 to 90 degrees. Subjective scores were higher in the nonsurgical group, with good to excellent results for 90% in the nonsurgical group and 88% in the surgically repaired group, suggesting that surgical intervention offered no benefit. Indelicato[39] also showed that patients treated with early motion returned to football 3 weeks earlier than did immobilized patients. In a subsequent study by Indelicato and associates,[40] they showed that a conservative approach in patients with complete MCL ruptures was successful in collegiate football players. All players were managed with a functional rehabilitation program, and 71% had good to excellent results.

Similar to Indelicato, both Reider and colleagues[41] and Jones and associates[42] found excellent outcomes in athletes with isolated grade III medial ligament injuries who were treated conservatively and agreed that nonoperative treatment of these lesions is justified. Reider and colleagues[41] studied 35 athletes who were treated with early functional rehabilitation for isolated grade III tears. Of these 35 athletes, 19 returned to full and unlimited activity in fewer than 8 weeks. At an average follow-up of 5.3 years, outcomes based on subjective and objective measurements were comparable with earlier investigations using a surgical repair. In 1985, Jones et al.[42] reported results for 24 high school football players who returned to competition at an average of 34 days. Management consisted of 1 week of immobilization followed by gradual range of motion and strengthening. The knee was tested weekly with valgus stress, and instability was reduced to grade 0 or 1 by 29 days. No increased incidence of reinjury was found the following spring.

Although Indelicato,[39] Fetto and Marshall,[34] Jones et al.,[42] and Reider et al.[41] found excellent results with nonoperative treatment, Kannus[24] studied 27 patients with grade III lesions at an average 9 years of follow-up. Patients were found to have poor outcomes (an average Lysholm score of 66) and degenerative changes on radiographs. Kannus[24] concluded that early surgical repair would prevent deterioration. A careful review of the patients showed that 16 of 27 had greater than a 2+ Lachman score, and 10 of 27 had anterolateral instability. Thus this study did not show that nonoperative treatment has poor outcomes but that associated injuries such as ACL injuries need to be addressed to prevent poor long-term outcome.

In recent more literature, the anatomic restoration of the medial knee structures has provided satisfactory outcomes. Lind et al.[18] described a technique to reconstruct the MCL and POL. The clinical results they published showed that 98% of their patients treated with this technique had normal or near normal International Knee Documentation Committee measures at follow-up of more than 2 years.[18]

LaPrade and associates[2] reported their technique and follow-up at an average of 1.5 years for reconstruction of the MCL and POL. Their outcomes showed improved International Knee Documentation Committee measures and decreased valgus opening on stress radiographs.

Combined injury to the MCL and ACL represents a completely different entity than an isolated MCL injury. The ACL is a primary restraint to anterior displacement and acts as a secondary stabilizer to valgus stress, especially in full extension. Conversely, the MCL is the primary restraint to valgus stress at 30 degrees of flexion. Therefore injury to the MCL and ACL results in both anterior and valgus instability and can significantly compromise knee function. Even though the apparent consensus is that a solitary MCL rupture can be treated nonoperatively, the optimal treatment for a concurrent ACL and MCL injury remains controversial. The extent of involvement of the posteromedial capsule and POL may help guide treatment strategies.

Two controversial studies regarding the management of combined ACL and MCL injuries have been reported in the literature. The first issue pertains to the various surgical options available for managing these injuries. Three principal surgical options exist: (1) surgical reconstruction and repair of both ligaments; (2) ACL reconstruction and nonoperative MCL management; and recently (3) operative management of MCL with nonoperative ACL treatment. ACL reconstruction with nonoperative management of the MCL remains the most popular option. The second controversial issue regarding combined injuries is whether early or late ACL reconstruction provides better functional and long-term results.

In years past, authors recommended surgical intervention for both ligamentous structures in concomitant ACL and MCL ruptures.[34,43,44] Fetto and Marshall[34] had 79% unsatisfactory outcomes in patients treated operatively for ACL and MCL tears. Even though studies have shown operative repair of all ligaments results in stable, functional knees, a high incidence of knee stiffness was found.[45-47] Other authors have stated that isolated operative MCL repair and nonoperative ACL reconstruction leads to good results. Hughston and Barrett[36] reported that 94% of their patients with combined ACL and MCL injury who were treated with only MCL reconstruction returned to their preinjury levels of athletic performance. They stated that the key to obtaining excellent results was reconstruction of the POL and posteromedial structures. Noyes and Barber-Westin[48] criticized the method used by Hughston and Barrett[36] method of reporting results and stated that the results may have been overly optimistic. However, Hughston[49] continued to report good results at 22 years of follow-up. In addition to Hughston, Shirakura and associates[50] reported excellent results in 14 patients with combined lesions but reconstruction of the MCL only; however, they did not report anteroposterior instability. Conversely, Frolke and coworkers[51] reported poor results with solitary MCL repair. They performed arthroscopically guided repair of the MCL, which led to functional stability in 68% of knees, but clinical testing of all 22 knees showed abnormal or severe abnormal examination findings.

Most authors suggest that nonoperative treatment of the MCL with reconstruction of the ACL provides good to excellent results. Shelbourne and Porter[52] demonstrated good to excellent results in 68 patients with ACL reconstruction and nonsurgical management of an MCL tear. They also showed that these patients achieved a greater range of motion and more rapid strength gains than did patients with surgical reconstruction and repair of both ligaments. Similarly, Noyes and Barber-Westin[48] demonstrated a higher incidence of motion problems when MCL and ACL were treated operatively, and they recommend arthroscopic reconstruction of the ACL with nonoperative management of the MCL after recovery of range of motion and muscle function. In a prospective randomized study, Halinen and associates[53] treated 47 consecutive patients with combined ACL and grade III MCL injuries. All patients underwent early ACL reconstruction within 3 weeks of injury. The MCL was treated operatively in 23 patients and nonoperatively in 24 patients. All patients were available for follow-up at a mean of 27 months. The nonoperative treatment of the MCL led to results similar to those obtained with operative treatment with respect to subjective function, postoperative stability, range of motion, muscle power, return to activities, and Lysholm score. Halinen and colleagues concluded that MCL ruptures did not need to be treated operatively when the ACL was reconstructed early.

In a retrospective study, Millett and colleagues[54] reported on 19 patients with a complete ACL injury and a minimal grade II MCL tear who underwent early ACL reconstruction and nonoperative treatment of the MCL. At 2-year follow-up, subjective evaluation showed a Lysholm score of 94.5 and a Tegner activity score of 8.4. Clinical examination revealed good range of motion and strength. None of the patients experienced graft failure or required subsequent surgery.

Another controversial issue regarding combined ACL and MCL injury is whether early or late ACL reconstruction provides optimal return of function and long-term results. Based on animal studies, MCL healing is adversely affected by ACL insufficiency,[55] and therefore it has been proposed that early ACL reconstruction will improve healing of the MCL. Both Halinen and colleagues[53] and Millett and associates[54] showed good subjective scores and minimal loss of motion complications with early ACL reconstruction (within 3 weeks). Conversely, Petersen and Laprell[56] demonstrated poorer results with early ACL reconstruction compared with late ACL reconstruction in combined injuries. All patients underwent nonoperative treatment of MCL injury, with early ACL reconstruction performed within 3 weeks of injury and late ACL reconstruction after a minimum of 10 weeks. The late reconstruction group had a lower rate of loss of motion and higher Lysholm scores compared with the early reconstruction group.

The literature supports nonoperative treatment of the MCL tear with surgical reconstruction of the ACL, and most surgeons are currently following this protocol. However, early versus late reconstruction continues to be a subject of debate, with studies supporting both points of view. Other factors such as preoperative and postoperative rehabilitation protocol along with bracing may need to be further analyzed to help assess whether early or late reconstruction is more beneficial.

Complications

Complications of MCL ruptures are rarely reported in the literature. Failure to diagnose associated ligament injuries, such as ACL, can lead to long-term instability and degenerative problems.[7,24] In addition, missed associated meniscal tears and articular cartilage defects can lead to continued pain. Failure to recognize and repair all injured medial and posteromedial structures may lead to residual instability.[7,8] Atrophy and arthrofibrosis are rare complications given the aggressive rehabilitation protocols with early motion and strengthening.[8] Infection is a rare complication with surgical reconstruction. Persistent pain and Pellegrini-Stieda lesions can occur after MCL sprains, usually near the femoral origin in the region of the medial epicondyle.[57] Treatment consists of a local injection or antiinflammatory medication and resection of the lesion maybe required for relief. In addition to pain, patients with femoral-sided lesions are more prone to have loss of motion and associated stiffness.[8,57]

Future Considerations

As with most topics within orthopaedic surgery, basic science knowledge is ever increasing. The avenues for future research are vast in the areas of chemistry, biology, and biomechanics. Our understanding of cellular processes allows us to alter the progression of injury or speed up the restoration of health.

Collagen healing is currently being investigated for the ligaments of the knee. Enzymatic processes in the inflammatory process of ligament injury and healing are plentiful. Research into the MCL and ACL response to a procollagen growth factor and transforming growth factor-β1 is ongoing.[58] This research is furthering the investigation into the role of procollagen processes of ligament healing.

The role of stem cells and angiogenesis factors in ligament healing are being investigated. Although angiogenesis plays a role in ligament healing, the details have yet to be borne out. A murine study of vascular endothelial growth factor showed that it does have a role in ligament healing. This same study demonstrated that stem cells also have a role in accelerating ligament healing.[59]

For a complete list of references, go to expertconsult.com.

Selected Readings

Citation: Wijdicks CA, et al: Structural properties of the primary medial knee ligaments. *Am J Sports Med* 38(8):1638–1646, 2010.
Level of Evidence: Cadaveric study
Summary: The two tibial attachments of the superficial medial collateral ligament (MCL) sustain clinically important loads, as do the central arm of the posterior oblique ligament and the deep MCL. Anatomic medial knee reconstructions may allow recreation of the unique stabilizing characteristics of these structures.

Citation: Marchant MH, Jr, et al: Management of medial-sided knee injuries, part 1: Medial collateral ligament. *Am J Sports Med* 39(5):1102–1113, 2011.

Level of Evidence: Clinical review

Summary: In this article the anatomy and biomechanics of medial-sided knee injuries are reviewed. Superficial medial collateral ligament and combined anterior cruciate ligament injuries are reviewed.

Citation: Tibor LM, et al: Management of medial-sided knee injuries, part 2: Posteromedial corner. *Am J Sports Med* 39(6):1332–1340, 2011.

Level of Evidence: Clinical review

Summary: In this article the anatomy and biomechanics of medial-sided knee injuries are reviewed. Posteromedial corner and combined posterior cruciate ligament injuries are reviewed.

Citation: Fanelli GC, Harris JD: Surgical treatment of acute medial collateral ligament and posteromedial corner injuries of the knee. *Sports Med Arthrosc Rev* 14:78–83, 2006.

Level of Evidence: Clinical review

Summary: In this article the current options for treatment and techniques for medial collateral and posteromedial corner injuries of the knee are reviewed.

Citation: Sims WF, Jacobson KE: The posteromedial corner of the knee: Medial-sided injury patterns revisited. *Am J Sports Med* 32:337–345, 2004.

Level of Evidence: III

Summary: The authors explain concepts with regard to medial-sided knee injuries that they believe to be important. Medial-sided knee injuries are underappreciated.

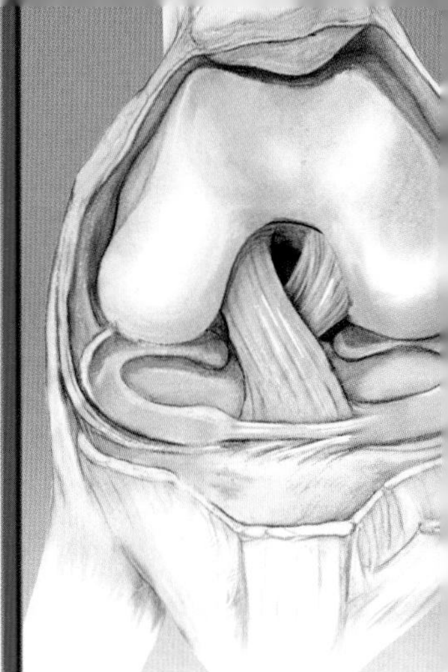

101

Lateral and Posterolateral Corner Injuries of the Knee

SCOTT M. ADAMS • MARK G. HAMMING • CLAUDE T. MOORMAN III

As understanding of the posterolateral corner (PLC) has increased, its significance to overall knee function and biomechanics has become clearer. Although it is a relatively uncommon injury, PLC injuries can have severe consequences for overall knee stability and function. Missed injuries may affect the outcome of surgeries to correct concomitant injuries. This chapter reviews the epidemiology, relevant anatomy, biomechanics, presentation, examination, imaging, and treatment of PLC injuries. Rehabilitation, potential complications, and future considerations for the management of these serious injuries are also discussed.

Isolated PLC injuries are relatively rare and have been reported to range from 1.6% to 7% of all knee injuries in persons who present for evaluation.[1-6] However, the true incidence is not fully known, because these injuries are believed to be underreported or often missed at the time of evaluation. In a review of 68 persons with PLC injuries, Pacheco et al. found that 72% were not correctly diagnosed at time of presentation to the hospital and 50% were still misdiagnosed by the time they were referred to a knee specialist.[7] This misdiagnosis may in part be due to the fact that understanding of the PLC has only recently improved. With recent advances, physicians are developing a better understanding of the anatomy, biomechanics, and mechanism of these injuries. Additionally, the effects of chronic deficiency on gait, level of activity, natural progression, and impact on the management of other injuries is becoming clearer. Finally, surgical techniques continue to evolve as the best way to treat these injuries continues to be debated.

Anatomy

An understanding of the PLC begins with an understanding of the relevant anatomy of the region. This anatomy is among the most complex around the knee. The PLC has been characterized by dynamic and static restraints, anatomic layers, and various structures with multiple names in the literature, thus making the use of consistent nomenclature difficult.

Layers of the Lateral Side of the Knee

Seebacher et al.[8] described the structures on the lateral side of the knee in three anatomic layers. The most superficial layer, layer 1, consists of the lateral fascia, iliotibial (IT) band, and the superficial portion of the biceps femoris tendon. The peroneal nerve, located posterior to the biceps, is located in the deepest aspect of layer 1. The intermediate layer, layer 2, consists of the retinaculum of the quadriceps and the proximal and distal patellofemoral ligaments. The deep layer, layer 3, includes the lateral part of the joint capsule, the lateral collateral ligament, the fabellofibular ligament, the coronary ligament, the popliteal tendon, and the arcuate ligament. Even when described in layers, Seebacher et al.[8] found anatomic variations within their dissected specimens.

Individual Structures

Recent descriptions have focused more on specific anatomic structures and their relation to the posterolateral knee, including the IT band, lateral collateral ligament, popliteus tendon, long and short heads of the biceps femoris, and several smaller structures (Fig. 101-1).

Iliotibial Band

The IT band, or IT tract, is composed of different layers and has at least four separate attachments at the knee.[9-12] The main component, the superficial layer, which covers much of the lateral side of the knee, has a wide attachment to Gerdy's tubercle. Additionally, it has an anterior component attaching to the patella called the iliopatellar band, which influences patellar tracking. The deep layer, a structure found on the medial aspect of the superficial layer, attaches to the lateral intermuscular septum of the distal femur. Distal to the lateral epicondyle of the femur, the deep layer blends with the superficial layer and attaches to Gerdy's tubercle.[12] The capsular-osseous layer, beginning at the lateral intermuscular septum of the femur, receives contributions from the lateral gastrocnemius and biceps femoris before inserting on Gerdy's tubercle. This layer also has attachments to the patella and can influence patellar tracking.[12] When viewed as a whole, the IT band is the first structure encountered during exposure for PLC reconstruction and serves as a stabilizer of the lateral side of the knee.

Fibular Collateral Ligament

With attachments on the fibular head and distal femur, the fibular collateral ligament (FCL; also known as the lateral collateral ligament) is a primary restraint to varus stress on the knee. Its fanlike attachment on the femur is in a bony depression 1.3 to 1.4 mm proximal and 3.1 to 4.6 mm posterior to the lateral epicondyle, but it does not actually attach to the epicondyle.[13,14] With an average length of 6.3 to 7.1 cm,

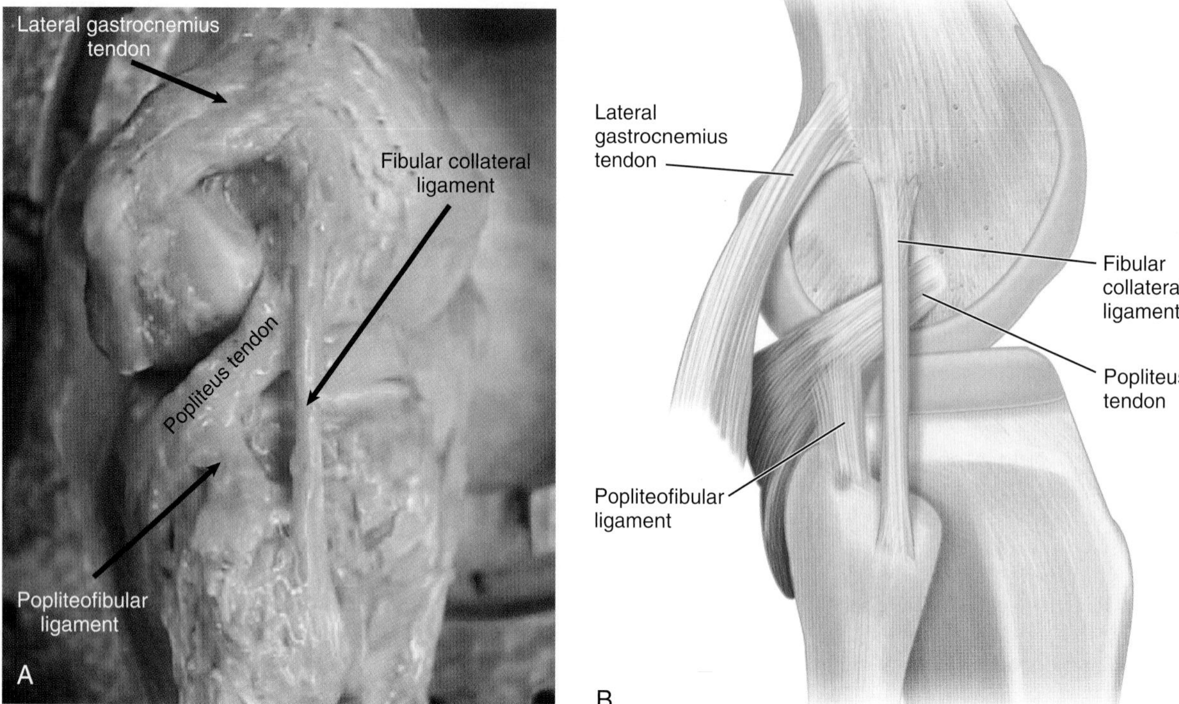

FIGURE 101-1 Image (**A**) and illustration (**B**) of the anatomy of the posterolateral corner and the relationships of individual structures to each other. *(From LaPrade RF, Ly TV, Wentorf FA, et al: The posterolateral attachments of the knee: a qualitative and quantitative morphologic analysis of the fibular collateral ligament, popliteus tendon, popliteofibular ligament, and lateral gastrocnemius tendon.* Am J Sports Med *31:854–860, 2003.)*

it traverses distally deep to the superficial layer of the IT band and attaches to the fibular head.[15-18] The tendon narrows as it courses distally to its narrowest point midway between the femoral and fibular attachments, where it measures 3.4 mm in an anteroposterior (AP) plane and 2.3 mm in a medial to lateral plane.[16] It then expands into its fanlike attachment on the lateral aspect of the fibular head, covering 38% of the width of the head, and is located 8.2 mm posterior and 28.4 mm distal to styloid process.[13,15,16] An understanding of FCL anatomy is essential to anatomic surgical reconstruction for both fibular and femoral tunnel placement.

Popliteus Tendon Complex

The popliteus begins on the posteromedial aspect of the tibia and courses proximally to insert in the popliteal sulcus on the lateral femoral condyle. At the level of the popliteal fossa, the muscle gives rise to the popliteus tendon, which then inserts into the popliteal sulcus. It is at this musculotendinous junction that the popliteofibular ligament attaches the popliteus to the fibula.[13] The tendon becomes intraarticular and runs medial to the FCL. It then inserts onto the femur typically 9.7 mm distal and 5.3 mm posterior to the lateral epicondyle,[14] which represents a distance of 18.5 mm between the femoral attachments of the two structures, a concept to take into consideration when planning a reconstruction.[13] In addition to its attachments on the femur and tibia, the popliteus contains popliteomeniscal fascicles that extend to the lateral meniscus, as well as attachments to the posterior capsule.

The popliteofibular ligament, originating at the musculotendinous junction of the popliteus, travels distally and laterally to insert on the fibular head.[13,17] With anterior and posterior divisions, the ligament provides a strong connection between the fibula and the popliteus.[19] The smaller anterior division attaches to the anteromedial aspect of the fibular styloid 2.8 mm from the tip of the styloid, whereas the larger posterior division attaches to the posteromedial aspect of the fibular styloid 1.6 mm distal to the tip of the styloid.[13] The true role of the popliteofibular ligament to overall stability has been debated. Some investigators propose that it is a primary stabilizer to varus stress, external tibial rotation, and posterior tibial translation.[20,21] However, others have found that it serves purely as a secondary stabilizer, serving a purpose if the FCL is transected.[22]

Biceps Femoris Muscle

Long Head

The long head of the biceps femoris muscle, originating at the ischial tuberosity, travels distally to the knee and forms two tendinous portions, the direct and anterior arms, with the direct arm attaching to the posterolateral fibular head and the anterior arm crossing lateral to the FCL and attaching to the lateral fibular head.[19] The anterior arm is separated from the FCL by the FCL-biceps bursa. This bursa, typically measuring 8.4 by 18 mm, is consistently found between the two structures and serves as a surgical landmark for identifying the FCL attachment to the fibular head.[18] In addition, the long head has three fascial attachments, the reflected arm and the lateral and anterior aponeurosis. The reflected arm travels superficial to the short head of the biceps femoris and inserts on the posterior aspect of the IT tract.[10,19]

Short Head

The short head of the biceps femoris, originating from the femur, travels distally at a 45-degree angle to the femur, where it splits into six components, including attachments to the long head of the biceps, the posterolateral aspect of the joint capsule, and the IT tract.[19] The attachment to the capsule (the "capsular arm") forms a large fascial sheath that includes the fabellofibular ligament.[17] Additionally, further distal, the short head attaches just lateral to the tip of the fibular styloid and a separate anterior arm travels proximal to the fibular styloid and medial to the FCL to attach posterior to Gerdy's tubercle.[17] The final component, the lateral aponeurotic expansion, attaches to the posteromedial aspect of the FCL.[19]

The long and short heads of the biceps femoris are innervated by different components of the sciatic nerve. The long head is innervated by the tibial component and the short head by the common peroneal nerve.

Fabellofibular Ligament

The fabellofibular ligament represents the most distal aspect of the capsular arm from the short head of the biceps femoris.[17] Originating from the fabella or fabella-analog, it courses distally to attach to the fibular styloid. It is thought to provide stability to the knee once it has reached close to full extension.[17]

Arcuate Ligament Complex

The arcuate ligament complex (also referred to as the *arcuate popliteal ligament* or *arcuate complex*), one of the more inconsistently referenced structures in the knee, is a Y-shaped structure consisting of medial and lateral limbs. Both limbs originate on the fibular styloid process. The lateral limb ascends proximally along the lateral joint capsule to insert on the lateral femoral condyle at the posterior joint capsule, whereas the medial limb courses over the musculotendinous junction of the popliteus, blends with the oblique popliteal ligament (ligament of Winslow), and then inserts variably onto the fabella, if present, or the posterior joint capsule.[8,19,23,24] The arcuate ligament complex, when present, is believed to be more accurately described as a variable confluence of several structures, including the posterior oblique, popliteofibular, fabellofibular, and short lateral ligaments, with the final appearance of a Y-shaped ligament complex.[25] It has been shown to contribute to the prevention of varus instability.[26]

Lateral Gastrocnemius Tendon

The lateral gastrocnemius tendon originates at the musculotendinous junction of the lateral gastrocnemius muscle and then courses proximally, first attaching to a fabella or fabella-analog before blending into the meniscofemoral portion of posterior capsule.[17] It ultimately attaches to the femur at the region of the supracondylar process 13.8 mm posterior to the fibular collateral attachment and 28.4 mm from the popliteus tendon attachment.[13]

Mid-Third Lateral Capsular Ligament

The mid-third lateral capsular ligament, a thickening of the lateral capsule of the knee, originates on the femur in an area around the lateral epicondyle and then travels distally and provides a capsular attachment to the lateral meniscus before inserting on the tibia between Gerdy's tubercle and the popliteal hiatus.[17,27] It is composed of meniscotibial and meniscofemoral ligaments. Clinically, the meniscotibial ligament is responsible for the Segond fracture, an avulsion of the lateral tibial plateau.[28,29] A Segond fracture can easily be seen on radiographs and magnetic resonance imaging (MRI) and is indicative of ligamentous injury to the knee.[27,29]

Neurovascular Structures

The peroneal nerve is intimately related to the structures of the PLC. As a result, the nerve is injured in 13% of PLC injuries.[26] In the popliteal fossa, the sciatic nerve splits to form the tibial and common peroneal nerves. The peroneal nerve courses distal and lateral to emerge from under the biceps femoris and then passes behind the fibular neck, ultimately passing deep to the peroneal longus.[30] The nerve is located approximately 15 mm from the joint capsule.[31]

The inferior lateral genicular artery is the main artery associated with the PLC. Originating from the popliteal artery, it is found along the posterior joint capsule proximal to the lateral meniscus. It continues laterally and passes anterior to the fabellofibular ligament and posterior to the popliteofibular ligament before traveling within the lateral capsular ligament along the lateral meniscus.[17]

Biomechanics

With its complex anatomy and its association with the function of other ligaments, the biomechanics of the PLC have proven difficult to determine and remain difficult to understand. In its most basic terms, the PLC serves to resist varus angulation, external tibial rotation, and posterior tibial translation. Through cadaveric sectioning studies, the role of individual structures has become clearer. Previous studies have identified the lateral collateral ligament, popliteus tendon, and popliteofibular ligament as being the key structures contributing to PLC function and stability.[32-36] Additionally, the PLC structures affect the function and loads seen on the cruciate ligaments (Fig. 101-2).

Role of PLC Structures to Varus Motion

The FCL is the primary restraint to varus stress. Sectioning of the FCL causes increases in varus motion in all degrees of knee flexion.[37] As long as the FCL remains intact, minimal change occurs in varus translation regardless of what o ther structures may be torn.[38] However, isolated sectioning of the popliteus tendon has shown small but significant increases in varus motion, but to a much smaller degree than isolated sectioning of the FCL.[39] Varus stress produces the greatest load on the FCL with the knee in 30 degrees of flexion, and the load subsequently decreases once the knee reaches 90 degrees of flexion, with an ultimate maximum tensile load of 295 to 309 N.[40-42] Once the FCL is torn, secondary structures assume the main restraint to varus motion, including the posterior cruciate ligament (PCL), popliteofibular ligament, posterior capsule, mid-third lateral capsule ligament, IT band, and popliteal tendon.[22,39,43,44] This primary function of the FCL is essential to consider during

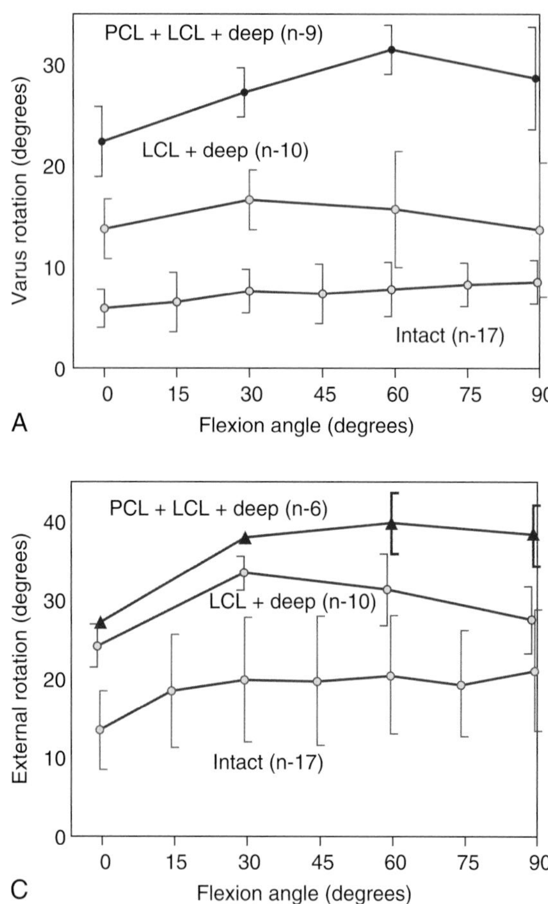

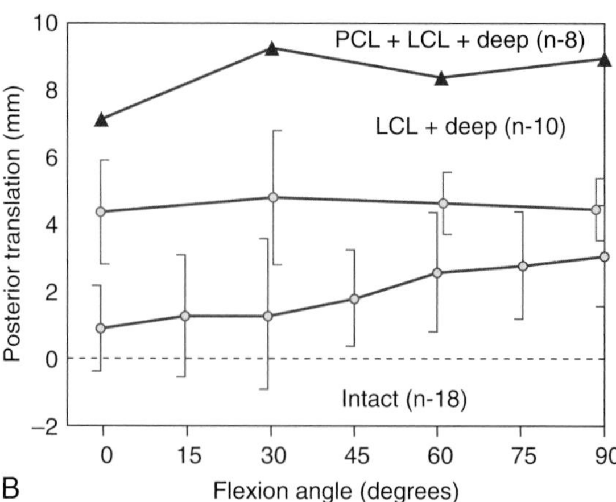

FIGURE 101-2 Sectioning studies showing motion versus knee flexion angle relative to contribution of the posterolateral structures and posterior cruciate ligament with respect to varus rotation (**A**), posterior translation (**B**), and external rotation stability (**C**). *LCL,* Lateral collateral ligament; *PCL,* posterior cruciate ligament; *deep,* popliteus-arcuate ligament complex. *(Modified from Gollehon DL, Torzilli PA, Warren RF: The role of the posterolateral and cruciate ligaments in the stability of the human knee: a biomechanical study.* J Bone Joint Surg Am *69:233–242, 1987.)*

reconstruction to recreate the main contributor to varus stability in the knee.

Role of the PLC Structures in Preventing External Rotation

The popliteus tendon and the popliteofibular ligament are the primary restraints to external rotation.[20-22] Isolated sectioning of the popliteus leads to significant increases in external rotation, and conversely, a reconstructed popliteus demonstrates significantly decreased external rotation compared with a sectioned specimen.[39] However, the FCL appears to have a greater contribution to external rotation stability than previously thought, especially at 30 degrees of knee flexion where the maximal load from external rotation forces is greater on the FCL than on the popliteus and popliteofibular ligament.[40] Consequently, it appears that the FCL plays a primary role in external rotation restraint when the knee is closer to full extension, and the popliteus and popliteofibular ligament assume responsibility with increasing degrees of knee flexion.

The PCL also affects external rotation resistance. The PLC and PCL work in concert to resist external rotation stresses. Isolated sectioning of the PCL does not affect external rotation motion of the knee if the PLC is intact.[38,43] As noted, the PLC experiences greatest external rotation moments at 30 degrees of knee flexion.[38,43] The PCL does not experience external rotation loads until 80 to 90 degrees of knee flexion, when it becomes a secondary stabilizer to external rotation, thus explaining why in the dial test, decreased external rotation at 90 degrees compared with 30 degrees of knee flexion suggests an intact PCL and an isolated PLC injury.[45]

Role of the PLC Structures in Preventing Anterior/Posterior Tibial Translation

Injured PLC structures have little effect on total anterior tibial translation if the anterior cruciate ligament (ACL) is intact.[36,38,43] The FCL, popliteus, and popliteofibular ligament each experience negligible force when subjected to an anterior drawer test in a knee with a competent ACL.[40] This finding is significant during the physical examination. In persons with an isolated PLC injury, findings of the Lachman test and anterior drawer test will be mostly normal because of the minimal impact of the PLC on anterior tibial translation. Slight differences in total translation may be found because sectioning the popliteus can cause up to a 2.6-mm increase of anterior translation.[39] However, the test should have a firm end point and very minimal clinical difference, although if the ACL is also torn, the combined ACL/PLC injury leads to significantly increased anterior tibial translation. Combined sectioning of the PLC and ACL causes an additional 7 mm of anterior translation,[34] which may lead to a more pronounced Lachman test during the physical examination.

Isolated PLC injuries can cause increased posterior tibial translation, even in the setting of an intact PCL.[36,38,43] This increase is small but significant, with the greatest increase occurring in the first 45 degrees of knee flexion. In the knee with a deficient PCL, the PLC assumes a major stabilizing role, with increases in force load of six to eight times that of the knee with an intact PCL, especially at higher degrees of knee flexion.[46] Total posterior tibial translation increases significantly, up to 20 to 25 mm, when both the PCL and PLC are torn and no longer resist posterior tibial translation.[38,47] Clinically, this finding is manifested in a more pronounced posterior drawer test than is found with isolated PCL tears, with a minimum of at least a grade 3 posterior drawer in the combined injury setting.[47]

Recent biomechanical studies have focused on the reconstruction of the cruciate ligaments in the setting of concomitant PLC injury to better explain the higher failure rate seen after cruciate ligament reconstruction in the knee with multiple ligament injuries. Graft rupture after ACL reconstruction has been reported to range from 1.8% to 10.4%, with an average rate of 5.8% reported in a recent review.[48] It is becoming increasingly clear that missed PLC injuries may contribute to a higher failure rate.[49-51] In response to varus load, ACL graft forces are increased with isolated FCL sectioning, and this force is further increased with varus and external rotation loads.[49] Additionally, concomitant reconstruction of the ACL and PLC decreases instability by allowing less anterior tibial translation, and instability was the major reason cited for poor subjective outcomes by patients with residual PLC injury after ACL reconstruction.[50,52]

In the setting of PCL injury, concomitant injury to the PLC is the most frequently associated injury and occurs in up to 60% of all PCL injuries.[53] A missed PLC injury can affect the success of PCL reconstruction.[53] In an isolated PCL injury, forces on the PCL graft resulting from external rotation loads, posterior tibial loads, or combined posterior and external rotation loads are similar to the native PCL. However, in the setting of residual PLC injury, forces acting on the PCL graft are increased during all loading conditions, with increases as much 150% on the reconstructed graft.[54] The increased load may predispose the PCL reconstruction to failure.

Classification

Classification systems have been created on the basis of the amount of instability and the location of the injury (Table 101-1). The American Medical Association initially standardized ligamentous injuries into grades I, II, and III based on the extent of injury and subsequent motion.[55] Hughston et al.[56] were the first to classify lateral side instability and identified six types of lateral compartment instability based on physical examination tests: anterolateral rotatory instability, posterolateral rotatory instability, combined anterolateral and posterolateral rotatory instability, combined anterolateral and anteromedial rotatory instability, combined posterolateral, anterolateral, and anteromedial rotatory instability, and straight lateral instability. These types were graded on the basis of various clinical exams as 1+, or minor, if the joint surfaces separated 5 mm or less; 2+, or moderate, if they separated 5 to 10 mm; and 3+, or severe, if they separated 10 mm or more. A classification system was developed by Fanelli and Feldmann[11] based on the location of the injury. Finally, injuries can be classified more simply as either stable or unstable, because it is instability that dictates surgical management.

TABLE 101-1

CLASSIFICATION SYSTEMS TO DESCRIBE POSTEROLATERAL CORNER INJURIES

System/Grade	Description
AMA	***Injury Severity***
I	Minimal tearing of ligament fibers, no increased motion
II	Partial tear of ligament, slight to moderate abnormal motion
III	Complete tear of ligament, loss of function and marked abnormal motion
Fanelli	***Structures Injured***
A	Popliteofibular ligament and popliteus tendon
B	Popliteofibular ligament, popliteus, and fibular collateral ligament
C	Popliteofibular ligament, popliteus, fibular collateral ligament, lateral capsule avulsion, and cruciate ligament disruption
Hughston	***Amount of Instability***
1+	Opening of 0-5 mm to varus stress
2+	Opening of 5-10 mm to varus stress
3+	Opening of 10+ mm to varus stress

History

Most PLC injuries are sustained during athletic competitions, motor vehicle accidents, and falls.[6,57-60] In one study, 65% of injuries were sports related, with 26% from motor vehicle accidents and 9% from falls.[7] A typical mechanism is a posterolaterally directed force to the anteromedial tibia, which leads to hyperextension and a varus force. Additional mechanisms include knee hyperextension or severe tibial external rotation in a partially flexed knee, and both contact and noncontact mechanisms have been reported.[61] An emerging mechanism that is increasing in frequency is injury during low-energy knee dislocation in obese persons. Azar et al.[62] reported on 17 obese persons with "ultra–low-velocity" knee dislocations, of which 50% had documented injury to the lateral-sided structures. In the United States alone, 35.7% of adults are considered obese, which is not only a major risk factor identified for these ultra–low-velocity knee dislocations but also increases the risk of limb-threatening neurovascular injury during dislocation.[62,63]

Concomitant Injury

PLC injuries are rarely isolated and are associated with concomitant injuries in 43% to 87% of patients.[2,3,35,26,60,64] These associated injuries commonly include ACL and PCL tears, as well as tibial plateau fractures. In the study by Gardner et al.[65] of operative tibial plateau fractures, 29% of the fractures had a complete FCL tear and 68% had injuries to the popliteofibular ligament and/or the popliteus tendon. Given that PLC injuries can occur in the setting of knee dislocations, in the case of multiple ligamentous injury, high clinical suspicion should be maintained for spontaneously reduced knee dislocation and subsequent neurovascular injury.

Physical Examination

In the acute setting, patients present after some form of trauma[6,57-60] and report pain, typically at the posterolateral aspect of the knee and at the fibular head.[2,61] They will have varying degrees of effusion. In a prospective study, LaPrade et al.[3] reported that 9.1% of patients presenting with a knee hemarthrosis had a PLC injury. Initially, depending on the degree of trauma, the basics of trauma care should be followed. First, a thorough primary survey consisting of airway, breathing, and circulation should be performed. During the secondary survey, a more detailed musculoskeletal examination can be completed. Gross deformity may suggest a knee dislocation. Recognizing a vascular injury is of paramount importance, and failure to do so can lead to amputation. In an acute setting, a detailed neurovascular examination should be performed. An ankle-brachial index score should be obtained, and any abnormal finding warrants additional workup and consultation. A thorough neurologic examination is necessary because of the high incidence of peroneal nerve injuries associated with PLC tears.[26] Particular attention should be given to peroneal nerve sensation, as well as ankle dorsiflexion, eversion, and great toe extension.[59]

In the chronic setting, patients often report pain at the medial joint line and/or lateral joint line, as well as at the posterolateral aspect of the knee.[26,59] However, with time, swelling and pain subside and instability becomes a primary complaint. This instability is most evident with the knee in extension and often presents as a varus or hyperextension-varus thrust during the stance phase of gait.[66] Patients experience difficulty ascending and descending stairs, may be seen walking with the knee in slight flexion or the ankle in equinus to alleviate these symptoms, and report having difficulty with twisting, pivoting, and cutting exercises.[35] One must also be mindful of the potential for a steppage gait if a foot-drop occurs from a concomitant peroneal nerve injury.[59]

For both chronic and acute cases, the physical examination should begin with an evaluation of the entire extremity, looking for areas of tenderness, ecchymosis, and deformity. As stated earlier, a detailed neurovascular examination is essential to evaluate for neurovascular injury. Overall limb alignment should be evaluated, because it is important to identify varus malalignment. This malalignment may not only exacerbate the instability but may also predispose a reconstruction to increased risk of failure.[57,67-69]

Next, examinations specific for ligamentous injury of the knee should be performed, which includes assessing for ACL, PCL, and MCL injuries. A thorough evaluation of the PLC is then pursued. In the series by DeLee et al.,[2] all patients had tenderness and swelling diffusely over the posterolateral joint. Point tenderness is often found at the fibular head.[2,61] Varus stress examination is paramount to a basic physical examination. This test should be performed with the knee in both full extension, as well as at 30 degrees of flexion. Varus instability in full extension is suggestive of a PLC injury and a PCL injury, whereas isolated instability at 30 degrees of flexion is more suggestive of an isolated PLC injury.[56] One must be sure that when testing at 30 degrees of flexion, a pure varus directed force is applied without external rotation of the tibia, which could contribute to false-positive examinations.[2] In a the series of PLC injuries to the knee reported by DeLee et al.,[2] the most sensitive examination technique was varus instability with the knee at 30 degrees of flexion.

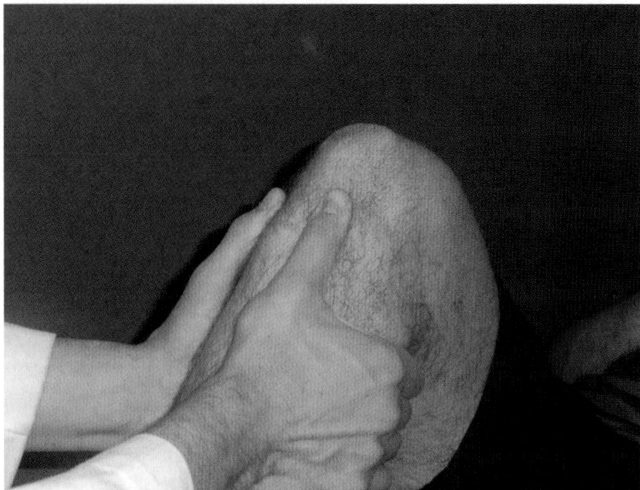

FIGURE 101-3 Posterolateral drawer test.

Other more specific tests for a PLC injury exist, including the posterolateral drawer test, the external rotation recurvatum test, the dial test, the standing apprehension test, and the reverse pivot shift.

The posterolateral drawer test has been described by having the physician flex the hip to 45 degrees and the knee to 80 degrees. The tibia is held in mild external rotation (approximately 15 degrees). With the examiner's thumbs on the tibial tubercle (Fig. 101-3), a posterior directed force on the proximal tibia will cause the tibial plateau to rotate posterolaterally on the femur.[2] The examiner should feel the posterolateral rotation.

The dial test is performed by positioning the patient either prone or supine with the knee at the edge of the examination table. If the patient is supine, an assistant must stabilize the knees to hold the patella in line.[70] When the knee is flexed to 30 degrees, the sole of the foot is externally rotated. The same maneuver is performed on the contralateral side (Fig. 101-4). A difference in external rotation of 10 to 15 degrees or more compared with the contralateral side is positive.[71] The same maneuvers are then performed at 90 degrees of knee flexion. A positive examination finding at 30 degrees of flexion indicates a PLC injury.[71] A positive examination finding at 30 degrees and 90 degrees of flexion raises suspicion for both a PLC injury and a PCL injury.[71] Tibial positioning during testing is important, because reduced tibial external rotation will be found on the dial test with a posteriorly subluxated tibia.[72,73] Therefore, when performing the dial test, an anterior force should be applied to the tibia if a concomitant PCL injury is suspected.[72,73] This full reduction of the tibia will allow for a more accurate estimate of tibial external rotation with dial testing.

The external rotation recurvatum test, described by Hughston and Norwood,[74] is performed by lifting the great toe of a patient in the supine position to observe the quantity of genu recurvatum (Fig. 101-5). The amount of recurvatum can be measured with a goniometer or the distance from the heel to the examination table.[26] One should also note differences in varus alignment and tibial external rotation.[70] The external rotation recurvatum test is less sensitive for PLC

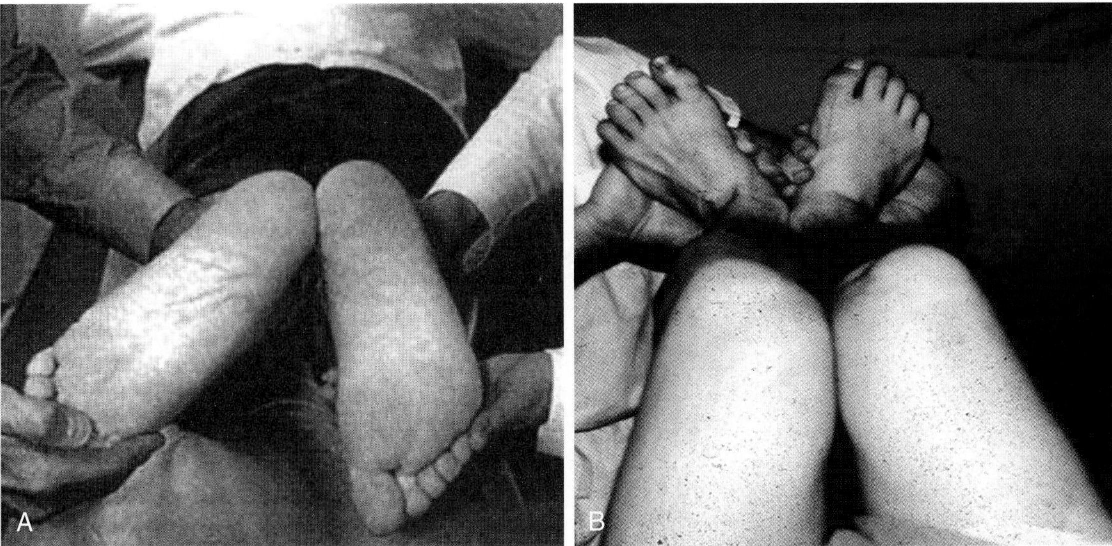

FIGURE 101-4 Dial test performed in the prone position (**A**) and the supine position (**B**).

injuries because it has been proposed that the intact anteromedial bundle of the ACL provides some stability with this maneuver.[2] For this reason, this test can be useful in identifying PLC injury with an ACL tear.[13,74] For identifying combined ACL/PLC injuries, this test has sensitivity of 100% but specificity of 30%.[13] One must be aware that this test has a high rate of false-negative findings in the setting of PLC injuries with intact ACLs.[13] It is seldom useful for isolated PLC injuries or combined PLC/PCL injuries.[75] Finally, an important consideration is that the posterolateral drawer test demonstrates instability in flexion, whereas the external rotation recurvatum test demonstrates instability in extension.[74]

The standing apprehension test (Fig. 101-6) is performed by having the patient stand with the knee at almost full extension. A force is the directed medially across the anterolateral femur.[59] To consider this test positive, the patient must feel an unstable sensation and rotation of the femur on the tibia must occur.[6] The utility of this examination should be placed in context with the remainder of the history and examination because it has the potential to be nonspecific.

The reverse pivot shift is another specific test for the PLC that is specific for the FCL, mid-third lateral capsular ligament, and popliteus complex.[26] To perform this maneuver, the knee is flexed to 45 degrees with a valgus stress transmitted through the externally rotated foot.[26] With subsequent extension of the leg, a subluxation is felt at approximately 25 degrees of flexion.[59] Biomechanically, the posteriorly subluxated lateral tibial plateau reduces at 20 to 30 degrees of flexion because the IT band changes from knee flexor to extensor.[35,76] False-positive rates have been reported to be as high as 35%, and thus careful comparison with the unaffected limb is essential.

Gait examination is more useful in the chronic injury setting. During ambulation, the patient may have the appearance of a varus thrust with a lateral tibial shift. These findings can be attributed to external rotation of the tibia during full

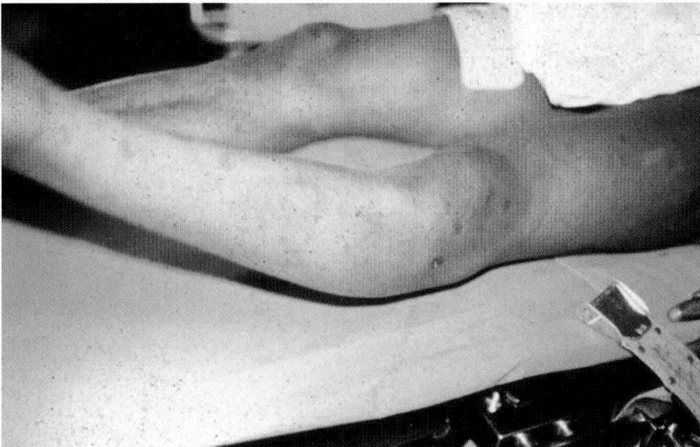

FIGURE 101-5 An example of the external rotation recurvatum test showing severe posterolateral corner injury.

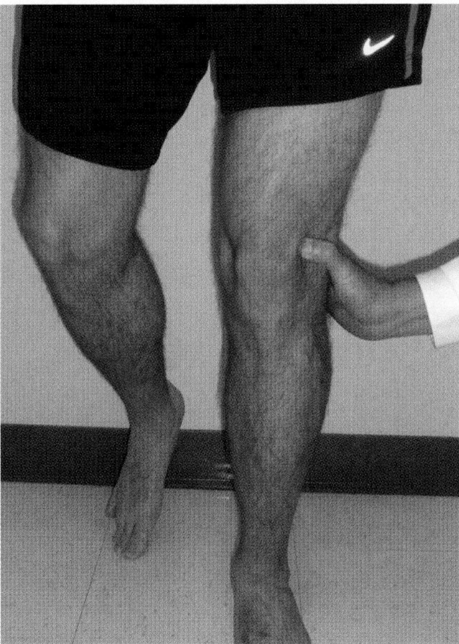

FIGURE 101-6 The standing apprehension test. As force is directed medially, the patient experiences instability and the examiner can feel the femur rotate on the tibia.

extension in the stance phase of the gait cycle. Previous authors liken this gait examination to a standing external rotation recurvatum test.[35] Furthermore, a hyperextension thrust gait can be present when loading the lower extremity during the early stance phase.[59] For this reason, some patients walk with a flexed knee.

The physical examination is critical in the detection of PLC injuries. Although modern imaging modalities are highly accurate for detecting injury to these structures, it is believed that they may be oversensitive for these injuries. Additionally, imaging cannot replace the physical examination for assessing clinical instability resulting from injury. Therefore the physical examination is the most important part of the workup to determine the need for operative intervention of PLC injuries. In essence, the examiner should trust the physical examination during the decision-making process.

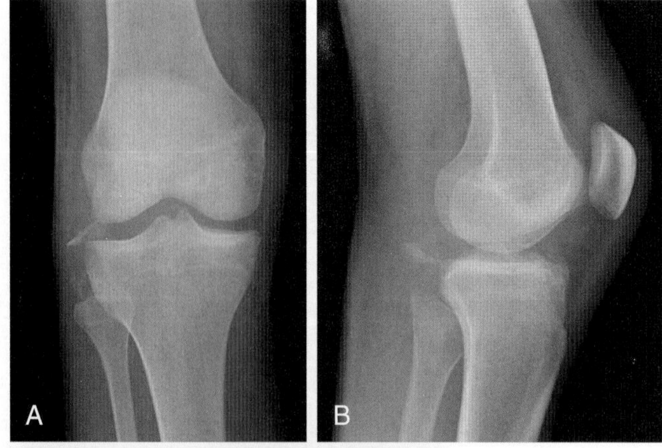

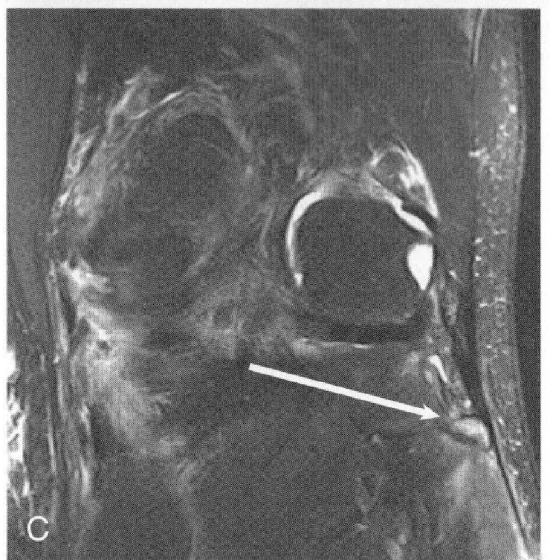

FIGURE 101-7 The arcuate sign as seen on anteroposterior (**A**) and lateral (**B**) radiographs. **C,** The arcuate sign (*arrow*) seen on coronal magnetic resonance imaging.

Imaging

Radiographs

Imaging initially begins with radiographs and may include standard AP, lateral, sunrise, and posteroanterior-flexion views. Radiographs are helpful in identifying tibial plateau fractures, Segond fractures, and avulsions of the fibular head. Additionally, they may reveal proximal tibiofibular joint dislocations, widening of the lateral joint surface, and arthritis. Evaluating for medial compartment arthritis is especially useful in the chronic setting. The "arcuate sign" refers to the radiographic finding of avulsion of the fibular styloid where the popliteofibular, fabellofibular, and arcuate ligaments attach, or it can represent a larger avulsion involving more of the fibular head that results from the pull of the biceps femoris and FCL, and it may be seen on a radiograph or MRI (Fig. 101-7).[77] Stress radiographs have been shown to aid in the diagnosis of PLC injuries.[78-80] Specifically, varus-stress radiographs with increased lateral joint space widening of 4.0 mm suggest isolated grade III PLC injury, widening of 6.6 mm suggests a combined PLC and ACL tear, and widening of 7.8 mm suggests PLC, ACL, and PCL injuries.[80] In a separate clinical study, lateral widening from varus stress totaled 18.6 mm for a complete injury and an average of 12.8 mm in partial injuries.[81] Therefore side-to-side comparisons can provide evidence of clinical laxity and warrant further clinical correlation to determine the need for surgical reconstruction. Additionally, in the chronic setting, AP full leg radiographs (hip to ankle) should be obtained to evaluate for varus malalignment.

Magnetic Resonance Imaging

MRI allows visualization of individual components of the PLC, including the IT band, FCL, biceps femoris tendon, and popliteus (Fig. 101-8).[23,82] LaPrade et al.[83] found that the accuracy of identifying torn individual structures ranges from 68% for the popliteofibular ligament to 95% for the FCL. Other studies have reported an ability to detect PLC injuries in 80% to 100% of the cases, especially if the MRI is performed in the acute setting.[8,84,85] MRI also identifies concomitant injuries such as tears of the cruciate ligaments, because isolated tears of the PLC are rare and most often occur in the setting of additional ligamentous injury (Fig. 101-9).[3] Additionally, similar to other ligamentous injuries, characteristic bone bruise patterns have been reported with PLC injuries, with the most common location being the anteromedial femoral condyle.[86] Although the complex anatomy of the PLC is better visualized on MRI, it remains difficult to determine clinically significant instability based on MRI findings alone. In an effort to simplify this diagnosis, it has been suggested that MRI evidence of injury to at least two structures, especially the popliteus, FCL, or posterior lateral joint capsule, is indicative of posterolateral rotatory instability and warrants a thorough clinical evaluation.[87]

Ultrasound

Ultrasound has emerged as an additional imaging modality for the evaluation of PLC injuries. This technique, which can be performed quickly and is noninvasive and inexpensive, has been shown to be useful in identifying the structures of the PLC.[88,89] Static ultrasound imaging has an overall sensitivity of 92% and a specificity of 75%, and dynamic ultrasound testing revealing greater than 10.5 mm of total lateral joint line width has sensitivity of 83% and a specificity of 100%.[90] Additionally, ultrasound has the ability to visualize dynamic processes and oblique structures, which are sometimes poorly visualized on MRI.

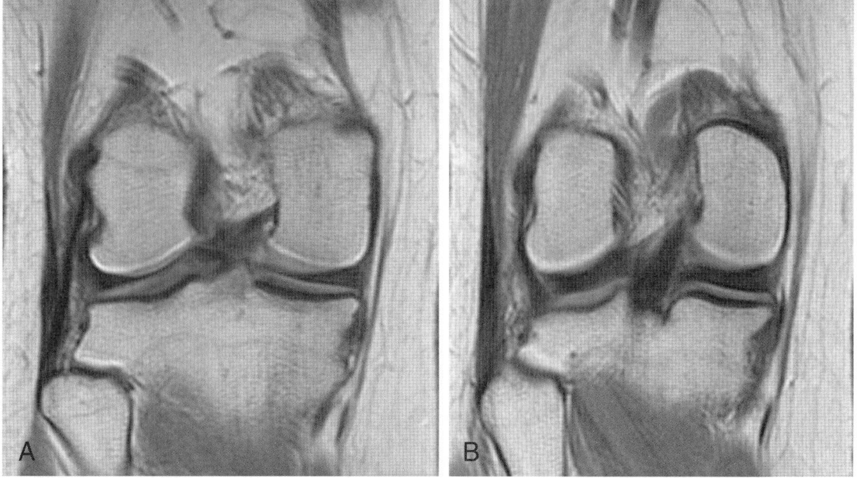

FIGURE 101-8 Coronal magnetic resonance imaging of the fibular collateral ligament and biceps femoris inserting on the fibula (**A**) and the popliteus and biceps femoris (**B**).

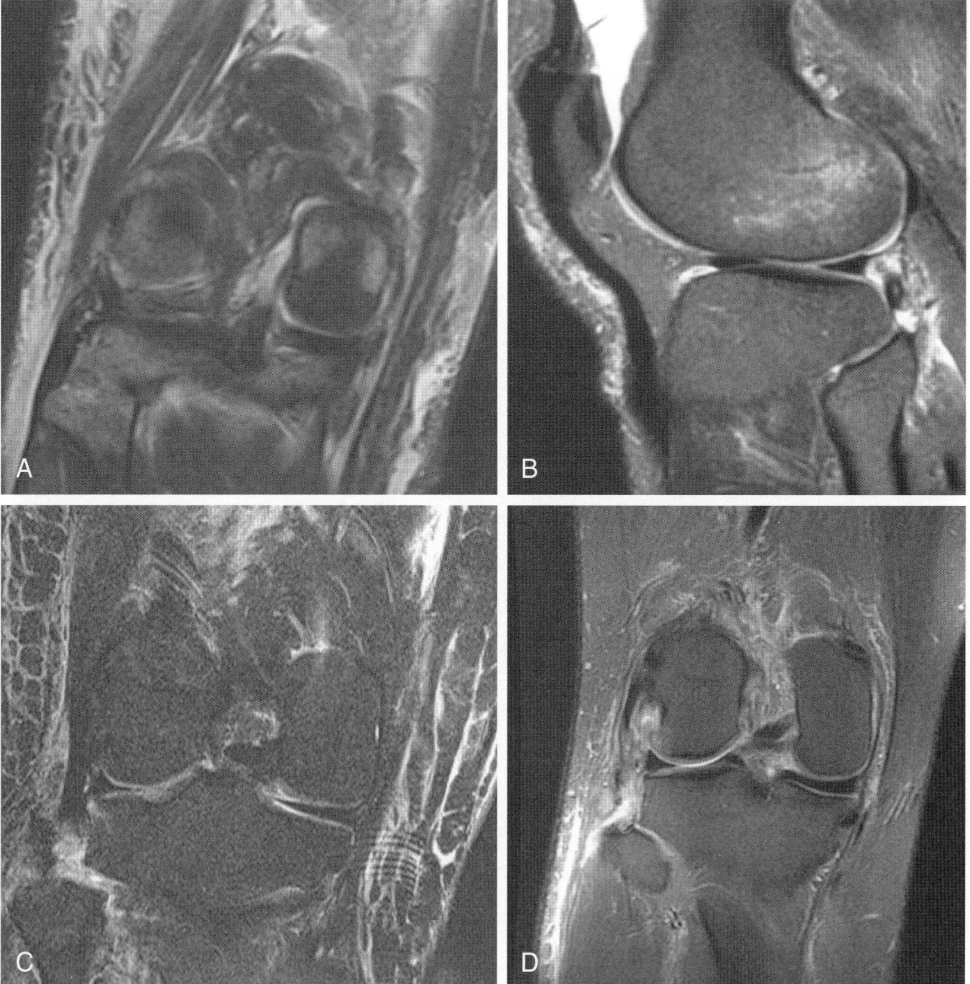

FIGURE 101-9 **A,** A tear of fibular collateral ligament near its femoral attachment with retraction of the ligament. **B,** The popliteus is torn and retracted. **C,** A tear of the biceps femoris. **D,** The fibular collateral is torn from its fibular insertion.

Treatment Options

Treatment is determined by the timing of the diagnosis, the extent of the injury, and the degree of subsequent instability.

Nonoperative Management

The decision to treat PLC injuries conservatively is based on the extent of injury and the presence of instability. Unstable joints warrant surgical intervention. Truly stable joints, which are based on examination after administration of an anesthetic, may be treated nonoperatively.

Surgical Considerations

The timing of surgery and the appropriate procedure for operative PLC injuries have long been debated. Treatment options consist of primary repair and reconstruction, whether "anatomic" or "nonanatomic" reconstruction techniques are used.

Diagnostic Arthroscopy

Diagnostic arthroscopy may assist in the diagnosis of PLC injuries, as well as any concomitant injuries in the knee. Arthroscopy is successful at identifying most injuries to the popliteus, coronary ligament, lateral meniscus, mid-third lateral capsular ligament, articular cartilage, and the cruciate ligaments, but it has less capability of identifying injuries to the popliteofibular ligament.[91,92] However, not all injuries to the popliteus identified during open dissection were visualized during arthroscopy.[92] Various arthroscopic findings have been described to suggest PLC injuries. The "lateral gutter drive-through" sign, signified as the ability to advance the arthroscope into the posterolateral compartment between a lax popliteus tendon and the lateral femoral condyle, suggests an avulsion of the popliteus off the femur.[93] The "drive-through sign," signified as greater than 10 mm of lateral compartment joint opening (Fig. 101-10), also suggests injury to the PLC.[91] The visualization of torn structures on diagnostic arthroscopy or the presence of either the drive-through sign or the lateral gutter drive-through sign should prompt close examination of the PLC to avoid missing subtle injuries.

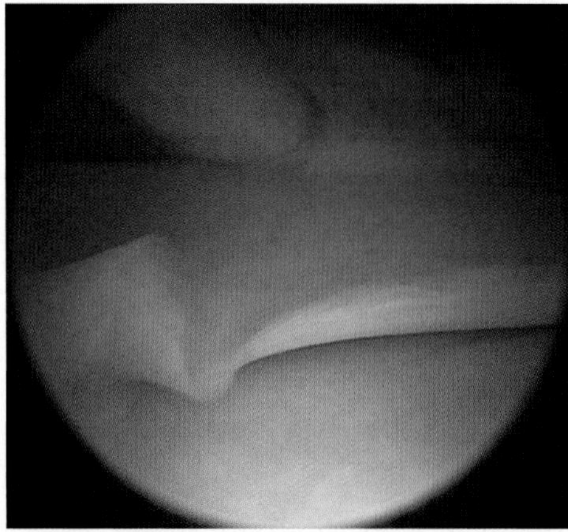

FIGURE 101-10 The lateral compartment "drive-through sign" consistent with a posterolateral corner injury. An opening greater than 10 mm is present between the tibia and femur (the femoral condyle is not visualized).

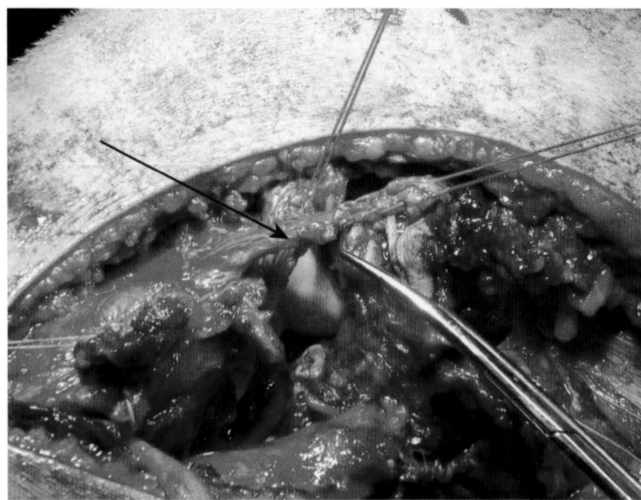

FIGURE 101-11 Preparing the fibular collateral ligament (*arrow*) for primary repair back to the femoral condyle. *(Courtesy Dean Taylor, MD.)*

Primary Repair

Debate continues over the merits of primary repair of structures. Historically, primary repair has been shown to be adequate for acute PLC injuries if performed in the first 3 weeks after an injury is sustained.[64,94] In this technique, avulsed structures are repaired directly to bone using suture anchors, nonabsorbable suture, bone tunnels, screw and washer constructs, or other fixation devices. However, recent studies have found that repair carries significantly inferior results compared with reconstruction, with up to a 40% failure rate in the setting of isolated repair.[95,96] Some experts advocate repair only if the injury is truly an isolated avulsion and no evidence is found of midsubstance injury.[97] Additionally, repair of avulsed structures can help augment the reconstruction procedures.[98]

Repair Techniques

For acute avulsions of the popliteus or FCL from their insertion on the femur (Fig. 101-11), repair may be performed by the recess procedure.[94] Originally described by Hughston, this technique uses small bone tunnels drilled at the anatomic insertion site of the avulsed structure. Initially, the structure is freed of adhesions, and its ability to be anatomically reduced is confirmed. Its proximal end is prepared with suture, which is then passed through the bone tunnel and tied on the medial side of the femur. Various techniques may be used for suture passing through bone, including cruciate ligament guides, Beath needles, or free-hand drilling. A second incision is made medially, and the suture is tied over a button and against the medial cortex of the femur. For concomitant injury, care must be taken to avoid interfering with cruciate ligament reconstruction tunnels.[99]

A similar technique may be used to repair structures back to their insertion on the fibular head. Whether the biceps femoris, the popliteus, or the FCL, the structure's insertion is initially identified and anatomic reduction is confirmed. Bone tunnels or suture anchors are used to secure the structure into its anatomic position. The popliteofibular ligament may be primarily repaired if the popliteus or FCL is uninjured.[97] For fibular head fractures, anatomic reduction and fixation is performed, addressing any concomitant avulsion injuries at the same time.

Reconstruction Techniques

Biceps Tenodesis

Initially described by Clancy, the biceps tenodesis attempts to recreate the FCL and popliteofibular ligament and to reinforce the posterolateral joint capsule.[100,101] A 12-cm lateral incision is made from 6 cm proximal to the lateral epicondyle down past Gerdy's tubercle. The lateral epicondyle is palpated and the IT band is split longitudinally over the epicondyle. The biceps tendon is freed of attachments to the lateral gastrocnemius muscle. Distally, the peroneal nerve is identified and freed of attachments to the biceps tendon to prevent tethering once the biceps is rerouted. Proximal excess muscle is removed from tendon to create a 6-cm tendinous portion at the level of the epicondyle. The lateral epicondyle is freed of soft tissue. The origin of the FCL is identified. A trough is made in the bone and a point 1 cm anterior to the lateral epicondyle is selected for drilling.[100-102] A 3.2-mm drill hole is made and a 6.5-mm screw and washer construct is selected. The proximal biceps tendon that had been freed of muscle is brought under the IT band and placed around the screw. The screw and washer are tightened to attach the tendon to the lateral femoral condyle. It is important to plan bone tunnels appropriately in the setting of multiligament reconstruction.[99] This nonanatomic technique requires that the distal biceps attachment to the fibula remains intact for tensioning purposes.

Split Biceps Tendon Transfer

In a modification to the technique described by Clancy, a portion of the biceps tendon is rerouted and attached via tenodesis to the epicondyle. This technique requires a stable proximal tibiofibular joint, intact attachments between the biceps tendon and the posterolateral capsule, and as previously described, the biceps attachment to the fibular head remains intact.[103] A lateral-based incision is made for exposure from the lateral epicondyle down to the fibular head. The peroneal nerve is identified, freed of adhesions, and protected throughout the repair. The IT band is split longitudinally over the epicondyle to expose the origin of the FCL and popliteus. The long head of the biceps is isolated and the anterior two thirds of the tendon is separated. This portion of the tendon is detached proximally, freed of excess muscle, brought medial to the IT band, and attached via tenodesis to an area 1 cm anterior to the lateral epicondyle using a screw and washer construct similar to that previously described. Tendon remaining after the tenodesis can be secured to the fibular head for additional reinforcement. The posterolateral capsule is then incised and attached to the newly rerouted tendon to augment the reconstruction with a posterolateral capsular shift.

Posterolateral Corner Sling Procedure

The PLC sling procedure, using autograft or allograft, creates an extraarticular sling extending from the posterior tibia to an area anterior and superior to the lateral femoral epicondyle.[104] With the knee flexed 45 degrees, an incision is made along the IT band from mid femur to a point distal to Gerdy's tubercle. The peroneal nerve is identified and protected. A plane between the lateral head of the gastrocnemius and the FCL is created and the gastrocnemius is retracted posteriorly. The popliteus and joint capsule are then identified, and the popliteus is mobilized and retracted posteriorly. A retractor is placed along the posterolateral aspect of the tibia. A 6- to 8-mm bone tunnel is created 1 to 1.5 cm below the articular surface of the tibia and medial enough to avoid violating the proximal tibiofibular joint. An allograft or autograft is passed through this tunnel from anterior to posterior and secured. The graft is brought proximal and secured to a point 1 cm anterior to the lateral femoral epicondyle using bone tunnels, suture anchors, or screw and washer constructs to complete the sling. An all-arthroscopic sling reconstruction of the popliteus tendon has been described.[105]

Proximal Tibial Osteotomy

In the setting of genu varum and a chronic PLC injury, a proximal tibial osteotomy (Fig. 101-12) has been shown to improve stability and, in the right patient population, can serve as the primary treatment for chronic posterolateral instability.[106] Additionally, it may serve as the initial procedure to correct malalignment in a two-stage approach to reconstruction. Both opening and closing wedge osteotomies have been described.[106,107] The goal of the osteotomy is the restore the mechanical axis to neutral or a slightly valgus position. Standard osteotomy techniques are used based on the surgeon's preference and experience. Arthur et al.[106] found that correction of the varus malalignment was sufficient to restore stability in 38% of their total study population (patients with PLC and other ligamentous injuries) and 67% of patients with isolated PLC injury, and thus a secondary procedure was not necessary.

Proximal tibial osteotomy has the potential to not only correct coronal malalignment but can also influence tibial slope (saggital alignment). An osteotomy to change coronal alignment has been used in the ACL- and PCL-deficient knee to affect stability. However, the impact of altering tibial slope to treat PLC injuries and instability remains controversial. It has been reported that in the combined PCL- and PLC-deficient knee, increasing tibial slope better stabilizes the joint and decreases forces on the PLC structures.[108] However, a biomechanical study showed that increasing the tibial slope in a knee with a combined PCL and PLC injury had no impact

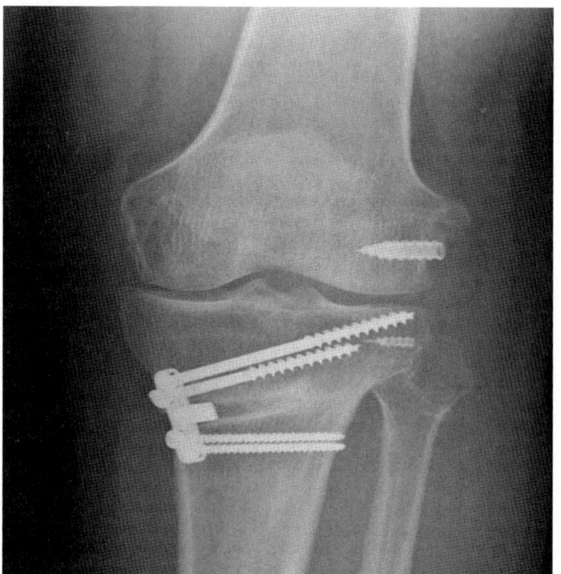

FIGURE 101-12 After presenting because of a failed posterolateral corner reconstruction, a proximal tibial osteotomy was performed and no additional reconstruction was required.

on stability during dial testing at 30 and 90 degrees and did not alter the reverse pivot shift test.[109]

Anatomic Reconstructions

Isolated Structure Reconstruction

Various techniques have been described for reconstructing individual structures, including the FCL, popliteus tendon, and popliteofibular ligament. In each case, an autograft or allograft may be used. Each procedure relies on a precise understanding of the anatomy of the PLC to accurately reconstruct the injured structure. A standard exposure is performed. The peroneal nerve is identified and protected. For the popliteus, the femoral origin of the popliteus is identified and cleared of soft tissue. A bone tunnel is created and an interference screw is used to secure the graft into the femur. The graft is passed distally to the posterolateral aspect of the tibia. Similar to the sling procedure previously described, an anterior-to-posterior bone tunnel is made in the tibia and the popliteus is passed from posterior to anterior and secured with interference screws. For the FCL, the femoral origin for the FCL is identified, a bone tunnel is created, and the graft is secured with an interference screw. A bone tunnel is then made in the proximal fibula (while protecting the peroneal nerve) and the graft is passed through this tunnel and brought back up to the femoral origin of the graft for additional fixation. The popliteofibular ligament can be reconstructed by extending the graft used to reconstruct the FCL through the same tibial tunnel that would be made for popliteus reconstruction after it exits the fibular tunnel.[110,111] When securing grafts in a fibular tunnel, the leg is placed in 30 degrees of knee flexion and a slight valgus stress is applied during fixation. Grafts in the tibial tunnel are secured with the knee in 60 degrees of flexion and with a similar valgus load applied.

Anatomic Reconstruction Technique

The anatomic reconstruction technique has been popularized by LaPrade et al.[111,112] In the orthopaedic literature, the "anatomic" technique has come to mean the inclusion of a tibial tunnel. After an initial lateral hockey stick incision is made, dissection is carried down to the IT band and the long head of the biceps femoris. The peroneal nerve is identified, and a neurolysis performed. A small incision is made through the anterior arm of the biceps femoris and dissection is carried down to the FCL, and its anatomic attachment to the fibula is identified and cleared from the bone. With use of a cruciate ligament tunnel guide, a 7-mm tunnel is made in the fibular head while protecting the peroneal nerve. The tibial tunnel is then drilled by first identifying relevant landmarks, including the starting point, which is an area just medial and distal to Gerdy's tubercle and the exit point of the tunnel, which is a small sulcus on the posterolateral tibial plateau at the level of the musculotendinous junction of the popliteus.[112] With use of a cruciate ligament tunnel guide and a guide pin, the tibial tunnel is drilled while protecting neurovascular structures. The IT band is then split over the lateral epicondyle of the femur. Dissection is carried down to the femoral attachment of the popliteus and FCL. Guide pins are placed through the attachment sites of each structure, and 9-mm tunnels are reamed. Previous prepared grafts with bone plugs are passed into these tunnels by using a passing stitch in the guide pin and bringing the pins out medial, and the plugs are secured with interference screws. The tendinous portion of the grafts have been tubularized and prepared for passage through the tunnels. One graft is then passed along the anatomic path of the popliteus and brought through the tibial tunnel in a posterior-to-anterior fashion. The second graft is passed along the anatomic path of the FCL and brought through the femoral tunnel from lateral to medial and then through the tibial tunnel from posterior to anterior. Interference screws are used for fixation in the tibia and fibula.

Fibula-Based Reconstruction

The focus of the fibula-based technique is reconstruction of the lateral collateral ligament and the popliteofibular ligament. This technique offers several advantages, including only needing a single hamstring autograft tendon, allowing for remaining native tissue to be preserved and incorporated into the reconstruction, and avoiding tunnels that could threaten a femoral tunnel created for ACL reconstruction in cases of concomitant injury. Additionally, it is relatively easy to perform and can be used in all settings of PLC injuries, including instances of associated tibiofibular dislocation. In this case, the tibiofibular joint is simply stabilized prior to proceeding with reconstruction. The fibula-based reconstruction is described in the Authors' Preferred Technique section.

Decision-Making Principles

The decision on how to ultimately treat a particular PLC injury depends on a number of factors, including the timing of the diagnosis, the extent of the injury, and the degree of subsequent instability.

Timing of Diagnosis

PLC injuries are classified as either acute or chronic. Typically, acute refers to treatment within 3 weeks from the time of injury, but some investigators include up to 6 weeks. Studies have shown that efforts should be made to treat PLC injuries acutely, assuming the patient and the knee are in a suitable condition for surgery, because acutely treated injuries have better outcomes than do chronically managed injuries.[6,35,59,64,79,94] Within the acute stage, structures are more easily visualized, scarring is not as prominent, and the tissue is more amenable to repair, if primary repair is to be attempted. However, as reconstructive techniques continue to improve, the timing of treatment is becoming less important, because reconstruction can effectively be performed in both the acute and chronic settings.

Nonoperative Management

The decision to treat a PLC injury nonoperatively must take into consideration the extent of the injury and the overall stability of the joint.

Grade I Injuries

Isolated grade I injuries are stable, and nonoperative treatment consistently produces good results.[6,57,61,64,113,114] The true outcome of these injuries is difficult to determine, because it is likely that many people do not seek treatment for isolated grade I injuries. These injuries are treated symptomatically. Physical therapy directed at quadriceps strengthening and range-of-motion exercises can begin almost immediately.

Grade II Injuries

The decision of how to treat grade II injuries is more difficult. Isolated grade II injuries with only mild abnormal joint motion typically respond well to nonoperative management but may result in some degree of residual instability.[6,57,61,64,113,114] For stable grade II injuries, management is similar to grade I injuries, and they are treated symptomatically. A similar physical therapy protocol may be used, but the patient should progress more slowly. For more severe grade II injuries and grade II injuries with concomitant ligamentous injuries, surgical intervention should be considered, which includes cases with concomitant ACL or PCL reconstruction because of the increased failure rate of these reconstructions in the setting of untreated PLC injuries.[49,50,52]

Grade III Injuries

Grade III injuries (those with significant instability) have universally inferior outcomes when treated conservatively compared with those treated surgically.[113-115] In each of these studies, conservatively managed grade III injuries were reported to have persistent instability, only fair outcomes, and increased rates of osteoarthritis. Similar to grade II injuries, concomitant cruciate ligament reconstructions have inferior outcomes in conservatively managed grade III PLC injuries.[49,50,52] For this reason, as in severe grade II injuries, surgical treatment is recommended to produce a more stable knee.

Repair Versus Reconstruction

Historically, it had been believed that primary repair within the acute setting produced good results and should be the primary treatment.[2,6,64,116] Repair consisted of identifying individual structures and securing avulsed structures to bone or performing side-to-side repair. However, recently, studies have started to cast doubt on the benefits of primary repair. Stannard et al.[95] found a 37% failure rate in acutely repaired knees. Levy et al.[96] identified a 40% failure rate of repair compared with 6% for reconstruction, and Geeslin and LaPrade[98] found superior results of combined repair and reconstruction. It has also been shown that the FCL and popliteus tendon have little healing potential, thus making primary repair less likely to be successful.[115] As a result, attempts at primary repair should be limited to the acute setting for structures with easily identified avulsions from bone without evidence of midsubstance injury and that are easily anatomically reduced with the knee in full extension.[57,97] Otherwise, reconstruction should be performed. Proponents of acute reconstruction also point out the ability for accelerated therapy and range-of-motion exercises compared with the need for longer immobilization for the repaired structures to heal.

AUTHORS' PREFERRED TECHNIQUE

For injuries that produce an unstable joint based on physical examination, we prefer a fibula-based reconstruction technique in both the acute and chronic settings.[117] The procedure is performed with the patient supine on the operating table. Initially, an examination is performed after administration of an anesthetic to confirm the diagnosis and recognize concomitant ligamentous injury. A tourniquet is placed on the upper thigh. A diagnostic arthroscopy is performed and intraarticular pathology is addressed, including articular cartilage injuries and meniscus tears. Typically, cruciate ligament reconstruction is performed at this time. After arthroscopy, the extremity is exsanguinated and the tourniquet is inflated. A semitendinosus tendon is harvested and prepared on the back table by tubularizing it and preparing each end with No. 2 nonabsorbable suture to facilitate graft passage.

A longitudinal incision is made on the lateral side of the knee centered on the lateral epicondyle proximally and between Gerdy's tubercle and the fibular head distally (Fig. 101-13). The incision is carried down to the iliotibial band with thick soft-tissue flaps preserved. The peroneal nerve is identified behind the biceps femoris, marked with a vessel loop, and protected throughout the procedure.

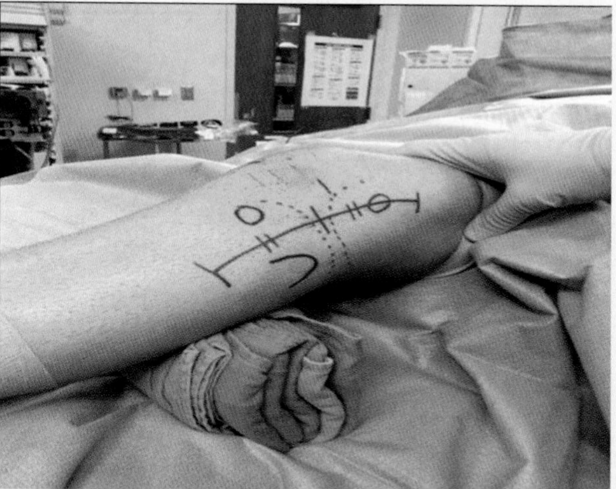

FIGURE 101-13 Surface anatomy for planning the incision to perform a posterolateral corner reconstruction on a left knee.

Next, exposure of the deep structures is performed through the three windows described by Terry and LaPrade.[19] In an acute injury, primary repair of individual structures can then be performed before proceeding with reconstruction with the use of direct sutures to bone, suture anchors, or screws and washers.

The femoral attachment of the FCL and the insertion of the popliteus are visualized. A point equidistant between these two structures is identified, and the soft tissue in this area is elevated off of bone (Fig. 101-14). A 6.5-mm screw and an 18-mm washer construct is used as an anchor and drilled appropriately. A countersink attached to the drill removes additional soft tissue and creates a bleeding bone bed to facilitate healing. An 18-mm washer is specifically chosen to help maintain the anatomic relationship of the femoral attachments of the popliteus and FCL, because they are 18.5 mm apart.[13] The screw, usually 30- to 35-mm long, is inserted until just enough protrudes to allow graft passage.

The peroneal nerve is then identified distally and a neurolysis is performed if necessary. It is protected with retractors and a tunnel is drilled anterior to posterior through the fibular head using a 6- to 7-mm acorn reamer over a guide wire 1 to 1.5 cm distal to the proximal tip of the fibular head (Fig. 101-15). The

Continued

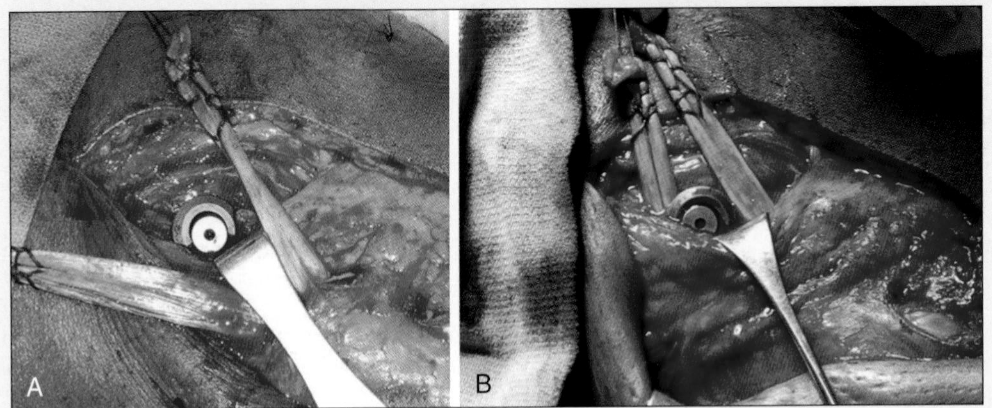

FIGURE 101-14 **A,** Graft passage through the fibular tunnel. **B,** Graft passage around the femoral washer.

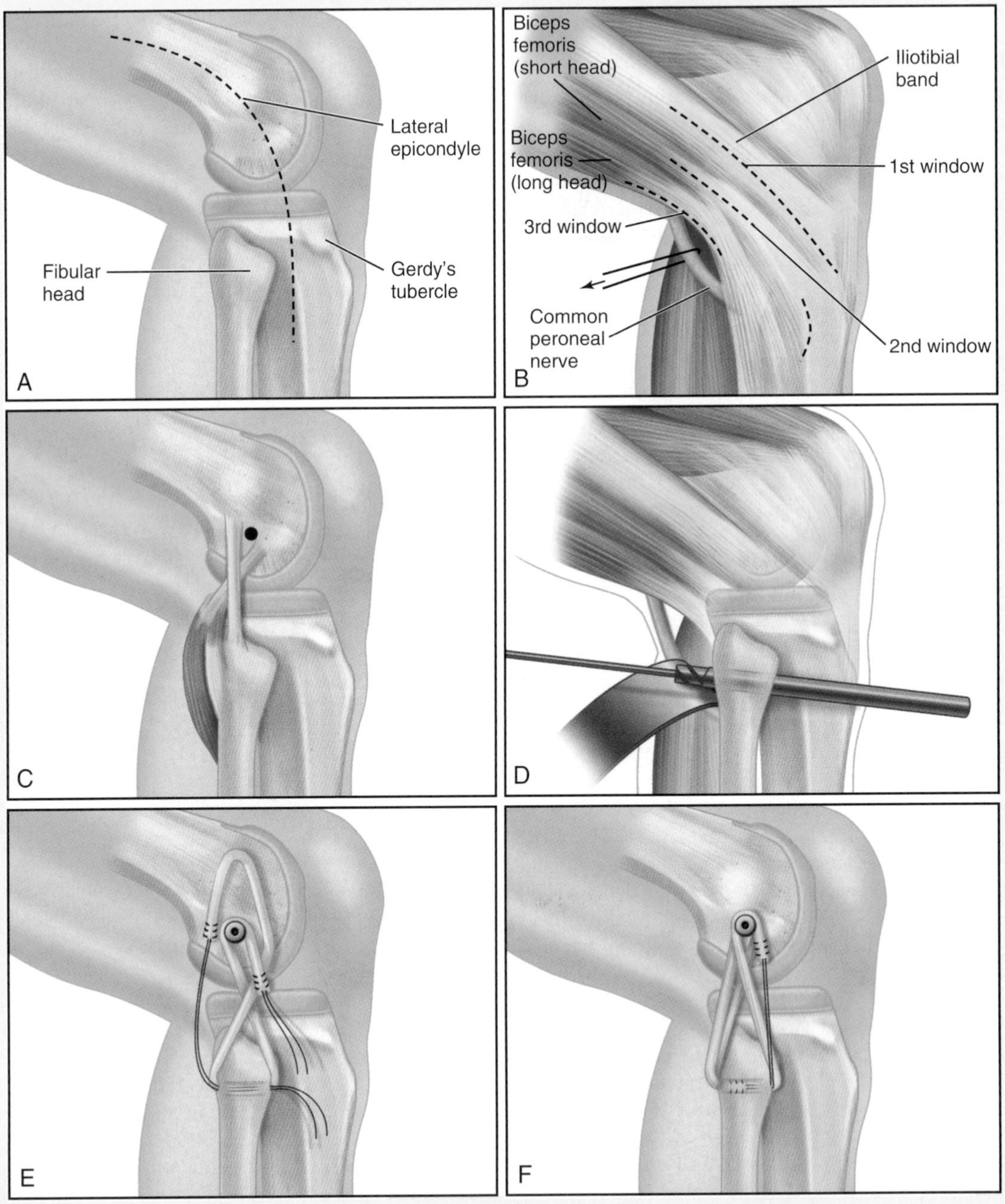

FIGURE 101-15 **A,** The longitudinal skin incision crosses the lateral epicondyle proximally and bisects Gerdy's tubercle and the fibular head distally. **B,** The lateral side of the knee is exposed through the three windows. **C,** The position of the femoral drill hole is at "ground zero," which is a point equidistant from the femoral attachment of the lateral collateral ligament and the insertion of the popliteus tendon. **D,** A 7-mm tunnel is drilled through the fibular head 1 to 1.5 cm from the proximal tip and superior to the point where the peroneal nerve crosses the neck of the fibular. **E** and **F,** The graft is passed through the fibula and around the washer and back through the tunnel (if length allows). *(From Larson MW, Moinfar AR, Moorman CT, III: Posterolateral corner reconstruction: fibular-based technique.* J Knee Surg *28[2]:163–166, 2005.)*

prepared semitendinosus graft is passed through this tunnel. A posterior limb is passed under the biceps femoris and under the IT band up to the screw on the femur. The anterior limb is passed under the IT band and up to just below the screw. The anterior limb does not pass around the screw so as to avoid excess soft tissue causing a more prominent screw and washer. The anterior limb is sutured to soft tissue just distal to the screw. The posterior limb is made longer than the anterior limb. The knee is flexed 30 degrees, valgus and internal rotatory forces are placed on the knee, and the screw and washer are tightened. The posterior limb is passed back through the tunnel in the fibular head. The passing sutures are then tied to each other and the graft limbs are sewn together for additional support.

The area is copiously irrigated. The tourniquet is let down and hemostasis is maintained. The incisions in the lateral capsule and IT bands are closed. The skin is closed and a bandage is applied. A hinged knee brace, locked in extension, is applied.

Surgical Pearls

- Use an 18-mm washer to restore the anatomic arrangement of the popliteus and FCL on the femur.
- In case of tibiofibular joint instability, drill a fibular tunnel for a graft before stabilizing the joint to avoid cutting the fixation device with the drill through the fibula.
- Minimize the amount of the graft under the washer to avoid prominent hardware.
- For obese patients, consider external fixation for added stability in the early postoperative period.
- When drilling for a femoral screw, dropping the hand slightly toward the ankle to allow a proximally directed screw will limit interference with ACL tunnels.
- Protection of the peroneal nerve is imperative during fibular tunnel preparation.

AUTHORS' PREFERRED TECHNIQUE

Proximal Tibial Osteotomy

In the setting of chronic varus malalignment, we perform an opening wedge osteotomy for deformity correction. Similar to the findings of Arthur et al.,[106] we have found that osteotomy alone can restore stability and PLC reconstruction is not always necessary (Fig. 101-16).

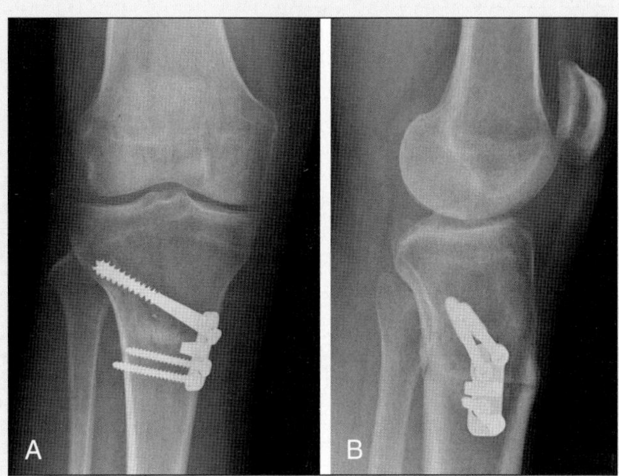

FIGURE 101-16 Final anteroposterior (**A**) and lateral (**B**) radiograph appearance of a completed high tibial osteotomy.

AUTHORS' PREFERRED TECHNIQUE

Proximal Tibiofibular Joint Instability

Proximal tibiofibular joint instability should be considered in the setting of PLC injury. Acute anterolateral dislocation, the most common form of instability, is frequently associated with injury to the FCL and biceps femoris tendon and results from injury to the anterior and posterior capsular ligaments.[118,119] The diagnosis can be made clinically and radiographically, with various tests and radiographic measures described.[119]

Proximal tibiofibular joint instability does not prevent a fibula-based reconstruction. The key is to identify the injury and stabilize the joint. Various techniques have been described throughout the literature. We use a suture fixation device technique for stabilization (Fig. 101-17). The incision created for PLC reconstruction is used. Dissection is carried down to the peroneal nerve. The nerve is identified and protected throughout. The suture device is passed across the fibula and into the tibia and finally deployed on the medial side of the tibia. It is tightened to the appropriate tension and tied over the fibula. A second device is deployed in a similar fashion. The knots are buried in soft tissue to avoid irritation of the peroneal nerve, or newer knotless devices may be used.

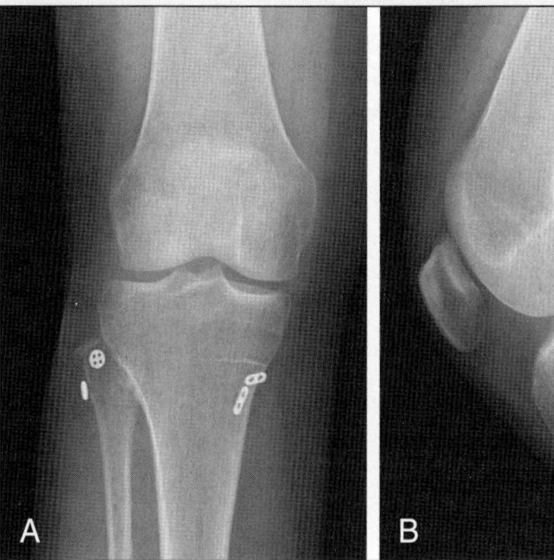

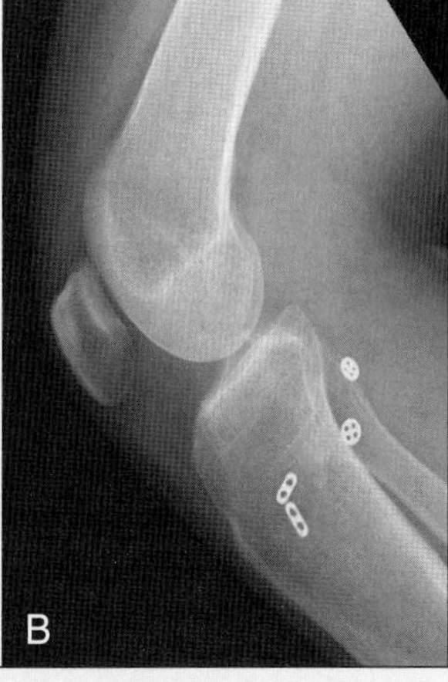

FIGURE 101-17 Anteroposterior (**A**) and lateral (**B**) radiographs showing proximal tibiofibular joint stabilization.

Postoperative Management

A four-phase rehabilitation protocol is used (Table 101-2). In phase I, typically in postoperative weeks 0 to 8, the goals are to protect the reconstructed structures, decrease inflammation and swelling, and carefully advance range of motion of the joint. Initially, the patient performs only toe-touch weight bearing for at least 6 weeks. The extremity is protected in a hinged knee brace locked in extension for 2 weeks. After 2 weeks, passive range of motion is begun as symptoms allow. Quadriceps sets are allowed and patella mobilization is performed. Hamstring contractions and stretching are avoided. Precautions are taken to specifically prevent tibial external rotation and varus stress. After 8 weeks, the brace is unlocked and active and passive range of motion is advanced as tolerated.

In phase II, typically during postoperative weeks 9 to 12, attempts are made to eliminate inflammation and swelling, obtain full range of motion, restore normal gait, and improve lower extremity strength. During this phase, more aggressive range-of-motion exercises are performed until full range of motion is achieved, which includes the use of a stationary bicycle. Closed kinetic chain quad strengthening begins, and cross-training machines may be used for conditioning. Gait mechanics are restored and proprioceptive exercises are performed.

In phase III, typically during postoperative weeks 13 to 24, attempts are made to increase strength to at least 85% of the contralateral limb, improve aerobic endurance, initiate plyometric exercises, and begin a running program. Modalities include using a spin bike, Cybex training, agility drills, and advanced proprioception exercises. Strengthening is continued. A return to running is initiated, initially using a treadmill, and is advanced to level, outdoor surfaces.

Phase IV is started once the extremity has reached greater than or equal to 85% of the strength of the contralateral limb and has results of a single-leg hop test greater than or equal to 85% of the contralateral limb, when no pain is experienced with forward running, agilities, jump training, or strengthening, and when the patient demonstrates good knee control with single-leg dynamic proprioceptive activities. This phase attempts to return the patient to full sport activities, to create equal strength, balance, proprioception, and power bilaterally, and to achieve a 100% global function rating. Exercises started in phase III are advanced, with a gradual increase in the level of participation in sport-specific activities, and the patient progresses to running on all surfaces without restriction.

Return to Play

Once the athlete has progressed to stage IV of the rehabilitation protocol, he or she begins sport-specific rehabilitation, conditioning, and training. Minimal data exist on PLC injuries in elite athletes, given their rare diagnosis.[120-122] In a retrospective review of National Football League players, Bushnell et al.[120] found that nine players over a 10-year period were diagnosed with isolated grade III fibular collateral ligament tears, and the four who underwent operative treatment and the five who were treated nonoperatively all returned to play in the NFL. In general, it may take at least a year for an athlete to return to a preinjury level of play. Extensive rehabilitation is required, and clearance from the treating physician must be obtained before returning to competitive training and sports. This decision is based on functional screening measures, strength testing, the knee's range of motion, absence of swelling, and painless sport-specific activities. Preoperatively, it is important to discuss the expected time frame for returning to sporting activities so the athlete has realistic expectations during the rehabilitation process.

Results

Numerous studies demonstrating the results of various techniques used to treat PLC instability have been published. Without a standardized outcome measure, it is difficult to

TABLE 101-2

FOUR-PHASE REHABILITATION PROTOCOL USED AFTER POSTEROLATERAL CORNER RECONSTRUCTION

Phase 1 (Weeks 0-8)	Phase 2 (Weeks 9-12)	Phase 3 (Weeks 13-24)	Phase 4 (Weeks 24+)
Restricted motion to promote healing (knee locked in extension for 2 weeks and then passive ROM 0-90 degrees with therapy after 2 weeks)	Obtain full knee ROM	Improve aerobic endurance, initiate plyometric exercises	Begin sport-specific functional motions
Toe-touch weight bearing for 6 weeks, and then gradual progression of weight-bearing status	Restore normal gait, initiate proprioception exercises	Initiate running program on level surfaces	Obtain equal balance and proprioception, gradually increase level of participation in sports
Quadriceps strengthening/patella mobilization	Continue strengthening, including closed kinetic chain exercises	Increase strength to at least 85% of the contralateral limb	Obtain equal bilateral lower extremity strength
Avoid hamstring stretches and external rotation/varus stress on the tibia	Eliminate residual swelling/inflammation	Have no pain with running, agility exercises, jumping, or strengthening	Pass all sport-specific functional screens and activities

ROM, Range of motion.

TABLE 101-3

CADAVERIC BIOMECHANICAL STUDIES OF POSTEROLATERAL CORNER RECONSTRUCTION

Study	Year	No. of Knees	Technique	Outcome
LaPrade et al.[111]	2005	10	Anatomic	No difference in external rotation stability between intact knee or reconstructed knee
Rauh et al.[123]	2010	10	Fibula based vs. anatomic	No difference in stability observed between either reconstruction technique
Apsingi et al.[124]	2009	10	Fibula based vs. anatomic	No difference in stability observed between either reconstruction technique
Nau et al.[125]	2005	10	Fibula based vs. anatomic	No difference in stability observed between either reconstruction technique

truly compare these various techniques. Additionally, the length of follow-up varies between the different studies, which can make one technique appear superior to another. Also, authors often use similar descriptive terms for techniques but offer a modification to a previously described technique of the same name. For example, within the literature, multiple authors describe an anatomic reconstruction, but great variability exists between the different anatomic techniques. In Tables 101-3[111,123-125] and 101-4,[67,95,96,106,113,126-130] studies indicating "fibular based" imply isolated tunnels in the fibula and femur, whereas studies indicating "anatomic" imply an additional tibial tunnel.

Complications

Complications may be separated into two categories: those resulting from the injury and those resulting from the surgery. As with any surgery, the risk of bleeding, infection, deep venous thrombosis, and prominent/painful hardware are associated with reconstruction of PLC injuries. Because injuries to the PLC more commonly occur with additional ligamentous injuries, they are often seen in the setting of knee dislocations and therefore may carry many of the same risks. In the setting of significant soft tissue injury or open wounds, infection and soft tissue healing can become a problem, and infection occurs

TABLE 101-4

RESULTS OF VARIOUS TECHNIQUES FOR POSTEROLATERAL CORNER RECONSTRUCTION

Study	Year	N	Mean Follow-up and Range (mo)	Mean Age and Range (yr)	Technique	Outcome
Kannus[113]	1989	23	99 (72-126)	34 (14-61)	Nonoperative management	Grade I and II: 82% returned to preinjury level of activity Grade III: 25% returned to preinjury level of activity
Levy et al.[96]	2010	10	34 (24-49)	Not reported	Repair	40% failure rate
Stannard et al.[95]	2005	57	24 (24-59)	33 (17-57)	Repair	37% failure rate
Arthur et al.[106]	2007	21	37 (19-65)	32 (18-49)	High tibial osteotomy	38% of patients stable after high tibial osteotomy only (no reconstruction needed)
Yoon et al.[126]	2006	25	39 (26-60)	33 (19-52)	Sling procedure	39% persistent excess laxity (12% external rotation, 28% varus laxity)
Kim et al.[101]	2003	46	40 (24-93)	35 (16-62)	Biceps tenodesis	17% with loss of stability at final follow-up
Yoon et al.[126]	2006	21	22 (12-41)	34 (21-64)	Anatomic	19% with greater than 1+ excess laxity
LaPrade et al.[127]	2010	54	53 (24-86)	32 (18-58)	Anatomic	5% recurrent instability requiring revision surgery
Jakobsen et al.[128]	2010	27	46 (24-86)	28 (13-57)	Anatomic	5% with rotatory instability and 5% varus instability
Camarda et al.[67]	2010	10	28 (18-40)	27 (16-47)	Fibular based	0% loss of stability, 10% overconstrained compared with uninjured side
Schechinger et al.[129]	2009	16	30 (24-75)	30 (19-61)	Fibular based + capsular shift	No functional instability, 25% with 1+ varus laxity
Khanduja et al.[130]	2006	19	67 (24-110)	30 (21-47)	Fibular based	26% with "residual minimal posterolateral instability" but not further defined

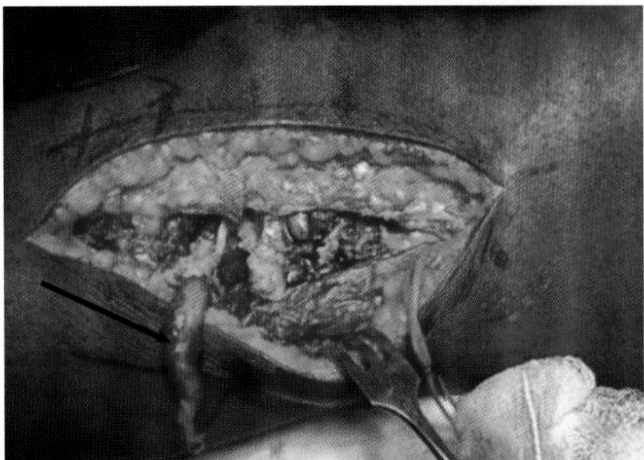

FIGURE 101-18 A peroneal nerve avulsion injury (*black arrow*) after a posterolateral corner injury. *(Courtesy Katherine Coyner, MD.)*

in up to 43% of open knee dislocations.[131] With its close proximity to the lateral joint capsule, common peroneal nerve injury is common and has been documented in 13% of patients with PLC injuries.[26,132] Nerve injury appears to be related to disruption of the distal attachment of the biceps tendon to the fibular head, causing the nerve to be displaced into an abnormal position, thus making it vulnerable to injury.[133] In the chronic setting, the risk of iatrogenic peroneal nerve injury may be increased because of the presence of more scar tissue, and subsequently, a more difficult neurolysis procedure (Fig. 101-18). Vascular injury, which requires immediate recognition and treatment, has been reported to occur in 12% to 64% of knee dislocations.[134,135] A detailed neurovascular examination is imperative, not only to identify limb-threatening emergencies, but to also identify neurologic deficit prior to surgical intervention, given the proximity of the peroneal nerve to the surgical field. Posttraumatic joint space narrowing after PLC reconstruction was reported to occur in 29% of patients followed up 4 years postoperatively, with most of those patients having evidence of early chondrosis at the time of initial surgery.[136] Joint stiffness, or arthrofibrosis, may also occur after these injuries and their reconstruction. Some period of immobilization is required to promote healing, which places the knee at risk for the development of arthrofibrosis. This risk can be decreased by determining, intraoperatively, a safe degree of flexion to allow in the early postoperative period and to perform patellar mobilization.[59] Iatrogenic fracture of the fibular head can occur during bone tunnel preparation if the guide pin is not appropriately placed prior to reaming. Painful hardware has been a problem with the tibial screw and washer construct in the past. Lower profile hardware may minimize this concern.

Future Considerations

Pediatric Posterolateral Corner Injuries

As the number of children playing sports increases and as more demands and expectations are placed on these adolescent athletes, the rate of injury is going to increase and may include a higher incidence of PLC injuries. Purely ligamentous injury is uncommon in the pediatric population, which is most often attributed to the ligament being stronger than the adjacent growth plate.[137,138] PLC injuries appear to be especially rare. In a review of 39 adolescents undergoing ACL reconstruction, despite 67% having concomitant injuries, none were diagnosed as having PLC injuries.[139] Case series have described isolated avulsions of the popliteus tendon and injuries to both the popliteus and FCL.[140-144] Von Heideken et al.[144] identified 23 reported cases of isolated pediatric PLC injuries in the literature, with most involving avulsion fractures at the femoral attachment of the popliteus and fibular collateral ligament. However, no extensive report on pediatric PLC injuries was found in the literature.

Given its rare incidence, treatment of isolated pediatric PLC injuries is not clear. Kannus and Jarvinen[145] reported on the nonoperative treatment of 33 adolescents with grade II and III ligament injuries, including five grade II and two grade III FCL injuries. The findings, which were not just specific to the LCL injuries, resembled those found in adults, with the grade II injuries doing well and the grade III injuries having poor results and persistent instability. It was recommended that the grade III injuries be treated surgically. However, the best way to surgically treat these injuries remains unclear. Additionally, surgical treatment in adolescents poses the additional risk of operating around the physis and risking growth disturbance. Complicating this situation is the fact that the one patient in the case series by Von Heideken et al.[144] who was treated nonoperatively was the only patient in whom a growth disturbance and angular deformity of the injured extremity developed. More research is necessary to better determine the best way to treat these rare injuries.

For a complete list of references, go to expertconsult.com.

Suggested Readings

Citation: Larson MW, Moinfar AR, Moorman CT, III: Posterolateral corner reconstruction: Fibular-based technique. *J Knee Surg* 18(2):163–166, 2005.
Level of Evidence: IV
Summary: The fibula-based technique for both acute and chronic posterolateral corner reconstruction is a successful way to restore stability, preserve native tissue to incorporate into the reconstruction, and minimize bone tunnels during combined reconstructions, and it is relatively easy to perform. The technique is thoroughly described.

Citation: LaPrade RF, Ly TV, Wentorf FA, et al: The posterolateral attachments of the knee: A qualitative and quantitative morphologic analysis of the fibular collateral ligament, popliteus tendon, popliteofibular ligament, and lateral gastrocnemius tendon. *Am J Sports Med* (31):854–860, 2003.
Level of Evidence: Cadaveric study
Summary: The femoral and tibial attachments for the major structures of the posterolateral corner have a consistent anatomic relationship to each other with consistently measurable distances between the various structures. It is important to consider these relationships and restore this anatomic relationship during reconstruction techniques.

Citation: Levy BA, Dajani KA, Morgan JA, et al: Repair versus reconstruction of the fibular collateral ligament and posterolateral corner in the multiligament-injured knee. *Am J Sports Med* 38(4):804–809, 2010.
Level of Evidence: III
Summary: Comparing the acute repair of structures with the reconstruction of the posterolateral corner revealed a much higher failure rate in the acute repair group, in which 40% failed compared with 6% in the reconstruction group. Reconstruction should be considered, even in the acute setting, because of the much higher rate of failure in the primary repair group.

Citation: LaPrade RF, Resig S, Wentorf F, et al: The effects of grade III posterolateral knee complex injuries on anterior cruciate ligament graft forces. *Am J Sports Med* 27(4):469–475, 1999.

Level of Evidence: Cadaveric study

Summary: Untreated grade III posterolateral corner injuries lead to significantly higher forces on the anterior cruciate ligament. Therefore, in the setting of combined injury, untreated grade III posterolateral corner injuries contribute to ACL graft failure because of this higher force experienced by the graft.

Citation: LaPrade RF, Wentorf FA, Fritts H, et al: A prospective magnetic resonance imaging study of the incidence of posterolateral and multiple ligament injuries in acute knee injuries presenting with a hemarthrosis. *Arthroscopy* 23:1341–1347, 2007.

Level of Evidence: II

Summary: Out of 331 patients with acute knee injuries presenting with a hemarthrosis, 9.1% of the entire group and 16% of the group diagnosed with ligament tears were found to have a posterolateral knee injury, and in more than 50% of these injuries, more than one posterolateral corner structure was involved. Posterolateral corner injuries may be more common than previously reported, and when present, they are usually associated with additional ligamentous injury.

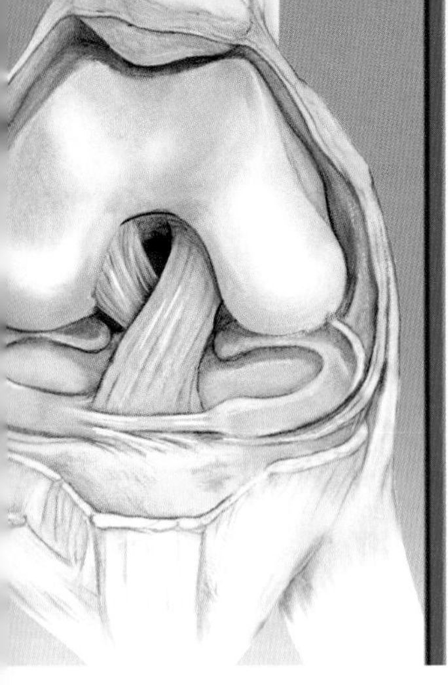

102

Multiligament Knee Injuries

ANDREW G. GEESLIN • ROBERT F. LAPRADE

Knee ligaments are responsible for providing the static stability of the knee, control of kinematics, and prevention of abnormal rotation and/or displacement that may damage the articular surfaces or the menisci. Multiligament knee injuries are rare and are estimated to account for 0.02% to 0.2% of orthopaedic injuries.[1] These injuries may spontaneously reduce or may present as an acutely dislocated knee requiring reduction. The diagnosis and management of multiligament injuries pose unique challenges to orthopaedic surgeons, and a wide spectrum of injury exists, ranging from two-ligament injuries such as a cruciate and collateral ligament rupture to a grossly unstable knee that requires spanning external fixation. Although the immediate concerns should be to determine the integrity of the neurovascular structures, other essential concepts include accurate identification of all injured structures, repair versus reconstruction, management of acute versus chronic injuries, single- versus two-stage surgery, and postoperative rehabilitation. During the past three decades, clinical outcome studies along with anatomic and biomechanical investigations have improved the management of these complex injuries.

History

In evaluating a patient who presents with knee pain or instability, the clinician must obtain a careful history of symptom onset, mechanism of injury, history of prior knee injuries, and previous operative and nonoperative treatments. Multiligament injuries associated with sports are considered low energy and are often isolated to the involved extremity, whereas those associated with automobile or motorcycle crashes are considered high-energy[2] and may be combined with other life-threatening injuries.

Acutely injured patients may be unable to ambulate because of swelling, pain, and instability. Determination of time since injury is crucial in patients who present with persistent dislocation because of the possibility of vascular injury and limb ischemia. Patients with chronic injuries may report mechanical symptoms including clicking, catching, or locking or may report instability on uneven ground, with cutting motions, and during activities of daily living. Neurologic deficits may be reported, including the presence of paresthesias in the common peroneal nerve distribution and a foot drop. Synthesis of this information will guide the clinician in the physical examination and selection of imaging studies.

Physical Examination

Examination of a patient with a suspected multiligament injury in the acute setting must include assessment of vascular status. If an arterial injury is suspected, an ankle-brachial index score should be determined; a score of less than 0.9 is an indication that advanced arterial imaging should be obtained.[3] Serial neurovascular examination and selective computed tomography angiography has been recommended; "hard signs" of ischemia warrant emergent vascular consultation.[4]

Neurologic status must also be assessed. The common peroneal nerve supplies motor innervation to the anterior (deep peroneal) and lateral (superficial peroneal) compartments of the leg, as well as the extensor hallucis brevis and extensor digitorum brevis (deep peroneal) on the dorsum of the foot. A 25% to 35% nerve injury rate has been reported in the knee dislocation population.[5] In a series of acute isolated or combined posterolateral corner (PLC) knee injuries in an orthopaedic sports medicine referral practice, 4 of 29 patients had a complete palsy of the common peroneal nerve and an additional 7 of 29 had a partial motor/sensory deficit.[6] Tibial nerve injuries may also occur in knee dislocations; although these injuries occur less frequently than common peroneal nerve injuries, they are more devastating.

Physical examination of knee stability is a repeatable method of predicting intraarticular pathology but may be more difficult in patients with acute injuries. It is important to examine both legs to assess for pathologic instability versus physiologic laxity. Multiligament injuries are not subtle on examination; however, attention to subtle findings will aid the clinician in determining which specific structures are injured. Anteroposterior stability should be assessed with the Lachman, pivot shift, and posterior drawer tests. The posterior sag and quadriceps active tests also aid in the evaluation of the posterior cruciate ligament (PCL).

Lateral and posterolateral knee injuries are typically combined with an injury to one or both of the cruciate ligaments.[6-8] In acute injuries, the patient may have tenderness to palpation at the fibular head. Examination maneuvers should include varus stress[9] at 0 and 20 degrees, reverse pivot shift, external rotation recurvatum,[10] and the dial test at 30 and 90 degrees. In a patient with a positive varus stress test at 30 degrees and negative findings at 0 degrees, an isolated fibular collateral ligament (FCL) tear is suspected. However, with multiligament injuries, the varus stress test will also be positive at 0 degrees. A positive dial test at both 30 and 90 degrees suggests a combined PCL and PLC injury.[11,12] A positive posterolateral drawer test reinforces findings consistent with a PLC injury but must be interpreted with caution, as discussed below.

Medial structures are evaluated with the valgus stress test at 0 and 20 degrees of flexion[13]; instability at full extension is indicative of a combined cruciate ligament injury. Assessment of medial compartment gapping at 20 degrees under a valgus stress primarily isolates the superficial medial collateral ligament (MCL). Evaluation of associated rotational abnormalities is assessed with anteromedial tibial rotation at 90 degrees of flexion and the dial test at 30 and 90 degrees of flexion.[14] Increased anteromedial rotation suggests a more extensive knee injury that includes the superficial MCL, as well as the posterior oblique ligament (POL) and deep MCL. The examiner must be careful to differentiate anteromedial from posterolateral tibial rotation during the dial test by palpation and visualization of tibial subluxation with the patient in the supine position.[14]

Gait assessment is an important component of the physical examination but may be compromised because of pain in persons with acute injuries. In subacute or chronic injuries, a varus thrust gait or foot drop may be observed in patients with combined lateral injuries. Patients with medial knee injuries may demonstrate a valgus thrust during the stance phase of gait, but this manifestation is less common and usually occurs in patients with genu valgus alignment.

Imaging

Radiographic examination of the knee for patients with a suspected multiligament injury should include standard anteroposterior and lateral views (Fig. 102-1), as well as weight-bearing flexion (Rosenberg) views.[15] These views allow visualization of tibial plateau, femoral condyle, or osteochondral fractures. Segond[16] and/or arcuate[17] fractures may be visualized with lateral/posterolateral injuries, and calcification near the MCL origin (Pellegrini-Stieda ossification) may be visualized in chronic medial-sided injuries. Baseline bilateral standing long-leg radiographs allow the clinician to determine the mechanical axis of the injured and contralateral extremities, which may have a significant impact on treatment decisions for chronic multiligament injuries.[18,19]

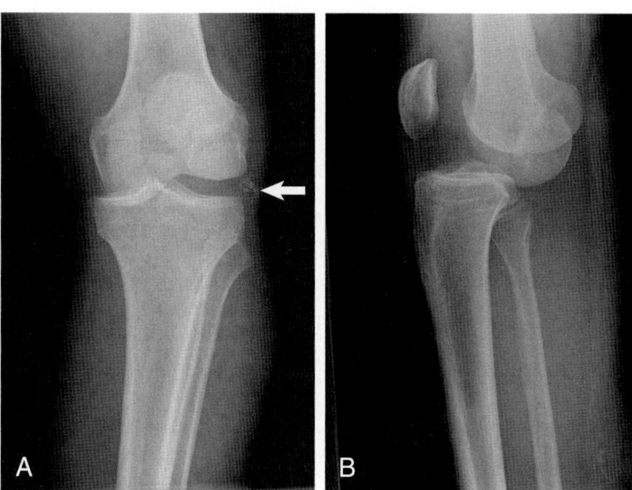

FIGURE 102-1 Anteroposterior (**A**) and lateral (**B**) radiographs demonstrating an acute left knee dislocation. An arcuate fracture is also visible on the anteroposterior radiograph (*arrow*).

Preoperative stress radiographs provide quantitative objective information on the stability to valgus and varus stress and should also be routinely obtained postoperatively. Biomechanical studies were performed to objectively quantify the amount of joint opening with varus[9] and valgus[13] stress; radiographic techniques were developed and tested by sequential sectioning in cadaveric knees with intact cruciate ligaments. Isolated sectioning of the FCL (simulating a grade III injury) resulted in an increase of 2.7 mm of lateral joint gapping at 20 degrees of flexion when compared with the contralateral knee. Sectioning of the FCL, popliteus tendon, and PFL (simulating a complete grade III PLC injury) was associated with lateral joint gapping of 4 mm at 20 degrees of flexion. Isolated sectioning of the superficial MCL (simulating a grade III injury) resulted in 3.2 mm of increased medial joint gapping at 20 degrees of flexion when compared with the contralateral knee. Increased medial joint gapping of 6.5 mm and 9.8 mm at 0 and 20 degrees of flexion, respectively, was associated with sectioning of the superficial MCL, deep MCL, and POL (simulating a complete medial knee injury).

Several imaging techniques have been developed to allow quantitative assessment of the integrity of the PCL and are especially useful in persons with chronic injuries. Stress radiographs have been described using the kneeling knee technique[20] and Telos device (Telos GmbH, Marburg, Germany)[21]; these two techniques have been reported to allow quantifying posterior displacement of the tibia and are superior to a physical examination and use of the KT-1000 arthrometer.[22]

Magnetic resonance imaging (MRI) has become part of the standard of care for evaluation of knee instability, especially in persons with acute injuries for whom examination may be limited by pain and swelling (Fig. 102-2). With high sensitivity and accuracy, MRI allows visualization of the cruciate and collateral ligaments, posteromedial corner and PLC,[23] bone marrow edema,[7,24,25] meniscal injuries, and cartilage lesions. Anteromedial femoral condyle bone bruises should alert the physician to a possible PLC injury.[7]

It is important to recognize common imaging findings associated with multiligament knee injuries. Plain radiographs may be negative in the acute setting if the patient is lying supine, and it may be difficult to obtain weight-bearing films. In chronic injuries, weight-bearing films may reveal varus or valgus gapping or loss of joint space and early findings of degenerative disease. Stress radiographs are especially useful to quantitatively assess stability of the PCL, medial complex, and posterolateral complex. In persons with acute injuries, MRI will reveal the status of the cruciate ligaments and allow assessment of the collateral structures if appropriate cuts and slice thickness are obtained. Classic bone bruises associated with ACL ruptures may be seen, as well as those associated with PLC injuries.

Decision-Making Principles

Patients with multiligament injuries are a heterogeneous group and may present with a variety of skin, bony,

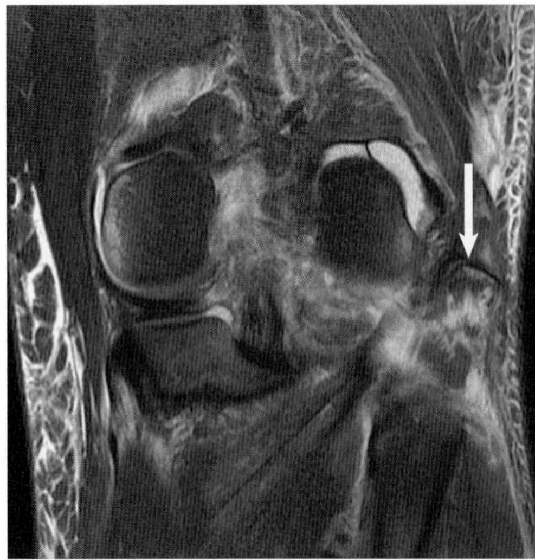

FIGURE 102-2 A coronal magnetic resonance image of a left knee injury with bicruciate rupture and a complete posterolateral corner injury including arcuate fracture *(arrow)* and grade III injury of the fibular collateral ligament, popliteus tendon, and popliteofibular ligament.

neurovascular, and ligamentous injuries. Although several general treatment algorithms have been developed, individualized treatment for the patient's specific knee injuries and concomitant injuries is necessary. Meniscus injuries should ideally be repaired, especially in the young patient, but may require a partial meniscectomy. Management of vascular injuries, open injuries, skin coverage, fracture treatment, and meniscus injuries will not be specifically discussed. Important considerations for treatment of multiligament injuries include operative versus nonoperative treatment, surgical timing, single- versus two-stage cruciate ligament reconstruction techniques, and repair versus reconstruction of collateral structures.

Knee ligament injuries have historically been classified with use of a grading scale that assesses sagittal (anteroposterior) and coronal (varus/valgus) plane[14,26] stability. Rotational stability does not have a formal classification system, although many injury types have been described.[27-29] Treatment must be based on the extent of injury to individual structures and the number of structures injured. Knee ligament injuries are often subjectively classified according to the original American Medical Association guidelines, rated as grade I, II, or III.[30] An additional classification system is based on the number and location of torn ligaments.[31]

Nonoperative Versus Operative Treatment

It must be recognized that multiligament knee injuries are rare and that few studies have been conducted that compare treatment strategies with a high level of evidence. Current literature favors surgical management of multiligament knee injuries,[32-34] whereas in early reports, nonoperative treatment was often recommended for "uncomplicated" cases (i.e., absence of vascular injury or fracture).[35,36] A recent review indicated improved outcomes in multiple subjective and objective facets for patients treated with an operation compared with those treated conservatively with immobilization.[34]

Surgical Timing

Several studies have evaluated the impact of surgical timing. However, interpretation of outcomes of surgically treated multiligament injuries is difficult because of the wide range of pathology within individual studies.[33] Irreducible knee injuries, open injuries, and popliteal vascular injuries necessitate emergent management. If the multiligament injury is associated with a high-energy trauma, overall medical status and serious concomitant extremity, torso, and head injuries may delay definitive treatment. Overlying skin injuries and associated plateau or femoral condyle fractures may necessitate delayed ligament reconstruction. These complicating factors will not be specifically evaluated; rather, the focus will be single-extremity multiligament injuries without concomitant injuries.

Timing of surgery is typically divided into one of the following three categories: acute (often defined as surgery within 3 weeks), chronic (often defined as surgery after 3 weeks), or staged (the index procedure is performed within 3 weeks of injury and second-stage surgery is delayed).[33] Harner et al.[37] reported improved subjective outcomes in acutely treated patients and no ultimate difference in range of motion; however, 4 of 19 patients with acutely reconstructed knees required manipulation for loss of flexion. Fanelli and Edson[38] reported on 35 patients with multiligament injuries and found no subjective differences (according to Tegner, Lysholm, and Hospital for Special Surgery knee ligament rating scales) or objective differences (according to use of the KT-1000 arthrometer) between the acute and chronic cohorts.

A recent systematic review of surgical treatment for multiligament injuries found increased anterior instability for patients treated acutely but no difference in posterior, varus, or valgus instability when compared with chronically treated injuries.[33] Additionally, flexion loss (>10 degrees), as well as the need to undergo a subsequent repeat operation for stiffness, were more frequent in acutely treated patients; no difference was found for extension. Lastly, patients treated with staged reconstructions had more "excellent" or "good" outcomes than did those treated acutely. As described later in this chapter, these findings may be difficult to interpret because many of these patients were treated with acute PLC repairs (which have been found to frequently fail) rather than reconstructions.

Persons with chronic multiligament injuries may present to the orthopaedic surgeon because of a failed index procedure, failed nonoperative management, or concomitant injuries that precluded acute surgical management of the multiligament injury. These patients may have varus malalignment, and a high-tibial osteotomy may be required to correct the mechanical axis prior to ligament reconstruction, because it has been reported as a cause of PLC repair or reconstruction failure.[39,40]

Cruciate Ligament Reconstruction

It is widely accepted that cruciate ligament injuries in patients with multiligament injuries require reconstruction. A biomechanical study by Veltri and colleagues[41] demonstrated the importance of reconstructing the cruciate ligaments in multiligament injuries. Options for anterior cruciate ligament (ACL) reconstruction in multiligament injuries include transtibial versus transportal drilling for femoral tunnels and autograft versus allograft; no known studies recommend double-bundle ACL reconstruction in these patients. The debate regarding the best PCL reconstruction technique to use in persons with multiligament injuries is similar to the debate for isolated injuries; graft fixation techniques, single- versus double-bundle technique, and transtibial tunnel versus tibial inlay technique. Few studies have been performed to compare cruciate ligament reconstruction techniques in the multiligament injury patient population; as such, surgeons must apply the principles used for reconstruction of isolated cruciate ligament injuries to this unique patient group.

Collateral Structures

Until recently it was believed that PLC structures could be successfully repaired if treated acutely. This practice has been challenged by outcomes studies that compare repair and reconstruction.[42,43] It has been biomechanically demonstrated that a deficient PLC leads to increased ACL[44] and PCL[45,46] graft forces; interestingly, Mook et al.[33] reported that more patients treated acutely for multiligament injuries underwent repairs rather than reconstructions of the PLC and suggest that repairs may have been insufficient to protect the ACL graft during healing. These findings may provide clinical evidence that reinforces the biomechanical principles of secondary stabilization between cruciate and collateral ligaments and may support the trend toward acute reconstruction, rather than repair, of PLC structures. As discussed later in this chapter, a gradual trend has occurred from local tissue transfers and acute repairs toward several different autograft or allograft tissue reconstruction techniques.

A well-defined and successful treatment algorithm for isolated grade III MCL injuries and those combined with ACL ruptures includes a short period of rest and edema control followed by physical therapy.[14] However, treatment of MCL injuries associated with bicruciate injuries is less well defined. Some authors advocate delayed cruciate reconstruction while the medial structures are protected with a brace and allowed to potentially heal. Other authors recommend acute repairs or reconstruction of medial structures, although a higher risk of arthrofibrosis is reported.

Graft Choice

Graft choice in multiligament injury reconstruction is determined by injury pattern, graft availability, and surgeon preference. Often surgeons prefer to use allografts when treating multiligament injuries because of multiple graft size options and the ability to avoid the increased operative time and donor site morbidity associated with harvesting the patellar and hamstring tendon, and possibly quadriceps tendon, grafts. Because of the heterogeneity of multiligament injuries, no conclusive studies are available to recommend a particular graft choice. Several techniques are discussed in the Treatment Options section, along with graft choices.

Special Considerations

Pediatric patients with multiligament injuries require special consideration because of their open physes and the potential risk of growth alteration with traditional ligament reconstruction. Physeal sparing techniques for ACL[47] and PCL[48] reconstruction have been described. Lateral and medial structures may be repaired via augmentation or recess procedures[6] or with use of suture anchors.

A recently defined type of knee dislocation has been termed *ultra–low velocity* and was described by Azar and colleagues.[49] These injuries are sustained by patients with a high body mass index as a result of falling from a standing height or tripping on objects, for example. Their treatment must be individualized based on medical comorbidities, patient expectations, preinjury activity level, and ability to comply with rigorous rehabilitation.

Conservative therapy with immobilization may be the only treatment suitable for elderly patients with multiligament injuries who have preinjury medical comorbidities.[50] Additionally, the presence of arthritis is a relative contraindication to multiligament reconstruction; in fact, most studies exclude patients with preexisting arthritis.

Treatment Options

Treatment recommendations for specific ligament injuries in this patient population are limited by the lack of comparative studies. No known studies have evaluated the impact of a specific cruciate ligament reconstruction technique on the outcomes of multiligament injuries. Repair versus reconstruction of collateral ligaments has been debated, but specific reconstruction methods have not been directly compared in clinical studies.

Acute Management

Every multiligament knee injury is unique, and a wide range of pathology exists. Most injuries are adequately stabilized in a knee immobilizer. However, some knees associated with a high-energy injury may remain subluxed in a knee immobilizer and require a spanning external fixator to achieve stability in the acute setting.

Anterior Cruciate Ligament

Although ACL reconstruction is recommended, the specific technique receives relatively little discussion in the context of multiligament injuries. Many authors have described single-bundle reconstruction using allograft or autograft with femoral tunnels created via a transtibial technique. Levy et al.[42] prefer to use a tibialis anterior allograft, Strobel et al.[51] recommend use of a hamstring autograft. Engebretsen et al.[1] initially preferred allografts for ACL reconstruction but changed their graft choice to a bone–patellar tendon–bone autograft. Harner et al.[37] prefer allograft bone–patellar tendon–bone but use an anteromedial portal drilling technique for ACL femoral tunnels rather than the transtibial technique as utilized by previous authors.

Posterior Cruciate Ligament

A review of treatment options for addressing PCL insufficiency in this patient population follows. It is generally accepted that PCL tears should be reconstructed in these patients, although the optimal technique has not yet been defined. A review of the causes of failure of a series of PCL reconstructions identified the importance of tunnel positioning and addressing concomitant collateral ligament instability.[19] However, investigators have not yet determined the role for the single- versus double-bundle technique and for transtibial versus tibial inlay graft placement.

Some studies have demonstrated that double-bundle PCL reconstructions restore native biomechanics[45,52]; however, relatively few studies have specifically described the detailed technique and associated outcomes of double-bundle PCL reconstructions in the multiligament injury population. Spiridonov et al.[53] recently described a double-bundle PCL reconstruction in seven patients with isolated PCL ruptures and 32 with multiligament injuries. Their technique includes two femoral tunnels and a single transtibial tunnel to anatomically reconstruct the anterolateral bundle (ALB) and posteromedial bundle (PMB). Because of the morbidity of graft harvest and the need for large collagen volume, the authors used allografts, specifically Achilles tendon, for the ALB and semitendinosus tendon for the PMB.

Several authors have described single-bundle PCL reconstructions in patients with multiligament injuries. Fanelli and Edson[38] recommend a single-bundle transtibial PCL reconstruction and report using either an autograft or allograft. Engebretsen et al.[1] describe a single-bundle transtibial PCL reconstruction; during the time of data collection, the investigators changed their graft source from allograft to hamstring autograft. Chhabra et al.[54] reported that approximately one third of patients with an acute multiligament injury have an intact PMB and meniscofemoral ligaments. They attempt to preserve these bundles and will perform a reconstruction of the ALB using an Achilles tendon allograft via a transtibial tunnel. In patients with complete ruptures of the entire PCL and patients with chronic injuries, the authors recommend double-bundle PCL reconstruction using an Achilles tendon allograft for the ALB and a semitendinosus autograft for the PMB.

A recent systematic review of the topic of transtibial versus tibial inlay technique for PCL reconstruction revealed a paucity of comparative outcomes studies and recommends surgeon preference as a reasonable factor for technique choice until further evidence is available.[55] Biomechanical studies have compared the two techniques, but it is difficult to apply their results to the multiligament injury population. Some investigators have recommended that the tibial inlay technique not be used for patients with multiligament injuries; however, this evidence is level V.[56] Stannard et al.[57] described a technique for double-bundle PCL reconstruction with a tibial inlay technique in patients with multiligament injuries. Their technique requires a single Achilles tendon allograft, split longitudinally, to reconstruct the ALB and PMB. Cooper and Stewart[58] described a single-bundle tibial inlay PCL reconstruction using either a bone–patellar tendon–bone autograft or allograft to reconstruct the ALB.

Medial/Posteromedial Structures

In a recent review, LaPrade and colleagues[14,59] underscored the importance of completely evaluating and treating the three main structures of the medial/posteromedial knee: the superficial MCL, deep MCL, and POL. When associated with multiligament injuries, most authors agree that grade III MCL injuries require treatment, often repair or reconstruction. A systematic review reported an absence of sufficient studies to allow formulation of evidence-based recommendations for treatment of MCL injuries in the multiligament injury population.[60] A general trend has been noted in the literature toward repair and/or reconstruction of medial knee injuries, which may be due to increased understanding of the anatomy and availability of biomechanically validated reconstruction techniques.

In early reports, Fanelli et al.[61] compared valgus stability in patients with bicruciate ruptures and medial-sided injuries. Bicruciate reconstructions were performed in all patients; two acutely presenting patients were treated with primary surgical repair of the MCL tears, and seven were treated with bracing to allow the MCL injury to heal with nonoperative treatment followed by subsequent bicruciate ligament reconstruction. More recently, Fanelli and Edson[38] describe an anterosuperior shift of the posteromedial capsule for repair of MCL injuries; when lesions are not amenable for repair, an autograft semitendinosus or allograft is used to reconstruct the superficial MCL and is accompanied by a capsular shift.

Lind et al.[62] described a rerouting of the ipsilateral semitendinosus tendon to reconstruct the superficial MCL and posteromedial structures in patients with multiligament injuries. The semitendinosus tendon was identified and harvested proximally but left intact at the pes insertion. A blind femoral tunnel, located at the isometric point of the MCL insertion, was created with a diameter equal to the size of the double-looped tendon. Additionally, a transtibial tunnel exiting 10 mm below the tibial plateau and posterolateral to the semimembranosus was drilled through the medial tibial plateau from anterior to posterior and reamed to the diameter of the semitendinosus tendon. The double-looped tendon was secured using interference screw fixation in the femur, pulled through the tibial tunnel, and secured with an additional interference screw.

LaPrade and colleagues[59] described an anatomically based and biomechanically validated[63] reconstruction of the medial knee structures.[64] Their technique reconstructs the POL and both the proximal and distal divisions of the superficial MCL. Two femoral and two tibial tunnels are created, and grafts are fixed in the tunnels with use of interference screws.

In a series of patients with knee dislocations, Harner et al.[37] describe repair or reconstruction of MCL injuries. Avulsions and midsubstance injuries were repaired with suture anchors and nonabsorbable sutures, respectively. Chronic injuries were treated with a reconstruction of the MCL using a semitendinosus autograft or Achilles tendon allograft.

Lateral/Posterolateral Structures

In contrast to the extraarticular medial structures, it is well recognized that grade III PLC injuries do not heal with bracing and can lead to significant morbidity without operative treatment. Recently reconstruction rather than repair of PLC injuries has been emphasized because of results of comparative outcomes studies. Early investigators reported good results with acute anatomic repair of PLC injuries; however, these patients were immobilized in a cast for 6 weeks postoperatively, and subjective outcomes scoring tools were not available.[65-67]

Fanelli and Edson[68] described a biceps tenodesis procedure combined with a posterolateral capsular shift. More recently, Stannard et al.[43] and Levy et al.[42] performed a mix of single- and dual-stage operations and found lower failure rates with reconstructions when compared with repairs of the PLC. Stannard et al.[43] performed a modified two-tailed technique with a tibialis anterior or posterior allograft for PLC reconstructions. This technique uses a single femoral tunnel at the isometric point along with a single fibular and tibial tunnel. Levy et al.[42] used a fibula-based technique with an Achilles tendon allograft, along with an anterodistal shift of the posterolateral capsule, to reconstruct the PLC.

LaPrade and colleagues recently reported on acute[6] and chronic[18] treatment of isolated and combined PLC injuries. All PLC and concomitant cruciate ligament tears were treated with a single-stage surgery. Acute avulsions of PLC structures were repaired with suture anchors or recess procedures; however, most acute PLC injuries were not amenable for repair and were treated with a complete anatomic PLC reconstruction of the FCL, popliteus tendon, and/or PFL. A minority of the patients in the chronic PLC injury study were found to have varus malalignment and required an opening wedge proximal tibial osteotomy to correct their mechanical axis before undergoing a soft tissue reconstruction. The remainder of the patients were treated with an anatomic reconstruction of the PLC with single-stage reconstruction of coexistent cruciate ligament tears.

AUTHORS' PREFERRED TECHNIQUE

Ligamentous Injuries

Our preferred technique for treatment of multiligament injuries is an anatomic single-stage reconstruction of the cruciate ligament(s) with concurrent treatment of medial/posteromedial and lateral/posterolateral supporting structures with anatomically based and biomechanically validated techniques. Grade III injuries to the medial and lateral structures require surgical treatment for patients with multiligament injuries with a repair and/or reconstruction when indicated. A repair of some structures may be possible in acute injuries with avulsions directly off bone; however, a reconstruction is required for acute injuries with midsubstance tears or inadequate tissue quality and for chronic injuries. It is the preference of the senior author to operate on patients with acute injuries within 3 weeks of injury to allow identification of injured structures and repair of meniscal pathology and extraarticular structures.

Preoperative Planning

Preoperative planning for treatment of multiligament injuries is critical because of the inherent complexity. The injury history, physical examination, and imaging studies will allow the surgeon to plan the details of the operation. The surgeon must be certain that all required equipment is available, including surgical instruments and any required allograft materials. Standard cruciate ligament reconstruction instruments including cannulated drill guides, eyelet-tipped passing pins, suture anchors, and cannulated interference screws (metallic or bioabsorbable) will be necessary. Appropriate graft harvesting instruments will be needed if the surgeon plans to use autografts; a graft preparation station will also be needed. A standard arthroscopic setup with 30- and 70-degree scopes will be necessary for evaluation and treatment of intraarticular injuries.

Patient Positioning

The patient is placed supine on the operating table, and after administration of an anesthetic, an examination is performed to confirm suspected ligamentous pathology. A leg holder is placed to allow sufficient access to the medial and lateral aspect of the injured extremity. A well-padded proximal thigh tourniquet is set in place but is not routinely used. The operative leg is prepped and draped free in the usual sterile fashion.

Extraarticular Injury Identification and Treatment

We recommend that open dissection for lateral and/or medial injuries be performed prior to arthroscopic examination, which will allow identification of injuries and assessment of tissue quality prior to arthroscopic fluid extravasation.

Lateral and Posterolateral Knee

A hockey-stick shaped incision centered over the posterior to mid portion of the iliotibial band is used to expose the lateral/posterolateral knee. The incision is positioned more posteriorly in patients with a planned autogenous patellar tendon graft harvest for concurrent ACL reconstruction to maintain a minimum of 6 cm between the two incisions. This incision is continued down through the skin and superficial tissues to the superficial layer of the iliotibial band. Posteriorly, the long and short heads of the biceps femoris are identified; palpation approximately 2 to 3 cm distal to the long head will usually allow identification of the common peroneal nerve. A neurolysis is then performed to release the nerve from scar tissue entrapment and safely isolate it from the surgical site (Fig. 102-3).

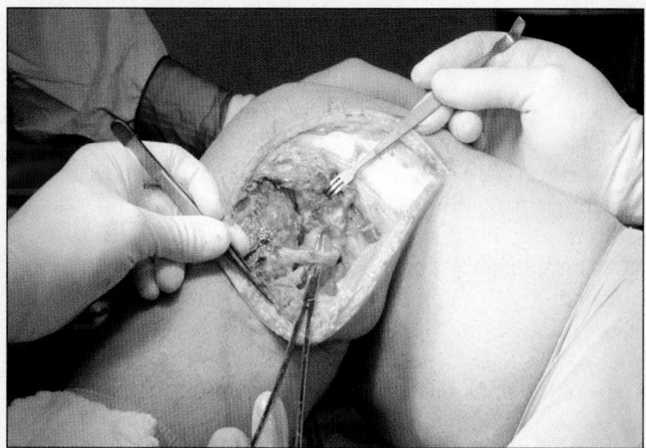

FIGURE 102-3 The open surgical approach to the posterolateral aspect of a left knee. The common peroneal nerve is elevated by the curved hemostat.

Continued

Avulsions of the biceps tendon are repaired with use of suture anchors with the knee in full extension. Arcuate avulsion fractures may be repaired with No. 5 nonabsorbable sutures passed through the proximal tendon and bony fragment and tied through drill holes in the fibula.[6]

Blunt dissection between the soleus and the lateral head of the gastrocnemius muscle will expose an interval through which the posteromedial aspect of the fibular head can be palpated. In this region the popliteofibular ligament (PFL) and musculotendinous junction of the popliteus tendon are found.

Next, an incision 1 cm proximal to the fibular head is made through the anterior arm of the long head of the biceps and the underlying biceps bursa. The distal aspect and insertion of the FCL can be identified through this incision, and a traction stitch is placed for upcoming identification of the proximal aspect of the ligament. Acute avulsions of the FCL directly from bone without intrasubstance stretch injuries, which usually occur in skeletally immature patients, may be repaired with use of suture anchors; however, the majority of FCL injuries are not amenable for repair and require a reconstruction. A fibular tunnel is drilled with use of a cruciate ligament aiming guide. The desired trajectory for anatomic graft placement is from the FCL attachment site of the lateral aspect of the fibular head to the posteromedial down slope of the fibular styloid. A retractor is placed medially to prevent iatrogenic injury to deep structures, and a guide pin is advanced; the tunnel is overreamed with a 7-mm reamer, and the entry and exit apertures are chamfered with a rasp.

Next, a tibial tunnel is created for passage and fixation of the PFL and popliteus tendon reconstruction grafts. The anterior tunnel aperture is located at the flat spot between Gerdy's tubercle and the tibial tubercle; an elevator is used to release the soft tissues from this region. The posterior tunnel aperture is located at the posterolateral aspect of the proximal tibia, slightly distal to the plateau. The previously identified popliteus musculotendinous junction, located 1 cm medial and 1 cm proximal to the fibular head reconstruction tunnel, is the landmark for the posterior aperture of the reconstruction tunnel. A cruciate ligament reconstruction aiming guide is used to create this tunnel; a retractor is placed posteriorly to protect against an erroneously placed guide pin. Accurate guide pin placement is confirmed by palpating posteriorly while cross-referencing with a blunt probe placed through the fibular tunnel.

Tension is then applied to the traction stitch in the FCL remnant to identify and evaluate the FCL femoral origin.[69] To allow direct visualization of the FCL and popliteus tendon attachment sites on the femur and prepare for potential tunnel drilling, a splitting incision is placed through the superficial layer of the iliotibial band from a point proximal to the lateral epicondyle and extended distally to Gerdy's tubercle. Next, a vertical incision through the lateral capsule allows identification of the femoral insertion of the popliteus tendon. Avulsions of the popliteus tendon directly from the femur without intrasubstance stretch injury or musculotendinous avulsion may be amenable for a recess procedure performed with the knee in full extension.[70] The creation of femoral tunnels for reconstruction of the FCL and popliteus tendon requires a thorough understanding of the anatomy (Fig. 102-4)[69] and is performed according to previously described techniques.[71] With use of a cruciate ligament aiming guide, two eyelet-tipped guide pins are aimed anteromedially to the adductor tubercle from the FCL and popliteus tendon attachment sites and advanced in a parallel fashion; tunnel orientation is important to avoid collision of the PLC tunnels with ACL reconstruction tunnels. The tunnels are then overreamed to a depth of 20 mm and a diameter of 9 mm (Fig. 102-5).

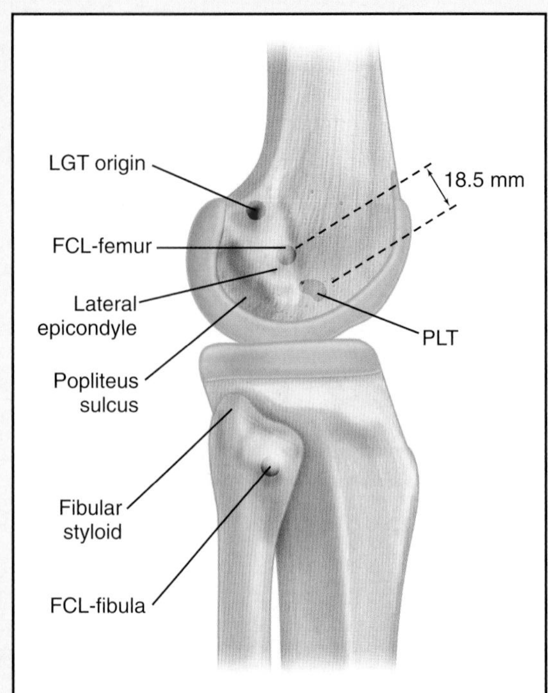

FIGURE 102-4 Attachments of key posterolateral knee stabilizing structures and associated bony landmarks. *FCL,* Fibular collateral ligament; *LGT,* lateral gastrocnemius tendon; *PLT,* popliteus tendon.

A split Achilles tendon allograft is prepared for the two limbs of the PLC reconstruction, and the grafts are secured in their femoral tunnels with 7 × 20 mm cannulated interference screws (Fig. 102-6). The FCL graft is passed through the fibular tunnel, but final fixation is delayed until the end of the procedure. Treatment of associated PLC structures is performed when indicated. Popliteomeniscal fascicle and coronary ligament tears are repaired with mattress sutures. Bony (Segond)[16] or soft tissue avulsions of the tibial attachment of the lateral capsular ligament[23] are repaired with suture anchors.[6]

Medial and Posteromedial Knee

The treatment of combined ACL/MCL injuries is well defined and will not be specifically discussed. The focus of this discussion is our preferred treatment of severe grade III medial ligamentous injuries combined with PCL or bicruciate ruptures, as well as possible associated lateral injuries. Surgical treatment is delayed until knee swelling decreases; medial tissues may be amenable for repair with augmentation, or a reconstruction may be required. Concurrent, rather than staged, cruciate ligament reconstruction is performed in all patients.

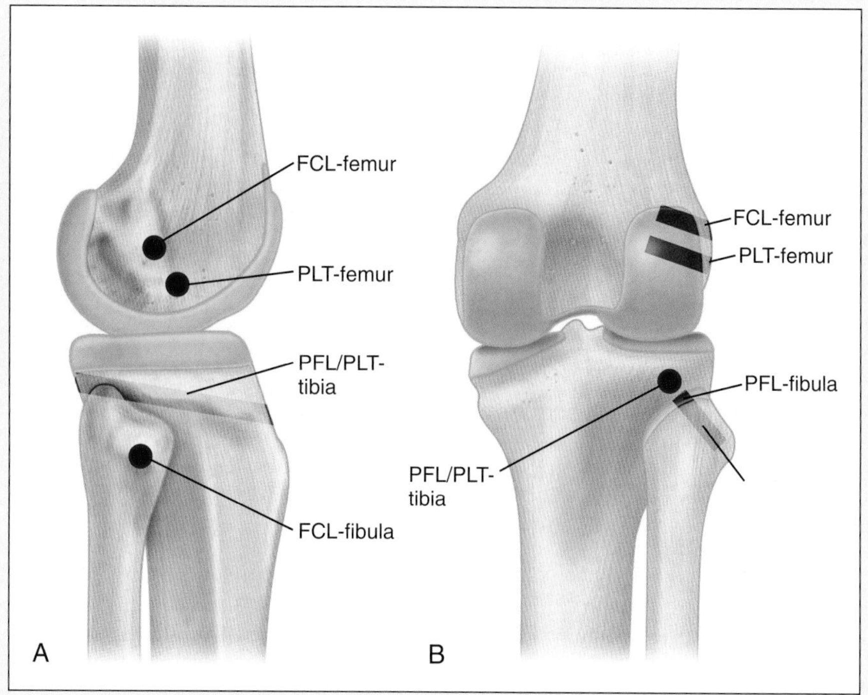

FIGURE 102-5 Lateral (**A**) and posterior (**B**) aspects of the knee demonstrating the position of bone tunnels for a complete reconstruction of the posterolateral corner of the knee. *FCL,* Fibular collateral ligament; *PFL,* popliteofibular ligament; *PLT,* popliteus tendon.

Exposure of the medial knee is performed via an anteromedial incision that extends distally from the region between the medial border of the patella and the medial epicondyle, to the region overlying the pes anserine tendons.[64] Next, the gracilis and semitendinosus tendon attachments are identified by incising the anterior border of the sartorial fascia. The semitendinosus tendon is removed with use of a standard tendon harvester and sectioned to create grafts of 16 cm and 12 cm for reconstruction of the superficial MCL and POL, respectively. Nonabsorbable sutures are used to tubularize each end, and the tendons are sized for 7-mm tunnels.

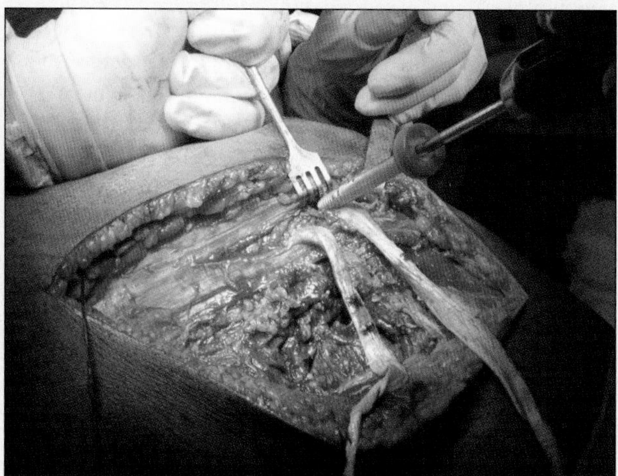

FIGURE 102-6 The intraoperative posterolateral aspect of the right knee demonstrating fixation of the posterolateral corner grafts in the femoral tunnels. An iliotibial band–splitting incision is visualized and an interference screw is advanced into the popliteus tendon femoral tunnel.

Within the pes anserine bursa, the superficial MCL distal tibial attachment is identified. Next, the superficial MCL is followed distally, and the tibial attachment is identified at the anteromedial proximal tibia. The superficial MCL has a proximal and distal tibial attachment; the distal attachment is approximately 6 cm distal to the joint line.[59] The tendon of the sartorius muscle is retracted distally and the largest portion of the POL, the central arm, is identified. The tibial attachment site of the POL central arm, with an underlying small bony ridge, can be found near the direct arm of the semimembranosus tendon.

Identification of the femoral attachments of the medial knee structures is often difficult because the bony and soft tissue landmarks are not as obvious as those on the posterolateral knee. The initial step is to identify the adductor magnus tendon and its distal attachment to the adductor tubercle (Fig. 102-7). This step will allow the surgeon to more accurately identify the medial epicondyle, the gastrocnemius tubercle, and the anatomic attachment sites of the superficial MCL and the POL (Fig. 102-8). The femoral attachment of the superficial MCL is approximately 6 mm posterosuperior to the medial epicondyle, and the POL femoral attachment is approximately 11 mm posterosuperior to the superficial MCL.[59] After identification of the femoral and tibial attachments of the superficial MCL and POL, guide pins are inserted and overreamed with a 7-mm cannulated drill and advanced to a depth of 30 mm. Allograft or a semitendinosus autografts are prepared (16 cm for the superficial MCL and 12 cm for the POL) and are fixed into the femoral tunnels using 7-mm

Continued

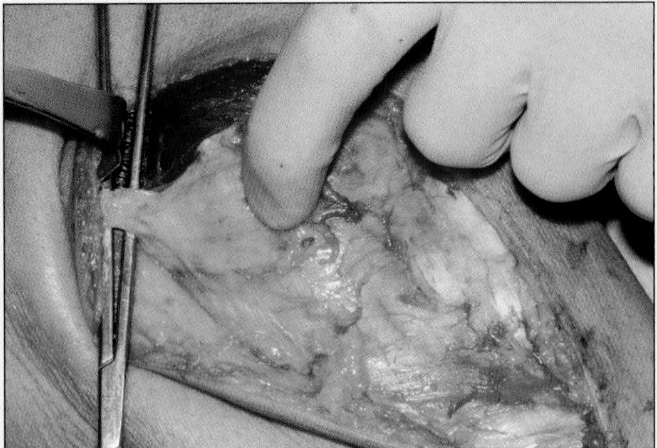

FIGURE 102-7 The open surgical approach for the medial aspect of a left knee. The adductor tendon is elevated by the hemostat and a gloved finger is shown palpating the medial epicondyle. The vastus medialis obliquus muscle is also visible.

bioabsorbable interference screws. Graft fixation in the tibial tunnels is delayed until the end of the procedure.

Intraarticular Injury Identification and Treatment

The arthroscopic portion of the surgery is delayed until after open dissection and injury identification to prevent arthroscopic fluid extravasation. Vertical inferomedial and inferolateral parapatellar portals are created and a standard arthroscopic assessment of the knee is performed. Varus and valgus stress is applied and the lateral and medial compartments, respectively, are observed for gapping (Fig. 102-9).

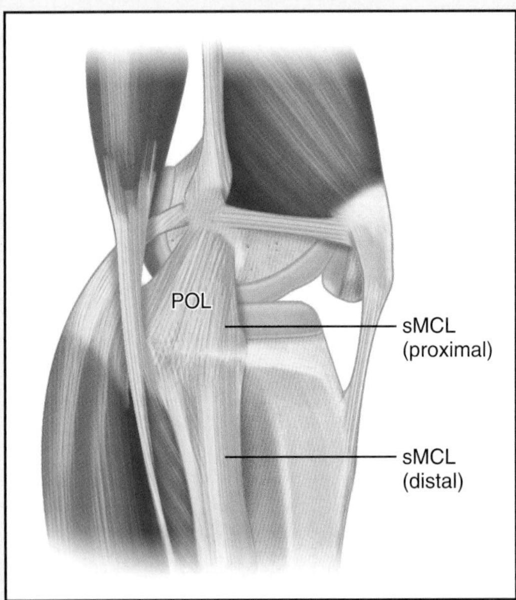

FIGURE 102-8 Anatomy of the medial aspect of the left knee. The posterior oblique ligament (*POL*) and superficial medial collateral ligament (*sMCL*) are demonstrated. *(From Coobs BR, Wijdicks CA, Armitage BM, et al: An in vitro analysis of an anatomical medial knee reconstruction.* Am J Sports Med *38[2]:339–347, 2010.)*

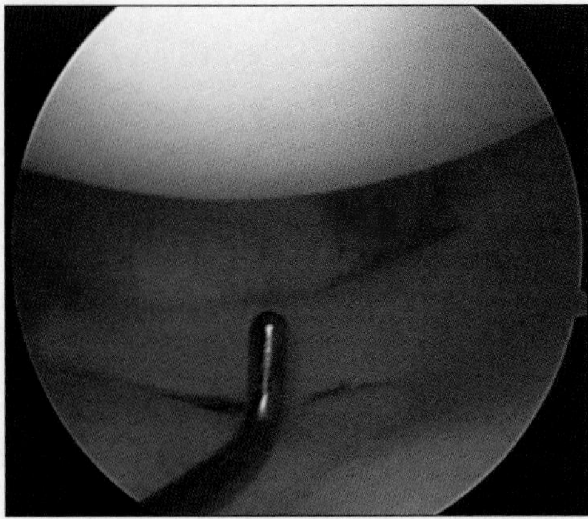

FIGURE 102-9 A lateral compartment "drive-through sign" is seen in this arthroscopic photograph in a patient with a posterolateral corner knee injury.

The articular cartilage surfaces are examined for lesions, and the meniscal roots and bodies are similarly assessed; meniscal tears are repaired if possible. Cruciate ligament injuries are addressed as discussed in the following sections.

Posterior Cruciate Ligament

An endoscopic double-bundle PCL reconstruction is preferred in patients with multiligament injuries. An Achilles tendon allograft is used for ALB reconstruction and a semitendinosus allograft is used for PMB reconstruction. The femoral attachments of these two bundles are identified with an arthroscopic coagulator. An additional portal is created through the posteromedial capsule to allow evaluation and debridement of the PCL tibial attachment. Debridement is continued until the popliteus muscle fibers are visualized. With use of a PCL guide, a guide pin is drilled from the anteromedial tibia, approximately 6 cm distal to the joint line, and exits at the PCL tibial attachment, approximately 1 cm distal to the joint line; pin placement is verified with intraoperative radiographs or fluoroscopy.

PCL reconstruction femoral tunnel creation is performed according to previously described techniques.[53] The ALB is positioned so that the aperture edge is adjacent to the articular cartilage margin at the top of the intercondylar roof and along the anterior aspect of the medial femoral condyle. An 11-mm tunnel is drilled to a depth of 25 mm. Similarly, a 7-mm PMB tunnel is created at the previously described location and reamed to a depth of 25 mm; a minimum 2-mm bone bridge is maintained between the two tunnels.

After femoral tunnel creation, the tibial tunnel is reamed. The previously placed tibial guide pin is used to advance a 12-mm headed reamer to create a complete tunnel exiting at the posterior tibia. The posterior tissues are protected against iatrogenic injury via retraction with a large curette placed through the posteromedial portal. To minimize the potential for cyclic graft failure due to friction against the tibial tunnel aperture, a "smoother" is passed through the tibial tunnel and out the anteromedial portal and cycled several times.

The grafts are then passed into their respective femoral tunnels endoscopically via the anterolateral arthroscopic portal. A 7-mm titanium screw is used to fix the ALB graft bone plug into its femoral tunnel, and a 7-mm bioabsorbable interference screw is used to fix the PMB soft tissue graft into its femoral tunnel. The ALB and PMB grafts are then pulled distally through the tibial tunnel, and the knee is cycled; tibial graft fixation is delayed until the end of the procedure.

Anterior Cruciate Ligament Reconstruction

A single-bundle anatomic ACL reconstruction is preferred for patients with multiligament injuries. A bone–patellar tendon–bone autograft or allograft is chosen based on the preference of the patient/surgeon and availability. The tibial attachment is identified, and residual tissue is debrided with the shaver. Next, the femoral attachment is similarly identified and debrided to identify the lateral intercondylar ridge. A burr hole is made to mark the midpoint of the ACL femoral attachment between the anteromedial and posterolateral bundles.

The femoral tunnel is created via the anteromedial portal technique. This closed socket femoral tunnel is created with a low-profile reamer prior to tibial tunnel reaming. This sequence allows for identification of the important regional anatomy of this tunnel prior to significant fluid extravasation from the joint. If there was no concurrent medial knee reconstruction incision or if an allograft was used, a 2-cm anteromedial tibial incision is centered approximately 35 mm distal to the joint and 10 mm anterior to the MCL. An ACL reconstruction guide is placed into the joint and centered over the native ACL attachment site; a guide pin is then advanced and the tunnel is reamed. The ACL graft is passed and fixed in the femoral tunnel. Tibial fixation is delayed until the end of the procedure.

Final Graft Fixation

The order of final graft fixation is important. To restore the central pivot of the knee, tibial fixation of the PCL grafts is performed according to previously defined techniques[53] once all associated ligament reconstruction grafts are fixed in their femoral tunnels. PLC grafts are secured next; care is taken to avoid overreducing the knee in patients with an associated medial knee injury. The FCL graft is passed through the fibula and fixed in its reconstruction tunnel at 20 degrees of knee flexion, in neutral rotation, and with a valgus reduction force on the knee. Next, the PLC grafts are passed anteriorly through the tibial tunnel, slack is removed from the grafts, and fixation of the popliteus tendon and PFL grafts is performed at 60 degrees of knee flexion, in neutral rotation, and with traction applied to the grafts (Fig. 102-10).

ACL graft tibial fixation is performed once the PLC grafts have been secured because of biomechanical evidence that fixation of the ACL graft prior to the PLC grafts can result in an external rotation deformity of the knee.[72] An interference screw is used in the tibial tunnel for fixation.

Graft fixation in the tibial tunnels is performed next for patients who underwent reconstruction of medial knee injuries (Fig. 102-11). The superficial MCL graft is passed into the tibial tunnel and tension is held while a varus moment is applied with the knee flexed to 20 degrees and in neutral rotation. At this position, the superficial MCL graft is secured

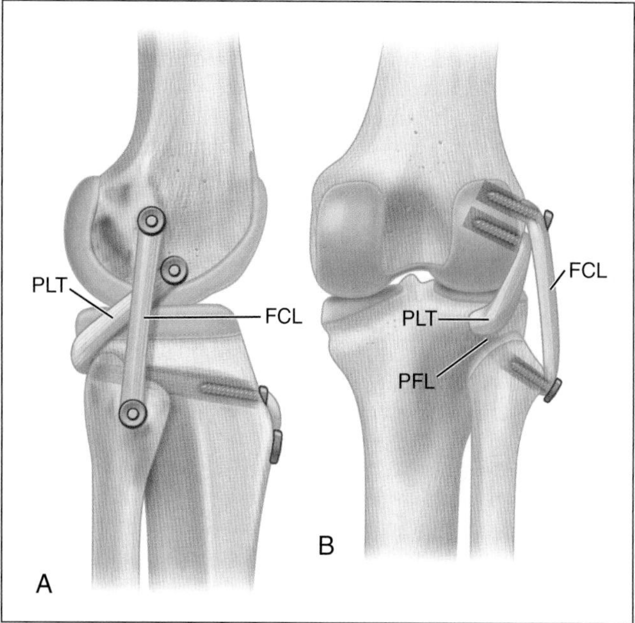

FIGURE 102-10 The lateral (**A**) and posterior (**B**) view of a posterolateral corner knee reconstruction are demonstrated in this illustration. The fibular collateral ligament (*FCL*), popliteus tendon (*PLT*), and popliteofibular ligament (*PFL*) grafts are shown.

with the interference screw. In a similar fashion, tension is applied to the POL graft via traction in full knee extension. The interference screw is inserted as a varus moment is applied with the knee held in extension and neutral rotation. A suture anchor is then used to recreate the proximal tibial superficial MCL attachment.

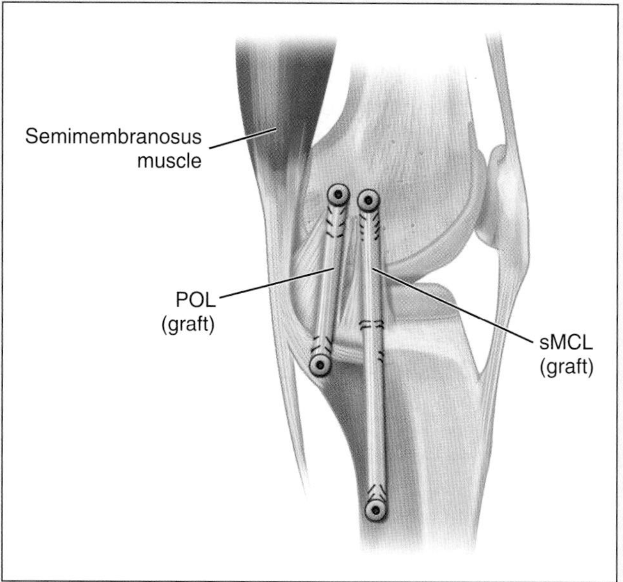

FIGURE 102-11 The medial aspect of the left knee with reconstruction grafts fixed in the femoral and tibial tunnels with interference screws. *POL,* Posterior oblique ligament; *sMCL,* superficial medial collateral ligament. *(From Coobs BR, Wijdicks CA, Armitage BM, et al: An in vitro analysis of an anatomical medial knee reconstruction.* Am J Sports Med *38[2]:339–347, 2010.)*

Postoperative Management

An important consideration in the treatment of multiligament injuries is postoperative rehabilitation and eventual return to play. These topics have received great attention for isolated ligament injuries, but less information is available for patients with multiligament injuries; as such, principles from the former must be applied to the latter. Two general approaches to postoperative care in multiligament injuries are immobilization versus early mobilization. A balance must be achieved between immobilization aimed at preventing the development of instability and early mobilization to minimize scar tissue and resultant range-of-motion deficits. Although a full discussion of various rehabilitation protocols is beyond the scope of this chapter, the basic preferences of several investigators are described below.

Noyes and Barber-Westin described a program of early protected range of motion in an attempt to limit arthrofibrosis.[73] They prescribed active assisted motion from 10 to 90 degrees six to eight times daily along with patellar mobilization for the first 4 weeks postoperatively. Between therapy sessions, the patient's knee was immobilized in a split cylinder cast to protect the reconstructed structures. After 4 weeks, the cast was changed to a hinged-brace and gradual increase in motion along with progression of weight bearing was then allowed.

A recent review of rehabilitation after reconstruction of multiligament injuries recommended complete immobilization with the knee locked in extension for the first 5 weeks after surgery.[74] For the first 6 weeks, the authors allow the patients to bear full weight while standing statically on both legs, but they must use crutches for ambulation and abstain from bearing weight on the operative leg. From postoperative weeks 5 to 10, the brace is unlocked and patients are allowed to perform passive knee flexion; isolated hamstring strengthening is strictly avoided during this period.

Harner et al.[37] also described their preferred surgical treatment and rehabilitation for patients with multiligament injuries. For the first 4 weeks, the knee is held in full extension via a locked knee brace, except during passive range-of-motion exercises at up to 90 degrees of flexion. Isolated hamstring contraction is avoided until 6 weeks after surgery. Partial weight bearing is allowed with the brace in full extension for the first 4 to 6 weeks and progresses thereafter.

In a recent systematic review, Mook et al.[33] evaluated the impact of postoperative rehabilitation on multiligament injury outcomes. Their findings indicate that early mobilization in acutely treated patients is associated with less posterior instability, varus/valgus laxity, and range-of-motion deficits when compared with immobilization after surgery. The apparent influence of early mobilization underscores the importance of a strong anatomic repair and/or reconstruction of posterolateral structures.

Wilkins[75] provided a detailed description of rehabilitation principles based on work by LaPrade and colleagues and describes early-phase rehabilitation (0 to 12 weeks) and late-phase rehabilitation (4 to 12 months). Similar to other authors, Wilkins recommends non–weight bearing for the first 6 weeks postoperatively, with occasional toe-touch weight bearing during showering and dressing activities; weight bearing is thereafter increased according to the protocol. For the first 2 weeks the brace is locked in full extension with the exception of therapy sessions where the patient is allowed knee motion within the "safe zone" as defined intraoperatively. Range of motion is then increased to 90 degrees until 4 weeks postoperatively and thereafter gradually progressed to goal of greater than or equal to 125 degrees. Because of posterior tibial translation associated with increasing flexion, isolated hamstring exercises are avoided for the first 4 months. Late-phase rehabilitation focuses on high-level balance training, sport-specific drills, and plyometric exercises and is initiated at approximately 4 months after surgery when the patient has regained full active range of motion, has resumed a normal gait, and has no signs of swelling.

Results

No level I studies are available on the topic of treatment and associated outcomes of surgical reconstruction of multiligament injuries. Most available studies are level III or IV, and unfortunately, evaluation of the results of some studies is limited by the heterogeneous patient mix. Often, isolated injuries were included in the analysis with multiligament injuries, and high-energy injuries in polytrauma patients may be reported along with low-energy injuries associated with sports. A summary of selected literature is provided in Table 102-1.

Complications

Complications can be discussed within the context of the initial injury or those associated with treatment. Vascular injuries are not infrequent in the setting of multiligament injuries, and although the reported incidence varies, a commonly referenced number is 32%.[76] Urgent vascular surgery consultation is required for suspected large vessel injury because prolonged ischemia may necessitate amputation. Peroneal nerve injuries are also common in the multiligament injury patient population, especially when combined with PLC injuries, and are estimated to occur at a rate of 25% to 35%.[5] A poor prognosis is associated with complete lesions, whereas most persons with incomplete nerve palsies often can be expected to recover. Treatment options include physical therapy with an ankle-foot orthosis, neurolysis, primary nerve repair, nerve grafting, and tendon transfers.[77] With high-energy injuries, infection and skin compromise may also occur; inevitably, definitive surgery will be delayed while skin concerns are addressed.

Complications may also be associated with treatment, whether nonoperative or operative. In both cases, persistent pain and instability may occur. If the initial treatment was nonoperative, the treatment is deemed a failure, and if the patient is a candidate, a chronic reconstruction may be required. If the initial treatment was operative, the patient may require revision reconstruction of all failed components.

Infection and bleeding can also occur with operative treatment. Incision and debridement with antibiotics and staged reconstruction may be necessary for infected cases. Bleeding may be the expected result of a difficult exposure, but attempts at adequate hemostasis must be obtained prior to closure. Bleeding may also occur because of iatrogenic injury to large vessels such as the popliteal artery that will necessitate immediate intervention by a vascular surgeon. Iatrogenic injury to

TABLE 102-1

SUMMARY OF SELECTED RECENT LITERATURE ON MULTILIGAMENT KNEE INJURIES

Study	Year	No. of Knees	Male (%)	Years of Follow-up, Average (Range)	Timing: No. of Patients (Time to Surgery)	Average Age (yr)	Injury Type (Schenck Classification)	Knee Function (Average Scores)	Physical Examination (Stability)
Levy	2010	28	Not given	Repair: 2.8 (2-4.1) Reconstruction: 2.3 (2-3.4)	Repair: 10 (5-33 days) Reconstruction: 18 (17-731 days)	*	KD I: 12 KD III: 10 KD IV: 44 KD V: 1	4/10 repairs failed 1/18 reconstructions failed IKDC: 79 (repair), 77 (reconstruction) Lysholm: 85 (repair), 88 (reconstruction)	IKDC objective at final follow-up: 0 repairs and 2 reconstructions had 1+ laxity to varus stress at 30° All patients were stable with the dial test at 30° and 90°
Engebretsen	2009	85	53	5.3 (2-9.9)	A: 50 (<2 wk) C: 35 Average: 14 mo	35.2	KD II-III: 88% KD IV: 12%	Lysholm: 83 IKDC 2000: 64	Lachman: 57% normal, 33% 1+ Pivot shift: 90% normal, 4% 1+ Posterior drawer: 26% normal, 57% 1+ Dial test: 86% normal, 11% 1+ Valgus: 60% normal, 30% 1+ Varus: 67% normal, 25% 1+
Strobel	2006	17	76	(2-5.5)	C: 17 (5-312 mo)	30.7	KD III: 17	IKDC: 71.8	Posterior drawer: 88% grade I or II, 12% grade III Lachman: 94% grade I or II, 6% grade III Posterolateral instability: 88% normal or nearly normal; 12% with residual instability
Stannard	2005	57	63	2.8 (2-4.9)	35 patients qualified for repair and were treated within 3 wk; 22 patients were chronic or had nonrepairable acute injuries	33	44 multiligament 13 isolated	Mean Lysholm, IKDC subjective repair success: 88.2, 59.8 Failed repair, s/p revision: 86.8, 63.6 Reconstruction success: 89.6, 56.1 Failed reconstruction, s/p revision: 92, 64.4	13/35 repairs failed; 12 underwent successful revision reconstruction 2/22 reconstructions failed IKDC objective: PLC repair success: 4 A, 14 B, 2 C, 1 D PLC repair failure: 3 A, 4 B, 4 C, 0 D PLC reconstruction success: 7 A, 9 B, 2 C, 2 D PLC reconstruction failure: 0 A, 1 B, 1 C, 0 D
Harner	2004	31	*	3.7 (2-6)	A: 19 (within 3 wk) C: 12 (5 wk-22 mo)	28.4	Acute: KD I: 3; KD II+: 16 Chronic: KD II: 7; KD III-L: 2; KD III-M: 3	Lysholm A: 91; C: 80 KOS ADL A: 91; C 84 Sports Activities Scale: A: 89; C: 69 Meyers: 10 excellent, 13 good, 5 fair, 3 poor	Lachman: 48% normal, 52% 1+ Posterior drawer: 71% 1+, 29% 2+ Varus stress: 30 degrees: 29% 1+, 6% 2+ Valgus stress 30 degrees: 16% 1+, 13% 2+
Fanelli	2002	35	74	(2-10)	A: 19 (<8 wk) C: 16 (3-26 mo)	*	KD II: 1 KD III-L: 19 KD III-M: 9 KD IV: 6	Lysholm: 91.2 HSS: 86.8	Lachman and pivot shift: 94% normal Posterior drawer: 46% normal, 54% 1+ Posterolateral stability: normal in 24%, "tighter than normal" in 76%

A, Acute; *C,* chronic; *HSS,* Hospital for Special Surgery; *IKDC,* International Knee Documentation Committee; *KD,* knee dislocation; *KOS ADLA,* Knee Outcome Survey Activities of Daily Living Scale; *PLC,* posterolateral corner; *s/p,* status postoperative.

the common peroneal nerve may occur during neurolysis or as a failure of adequate neurolysis prior to ligament reconstruction. However, adequately exposed and carefully handled nerves may still be associated with foot drop if the initial injury was severe. As with any surgery, deep vein thrombosis may occur; adequate prophylaxis is essential, especially in older and obese patients.

General causes of ligament reconstruction failure may include lack of incorporation of allografts, unrecognized or untreated ligament lesions, or technical concerns due to the repair technique or reconstruction tunnel placement. A persistent postoperative effusion may occur in some patients and will necessitate delaying progression of the rehabilitation protocol.

Future Considerations

Because of the rarity of multiligament injuries and the variation of severity and presence of concomitant injuries, studies with a high level of evidence are limited. Additional clinical studies are necessary to make definitive recommendations on operative timing, surgical technique, and rehabilitation. Level I studies with randomization of surgical treatment may seem impractical because of the complexity of these injuries and the treatment preferences of particular surgeons. However, prospective multicenter studies with treatment outcomes assessed in a standardized method with validated subjective evaluations and unbiased objective measurements of stability and function would significantly benefit the multiligament injury evidence base.

In the past one to two decades, several ligament reconstruction techniques have been developed and tested in persons with isolated ligament injuries. However, few studies address the biomechanics of multiligament injuries and subsequent ligament reconstruction. Additionally, laboratory and clinical studies may evaluate the role of biologic treatments such as stem cells and applied growth factors including platelet-rich plasma therapy in the setting of multiligament reconstruction.

For a complete list of references, go to expertconsult.com.

Suggested Readings

Citation: Mook WR, Miller MD, Diduch DR, et al: Multiple-ligament knee injuries: A systematic review of the timing of operative intervention and postoperative rehabilitation. *J Bone Joint Surg Am* 91A(12):2946–2957, 2009.

Level of Evidence: III

Summary: Mook and colleagues performed a systematic review of the literature on multiple-ligament knee injuries to assess the impact of surgical timing and postoperative rehabilitation. The study included 24 retrospective studies and revealed several findings regarding the impact of these two factors on subjective and objective outcomes, which are discussed, with the associated limitations.

Citation: Engebretsen L, Risberg MA, Robertson B, et al: Outcome after knee dislocations: A 2-9 years follow-up of 85 consecutive patients. *Knee Surg Sports Traumatol Arthrosc* 17(9):1013–1026, 2009.

Level of Evidence: IV

Summary: Engebretsen and colleagues report outcomes and surgical technique for 85 patients after knee dislocation. At final follow-up, the median Lysholm score was 83, knee function was found to be lower in patients who sustained high-energy compared with low-energy trauma, and 87% of injured knees had Kellgren and Lawrence grade 2 or higher compared with 35% of the uninjured knees.

Citation: Harner CD, Waltrip RL, Bennett CH, et al: Surgical management of knee dislocations. *J Bone Joint Surg Am* 86A(2):262–273, 2004.

Level of Evidence: III

Summary: The authors describe their surgical technique and associated outcomes for 33 patients with multiligament knee injuries. Importantly, they found that acutely treated patients had higher subjective scores and improved objective knee stability.

Citation: Fanelli GC, Edson CJ: Arthroscopically assisted combined anterior and posterior cruciate ligament reconstruction in the multiple ligament injured knee: 2- to 10-year follow-up. *Arthroscopy* 18(7):703–714, 2002.

Level of Evidence: III

Summary: Surgical technique and associated outcomes for 35 patients with multiligament injuries are reported. Nineteen patients were treated within 8 weeks and 16 patients were treated chronically; no significant subjective or objective differences were found between the two groups.

Citation: Stannard JP, Brown SL, Farris RC, et al: The posterolateral corner of the knee: Repair versus reconstruction. *Am J Sports Med* 33(6):881–888, 2005.

Level of Evidence: II

Summary: Stannard and colleagues performed a cohort study comparing PLC repair versus reconstruction in combination with treatment of multiligament knee injuries. The failure rate for repairs of the PLC was significantly higher than for reconstructions.

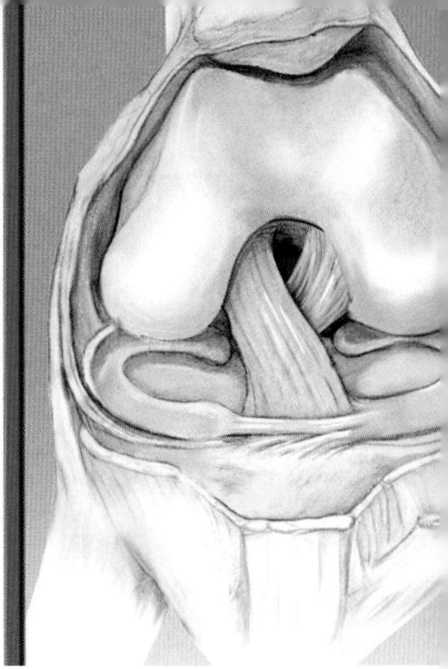

103

Knee Arthritis

CATHERINE HUI • STEPHEN R. THOMPSON • J. ROBERT GIFFIN

Knee osteoarthritis (OA) is an extremely common cause of disability. The etiology is multifactorial, but joint injury is an prevalent cause of OA in the knee.[1,2] Studies have shown that meniscal injury requiring a meniscectomy alters knee biomechanics and leads to gonarthrosis.[3] Anterior cruciate ligament (ACL) rupture, a frequently seen and often devastating injury, is characteristically associated with meniscal and chondral injuries.[4] Further deterioration of the joint related to multiple subluxation episodes over time leads to gonarthrosis that typically affects the medial compartment and results in varus deformity.[5-9]

History

A thorough history rules out systemic causes of pain such as rheumatoid or other inflammatory arthritides, as well as referred hip pain or radiating pain resulting from degenerative disk disease. Patients with knee OA usually present with pain. Other symptoms include catching, locking, swelling, and decreased motion.[1,10,11] Instability is a frequent complaint, but in general it represents quadriceps weakness rather than true ligamentous instability.[12] Patients with chronic ACL deficiency in whom medial compartment gonarthrosis with subsequent varus deformity has developed may experience pain and/or instability. However, in these patients pain is the most common presenting symptom, and instability may not be present as a result of the constraint acquired through the degenerative process and the development of a "cupula" from posteromedial tibial wear.[8] Table 103-1 outlines key questions for patients presenting with knee OA.

Physical Examination

A systematic approach to the physical examination of the knee includes inspection, palpitation, range of motion (ROM), and special tests when appropriate. A comparison of the affected and nonaffected limbs, an examination of the joints above and below the affected knee, and an assessment of the patient's distal neurovascular status are routine components of the physical examination.[13,14]

The inspection begins with an evaluation of limb alignment both while the patient is standing and walking. Varus, valgus, or neutral alignment is noted, as well as an antalgic or Trendelenburg gait or a thrust (i.e., a dynamic change in the deformity with weight bearing).[13,15] If possible, the patient should perform a full squat and the duck walk (Childress sign). Pain with either or both of these activities suggests a meniscal tear.[16] Any previous incisions are noted.

With the patient seated and his or her knees flexed over the edge of the table, patellar position and quadriceps asymmetry, if present, are determined. Quadriceps reflex inhibition due to knee injury and effusion frequently leads to quadriceps atrophy.[17,18]

An effusion, which is characterized by asymmetry in the peripatellar groove on either side of the patella, is confirmed with the swipe test. This test is performed with the patient in the supine position with his or her legs extended and relaxed. The examiner strokes the medial side starting just below the joint line and moving toward the suprapatellar pouch and then does the same on the lateral side while observing for a fluid-wave bulge medially. The presence of a fluid wave indicates a positive swipe test and confirms a small to medium intracapsular effusion.[14]

The patellar ballottement test identifies a moderate to severe effusion. With the knee in full extension, the examiner compresses the patella toward the trochlea and then releases it. If fluid is present, the patella will feel as if it is floating.[14]

Palpation of the knee structures is performed in a methodical fashion and guided by the suspected diagnosis. The temperature of the knee to touch is compared with that of the opposite knee. Increased warmth suggests the presence of inflammation. It is important to determine the point of maximal tenderness. Generally, the area anticipated to be most tender is palpated last so that the patient is not guarding during the remainder of the examination.[14]

ROM compared with the contralateral knee is measured. Patellar tracking during ROM is palpated, as well as crepitus (a palpable grating sensation) during flexion and extension, with particular attention to its specific location.[14] Finally, the patient is asked to perform a straight leg raise to assess quadriceps strength and extensor mechanism function.[14]

Special tests are then performed, including an assessment of cruciate and collateral stability (see Chapter 92). These tests are particularly important to detect the presence of a chronically deficient ACL.

Imaging

Radiographs taken during weight bearing are the gold standard for imaging any knee condition, especially OA. The standard radiographic knee series includes the following views: bilateral standing anteroposterior (AP); bilateral

TABLE 103-1

KEY QUESTIONS FOR PATIENTS PRESENTING WITH KNEE OSTEOARTHRITIS

Question	Patient Response
Identification	Age, occupation
Chief complaint	Pain/clicking/locking/swelling/decreased motion/instability
History of presenting illness	Pain history
	W: Where is most of the pain located? (point with finger)
	W: When did it start?
	Q: Quality of the pain; does it radiate?
	Q: Quantity of pain
	A: Aggravating factors
	A: Alleviating factors
	A: Associated symptoms
	Associated trauma or injury?
	Mechanism of injury
	Date
	Treatment
Treatments to date	Analgesics, NSAIDs, bracing, physiotherapy, injections, surgery
Functional status	Walking tolerance (No. of blocks) that is limited by knee symptoms
	Sleep disturbance
	Pain at rest
	ADLs
	Sports
Expectations	Return to physical work
	Return to sports and activities
	Level of competition?
	High-impact versus low-impact activities?

ADLs, Activities of daily living; *NSAIDs,* nonsteroidal antiinflammatory drugs.

standing 45-degree posteroanterior (PA) flexion; and lateral and skyline of the affected knee. The specific purpose of the two standing films is to identify joint space narrowing compared with the nonaffected knee.[19-21]

The weight-bearing 45-degree PA flexion radiograph was first described by Rosenberg et al.[21] in 1988 and is often referred to as the *Rosenberg view* (Figure 103-1). The authors noted that some patients for whom no joint space narrowing was visible on standing full-extension AP views often were found to have areas of significant cartilage wear at the time of arthroscopy. As the knee is flexed during the stance phase of gait, the femorotibial contact area moves posteriorly and decreases in size so that force per unit area loading of the knee is increased. Therefore the flexed knee is much more susceptible to chondral damage and subsequent OA. Furthermore, in patients with ACL deficiency, the altered knee biomechanics lead to increased posteromedial wear, particularly on the tibia. For these reasons, the Rosenberg view has better sensitivity and specificity than the conventional standing AP radiograph in detecting joint space narrowing and OA.[20,21]

If joint space narrowing is observed on the standard knee series, a standing hip to ankle radiograph should be obtained to assess limb alignment (Fig. 103-2). This view is critical for decision making and surgical planning.[22-24] A line from the center of the hip to the center of the ankle defines the mechanical axis in the coronal plane.[25] This line generally passes through the center of the knee in a neutrally aligned limb. Any deviation from this point is considered malalignment. If the line falls toward the medial side of the knee, the limb is in varus alignment, and if the line falls toward the lateral side of the knee, the limb is in valgus alignment.[26]

Sagittal plane alignment is determined by measuring the posterior tibial slope. This angle is defined by a line perpendicular to the middiaphysis of the tibia and the posterior inclination of the tibial plateau on a lateral radiograph.[27]

Radiographs also identify signs and severity of OA (e.g., osteophytes, joint space narrowing, subchondral sclerosis, and subchondral cysts), which areas of the knee are affected, limb alignment, posterior tibial slope, patellar height, previous fracture, deformity, and previous surgery, as well as previous implants used and the location of the implants.

Magnetic resonance imaging (MRI) is a commonly ordered investigation in patients who present with knee conditions. However, most of the information required for decision making in patients with knee OA can be gathered from a proper history, physical examination, and the aforementioned radiographs.[19] Bhattacharyya et al.[28] reviewed radiographs and MRI images in 154 patients (men ≥45 years; women ≥50 years) with symptomatic and asymptomatic knee OA. The groups were similar in age. However, patients in the symptomatic OA group had significantly higher body mass index (BMI) scores. The authors found that meniscal tears were highly prevalent in both asymptomatic (76%) and symptomatic (91%) cases of knee OA. Increased radiographic evidence of OA was associated with an increased rate of meniscal tears. No significant difference in pain and function was found on visual analog scale or Western Ontario and McMaster Universities Osteoarthritis Index (WOMAC) scores between patients with and without a medial or lateral meniscal tear in the osteoarthritic group. Ultimately, the etiology of pain in patients with knee OA is multifactorial and can include cartilage lesions, synovial inflammation, and periarticular muscle strains. The investigators concluded that there is no indication for routine use of MRI for the evaluation and management of patients with OA of the knee.[28]

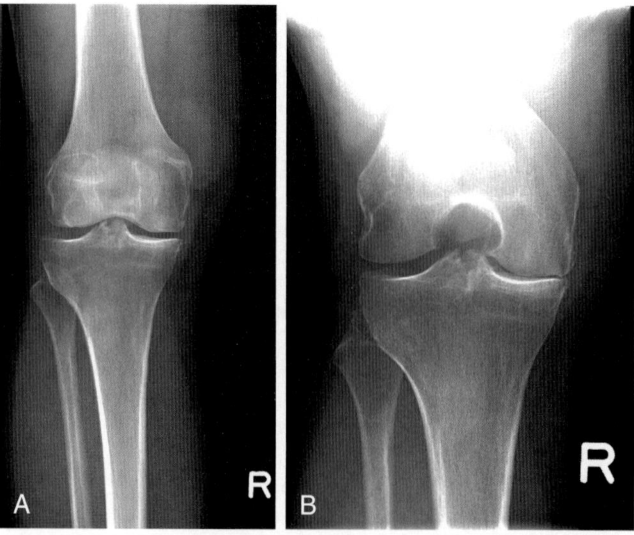

FIGURE 103-1 **A,** A conventional standing anteroposterior radiograph of the right knee with no visible joint space narrowing. **B,** A "Rosenberg view" of the same knee shows evidence of joint space narrowing and osteoarthritis.

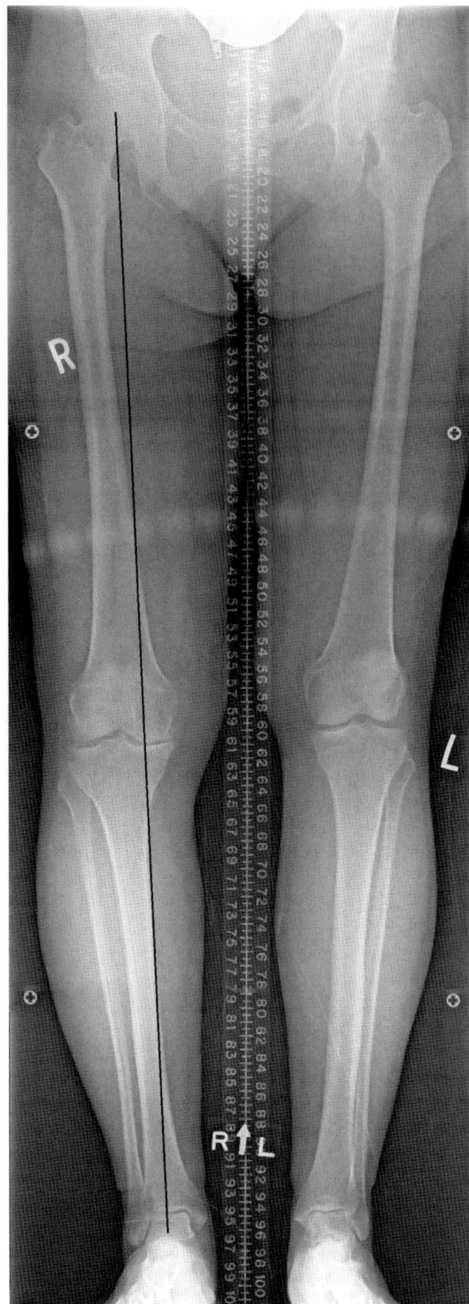

FIGURE 103-2 This standing hip to ankle radiographic view is critical in decision making and surgical planning. A line from the center of the hip to the center of the ankle defines the mechanical axis in the coronal plane. In a neutrally aligned limb, this line passes through the center of the knee. Any deviation from this point is considered malalignment. Here the line falls toward the medial side of the knee, indicating varus alignment of the limb.

Treatment Options

Figure 103-3 shows possible treatment options, from least invasive to most invasive.

Nonoperative Treatment Options

Education and Activity Modification

The natural history of OA is a waxing and waning course, with days when symptoms are manageable and days when symptoms seem to worsen. Patients should be educated about self-management techniques, including lifestyle and activity modification. Encouraging patients to take responsibility for their condition allows them to actively participate in their care and has been shown to improve symptoms.[29,30]

Weight Loss

Patients with symptomatic knee OA who have a BMI score of more than 25 kg/m^2 should be encouraged to lose weight through diet and exercise. Studies have shown an improvement in overall clinical function in the WOMAC function subscale with weight loss.[29,30] Other studies have shown that weight reduction decreases the knee joint load per step at a ratio of 1 lb lost to a 4-lb reduction in knee-joint load per step.[31,32] Not only does weight loss have a beneficial effect on symptoms of knee OA, but it also encompasses whole-body health benefits that cannot be overlooked.

Low-Impact Exercise

Multiple studies have shown that low-impact exercise, such as walking, biking, and using an elliptical trainer, have the beneficial effects of decreasing pain and disability in patients with knee OA.[29,30] The American Geriatrics Society recommends a minimum of 20 to 30 minutes of physical activity per day, two to five times per week, for persons with OA.[33]

Analgesic Medications

Patients who have a symptomatic osteoarthritic knee should be encouraged to use acetaminophen for pain relief. Studies comparing use of acetaminophen (≤4 g/day) with a placebo have shown significant benefit in pain relief without any significant adverse effects.[29,30]

Nonsteroidal Antiinflammatory Drugs

In patients who have no risk factors for gastrointestinal disease, nonsteroidal antiinflammatory drugs (NSAIDs) may be prescribed for pain relief. Studies have shown a statistically significant, favorable clinical response with the use of NSAIDs versus acetaminophen. Consideration for additional gastroprotective medication along with nonselective NSAID medication or cyclooxygenase-2 inhibitors is recommended. Topical NSAID medication has been shown to improve pain, stiffness, and function and should also be considered.[29,30]

Braces

The use of an unloader knee brace may be a cost-effective adjunct to treatment and a reasonable option to help decrease symptoms and increase function in patients with knee OA.[34,35] This type of brace functions by helping to transfer the weight-bearing forces from the worn to the unworn part of the knee. Although it can be used for either varus or valgus deformities, it has been primarily studied in patients with medial compartment OA (MCOA). In a study by Kirkley et al.,[35] a varus unloader brace was shown to have significant benefit compared with a neoprene sleeve or medical management alone in decreasing pain and improving function. The authors recommended its use in patients with symptomatic unicompartmental OA who have a correctable deformity and an average-sized leg.[35] Also, the use of an unloader brace may help determine if the patient will have any benefit from a limb realignment procedure. A further advantage of bracing relates to proprioception. Studies have shown that patients with knee

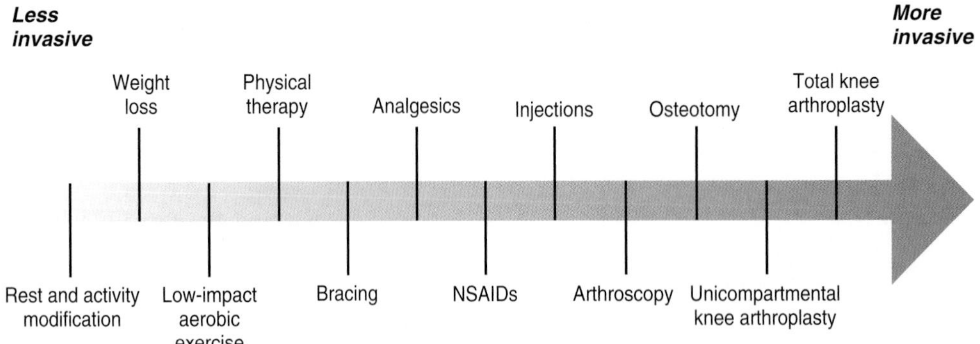

FIGURE 103-3 Treatment options from least to most invasive for patients with symptomatic osteoarthritis of the knee. *NSAIDs,* Nonsteroidal antiinflammatory drugs.

OA have decreased proprioception. Kirkley et al.[35] report that knee braces offer a proprioceptive benefit. The disadvantages to bracing are compliance, difficulty in obtaining a proper fit, and cost.

Physical Therapy

Quadriceps-strengthening exercises have been shown to provide a significant benefit for symptomatic pain relief. The use of ROM and stretching exercises has not been studied extensively, and their clinical effect is unknown. However, flexibility and motion exercises appear to have no adverse effects and offer many health benefits.[36-38]

Injections

Intraarticular corticosteroid injections may be prescribed for short-term relief of acute pain due to an arthritic "flare-up." Studies have shown that the mean duration of the effect of a corticosteroid injection is 1 week.[39-41] On the other hand, the benefit of viscosupplementation with hyaluronic acid injections has not been completely established. High-quality studies are scarce, and previous studies have had problems with bias and unclear significance of the selected outcomes. Although a clear recommendation cannot be made for viscosupplementation, in general it seems to provide a positive trend in clinical effect with minimal adverse effects and therefore may be used in selected patients.[42]

Treatment Not Recommended

Several treatment options such as glucosamine and/or chondroitin, lateral heel wedges, and needle lavage have historically been prescribed as nonoperative treatment options for patients with symptomatic OA of the knee. However, a sufficient number of high-quality studies have shown that glucosamine hydrochloride and/or chondroitin sulphate have no clinical benefit compared with placebo.[42] Likewise, no good evidence exists to support the prescription of lateral heel wedges for MCOA of the knee.[43] Lastly, studies recommending needle lavage have been of poor quality, and the procedure has not been shown to have any lasting benefit.[44,45]

Operative Options

Arthroscopy

Arthroscopic lavage, debridement, and/or meniscectomy are not recommended in patients whose primary symptom is pain. In 2002 Moseley et al.[46] conducted the first of two randomized controlled studies of the effect of arthroscopic surgery in patients with OA of the knee who presented with knee pain. They compared arthroscopic surgery with arthroscopic lavage and "sham" surgery in 180 patients and found that results of arthroscopic surgery were no better than those of sham surgery at a follow-up of 2 years.[46] In 2008 Kirkley et al.[1] conducted another randomized controlled trial with 188 patients in which arthroscopic surgery was compared with optimized physiotherapy and medical management. These investigators specifically addressed several weaknesses of the study by Moseley et al.,[46] which included the use of a nonvalidated outcome measure and the lack of generalizability of their results. This study also showed no difference among the three groups in WOMAC or Short Form (SF)-36 scores at 2 years after surgery. Dervin et al.[46a] studied the ability of two groups of surgeons to independently predict the outcome of arthroscopic debridement based on clinical symptoms, signs, and plain radiography. One hundred twenty-six patients were followed up for 2 years subsequent to failure of medical management and arthroscopic debridement. Fifty-six patients (44%) reported a clinically important reduction in pain on the WOMAC pain scale. Furthermore, they found that physicians correctly predicted outcome only 59% or less of the time.[1]

Arthroscopic surgery is not recommended in patients with documented knee OA. Expert opinion suggests that arthroscopy should be considered only in cases in which mechanical symptoms rather than pain are the chief complaint.[47]

Osteotomy

An osteotomy is a bony realignment procedure for unicompartmental arthritis of the knee. The biomechanical principle of osteotomy is to redistribute the weight-bearing forces from the worn to the unworn compartment of the knee to relieve pain and slow disease progression.[48-53] The most frequently seen deformity is varus alignment due to MCOA, with isolated lateral compartment OA one eighth as common as isolated MCOA. The majority of osteotomies are performed on the proximal tibia to treat MCOA. Biopsy and second-look arthroscopic and other open procedures have shown that there is regrowth of fibrocartilage in the worn medial compartment with a predilection for the ulcerated regions of wear in the weight-bearing portion of the medial femoral condyle.[54-57] Box 103-1 outlines the indications for an osteotomy.

Medial Compartment Osteoarthritis

Both medial opening wedge high tibial osteotomy (HTO) and lateral closing wedge HTO have been used to successfully

BOX 103-1 Indications for an Osteotomy

Malalignment + Arthrosis
Malalignment + Instability
Malalignment + Arthrosis + Instability
Malalignment + Meniscal/Cartilage Transplant ± Instability

treat MCOA (Fig. 103-4). The advantages and disadvantages of each technique are outlined in Table 103-2.

Medial Opening Wedge HTO. Historically, along with the points shown in Table 103-2, the concerns with medial opening wedge HTO have been prolonged immobilization and restricted weight bearing, both of which have a significant impact on the patient's quality of life. Recent improvements in implant technology have led to the development of locking plates for HTO. These devices are much stronger than previous nonlocking implants and allow weight bearing as early as 2 weeks after surgery with no loss of correction of the osteotomy and no delayed union or nonunion.[58,59] Another concern with medial opening wedge HTO is the morbidity associated with the harvesting of iliac crest bone graft required to fill the osteotomy. However, several recent studies have reported that an autograft, an allograft, and even no graft for corrections of 8 mm or less have produced good results, with union occurring by 12 weeks after surgery.[60]

Lateral Closing Wedge HTO. Coventry[61] first described the technique of lateral closing wedge HTO in 1965. Advantages and disadvantages are described in Table 103-2. Currently, our only indication for this procedure is a previous successful lateral closing wedge HTO in the contralateral limb.

Other Techniques. Less commonly used tibial osteotomy techniques include the dome osteotomy and external fixation. These techniques are recommended for deformities greater than 25 degrees, as well for those that require gradual rather than acute correction, as in skeletally mature patients with Blount disease or in younger patients with idiopathic genu varum.[62-65]

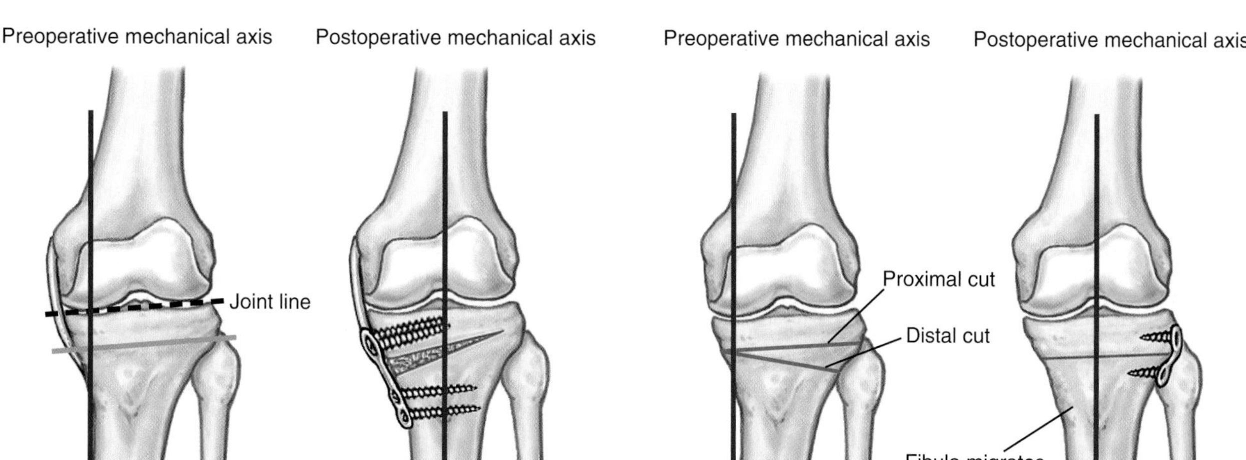

FIGURE 103-4 Basic principles of opening wedge (**A**) and closing wedge (**B**) high tibial osteotomies.

TABLE 103-2

MEDIAL OPENING WEDGE VERSUS LATERAL CLOSING WEDGE HIGH TIBIAL OSTEOTOMY

	Advantages	Disadvantages
Medial opening wedge	The procedure is technically easier to perform (requiring just one bone cut) It provides the ability to achieve a predictable correction in coronal and sagittal planes It can be combined with other procedures such as ligamentous reconstruction with relative ease It restores bone stock	Healing in distraction leads to more potential problems with delayed and nonunion The tibial slope may be difficult to maintain
Lateral closing wedge	Healing in compression leads to fewer problems with delayed and nonunion It provides favorable alterations in the tibial slope to treat chronic anterior cruciate ligament deficiency	The procedure is technically more difficult for inexperienced surgeons • Peroneal nerve • Proximal tibiofibular joint It decreases bone stock It makes future total knee arthroplasty more technically challenging

Lateral Compartment OA

Lateral compartment OA can be caused by pathology on the femoral or tibial side of the knee. The osteotomy should be performed at the site of the cause of the deformity.

Proximal Tibial Osteotomies. The results of proximal tibial varus osteotomies have not equaled those of proximal tibial valgus osteotomies. A concern remains that proximal tibial osteotomies for lateral compartment OA will cause joint line obliquity greater than 10 degrees, leading to lateral subluxation of the tibia. Another concern is that medial collateral ligament (MCL) laxity occurs if the wedge is taken above the MCL insertion. However, a role still exists for proximal tibial osteotomy in the valgus knee. This role includes small corrections of 12 degrees or less that avoid excessive joint line obliquity in persons with posttraumatic OA for whom the deformity is primarily at or below the joint. If the deformity is primarily in the femur or the correction is greater than 12 degrees, a distal femoral osteotomy should be considered.[66,67]

Distal Femoral Osteotomies. A distal femoral varus osteotomy is an appropriate procedure for patients with valgus deformity of the femur, such as a hypoplastic lateral femoral condyle, or if the required correction is greater than 12 degrees.[23] Again, this procedure can be a medial closing wedge or a lateral opening wedge osteotomy. The advantages and disadvantages of each procedure are similar to those listed for opening and closing wedge proximal tibial osteotomies in persons with MCOA (see Table 103-2). One additional advantage of a lateral opening wedge distal femoral osteotomy is that the correction can be tailored to the desired amount of varus. On the other hand, the medial closing wedge technique using a 90-degree blade plate typically results in a tibiofemoral angle correction of 0 degrees and a mechanical axis correction of 6 degrees varus.[66] Whether tailoring the correction with a lateral opening wedge technique is superior to using the medial closing wedge technique with regard to long-term outcome has yet to be determined.

Knee Instability

Knee instability can be due to both bony and soft tissue factors. Ligamentous causes are the most common. However, altered tibial slope in the sagittal plane occurring in isolation as a result of a tibial physeal arrest or in combination with ligamentous insufficiency can also cause anterior-posterior instability. In such cases, the condition must be corrected to create a stable joint before ligamentous reconstruction, and a combined ligamentous and bony procedure should be considered to decrease the risk of graft failure.[5,8,68] Normally the posterior tibial slope is 10 degrees ± 3 degrees.[27] A posterior tibial slope greater than 13 degrees results in anterior tibial translation and altered joint biomechanics, as well as meniscal load sharing, leading to increased chondral wear. Similarly, a posterior tibial slope of less than 7 degrees (relative decreased slope) is also considered abnormal and leads to posterior translation of the tibia and may have a similar outcome.[69] When these conditions are symptomatic, they should be addressed with an osteotomy to improve the bony stability. Osteotomies for sagittal plane deformities are usually approached anteriorly with either an anterior closing wedge osteotomy for increased tibial slope or an opening wedge osteotomy for decreased slope.[70]

Combined Instability and Pain

Patients with chronic ligament deficiency may present with pain, instability, or both characteristics. Patients most commonly have chronic ACL deficiency. However, posterior cruciate ligament and posterolateral corner insufficiency may also be present. It has been shown that in patients with instability and malalignment, soft tissue ligamentous reconstruction is at risk of failure because of the malalignment.[5,68] Therefore an osteotomy to correct the malalignment followed by simultaneous or staged ligamentous reconstruction should be considered.[8]

In patients whose primary symptom is instability with mild or moderate medial compartment degeneration, an osteotomy alone may not prove beneficial. Although ligament reconstruction alone has been shown to be successful,[9,71,72] it does not address the malalignment, predictably alleviate any symptoms of pain, or offer any chondroprotection to the damaged medial compartment. In these patients, an osteotomy to address pain combined with a simultaneous or staged soft tissue procedure to address ligament deficiency should be considered.

In patients presenting with chronic ACL deficiency, treatment options include lateral closing wedge osteotomy or combined HTO and ACL reconstruction. A lateral closing wedge osteotomy favorably decreases the tibial slope, which helps improve instability related to ACL deficiency. A medial opening wedge osteotomy tends to change tibial slope in an unfavorable direction, and therefore combined procedures should be considered.[48,50,73] Previous studies have described combined HTO and ACL reconstruction as simultaneous or staged procedures, with the osteotomy usually performed first.[68,74] Simultaneous medial opening wedge HTO and ACL reconstruction allows for biplanar correction of the knee deformity with restoration of ligamentous support in one operation and results in improvements in both bony and soft tissue support, which in theory leads to improved overall knee joint function.[6,75-77]

Return to Sport After an Osteotomy

The true benefit of an osteotomy is that is allows unrestricted activity while preserving the knee joint. Multiple studies have shown that HTO affords young, active patients with OA the ability to return to recreational sports and to maintain an active lifestyle.[78,79] Van Raaij et al.[80] found that HTO postpones primary total knee arthroplasty (TKA) for a median of 7 years in this group of patients.

Patient Satisfaction After HTO

With careful patient selection, satisfaction after HTO is very high. Hui et al.[81] showed that at a mean follow-up of 12 years, 85% of a cohort of 397 patients who underwent lateral closing wedge HTO were enthusiastic or satisfied and 84% would have the same surgery again. Similarly, at a mean of 6.5 years after surgery, Tang and Henderson[82] reported patient satisfaction of 76%, with 90% of patients saying they would choose the same surgery again.

Arthroplasty

Medial Compartment Osteoarthritis

For many years, unicompartmental knee arthroplasty (UKA) has been performed to treat isolated MCOA. The potential benefits of UKA compared with TKA are lower perioperative morbidity, less blood loss, maintenance of normal knee kinematics, and quicker patient rehabilitation and recovery.[83] Controversies remain regarding a fixed bearing versus mobile bearing implant design, but both have shown good long-term success.[84-86] However, concern remains regarding the durability of UKA in younger patients.[87]

Tricompartmental Osteoarthritis

In patients presenting with severe tricompartmental osteoarthritis, the gold standard is a TKA. This procedure offers long-term, predictable pain relief. TKA for symptoms other than pain, such as stiffness, swelling, or instability, has unpredictable outcomes and is not recommended.[88]

Combined Instability and Pain

Historically, ACL insufficiency has been a contraindication to UKA because of concerns relating to increased anterior tibial translation and altered knee biomechanics with subsequent increased lateral compartment arthrosis and polyethylene wear resulting from posterior loading of the implant and ultimate prosthesis failure. Recently, combined UKA using the Oxford prosthesis (Biomet, Oxford, UK) and ACL reconstruction has been performed to address both instability and pain related to MCOA. However, controversy remains regarding implant survival in this subgroup.[89,90] Lateral UKA is contraindicated in patients with ACL insufficiency because of increased lateral compared with medial compartment mobility, which leads to even more abnormal contact pressures and a potentially higher rate of failure.[91]

Return to Sport After Arthroplasty

Parratte et al.[87] reviewed data for 31 patients who underwent UKA at a mean age of 46 years (range, 41 to 49 years) and who were allowed unrestricted activity after surgery (data for a total of 35 knees were reviewed). At a mean follow-up of 9.7 years (range, 5 to 16 years), 75% had returned to manual work at the same level as before surgery, 60% had returned to the same level of participation in sports, and 30% were participating in sports at a lower level. Ten percent were unable to return to their sport. The authors acknowledge that revision for polyethylene wear remains the main concern.[87] In a biomechanical study, Kuster[92] previously demonstrated that running and jumping produces surface loads that exceed the limits of polyethylene resistance. The general recommendation for return to sport after an arthroplasty is low-impact activities such as cycling, bowling, swimming, scuba, golf, skating, cross-country skiing, weight lifting, dancing, and walking.[93]

Decision-Making Principles

Management of patients with knee OA should be individualized. Physiologic rather than chronologic age should be considered, along with the patient's goals and expectations. Patient education is paramount to successful management of these patients. Figure 103-5 outlines the treatment algorithm for patients presenting with knee OA. Management always begins with nonoperative treatment and progresses from less invasive to more invasive options (Fig. 103-3).

Medial Compartment Osteoarthritis

Several factors need to be considered when deciding the best surgical treatment for patients with isolated MCOA of the knee for whom conservative management has failed. Table 103-3 outlines the indications for HTO versus UKA versus TKA in these patients.

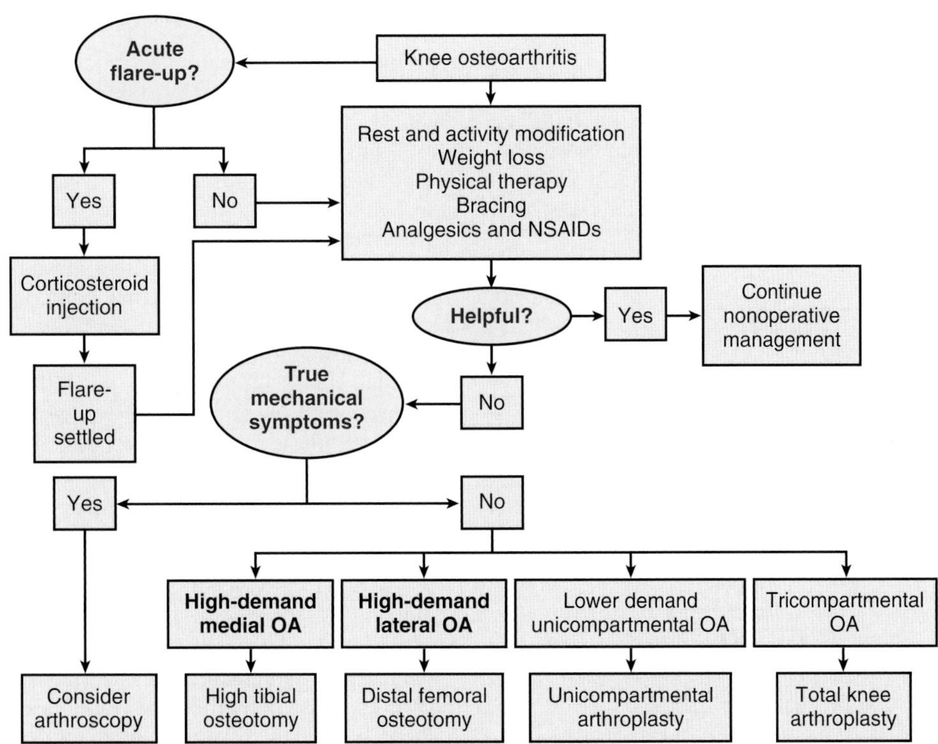

FIGURE 103-5 A treatment algorithm for patients with knee osteoarthritis (OA). *NSAIDs,* Nonsteroidal antiinflammatory drugs.

TABLE 103-3

INDICATIONS FOR SURGERY IN PATIENTS WITH MEDIAL COMPARTMENT OSTEOARTHRITIS OF THE KNEE

	HTO	UKA	TKR
Age*	≤65 yr	≥55 yr	≥65 yr
Activity level	High	Low	Low
Body mass index	Any	<30	<30
Malalignment	5°-20°	0°-5°	Any
AP instability	Any	None†	Any‡
ML instability	≤Grade II	None	Any‡
ROM	Arc ≥120°	Arc ≥90°	Any
MCOA	Any	Any	Any
PFOA	≤Grade II§	≤Grade II§	Any
LCOA	Any	Any	Any

AP, Anteroposterior; *HTO,* High tibial osteotomy; *LCOA,* lateral compartment osteoarthritis; *MCOA,* medial compartment osteoarthritis; *ML,* mediolateral instability; *PFOA,* patellofemoral osteoarthritis; *ROM,* range of motion; *TKR,* total knee replacement; *UKA,* unicompartmental knee arthroplasty.
*Physiologic age should be considered here.
†Long-term results of combined anterior cruciate ligament reconstruction and UKA have not been established.
‡Increasing instability requires increased component constraint.
§For MCOA, the patient may have up to grade II PFOA if no patellofemoral symptoms are present.

Lateral Compartment Osteoarthritis

In general, lateral compartment OA is better tolerated than MCOA. The treatment algorithm for patients with symptomatic lateral compartment OA of the knee for whom conservative management has failed is shown in Figure 103-6. The lateral compartment UKA procedure remains controversial and is not recommended until longer term results are reported.

Chronic ACL Insufficiency

Figure 103-7 outlines the treatment algorithm for patients who present with symptomatic instability and pain caused by chronic ACL insufficiency. Use of UKA in patients with chronic ACL insufficiency with or without combined ACL reconstruction is controversial and is not recommended.

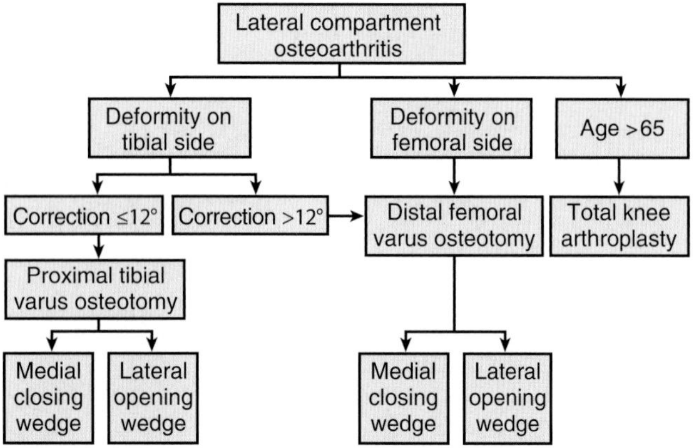

FIGURE 103-6 A treatment algorithm for patients with lateral compartment knee osteoarthritis.

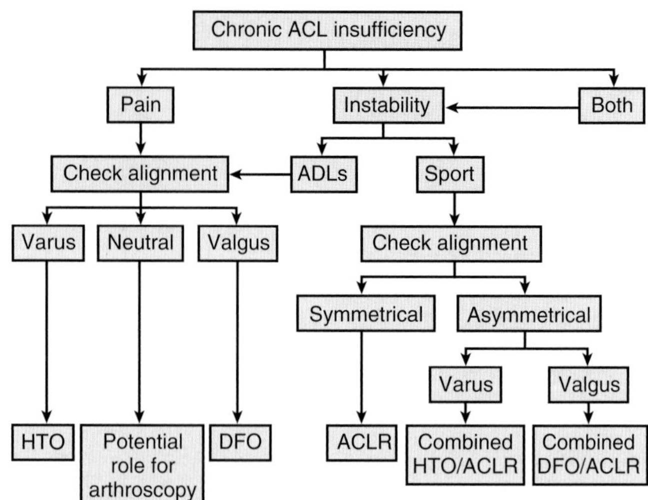

FIGURE 103-7 A treatment algorithm for patients with chronic anterior cruciate ligament (ACL) insufficiency and osteoarthritis. *ACLR,* Anterior cruciate ligament reconstruction; *ADLs,* activities of daily living; *DFO,* distal femoral osteotomy; *HTO,* high tibial osteotomy.

AUTHORS' PREFERRED TECHNIQUE

Medial Collateral Osteoarthritis

Our preferred technique for physiologically young patients with MCOA who place a high demand on their knees is a medial opening wedge HTO. We use a modification of the technique previously described by Puddu and Franco.[94] Preoperative planning is critical to osteotomy surgery and begins with a determination of limb alignment in both the coronal and sagittal planes.

Postoperative Management

The most important aspect of rehabilitation after an HTO is ROM. Early postoperative knee ROM exercises promote healing and articular cartilage nourishment, as well as lower limb neuromuscular function. Normal weight bearing is encouraged as soon as possible to help with bone turnover and healing.[96] With the advent of locking plate technology, partial weight bearing can commence at 2 weeks after surgery, and full weight bearing is usually achieved by 6 weeks. Several recent studies have shown that early weight bearing with locking plates does not negatively affect limb alignment, loss of correction, and delayed/nonunion.[58,59]

Table 103-4 outlines our rehabilitation protocol after uncomplicated medial opening wedge HTO using a locking plate. Each phase in this regimen builds on the previous one, and every patient should be treated on an individual basis based on the type of surgery he or she underwent. For example, if concomitant procedures such as ligament reconstruction, microfracture, or meniscal transplant are performed, the rehabilitation program should be altered with these procedures in mind. If a nonlocking plate is used, the approximate timelines need to be adjusted accordingly.

Return to sport and activity is permitted when radiographic and clinical evidence shows bone healing and when the patient has regained muscle bulk and control of the newly

Text continued on p. 1239

AUTHORS' PREFERRED TECHNIQUE

Medial Opening Wedge HTO

Preoperative Planning

1. Obtain the following radiographs of both limbs: standing anteroposterior (AP) in full extension, standing 30-degree posteroanterior, lateral, skyline, and standing hip to ankle.
   - Assess lateral and patellofemoral osteoarthritis (OA).
   - Measure patellar height.
   - Measure the posterior tibial slope.
2. Plan the osteotomy. We typically use the technique previously described by Dugdale et al. (Figure 103-8).[95]
   - Measure the width of the tibial plateau.
   - Determine the correction point at 62.5% across the plateau from the medial edge. This point lies slightly lateral to the tip of the lateral tibial spine and equates to 3 degrees to 5 degrees of mechanical valgus (Figure 103-8, *A*).
   - Draw a line from the center of the femoral head to the 62.5% correction point (ȧ) and another line from the center of the ankle to this point (ḃ) (Figure 103-8, *B*).
   - Draw the intended osteotomy from the junction of the proximal tibial metadiaphysis (~4 cm from the top of the medial tibial plateau) to the top of the fibular head (ė) and measure the length of the osteotomy (Fig. 103-8, *C*).
   - Transpose the intended osteotomy line (ė → ë) over the top of line ḃ (Fig. 103-8, *D*).
   - Draw a line (l) perpendicular to the top of line ë across to line ȧ. Measure the length of this line. This line serves as the base of an isosceles triangle and is the intended wedge size of the osteotomy (Fig. 103-8, *E*).

Diagnostic Arthroscopy

1. Examine the lateral and patellofemoral compartments.
   - If Ahlbäck grade II or III degeneration is present in the lateral compartment, consider correcting the weight-bearing line to 50% the distance across the width of the tibial plateau rather than to the 62.5% point.
   - If Ahlbäck grade IV degeneration is present in the lateral compartment, abandon the osteotomy and consider total knee arthroplasty at a later date.
   - If Ahlback grade IV degeneration is present in the patellofemoral joint, consider a concomitant tibial tubercle osteotomy.

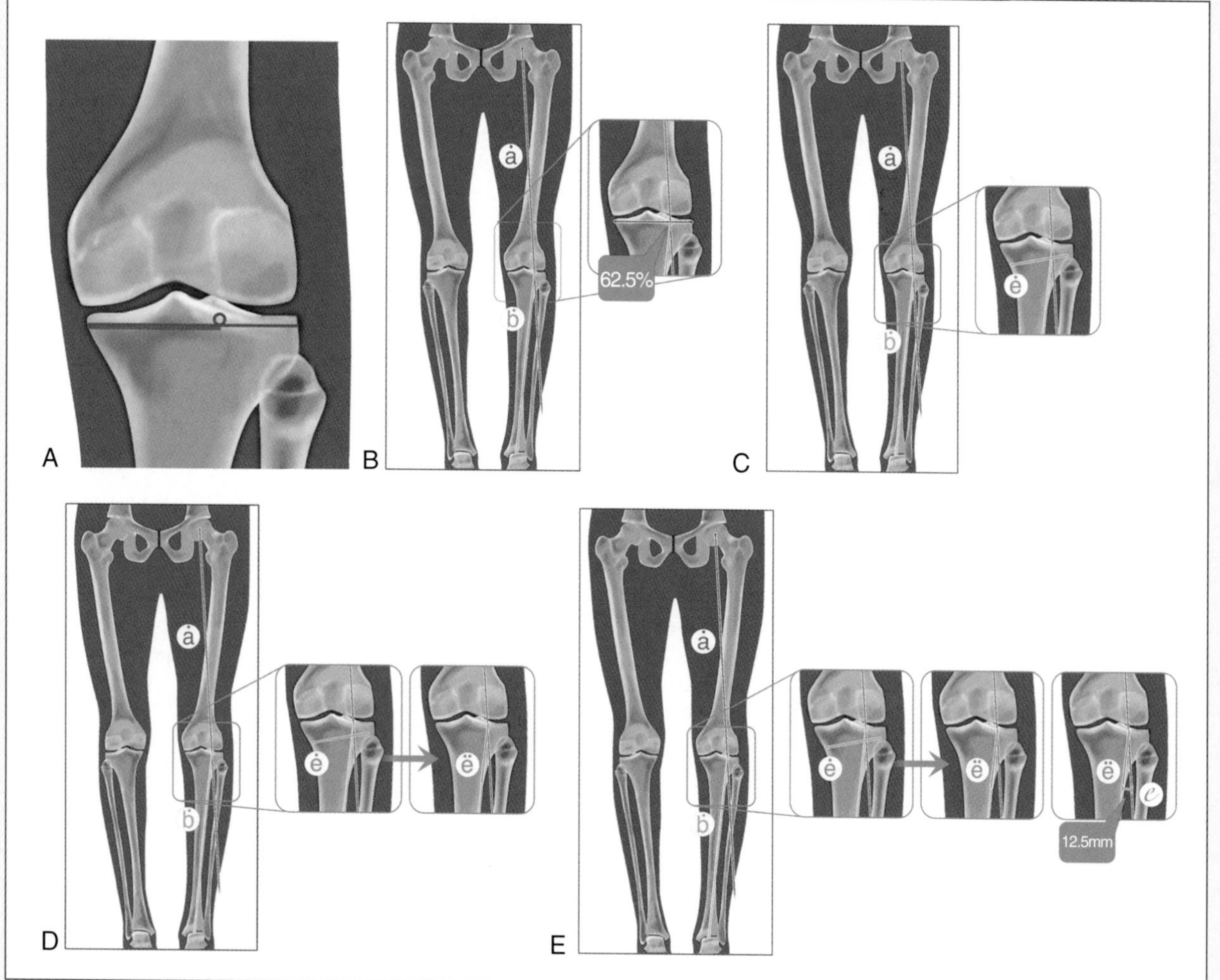

FIGURE 103-8 The trigonometric method for planning the osteotomy size for an opening wedge high tibial osteotomy.

Continued

2. Perform any meniscal work or debridement as required.
3. A 5-cm longitudinal incision is made starting 1 cm distal to the medial joint line midway between the tibial tubercle and the posteromedial border of the tibia (Fig. 103–9, *A*).
4. Expose the sartorial fascia and open it at the top of the pes anserine. Retract the pes tendons distally. Sharply release the pes from its insertion onto the tibia to expose the superficial medial collateral ligament (MCL).
5. Identify the posteromedial border of the tibia and, using electrocautery, make a 1- to 1.5-cm longitudinal incision along this border in line with the fibers of the superficial MCL.
6. Using a Cobb elevator, bluntly lift the gastrocnemius off the posterior aspect of the tibia, making sure to stay on the bone.
7. Insert a finger into this interval to ensure the dissection has been carried out across the entire width of the tibia and insert a blunt retractor to protect the neurovascular structures.
8. Next, identify the medial border of the patellar tendon and the interval between the tibia and patellar tendon bursa. Place a retractor into this interval.
9. Obtain an AP image of the knee in line with the posterior tibial slope (at approximately 10 degrees of knee flexion).
10. Place a guide pin along the anterior border of the superficial MCL at the junction of the metadiaphysis of the proximal tibia. Under fluoroscopy, direct the pin toward the top of the fibular head to a point approximately 1 cm below the lateral joint line.
11. Place a large osteotome beneath the pin and adjust it so that it is in line with the posterior tibial slope on an AP image of the knee. With the knee and the osteotome in plane with the posterior tibial slope on the fluoroscopic image of the knee, the plane of the osteotomy will match the posterior tibial slope of the patient. This step is critical (Fig. 103-9, *C*).
12. Mark the position of the osteotome with a marking pen followed by electrocautery (Fig. 103-9, *D*). If a tibial tubercle osteotomy is required, mark the osteotomy line 1 cm short of the tibial tubercle (see the Concomitant Tibial Tubercle Osteotomy section in this box for details).
13. Cut the tibial cortex with a small oscillating saw blade between the tibial tubercle and the posteromedial tibial border (Fig. 103-9, *E*). It is imperative that the angle of the saw blade be in plane with the posterior tibial slope, similar to the osteotome in step 11. The osteotomy is made below the guide pin to avoid proximal migration of the osteotomy into the joint.
14. The osteotomy is advanced toward the lateral tibial cortex using small, thin, flexible osteotomes (Fig. 103-9, *F*).
15. Graduated solid osteotomes are then used, starting with the broadest, which is usually advanced to two thirds the width of the osteotomy. A narrow osteotome is then used along the posterior tibial cortex and is advanced to approximately 1 cm from the lateral tibial cortex under fluoroscopic guidance. Again, it is critical for the plane of the osteotomy to mimic the posterior tibial slope (Fig. 103-9, *G*).
16. Check the mobility of the osteotomy by applying a valgus force across the osteotomy. It should open easily. If it does not open easily, step 15 should be repeated until the osteotomy opens without difficulty to the desired wedge size.
17. Insert both blades of an osteotome jack approximately two thirds across the osteotomy and gradually open the jack to the desired correction (Fig. 103-9, *H*).
18. At this point, check that the osteotomy is trapezoid in shape (i.e., narrower anteriorly and wider posteriorly because the tibia is a triangular-shaped bone). A rectangular-shaped osteotomy indicates that the posterior tibial slope has been altered.
19. Insert the osteotomy wedge trial to the desired correction and confirm that the limb is in valgus alignment (Fig. 103-9, *I*).
20. With the wedge trial holding the osteotomy open, insert the plate into the osteotomy site. Bend the plate as required to fit the shape of the tibia. Once the plate is inserted, remove the wedge trial.
21. Secure the plate with three locking cancellous screws above and three locking cortical screws below. The screws should be directed away from the osteotomy (Fig. 103-9, *J*).
22. Mix corticocancellous allograft bone chips with 1 g of vancomycin powder. Insert and pack the mixture into the osteotomy with a bone tamp. Note that bone grafting is optional for corrections of 7.5 mm or less (Fig. 103-10).
23. Repair the pes anserine over the top of the plate.
24. Insert a drain to exit separately from the incision.
25. Close the skin over the top of the drain.
26. Apply a hinged knee brace locked in full extension.

Concomitant Tibial Tubercle Osteotomy

Indications for a concomitant tibial tubercle osteotomy (TTO) are (1) large corrections >12.5 mm and (2) severe patellofemoral osteoarthritis.

1. If a TTO is required, mark the osteotomy line 1 cm short of the tibial tubercle in step 12. It is important that the thickness of the TTO be 1 cm proximally to avoid fracture.
2. From this point, mark a line exiting the anterior tibial cortex approximately 3 cm distally using electrocautery. For a larger correction, the length of the TTO should be extended to allow enough room for adequate fixation because the tubercle will translate superomedially with the opening of the osteotomy.
3. After the osteotomy cut has been made, make a flat TTO cut along the previously marked line with the small oscillating saw from medial to lateral. It is important that the cut be flat to allow appropriate translation of the tubercle when the osteotomy is distracted.
4. Proceed with steps 14 to 22 as previously outlined.
5. Just before closure (step 23), secure the TTO with one or two 4.5-mm cortical screws from an anterior to posterior direction. It is important to countersink these screws to avoid screw prominence anteriorly.

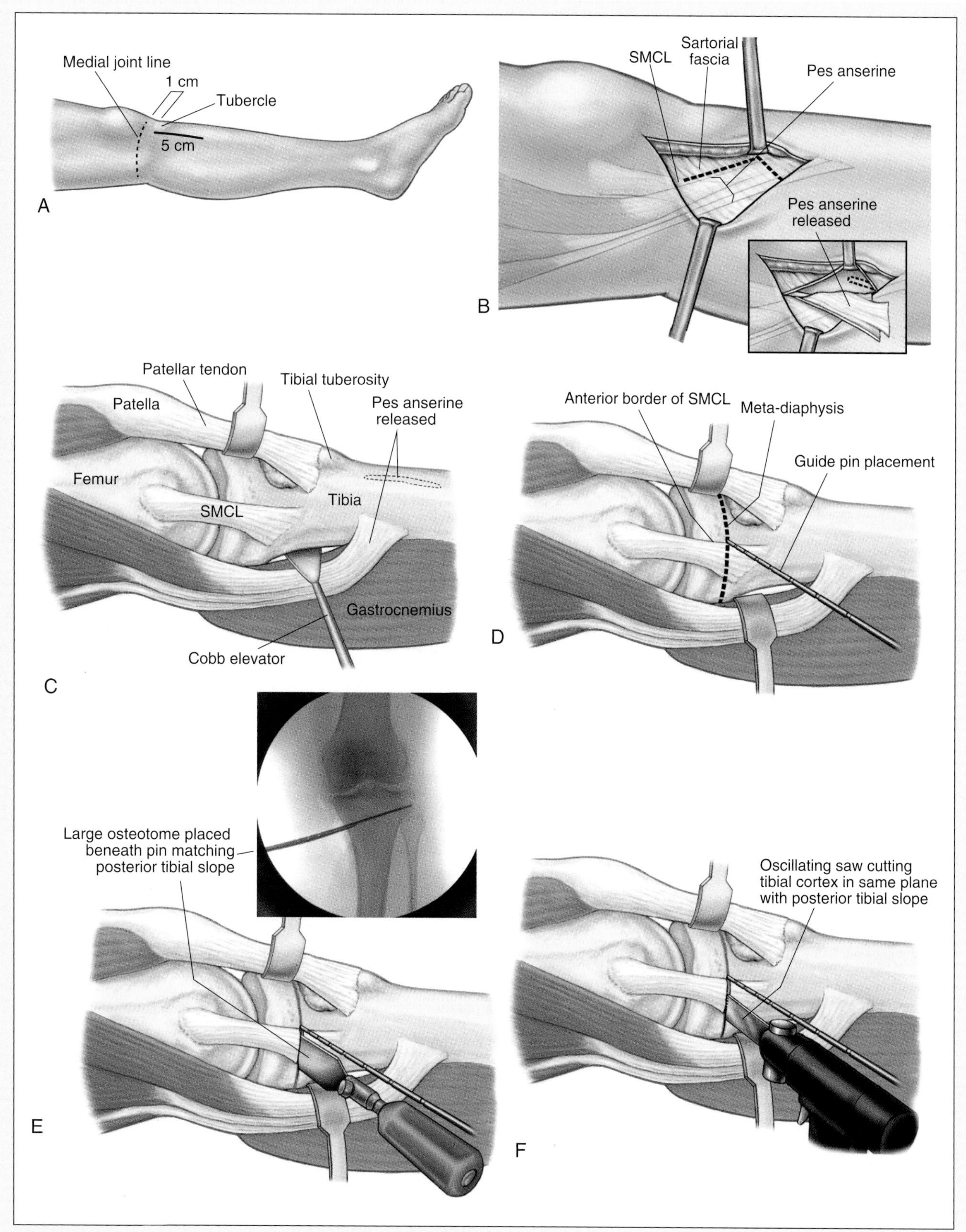

FIGURE 103-9 A large osteotome is placed beneath the pin and adjusted so that it is in line with the posterior tibial slope on an anteroposterior image of the knee. With the knee and the osteotome in plane with the posterior tibial slope on the fluoroscopic image of the knee, the plane of the osteotomy will match the posterior tibial slope of the patient. This step is critical. *SMCL,* Superficial medial collateral ligament.

Continued

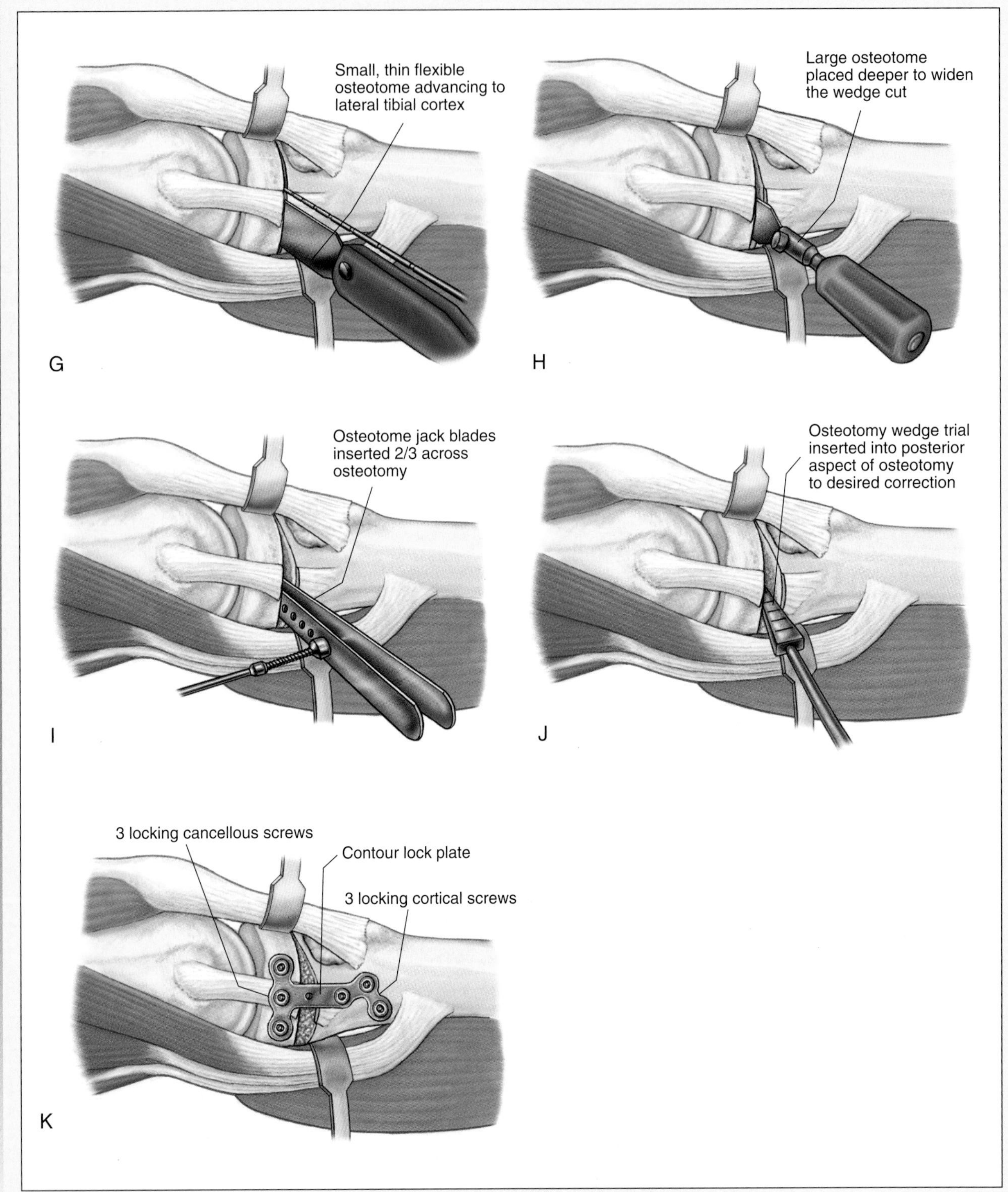

FIGURE 103-9, cont'd

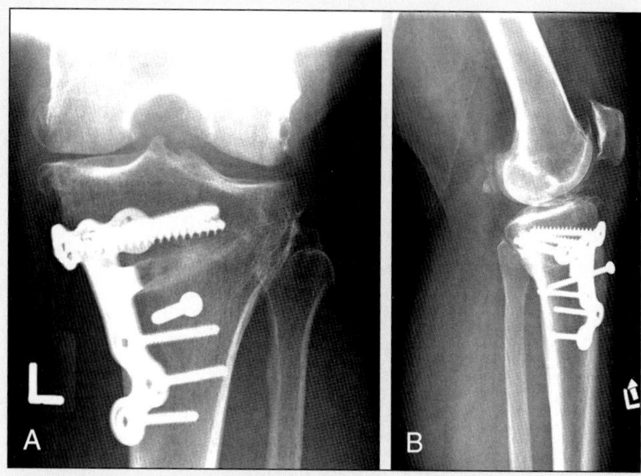

FIGURE 103-10 Anteroposterior (**A**) and lateral (**B**) radiographs demonstrating a completed medial opening wedge high tibial osteotomy with a tibial tubercle osteotomy.

aligned limb. Timing of return to play depends on the individual patient, his or her type of surgery, and his or her sport or activity. Return to play can occur in as few as 6 months or as many as 18 months after surgery. Most patients are able to return to the sport they previously played. However, some patients may never be able to return at the same level.[78,79]

Results

The mid- and long-term outcomes of HTO for MCOA of the knee have been well established and are shown in Table 103-5.[81,82,97-102] Fewer, smaller studies reporting the outcomes of distal femoral osteotomies for lateral compartment OA of the knee are available (Table 103-6).[103-112] Lateral

TABLE 103-4

POSTOPERATIVE REHABILITATION GUIDELINES AFTER A MEDIAL OPENING WEDGE HIGH TIBIAL OSTEOTOMY

Phase	Approximate Timeline	Guidelines	Restrictions
1 (Immediate postoperative)	Day of surgery to 2 wk	Manage pain and swelling Start ROM exercises (may come out of brace) Activate quadriceps	Brace is worn full time except during exercises (locked in extension) Feather/touch weight bearing
2 (Early postoperative)	2-6 wk	Regain full ROM (especially extension) Gait retraining → progress to WBAT Stationary bike with low resistance Core/proximal muscle/quadriceps strengthening	Brace is worn full time except during exercises (fully unlocked)
(Muscle strengthening and control)	6 wk–3 mo	Normal gait—no limp Continue strengthening Stretching and flexibility Increase cardiovascular fitness with low-impact exercise Balance and proprioception exercises (e.g., wobble board) Pool work (e.g., water running)	Brace is off Low-impact activities
4 (Neuromuscular retraining and return to normal function)	3-6 mo	Begin neuromuscular training exercises Continue strengthening Progress to resistance on gym equipment and maintain cardiovascular fitness May ride normal bicycle	
5 (Return to sport and activities)	6-12 mo	Progress to neuromuscular training exercises May progress to higher impact activities Gradual return to all activities, including sports	No restrictions

ROM, Range of motion; *WBAT,* weight bearing as tolerated.

TABLE 103-5

LONG-TERM OUTCOMES OF A HIGH TIBIAL OSTEOTOMY FOR MEDIAL COMPARTMENT OSTEOARTHRITIS

Study	Year	No.	Mean Follow-up (Yr) (Range)	Mean Age (Yr)	Technique	Outcomes
Hui et al.[81]	2011	455 patients	12 (1-19)	50	LCW	95% survival 5 yr 79% survival 10 yr 56% survival 15 yr
Saragaglia et al.[97]	2011	110 patients (124 knees)	10.4 (8-14)	53.3	MOW	88% survival 5 yr 74% survival 10 yr
DeMeo et al.[98]	2010	20 patients	8.3 (2-14)	49.4	MOW	70% survival 8 yr
Akizuki et al.[99]	2008	132 patients	16 (16-20)	63	LCW	98% survival 10 yr 90% survival 15 yr
Gstöttner et al.[100]	2008	111 patients (132 knees)	12 (1-25)	54	LCW	80% survival 10 yr 66% survival 15 yr
Tang and Henderson[82]	2005	67 knees	6.5 (1-21)	49	LCW	75% survival 10 yr 67% survival 15 yr
Naudie et al.[101]	2004	85 patients (106 knees)	14 (10-22)	55	LCW	95% survival 5yr 80% survival 10 yr 65% survival 15yr
Hernigou et al.[102]	1987	184 patients (250 knees)	11.5 (10-13)	60.3	MOW	90% good/excellent 5 yr 45% good/excellent 10 yr

LCW, Lateral compartment wedge; *MOW,* medial opening wedge.

compartment OA is less common than medial compartment disease, and frequently patients with lateral compartment OA have an inflammatory arthropathy that precludes realignment procedures.

Although numerous large, long-term studies of closing wedge proximal tibia and distal femoral osteotomies have been performed, fewer studies of the opening wedge osteotomy exist. Hernigou et al.[102] published the largest study on medial opening wedge HTO in 1987 with a mean follow-up of 11.5 years. Outcomes of lateral opening wedge distal femoral osteotomies have been reported in small case series with short-term follow-up periods.[103,104]

Complications

Complications of HTO can be categorized as intraoperative, early postoperative, or late postoperative. Table 103-7[65,113-115] outlines the most common complications and their management. Complications after a distal femoral osteotomy are very similar to those that occur after a proximal tibial osteotomy.

TABLE 103-6

LONG-TERM OUTCOMES OF A HIGH TIBIAL OSTEOTOMY FOR LATERAL COMPARTMENT OSTEOARTHRITIS

Study	Year	No.	Mean Follow-up (Yr) (Range)	Mean Age (Yr)	Technique	Outcomes
Sternheim et al.[103]	2011	41 patients (45 knees)	13.3 (3-25)	46.2	MCW	90% survival 10 yr 79% survival 15 yr 21.5% survival 20 yr
Puddu et al.[104]	2009	30 patients	– (4-12)	52	LOW	82% good/excellent
Das et al.[105]	2008	12 patients	74 mo* (51-89)	52	LOW	58% good/excellent
Backstein et al.[106]	2007	38 patients (40 knees)	10 (3-20)	44	MCW	82% survival 10 yr 45% survival 15 yr
Wang and Hsu[107]	2006	30 patients	8 (5-14)	53	MCW	87% survival 10 yr
Gross and Hutchison[108]	2000	20 patients (21 knees)	11 (5-20)	56	MCW	83% survival 4 yr 64% survival 10 yr
Marti et al.[109]	2000	15 patients	– (1-14)	59	MCW	73% good results
Finkelstein et al.[110]	1996	20 patients (21 knees)	11 (8-20)	59	MCW	64% survival 10 yr
Healy et al.[111]	1988	21 patients (23 knees)	4 (2-9)	56	MCW	83% good/excellent
McDermott et al.[112]	1988	24 patients	4 (2-11.5)	52	MCW	92% good results (most improvement in pain)

LOW, Lateral opening wedge; *MCW,* medial compartment wedge.
*Telephone follow-up of functional Hospital for Special Surgery and Lysholm score.

TABLE 103-7

COMPLICATIONS ASSOCIATED WITH HIGH TIBIAL OSTEOTOMY SURGERY

Complication	Osteotomy	Frequency (%)	Management
Intraoperative			
Intraarticular fracture	MOW	7-18.2	Determine if additional fixation required Consider changing weight-bearing status postoperatively
Fracture of opposite cortex	MOW LCW	4.3	No additional procedure required (MOW) Additional fixation required (LCW)
Peroneal nerve injury	LCW	2-16	Most commonly neurapraxia—monitor and consider NCS and EMG 6 wk after surgery if no sign of improvement Tag ends of nerve and consult plastic surgeon if patient has direct nerve injury
Vascular injury	All	0.4	Gain proximal and distal control of vessel if possible Call vascular surgeon
Early Postoperative			
Undercorrection/ overcorrection	All	–	Revision osteotomy
Hematoma	All	10.2	Preventable with insertion of drain Irrigation and debridement if associated with prolonged drainage
Infection	All	2.3-81	Antibiotic therapy Regular pin site care with external fixator
VTE	All	1.3-9.8	No routine prophylaxis required—encourage mobilization Consider prophylaxis with LMWH in high-risk patients Prophylaxis with 6 wk of Coumadin in patients with known history of VTE
Stiffness	All	3	Preventable with early ROM Physiotherapy Consider manipulation with the patient anesthetized once the osteotomy has united Consider arthrolysis if severe
Compartment syndrome	All	2-2.6	Emergent compartment release
Late Postoperative			
Delayed union	MOW	4.3	Rule out infection Bone graft osteotomy site
Nonunion	MOW	0.7-4.4	Rule out infection Bone graft osteotomy site
Pseudoarthrosis	MOW	0.7-4.4	Rule out infection Bone graft osteotomy site
Hardware irritation	All	4.3	Implant removal
Loss of correction	All	4.4-15.2	Revision osteotomy
Failure of fixation	All	4.4-16.4	Revision osteotomy
Patella baja	All	7.6-8.8	Consider simultaneous TTO for MOWHTO corrections ≥12.5 mm Early ROM

EMG, Electromyography; *LCW,* lateral closing wedge; *LMWH,* low molecular weight heparin; *MOW,* medial opening wedge; *MOWHTO,* medial opening wedge high tibial osteotomy; *NCS,* nerve conduction study; *ROM,* range of motion; *TTO,* tibial tubercle osteotomy; *VTE,* venous thromboembolism.

Data from references 65, 113, 114, and 115.

Summary

Knee OA is a common condition encountered by all physicians. Arthritis in an athlete can be particularly difficult to treat, given the high demands that athletes place on their bodies. Because opening wedge osteotomies have emerged as the preferred method of surgical management, future studies should focus on determining the long-term outcomes in larger numbers of patients. Additionally, better defining the success of early weight bearing after locking-plate HTO will be vital.

Conservative management should be the first line of therapy. Surgical intervention is considered in patients who have exhausted conservative therapies. Joint-preserving osteotomy procedures are recommended in active persons with unicompartmental OA. TKA is a successful procedure reserved for less active persons or those with tricompartmental arthritis.

For a complete list of references, go to expertconsult.com.

Suggested Readings

Citation: Bhattacharyya T, Gale D, Dewire P, et al: The clinical importance of meniscal tears demonstrated by magnetic resonance imaging (MRI) in osteoarthritis of the knee. *J Bone Joint Surg Am* 85A(1):4–9, 2003.

Level of Evidence: I

Summary: Meniscal tears are highly prevalent in both asymptomatic and clinically osteoarthritic knees of older persons. Because osteoarthritic knees with a meniscal tear are not more painful than those without a tear and the meniscal tears do not affect functional status, magnetic resonance imaging should not be routinely ordered for patients with osteoarthritis of the knee.

Citation: Coventry M: Osteotomy of the upper portion of the tibia for degenerative arthritis. *J Bone Joint Surg* 47:984–990, 1965.
Level of Evidence: IV
Summary: In this classic article, Coventry describes his original lateral closing wedge high tibial osteotomy technique and his encouraging results in a case series of 32 patients with varus osteoarthritis of the knee.
Citation: Dugdale TW, Noyes FR, Styer D: Preoperative planning for high tibial osteotomy. The effect of lateral tibiofemoral separation and tibiofemoral length. *Clin Orthop Relat Res* 274:248–264, 1992.
Level of Evidence: IV
Summary: This article describes how to preoperatively plan the correction required during high tibial osteotomy surgery to restore the weight-bearing line (center femoral head to center tibiotalar joint) to a point 62.5% across the width of the tibial plateau.
Citation: Felson D, Zhang Y, Anthony J, et al: Weight loss reduces the risk for symptomatic knee osteoarthritis in women: The Framingham study. *Ann Intern Med* 116(7):535, 1992.
Level of Evidence: IV
Summary: In this report on a large case series with long-term follow-up, it is shown that weight loss reduces the risk for symptomatic osteoarthritis in women.
Citation: Hernigou P, Medevielle D, Debeyre J, et al: Proximal tibial osteotomy for osteoarthritis with varus deformity. A ten- to thirteen-year follow-up study. *J Bone Joint Surg Am* 69A(3):332–354, 1987.
Level of Evidence: IV
Summary: This article includes the longest published follow-up of patients undergoing opening wedge high tibial osteotomy for varus osteoarthritis of the knee and shows good success at a mean of 11 years after surgery.
Citation: Kirkley A, Birmingham TB, Litchfield RB, et al: A randomized trial of arthroscopic surgery for osteoarthritis of the knee. *N Engl J Med* 359(11): 1097–1107, 2008.
Level of Evidence: I
Summary: In this article it is reported that arthroscopic surgery for osteoarthritis of the knee provides no additional benefit to optimized physical and medical therapy.
Citation: Moseley JB, O'Malley K, Petersen NJ, et al: A controlled trial of arthroscopic surgery for osteoarthritis of the knee. *N Engl J Med* 347(2):81–88, 2002.
Level of Evidence: I
Summary: In this article it is reported that the outcomes after arthroscopic lavage or arthroscopic debridement were no better than those after a placebo procedure in patients with knee osteoarthritis.
Citation: Richmond J, Hunter D, Irrgang J, et al: Treatment of osteoarthritis of the knee (nonarthroplasty). *J Am Acad Orthop Surg* 17(9):591–600, 2009.
Level of Evidence: I
Summary: This article provides American Academy of Orthopaedic Surgeons–approved evidence-based clinical practice guidelines for the appropriate nonoperative treatment of knee osteoarthritis.
Citation: Rosenberg TD, Paulos LE, Parker RD, et al: The forty-five-degree posteroanterior flexion weight-bearing radiograph of the knee. *J Bone Joint Surg Am* 70A(10):1479–1483, 1988.
Level of Evidence: IV
Summary: In this article it is reported that posteroanterior weight-bearing radiographs with the knee at 45 degrees of flexion were more accurate, more specific, and more sensitive than conventional extension weight-bearing anteroposterior radiographs.

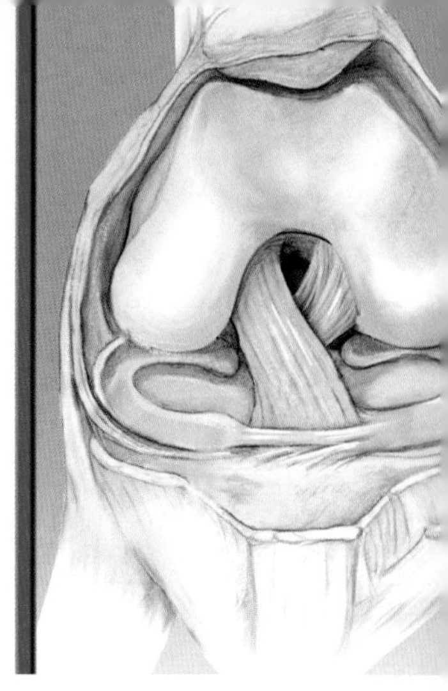

104

Patellar Instability

ERIC W. TAN • ANDREW J. COSGAREA

Patellar instability is a broad topic that encompasses a continuum of patellar abnormalities ranging from asymptomatic maltracking to debilitating recurrent dislocations. To address this complex topic, it is important to first define several terms. During the normal knee flexion cycle, the patella tracks in the center of the trochlea of the distal femur. *Maltracking* occurs when the course of the moving patella deviates from the bony constraints of the trochlear groove. Maltracking may or may not be symptomatic. The term *subluxation* is used to describe a specific episode in which the patella abruptly leaves the trochlear groove. Subluxation episodes are usually transient and uncomfortable. When the patella displaces completely from the trochlear groove, it is considered a *dislocation*. First-time dislocation episodes are typically the result of indirect or direct trauma. After dislocating, the patella may spontaneously reduce, or a manual reduction may be necessary. Chronic patellar dislocation describes the rare situation in which the patella remains dislocated for months or years. In the acute setting, a patella dislocation usually causes substantial pain and morbidity. Patients with *recurrent* patellar instability episodes, whether subluxation or dislocation, usually have demonstrable risk factors. Patients with abnormal skeletal anatomy, defined as *malalignment,* are predisposed to maltracking and instability. Similar to maltracking, malalignment implies a deviation from normal biomechanics or anatomy, but it does not always result in patellar instability.

Patellar dislocations represent 2% to 3% of all knee injuries and are the second most common cause of traumatic knee hemarthrosis.[1,2] The annual risk of a first-time patellar dislocation is 5.8 per 100,000.[3] Although most persons who experience a first-time dislocation will have no further instability, the literature reports a recurrence rate of 15% to 60% and an annual risk of recurrence of 3.8 per 100,000.[3-7]

Despite the prevalence of patellar instability, ideal management recommendations remain controversial, and evidence-based literature is limited. The great variability of patellar pathologies and patient symptoms makes it difficult to form global treatment recommendations. A thorough understanding of the specific patellar abnormality, the level of functional disability, and the patient's desired activity level must be taken into account when evaluating and assessing a patient with patellar instability. Identification and correction of anatomic and biomechanical risk factors form the basis for developing successful nonoperative and operative treatment strategies.

History

In the assessment of a patient with patellar instability, it is imperative to determine the mechanism of injury. Sports-related activities account for 61% to 72% of first-time dislocations.[3,8] Patellar instability may result from direct trauma to the medial knee or, more frequently, an indirect injury, such as when the leg rotates around a planted foot (Fig. 104-1). In most cases of patellar dislocation, the patella will spontaneously reduce. Often, patients will report feeling the knee "give way" and the kneecap "pop" or "clunk" in or out of place. They may describe an abnormal shape to the inside of the knee, sometimes confusing the prominent medial femoral condyle for what they mistakenly think is a medially dislocated patella. Patients may state that the patella reduced when they extended their knee or that they pushed it back into place. Swelling will develop soon after the injury in most patients unless their patella is very unstable; in those cases, subsequent swelling and pain may be minor or absent.

It is important to distinguish pain secondary to patellar instability from that of other patellofemoral disorders. Patellofemoral pain syndrome (PFPS) is the most common cause of anterior knee pain and can be confused with patellar instability. Patients with PFPS typically describe anterior knee pain exacerbated by prolonged sitting or when descending the stairs. The pain may be bilateral, or it may change from one knee to the other over time. In addition, the patients may feel like the knee is "unstable," but when questioned carefully, they do not describe the same mechanisms of injury that would result in frank instability or they do not experience episodes in which the patella actually leaves the trochlear groove. Distinguishing between the two clinical entities is imperative because isolated PFPS is rarely treated successfully by surgical means. Furthermore, it is not uncommon for patients with instability to also experience PFPS.

Pain may also be the result of complex regional pain syndrome. The classic presentation is an exaggerated pain response, burning in nature, with intolerance to cold stimuli.[9] The pain is typically continuous, deep, diffuse, and nonanatomic in distribution. Complex regional pain syndrome may also result in decreased patellar mobility, tenderness and hypersensitivity of the patella and retinacula, changes in skin temperature and color, and associated hair growth.[10] Finally, localized pain can be the result of a neuroma, in which case

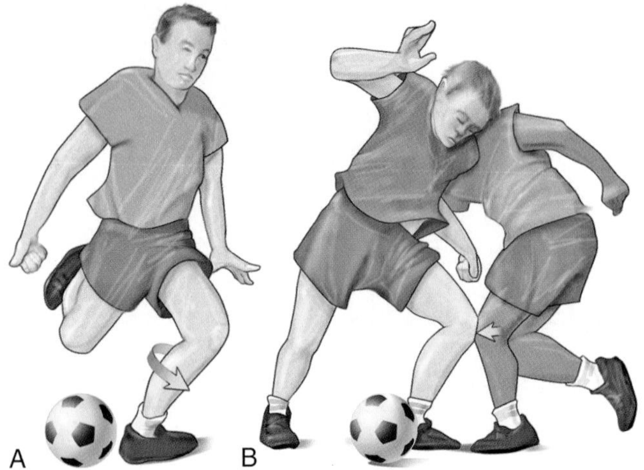

FIGURE 104-1 Mechanisms of acute patellar dislocation. A noncontact dislocation occurs by external rotation of the lower leg relative to the body (**A**), whereas contact injuries are caused by a direct blow to the medial side of the knee (**B**). *(Modified from The Cleveland Center for Medical Art & Photography, Copyright 2008.)*

it typically causes burning or sharp, stabbing pain in the distribution of the affected cutaneous nerve. Other causes of anterior knee pain include osteochondritis dissecans of the patella or trochlea, patellofemoral osteoarthritis, patellar or quadriceps tendinosis, or pigmented villonodular synovitis.

Physical Examination

Pertinent Bony Anatomy

Lower extremity alignment is determined primarily by the relationship between the femur and tibia. Abnormalities in the position and relationship of these bony structures result in malalignment that can predispose patients to patellar instability. Normally, the knee has a tibiofemoral angle of approximately 5 to 7 degrees of valgus.[11,12] With excess knee valgus, or genu valgum, the mechanical pull of the quadriceps muscle changes, increasing the normal laterally directed force vector on the patella. The rotation of the femur and tibia also influences patellar stability. Normally, the femoral neck has 7 to 20 degrees of anteversion and the tibia has 15 degrees of external rotation (Fig. 104-2).[13,14] Increases in femoral anteversion and external tibial torsion will further increase the laterally directed forces on the patella.

The patella is a sesamoid bone within the extensor mechanism of the knee that articulates with the distal femur. It is stabilized superiorly and inferiorly by the quadriceps and patellar tendons, respectively, and medially and laterally by the ridges of the femoral trochlea. At the distal end of the femur is the trochlea, which articulates with the patella and provides a bony restraint to excessive medial and lateral translation. The lateral trochlear ridge, which is typically larger, more proximal, and more anterior than the medial trochlear ridge, helps keep the patella centered in the trochlea by resisting pathologic lateral patellar excursion.[15] Anatomic variations (including trochlear dysplasia, resulting in a shallow trochlear floor relative to the medial and lateral condyles) and hypoplasia of the lateral condyle decrease the resistance to lateral patellar translation. Under normal conditions, the patella "engages" in the trochlea at 20 degrees of flexion. Patients with a relatively longer patella tendon, called patella alta, have less osseous stability because more knee flexion is required before the patella is "engaged" and stabilized by the bony constraints of the trochlear groove. In addition, patients with patella alta have a decreased patellofemoral contact area compared with patients who have knees of normal patellar height.[16-18]

The bony anatomy of the tibia and foot also affects patellar instability. Normally, the tibial tuberosity is approximately 9 to 13 mm lateral to the center of the patella.[19,20] This relationship changes during the knee flexion arc in most patients. The distance is greatest during terminal knee extension in part because of the "screw home mechanism," where the tibia externally rotates on the femur.[21-23] Any further lateralization of the tuberosity relative to the center of the patella will result in an increase in the laterally directed force on the patella. Furthermore, hindfoot valgus and excessive pronation of the foot place a valgus force on the knee, which also increases the laterally directed force on the patella.[24]

Pertinent Soft Tissue Anatomy

The quadriceps complex, consisting of the rectus femoris, vastus lateralis, vastus intermedius, and vastus medialis muscles, is the most important dynamic stabilizer of the

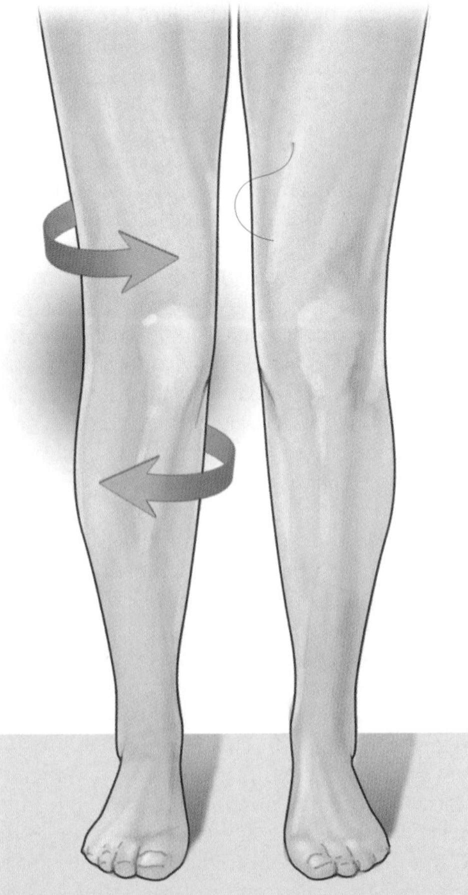

FIGURE 104-2 Torsion of the femur and/or tibia. *(Modified from The Cleveland Center for Medical Art & Photography, Copyright 2008.)*

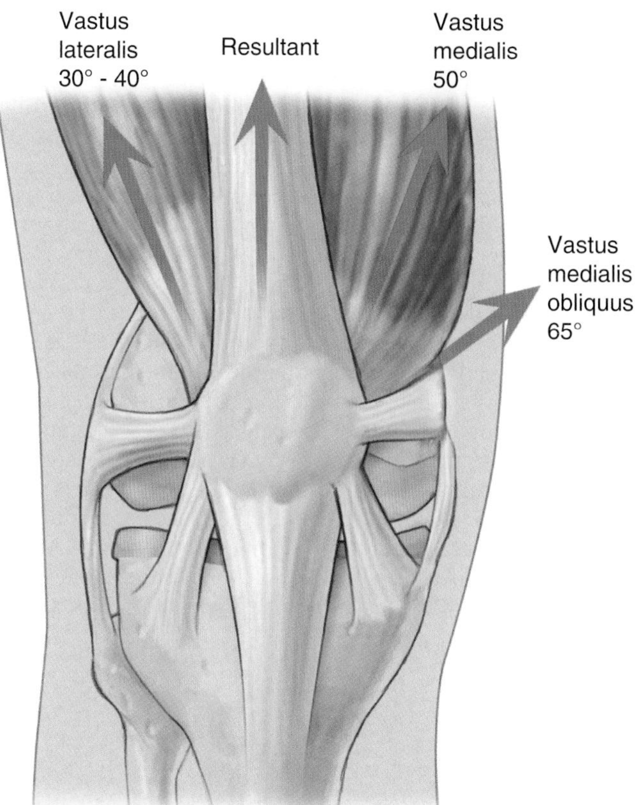

FIGURE 104-3 Quadriceps musculature. *(Modified from The Cleveland Center for Medical Art & Photography, Copyright 2008.)*

patella (Fig. 104-3). All four muscles converge in the distal thigh and insert through the quadriceps tendon at the proximal pole of the patella. Each of the individual muscles contributes a different force vector based on its angle of insertion. The vastus medialis and lateralis muscles provide additional connections to the tibia through attachments to the medial and lateral patellar retinacula, respectively. The vastus medialis oblique (VMO) is a distinct part of the vastus medialis muscle that originates off of the lateral intermuscular septum and inserts at a high angle, up to 65 degrees, on the proximal third of the medial border of the patella.[25] The VMO is an important medial patellar stabilizer that counterbalances the pull of the vastus lateralis muscle.[26,27] In addition, the VMO may exert a force on the medial patellofemoral ligament (MPFL), adding additional medial stability to the patella.[28,29] Atrophy, hypoplasia, and impaired motor control of the VMO will therefore result in decreased opposed activity of the vastus lateralis muscle, producing increased lateral patellar displacement.[30] The dynamic muscular stabilizers can compensate to some degree for anatomic bony and soft tissue deficiencies that predispose to patellar instability. Conversely, weakness of the dynamic stabilizers may predispose athletes to patellar instability episodes during athletic activities even if they have "normal" anatomy and tracking under less stressful circumstances.

The primary soft tissue static stabilizers of the patella are the patellofemoral, patellotibial, and patellomeniscal ligaments (Fig. 104-4). Studies have shown that the MPFL is the primary passive soft tissue restraint on the medial side of the patella, contributing 50% to 60% of the total restraining force against lateral patellar displacement.[31-34] Importantly, the MPFL is almost always disrupted in first-time patellar dislocations.[29,35,36] The MPFL has been shown to be a distinct structure in the knee.[31,37-39] The exact origin of the MPFL is controversial, but it appears to be in the saddle between the adductor tubercle and medial epicondyle of the femur.[40,41] From its attachment near the medial epicondyle, the ligament then courses anteriorly and laterally, inserting on the proximal two thirds of the medial border of the patella. It is 4.5 to 6.4 cm long and 1.9 cm wide, with a tensile strength of 208 N.[39,42,43]

Examination Overview

Acute Patellar Instability Episode

Clinical assessment of a patient who has recently sustained an episode of patellar instability can be difficult. Knee range of motion is usually limited because of soft tissue swelling and joint effusion, and patients have difficulty relaxing for examination because of pain and fear. Aspiration of a joint effusion is occasionally indicated for comfort. The presence of hemarthrosis suggests one of a limited number of injuries to the knee, including ligamentous or meniscal tears, patellar dislocations, and intraarticular fractures.[44,45] The ligamentous, bony, and muscular structures of the knee should be systematically examined. Palpation along the course of the

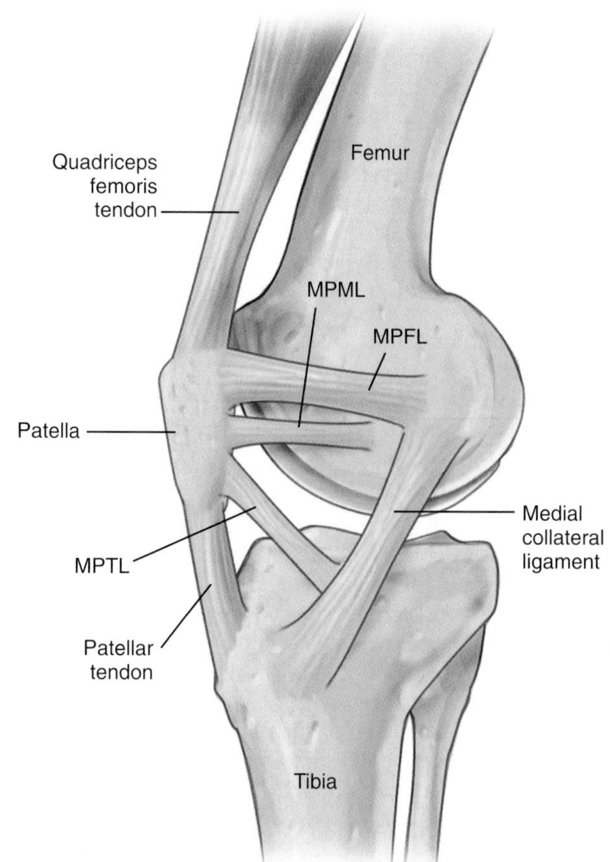

FIGURE 104-4 Medial patellofemoral ligaments. *MPFL,* Medial patellofemoral ligament; *MPML,* medial patellomeniscal ligament; *MPTL,* medial patellotibial ligament. *(Modified from The Cleveland Center for Medical Art & Photography, Copyright 2008.)*

quadriceps, VMO, medial retinaculum, and MPFL is necessary to localize any site of failure. The MPFL will be tender at its site of rupture, which can be anywhere along the course from the medial epicondyle to the patella. Tenderness at the medial epicondyle, the most common site of MPFL failure, is called the Bassett sign.[46] Pain and tenderness at the inferior pole of the patella may represent tendinosis or an incomplete or complete patellar tendon tear. Similarly, tenderness at the superior patellar pole may represent quadriceps tendinosis or tendon failure. The competence of the extensor mechanism is confirmed by asking the patient to extend his or her knee against resistance from a flexed position. Rarely, osteochondral or chondral loose bodies may be palpated in the suprapatellar pouch or medial and lateral gutters. Concomitant injury to the collateral or cruciate ligaments or meniscus can be determined with use of the standard ligamentous and meniscal tests. Resolution of acute pain and swelling allows for a more comprehensive examination.

Standing Examination and Gait Testing

With the patient standing, the lower extremity is visualized. Malalignment abnormalities, including genu valgum, pes planus, hindfoot valgus, and pronation of the foot, may be identified. Patients may have "squinting patella" (patellae that point toward each other) as a result of increased femoral anteversion. In addition, core strength testing is performed. A single-leg squat test is used to assess hip strength and trunk control by requiring the patient to slowly lower the body over a single planted foot.[47] Poor control suggests core and hip rotation weakness that can predispose to instability. Gait testing provides insight into the dynamic factors influencing patellar tracking. A "kneeing-in" gait may be the result of increased femoral anteversion, external tibial torsion, or foot pronation.[48,49] These anatomic abnormalities, combined with core and hip rotation strength deficits, lead to the development of a valgus thrust, which generates an external rotation moment about the knee, resulting in a dramatic lateral force on the patella.[50]

Sitting Examination: J Sign

The J sign refers to the shape of the track that the patella follows as the knee extends from a flexed position. As the patient extends the knee from 90 degrees of flexion, the patella will move laterally as it passes the proximal-most portion of the lateral trochlear ridge, which usually happens at approximately 20 degrees of knee flexion; however, it occurs earlier (at a greater flexion angle) in patients with patella alta. The presence of a J sign may be a normal variant, especially if seen bilaterally in asymptomatic patients. In patients with patellar instability, a positive J sign has been associated with lateral retinacular tightness or medial retinacular insufficiency, VMO deficiency, soft tissue imbalance, and patella alta and hypoplastic lateral condyle.[24,51] The precise cause and clinical significance of the J sign, particularly in asymptomatic patients, remains unclear.

Supine Examination

Muscle bulk, especially of the VMO, should be evaluated for evidence of atrophy or hypoplasia. Strength deficits are determined by asking the patient to extend the knee against resistance. Positioning of the tibial tuberosity relative to the center of the patella is visualized and compared with the other knee. A hip examination, including muscle strength testing and range of motion, should be performed. Tightness of the iliotibial band is examined with use of Ober's test.[52] An excessively tight ITB can cause increased tension in the lateral retinaculum, resulting in patellar maltracking and instability.[53]

Quadriceps Angle

The quadriceps angle, or Q angle, is measured as the angle between the vector of action of the quadriceps tendon and the patellar tendon. Clinically, the measurement is taken as the angle between lines from the anterior superior iliac spine of the pelvis to the middle of the patella and from the middle of the patella to the tibial tuberosity (Fig. 104-5). A larger Q angle theoretically results in a greater laterally directed force on the patella on contraction of the quadriceps muscle. Normal Q angles in males and females range from 8 to 16 degrees and 15 to 19 degrees, respectively, in the supine position and 11 to 20 degrees and 15 to 23 degrees, respectively,

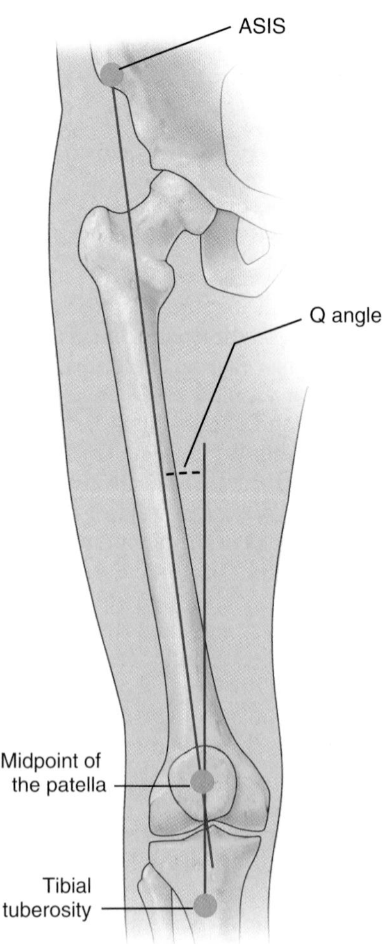

FIGURE 104-5 The quadriceps angle (Q angle) formed by the intersection of a line from the anterior superior iliac spine (*ASIS*) to the midpoint of the patella, with a line from the midpoint of the patella to the midpoint of the tibial tuberosity. *(Modified from Livingston LA, Mandigo JL: Bilateral Q angle asymmetry and anterior knee pain syndrome.* Clin Biomech [Bristol, Avon] *14[1]:7–13, 1999.)*

in the standing position.[51,54,55] Q-angle measurements vary widely as a result of differences in measurement techniques (supine, standing, sitting, and knee flexion angle) and poor inter- and intraobserver reliability.[24,56-60] Failure to precisely identify the center of the patella or to keep the leg in neutral rotation may also lead to inaccurate measurements of the Q angle.[61,62] In addition, patients with patella alta, a positive J sign, or persistent patellar subluxation or dislocation may have falsely low Q angles. Although it has been typically accepted that higher Q angles are associated with a higher risk of patellar instability or pain, this phenomenon has not been consistently found in the literature.[8,63-67] In fact, Sanfridsson et al.[68] found lower Q-angle values in patients with a history of patellar instability, and Cooney et al.[69] showed a negative relationship between the quadriceps angle and the tibial tuberosity–trochlear groove (TT-TG) distance. Therefore the usefulness of the Q angle remains controversial, and clinicians must be mindful that the Q angle is only one piece of information; the Q angle alone should not dictate treatment for a patient.

Patellar Tilt Test

The patellar tilt test is used to evaluate the lateral soft tissue restraints, including the lateral retinaculum and the iliotibial band. With the knee fully extended and the quadriceps relaxed, the examiner lifts the lateral border of the patella (Fig. 104-6). If the patella does not correct to at least neutral with the anterior surface of the patella parallel to the floor, it suggests tight lateral structures.[70,71]

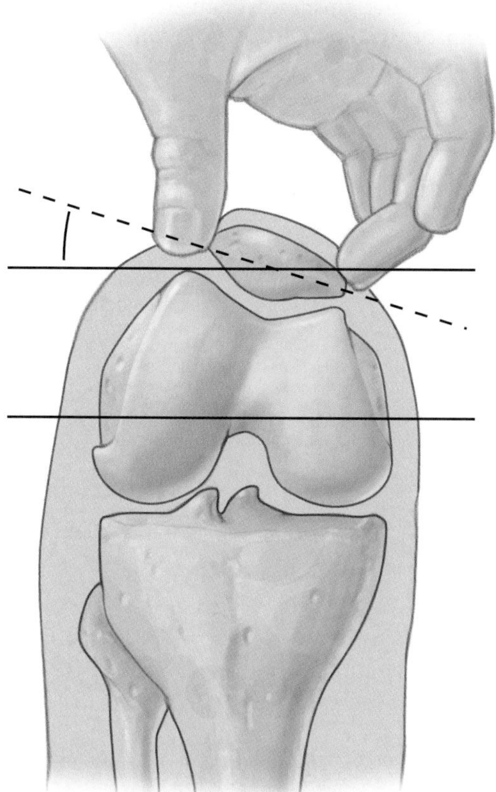

FIGURE 104-6 Patellar tilt test. *(Modified from The Cleveland Center for Medical Art & Photography, Copyright 2008.)*

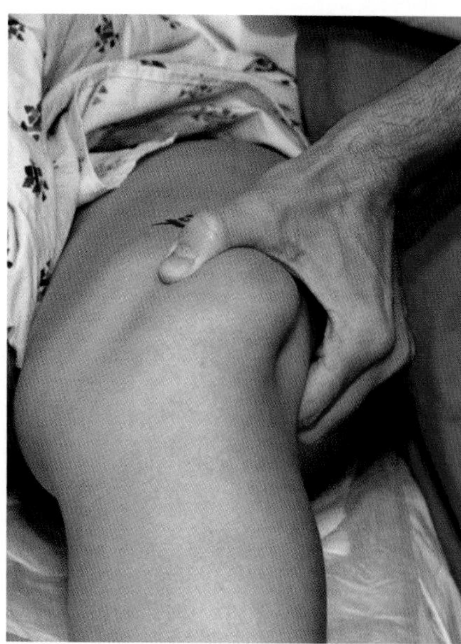

FIGURE 104-7 Patellar glide test. Note that the patella is displaced laterally.

Patellar Glide Test

The integrity of the medial and lateral structures can be assessed with the patellar glide test. With the knee in full extension and the quadriceps relaxed, the patella is translated medially and laterally (Fig. 104-7). Using the width of the patella divided into quadrants, the amount of patellar glide is reported as the number of quadrants worth of translation that the patella exhibits on examination (i.e., if the patella translates a distance equivalent to 75% of the patellar width, the patellar glide would be graded as 3). With a laterally directed force, a patellar glide grade of 3 or 4 may suggest a deficiency in the medial soft tissue patellar restraints, mainly the MPFL, and a medial translation of one quadrant or less suggests tightness of lateral structures.[24,71] However, the clinician should compare the patellar mobility to the asymptomatic knees because increased patellar glide bilaterally is more indicative of generalized hyperlaxity and does not necessarily mean that the patient has patellar instability. The patellar glide test is also subject to a high degree of interobserver variability.[72] Although measurement instruments have been developed to allow for improved inter- and intraobserver reliability, they are not routinely used in clinical practice.[56,73]

Patellar Apprehension Test

The most commonly used provocative test for determining patellar instability is the apprehension test. The test is positive if the patient has a feeling similar to a subluxation or dislocation episode as the patella is manually translated laterally while the quadriceps is relaxed.[74,75] Importantly, it is the apprehension, not the presence of pain alone, that makes the test positive. Although lateral patellar instability is more common, medial patellar instability may occur, especially in the setting of previous patellar realignment surgery. Medial subluxation of the patella is evaluated using the Fulkerson relocation test.[76] While the patient is supine with the knee extended, the patella is manually displaced medially. With knee flexion, the patella falls into the trochlea. The test is positive if relocation of the patella reproduces pain or a sense of instability.

Prone Examination

Femoral anteversion is measured using Craig's test.[77] The patient is placed prone, and the knee is flexed to 90 degrees. While the greater trochanter is palpated, the leg is rotated until the greater trochanter is positioned as far laterally as possible, placing the head into the center of the acetabulum. The angle between an imaginary vertical line and the axis of the tibia is the amount of femoral anteversion present.

Imaging

Radiographs

The standard series of conventional radiographs includes standing anteroposterior, lateral at 30 degrees of flexion, tunnel, and sunrise views. These views may reveal persistent subluxation, osteochondral fractures, and abnormal anatomy of the knee, including patellar positioning and trochlear morphology. The anteroposterior radiograph is useful for examining the tibiofemoral alignment in addition to identifying bipartite patella and patellar fractures. Assessment of tibiofemoral arthritis is also best assessed using this view. The tunnel view radiograph is helpful in identifying the presence of loose bodies or osteochondritis dissecans lesions in the knee.

The sunrise or axial radiograph is usually obtained in 45 degrees or more of knee flexion. This view is most useful for identifying displacement of the patella from the normal location in the trochlear groove. It may also show the bony irregularities of the lateral trochlear ridge or medial facet of the patella that can occur with patellar dislocations. Occasionally, a loose body in the lateral gutter will be apparent only on axial views. The Merchant view is obtained with the knee flexed 45 degrees over the end of the table and the x-ray beam angled 30 degrees downward.[78] Measurement of the sulcus angle on this view is one way to characterize trochlear dysplasia. The sulcus angle is measured as the angle between two lines originating from the deepest part of the femoral trochlear to the highest points of the medial and lateral condyles. Values greater than 145 degrees suggest trochlear dysplasia.[79]

Relative patellar height is best assessed on a lateral radiograph obtained with the knee flexed to 30 degrees. Patella alta is associated with patellar instability.[17,80] A more proximally situated patella requires a greater degree of knee flexion before it engages the bony constraints of the trochlea of the femur. Various methods of assessing relative patellar height have been described (Table 104-1),[81-85] including the Insall-Salvati,[86] modified Insall-Salvati,[87] Blackburne-Peel,[88] Caton-Deschamps,[89] and Labelle-Laurin[90] indices. The Blackburne-Peel ratio was found to be the most reproducible with the least interobserver error.[91,92] It is defined as the ratio of the perpendicular distance from the lower articular margin of the patella to the tibial plateau divided by the length of the articular surface of the patella.[88] A ratio of 0.8 is considered normal, whereas values above 1.0 indicate patella alta. Compared with the other indices of patellar height, the Blackburne-Peel ratio relies on consistent osseous landmarks rather than the variable anatomy of the patella and location of the tibial tuberosity.

Trochlear dysplasia, another known risk factor of patella instability, is best evaluated on a true lateral radiograph.[34,93-95] Three anterior lines are important in determining the trochlear morphology: the most anterior line is the medial femoral condyle, the middle line is the lateral femoral condyle, and the remaining line is the floor of the trochlea (Fig. 104-8). Normally, the line of the lateral ridge terminates proximal to the line of the medial ridge. However, a shallow, flattened trochlea will cause the trochlear line to prematurely cross the anterior aspect of the femoral condyles, known as the crossing sign.[94] Dejour et al.[94] reported the presence of the crossing sign in 96% of patients with history of a true patellar dislocation compared with 3% in the control group. The presence of a supratrochlear spur (trochlear prominence) and double contour (medial condyle hypoplasia) are additional findings of trochlear dysplasia.

Additional quantitative measurements of trochlear dysplasia can be made, including trochlear bump and depth. Using a true lateral radiograph, a straight line is drawn tangential to the anterior femoral cortex. The trochlear floor may be anterior, posterior, or flush with the anterior femoral cortex, forming the trochlear bump.[94] The size of the bump can be measured; positive values indicate anterior positioning of the

TABLE 104-1

DIFFERENT INDICES OF PATELLAR HEIGHT

Measurement	Normal	Alta	Baja
Insall-Salvati[86]	1.0	>1.2	<0.8
Modified Insall-Salvati[87]	–	>2.0	–
Blackburne-Peel[88]	0.8	>1.0	<0.5
Caton-Deschamps[89]	<1.2	>1.2	<0.6
Labelle-Laurin[90]	Visual	Visual	–

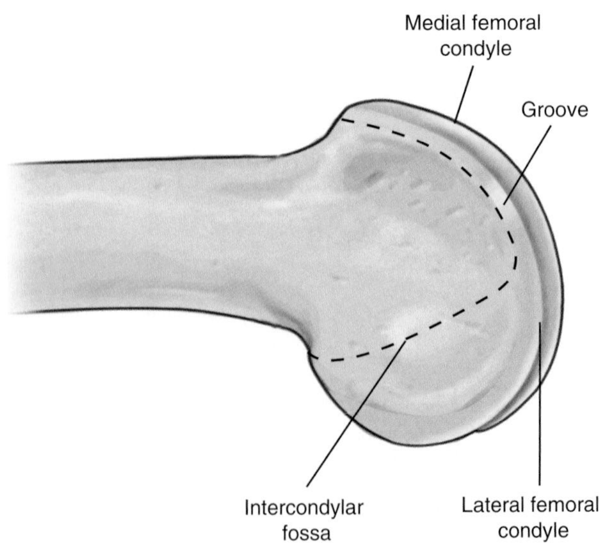

FIGURE 104-8 Lateral view of the knee for trochlear dysplasia. *(Modified from The Cleveland Center for Medical Art & Photography, Copyright 2008.)*

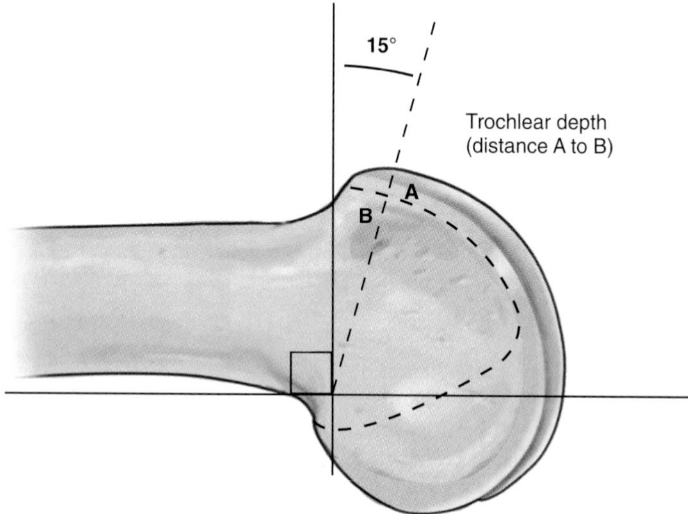

FIGURE 104-9 Trochlear depth. *(Modified from The Cleveland Center for Medical Art & Photography, Copyright 2008.)*

trochlear floor relative to the anterior femoral cortex, which suggests a shallow trochlea. In the normal knee, the value of the trochlear bump is near zero (i.e., the anterior femoral cortex is flush with the trochlear floor). However, in one study values of more than +3 mm were present in 66% of patients with objective patellar instability.[94] Trochlear depth is the distance between the trochlear floor and most anterior condylar contour line measured along a line 15 degrees from the perpendicular to the tangent of the posterior femoral cortex (Fig. 104-9). Trochlear depth measurements less than 4 mm were found in 85% of knees with patellar instability compared with only 3% of control subjects.[94]

A classification of trochlear dysplasia has been developed using information from the lateral and axial radiographs (Fig. 104-10).[96] Type A dysplasia is characterized by a shallow trochlear without any changes to trochlear morphology. This type is seen as a crossing sign on the lateral radiograph and sulcus angle greater than 145 degrees on the axial view. Type B dysplasia is characterized by a supratrochlear spur on the lateral view and a flat or convex trochlear on the axial view. Type C dysplasia is present when a crossing sign and double contour are present on lateral radiographs, with medial condyle hypoplasia on axial radiographs. Type D dysplasia represents the most severe form of dysplasia, characterized by a crossing sign, supratrochlear spur, and double contour on the lateral view in addition to asymmetry of the trochlear facets, with a cliff between them on the axial view.

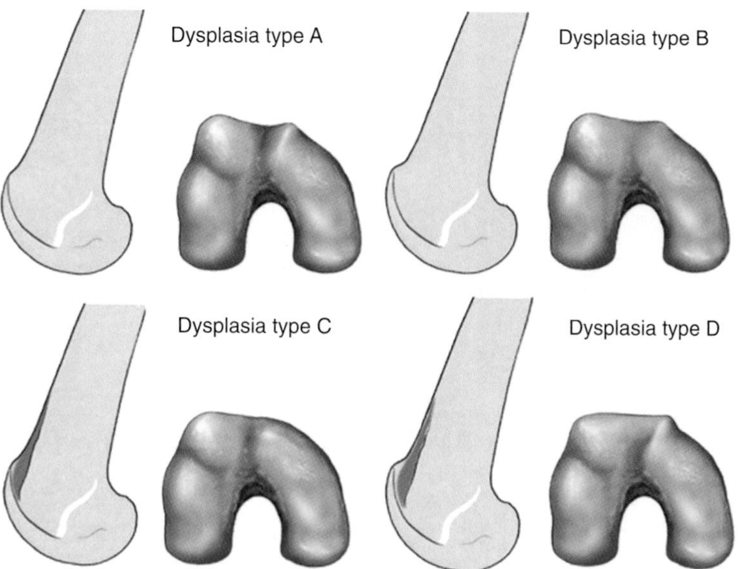

FIGURE 104-10 Dejour's classification of trochlear dysplasia. Type A: crossing sign (flat or convex trochlea). Type B: crossing sign and supratrochlear spur. Type C: crossing sign and double contour. Type D: crossing sign, supratrochlear spur, double contour, and sharp step-off of the trochlea. *(Modified from Grelsamer RP, Dejour D, Gould J: The pathophysiology of patellofemoral arthritis.* Orthop Clin North Am *39[3]:269–274, 2008.)*

Computed Tomography

One major limitation of radiographs is the inability to obtain axial images of the patellofemoral joint at angles from 20 degrees of knee flexion to full extension. Computed tomography (CT) imaging allows for great osseous detail and improved accuracy of the measurements compared with those made on conventional radiographs. Patellar tilt is measured as the angle between a line going through the patellar axis and a line tangential to the posterior condyles. Angles greater than 20 degrees are present in more than 80% of patients with patellar instability.[93,94]

In addition, CT imaging may used to quantify lateralization of the tibial tuberosity, known as the TT-TG distance. Superimposing an axial CT image of the tibial tuberosity and the trochlear groove, the TT-TG distance is that between the center of the tuberosity and groove in a line parallel to the posterior femoral condyles (Fig. 104-11). A TT-TG distance of more than 15 to 20 mm is associated with patellar instability.[94,97-99]

CT imaging also allows for three-dimensional reconstructions to be performed, providing a better spatial understanding of the knee anatomy. Furthermore, dynamic CT has been used to assess patellar tracking, allowing visualization of the patellofemoral joint through clinically relevant ranges of motion.[100] Although studies of patellar instability using dynamic imaging modalities to date have been limited, this imaging protocol has become more widespread in the clinical setting and will likely enhance our understanding of the static and dynamic properties of the patellofemoral joint and guide therapeutic recommendations.

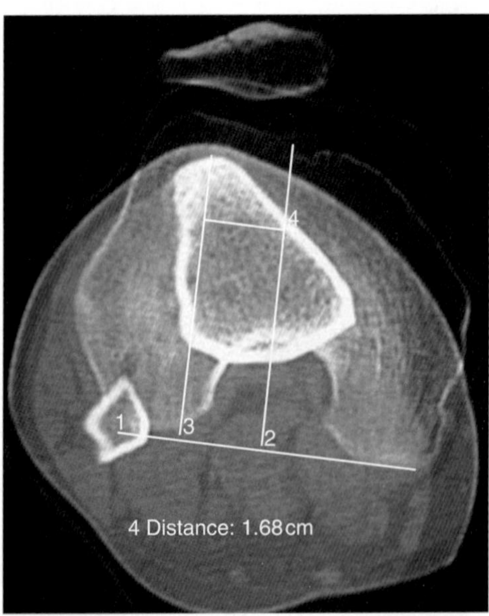

FIGURE 104-11 A computed tomography scan showing the technique of measuring the tibial tuberosity–trochlear groove distance (TT-TG). The image of the trochlear groove is superimposed on the image of the tibial tuberosity using the digital radiology software. A line parallel to the posterior femoral condyles is drawn (*line 1*). A perpendicular to line 1 is then taken through the central portion of the trochlea (*line 2*) and through the tibial tuberosity (*line 3*). The difference between line 2 and line 3 (i.e., *line 4*) is the TT-TG. In this case, it is 1.68 cm. *(Modified from Bicos J, Fulkerson JP, Amis A: Current concepts review: the medial patellofemoral ligament.* Am J Sports Med *35[3]:484–492, 2007.)*

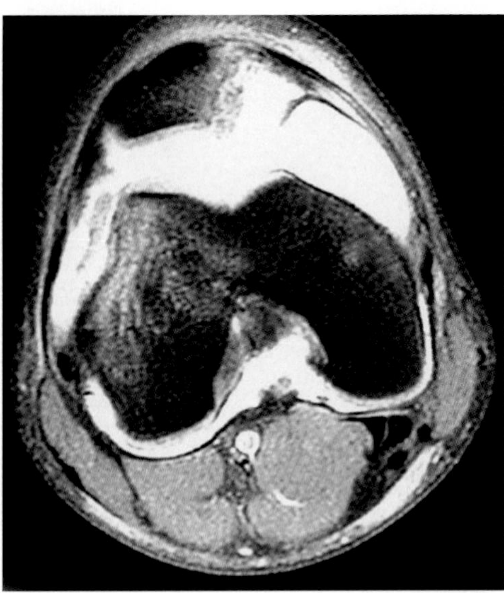

FIGURE 104-12 An axial magnetic resonance imaging scan after acute lateral patellar dislocation shows knee effusion, bony bruising of the lateral femoral condyle and medial patellar facet from impaction, and disruption of the patellar attachment of the medial patellofemoral ligament.

Magnetic Resonance Imaging

Magnetic resonance imaging (MRI) provides additional imaging details not seen on conventional radiographs and CT imaging. MRI allows assessment of the articular cartilage, trochlear geometry, and soft tissue structures, including the MPFL.[35,101,102] The classical MRI findings after an acute episode of patellar instability include impaction injury to the lateral femoral condyle, osteochondral damage to the medial patella facet, and disruption of the medial retinaculum and MPFL (Fig. 104-12).[103] MRI is 85% sensitive and 70% accurate in detecting injury to the MPFL.[36] Characterization using MRI of trochlear dysplasia and localization of an MPFL rupture, if present, may be helpful in cases when MPFL repair is contemplated.[104] Furthermore, MRI can be used effectively to calculate the similar measurements made on radiographs and CT imaging, including TT-TG distance, without radiation exposure.[105,106] Kinematic MRI has been used to evaluate patellofemoral tracking.[107-110] The use of kinematic MRI in the clinical setting remains limited as a result of a lack of availability.

Decision-Making Principles and Treatment Options

Treatment of patellar instability must be patient-specific. Historically, a plethora of rehabilitation regimens and surgical procedures have been described.[16,48,96,111-118] Important details from the history, physical examination, and imaging studies will help the clinician determine which treatment options are most suitable for each patient.

Acute Patellar Instability Episode

During the acute phase after a patellar injury, regardless of whether it is a first-time or recurrent injury, the immediate goals of management are to provide relief of symptoms. Relative rest, light compression, and elevation are the initial interventions. Most patients benefit from the use of crutches to limit weight bearing. Pain is generally well controlled with cryotherapy and over-the-counter analgesic medications. A knee immobilizer may be used with patients who are particularly unstable or uncomfortable, followed by a more functional hinged brace within the first 1 to 2 weeks as symptoms allow. Knee aspiration is helpful in relieving pain for some patients with a tense hemarthrosis. Heel slides and quadriceps activation exercises may be initiated within days of the injury, depending on the severity of pain, soft tissue swelling, and effusion. Conventional radiographs should be obtained to look for fractures or large osteochondral loose bodies. MRI may be used selectively to assess the status of the extensor mechanism and to rule out concomitant intraarticular abnormality. Formal referral to a physical therapist allows for a supervised functional progression back to normal sedentary activities in days to weeks and to athletic activities in weeks to months.

Subacute, First-Time Patellar Instability Episode

Nonsurgical treatment remains the mainstay of therapy for first-time episodes of patellar instability.[2,119] Protocols vary, ranging from a simple period of immobilization to those that involve rapid rehabilitation. Proponents of immobilization suggest that it will help facilitate healing of the torn MPFL. Proponents of early mobilization argue that it helps prevent stiffness and muscle atrophy. In most cases, it is appropriate to initially immobilize the knee for several days and then begin range-of-motion exercises once the quadriceps muscle function returns. Rehabilitation protocols typically include strengthening of the quadriceps, gluteal, and core muscles. Taping and bracing of the patella have been theorized to provide patellar stability by increasing the strength of the quadriceps muscle and by activating the VMO earlier than the vastus lateralis muscle during use of stairs.[112,120,121] However, Muhle et al.[122] showed no effect of patellar realignment bracing on patellar positioning. Regardless of the specific nonoperative intervention used, recurrence rates of 15% to 60% have been reported.[3-7,114]

Some authors have advocated surgical repair of the MPFL after a first-time dislocation,[2,4,5,7,111,123-127] but the benefit remains unclear. To date, few studies have compared nonoperative versus operative treatment in persons with first-time patellar dislocations.[2,4,5,7,111,123-127] In most studies, no major differences were found in postoperative episodes of instability, activity level or function, and subjective patient measures. Camanho et al.[4] and Bitar et al.[111] have advocated primary surgical intervention, having demonstrated higher Kujala outcome scores and lower rates of recurrence in patients undergoing MPFL repair and reconstruction, respectively.

Well-accepted indications exist for surgical intervention in the acute setting, however, including an irreducible patellar dislocation and a large or displaced osteochondral fracture with an associated loose body.[2] Other relative indications for surgery include disruption of the quadriceps or VMO and the presence of an associated ligamentous, chondral, or meniscal injury. Many clinicians would consider repairing the torn MPFL if surgery was indicated after a first dislocation for other reasons. Additional high-quality studies are needed to delineate the role of primary surgical intervention in the treatment of first-time episodes of patellar instability.[128]

Subacute, Recurrent Patellar Instability Episode

For patients with recurrent patellar instability, surgical stabilization becomes a more compelling option. Rehabilitation programs still may be successful for persons without evidence of mechanical or structural anomalies that would require surgical correction[48,129]; however, we are unaware of any studies that have formally assessed the effect of different rehabilitation programs on recurrent patellar instability.

When comprehensive nonoperative treatment fails, surgical intervention is usually recommended. With the use of information from the history, physical examination, and imaging studies, a patient-specific surgical solution can be developed. The goal of surgical intervention is to "individualize, customize, and normalize" a solution tailored to the unique pathologic condition that is leading to the recurrent instability.[48] In most cases, patients undergo a medially based soft tissue repair or reconstruction or a proximal tibial bony realignment procedure. Medial soft tissue procedures, such as MPFL reconstruction, focus on stabilization by reestablishing the deficient medial soft tissue checkrein. Tibial tuberosity osteotomy (TTO) procedures result in realignment of the abnormal bony anatomy. Surgical modification of the position of the tibial tuberosity changes the forces applied to the patella through the patella tendon, allowing the surgeon to customize the procedure so as to address maltracking and unload specific areas of articular cartilage that are experiencing excessive pressure. One or both of these surgical procedures may be used, depending on the needs of the patient.

Alternative procedures have been described with varied results. Isolated lateral retinacular release has been shown to be effective in reducing patellar tilt but not in treating recurrent instability, and excessive lateral release has been associated with increased rates of recurrent instability.[130,131] Lateral retinacular release is therefore recommended as an adjunct to other patellar stability procedures in patients with a tight lateral retinaculum. A number of proximal soft tissue surgeries have been described, including medial reefing (i.e., tightening of medial structures), VMO advancement (i.e., reattachment of the VMO more distally and laterally on the patella), and the Galleazzi procedure (i.e., passage of the semitendinosus tendon through a tunnel from the medial side of the patella).[48,132-135] Many of these procedures have had very good results over the years and continue to be used successfully today. One attribute that all of these procedures seem to have in common is that they recreate the medial soft tissue restraint to excessive lateral translation.

Other surgical procedures have been developed to address bony malalignment. Operations that deepen the trochlea (trochleoplasty) or elevate the anterior portion of the lateral femoral condyle (trochlear osteotomy) were developed to treat trochlear dysplasia.[15,96,136,137] They have been used extensively in Europe, and in some cases have demonstrated excellent early results.[99,138-140] These trochlear procedures help improve radiographic indices of trochlear dysplasia and lateral stability, but they may also result in postoperative stiffness and patellofemoral arthrosis.[99,138,139,141-144]

Another less common approach has been to address malalignment using femoral osteotomies.[145-148] Excessive femoral anteversion can be corrected with a proximal derotation osteotomy, most frequently in the pediatric population. Excessive valgus alignment can be corrected through distal femoral osteotomies. Although femoral osteotomies have the advantage of directly correcting femoral malalignment, the procedures are associated with greater morbidity compared with knee-based osteotomies and soft tissue reconstructions and should be recommended selectively.

AUTHORS' PREFERRED TECHNIQUE

Medial Patellofemoral Ligament Reconstruction

Injury to the MPFL is considered the essential lesion in recurrent lateral patellar dislocations.[31,35,42,149] MPFL reconstruction provides a reliable method for treating patellar instability in patients without marked bony malalignment. A variety of techniques have been described using different graft sources and a multitude of fixation techniques,[111,116,117,150-155] but initial enthusiasm has been tempered somewhat by recent descriptions[156-158] of complications related to the surgical technique.

Surgical Technique

Positioning and Preparation

- Supine position on the operating room table
- Induction of general or regional anesthesia
- Administration of prophylactic intravenous antibiotics before making the incision
- Examination of both knees after induction of anesthesia
  - Comprehensive ligamentous examination
  - Glide test to determine competence of soft tissue restraints
  - Tilt test to assess for lateral retinacular tightness
- Placement of a tourniquet on the proximal thigh of the affected leg
- Placement of a padded valgus bar on the operating room table just distal to the tourniquet
- Placement of a thigh-high compressive stocking on the contralateral leg

Diagnostic Arthroscopy

- Observation for loose bodies or meniscal abnormality
- Patellofemoral joint evaluation
  - Assessment of the articular surface of the patella and trochlea for any chondral lesions
  - Evaluation of patellar tracking in the trochlear groove during flexion and extension
- Chondral damage addressed with debridement or repair techniques, as indicated.
- The location and severity of chondral damage is used to determine if a TTO is indicated.
- Arthroscopic lateral retinacular release if the lateral retinaculum is clinically and radiographically determined to be tight.
- If a concomitant TTO is needed, it should be performed before the MPFL reconstruction.

Graft Harvest

Hamstring autografts are the preferred graft for most patients. Although smaller than the semitendinosus tendon, even the gracilis tendon is substantially stronger than the native MPFL.[42] Allograft tendons are typically reserved for revision cases or for patients with connective tissues disorders (e.g., Ehlers-Danlos syndrome).

- The leg is exsanguinated with an Esmarch bandage and the tourniquet is inflated.
- A short, longitudinal incision is made over the pes anserine insertion.
- The sartorial fascia is incised and everted to expose the gracilis and semitendinosus tendons.
- The gracilis or semitendinosus tendon is dissected from the sartorial fascia and tagged.
- The tendon is harvested with a tendon stripper and placed on a separate table.
- Muscle and soft tissue debris are removed from the graft.
- No. 2 FiberLoop (Arthrex Inc., Naples, FL) is woven through the patellar end of the graft in a locking fashion.

Patellar Tunnel

- A 2-cm longitudinal incision is made along the medial border of the patella.
- A short 2.5-mm Kirschner wire (K wire) is drilled from medial to lateral, just proximal to the patellar equator, between the anterior cortical and posterior articular surfaces.
- Positioning of the K wire is confirmed with lateral fluoroscopic imaging.
- The K wire is exchanged with a full-length 2.4-mm eyelet K wire.
- The eyelet K wire is overdrilled with a 5.0-mm cannulated drill to a depth of 15 mm (Fig. 104-13).
- One K wire is drilled transversely through the tunnel to the lateral side, exiting the skin.
- One suture from the graft is placed in the K-wire eyelet before it is pulled through to the lateral side.
- A second K wire is then placed through the blind tunnel, diverging from the first K wire so that it exits from the superolateral arthroscopy portal.
- The second graft suture is placed into that eyelet (Fig. 104-14).
- The first suture is retrieved through the superolateral portal with a right angle clamp.
- The graft is docked into the blind patella tunnel by pulling on the suture pair.
- The sutures are tied directly over the lateral border of the patella.
- Fixation is confirmed by aggressive manual traction on the femoral end of the graft.

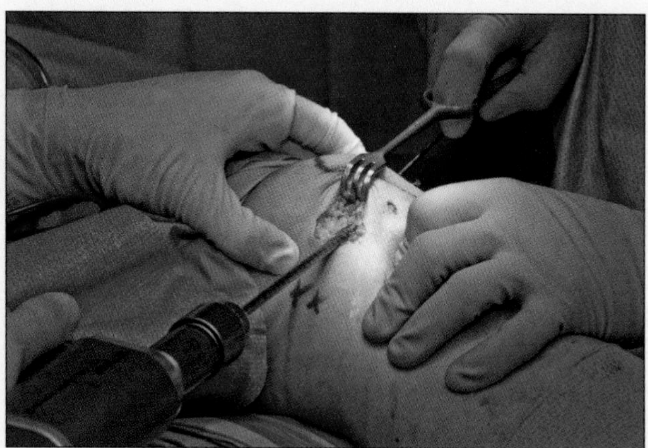

FIGURE 104-13 The patellar tunnel is drilled with a cannulated drill bit.

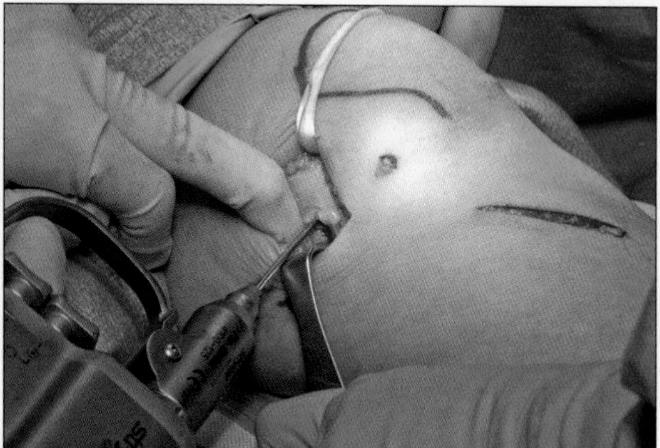

FIGURE 104-15 A K wire is placed just anterior to the medial femoral epicondyle.

Femoral Tunnel

- An incision is made just anterior to the medial femoral epicondyle.
- A short 2.5-mm K wire is placed immediately anterior to the medial femoral epicondyle (Fig. 104-15).
- Positioning of the wire is confirmed with lateral fluoroscopy.
- The free graft end is passed through a soft tissue tunnel between the medial retinaculum and capsular layers and then wrapped around the base of the K wire.
- Isometry of the graft is assessed by holding traction on the end of the graft as the knee is flexed and extended.
- The position of the K wire can be modified as necessary for appropriate isometry of the graft.
- The short 2.5-mm K wire is removed and replaced with a 2.4-mm full-length K wire.
- The K wire is drilled in a slight anterior and proximal direction so that it safely avoids the peroneal nerve.
- The K wire is overdrilled with a 6.0-mm cannulated drill bit to a depth of 20 mm.
- The graft is cut 2 cm longer than the distance from the patella to the femoral tunnel.

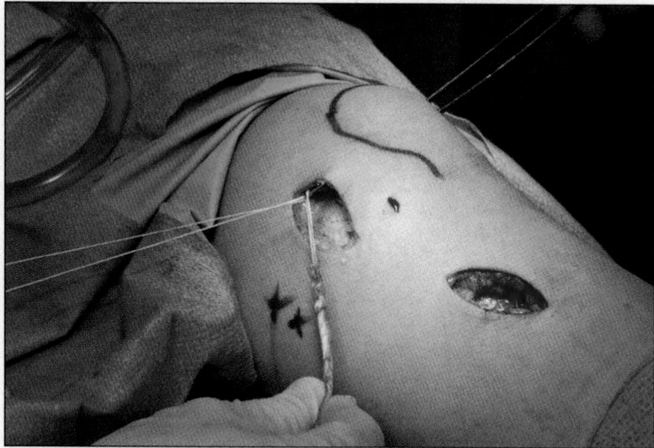

FIGURE 104-14 The graft pulled into the blind patellar tunnel.

- A No. 2 nonabsorbable suture is woven through the end of the graft, with a small loop remaining at the distal end.
- A No. 5 nonabsorbable suture is passed through the loop, creating a pull-through suture.
- Both suture ends of the No. 5 suture are passed through the eyelet of the K wire, which is then pulled out the lateral side of the femur, docking the graft into the blind femoral tunnel.

Graft Fixation

- The surgeon applies tension to the graft by pulling on the free ends of the No. 5 pull-through suture exiting the lateral thigh.
- Graft isometry is determined by feeling the tension in the No. 5 pull-through suture as the knee is taken through a full range of motion.
- The graft is fixed at the knee flexion angle corresponding to the greatest graft tension, ensuring that the patella is not overconstrained.
- Patellar glide is measured in full extension, with an attempt to reproduce the same amount of translation on the contralateral knee.
- Once the appropriate graft length has been determined, a bioabsorbable, cannulated femoral interference screw (7 × 23 mm) is inserted to just below the cortical surface (Fig. 104-16).
- After femoral fixation, the patella should no longer be dislocatable, and there should be a firm end point to lateral patellar translation.
- The No. 5 pull-through suture can then be removed from the lateral side of the knee.

Closure

- At the harvest site, the sartorial fascia is repaired with No. 0 absorbable sutures.
- Standard closure is used for the incisions and portals.
- Local anesthetic is injected around the incisions and portal.
- Sterile dressings are applied, followed by a cryotherapy unit, a thigh-high compressive stocking, and a hinged knee brace locked in full extension.

Continued

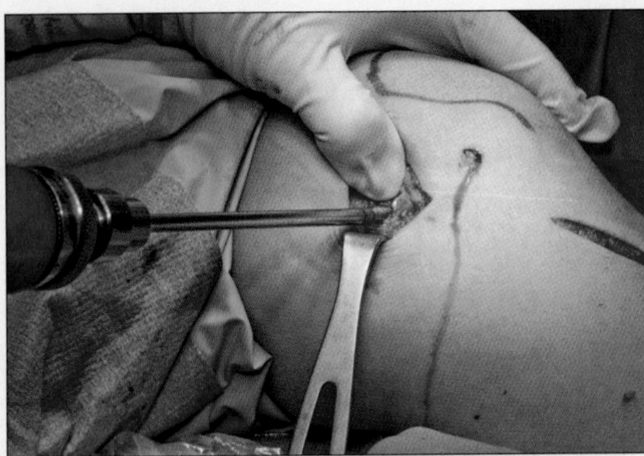

FIGURE 104-16 The graft is secured in the blind femoral tunnel using an absorbable interference screw.

Postoperative Management

- Patients are discharged with crutches and allowed touch-down weight bearing with the brace locked in extension. They are instructed to perform quadriceps sets, straight-leg raises, and ankle pumps.
- After 1 week, patients are advanced to 25% weight bearing with the brace locked in extension. Knee range-of-motion, quadriceps strengthening, and flexion exercises are initiated. Formal physical therapy sessions are prescribed three times per week for the next 12 weeks.
- After 2 weeks, the sutures are removed and patients are allowed to bear full weight as tolerated with the brace locked in extension. No restriction is placed on range of motion.
- After 4 weeks, patients are expected to have at least 120 degrees of knee flexion.
- After 6 weeks, the brace is discontinued, and most patients will have regained full motion.
- By 2 months, patients may begin using the treadmill and elliptical machine.
- By 3 months, patients begin jogging and sport-specific drills as tolerated.
- Patients generally return to sports by 4 to 6 months.

Results

Previous studies have shown that MPFL reconstruction has a success rate of 70% to 100%, with very few cases of recurrent subluxation or dislocation.[150,151,154,155,158-163] Most recently, Deie et al.[152] showed good outcomes with MPFL reconstruction in 31 knees with recurrent patellar instability. Range of motion, Kujala scores, and radiographic indices all improved with surgical intervention. Of the 31 knees, only one showed postoperative signs of apprehension. No postoperative episodes of patellar dislocation were reported. Despite seemingly excellent results, most of the outcomes data on MPFL reconstruction are limited by small sample sizes and short-term follow-up.[150] In addition, the surgical techniques described and the grafts used in previous MPFL studies are varied, making generalization regarding the outcomes of MPFL reconstruction difficult. Larger randomized controlled studies examining the specific type of MPFL reconstruction are needed to determine the true efficacy of MPFL reconstruction.

Complications

As with other ligament reconstruction procedures, positioning of the bony tunnels and tensioning of the graft are crucial to the success of MPFL reconstruction. Malpositioning of the femoral (Fig. 104-17) or patellar tunnels and excessive graft tension are associated with serious potential complications, including medial patellofemoral articular overload, iatrogenic medial subluxation, and recurrent lateral instability.[48,156,157,164] The use of fluoroscopy during tunnel placement can help minimize malpositioning. Careful attention to surgical technique will ensure that appropriate MPFL graft tension is achieved (Box 104-1). In addition, confirmation of full knee range of motion before and after graft fixation can help ensure that the graft is not too tight. Other reported complications include wound-healing problems, hemarthrosis, implant pain, loss of motion, and arthrofibrosis.[37,151,155,160,163] Patellar fractures through a patellar bone bridge or after violating the anterior cortex have also been reported.[125,165]

Results

Excellent to good outcomes have been reported in 80% to 95% of patients.[170,173-177] Long-term studies have shown

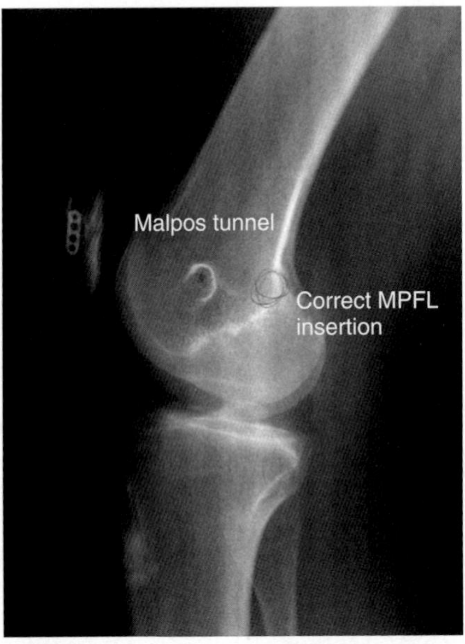

FIGURE 104-17 A lateral radiograph showing an anteriorly and proximally positioned femoral tunnel in a 20-year-old woman after an autograft medial patellofemoral ligament (*MPFL*) reconstruction. Recurrent lateral instability developed. *Malpos,* Malpositioned. *(From Bollier M, Fulkerson J, Cosgarea A, et al: Technical failure of medial patellofemoral ligament reconstruction.* Arthroscopy *27[8]:1153–1159, 2011.)*

AUTHORS' PREFERRED TECHNIQUE

Tibial Tuberosity Osteotomy

TTO changes the distal insertion of the patellar tendon, which leads to realignment of the extensor mechanism and can result in improved patellar tracking, changing the patellofemoral contact pressures, and correcting the patellar height index.[96] Depending on the type of malalignment present, various transfer procedures have been described.[166-169] Isolated medialization of the tibial tuberosity, known as the Elmslie-Trillat procedure, is performed to medialize the patellar tendon. It is indicated for patients with a history of recurrent instability and excessive lateralization of the tuberosity but minimal articular cartilage damage. Anteromedialization, best known as the Fulkerson osteotomy, is indicated in patients with recurrent instability, a lateralized tuberosity, and chondral damage over the lateral or distal patellofemoral joint.[170] The goal of the surgical procedure is to correct excessive lateral forces and to unload joint surface areas that have been damaged. Both of these procedures can be modified to displace the tuberosity distally at the time of screw fixation. Distalization of the tibial tuberosity may be used to correct for instability believed to be related to patella alta or to reduce distal patellar articular cartilage contact forces.[171,172]

Surgical Technique

Positioning and Preparation

- Supine position on the operating room table
- Induction of general or regional anesthesia
- Administration of prophylactic intravenous antibiotics before the incision is made
- Examination of both knees after anesthesia is induced
  - Comprehensive ligamentous examination
  - Glide test to determine competence of soft tissue restraints
  - Tilt test to assess for lateral retinacular tightness
- Placement of a tourniquet on the proximal thigh of the affected leg
- Placement of a padded valgus bar on the operating room table just distal to the tourniquet
- Placement of a thigh-high compressive stocking on the contralateral leg

Diagnostic Arthroscopy

- Diagnostic arthroscopy to evaluate for loose bodies or meniscal abnormality.
- Patellofemoral joint evaluation
  - Assessment of the articular surface of the patella and trochlea for any chondral lesions
  - Evaluation of the patellar tracking in the trochlear groove during flexion and extension
- Chondral damage is addressed with debridement or repair techniques, as indicated.

Exposure

- The leg is exsanguinated and the tourniquet is inflated.
- An incision is made from the inferolateral portal to a point that is just lateral to the anterior tibial crest, 6 cm distal to the tibial tuberosity.
- An open lateral retinacular release or retinacular lengthening is performed if the lateral retinaculum was clinically and radiographically determined to be tight.
- The medial and lateral borders of the patellar tendon are exposed.
- Using a scalpel and periosteal elevator, the anterior compartment muscles are sharply dissected off the anterolateral border of the proximal tibia.
- The medial border of the shingle is defined using sharp dissection and elevation of the periosteum along the medial tibial crest.

Shingle Preparation

- A series of 2.5-mm drill bits are drilled from medial to lateral.
  - If only medialization is desired, a 0-degree angle (parallel to the floor) is used.
  - If concomitant anteriorization is desired, the angle from anteromedial to posterolateral is generally 45 degrees but may be as high as 60 degrees.
- Soft tissue retractors are used to protect the soft tissues and neurovascular structures from the drill bits as they exit the posterolateral tibial cortex.
- Each drill bit is placed 1 cm distal and parallel to the previous drill bit.
- The most distal drill bit is just through the anterior cortex, approximately 6 cm distal to the patellar tendon attachment, creating a shingle that converges toward the anterior cortex distally.

Osteotomy

- A 0.25-inch straight osteotome is used to connect the holes between the drill bits on the medial side of the shingles.
- A 0.25-inch curved osteotome is used to connect the holes between the drill bits on the lateral side of the shingle (Fig. 104-18).

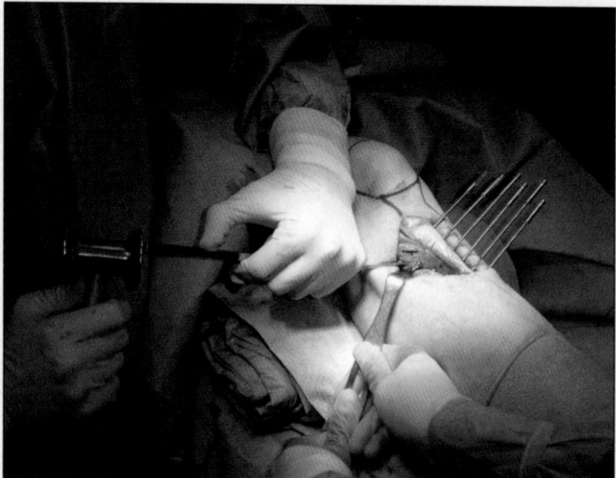

FIGURE 104-18 A 0.25-inch curved osteotome is used to connect the drill holes on the lateral side of the shingle.

Continued

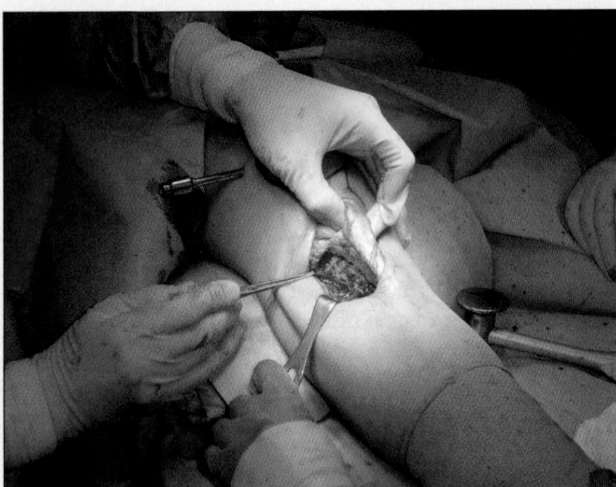

FIGURE 104-19 After the osteotomy is completed, the shingle is translated anteriorly and medially.

- Every other drill bit is then removed, and a 0.5-inch straight osteotome is used to connect the holes between the remaining drill bits.
- To complete the proximal transverse cut on the shingle, the patella tendon is retracted and a 0.25-inch straight osteotomy is passed from anteromedial to posterolateral parallel to the most proximal drill bit.
- Finally, a 1-inch osteotome is passed from the medial side of the shingle to complete the osteotomy.
- A gentle prying motion is used to mobilize the shingle without fracturing the distal hinged attachment (Fig. 104-19).

Shingle Fixation

- A bolster is placed proximal to the knee joint so that the neurovascular structures are not pressed against the posterior tibial cortex.
- Preliminary fixation is achieved by passing three 2.5-mm drill bits through the shingle and into the posterior cortex of the tibia.
- The knee is taken through its full range of motion to assess patellar tracking. The shingle may be moved as needed to improve tracking.
- Screw length and positioning are confirmed with lateral fluoroscopy.
- Each drill bit is removed, the bone is tapped, and the shingle is overdrilled with a 3.5-mm drill bit.
- 3.5-mm bicortical screws of appropriate length are placed. Position and length are confirmed with fluoroscopy.
- A bone graft is harvested from the lateral side of the shingle and digitally packed under the medial overhang of the shingle.

Closure

- The periosteum over the medial tibia crest is repaired with absorbable No. 0 suture (Fig. 104-20).
- The anterior compartment muscles are repaired to the tibia using absorbable No. 0 suture.
- A 0.1875-inch drain is placed at the surgical site in the subcutaneous space and exiting the superolateral portal.
- Standard closure is performed, and a local anesthetic is injected around the incisions and portal.
- Sterile dressings are applied, followed by a cryotherapy unit, a thigh-high compressive stocking, and a hinged knee brace locked in full extension.

Postoperative Management

- The drain is removed before discharge, if appropriate.
- Patients are discharged with crutches and are restricted from any weight bearing, with the brace locked in extension. They are instructed to perform quadriceps sets, straight-leg raises, and ankle pumps.
- After 2 weeks, the sutures are removed and patients are allowed to bear one third of body weight with the brace locked in extension. Range of motion is not restricted. Formal physical therapy sessions are prescribed three times per week for the next 12 weeks.
- After 4 weeks, patients are allowed to progress to two thirds body weight. They are expected to have at least 100 degrees of knee flexion.
- After 6 weeks, patients progress to full weight bearing.
- After 7 weeks, use of the brace is discontinued, and most patients will have regained full motion.
- By 3 months, most patients will begin using the treadmill and elliptical machine.
- By 4 months, patients begin jogging and transition to sport-specific drills as tolerated.
- Patients generally return to sports by 6 to 8 months.

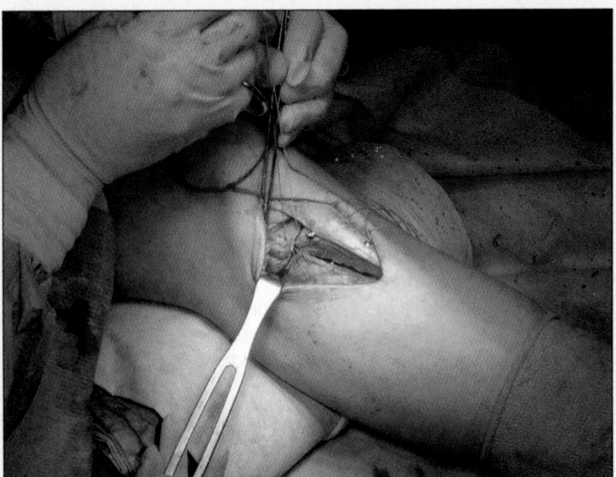

FIGURE 104-20 After fixation of the shingle with three 3.5-mm bicortical screws, the anterior compartment muscles are sutured back to the tibia.

BOX 104-1 Pearls for Setting Appropriate Medial Patellofemoral Ligament Graft Tension

1. In full extension, the patella is not centered in the trochlear groove, and estimating correct MPFL tension/length is difficult.
2. Have an assistant hold the lateral border of the patella flush with the lateral trochlea in 30 degrees of knee flexion while tension is placed on the graft. This maneuver prevents overtightening of the MPFL graft.
3. Place tension on the MPFL with the knee in 60 degrees of knee flexion with the patella fully centered in the trochlear groove, which is when the MPFL is at its maximal length. A checkrein to lateral translation will exist without placing too much tension on the patella.
4. The goal is to not overtighten the MPFL graft. The MPFL graft should guide the patella into the trochlear groove during early knee flexion. The patella should engage and center in the trochlear groove at 20 to 30 degrees of knee flexion.

MPFL, Medial patellofemoral ligament.
From Bollier M, Fulkerson J, Cosgarea A, et al: Technical failure of medial patellofemoral ligament reconstruction. *Arthroscopy* 27(8):1153–1159, 2011.

maintenance of patellar stability with rates of recurrent patellar instability between 8% and 15%.[177-180] However, some patients appear to have a high rate of postoperative patellofemoral pain and arthritis.[181,182] Pidoriano et al.[170] showed that the pattern of preoperative chondral damage correlated with clinical results after anteromedialization of the tibial tuberosity. As expected, patients with distal and lateral lesions improved after surgery, whereas patients with medial, proximal, or diffuse lesions did poorly. To our knowledge, no randomized controlled studies have been performed to examine the efficacy of TTO compared with alternative stabilization techniques.

Complications

TTO causes an alteration of the presurgical knee biomechanics, resulting in a predictable change in joint surface loading. Anteriorization of the tibial tuberosity increases proximal patellar loading and decreases inferior pole loading. Medialization increases medial loading and decreases lateral loading. Based on these principals, the surgeon can predict how patellofemoral loading patterns may be surgically altered. In accordance with these principles, patients with proximal patellar lesions may be adversely affected by anteriorization, and patients with medial lesions may be adversely affected by medialization. Additionally, overmedialization of the tubercle increases patellofemoral contact pressures, which may result in patellofemoral osteoarthritis.[182-185]

Postoperative fractures of the proximal tibia or tibial tuberosity shingle have also been described.[186-188] It is unclear what changes in joint surface loading occur after distalization or trochlear osteotomy. Recent work has suggested that in addition to the patellofemoral joint surface loading changes that occur, anteromedialization of the tibial tuberosity causes changes in the presurgical tibiofemoral compartment loading.[189] These findings have implications regarding the potential for the development of osteoarthritis and will require long-term clinical studies before we fully understand the consequences. Additional complications have been reported, including pseudarthrosis, nonunion, malunion, wound complications, postoperative bleeding requiring intervention, compartment syndrome, painful hardware, and saphenous vein and nerve injury.[177,190,191]

Future Considerations

The diagnosis and treatment of patellar instability remain a complex challenge. Each patient with patellar instability is unique, and his or her specific abnormality must be identified so that treatment plans can be individualized to produce the best outcomes. Despite numerous studies examining the treatment of patellar instability, high-quality outcomes data are limited and lacking. Randomized controlled studies and studies with larger sample sizes and long-term follow-up are needed to delineate the role of nonoperative and surgical management. Additional biomechanical studies should provide insight regarding the surgical procedures that will best correct patellar instability and unload damaged articular surfaces. Finally, surgical techniques must be standardized to make studies comparable.

For a complete list of references, go to expertconsult.com.

Suggested Readings

Citation: Buckens CFM, Saris DBF: Reconstruction of the medial patellofemoral ligament for treatment of patellofemoral instability: A systematic review. *Am J Sports Med* 38(1):181–188, 2010.
Level of Evidence: II
Summary: In this review of 14 articles, generally excellent outcomes are shown for medial patellofemoral ligament reconstruction. However, conclusions are limited by small sample sizes, short-term follow-up, use of various adjunct procedures, and lack of standardization of reconstructive surgical procedures.

Citation: Colvin AC, West RV: Patellar instability. *J Bone Joint Surg Am* 90A(12):2751–2762, 2008.
Level of Evidence: N/A
Summary: In this comprehensive overview of the evaluation and management of patellar instability, anatomic and radiographic findings are reviewed in addition to nonoperative and operative treatment options for first-time and recurrent instability episodes.

Citation: Pidoriano AJ, Weinstein RN, Buuck DA, et al: Correlation of patellar articular lesions with results from anteromedial tibial tubercle transfer. *Am J Sports Med* 25(4):533–537, 1997.
Level of Evidence: III
Summary: This retrospective study shows that the pattern of preoperative chondral damage correlates with clinical results after anteromedialization of the tibial tuberosity. Patients with distal and lateral lesions improved after surgery because those areas were unloaded by the surgical procedure.

Citation: Smith TO, Song F, Donell ST, et al: Operative versus non-operative management of patellar dislocation. A meta-analysis. *Knee Surg Sports Traumatol Arthrosc* 19(6):988–998, 2011.
Level of Evidence: II
Summary: This metaanalysis, including five randomized controlled studies and six nonrandomized controlled studies, shows that operative management of patellar dislocation is associated with a significantly higher risk of patellofemoral joint osteoarthritis ($P = .04$) but a significantly lower risk of subsequent patellar dislocation compared with nonsurgical management ($P < .01$). However, findings are limited by statistically significant publication bias, issues related to the methodologic quality of the evidence base, and the variety of surgical interventions used.

Citation: Stefancin JJ, Parker RD: First-time traumatic patellar dislocation: a systematic review. *Clin Orthop Relat Res* 455:93–101, 2007.
Level of Evidence: II
Summary: The authors review 70 articles to make evidence-based recommendations on the diagnosis and treatment of first-time traumatic patellar dislocations. They recommend initial nonoperative management for patients, with operative intervention reserved for specific indications, including osteochondral fractures, second dislocation, or a lack of improvement after appropriate rehabilitation.

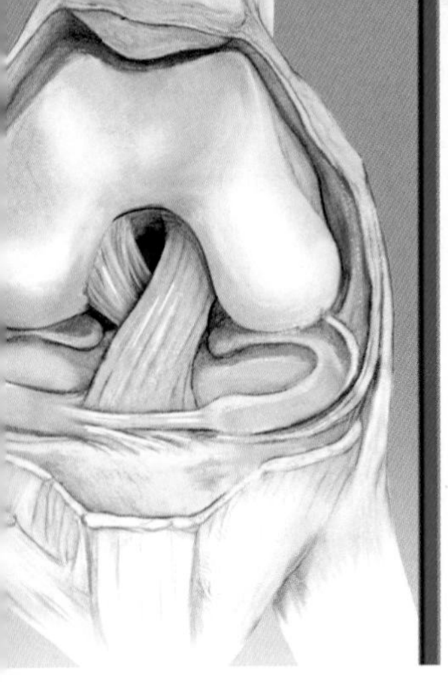

105

Patellofemoral Pain

BRETT W. McCOY • WAQAS M. HUSSAIN • MICHAEL J. GRIESSER • RICHARD D. PARKER

Overview of Pathologies

Patellofemoral pain is a common musculoskeletal ailment in active adolescents and adults. The incidence may be as high as 50% in some populations.[1] Patellofemoral pain, which is also known as anterior knee pain, is attributable to multiple etiologies, and despite being commonplace, it often results in consternation for clinicians as they attempt to accurately diagnose and efficiently treat it. Whereas most chapters in this book address specific disease processes, the topic of "patellofemoral pain" reflects the broad application of this term as a generic descriptor for various causes of pain in a particular location. The reason for this generic description is multifactorial but includes the similarity in clinical presentation among different etiologies, the elusiveness in defining the exact focus of pain based on simple diagnostic studies, and the similarity in treatment protocols, which often emphasize early nonsurgical management.

A subset of patients with patellofemoral pain have no definable pathology. This process has been described by different names, including patellofemoral pain syndrome and idiopathic anterior knee pain. It is important to note that these terms to some extent are diagnoses of exclusion and should not be used to mislabel a definable disease process. It is also a misnomer to attribute all patellofemoral pain to "chondromalacia" because in many cases no chondral pathology exists.

Anatomic Considerations

The anterior aspect of the knee has several unique properties that serve as a predisposition for pain. First, the patellofemoral joint experiences joint reaction forces that become higher as the knee flexion angle increases (Fig. 105-1).[2] Squatting and jumping have been reported to create forces 7.6 times and 12 times body weight, respectively.[3,4] The anterior aspect of the knee also provides significant sensory feedback. Dye[5] underwent arthroscopy without anesthesia and reported the highest subjective pain sensation in the anterior synovium, fat pad, and joint capsule. Interestingly, structures that commonly require intervention (e.g., the menisci, articular cartilage, and ligaments) were much less sensitive.[5] Dye and colleagues[5] also reported accurate spatial localization to palpation in the anterior structures (Fig. 105-2), which correlates with previous findings about the relatively high concentration of type IVa afferent nerve fibers in the patellar ligament and retinaculum.[6]

Entheses are defined as the insertion sites between tendon and bone. A recent study noted adipose tissue at multiple entheses and stressed that this common occurrence is not a pathologic process.[7] The investigators noted a rich innervation of this adipose tissue and suggested a role in mechanosensory feedback. Although it is commonly implicated in pain syndromes, this innervation may serve an important function in normal knee physiology. In certain pathologic conditions, a proliferation of nociceptive axons and an increase in neural growth factor may be found.[8,9] The subchondral bone is also richly innervated, and thus any pathology involving trauma or edema to this area would likely prove noxious.

Malalignment is a commonly proposed mechanism for patellofemoral pain.[10,11] A significant amount of literature questions a link between malalignment and patellofemoral pain, however.[12-14] The common occurrence of pain at rest is an argument against malalignment as a major component of most anterior knee pain.[15] Dye[12] proposed that pain is from a loss of tissue homeostasis. The loads encountered may reach the limitation of some of the soft tissue structures. Increased intraosseous pressure in the patella with resultant tissue ischemia has also been proposed.[16] Some studies support altered vascular flow (arterial and venous) and concomitant degenerative conditions.[17-19] However, it is difficult to assess if these changes are primary or secondary in nature.

History

Patients with patellofemoral conditions should be stratified into those experiencing pain and those experiencing instability. Admittedly some overlap occurs, but patients commonly endorse either a chief complaint of instability with reasonable pain resolution after the acute incident or significant pain with no symptoms of instability. This determination is a useful initial stratification tool. The temporal relationship of the patient's symptoms also helps aid in diagnosis. Much of the acute pathology (e.g., extensor mechanism disruption, patellar fractures, and instability) is addressed in other chapters. Activity-related chronic pain is a common clinical scenario that encompasses multiple disorders and has a broad differential diagnosis (Table 105-1). This chapter focuses predominantly on these processes, and the clinical parameters specific to certain etiologies are reviewed in greater detail.

For patients with activity-related chronic pain (without acute trauma), the discomfort commonly occurs while ascending or descending stairs, with deep squats, or while sitting for

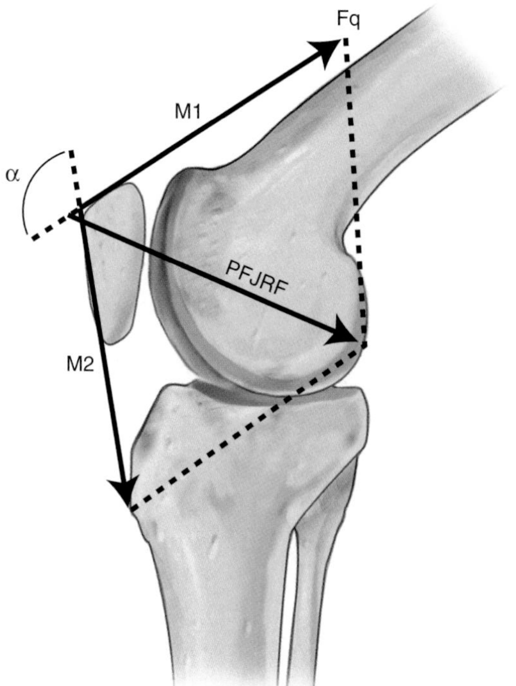

FIGURE 105-1 The patellofemoral joint reaction force (*PFJRF*) becomes higher as the knee flexion angle increases. In complete extension, M1 and M2 are in opposite directions, but in the same plane; the resultant PFJRF is almost zero. As flexion increases, M1 and M2 converge, and the vector PFJRF increases. *(From Scott WN, editor:* Insall & Scott Surgery of the Knee, *ed 5, Philadelphia, 2012, Elsevier.)*

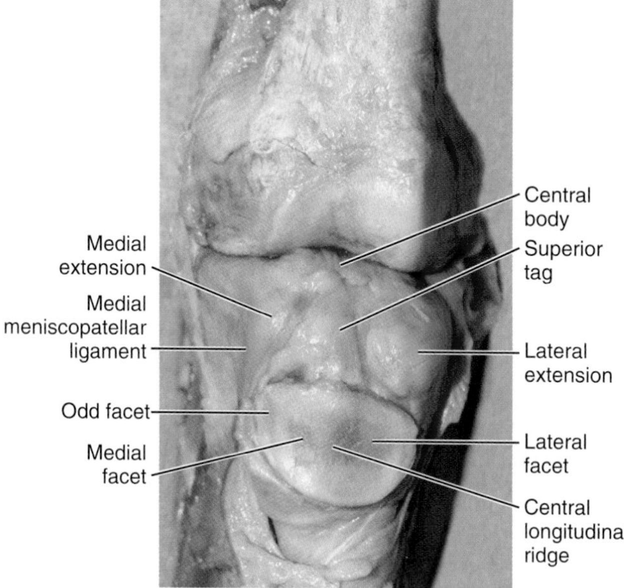

FIGURE 105-2 Posterior anatomy of the patella with adjacent capsular thickenings and fat pads with the medial and lateral meniscopatellar ligaments. *(From Noyes FR, editor:* Noyes' Knee Disorders: Surgery, Rehabilitation, Clinical Outcomes, *Philadelphia, 2010, Elsevier.)*

prolonged periods. It is common to have the symptoms bilaterally (in one study of adolescents with anterior knee pain, bilateral symptoms were described by approximately two thirds of subjects).[20] Patellofemoral pain is also common during periods of increased activity, such as during high-intensity training with military recruits.[21]

Physical Examination

In all patients presenting with knee pain (particularly patellofemoral pain), the physical examination should include an assessment for hip pathology. This assessment is particularly important for adolescents with anterior knee and distal thigh pain. Conditions such as slipped capital femoral epiphysis often present with knee pain as the chief complaint. One study demonstrated a 52% missed diagnosis rate and a referral delay of 76 days after primary care visitation for patients with slipped capital femoral epiphysis.[22] A simple logroll examination should not provoke pain in the patient with patellofemoral pathology. An alternative examination can be performed with the patient seated at the edge of the examination table and the knee flexed to approximately 90 degrees. The examiner can rotate the hip into internal and external rotation by moving the foot and ankle in a pendulum motion (abduction/adduction). If pain is felt at the extremes of motion either in the groin, thigh, or knee, then a strong consideration should be given to pathology of the hip joint.

TABLE 105-1

DIFFERENTIAL DIAGNOSIS OF PATELLOFEMORAL PAIN

Acute Pain	Activity-Related Chronic Pain	Constant Pain
Extensor mechanism disruption	Degenerative processes	Complex regional pain syndrome
Fracture patella (including avulsion fractures)	Inflammatory arthropathies	Neuroma
Chondral injury	Overuse injuries: tendonitis, insufficiency fractures	Oncologic process (some)
Patellar instability	Chondral lesion: traumatic, osteochondritis dissecans	
Loose body	Osteochondroses: Osgood-Schlatter disease, Sinding-Larsen-Johansson disease	
Infection	Iliotibial band syndrome	
Hip pathology	Synovial fat pad impingement	
Slipped capital femoral epiphysis	Symptomatic plica	

It is important to note that many variations exist in patellofemoral anatomy. These variations are evident during examination and may predispose a patient to patellofemoral pain; however, it is important to note that few, if any, examination findings are highly specific for a diagnosis in the differential diagnosis for patellofemoral pain. Malalignment is not pathognomonic for anterior knee pain. The examination findings are a portion of the complex clinical picture commonly encountered in the patient with anterior knee pain.

Global

The association of chronic pain and pain syndromes with the patellofemoral region requires an awareness of psychological and social factors. A component of anxiety or an exaggerated emotional response should be considered when evaluating treatment plans and determining prognosis. J.T. Andrish (personal communication, Cleveland Clinic, Cleveland, Ohio, 2011) noted a somatization of pain as a result of sexual or physical abuse in female adolescents with patellofemoral pain. This consideration is important in patients without significant structural pathology or who have failed to respond to multiple interventions.

Inspection

Gross inspection identifies limb alignment, prior incisions, gross atrophy, and large effusions and may demonstrate vasomotor changes associated with complex regional pain syndrome. Standing examination allows for evaluation of limb alignment and rotation profile. Patients with increased femoral anteversion and genu valgum may be at an increased risk for patellofemoral pain. A seated examination with the legs hanging off the end of the examination table provides a rough assessment of the Q angle. The Q angle is a measurement from the anterior superior iliac spine to the center of the patella and then from the center of the patella to the tibial tuberosity (Fig. 105-3). It is important to appreciate that the Q angle may be affected by the relationship of the proximal femur and the amount of knee flexion (Figs. 105-4 and 105-5). An elevated Q angle may predispose the patient to anterior knee pain, although significant variability exists. A flexion/extension cycle helps assess patellar tracking. A J sign is noted when the patella deviates laterally when the knee reaches terminal extension, and thus the Q angle may be less accurate in full extension in a patient with a positive J sign. Patients with external tibial torsion of foot pronation may experience increased patellofemoral pain.

Gait monitoring may help with patellar tracking and determining excessive femoral anteversion, as well as an awareness of global deficiencies in the kinetic chain. These factors may provide information regarding patellar instability, which is addressed in greater depth in Chapter 104. It is important to include an assessment for instability in the examination of patients with patellofemoral pain to determine any causal relationship between the two.

Palpation

Many of the involved structures (e.g., the fat pad, quadriceps and patellar tendon attachments to the patella, retinaculum/patellofemoral ligaments, and tibial tubercle) can be palpated with reasonable ease and can aid in localizing the focus of pain. In one study, 98% of adolescent patients with patellofemoral pain experienced pain with palpation over the medial patellofemoral ligament.[23] An appreciation of the different diagnoses helps the examiner with this portion of the examination by identifying which locations are commonly painful (e.g., the patellar/quadriceps tendons, iliotibial [IT] band, tibial tuberosity, infrapatellar fat pad, menisci, and retinaculum).

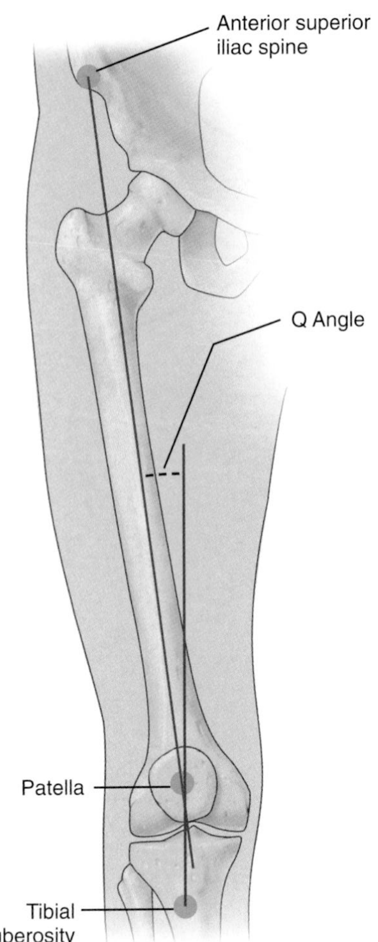

FIGURE 105-3 Q angle. *(Modified from Livingston LA, Mandigo JL: Bilateral Q angle asymmetry and anterior knee pain syndrome,* Clin Biomech [Bristol, Avon] *14[1]:7–13, 1999.)*

Range of Motion

Fulkerson[24] advises a prone examination to compare knee flexion, and any discrepancy would be attributable to quadriceps tightness. The motion should be symmetric and approach the gluteal crease. Decreased extension can be determined in the supine, prone, or standing positions by requesting that the patient straighten his or her legs completely and assessing them from a lateral position. If genu recurvatum is possible, this characteristic can be determined in the standing or supine position by attempting to hyperextend the knee while supporting the thigh just cephalad. Crepitus is common during range of motion testing in both symptomatic and asymptomatic patients.

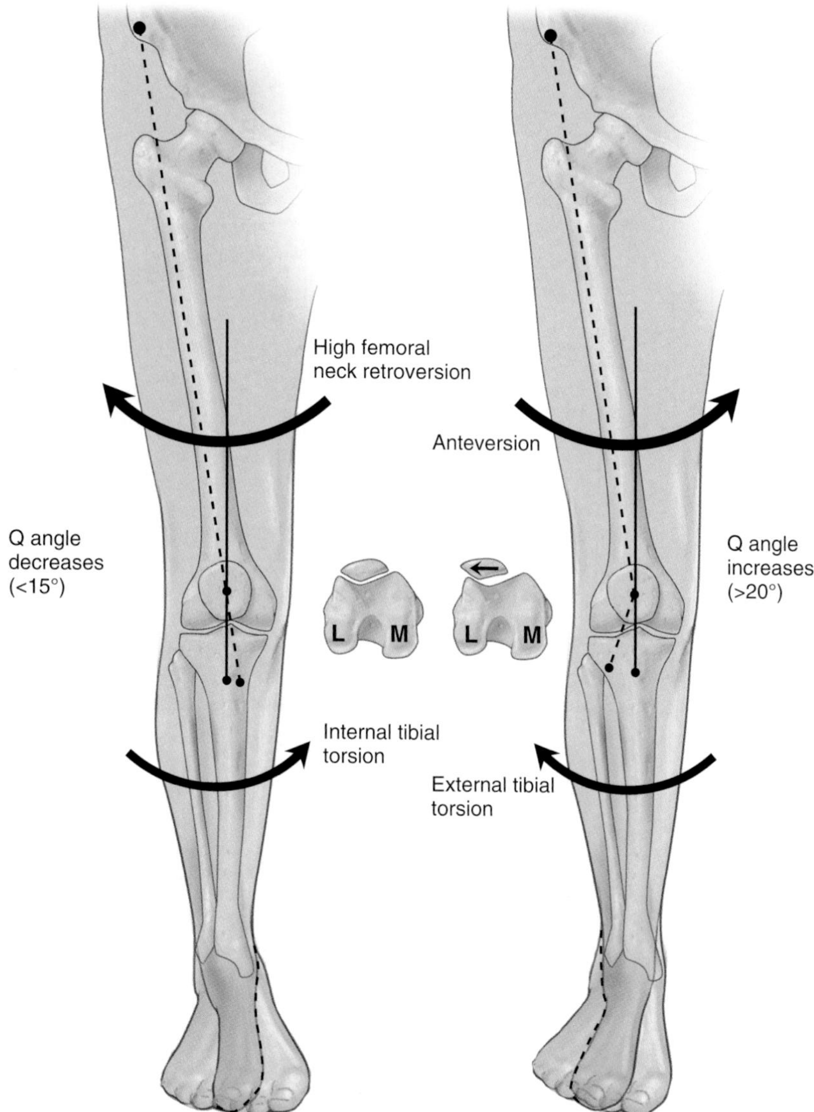

FIGURE 105-4 High femoral neck retroversion rotates the distal end of the femur externally. In combination with internal tibial torsion, the Q angle is decreased. Patellar tracking is improved, and patellofemoral sulcus alignment is normal. High femoral neck anteversion rotates the distal end of the femur internally. In combination with external tibial torsion, the Q angle is increased. Patellar tracking is compromised, and the patella tends to track laterally. *(From Tria AJ, Jr, Klein KS:* An Illustrated Guide to the Knee, *New York, 1992, Churchill Livingstone.)*

Provocative Tests

Pressure applied in various manners to the patella has different names, including patellar grind, patellar compression, or the Clarke sign. The first mention of patellar grind was by Owre[25] in 1936:

> *Pressure-pain over the patella is tested by clasping the patella with the thumb and index finger of each hand with the remaining fingers resting against the thigh and leg. While the patient lies with the leg relaxed and extended, the patella is pressed against the medial and lateral femoral condyles. By moving the patella in an upward and down-ward direction the greater part of the surface cartilage may be examined in this manner. In some cases, pain is elicited on the slightest pressure of the patella against the condyle, at other times considerable pressure must be exerted to obtain a positive response of an unpleasant sensation.*

This test was described as positive in patients with retropatellar chondral pathology. Other variations of the grind test or Clarke sign (or test) involve application of pressure on the superior border of the patella (with the web space of the thumb) while asking the patient to contract the quadriceps muscles. In a study that examined the Clarke sign in patients undergoing arthroscopy and in which direct visualization was used as the gold standard for chondral pathology, the authors noted very poor diagnostic value (sensitivity 0.39, specificity 0.67, and positive predictive value 0.25) and further indicated that a literature search identified multiple issues pertaining to this test, and thus they recommend that it not be a part of a routine examination.[26]

A more gently applied posterior force to the patella during flexion and extension may elicit crepitus and pain in patients with chondral pathology (Fig. 105-6). This test may help identify the location of pathology, because a more distal lesion will be painful in early flexion as the patella engages the

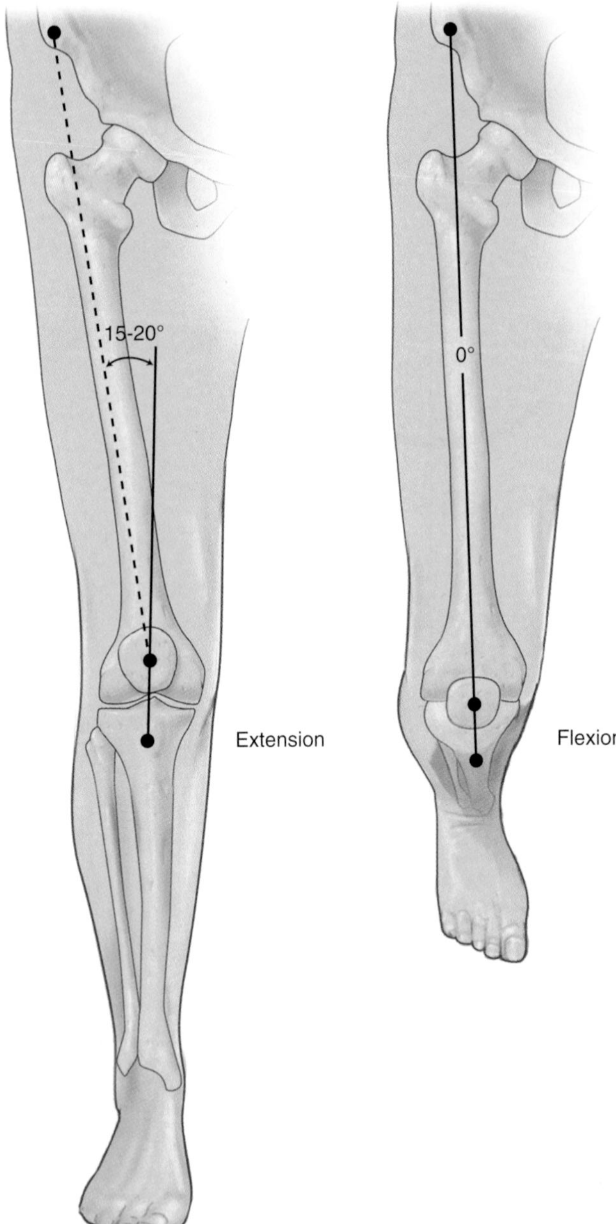

FIGURE 105-5 Flexion of the knee decreases the Q angle as the result of internal tibial rotation. *(From Tria AJ Jr, Klein KS:* An Illustrated Guide to the Knee, *New York, 1992, Churchill Livingstone.)*

trochlea, whereas a more proximal lesion will be painful at greater degrees of knee flexion (Fig. 105-7).

Patellar instability testing is discussed in greater detail in Chapter 104. The patellar apprehension test is performed by application of a laterally directed pressure to the medial aspect of the patella with both thumbs in approximately 30 degrees of flexion. The test is positive if the patient experiences apprehension that the patella may dislocate laterally. The sensitivity of this test was noted to be 0.39 in one study.[27] However, in a study evaluating patients with patellofemoral pain, apprehension testing elicited pain in 89% of patients at the focus of pressure, and thus it is important to appreciate that although patients with patellofemoral pain may experience pain during

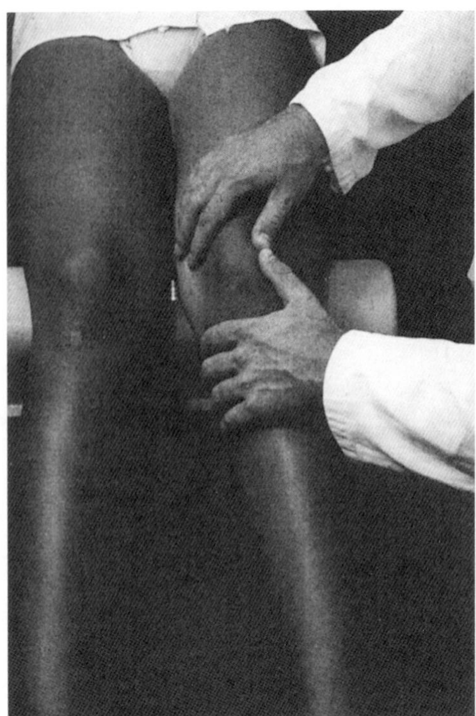

FIGURE 105-6 The patellar compression test. With the knee flexed slightly to engage the patella in the femoral trochlea, direct compression is applied to the patella. *(From Scott WN, editor:* Insall & Scott Surgery of the Knee, *ed 5, Philadelphia, 2012, Elsevier.)*

apprehension testing, this pain does not represent a positive test for instability. Manipulation of the patella in the transverse plane may reveal a tight retinaculum, as evidenced by a lack of motion (Fig. 105-8). The patellar tilt test should also be performed as an assessment for a tight retinaculum and may have some utility in determining possible interventions.[28]

Diagnostic Studies

Standard radiographs help detect pathologic processes such as degenerative changes, certain osteochondroses, calcified loose bodies, osteochondritis dissecans (OCD), and some neoplasms. They also provide information regarding

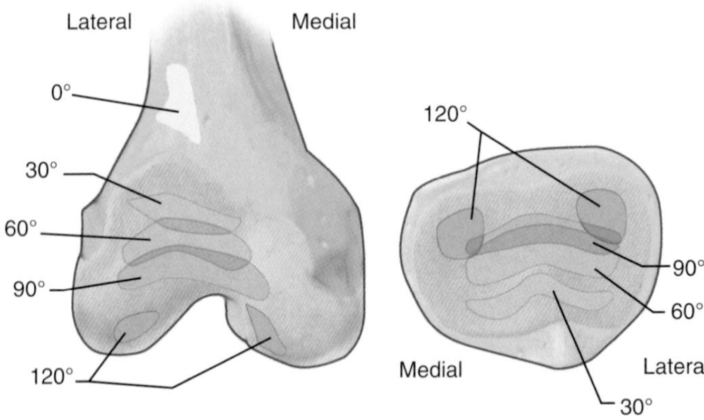

FIGURE 105-7 The patellofemoral joint contact areas according to the knee flexion angle. *(From Scott WN, editor:* Insall & Scott Surgery of the Knee, *ed 5, Philadelphia, 2012, Elsevier.)*

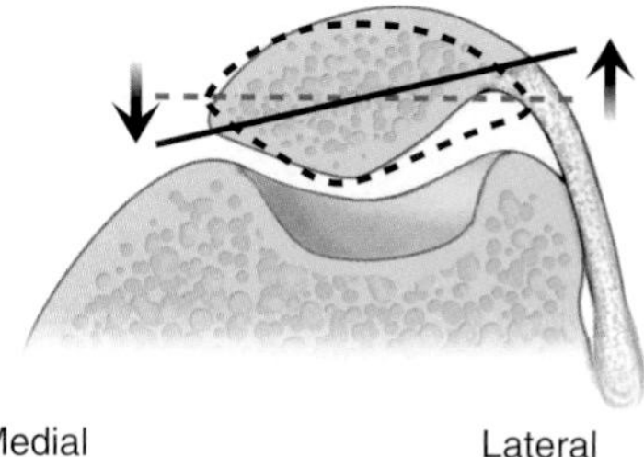

FIGURE 105-8 The passive patellar tilt test. In full extension, the transverse axis of a normal patella tilts beyond the horizontal. The inability to perform this maneuver may indicate an excessively tight lateral retinaculum. *(From Scott WN, editor:* Insall & Scott Surgery of the Knee, *ed 5, Philadelphia, 2012, Elsevier.)*

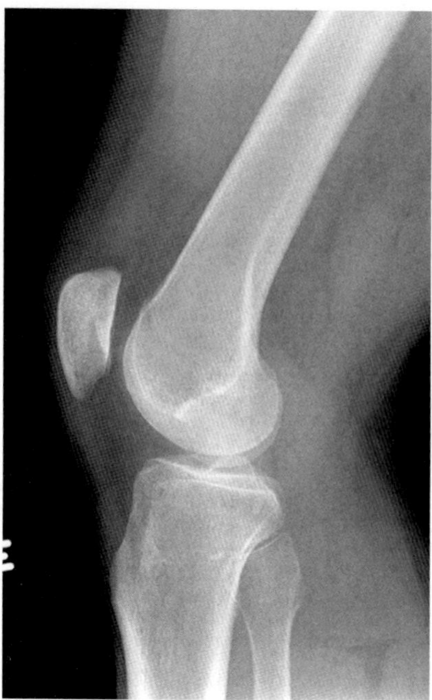

FIGURE 105-9 Lateral radiograph of the knee.

alignment and subtle anatomic variations. Standard views include weight-bearing anteroposterior and lateral views, as well as an axial view. The lateral radiograph is useful for determining patellar height (Fig. 105-9). Patients with patella alta may have a predisposition to instability, whereas patients with patella baja may encounter increased patellar load and the subsequent risk of degenerative conditions.

An axial radiograph commonly obtained is the Merchant view (Fig. 105-10).[29] It is taken with the knee flexed to 45 degrees and the x-ray beam projected 30 degrees caudad from the long axis of the femur (see Fig. 105-10).[29] It is important to note that the patella engages the trochlea in flexion greater than approximately 20 degrees and that this view is not an accurate representation of the relationship between the patella and the femur in full extension or slight flexion. Murray et al.[30] demonstrated that the lateral and axial views are the most useful views for evaluating instability and noted a high sensitivity of the lateral view for detecting prior dislocation; thus a normal lateral radiograph can help rule out instability as a component of anterior knee pain in some patients. The axial view is also useful for evaluating patellar tilt and

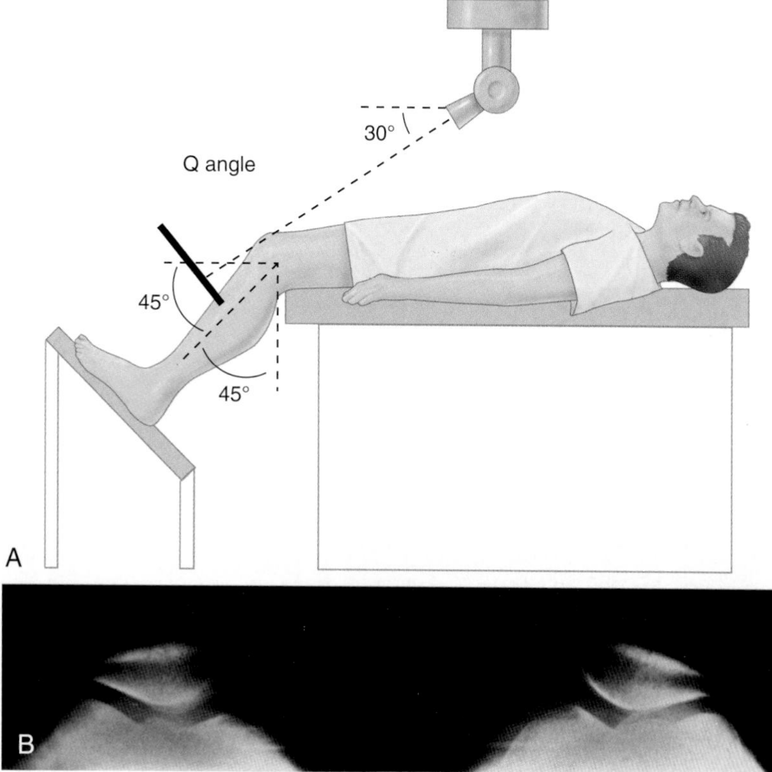

FIGURE 105-10 Merchant view. **A,** Technique. **B,** A normal Merchant view. Patellofemoral alignment is normal bilaterally, and the osseous structures and articular cortices are normal. *(From Scott WN, editor:* Insall & Scott Surgery of the Knee, *ed 5, Philadelphia, 2012, Elsevier.)*

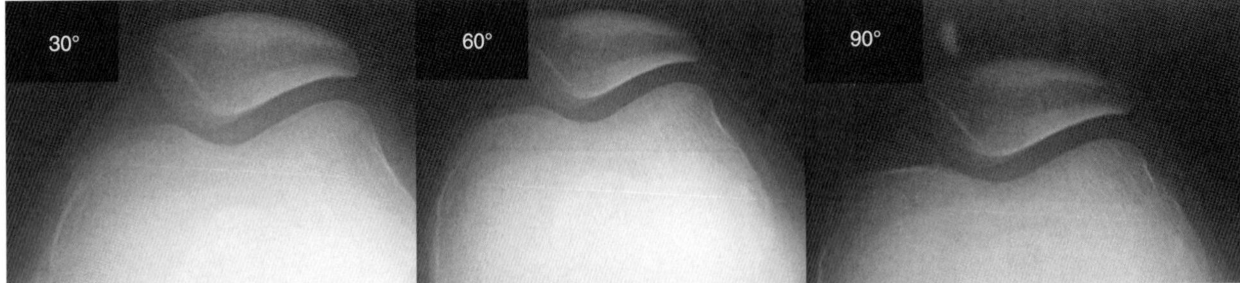

FIGURE 105-11 Axial views performed at 30, 60, and 90 degrees of knee flexion. Note how the trochlear shape changes as flexion increases and the medial facet seems bigger. It is not necessary to routinely perform 60- and 90-degree flexion radiographs in common patellofemoral disorders. *(From Scott WN, editor:* Insall & Scott Surgery of the Knee, *ed 5, Philadelphia, 2012, Elsevier.)*

subluxation. Different parameters have been defined, and the clinical utility of these parameters remains uncertain (Fig. 105-11). When evaluating axial radiographs, it is important to note that the sulcus of the trochlea lies lateral to the midline of the femoral condyles and is not completely centered as previously thought.[31] Magnetic resonance arthrograms further confirmed that articular congruity may exist even when osseous incongruity appears on plain radiographs.[32]

Computed tomography (CT) has utility in evaluating instability by helping determine the relationship of the patella and the trochlear groove, as well as identifying trochlear dysplasia. It is used to measure the tibial tuberosity–trochlear groove distance (the discussion of these topics is addressed in separate chapters). Indications for CT scans in patients without instability are limited. Magnetic resonance imaging (MRI) is the modality of choice for evaluating chondral pathology because plain radiographs have limited utility (Fig. 105-12). MRI is also commonly used to diagnose or rule out intraarticular pathology. One study demonstrated that edema in the superolateral fat pad on MRI correlates with other anatomic parameters (e.g., trochlear morphology and patellar alignment) suggestive of patellar maltracking or impingement in the young, symptomatic patient.[33] Radionuclide scanning can be used to identify occult fractures or insertional tendinopathies. Diffuse uptake can also be seen in persons with complex regional pain syndrome.

Specific Conditions

Idiopathic Anterior Knee Pain/ Patellofemoral Pain Syndrome

Many patients have no definitive causative lesion for patellofemoral pain. This situation is commonly encountered in the overuse type of injury. The practitioner may find some potentially predisposing factors on physical examination or with imaging (e.g., quadriceps atrophy, hamstring tightness, or a high Q angle). In a prospective study, patients with a hypermobile patella had a higher incidence of anterior knee pain, and in a separate study this examination finding correlated with a worse prognosis for patients with patellofemoral pain.[34,35] However, these findings are common in patients with no anterior knee pain. This type of condition has been referred to by several names, including *anterior knee pain, patellofemoral pain syndrome,* and *idiopathic anterior knee pain.* These terms are generally diagnoses of exclusion, and this lack of objective criteria means that inclusion and exclusion criteria have significant limitations. Thus significant variability and limitations relating to patellofemoral pain exist in the literature. Validated diagnostic criteria and outcome measures do not exist at this time.

The natural history of idiopathic anterior knee pain has decent long-term results (71% improvement at 16 years).[36] In

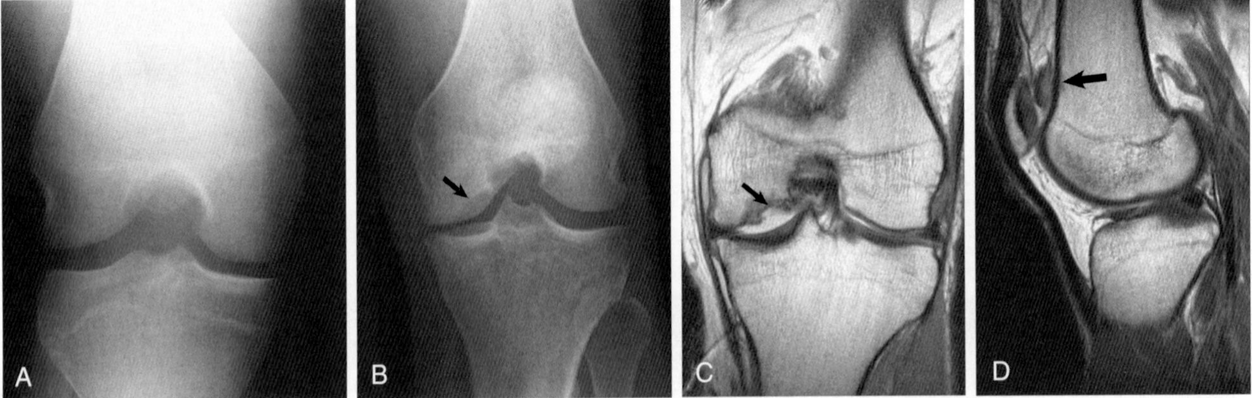

FIGURE 105-12 Tunnel view. **A,** A normal tunnel view demonstrates the posterior aspect of the femoral condyles, the tibial spines, the articular surfaces of the tibial plateau, and the intercondylar notch. **B,** A tunnel view from a different patient demonstrating an ovoid area of lucency at the inner margin of the medial femoral condyle *(arrow)* that is suspicious for osteochondritis desiccans. Coronal **(C)** and sagittal proton density **(D)** magnetic resonance imaging confirms the large osteochondral defect *(arrow)* with a completely displaced osteochondral fragment located in the suprapatellar joint recess *(arrow). (Case courtesy the Hospital for Special Surgery, New York, NY. From Scott WN, editor:* Insall & Scott Surgery of the Knee, *ed 5, Philadelphia, 2012, Elsevier.)*

a study of military recruits, 15% had pain during initial training. At 6-year follow-up (3 years after returning to civilian life), 50% still experienced some pain, but only 8% described it as severe pain.[21] The treatment of patellofemoral pain syndrome focuses on physiotherapy, bracing, and pharmacotherapy. Systematic reviews have failed to demonstrate that any of these modalities decrease pain in a meaningful fashion.[37,38] For patients who have significant disability with use of conservative treatment modalities, arthroscopy can be considered for diagnostic and therapeutic reasons. Patellar denervation has been described using electrocautery[39] and can be accomplished via an anterolateral, anteromedial, and superior portal (either medial and lateral). This procedure should be applied sparingly, and we strongly urge the clinician to search for other diagnoses before labeling a condition as idiopathic anterior knee pain or patellofemoral pain syndrome.

Chondromalacia

With regard to chondromalacia, please refer to the discussion of OCD, as well as Chapters 97 and 103.

Synovial Impingement Syndromes

Impingement is a common cause of patellofemoral pain. The offending structures are plicae or the infrapatellar fat pad. The plicae are embryologic remnants that are normal anatomic structures. The determination of pathologic versus normal plica is difficult.[40] The medial plica is most commonly symptomatic (Fig. 105-13).[41] This plica was shown to be present in approximately 80% of the population in one cohort.[42] Patients describe activity-related pain that worsens with flexion and is relieved with extension. With a hypertrophic plica, a thick palpable cord may be present. Both flexion and extension tests have been described to aid in the diagnosis of pathologic plicae, but they are of limited utility.[43] MRI may detect a prominent plica, but no study has demonstrated a role for determining pathologic versus normal plicae. Chondral pathology of the medial femoral condyle has been noted in cases of severe plicae, and this pathology may be appreciated on MRI.[44]

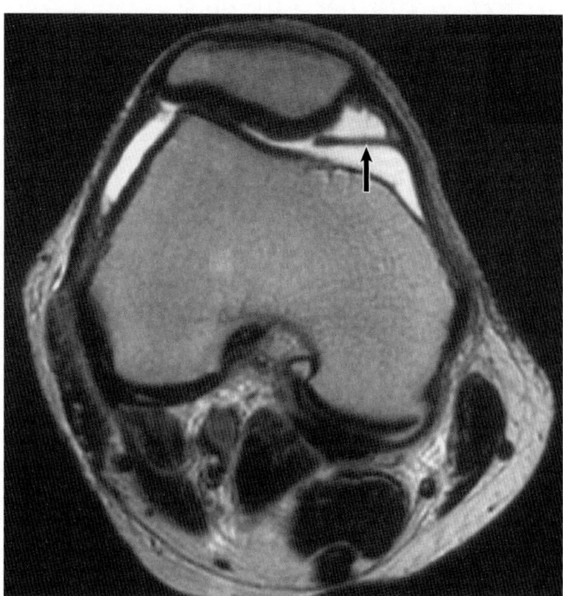

FIGURE 105-13 An axial magnetic resonance image with a low-signal, thick medial patellar plica *(arrow)* that is highlighted by the large effusion. *(From Scott WN, editor:* Insall & Scott Surgery of the Knee, *ed 5, Philadelphia, 2012, Elsevier.)*

The treatment of symptomatic plicae should begin with conservative modalities, including activity modification, use of antiinflammatory medications, physiotherapy (focused primarily on stretching), and corticosteroid injections. This treatment is reported to succeed in fewer than half of the patients affected.[45] However, significant variability exists in the diagnostic criteria, and thus results should be interpreted cautiously. For patients who do not respond to nonoperative treatment, arthroscopy with plica excision is a straightforward option with low associated morbidity. In patients with associated cartilage degeneration, midterm results support plica excision.[46] The procedure should include a thorough evaluation for other pathology.

The infrapatellar fat pad was implicated in anterior knee pain by Hoffa[47] in 1904. As previously mentioned, this area has a rich innervation and thus can result in significant pain. This area may become swollen and tender to palpation. The Hoffa maneuver involves applying pressure just medial and lateral to the patellar tendon (separately) and extending the knee, which may elicit either pain or apprehension. Plain radiographs are of limited utility because this diagnosis is predominantly clinical. Some evidence indicates that MRI may aid in the diagnosis, and use of MRI may become more relevant with the advent of more powerful MRI machines.[33,48]

The treatment of fat pad impingement is similar to the initial treatment for symptomatic plica. The modalities include activity avoidance, physiotherapy, cryotherapy, and transcutaneous electrical nerve stimulation. For patients who do not respond to conservative modalities, surgical excision has been described.[48-50] We recommend this treatment only when the patient has exhausted all nonoperative modalities.

Intraosseous Hypertension of the Patella

Increased intraosseous pressure has been described in the femur and tibia of painful knees by Arnoldi and colleagues.[51] These investigators later correlated knee pain with increased pressure in the patella. It has been suggested that this phenomenon may be related to decreased venous outflow based on intraosseous phlebography.[52] The diagnostic criterion for patellar hypertension is an increase in intraosseous pressure of greater than 25 mm Hg with sustained knee flexion. Schneider and colleagues[53,54] reported on a series of patients with patellofemoral pain that failed to respond to conservative measures. After administration of a local anesthetic a "provocation test" was performed (i.e., the reproduction of symptoms by raising the intraosseous pressure), and patients underwent intraosseous drilling and decompression. In this series at 1-year follow-up, 88% of subjects had an objective decrease in pressure measurement.[53] A subsequent publication demonstrated improved clinical outcome scores (the Visual Analog Scale score decreased from 7.6 to 2.1) with this treatment protocol in a 3-year follow-up.[55] The validity of this diagnosis is debated; however, it does appear in several series that patellar drilling and decompression may benefit patients who fail to respond to conservative treatment for patellofemoral pain. It remains unclear if this diagnosis is the primary pathology or if it is secondary to other disease processes (including lateral patella compression syndrome).

Lateral Patella Compression Syndrome

Ficat[56] originally described lateral patellar compression syndrome. The etiology is thought to be a tight lateral retinaculum. Patients report pain while ascending or descending stairs and may have a positive theatre sign (i.e., pain with prolonged sitting). They do not present with a history of instability. As the condition progresses, if chondral wear occurs, the clinical picture may evolve (e.g., effusions, loose bodies, mechanical symptoms, or a degenerative picture).

On examination these patients have pain with patellar compression testing (especially in the lateral aspect). They do not exhibit excessive patellar mobility because the retinaculum is tight, and the examiner may have difficulty everting the lateral patellar edge above parallel to the floor, indicative of a tight lateral retinaculum (pain may also be replicated). The amount of medial patellar glide is generally less than two quadrants. These patients may also have subtle findings of an increased Q angle, a tight IT band, and foot pronation. Axial radiographs demonstrate increased patellar tilt and a decreased lateral patellofemoral angle.

The treatment of this condition should primarily focus on nonoperative modalities to decrease inflammation, including use of nonsteroidal antiinflammatory drugs, activity modification, and physical therapy. Modalities to help loosen the lateral retinaculum and IT band are useful adjuncts. For patients who fail to respond to conservative modalities and still have significant functional limitation, surgery can be considered. This condition remains one of the few indications for an isolated lateral release. We generally perform this procedure arthroscopically with electrocautery and begin approximately 1 cm superior to the patella and carry out the release down to the anterolateral portal. Other authors have recommended a longer release, but it is important not to create iatrogenic instability.[57] If any evidence of patellar hypermobility exists, then an open lateral retinacular lengthening procedure should be considered.

Osteochondroses

Overview

Osteochondrosis is defined as any disease that affects the progress of bone growth through necrosis of bone tissue. The disease results from disordered endochondral ossification of a previously normal developing epiphysis.[58] The inflammation that is typically seen with overuse injuries in adults is found in a different location in an immature patient. Young athletes present with reports of pain localized to a specific region of the knee, classically at the origin or insertion of a tendinous structure, whereas in mature persons the advanced radiographic findings are consistently within the tendon itself. The area of the apophysis is the "weak link" in the young athlete and sustains the stresses associated with repetitive activities.

In the extensor mechanism complex, a variety of osteochondroses are found, most notably at the tibial tubercle, infrapatellar region, or the superior pole of the patella. The eponyms used for these osteochondroses are well known.

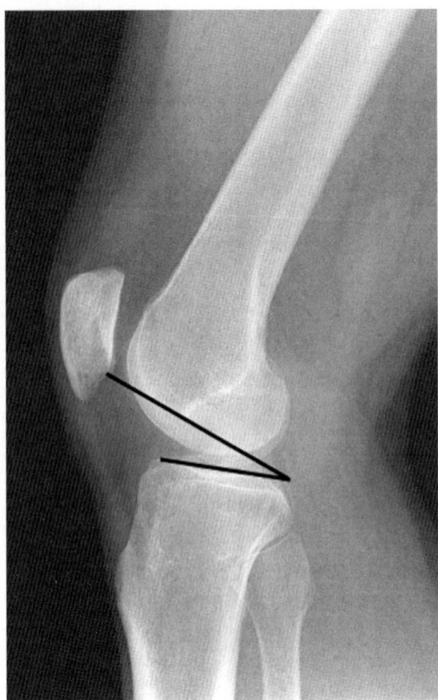

FIGURE 105-14 A lateral radiograph demonstrating the plateau-patella angle (normal range, 21 to 29 degrees).

Much has been written with regard to Osgood-Schlatter and Sinding-Larsen-Johansson disease, which affect the tibial tubercle and distal pole of the patella, respectively (Figs. 105-14 and 105-15).[59] These entities are found in persons undergoing rapid growth who participate in athletic activities. The onset of symptoms of both conditions directly correlates with periods of rapid growth. Extraarticular osteochondroses of the patella should not be confused with OCD of the patella. OCD is a lesion that affects the subchondral bone and leads to subchondral delamination or sequestration.

Osgood-Schlatter Disease

Osteochondrosis of the tibial tubercle was first recognized in the early 1900s, and Osgood and Schlatter were credited with identifying this condition.[60] They described the disease as occurring in children who place stress on the developing tubercle via force from the patellar tendon during periods of rapid growth. Other investigators theorized that the maturing tubercle is partially or completely avulsed. The authors distinguished this entity from a tibial tubercle avulsion fracture and stressed that the condition occurs as a result of repetitive loading of the area. This description is the classic description of traction apophysitis.

Osgood-Schlatter disease was originally reported to be more common in males than in females.[61,62] However, with the increasing number of young female athletes, the condition is now being seen at similar rates among males and females. Females present with symptoms earlier, generally between the ages of 10 and 13 years, as opposed to males, who present with the condition between the ages of 12 and 14 years, correlating with periods of rapid growth.[63] The incidence in nonathletic adolescents has been quoted as 4.5%, as opposed to 21% in the active adolescent population.[61] Osgood-Schlatter disease occurs bilaterally in 20% to 30% of patients.[64]

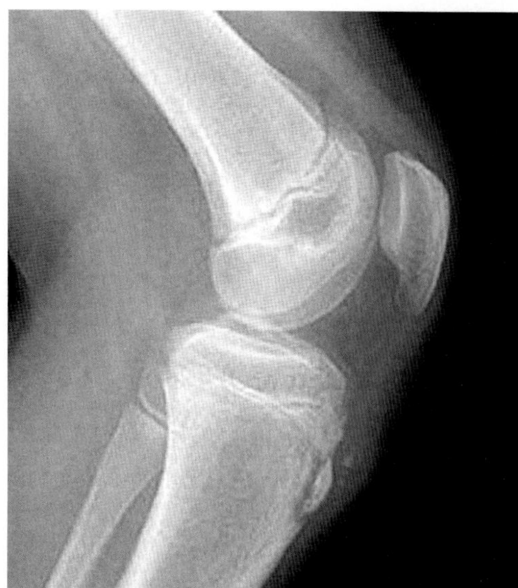

FIGURE 105-15 Osgood-Schlatter disease of the tibial apophysis.

Etiology

The etiology of Osgood-Schlatter disease has been investigated, but no definitive answer has been determined. The condition occurs exclusively in adolescents during periods of rapid growth. During this time, an imbalance of growth between the bone and the muscle unit may lead the apophysis to become more susceptible to overuse injury.[65] Investigators have evaluated a variety of anatomic factors that may predispose to the condition. Patella alta has been associated with Osgood-Schlatter disease, but no definitive predisposition has been established.[61] A single study evaluating radiographs in patients with and without Osgood-Schlatter disease associated patella alta with the condition; however, some limitations were noted in the assessment of the patellar height on plain radiographs.[66] A later investigation attempting to link patella alta, Osgood-Schlatter disease, and tibial tubercle avulsion fractures showed no association among the three.[67] One study that has shown a significant anatomic variant in these patients focused on the patellar angle.[68] The patellar angle is the angle between the articular surface and the inferior pole of the patella (Fig. 105-14). This angle is also referred to as the *plateau-patella angle* (with a normal range of 21 to 29 degrees). Persons with the condition showed a smaller patellar angle, which the authors associated with a need for greater quadriceps force to perform similar activities.[68]

Although the maturation of the tibial tubercle predisposes to this condition, repetitive microtrauma has been seen as an integral part of the disease process, because persons who are less active develop the condition at an exponentially lower rate.[61] A single event such as a forceful jump or direct contact with repeated kneeling can aggravate the syndrome. It is believed that repetitive, submaximal stresses acting on the immature patellar tendon-tibial tubercle junction lead to minor avulsion and attempts at repair. These findings define Osgood-Schlatter disease.[62] This description of causality attempts to highlight the requirement of a developing tubercle and an active adolescent.

Diagnosis

The clinical presentation of Osgood-Schlatter disease consists of reports of activity-related pain focused over the tibial tubercle and distal patellar tendon that worsens with running, jumping, or kneeling. This pain may be accompanied with swelling over the area. Activities such as basketball, volleyball, gymnastics, and soccer that include running and jumping and load the knee in flexion, leading to an eccentric quadriceps contraction, seem to predispose adolescents to this condition.

Tenderness, swelling, and prominence of the tibial tubercle, particularly in the distal half, are often found on physical examination. Patients may walk with an antalgic gait, which is often noticed by the parent rather than the individual. Acute cases can present with an extensor lag, confusing the diagnosis and raising concern for a tibial avulsion fracture. Passive range of motion of the knee is usually full, and knee effusions are not seen. Quadriceps and hamstring tightness is common, with some investigators postulating that it is part of the cause. The differential diagnosis of Osgood-Schlatter disease includes avulsion fracture of the tibial tuberosity, patellofemoral stress syndrome, pes anserinus bursitis, Sinding-Larsen-Johansson disease, and infection.

Plain radiographs of the effected knee are useful for evaluation of the tibial tuberosity. The lateral radiograph of the knee is most useful in assessing the extensor mechanism (Fig. 105-15). The apophysis can show separation or fragmentation of the tibial tubercle. Enlargement of the tubercle may also be seen. Soft tissue swelling can also be appreciated, along with thickening of the patellar tendon.[61] Ultrasound has been studied and used in some institutions for diagnosis of Osgood-Schlatter disease.[69] Because of the high level of operator dependence, this modality is not widely recommended. MRI is appropriate for cases in which the extent of soft tissue swelling or tubercle prominence is unusual.

Natural History

A handful of studies have followed the natural history of Osgood-Schlatter disease.[61,70,71] Krause et al.[70] reported on the natural history of Osgood-Schlatter disease in 50 patients treated nonoperatively versus operatively. The majority of patients seen in adulthood for follow-up had no residual symptoms, regardless of treatment. Krause et al.[70] concluded that two groups of patients could be stratified by retrospectively evaluating the presentation and progression of the disease. The group of patients without radiographic abnormalities (such as fragmentation and irregular ossification) had minimal symptoms in adult life. Natural history investigations have all shown no increased incidence of patellar instability, anterior knee pain, or premature proximal tibial growth arrest in patients with Osgood-Schlatter disease.[61,70,71]

A recent study looked at the utility of injection-related therapies such as hyperosmolar dextrose, which showed beneficial effects.[72] Additionally, several recent studies have examined surgical treatment of unresolved Osgood-Schlatter disease with reasonable success.[73-76] The unifying theme among proposed surgical treatments is resection of the tubercle prominence subperiosteally or ossicle excision.

AUTHORS' PREFERRED TECHNIQUE

Osgood-Schlatter Disease

The treatment of Osgood-Schlatter disease is guided by the severity of symptoms. As evidenced by the natural history, this syndrome is generally a self-limited condition.[70] Improvement can be gradual, which should be stressed to the patient and family. A period of 12 to 18 months can pass before the complete resolution of symptoms occurs, which correlates with the time needed for closure of the epiphysis. Although most patients continue with their athletic endeavors, the severity of pain in some persons leads to a change in position or even in sport. Nonoperative management includes activity restriction or adjustment and proper padding of the tubercle to avoid painful symptoms. Additionally, use of nonsteroidal antiinflammatory drugs, ice, and physical therapy can play an important role.[77-79] Severe pain should lead the clinician to recommend a short time of absolute sport restriction until symptoms improve, which may include a brief period of immobilization. Pain that does not resolve with activity restriction should be investigated further for other etiologies. Nonimpact activities, as well as hamstring and quadriceps flexibility exercises, maintain knee range of motion and may quicken recovery. Injections over the site of discomfort are contraindicated.

For patients whose symptoms do not improve, surgical intervention can be successful. The two most common procedures performed are ossicle excision and tibial tubercle prominence resection.[71,80] Ossicle excision is performed by creating a longitudinal split in the patellar tendon and enucleating the fragment. The success rate of this procedure has been reported to be 93%. It is most useful in patients who have a distinct separate ossicle in the proximal aspect of the tibial tubercle that is painful with direct contact.[71] Tubercle prominence resection has also shown good results in recalcitrant cases of Osgood-Schlatter disease.[73,74,76,81,82] The patients who require surgery should have symptoms for longer than 1 year and have allowed significant time to elapse since physeal closure. The greatest success is in persons who have pain with activities and particularly with kneeling.[81]

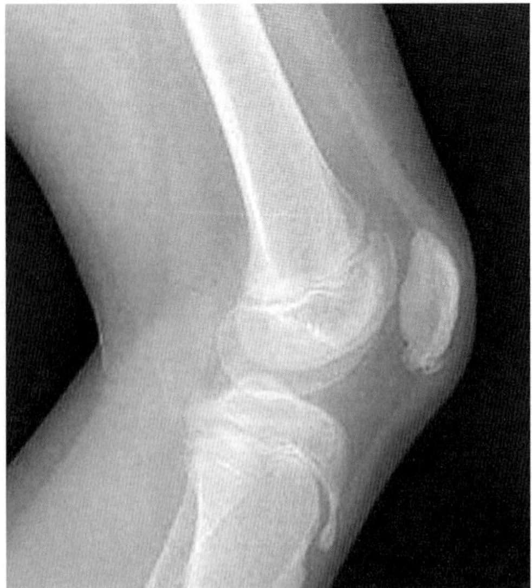

FIGURE 105-16 Sinding-Larsen-Johansson disease.

Sinding-Larsen-Johansson Disease

Osteochondrosis of the inferior pole of the patella was first described in the early 1920s. Similar to Osgood-Schlatter disease, this syndrome affects the maturing active adolescent and occurs in females at a younger age than males, which is attributable to earlier skeletal maturity.[83]

The symptoms are similar to those of Osgood-Schlatter disease (i.e., activity-related pain over the inferior pole of the patella and pain with running and jumping sports). The examination shows point tenderness at the inferior patella–patellar tendon junction with variable amounts of swelling in this location. The remainder of the examination is often normal. Calcification at this location is found in chronic cases of Sinding-Larsen-Johansson disease. A palpable gap in the location of the patella–patellar tendon junction should lead to suspicion of a patellar sleeve fracture. This step-off, along with the inability to perform a straight leg raise, is the classic presentation.[84] Assessment for tibial tubercle pain and prominence should be performed to differentiate this condition from Osgood-Schlatter disease. Although rare, the diagnosis of both of these entities has been reported.[85,86] Traditionally, Sinding-Larsen-Johansson is seen in slightly younger persons because the maturation of the inferior pole of the patella occurs prior to that of the tibial tuberosity.

Radiographic assessment includes anteroposterior, lateral, and Merchant views of both knees in the adolescent. Calcification or ossification of the inferior pole of the patella can often be identified (Fig. 105-16). Additionally, ultrasound has also been used as a diagnostic tool for this condition, and although successful, it has not yet achieved widespread acceptance.[69]

AUTHORS' PREFERRED TECHNIQUE

Sinding-Larsen-Johansson Disease

Sinding-Larsen-Johansson disease is a self-limited condition. The resolution of symptoms follows the full maturation of the inferior pole of the patella, which takes a period of 12 to 18 months. Management is similar to that for Osgood-Schlatter disease (i.e., activity modification, use of ice and antiinflammatory medications, and physical therapy). Patients are allowed to participate in sports as symptoms improve. Late sequelae of the disease are few, with one report of a fracture through a previously united Sinding-Larsen-Johansson ossicle.[87] No recent reports regarding new forms of treatment have emerged in the literature.

Superior Pole Osteochondrosis

Although they are rare, superior pole osteochondroses have been reported in the literature.[88-90] The condition can be distinguished from bipartite changes in the patella by both radiographic appearance and clinical symptomatology. The largest case series by Batten et al.[89] described the condition in six active male patients all between 10 and 11 years of age. The location of their discomfort was the anterior portion of the knee, not specifically the proximal pole. Upon radiographic investigation, the proximal pole of the patella showed fragmentation similar to that seen in Sinding-Larsen-Johansson disease. Grogan et al.[91] reported on seven cases of proximal pole fragmentation that they believed were avulsion injuries due to direct trauma. They found these cases to be similar in appearance and presentation to avulsion injuries to the distal pole of the patella and tibial tuberosity. Tyler and McCarthy[88] assessed the histologic change that occurs in these patients and found osteonecrosis with reparative changes, similar to those seen in persons with Sinding-Larsen-Johansson and Osgood-Schlatter disease.

Osteochondrosis of the proximal pole of the patella typically presents with anterior knee pain that may be poorly localized.[89] Pain may be reproduced with palpation over the proximal area of the patella. Individuals may also have symptoms of other extraarticular osteochondroses.[89] Radiographic changes may be indicative of the chronicity of symptoms. No reports have been made of operative interventions because this process is self-limiting. Although our understanding of this condition is limited because of its rarity, the principles of nonoperative management lead to resolution of this syndrome. No recent literature has emerged regarding new treatment modalities.

Osteochondritis Dissecans of the Patella

OCD is a disease process first described by Sir James Paget, and its etiology continues to challenge investigators. Theories include ischemia or endochondral ossification defects.[92] The condition was given the name "osteochondritis dissecans" by Koenig.[93] At the time, Koenig believed that these lesions developed as a result of trauma and deteriorated because of subsequent inflammation. Although he later acknowledged that his theory was flawed, the name continued to be used even though the inflammatory process is not the cardinal cause of the abnormality. The condition was first recognized in the knee but subsequently has been described in a number of joints, including the ankle, elbow, and hip.

Rombold first described OCD of the patella in 1936. Although quite uncommon, it must remain in the differential diagnosis of anterior knee pain. Similar to OCD in other areas, the differentiation of juvenile, adolescent, and adult types of lesions is necessary to follow an appropriate treatment algorithm.[94] The juvenile type of OCD is found in patients with completely open physes. The adolescent category includes patients who are in the process of physeal closure. Adult lesions are found in patients with fully closed physes.

The lateral posterior portion of the medial femoral condyle is the classic location, comprising 70% to 80% of all OCD lesions of the knee joint.[92] Patellar lesions are rare, making up 5% to 10% of knee lesions.[95] The defect is most commonly located in the distal half of the patella.[60,95] Desai et al.[95] reported that more than 85% of lesions are found in the inferomedial area of the patella. The incidence of bilateral lesions is approximately 20% and is more common in males in their second and third decades.[60]

Etiology

The true cause of OCD is unknown, although most theories center on an initial traumatic event followed by repetitive microtrauma that leads to subchondral delamination and sequestration on convex articular surfaces.[92,94] In evaluating the pathology of these lesions, ischemia is an overwhelming finding.[92,96,97] A number of investigators have associated macrotrauma from sport-related injuries to OCD lesions of the knee. Patellar subluxation or dislocation was associated with OCD lesions of the patella in a number of studies.[95,98,99] Another associated finding is a flattened articular surface of the patella as described by Bruns et al.[100] Although this study and others have described associations, no distinct cause of OCD of the patella can be delineated.

Diagnosis

Patients with OCD lesions in the knee often present with nonspecific, poorly localized knee pain that is related to activity. An association with recent trauma is often made by the patient but is frequently incidental. Reports of intermittent knee effusions, mechanical symptoms, or stiffness are common. The classic range has been reported as 12 to 40 years of age.[95,101,102] A familial predisposition has not been reported, although medical conditions such as chronic renal disease or malignancy have been associated with the condition.

The physical examination varies depending on the status of the lesion. Unstable lesions may result in joint effusion or limitations in range of motion. Patellar apprehension and translational testing creates discomfort in the setting of patellar OCD. Crepitus can also be appreciated in most of these patients.[103] Gait can be affected; Wilson[104] has described patients with medial femoral condyle lesions who walk with an external rotation gait. Pain has been theorized to occur in these patients when the tibial spine impinges against the lesion. Discomfort with forced internal rotation of the tibia should raise suspicion for a medial femoral condyle lesion. No connection between patellar alignment and OCD has been reported in the literature.

Standard imaging of the knee is ordered when OCD is suspected, with the addition of a tunnel view useful for lesions of the femoral condyle. Diagnosing patellar OCD can be difficult, and skyline and lateral radiographs are the most useful in making the diagnosis.[101,102] The affected area typically shows an area of lucency with subchondral sclerosis in chronic lesions. CT and MRI both provide further detail, with MRI delineating fluid in the area of the lesion and CT demonstrating regions of sclerosis. Healing defects can also be evaluated with use of these measures. Fluid shown behind a lesion on MRI is suggestive of delayed union. Finally, cartilage changes can be seen on MRI, with new sequencing techniques becoming more reliable in identifying them.

Natural History

The progression of OCD lesions is dependent on the age and maturity of the patient. Patients with open physes have the greatest potential for healing of these defects. Lesions can heal to a variable degree in adolescent patients with closing physes.[94,105-108] Mature patients often experience some degree of degenerative changes in relation to the lesion.

AUTHORS' PREFERRED TECHNIQUE

Osteochondritis Dissecans of the Patella

Traditionally, patellar OCD lesions are discovered when they produce significant anterior knee pain or mechanical symptoms. In these situations, nonoperative management may fail. A variable course of activity modifications can lead to healing of a patellar lesion, although the likelihood of success is directly related to the immaturity of the patient's skeleton. In patients with an immature skeleton, patellar defects may heal after 8 weeks of immobilization in a cast. The patient and family need to be instructed that the period for healing can be prolonged and may take up to 12 months in some persons. If a lesion is discovered incidentally, a patient with an immature skeleton should be informed of the condition and observed. Activity modifications in this subset of patients are unnecessary and should only be implemented if the lesion becomes symptomatic.[101]

Fragment excision or removal of a loose body is a common intervention for many OCD lesions. A small fragment in a non–weight-bearing portion of the knee joint can be appropriately treated in this fashion. Typically, lesions in the patella are in weight-bearing portions of the articulation.[95,102] Excision is appropriate for small lesions or fragments without appropriate subchondral bone. Chronic lesions may appear sclerotic on evaluation, and a sclerotic fragment or bed creates a poor environment for healing and typically leads to fragment excision. When this modality is chosen, an arthroscopic approach can be used. The fragment, if loose, should be located. Once it is removed, the bed of the lesion can be debrided of any fibrous tissue. Drilling or microfracture of the region can be performed to elicit a vascular response. When microfracture fails, osteochondral transplantation or autologous chondrocyte implantation can be a consideration. Numerous reports have shown that excision with base debridement can relieve pain and help patients return to their activities of daily living.[60,98,103] After the initial 6 weeks of protected weight bearing and restricted motion, full motion is allowed and strengthening is initiated.

Lesions that remain in their anatomic location (Fig. 105-17) can be treated with in situ drilling, fixation, or grafting with fixation. In situ drilling is reserved for patients for whom nonoperative management has failed. These closed, stable lesions can be approached in an antegrade or retrograde fashion. Retrograde drilling preserves the articular cartilage surface and is preferred by many clinicians.[109,110] An anterior cruciate ligament guide can be used to ensure appropriate tracking. The drill is advanced to the subchondral articular margin. The number of passes performed is dependent on the size of the lesion, with tracks being approximately 3 to 5 mm apart. With a closed stable lesion, full range of motion and closed-chain exercises are begun within a few days. Patients remain on crutches with weight bearing in extension for 4 weeks.

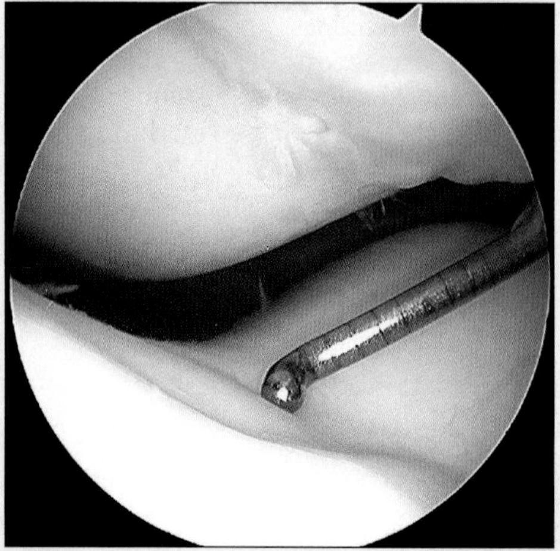

FIGURE 105-17 Osteochondritis dissecans of the trochlea (grade I).

Lesions that are in an appropriate position but unstable can be fixed in situ. At surgery, arthroscopic probing of these defects shows a closed, unstable lesion. Again, a retrograde or antegrade approach can be used for fixation. Matava and Brown[111] reported a technique in which bioabsorbable pins are used in a retrograde fashion to fix patellar OCD lesions. One limb of a ring forceps is introduced arthroscopically to stabilize the lesion. The opposite limb is placed on the skin overlying the patella and clamped to provide compression on the area. An incision is made within the ring and the pins are introduced in a retrograde fashion. Sekiya et al.[112] presented a case report with a similar retrograde technique to allow for fixation without compromising the articular surface. Antegrade techniques have also been successful and are often needed when a lack of subchondral bone is involved in the lesion. A variety of devices can be used for fixation, from darts to small metallic screws. Both metallic and biologic implants have limitations.[113,114] Outcomes of in situ fixation are related to the size of the lesion and the maturity of the patient. The postoperative rehabilitation is similar to that for in situ drilling, although the rehabilitation may progress at a slower rate.

In situ bone grafting with fixation is used for lesions that are unstable and that provide a window for access to the subchondral bone. In these cases where the lesion is open and loss is observed, an autologous bone graft can be placed in the defect. Appropriate debridement of fibrous tissue at the base is first performed, followed by placement of the graft. Weight bearing in extension with crutches for 6 to 8 weeks is recommended. Advancement in strengthening and return to athletic activities is graduated thereafter.

Open reduction and internal fixation is reserved for large, unstable lesions that are partially or completely detached. The fragment must have potential for healing without significant evidence of sclerosis. The base of the lesion also must show some evidence of healing potential after debridement of any fibrous tissue. Lesions without macroscopic evidence of healthy articular cartilage should not be replaced. The fragment can then be fixed to its original position using a variety of devices. Both retrograde and antegrade techniques are appropriate for fixation. Kocher et al.[115] have reported an 85% rate of success with operative fixation in juvenile patients with OCD of the knee. Although patients had mostly condylar lesions, the significance of this study was found when investigating lesions that were fully detached. All six fully detached lesions healed with fixation. Clinicians therefore should reconsider fragment excision or removal carefully in this subset of patients for large lesions. The rehabilitation protocol for open reduction and internal fixation is similar to that of in situ fixation as mentioned earlier.

Salvage techniques for problematic OCD lesions of the patella include osteochondral grafting, autologous chondrocyte implantation (ACI), and mosaicplasty (Fig. 105-18). These interventions are performed in patients who have large symptomatic unstable lesions that are unsalvageable. Some recent evidence has emerged that ACI may improve short-term function in adolescents and young adults with patellofemoral OCD.[116-118] Additionally, recent evidence of the benefit of mosaicplasty in patellar lesions has emerged.[119] However, only one of these studies reported follow-up beyond 26 months.[118] Although they offer potential benefits compared with other treatments, ACI and mosaicplasty for patellofemoral chondral injuries have been disappointing when compared with condylar interventions.

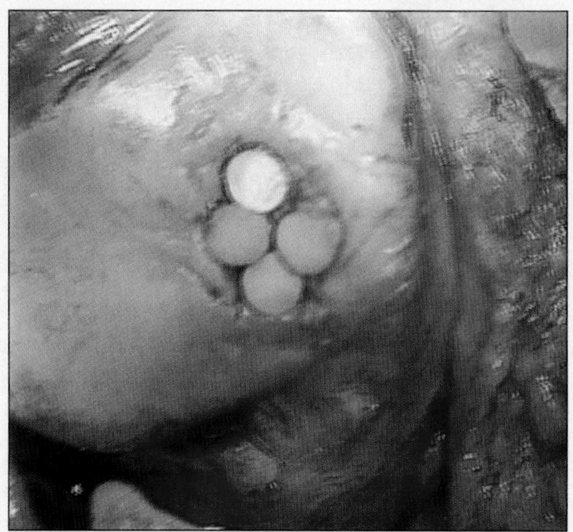

FIGURE 105-18 Osteochondritis dissecans defect of the patella treated with osteochondral transplantation.

Tendinopathies

For information on tendinopathies, see Chapter 106.

Complex Regional Pain Syndrome

Reflex sympathetic dystrophy was suggested as a cause of some anterior knee pain by Merchant[10] in 1988. Specific to anterior knee pain, scintigraphy has been demonstrated to aid in the diagnosis of sympathetically mediated pain, and a sympathetic blockade may be a useful treatment modality.[120] The discussion of complex regional pain syndrome is beyond the scope of this chapter, but it is an important consideration in the differential diagnosis for chronic patellofemoral pain and is discussed in greater length in Chapter 23.

For a complete list of references, go to expertconsult.com.

Suggested Readings

Citation: Dye SF: The pathophysiology of patellofemoral pain: A tissue homeostasis perspective. *Clin Orthop Relat Res* 436:100–110, 2005.

Level of Evidence: V

Summary: In this article, the authors evaluate the perspective that tissue homeostasis such as intraosseous hypertension is the etiology of patellofemoral pain in contrast to structural abnormalities.

Citation: Dye SF, Vaupel GL, Dye CC: Conscious neurosensory mapping of the internal structures of the human knee without intraarticular anesthesia. *Am J Sports Med* 26(6):773–777, 1998.

Level of Evidence: V

Summary: In this article, the authors report the case of a physician who underwent knee arthroscopy without use of an anesthetic, and the degree of noxious stimulus in various locations is noted.

Citation: Kodali P, Islam A, Andrish J: Anterior knee pain in the young athlete: diagnosis and treatment. *Sports Med Arthrosc* 19(1):27–33.

Level of Evidence: V

Summary: In this review article, the various etiologies and treatments of anterior knee pain are discussed.

Citation: Pihlajamaki HK, Visuri TI: Long-term outcome after surgical treatment of unresolved Osgood-Schlatter disease in young men: Surgical technique. *J Bone Joint Surg Am* 92A(Suppl 1 Pt 2):258–264.

Level of Evidence: IV

Summary: In this article, a case series is described with follow-up of patients with Osgood-Schlatter disease who did not respond to conservative management and subsequently underwent operative intervention. In this series, 87% of subjects had no activity limitation with activities of daily living and 75% returned to their preoperative athletic level.

Citation: Witvrouw E, Lysens R, Bellemans J, et al: Intrinsic risk factors for the development of anterior knee pain in an athletic population. A two-year prospective study. *Am J Sports Med* 28(4):480–489, 2000.

Level of Evidence: II

Summary: In this description of a prospective cohort study, 282 athletic patients were followed up to evaluate risk factors for anterior knee pain. The authors noted a significant correlation between the incidence of patellofemoral pain and patients with a shortened quadriceps muscle, an altered vastus medialis obliquus muscle reflex response time, decreased explosive strength, and a hypermobile patella.

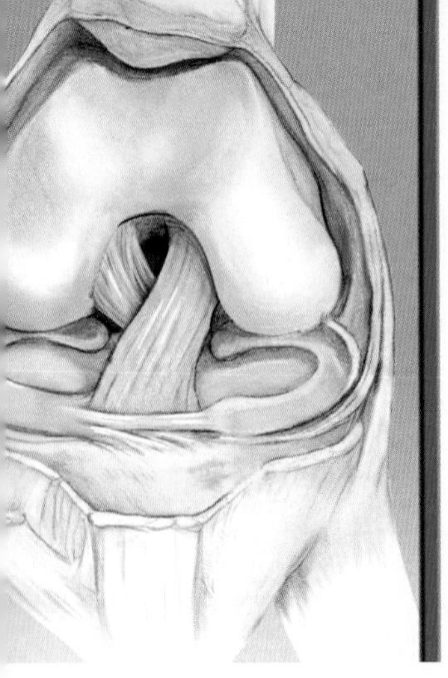

106

Extensor Mechanism Injuries of the Knee

MICHAEL J. GRIESSER • WAQAS M. HUSSAIN • BRETT W. McCOY • RICHARD D. PARKER

Patellar and Quadriceps Tendinopathies and Ruptures

The patellofemoral articulation encounters one of the highest joint reaction forces in the body. Competent patellar and quadriceps tendons are essential for proper function, and these structures contribute to the extensor mechanism. It is important to have a firm understanding of the anatomy and biomechanics of this complex to provide a rationale for sound treatment.

Disease of the extensor mechanism tendons may manifest as tendinosis, tendinitis, or rupture. An orthopaedist must have a thorough understanding of the pathophysiology of these structures because a correct and prompt diagnosis influences treatment options and resultant rates of success. Tendinopathies can occur in the presence of systemic diseases and endocrinopathy and in conjunction with certain medications and hormonal supplementation. As a result, it is important to not only understand the classic presentation of problems affecting these structures but also to maintain a wide diagnostic differential when evaluating these problems.

Advances in imaging continue to assist in the evaluation and treatment of disease. An understanding of the techniques and anticipated radiographic features of these methods is essential. In combination with clinical findings, these studies may not only confirm pathology but can offer options for therapeutic measures and surgical planning.

Extensor mechanism problems affect both adults and children. Certain injuries are more likely to be found in particular age groups and populations. Treatment options in each of these groups depend on age, activity, and diagnosis. Operative and nonoperative treatment plans can be tailored based on these characteristics, and an effective physician must understand the options and indications for both.

Athletes with extensor mechanism injuries often ask, "When can I return to play?" Thus it is important for each sports medicine physician to have an activity-specific understanding of the stresses and effects on healing related to exercise.

Relevant Anatomy and Biomechanics

Anterior knee pain is one of the most common clinical complaints in all age groups and can affect as many as 25% of athletes. The extensor mechanism is composed of the quadriceps, patella, and patellar tendon (or patellar ligament) because of its function of connecting bone to bone. To minimize confusion, the structure are uniformly referred to as the *patellar tendon* throughout this chapter. Pathology and disability can be derived from any of these structures, as well as the corresponding articular surfaces on the underlying patella and the complementary trochlear groove.

The patella has static stabilizers, including the quadriceps and patellar tendon; osseous anatomy created by the congruence of the patella within the trochlear groove; medial and lateral retinacular structures; and associated ligaments, including the medial patellofemoral (MPFL) and patellomeniscal ligaments. Desio et al.[1] have elaborately described the MPFL and its influence on restraint from lateral subluxation at 20 degrees of knee flexion.

The patella is also surrounded by dynamic stabilizers, which work together to yield balance and function. These structures include the rectus femoris, vastus lateralis, vastus intermedius, and vastus medialis, including the vastus medialis obliquus. Each of these muscles is innervated by the femoral nerve, which is composed of the posterior divisions of the second, third, and fourth lumbar spinal nerves. The direct head of the rectus femoris originates at the anterior inferior iliac spine, whereas the reflected head begins superior to the acetabulum.[2,3] It therefore crosses both the hip and knee and can serve to flex the thigh and extend the lower leg. The remaining three muscles of the quadriceps femoris include the vastus lateralis, which originates from the lateral lip of the linea aspera and lateral surface of the greater trochanter; the vastus intermedius, which originates from the anterior aspect of the femoral shaft; and the vastus medialis, which originates from the medial lip of the linea aspera and the distal aspect of the intertrochanteric line.

The quadriceps tendon is a confluence of these individual insertions and attaches to the proximal pole of the patella, enveloping it on three sides as it advances from proximal to distal. The tendon has an ample vascular supply but contains an avascular portion in the deep aspect of the tendon that measures approximately 1.5 × 3 cm.[4] Arteries from the descending branches of the lateral femoral circumflex, the descending geniculate, and the medial and lateral superior geniculate arteries provide the tendon with nourishment.[2,3,5]

The patellar tendon is a continuation of the quadriceps tendon beyond the distal pole of the patella and inserts on the tibial tuberosity.[3,5,6] The blood supply of the patellar tendon is not as rich as that of the quadriceps. Nonetheless, it is supplied by vessels from the infrapatellar fat pad, as

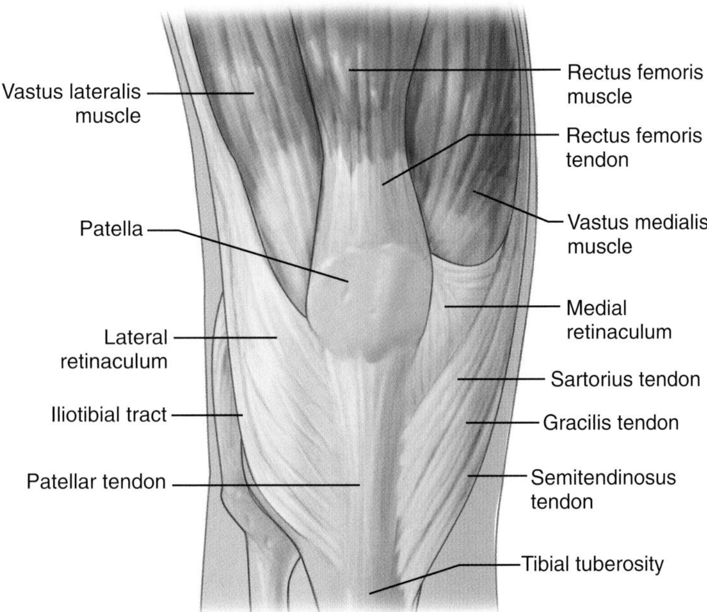

FIGURE 106-1 Normal anatomy of the extensor mechanism of the knee. *(Modified from Matava MJ: Patellar tendon ruptures.* J Am Acad Orthop Surg *4[6]:287–296, 1996.)*

well as the inferior medial and lateral geniculate arteries (Fig. 106-1).

Biomechanics

The knee consists of three compartments: the medial and lateral femorotibial and the patellofemoral articulations or joints. The patella increases the extensor moment arm by transmitting the longitudinal contractile force at a greater distance from the knee axis of rotation (Fig. 106-2).[7] The efficiency of the extensor mechanism increases 1.5 times through this advantage. Patellofemoral contact initiates at 10 degrees of flexion and shifts distally to proximally with increasing degrees of flexion (Fig. 106-3).[7] Weakness of the quadriceps musculature can lead to increased stress and strain throughout the tendons. Ascending stairs can increase forces within the patellar tendon by 3.2 times body weight, and the greatest forces on the structure occur at about 60 degrees of knee flexion.[5,8,9]

Huberti and colleagues[10] described a concept referred to as the *extensor mechanism force ratio*. This ratio is the fraction of the force found in the patellar tendon (distal) divided by the quadriceps tendon (proximal)[5,10] and is greater than 1.0 when the knee is in less than 45 degrees of flexion. With smaller degrees of flexion, the distal pole of the patella is articulating with the trochlear groove. At this point, the quadriceps tendon has a mechanical advantage. Conversely, with knee flexion angles greater than 45 degrees, the patellar articulation with the trochlea is more proximal and allows for the patellar tendon to have the primary mechanical advantage.[5,10] This concept explains the position of knee flexion related to the likelihood of tendon failure. At a position of knee flexion less than 45 degrees, the quadriceps tendon is more likely to be injured. On the other hand, with the extremity in greater than 45 degrees of flexion, the patellar tendon is at higher risk for tensile failure.

Tendon Structure

Tendon is a complex material consisting of collagen fibrils embedded in a matrix of proteoglycans. Both quadriceps and patellar tendons are mainly composed of water in the extracellular matrix. However, the predominant cell type found within tendons is the fibroblast. This cell is present in the spaces between the parallel collagen bundles (Fig. 106-4).[9]

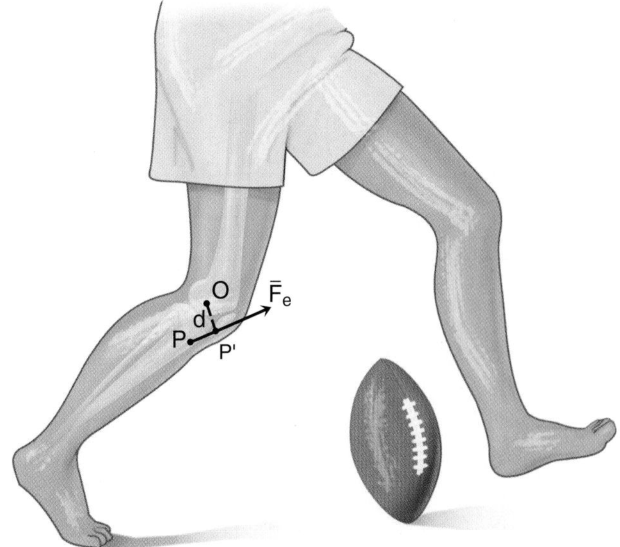

FIGURE 106-2 Patellar biomechanics.

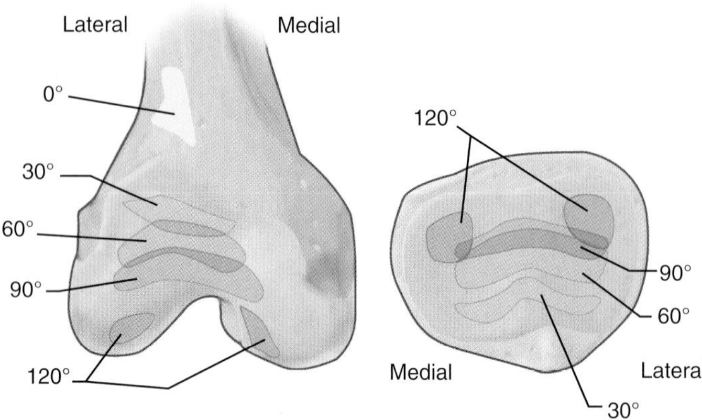

FIGURE 106-3 Patellar contact areas according to degrees of knee flexion. *(From Scott WN, editor:* Insall & Scott Surgery of the Knee, *ed 5, Phladelphia: 2012, Elsevier.)*

Tendon is composed primarily of type I collagen and contains a high concentration of glycine, proline, and hydroxyproline.[9] The secondary structure of collagen is related to the arrangement of each chain in a left-handed configuration. The tertiary structure refers to three collagen chains combined into a collagen molecule. Likewise, the quaternary structure is related to the organization of collagen molecules into a stable, low-energy biologic unit based on the association of its amino acids with adjacent molecules. This quarter-stagger arrangement of adjacent collagen molecules results in oppositely charged amino acids being aligned.[9] A great deal of energy is required to separate these molecules, accounting for the overall strength of this structure (Fig. 106-5).

Tendon possesses one of the highest tensile strengths of any soft tissue in the human body for two reasons. First, it is composed of collagen, which is one of the strongest fibrous proteins in the body. Second, tendon collagen fibers are arranged parallel to the direction of the tensile force.[9] The elastic modulus of human tendon ranges from 1200 to 1800 megapascals (MPa), the ultimate tensile strength ranges from 50 to 105 MPa, and the ultimate strain ranges from 9% to 35%.[9]

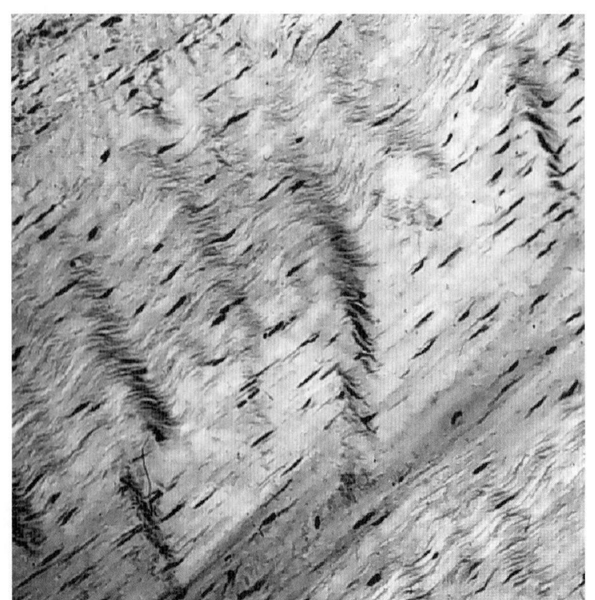

FIGURE 106-4 Histologic features of a normal patellar tendon with the typical collagen crimp pattern.

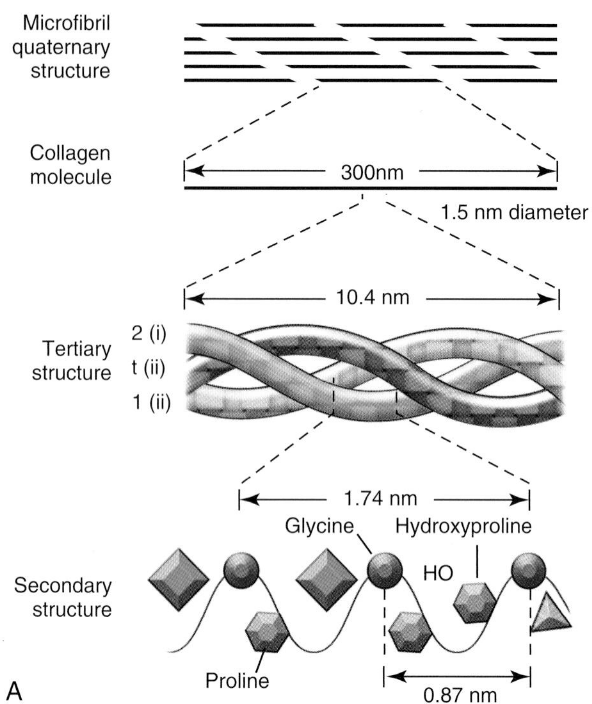

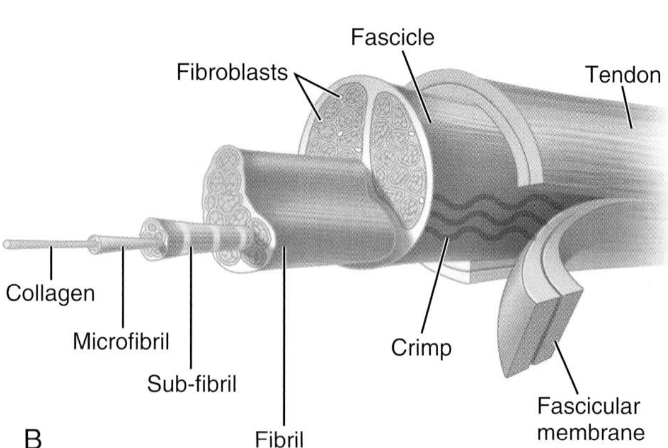

FIGURE 106-5 Schematic drawings of the structural organization of collagen into the microfibril. *(Modified from Woo SL, An KN, Arnoczky SP, et al: Anatomy, biology, and biomechanics of tendon and ligament. In Buckwalter JA, Einhorn TA, Simon SR, editors:* Orthopaedic basic science: Foundations of clinical practice, *Rosemont, IL, 2007, American Academy of Orthopaedic Surgeons.)*

Pathophysiology of Tendon Injury

The specific details of tendon injury continue to be investigated. Tendons can become injured as a result of direct trauma with laceration or contusion or indirect trauma through tensile overload. However, it is generally accepted that healthy tendons do not rupture. In a situation in which there is tensile overload of the extensor mechanism, the forces most often result in a transverse fracture of the patella.[11]

Research into the understanding of tendinopathy continues to advance, but it remains one of the most difficult challenges in sports medicine to manage. Its pathogenesis consists of repetitive chronic overloading, ischemia with reperfusion injury, microtrauma, hypoxia, aging, and hyperthermia. These factors can be correlated with skeletal maturity, anatomic location, vascularity, and magnitude of applied forces.

Most tendons are able to withstand tensile forces larger than those exerted by muscles or sustained by bones. Therefore these types of injuries often result in avulsion fractures or tendon disruption at the musculotendinous junction.[9] Midsubstance tendon ruptures are less commonly seen and often occur within the context of preexisting pathology. Kannus and Jozsa[12] studied specimens obtained from the biopsy of spontaneously ruptured Achilles or biceps tendons in 891 patients. Age- and sex-matched control specimens were obtained for comparison, and no normal structures were seen in spontaneously ruptured tendons.[12] Characteristic histopathologic patterns in the ruptured tendons included hypoxic degenerative tendinopathy, mucoid degeneration, tendolipomatosis, and calcifying tendinopathy, either in isolation or combination.[12,13] These changes were also found in 34% of the control tendons, which is less often than in pathologic specimens.

Mechanical testing performed on the patellar tendon has shown tensile strains to be less midsubstance than at the origin and insertion sites on the patella and tibial tuberosity.[9,14] Woo et al.[9,14] demonstrated that at peak load just prior to tendon failure, the end-region strain at the insertion site is three to four times than that seen in the mid body. Thus healthy tendon rarely fails within its substance,[5,9,14] and if this occurs, the physician must consider external factors such as metabolic derangements (Box 106-1).

Metabolic abnormalities have been shown to influence the physiologic status and biomechanical function of tendons. These conditions can be innate, induced, or iatrogenic. Conditions such as diabetes mellitus can compromise the blood supply and limit the reparative ability of a structure after injury. Metabolic conditions such as gout, renal failure, hypothyroidism, and chondrocalcinosis can lead to tendinopathy and ruptures.[15-22] Also, local and systemic corticosteroid injections have been shown to limit the inflammatory phase of healing.[23] Tendon ruptures have been documented after the administration of these agents.[24]

Other drugs have been associated with tendon disease. Fluoroquinolone antibiotics, such as levofloxacin and ciprofloxacin, have been shown to alter the extracellular matrix in tendons and can influence healing after injury.[25,26] Ciprofloxacin also induces interleukin-1β–mediated matrix metalloproteinase-3 release.[27,28] Matrix metalloproteinases are a family of proteolytic enzymes that have the ability to degrade the extracellular matrix network and facilitate tissue remodeling.[29-31] Fluoroquinolones can also inhibit tenocyte metabolism, reducing cell proliferation and collagen and matrix synthesis.[25,32] Additionally, investigations have noted decreased biomechanical properties of healing patellar tendon with administration of antiinflammatory drugs compared with acetaminophen and controls.[33]

BOX 106-1 Conditions Associated with Occult Tendinopathy

Hyperparathyroidism
Calcium pyrophosphate deposition
Diabetes mellitus
Steroid-induced tendinopathy
Fluoroquinolone-induced tendinopathy
Osteomalacia
Chronic renal insufficiency
Gout
Uremia
Systemic lupus erythematosus
Rheumatoid arthritis

Cyclic tensile loading of tendons is required to maintain normal tendon health.[13] This repetitive mechanical loading of a tendon leads to a cellular response that can either be adequate, leading to adaptation, or inadequate, leading to transient weakness. This process is referred to as *mechanobiology* or *mechanotransduction* and couples tendon stretch with a cellular biologic response. Excessive mechanical stretch stimulates an anabolic response, whereas normal stimuli promote a catabolic response. Continued loading in the face of a weakened tendon can lead to an accumulation of injury, thus inhibiting the healing capacity and resulting in an overuse injury.[13] The adaptive and reparative ability of tendon can be overcome when it is repeatedly strained at 4% to 8% of its original length.[5] This stress may result in microscopic or macroscopic injuries to the collagen fibrils, noncollagenous matrix, and microvasculature, resulting in inflammation, edema, and pain.[5]

Tendon pathology has been defined in terms of *tendinitis* and *tendinosis*. Tendinitis refers to the presence of inflammatory cells, which can be noted on histologic evaluation. Early pathologic alterations that occur in the presence of repetitive microtrauma to the patellar tendon include inflammatory cell invasion, resultant tissue edema, and fibrin exudation in the paratenon,[5] which is referred to as *paratenonitis*. Maffulli and colleagues[27,28] recommended use of the term *tendinopathy* as a generic descriptor of these clinical conditions described in Table 106-1. They believe that the terms *tendinosis* and *tendinitis* should be reserved for use after histopathologic examination.[27,28] Continued microtrauma can overwhelm reparative capabilities, leading to chronic inflammation. This process results in fibrosis and thickening of the paratenon and chronic peritendinitis. The development of tendinosis is thought to result from chronic peritendinitis and is characterized by histopathologic findings of mucoid degeneration, tendolipomatosis, and calcifying tendinopathy, either alone or in combination.[12,13]

Yuan et al.[34] and Cook et al.[35] presented evidence that the earliest identifiable morphologic changes in tendinosis occur in tenocytes and not collagen fibers. Microscopic evaluation of degenerative tendons demonstrate a paucity of inflammatory cells, tenocyte morphology and density changes, accumulation of glycosaminoglycans, and collagen fiber thinning and disarray with or without neurovascular proliferation.[13,35-40]

Apoptosis may also play a significant role in tendinosis. Yuan et al.[34] demonstrated excessive apoptosis in ruptured human rotator cuff specimens. Likewise, Lian et al.[36] performed a similar study on biopsy specimens in patients with patellar tendinopathy diagnosed clinically and confirmed with magnetic resonance image (MRI). They found that the samples with tendinopathy displayed increased cellularity

TABLE 106-1

CLASSIFICATION OF TENDON DISORDERS

New	Old	Definition	Histologic Findings	Clinical Signs and Symptoms
Paratenonitis	Tenosynovitis Tenovaginitis Peritendinitis	Inflammation of only the paratenon whether or not it is lined by synovium	Inflammatory cells in paratenon or peritendinous areolar tissue	Cardinal inflammatory signs: warmth, swelling, pain, crepitation, local tenderness, and dysfunction
Paratenonitis with tendinosis	Tendinitis	Paratenon inflammation associated with intratendinous degeneration	Same as above, with loss of tendon, collagen fiber disorientation, and scattered vascular ingrowth but no prominent intratendinous inflammation	Same as above, often with a palpable tendon nodule, swelling, and inflammatory signs
Tendinosis	Tendinitis	Intratendinous degeneration due to atrophy (e.g., aging, microtrauma, or vascular compromise)	Noninflammatory intratendinous collagen degeneration with fiber disorientation, hypocellularity, scattered vascular ingrowth, occasional local necrosis, or calcification	Often a palpable tendon nodule that may be asymptomatic but may also be point tender; swelling of the tendon sheath is absent
	Tendon strain or tear	Symptomatic overload of the tendon with vascular disruption and inflammatory repair response	Three recognized subgroups: each displays variable histologic characteristics from purely inflammation with acute hemorrhage and tear to inflammation superimposed on preexisting degeneration, to calcification and tendinosis changes in chronic conditions; in the chronic stage, it may be (1) interstitial microinjury, (2) central tendon necrosis, (3) frank partial rupture, or (4) acute complete rupture	Symptoms are inflammatory and proportional to vascular disruption, hematoma, or atrophy-related cell necrosis; symptom duration defines each subgroup: A: Acute (<2 wk) B: Subacute (4-6 wk) C: Chronic (>6 wk)

compared with controls and also contained a higher number of apoptotic cells.[36]

Evaluation of Quadriceps and Patellar Tendinosis

History

Isolated quadriceps tendinopathy has not been well described in the contemporary literature and is often mentioned in the context of bilateral involvement due to underlying medical comorbidity. A few reports have been made of sequelae due to calcific tendinitis leading to chronic enthesopathic changes, and in some cases, bilateral tendon rupture.[41] Likewise, as we further detail in this chapter when discussing the treatment of patellar tendon disease, Doppler ultrasound-guided sclerosing agents have also been explored as investigative options for treating bilateral quadriceps tendinopathy.[42]

Most publications describing extensor mechanism pathology focus on the patellar tendon. Patellar tendinosis, or jumper's knee, results from microtears of the patellar tendon followed by a chronic inflammatory response. It is an injury that follows excessive use and is commonly seen in athletes who participate in sports that involve jumping, kicking, or leaping, such as volleyball and basketball.[43] Thus it is important to obtain a history of athletic activity from each patient.

Zwerver et al.[44] noted that in nonelite athletes the prevalence of jumper's knee varied between 14.4% and 2.5% for different sports, and males were twice as likely to be affected. They also identified sport-specific loading characteristics, a higher body weight, a taller stature, and younger age as risk factors for the development of patellar tendinitis.[44] Lian et al.[45] studied the prevalence of jumper's knee among elite athletes and demonstrated the likelihood of developing tendinopathy while participating in various sports. Cyclists had a zero incidence, whereas male basketball and volleyball players demonstrated a prevalence of 32% and 44%, respectively. Players routinely exhibited symptoms lasting longer than 2 years, and affected athletes had significant pain and functional losses.[45] Hägglund et al.[46] recently studied the epidemiology of patellar tendinopathy in elite male soccer players. Between 2001 and 2009, the investigators followed up on 51 European soccer clubs from the Swedish First and European Football Associations Champions leagues; 1.5% of all injuries consisted of patellar tendinopathies, and each season, 2.4% of players were affected. Additionally, the investigators noted no significant differences with regard to prevalence or incidence between play on artificial or natural turf.[46]

Ferretti et al.[47,48] demonstrated a linear relationship between training volume and the prevalence of tendinopathy among volleyball players. They also demonstrated a higher prevalence of tendinopathy among players who trained on a harder surface. Backman and Danielson[49] performed a 1-year prospective study investigating the correlation between low ankle dorsiflexion range and an increased risk of patellar tendinitis in junior elite basketball players. They postulated that a decrease in ankle motion may predispose players to the development of tendinitis because of higher level compensatory energy absorbed by the patellar tendon. They concluded that low ankle dorsiflexion is a risk factor for the development of tendinitis in basketball players and that 36.5 degrees was found to be the best cutoff in regard to screening for persons at risk.[49]

Symptoms may occur in young adults undergoing a rapid phase in growth. In these cases, a relative discrepancy in tendon length may be found compared with adjacent bony structures. This finding occurs when the tendon does not lengthen as quickly as the bones to which it is attached.[43]

Commonly, patients report discomfort in the distribution of the patellar tendon. Traditionally, pain in persons with tendinopathy has been attributed to inflammation. However, Khan et al.[50] reported that chronically painful Achilles and patellar tendons showed no evidence of inflammation, and many tendons with intratendinous lesions detected on MRI or ultrasound were asymptomatic. Different causes have been proposed to explain the origin of pain in degenerative tendons, including elevated concentrations of glutamate, prostaglandin E_2,[51-54] and substance P[55,56] in symptomatic persons.

Physical Examination

A patient may have tenderness over the patellar tendon and signs of inflammation, such as redness, swelling, warmth, and crepitation. Pain is often centered on the distal patellar pole and the proximal part of the patellar tendon. Tenderness to palpation may be present with the knee in extension and absent with the knee in flexion. The patient may have a feeling of "bogginess" centered over the tendon itself[5] and may also have pain with resisted extension and with full passive flexion.[43]

Blazina et al.[57] established a classification for patellar tendinopathy. In stage 1, pain is present only after activity. In stage 2, pain is present at the beginning of activity, disappears after a warm-up, but may reappear with fatigue. In stage 3, pain is constant, both at rest and with activity. In stage 4, the patellar tendon is completely ruptured.[5,57]

Imaging

Imaging is not routinely necessary for the treatment of patellar or quadriceps tendinosis. However, plain radiographs should be obtained in the initial evaluation of all patients with patellar tendinitis. One should be alert for the presence of traction osteophytes at the distal pole of the patella, tendon calcification, and even decreased bone mineral density at the sites of attachment. Other modalities such as ultrasound and MRI are used when nonoperative treatments have failed to produce anticipated improvements or when planning surgical intervention. Ultrasound evaluations can demonstrate a hypoechoic signal within the fibers of the patellar tendon.[43,58] Warden et al.[59] performed MRI and grayscale and color Doppler ultrasound on 30 patients with clinically diagnosed patellar tendinopathy and 33 activity-matched asymptomatic control subjects. These investigators concluded that ultrasonography was more accurate than MRI in confirming clinically diagnosed patellar tendinopathy. They added that combining grayscale and color Doppler ultrasound best confirms clinically diagnosed patellar tendinopathy because of the high sensitivity of grayscale and the strong likelihood that symptomatic persons would demonstrate a positive color Doppler test (Fig. 106-6).[59]

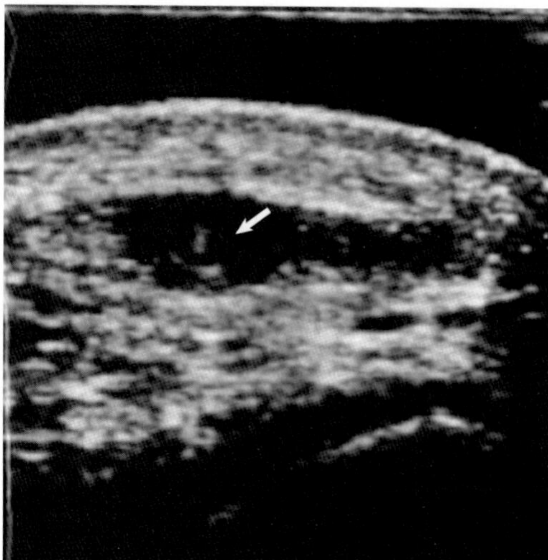

FIGURE 106-6 Ultrasound of a knee and patellar tendon. The *arrow* points to a hypoechoic region of the patellar tendon.

Sagittal MRI may demonstrate thickening of the patellar tendon, especially on the posterior, central, or medial aspects (Fig. 106-7).[60,61] MRI may also demonstrate foci of abnormal signal intensity in the posterior portion of the proximal patellar tendon (Fig. 106-8). Furthermore, absence of abnormality on T2-weighted images can suggest that nonoperative treatments may be more effective.[5]

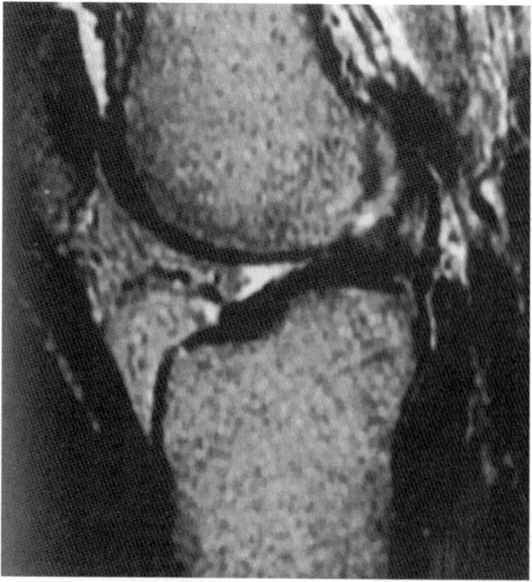

FIGURE 106-7 A magnetic resonance image of the knee showing thickening of the patellar tendon.

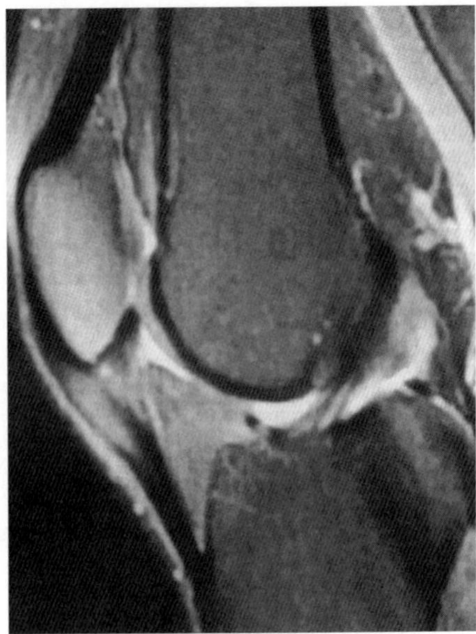

FIGURE 106-8 A magnetic resonance image of the knee showing high signal intensity within the tendon.

Treatment Options

Nonoperative

Various recommendations have been suggested in the management of acute and chronic tendon disorders. However, few well-constructed studies have been performed to demonstrate the efficacy of these treatments. Initial management includes activity modification, the initiation of active rest, the use of antiinflammatory medications, and the administration of cryotherapy. Stretching and isometric strengthening of the quadriceps should be started immediately.[43] However, isotonic or isokinetic exercises should only begin once symptoms have improved.

Operative

When nonoperative means have failed to produce improvement in symptoms and imaging studies confirm evidence of intratendinous degenerative changes, operative intervention may be considered. One option is to split the tendon longitudinally and excise the gelatinous material between normal fibers.[43,58] The remainder of the tendon should be closed with absorbable suture. Roels et al.[62] presented a series of 10 subjects with this technique, and all patients were able to return to sports.

Decision-Making Principles

Bahr et al.[63] performed a randomized controlled trial on surgical treatment versus eccentric training for patellar tendinopathy. Thirty-five patients (40 knees) with grade 3 patellar tendinopathy were randomly assigned to surgical or eccentric strength training. No advantage was demonstrated for operative treatment compared with eccentric exercise. The authors concluded that eccentric training should be initiated for 12 weeks before an open tenotomy is considered.[63]

When persons present with a history and physical examination consistent with patellar tendinitis, the first step is to obtain plain radiographs of the knee. We examine the images carefully for the presence of osteoarthritis, patellar malpositioning, or spur formation. However, the radiographs typically do not change our first step of treatment. We also consider obtaining an MRI of the knee based on the severity and duration of symptoms. These images help us to determine prognosis and likelihood of recovery. Patients with pain and obvious osteophyte formation at the distal pole of the patella are less likely to recover after nonoperative intervention.

After the initiation of physical therapy, a clinical reevaluation at 6 weeks is routine. This appointment is made for patient reassurance and evaluation of compliance with the treatment regimen. Correspondence with the physical therapist assists in making subsequent recommendations. Improvement at 6 weeks is a good indicator of future clinical success, but failure to improve offers no insight. A full 3 months of therapy should be completed as previously outlined to improve symptoms.

AUTHORS' PREFERRED TECHNIQUE

Patellar Tendinitis

If nonoperative interventions fail to produce clinical improvement, a discussion outlining surgical options and the risks and benefits of each procedure may be appropriate. Our preferred treatment of refractory patellar tendinitis is to perform a midline incision centered over the proximal third of the patellar tendon. We essentially perform a patellar tendon harvest with excision of the diseased portion of the tendon as if we were obtaining a tissue for an anterior cruciate ligament (ACL) reconstruction with an autologous bone–patellar tendon–bone (BTB) graft. Based on the location of the tendinopathy, we may or may not include the opposite bone-tendon interface. If disease is proximal only, we focus the harvest at this location and remove only the isolated area involved.

Postoperative Management

Postoperative management is based on the same guidelines that accompany patellar tendon repair and are outlined in the next section. These guidelines consist of early mobilization with full weight bearing after primary repair of the excised portion of the tendon.

Return to Play

Although most operatively treated injuries end an athlete's playing season, return to play the following season is common. Far more commonly, given the subacute nature of the problem, athletes are able to complete their current season with appropriate nonoperative recommendations and treatments and contemplate the necessity of surgical intervention during the off-season.

Results

Panni et al.[64] performed a clinical cohort study of 42 patients with patellar tendinopathy. After 6 months of nonoperative treatment as previously outlined, 33 patients (79%) showed symptomatic improvement and were able to return to sports.[64] Kon et al.[65] published a prospective study of 20 male athletes with a mean history of 20.7 months of pain and noted no adverse reactions and improved outcomes with the administration of platelet-rich plasma (PRP) in patients with chronic patellar tendinitis. Likewise, Gosens et al.[66] showed that patients treated with PRP injections for patellar tendinopathy displayed significant improvement, but patients previously treated with other modalities including cortisone, ethoxysclerol, or surgical management did not display significant improvement. Despite these positive results, overall concerns for lack of standardization among study protocols, delivery mechanisms, and separation techniques have generated mixed reviews regarding the efficacy of this treatment.[67] In regard to ACL reconstruction, de Almeida et al.[68] performed a prospective randomized controlled trial of 27 patients, of whom 12 received PRP in the patellar tendon donor site after graft harvest for ACL reconstruction. MRI was used to assess healing 6 months after surgery, and questionnaires were distributed. The authors concluded that PRP had a positive effect on the harvest site based on MRI and reduced pain in the immediate postoperative period.[68]

Additionally, ultrasound-guided sclerosis has also been explored as a nonoperative adjunct. Hoksrud and Bahr[69] investigated the effects of scleroring treatments for patellar tendinitis at a mean of 44 months after the procedure. They concluded that polidocanol was effective for the majority of patients, but one third of their subjects elected to seek additional treatment through arthroscopic surgery during the study period.[69] After this investigation, Hoksrud et al.[70] also performed an additional prospective trial investigating sclerosing treatment on patellar tendon pain and function in 101 patients. They recruited subjects clinically diagnosed with jumper's knee and neovascularization evident on power Doppler ultrasound in areas corresponding with pain. The subjects received up to a maximum of five ultrasound-guided injections of polidocanol at 4- to 6-week periods. The authors concluded that the treatment resulted in moderate improvement in knee function and pain. Despite this benefit, they noted that the majority of patients continued to have reduced function and significant pain 2 years after treatment.[70]

Clarke et al.[71] have recently investigated the use of the injection of laboratory-amplified tenocyte-like cells for the treatment of patellar tendinopathy. They studied 60 patellar tendons in 46 patients with refractory symptoms and compared the outcomes of injecting collagen-producing cells derived from dermal fibroblasts suspended in plasma with plasma alone. They concluded that injection of the skin-derived tendonlike cells is a safe option for short-term treatment of patellar tendinopathy and demonstrated greater improvement in pain and function compared with plasma alone.[71]

Panni et al.[64] treated nine patients with Blazina stage 3 tendinopathy who had not responded to nonoperative management with surgical removal of degenerative tendon, placement of multiple longitudinal tenotomies, and drilling of the distal pole of the patella. At a mean of 4.8 years, clinical results were good to excellent in all patients.[64]

Shelbourne et al.[72] performed a similar study investigating 16 elite athletes with 22 symptomatic and MRI-documented cases of patellar tendinitis who did not respond to nonoperative management. These patients underwent excision of the necrosis with placement of longitudinal cuts in the tendon to stimulate healing. Subjective improvement was noted in all 16 athletes when they were examined at a mean of 8.1 months. Fourteen of 16 patients (87.5%) were able to return to sport at the same level of intensity.[72]

Arthroscopic patellar tenotomy has been advocated based on a retrospective outcome study[73] (see Fig. 106-9 for a treatment algorithm). Likewise, arthroscopic debridement has also recently been investigated. Pascarella et al.[74] noted that although open surgery is typically recommended for persons who have not responded to nonsurgical management, arthroscopy may be considered a safe and effective option. They studied 73 knees in 64 patients (of whom 27 were professional athletes) who underwent debridement of Hoffa's body posterior to the patellar tendon, debridement of the abnormal tendon, and excision of the distal pole of the patella. The investigators concluded that arthroscopic surgery provided significant improvement with regard to symptoms and function with maintained benefits for at least 3 years. However, they also noted that some patients were unable to return to sport at their preinjury level, and even if they did, they participated with symptoms.[74]

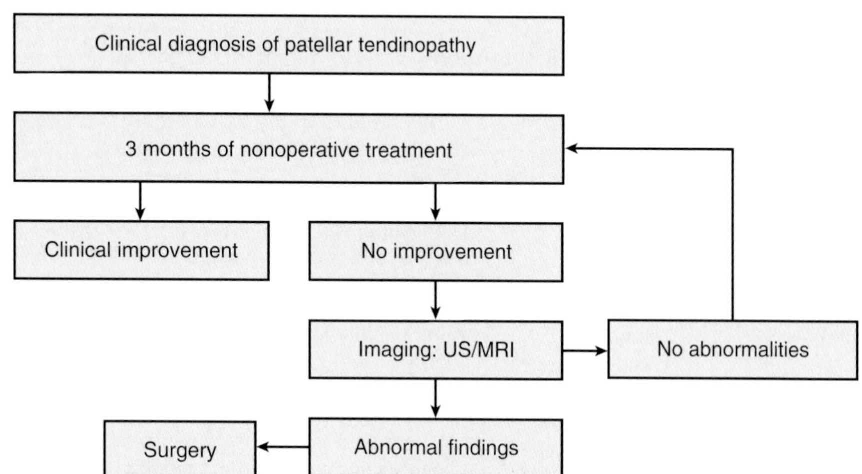

FIGURE 106-9 Treatment algorithm for patellar tendinopathy. *US,* Ultrasound; MRI, magnetic resonance imaging.

Complications

Complications can occur, and as with most surgical procedures, include considerations such as infection, stiffness, pain refractory to treatment, and the need for further surgery. Most of these complications can be minimized with meticulous surgical technique and appropriate rehabilitation principles.

Future Considerations

Other investigative modalities include extracorporeal shockwave therapy, pulsed magnetic fields, direct current applied to tendons, laser therapy, radiofrequency ablation, administration of cytokines and growth factors, gene therapy, bone morphogenic protein–12, gene transfers, and tissue engineering with mesenchymal stem cells.[27]

Recently, PRP therapies have attracted great attention and offer an additional nonsurgical option for treatment of tendinitis. Emerging research focusing on patellar tendinitis has yielded promising outcomes.

Classification of Quadriceps and Patellar Tendon Ruptures

Although ruptures of the patellar and quadriceps tendons occur with relative infrequency, they are serious injuries that require surgical intervention in an effort to restore essential function. Ruptures in patellar tendons are thought to occur less frequently than in quadriceps tendons.[75] They are usually seen in patients younger than 40 years,[76] whereas quadriceps ruptures are more common in patients older than 40 years and are often associated with underlying medical conditions. Galen is credited with first describing a patient with a ruptured extensor mechanism. This injury was sustained as a result of a "wrestling match."[76] McBurney was the first to publish a single case in 1887.[76] He described a 50-year-old man who was struck by the edge of a heavy box just above the patella. The patient's ruptured quadriceps tendon was sutured successfully with catgut and silver wire.[76]

Spontaneous ruptures tend to occur in elderly patients with minimal trauma as a result of degenerative changes related to aging.[77] Additionally, preexisting medical problems such as chronic steroid use,[78] rheumatoid arthritis, and diabetes mellitus may act as predisposing factors.[79] Anabolic steroid use is also associated with an increased risk for tendon ruptures.[80-82] Recently, an association between androstenediol supplements and tendon rupture was presented.[82]

In addition, polymorphisms in genes coding for collagen may be implicated in tendon rupture. Galasso et al.[83] described a case report of a patient with collagen type V alpha 1 polymorphism who incurred spontaneous, simultaneous quadriceps tendon ruptures. Compared with three sex- and age-matched control subjects, histologic analysis of his tissue revealed a significant reduction in type V collagen and an alteration in collagen structure.[83]

Patellar tendon rupture is the third most common cause of disruption of the extensor mechanism of the knee, following patellar fracture and quadriceps tendon rupture.[78] Zernicke et al.[84] estimated that a force of 17.5 times body weight is required to cause rupture in healthy patients, supporting the notion that normal tendons do not tear.

It is important to establish prompt diagnoses for patellar and quadriceps tendon disruptions because of the consequences of neglected injuries. Accentuated scar tissue formation, tendon shortening and retraction, and muscular atrophy are all problems encountered with chronic tears.[75,76,78,85,86]

No widely accepted classification system exists for patellar tendon or quadriceps tendon ruptures. Clinically, it is helpful to group them based on the location, configuration, and chronicity of rupture (Table 106-2).

Evaluation of Quadriceps and Patellar Tendon Ruptures

History

Patellar and quadriceps tendon ruptures may be difficult to diagnose. Siwek and Rao[76] performed a retrospective analysis of 36 quadriceps tendon and 36 patellar tendon ruptures. They found that 38% of these injuries were initially misdiagnosed.[76,87] Diagnosis may be more difficult when the injury is accompanied by hemarthrosis, which can mask the presence

TABLE 106-2

CLASSIFICATION OF PATELLAR TENDON OR QUADRICEPS TENDON RUPTURES

Ruptured Tendon	Age Seen (yr)	Causes of Injury	Diagnosis	Treatment
Patella	Usually <40	Traumatic; underlying tendinopathy	Pain: inability to perform a straight-leg raise Radiographs: patella alta Ultrasound: gap Magnetic resonance imaging: increased signal intensity within the tendon indicating gap formation	Early primary reconstruction; if delayed diagnosis, can perform delayed reconstruction
Quadriceps	Usually >40	Traumatic; underlying tendinopathy	Pain: inability to perform a straight-leg raise Radiographs: patella baja Ultrasound: gap Magnetic resonance imaging: increased signal intensity within the tendon indicating gap formation	Early primary reconstruction; if delayed diagnosis, can perform delayed reconstruction

of a suprapatellar gap.[86] As a result, one must maintain a high index of suspicion with regard to injuries around the knee. Diagnostic failure rates of 10% to 50% have been reported, and delays in diagnosis have ranged from days to months.[76,88-90]

Bottoni et al.[87] reported that the mechanism of injury is deceleration with the knee fixed in a semiflexed posture accompanied by a strong contraction against a planted foot or lower leg. Patients with patellar tendon rupture often describe a pop or tearing sensation.[87] The pain associated with a quadriceps tendon rupture is described as an immediate, intense tearing sensation at the time of rupture.[86] Immobilization of the extremity in extension provides pain relief.

Physical Examination

Physical examination of a quadriceps tendon rupture presents with a triad of pain, inability to actively extend the knee, and a palpable suprapatellar gap.[86,89-91] Patients are unable to actively extend the knee but may be able to maintain extension against gravity through an intact retinaculum. Knee aspiration with an intraarticular local anesthetic can relieve pain and permit an adequate physical examination and diagnosis.[86] A suprapatellar gap or palpable depression just superior to the patella is pathognomonic for quadriceps tendon rupture (Fig. 106-10).[86]

Imaging

Various imaging modalities may be useful in the diagnosis of patellar and quadriceps tendon ruptures. Plain anteroposterior and lateral radiographs should be obtained initially to evaluate for fracture, osteochondral injuries, or patellar dislocations. Associated findings on radiographs may include the obliteration of the quadriceps or patellar tendon shadows, calcific densities at the proximal or distal patellar poles, and patellar height alterations due to the disruption of the tethering effect of the noninjured tendon.

The Insall-Salvati ratio has been used as a method to determine patellar height. This measurement carries higher intraobserver and interobserver variability. This ratio is calculated by dividing the patellar tendon length by the greatest diagonal distance of the bony patella and should equal 1. This measurement has a relatively low rate of reproducibility compared with other measurement techniques (Fig. 106-11).

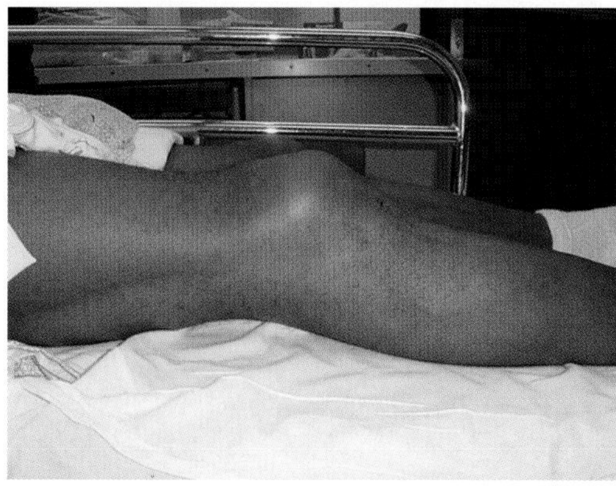

FIGURE 106-10 A patient with a rupture.

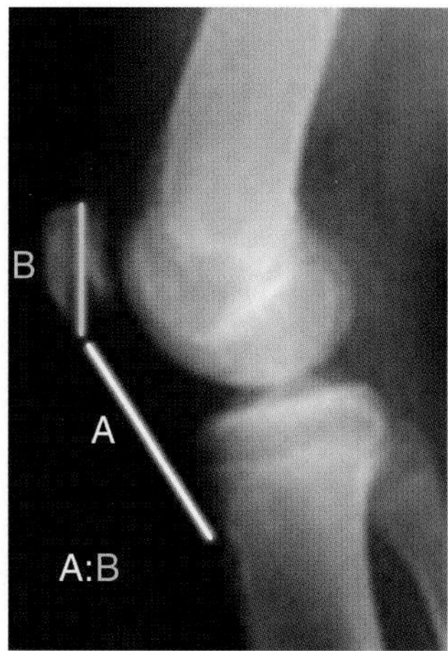

FIGURE 106-11 The Insall-Salvati ratio.

Clinically, the Blackburne-Peel method of measuring patellar height yields a lower interobserver variability and lacks positional influences because of flexion of the knee from 30 to 50 degrees.[92,93] This technique measures a perpendicular distance from a line drawn along the tibial plateau to the inferior articular margin of the patella. This length is divided with the length of the articular surface of the patella. Normal values for males and females are 0.805 and 0.806, respectively (Fig. 106-12).

With disruption of the patellar tendon, proximal migration of the patella occurs, resulting in a higher Insall-Salvati ratio (>1) and Blackburne-Peel measurement (>0.805) (Fig. 106-13). With disruption of the quadriceps tendon, a distal migration of the patella occurs, resulting in a lower Insall-Salvati ratio (<1) and Blackburne-Peel measurement (<0.805). An associated anterior tilt of the patella away from the trochlear groove may also be observed (Fig. 106-14).

High-resolution ultrasonography has been shown to be an effective means of evaluating both the patellar and quadriceps tendons in acute and chronic tendon injuries.[75,86] MRI is the most sensitive test available to evaluate the injured quadriceps and patellar tendons.[75,86] It also provides accurate information

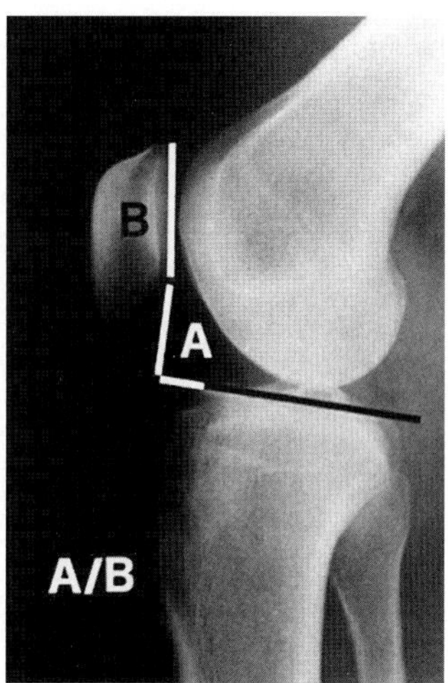

FIGURE 106-12 The Blackburne-Peel method of measuring patellar height.

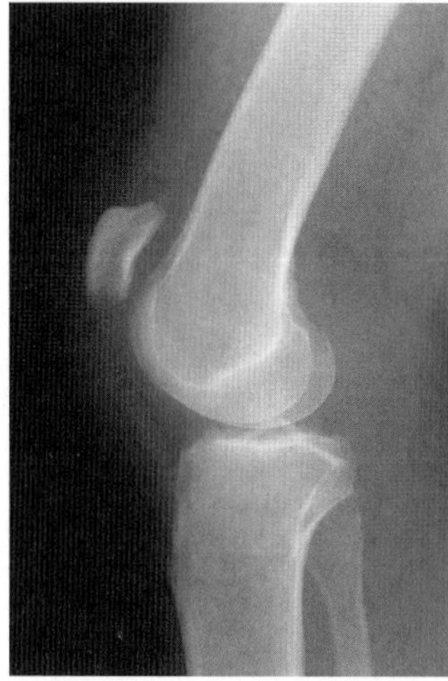

FIGURE 106-13 A lateral radiograph of a patellar tendon rupture.

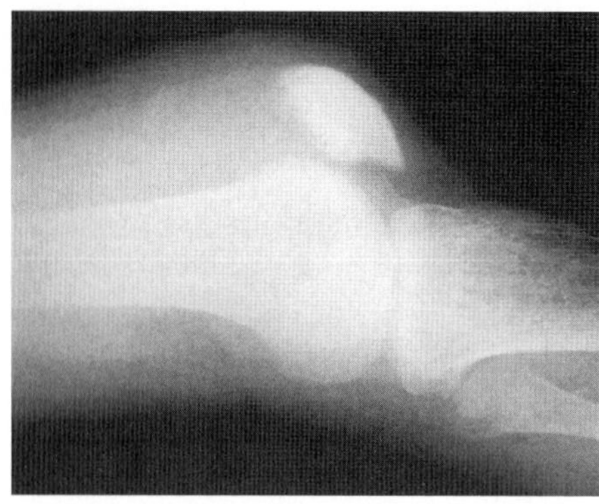

FIGURE 106-14 A lateral radiograph of a quadriceps tendon rupture.

about the location of injury, providing insight on how to approach repair or reconstruction. Routine use of MRI is primarily limited by cost (Fig. 106-15).

Treatment Options

Nonoperative

Incomplete ruptures of quadriceps and patellar tendons may be treated nonsurgically. Accurate diagnosis is essential, and immobilization in extension for 3 to 6 weeks is recommended.[86,87] Gradual knee flexion after this initial period of immobilization is advocated once the patient achieves good quadriceps muscle control and is able to perform a straight-leg raise without discomfort.[86]

Operative

Complete ruptures of quadriceps and patellar tendons require operative intervention. A delay in surgery can lead to complications associated with poorer outcomes. Surgical intervention for acute ruptures involves a simple end-to-end repair with or without a reinforcing cerclage of nonabsorbable suture, tape, or wire.[75]

Although midsubstance tears are less common, they can usually be repaired through reapproximation with heavy nonabsorbable suture.[87] More commonly, the disruption occurs at the patella. In this situation, a series of Krackow stitches[94] should be placed in either the distal quadriceps or proximal patellar tendon, depending on the rupture type. A recent study demonstrated that applying pretension to the Krackow stitch–tendon construct did not result in a clinically important decrease in tendon gapping.[95] In the case of a patellar tendon rupture, a small groove or trough may be made at the nose of the patella to allow the tendon to settle into a bleeding bony bed. The Krackow sutures can then be passed through drill holes in the patella. An ACL guide may be used to facilitate drill and suture passage through the patella. Augmentation with hamstring tendons may also be considered in certain cases.

Neglected and recurrent ruptures are more difficult to manage. In the case of a neglected patellar tendon rupture, the surgeon must be aware of patellar mobility, height, and likelihood of return to its native position in the trochlea. Augmentation with fascia lata or hamstring tendons has been advocated in these situations (Figs. 106-16 and 106-17).[75]

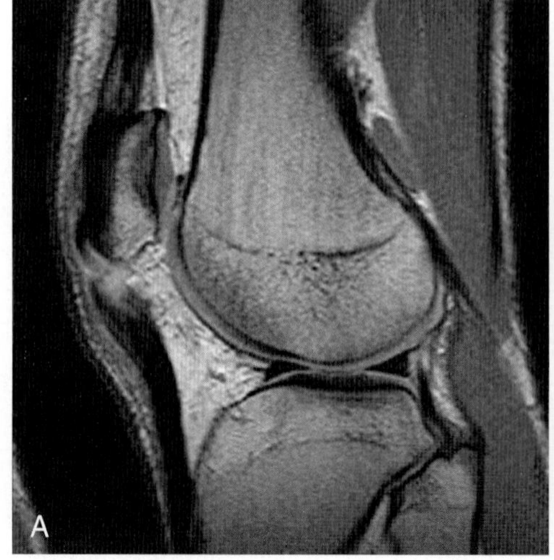

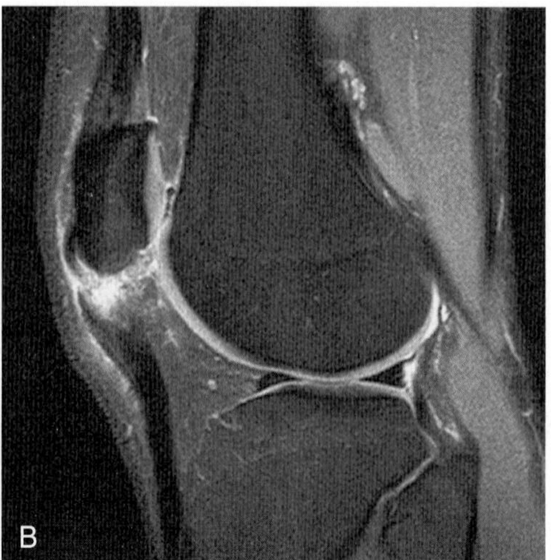

FIGURE 106-15 A and B, Magnetic resonance images of patellar tendon disruption.

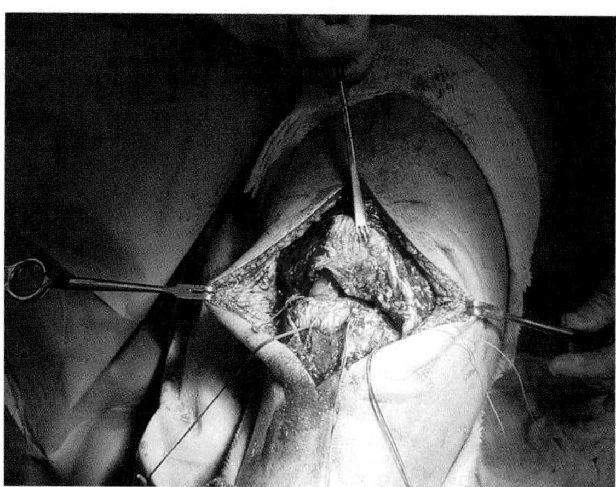

FIGURE 106-16 Quadriceps tendon rupture repair.

AUTHORS' PREFERRED TECHNIQUE

Primary Patellar and Quadriceps Tendon Repairs

We prefer to use a standard anterior incision to allow full exposure of the extensor mechanism. Commonly, ruptures occur adjacent to the patella, which enables the use of a locking Krackow-type suture in the residual tendon with free sutures exiting its end. A bony trough is created in either the distal or proximal pole of the patella to allow the tendon stump to lie adjacent to a bleeding base. A nonabsorbable suture (No. 2 FiberWire, Arthrex, Naples, FL) is passed through longitudinal drill holes in the patella and tied.

Decision-Making Principles

Most patients who undergo a primary repair of patellar or quadriceps tendon ruptures relatively soon after the injury can expect good to excellent results.[75,86] Timing of the repair does appear to correlate with overall outcome. Most studies advocate a 1-week time frame as optimal for performing the repair.

No large series have evaluated the outcome of chronic neglected patellar tendon disruptions. Alternatively, Konrath et al.[88] studied 51 quadriceps tendon repairs in 39 patients. Most patients were satisfied and were able to return to their previous state of employment. Interestingly, these investigators found no correlation between the length of time from tendon rupture to surgical repair and final strength, functional score, or activity score.[86,88]

Benner et al.[96] recently studied the results of patients with patellar tendon ruptures after ACL reconstruction with patellar tendon autograft, comparing outcomes between ipsilateral and contralateral graft harvest. Patellar tendon ruptures occurred in six patients with an ipsilateral graft (0.24%) and seven patients with a contralateral graft (0.25%). These investigators noted no significant differences in the incidence of patellar tendon rupture between ipsilateral and contralateral groups.[96]

Postoperative Management

Langenhan et al.[97] recently published a study investigating clinical outcomes exploring functional versus restrictive postoperative rehabilitation protocols after quadriceps tendon repair. Sixty-six consecutive patients undergoing primary unilateral quadriceps tendon repair were treated with either early functional or restrictive postoperative rehabilitation. These investigators concluded that early mobilization with full weight bearing after primary repair is safe and does not lead to inferior outcomes or more complications.[97]

Return to Play

Boublik et al.[98] studied patellar tendon ruptures in National Football League players, exploring surgical repairs of isolated ruptures and return to sport. These investigators identified 24 ruptures in 22 players over a 10-year period and noted that 11 of the 24 injuries presented with antecedent symptoms and most commonly were caused by an eccentric load to a contracting extensor mechanism. Three of the cases were associated with a concomitant ACL rupture, and players with 19 of the 24 injuries were able to return to play for at least one National Football League game. Of the players who returned, more were selected earlier in the draft, and the

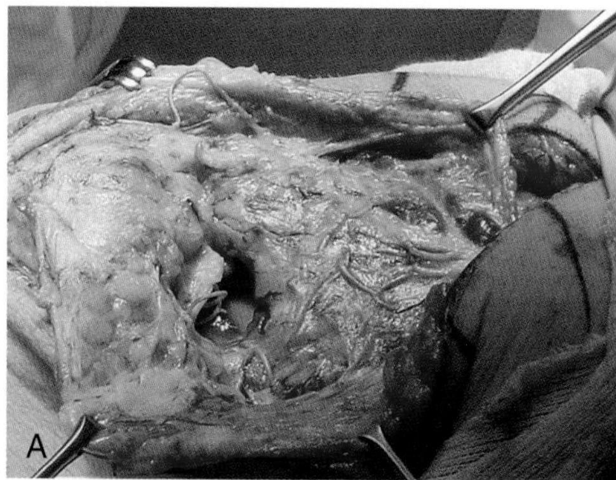

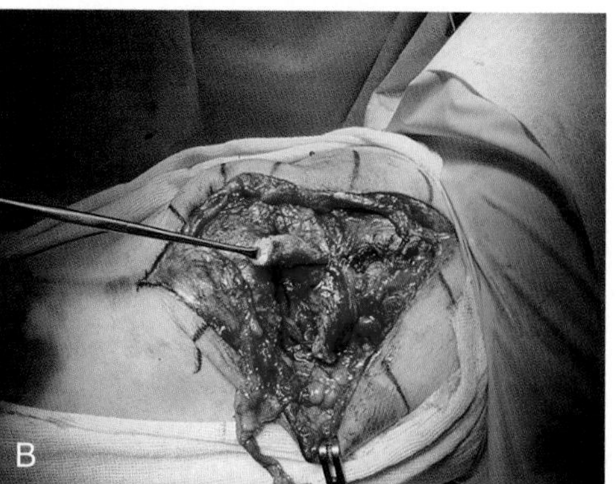

FIGURE 106-17 Recurrent quadriceps tendon rupture. **A,** Recurrent quadriceps rupture. **B,** The Codivilla method of quadriceps tendon lengthening and repair.

average number of games played totaled 45.4, ranging from 1 to 142. The authors concluded that although this injury may end a player's season, repair of isolated ruptures may allow for return to play the following season.[98]

Results

Most patients who undergo a primary repair of patellar or quadriceps tendon ruptures relatively soon after the injury can expect good to excellent results.[75,86] Matava[75] and Ilan et al.[86] demonstrated that no relationship appears to exist between the configuration of the rupture, the method of repair, and the clinical outcome. However, the timing of the repair did appear to correlate with overall outcome. Most studies advocate a 1-week time frame as optimal for performing the repair.

Complications

The most common complications after patellar and quadriceps tendon repairs and reconstructions are diminished quadriceps strength and loss of knee flexion. Of particular concern is that patients may have difficulty obtaining full knee flexion. West et al.[99] investigated the outcomes of early motion after quadriceps and patellar tendon repairs protected with a "relaxing suture." They concluded that this single-suture augmentation is strong enough to permit early motion, full weight bearing, and brace-free ambulation.[99] Other complications that can be encountered with surgery relate to the risks of the procedure itself, including infection, bleeding, recurrent rupture, wound dehiscence, deep venous thrombosis, myocardial infarction, and stroke.

Future Considerations

Future research and considerations will likely focus on biologic enhancement of tendon repair and are outlined in the previous "Future Considerations" section regarding tendinopathies.

Patellar Fractures

Patella fractures are relatively uncommon, constituting about 1% of all skeletal injuries.[100] They are usually the result of significant trauma and do not commonly occur through participation in sports. The mechanism of injury is either a direct blow to the patella or an indirect force transmitted to the patella through the extensor mechanism.[101] The various fracture patterns are usually representative of the injury mechanism. These fractures can be broadly divided into displaced and nondisplaced fractures.

Both nonoperative and operative management may be used with good outcomes depending on the age and activity level of the patient, the fracture pattern, and the amount of displacement. Multiple techniques have been described for the surgical treatment of displaced fractures. The fundamental principles of this treatment include anatomic reduction and rigid internal fixation allowing early knee motion and rehabilitation.

Anatomy and Biomechanics

The patella is the largest sesamoid bone in the body. It ossifies from a single center that usually appears in the second or third year, but its appearance may be delayed until the sixth year. Rarely the bone is developed by two centers, placed side by side. Ossification is completed around the age of puberty, and incomplete ossification may result in a bipartite patella.

The patella is a flat triangular bone with a base or a thick superior border that provides an attachment for the quadriceps tendon. The medial and lateral borders, which are thinner and converge distally, provide attachments for the vastus lateralis and medialis. The apex is pointed and provides an origin for the patellar tendon. The posterior articular surface is divided by a vertical ridge and then again into thirds by two horizontal prominences. The lateral facet is larger than the medial facet. The lower facets engage with the trochlear groove in early flexion followed by the middle and then the upper facets with increased range of motion. In full flexion, the most medial aspect of the patellar articular surface, designated the crescentic or odd facet, is the main contact point. Patellofemoral contact is initiated at about 20 degrees of flexion, and the patella undergoes approximately 7 cm of excursion from extension to full flexion. The forces generated across the patellofemoral joint are tremendous, ranging from half of body weight for normal walking to nearly eight times body weight for jumping from a small height.[102] The articular surface of the patella is the thickest in the body, averaging more than 1 cm in thickness.

The blood supply to the patella is from a vascular anastomotic ring lying in a thin layer of loose connective tissue covering the rectus expansion (Fig. 106-18). The main vessels contributing to this anastomotic ring are the supreme geniculate, medial superior geniculate, medial inferior geniculate, lateral superior geniculate arteries, and anterior tibial recurrent artery. Nutrient vessels pass obliquely into the anterior surface of the patella from this complex network. Disruption of this supply by injury or surgical dissection can result in avascular necrosis. Rates of 3.5% to 24% have been reported after patellar fracture.[103]

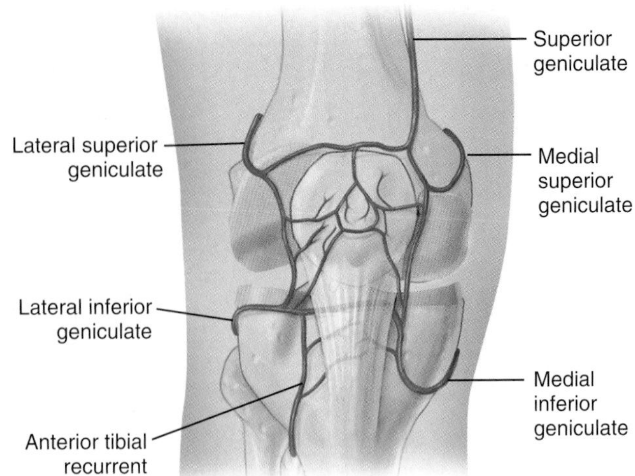

FIGURE 106-18 Schematic arterial blood supply to the patella.

Classification

Fracture patterns of the patella are classified by their configuration and are usually consistent with the mechanism of injury. Indirect forces typically produce nondisplaced or minimally displaced transverse fractures of the central or distal third and, uncommonly, a vertical fracture. Blunt injury to the patella either from a direct blow or from a fall onto the flexed knee produces a comminuted stellate fracture pattern.

Evaluation

History

Patellar fractures result from either an indirect force applied through strong contraction of the extensor mechanism against a flexed knee or from a direct force, such as a fall or blunt trauma to the anterior patella. The subcutaneous location of this bone places it at risk for injury from direct impact. Traumatic separation of a bipartite patella can also occur,[104] and patients with this condition may have an antecedent dull ache or pain prior to the traumatic episode. Patients with patella fractures usually present with a painful, swollen knee after either direct trauma or a fall in which an attempt is made to stop suddenly. Weight bearing is painful and, depending on the competence of the medial and lateral retinacula, the patient may or may not be able to extend the knee.

Reports of patella fractures after ACL reconstruction using a BTB autograft have been reported in the literature.[105] Stein et al.[106] cited a fracture incidence of 1.3% in 618 consecutive patients undergoing ACL reconstruction with single-incision BTB autograft of the donor knee. These investigators demonstrated no difference in the outcome of these patients, with minimal residual sequelae.[106] Another recent report from Lee et al.[107] demonstrated two patellar fractures in 1725 consecutive patients undergoing primary ACL reconstruction with a BTB graft. Both patients healed with a satisfactory outcome.

Physical Examination

Localized tenderness and a hemarthrosis are typically present. It is important to examine the skin around the knee for abrasions and lacerations. Because of the superficial position of the bone,[101] intraarticular communication must be explored and ruled out. With a displaced fracture, a gap between the two fragments may be palpated. The integrity of the extensor mechanism also needs to be evaluated. On occasion, a patient may be limited by pain, and an aspiration of the hemarthrosis followed by an injection of intraarticular local anesthetic can be performed for further evaluation.

Imaging

Most patellar fractures can easily be diagnosed with standard radiographs (Fig. 106-19). Radiographic evaluation includes anteroposterior, lateral, and Merchant views. The anteroposterior view is used to assess for fragmentation, but visualization can be difficult because of overlap of the distal femur. The lateral view best reveals the degree of comminution or separation between the fragments. Likewise, some vertical and osteochondral fractures may be best seen on tangential or Merchant views. Osteochondral, marginal, and especially chondral injuries are more accurately evaluated with MRI. Other diagnostic studies, including computed tomography and bone scans, have been described but provide little additional clinical value. Bone scans have been reported to be helpful in evaluating patellar stress fractures in athletes.[108]

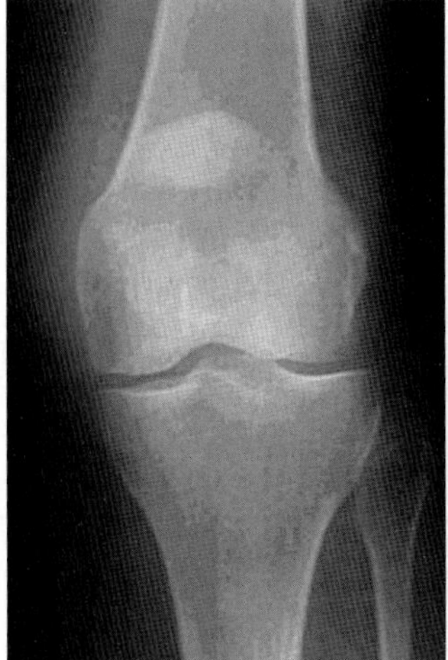
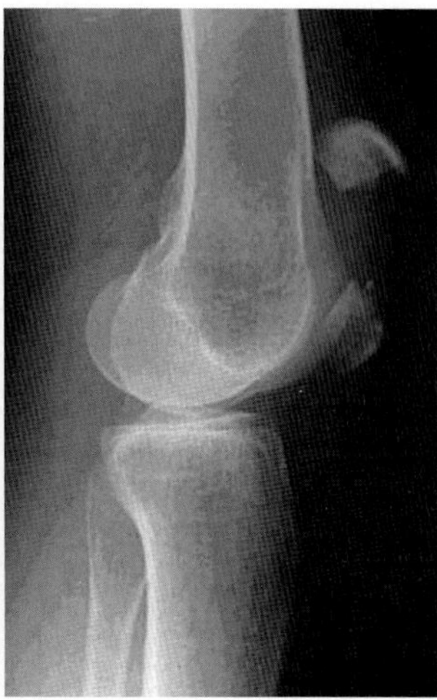

FIGURE 106-19 A significantly displaced patellar fracture with disruption of the extensor retinaculum.

A bipartite patella can be confused with an acute fracture and must be considered when radiographs reveal a small fragment separated from the main portion of the patella. In most cases these secondary ossification centers are located in the superolateral pole. The separation is minimal, and the borders are usually smooth. Contralateral radiographs may be of assistance if a variant is present.

Treatment Options

Nonoperative

Initial treatment of patellar fractures should include splinting in extension and application of ice. The indications for nonoperative management include nondisplaced fractures with an intact articular surface. The patient should have minimal displacement of fragments (<2 to 3 mm) (Fig. 106-20). Patients must also demonstrate a preserved extensor mechanism. The retinacula on either side of the patella should not be torn as evidenced by the patient's ability to maintain extension against gravity. Lastly, elderly patients who are poor surgical candidates and debilitated patients with poor bone quality should be treated without surgery.

Nonoperative treatment consists of casting in extension for up to 6 weeks. After initial splinting, the fracture is immobilized in a cylinder cast from the ankle to the groin. Weight bearing as tolerated is allowed, and performance of quadriceps exercises is encouraged during casting to limit atrophy. A loss of terminal extension or persistent lag is not uncommon, but this problem is rare in the elderly population. A study on nonoperative treatment of patella fractures displaced by more than 1 cm in elderly patients treated without surgery revealed satisfactory outcomes in 9 of 12 patients.[109]

Operative

When operative treatment is considered, the goal should be an anatomic reduction and rigid internal fixation allowing early motion. The technique of patella fixation is a topic of considerable controversy. Anatomic restoration of the

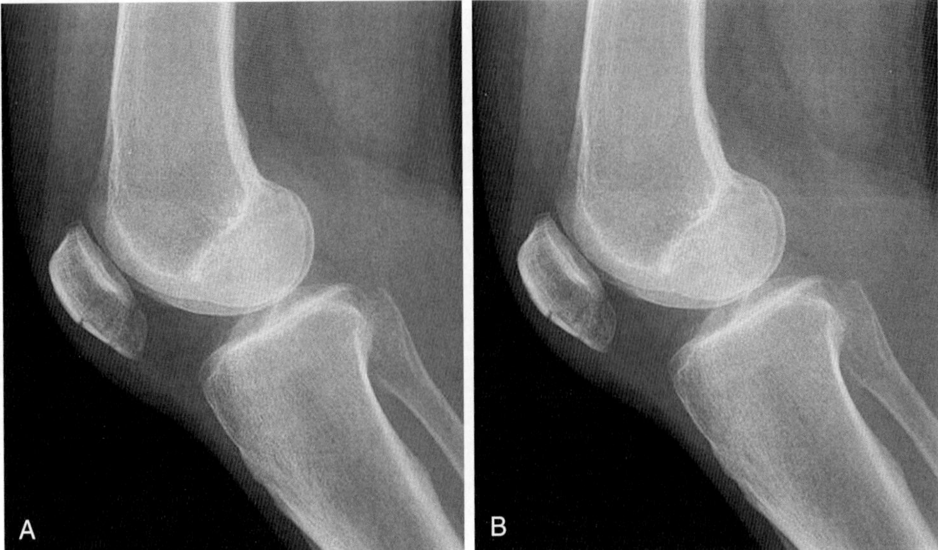

FIGURE 106-20 A nondisplaced fracture amenable to nonoperative treatment.

fragments with stabilization by screws or wires provides the strongest construct.

Skin integrity is an important consideration. Abrasions and lacerations should be closely scrutinized for joint communication. Open fractures should be treated with immediate irrigation and debridement followed by operative fixation if indicated. Timely surgical intervention is recommended if skin abrasions or superficial lacerations are present. If lacerations become infected, surgical repair should be delayed 7 to 10 days. Postoperative swelling can also present problems because of the lack of soft tissue coverage over the patella. Skin and subcutaneous necrosis due to swelling can result in a need for skin grafting or flap coverage. Meticulous skin-handling techniques and postoperative extremity elevation should be used to help prevent these complications.

Both transverse and longitudinal incisions have been used for exposure and repair of the patella and retinacula. A midline longitudinal incision allows excellent exposure and does not compromise the skin if future operations are required. A concomitant retinacular injury usually allows excellent visualization of the articular surface during reduction. The lateral retinaculum can be incised longitudinally to allow for better exposure if necessary.[110] Digital palpation of the chondral surface during reduction and fixation can confirm anatomic articular surface alignment.

Of historical importance, external patellar fixation was originally described by Malgaigne but abandoned. Liang and Wu[111] reported good or excellent results in 26 of 27 patients treated with an external compression fixator attached by transverse percutaneous pins. No osteomyelitis developed, and 80% of patients regained knee motion equal to that on the uninjured side.

Stabilization of bony fragments can be accomplished by cerclage wire, tension-band techniques, or interfragmentary lag screw fixation. Berger first described circumferential cerclage wiring to reduce bone fragments.[111a] Indirect reduction is obtained through compression as tension is applied to the wire. Bandi and Müller[112] advocated the tension-band wiring technique whereby two Kirschner wires are passed longitudinally through the patella. Around these wires, a heavy-gauge wire is applied in a figure-eight fashion and tightened over the anterior surface of the bone. The Kirschner wires provide an anchor against which the figure-eight wire is tensioned. Biomechanical evaluation has found that this configuration produces a compression effect on the articular surface with knee flexion.[113]

Lag screw fixation of larger fragments can be used alone or in conjunction with tension-band techniques. Two large fragments can be rigidly fixed with parallel lag screws, or several smaller fragments can be stabilized with lag screws, followed by tension banding. Another technique reported by Berg[114] incorporates the use of cannulated screws through which a wire is passed and then secured in a figure-eight fashion. This technique has the advantage of applying both compression through the lag screws and the tension-band technique while maintaining a low profile. Because of the subcutaneous position of the patella, hardware placed to stabilize fractures often requires subsequent removal after successful stabilization. To avoid hardware complications, heavy-gauge suture has been advocated as an alternative to wire. Tension-band techniques using braided heavy polyester sutures have demonstrated promising results comparable to using wire.[115] Alternative techniques have been described to obtain stable fixation. The use of biodegradable wires and screws has not compared favorably with conventional fixation. If equivalent fixation can be obtained, the need to remove hardware can be obviated. With respect to plates, Thelen et al.[116] also studied the use of bilateral polyaxial 2.7-mm fixed-angle plates for fracture stabilization in a sawbones model and concluded that both the plate fixation and cannulated screws with tension wiring maintained better reduction than did traditional tension-band wiring.

Fractures involving the distal pole of the patella can be treated with internal fixation of the fragment or by excision and reattachment of the patellar tendon. Veselko and Kastelec[117] compared osteosynthesis with a basket plate against distal pole resection. Internal fixation allowed for early mobilization, weight bearing, and overall better results than did distal pole excision.

When the fracture is multifragmented, all attempts should be made to conserve the patella. After patellectomy, extensor lag, weakness, malalignment, and restricted motion are common problems. Quadriceps strength is reduced by 20% to 60% and tibiofemoral forces can increase up to 250%, leading to early degeneration of the tibiofemoral joint.[118] Primary reconstruction of the patella is recommended in multifragmentary fractures. If the outcome is poor, patellectomy should be considered because early intervention results in better outcomes than delayed treatment.[119] If a total patellectomy is performed, one should consider advancing the vastus medialis obliquus muscle over the closed defect for improved outcomes.[120]

Decision-Making Principles

Decision-making principles should be based on appropriate interpretation of the fracture pattern and preservation of the patella as previously discussed in the "Treatment Options" section.

AUTHORS' PREFERRED TECHNIQUE

Patellar Fractures

Our preferred treatment is based on the configuration of the fracture patterns. If at all possible, we prefer to save as much of the patella as we can. We prefer rigid, strong fixation and favor tension-band wiring whenever possible and typically secure fixation through an open midline incision. We are aggressive in terms of surgical fixation because of the desire for early motion and rehabilitation.

Postoperative Management

For nondisplaced fractures, the knee is immobilized in a locked extension brace and the patient can bear partial weight on crutches for 6 weeks. Quadriceps exercise is continued during this period, after which the knee is mobilized to regain its range of motion.

During internal fixation, the knee is flexed to determine the safe degree of motion that does not disrupt the construct. A hinged brace is applied and the patient is allowed to bear weight as tolerated. The knee is mobilized through the predetermined range twice a day. Both quadriceps and hamstring muscles are continuously strengthened throughout the recovery period.

Return to Play

Athletes are permitted to return to play when healing of the tendon is complete and they have achieved appropriate range of motion and strength compared with the uninjured side. Most athletes are able to return to play after the fracture has consolidated and they have regained approximately 90% of quadriceps strength. Most are able to return to play within 6 to 9 months. Despite improved surgical techniques and rehabilitation protocols, athletes often have a difficult time returning to their preinjury level of competition.[121]

Results

Lebrun et al.[122] studied functional outcomes after operatively treated patella fractures in a cohort of trauma patients with a mean follow-up of 6.5 years and functional testing. Based on outcomes measures, these investigators concluded that significant symptomatic complaints and functional deficits persisted. They suggested that surgeons counsel patients on expectations for long-term pain and function and underscore our current limitations in fracture management.[122]

Complications

Significant complications may occur with fractures of the patella. Patella baja can occur, especially after prolonged immobilization. Early range of motion of the knee reduces this occurence.[123] Arthrofibrosis can also be reduced with early mobilization.

Skin necrosis is an uncommon but serious complication. Careful examination of the skin is required, and when its viability is in doubt, it is best to delay surgery for up to 10 days. Skin necrosis is managed by covering the defect with a local medial gastrocnemius flap or a free muscle flap.

Surgical site infections may occur in open injuries or as a result of skin necrosis. Wound debridement with appropriate soft tissue coverage and intravenous antibiotics often proves successful in eradicating the infection. A stable construct in the milieu of an infection should be left in situ. However, if the fixation is unstable, then all hardware should be removed until the infection is eradicated.

Hardware failure is most often the result of poor surgical technique. Failure to achieve an anatomic reduction may lead to nonunion and subsequent implant breakage.

Future Considerations

As with tendinopathies and tendon rupture healing discussed previously, future research and considerations should focus on biologic enhancement of patellar bone healing, which may allow earlier mobilization and possibly improved results.

For a complete list of references, go to expertconsult.com.

Suggested Readings

Citation: Zwerver J, Bredeweg SW, van den Akker-Scheek I: Prevalence of Jumper's knee among nonelite athletes from different sports: A cross-sectional survey. *Am J Sports Med* 39:1984–1988, 2011.
Level of Evidence: II
Summary: The prevalence of jumper's knee is high among nonelite athletes and varies between 14.4% and 2.5% for different sports. It is almost twice as common among male nonelite athletes compared with female athletes. Different sport-specific loading characteristics of the knee extensor apparatus, a younger age, a taller body stature, and higher body weight seem to be risk factors associated with patellar tendinopathy.

Citation: Hagglund M, Zwerver J, Ekstrand J: Epidemiology of patellar tendinopathy in elite male soccer players. *Am J Sports Med* 39:1906–1911, 2011.
Level of Evidence: II
Summary: Although mainly mild in nature, patellar tendinopathy is a fairly common condition in elite soccer players, and the recurrence rate is high. Exposure to artificial turf did not increase the prevalence or incidence of injury. A high total amount of exposure was identified as a risk factor for patellar tendinopathy.

Citation: Sheth U, Simunovic N, Klein G, et al: Efficacy of autologous platelet-rich plasma use for orthopaedic indications: A meta-analysis. *J Bone Joint Surg Am* 94A:298–307, 2012.

Level of Evidence: II
Summary: The current literature is complicated by a lack of standardization of study protocols, platelet-separation techniques, and outcome measures. As a result, uncertainty exists about the evidence to support the increasing clinical use of platelet-rich plasma and autologous blood concentrates as a treatment modality for orthopaedic bone and soft tissue injuries.
Citation: de Almeida AM, Demange MK, Sobrado MF, et al: Patellar tendon healing with platelet-rich plasma: A prospective randomized controlled trial. *Am J Sports Med* 40(6):1282–1288, 2012.
Level of Evidence: I
Summary: Platelet-rich plasma had a positive effect on patellar tendon harvest site healing as demonstrated by magnetic resonance imaging after 6 months and also reduced pain in the immediate postoperative period.
Citation: Hoksrud A, Bahr R: Ultrasound-guided sclerosing treatment in patients with patellar tendinopathy (jumper's knee). 44-month follow-up. *Am J Sports Med* 39:2377–2380, 2011.
Level of Evidence: IV
Summary: Sclerosing treatment with polidocanol was effective for the majority of the patients. Nevertheless, one third elected to seek additional treatment through arthroscopic surgery during the 44-month follow-up period.
Citation: Boublik M, Schlegel T, Koonce R, et al: Patellar tendon ruptures in National Football League players. *Am J Sports Med* 39:2436–2440, 2011.
Level of Evidence: IV
Summary: Patellar tendon ruptures can occur in otherwise healthy professional football players without antecedent symptoms or predisposing factors. The most common mechanism of injury is eccentric overload. Close attention should be paid to stability examination of the knee given the not uncommon occurrence of concomitant anterior cruciate ligament injury.
Citation: Melvin JS, Mehta S: Patellar fractures in adults. *J Am Acad Orthop Surg* 19:198–207, 2011.
Level of Evidence: V
Summary: Surgical fixation is recommended for fractures that either disrupt the extensor mechanism or demonstrate greater than 2 to 3 mm of step-off and greater than 1 to 4 mm of displacement. Anatomic reduction and fixation with a tension-band technique is associated with the best outcomes; however, symptomatic hardware is a frequent complication.

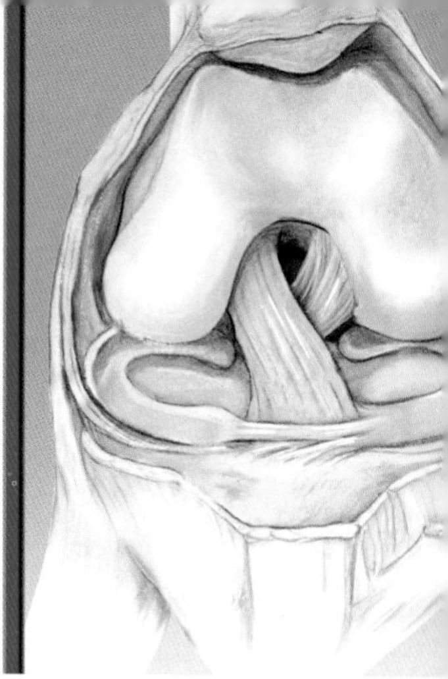

107

Loss of Knee Motion

K. DONALD SHELBOURNE • HEATHER FREEMAN

Full range of motion (ROM) in the knee joint is critical for optimal function. A slight loss of knee motion can cause limited function and pain, and a more severe loss of knee motion will lead to significant impairment and disability. For optimum function, the knee should have ROM and strength that is symmetric to the opposite, normal knee. When something causes a loss of normal knee motion, a cascade of events often occurs, beginning with relative disuse of the involved lower extremity, increased pain, and subsequent loss of strength.

Loss of knee motion can occur for many reasons, including acute knee injury, lack of appropriate rehabilitation after a surgical procedure or an injury, arthrofibrosis (which commonly occurs after anterior cruciate ligament [ACL] reconstruction or lower extremity fractures), relative disuse due to injury or degenerative joint disease, displaced bucket-handle meniscus tears, or mucoid degeneration of the ACL or posterior cruciate ligament (PCL). Clinicians should be vigilant about detecting loss of ROM of the knee in any patient with knee pain or injury because by restoring normal, symmetric knee motion first, followed by restoring symmetric strength, many symptoms may subside or abate, negating the need for further surgical intervention. Use of this proactive approach helps patients avoid problems in the short term after a knee injury or surgery, and some evidence indicates that it may also prevent long-term problems, including knee osteoarthritis.[1-3]

Early intervention for ROM loss requires early detection. To identify loss of knee motion, the opposite, normal knee must also be examined to establish a baseline for comparison, and the examination must include an assessment of knee hyperextension. Unfortunately, this step is sometimes overlooked. A recent study found that in patients who were seeking a second opinion for their knee problem, only 37% of them reported having their opposite, normal knee physically touched during the physical examination.[4]

This chapter provides an overview of the diagnosis and treatment for loss of ROM of the knee. The reasons for loss of knee motion and thus the treatments are wide ranging. However, common themes regarding effective treatment remain the same regardless of the specific cause of loss of knee motion. Most cases of loss of knee motion can be effectively treated without surgery if proper rehabilitation is performed. In some cases, such as arthrofibrosis or displaced bucket-handle meniscus tears, surgical intervention is necessary to remove a mechanical block to knee ROM. The surgical treatment for arthrofibrosis after ACL reconstruction is outlined in detail in this chapter. The principles of rehabilitation for loss of knee motion remain the same whether or not surgical intervention is a part of the treatment plan, and these rehabilitation principles are discussed in this chapter.

History

Patients with loss of knee motion may present with varying subjective histories. It is important to determine how long the ROM loss has been present. This information can be difficult to elicit from patients because they are often unaware that their ROM is lacking, so we ask patients how long they have felt like they have had a bad knee. Generally speaking, the longer the ROM loss has been present, the more slowly it may respond to treatment. However, long-term ROM loss does not always mean that more aggressive forms of treatment are necessary; rather, it is important for both the clinician and patient to understand that progress may occur at a slower pace.

In patients who have had previous knee surgery, it is important to obtain pertinent details about the surgical procedure. When loss of motion is present it is perhaps even more important to ascertain what, if any, pre- and postoperative rehabilitation was performed. In our experience, many patients with persistent pain after a knee arthroscopy or other knee surgery have loss of knee motion that was likely present before surgical intervention but was overlooked and not treated.

In patients who have not had a previous knee surgery, a careful subjective history can often identify a precipitating injury that may not have seemed significant at the time but may have led them to begin favoring their knee. When patients favor their knee, they stand with their weight shifted away from the involved lower extremity, holding the knee slightly bent. Over time, this habit slowly leads to increasing amounts of knee extension loss. Without full terminal knee extension, it is not comfortable to stand with the body weight shifted toward the involved knee because the patient loses the ability to "lock out" the knee, and therefore they cannot relax the quadriceps muscles during stance as they can for the opposite, normal knee. This scenario feeds the vicious cycle of disuse, increased pain, and further loss of strength.

Other times the subjective history reveals a significant injury to which the patient can attribute the ROM loss with certainty. A displaced bucket-handle meniscus tear blocks the intercondylar notch, resulting in the inability to fully extend the knee. Although this scenario may not always be caused by a specific injury, patients can usually identify exactly when this mechanism occurred and report that their knee feels "locked."

When a patient does not have a history of a specific injury, the ROM loss may be associated with degenerative joint disease. Another potential cause of ROM loss is mucoid degeneration of the cruciate ligaments, most commonly the ACL. This pathology presents as a gradual loss of knee flexion combined with posterolateral knee pain. An effusion is usually not present.

Physical Examination

The physical examination for any knee problem should include a careful assessment of the knee ROM of both knees, including an assessment of knee hyperextension. The uninvolved knee should always be examined before the involved knee; this examination is important to establish a baseline of what the ROM should be for the involved knee. It is also important that both knees be fully exposed (to the level of the mid thigh) for the examination.

Knee extension (including hyperextension) is assessed in two ways. First, the examiner should perform a passive assessment of hyperextension (Fig. 107-1). The examiner stabilizes the thigh on the examination table with one hand, while the other hand passively lifts the heel off the table, assessing the amount of movement available and the quality of the end feel. When ROM is limited, the patient should be asked if the discomfort is perceived posteriorly or anteriorly when a stretch is applied. Posterior discomfort indicates capsular and soft tissue tightness, whereas anterior discomfort may indicate an intraarticular mechanical blockage. Second, knee extension should be measured with the patient lying supine, with both heels propped up on a 6- to 8-inch bolster, allowing the knees to fall into hyperextension. This position allows for visual assessment of knee extension symmetry, as well as goniometric measurement of knee extension.

It is important to note that knee hyperextension is normal. DeCarlo and Sell[5] studied a group of healthy young athletes and found that 95% of males and 96% of females have some degree of knee hyperextension. The mean knee hyperextension was 5 degrees for males and 6 degrees for females. Therefore treatment to restore normal knee ROM should include restoration of hyperextension when it is present in the opposite knee.

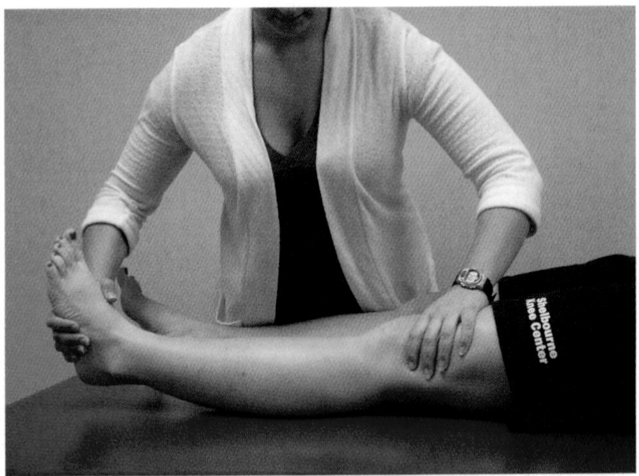

FIGURE 107-1 Passive assessment of knee hyperextension.

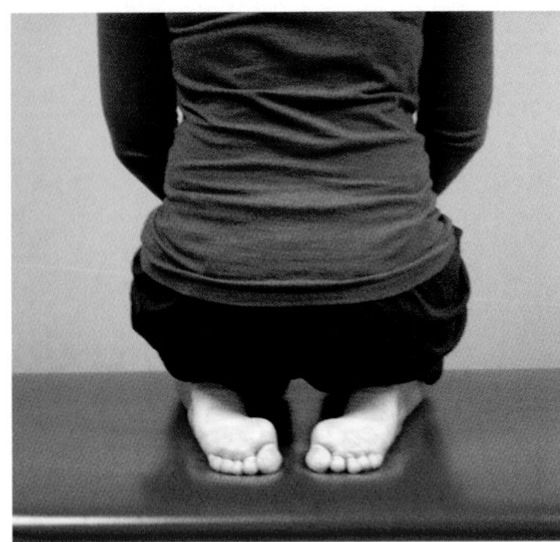

FIGURE 107-2 Full knee flexion can be assessed by asking the patient to sit on his or her heels. If knee flexion is lacking in one knee, the patient shows a lateral pelvic tilt away from the involved knee.

Knee flexion is assessed with the patient lying supine or in a long-sitting position. The patient should be asked to grasp the front of his or her ankle with both hands (or use a towel looped around this area if necessary) and pull the heel as far as possible toward the buttocks. Goniometric measurement can be made once maximal flexion is reached. Another method for assessing knee flexion is to ask the patient to sit on his or her heels (Fig. 107-2). Patients with full flexion of both knees are able to comfortably sit back onto their heels without any pelvic tilt. Knee flexion loss leads to minor to severe tilting of the pelvis away from the involved extremity. This method of assessing flexion is also very helpful for patients to self-assess their knee flexion and adjust their activity levels accordingly.

For the purposes of this chapter, we focus on the examination for ROM deficits, but a full knee examination should also be performed, including observation of gait, observation for disuse of the lower extremity when arising from a chair or with habitual standing postures, observation of patella alignment and mobility, palpation for crepitus, assessment for a joint effusion, and special testing for meniscal pathology and ligamentous laxity.

Imaging

Bilateral radiographs, including weight-bearing posteroanterior, lateral, and Merchant[6] views, are routinely obtained. Again, even in the absence of bilateral symptoms, it is important to obtain bilateral radiographs to provide a baseline for comparison with the involved knee.

When osteoarthritis is suspected, we also recommend obtaining an anteroposterior view. A study by Rosenberg and colleagues[7] showed that the posteroanterior view is more sensitive for detecting joint space narrowing of the tibiofemoral

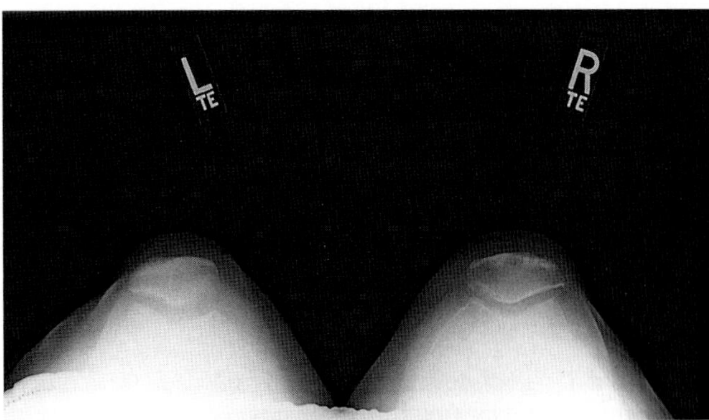

FIGURE 107-3 A Merchant view radiograph showing disuse osteopenia of the right patella after relative disuse of the right lower extremity for an extended period.

joint. This view is more sensitive because it is taken with the knees bent to a 45-degree angle, allowing for weight bearing with the tibiofemoral joint aligned in a position where more cartilage degeneration is likely. The anteroposterior view is not as sensitive for detecting joint space narrowing but provides information regarding the amount of joint space remaining when the knee is in a fully extended position.

In cases of long-standing ROM loss, the Merchant view radiograph can provide useful information by providing a visual comparison of the bone density of the patellae. When a patient has been favoring one knee for any considerable length of time, disuse osteopenia is evident on the Merchant view (Fig. 107-3).

In patients with severe ROM loss, it is important to observe for signs of patella baja on the lateral-view radiographs. Again, comparison with the opposite knee is important to determine the height of the patella compared with Blumensaat's line and the apparent length of the patellar tendon based on measurements from the inferior pole of the patella to the tibial tubercle. Although normal ranges have been established for each of these measurements, what is normal for each patient varies and should be based on the measurements for the uninvolved knee.

Magnetic resonance imaging (MRI) is useful when arthrofibrosis is present. In patients with arthrofibrosis types 1 or 2, the MRI can help identify the presence of a cyclops lesion, which is commonly present in patients with arthrofibrosis after ACL reconstruction. In persons with arthrofibrosis types 3 or 4, the MRI provides valuable insight about the extent of scar tissue formation in the fat pad.

Decision-Making Principles

Despite the wide range of pathologies that can cause limited knee ROM, a vast majority of cases of limited knee motion can be effectively treated with a directed rehabilitation program. One exception to this is in the case of a displaced bucket-handle meniscus tear, which would need to be arthroscopically reduced and removed or repaired.

Another condition to consider is arthrofibrosis, particularly in patients who have had any previous knee surgeries, including ACL reconstruction, but also fractures around the knee. Arthrofibrosis is an abnormal proliferation of fibrotic tissue in the knee joint. The fibrotic tissue is commonly found in the extrasynovial space anteriorly in a fibrotic fat pad or near the intercondylar notch, presenting as a cyclops lesion at the base of the reconstructed ACL. Arthrofibrosis can cause a loss of knee extension alone, or knee extension and flexion may both be limited. Shelbourne et al.[8] developed a classification for arthrofibrosis to help guide treatment (Table 107-1). Most patients with type 1 arthrofibrosis respond to nonoperative rehabilitation and do not need surgery, but most cases of types 2, 3, or 4 require a combination of rehabilitation and operative treatment to achieve satisfactory results. In these patients, pre- and postoperative rehabilitation is a vital component of the treatment process. In nearly all other cases of knee ROM loss that were not caused by a previous surgery, a directed rehabilitation program completed under the supervision of a well-trained knee therapist resolves significant deficits and provides a corresponding improvement in function.

Not all rehabilitation programs are designed the same way, but the foundation of a rehabilitation program for limited knee motion should be to work on regaining symmetry in three distinct, sequential phases: (1) knee extension, (2) knee flexion, and (3) knee strength. Our experience has shown us that these phases of rehabilitation should not overlap; rather, one should focus only on extension ROM until symmetry is restored, and then shift toward working on flexion ROM while maintaining full extension. Finally, once full ROM symmetry is achieved, unilateral strengthening exercises should be initiated until strength symmetry is restored. This rehabilitation program is described in greater detail in the "Authors' Preferred Technique" and "Postoperative Management" sections.

If ROM progress plateaus before symmetric knee extension is achieved, surgical intervention may be needed to remove a mechanical blockage to extension. When degenerative joint disease is present, the mechanical blockage may be caused by an osteophyte on the anterior tibia or near the intercondylar notch.

TABLE 107-1

CLASSIFICATION OF ARTHROFIBROSIS

Type	Knee Flexion	Knee Extension	Other Features
1	Normal	≤10° deficit*	Able to fully extend with overpressure
2	Normal	>10° deficit*	Unable to fully extend with overpressure
3	≥25° deficit*	>10° deficit*	Decreased medial/lateral patellar mobility
4	≥30° deficit*	>10° deficit*	Patella infera evident on radiographs

From Shelbourne KD, Patel DV, Martini DJ: Classification and management of arthrofibrosis of the knee after anterior cruciate ligament reconstruction. *Am J Sports Med* 24:857–862, 1996.

*All range of motion deficits are based on comparison with the range of motion of the normal, uninvolved knee.

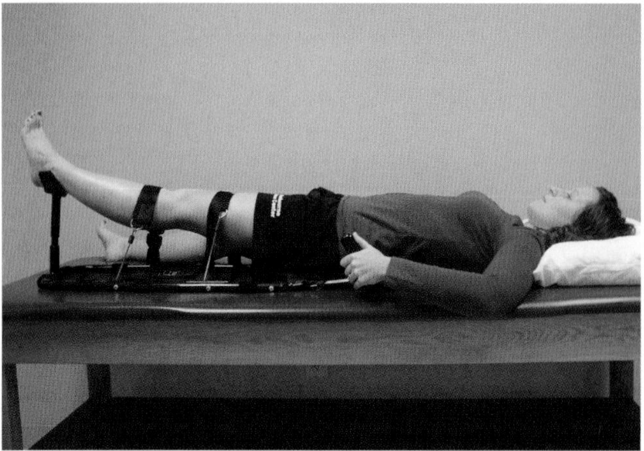

FIGURE 107-4 A passive knee extension device is used to restore symmetric knee extension, including hyperextension. The patient lies supine and controls the intensity of the stretch with a hand-held crank. The stretch is performed at least two to three times per day for 10 to 15 minutes per session.

Mucoid degeneration of the ACL is a rare condition but presents with a classic history. Patients with this condition are typically middle aged and report an insidious onset of gradual loss of knee flexion accompanied by posterolateral knee pain. Some knee extension loss may be present, but it is usually mild and easily resolves with rehabilitation using either a towel stretch or a passive knee extension device (Elite Seat, Kneebourne Therapeutics, Inc., Noblesville, IN) (Fig. 107-4). The appearance on MRI is often described as a "celery stalk" feature, with a striated appearance on T2-saturated images indicating fluid between the ACL fibers. An enlarged, bulbous area is usually present proximally (Fig. 107-5). Literature on this topic is sparse and mostly includes case reports regarding debridement or resection of the ACL, but residual instability has been an undesirable aftereffect of this procedure.[9,10] We have found that this condition responds favorably to oral or injected steroids and rehabilitation using the principles described in detail later in this chapter.

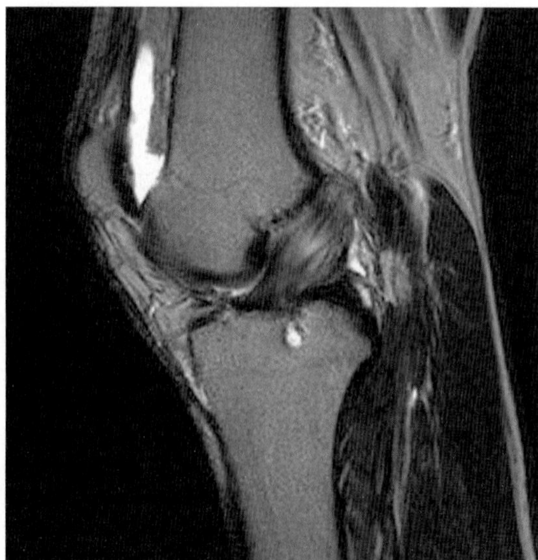

FIGURE 107-5 A magnetic resonance image showing mucoid degeneration of the anterior cruciate ligament.

Treatment Options

Nonsurgical treatment with a carefully planned rehabilitation program is the first line of treatment for most patients with loss of knee ROM. As discussed in the previous section, surgery may be necessary in some cases to allow full, symmetric ROM to be regained, particularly in cases of type 2, 3, or 4 arthrofibrosis after an ACL reconstruction or when a bucket-handle meniscus tear becomes displaced and is blocking the intercondylar notch.

The following surgical interventions have been described for loss of knee motion: anterior interval release,[11] notchplasty and/or removal of a cyclops lesion,[12] posterior capsular release,[13,14] peripatellar release, and manipulation with the patient under anesthesia.[15]

The anterior interval is defined as the space posterior to the patellar tendon and extending to the anterior tibia and transverse meniscal ligament. Trauma to the infrapatellar fat pad can lead to fibrotic formation in this area of the knee, limiting both knee extension and flexion. This presentation is most commonly seen in patients who have undergone arthroscopic ACL surgery, with fat pad trauma occurring as a result of repeatedly passing instruments through the fat pad. Although arthroscopic ACL surgery is believed to be less traumatic for the patient, the trauma to the fat pad is underestimated. Fat pad trauma can lead to fat pad fibrosis, and in its most severe form, fibrosis in this area can lead to infrapatellar contracture syndrome, which further limits patellar mobility and knee flexion.[16] If full knee flexion is not emphasized immediately after surgery, patellar mobility decreases and permanent flexion deficits may occur. Anterior interval release can be performed arthroscopically with use of a 30-degree scope and portals that are slightly farther away from midline than usual to allow for better visualization of this area.[11] Abnormal tissue may be removed with a basket forceps, meniscal shaver, or electrothermal probe.

Under normal circumstances, the ACL and PCL fit perfectly within the intercondylar notch, completely occupying this space when the knee is in terminal extension. Occasionally after ACL reconstruction, a mismatch occurs between the size of the graft and the width of the intercondylar notch, or a cyclops lesion[17] forms, blocking full knee extension. A cyclops lesion is a fibrous nodule that forms on the anterior aspect of the ACL graft (Fig. 107-6). We theorize that this

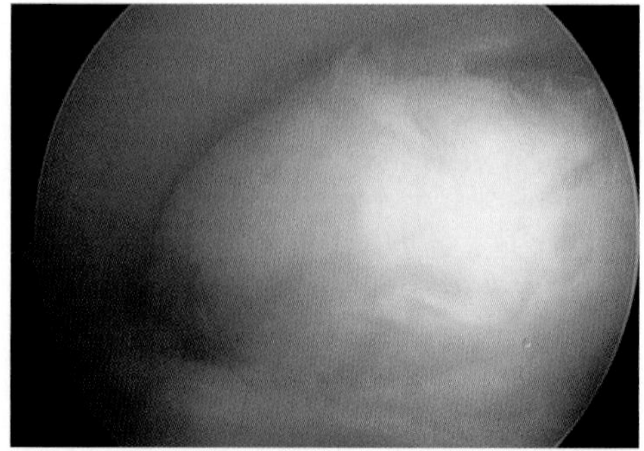

FIGURE 107-6 An arthroscopic view of a cyclops lesion on the anterior aspect of the anterior cruciate ligament graft.

complication can be prevented after ACL reconstruction by ensuring that full, symmetric knee extension is restored prior to and immediately after surgery. These lesions can be carefully excised during arthroscopy until terminal extension is regained. If the intercondylar notch width is not adequate to handle the size of the ACL graft and the PCL, a notchplasty can also be performed.

When knee extension has been lacking for a longer duration of time, the posterior capsule becomes tight. Arthroscopic release of the posterior capsule has been described by LaPrade et al.[13] and Mariani.[14] Another option is to use a more aggressive approach to rehabilitation that focuses on knee extension by using a passive knee extension device (Elite Seat, Kneebourne Therapeutics, Inc.) (see Fig. 107-4). Use of a long-duration stretch of 10 to 15 minutes per session several times each day can eventually improve posterior capsular mobility and restore full knee extension compared with the opposite knee.

Decreased patellar mobility has been treated with release of the medial and/or lateral retinaculum and the suprapatellar pouch.[18,19] Care must be taken to provide adequate release without overreleasing these structures and inducing patellar instability.[18]

Manipulation with the patient under anesthesia has been described to regain knee extension and/or knee flexion.[15] Manipulation of the knee can effectively improve knee motion, but it does not directly approach the knee problem selectively, and there is a risk of supracondylar femur fracture, patellar tendon rupture, and neurologic or vascular injury.

Many surgeons use more than one of these techniques in combination based on the location of the adhesions and the degree of ROM limitation that is present.

AUTHORS' PREFERRED TECHNIQUE

Loss of Knee Motion

It is important to emphasize that surgical treatment is only one part of the process for treating knee ROM loss and that surgical intervention is not always needed. For optimal results, patients must first maximize their knee ROM with a directed rehabilitation program, and if surgery is needed, a focused postoperative rehabilitation program is used to further maximize knee motion. In fact, we now require all patients undergoing surgery for arthrofibrosis to use a passive knee extension device (see Fig. 107-4) several times daily before and after surgery to maximize results. In past years, extension casting was used on the operating room table and followed by serial extension casting as an outpatient to provide a low-load, long-duration stretch; however, this treatment was difficult to implement because of the postoperative hemarthrosis that developed and the frequency of outpatient visits required for serial casting. Instead, we now have the patient perform several stretching sessions each day in the passive knee extension device and have found that this technique is highly effective and more cost- and time-efficient.[20]

When surgical intervention is needed to treat arthrofibrosis, the lead author uses a step wise process to address the specific areas of fibrosis that have developed in the knee. This section addresses the surgical treatment of arthrofibrosis, specifically arthrofibrosis that develops after ACL reconstruction. This approach is based on the classification of arthrofibrosis shown in Table 107-1 and has been previously described.[8]

Arthroscopy is performed after general anesthesia is induced and after the knee is injected with 20 mL of 0.25% bupivacaine and epinephrine. Knee ROM and patellar mobility are evaluated once general anesthesia is achieved and are reassessed throughout the surgical procedure to determine if additional surgical steps are needed to remove mechanical blockages to knee extension and flexion.

To improve visibility of the anterior aspect of the knee joint, standard medial and lateral portals are used, but the position of the portals is adjusted to be more proximal and slightly farther medial and lateral, respectively.

The first step is to examine the area anterior to the proximal tibia. If extrasynovial scar tissue has formed in this area, a blunt trocar is used to loosen the scar between the posterior aspect of the patellar tendon and the anterior aspect of the tibia. A basket forceps and meniscal shaver may be used to excise scar tissue in this area. One should ensure that the entire area from the anterior horns of the medial and lateral menisci down to the upper tibia is free of extrasynovial scar tissue. Patients with type 2, 3, or 4 arthrofibrosis often have scar formation in this area of the knee (Fig. 107-7).

Second, examine the intercondylar notch for signs of impingement, including the base of the ACL where a cyclops lesion may form (see Fig. 107-6). In patients with type 1 arthrofibrosis, this area is typically the only area of mechanical blockage causing ROM loss; this lesion is located inside the synovium and is not part of the fat pad (Fig. 107-8). The knee must be placed through a ROM into full, terminal extension to determine if the ACL fits in the intercondylar notch without any sign of impingement (Fig. 107-9). Excision or ablation can be used to remove scar tissue that has formed in this area. If needed, a notchplasty may be performed to allow the ACL to fit within the intercondylar notch so the remaining knee extension that needs to be regained after surgery can be achieved with the passive knee extension device.

Fibrosis of the infrapatellar fat pad and/or the joint capsule is usually associated with type 3 or 4 arthrofibrosis. After using a blunt probe to establish a plane between the patellar tendon and the scar tissue, the scar tissue should be removed

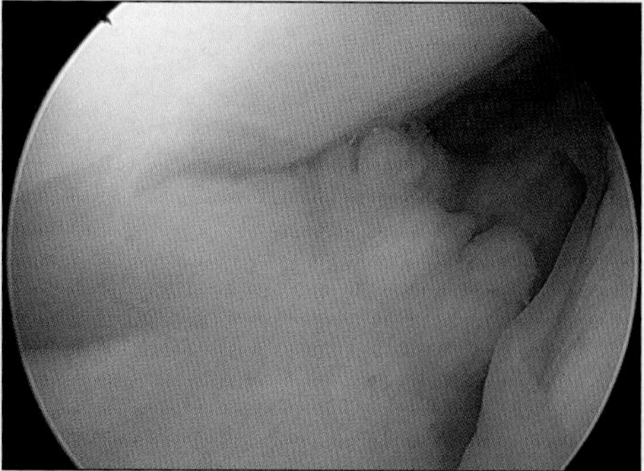

FIGURE 107-7 An arthroscopic view of anterior scar tissue extending into the medial compartment.

Continued

distally to the level of the upper tibia and anteriorly to the horns of the menisci. When the joint capsule is fibrotic, excision of the fibrotic capsule can be performed up to the insertion of the vastus medialis oblique and vastus lateralis muscles, which improves mobility of the patella and patellar tendon.

Patients with type 4 arthrofibrosis are not likely to regain full, symmetric knee flexion because of the shortening of the patellar tendon. However, in patients with type 3 or 4 arthrofibrosis, a manipulation is performed to maximize knee flexion. We do not recommend forceful manipulation for knee extension because most of the knee extension loss is due to either mechanical blocks that can be selectively removed and/or posterior capsular tightness that can be slowly stretched out during the course of postoperative rehabilitation.

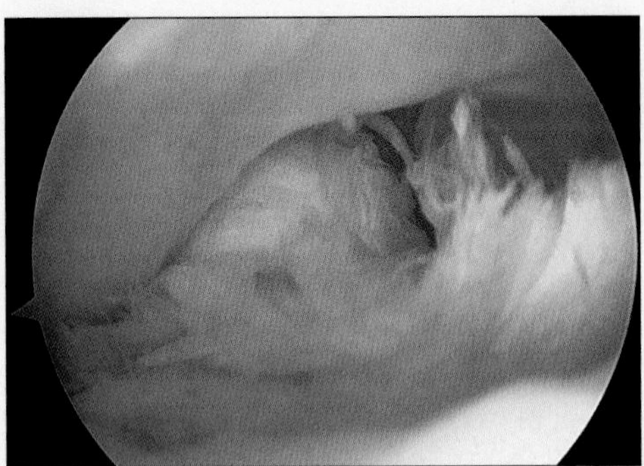

FIGURE 107-8 An arthroscopic view of the same knee depicted in Figure 107-7, showing the intercondylar notch area with the knee in about 30 degrees of flexion. Scar tissue that is visible anterior to the ACL graft gets impinged when the knee is placed in full extension.

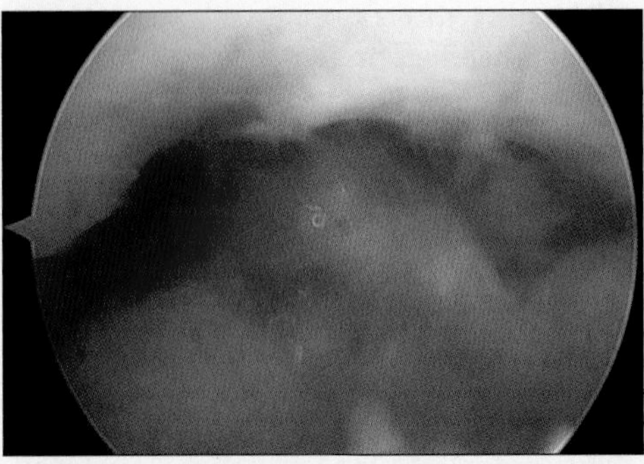

FIGURE 107-9 An arthroscopic view after debridement of scar tissue (in the same knee as depicted in Figures 107-7 and 107-8) shows a good fit of the anterior cruciate ligament graft in the intercondylar notch.

Postoperative Management

The primary goals of postoperative treatment are to prevent a hemarthrosis and achieve/maintain full terminal extension, symmetric to the opposite knee. Once the mechanical block to extension has been removed, immediate emphasis on full knee extension is needed to stretch the posterior capsule and allow the patient to regain full, symmetric knee extension. To regain knee ROM, we have found that it is best to work only on knee extension first until symmetry is restored, and then switch the focus of rehabilitation to knee flexion exercises during the next phase.

Patients remain in the hospital overnight as a 23-hour stay after surgery. Continuous intravenous administration of ketorolac is used for pain control and prevention of swelling. Antiembolism stockings and a cold/compression device (Cryo/Cuff, DJO Inc., Vista, CA) are used at all times starting immediately after surgery to prevent a hemarthrosis. The knee is placed in a continuous passive motion (CPM) machine set from 0 to 30 degrees, but the primary purpose of the CPM is to elevate the knee above the level of the heart (Fig. 107-10).

Knee extension exercises are performed three to four times per day to ensure that full terminal knee extension is maintained. When the knee is in full terminal extension, the intercondylar notch is completely filled by the ACL and PCL, which prevents formation of fibrotic tissue near this notch. Knee extension exercises consist of using the passive knee extension device (see Fig. 107-4), towel stretch (Fig. 107-11), active heel lift (Fig. 107-12), heel prop stretch, and straight-leg raises. The active heel lift and straight-leg raise exercises are used to improve quadriceps muscle control and active terminal knee extension, which is important for long-term maintenance of full, symmetric knee extension.

Patients are discharged home but continue to follow the previously outlined protocol for the first 5 postoperative days. Patients are instructed to remain lying down with their knee elevated in the CPM machine and to use the cold/compression device at all times, except when ambulating to and from the bathroom. This component of the protocol is vital to prevent the development of a hemarthrosis. Prevention of a hemarthrosis allows good quadriceps muscle control, which helps regain/maintain full knee extension and consequently allows for knee flexion deficits to be addressed sooner.

After the first postoperative week, patients continue to focus on the same rehabilitation goals but may gradually begin to return to normal daily activities. They are encouraged

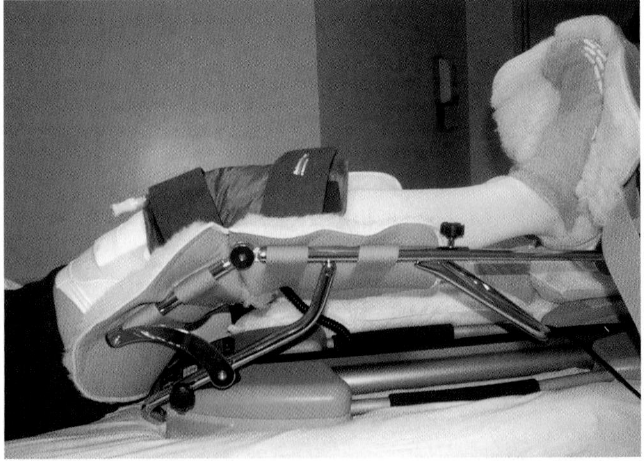

FIGURE 107-10 A continuous passive motion machine is used in the early postoperative phase to help prevent a hemarthrosis by keeping the knee above the level of the heart. A cold/compression device is also applied to the knee.

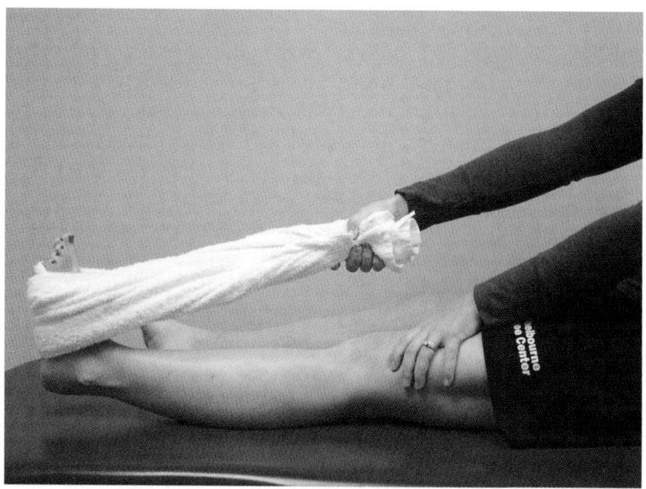

FIGURE 107-11 The towel stretch exercise for knee extension.

to use the cold/compression device at least 3 times a day for 30 minutes or more frequently if necessary to control swelling. During this phase of rehabilitation, it is important to educate patients about habits they need to work on to use their involved knee normally throughout the day and encourage full knee extension during daily activities. We call these extension habits. For the sitting extension habit, patients are advised to sit with their knee fully extended and their heel propped up on their other foot, allowing the knee to fall into full extension. The standing extension habit involves having the patient shift his or her weight onto the involved lower extremity, locking the knee out straight. This exercise encourages full knee extension and normal use of the involved lower extremity during activities of daily living. In addition, it maintains the newly achieved posterior capsular stretch and full contact of the femur, tibia, and ACL in terminal extension.

The speed at which each patient is ready to progress to the next phase of rehabilitation varies considerably based on the chronicity and extent of knee motion loss present. Once full, symmetric knee extension is regained and the patient can easily perform an active heel lift, knee flexion exercises are begun. In cases of more severe knee flexion loss, we begin with a wall slide exercise (Fig. 107-13). Heel-slide exercises are the primary exercise used to improve knee flexion, with a 5-second hold and 10 to 15 repetitions performed per exercise session. Full knee flexion is achieved when the patient can sit on his or her heels without tilting the pelvis laterally (see Fig. 107-2). Patients must be instructed regarding ways to monitor their knee extension closely, and knee flexion exercises should be put on hold if any loss of knee extension occurs.

Low-impact exercise using a bike or elliptical machine may be slowly introduced at this point. We recommend starting without any resistance and gradually increasing the time of the workout by 2 to 3 minutes according to the ability of the patient. ROM must be closely monitored and low-impact exercise should be stopped if the patient begins to lose motion.

Once full, symmetric knee flexion and extension are achieved and maintained, the rehabilitation focus shifts to a unilateral strengthening program to restore strength symmetry. We have found that trying to work on strength in the knee before full extension and flexion have been achieved is difficult because strengthening exercises frequently cause swelling and loss of ROM when they are performed on a stiff knee, thus defeating the purpose of the early phases of rehabilitation.

Loss of knee motion is often associated with significant strength deficits as a result of disuse. We recommend performing isokinetic testing of the quadriceps muscle group to quantify the amount of strength loss compared with the noninvolved knee. We consider strength to be symmetric when it is within 10% of the opposite, normal knee. We recommend using a high number of repetitions and low resistance for single leg press, single knee extension, and step-down exercises to achieve this goal. As with the other phases of the rehabilitation program, care must be taken to ensure that ROM loss does not occur once strengthening exercises commence. If the patient begins to lose knee motion, one should back off from the strengthening exercises until full ROM is restored, and then slowly introduce strengthening exercises again.

Patients who are treated nonoperatively for knee ROM loss follow the same rehabilitation program and progression,

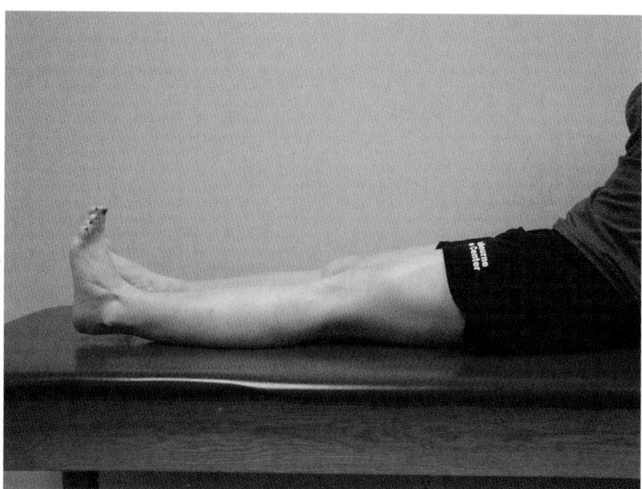

FIGURE 107-12 The active heel lift exercise consists of having the patient contract his or her quadriceps muscle group to actively raise the heel off the table, achieving active terminal knee extension.

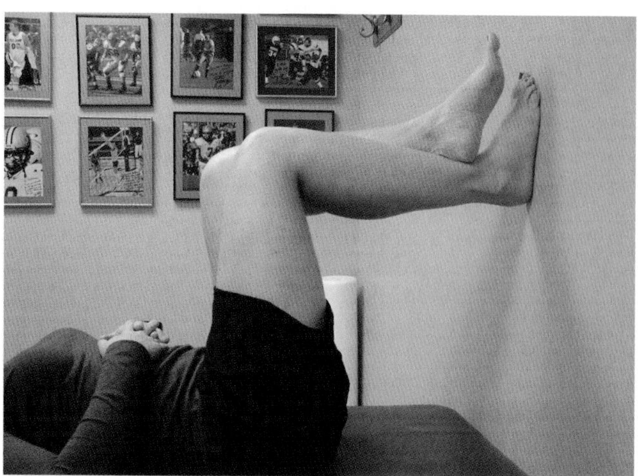

FIGURE 107-13 The wall slide exercise is helpful in regaining knee flexion in patients with more severe knee flexion loss.

except for the surgery-specific measures such as the use of a CPM, antiembolism stockings, and a period of relative bed rest. We are finding that in a large number of patients who come to us for a second opinion, their knee ROM loss was overlooked and not treated by the previous physician and/or therapist. By carefully examining both knees and using the previously outlined treatment principles, many cases of anterior knee pain or generalized knee pain can be addressed effectively without surgery.

Return to Sports

Participation in impact activities, such as running and jumping, is not encouraged until full ROM and strength symmetry are restored. Once these goals are reached, impact activities may be gradually introduced on an every-other-day basis. We recommend using a functional sports progression in which speed and change of direction are gradually increased based on the patient's tolerance. After the patient is comfortable performing individual speed and agility drills, individual sport-specific drills are introduced, followed by drills against a defender, and finally scrimmage and game situations are permitted. Close monitoring of knee extension and knee flexion must be performed on a daily basis to detect any loss of motion early and adjust activity levels accordingly. Patients should be instructed to monitor their own ROM by assessing end feel of the towel stretch exercise and sitting on their heels.

Results

Because arthrofibrosis is a difficult complication to treat, prevention of this problem is the best treatment. The lead author coauthored a published series of 33 patients treated with the previously outlined protocol for arthrofibrosis.[20] The study group included 19 women and 14 men, with a mean age of 31 years. All of these patients were seen in our center after arthrofibrosis developed following knee surgery performed elsewhere, and 27 of these patients experienced arthrofibrosis after an ACL reconstruction. The mean preoperative ROM was 0-8-117 degrees (hyperextension-extension-flexion) for the involved knee compared with 5-0-147 degrees for the uninvolved knee. At a mean of 8.6 months after surgery, the mean involved knee ROM improved to 3-0-134 degrees. The mean subjective scores on the International Knee Documentation Committee (IKDC) survey improved from 45.3 to 67.1 ($P <$ .01), and the patients who achieved normal ROM according to IKDC criteria (knee extension within 2 degrees and knee flexion within 5 degrees of the opposite knee) also had the highest subjective scores. Although these patients showed significant improvement after treatment, the results are still not nearly as good as they could have been if this ROM problem had been prevented and arthrofibrosis had not developed.

Another study looked at patients who did not have arthrofibrosis but were diagnosed with a deconditioned knee, including at least 5 degrees of extension loss compared with the opposite knee.[21] This group of patients included 25 men and 25 women with a mean age of 53.2 years. Osteoarthritis was the underlying pathology in 41 of the 50 patients, and 7 had undergone previous arthroscopy without rehabilitation. All patients were treated nonoperatively with the previously described rehabilitation program. After 3 months of rehabilitation and a guided home exercise program, the mean side-to-side deficit in knee extension improved from 10 to 3 degrees ($P <$ .01), and the mean side-to-side deficit in knee flexion improved from 19 to 9 degrees. Correspondingly, the IKDC subjective scores increased as ROM improved, with a mean at initial evaluation of 34.5 points, improving to 70.5 points 12 months later. This study shows how severe loss of ROM in nonoperative patients can be improved greatly with rehabilitation, and correspondingly, subjective scores and function also improve. Without carefully examining each patient with knee pain, slight ROM loss that is contributing to the patient's knee symptoms can be overlooked, and unnecessary knee surgery may be performed.

Complications

As mentioned earlier, a vast majority of patients with knee ROM loss can be treated nonoperatively, especially when the ROM loss is detected early. Very few complications are associated with nonoperative treatment methods. An increased risk of complications is found in cases that are more advanced and require surgical intervention. As with any surgical procedure, the risk exists for infection, wound-healing problems, deep venous thrombosis, nerve injury, vascular injury, iatrogenic chondral injury, and development of a hemarthrosis. Manipulation is associated with a risk for supracondylar femur fracture or neurovascular injury. The risk of these complications can be minimized with careful surgical techniques, appropriate portal placement, and closely supervised perioperative care and rehabilitation.

Future Considerations

We believe that the detrimental effects of knee ROM loss have been underestimated. In the short term, patients with loss of knee ROM might feel fine, but this condition can lead to problems in the future, just as a patient with high blood pressure or high cholesterol may feel fine now, but without early identification and treatment of these medical issues, more serious problems are known to occur with time. We believe that restoration of full, symmetric knee ROM is critical after any knee surgery. Secondarily, any loss of knee ROM must be identified early and proper treatment should be initiated. As a medical community, we are just beginning to understand the potentially devastating consequences of loss of knee ROM on long-term function.

Several studies have found a link between loss of normal knee motion and osteoarthritis after ACL reconstruction.[2,3,22] The development of osteoarthritis after ACL reconstruction is often attributed to meniscal damage or articular cartilage damage associated with the ACL injury, and evidence exists to support this association.[3,23-32] However, the results of two recent studies indicate that the loss of normal knee ROM is associated with lower subjective scores and an increased incidence of radiographic arthritic changes. The impact is even greater when ROM loss is combined with meniscal or articular cartilage damage.[2,22] One reason that loss of motion may have been overlooked in the past is that long-term follow-up of a minimum of 5 to 10 years is required for these trends to become evident in the data, and many studies in the orthopaedic literature do not include follow-up times that are long enough to detect these long-term changes. Another potential reason that this factor may not be as well recognized in the literature is that precise measurements of knee ROM must be made and compared with the opposite, normal knee to detect smaller side-to-side differences that may still be significant enough to affect function but could be easily overlooked with a cursory evaluation of knee ROM.

Outside the context of ACL reconstruction, several other studies have found a relationship between ROM loss and abnormal findings of radiographs.[33-35] Although these studies were not designed to determine cause and effect, they interpreted loss of motion to be an indication of the extent of osteoarthritis. Current clinical reasoning seems to be that the presence of osteoarthritis leads to a loss of ROM, but is it possible that the loss of knee ROM could predispose the joint to arthritic changes? Another common thought seems to be that it is not possible to improve ROM in the arthritic knee, but our experience and research have shown us that although the progress may occur more slowly, knee ROM can be improved in arthritic knees and is often accompanied by improvements in pain and function.[21] Further research is needed in this area, but careful assessment of every patient and early recognition and treatment of knee ROM loss can prevent long-term deficits that are detrimental to the patient's functional outcome.

For a complete list of references, go to expertconsult.com.

Suggested Readings

Citation: Biggs-Kinzer A, Murphy B, Shelbourne KD, et al: Perioperative rehabilitation using a knee extension device and arthroscopic debridement in the treatment of arthrofibrosis. *Sports Health* 2:417–423, 2010.

Level of Evidence: IV

Summary: The authors provide a case series report of 33 patients who underwent arthroscopy and a perioperative rehabilitation program for the treatment of arthrofibrosis. Details of the pre- and postoperative rehabilitation are clearly described.

Citation: Kim DH, Gill TJ, Millett PJ: Arthroscopic treatment of the arthrofibrotic knee. *Arthroscopy* 20(suppl 2):187–194, 2004.

Level of Evidence: V

Summary: The authors of this article provide a comprehensive description of the many potential causes of range of motion loss in the knee and a detailed, systematic approach to arthroscopic treatment based on the specific area(s) of pathology.

Citation: Lintz F, Pujol N, Boisrenoult P, et al: Anterior cruciate ligament mucoid degeneration: A review of the literature and management guidelines. *Knee Surg Sports Traumatol Arthrosc* 19:1326–1333, 2011.

Level of Evidence: IV

Summary: The authors of this article provide a systematic review of the current literature on mucoid degeneration of the ACL, describing the clinical features of this disease, epidemiology, appearance on imaging studies and arthroscopic examination, and treatment options.

Citation: Shelbourne KD, Freeman H, Gray T: Osteoarthritis after ACL reconstruction: The importance of regaining and maintaining full range of motion. *Sports Health* 4(1):79–85, 2012.

Level of Evidence: IV

Summary: The authors of this article provide a review of the current literature with regard to the association between range of motion loss and osteoarthritis after ACL reconstruction and discuss the potential long-term benefits of achieving and maintaining full symmetric range of motion early after anterior cruciate ligament surgery.

Citation: Shelbourne KD, Wilkens JH, Mollabashy A, et al: Arthrofibrosis in acute anterior cruciate ligament reconstruction: the effect of timing of reconstruction and rehabilitation. *Am J Sports Med* 19:332–336, 1991.

Level of Evidence: IV

Summary: The effects of timing of surgery and rehabilitation programs (accelerated vs. nonaccelerated) used in conjunction with anterior cruciate ligament reconstruction were investigated in this retrospective review of 169 patients. A lower incidence of arthrofibrosis was found when surgery was delayed by at least 3 weeks from the time of injury.

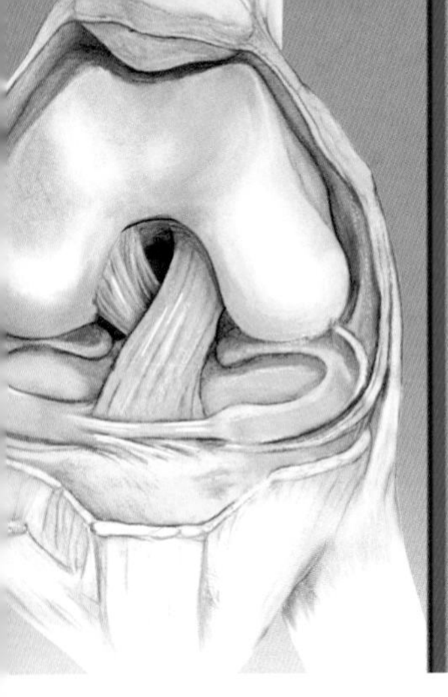

108

Vascular Problems of the Knee

NIMA NASSIRI • PETER LAWRENCE

The most common source of pain and dysfunction in the lower limb of the athlete is musculoskeletal in origin; nevertheless, vascular pathology may also present in a similar fashion. Sports that involve frequent repetitive motions or high-impact collisions have the highest incidence of vascular pathology.

Vascular issues in athletic patients may be difficult to diagnose for several reasons. First, most athletes are young and otherwise in good health, making vascular disease an unlikely concern in the differential diagnosis. Second, an injured athlete's signs and symptoms may have plausible musculoskeletal etiologies, which could present in an identical fashion. Provocative testing and appropriate imaging are thus often required for the diagnosis of underlying vascular pathology. Third, a clinician may not be entirely comfortable with the typical presentation of vascular pathology in the lower limbs, details of the vascular physical examination, and inclusion criteria for vascular pathology in the differential diagnosis.

Underlying vascular issues should be suspected in any athlete who presents with limb pain, early-onset fatigue, limb swelling, limb discoloration, or skin color changes.[1] Familiarity with provocative physical examination maneuvers and imaging modalities is essential to confirm most vascular diagnoses. Moreover, simulation of an athlete's sport-specific positioning, motions, and level of exertion during vascular testing can uncover underlying pathology and can mean the difference between confirming or missing the diagnosis.

Vascular pathology that remains undetected for a prolonged period may have devastating consequences for the athletic patient, including retirement, loss of limb function, or even limb amputation. Consequently, familiarization with the spectrum of traumatic and nontraumatic vascular knee injuries may facilitate early detection, diagnosis, and treatment and provide an improved prognosis for the athletic patient. The intent of this chapter is to review common vascular knee injuries in athletes and provide sports medicine practitioners with a reference for the presentation, evaluation, and clinical management of lower extremity sports-related vascular injuries, including a guide to return to sports when appropriate.

Knee Dislocations

Tibial-femoral knee dislocation is a severe injury with the potential for limb-threatening vascular compromise. Although historically traumatic knee dislocations are considered to be rare injuries, in recent years they have been reported more frequently.[2-4] The popliteal vessels, which cross the popliteal fossa, anchored above and below the joint by the adductor hiatus and the soleus muscle, respectively, are particularly vulnerable to injury from knee dislocation (Fig. 108-1). Knee dislocations are defined in terms of the tibial displacement with respect to the femur and can be characterized as anterior, posterior, lateral, and rotatory.

Anterior Knee Dislocations

Anterior dislocations are the most common, constituting 50% to 60% of all knee dislocations.[2,4,5] Forced hyperextension is the primary mechanism of injury causing anterior dislocation of the knee. In his 1963 landmark study, Kennedy[3] reproduced anterior knee dislocations using cadaver knee specimens subjected to various degrees of hyperextension and elucidated the vascular trauma incurred during forced hyperextension. Rupture of the popliteal artery occurs at an average of 50 degrees of hyperextension. However, at angles below the threshold of arterial rupture, stretching that results in injuries to the tunica intima, contusion, laceration, transection, or avulsion of the popliteal vessels may still occur. Intimal tearing increases the likelihood for arterial occlusion and thrombosis.[2] The poor collateral circulation surrounding the knee joint, as well as the soft tissue injury, further increases the risk for ischemia as a result of acute popliteal occlusion.[6,7] Damage to the popliteal artery occurs in 40% of anterior knee dislocations.[2,5,8] Moreover, stretching of the tibial nerve within the popliteal fossa may cause paresthesia in the lower leg, which is often a finding associated with knee dislocation and popliteal artery injury.

Posterior Dislocation of the Knee

Posterior dislocation of the tibia on the femur accounts for approximately 33% of knee dislocations and may also be a source of potential neurovascular injury.[8] Kennedy's hallmark study revealed that much greater forces are required to induce posterior knee dislocations compared with the anterior knee dislocations,[3] such as those that occur in the classic "dashboard injury."

Injury to collateral ligaments in association with damage to the PCL results in posterior dislocation and multidirectional instability that increases the likelihood of damage to the neurovascular structures within the popliteal fossa. Green and

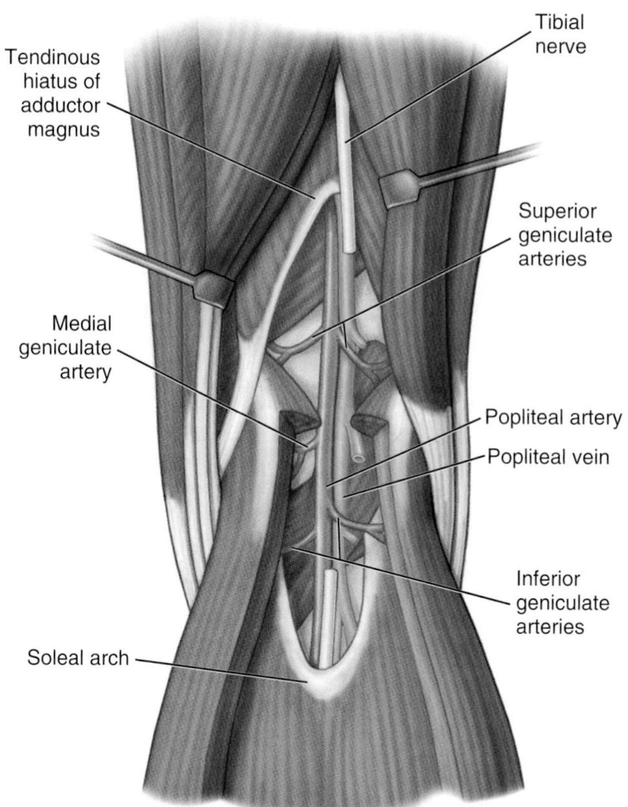

FIGURE 108-1 Anatomy of the popliteal artery. The popliteal artery crosses the popliteal fossa and is anchored above by the adductor hiatus and below by the soleus muscle.

Allen[8] reported that 44% of posterior dislocations had associated injury to the popliteal vessels. Posterior displacement of the tibia directly translates force onto the popliteal artery and vein, with a high likelihood of vessel transection.

Vascular Injury from Knee Dislocation

When knee dislocation is diagnosed or suspected, one of the primary jobs of the clinician is to determine if concomitant injury to the popliteal artery and/or vein has occurred. Failure to recognize popliteal artery injury and restore vessel continuity after knee trauma is a potential cause of lower extremity amputation. Consequently, early recognition of vascular injury remains paramount for limb salvage. During a knee dislocation, the popliteal vessels are at risk for injury because of their anatomic location (Fig. 108-1). The superficial femoral artery traverses past the tendinous hiatus of the adductor magnus muscle and continues as the popliteal artery. Five smaller collateral vessels branch off of the popliteal artery as it crosses the knee joint within the popliteal fossa: the medial and lateral superior geniculate, middle geniculate, and medial and lateral inferior geniculate arteries. The popliteal artery exits the popliteal fossa anchored below the knee joint by the soleal arch before dividing into the anterior and posterior tibial arteries. The genicular arteries form an intricate network of collateral vessels surrounding the contiguous ends of the femur and tibia. This circumpatellar network is divided into superficial and deep plexuses. The superficial plexus is located between the fascia and skin and forms three well-defined arches, one above the upper border of the patella and two below the patella. The deep plexus forms a close network of vessels that surround the articular surfaces of the femur and tibia. The network of genicular anastomoses provides the leg with collateral circulation, which is abundant in number but small in vessel caliber. Frequently the collateral vessels are injured or disrupted in conjunction with the popliteal artery during knee dislocation as a result of soft tissue injury.

The anterior and posterior tibial veins converge to form the popliteal vein at the lower border of the popliteus muscle. Occasionally the popliteal vein is duplicated and present on both the medial and lateral aspects of the popliteal artery. Proximal to the popliteal fossa, the popliteal vein traverses the adductor hiatus and continues as the femoral vein.

Clinical Presentation

Injury to the popliteal artery has been reported to occur in approximately 30% of all complete knee dislocations.[8-11] Types of arterial damage sustained during dislocations of the knee may include injury to the tunica intima, avulsion injury, occlusions, aneurysm generation with secondary thrombosis, embolization, rupture, and transection. Although trauma to the popliteal vessels is easily detected in cases of open knee injuries, identification of neurovascular injury as a result of blunt knee dislocation or instability may be delayed or missed entirely. Clinical indicators of vascular trauma after knee dislocation are classified as hard or soft signs (Table 108-1). Hard signs demand immediate vascular repair and include pulse deficits, acute limb ischemia, active hemorrhage, and pulsatile hematoma.[12] Hallmark signs of acute limb ischemia include pain, paresthesia, loss of sensation or motor function, pallor, and pulselessness in the distal extremity of the affected limb. In the presence of these hard signs, a diagnosis of vascular injury is strongly suggested, and treatment should involve immediate vascular repair. Alternatively, soft signs of injury to the popliteal artery after knee dislocation warrant further diagnostic evaluation and monitoring. These signs include small hematomas, reduced pedal pulses and ankle pressures, neural deficits from injury to the tibial nerve or its branches, and early hemorrhaging that has ceased. When soft signs are

TABLE 108-1

INDICATORS OF POPLITEAL VESSEL COMPROMISE DURING THE VASCULAR PHYSICAL EXAMINATION

Type of Sign	Indicator
Hard	Pulse deficits in pedal pulses with an ankle brachial index <0.5
	Distal ischemia (pain, paresthesia, pallor, and other symptoms of acute ischemia)
	Active hemorrhage and pulsatile bleeding
	Expanding hematoma
	Evidence of compartment syndrome
Soft	Small hematoma that does not change in size
	Hemorrhage that has ceased
	Reduced ankle pressure <0.9 but >0.5
	Neural deficits from injury to the tibial nerve

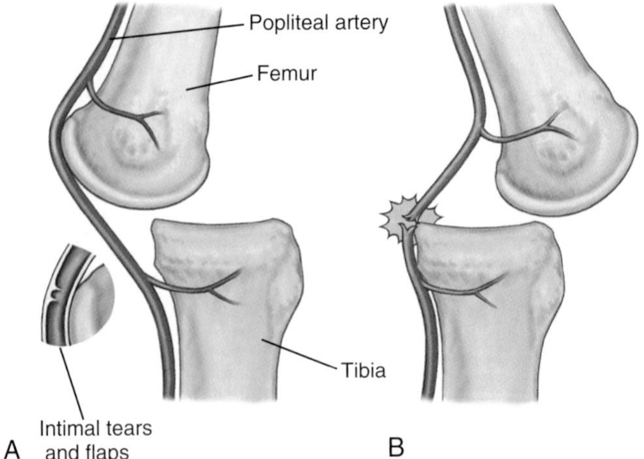

FIGURE 108-2 Mechanisms of popliteal artery injury after knee dislocation. Posterior knee dislocations (**A**) and anterior knee dislocations (**B**) stretch the popliteal artery.

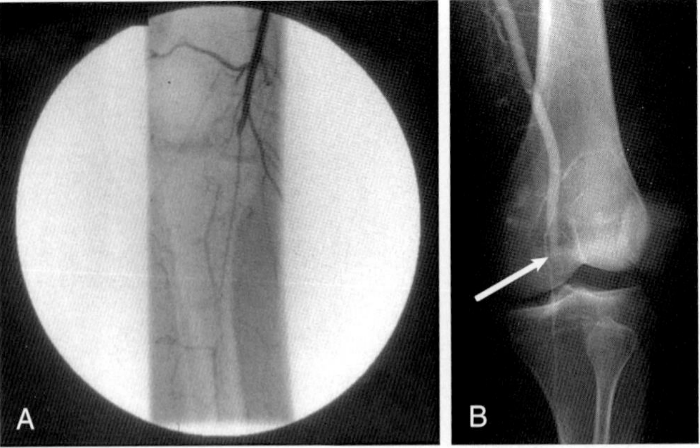

FIGURE 108-3 Arterial injury after a knee dislocation. **A,** Anterior dislocation of the knee causes occlusion at the popliteal-tibial artery junction. **B,** A coronal view of the lower extremity angiogram after posterior knee dislocation reveals an occluded popliteal artery (arrow). *(**A,** From Seroyer ST, Musahl V, Harner CD: Management of the acute knee dislocation: the Pittsburgh experience,* Int J Care Injured *39:710-718, 2008. **B,** From Kapur S, Wissman RD, Robertson M, et al: Acute knee dislocation: review of an elusive entity,* Curr Probl Diagn Radiol *38:237-250, 2009).*

present, imaging of the popliteal vessels is required to assess the extent of vascular trauma.

Vascular injuries associated with knee dislocations result from excessive stretching or transection of the popliteal vessels (Fig. 108-2). Common vascular injuries following anterior knee dislocations include intimal tears and the formation of intimal flaps. In such patients, blood flow through the artery may not be appreciably altered, and consequently patients may present without any hard signs of vascular trauma. Nevertheless, the presence of intimal tears and flaps increases the risk of thrombosis and embolization. Moreover, extensive intimal injuries accelerate vessel wall damage over time, and patients who initially lack symptoms of vascular compromise may begin to exhibit diminished popliteal flow. Some authors suggest that posterior knee dislocations more commonly result in transection of the popliteal artery, with resultant acute limb ischemia.[13] Blood flow through the popliteal artery becomes significantly diminished (Fig. 108-3), and patients present with immediate hard signs of vascular injury such as active hemorrhage, expanding hematoma, bruits in the distal arterial circuitry, and signs of acute ischemia such as pain, paresthesia, poikilothermia, pallor, and pulselessness. These signs indicate significant vascular compromise that demands immediate operative intervention and vascular repair.

Physical Examination and Testing

The high rate of popliteal artery injury associated with knee dislocations, combined with the possibility of delayed presentation of symptoms of vascular trauma as a result of knee dislocation, demands that diagnostic evaluation for vascular integrity be performed for all patients suspected of having a knee dislocation. The diagnosis of knee dislocation itself is based on the mechanism of injury obtained from the history, physical examination, and radiographic findings. Frequently, patients may present with the knee already reduced.[5] Because the risk for arterial injury is the same in both the reduced and dislocated knee,[10] clinical suspicion of popliteal artery damage should remain high in such patients. Absence of hemarthrosis in patients suspected of having had a knee dislocation does not decrease the risk for vascular injury.

Diagnostic evaluation of vascular integrity in the lower limb is critical to determining a method of treatment (Fig. 108-4). Serial measurements of pulse quality in both the posterior tibial and dorsalis pedis arteries should be performed because the pulse may be diminished or absent after an upstream arterial injury. Studies reveal that clinical evaluation of peripheral pulses accurately identifies the existence of vascular lesions after knee dislocation with a specificity of 91%.[14,15] Although the presence of pulse abnormalities is sufficient to rule in the existence of vascular lesions, a low sensitivity of 79% means that vascular injury may exist in the absence of peripheral pulse deficits.[15,16] In addition to digital

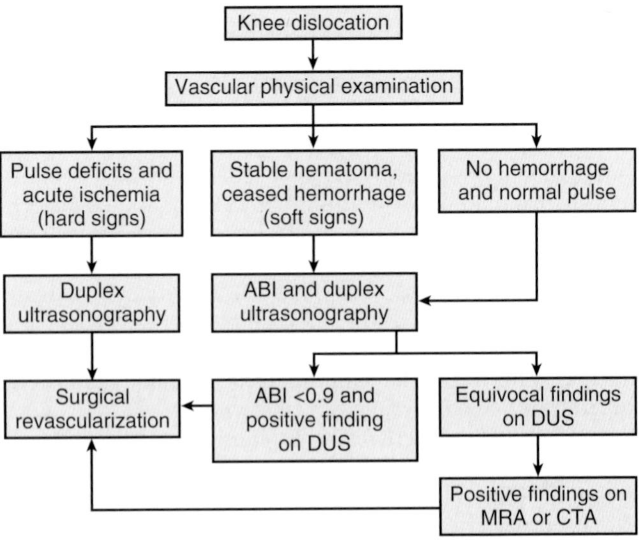

FIGURE 108-4 Algorithm to determine the extent of vascular pathology associated with knee dislocations. *ABI,* Ankle brachial index; *CTA,* computed tomographic angiography; *DUS,* duplex ultrasonography; *MRA,* magnetic resonance angiography.

pulse evaluation, serial measurements of the ankle brachial index (ABI) enable the clinician to qualitatively assess deficits in distal perfusion induced by vascular trauma. ABI values <0.9 indicate the presence of vascular injury requiring surgical intervention with 95% to 100% sensitivity and 80% to 100% specificity.[17]

Imaging

In patients presenting with pulse abnormalities and associated ischemic syndrome, surgical intervention and revascularization is the primary priority, and imaging may be performed to determine the location and severity of vascular compromise. In this context, imaging aids in determining the surgical approach and should be performed in the operating room to minimize warm ischemia time. Previous studies have found that approximately 3 hours are saved when arteriographic imaging is performed in the operating arena.[18] In patients with pulse abnormalities in the absence of ischemia, imaging is mandatory to determine if intervention and vascular repair are required.

Historically, arteriography has served as the gold standard for symptomatic vascular lesions after knee dislocation. This form of imaging allows the examiner to identify the location and extent of injury and the presence of intimal flap tears both within the popliteal artery and its distal branches. However, the invasive nature of angiography has led to a trend in recent years toward less invasive and safer imaging modalities. Moreover, arteriography is not fully reliable as an imaging tool. Studies have reported 1% to 6% false-negative rates, which can delay patient treatment, and 2.4% to 7% false-positive rates, which can result in unnecessary surgical intervention.[14,19,20] In the Lower Extremity Assessment Project study, it was reported that patients with hard signs of vascular injury can be treated effectively without arteriographic imaging before surgery.[21]

In recent years, duplex ultrasonography has become a mainstay of the rapid evaluation of vascular pathology resulting from suspected popliteal artery injury and can be used to analyze flow through the popliteal vessels in real time in the emergency department or operating room (Fig. 108-4). Studies assessing the diagnostic value of duplex scanning as a means of noninvasive imaging in persons with lower limb trauma reported a diagnostic sensitivity of 95%, a specificity of 99%, and a diagnostic accuracy of 98%.[22] The rapidity with which duplex scanning can be performed makes it an ideal tool for visualization of vascular trauma, particularly in patients with vascular compromise who are awaiting operative intervention.

Computed tomographic angiography (CTA) and magnetic resonance angiography (MRA) also can be used to visualize intimal tears when duplex ultrasound results are equivocal.

Treatment Options

Warm ischemia time remains the single most important variable that determines functional outcome in patients with a popliteal artery injury resulting from knee dislocation.[21] Prompt diagnostic evaluation, including imaging to determine the extent of vascular injury, and operative intervention to restore adequate distal perfusion in the hypoperfused patient are essential for successful treatment and limb salvage. Warm ischemia times greater than 6 hours can cause irreversible neurologic injury and muscle necrosis distal to the site of blood flow obstruction, and the rate of amputation in patients who experience a delay in arterial reconstruction exceeding 8 hours has been reported to be 85%.[5,11] Consequently, any delay of imaging and immediate intervention in cases of limb ischemia increases morbidity and worsens patient prognosis.

Immediate surgical repair is obligatory as soon as vascular trauma is confirmed. The principles of surgical intervention in patients with popliteal artery injuries include (1) rapid restoration of arterial blood flow to the distal extremity, (2) removal of thrombus in the distal artery, and (3) alleviation of compartment syndrome, which may exacerbate distal ischemia. Whether vascular or orthopaedic reconstruction should be performed first remains an area of debate, with the appropriate sequence of repair depending on the time course of injury and the severity of the ischemia. If the patient presents with prolonged warm ischemia time or severe deficits in distal perfusion, prompt vascular repair and restoration of arterial flow is indicated before orthopaedic management. In such cases, however, secondary orthopaedic procedures may damage newly repaired vascular structures. Consequently, the order of repair should be determined on a case-by-case basis, with special consideration given to the extent and severity of ischemia in the presenting patient.

Reconstruction of the popliteal artery can be achieved through either posterior or medial approaches. The posterior approach allows for greater visualization of structures within the popliteal fossa and is more ideally suited for treatment of lesions of the midpopliteal artery, whereas the medial approach allows easier access to distal structures of the popliteal fossa and is associated with more rapid postsurgical healing. The type of surgical repair performed depends on the extent of vascular injury and may include lateral repair, end-to-end arterial repair with interposition vein graft, repair of intimal injury by vein patch, or bypass by saphenous vein grafting.[13] The majority of popliteal artery repairs that result from knee dislocations require venous grafting. Venous patches are used to provide structural integrity in cases of intimal tears and flaps, and greater saphenous vein grafts from the contralateral leg are used for extensive arterial resection. End-to-end repair of the popliteal artery through a posterior approach requires the least dissection of the popliteal artery and surrounding soft tissue. If the popliteal vein is also damaged after knee dislocation, venous repair is required and can be accomplished by lateral repair or interposition vein grafts.[13,23] Failure to repair venous injuries is associated with an increased risk of lower extremity edema, thrombosis, and embolization, as well as limb loss. If ischemia has been present for several hours, a fasciotomy is mandatory to prevent compartment syndrome. Fasciotomy is required in the treatment of 50% to 80% of patients with injury to the popliteal artery and is associated with a significant improvement in the rate of limb salvage.[18,24] Primary amputation is rarely indicated and is only used when extensive muscle necrosis is present in the distal extremity. Typically, warm ischemia times exceeding 6 hours are associated with a dramatic increase in the rate of eventual limb amputation.[21]

Although historically all popliteal artery injuries resulting from knee dislocations have been repaired through open surgical methods, in some studies authors have reported the successful treatment of blunt popliteal artery injuries and

AUTHORS' PREFERRED TECHNIQUE

Popliteal Artery Repair in Knee Dislocation

I. Initial examination
  A. Patient history and presentation
  B. Examination of pedal pulses on both the affected and contralateral limb
  C. Bilateral ankle brachial index measurements
  D. Imaging of the popliteal space using duplex ultrasonography
II. In patients presenting with hard signs of vascular injury, no further imaging is required and immediate surgical intervention is warranted
III. In patients presenting with soft signs of vascular injury or if the duplex scanning yields equivocal results, further imaging via magnetic resonance angiography and computed tomographic angiography scanning is necessary to establish treatment protocol
IV. Open surgical intervention
  A. With the patient lying prone, an S-shaped incision is made in the popliteal region
    • The posterior approach is preferred over the medial approach because it facilitates greater access to the neurovascular structures of the popliteal fossa with the least amount of soft tissue dissection and sparing of the saphenous vein
  B. Skin flaps are raised to expose underlying deep fascia, which is then transected longitudinally
    • Care should be taken to avoid transection of the median cutaneous sural nerve
  C. The tibial nerve is encountered first and mobilized
  D. The popliteal vein passes through the medial and lateral heads of the gastrocnemius muscle deep in the popliteal fossa
  E. The popliteal artery lies deeper in the popliteal space and can be followed distally
V. Arterial reconstruction is required if evidence of significant intimal injury, stenosis, occlusion, thrombosis, or laceration is observed
  A. Placement of a short interposition vein graft, which is usually harvested from the ipsilateral lesser saphenous vein or contralateral saphenous vein
  B. An alternative is a short venous bypass graft with exclusion of the occluded artery to avoid thromboembolism

acutely ischemic distal lower extremities with use of endovascular techniques.[25,26] Proponents of endovascular repair in cases of blunt popliteal artery injury cite the usefulness of a percutaneous approach in cases in which extensive soft tissue damage to the surrounding structures of the popliteal fossa may complicate open repair. Endovascular techniques allow for visualization of the injury site, removal of any associated thrombus, protection against distal embolization, and repair of an intimal lesion. However, the durability of covered stents and endografts in the popliteal location, where excessive motion occurs, has not been established.

Postoperative Management

Postoperative follow-up should include focused physical examinations with special attention to distal perfusion. Ankle pressures, ABI measurements, and duplex scanning should be performed to assess blood flow through the reconstructed artery within the popliteal fossa. Use of other imaging modalities such as computed tomography (CT)/CTA and magnetic resonance imaging (MRI)/MRA are generally not recommended unless symptoms of graft occlusion or diminished blood flow reappear. Follow-up should be scheduled within 4 to 6 weeks after surgery and twice annually within the first year. In subsequent years, annual follow-up is sufficient to ensure graft patency.

Complications

Postoperative complications after popliteal artery repair are centered on evaluation for delayed compartment syndrome, graft patency, maintenance of tension-free healing, and prevention of postsurgical deep vein thrombosis (DVT). Antiplatelet medications are typically prescribed for patients to prevent postsurgical graft thrombosis. Patency of the vein graft may be compromised by stenosis at the sites of venous graft-artery interface. Postsurgical follow-up should include physical examination and imaging via duplex ultrasonography to ensure graft patency and appropriate healing.

Popliteal Artery Entrapment Syndrome

Popliteal artery entrapment syndrome (PAES) is characterized by the extrinsic compression of the popliteal vessels by the musculotendinous structures of the popliteal fossa. Anomalies in the embryologic development and migration of the medial head of the gastrocnemius muscle generate anatomic variants that entrap the popliteal vessels and tibial nerve.[27] PAES is usually a congenital abnormality, with estimates of its frequency reported between 0.62% to 3.5% of the population,[28,29] but functional PAES may occur in the absence of any embryologic or anatomic abnormality. In persons with functional PAES, the popliteal vessels become impinged from physiologic hypertrophy of the gastrocnemius, soleus, plantaris, or semimembranosus muscles.[30,31] Functional PAES is particularly prevalent in well-conditioned athletes.

History

Entrapment of the popliteal artery was first documented by 1879 by an Edinburgh medical student, Anderson Stuart, who described an abnormality in the course of the popliteal artery in the amputated limb of a patient with gangrene.[32] Nearly 50 years later, Louis Dubreuil-Chambardel described separation of the popliteal vessels by an accessory gastrocnemius muscle in a patient.[33] Although entrapment of the popliteal artery has been documented for more than a century, it was not until the mid 1960s that the term *popliteal artery entrapment syndrome* was first used by Love and Whelan[27] to define a clinical presentation. In 1985, Rignault et al.[30] presented the first case report of functional entrapment syndrome caused by hypertrophy of the gastrocnemius in an "intensively trained athlete."

After these initial reports, numerous publications documented the clinical progression of PAES in further detail. Studies have estimated that approximately 60% of young patients who present with intermittent claudication have PAES.[34]

Classification

Originally, Insua et al.[35] presented the first classification system for PAES based on variations of the course of the popliteal artery in relation to the medial head of the gastrocnemius muscle. A simplified classification scheme for PAES, provided by Delaney and Gonzalez,[36] was proposed and consisted of four subtypes. Modifications to the Delaney scheme by Rich et al.[37] in 1979 yielded a five-subtype system that included impingement of both the popliteal artery and vein (Fig. 108-5). Lastly, with the documentation of functional PAES by Rignault and colleagues[30] in 1985, a sixth subtype was added to facilitate the classification of patients presenting with symptoms of PAES in the absence of any overt anatomic variation or developmental abnormality. The current six-subtype classification system is the most widely accepted system among clinicians.

Type I: Type I is the most common variant of PAES and is characterized by a significant medial shift of the popliteal artery with normal positioning of the medial head of the gastrocnemius muscle.[38] This type of arterial entrapment occurs when the popliteal artery completes its development before the embryologic migration of the medial head of the gastrocnemius muscle. Consequently,

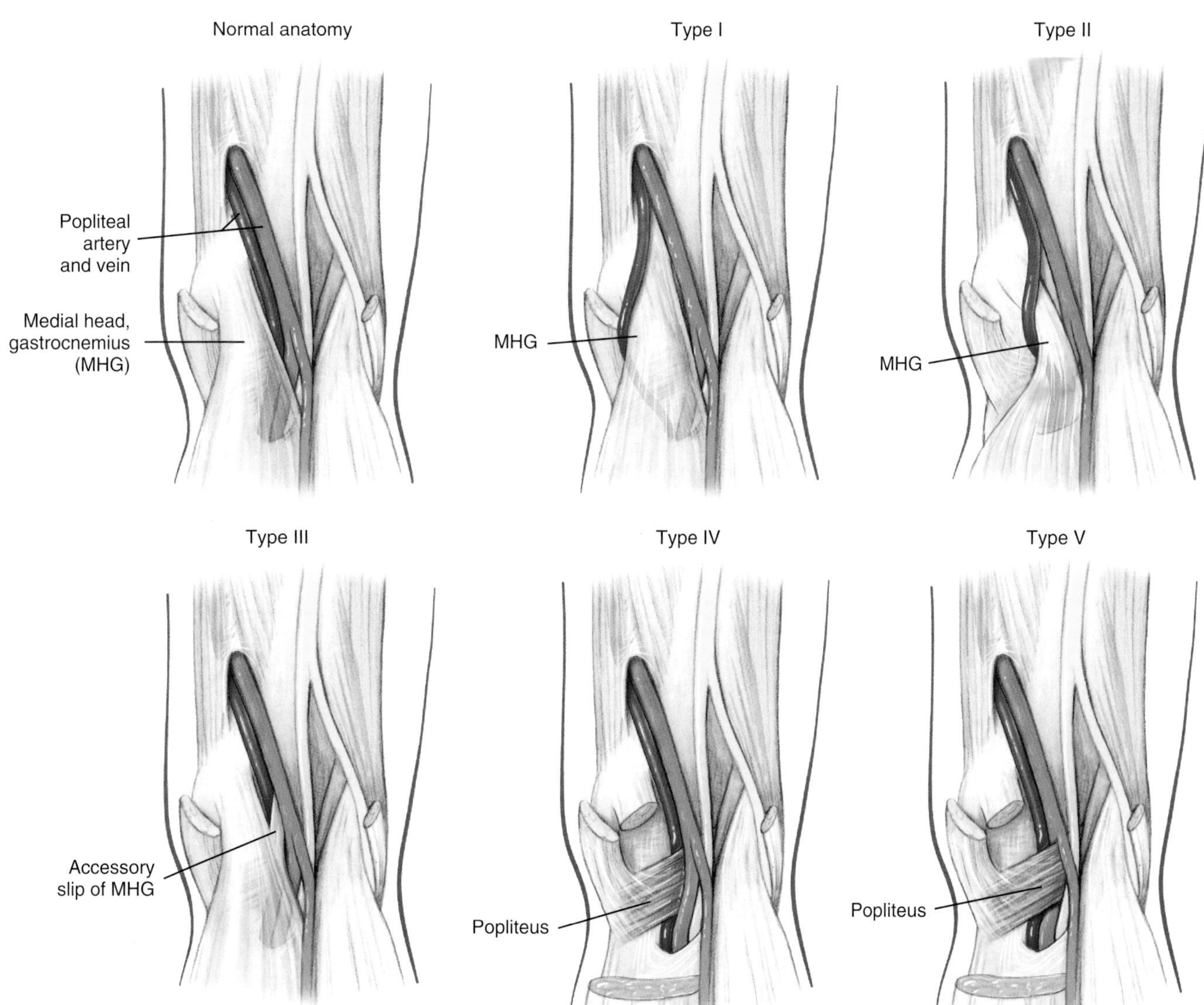

FIGURE 108-5 The popliteal artery entrapment syndrome (PAES) classification scheme. Normal anatomy of the popliteal fossa and the classification types of PAES are shown.

as the medial muscle head completes its migration, it sweeps the popliteal artery medially.[39]

Type II: In type II popliteal artery entrapment, the popliteal artery is shifted medially to a lesser degree than its type I counterpart, and the medial head of the gastrocnemius expresses variable attachment to either the lateral aspect of the medial femoral condyle, the intercondylar area, or the lower femur superior to the condyle.[38] Type II entrapment occurs when the distal popliteal artery forms prematurely and temporarily arrests the migration of the medial head of the gastrocnemius. Consequently, the popliteal artery is medially displaced relative to an abnormally positioned medial head of the gastrocnemius.

Type III: Type III popliteal entrapment results from abnormal mature muscle slips or fibrotendinous bands that branch off the medial head of the gastrocnemius muscle, slip between the popliteal artery and vein, and attach to either the medial or lateral femoral condyle. These accessory tissues are derived from the embryologic remnants of the migrating medial head, and in the adult, they persist posterior to the popliteal artery. As a result, the popliteal artery becomes separated from the popliteal vein and entrapped between the two layers of musculotendinous tissue.

Type IV: Type IV popliteal entrapment occurs when the axial artery, the embryologic precursor of the tibial arteries, persists as the mature distal popliteal artery. Consequently, the artery remains in its embryologic position and is compressed as it passes deep to the popliteus muscle or associated fibrous bands.

Type V: Type V popliteal entrapment can occur via any of the aforementioned mechanisms but is unique in that both the popliteal artery and vein are entrapped and compressed. Impingement of both popliteal vessels is estimated to occur in 10% to 15% of all cases of popliteal entrapment.[39-41]

Type VI: Functional popliteal entrapment occurs in patients in the absence of any anatomic or developmental abnormality. Although the exact mechanism of popliteal entrapment in this subtype of patients remains to be elucidated, it is believed that hypertrophy of the medial head of the gastrocnemius compresses the posteromedial aspect of the popliteal artery, resulting in physiologic occlusion of the artery during plantar flexion or extension.[30,31,38] Some investigators have proposed that a more lateral attachment of the medial head of the gastrocnemius within physiologic normal limits may predispose a person to functional popliteal entrapment upon hypertrophy of the gastrocnemius as a result of lower limb exercise.[38,42]

Clinical Presentation

The hallmark of PAES is a young, active, and otherwise healthy person with intermittent claudication of the calf and foot. Approximately 60% of patients with symptoms of PAES are younger than 30 years, and the syndrome has a significant predilection for the male sex, with approximately 80% of all reported cases occurring in men.[1,41] In more than a fourth of all cases, PAES is simultaneously present in both lower extremities.[38] Participation in sports such as basketball, football, rugby, and martial arts is most commonly associated with popliteal entrapment.

Intermittent claudication of the calf or foot is the most common symptom and is reported to occur in 69% to 90% of patients with PAES.[34,43,44] In rare cases, symptoms may present in an atypical fashion, such as the onset of claudication after standing or walking, which improves with running.[45,46]

In addition to claudication, patients may present with symptoms such as coldness, pallor, or loss of sensation in the lower extremities. Because the tibial nerve travels adjacent to the popliteal artery through the popliteal fossa, all cases of PAES may potentially impinge the nerve and result in paresthesia in the distal extremity. In fewer than 10% of patients with PAES, concomitant symptoms of critical limb ischemia (CLI) may exist.[39,47] Signs and symptoms of CLI include paresthesia, pallor of the foot and toes, ischemia, pain upon resting, and tissue necrosis. Importantly, PAES results from the extrinsic compression of the popliteal artery rather than intrinsic occlusion from atherosclerosis, as observed in patients with peripheral arterial disease. Consequently the patient with PAES who has signs and symptoms of CLI will lack the diffuse atherosclerosis observed in patients with end-stage peripheral arterial disease. Acute limb ischemia is rare in patients with PAES.[39] A patient with PAES who has venous involvement may also report calf and ankle swelling.

In most cases, pedal pulses are palpable and normal at rest in a patient with PAES, provided that compression of the popliteal artery has not progressed to a state of chronic occlusion. Blood flow through the lumen of the popliteal artery is significantly attenuated upon compression. Stress maneuvers such as active plantar flexion or dorsiflexion of the foot against resistance temporarily stenoses the otherwise patent lumen of the popliteal artery in the patient with PAES and results in diminished pedal pulses.[38] Left untreated, the constant compressive stimuli may compromise the structural integrity of the popliteal artery and cause chronic occlusion.

In approximately 12% of cases, poststenotic dilatation of the popliteal artery may occur after compression.[39] In such patients, degeneration of the popliteal artery increases the likelihood of aneurysm formation; popliteal aneurysms in these otherwise young and healthy persons can be a source of distal embolization. Studies report that between 20% and 30% of patients with popliteal artery aneurysm in conjunction with PAES experience an embolic event in the absence of intervention.[40,48] Alternatively, distal emboli may also result from focal thrombus formation secondary to arterial degeneration in a normal-caliber entrapped artery.[42]

Physical Examination and Testing

In most diagnostic cases, a detailed patient history and thorough physical examination are sufficient to include or exclude PAES as a differential diagnosis. If popliteal entrapment is suspected, provocative testing and noninvasive diagnostic evaluations should be performed to both confirm the diagnosis and determine the severity of the entrapment. Initial testing includes a thorough assessment of the pulses in the femoral, popliteal, posterior tibial, and dorsalis pedis arteries in both the affected and contralateral limb. Because PAES is characterized by intermittent claudication, pulses should also be qualitatively evaluated as the patient performs dynamic provocative maneuvers. Traditionally, these maneuvers include active plantar flexion and dorsiflexion of the ankle against resistance with the knee in full extension.[47] In the late stages of PAES, a collateral network gradually develops as a result of extrinsic popliteal artery occlusion, and thus the foot appears normal, even when pulses are absent.

Resting and postexertional ABIs help confirm the diagnosis of PAES. An ABI value greater than 1 is considered normal, and thus an ABI value <0.9 suggests arterial stenosis/occlusion. In persons with PAES, claudication typically develops after exercise or exertion in the lower limbs. ABI values should reflect this phenomenon and may be normal at rest but less than 1 upon stress testing.

In conjunction with examining the arterial circulation, a thorough venous evaluation should also be performed in the patient suspected of having PAES. Signs of venous obstruction in the popliteal fossa include swelling, cyanosis, and distention of the superficial veins of the distal extremities of the lower limbs. The presence of these signs supports the diagnosis of PAES, specifically type V.

Imaging

In addition to physical examination and provocative testing, imaging is an important diagnostic tool used to confirm a definitive diagnosis of PAES. Both noninvasive and invasive imaging protocols may be used in the evaluation of a patient with PAES. Noninvasive imaging modalities include duplex ultrasonography, CT, and MRI.

Duplex Ultrasonography

Duplex scanning allows real-time visualization of the popliteal artery (Fig. 108-6). It is obtained as the patient performs dynamic provocative maneuvers and provides a qualitative measure of the degree of stenosis. A 50% decrease in the peak systolic velocity through the popliteal artery during active plantar flexion is considered diagnostic of PAES.[47] Although a positive duplex test upon provocative maneuvers supports the diagnosis of PAES, further imaging studies should be performed before surgical intervention. Studies measuring peak systolic velocities through the popliteal artery have reported high rates of compression (53% to 72%) in healthy patients without PAES.[41,49,50] Such high rates of false-positive results suggest that duplex testing overestimates the actual rate of popliteal artery compression. Consequently, positive findings on duplex scanning should raise clinical suspicion of PAES but warrant use of other imaging modalities.

MRI and MRA

In recent years, the MRI/MRA imaging modalities have emerged as highly accurate and minimally invasive tools for the diagnosis and evaluation of PAES. Similar to CT/CTA, MRI/MRA imaging allows for the visualization of anatomic and functional relationships between structures within the popliteal fossa. Also analogous to a CT scan, MRI is noninvasive and able to differentiate between anatomic abnormalities with similarly presenting pathologies. Unlike CTA, the contrast dye used during MRA imaging is not nephrotoxic. Moreover, studies have demonstrated the superiority of MRI compared with ultrasound and CT-based imaging modalities in the diagnosis of PAES because it better facilitates visualization of the muscular anatomy (Fig. 108-7). Most studies suggest that MRI/MRA be used as the principal diagnostic tool for the evaluation of young patients who present with symptoms of PAES.[51] As with all of the other imaging modalities, MRI/MRA for PAES should be performed in both resting conditions and under active plantar flexion against resistance (see Fig. 108-7). In this way, subtle popliteal entrapment that would otherwise be overlooked on neutral imaging may be identified.

CT and CTA

CT/CTA currently plays an alternative role as a diagnostic tool in the evaluation of patients suspected of having PAES. CT scanning also allows for the visualization of the many structures within the popliteal fossa, specifically revealing the anatomic relationship between the popliteal artery and surrounding bony, tendinous, and muscular structures. In addition to elucidating relationships between structures in the

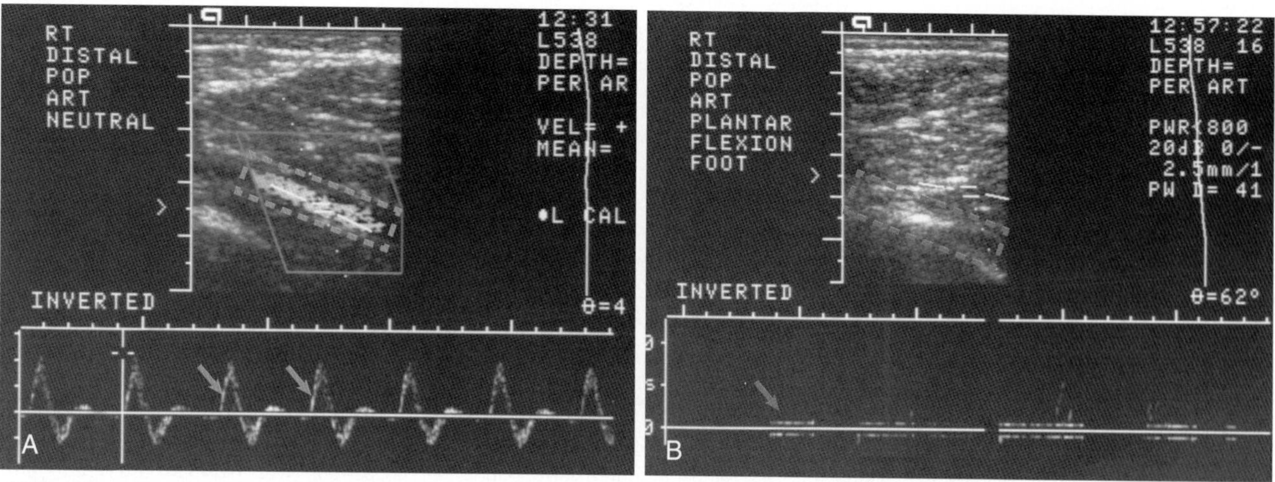

FIGURE 108-6 Duplex ultrasonography (DUS) in a 49-year-old man with right popliteal artery entrapment syndrome. **A,** DUS of the right popliteal fossa with the leg in neutral position shows a normal triphasic waveform (*arrows*). **B,** DUS obtained with plantar flexion of the right foot shows compression of the popliteal artery and diminished flow (*arrow*). *(From Macedo TA, Johnson CM, Hallett JW Jr, et al: Popliteal artery entrapment syndrome: role of imaging in the diagnosis,* AJR Am J Roentgenol *181[5]:1259-1265, 2003.)*

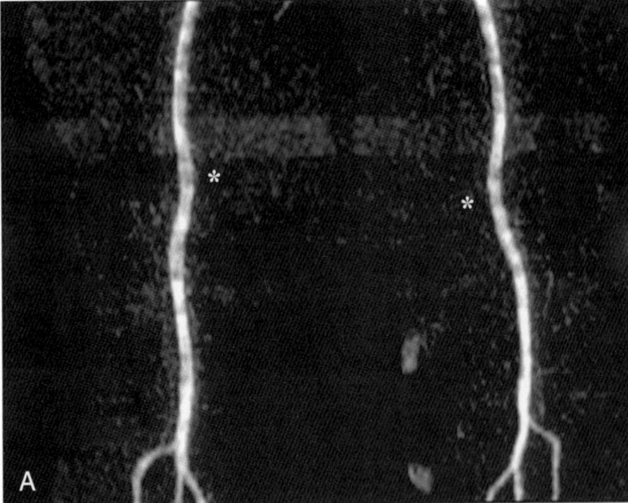

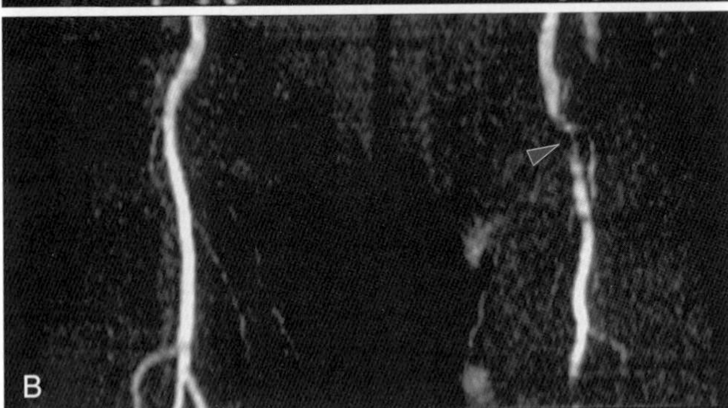

FIGURE 108-7 Imaging in a patient with popliteal artery entrapment syndrome. **A,** Time-of-flight magnetic resonance angiography (MRA) of the popliteal arteries in the neutral position shows normal arterial flow. Medial deviation along the path of both popliteal arteries is observed (*asterisks*). **B,** Time-of-flight MRA of the popliteal arteries with active plantar flexion of the feet shows near occlusion (*arrowhead*) of the left popliteal artery and no change in the right leg.

popliteal fossa, CT/CTA can be used to reveal focal sites of arterial stenosis, occlusion, thrombosis, or degeneration (Fig. 108-8). As with the other imaging modalities, CT/CTA scans should be obtained while the patient is in both a neutral state and during active plantar flexion against resistance. In contrast to duplex ultrasonography and angiography, both limbs can be evaluated simultaneously with CT/CTA scanning, thereby eliminating concern about the possibility of bilateral entrapment.[52-55] Lastly, CTA can be used to differentiate between pathologies with otherwise similar clinical presentations, such as adventitial cystic disease and a popliteal artery aneurysm.

Angiography

Historically, contrast angiography has served as the gold standard in diagnosing PAES. As with noninvasive imaging modalities, provocative maneuvers are required when performing angiography to reveal the popliteal entrapment. In the absence of provocative testing, angiography has a low sensitivity for PAES and may indicate that a popliteal artery is healthy despite underlying pathology. Diagnosis of PAES on the basis of angiography is indicated when at least two of the following imaging features are present (Fig. 108-9)[39]:

1. Medial displacement of the proximal popliteal artery
2. Segmental stenosis of the midpopliteal artery
3. Poststenotic dilatation of the popliteal artery

Contrast angiography also allows for visualization of the tibial artery and is useful in cases of embolization resulting from popliteal aneurysm or a thrombogenic popliteal artery caused by entrapment.

Although angiography is an effective diagnostic tool for the evaluation of patients suspected of having PAES,[38,56] many concerns have been raised with regard to this imaging modality. Angiography is a fundamentally invasive procedure, and as such, it carries an increased risk of potential complications from arterial catheterization. Although in healthy persons the dye is cleared with relative ease, it may be a source of significant morbidity in patients with renal insufficiency. Angiography also does not evaluate muscular abnormalities. With the advent of CTA and MRA imaging methods, angiography is no longer used as a staple for the diagnosis of PAES; rather, these higher specificity and less invasive imaging modalities are now favored.[51] Angiography is used in conjunction with treatment, however, such as when thrombolysis of distal emboli is performed.

Treatment Options

Surgical intervention is the primary treatment option for symptomatic PAES and is warranted in almost all cases. The

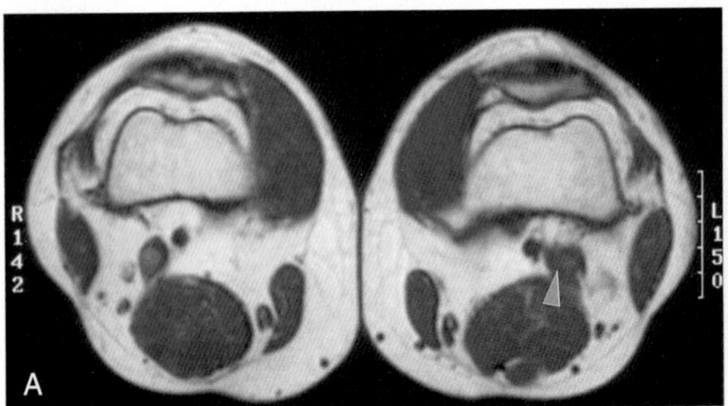

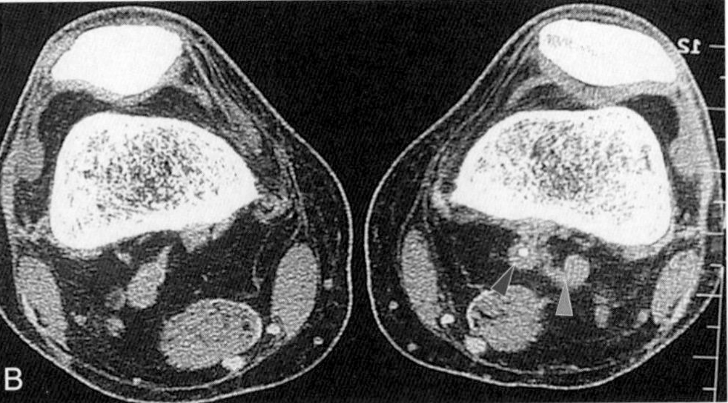

FIGURE 108-8 Axial magnetic resonance imaging (MRI) and computed tomography (CT) in patients with popliteal artery entrapment syndrome. **A,** T1-weighted MRI reveals abnormal muscle slip (*orange arrowhead*) between popliteal vessels. The contralateral image shows normal anatomy. **B,** Bilateral CT angiography of the lower extremities shows an abnormal muscle band (*orange arrowhead*) from the medial head of the gastrocnemius muscle with significant occlusion of the right popliteal artery (*blue arrowhead*). The contralateral extremity shows normal anatomy.

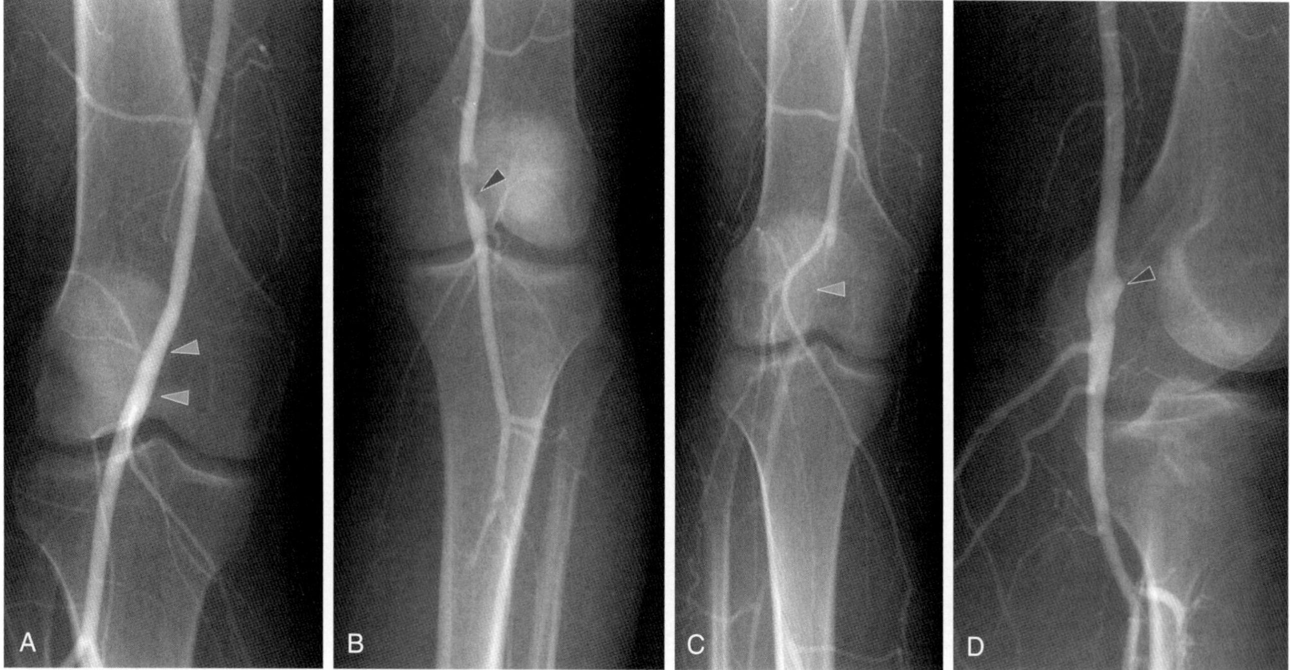

FIGURE 108-9 Angiographic findings encountered with popliteal artery entrapment syndrome (PAES). **A,** The angiogram of a 34-year-old woman with PAES shows medial deviation of the popliteal artery (*orange arrowheads*). **B,** The angiogram of a 21-year-old man with PAES shows nonocclusive acute thrombus of the popliteal artery (*blue arrowhead*) with embolization to the distal tibial artery. **C,** The angiogram of a 34-year-old woman with PAES shows occlusion of the popliteal artery (*orange arrowhead*). **D,** The angiogram of a 37-year-old man with PAES shows a popliteal artery aneurysm (*blue arrowhead*).

basic goals of surgical intervention in the treatment of PAES are threefold: (1) relieve the neurovascular structures from entrapment, (2) restore normal blood flow and distal perfusion, and (3) restore normal anatomy.[41]

The degree of surgical complexity for an individual patient depends on the anatomy within the popliteal fossa and the integrity of the popliteal vessels. At an early clinical stage, the popliteal artery, although entrapped, remains physiologically normal. In the absence of arterial disease, surgical therapy limited to musculotendinous release is sufficient to restore normal anatomy and blood flow through the popliteal vessels. Musculotendinous release is achieved by myotomy of the medial head of the gastrocnemius muscle, as well as by excision of any abnormal muscle slips and tendinous bands that contribute to the entrapment (Fig. 108-10). Symptomatic patients with PAES who have normal popliteal vessels and are treated with surgical myotomy have been shown to return to prior levels of athletic activity, do not require additional intervention, and maintain popliteal artery patency throughout a 10-year follow-up.[38]

A posterior or medial surgical approach may be used to perform musculotendinous release and decompression of the popliteal artery, although the posterior approach is more widely used and provides the surgeon with greater operative flexibility and a wider window for identification of anatomic abnormalities.[57] The approach is performed by making an S- or Z-shaped incision in the prone patient. Once the neurovascular structures of the popliteal fossa and the anomalous anatomy are identified, the medial head of the gastrocnemius and any contributing muscle flaps and tendinous bands are released from their attachments. Reattachment of the medial muscle head after myotomy is usually not necessary because no measurable postsurgical loss of strength is observed after its release.[58]

The major advantage of the medial calf approach is a more rapid postsurgical recovery compared with the posterior approach. Proponents of the medial approach highlight its utility in long-segment occlusions of the popliteal artery.[58] However, the medial approach has significant disadvantages that limit its applicability. Specifically, identification and adequate exposure of the various anatomic structures of the popliteal fossa are more difficult to accomplish through the medial approach. Accordingly, the medial approach is associated with a higher rate of missed entrapment and recurrent entrapment.[39]

The natural history of PAES involves progressive popliteal arterial degeneration and fibrosis with eventual thrombosis and occlusion. Marked thickening of the arterial wall at the site of entrapment or poststenotic dilatation and aneurysm formation are additional signs of chronic arterial compression. In the presence of such findings, operative intervention must include, in addition to entrapment release, arterial resection and bypass using a saphenous vein graft. Once a popliteal artery has become occluded, dilated, or thrombosed, it should be resected and replaced with an autogenous conduit.[39,41] The posterior approach is useful in cases requiring popliteal artery reconstruction.

Type VI functional popliteal entrapment results from hypertrophy of the medial head of the gastrocnemius muscle and can, in time, cause arterial degeneration as a result of chronic entrapment. In a symptomatic patient with functional PAES, surgical intervention is indicated. Surgical decompression involves transection of the compressive portion of the medial head of the gastrocnemius muscle and should be

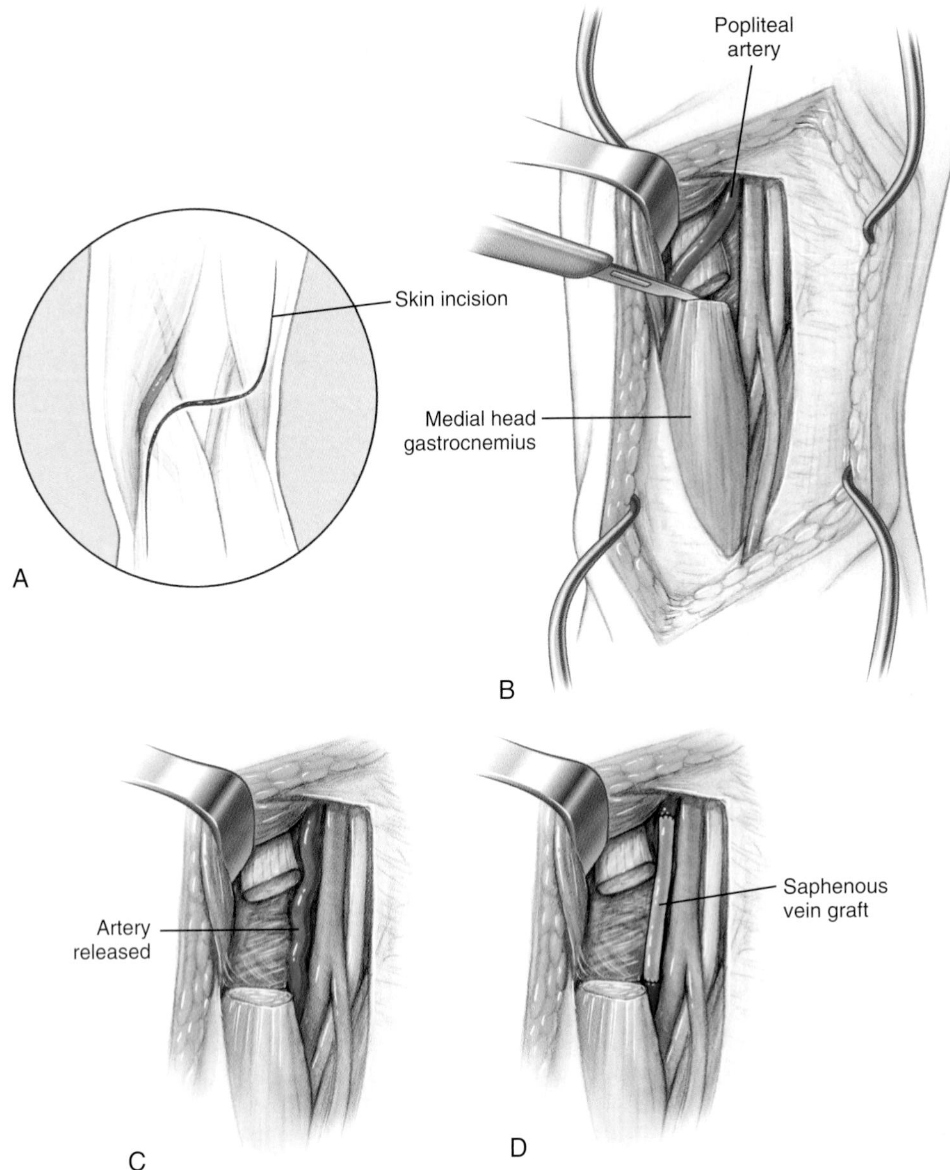

FIGURE 108-10 The operative approach for treating popliteal artery entrapment syndrome. **A,** An S-shaped incision for the posterior surgical approach to the popliteal fossa. **B,** Operative exposure showing type I popliteal artery entrapment and subsequent sharp division of the medial head of the gastrocnemius. **C,** Successful release of the undamaged popliteal artery (the muscle will not need to be reattached). **D,** Successful saphenous vein bypass of the injured popliteal artery after myotomy (if indicated by imaging and operative investigation).

performed through a posterior approach. Release of the entire tendon from its attachment is usually not necessary because these patients lack an anatomic abnormality.

Endovascular therapies for the treatment of PAES have limited value because of their inability to alter the extrinsic muscle compression in the popliteal fossa. Some studies report the use of initial endovascular intervention via balloon angioplasty and thrombolysis followed by myotomy several weeks later.[59] However, benefits of this approach are largely speculative. An inability to relieve the underlying source of popliteal compression raises the risk of reocclusion after endoluminal therapy. Consequently, open surgery remains the gold standard for correcting anatomic abnormalities and restoring arterial flow in the patient with PAES.

Postoperative Management

In the absence of arterial occlusion or signs of vessel degeneration, musculotendinous release and decompression are sufficient to alleviate claudication and restore adequate blood flow.[38] Postoperative recovery is based primarily on wound healing, and as mentioned earlier, it is more rapidly achieved with the medial surgical approach. Reports suggest that patients who begin postoperative physical therapy early and within an appropriate time frame experience better outcomes compared with patients who do not participate in physical therapy.[60] Patients can be discharged from the hospital once they are ambulatory with crutches, usually 1 to 2 days after surgery.

AUTHORS' PREFERRED TECHNIQUE

Popliteal Artery Entrapment Syndrome

I. Patient evaluation and exposure of soft tissue structures of the popliteal fossa are achieved as described in the Authors' Preferred Technique box in the Knee Dislocation section.

II. Decompression of the popliteal entrapment via myotomy
   A. Type I to V
      - Divide the medial head of the gastrocnemius from its posterior attachment to the femoral condyles
      - Resect any accessory muscle or tendinous tissue contributing to popliteal artery entrapment
      - It is not necessary to reattach the muscle
   B. Type VI
      - Excision of the segments of the medial head of the gastrocnemius muscle that are compressing the popliteal artery, with preservation of the tendinous attachment to the posterior femoral condyle

III. Popliteal artery reconstruction is required if evidence of chronic high-grade stenosis, occlusion, or thrombosis is found
   A. Resection of degenerated and thrombosed artery
   B. Placement of a short interposition vein graft, usually harvested from the ipsilateral lesser saphenous vein
   C. A short venous bypass graft can be performed as an alternative with exclusion of the occluded artery to avoid thromboembolism
   D. If poststenotic dilatation/aneurysm is present, arterial resection followed by vein graft replacement is mandatory to avoid later development of an aneurysm

Criteria for Return to Play

A return to a full level of athletic activity can be achieved after treatment of PAES. Patients who require arterial reconstruction in addition to decompression have longer recovery times than do patients who undergo decompression alone. Factors that determine the rate of recovery include wound healing, return of limb strength and flexibility, adequate distal perfusion as a result of decompression, and graft patency after arterial reconstruction. Before the athlete can return to play, restoration of blood flow and vessel patency should be evaluated through physical examination, ABI, and duplex ultrasonography at rest and as provocative maneuvers are performed. CTA, MRA, and angiography are usually not necessary unless symptoms of claudication persist or recur. Recovery commonly takes 6 to 8 weeks, and then moderate strengthening exercises may be initiated. After an initial strengthening regimen is completed, preoperative levels of activity and strength training may be resumed. Once full return to physical activity is achieved, follow-up should be performed every 4 to 6 months for the first year and annually thereafter.

Complications

Postoperative complications are usually minimal after myotomy alone with decompression of the entrapped artery, and patients typically return to prior levels of athletic activity without requiring additional interventions. Patients with popliteal occlusion, degeneration, or aneurysm as a result of chronic compression require arterial resection and replacement in addition to a myotomy. Such patients have a higher risk of potential complications. Patients for whom arterial reconstruction is performed should be treated with antiplatelet drugs, such as aspirin. The potential for postsurgical graft failure and acute graft thrombosis also exists and is a potential source of postoperative morbidity. Because stenosis of the vein graft at the proximal and distal anastomosis also may occur, patients should be followed up closely with physical examination, ABI testing, and duplex ultrasonography to monitor the integrity of the graft. When vein graft stenosis is symptomatic or greater than 60%, balloon angioplasty is indicated.

For a complete list of references, go to expertconsult.com.

Suggested Readings

Citation: Perlowski AA, Jaff MR: Vascular disorders in athletes. *Vasc Med* 15(6):469–479, 2010.

Level of Evidence: II (prognostic studies)

Summary: Physical examination and imaging of an athlete suspected of sustaining a vascular injury should be performed with the patient in both neutral and provocative positions specific to the suspected vascular injury to fully expose underlying pathology. Proper use of noninvasive diagnostic studies such as duplex ultrasonography, computed tomography, and magnetic resonance imaging can ensure prompt and accurate diagnosis. A multifaceted approach to the diagnosis and treatment of an athlete affected by vascular disease allows for faster recovery and a return to previous levels of activity.

Citation: Green NE, Allen BL: Vascular injuries associated with dislocation of the knee. *J Bone Joint Surg Am* 59A(2):236–239, 1977.

Level of Evidence: I (prognostic/therapeutic study)

Summary: A combined retrospective and prospective study of 245 cases reveals a high incidence of injury to the popliteal artery as a result of knee dislocation. Vascular intervention and repair must be performed within 6 hours from the time of injury to prevent ischemic injury and avoid amputation. In 95% of cases in which patients did not receive prompt treatment, either amputation was necessary or ischemic changes occurred.

Citation: Varnell RM, et al: Arterial injury complicating knee disruption. Third place winner: Conrad Jobst award. *Am Surg* 55(12):699–704, 1989.

Level of Evidence: I (diagnostic study)

Summary: A retrospective study of 30 patients with either knee dislocation or severe knee ligamentous disruption revealed no significant difference in the frequency of major or minor vascular abnormalities between the two groups. Doppler pressure measurements were highly predictive of major arterial trauma in both groups. Arterial injury can occur with both dislocation and ligament injury of the knee, and Doppler flow measurements should be assessed in all cases of suspected vascular injury.

Citation: Bynoe RP, et al: Noninvasive diagnosis of vascular trauma by duplex ultrasonography. *J Vasc Surg* 14(3):346–352, 1991.

Level of Evidence: I (prognostic/diagnostic study)

Summary: In a prospective evaluation of a large number of patients with potential vascular injury in the neck and extremities, duplex ultrasonography had more than 90% sensitivity, specificity, and overall accuracy in detecting vascular pathology. Duplex ultrasonography has no interventional risks and is a rapid and cost-effective method of screening patients with suspected vascular trauma in the neck and extremities.

Citation: Levien LJ, Veller MG: Popliteal artery entrapment syndrome: more common than previously recognized. *J Vasc Surg* 30(4):587–598, 1999.

Level of Evidence: I (therapeutic study)

Summary: A retrospective analysis of patients with unequivocal evidence of popliteal artery entrapment syndrome suggests that surgical intervention is required in all confirmed cases of popliteal entrapment (types I, II, III, and IV). Approximately 50% of the normal population may display transient popliteal compression in the extremes of limb movement. Consequently, surgical decompression in patients with functional popliteal entrapment is indicated only if discrete and typical symptoms are present. If the patient has significant degeneration or occlusion of the popliteal artery, complete replacement with a vein graft is indicated.

Citation: di Marzo L, Cavallaro A: Popliteal vascular entrapment. *World J Surg* 29(Suppl 1):S43–S45, 2005.

Level of Evidence: II (prognostic/therapeutic studies)

Summary: Signs and symptoms of claudication in a young patient should always raise suspicion of popliteal artery entrapment. The higher specificity and sensitivity of computed tomography and magnetic resonance imaging in evaluating the popliteal vessels represents a valid alternative to the more invasive digital angiography. Current studies encourage the identification of patients with popliteal artery entrapment syndrome at an early stage. The only parameter influencing the long-term outcome of patients with popliteal artery entrapment is age at presentation.

SECTION 8

Leg, Ankle, and Foot

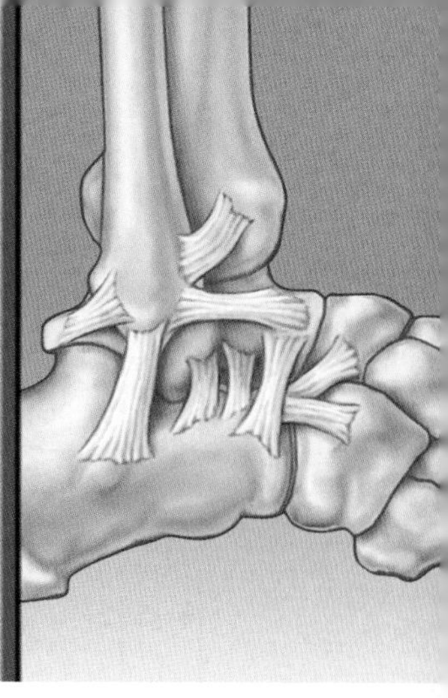

109

Foot and Ankle Biomechanics

ANDREW HASKELL

This section discusses the relationship between the joints of the foot and ankle and their interconnection to the lower extremity. Motion of various foot and ankle segments (kinematics) and the forces experienced by the lower extremity (kinetics) are explored over the gait cycle. Special attention is given to the biomechanical mechanism by which the components of the foot and ankle interact. The biomechanics of walking are compared with running, and clinical correlations are made throughout the chapter.

Gait consists of a cyclical set of motions between the heel strike of one step and the heel strike of the same foot on the subsequent step. A single cycle can be divided into a stance phase and a swing phase. During walking, the stance phase is further divided into periods of double- and single-limb support (Fig. 109-1). The stance phase of walking can be divided into three intervals: the first interval extends from initial heel strike to the foot laying flat on the floor; the second interval occurs as the body passes over the flat foot; and the third interval extends from the beginning of ankle joint plantar flexion as the heel rises from the floor to when the toes lift from the floor. Changes in the gait cycle during running are illustrated in Figure 109-2. During walking, one foot is always in contact with the ground; as the speed of gait increases, a transition occurs with incorporation of a float phase during which both feet leave the ground. Rather than a period of double-limb support as occurs during walking, a period occurs with no limb support (the float phase) during running. As the speed of gait continues to increase, the stance phase, both in real time and in percentage of the gait cycle, decreases.

The functions of the ankle, subtalar, transverse tarsal, and metatarsophalangeal joints interrelate closely to fulfill the varying requirements of the foot during bipedal walking and running. At initial ground contact, a complex set of energy absorption mechanisms helps lessen the shock wave that propagates up the axial skeleton. Later in stance, passive and active mechanisms alter the structure of the foot to provide the body with a stable platform and to functionally elongate the stance limb, allowing for a greater stride length. During walking, the toes are lifted from the floor, whereas in athletics, forceful push-off facilitates rapid acceleration and deceleration, direction change, and jumping.

The linkage between the ankle joint, subtalar joint, transverse tarsal joint, metatarsophalangeal joints, and plantar aponeurosis should be emphasized further. The terms *pronation* and *supination* describe a coordinated series of movements linking the joints of the ankle and foot. It is this linked series of movements that enable the athlete to absorb the forces of impact, yet create a rigid platform from which to push off (Table 109-1). The function of the plantar aponeurosis, the transverse metatarsal break, and the muscles of the leg and foot enhance these joint motions further.

The stresses applied to the joints of the foot and ankle vary greatly from normal walking to athletics. The stresses can be repetitive, as in a long-distance runner, or impulsive, as occurs in the push-off foot of a shot-putter. The vertical force involved in running is 2 to 2.5 times body weight compared with 1.2 times body weight in walking[1] and can be higher for many sports with extreme push-off, such as a football lineman engaged in blocking or a basketball player engaged in rapid accelerating and jumping activities (Fig. 109-3). The nature of these forces depends on the activity and includes vertical force, fore and aft shear, side-to-side shear, and torque forces. These forces are measured in a variety of ways, including force plate analysis or thin film pressure transducers placed in a shoe.[2] The foot and ankle complex must be supple enough to absorb impact and rigid enough to transmit muscle forces, or injuries such as sprains, strains, stress fractures, and fascial tears may result. Athletic training can help attenuate these forces and minimize the risk of injury.[3]

Dysfunction of the foot and ankle complex may result in an altered gait pattern, declining athletic performance, and compensatory changes in the knee and hip joints. The ankle and subtalar joint complex function as a universal joint, linking pelvic, thigh, and leg rotation to hindfoot motion and longitudinal arch stability, which allows the ankle joints to compensate for some degree of dysfunction in the hindfoot and vice versa. Athletics, however, require maximum performance from these systems, and dysfunction of ankle and foot mechanics often leads to pain, injury, and loss of performance.

Ankle Joint

The ankle joint allows sagittal plane motion of 20 degrees of dorsiflexion to 50 degrees of plantar flexion, with marked variability between individuals, along an axis running between the tips of the malleoli. The trochlear surface of the talus rotates around this axis, as would a section from a cone whose apex is based medially (Fig. 109-4).[4]

The talus is stabilized within the ankle mortise by bony and soft tissue restraints. The congruity of the ankle mortise

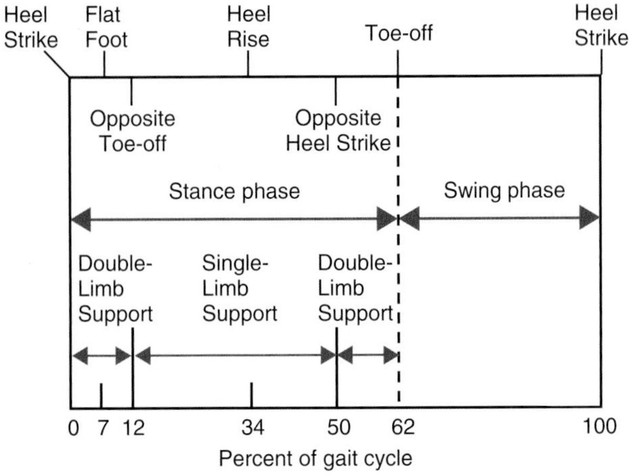

FIGURE 109-1 The walking cycle. The gait cycle during walking is divided into stance and swing phases. The stance phase constitutes periods of double-limb support and single-limb support. In contrast, running does not include a period of double-limb support but instead has a float phase during which neither limb is in contact with the ground. *(From Haskell A, Mann RA: Biomechanics of the foot and ankle. In Coughlin MJ, Saltzman CL, Anderson RB, editors:* Mann's surgery of the foot and ankle, *ed 9, Philadelphia, 2014, Elsevier.)*

leads to considerable inherent bony stability.[5,6] Ligament support includes the deltoid ligament medially[7] and three separate ligamentous bands laterally: the anterior and posterior talofibular ligaments and the calcaneofibular ligament.[8] The anterior talofibular ligament is taut with the ankle joint in plantar flexion, and the calcaneofibular ligament is taut with the ankle joint in dorsiflexion (Fig. 109-5).[4] The anterior

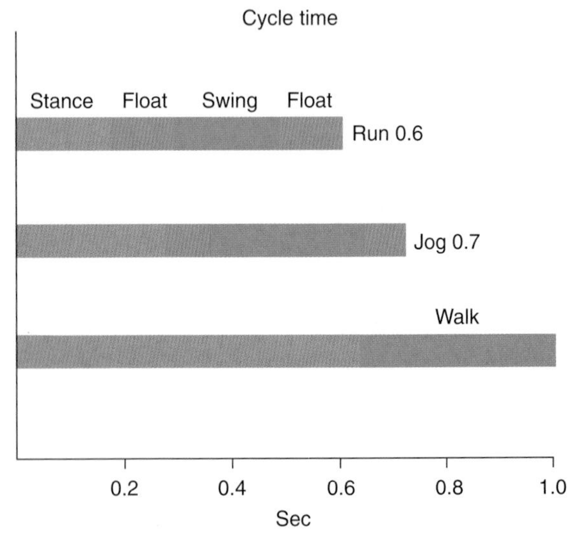

FIGURE 109-2 Variations in the gait cycle. The stance phase of walking is greater than 50% of the total gait cycle. As the transition to jogging is made, a float period is incorporated during which neither foot is in contact with the ground. As running speed increases, stance phase decreases and the float phase increases. In the illustration, the walking pace is 16 minutes per mile, jogging is 9 minutes per mile, and running is 5 minutes per mile. *(From Haskell A, Mann RA: Biomechanics of the foot and ankle. In Coughlin MJ, Saltzman CL, Anderson RB, editors:* Mann's surgery of the foot and ankle, *ed 9, Philadelphia, 2014, Elsevier.)*

TABLE 109-1

COMPARISON OF FOOT CHARACTERISTICS BASED ON FOOT POSITION

	FOOT POSITION	
	Pronation	**Supination**
Joint position	Ankle dorsiflexion Subtalar eversion Transverse tarsal abduction	Ankle plantarflexion Subtalar inversion Transverse tarsal adduction
Arch stiffness	Supple	Rigid
Gait cycle	Heel strike	Flat foot to toe-off
Function	Energy absorption	Energy transfer to ground

talofibular ligament is injured most frequently during ankle sprains, in part because the ankle has less intrinsic bony stability in plantar flexion when this ligament is under tension.[9] Injuries to the calcaneofibular ligament are frequently seen in conjunction with anterior talofibular ligament sprains.

Two series of dorsiflexion and plantar flexion occur during the gait cycle. At heel strike, the dorsiflexed ankle rapidly plantarflexes. This motion ends with the foot flat, after which progressive dorsiflexion occurs. Dorsiflexion reaches a maximum at 40% of the walking cycle, when plantar flexion begins as the heel rises, and continues until toe-off, when dorsiflexion occurs again during the swing phase (Fig. 109-6).

The force applied across the ankle joint during walking is approximately 4.5 times body weight.[10] This maximum stress occurs just before and just after the onset of plantar flexion of the ankle joint as the body moves over the stance limb. If this force were extrapolated to running, in which the ground reaction force is more than double that of walking, we would see stress across the ankle joint that approaches 10 times body weight.

Muscle control of the ankle joint can be divided on the basis of the anterior and posterior leg muscle compartments. The lateral compartment muscles function with the posterior compartment. During normal walking, the anterior compartment muscles become active late in the stance phase and in

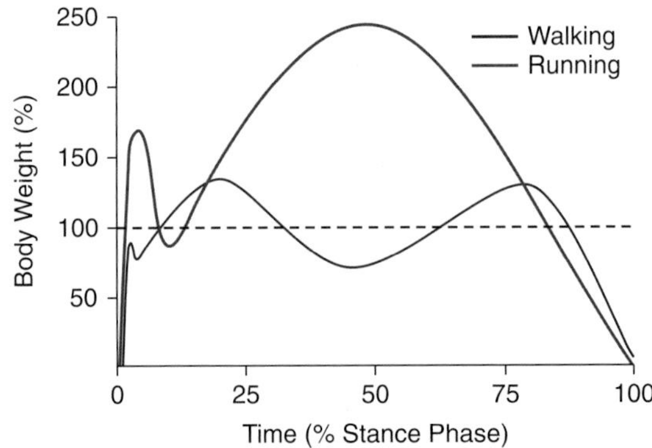

FIGURE 109-3 Comparison of vertical ground reaction force for walking (*blue line*) versus jogging (*red line*). The horizontal axis is scaled as a percentage of the total time in the stance phase for walking (0.6 seconds) and running (0.24 seconds). The vertical axis is shown as a percentage of body weight.

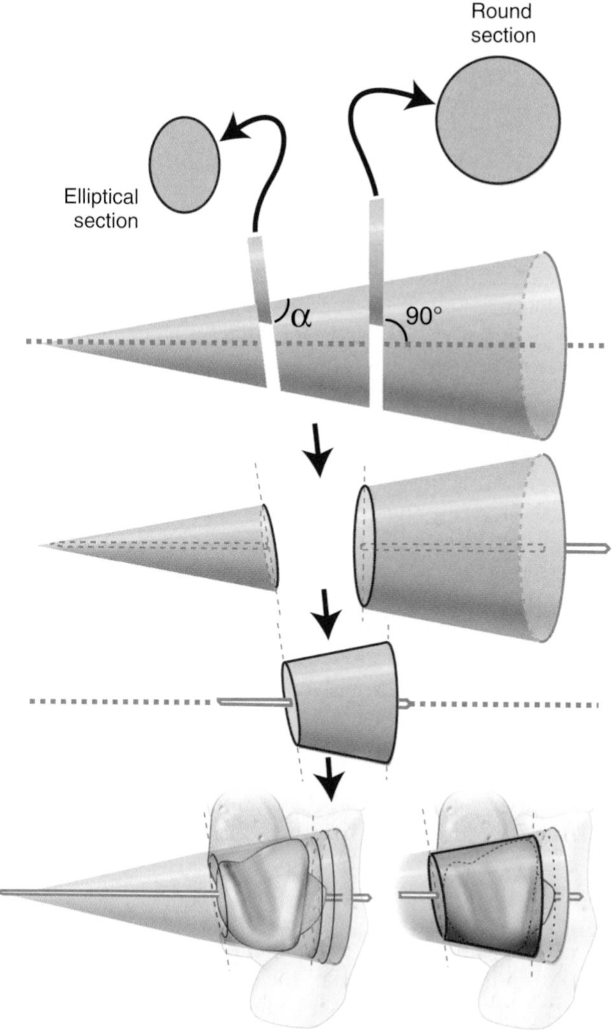

FIGURE 109-4 The trochlear surface of the talus is a section from a cone. The apex of the cone is directed medially, and the open end is directed laterally. *(From Stiehl JB, editor:* Inman's joints of the ankle, *ed 2, Baltimore, 1991, Williams & Wilkins.)*

the swing phase to bring about dorsiflexion of the ankle joint by a concentric (shortening) contraction (see Fig. 109-6).[11] This muscle group remains active after heel strike to control the rapid plantar flexion of the ankle joint that occurs by an eccentric (lengthening) contraction. This eccentric contraction during plantar flexion helps dissipate the forces on the limb at initial ground contact. The anterior compartment becomes electrically silent by the time the foot is flat. The posterior compartment muscles are active after the foot is flat (15% to 20% of gait cycle), during which time the ankle joint is undergoing dorsiflexion, and they remain active until about halfway through the cycle, at which time approximately 50% to 60% of ankle joint plantar flexion has occurred.[12] This muscle group initially undergoes an eccentric contraction controlling forward movement of the tibia over the foot, then a concentric contraction when plantar flexion begins. The electrical activity of the posterior calf group ceases before full plantar flexion has occurred, indicating that the last portion of plantar flexion is a passive phenomenon.

As the speed of gait increases to steady running and sprinting, several changes occur. The ankle joint starts in slight dorsiflexion and, at heel strike, remains dorsiflexed (see Fig. 109-6). The tibia moves forward and the foot-flat position is achieved. As running speed increases, the magnitude of the motion increases, the duration of stance phase reduces significantly, and the period of double-limb support gives way to a period lacking limb support. The electrical activity of the anterior compartment still begins late in stance and continues through swing, but during running it lasts through about the first third of the stance phase. The posterior calf muscles show a significant change in their activity in that they become active late in the swing phase and remain active until about halfway

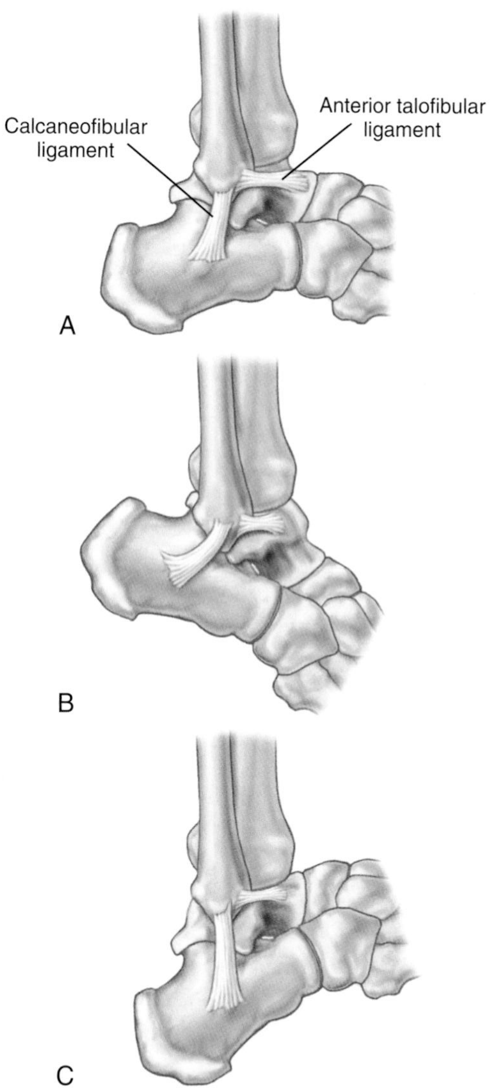

FIGURE 109-5 Calcaneofibular (**A**) and anterior talofibular (**B**) ligaments. **A,** In plantar flexion, the anterior talofibular ligament is in line with the fibula, thereby providing most of the support to the lateral aspect of the ankle joint. **B,** When the ankle is in neutral position, both the anterior talofibular and the calcaneofibular ligaments support the joint. The obliquely placed structure depicts the axis of the subtalar joint. It should be noted that the calcaneofibular ligament parallels the axis. **C,** When the ankle joint is in dorsiflexion, the calcaneofibular ligament is in line with the fibula and supports the lateral aspect of the joint. *(Modified from Stiehl JB, editor:* Inman's joints of the ankle, *ed 2, Baltimore, 1991, Williams & Wilkins.)*

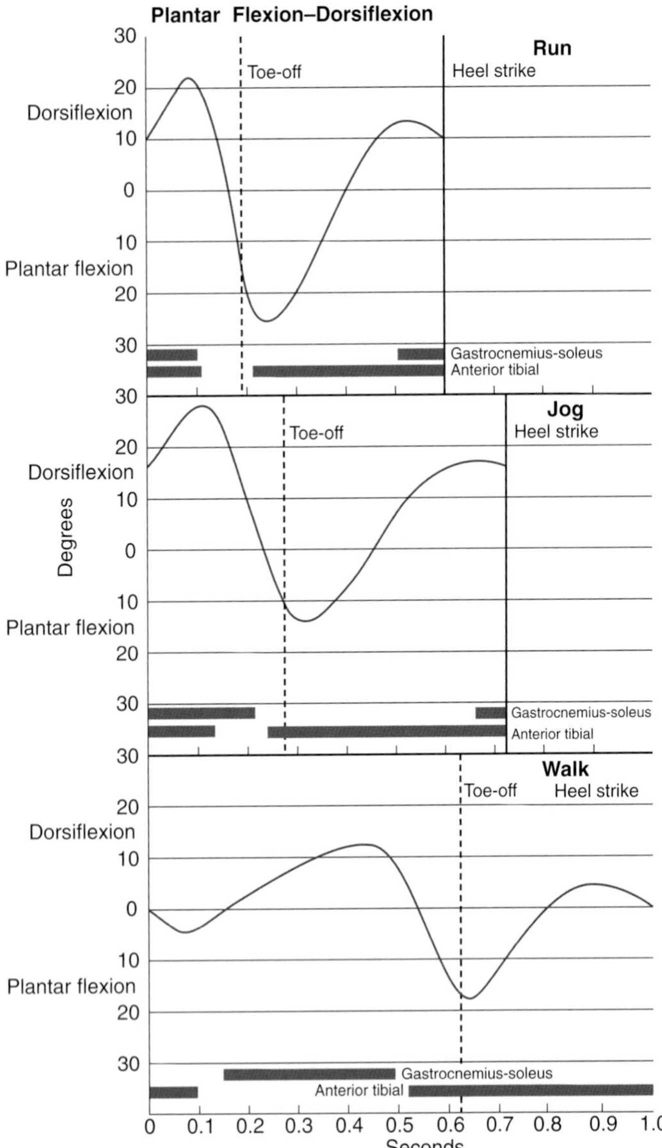

FIGURE 109-6 Ankle joint range of motion for walking, jogging, and running. The muscle function of the anterior and posterior compartment is noted on the bottom of the graph. *(From Mann RA: Biomechanics of running. In American Academy of Orthopaedic Surgeons:* Symposium on the Foot and Leg in Running Sports, *St. Louis, 1982, CV Mosby.)*

through ankle joint plantar flexion.[13] This increased activity in the posterior calf musculature probably results in increased stability of the ankle joint at the time of initial ground contact.

Recently, an interest in running styles more amenable to bare feet or shoes with minimal heel padding[14] has led to exploration of kinematic and kinetic differences when compared with the heel-strike pattern of running. Shoes with padded heels allow for a heel-strike pattern of running, whereas athletes who run barefoot land with more plantar flexion at the ankle, striking either the midfoot or forefoot first. Midfoot or forefoot strike patterns are associated with shorter stride length and higher stride frequency.[14,15] Flatter foot placement at touchdown correlates with lower peak heel pressures but significantly higher leg stiffness during the stance phase.[15,16] Tibial internal rotation excursion is similar.[17] Plantar flexor force output is greater in forefoot striking than in rearfoot striking and in barefoot than in shod running, although Achilles tendon strain was lower while running barefoot than while running when wearing a standard shoe.[18] Comparison of running with forefoot and rearfoot strike patterns finds similar oxygen uptake and internal mechanical work, with reports of increased metabolic demand in shod runners explained by an approximately 1% increase in metabolic demand for each 100 g of added shoe weight.[15,18,19] Despite no difference in internal work, an increase in external and total mechanical work occurs in forefoot strike runners, which perhaps is explained by higher storage and release of energy in the elastic structures of the lower leg.[15,20] Another way to look at this issue is that traditional shoes with padded heels attenuate the foot-ground impact, which may decrease the storage and restitution of elastic energy capacity and result in lower net efficiency in shod running compared with minimal-shoe running.[15,18]

Study of the strike pattern in running has also focused on possible practical differences, including comparison of injury rates and performance. The lack of difference in energy expenditure between the two styles of strike pattern is borne out in a study of marathon runners, which found no association between strike pattern and race time. Incidentally, a large number of runners switched from a midfoot pattern at 10 km to a heel strike pattern at 32 km, perhaps related to fatigue or pace.[21] In a study of 52 middle- and long-distance collegiate runners, it was found that runners with rearfoot strike patterns (two thirds of the group) had approximately twice the rate of repetitive stress injuries than did runners who habitually had a forefoot strike, although a number of other covariates were present, including gender, race distance, and average miles per week. Traumatic injury rates were not significantly different between the two groups.[22] Anecdotal reports suggest forefoot striking may help people with chronic exertional compartment syndrome,[23] but it may be associated with the development of metatarsal stress fractures.[24]

Although we speak of ankle joint dorsiflexion and plantar flexion, only about half of this motion comes from the ankle joint; the remainder comes from the movement occurring within the subtalar and transverse tarsal joints.[25] If motion of the ankle joint is diminished (perhaps from an anterior impingement), degenerative changes occur within the joint, or fusion occurs, the subtalar and transverse tarsal joints compensate for the lost motion. If degenerative changes occur within the subtalar or transverse tarsal joints, any loss of ankle joint motion is magnified. This compensatory increase in motion of the neighboring joints is nonphysiologic and often leads to pain, loss of function, and degenerative changes over time.[26]

Subtalar Joint

The subtalar joint complex permits inversion and eversion. The axis of the subtalar joint is variable but is approximately 42 degrees to the horizontal plane and passes from medial to lateral at about 16 degrees (Fig. 109-7).[10,27] The range of motion of the subtalar joint allows approximately 30 degrees of inversion and 15 degrees of eversion, although measurement of subtalar joint motion is difficult. Although the overall pattern of motion appears to be consistent, the magnitude of motion varies considerably between persons.[28]

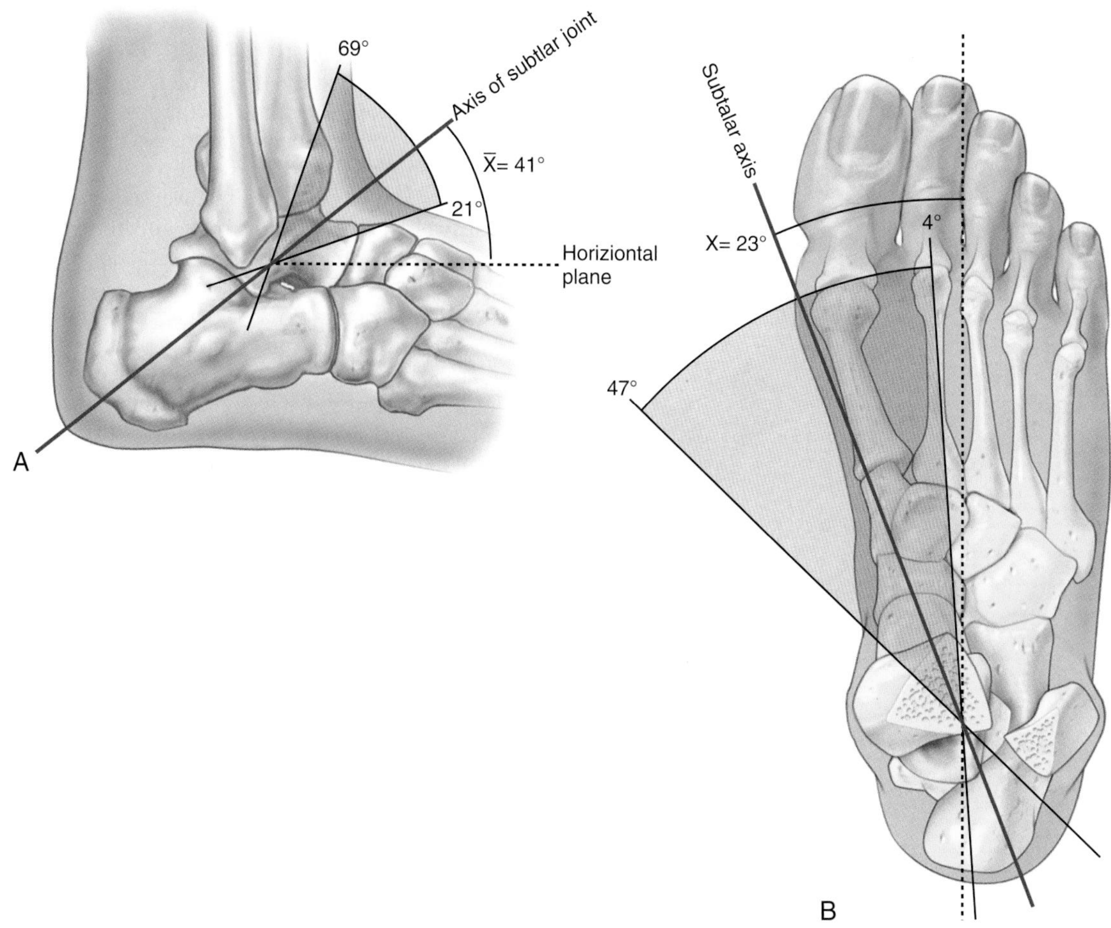

FIGURE 109-7 Variations in the subtalar joint axes. In the horizontal plane (**A**), the axis approximates 45 degrees and (**B**) passes about 23 degrees medial to the midline. *(**A** and **B** modified from Isman RE, Inman VT: Anthropometric studies of the human foot and ankle.* Bull Prosthet Res *10:97, 1969.)*

The subtalar joint, which is stabilized primarily by the joint configuration and the interosseous ligament, is less constrained than the ankle.[29,30] When the long axis of the tibia passes medial to the obliquely placed subtalar joint axis, subtalar joint eversion ceases because of the configuration of the joint surfaces and the interosseous ligament. When the weight-bearing line is lateral to the subtalar joint axis, inversion stability depends on lateral ligament support and active muscle function.

The subtalar joint has been likened to an oblique hinge that functions to translate motion between the transverse tarsal joint distally and the ankle joint and leg proximally (Fig. 109-8).[31,32] This linkage is important for energy dissipation at heel strike, which is largely a passive mechanism. At the time of initial ground contact during walking, the slightly inverted subtalar joint undergoes rapid eversion, the tibia undergoes internal rotation, the transverse tarsal joints become supple, and the medial longitudinal arch flattens. This linkage is also important for efficient energy transfer during heel rise and toe-off, which involves both passive and active mechanisms. During the flatfoot phase, the subtalar joint undergoes progressive inversion, which reaches a maximum at toe-off. This movement increases the stability of the transverse tarsal joints and medial longitudinal arch, stiffening the foot and allowing it to act as a rigid extension of the leg. Pelvis rotation causes an external rotation torque, which is transmitted from the lower extremity across the ankle joint and is translated by the subtalar joint into hindfoot inversion. The plantar aponeurosis mechanism and the oblique metatarsal break enhance the inversion, as described below.

To best appreciate how various muscles affect the subtalar joint, examine the size and location of the muscles in relation to the subtalar joint axis (Fig. 109-9). In general, muscles with tendons passing medial to the axis produce inversion, whereas tendons passing laterally produce eversion, although the function of the muscles on the axis is affected by the starting position of the subtalar joint. The main invertors are the tibialis posterior and the gastrocnemius-soleus complex, and the main evertor is the peroneus brevis and, to a much lesser extent, the peroneus longus, which is mainly a plantar flexor of the first metatarsal. The tibialis anterior lies on the subtalar joint axis and provides little influence on the neutral subtalar joint. However, it is the only functioning muscle at heel strike and may resist eversion of the initially inverted subtalar joint. The inversion that occurs during the last half of stance is due to the passive mechanisms noted previously, along with the input from the gastrocnemius-soleus complex and the tibialis posterior muscle. The patient who lacks posterior tibial tendon function cannot initiate standing on tiptoe but can maintain the position when it is achieved. It can be concluded that posterior tibial tendon function is necessary to initiate inversion and that the gastrocnemius-soleus complex is

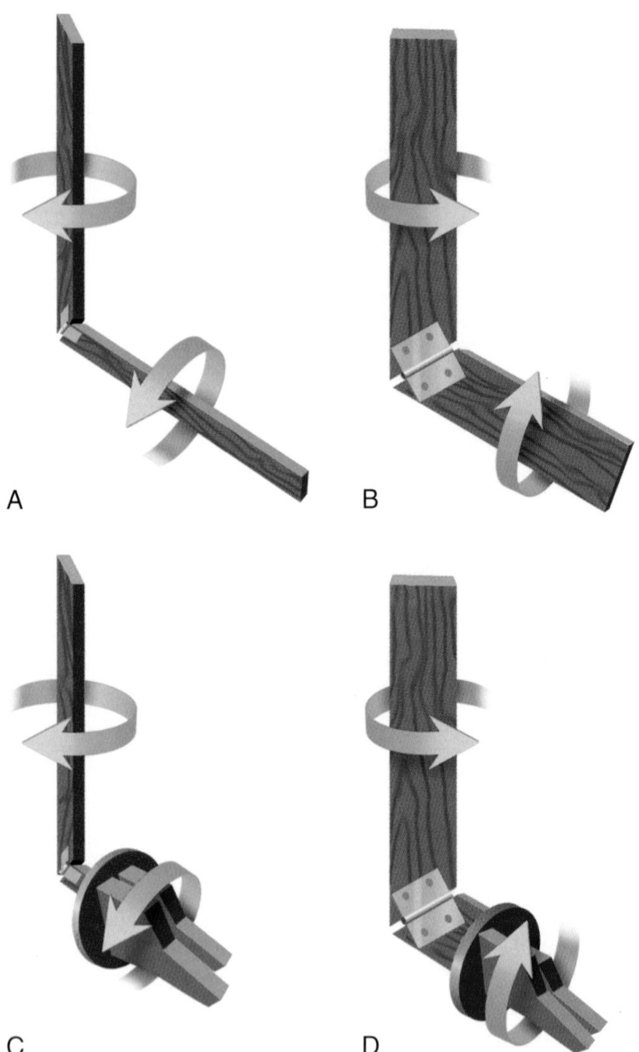

FIGURE 109-8 The mitered hinge effect of the subtalar joint. The subtalar joint acts as a mitered hinge, linking motion between the calcaneus below and the tibia above (**A** and **B**). The model also demonstrates flattening and elevation of the longitudinal arch. Flattening of the longitudinal arch occurs at the time of heel strike with eversion of the calcaneus and internal rotation of the tibia (**A** and **C**). Elevation and stabilization of the longitudinal arch are associated with the outward rotation of the tibia, causing inversion of the calcaneus and locking of the transverse tarsal joint (**B** and **D**). *(Adapted from Mann RA, Haskell A: Biomechanics of the foot and ankle. In Coughlin MJ, Mann RA, Saltzman CL, editors:* Surgery of the foot and ankle, *ed 8, Philadelphia, 2007, Elsevier.)*

necessary to maintain it. During running, the posterior calf muscles become active late in swing phase and remain active through most of stance (see Fig. 109-6). Besides providing stability to the ankle joint, these muscles contribute to inversion of the subtalar joint before initial ground contact.

If the motion in the subtalar joint is restricted, its ability to translate rotation proximally and distally is impaired, placing increased stress on the ankle and transverse tarsal joints. For example, talocalcaneal coalition can lead to a spastic peroneal flatfoot or ball-in-socket ankle because of the lack of subtalar motion. The degree of ankle joint dorsiflexion and plantar flexion also is affected, and the ankle can become arthritic from the abnormal stresses.[33]

People with flat feet have increased eversion of the subtalar joint during stance (Fig. 109-10). This eversion translates to increased tibial internal rotation, which can affect knee alignment, patellofemoral tracking, or the hip in selected cases. The theory behind orthotic use for many conditions involving the foot, ankle, knee, hip, and back is the effect they have on the linkage system within the lower extremity. The use of a medial heel wedge, whether built into the shoe or within an orthotic device, may influence the rotation of the subtalar joint.[34] Recall that at the time of initial heel contact with the ground, rapid eversion of the subtalar joint and flattening of the longitudinal arch occur. Buildup of material along the medial arch that prevents some of this rotation from occurring, in theory, decreases the degree of internal rotation being transmitted to the lower extremity, which may have a beneficial effect on the forces across the ankle, knee, and hip. For instance, a runner with chronic knee pain may be helped by an orthotic device that limits eversion of the calcaneus, which in turn diminishes internal rotation of the tibia and affects the patellofemoral joint. However, reliable data to support this theory are lacking, and the benefit may in part be psychological.[35] Soft orthoses and compliant shoe material help absorb the impact of initial ground contact. For persons engaged in repetitive sports, such as long-distance running, a material that helps to absorb some of this impact could be beneficial if the athlete is having problems such as heel pain, metatarsalgia, or shin splints. However, softer material paradoxically can lead to greater vertical impact when landing from jumps as the athlete attempts to improve balance and stability.[36]

Transverse Tarsal Joint

The transverse tarsal joint, consisting of the talonavicular and calcaneocuboid joints, lies distal to the subtalar joint and is influenced strongly by subtalar position.[37] The transverse tarsal joint moves in adduction and abduction and is measured with the calcaneus in a neutral position of slight valgus and the forefoot parallel to the floor. Normal motion is approximately 20 degrees of adduction and 10 degrees of abduction. The forefoot may also rotate into supination (forefoot varus) or pronation (forefoot valgus) through the transverse tarsal joint. Normally, forefoot rotation is neutral with the hindfoot held in a neutral position of slight valgus but may be fixed in a rotated position in people with long-standing planovalgus or cavovarus deformities.

The main support of the joint complex is ligamentous, but its stability is largely determined by subtalar joint position. When the calcaneus is in an everted position, the axes of the transverse tarsal joint are parallel, permitting motion to occur about this joint system. During normal walking, this phenomenon occurs at heel strike, creating a flexible foot to absorb the energy of impact. When the calcaneus is inverted, the axes of the transverse tarsal joint are nonparallel, creating a stable joint system (Fig. 109-11).[37] This situation occurs at heel rise and toe-off, creating a rigid foot to effectively lengthen the limb and assist in propulsion during running.

Impairment of the transverse tarsal joint impairs subtalar joint motion because for subtalar motion to occur, rotation must occur about the talonavicular and calcaneocuboid joints. If an isolated arthrodesis of the talonavicular joint is carried out, most subtalar joint motion is lost.[38] When performing arthrodeses in the area of the hindfoot, sparing the

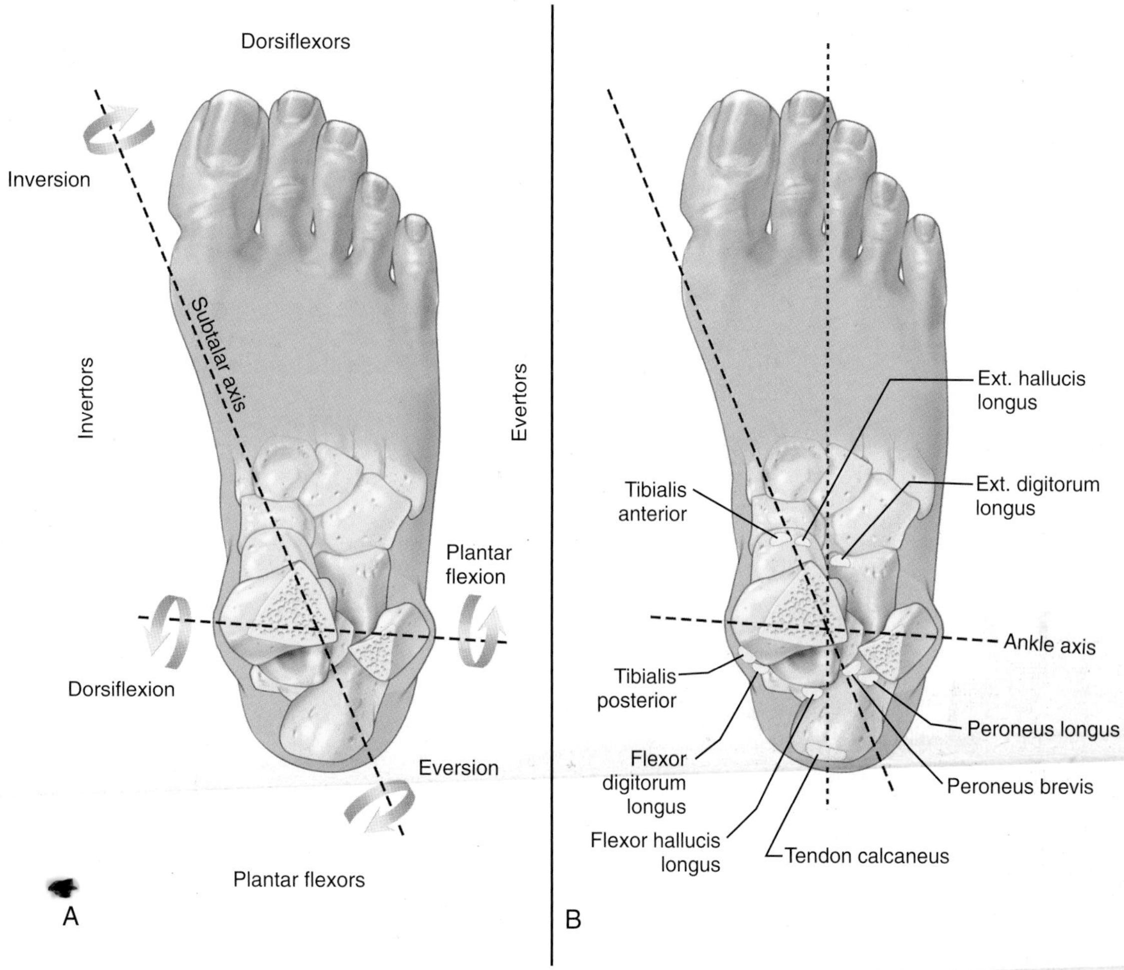

FIGURE 109-9 **A,** The location and the types of rotation that occur about the ankle and the subtalar axes. **B,** The relationship of the various extrinsic muscles about the subtalar and ankle joint axes. *Ext,* Extensor. *(From Haskell A, Mann RA: Biomechanics of the foot. In American Academy of Orthopaedic Surgeons:* Atlas of orthoses and assistive devices, *Philadelphia, 2008, Elsevier.)*

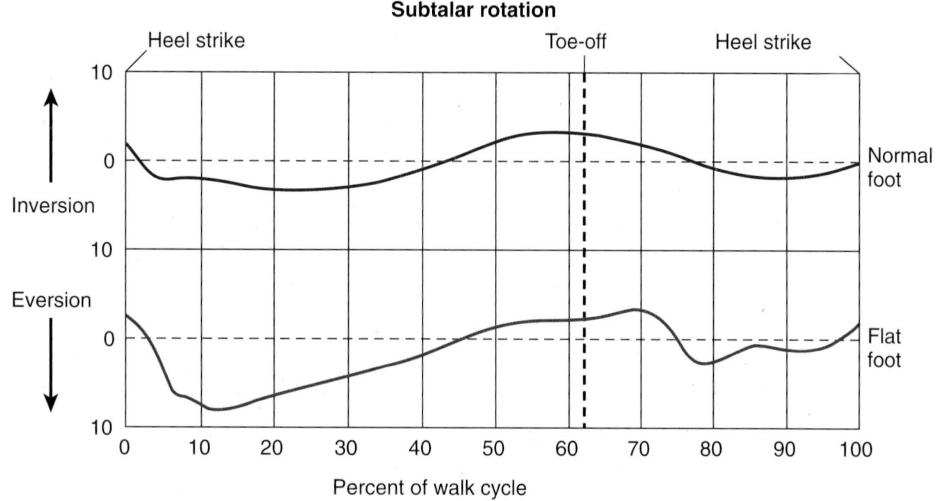

FIGURE 109-10 Subtalar joint motion in a person with a normal foot and in a flatfooted person. *(Data from Wright DG, Desai ME, Henderson BS: Action of the subtalar and ankle joint complex during the stance phase of walking.* J Bone Joint Surg Am *46A:361, 1964.)*

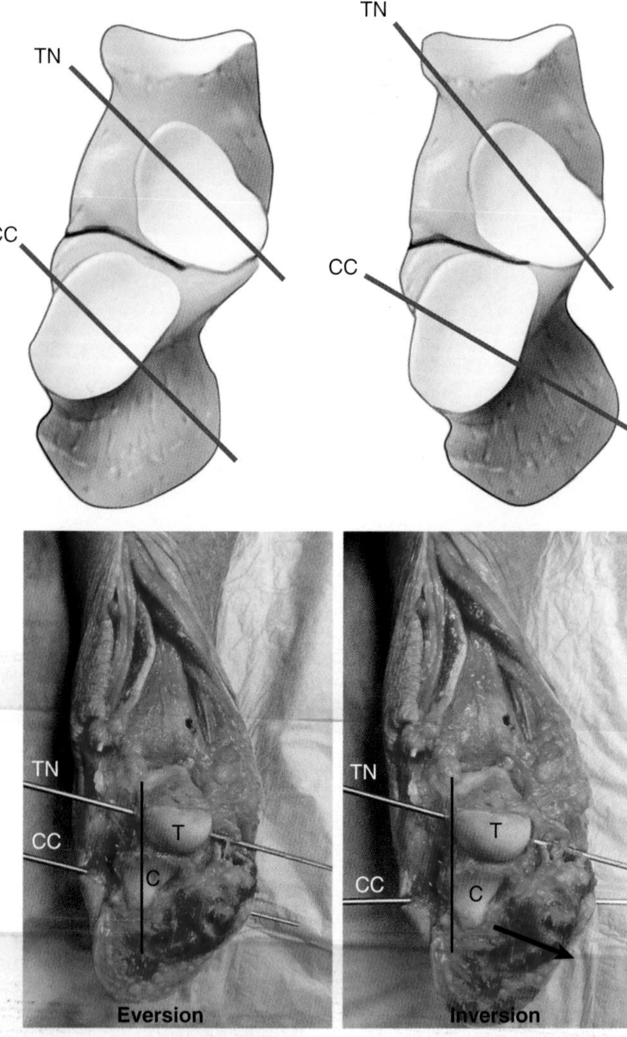

FIGURE 109-11 The function of the transverse tarsal joint as described by Elftman. When the calcaneus is in eversion, the resultant axes of the talonavicular (*TN*) and calcaneocuboid (*CC*) joints are parallel or congruent. When the subtalar joint is in an inverted position, the axes are incongruent, giving increased stability to the midfoot. *T,* Talar articular surface of the TN joint; *C,* calcaneal articular surface of the CC joint. *(Modfied from Haskell A, Mann RA: Biomechanics of the foot and ankle. In Coughlin MJ, Saltzman CL, Anderson RB, editors:* Mann's surgery of the foot and ankle, *ed 9, Philadelphia, 2014, Elsevier.)*

talonavicular joint when appropriate usually results in a more functional foot.

Windlass Mechanism and Metatarsal Break

The function of the plantar aponeurosis during gait is often described by comparing it with a windlass mechanism. The plantar aponeurosis arises from the tubercle of the calcaneus and inserts into the base of the proximal phalanges (Fig. 109-12). After heel rise, the metatarsophalangeal joints dorsiflex, tightening the plantar aponeurosis. This mechanism depresses the metatarsal heads, elevates and stabilizes the longitudinal arch, and helps bring the calcaneus into an inverted position (Fig. 109-13).[39] The inverted calcaneus causes the transverse tarsal joint axes to diverge, helping stabilize the midfoot at toe-off.

The oblique metatarsal break is created by the lateral slope formed by the metatarsophalangeal joints two through five (Fig. 109-14).[18] This oblique line creates a camlike action as the body weight is brought over the metatarsal heads, further enhancing external rotation of the lower extremity and inversion of the calcaneus.

Turf-toe injuries are common in athletes and can lead to stiffness in the first metatarsophalangeal joint or result in hallux rigidus, a degenerative arthritis of the first

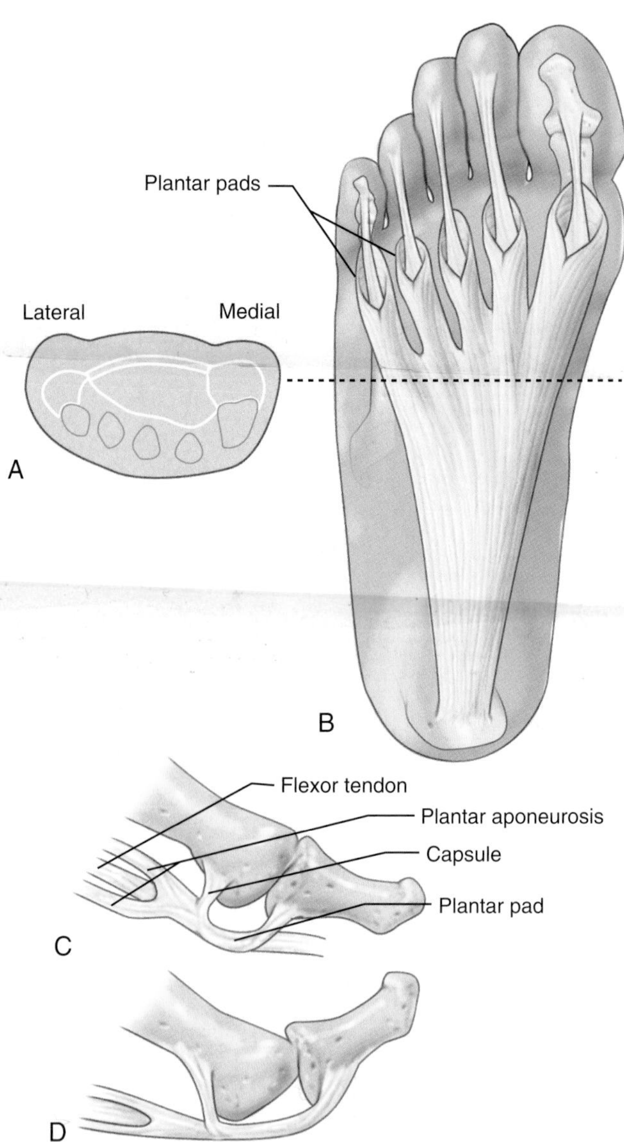

FIGURE 109-12 Plantar aponeurosis. **A,** Cross-section. **B,** The plantar aponeurosis originates from the tubercle of the calcaneus and passes forward to insert into the base of the proximal phalanges. The aponeurosis divides, permitting the long flexor tendon to pass distally. **C,** Components of the plantar pad and its insertion into the base of the proximal phalanx. **D,** Extension of the toes draws the plantar pad over the metatarsal head, pushing it into plantar flexion. *(From Mann RA, Haskell A: Biomechanics of the foot and ankle. In Coughlin MJ, Mann RA, Saltzman CL, editors:* Surgery of the foot and ankle, *ed 8, Philadelphia, 2007, Elsevier.)*

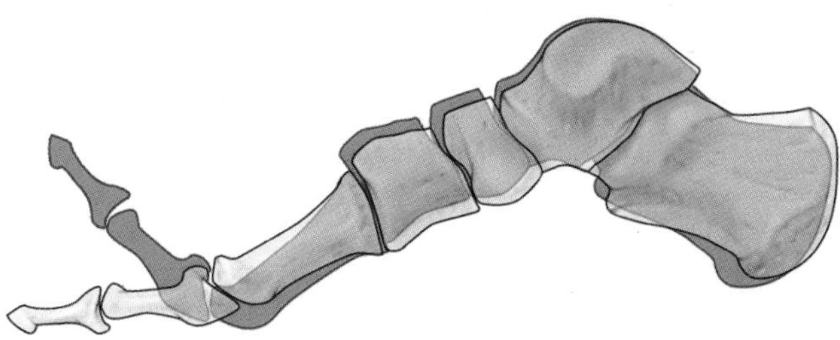

FIGURE 109-13 The function of the plantar aponeurosis. The black outline shows the medial column with the foot at rest. The red figure shows the medial column with the first ray dorsiflexed. Note that dorsiflexion of the metatarsophalangeal joints tightens the plantar aponeurosis, which results in depression of the metatarsal heads, elevation and shortening of the longitudinal arch, inversion of the calcaneus, and elevation of the calcaneal pitch.

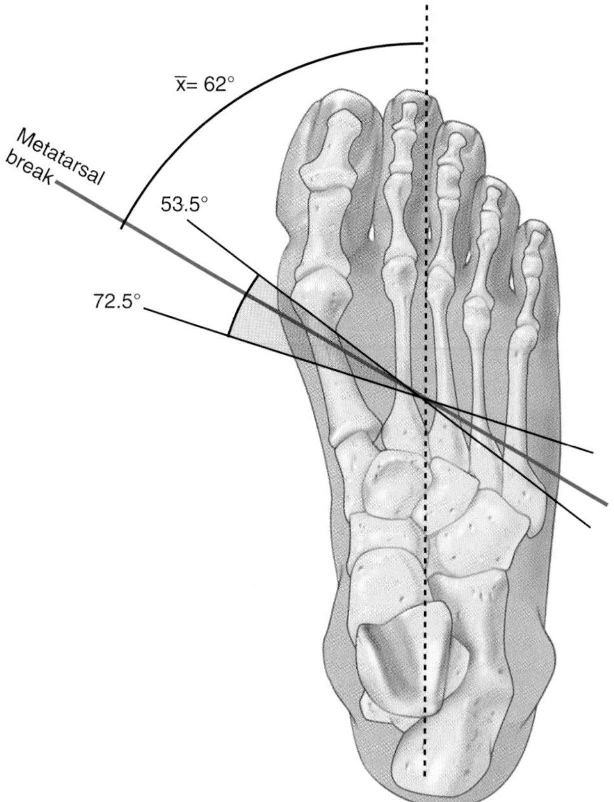

FIGURE 109-14 The metatarsal break passes obliquely at an angle of about 62 degrees to the long axis of the foot. *(Modfied from Isman RE, Inman VT: Anthropometric studies of the human foot and ankle.* Bull Prosthet Res *10:97, 1969.)*

metatarsophalangeal joint. Loss of first metatarsophalangeal joint dorsiflexion prevents normal function of the windlass mechanism and metatarsal break. This situation frequently leads to external rotation of the foot during gait to relieve the stress across the involved area and can cause compensatory changes throughout the lower extremity.

For a complete list of references, go to expertconsult.com.

Suggested Readings

Citation: Hof AL, Elzinga H, Grimmius W, et al: Speed dependence of averaged EMG profiles in walking. *Gait Posture* 16:78–86, 2002.
Level of Evidence: I
Summary: Twenty subjects walked on treadmills at varying speeds while electromyographic (EMG) data were collected from a large number of muscles. The EMG activity of a muscle or functional muscle group can be described by a linear equation representing a fixed component and a component that varies with speed. This finding supports the concept of a central pattern generator for human locomotion.

Citation: Hreljac A: Determinants of the gait transition speed during human locomotion: Kinematic factors. *J Biomech* 28:669–677, 1995.
Level of Evidence: I
Summary: Twenty subjects walked and ran on treadmills at varying speeds while biomechanical measurements were made. Preselected parameters were tested against predefined criteria as possible determinants of why runners transition from walking to running. Maximum ankle angular velocity met the criteria most closely, followed by maximum ankle angular acceleration. The authors hypothesize that gait transition from walking to running is made to protect the ankle dorsiflexors, which are functioning at near-maximum capacity during fast walking.

Citation: Nilsson J, Thorstensson A, Halbertsma J: Changes in leg movements and muscle activity with speed of locomotion and mode of progression in humans. *Acta Physiol Scand* 123:457, 1985.
Level of Evidence: I
Summary: Twelve subjects walked and ran at preset speeds on a treadmill while biomechanical measurements were made. The peak amplitude of the vertical ground reaction force in walking increased from 1.0 to 1.5 times body weight and during running increased from 2.0 to 2.9 times body weight as speed increased. Running has a shorter support phase duration and increased vertical peak force compared with walking.

Citation: Squadrone R, Gallozzi C: Biomechanical and physiological comparison of barefoot and two shod conditions in experienced barefoot runners. *J Sports Med Phys Fitness* 49:6–13, 2009.
Level of Evidence: I
Summary: Eight experienced barefoot runners ran on a treadmill barefoot, with minimal running shoes, and with traditional running shoes while biomechanical and physiological measurements were taken. When running barefoot, the foot strikes with more plantar flexion at the ankle, which was associated with reduced impact forces, shorter stride length and contact times, and greater stride frequency.

Citation: Wülker N, Stukenborg C, Savory KM, et al: Hindfoot motion after isolated and combined arthrodeses: Measurements in anatomic specimens. *Foot Ankle Int* 21:921, 2000.
Level of Evidence: I
Summary: Eight cadaveric specimens were used to compare motion of the hindfoot joints before and after selective arthrodeses. Isolated subtalar fusion diminished talonavicular joint motion to one third of baseline but did not affect calcaneocuboid joint motion. Isolated talonavicular joint fusion reduced subtalar and calcaneocuboid joint motion to one quarter of baseline. Isolated calcaneocuboid joint fusion did not affect talonavicular or subtalar joint motion.

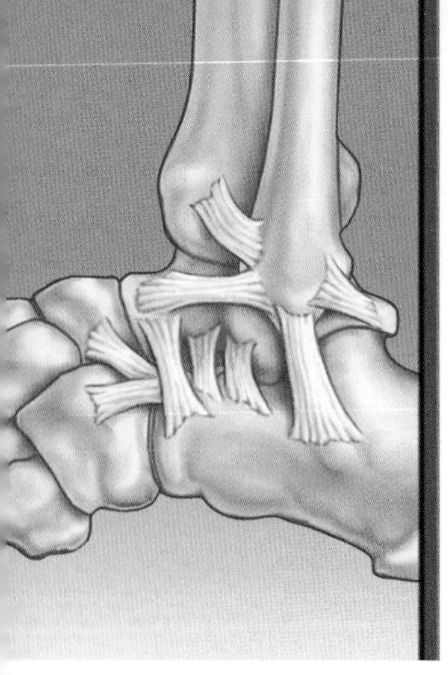

110

Leg, Ankle, and Foot Diagnosis and Decision Making

ANISH R. KADAKIA

Overview of Pathologies

Evaluation of conditions of the foot and ankle is facilitated by the relative subcutaneous location of the major bony, tendinous, and neurovascular structures. This ease of palpation is offset by the complex anatomy of the foot and ankle that transmits up to four times body weight during running and must act as a stable platform during gait. This difficulty is exemplified by a patient with a report of heel pain, in which case one would presume that the ease of palpation of the calcaneus and adjacent structures would facilitate the diagnosis. However, in the case of a chronic Achilles tendon rupture, the patient may have no tenderness with a focal examination, and the diagnosis may only be made by obtaining an appropriate history combined with findings of increased passive dorsiflexion and weak plantar flexion compared with the contralateral lower extremity. The goal of this chapter is to provide a framework for approaching cases of foot and ankle pain commonly seen in athletes.

Chronic exertional compartment syndrome is a condition that occurs in athletes and persons involved in repetitive exertional/loading activities. It is most commonly seen in the lower extremities of distance runners. The pain worsens over the course of the activity and requires premature cessation of exercise, followed by resolution after rest. The underlying cause of the pain has not been definitively determined. The presumed etiology is increased osmotic pressure and edema that results in increased intracompartmental pressure, causing occlusion of the microvasculature and ischemic pain. In contrast to acute compartment syndrome, this condition is not a surgical emergency.

Athletes may experience chronic lower limb pain, which may be attributable to peripheral nerve entrapment. Compared with other problems of the lower limb, this entity is quite rare, with a heterogeneous group of nerve disorders that present with often vague and diffuse locations of pain. The difficulty of properly understanding the entire spectrum of peripheral nerve entrapments may lead to misdiagnosis or underdiagnosis. Adequate treatment of peripheral nerve entrapment requires a proper understanding of the anatomic course, the possible causes, precise identification of the involved nerve, and a clear determination of the location of compression.

Acute ankle ligament injuries are very common; an ankle sprain occurs in an estimated one in every 10,000 persons each day. The lateral ligamentous complex is the most commonly injured. In addition to a simple lateral ankle sprain, a multitude of ligamentous injuries can occur in the foot and ankle, and failure to recognize and appropriately identify these entities may lead to significant morbidity for these patients. With respect to the ankle, this includes syndesmotic injuries (high ankle sprains) and medial (deltoid) ligament injuries. Ankle and subtalar dislocations are not solely caused by high-energy injuries and can occur simply from sliding into a base while playing baseball. A diagnosis of a "foot sprain" is not sufficient to initiate treatment given that some injuries require operative intervention. Sprains of the hindfoot can be associated with fractures of the anterior process or disruption of the stability of Chopart's joint. Both of these injuries respond poorly if aggressive treatment is begun, as is common for a lateral ankle ligament injury. Lisfranc injuries involve disruption of the stabilizing ligaments of the midfoot and are commonly associated with American football or soccer. Any patient who presents with midfoot pain and swelling after an injury should be presumed to have an injury to the tarsometatarsal joint complex, and all efforts should be made to rule out the diagnosis before functional nonoperative treatment is initiated. Rupture of the stabilizing plantar ligaments of the great toe, known as turf toe, can be particularly disabling and has the potential to end the career of a high-level athlete.

Injuries to the tendons that cross the ankle joint range from simple tendonitis to frank rupture. Along the anterior aspect of the ankle, the anterior tibial tendon is most commonly involved, with the extensor hallucis longus and extensor digitorum longus typically involved only in the setting of a traumatic laceration. Anterior tibial tendonitis most commonly involves the insertion of the tendon at the medial cuneiform, with a rupture occurring both at midsubstance or at the insertion. Unlike patients with injuries to the Achilles tendon, patients with rupture of the anterior tibial tendon do not commonly present acutely, and this delayed presentation creates difficulty with surgical reconstruction. Sports that involve explosive push-off are popular both with youth and patients who are older than 30 years and are a common inciting factor in ruptures of the Achilles tendon. Repetitive high-energy loading of the ankle as experienced during running or jumping may lead to excess strain on the both the Achilles and posterior tibial tendons. In these cases, the subcutaneous nature of the tendons greatly facilitates the diagnosis because localized swelling in the area of the foot and ankle is rarely a benign process. In the setting of posterior tibial tendon disease, patients may also note the presence or worsening of a flatfoot deformity. The flexor hallucis longus (FHL), in contrast, is the deepest tendon within the posterior ankle and may not present with subcutaneous swelling. The association with repetitive plantar flexion and injuries to the FHL should guide the examiner to perform more provocative testing to obtain the diagnosis after eliciting this history.

Osteochondral lesions of the talus and tibia (OLTs) can be particularly difficult to treat in the athletic population. To make an accurate diagnosis, knowledge of the functional consequence of the OLTs is required. These lesions may present with a sense of instability or giving way for the patient that can be easily confused with chronic ankle instability. Persons with OLTs commonly have additional pain and swelling between episodes, in addition to possible episodes of locking of the ankle joint. Given that plain radiographs may not clearly demonstrate an OLT, eliciting an accurate history and performing a thorough physical examination are crucial in determining the next most appropriate step in the care of the patient. Articular injuries are not isolated to the talus or tibia and commonly occur in the second metatarsal, known as *Freiberg's infraction*. However, focal cartilage defects may also occur in the third metatarsal head and the first metatarsal head. Failure to recognize these conditions may lead to continued pain for the athlete and inability to play, in addition to possibly accelerating articular injury, leading to arthrosis. Pain and swelling of the joints without a clearly defined radiographic etiology raises the likelihood of this diagnosis.

Heel pain is a frequent complaint in athletes. Although heel pain rarely leads to surgical intervention, it can be very disabling and can be successfully treated if the correct diagnosis is made. Many patients with plantar heel pain may have tenderness over the plantar fascia, but this finding in and of itself does not complete the examination and permit a diagnosis to be made. In some cases, a concomitant calcaneal stress fracture, fat pad atrophy, or compression of the first branch of the medial plantar nerve may exist, requiring alteration of the treatment. Such alteration is most crucial in patients who fail to experience relief after a reasonable period of nonoperative treatment. The practitioner should always question the initial diagnosis in the setting of persistent pain to minimize the risk of pursuing an inappropriate treatment course.

Pain within the lesser forefoot is termed *metatarsalgia*; however, metatarsalgia is a descriptive term of the location of the pain and does not offer any true diagnostic information. Metatarsalgia may be the result of multiple etiologies, ranging from instability of the first tarsometatarsal to Freiberg's infraction, Morton's neuroma, plantar plate rupture, or an equinus contracture. Complicating the diagnosis is that multiple factors may contribute to the pain and each one must be addressed to achieve success. Pain within the sesamoid complex should be aggressively treated nonoperatively because an early stress fracture is difficult to differentiate from sesamoiditis at initial presentation. In this case, the clinical symptom of sesamoid pain is easy to make given the subcutaneous position of the bone; however, the underlying root cause is more difficult to determine even with advanced imaging. Therefore aggressive treatment, although cumbersome, can minimize the risk of long-term pain and discomfort, which is extremely disabling for the athlete.

History

Obtaining a thorough history not only provides information regarding the cause of the complaint but also aids in constructing a focused physical examination that maximizes the information gathered given the time constraints of the practitioner. The location of the complaint is one of the most useful aspects of the history in determining the cause. Having a patient use a single digit to locate the point of maximal tenderness and/or swelling greatly facilitates determination of the correct diagnosis. A working knowledge of the subcutaneous anatomy of the foot and ankle is required to gain the most information from this maneuver. The inability to localize a specific site also provides valuable information that the underlying cause may be neurologic, autoimmune, or medication related. Pain over the entire lateral aspect of the foot, for example, is more likely related to the sural nerve than the peroneal tendons or the fifth metatarsal. The concomitant sensation of a "pop" or the sense that something is moving out of place along with the painful episodes is associated with FHL stenosing synovitis (posterior), peroneal subluxation (lateral), or posterior tibial subluxation (medial).

When obtaining the history, rather than using a repetitive list of questions, the questions should be adapted to the patient's responses. For example, when inciting factors are elicited and the patient reports onset during exercise, the examiner should consider exertional compartment syndrome, with follow-up questions to determine if the severity increases with duration of exercise, if pain ceases after rest, and if pain is not present during activities of daily living to corroborate the diagnosis. Pain after a period of immobility is common in persons with inflammatory etiologies, such as tendonitis, arthritis, and plantar fasciitis. Persons with stress fractures, on the other hand, have minimal pain after immobility; in contrast, the pain gets worse over time, and the pain does not cease with rest as would occur with exertional compartment syndrome.

Clearly defining the exact activity that causes the pain is helpful. For example, many dancers experience foot and ankle pain, and determining whether they are ballet dancers engaging in en-pointe activity (leading to FHL synovitis) or ballroom dancers (who often have sesamoiditis) leads the examiner toward the most likely etiology. Not only is the particular activity critical in determining the diagnosis, it also plays an important role in determining the timing and type of surgical intervention that would be appropriate. In the case of ballet dancers, for whom maximum mobility is critical to their career, hallux valgus surgery is avoided and more minimally invasive techniques involving arthroscopy should be used to minimize stiffness. Conversely, in athletes for whom stability is more critical than flexibility, retention of hardware for syndesmotic and tarsometatarsal injuries is considered.

Initiation of a new activity or modification of activity such as an increase in intensity or duration is commonly noted in the setting of tendonitis and stress fractures. Additionally, alteration of shoe wear can be temporally related and may contribute to the cause of the discomfort, especially given the rise in the popularity of minimalist shoes and their association with metatarsal stress fractures. Stress fractures and acute tendonitis are also commonly seen in runners who are training for a marathon as they increase their duration to gain endurance. Regardless of the length of time patients have participated in the activity, they can still experience overuse injuries as a result of a deformity such as a cavovarus foot or biologic factors such as osteopenia or vitamin D deficiency. Pain associated with activity on uneven surfaces such as grass or gravel is related to the subtalar and transverse tarsal joints and is commonly noted in patients with sinus tarsi syndrome. Increased pain with use of stairs, particularly with descent, is noted in patients with Achilles tendon disease, given the strain placed across the tendon during the eccentric contraction needed to stabilize the body. In patients with plantar fasciitis or fat pad atrophy, running on a rubber surface may be preferable to running on a hard surface such as asphalt or concrete, as opposed to patients with stress fractures, who would not note a significant difference.

In addition to pain and swelling, the presence of mechanical symptoms must be determined. A sense of instability or frank episodes of giving way may be related to a multitude of causes. Paroxysmal instability that occurs without cause is most likely the result of an OLT or a loose body. Locking or catching of the ankle is indicative of a loose body or unstable osteochondral flap. A sense that the ankle feels loose associated with episodes of giving way is more likely related to laxity of the lateral collateral ligaments. Peroneal tendon disease can lead to instability because the role of these tendons as a secondary stabilizer is compromised. In these cases, however, the complaint is commonly associated with pain and swelling along the posterolateral aspect of the ankle. These conditions may occur concomitantly, and therefore even when a positive response is elicited for one diagnosis, the practitioner must further question the patient regarding other additional causes.

In cases of trauma, determining the mechanism of injury greatly facilitates the diagnosis; however, many patients are unable to recall the details of the injury. Although no mechanism creates the same injury in all cases, a common pattern does exist. For example, an inversion injury of a plantar-flexed foot without external force most commonly disrupts the lateral collateral ligaments of the ankle, creating an ankle sprain. Getting struck by another player while the foot is in a plantar-flexed position increases the risk of a tarsometatarsal (Lisfranc) injury. Disruption to the syndesmosis occurs with an external rotation force coupled with axial loading to a dorsiflexed and externally rotated foot. This mechanism may be seen in sports that require frequent alteration of direction at high speeds such as basketball, American football, and soccer. Explosive push-off as seen in tennis or basketball is associated with a rupture of the Achilles tendon. Additionally, patients may state that they heard an audible pop or gunshot-type sound and felt as if they were kicked in the back of the leg. Hyperdorsiflexion of the great toe is directly linked to turf-toe injuries.

Neurologic reports of numbness, tingling, or burning should be elicited. Radiating pain from proximal to distal or less commonly from distal to proximal (the Valleix phenomenon) can occur as a result of nerve entrapment and is less likely to be the result of a musculoskeletal etiology. Transient numbness or even foot drop with exercise may occur in patients with exertional compartment syndrome. The transient nature of the symptom and the direct correlation to activity differentiate these symptoms from nerve entrapment, with which the symptom is present at rest. A prior history of surgery will guide the practitioner to examine the incisions carefully to determine possible iatrogenic causes of the neurologic symptoms. Failure to obtain relief with antiinflammatory medication is common in patients with nerve disorders.

Obtaining a complete history includes not only a detailed discussion of the chief complaint but must include a review of the patient's medical and surgical history in addition to current medications and prior thrombosis or thrombosis in family members. Clearly, a patient with an autoimmune disease requires alteration of the treatment plan because medical management must be optimized before considering any surgical intervention. Current fluoroquinolone use, although common knowledge to the medical community, may not be recognized by the patient and is associated with tendonitis, particularly of the Achilles tendon. Diffuse musculoskeletal pain or muscle tenderness may be related to the use of cholesterol-lowering statin medications and should be considered in cases without a clearly identifiable cause. Patients with diabetes should be examined for sensory neuropathy and may require prolonged periods of non–weight bearing compared with persons who are not diabetic. In patients with a history of thrombosis, consideration of the use of antithrombotic medication is critical when proposing immobilization for acute injuries.

Physical Examination

The examination should begin with the patient seated, with exposure of both lower extremities distal to the knee. Visual inspection for swelling quickly guides the examiner to possible areas of pathology. The location of the swelling is correlated with common disease processes. For example, posteromedial swelling is related to the posterior tibial tendon; swelling that is directly posterior is related to the Achilles tendon; posterolateral swelling relates to the peroneal tendons; swelling in the dorsal medial midfoot relates to the anterior tibialis; and swelling of the central forefoot can be attributed to a stress fracture (Fig. 110-1). In the setting of trauma, if the patient can be examined quickly after the injury, the focal area of swelling helps to determine the site of the injury.

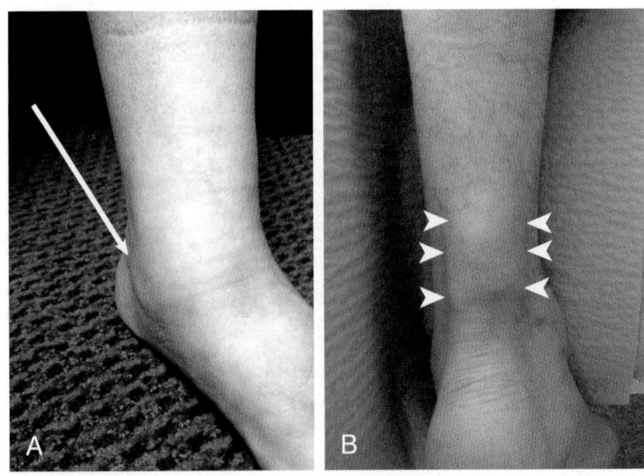

FIGURE 110-1 **A,** Posteromedial swelling (*arrow*) in a patient with acute posterior tibial tendonitis. Note the loss of contour of the medial malleolus. **B,** Swelling and thickening of the posterior aspect of the heel (*arrowheads*) that is consistent with Achilles tendinosis.

However, in a delayed presentation more than 24 hours after the injury, the swelling is typically diffuse, limiting the effectiveness of this finding. Asymmetric circumferential swelling of the leg after an injury or surgery may indicate the presence of a thrombosis and should be further evaluated, because the injury itself typically does not cause circumferential edema of the entire leg. The presence of any abnormal bony or soft tissue prominences should be noted. Although such prominences can be the result of a benign or malignant tumor, in some cases a posttraumatic deformity may be the cause. Classically, this posttraumatic deformity can be seen after a rupture of the anterior tibial tendon, and patients may present with a "pseudotumor" along the anterior ankle as a result of proximal migration of the tendon (Fig. 110-2). Further motor examination will clearly determine the diagnosis and avoid an inappropriate workup.

The presence of ecchymosis typically correlates with the area of injury. Plantar midfoot ecchymosis is highly indicative of a Lisfranc injury (Fig. 110-3). However, the presence of ecchymosis can be difficult to interpret in the delayed setting because blood tracks through the subcutaneous tissue after injury, as is commonly seen with distal forefoot ecchymosis after an ankle sprain. In the setting of an Achilles tendon rupture, bruising is commonly noted along the posterior superior calcaneus and not directly at the site of rupture given the dependent position of the limb. An understanding of this phenomenon can guide the examiner to look for a more proximal site of injury after identifying distal ecchymosis, such as with a Thompson test in this case. Further inspection for prior surgical scars can identify possible sites of nerve injury or entrapment. Although more relevant when examining for deformity, the presence of a callus formation notes an area of focal overload. In the athlete, a callus over the fifth metatarsal base and head is suggestive of a cavovarus deformity and is important to consider when treating ankle sprains, instability, fifth metatarsal fractures, and peroneal tendon disease. Diffuse callus formation over the plantar forefoot may suggest an equinus contracture, which must be addressed when treating patients with metatarsalgia.

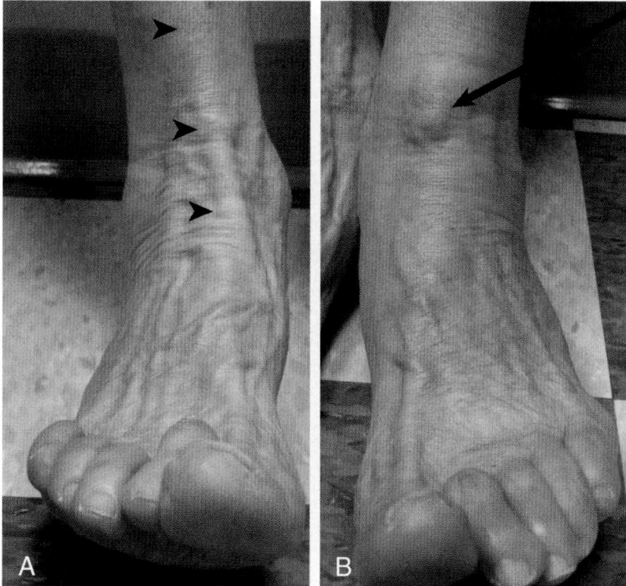

FIGURE 110-2 A patient with a chronic rupture of the left anterior tibial tendon. He was referred for a "mass" on the left ankle (**B;** *arrow*). The clear asymmetry from the intact anterior tibial tendon (**A;** *arrowheads*) with attempted dorsiflexion is consistent with an anterior tibial tendon rupture.

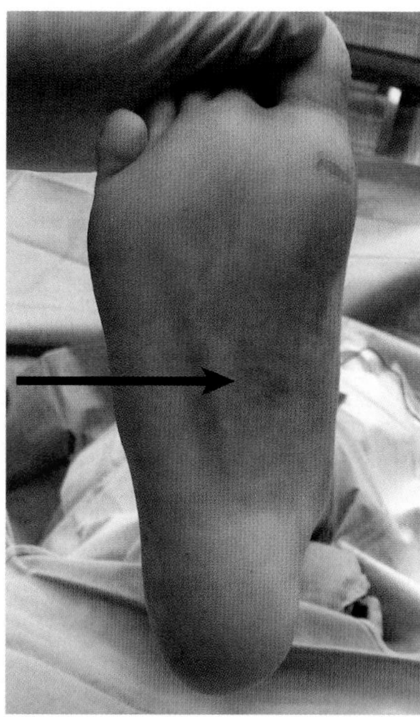

FIGURE 110-3 Plantar ecchymosis (*arrow*) in the setting of a midfoot injury should raise the suspicion of a Lisfranc injury.

Although evaluation of gait and alignment is important, this evaluation can be deferred in the setting of acute trauma to prevent further injury and decrease patient discomfort. The presence of a cavovarus deformity with an elevated longitudinal arch with hindfoot varus and a plantar-flexed first ray must be recognized and addressed when treating the previously described associated conditions to decrease the risk of recurrence (Fig. 110-4). The presence of pes planus with collapse of the longitudinal arch and hindfoot valgus may be seen as a normal condition, resulting from posterior tibial tendon dysfunction or chronic Lisfranc injuries. Comparison with the contralateral lower extremity is critical to help identify subtle differences, especially in cases in which the patient may already have congenital pes planus (Fig. 110-5). Abnormal gait patterns can clearly indicate the pathologic process. Steppage gait with increased knee and hip flexion during the swing phase occurs as a result of foot drop and may be seen with an anterior tibial tendon rupture or peroneal nerve palsy. A calcaneus gait pattern with increased dorsiflexion during heel strike occurs with triceps surae weakness after a chronic Achilles rupture. Pain with weight bearing results in an antalgic gait with a shortened stance phase on the affected limb.

To minimize the discomfort of the patient, palpation for the site of maximum tenderness in addition to provocative testing is deferred until the end of the examination. Tactile examination begins with a vascular evaluation to assess the dorsalis pedis and posterior tibialis pulses. Although this evaluation can become routine, special attention is required after severe trauma such as an ankle or hindfoot dislocation and in any patient who may require surgical intervention. A sensory examination of the five peripheral nerves that innervate the foot should follow. These nerves include the deep

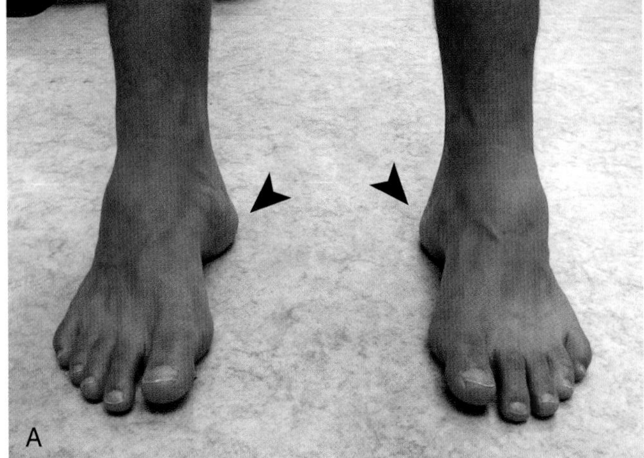

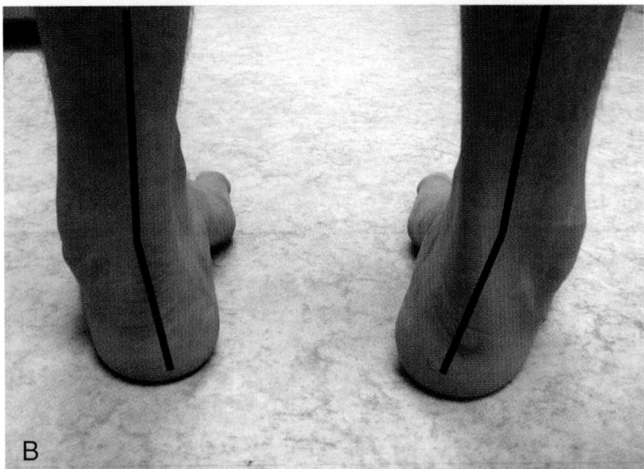

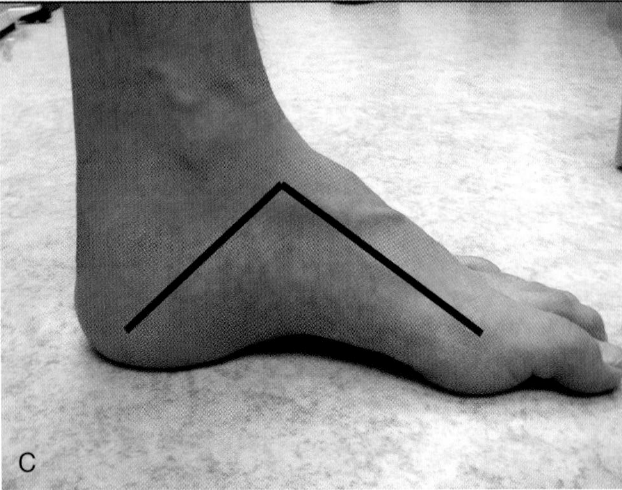

FIGURE 110-4 **A,** Frontal view of a patient with a cavovarus deformity. In patients with this deformity, the posteromedial aspect of the heel (*arrowhead*) is clearly visible. The varus hindfoot deformity can be viewed from the posterior aspect (**B**), and in severe cases, none of the lesser toes is visible. From the medial aspect (**C**), the cavus aspect of the deformity can be visualized.

peroneal nerve (first web space), superficial peroneal nerve (dorsal foot), saphenous nerve (medial ankle), sural nerve (lateral foot), and tibial nerve (plantar foot; Fig. 110-6). After acute ankle sprains, decreased sensation over the course of the superficial peroneal nerve is not uncommon as a result of traction injury. If neuroma is a concern, provocative testing of the suspected nerve can be performed. Compression of the nerve at the suspected site of injury should reproduce the patient's symptoms. To adequately test the nerve, the compression should be held for 30 seconds. In the setting of a postsurgical neuroma, the site of injury is clearly identified by the scar. However, in suspected atraumatic neuroma formation, knowledge of the common sites of compression guide the examination: the distal third of the anterolateral tibia, superficial peroneal nerve; the tarsal tunnel, the tibial nerve; the dorsal hindfoot and midfoot, the deep peroneal nerve; and the second or third web space, the interdigital nerves. Compression of the abductor hallucis muscle increases the pressure on the first branch of the lateral plantar nerve and is important to perform when evaluating heel pain.

Motor testing involves assessment of individual muscles and can provide information regarding the status of tendon integrity and neurologic innervation. Isolated weakness of a single muscle is most likely related to a discontinuity of the tendon (Fig. 110-7). Neurologic causes of muscle weakness involve more than muscle groups and may be associated with a concomitant sensory deficit. Given that most of the tendons of the foot and ankle cross distal to the ankle joint, an isolated tendon injury may not result in complete loss of active mobility. Relative weakness compared with the contralateral limb is very useful to determine subtle weakness. In the setting of a complete rupture of the Achilles tendon, plantar-flexion power to resistance (4-5) may still be present as a result of the multiple tendons that cross posterior to the ankle joint. Having the patient push against resistance with the contralateral hand palpating for the tested tendon can determine continuity and additionally assess for tendon disease if the patient reports pain during the maneuver. Subtle weakness may be difficult to discern with a manual resistance examination because of the strength of the lower extremity. Fatigue testing

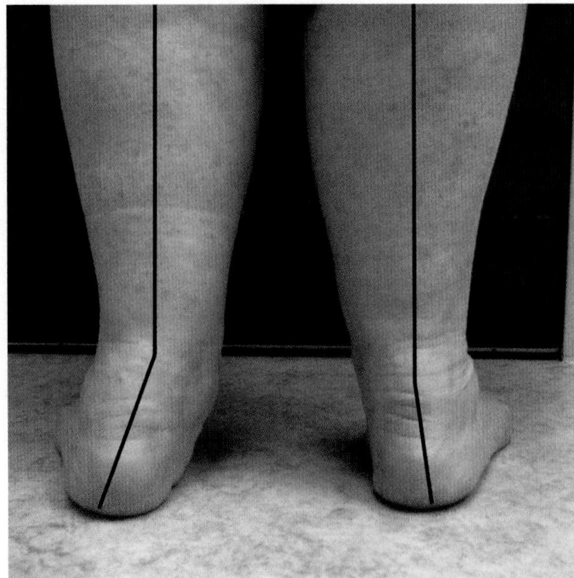

FIGURE 110-5 This patient has a history of bilateral pes planus but presented with increased pain in the left lower extremity. The increased severity of the valgus on the left leg is clearly demonstrated when compared with her unaffected right leg. This finding is consistent with posterior tibial tendon dysfunction in most cases.

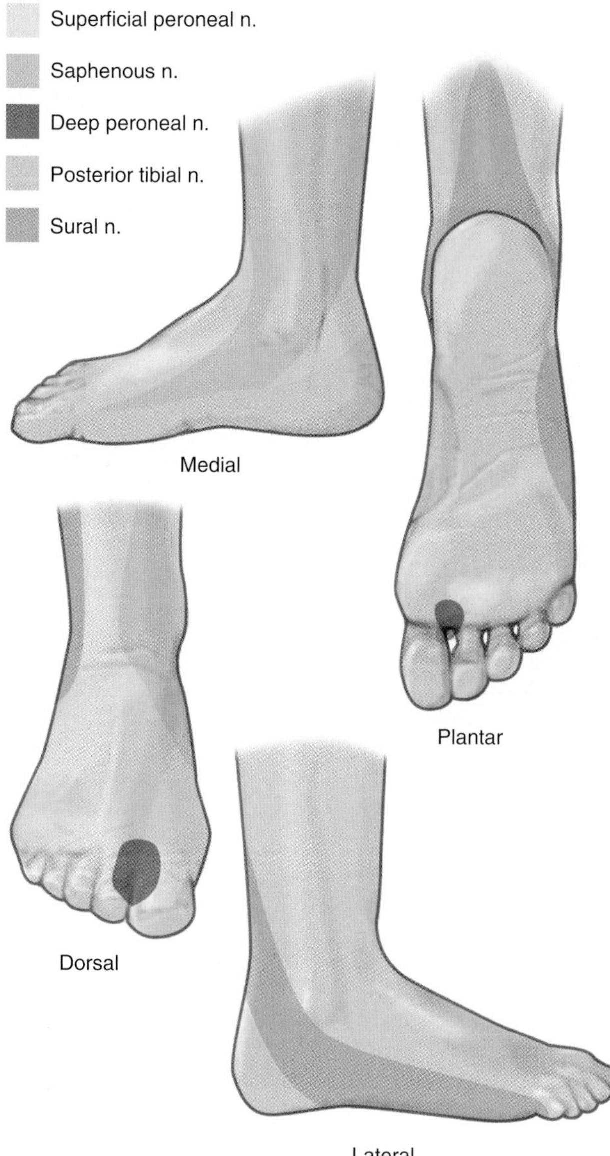

FIGURE 110-6 Sensory nerve distribution of the ankle.

is useful in these cases, such as the repeated single-limb heel rise for the evaluation of the posterior tibial tendon (Fig. 110-8). The single-limb heel rise examination is also valuable when assessing strength in the setting of a chronic Achilles tendon rupture. Subtle anterior tibial tendon weakness may be tested with heel walking.

Both passive and active range of motion should be compared with the contralateral side. Combining active range of motion with a motor examination minimizes repetition. The rate of variability of normal motion of the joints of the foot and ankle is high, with no defined absolute normal. Asymmetry between extremities or pain at the extremes of motion is more relevant than the absolute value. Typically, dorsiflexion is evaluated with an interest in the amount of restriction of motion resulting from a gastrocnemius or Achilles contracture (Fig. 110-9). Importantly, however, increased motion is just as valuable, because this finding is seen with a chronic Achilles tendon rupture and may be the primary clue to the diagnosis (Fig. 110-10). Maximal range of motion of the ankle is 10 to 23 degrees of dorsiflexion and 23 to 48 degrees of plantar flexion (Fig. 110-11). Maximal range of subtalar inversion is 5 to 50 degrees and eversion is 5 to 26 degrees (Fig. 110-12). Maximal range of motion for the first metatarsophalangeal joint (great toe) is 45 to 90 degrees of dorsiflexion and 10 to 40 degrees of plantar flexion (Fig. 110-13). Although active range of motion after trauma may be significantly restricted, passive range of motion should be present, although reduced. In the case of a severe restriction of motion or a locked joint, the risk of a dislocation or subluxation is present and must be evaluated with further imaging. Pain, grinding, or crepitus during passive range of motion testing is consistent with articular cartilage degeneration from loose bodies or arthritis. Triggering during passive stretching of the tendon is a result of stenosing tenosynovitis that is associated most commonly with the FHL in the foot and ankle.

Palpation for the sites of tenderness can quickly provide information for diagnosis in cases of trauma, tendon disorders, and arthritis. However, palpation may cause significant pain for the patient if it is performed at the beginning of the examination, preventing the completion of a proper evaluation. Additionally, although palpation may be an easy way to

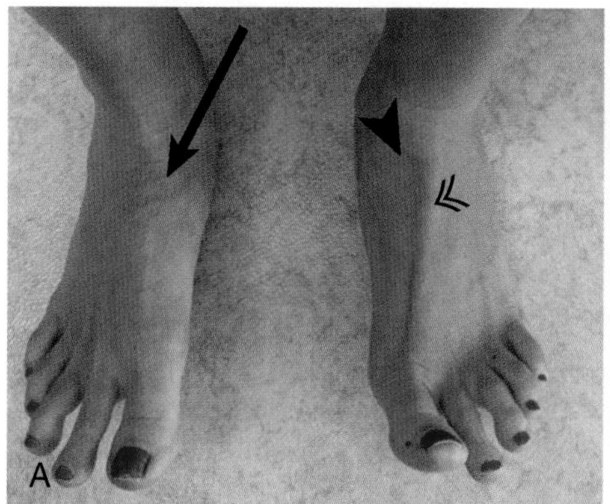

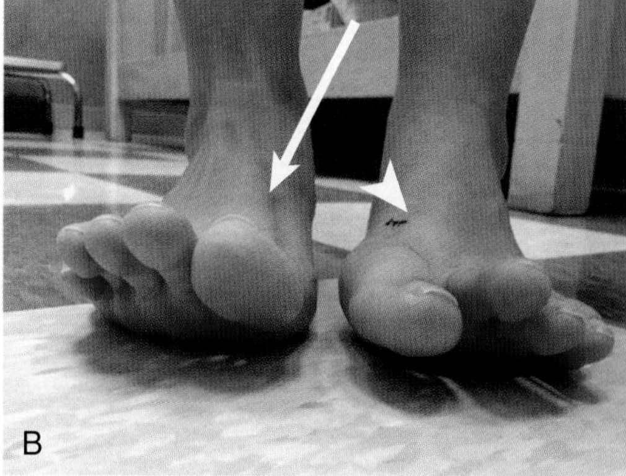

FIGURE 110-7 **A,** Chronic rupture of the anterior tibial tendon on the left lower extremity. The lack of function of the tendon is clearly seen (*black arrowhead*) when compared with taut anterior tibialis (*black arrow*) on the right leg. Additionally, the function of the extensor hallucis longus (EHL; *black double arrow*) and extensor digitorum longus rule out the possibility of a proximal neurologic etiology. The extensor recruitment allows the patient to perform active dorsiflexion. A follow-up examination with heel walking will demonstrate fatigue of the left leg compared with the right. **B,** Traumatic laceration to the dorsum of the foot with a lack of function of the EHL (*white arrowhead*), which is made more clear when compared with the normal contralateral foot (*white arrow*).

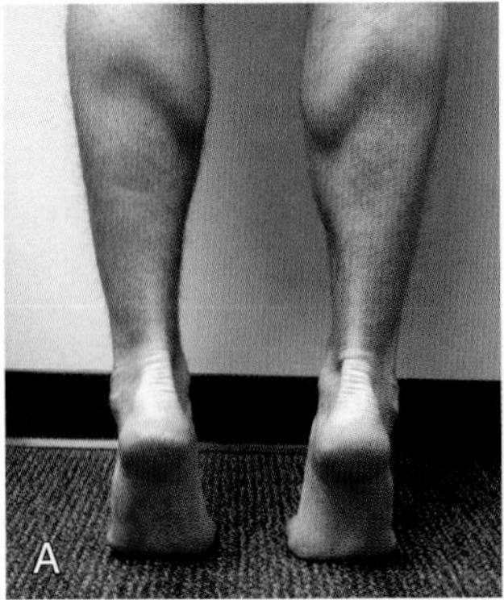

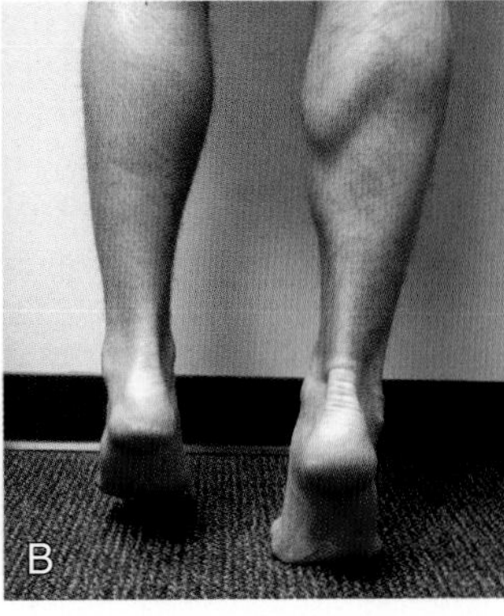

FIGURE 110-8 Strength testing of the posterior tibial tendon with a double-limb heel rise (**A**) will be unable to detect dysfunction because the patient can compensate with the unaffected limb. To isolate the affected posterior tibial tendon, the patient must elevate the unaffected limb and perform the maneuver with only the affected extremity (**B**). This test is valid only for function of the posterior tibialis if the Achilles tendon is intact.

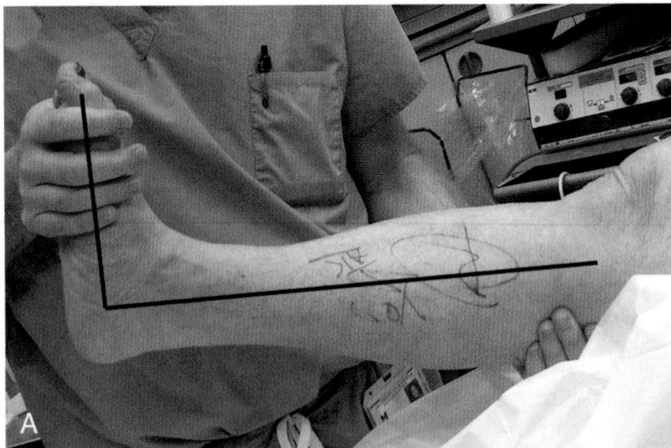

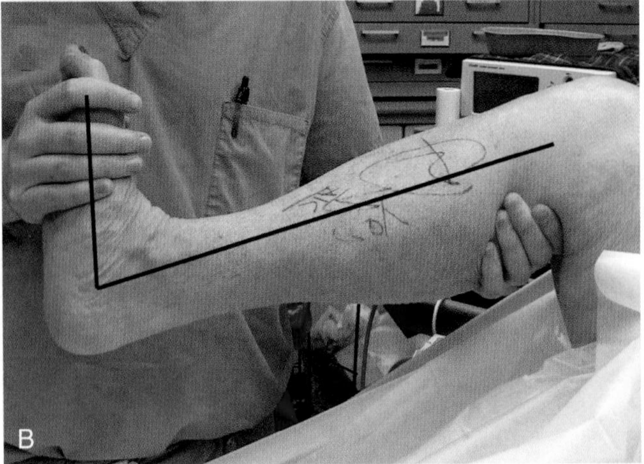

FIGURE 110-9 **A,** Dorsiflexion of the ankle with the knee in extension does not achieve flexion past neutral. **B,** With knee flexion the contribution of the gastrocnemius is eliminated, with a resultant increase in dorsiflexion, which is consistent with an isolated gastrocnemius contracture. If no increase in motion occurs, both the gastrocnemius and soleus are contracted, and lengthening of the Achilles tendon is required for correction.

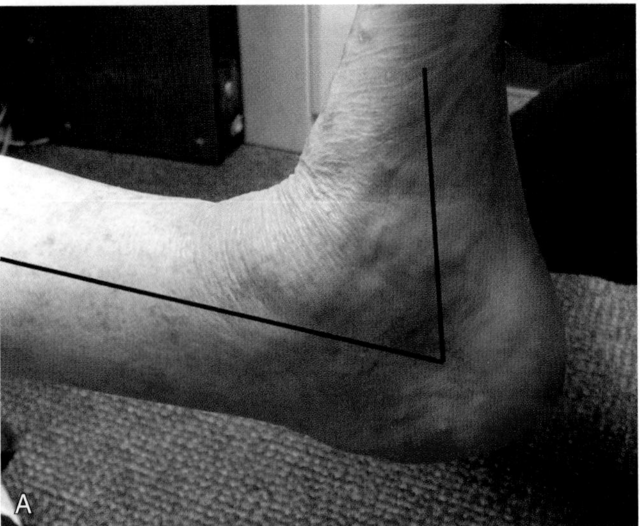

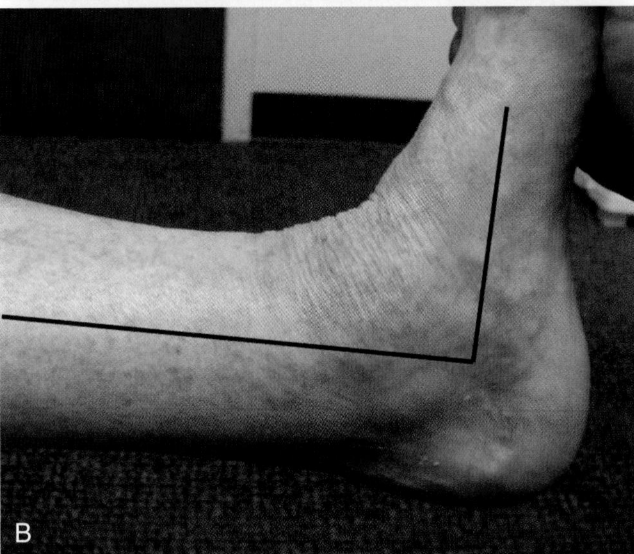

FIGURE 110-10 This patient presented with heel pain and difficulty walking on stairs with the affected lower extremity. Note the hyperdorsiflexion of the affected ankle (**A**) compared with the uninjured side (**B**). Given the chronicity of the presentation, no clear defect may be palpable in these cases. Follow-up testing with manual strength examination and single-limb heel testing is appropriate to demonstrate weakness and thus corroborate the diagnosis of a chronic Achilles rupture.

determine the diagnosis is many cases, it is not extremely helpful in the evaluation of instability, chronic tendon ruptures, exertional compartment syndrome, and neurologic disorders. A thorough knowledge of the subcutaneous anatomy of the foot and ankle greatly facilitates the usefulness of the examination. When evaluating patients with a suspected injury, such as an ankle sprain, palpation should be performed in a centripetal fashion to identify other areas of concomitant injury. Additionally, the amount of pressure used should be minimal to avoid harm and discomfort to the patient. In contrast, when performing the examination for chronic conditions, deeper palpation may be required to identify the areas of concern. Comparison with the contralateral lower extremity is crucial because many areas are tender to palpation in a normal patient, and a relative increase in

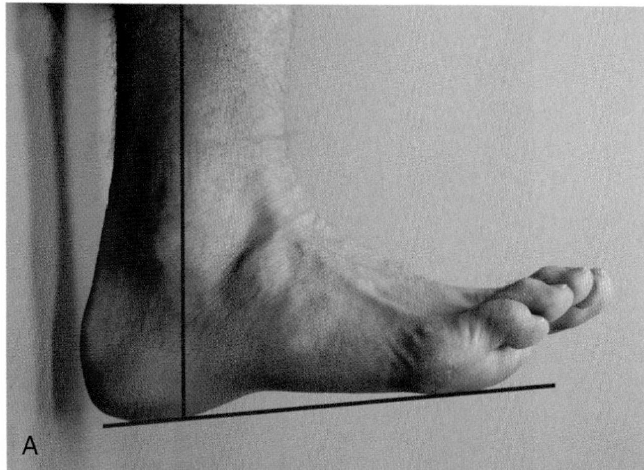

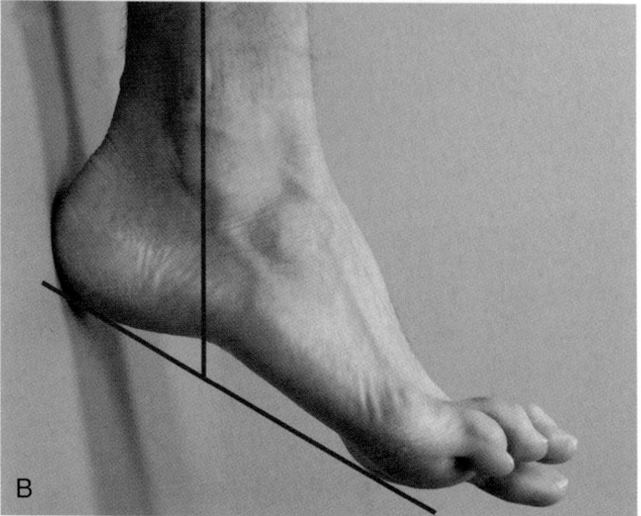

FIGURE 110-11 Dorsiflexion of the ankle (**A**) is typically 25% to 50% the magnitude of plantar flexion (**B**). This difference partially accounts for why a small decrease in the absolute dorsiflexion is implicated in many pathologic conditions of the foot and ankle. A 5-degree loss of motion may result in a 50% loss of functional dorsiflexion for the patient.

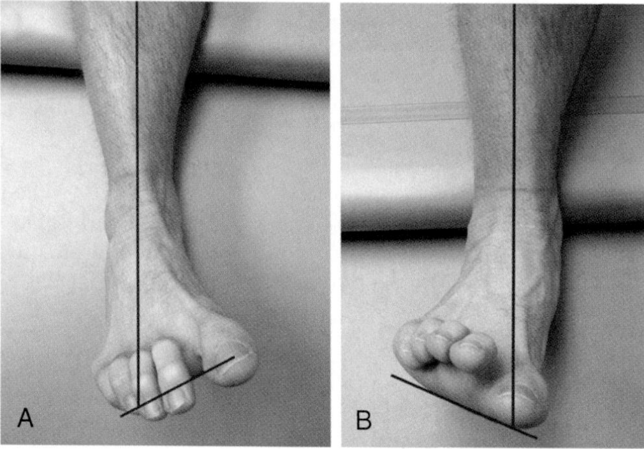

FIGURE 110-12 Inversion of the hindfoot (**A**) is greater than eversion (**B**). This asymmetry partially accounts for why a pes planus deformity is better tolerated than a pes cavus deformity, because the foot has limited eversion capacity to compensate for hindfoot varus.

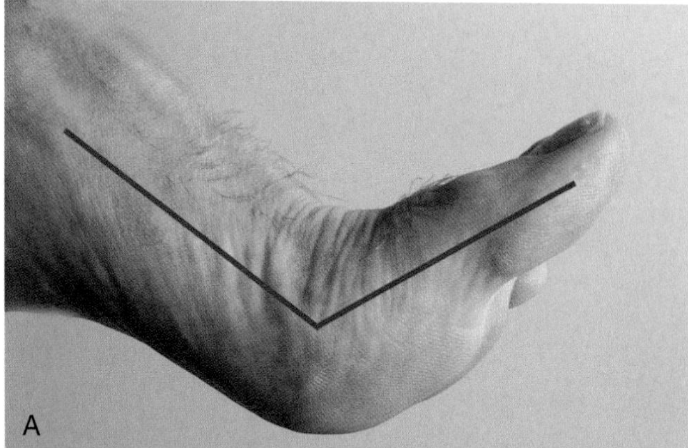

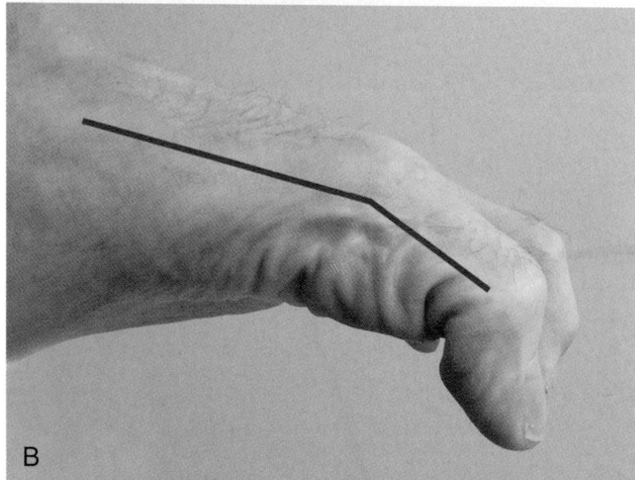

FIGURE 110-13 Dorsiflexion of the first metatarsophalangeal (MTP) joint (**A**) is greater in magnitude and more critical to function than is plantar flexion of the first MTP joint (**B**).

discomfort provides more valuable information. The sinus tarsi is a particularly sensitive spot, and unless both extremities are examined and compared, the presence of pain with palpation is a nondiagnostic finding.

Stability of the lateral ankle ligaments can be assessed with the anterior drawer and varus talar tilt tests. The anterior drawer test is performed with anterior pressure on the hindfoot with the ankle in plantar flexion, which evaluates the anterior talofibular ligament (Fig. 110-14). The varus stress test is performed with inversion of the ankle in dorsiflexion to evaluate the calcaneofibular ligament (Fig. 110-15). Signs of ligamentous laxity should be tested, because these signs guide surgical treatment (Fig. 110-16). Stability testing is not isolated to the ankle and can also be performed for the hindfoot, midfoot, and forefoot joints. Stabilization of the hindfoot with dorsiflexion and plantar-flexion stress placed on the first metatarsal subjectively evaluates the first tarsometatarsal. The "vertical Lachman" test for lesser metatarsophalangeal instability is important to perform in the setting of forefoot pain. The hindfoot is difficult to examine for stability given the amount of mobility that is normally present; however, use of fluoroscopy during the examination for suspected instability of the subtalar or Chopart joints increases the yield from stress testing because subluxation of the joints can be directly visualized.

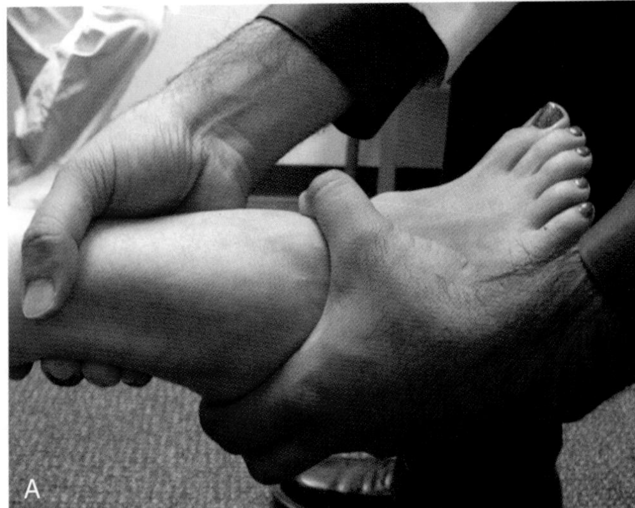

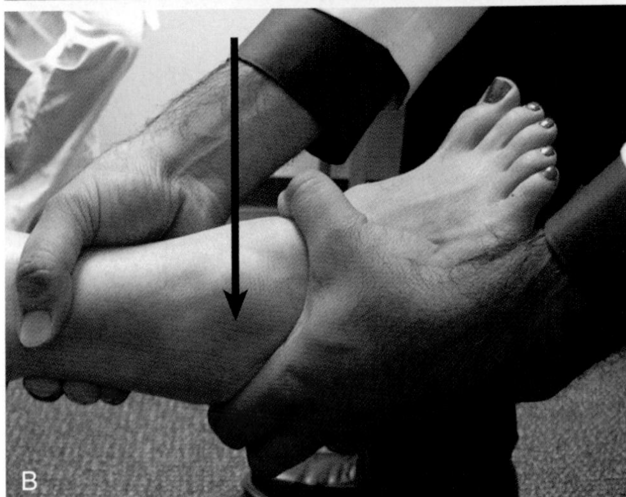

FIGURE 110-14 To perform the anterior drawer test, one hand stabilizes the anterior distal tibia while the other is cupped around the posterior calcaneus (**A**). The heel is translated anteriorly with respect to the tibia, and any subluxation should be noted (**B**). Note the sulcus that is created over the anterolateral ankle with an unstable ankle (*arrow*).

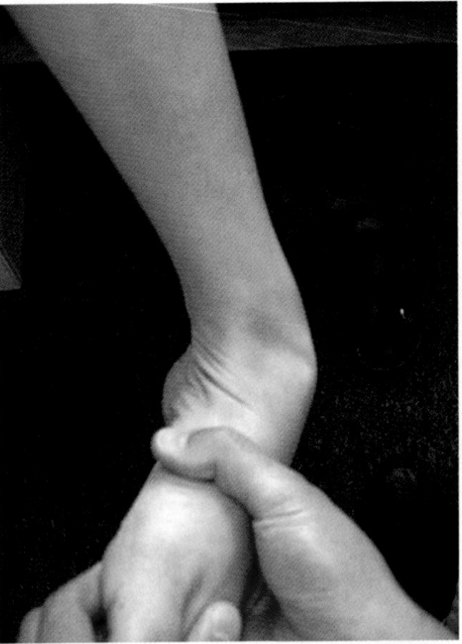

FIGURE 110-15 The inversion stress test in a patient with severe laxity of the calcaneofibular ligament.

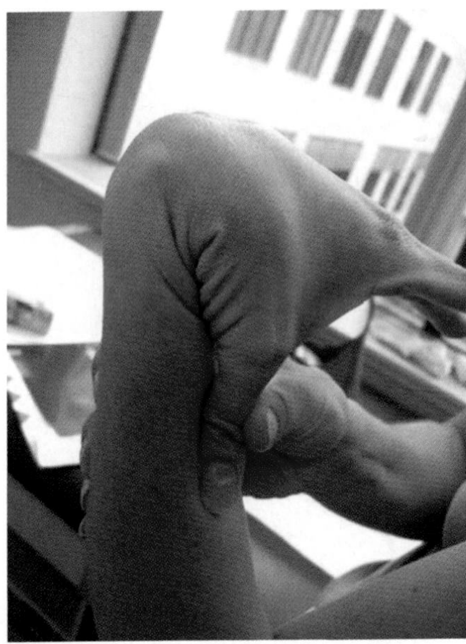

FIGURE 110-16 Patients with hyperlaxity are easily able to flex the wrist and place the thumb on the volar forearm.

After a thorough physical examination of the lower extremities is conducted, further provocative testing (covered in detail in other chapters in this section) can be performed to evaluate specific suspected conditions. For example, a midcalf compression test and external rotation stress testing may be required to evaluate for a possible syndesmotic injury in a patient with lateral ankle swelling and pain after trauma. This specific test would not be indicated if midfoot swelling and pain were present, in which case stress testing of the midfoot along with a single-limb weight-bearing examination would be performed for evaluation of a Lisfranc injury. When evaluating a patient with a foot and ankle complaint, in many cases, a thorough history and physical examination is sufficient to determine the diagnosis without the need for further imaging.

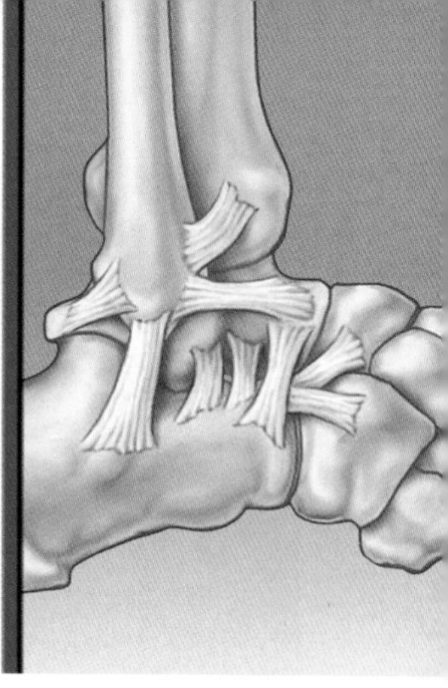

111

Imaging of the Foot and Ankle

ANISH R. KADAKIA

Radiographs

Radiographs are often the initial imaging study performed for any patient presenting with a problem related to the foot and ankle. Radiographs are clearly beneficial when evaluating for suspected arthritis, osteonecrosis, tumors, nonunion, or trauma. In addition, the alignment of the ankle and foot may contribute to the presenting complaint even if the radiographs being viewed are free of pathologic abnormalities. To appropriately evaluate the osseous structures and alignment of the foot, the radiographs should be obtained with weight bearing in all cases, except when a fracture may be suspected (Figs. 111-1 to 111-3). Specifically, in the setting of a suspected Lisfranc injury, if the initial non–weight-bearing radiographs are negative, follow-up weight-bearing films should be ordered to evaluate for diastasis of the tarsometatarsal joints.

Computed Tomography

The most current generation of multidetector computed tomography (CT) scanners are capable of providing high-resolution images in all imaging planes and are superb for evaluating the extent and location of intraarticular fractures in the area of the ankle and hindfoot. Given the difficulty in assessing joint congruity in the hindfoot, follow-up CT imaging is recommended in this setting to better appreciate the fracture pattern and joint congruity. Cystic osteochondral defects of the talus are excellently visualized with this modality to accurately calculate the size of the lesion and guide preoperative planning. It is also an excellent method of assessing bony healing, including evaluation of fractures and arthrodeses. Sufficient data are available to suggest that determination of the percentage of bony trabeculation across an arthrodesis site in the ankle and hindfoot is grossly underestimated with plain radiography. The administration of intraarticular contrast material followed by CT imaging through the ankle (CT arthrography) is an accurate means of assessing internal derangement in patients who have a contraindication to magnetic resonance imaging (MRI).

Ultrasound

The primary advantage of ultrasound compared with MRI is the ability to evaluate the tendinous structures in a dynamic fashion.[1] Ultrasound is the imaging modality of choice for the evaluation of peroneal tendon subluxation. The evaluation for tendon apposition in the setting of an Achilles tendon rupture or for evaluation of flexor hallucis longus (FHL) stenosing tenosynovitis are examples of when the ability to perform a dynamic examination is critical. Advantages include a relative cost saving compared with MRI and improved localization of soft tissue structures for injection. A limitation of ultrasound is that visualization of the affected structure may prove more difficult in patients with a high amount of subcutaneous fat.[2] Additionally, the clinician is reliant upon the interpretation of the radiologist and the skill of the ultrasonographer for the determination of the pathologic findings. Good communication between the clinician and the radiologist is critical to ensure that the radiologist has an understanding of the exact clinical concern so the examination can be tailored appropriately.

Magnetic Resonance Imaging

MRI is well accepted as the primary noninvasive imaging modality for providing a global assessment of the foot and ankle and is very accurate for the evaluation of cartilaginous, tendon, ligament, and bony abnormalities. MR arthrography of the ankle can be used to obtain a more precise evaluation of articular cartilage injuries to the talar dome or tibial plafond.[3] T1-weighted fat-saturated images are key to evaluate the gadolinium contrast material in the joint. These images show the contrast to the greatest advantage. Because evaluation of bone marrow is also critical, T1-weighted non–fat-saturated images are also essential. T1-weighted images in general are superior to evaluate the anatomy, bone marrow, hemorrhage, masses, fat, and fatty infiltration of muscles. Proton density or intermediate images are high resolution and therefore important in the evaluation of ligaments, tendons, and small structures such as cartilage.[3] T2-weighted images are the best sequence to evaluate for fluid, edema, joint effusions, muscle, and soft tissue injuries. Fluid sensitivity is increased with use of fat saturation.[4]

Dedicated foot and ankle coils or smokestack coils are critical in obtaining high-quality imaging of foot and ankle disorders. Images are performed in the sagittal, axial, and coronal imaging planes. When ordering an MRI, the specific area of concern should be communicated to the radiologist. Given that the smallest field of view optimizes image quality, an MRI scan that captures the entire foot and ankle will compromise the quality of the foot images. Additionally, specific protocols may exist for the forefoot versus the hindfoot, and

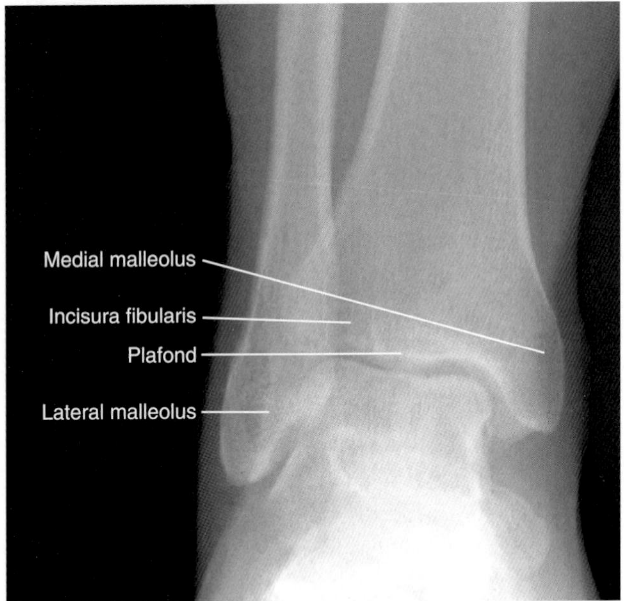

FIGURE 111-1 An anteroposterior standing radiograph of the ankle. *(From Miller M, Hart J, MacKnight J, editors:* Essential orthopaedics, *Philadelphia, 2008, Elsevier.)*

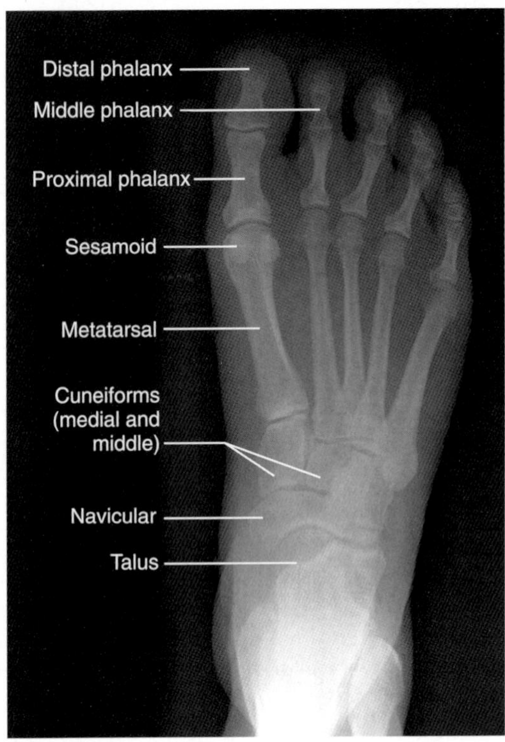

FIGURE 111-3 An anteroposterior standing radiograph of the foot. *(From Miller M, Hart J, MacKnight J, editors:* Essential orthopaedics, *Philadelphia, 2008, Elsevier.)*

therefore the specific site of the pathologic condition should be stated to ensure that the appropriate MRI protocol is used.

Imaging of Tendons

Given a tendon's lack of fluid, a normal tendon has low signal intensity on all imaging sequences (Fig. 111-4). Axial cuts are the most useful to determine the presence and extent of tenosynovitis and tendinosis. Coronal imaging, although complementary, provides the least information. An area of focal thickening is not a normal finding.

Achilles Tendon

Disorders of the Achilles tendon are diagnosed with relative ease as a result of the subcutaneous nature of the tendon. The presence of tendinosis is noted by focal thickening of the tendon that moves in conjunction with the tendon, as opposed to paratenonitis. The primary utility of MRI is to determine the precise location and affected volume of the tendon for preoperative planning. Increasingly, with nonoperative management of Achilles tendon ruptures demonstrating good results with functional rehabilitation, MRI is very useful to determine if adequate apposition is obtained with plantar flexion of the ankle after the cast has been placed as an alternative to ultrasonography.

Normal Appearance

The primary evaluation of the Achilles tendon is performed with use of a combination of T1- and T2-weighted axial and sagittal images. The tendon has a near uniform thickness and flattens out distally as it inserts into the calcaneus. The tendon

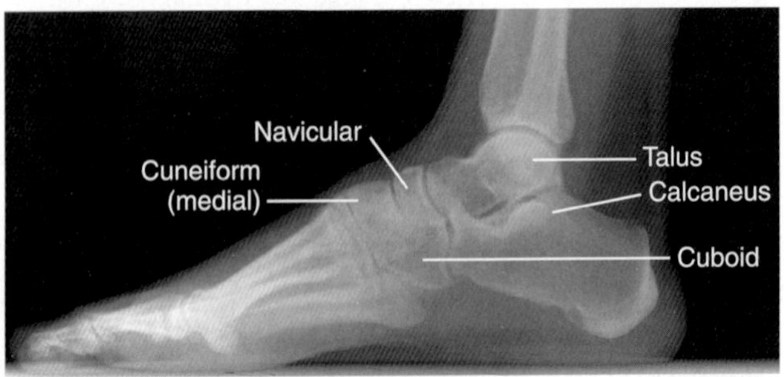

FIGURE 111-2 A lateral standing radiograph of the foot. *(From Miller M, Hart J, MacKnight J, editors:* Essential orthopaedics, *Philadelphia, 2008, Elsevier.)*

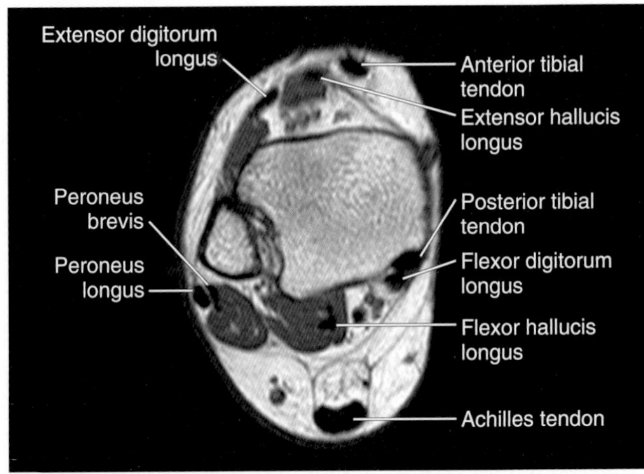

FIGURE 111-4 An axial T1-weighted magnetic resonance image of the distal leg. The tendons at this level are denoted.

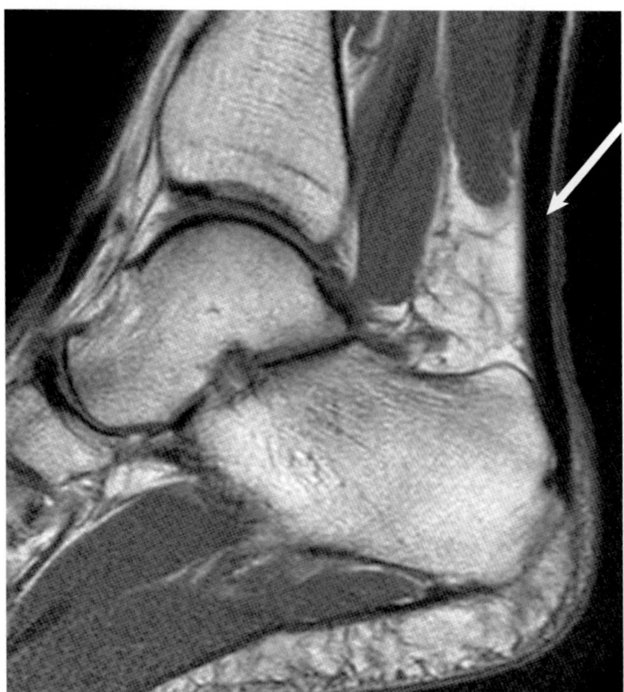

FIGURE 111-5 A T1-weighted image of a normal Achilles tendon. Note the uniform thickness and the low signal intensity of the tendon (*arrow*). *(From Joos D, Tran N, Kadakia AR: Achilles tendon disorders. In Miller MD, Sanders TG, editors:* Presentation, imaging and treatment of common musculoskeletal conditions, *Philadelphia, 2011, Elsevier.)*

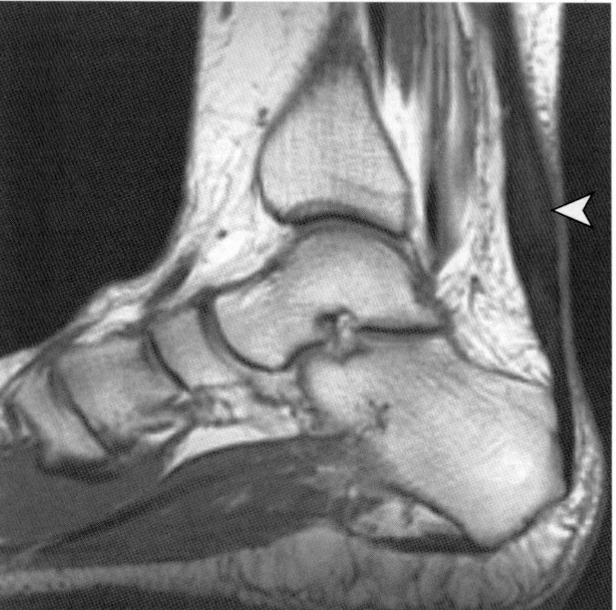

FIGURE 111-6 A T1-weighted magnetic resonance image of a patient with noninsertional Achilles tendinosis. Note the intermediate signal intensity and fusiform thickening of the tendon (*arrowhead*). *(From Joos D, Tran N, Kadakia AR: Achilles tendon disorders. In Miller MD, Sanders TG, editors:* Presentation, imaging and treatment of common musculoskeletal conditions, *Philadelphia, 2011, Elsevier.)*

should be taut and parallel when comparing the anterior and posterior margins of the tendon (Fig. 111-5). A flat or concave anterior margin is normal. The normal anteroposterior diameter on axial or sagittal imaging is 7 mm.

Direct MRI Signs of Disease

Intermediate or high signal intensity on either a T1- or T2-weighted image with continuity of the tendon is indicative of Achilles tendinopathy. Fusiform thickening of the tendon noted on T1-weighted sagittal imaging is diagnostic of Achilles tendinosis (Fig. 111-6). High signal intensity on a T2-weighted image that is as bright as fluid is suggestive of a more acute process and is sometimes referred to as a "partial tear." Calcification of the Achilles insertion is easily visualized on T1-weighted sagittal images and is diagnostic of insertional Achilles tendinopathy. A teardrop fluid signal (high intensity) anterior to the Achilles tendon at the level of the calcaneus is suggestive of retrocalcaneal bursitis (Fig. 111-7). Fluid signal (high intensity) posterior to the Achilles tendon itself is suggestive of retro Achilles bursitis. A fluid signal defect (high intensity) within the Achilles tendon on both T1- and T2-weighted fat-saturated images is indicative of an acute rupture (Fig. 111-8).

Indirect MRI Signs of Disease

High signal intensity on T1- or T2-weighted fat-saturated imaging of the Kager fat pad is suggestive of paratenonitis. A wavy or retracted appearance of the tendon on T1- or T2-weighted fat-saturated imaging is highly suggestive of an Achilles rupture.

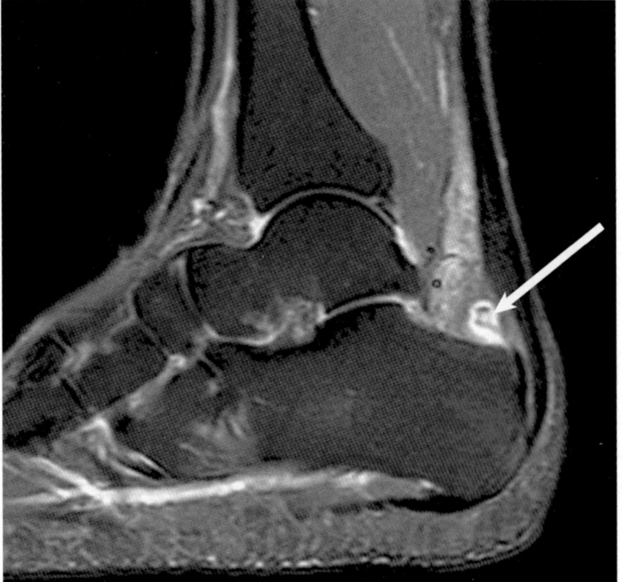

FIGURE 111-7 A T2-weighted fat-saturated image with a teardrop high signal intensity immediately anterior to the Achilles at the level of the calcaneus is consistent with retrocalcaneal bursitis (*arrow*). *(From Joos D, Tran N, Kadakia AR: Achilles tendon disorders. In Miller MD, Sanders TG, editors:* Presentation, imaging and treatment of common musculoskeletal conditions, *Philadelphia, 2011, Elsevier.)*

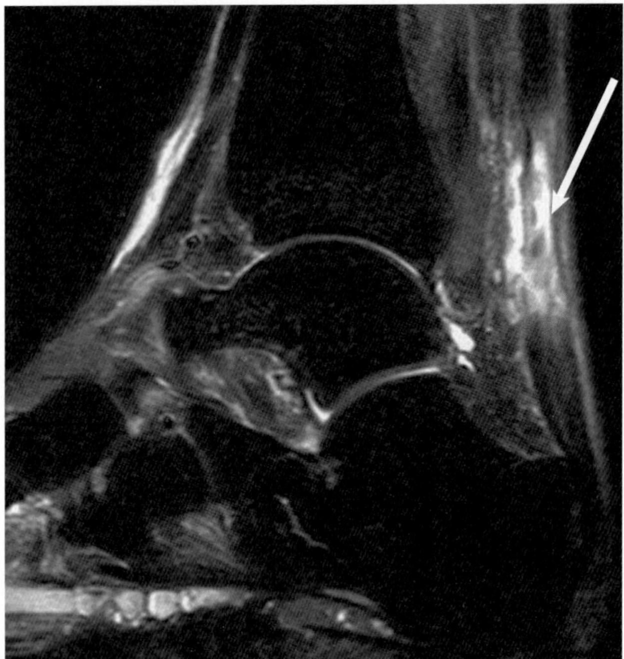

FIGURE 111-8 A T2-weighted magnetic resonance image of an acute Achilles rupture. Note the high signal intensity (*arrow*) that completely disrupts the low signal of the Achilles tendon. *(From Joos D, Tran N, Kadakia AR: Achilles tendon disorders. In Miller MD, Sanders TG, editors:* Presentation, imaging and treatment of common musculoskeletal conditions, *Philadelphia, 2011, Elsevier.)*

Pitfalls

A small amount of increased signal intensity near the insertion of the Achilles tendon represents interposed fat and is normal; it should not be confused with insertional tendinosis. The plantaris tendon can be intact in the presence of an Achilles rupture and should not be confused with a partial tear or intact Achilles tendon.

Posterior Tibial Tendon

Routine use of advanced imaging to determine of the presence of posterior tibial tendon disease is not required. Given the associated flatfoot deformity and subcutaneous position of the tendon, physical examination plays the major role in the diagnosis. However, in cases of suspected tenosynovitis or posttraumatic or sudden-onset flatfoot, and in patients in whom possible debridement and retention of the tendon is being considered, MRI is an excellent adjunct. Isolated debridement and retention of the tendon is typically considered only in the setting of tenosynovitis without intrinsic disease. In the setting of tendinosis, retention of the posterior tibial tendon with an associated tendon transfer will improve the postoperative inversion strength but carries the risk of persistent pain and should be performed with caution.

Magnetic Resonance Imaging

Normal Appearance

Axial cuts are the most useful in evaluating the posterior tibial tendon. Ideally the patient should be positioned prone with the foot plantar flexed to place the tendons in a more linear position and reduce the "magic angle" effect. The posterior tibial tendon should be of uniform thickness throughout its length (Fig. 111-9).

Direct MRI Signs

The presence of fluid (high signal intensity) adjacent to the posterior tibial tendon on T2-weighted imaging is sensitive for tenosynovitis (Fig. 111-10). This finding is not specific and is seen in 22% of asymptomatic persons. A focal area of increased signal on T2-weighted images, known as a *punctate signal,* corresponds to a small intrasubstance tear. A focal area of increased signal intensity within the substance of the tendon that extends to the tendon surface on T1-weighted imaging and corresponding high signal intensity on T2-weighted imaging is consistent with a tear.[5] Complete absence of the posterior tibial tendon or replacement of the normal tendon location with high signal intensity on T2-weighted imaging indicates a rupture. Replacement or infiltration of the normally low signal intensity of the tendon with intermediate (gray) signal is consistent with tendinosis (Fig. 111-11). A small tendon caliber (smaller diameter than the flexor digitorum longus) is consistent with atrophic tendinosis and can be seen on any axial imaging sequence.

Indirect MRI Signs

Periretinacular soft tissue edema and thickening of the flexor retinaculum on any imaging sequence is suggestive of disease. Soft tissue edema adjacent to the flexor retinaculum can be seen on T2-weighted imaging. High signal intensity within the medial malleolus without a prior history of trauma may

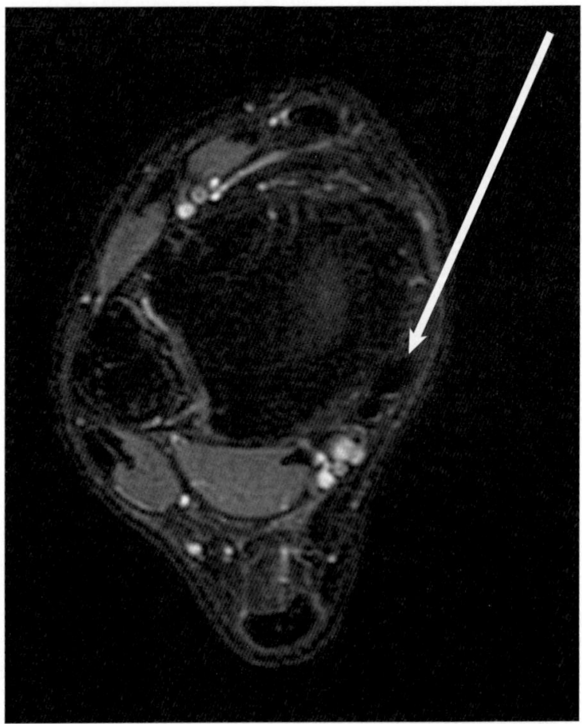

FIGURE 111-9 An axial T2-weighted image of the posterior tibial tendon (*arrow*). The tendon is normal with a low signal appearance (dark) and lack of presence of fluid within the tendon sheath. *(From Joos D, Kadakia AR: Flexor tendon disorders. In Miller MD, Sanders TG, editors:* Presentation, imaging and treatment of common musculoskeletal conditions, *Philadelphia, 2011, Elsevier.)*

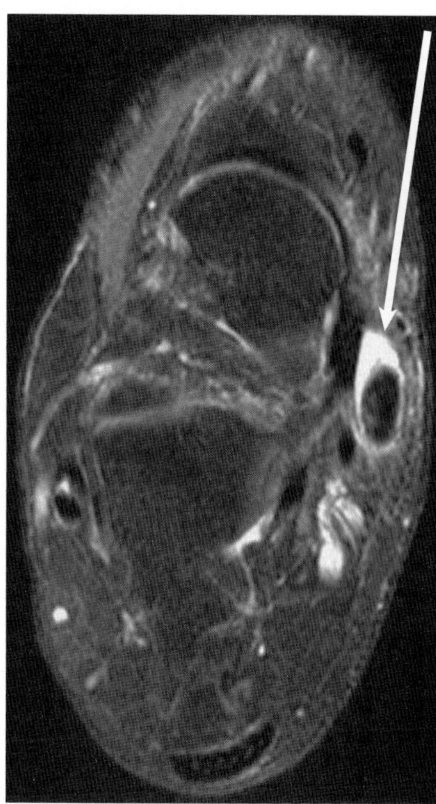

FIGURE 111-10 An axial T2-weighted image of a patient with tenosynovitis of the posterior tibial tendon. Note the high signal intensity (fluid) adjacent to the tendon (*arrow*). *(From Joos D, Kadakia AR: Flexor tendon disorders. In Miller MD, Sanders TC, editors:* Presentation, imaging and treatment of common musculoskeletal conditions, *Philadelphia, 2011, Elsevier.)*

also be seen. High signal intensity noted on T2-weighted imaging within the accessory navicular can be present.

Pitfalls

A small amount of fluid within the tendon sheath can be normal; correlation with intrasubstance increased signal intensity is more specific for tendon disease.

Flexor Hallucis Longus

FHL tendinopathy has classically been described as a disorder in female ballet dancers, in whom constant ankle hyper plantar flexion can cause FHL irritation at its entrance to the flexor retinaculum. Recently it has been noted to affect other patients with chronic foot or ankle pain who often initially were diagnosed with other foot or ankle pathologic conditions. Ultrasound can be effective in determining the presence of dynamic entrapment of the FHL within the fibro-osseous tunnel. MRI is also particularly useful to evaluate for synovitis, the extent of tendon degeneration, and edema within the os-trigonum, which can be associated with this condition.

Magnetic Resonance Imaging

Normal Appearance

Sagittal cuts are a useful adjunct when evaluating the FHL as it passes under the sustentaculum tali to the forefoot. Ideally the patient should be positioned prone with the foot plantar flexed to place the tendons in a more linear position and reduce the "magic angle" effect. The tendon has a very low lying muscle belly that is normally present at the level of the ankle.

Direct MRI Signs

MRI findings of tendinosis as outlined previously, with increased signal intensity within the tendon or tears of the tendon, are rarely seen in the FHL. The presence of fluid (high signal intensity) on T2-weighted imaging is diagnostic of FHL tenosynovitis. The most common location is posterior to the talus within the fibro-osseous tunnel (Fig. 111-12). However, it can also occur in the midfoot at the knot of Henry or distally at the level of the first metatarsophalangeal joint as it passes between the sesamoids. Careful inspection of the entire length of the FHL should be performed from the ankle to the insertion into the distal phalanx because compression can occur in the ankle, midfoot, and forefoot. The presence of fluid proximal and distal to the tendon at the level of the fibro-osseous tunnel posteriorly is diagnostic of stenosing tenosynovitis.[6] The severe compression limits the fluid from entering the tunnel.

Indirect MRI Signs

High signal intensity within the os-trigonum on T2-weighted imaging should prompt close inspection of the FHL because

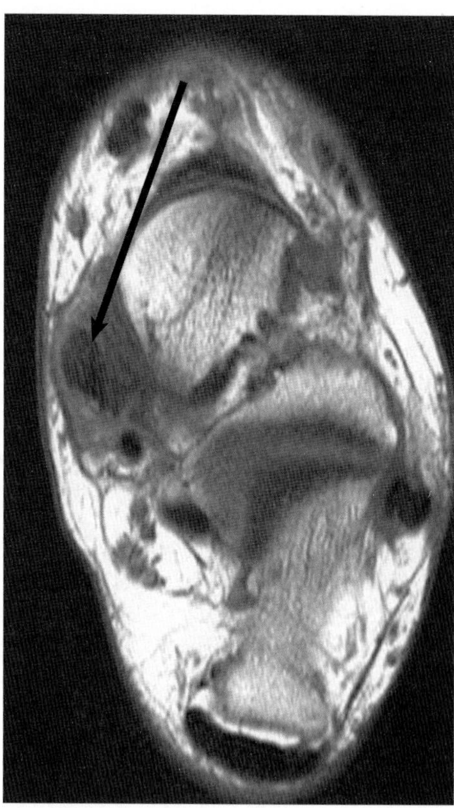

FIGURE 111-11 An axial T1-weighted image with infiltration of the normally low signal intensity of the posterior tibial tendon with intermediate (gray) signal (*arrow*). *(From Joos D, Kadakia AR: Flexor tendon disorders. In Miller MD, Sanders TC, editors:* Presentation, imaging and treatment of common musculoskeletal conditions, *Philadelphia, 2011, Elsevier.)*

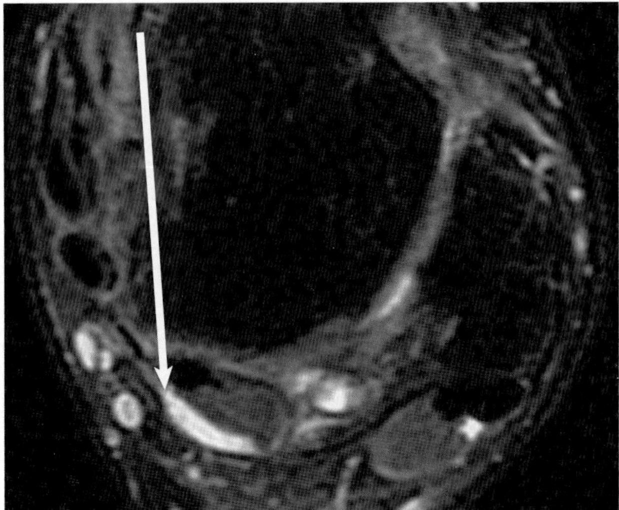

FIGURE 111-12 An axial T2-weighted image with high signal intensity (*arrow*) adjacent to the flexor hallucis longus at the posterior aspect of the talus. *(From Joos D, Kadakia AR: Flexor tendon disorders. In Miller MD, Sanders TC, editors:* Presentation, imaging and treatment of common musculoskeletal conditions, *Philadelphia, 2011, Elsevier.)*

both FHL synovitis and os-trigonum syndrome can occur simultaneously.

Pitfalls

Failure to inspect the entire length of the tendon can lead one to miss the less common but symptomatic compression of the FHL within the knot of Henry and sesamoid complex.

Peroneal Tendons

Intrinsic disorders of the peroneal tendons include tenosynovitis, tendinosis, tendon tears, and painful os peroneum syndrome. Additionally, symptomatic subluxation or intrasheath subluxation may be present, producing pain in addition to instability. Chronic subluxation of the tendons increases the risk of developing degenerative tears of the tendons as a result of the mechanical trauma from the posterolateral fibrocartilaginous ridge of the fibula. Ultrasound can be a very effective tool for examination of the peroneal tendons, specifically in the setting of intrasheath subluxation, where subjective "snapping" may be the only appreciable finding. MRI is very useful when considering operative intervention to determine the presence of synovitis, tendinosis, tears, a low-lying muscle belly of the brevis, and a peroneus quartus, in addition to visualizing the concavity of the fibular groove.

Magnetic Resonance Imaging

Normal Appearance

The primary evaluation of the peroneal tendons is performed using a combination of T1- and T2-weighted axial images. The peroneus quartus is a normal muscle variant encountered in 13% to 26% of patients. It will appear as a third tendon within the peroneal tendon sheath (Fig. 111-13). The common insertion is the calcaneus, although multiple variants have been noted. A flat or convex fibular groove is associated with peroneal tendon disorders, but a flat groove is seen in more than two thirds of normal persons.

Direct MRI Signs

As measured on axial imaging, abnormal thickening of the peroneal tendon is noted if the tendon has a larger diameter than the posterior tibial tendon. Intermediate signal intensity within the peroneal tendons noted on three consecutive T1-weighted proton density–weighted images is 92% sensitive for the detection of clinically relevant peroneal tendon disorders (Fig. 111-14).[7] Fluid within the peroneal tendon sheath noted on T2-weighted imaging is a nonspecific finding that can be seen commonly in asymptomatic persons. However, the presence of circumferential fluid within the peroneal tendon sheath of greater than 3 mm in width is highly suggestive of clinically relevant peroneal tenosynovitis. The presence of a bisected or split peroneus brevis on either T1- or T2-weighted imaging is diagnostic of a tear (Fig. 111-15). A split that does not extend across the full width of the tendon is a partial tear.

Indirect MRI Signs

Irregular contour of the tendons on either T1- or T2-weighted imaging is suggestive of a peroneal tendon tear. The presence of a "C-shaped" peroneus brevis with the arms extending

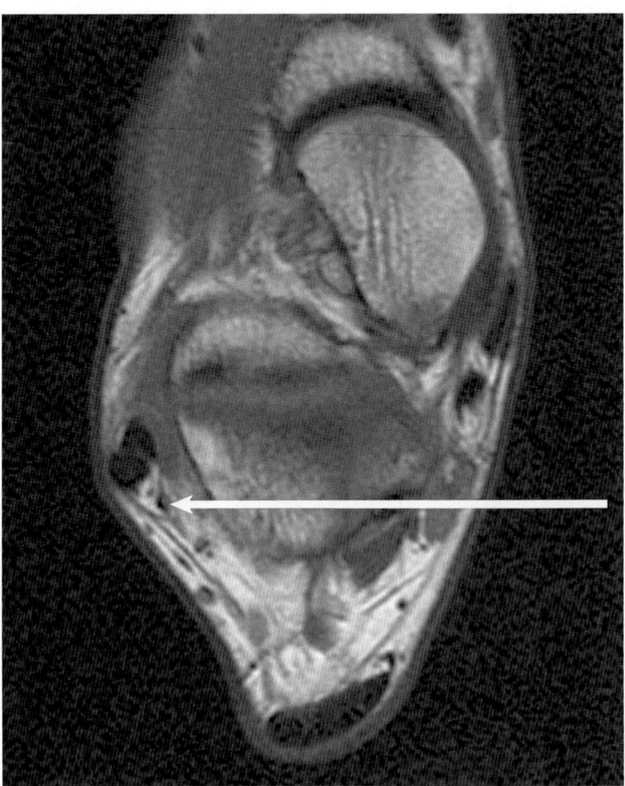

FIGURE 111-13 A T1-weighted axial image of the ankle highlighting the presence of a peroneus quartus (*arrow*). The tendon is a small-caliber low signal intensity structure located posterior within the peroneal retinaculum. Proximally the tendon has its own muscle belly and typically will insert on the calcaneus. *(From Joos D, Kadakia AR: Peroneal tendon disorders. In Miller MD, Sanders TC, editors:* Presentation, imaging and treatment of common musculoskeletal conditions, *Philadelphia, 2011, Elsevier.)*

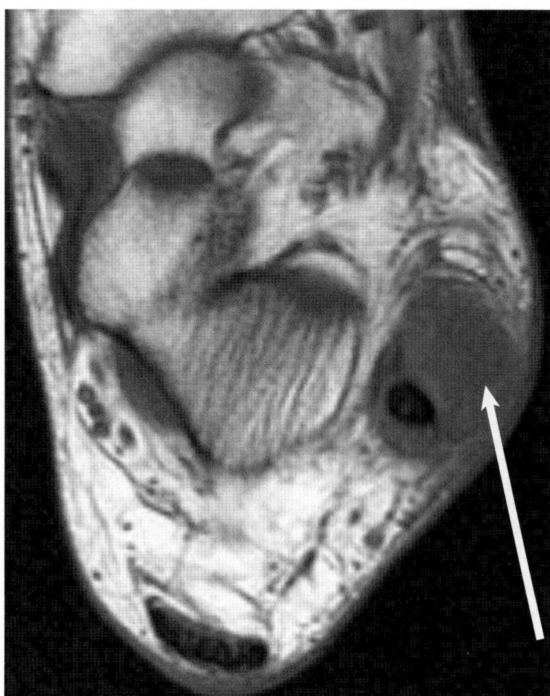

FIGURE 111-14 A T1-weighted axial image with intermediate signal intensity in the location of the peroneus brevis. This finding was noted on multiple axial images, consistent with severe tendinosis of the peroneus brevis (*arrow*). Obvious thickening of the tendon is also noted. The normal peroneus longus is noted posterior to the pathologic brevis. *(From Joos D, Kadakia AR: Peroneal tendon disorders. In Miller MD, Sanders TG, editors:* Presentation, imaging and treatment of common musculoskeletal conditions, *Philadelphia, 2011, Elsevier.)*

posteriorly around the peroneus longus is consistent with a tear. Thickening or attenuation of the lateral collateral ligaments warrants careful examination of the peroneal tendons because the two conditions commonly coexist. A peroneal tubercle that is greater than 5 mm is an uncommon finding in normal persons and can be associated with peroneus longus synovitis and rupture. A "low-lying" muscle belly of the peroneus brevis is associated with peroneal tendon disease. Although the muscle belly can extend to the tip of the fibula in one third of normal persons, it rarely extends 1 cm past the fibular tip.

Pitfalls

Increased fluid signal within the tendons can be noted as they course around the distal fibula and is termed the *magic angle phenomenon*.[8] This signal is normal and should not be confused with a pathologic finding. The presence of intermediate signal intensity or fluid is a very common finding in healthy persons. MRI alone is specific for the diagnosis of peroneal tendon disease and must be used only as an adjunct with a good clinical examination to prevent misdiagnosis. The presence of a peroneus quartus should not be mistaken as a split tear of the peroneal tendons. The tendon has its own muscle mass, and the tendon structure of the longus and the brevis will be normal. Bifurcated or trifurcated tendon slips can be differentiated from a tear by the presence of the slip within the muscle proximal to the ankle joint.

Anterior Tibial Tendon

MRI and dynamic ultrasound are the two most common imaging studies used to confirm the diagnosis of a rupture of the tendon. MRI is excellent to determine the extent of disease in a patient with insertional tendinosis. If the clinical situation is obvious based on the history and physical examination, further imaging is not necessary. However, if surgical intervention is planned, these studies are useful for preoperative planning.

Magnetic Resonance Imaging

Direct MRI Signs

Discontinuity of the tendon is consistent with a complete tear of the tendon (Fig. 111-16). Intermediate signal intensity within an extensor tendon noted on consecutive T1-weighted proton density–weighted images with an increased tendon diameter is sensitive for tendinosis (Fig. 111-17).[9] Tendon thickness of greater than 5 mm within the distal 3 cm of the anterior tibial tendon is 94% sensitive in the diagnosis of tendinosis. Increased signal intensity on both T1- and T2-weighted imaging without discontinuity of the tendon is diagnostic of a partial tear.[9]

Indirect MRI Signs

Dorsal osteophyte formation along the midfoot or hindfoot can be associated with an attritional anterior tibial tendon tear.

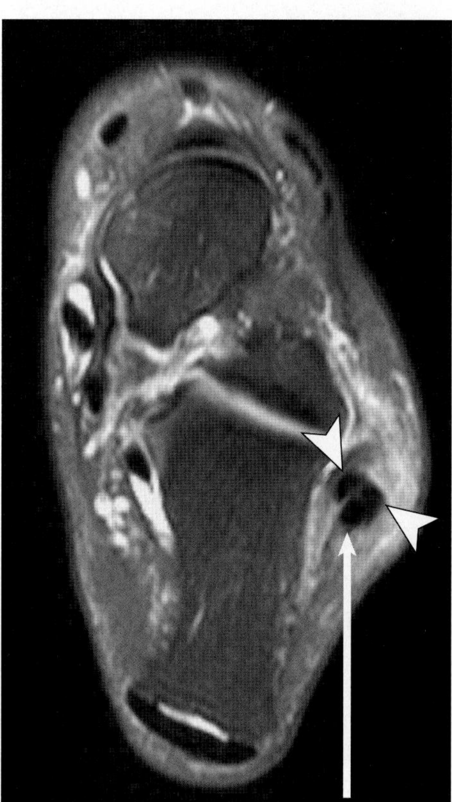

FIGURE 111-15 A T2-weighted axial image of a longitudinal split tear of the brevis (*arrowheads*). The normal peroneus longus (*arrow*) lies posterior to the split brevis. *(From Joos D, Kadakia AR: Peroneal tendon disorders. In Miller MD, Sanders TG, editors:* Presentation, imaging and treatment of common musculoskeletal conditions, *Philadelphia, 2011, Elsevier.)*

Pitfalls

Review of only T1-weighted imaging may lead to a misdiagnosis of a ganglion as tendinosis, because it will appear as intermediate signal intensity. This appearance is easily differentiated from tendinosis on T2-weighted imaging by the high signal intensity (fluid) of the ganglion that is not seen with tendinosis.

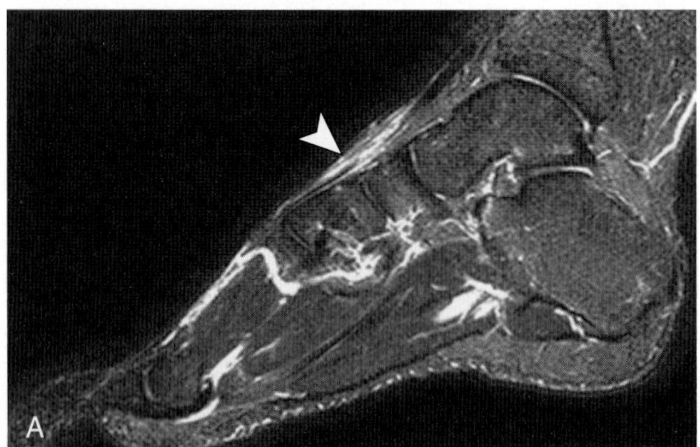

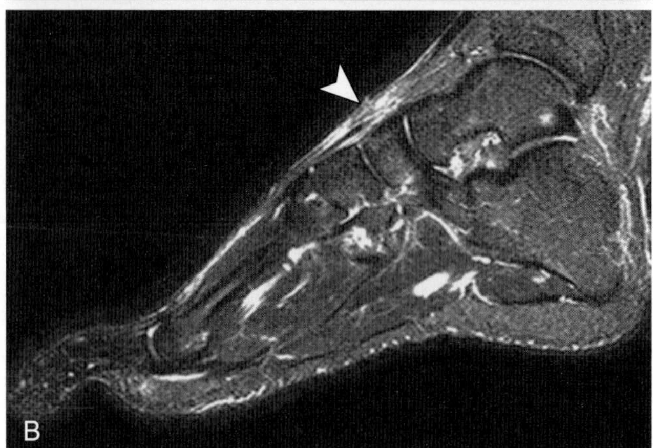

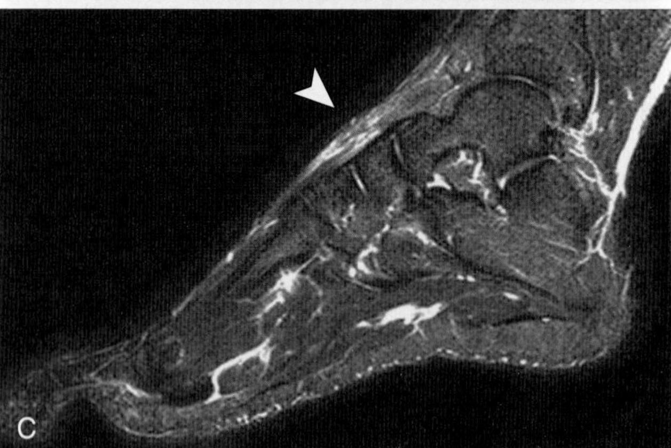

FIGURE 111-16 Three consecutive sagittal T2-weighted images in a patient with a laceration of the extensor hallucis longus (EHL). The EHL distal stump is identified (**A,** *arrowhead*). **B,** The site of rupture (*arrowhead*); note the rounding off of the cut edge. **C,** Edema (*arrowhead*) and lack of the tendon that has retracted proximally. *(From Joos D, Kadakia AR: Extensor tendon disorders. In Miller MD, Sanders TG, editors:* Presentation, imaging and treatment of common musculoskeletal conditions, *Philadelphia, 2011, Elsevier.)*

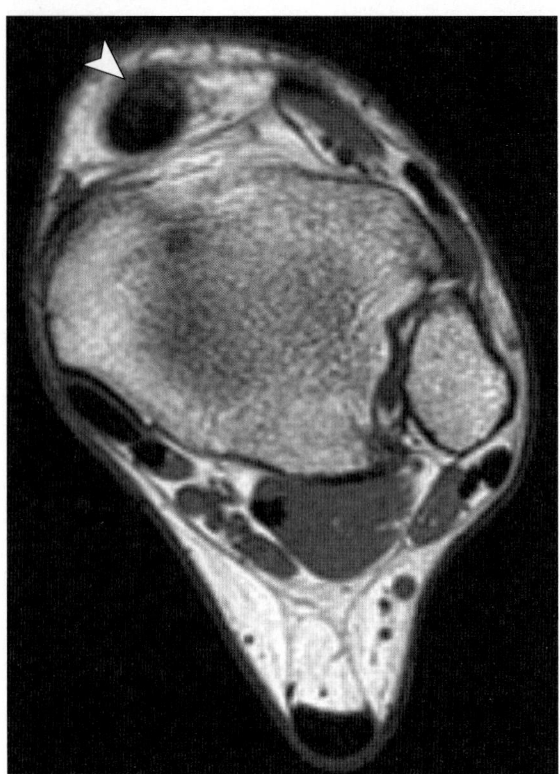

FIGURE 111-17 An axial T1-weighted image of a patient with severe tendinosis of the anterior tibial tendon (*arrowhead*). The tendon is thickened with significant intermediate signal present that is obliterating the normal architecture of the tendon. *(From Joos D, Kadakia AR: Extensor tendon disorders. In Miller MD, Sanders TG, editors:* Presentation, imaging and treatment of common musculoskeletal conditions, *Philadelphia, 2011, Elsevier.)*

Imaging of Ligaments

Magnetic Resonance Imaging

Normal Appearance

The ankle ligaments are uniformly low in signal intensity on all imaging sequences. The anterior talofibular ligament is best seen in the axial plane on proton density and proton density fat-saturated images as a thin linear structure (Fig. 111-18). The calcaneofibular ligament is well visualized in the axial and coronal planes. The syndesmotic ligaments are best seen in the axial plane.

Direct MRI Signs

Acute ligamentous injuries are classified by MRI as grade I, II, or III. Grade I injuries will demonstrate edema (but not discrete fluid) around the ligament. Grade II injuries will have increased signal within the ligament, consistent with a partial-thickness tear. Fluid can also be present around the ligament. In the setting of a grade III injury, complete disruption of the ligament will be noted by the absence or discontinuity of the ligament. Avulsion fractures may be seen at the site of ligament insertion.

Remote or chronic ligament injuries, sprains, and tears have characteristic appearances on MRI. The previously injured ligament may be increased in signal, wavy, thickened, and attenuated or absent (see Figs. 111-7 and 111-8).[10]

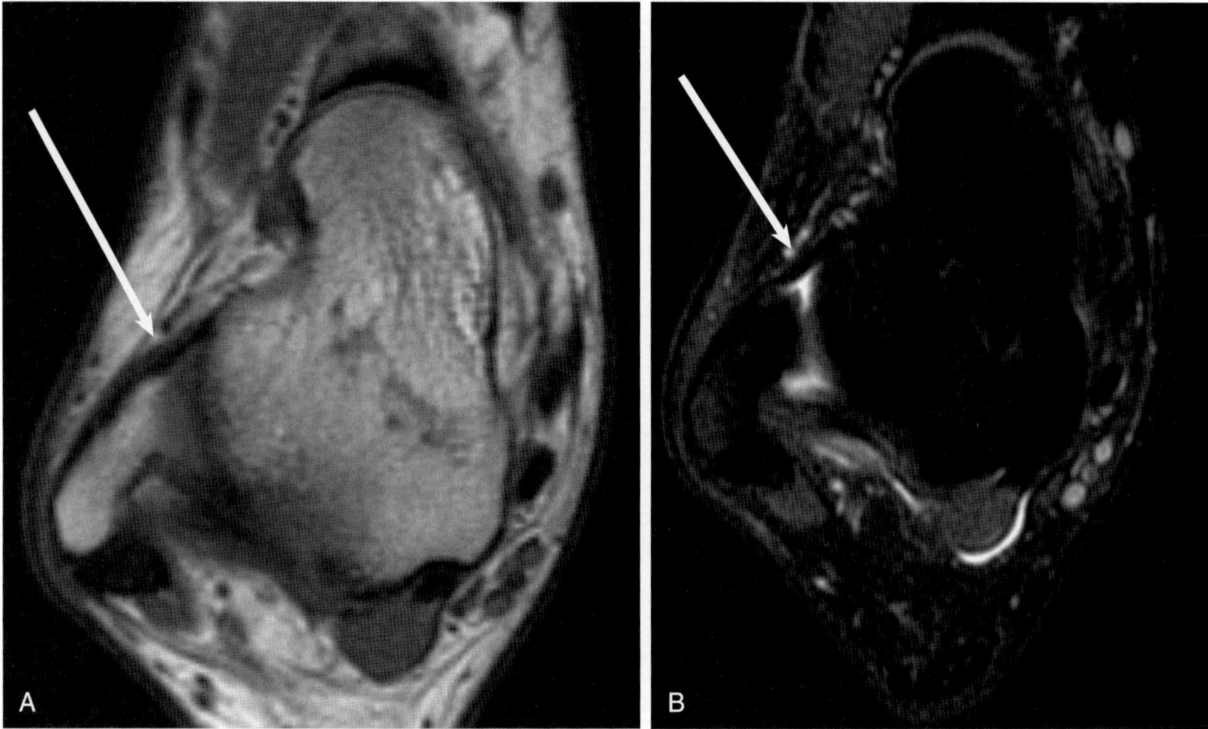

FIGURE 111-18 Axial T1-weighted (**A**) and T2-weighted fat-saturated (**B**) images demonstrating the anterior talofibular ligament (*arrow*). The ligament is low in signal intensity, of uniform thickness, and taut. *(From Joos D, Sabb B, Tran NK, et al: Acute ankle ligament injuries. In Miller MD, Sanders TG, editors:* Presentation, imaging and treatment of common musculoskeletal conditions, *Philadelphia, 2011, Elsevier.)*

Typically no soft tissue edema surrounds the remotely torn ligament, which helps one distinguish between an acute and chronic injury.

Not only is MRI accurate at evaluating the ankle ligaments, but it can also help rule out or occasionally rule in other pathologic conditions. Osteochondral lesions of the talus and syndesmotic injuries can be difficult to distinguish from post-sprain instability. MRI is quick to identify most of these confounding processes.

Indirect MRI Signs

Indirect syndesmotic injury may be noted by a linear fluid signal 1.25 cm/1.5 cm on T2-weighted fat-saturated images consistent with injury. This finding is not pathognomonic but is highly suggestive in the setting of trauma. The presence of an ankle effusion, especially when joint fluid leaks out of the joint capsule, is indicative of a tear of the anterior talofibular ligament. Bone marrow edema of the distal fibula or talar insertion of the anterior talofibular ligament can be present. Bone marrow edema of the medial malleolus and talar insertion of the deltoid ligament may also be seen.

Pitfalls

Fluid in the peroneal tendon sheath can be a secondary sign of calcaneofibular ligament (CFL) injury; however, peroneal tenosynovitis can incite surrounding edema (peritendinitis) and result in the appearance of a CFL sprain (a pseudosprain of the CFL). A couple of important exceptions exist to the rule that the ligaments are dark on all conventional MRI sequences. In particular, the deltoid ligament and the posterior talofibular ligament are usually intermediate to bright on T2-weighted fat-saturated images. This normal appearance can be misinterpreted as an acute or chronic ligament sprain. Meniscoid lesions can be easily overlooked on imaging studies. One must be vigilant and systematic in the evaluation of the imaging to correctly establish this diagnosis by imaging. The lesion can be a source of pain for the patient and should be debrided if surgical intervention is performed.

Osteochondral Lesions

Osteochondral lesions of the talus (OLTs) may be visualized on plain radiographs as a result of an associated fracture of the subchondral bone or a cystic defect. However, these findings are not universally present and thus in cases of chronic injuries with mechanical symptoms, such as locking or giving way, or a feeling of instability of the ankle joint, in addition to pain and persistent swelling, MRI is the imaging modality of choice to visualize the articular surface and subchondral bone. However, caution is necessary because the presence of abnormal findings on MRI, especially within the medial talar dome, may not be the causative factor for the patient's complaint. Combining the information from the history and physical examination along with the MRI findings is critical prior to recommending surgical intervention for an OLT.

Magnetic Resonance Imaging

Normal Appearance

The talus is normally bright on T1-weighted images and is dark on the T2-weighted fat-saturated images. Because the cartilage of the talus is thin, it is sometimes difficult to see on conventional MRI sequences. However, when an osteochondral lesion is present, the effect on the subchondral bone is very apparent. MRI allows multiplanar imaging of the talus for localization and characterization of OLTs. MRI has been proven itself sensitive and specific in the diagnosis of OLTs.

Direct MRI Signs

The lesions can be located anywhere in the talar dome (but most often in the lateral or medial aspect of the talus, in its midportion from anterior to posterior; Fig. 111-19). The lesions are typically dark on T1-weighted images and variable on T2-weighted fat-saturated images. Signs of instability include fluid undercutting the lesion, a cystic lesion, or a high intensity T2-weighted fat-saturated signal at the interface between the lesion and the underlying talus and partial or complete separation of the fragment from its normal location (Fig. 111-20).[11] Cystic lesions appear as a bright fluid-filled area beneath the subchondral bone on T2-weighted imaging.

Indirect MRI Signs

Intraarticular bodies must be scrutinized, and one would have to assess for talar dome donor sites. One of earliest signs of OLT is decreased T1-weighted signal, often without significant increased T2-weighted fat-saturated signal or any cartilage defect.[11]

Pitfalls

Early OLT may only appear as low T1-weighted signal intensity and should not be confused with posttraumatic edema or early osteoarthritis (OA). OA can also result in osteochondral abnormalities in the talus. This process is separate and occurs by a different mechanism. One pitfall is to have a patient with OA mistakenly diagnosed as having OLT; the treatment of osteochondral lesions in OA is not the same as the treatment of OLT in a younger nonarthritic patient. One way to help make the distinction is to evaluate the joint for overall changes of OA, including osteophyte, joint space narrowing, and changes of the associated tibial plafond.

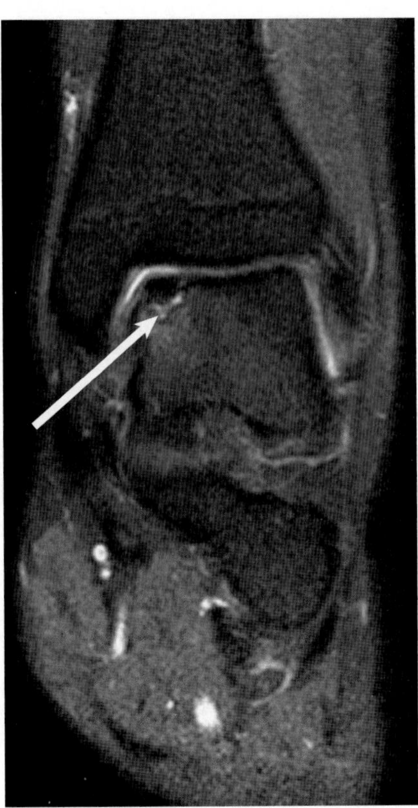

FIGURE 111-20 A patient with an unstable osteochondral lesion of the talus. The bright fluid undercutting the lesion is well visualized on the fluid-sensitive T2-weighted fat-saturated image (*arrow*). Fluid interposing between the osteochondral lesion of the talus and the talus is an excellent indicator of instability. *(From Joos D, Sabb B, Kadakia AR: Osteochondral lesions. In Miller MD, Sanders TG, editors:* Presentation, imaging and treatment of common musculoskeletal conditions, *Philadelphia, 2011, Elsevier.)*

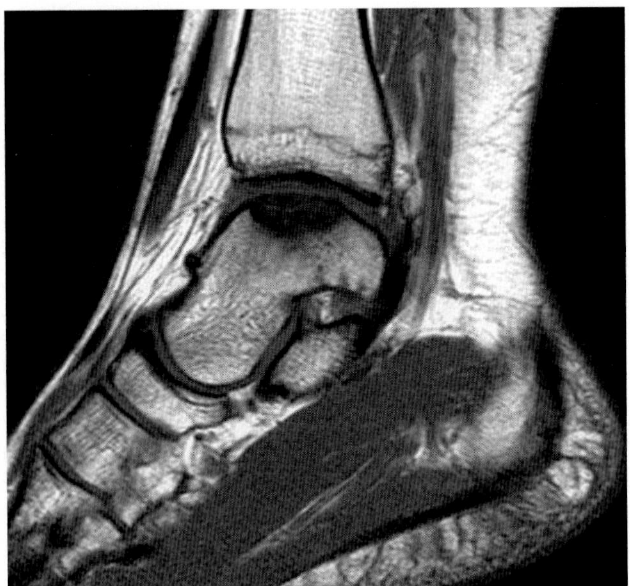

FIGURE 111-19 Sagittal magnetic resonance imaging demonstrating the most common central location of osteochondral lesions. The lesion has the typical dark appearance on T1-weighted imaging. *(From Joos D, Sabb B, Kadakia AR: Osteochondral lesions. In Miller MD, Sanders TG, editors:* Presentation, imaging and treatment of common musculoskeletal conditions, *Philadelphia, 2011, Elsevier.)*

Nerve Entrapment

Entrapment or compression of the peripheral nerves at the foot and ankle are common and often unrecognized causes of pain and disability. These disorders are diagnosed primarily by clinical examination and adjunctive nerve testing if such testing is believed appropriate. The use of ultrasound has been advocated by some authors in the diagnosis and as a localizing aid for injection of Morton neuromas. The primary role of MRI in the treatment of nerve compression disorders is to rule out a mass-occupying lesion, most commonly in the setting of suspected tarsal tunnel. Routine use of MRI in the evaluation of nerve disorders is not advocated.

Magnetic Resonance Imaging: Interdigital Nerve

Normal Appearance

The nerve should appear circular and less than 3 mm in width.

Direct MRI Signs

Coronal T1-weighted imaging is most useful for evaluation of the presence of a Morton neuroma. Use of contrast-enhanced T2-weighted imaging can be used to ensure that the mass is a neuroma, differentiating it from other lesions. The neuroma should appear as an ovoid or dumbbell-shaped plantar mass (inferior to the intermetatarsal ligament) between the metatarsal heads (Fig. 111-21). Neuromas will appear with low to intermediate signal intensity on T1- and T2-weighted imaging. Although MRI can aid in the diagnosis of a neuroma, the sensitivity has been reported as 76% to 87% with surgical confirmation as the gold standard. Surgically confirmed neuromas have been shown to have a high association with widths greater than 5 mm.

Indirect MRI Signs

The neuroma must be visualized directly to be diagnosed.

Pitfalls

Intermetatarsal bursitis is differentiated from a neuroma by its small size (<3 mm) and high signal intensity on T2-weighted imaging, consistent with fluid.

Magnetic Resonance Imaging: Tarsal Tunnel

Normal Appearance

The normal appearance of the tarsal tunnel should demonstrate the contents of the tarsal tunnel without any evidence of a mass-occupying lesion. The normal contents of the tarsal tunnel will be noted with a thin overlying flexor retinaculum. Axial imaging provides the most information (Fig. 111-22).

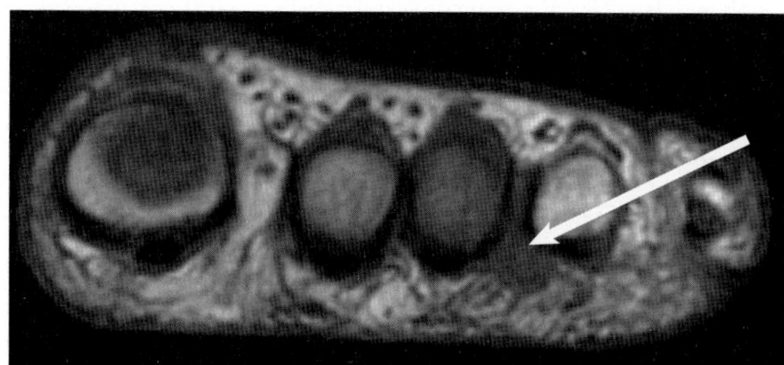

FIGURE 111-21 A coronal T1-weighted image of a Morton neuroma (*arrow*). Note that the neuroma is pear shaped and is plantar to the intermetatarsal ligament. *(From Seybold J, Kadakia AR: Nerve entrapment syndromes. In Miller MD, Sanders TC, editors:* Presentation, imaging and treatment of common musculoskeletal conditions, *Philadelphia, 2011, Elsevier.)*

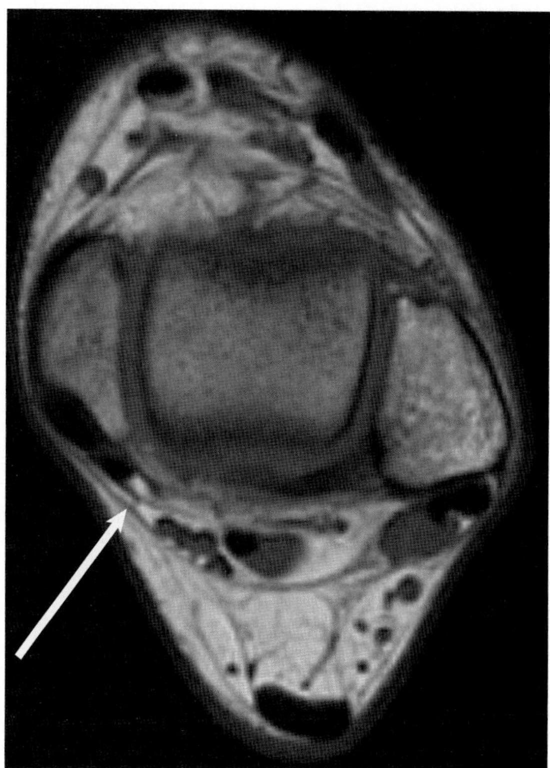

FIGURE 111-22 An axial T1-weighted image of a normal tarsal tunnel. The flexor retinaculum can be visualized (*arrow*) as a thin hypoechoic band. The contents of the tarsal tunnel are easily visualized without any mass-occupying lesion. *(From Seybold J, Kadakia AR: Nerve entrapment syndromes. In Miller MD, Sanders TC, editors:* Presentation, imaging and treatment of common musculoskeletal conditions, *Philadelphia, 2011, Elsevier.)*

Direct MRI Signs

The most common MRI finding in the setting of tarsal tunnel is a mass-occupying lesion. These lesions include neurofibrosarcoma, neurilemoma, ganglion, hemangioma, venous varicosities or dilated posterior tibial veins (Fig. 111-23), FHL tenosynovitis with fluid within the tendon sheath, and hypertrophy of the abductor hallucis.

Indirect MRI Signs

Flattening of the tibial nerve suggests tarsal tunnel syndrome, and a mass-occupying lesion should be sought.

Plantar Fasciitis

MRI is not required to obtain the diagnosis of either planar fasciitis or fibromatosis. The primary use is to rule out other conditions such as a calcaneal stress fracture, plantar fascia rupture, neoplasm, and Baxter's neuritis.

Magnetic Resonance Imaging

Normal Appearance

Sagittal and coronal imaging is superior for visualization of the plantar fascia. The ligament should appear hypoechoic on all sequences, and the maximum thickness is no greater than 4 mm.

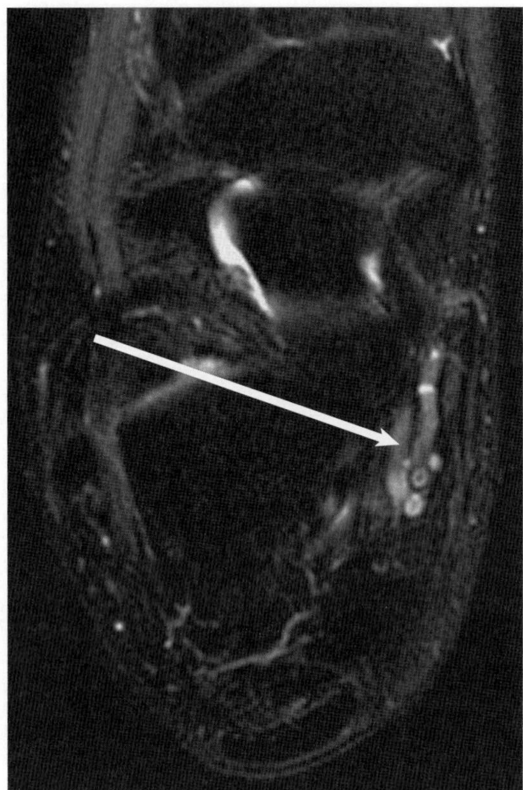

FIGURE 111-23 An axial T2-weighted fat-saturated image of venous varicosities (*arrow*) within the tarsal tunnel. These varicosities appear as torturous high signal intensity structures. *(From Seybold J, Kadakia AR: Nerve entrapment syndromes. In Miller MD, Sanders TG, editors:* Presentation, imaging and treatment of common musculoskeletal conditions, *Philadelphia, 2011, Elsevier.)*

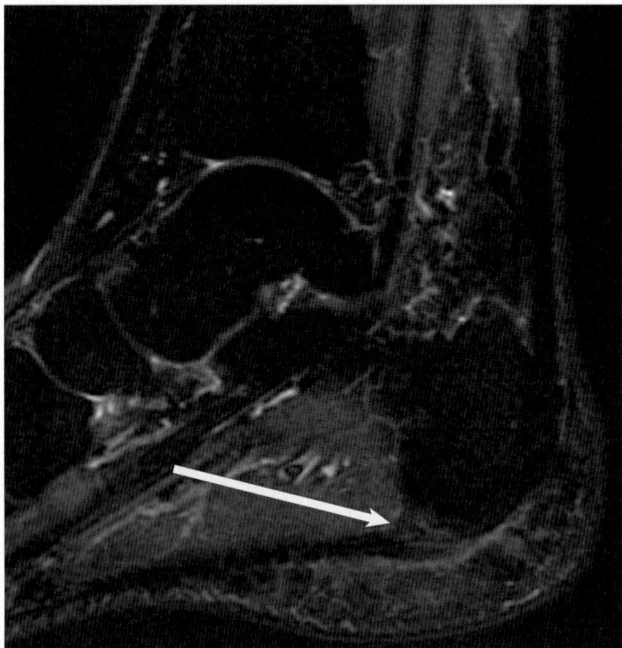

FIGURE 111-24 A sagittal T2-weighted image demonstrating increased signal at the origin of the plantar fascia (*arrow*) in a patient with plantar fasciitis. *(From Seybold J, Kadakia AR: The plantar fascia. In Miller MD, Sanders TG, editors:* Presentation, imaging and treatment of common musculoskeletal conditions, *Philadelphia, 2011, Elsevier.)*

Direct MRI Signs

Thickening of the plantar fascia (7 to 8 mm) at the insertion is seen with fasciitis. Increased signal intensity at the insertion of the fascia seen best on T2-weighted or short tau inversion recovery sequences (Fig. 111-24). Plantar fascia rupture is noted by high signal intensity (fluid) at the proximal aspect of the plantar fascia with complete discontinuity from the calcaneal origin. Plantar fibromatosis can be identified by a single or multiple subcutaneous nodules that are not commonly greater than 3 cm in diameter.

Indirect MRI Signs

Increased signal intensity at the calcaneal insertional site is suggestive of plantar fasciitis, along with surrounding subcutaneous edema. With plantar fibromatosis, no reactive edema is usually noted.

For a complete list of references, go to expertconsult.com.

Suggested Readings

Citation: Recht MP, Donley BG: Magnetic resonance imaging of the foot and ankle. *J Am Acad Orthop Surg* 9:187–199, 2001.

Level of Evidence: V

Summary: The authors provide an excellent overview of the normal and pathologic findings noted with magnetic resonance imaging of the foot and ankle. The inclusion of excellent figures aids in the usefulness of this review.

Citation: Feighan J, Towers J, Conti S: The use of magnetic resonance imaging in posterior tibial tendon dysfunction. *Clin Orthop* 365:23–38, 1999.

Level of Evidence: III

Summary: The authors present an excellent review of the appropriate technique and abnormalities noted on magnetic resonance imaging of posterior tibial tendon dysfunction. Supplemental cases provide additional clarification.

Citation: Lo LD, Schweitzer ME, Fan JK, et al: MRI imaging findings of entrapment of the flexor hallucis longus tendon. *Am J Roentgenol* 176:1145–1148, 2001.

Level of Evidence: III

Summary: The authors provide a retrospective review of the variable imaging findings noted in patients with flexor hallucis longus tendon entrapment. The authors provide a thorough discussion of the multiple causes for this disorder and their relevant imaging findings.

Citation: Kijowski R, De Smet A, Mukharjee R: Magnetic resonance imaging findings in patients with peroneal tendinopathy and peroneal tenosynovitis. *Skeletal Radiol* 36:105–114, 2007.

Level of Evidence: III

Summary: The authors of this excellent study compare the magnetic resonance imaging findings of patients who have peroneal disease with the findings of persons who do not have any pathologic abnormality. The authors were able to conclude that intermediate signal was required on three consecutive images to be consistent with disease and that circumferential fluid of greater than 3 mm in maximal width is sensitive for peroneal tenosynovitis.

Citation: Mengiardi B, Pfirrmann CW, Vienee P, et al: Anterior tibial tendon abnormalities: MR imaging findings. *Radiology* 235:977–984, 2005.

Level of Evidence: III

Summary: The authors of this excellent study compare the magnetic resonance imaging findings in patients who have known disease of the anterior tibial tendon with findings in age-matched control subjects. The authors concluded that thickening of greater than or equal to 5 mm and diffuse signal intensity abnormality within 3 cm of the insertion is consistent with anterior tibial tendinosis.

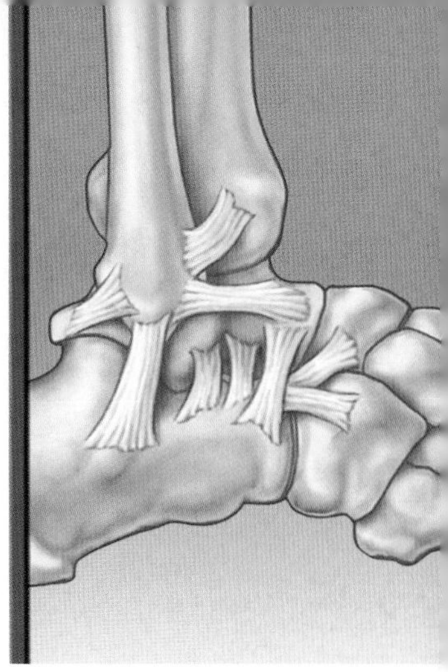

112

Leg Pain and Exertional Compartment Syndromes

BRITT MARCUSSEN • CHRISTOPHER HOGREFE • ANNUNZIATO AMENDOLA

Exertional leg pain is a common problem encountered in recreational and competitive athletes. In runners, 45% or more experience an injury in any given year, with one in seven seeking medical treatment.[1] Clinically, it can be a challenge to determine the exact cause of exercise-induced leg pain. The differential diagnosis is broad and includes etiologies such as medial tibial stress syndrome (MTSS), stress fracture, chronic exertional compartment syndrome (CECS), muscle strains, fascial hernias, tumors, and vascular and neurologic causes (Box 112-1).

Activity-induced acute compartment syndrome associated with military training has been well known and described in the literature since the early 1950s.[2-4] In the arena of sport, Mavor[5] first reported a case of CECS in a professional soccer player who had recurrent anterior leg pain and muscle herniation. The player was treated with a fasciotomy and fascia lata grafting with complete resolution of his symptoms, and he resumed his high level of sporting activity. In 1975, Reneman[6] was the first to identify increases in intracompartmental pressures in athletes with suspected CECS.

CECS is a condition that occurs in athletes and persons involved in repetitive exertional/loading activities. Most commonly it is seen in the lower extremities of distance runners. However, it can occur in athletes who participate in a wide variety of sports, including basketball, skating, and soccer.[7-9] Although the leg is the most common location, it also has been described in the foot, forearm, and thigh.[10-12]

Epidemiology

The incidence of the various causes of exertional leg pain varies widely, likely because of the difficulty in making a firm diagnosis in many cases. MTSS and CECS account for the majority of the cases of exercise-induced leg pain. MTSS represents between 13% and 42% of these cases, whereas CECS is reported to account for 27% to 33%.[13,14] Other common causes include stress fractures and nerve entrapments.[14-18]

With regard to the population affected, in a series of 100 patients with CECS, Detmer et al.[19] reported that it occurs primarily in young patients with a mean age of 26 years. Detmer et al.[19] also reported that the mean time to diagnosis was 22 months and that the CECS was bilateral in 82 of 100 cases.

Anatomy

Four muscle compartments are present in the lower extremity (Fig. 112-1). Each compartment is bound by bone and sits within its own investing fascia. In the case of CECS, the anterior compartment is most commonly involved (45%), followed by the deep posterior compartment (40%). In a significant portion of these cases, both the anterior and posterior compartments can be symptomatic simultaneously. The lateral compartment and superficial posterior compartment are much less likely to be affected, representing 10% and 5% of the involved compartments, respectively.[20] It should be noted that some authors have advocated that a separately functioning compartment be recognized for the tibialis posterior; however, such a compartment has not been shown to be a consistent anatomic finding.[21]

Each compartment contains one or more muscles and one major neurovascular structure (Box 112-2). The anterior compartment, which is the most commonly involved in CECS, contains the extensor hallucis longus, extensor digitorum longus, tibialis anterior, and peroneus tertius muscles and the anterior tibial and deep peroneal nerves. The lateral compartment contains the peroneus longus and brevis muscles, along with the superficial peroneal nerve. The deep posterior compartment contains the flexor hallucis longus, flexor digitorum longus, and posterior tibial muscles, as well as the posterior tibial and peroneal arteries and veins, in addition to the posterior tibial nerve. The superficial posterior compartment contains the gastrocnemius and soleus muscles; it is the least likely of all the compartments to be involved, because the fascia over this compartment is very thin and pliable.

Only two compartments contain significant vascular structures. The anterior compartment contains the anterior tibial artery and vein, which terminate in the dorsalis pedis vessels. The deep posterior compartment contains the posterior tibial artery and vein and the peroneal artery and vein, which terminate in the medial and lateral plantar vessels.

The superficial peroneal nerve exits the fascia from the lateral compartment, adjacent to the intramuscular septum, 11 cm proximal to the tip of the fibula. At this point, herniations may occur that can produce symptoms of CECS or nerve entrapment.

BOX 112-1 Differential Diagnosis of Leg Pain in Athletes

Muscle and Tendon
Chronic exertional compartment syndrome
Muscle strains
Fascial hernias
Tendinopathy

Bone
Medial tibial stress syndrome
Stress fracture

Vascular
Popliteal artery entrapment syndrome
Intermittent claudication
Venous insufficiency

Neurologic
Peripheral or central nerve entrapment or impingement
Referred pain from proximal joints (hip and knee)

Tumor

Infection

Pathophysiology

The cause of pain in persons with CECS is unclear, and the definite pathophysiology is also obscure. Consider that normal muscle physiology allows up to a 20% increase of muscle volume during exercise,[22,23] which is reflected in an increase in the intracompartmental pressures even in normal, asymptomatic persons.[24] This increase in the intracompartmental pressures may be due to increased blood volume from increased blood flow, or it may reflect muscle fiber swelling and fluid retention in the muscle.

It is generally accepted that exercise-induced biomechanical overload (e.g., dynamic exercise resulting in muscle contraction) produces increased pressure in an unyielding osseofascial compartment of the leg.[25,26] The proposed underlying pathophysiology behind the increase in pressure includes arterial spasm, capillary obstruction, arterial venous collapse, venous outflow obstructions, muscle hypertrophy, fascial inflexibility, and a release of protein bonds that results in increased osmotic pressure and edema.[27-29] The resulting high pressure has been proposed to result in microvascular occlusion and ischemic pain. Theoretically, arterial inflow reaches the vascular bed in muscle only during relaxation between contractions, leading to an eventual increase in muscle relaxation pressure. The end result, at least mechanistically, is ischemic pain and impaired muscle function.[30] However, no histochemical evidence has been found to support ischemic damage,[27] which raises the question of whether the increased pressure is a consequence, not the cause.[28]

Additional factors or associations shed light on the pathophysiology of CECS. Use of anabolic steroids and eccentric exercises induces muscular hypertrophy, increases intracompartmental pressures, and decreases fascial elasticity, all of which may predispose a person to the development of CECS. Posttraumatic soft tissue inflammation, myofascial scarring, and venous hypertension also may all contribute to the pathophysiology of CECS.[30] In addition, sympathetic blockade has been shown to reduce pain, inferring that some vascular spasms may occur as a result of sympathetic stimulation.[31]

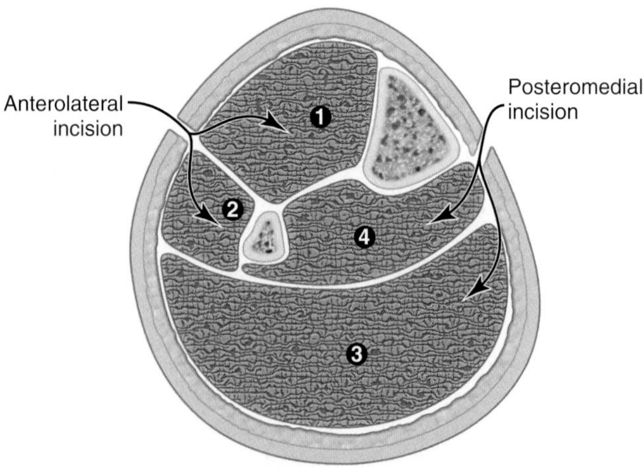

FIGURE 112-1 A cross-sectional diagram of the leg demonstrating the compartments and the location for medial and lateral fascial incisions. *1,* Anterior compartment; *2,* lateral compartment; *3,* superficial posterior compartment; *4,* deep posterior compartment.

Classification

Compartment syndromes may be classified as either acute or chronic. Acute compartment syndromes represent a surgical emergency that can result in devastating injury with loss of function and potentially the loss of a limb. The vast majority involve men (91%, with an average age of 32 years) and are typically associated with trauma (36% involve tibial diaphyseal fractures) or an ischemic event.[32] They have also been described in the setting of exercise (particularly when untrained persons initiate a training program), with increases

BOX 112-2 Anatomic Structures of the Four Compartments of the Leg

Anterior
Tibialis anterior muscle
Extensor hallucis longus muscle
Extensor digitorum longus muscle
Peroneus tertius muscle
Anterior tibial artery and vein
Deep peroneal nerve

Lateral
Peroneus longus and brevis muscles
Superficial peroneal nerve

Superficial Posterior
Gastrocnemius and soleus muscles
Sural nerve

Deep Posterior
Flexor hallucis longus muscle
Flexor digitorum longus muscle
Posterior tibialis muscle
Posterior tibial artery and vein
Peroneal artery and vein
Posterior tibial nerve

or changes in a training program, or with athletic injuries.[33-35] The immediate management of these injuries involves wide surgical decompression to avoid serious and long-term sequelae.

On the other hand, exertional compartment syndromes are less severe. They are symptomatic only during exercise and slowly resolve after the cessation of activity. They generally do not require acute surgical decompression unless they convert to a more acute syndrome.

No classification system has been developed or is in common use for CECS. Typically, the specific compartments involved are simply described. A high incidence of bilaterality also occurs, which is reported to be from 50% to greater than 80%, although it is not necessarily the case that the same compartment is affected within each limb.[36,37]

History

The clinical history is the key to differentiating CECS from other forms of exertional leg pain. Clinically, CECS often presents with exertional leg pain after a change in training intensity or volume.[15] It typically occurs after a stereotypic exercise duration or intensity.[13,16,38] Changes in footwear or training surface have also been implicated.[39] Pain at rest should alert the clinician to search for other causes. Patients may also report paresthesias and in some cases weakness related to compression of the nerve passing through the affected compartment. These key features can often help differentiate CECS from MTSS and stress fracture, two other common causes of exertional leg pain. The presentation is usually in young, healthy athletes, most commonly bilaterally. Unilateral involvement should lead the physician to rule out anatomic or unilateral biomechanical abnormalities, as previously mentioned.

The sensation the athlete experiences is often described as a pressure, fullness, burning, or crampy-type pain. If the athlete continues to exercise at increased intensity, the pain is typically progressive, and inevitably the athlete will not be able to continue to exercise. The pain abates with a decrease in intensity or, more likely, cessation of the provocative activity often after, again, a stereotypical brief period. Athletes can often predict at what point or intensity symptoms occur. Dysesthesia and weakness corresponding to the affected compartment can occur. Symptoms typically return with subsequent exercise sessions that are of similar intensity or duration.[13,16,38] In extreme circumstances, when the athlete continues to compete through the pain, acute compartment syndrome and rhabdomyolysis can occur.[33,40]

Physical Examination

Unlike with stress fractures and MTSS, the other two most common causes of exertional leg pain, tenderness with palpation is usually not found in persons with CECS. Thus if no palpable areas of tenderness are present, further examination after engaging the athlete in the provocative activity is mandatory. Tenderness, when present after exercise, is typically diffuse over the involved muscle group. Swelling or increased tissue tension may be detectable. Muscle herniations are not uncommon, especially at the exit site for cutaneous nerves.[41] As previously noted, when symptoms are severe, dysesthesia and motor weakness may be clinically apparent.

Knowledge of the anatomy of the nerve distributions and nerve functions can sometimes assist in the diagnosis of CECS. When the anterior compartment is involved, compression of the deep peroneal nerve can occur. This compression can result in dysesthesias over the dorsum of the foot (particularly the web space of the great toe), foot drop, or the sensation of loss of ankle control.[42] When the lateral compartment is affected, weakness of foot eversion and/or loss of sensation over the anterolateral shin and dorsum of the foot may be present. With deep posterior compartment involvement, weakness of the foot muscles and loss or abnormal sensation on the plantar aspect of the foot may be present.

Imaging

When the diagnosis is unclear, radiographs, bone scans, and/or magnetic resonance imaging (MRI) may be obtained. Findings of these studies are generally normal in CECS. Their value lies in identifying or excluding other causes of exertional leg pain (e.g., stress fractures). Vascular studies such as pre- and postexercise ankle brachial indexes, arteriograms, or MRI with or without arthrography can be performed to differentiate CECS from popliteal artery entrapment.

Noninvasive testing has been used to assist in the diagnosis of CECS as well. MRI has been performed in the acute setting. The affected compartment shows increased signal intensity on T2-weighted images associated with CECS that resolves with rest.[43,44] This increased signal is secondary to the recruitment of muscle fibers during activity that results in increased interstitial water content, independent of vascular patency (Fig. 112-2).[45] Near-infrared spectroscopy has also been used. It demonstrates decreased tissue oxygenation and delayed reoxygenation after exercise in persons with CECS.[46,47]

Decision-Making Principles

Ultimately, CECS, like acute compartment syndrome, continues to be a clinical diagnosis. When the clinical diagnosis is in doubt, intracompartmental pressure testing remains the standard diagnostic test. Numerous devices, techniques, and protocols have been used.[48] Studies have monitored pressures at rest, during exercise, and after exercise.[30,48,49] However, the difficulty of measuring pressures during exercise makes it impractical in most settings. The most widely cited criterion for the diagnosis of CECS comes from Pedowitz et al.[50] (Table 112-1). Preexercise pressures greater than 15 mm Hg and 1-minute and 5-minute postexercise pressures greater than 30 mm Hg and 20 mm Hg, respectively, are considered

TABLE 112-1

MODIFIED PEDOWITZ CRITERIA

Time	Pressure Measurement
Before exercise	>15 mm Hg
1 min after exercise	>30 mm Hg
5 min after exercise	>20 mm Hg

From Pedowitz RA, Hargens AR, Mubarak SJ, et al: Modified criteria for the objective diagnosis of chronic compartment syndrome of the leg. *Am J Sports Med* 18(1):35-40, 1990.

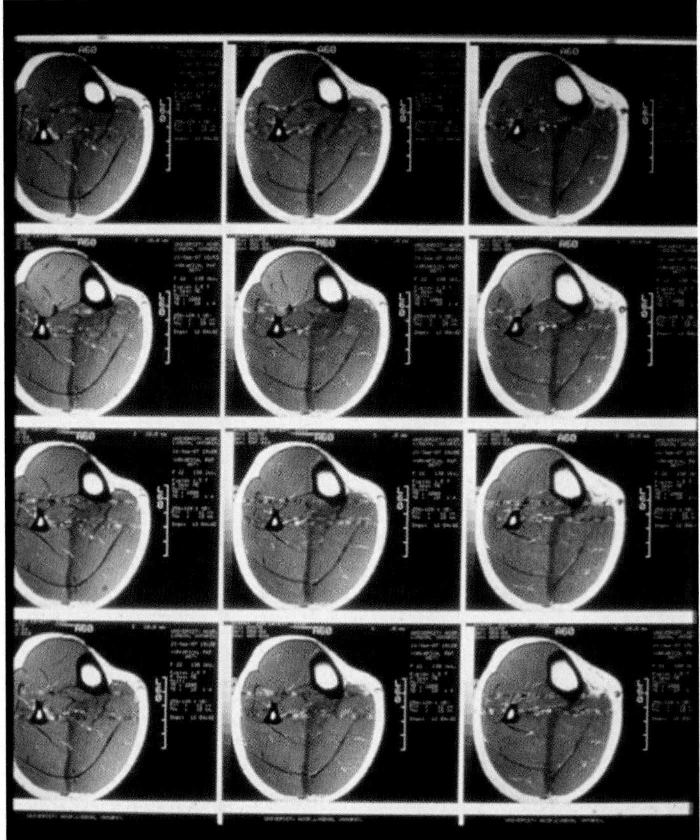

FIGURE 112-2 Magnetic resonance imaging findings in a person with chronic exertional compartment syndrome involving the anterior compartment musculature before exercise (*top row*), 5 minutes after exercise (*second row*), 10 minutes after exercise (*third row*), and 15 minutes after exercise (*fourth row*).

abnormal. However, in two recent literature reviews in which studies on compartment pressure testing were evaluated, limitations associated with the use of the current criteria were noted.[30,49] The authors of both reviews point out that protocols generally have a lack of standardization, validated control groups are lacking, and a significant degree of overlap exists in pressures recorded between control groups and symptomatic groups. On the basis of their systematic review, Aweid et al.[30] noted that the only time point at which significant overlap did not occur between the symptomatic and control groups is 1 minute after exercise. At that point, pressures greater than 27.5 mm Hg are highly suggestive of CECS.

Compartment Testing

Compartment pressures can be reliably measured with use of the Stryker Intra-Compartmental Pressure Monitor (Stryker Orthopaedics, Mawah, NJ). This device has been validated with in vitro models possessing known pressures.[51] The Stryker Intra-Compartmental Pressure Monitor can be used for continuous monitoring but is more commonly used for intermittent monitoring with percutaneous needle penetration into the compartment. Various types of needles can be used (e.g., slit catheters, side port needles, and straight needles), but the current evidence suggests that the slit catheter is the most accurate. Although straight needles are commonly used, they tend to overestimate the pressure.[48]

The patient should be placed supine on a table for the pressure measurements. The location where the measurements will be taken is marked on the skin in indelible ink; the skin is then anesthetized with a local anesthetic and prepped in an aseptic fashion. The monitor device should be held horizontally and set at zero before each pressure reading. No standard angle of entry has been agreed upon, but an angle of 45 degrees to the skin is reproducible, minimizes discomfort, and permits a reasonable depth.[48] Anterior and lateral compartments are measured at their midbellies directly through independent skin puncture wounds, whereas the superficial and deep compartments are measured through the same skin puncture wound, with further penetration for the deep compartments. With each pressure measurement, a small amount of fluid is injected, and the reading is recorded. As previously described, some investigators advocate the use of the modified Pedowitz criteria (see Table 112-1) to confirm the presence of CECS in the involved compartments, whereas Aweid et al.[30] offer alternative diagnostic criteria.

The role and impact of ultrasound guidance in compartment testing have been analyzed. Wiley and colleagues[52] have shown that ultrasound-guided insertion provides a safe, reliable, and reproducible method for proper needle placement in the deep tibialis posterior compartment. Despite this evidence, it does not appear that ultrasound guidance is indicated for routine deep and superficial posterior leg compartment pressure testing. The accuracy in testing both types of compartments is similar, regardless of the experience of the investigator.[53]

Lastly, bilateral compartment testing should be considered. Conservative estimates of bilateral CECS range from 50% to greater than 80%, as previously noted, with some investigators approximating the incidence at 90%.[36,37]

Treatment Options

The treatment of CECS can include either conservative or surgical measures. Although the evidence is lacking with respect to the success of nonoperative treatment, the initial management is generally to attempt nonoperative measures. Specific recommendations are largely based on case series and expert opinion. Therefore, because of the lack of definitive diagnostic criteria, the clinical history and physical examination remain paramount in making the diagnosis, and compartment pressure testing should be performed for confirmation. If the pressures are normal or if the history is inconsistent (e.g., the presence of non–exercise-induced pain), the diagnosis should remain in question, and operative intervention should be discouraged.

Nonoperative treatments such as physical therapy, use of antiinflammatory agents, stretching and icing, and orthotics can be used in the initial management of suspected CECS. However, relative or complete rest from the inciting activity is often also necessary.

Prior to return to activity, both intrinsic and extrinsic factors that may be contributing to the symptoms must be addressed and corrected. Modifiable extrinsic factors may include changes to the training surface, shoe design, and the training program itself.

Stretching and strengthening programs can address potential mechanical factors related to the lower limb and core. Gait modifications may be used to alter the biomechanical forces traveling through the affected compartment.[54-56]

In a recent study of 10 patients with CECS, a 6-week forefoot-strike running intervention was implemented. This resulted in decreased postrunning lower leg intracompartmental pressures. Surgical intervention was avoided in all of these patients.[56] Other methods used have included deep tissue massage, myofascial release, and ultrasound. If the response to conservative measures does not allow the athlete to return to the desired level of activity, operative treatment should be considered. An adequate trial of conservative measures is generally considered to be in the range of 3 to 6 months.[16,19,20,57]

Surgical treatment entails a fasciotomy, with or without fasciectomy, and resection of any facial bands. When a facial herniation is present, it must be included in the release to avoid recurrent symptoms that can occur if it is neglected. When surgery is pursued, all symptomatic compartments should be addressed with surgical release. Previously, persons with anterior symptoms had anterior and lateral compartments released. However, Schepsis and colleagues[57] found that, in patients with complaints isolated to the anterior compartment, release of the anterior compartment alone produced results equal to those of a combined anterior and lateral compartment release. It is now generally accepted that surgical release should be performed only for the symptomatic compartments. Open and subcutaneous techniques are described. Current trends are for limited incision techniques with a rapid return to weight bearing, motion, and resumption of activity. As with conservative measures, no controlled trials that directly compare surgical techniques have been performed. Regardless, success rates are generally high, in the 80% to 90% range.[58-68]

AUTHORS' PREFERRED METHOD

Decision Making for Fasciotomy

The ideal surgical candidate for fasciotomy is an otherwise healthy patient who has bilateral exercise-induced pain only that is always relieved by rest and is reproducible. The patient can clearly state when the pain comes on, how long it takes to resolve after the cessation of exercise, and that the pain occurs every time exercise is performed. If the patient has elevated resting pressures greater than 15 mm or immediate postexercise pressures are greater than 30 mm, the diagnosis is confirmed. If the patient has an inconsistent history, pain at rest, unilateral symptoms, tenderness, or abnormal findings of a neurological examination at rest, the senior author (AA) has concerns regarding surgical intervention. Investigation should continue to make the definitive diagnosis. If the diagnosis has been confirmed, we perform bilateral surgery: anterior compartment release alone for anterior compartment syndrome, both anterior and lateral releases for anterolateral compartment syndrome, and posterior fascial release (tibialis posterior, flexor hallucis longus, flexor digitorum longus [FDL], and soleal bridge) for posterior compartment syndrome.

Anterior and Lateral Compartment Release

We prefer to use a double-incision technique similar to that described by Rorabeck and colleagues[67] to avoid injury to the superficial peroneal nerve by direct exposure rather than blind fascial release. The anterior intermuscular septum is usually superficially located and centered between the palpable anterior border of the tibia and the lateral border of the fibula. Two longitudinal incisions, 2 to 3 cm long, are centered over the intermuscular septum (IMS) at the junctions of the proximal/middle and middle/distal thirds of the leg (Fig. 112-3). The superficial peroneal nerve exits the lateral compartment fascia 11 cm from the distal tip of the fibula. The distal incision should be centered at this point to allow for direct visualization and protection of the nerve. They are carried down full thickness to the muscle fascia. The IMS and superficial peroneal nerve can be easily identified. Using finger dissection, the plane is developed between the muscle fascia and subcutaneous fatty tissues from the knee to the ankle. One channel is made over each compartment to avoid making

Continued

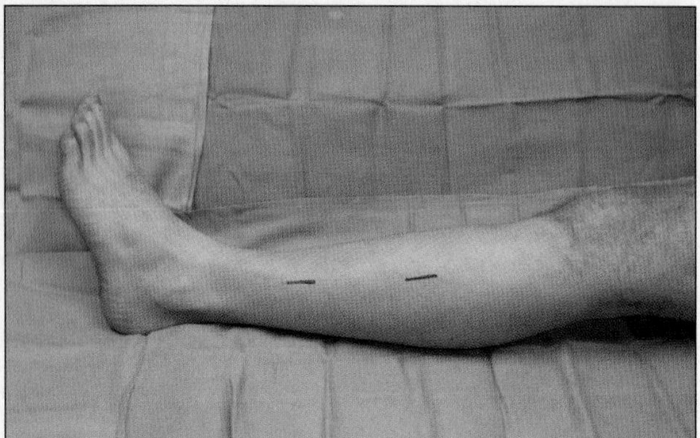

FIGURE 112-3 Skin markings for the anterior and lateral compartment double-incision technique. Incisions are placed along the intermuscular septum, located about midway between the subcutaneous anterior border of the tibia and the subcutaneous lateral border of the fibula. The distal incision is centered over the exit of the superficial peroneal nerve, about 10 cm from the ankle joint line. The proximal incision is centered 10 cm distal to the proximal fibula.

a large subcutaneous space and to minimize the occurrence of a seroma. The superficial peroneal nerve and any branches are visualized through the distal incision (Fig. 112-4) and are protected throughout the procedure. The nerve is released if its exit from the fascia is believed to be tight.

A small longitudinal incision is then made into the anterior and lateral fascia 1 cm on either side of the IMS at both incisions (Fig. 112-5). From the proximal incision, the anterior and lateral compartment fasciotomy is carried out proximally (Fig. 112-6). We prefer to use 8- and 12-inch Metzenbaum scissors, but a fasciotome may also be used. The distal incision is then used to carry the fasciotomies distally to the level of the superior extensor retinaculum. Using either the proximal or distal incisions, the fasciotomies are connected. The advantages of the double-incision technique include easier access to the anterior and lateral compartment fascia adjacent to the IMS and confirmation of a complete fasciotomy. When this technique is used, we strongly recommend not proceeding with the fasciotomy until the subcutaneous tissue has been separated from the fascia, which decreases the risk of injury to the subcutaneous structures, makes passage of the instrument much easier, and allows distal inspection to confirm a complete fasciotomy.

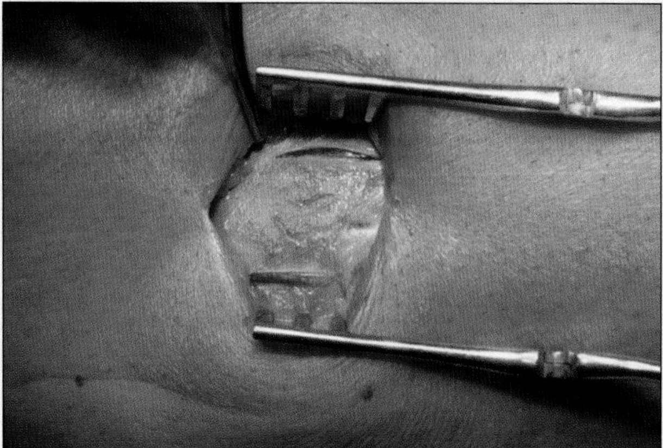

FIGURE 112-5 Fascial incisions for anterior and lateral compartment releases. Note the intermuscular raphe between the incisions.

Posterior Compartment Release

We use a single-incision technique for release of the superficial and deep posterior compartments. The incision is located 1 cm posterior to the posterior subcutaneous border of the tibia. It is centered at the level of the distal gastrocnemius curve and is 8 to 10 cm long (Fig. 112-7). The long saphenous nerve and vein are usually in the center of the field and are easily identified on the posteromedial border of the tibia. Proximally, the flexor digitorum longus occupies this position. A small vertical incision is made at the osseofascial junction, and then, using Metzenbaum scissors and staying directly on the posterior border of the tibia, the fascia is released to the level of the tibialis posterior tendon. The surgeon's finger should follow the instrument to ensure a complete release. The release is then taken proximally. The soleus will be encountered in the proximal one third of the tibia at the soleus bridge. Release of this stout structure must be complete

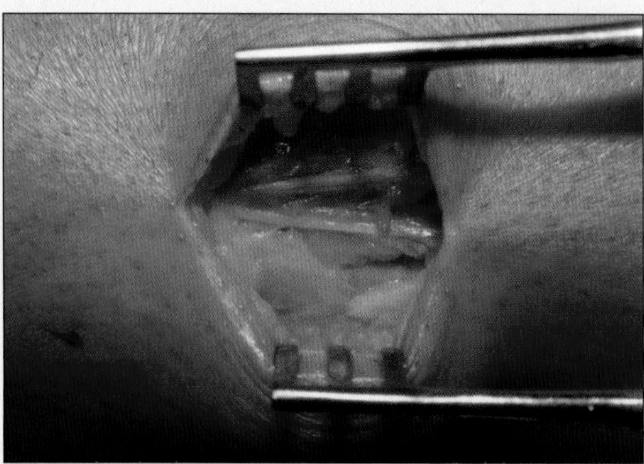

FIGURE 112-4 The superficial peroneal nerve in the distal incision.

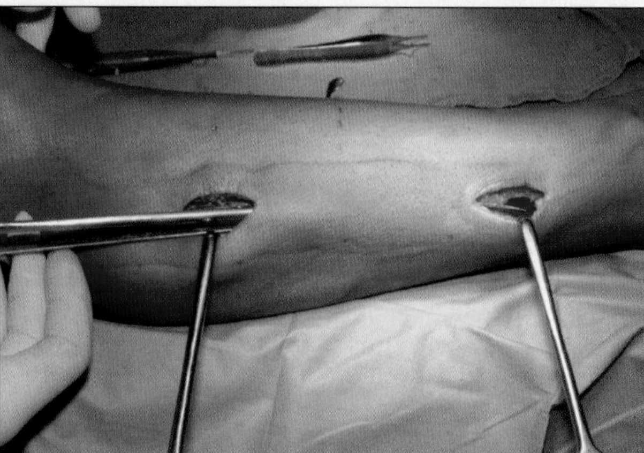

FIGURE 112-6 A fasciotomy is performed using long Metzenbaum scissors in a push-cut fashion. The nerve is visualized directly and protected in the distal incision.

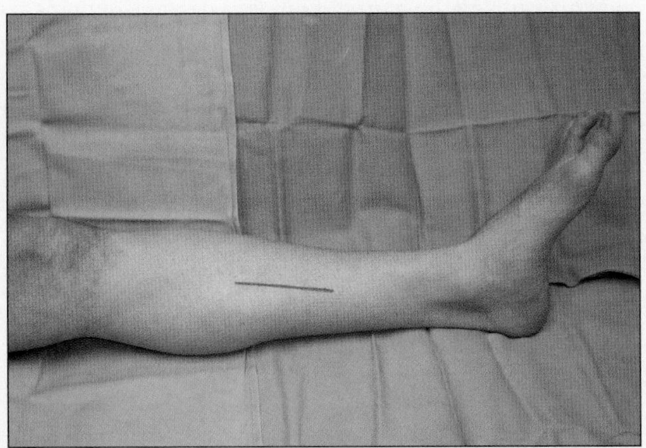

FIGURE 112-7 Skin marking for posterior compartment releases. A 10-cm incision is located along the posteromedial subcutaneous border of the tibia, centered at the distal insertion of the gastrocnemius muscle.

because it also represents the proximal confluence of the flexor hallucis longus and FDL fascia, facilitating the release of the deep posterior compartment. A Bristow or wide elevator is then used to release the tibialis posterior muscle off the tibia, completing the release of the tibialis posterior compartment (Fig. 112-8). We have found this technique effective in releasing the deep posterior compartments. Remaining on the posterior aspect of the tibia throughout the release ensures safety of the posterior tibial neurovascular bundle, which is posterior to the tibialis posterior and FDL. Verification of an adequate release by digital examination is of the utmost importance. After the anterior or posterior releases are performed, the tourniquet is released and hemostasis is obtained. The subcutaneous tissues are closed, and the skin is sutured using a subcuticular stitch. A sterile dressing and a compression bandage are applied to both legs. As mentioned, most patients have bilateral symptoms and hence undergo bilateral procedures. Patients with anterior and posterior symptoms have both compartments released.

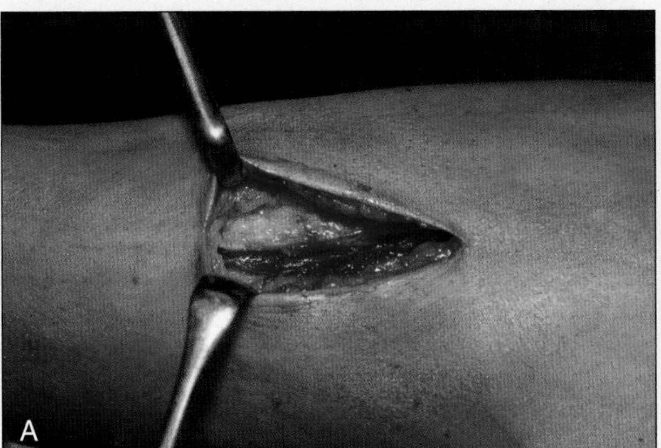

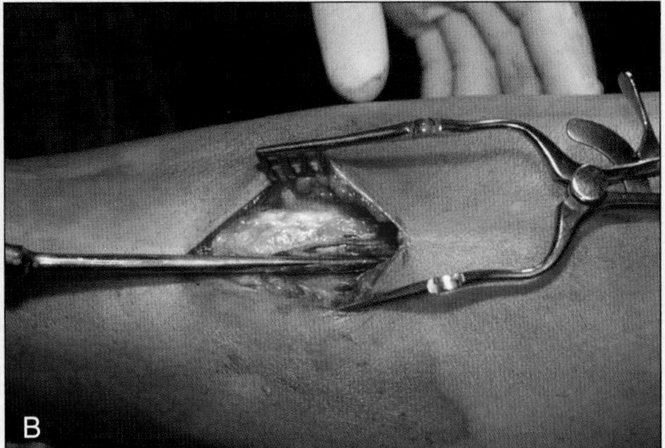

FIGURE 112-8 **A** and **B,** Fascial incisions for posterior compartment releases. The muscle fascia is taken directly off the posteromedial border of the tibia.

Postoperative Care

Weight bearing is initiated immediately after surgery, with crutches discontinued as tolerated, generally within the first week. Early passive and active range of motion exercises are implemented after surgery to prevent fascial scarring.[13,16,20,69] During the first 2 days, patients follow a PRICE (protection, rest, ice, compression, and elevation) protocol, as well as anterior and posterior stretching (toe pointing) three to six times per day. Postoperative compressive dressings should be left in place for the first 2 days. From the third day to the 2-week follow-up visit, patients perform aggressive anterior and posterior compartment stretches three times per day and increase their walking distance. Once they are weaned from crutches, nonimpact activities such as hydrotherapy, stationary cycling, and elliptical training are initiated. After 2 weeks, the wounds are checked, the sutures are removed, and a formal physical therapy regimen of stretching and functional return to sport-specific activity is begun. Low-impact stationary bicycling, treadmill or track walking, and/or hydrotherapy can be started.[70] When strength and control of the ankle and foot are regained, functional training can begin, usually by 4 to 6 weeks. At that point, running may be implemented, with speed and agility drills added during the eighth week.[13,20,69]

No objective criteria exist for return to play after fascial release for CECS. The timing of return to play is based on satisfactory completion of the progression outlined in the preceding section. In summation, the athlete should be nearly pain free, have demonstrated acceptable strength and endurance, and be able to replicate the demands of practice and play in the therapy sessions. A general guideline for full return to athletic activities is 8 to 12 weeks after surgical intervention.

Results

To date, the operative and nonoperative treatment of CECS has not been studied in controlled trials. Additionally, no studies have been performed to compare the efficacy and/or outcomes of the different surgical procedures. Most surgical procedures report a high rate of satisfaction and return to unlimited physical activity, with 60% to 100% rates of relief.[58-68] De Fijter and associates[61] reported a 96% return to unlimited exercise in 118 military personnel after a percutaneous fasciotomy, with an average follow-up of 62 months. Raikin and colleagues[66] reported bilateral simultaneous releases in 16 patients; 16 months after surgery, 14 patients were pain free and all returned to sports an average of 10.7 weeks after surgery. Moushine and coworkers[65] reported the cases of 18 consecutive athletes treated with the two-incision fasciotomy technique, all of whom had returned to full sporting activity at the 2-year follow-up, with an average return to sporting activity of 25 days.

Howard and colleagues[63] reported slightly less favorable results of 68% pain relief, but when stratified by compartment, patients with anterior release had 81% relief, whereas posterior release yielded 50% relief. Slimmon and associates[68] also had less favorable outcomes using a single-incision technique. They reported 60% good or excellent results in patients undergoing a single operation, with 58% of patients exercising at a lower level than before the development of symptoms.[68] Hutchinson and coworkers[71] demonstrated incomplete releases with a single-incision technique, which may account for the less favorable outcomes. Although Schepsis and colleagues[59] found that releasing only the involved compartments versus both the anterior and lateral compartments yielded identical results, the release of both compartments resulted in a delay of return to sport by more than 3 weeks on average (11.4 vs. 8.1 weeks).[59] In conclusion, minimally invasive, percutaneous, and single- and double-incision techniques are all currently used. Evidence shows that single-incision techniques yield inferior results compared with double-incision techniques.[68]

Overall, surgical treatment of CECS has a high rate of satisfactory outcome and return to sporting activities with a relatively low complication rate. When an accurate diagnosis of CECS has been made, the patient wishes to undergo surgical treatment, and modification of activity is unacceptable, fasciotomy of the affected compartments may be recommended. In this context relative to CECS, excellent results can be achieved if the procedure is performed properly.

Complications

Reported complications have included hematoma or seroma formation (9%), superficial peroneal nerve injury (2%), anterior ankle pain (5%), and recurrence of symptoms (2%).[61] Theoretical concerns have been expressed in the vascular surgery literature regarding the function of muscles and their compartments in the return of fluids in dependent limbs. This concern, in turn, raised the possibility of venous insufficiency after fascial release. However, no documented cases with clinically significant findings have been reported to date.[72]

Recurrence after a fasciotomy for CECS has been reported in several studies. Only one study has been published on the surgical treatment for recurrent CECS.[73] In this situation, careful dissection, release of nerve entrapment, and fasciectomy are essential, and the results are not as predictable as with the primary surgery.[73]

For a complete list of references, go to expertconsult.com.

Suggested Readings

Citation: Blackman PG: A review of chronic exertional compartment syndrome in the lower leg. *Med Sci Sports Exerc* 32(3 Suppl):S4–10, 2000.
Level of Evidence: III
Summary: Chronic exertional compartment syndrome in the lower leg has been described as early as 1956. In this review the author describes the five relevant anatomic compartments and the important clinical features upon presentation that are used in the diagnosis.

Citation: Clanton TO, Solcher BW: Chronic leg pain in the athlete. *Clin Sports Med* 13(4):743–759, 1994.
Level of Evidence: III
Summary: The authors provide an excellent review of chronic leg pain in athletes. The review covers the history, examination, various presentations, and appropriate use of diagnostic studies when evaluating athletes with leg pain.

Citation: Wilder RP, Sethi S: Overuse injuries: Tendinopathies, stress fractures, compartment syndrome, and shin splints. *Clin Sports Med* 23(1):55–81, 2004.
Level of Evidence: III
Summary: The authors of this article discuss common overuse injuries of the lower leg, ankle, and foot: tendinopathies, stress fractures, chronic exertional compartment syndrome, and shin splints.

Citation: Edwards P, Myerson MS: Exertional compartment syndrome of the leg: Steps for expedient return to activity. *Phys Sports Med* 24(4):31–46, 1996.
Level of Evidence: III
Summary: The authors describe a stepwise approach to the patient with suspected exertional compartment syndrome. The article covers diagnosis, nonoperative treatment, and operative treatment.

Citation: Styf J, Körner L, Suurkula M: Intramuscular pressure and muscle blood flow during exercise in chronic compartment syndrome. *J Bone Joint Surg Br* 69B(2):301–305, 1987.
Level of Evidence: IV
Summary: In nine patients with chronic compartment syndrome, the intramuscular pressure and muscle blood flow during constant dynamic exercise were studied via the microcapillary infusion method and the 133-xenon clearance technique. The authors' analysis suggested that chronic compartment syndrome is due to increased muscle relaxation pressure during exercise, which causes decreased muscle blood flow, leading to ischemic pain and impaired muscle function.

Citation: Slimmon D, Bennell K, Brukner P, et al: Long-term outcome of fasciotomy with partial fasciectomy for chronic exertional compartment syndrome of the lower leg. *Am J Sports Med* 30(4):581–588, 2002.
Level of Evidence: IV
Summary: In this review of 50 patients who underwent a single operation, 60% (30) reported an excellent or good outcome for the treatment of exertional compartment syndrome. The authors noted that average pain and pain on running were significantly reduced, although some subjects still reported considerable levels of pain, and that patients should be counseled that they may not be able to return to their preinjury level of exercise or remain pain free.

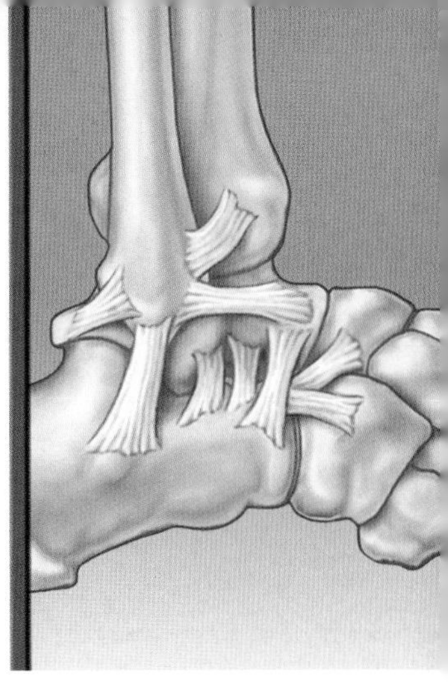

113

Peripheral Nerve Entrapment Around the Foot and Ankle

NORMAN ESPINOSA

Athletes may have chronic lower limb pain, which can be caused by peripheral nerve entrapment. Compared with other problems of the lower limb, this entity is quite rare, with a heterogeneous group of nerve disorders and multiple, sometimes very complex, causes and clinical presentations. Even for a perceptive clinician, distinguishing between the different medical causes may be difficult given that many of their presenting features overlap. The difficulty of understanding the entire spectrum of peripheral nerve entrapments may lead to misdiagnosis or underdiagnosis, with an inherent risk of potential patient mismanagement. This scenario can be frustrating for both the athlete and the treating physician. However, the approach to the problem can be facilitated with use of a structured algorithm. Adequate treatment of peripheral nerve entrapment requires a proper understanding of the anatomic course and the possible causes, precise identification of the involved nerve, and clear determination of the location of compression. When adhering to the presented diagnostic rules, an optimal treatment strategy can be formulated that should always be tailored to the athlete's condition and needs. This chapter provides an overview of the most important peripheral nerve entrapment syndromes found around the foot and ankle, with a specific focus on athletes.

Sural Nerve Entrapment

Because of its use in reconstructive surgery as a nerve graft, the sural nerve has become a well-investigated peripheral human nerve.[1-5] In 1974 Pringle and coworkers[6] were the first to report on the entrapment neuropathy of the sural nerve and its clinical sequelae. This pathologic condition may affect athletes who run but also other persons dedicated to sports.[4,7] The sural nerve is purely sensory and provides sensation to the posterolateral part of the distal one third of the leg and the lateral border of the foot, including the lateral aspect of the heel and the fifth toe (Fig. 113-1).[8,9] Communicating branches may expand the region of sensible innervation, extending it up to the third and fourth web space. Anatomically, in 80% of cases it arises from the distal union of the medial sural cutaneous branch of the tibial nerve and the peroneal communication branch of the common peroneal nerve. In 20% of persons the peroneal communicating branch is missing.[10,11] In those cases the sural nerve arises as a branch from the medial sural cutaneous nerve. The medial sural nerve runs between the heads of the gastrocnemius muscle and penetrates its deep aponeurosis halfway up the leg. Anatomically, the peroneal nerve anastomoses with the sural nerve. The sural nerve progresses down the border of the Achilles tendon. First it runs in midline with the calf and then, approximately 10 cm above the calcaneal tuberosity, it crosses the Achilles tendon and is positioned laterally (Fig. 113-2). Then the sural nerve runs approximately 1.5 cm posterior and inferior to the tip of the fibula to end up at the lateral side to the fifth metatarsal.[8]

Sural nerve entrapment may happen anywhere in its course. Common sites include the lateral aspect of the heel or foot.[12] Trauma plays a significant role as a risk factor for sural nerve entrapment. Recurrent ankle sprains can cause stretching of the nerve and result in structural damage.[4] General edema after trauma can cause external compression and impair nerve function. In addition, fractures of the base of the fifth metatarsal and ganglions of the peroneal sheaths or calcaneocuboid joint can cause nerve injury.[13-15] Prior surgery at the posterior calf, Achilles tendon repair (especially percutaneous),[15] posterolateral portals of arthroscopy (Fig. 113-3),[16,17] calcaneal osteotomies, ankle ligament reconstructions,[18] peroneal tendon repairs,[19] exposure for subtalar fusion, traction, and any scar are believed to be risk factors resulting in lesion or entrapment of the sural nerve. Less commonly, sural nerve entrapment within the gastrocnemius has been reported in the literature.[20]

History

Patients may note radiating and tingling symptoms. Chronic burning, numbness, paresthesia, or aching may be present along the course of the sural nerve, specifically at the posterolateral aspect of the leg, and might worsen during the night or with physical activity (e.g., running).

Physical Examination

Occasionally the spot of maximum pain enables the identification of the entrapment, and thus examination of the entire course of the sural nerve must be performed. Local tenderness and a positive Tinel sign are identified. Inspection for possible scars from previous surgeries is mandatory. Local anesthetic injections at suspected areas help establish the diagnosis.

S1-S2 nerve root impingement should be evaluated with a thorough lumbosacral assessment. Exertional compartment syndrome, popliteal artery entrapment, ankle sprains, and Achilles tendon disease can mimic neural entrapment.[21-23]

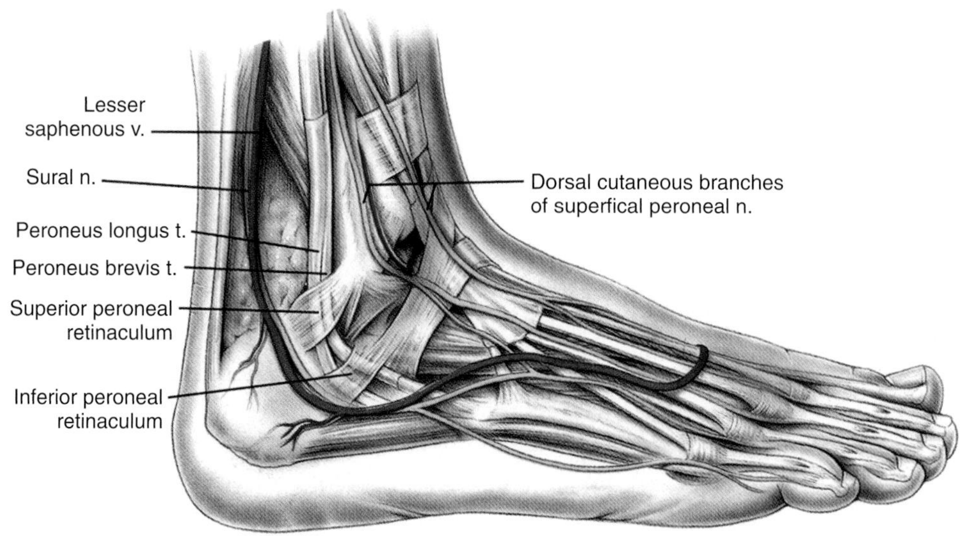

FIGURE 113-1 The anatomy of the lateral aspect of the foot and ankle. *n.,* Nerve; *t.,* tendon; *v.,* vein. *(From Ferkel RD, Weiss RA: Correlative surgical anatomy. In Ferkel RD, Whipple TL, editors:* Arthroscopic surgery: The foot and ankle, *Philadelphia, 1996, Lippincott-Raven.)*

Imaging

Plain radiographs may rule out an osseous malformation that can result in compression of the nerve (e.g., hypertrophic callus formations after a fracture). Some authors recommend stress views in the presence of hyperlaxity or chronic lateral ankle instability; however, the large variability in tibiotalar and anterior drawer values in both injured and noninjured ankles mitigates their value for routine use.[24] Magnetic resonance imaging (MRI) is useful to evaluate the nerve tissue and to identify a space-occupying mass.[25] Although computed tomography (CT) provides less detail in terms of soft tissue contents, it can be a useful adjunct when physical

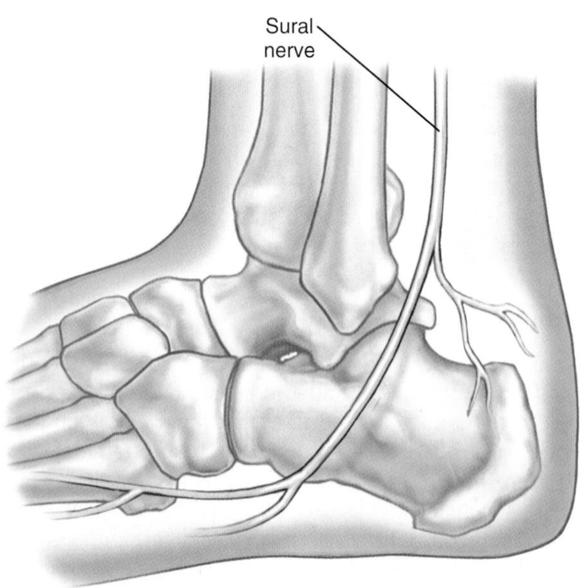

FIGURE 113-2 The course of the sural nerve.

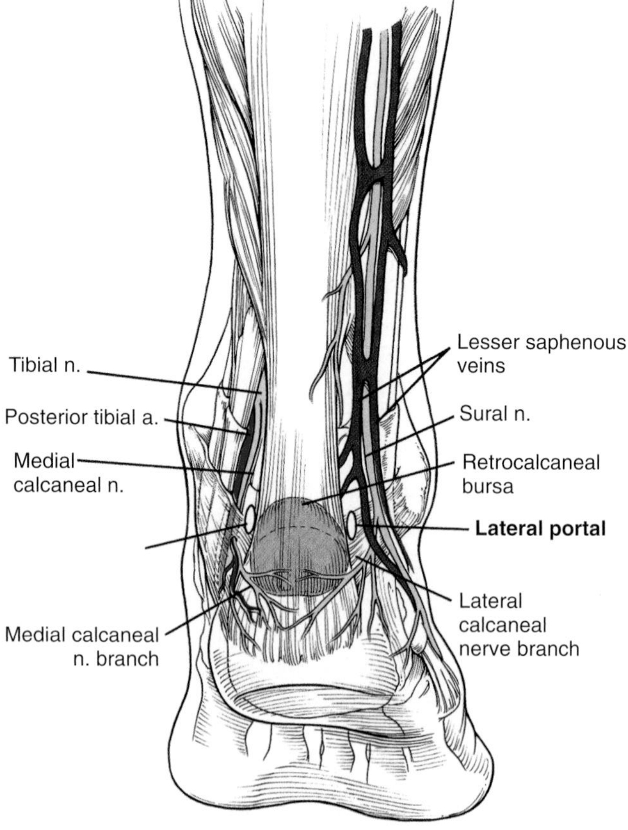

FIGURE 113-3 The posterior anatomy of the hindfoot with regard to arthroscopic portals. The sural nerve can be injured when inserting the scope through the posterolateral portal. *a.,* Artery; *n.,* nerve. *(From Ferkel RD, Weiss RA: Correlative surgical anatomy. In Ferkel RD, Whipple TL, editors:* Arthroscopic surgery: The foot and ankle, *Philadelphia, 1996, Lippincott-Raven.)*

examination suggests that an osseous structure is contributing to impingement or compression of a peripheral nerve or neurovascular bundle.[26]

Treatment Options

Conservative Treatment

Conservative measures should be determined according to the underlying pathomechanism. Chronic ankle instability can be addressed by bracing or application of orthotics. When using those measures, it is important to ensure that no external compression is applied to the nerve. In cases of external compression such as chronic lymphatic edema, this compression should be treated first. Isolated sural neuralgia might respond to vitamin B6, nonsteroidal antiinflammatory drugs (NSAIDs), gabapentin, tricyclic antidepressants, Lidocaine patches, and/or topically applied analgesic creams.[4]

Surgical Treatment

Surgical treatment is warranted when conservative measures have failed. The surgical options include sural neurolysis or neurectomy. In case of revision nerve surgery, a neurectomy with burial into healthy soft tissues or bone might be preferred rather than pure neurolysis. However, patients must be counseled about the limited results obtained with revision nerve surgery. Incisions vary according to the presence of previous incisions, the location of neuroma or entrapment, and the type of possible additional operation performed.

AUTHOR'S PREFERRED TECHNIQUE

Sural Nerve Entrapment

The patient is placed in the lateral decubitus or prone position. Both positions allow adequate access to the entire course of the sural nerve. A 10-cm skin incision is made over the area of maximum tenderness (this area should be assessed prior to surgery without use of an anesthetic). The sural nerve is identified and the compressive structure is released and/or removed. Excessive soft tissue resection should not be performed. Resection of fat away from the sural nerve should be avoided because such resection can lead to excessive scarring and thus to a potential recurrence of entrapment.

When considering a neurectomy, the nerve should be identified and dissected further distally and proximally. The nerve can then either be stripped or transected (Fig. 113-4). The stump can be buried into soft tissue, such as muscle, or into bone. Burial into bone can be difficult. To facilitate burial into bone, two perpendicular small unicortical drill holes (2.5 mm) are made through the cortex of the bone (e.g., the fibula). The nerve stump is inserted into one end of the bone while a suction device is placed into the other drill hole, and suction is used to draw the nerve into the bone. It is now possible to suture the epineurium onto the periosteum. One should ensure that no tension is placed on the nerve while moving the ankle up and down together with simultaneous observation of the structures involved.

I do not use vein-wrapping procedures in cases of sural nerve entrapment because of the reasonable results obtained with a neurectomy.

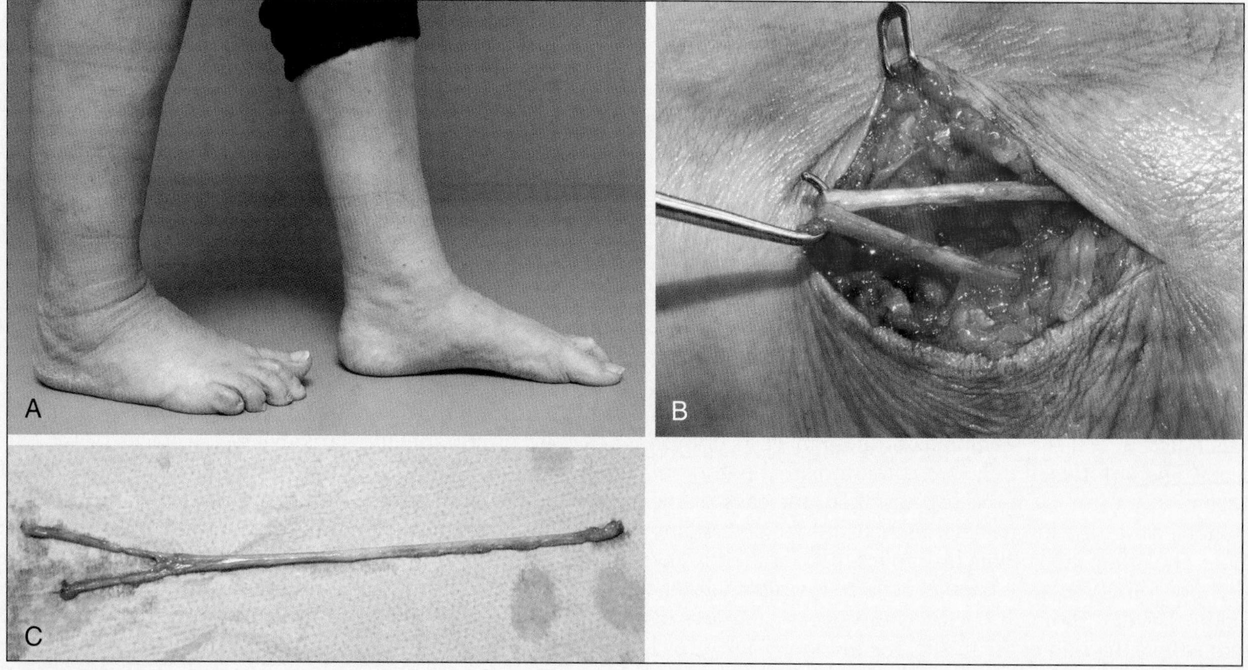

FIGURE 113-4 **A,** The right foot and leg of a 55-year-old patient who had previously been treated with a calcaneal osteotomy. Unfortunately, therapy-refractory pain developed along the course of the sural nerve. **B,** The nerve was approached over its point of maximal tenderness. Intraoperative findings revealed that the bifurcation has been entrapped and damaged. **C,** The resected sural nerve.

Postoperative Management

A cast is applied to the lower limb and is worn for 1 week. The cast should be in a neutral position. Walking with crutches is recommended for 1 week. After 1 week, gradual resumption of weight bearing is allowed as tolerated in a boot for 3 weeks. Physical therapy, including range of motion exercises and wobble-board training, is begun. Full athletic training can be resumed 4 to 6 weeks after the operation. In case of extensile surgery affecting a joint or including complex osteotomies, a boot should be worn for 4 weeks and training should not be resumed before 8 weeks after the operation.

Results

When space-occupying lesions are present, resection yields satisfactory symptomatic relief. Decompression of the sural nerve by excision of ganglia with neurolysis could be curative.[7] Posttraumatic bony impingement for sural nerve entrapment can be addressed by restoring anatomy. Gould and Trevino[13] described three cases of fractures of the base of the fifth metatarsal with dorsal displacement of the fracture fragment and tenting of the sural nerve. After reduction of the fracture fragment and neurolysis, all patients improved within several months. In a study performed by Fabre et al.,[7] 13 athletes (18 limbs) were treated for sural nerve entrapment. Nine limbs had excellent results, eight limbs had good results, and one limb had a fair result at the time of follow-up. Ten patients had cessation of calf pain. However, in patients in whom prior surgical scarring or injury is the cause of the entrapment, the results of nerve release are less predictable, and resection and burial may ultimately be required even though a true neuroma is not present. In the presence of a neuroma, resection of the damaged nerve and burial into healthy tissue (e.g., muscle or bone) can improve symptoms. In cases of ankle instability, lateral ankle ligament reconstruction without nerve release could be enough to help the patients reduce pain and discomfort and is a reasonable option if a neuroma is not present.[27]

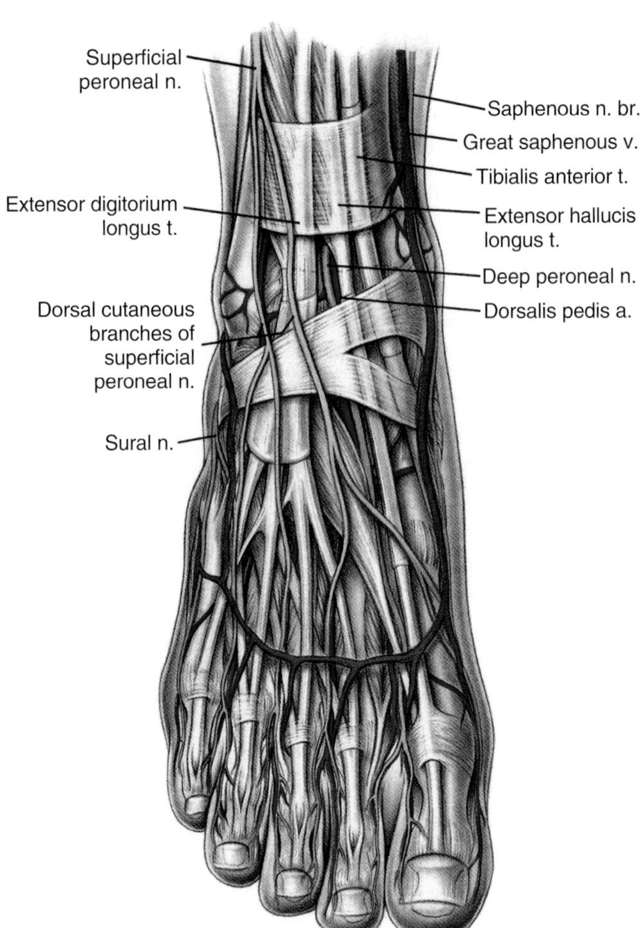

FIGURE 113-5 The anatomy of the dorsum of the foot. *a.*, Artery; *n.*, nerve; *n. br.*, nerve branch; *t.*, tendon; *v.*, vein. *(From Ferkel RD, Weiss RA: Correlative surgical anatomy. In Ferkel RD, Whipple TL, editors:* Arthroscopic surgery: The foot and ankle, *Philadelphia, 1996, Lippincott-Raven.)*

Saphenous Nerve Entrapment

Saphenous nerve entrapment is rare.[4] The saphenous nerve is the longest sensory branch of the femoral nerve and arises from the L1-L3 nerve roots. The nerve leaves the femoral triangle to enter the adductor canal (or the subsartorial canal of Hunter) together with the femoral artery and vein. The walls of the canal consist of the vastus medialis and adductor longus muscles, and the membrane of these muscles bridges the roof. The sartorius muscle covers the proximal portion of the canal and also covers the two terminal branches of the saphenous nerve, the infrapatellar branch and the descending branch. The infrapatellar branch supplies the sensation to the medial portion of the knee joint and the overlying anteromedial skin. The descending branch accompanies the saphenous vein to supply the skin of the medial leg and foot (Figs. 113-5 and 113-6).[10,11,28]

Entrapment occurs at the subsartorial fascia just proximal to the femoral condyle.[29,30] Local trauma can damage the nerve. Harvesting the saphenous vein for cardiac or vascular surgery can potentially lead to damage to the saphenous nerve.[31] Other causes include angulation, stretch, pressure, and friction.

History

Saphenous nerve entrapment can present with a variety of different symptoms. As a rule, symptomatology depends on the site of entrapment. Proximal involvement of the saphenous nerve, that is, the infrapatellar branch, could result in atypical or refractory knee pain.[29] Flexion of the knee joint might worsen the symptoms. Some patients receive incorrect knee treatment with application of a constricting brace because of missed or neglected saphenous nerve entrapment, and they report having pain. Patients may report claudicant or exercise-related medial leg or knee pain. This syndrome has been observed in cyclists and rowers. With distal involvement of the saphenous nerve, patients may feel pain, numbness, or paresthesias localized to the medial side of the leg or foot (typically proximal to the first metatarsophalangeal [MTP] joint).

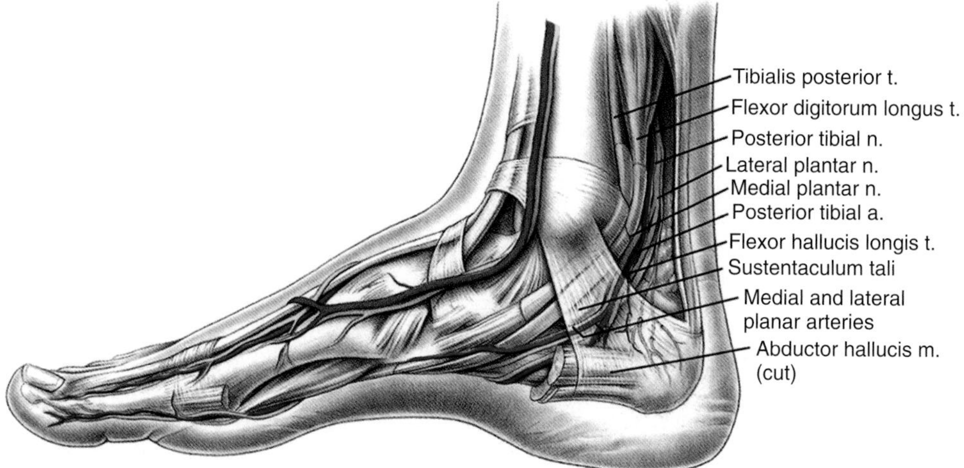

FIGURE 113-6 The anatomy of the medial aspect of the foot and ankle. *a.*, Artery; *m.*, muscle; *n.*, nerve; *t.*, tendon. *(From Ferkel RD, Weiss RA: Correlative surgical anatomy. In Ferkel RD, Whipple TL, editors:* Arthroscopic surgery: The foot and ankle, *Philadelphia, 1996, Lippincott-Raven.)*

Physical Examination

The nerve should be palpated along its anatomic course starting proximally from the medial condyle of the femur and traced down the medial side of the leg and the foot. Tenderness to palpation along the course of the nerve is the hallmark of diagnosis. Tenderness at the subsartorial fascia might be found, and it might be associated with a reproducible Tinel sign at the site of entrapment.[32] Relief of pain with injection of a local anesthetic suggests localization of a more precise site of entrapment.

It is possible to use nerve conduction studies to assess the main branch of the saphenous nerve or the terminal branches.[33] However, routine testing may not yield useful results in patients with significant subcutaneous adipose tissue or swelling of the extremity.[34]

Electromyography for suspected saphenous nerve impingement should include testing of the adductor longus and quadriceps muscles. Although electromyography is expected to be negative in persons with saphenous nerve entrapment, it could be helpful to assess the presence of radiculopathy.[35]

Imaging

Conventional radiographs help identify posttraumatic and primary impingement on the nerve. Advanced diagnostic studies such as MRI or CT are not routinely indicated but can be considered to more clearly elucidate bony structures surrounding the course of the nerve (with CT) or for preoperative planning and more precise localization of impingement in cases refractory to conservative measures.

Treatment Options

Conservative Treatment

Nonoperative treatment encompasses removal of any extrinsic factors that could lead to saphenous nerve entrapment. Activity modifications and physical therapy (including strengthening exercises and proprioception) may help reduce pain. NSAIDs, topical analgesic agents, and systemic nerve modulators have been recommended for persons with saphenous nerve entrapment syndrome.[32] Local injections of anesthetics with or without steroids could alleviate pain. Romanoff et al.[30] reported an 80% success rate after a series of injections in 30 patients without application of steroids. However, if these measures do not improve the symptoms, surgery should be considered.

Surgical Treatment

Surgical treatment includes decompression, neurectomy, and neurolysis. Decompression is preferred and can be achieved via release of the anterior aspect of the Hunter canal and dissection of the saphenous nerve fibers from the surrounding sartorial fascia. Local nerve release may be necessary for more distal entrapments.

The best management for the transected proximal nerve is to bury and secure the nerve within an adjacent muscle belly. The nerve can also be compressed as it travels between the sartorius and gracilis muscles near their insertion. The nerve can either be released or divided in this region. Probably the most frequently seen problem in the sporting population is a neuroma of the infrapatellar branch, which can be irritated by repetitive movement of the knee or by direct pressure producing symptoms from the neuroma. Surgical treatment is simple. A straight incision is made over the neuroma, which is then excised, dividing the infrapatellar branch fairly proximally. In my experience, simple transection and placing it into muscle is all that is required.

Results

A reduction or elimination of pain can be expected in 60% to 80% of cases.[34] However, a large number of patients might still require a neurectomy. Debate is ongoing about whether neurolysis of the nerve or neurectomy achieves the best results. The chief problem with division of the saphenous nerve is the resulting distal anesthesia, with subjective discomfort in some patients. On the other hand, simple neurolysis includes complete fascial band release around the saphenous nerve with potential scar tissue formation, which could itself lead to new entrapment of the nerve. Worth et al.[36] showed that in 15 patients with saphenous nerve entrapment, complete relief was achieved in 13 knees after a neurectomy. The authors concluded that a neurectomy provides a more predictable result than does neurolysis. A neurectomy is best performed proximal to the fascia in the canal between the vastus medialis and adductor magnus.[34]

In a study by Koppel and Thompson, two patients had relief of symptoms 24 hours after decompression. However, because they were not followed up for a longer period, interpretation of these results is maximally limited. Dellon et al.[36a] reported the results of a neurectomy in 70 patients. Sixty-two of these patients were treated with a neurectomy of the infrapatellar branch. Eighty-four percent had improvement of pain according to the visual analogue scale.

Tarsal Tunnel Syndrome

Tarsal tunnel syndrome, an entrapment neuropathy involving the tibial nerve, was first described by Lam in 1962.[37] It is relatively uncommon in athletes and thus may be misdiagnosed or not diagnosed. Although patients with this syndrome who are not athletes are often middle aged to elderly with an equal distribution among male and female patients, in athletes who have this syndrome, the patients are younger with a female preponderance.[37-39]

The tibial nerve arises from the sciatic nerve. The tarsal tunnel is located behind the medial malleolus (see Fig. 113-6). Its borders are created by the tibia anteriorly, the posterior process of the talus and calcaneus laterally, and the flexor retinaculum medially. The flexor retinaculum is confluent with the sheaths of the posterior tibial tendon, the flexor hallucis longus tendon, and the flexor digitorum longus tendon. The flexor retinaculum and the abductor hallucis both are frequent sites of compression.[11] More recently, Singh and Kumar[40] were able to demonstrate three well-defined fascial septae in the sole of the foot. Two of these septae represented potential sites of compression of the posterior tibial nerve and its branches and were distinct when compared with the classic entrapment sites. In most of the cases (93%), the tibial nerve splits into three major branches within the tarsal tunnel: the medial plantar nerve, the lateral plantar nerve, and the medial calcaneal branch. The medial calcaneal branch arises from the tibial nerve in 75% of cases, and in 25% of cases it arises from the lateral plantar nerve. The calcaneal branches originate proximal to the tarsal tunnel in 39%, within the tarsal canal in 34%, and distal to the tunnel in 16% (Fig. 113-7).

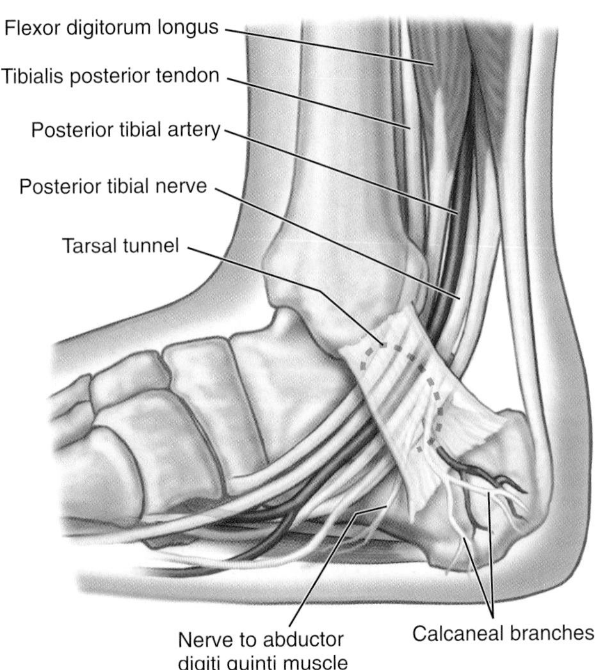

FIGURE 113-7 The course of the tibial nerve and its branches in the distal aspect of the lower limb and ankle.

Causes

A specific cause can be identified in approximately 60% to 80% of patients.[4,34,41] Table 113-1 provides a synopsis of the possible causes based on the work of Cimino.[42] Engorged varicose veins,[43] systemic diseases,[44] neurilemoma (i.e., a benign nerve sheath tumor),[45] pigmented villonodular synovitis,[46] lipomas, synovial cysts, intraneural degenerative cysts, ganglion cysts (flexor hallucis longus tendon sheaths), and accessory muscles[47] all can result in tibial nerve entrapment.

Postural deformities or mechanical abnormalities may contribute to the development of tarsal tunnel syndrome.[2,42,48-55] Hindfoot valgus (8% of cases) and deltoid ligament

TABLE 113-1

CAUSES OF TARSAL TUNNEL SYNDROME

Cause	No. of Cases
Idiopathic	25
Traumatic	21
Varicosities	16
Heel varus	14
Fibrosis	11
Ganglion	10
Diabetes	3
Obesity	3
Tight tarsal canal	3
Hypertrophic abductor hallucis	3
Rheumatoid arthritis	3
Lipoma	2
Anomalous artery	1
Acromegaly	1
Ankylosing spondylitis	1
Regional migratory osteoporosis	1
Flexor digitorum accessorius longus	1
Subtotal	122
Causes not reported	64
Total	**186**

From Cimino WR: Tarsal tunnel syndrome: Review of the literature. *Foot Ankle* 11(1):47–52, 1990.

insufficiency can result in stretching of the tibial nerve and compression. More frequently hindfoot varus (11%) with a hyperpronated forefoot is often associated with tarsal tunnel syndrome.[56] Rosson et al.[57] found that (1) pronation and plantar flexion significantly increased pressures in the medial and lateral plantar tunnels to levels sufficient to cause chronic nerve compression, (2) a tunnel release and septum excision significantly decreased those pressures, and (3) compared with cadaver pressures, patients had similar tarsal tunnel pressures but higher lateral plantar tunnel pressures in some positions.

History

Symptoms can range from burning and shooting sensations followed by paresthesia to disturbances in temperature perception to mild loss of sensation or tingling over the heel and sole of the foot.[56] Athletes presenting with tarsal tunnel syndrome often report plantar pain and discomfort at the medial ankle, with both being aggravated during sprinting, jumping, and certain martial sports. The symptoms are usually worse during activities and improve while resting. Some patients report pain during the night.

Physical Examination

Because of their implications regarding selection of treatment, any postural deformity should be ruled out (e.g., hindfoot valgus or varus). The entire course of the tibial nerve and its branches must be carefully palpated, and irritability, tingling, and any other discomfort should be sought. Occasionally, the Valleix phenomenon can be reproduced (i.e., tenderness proximal and distal to the entrapment site). Focusing on sensory examination alone is not sufficient because patients frequently do not have sensory loss at the plantar aspect of the foot.[41] Sensory testing of distal sensory branches using the Semmes-Weinstein monofilaments or two-point discrimination can reveal tibial nerve deficits. Motor weakness is difficult to evaluate, especially when assessing the intrinsic muscles. At times, and in cases of chronic tarsal tunnel syndrome, weakness of the abductor hallucis and abductor digiti quinti muscles might be present as reflected by atrophy. Moving the ankle into maximum dorsiflexion or the heel into eversion may increase symptoms as a result of increased tension on the tibial nerve.[58]

Electrodiagnostic studies (e.g., nerve conduction studies, amplitude measurement, motor-evoked potential, fibrillation potentials, and sensory conduction velocities) are recommended to confirm a clinically suspected tarsal tunnel syndrome and to rule out any other neuropathy in the foot. Of all the electrodiagnostic studies, the sensory nerve conduction velocity is believed to be the most accurate study. The sensitivity is reported to be approximately 90%.[54,58,59-62] However, in the presence of a positive history and physical examination, normal findings of an electrodiagnostic study do not exclude the diagnosis of tarsal tunnel syndrome.

Imaging

Conventional radiography (including weight-bearing anteroposterior views of the ankle and dorsoplantar and lateral views of the entire foot) may help detect possible osseous alterations that could predispose to tarsal tunnel syndrome (e.g., malunited fractures of the hindfoot or coalitions). Hindfoot alignment views help estimate the amount of deformity and prepare for any corrective intervention (e.g., supramalleolar or calcaneal osteotomies).[63,64]

If the clinician has any suspicion of a space-occupying lesion, MRI should be taken into consideration. In a study performed by Frey and Kerr,[65] 88% of patients with suspicious tarsal tunnel syndrome revealed that a pathologic condition could be found. However, although imaging signs of direct tibial nerve dysfunction can sometimes be found, it is more likely that the tibial nerve will appear normal on imaging when no specific focal masses are present.[66]

Decision-Making Principles

In the absence of any lesion that could lead to nerve entrapment, nonoperative measures are recommended as the first line of treatment. If no improvement occurs despite use of adequate nonoperative measures, then simple tarsal tunnel release may be warranted. However, in the presence of a space-occupying lesion within the tarsal tunnel, surgical treatment is preferred. An operation should be performed to remove the mass that compresses the tibial nerve. A specific deformity or adjacent disease that is responsible for any tarsal tunnel symptoms should be addressed and either resected or corrected to achieve realignment of the hindfoot and forefoot, respectively.

Treatment Options

Conservative Treatment

Nonoperative measures include administration of NSAIDs to reduce the inflammatory response, oral vitamin B6, and tricyclic antidepressants (e.g., Imipramine, nortriptyline, desipramine, and amitriptyline). In addition, selective serotonin reuptake inhibitors (e.g., sertraline, paroxetine, or duloxetine) or antiseizure drugs (e.g., gabapentin, topiramate, pregabalin, or carbamazepine) can be used to improve symptoms.[56] Currently no clear guidelines for administration are available in the literature. Schon and Mann[66a] recommend using NSAIDs, vitamin B6, 100 mg twice a day, and either amitriptyline (starting with 25 mg at night and gradually increasing to up to 75 mg per night for several months), gabapentin (starting with 75 mg twice a day and progressing up to 150 mg over 2 to 3 weeks) or pregabalin (starting with 100 mg or 300 mg at night and augmenting up to 900 mg three times a day if it is not effective enough at lower dosages). Patients who are uncomfortable with the administration of those medications may be referred to a neurologist. Physical therapy (including desensitization therapy) is useful and might serve to break up scar tissue within the tunnel to assist in mobilization of the constricted nerve. Stretching exercises should be avoided because they could aggravate tibial nerve symptoms.[67]

Local steroid injection into the area of the tibial nerve and the use of stirrup braces, off-the-shelf boot braces, or a short-leg walking cast may be successful means to treat tarsal tunnel syndrome. In case of any postural abnormality, orthotics could be used to place the foot in a more plantigrade position and to unload the medial longitudinal arch.[54,56,68]

Surgical Treatment

AUTHORS' PREFERRED TECHNIQUE

Tarsal Tunnel Syndrome

The patient is placed in the supine position. A tourniquet is used and inflated up to 280 mm Hg. Alternatively, no tourniquet is used. The advantage of using a tourniquet is that veins and arteries can easily be visualized during surgery and thus proper hemostasis can be performed.

A curved incision starting 10 cm proximal to the tip of the medial malleolus and 2 cm posterior to the tibial margin is performed and directed distally, crossing the course of the posterior tibial tendon to end up over the midportion of the abductor hallucis longus muscle (Fig. 113-8, *A*). The flexor retinaculum is exposed, and the retinaculum is released. In the distal aspect of the tarsal tunnel, the retinaculum becomes dense and taut. Therefore, to avoid any other underlying neurovascular structure, a curved clamp can be inserted and the retinaculum incised. After release of the retinaculum, the tibial nerve is explored proximally by blunt dissection and traced distally until reaching the bifurcation of branches. The medial plantar nerve is followed distally around the medial malleolus and beneath the abductor hallucis muscle belly (Fig. 113-8, *B*). At this point a fibrous tunnel or septum needs to be split to release the nerve branch. Care is necessary because large veins accompany the nerve on its course distally into the foot. The lateral plantar nerve is traced distally and slightly posterior to the medial malleolus. Quite frequently the nerve can be identified at the edge of the abductor hallucis. The superficial fascia over the muscle is released. The abductor is reflected plantarly and the deep fascia of the abductor released to relieve the first posterior branch of

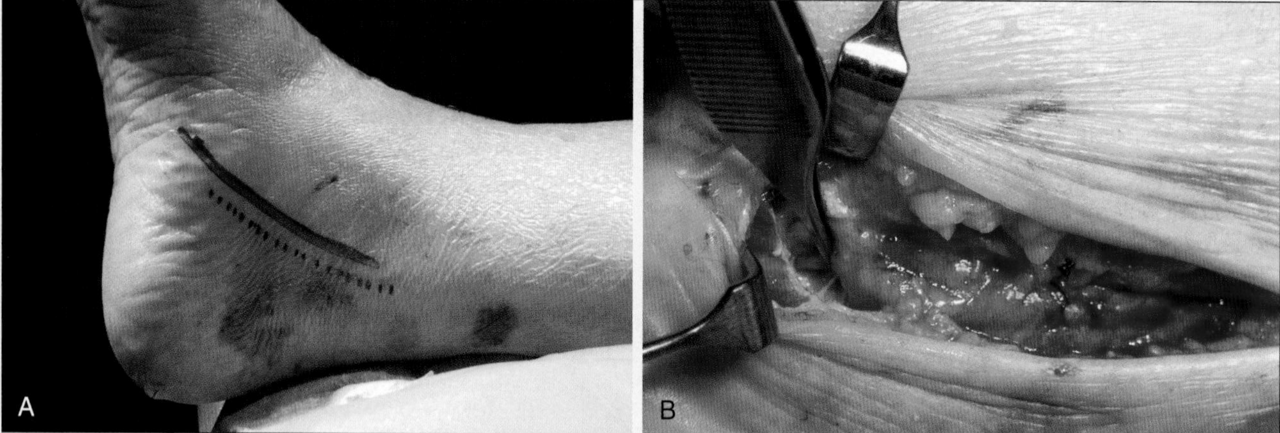

FIGURE 113-8 **A,** The surgical approach to the tarsal tunnel is outlined. Depending on the nerve branches involved, a slightly more anterior or posterior position of the skin incision should be chosen. In this case a position a little bit more anterior has been chosen to release the main tibial nerve. **B,** The tarsal tunnel has been released and the tibial nerve has been decompressed.

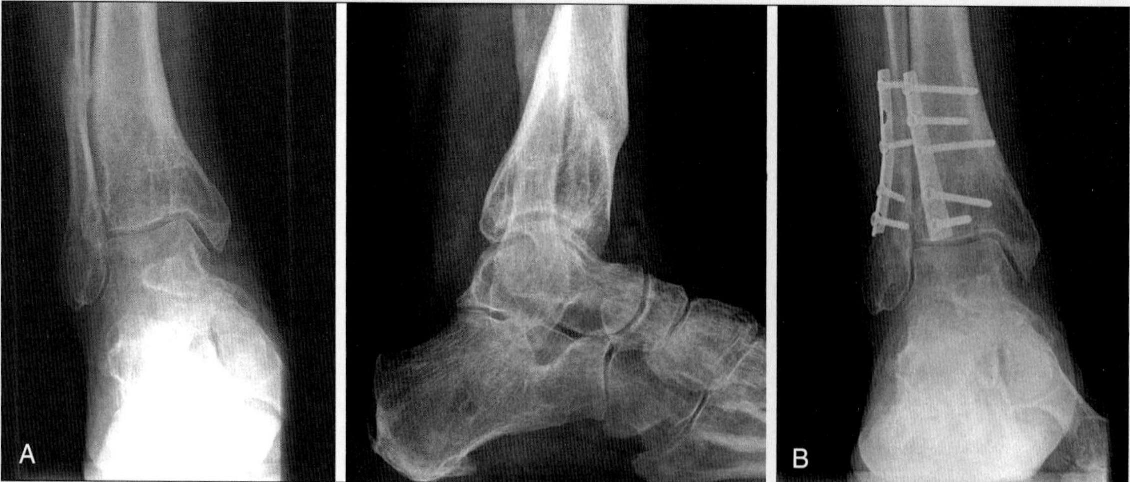

FIGURE 113-9 **A,** A 64-year-old male patient who had both posttraumatic ankle arthrosis and tarsal tunnel syndrome. To compensate for the clearly visible varus deformity, the patient exerted too much eversion at the subtalar joint, with subsequent stretching of the tibial nerve. **B,** The postoperative radiographs. A supramalleolar osteotomy has been performed, along with a tarsal tunnel release. One year after surgery the patient was completely pain free and very satisfied. Realignment resulted in unloading of the ankle as well as the subtalar joint.

the lateral plantar nerve. The lateral plantar nerve provides the nerve to the abductor digiti minimi muscle. Frequently this nerve leaves the lateral plantar nerve before the latter passes under the abductor hallucis muscle belly. The medial calcaneal branch is identified. Any constricting tissue should be released. When additional hindfoot alignment is present, this should be corrected (Fig. 113-9). After tarsal tunnel release, it is necessary to release the tourniquet prior to closure and obtain meticulous hemostasis to prevent new compression.

In cases of so-called *adhesive neuralgia* (i.e., pain from a nerve scarred to surrounding tissue), a revision nerve release should be performed first. This procedure is very delicate because the nerve could be tethered very closely to the scar and thus be damaged during preparation. The saphenous vein is harvested and its small side branch vessels are tied off. Usually the entire saphenous vein must be harvested up to the knee. The ends of the vein are tied and the vein is filled with a Marcaine and saline solution. Afterward the vein is cut longitudinally and wrapped around the nerve. The inner lumen should be placed to the side of the nerve. Each turn is secured by means of a simple suture using 7-0 Vicryl. After wrapping, the surgeon must ensure that no binding of the wrap and nerve is present.

Postoperative Management

After complete decompression of the tibial nerve, a non–weight-bearing short leg cast should be applied in neutral position for 2 weeks. Afterward the cast is removed and the patient is encouraged to return to activities of daily living without having any rehabilitation. Return to sports activities is allowed 3 months after the operation.

Results

When a well-localized lesion is present (e.g., a lipoma or ganglion), the clinical results are quite satisfactory in terms of symptomatic relief. Simple tarsal tunnel release is successful in approximately 75% of all patients. Twenty-five percent obtain little or no relief. Many studies in the literature prove the unpredictable character of surgically performed tarsal tunnel release.[50,69-71]

In a review of 24 articles that included 122 patients, Cimino[42] was able to show that in 91% of all cases a good and improved result was achieved after tarsal tunnel release. Seven percent had poor results, and in 2% a recurrence had been found. Kinoshita et al.[49] treated 41 patients and found no functional deficit after a minimal follow-up of 24 months. The same author presented the results after tarsal tunnel release in athletes after a mean follow-up of 59 months. Twenty-two percent (4 of 18 patients) were not able to return to their preoperative athlete level.[50] Sammarco and Chang[72] presented results of 62 patients who have been treated. The duration of symptoms averaged 31 months. After a mean time interval of 9 months, the patients were able to return to their former activity level.[72] Kim et al.[73] have performed one of the largest studies on this topic. After a mean follow-up time of 33 years, 135 cases have been reviewed. Among these cases, 94 included tibial nerve lesions without discontinuity that were treated with neurolysis.[73] Eighty-one percent (76 patients) of those patients had a good to excellent result. Similar results have been presented by Carrel and coworkers[74] in a series of 200 patients.

Lateral Plantar Nerve Entrapment

One of the problems with lateral plantar nerve entrapment (including the calcaneal branches) is that it could mimic nonspecific heel pain, misleading physicians and thus resulting in great annoyance of patients and practitioners as well.[75] The diagnosis is mainly based on clinical findings. Among all patients who experience chronic unresolving heel pain, up to 20% are thought to have an entrapment of the first branch of the lateral plantar nerve. No predominance is found regarding the activity level of the affected persons. Most frequently, runners and joggers are affected by this type of disease, with a young and male preponderance (80% to 90%).[76] Other sports activities related to the problem include soccer, dance, baseball, basketball, and tennis.

Anatomically, the first branch of the lateral plantar nerve runs between the fascia of the abductor hallucis muscle and the quadratus plantae in an oblique direction. The first branch then divides into three branches that innervate the periosteum of the medial process of the calcaneal tuberosity, the flexor digitorum brevis muscle, the plantar ligament, and the abductor digiti minimi muscle.[10]

In contrast, the calcaneal branches of the lateral plantar nerve provide sensation to the medial aspect of the calcaneus. The medial calcaneal nerve originates from the medial plantar nerve. Approximately 70% of medial calcaneal nerves originate proximal to the tarsal tunnel, and 60% of them reveal multiple branches. Chronic heel pain may be due to problems located at the calcaneal branches.[76-79]

Przylucki and Jones[79a] and Baxter[80] both located the site of entrapment of the first branch of the lateral plantar nerve between the fascia of the abductor hallucis muscle and the medial plantar margin of the quadratus plantae. Excessive pronation can cause stretching of the nerve branch. Edema within the abductor hallucis muscle as a result of repetitive stress or inflammation from chronic pressure can augment pressure within the compartment and compromise the nerve as it courses underneath the plantar ligament or at the osseous canal between the calcaneus and the flexor digitorum brevis. Other causes encompass hypertrophy of the quadratus plantae muscle or accessory muscles, and abnormal bursae and phlebitis within the venous plexus have been described to be the cause of entrapment neuropathy (see Fig. 113-7).[75,81-83]

Calcaneal nerve branch entrapment might occur as a result of calcaneal neuromas or true medial calcaneal nerve neuroma (as a result of transection from a previous surgery). Rarely, accessory muscles of the soleus muscles or flexor hallucis longus muscle result in overstretching and entrapment of the nerves beneath the muscle masses.[77]

History

More proximal and distal nerve entrapments must be excluded. Patients report chronic heel pain, which is aggravated during walking and running. Patients may report heel pain in the morning when taking their first few steps. The pain radiates from the medial inferior aspect of the heel proximally into the medial area of the ankle or laterally and plantar into the foot.[34,56] In contrast to patients with plantar fasciitis, whose pain is more directly plantar, the presence of a more medial location of pain is typical for this condition.

In cases of calcaneal nerve entrapment, the diagnosis is a bit more difficult to establish because variation exists regarding location, origin, and course. Nonetheless, physicians are confronted with the fact that sometimes a medial calcaneal nerve branch might arise from the medial plantar nerve.

Physical Examination

Tenderness (i.e., reproducible symptoms and radiation of pain proximally and distally from the spot) over the first branch of the lateral plantar nerve deep to the abductor hallucis muscle is highly suspicious for the presence of lateral plantar nerve entrapment. Patients may also have pain over the origin of the plantar fascia, which does not rule out concomitant compression of the first branch of the lateral plantar nerve.

Imaging

The same imaging techniques presented for the tarsal tunnel syndrome could be applied for lateral plantar nerve entrapment. However, it should be pointed out that clinical examination is crucial to establish the correct diagnosis.

The following differential diagnoses should be considered in patients with lateral plantar nerve entrapment:

- Plantar fasciitis
- Fasciitis or tendinitis of the origin of the abductor hallucis muscle
- Periostitis
- Stress fracture of the calcaneus
- Tarsal tunnel syndrome
- Systemic arthritides

Decision-Making Principles

The problem of lateral plantar nerve entrapment is that it is often misdiagnosed or not diagnosed. Many patients are treated for plantar fasciitis instead of the nerve disease, and thus the delay until proper treatment is initiated can be up to 2 years after the initial presentation of symptoms. In case of a highly suspicious clinical finding or in patients who have not responded to nonoperative management after 6 to 12 months, surgery might be warranted.

Treatment Options

Similar to the treatment strategies presented for tarsal tunnel syndrome, nonoperative measures to improve the condition in athletes experiencing lateral plantar nerve entrapment include rest, NSAIDs, contrast baths, ice massage, physical therapy, and steroid injections. A shock-absorbing heel pad could help diminish inflammation and pressure. Excessive pronation can be inhibited by means of orthotic devices. Conservative treatment should be used for 12 to 18 months because more than half of patients require more than 6 months before maximum improvement is achieved.[4] Surgical management is described in the box below.

AUTHORS' PREFERRED TECHNIQUE

Lateral Plantar Nerve Entrapment

The patient is placed in the supine position. I use a tourniquet at the ankle. A 5-cm skin incision is made along the course of the lateral plantar nerve (medially over the heel over abductor hallucis muscle; Fig. 113-10). Subcutaneous dissection is followed by incision and splitting of the superficial fascia of the abductor hallucis muscle. The abductor hallucis muscle is reflected plantarly by means of a small retractor; with this technique the deep fascia can be visualized and released. The muscle is then reflected superiorly and the remainder of the deep fascia (where the nerve gets entrapped) is released. Sometimes the medial aspect of the plantar fascia must be released to identify the proper fascial plane between the deep abductor fascia and plantar fascia.

In cases of calcaneal nerve entrapment, the lateral plantar nerve needs to be traced deep and distally into the heel. The calcaneal nerve branches are located superficial to the abductor muscle. The large nerve branch ramifies into the skin of the medial and plantar aspect of the heel. Accessory muscles need to be resected at their bulky portion.

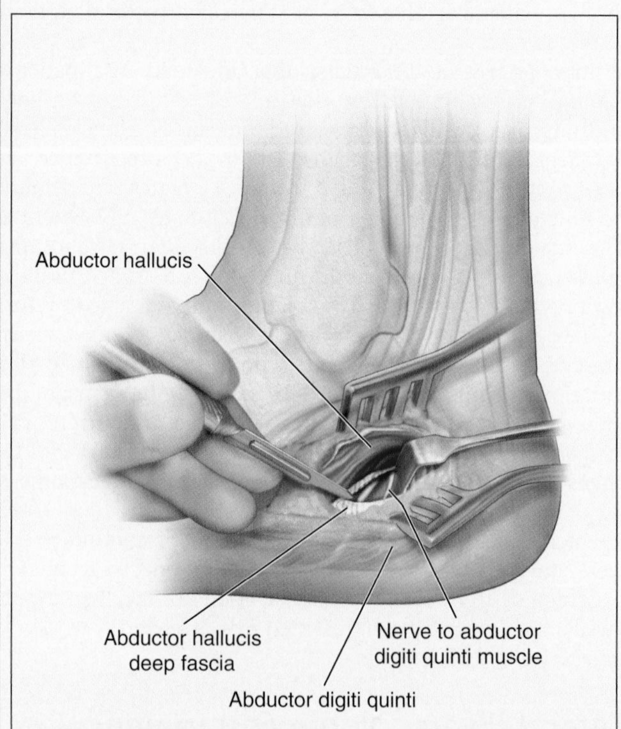

FIGURE 113-10 The surgical approach to the lateral plantar nerve and its branches.

Postoperative Management

The foot is placed in a cast in neutral position. The cast is worn for 2 weeks and the patient should not bear weight during this time. The sutures are removed 2 weeks after the operation and the patient is then allowed to bear weight as tolerated. Return to sports might be possible 10 to 12 weeks after undergoing surgery.

Results

Baxter and Pfeffer[84] reported excellent and good results in 89% of patients and complete resolution in 83% of patients. Watson and coworkers[85] presented similar results (88% good to excellent), but in conjunction with a partial plantar fasciotomy. In their study, 7% reported fair results and the remainder had a poor outcome. The mean time until resumption of sports activities was found to average 3 months for athletes.[4]

Limited information is available in the literature regarding surgical treatment of entrapped calcaneal nerve branches. However, Schon[86] and Gould[41] reported good to excellent results in 75% of cases.

Complications

Notable complications are reported in the literature. Inadvertent transection of the medial calcaneal nerve results in numbness along the medial and plantar aspect of the heel and, in the worst case, could promote the development of a painful neuroma. However, although potential nerve injuries can occur, the overall rate is low. In the study presented by Watson et al.,[85] one case of wound dehiscence (1%) was found and one patient (1%) experienced a deep vein thrombosis.

Medial Plantar Nerve Entrapment

The incidence or demographic predilection of medial plantar nerve entrapment is not known. Among athletes, joggers are mostly affected, which is how this pathologic entity gained its eponym: jogger's foot. Dancers and gymnasts may also experience medial plantar nerve entrapment.

Anatomically, the medial plantar nerve courses underneath the flexor retinaculum and then deep to the abductor hallucis muscle. It then runs on the plantar surface of the flexor digitorum longus muscle while traversing the knot of Henry. Along the tendon of the flexor digitorum longus tendon, it spreads into its branches.[11]

Henry's knot is the typical site of compression and entrapment. Hyperpronation or excessive valgus while walking or running stresses the region of Henry's knot. Additionally, external compression through medial arch supports could compress the medial plantar nerve.[34,87]

History

Patients often report shooting pain along the medial longitudinal arch, sometimes radiating into the medial three toes and proximally into the ankle; the pain is often worse when running. At times, especially after exercise, sensation can be impaired.

Physical Examination

Inspection allows judging of any postural abnormality, such as hindfoot valgus. Palpation along the medial plantar nerve may reproduce medial arch pain possibly associated with radiation, dysesthesia, and/or paresthesia to the medial three toes. Sometimes it may be difficult to distinguish between neuralgia and tendinitis. Heel rise or eversion of the heel tightens the adductor hallucis brevis muscle and aggravates symptoms.

Imaging

See the section on imaging for tarsal tunnel syndrome.

Decision-Making Principles

Based on the current leading opinions of experts in this field, once medial nerve entrapment has been diagnosed, it should be treated surgically rather than conservatively.

Treatment Options

Conservative Treatment

Measures include removal of disturbing or compressive orthotic devices and adjustment of the athlete's training.

Surgical Treatment

The patient is placed in a supine position. A 6- to 10-cm skin incision is made plantar to the talonavicular joint and parallel to the floor. The superficial fascia of the abductor hallucis muscle is split and the muscle is reflected plantarly followed by release of the deep fascia. The knot of Henry needs to be exposed and the naviculocalcaneal ligament released.

Postoperative Management

The foot is placed in a cast in neutral position for 2 weeks and the patient should not bear weight on the foot during this time. The sutures are removed 2 weeks after the operation and the patient is then allowed to bear weight as tolerated. Return to sports might be possible 10 to 12 weeks after the operation.

Superficial Peroneal Nerve Entrapment

Entrapment of the superficial peroneal nerve is a rare condition and was first described by Henry in 1945.[88,89] The typical athlete affected by superficial peroneal nerve entrapment is a runner with an average age of less than 30 years. No gender preponderance has been identified. Superficial peroneal nerve entrapment may also occur in persons performing stop-and-go sports activities. Approximately 25% of patients reveal a traumatic event before symptoms commence (most often an ankle sprain).[90]

The superficial peroneal nerve is a branch of the common peroneal nerve. It provides motor innervation to the peroneus longus and brevis muscles along its course within the anterolateral compartment. Approximately 10 cm above the tip of the fibula, the nerve pierces the fascia and becomes subcutaneous. It then divides into two branches (the intermediate and the medial dorsal cutaneous nerves), which provide

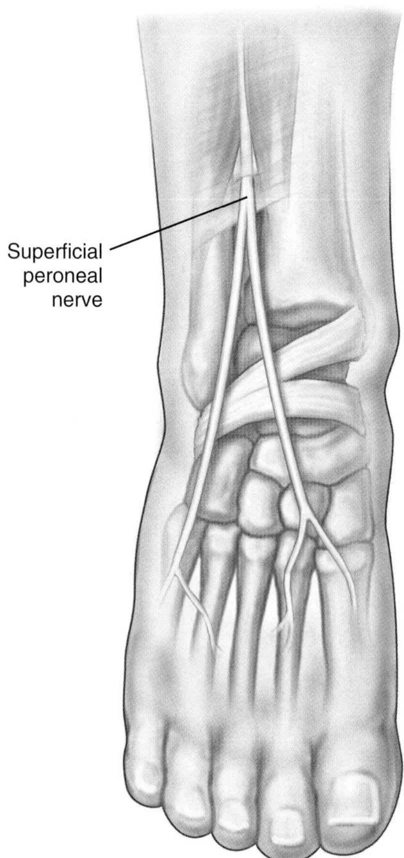

FIGURE 113-11 A frequent site of superficial peroneal nerve entrapment is the spot where the nerve pierces the fascia to become anterior.

sensation to the dorsum of the foot (including the medial distal aspect of the greater toe to fifth toe; see Figs. 113-1 and 113-5).[91]

The site where the superficial peroneal nerve exits the fascia is a typical location of entrapment (Fig. 113-11).[92] In addition, chronic ankle sprains could lead to stretching of the superficial peroneal nerve and induce a focal lesion.[93] The presence of exostoses or osteochondromas may result in impingement anywhere along the course of the nerve. Other causes include entrapment within scar tissue after previous anterior compartment fasciotomy, direct hit by blunt trauma, ganglion formations, fibular fractures (including iatrogenic damage to the nerve as a result of surgery), exertional compartment syndrome, fascial defects,[88] syndesmotic sprains, lower extremity edema, neoplasia, and idiopathic causes.[4] Postural deformities, such as hindfoot varus, result in greater risk of sustaining ankle sprains or may predispose the person to chronic ankle instability.

History

Affected persons report a long-standing history of pain similar to an ankle sprain that failed to resolve; this pain is found over the anterolateral border of the shank (the mid to distal third) and might radiate down over the dorsum of the foot. The latter can be a single symptom without the presence of pain at the anterolateral border of the shank. Approximately one third of patients report numbness and paresthesia along the course of the superficial peroneal nerve. Pain is often aggravated with physical activity, such as jogging, walking, running, kneeling, and squatting. Twenty-five percent of patients have a positive history of prior ankle sprains or chronic ankle instability.[94]

Physical Examination

Before assessing the lower limb, examination of the lumbar spine is required to rule out any spinal disorder that could be responsible for leg pain (e.g., disk herniation). The lower leg should be inspected for any varus deformity or scar that could indicate a potential site of nerve entrapment. Proximal entrapment of the common peroneal nerve is examined by palpating the subcapital region of the fibular head. To identify any entrapment at the fascial exit of the superficial peroneal nerve, the examiner palpates the anterolateral region of the calf approximately 10 cm proximal to the tip of the fibula. Paresthesia and numbness after external compression are suggestive for entrapment. In addition, three tests to identify possible superficial nerve entrapment could help to assess[89] (1) active dorsiflexion and eversion against resistance while the nerve impingement site is palpated; (2) plantar flexion and inversion against resistance without pressure over the nerve; and (3) plantar flexion and inversion against resistance with pressure along the course of the nerve.[92,95-97]

Localized injection of anesthetic at the site of maximal tenderness could be a diagnostic and therapeutic measure.

Nerve conduction studies in the superficial peroneal nerve are performed in a standardized fashion, and positive results are obtained in nearly 98% of patients. Nerve conduction studies should be reserved for situations in which the diagnosis is in question. However, studies have shown reproducible and consistent changes to conduction velocity in the superficial peroneal nerve in cases of impingement. Other studies have shown increased latencies and attenuation of action potentials. Be aware that normal nerve conduction studies do not rule out superficial peroneal nerve involvement and must be seen as an adjunctive tool in establishing the diagnosis.

Imaging

A standardized workup includes anteroposterior and lateral views of the entire lower leg to assess bony impingement as a result of injury or prior fracture. A CT scan may provide more detailed information if bony involvement in the impingement is suspected after plain radiography. MRI can be useful to define soft tissue involvement and might be used to examine the passage of the nerve through the crural fascia or to assess nerve-compressing soft tissue lesions. Ultrasound can be helpful to identify a cystic mass impinging on the nerve. Because the superficial peroneal nerve does not have an accompanying vascular structure, it can be difficult to localize with MRI or ultrasound without a good appreciation of its expected anatomic course.

Decision-Making Principles

The superficial peroneal nerve is less responsive to conservative treatment than is the deep peroneal nerve. However, once entrapment of the superficial peroneal nerve is diagnosed, nonoperative measures should be tried first before embarking on surgical treatment. No recommendations are available regarding how long conservative measures should be tried. It is my experience that one should wait at least 6 months before deciding whether surgery is warranted.

Treatment Options

Conservative Treatment

Nonoperative measures include strengthening exercises of the peroneal muscles and should focus on range of motion. To prevent inversion of the ankle, a supportive ankle brace or lateral heel and sole wedges in the shoe could be applied to reduce the varus thrust. Occasionally dorsiflexion night splints can be of benefit. Cortisone injections with or without the addition of local anesthetic agents may help reduce symptoms. However, the latter can never be seen as a causal cure.[3,4,89,90,94]

Surgical Treatment

If conservative treatment fails, surgery is warranted. In such a case, superficial nerve release is performed. Release of the nerve is performed at its site of entrapment, and therefore no specific type of surgery can be proposed in this chapter. However, my technique of nerve decompression is described in the box below.

AUTHORS' PREFERRED TECHNIQUE

Superficial Peroneal Nerve Entrapment

The patient is placed in the lateral decubitus or supine position. The more distal and anterior the site of entrapment, the more supine the placement of the patient. A 10-cm skin incision is made over the area of maximum tenderness (this area should be assessed before surgery without anesthesia). The nerve is identified and the compressive structure is released and/or removed (Fig. 113-12). I always release the fascia—a common site of entrapment or compression—to relieve the nerve.

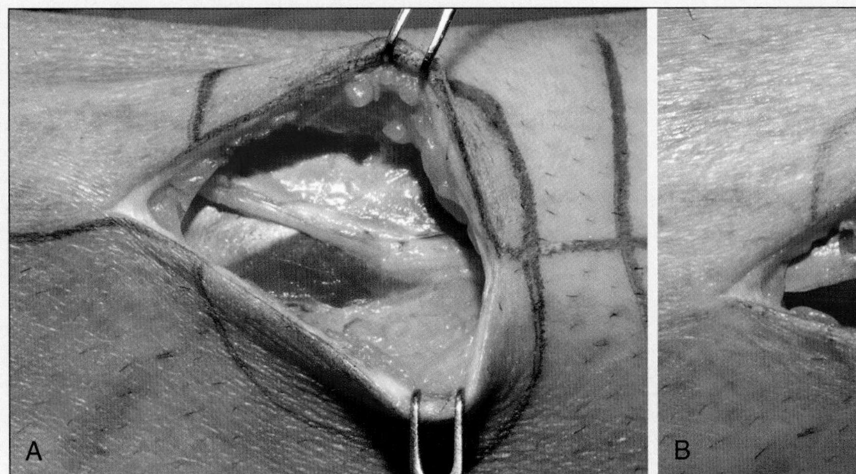

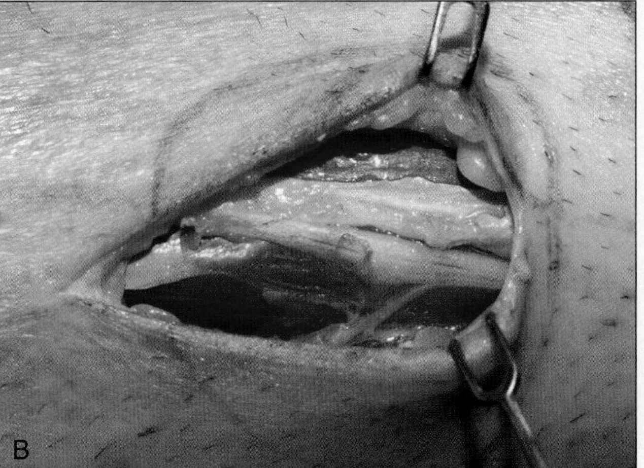

FIGURE 113-12 **A,** A fascial entrapment of the superficial peroneal nerve within a scar that has developed as a result of previous surgery (endoscopic compartment release). **B,** After release of the scar tissue, fasciotomy, and careful mobilization of the nerve.

Postoperative Management

The patient wears a compressive wrap or splint for 2 weeks until the sutures are removed. The patient is allowed to ambulate as tolerated 3 to 4 days after surgery. Three weeks after the operation, activities can be resumed. Return to sports may take up to 8 and 12 weeks.

Results

Although decompression of the superficial nerve yields improvement in 75% of patients, the results are less predictable for athletes. Styf[89] reported that only 9 of the 19 patients in his series were completely satisfied with the procedure. It appears that chronic irreversible damage to the nerve can occur in this condition. In case of persisting symptoms after release, repeat exploration and transection and burial into muscle as well should be considered.[89]

Deep Peroneal Nerve Entrapment

Historically, Kopell and Thompson[98] first described entrapment of the deep peroneal nerve in 1960. Marinacci[99] termed the pathologic findings "anterior tarsal tunnel syndrome" with involvement of either the motor or sensory component. Typically, runners are the affected population.[3,100,101]

The course of the deep peroneal nerve is complex and deserves specific attention. As a branch of the common peroneal nerve, it tracks within the proximal third of the calf and lies between the muscle bellies of the tibialis anterior and

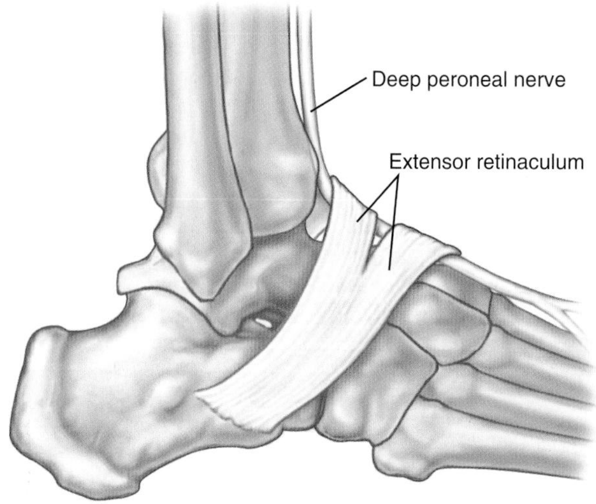

FIGURE 113-13 The deep peroneal nerve can become entrapped under the inferior extensor retinaculum.

extensor digitorum longus muscles. The anterior tibial artery accompanies the nerve. When entering the distal third of the calf, the nerve runs between the extensor hallucis and extensor digitorum longus (5 cm above the joint line), secondary to the oblique path of the extensor hallucis longus tendon that travels medially. The deep peroneal nerve provides motor innervation to the tibialis anterior, the extensor digitorum communis, and the extensor hallucis longus muscles. At the level of the ankle joint, the nerve sends a branch to the extensor digitorum brevis muscle while the other sensory branch delivers sensation to the first web space (see Fig. 113-5).[10,11,102]

Most commonly the sensory branch of the deep peroneal nerve gets entrapped underneath the inferior extensor retinaculum (Fig. 113-13) and is the site of the so-called *anterior tarsal tunnel syndrome*. Entrapment may also occur at the superior edge of the inferior extensor retinaculum and at a location where the extensor hallucis longus tendon crosses the nerve. Osteophytes at the talonavicular joint, pes cavovarus, improper footwear (e.g., tight ski boots) and trauma (repetitive ankle sprains) are possible causes for deep peroneal nerve entrapment.[103-111]

History

In general, patients report dorsal foot pain and disturbances of sensation at the first web space. The classic anterior tarsal tunnel syndrome is characterized by pain or burning sensations over the dorsum of the foot and may result in atrophy and weakness of the extensor digitorum longus muscle. A few patients report paresthesia in the first dorsal web space. Symptoms may be aggravated by physical activity, especially with the foot held in plantar flexion, a position that places stretch on the nerve and compresses the contents of the anterior tarsal tunnel against the dorsal aspect of the talonavicular joint. The pain resolves with rest. Pain at night has been described.[105] These symptoms can also be seen in patients with exertional anterolateral compartment syndrome, and this condition can be an underlying cause of nerve compression exacerbated with activity.[112] Pain might be associated with specific footwear or a specific activity.

Physical Examination

Palpation along the course of the deep peroneal nerve may reveal the spot of highest nerve irritation and identifies any alteration of sensation. In addition, the presence of osteophytes and other foot abnormalities should be evaluated.[34] The proximal course of the nerve near the fibular neck should also be examined because tenderness is often elicited with percussion (the Tinel sign) at the site of entrapment or along the course of the nerve distally. Forceful plantar flexion and inversion of the ankle stretches the nerve and decreases the available space in the anterior tarsal tunnel, resulting in compression of the nerve against the floor of the tunnel. This maneuver may provoke symptoms over the dorsum of the foot.[107,113] A careful motor examination is also indicated, as previously mentioned. The subtle weakness caused by decreased innervation or loss of innervation to the extensor digitorum brevis is often difficult to appreciate. Palpating the extensor digitorum brevis during active dorsiflexion of the toes may detect loss of the contribution of this muscle.

Electrodiagnostic studies may be useful in diagnosing deep peroneal nerve entrapment and determining involvement of the extensor digitorum brevis (indicating a lesion proximal to the inferior retinaculum).[114] Electrodiagnostic studies are able to reveal increased latency and reduced motor recruitment of the extensor digitorum brevis muscle. However, in a study performed by Rosselle et al.[114a] abnormal signals have been found in approximately 76% of asymptomatic persons, along with decreased extensor digitorum brevis motor recruitment in 38% of asymptomatic persons.

In patients in whom an exercise-induced compartment syndrome is suspected, exercise testing with or without measurement of compartment pressures should be considered.

Imaging

Plain radiographs are able to demonstrate the presence of dorsal osteophytes (on the lateral view of the foot), particularly at the talonavicular joint, which could impinge against the nerve or lead to space obliteration in the anterior ankle compartment. Conventional radiographs can also help detect fractures, bone fragments, or soft tissue swelling near the course of the nerve. MRI has a limited role in diagnosis of the condition but becomes important when the problem is believed to be a result of impingement from an adjacent mass.[25,66,115]

Treatment Options

Conservative Treatment

The goal is to reduce pressure or eliminate compressive forces at the dorsum of the foot that could harm the deep peroneal nerve. Conservative treatment usually includes proper footwear adaptation (i.e., it should be accommodative, avoiding any external pressure over the nerve). NSAIDs, vitamin B6, tricyclic antidepressants, gabapentin, Lidocaine patches, or analgesic creams (e.g., Capsaicin) can modulate nerve pain. Corticosteroid injections have been reported to be useful to reduce nerve irritation. Sometimes orthotics should be considered to correct flexible flatfoot deformities.[90,116]

Surgical Treatment

AUTHORS' PREFERRED TECHNIQUE

Deep Peroneal Nerve Entrapment

The patient is placed in a supine position on the operating table. Before surgery the maximum point of tenderness should be assessed and marked with a pen so the correct spot is decompressed. A 5- to 10-cm skin incision is made. In cases of classic anterior tarsal tunnel syndrome, the retinaculum is released. Release should be performed at the site of compression and not more—that is, the entire retinaculum should not be released, because this maneuver could result in bowstringing of the anterior tibial or other extensor tendons. A Z-shaped incision of the retinaculum allows lengthening and tension-free closure. Any bony exostosis must be removed. Any hindfoot deformity should be corrected. In addition, if ankle instability is present, ankle ligament reconstruction combined with a lateralizing calcaneal osteotomy should be considered. In cases of anterior compartment syndrome, a fasciotomy should be performed. If the extensor hallucis brevis is the cause of nerve entrapment, a segmental resection of the muscle belly is needed along with release of the deep fascia in the midfoot.

Postoperative Management

The lower limb is put into a cast for 1 week. The cast should be applied in a neutral position. Walking with crutches is recommended for 1 week. After that period, gradual resumption of weight bearing is allowed as tolerated. Training can be resumed 4 to 6 weeks after the operation. When an extensive surgical procedure is performed, a boot should be worn for 4 weeks and training resumed 8 weeks after the operation.

Results

Surgical decompression might yield excellent and good results in approximately 80% of patients, but approximately 20% do not improve at all.[117] However, structural nerve damage is related to poor outcomes, and simple decompression may not be enough to resolve symptoms. In the latter case, nerve resection might be an option. Resection and translocation of the nerves into the anterolateral compartment yields excellent results in more than 80% of patients. Segmental resection of the extensor hallucis brevis together with a transfer to the extensor hallucis longus yields good to excellent pain relief more than 6 months after the operation. Liu et al.[111] have reviewed 10 patients who have been treated for deep peroneal nerve entrapment or its branches and have studied the anatomy of the tunnel in 25 adult feet. Results of operative decompression in nine feet of eight patients were successful at follow-up of 1.5 and 4 years.[111]

Interdigital Neuralgia (Morton's Neuroma)

The clinical symptoms of interdigital neuroma were first described by Civinni in 1835 and thereafter by Durlacher.[118] Morton, whose name is attached to the condition, mistakenly attributed the cause to a pathologic fourth MTP joint and noted relief of symptoms with resection of the fourth metatarsal head. The term "neuroma" is incorrect and, in my opinion, the condition should instead be called interdigital neuralgia. The nerve is the structure that is affected because of perineural fibrosis. Interdigital neuralgia is a common condition found in daily orthopaedic practice; it has the potential of becoming very debilitating, impairing quality of life. Its incidence has been calculated to be 50.2 for men and 87.5 for women with regard to the annual age standardized rates per 100,000 of new presentations in primary care. Interdigital neuromas are frequently found to be unilateral, but 15% of patients experience a bilateral occurrence. The simultaneous development of two adjacent interdigital neuromas in the same foot occurs in only 3% of patients. Twice as many neuromas are found in the third web space as in the second web space. Interdigital neuromas in the fourth web space are rare.

Although many studies support the hypothesis of entrapment neuropathy beneath the transverse metatarsal ligament, other factors are also able to promote the formation of a primary interdigital neuroma, resulting in uncertainty about its cause. Thus a multifactorial process must be considered more likely. Anatomic, traumatic, and extrinsic causes all have been discussed as promoting the development of an interdigital neuroma. In addition, some conditions could mimic symptoms seen in patients with interdigital neuroma.[119,120] Therefore, before embarking on any treatment, it is important to identify the exact cause of a symptomatic interdigital neuroma. Identifying the cause is even more important and complex in the presence of a recurrent interdigital neuroma.

Pathomechanism and Etiologies

The hypothesis of intrinsic nerve disease beyond simple compression by the intermetatarsal ligament is well accepted.[121] On an ultrastructural level, the nerve undergoes the following alterations: thickening of the perineurium and deposition of amorphous eosinophilic material built up by filaments of tubular structures; demyelinization and degeneration of nerve fibers without signs of Wallerian degeneration; local initial hyperplasia of unmyelinated nerves followed by degeneration; intraneural fibrosis and sclerohyalinosis; and increase of elastic fibers within the stroma. Those changes are induced either by anatomic, traumatic, or extrinsic factors, which will be discussed in detail.[122,123]

Anatomic factors include variants with communicating branches within the third web space connecting the lateral plantar nerve and medial plantar nerve that result in a thickening of the common digital nerve. However, the frequency of such communicating branches has only been found to be about 28%.[78,124] As such, it cannot be the solitary explanation for interdigital neuroma. In addition, the degree of mobility of the first medial three rays in relation to the lateral two rays also plays a role in the development of an interdigital neuralgia. Similar to the hand, the mobility for the lateral two rays is greater when compared with the medial three rays that are firmly attached to the cuneiforms. The greater mobility between the fourth and third ray could result in higher strains and stresses within the nerve and underneath the intermetatarsal ligament. Nevertheless, this type of theory is negated by the fact that interdigital neuralgia could also be found in the second web space.[125] Hyperextension of the toes leads to increased plantar depression of the metatarsal heads. The nerve is tethered and squeezed underneath the intermetatarsal ligament. People with excessive hyperextension at the MTP joints have an 8 to 10 times higher incidence of interdigital neuroma. Other factors include trauma, which might occur in runners, dancers, and athletes in other sports. The increased incidence in those athletes is explained by exposure to repetitive stresses exerted at the metatarsal region.[126] Besides this acute trauma, crush injuries or direct penetration of the forefoot by a sharp object must be included in the differential diagnosis.

Besides anatomic and traumatic factors, extrinsic causes should be discussed. A mass below or above the ligament can apply abnormal pressures on the common interdigital nerve. Such a mass encompasses an inflamed bursa, a ganglion, or a synovial cyst that arises from the MTP joint and a lipoma from the plantar aspect of the foot.[121] Degeneration of the MTP joint can result in a local inflammatory response. In addition, the capsule attenuates and the proximal phalanx of the third toe deviates medially. As a result, the third metatarsal head is pushed laterally against the fourth metatarsal head, compressing the bursa and obliterating the third web space. MTP joint instability itself can exert traction on the capsule and the nerve, inducing pain in approximately 10% to 15% of patients.[127] Ultimately, the intermetatarsal ligament itself is thickened.

Athletes who have sustained a fracture of the metatarsal head and/or neck region that resulted in malunion and altered pressure distribution of the forefoot could also experience interdigital neuralgia.

History

Generally, a thorough history helps one perform a proper clinical examination and make the correct diagnosis. Most patients report plantar pain that is increased when walking (92%) but relieved when either resting (89%) or removing footwear (70%). The pain usually is characterized as burning, tingling, or electric with radiation into the involved toes (62%). Numbness is less frequently reported (40%).[125]

Physical Examination

The foot is grasped with both hands and the plantar interspaces are palpated starting proximal to the metatarsal heads and proceeding more distally. Reproducible pain and paresthesias are highly suspect for the presence of an interdigital neuroma. The Mulder click sign consists of milking the small mass of nerve and bursal tissue between the involved metatarsal heads with alternating thumb and forefinger pressure while simultaneously compressing these same metatarsal heads.[128] The mini-Lachman test is performed to evaluate the MTP joints for possible instability.[129]

Local injection of 1 to 2 mL of local anesthetic into the affected web space may provide pain relief. However, the finding should be interpreted with caution, because a positive result does not habitually reflect the presence of an interdigital neuralgia. Other abnormalities, such as inflammatory processes, MTP joint instability, or degeneration of the plantar plate and/or joint capsule can mimic symptoms of interdigital neuralgia. The result of local injection therefore must always be correlated with the clinical and radiographic findings.

Electrodiagnostic studies are only indicated when a peripheral neuropathy or radiculopathy is suspected.

Imaging

Findings of conventional radiography (standing and weight-bearing dorsoplantar and lateral views of the foot) are often normal but serve to identify any osseous abnormality, subluxation or dislocation of the MTP joints, degenerative or arthritic changes within the MTP joints, or possible evidence of a foreign body (such as fracture fragments).[130]

Debate continues about whether ultrasonography or MRI should be used to diagnose interdigital neuralgia.[131] Ultrasound is user dependent and may result in lower sensitivities and specificities when performed by inexperienced personnel. However, in experienced hands, ultrasound yields a high sensitivity (91% to 100%) and specificity (83% to 100%).[132] More recently, Symeonidis and coworkers[133] were able to demonstrate that ultrasound could lead to overdiagnosis with a high rate of incidental findings in an asymptomatic population having interdigital nerve enlargement. The authors concluded that ultrasound is unreliable unless it is correlated with an equivocal clinical examination and that clinical examination alone remains the gold standard in assessing interdigital neuralgia.[133]

MRI is the primary diagnostic tool to assess interdigital neuralgia and is often used to identify or exclude other pathologic conditions in the forefoot. Recently, Lee[134] presented a retrospective analysis to compare the diagnostic accuracy of both ultrasonography and MRI for the assessment of primary interdigital neuroma. The data were correlated with the surgical and pathologic findings. The detection rate of primary Morton neuroma was 79% for ultrasonography and 76% for MRI. However, even MRI can lead to misinterpretation of the results. Zanetti et al.[134a] and Biasca et al.[134b] were able to demonstrate a 30% prevalence of interdigital neuromas in an asymptomatic population. After comparing their results with a symptomatic group, they concluded that a mass suggestive of interdigital neuroma and larger than 5 mm could be seen as a true interdigital neuroma. Thus even in the presence of highly sophisticated imaging technology, only the combination of symptoms and positive imaging can help establish the correct diagnosis.[135-137]

Decision-Making Principles

In general, only symptomatic athletes should undergo treatment. My preferred algorithm is to start with a conservative (i.e., nonoperative) treatment, which should be continued for at least 6 months. In case of failure, surgical resection should be considered. Generally speaking, smaller sized lesions are more amenable to conservative treatment, whereas larger ones may be treated surgically.

Treatment Options

As previously mentioned, conservative and surgical treatment strategies attempt to resolve pain. Usually nonoperative management should be continued for at least 6 months before embarking on surgery. Although many patients are successfully treated with conservative measures, approximately 70% elect surgical treatment over time because they do not want to have their lives dominated by their foot problem. When selecting surgery, patients must be advised that the success rate after resection rarely exceeds 90% and thus remains limited.

Conservative Treatment

The goal of nonoperative treatment is to alleviate the pressure underneath the metatarsal heads, that is, to achieve proper decompression within the affected web space. This goal is best achieved by means of footwear modifications, including fitting the foot into wide, soft, laced shoes. Soft-heeled shoes are preferred. A metatarsal bar or pad elevates the metatarsal heads and reduces the forefoot pressure. A local injection of a mixture containing Lidocaine and corticosteroids may be added after shoe modifications have been introduced. The effect of combined shoe adaptation and local injections of local anesthetics and steroids is better than the sole use of shoe modifications. However, adverse effects of corticosteroid injections must be kept in mind, which include subcutaneous tissue atrophy and discoloration of the skin, increased wound breakdown, and disruption of the MTP joint capsule with resulting joint instability. When surgery is considered, it should not be performed within 4 weeks after the local injection of steroids.

Radiofrequency ablation and alcohol injections have been reported to be less traumatic, but the literature remains inconclusive. The use of ethanol injection in the treatment of symptomatic interdigital neuralgia remains inconclusive. Recent studies indicated that more than 90% of patients experienced partial or total symptomatic relief after ultrasound-guided injections with alcohol (70% carbocaine-adrenaline and 30% ethylic alcohol).[138-140] Another study showed a high failure rate after local alcohol injections without ultrasound guidance. The authors concluded that alcohol injections that are not guided by ultrasound are not efficacious, and they have abandoned the use of such injections in their clinic.[118]

Surgical Treatment

Nerve Resection

An interdigital neuroma can be excised either through a plantar or dorsal approach. A more recent investigation found no statistically significant differences between plantar and dorsal approaches in terms of outcomes or complications. However,

AUTHORS' PREFERRED TECHNIQUE

Morton's Neuroma: Nerve Resection

I almost always use the dorsal approach. An incision is made in the dorsal aspect of the foot, starting in the web space over the affected common interdigital nerve. The length of the incision varies but averages 3 cm. The dorsal digital nerves are avoided. The incision is deepened through the subcutaneous tissue. The innominate fascia is explored and incised. Afterward a laminar spreader is placed beneath the metatarsal heads (Fig. 113-14, *A*). After spreading, the transverse metatarsal ligament becomes taut and can be split. The spreader is placed a little deeper beneath the metatarsal heads. The nerve is exposed at its proximal aspect. The nerve is traced proximally until it enters intrinsic musculature; then the common digital nerve is cut proximal to the metatarsal heads. The nerve is then dissected out distally past the bifurcation and excised (Fig. 113-14, *B*). One must be sure to remove any accessory branch to either the common or interdigital nerves. The nerve specimen should be sent for histologic examination.

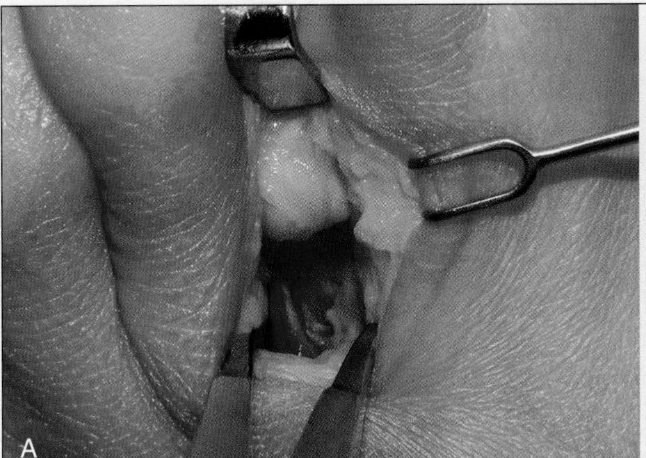

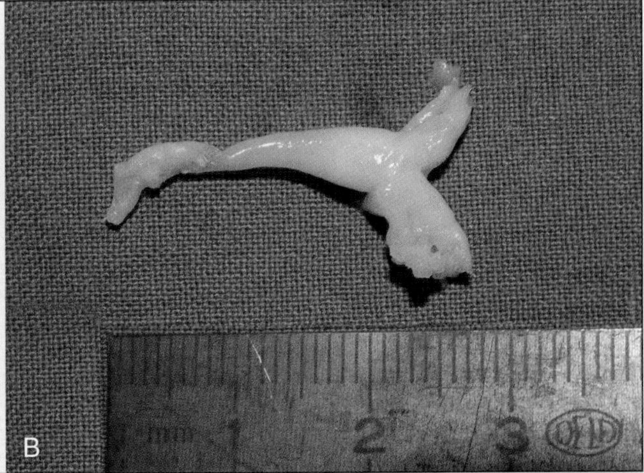

FIGURE 113-14 **A,** The dorsal approach to the intermetatarsal web space. A 3-cm skin incision is made. After transection of the innominate fascia and the transverse ligament, the enlarged interdigital nerve appears. To improve visualization, a laminar spreader is inserted. **B,** The resected nerve. The common interdigital nerve stump can be appreciated on the left. The bifurcation is visible on the right.

supporters of the dorsal approach claim that fewer problems are observed with scar formation. If a keloid develops from any plantar incision, the symptoms can become very difficult to treat.[141,142] I prefer the dorsal approach to treat primary intermetatarsal neuralgia. In case of revision, sometimes a plantar approach is needed, because this approach allows for extensile exposure of the nerve proximally. In the case of revision, the risk of a painful plantar scar is outweighed by the need to ensure adequate resection of the nerve.

Postoperative Management

Patients are allowed to ambulate in a postoperative and stiff-soled shoe for 2 weeks. The sutures are removed 2 weeks after the operation. After 3 to 5 weeks after the operation, the patient can start to work on active and passive range of motion exercises. Return to sports might take up to 6 weeks.

Results

Mann and Reynolds[125] reported that 71% of patients were essentially asymptomatic, 9% were significantly improved, 6% were marginally improved, and 14% resulted in failure. Coughlin and Pinsonneault[143] reported an average good to excellent satisfaction rate of 85%, but 65% were pain free with minor or major footwear restrictions. Akermark et al.,[141] Giannini et al.,[144] and Benedetti et al.[145] have reported similar results. Akermark and co-workers[141] did not find any difference in using the plantar or dorsal approach.

Complications

In patients who have received multiple steroid injections before surgery, soft tissue conditions can be critical, raising the risk of possible wound-healing problems and infection. Resection of adjacent web space neuromas could lead to vascular compromise or deprivation, resulting in increased risk of frostbite in the winter. In case of excessive soft tissue resection during surgery, vascular compromise could theoretically result in necrosis of the involved toe, requiring amputation. A few patients might experience complex regional pain syndrome type 2 after resection of the neuroma.

When using the plantar approach, the incision must be kept strictly between the metatarsals. An improper incision placement is unforgiving. The incision is carried out through the subcutaneous tissue. The common digital nerve is exposed and traced down to the bifurcation. The nerve branches are cut and the specimen sent for pathologic examination.

Surgical neurolysis offers an alternative to nerve resection and can be performed endoscopically or in an open manner. Okafor et al.[146] noted that 72% of patients had complete resolution of pain. In combination with forefoot deformity, the results appeared to deteriorate. Further investigations are needed to judge the true value of neurolysis. However, given that recurrence rates up to 77% have been reported in the literature, neurolysis is not currently recommended by the authors.[146]

For a complete list of references, go to expertconsult.com.

Suggested Readings

Citation: Akermark C, Crone H, Saartok T, et al: Plantar versus dorsal incision in the treatment of primary intermetatarsal Morton's neuroma. *Foot Ankle Int* 29(2):136–141, 2008.
Level of Evidence: III (retrospective, comparative study)
Summary: Regardless of whether a dorsal or plantar approach was chosen for the surgical treatment of painful Morton's neuroma, the clinical and patient satisfaction was comparable among the groups. The authors found significant differences in favor of plantar incisions with regard to residual sensory loss and the number of complications.

Citation: Espinosa N, Seybold JD, Jankauskas L, et al: Alcohol sclerosing therapy is not an effective treatment for interdigital neuroma. *Foot Ankle Int* 32(6):576–580, 2011.
Level of Evidence: IV (retrospective case series)
Summary: In the clinical setting without ultrasound-controlled guidance, alcohol injections for the treatment of painful intermetatarsal Morton's neuroma are not effective.

Citation: Kim DH, Ryu S, Tiel RL, et al: Surgical management and results of 135 tibial nerve lesions at the Louisiana State University Health Sciences Center. *Neurosurgery* 53(5):1114–1124, 2003.
Level of Evidence: IV (retrospective case series)
Summary: In 33 years of clinical and surgical experience with tibial nerve lesions, the authors were able to demonstrate excellent outcomes after surgical exploration and repair. The best results were obtained in patients who had recordable nerve action potentials treated by external neurolysis, whereas patients with larger nerve lesions in continuity or repeat operations as a result of tarsal tunnel syndrome did less well.

Citation: Sammarco GJ, Chang L: Outcome of surgical treatment of tarsal tunnel syndrome. *Foot Ankle Int* 24(2):125–131, 2003.
Level of Evidence: IV (retrospective case series)
Summary: After an average follow-up of 5 years, 108 ankles were reviewed with regard to surgical treatment of tarsal tunnel syndrome. Patients who experienced symptoms for less than 1 year before surgery showed higher outcome scores than did those with long-standing symptoms.

Citation: Zanetti M, Ledermann T, Zollinger H, et al: Efficacy of MR imaging in patients suspected of having Morton's neuroma. *AJR Am J Roentgenol* 168(2):529–532, 1997.
Level of Evidence: II (prospective, diagnostic study)
Summary: Thirty-two patients were prospectively enrolled in this study. In 16 of the 32 patients, additional surgical evaluation of the intermetatarsal spaces was performed. The authors concluded that magnetic resonance imaging is accurate in diagnosing Morton's neuroma and assessing correct localization.

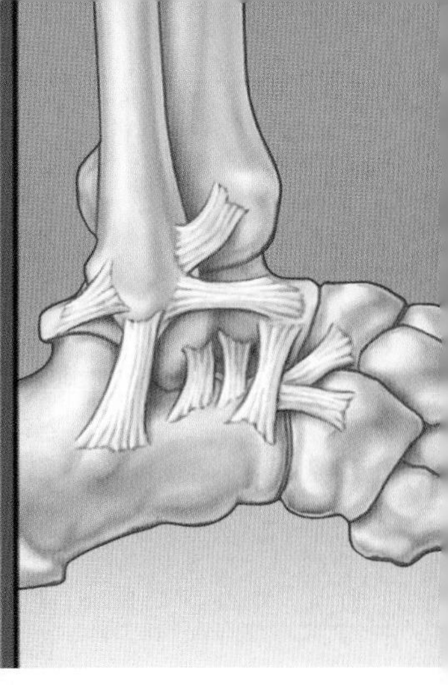

114

Ankle Arthroscopy

REBECCA CERRATO • JOHN CAMPBELL • RACHEL TRICHE

Historically, the ankle joint was believed to be unsuitable for arthroscopy because intraarticular access of this joint is narrow.[1] Takagi[2] and later Watanabe[3] described techniques and pioneered the use of arthroscopy in the examination of the ankle. Compared with open arthrotomy, arthroscopy has recognized benefits of shortened recovery times and limited surgical morbidity. Today, arthroscopy of the foot and ankle has evolved from simply a diagnostic tool to a versatile treatment modality for a variety of pathologies.

It is important to understand the surface and superficial anatomy in the area of the ankle to minimize the risk of damage to the surrounding structures when performing ankle arthroscopy. Important landmarks to identify include the tibialis anterior tendon, the peroneus tertius tendon, the level of the joint line, the superficial peroneal nerve and its branches, and the great saphenous vein. It is also important to understand the location of the deep peroneal nerve and dorsalis pedis artery as they cross the anterior ankle joint. The branches of the superficial peroneal nerve are most commonly injured during this procedure.[4] These branches can be identified and marked prior to the procedure by plantar flexing and inverting the foot.

The anteromedial, anterolateral, and posterolateral portals are most commonly used for ankle arthroscopy. Anterior portal options include the anteromedial, anterolateral, anterocentral, and accessory anteromedial and anterolateral portals. The anteromedial portal is made just medial to the tibialis anterior tendon at the level of the joint line. Confirmation of planned portal placement is recommended with use of an 18-gauge needle to localize and insufflate the joint with approximately 10 mL of saline solution before creating the portal. All portals should be created by making a small incision with a scalpel through the skin only and then using a blunt instrument such as a mosquito clamp to spread the soft tissue down to the capsule. Once the soft tissue is safely cleared, the capsule can be penetrated. This technique helps minimize the risk of damage to overlying structures. An accessory anteromedial portal can be created 1 cm anterior and 0.5 to 1 cm inferior to the medial malleolus.

The anterolateral portal is created under direct visualization once the arthroscope has been introduced through the anteromedial portal. A needle is once again used to confirm portal placement at or just above the level of the joint lateral to the peroneus tertius tendon. The needle can be used to confirm that the portal will allow adequate access to the area being treated before making the skin incision. An accessory anterolateral portal can be placed 1 cm anterior to and at the level of the tip of the distal fibula.

The anterocentral portal carries increased risk of neurovascular damage and thus is not commonly used.[5] It is located between the extensor digitorum tendons, with the deep peroneal nerve and dorsalis pedis artery just medial to this portal, coursing between the extensor hallucis and extensor digitorum communis tendons.

Posterior portals options include posterolateral, trans Achilles, and posteromedial (Fig. 114-1). A posterolateral portal is placed just lateral to the Achilles tendon approximately 1 to 1.5 cm proximal to the tip of the distal fibula. This portal can be established under direct visualization if anterior arthroscopy is being performed. If hindfoot endoscopy is being performed, this portal should be established first, followed by the posteromedial portal. The trans Achilles portal can be established at or just below the joint level through the midportion of the tendon but is less favored because of Achilles tendon morbidity and increased difficulty with instrument manipulation. The posteromedial portal risks damage to the posterior tibial artery and tibial nerve, as well as the calcaneal nerve and branches. If used, it is placed medial to the Achilles tendon at the joint level after establishing the posterolateral portal. After a small skin incision is made, a blunt instrument such as a mosquito is directed toward the arthroscope and "walked down," maintaining contact with the arthroscope until bone is palpated. The lens of the arthroscope is directed laterally to protect it until the mosquito reaches the bone, at which point the lens can be turned medially to visualize the introduction of an instrument, usually a motorized shaver, through the newly established portal.

Soft Tissue Conditions Amenable to Arthroscopy

It is estimated that 3% of all ankle sprains lead to anterolateral impingement.[6] Wolin et al.[7] were the first to describe the pathology. They described a mass of hypertrophied fibrocartilaginous scar tissue that originated from the anterior talofibular ligament and rested in the lateral gutter. They coined the term *meniscoid lesion* because of its similar appearance to a knee meniscus. Bassett et al.[8] described another cause of impingement after an inversion sprain. The distal fascicle of the anteroinferior tibiofibular ligament can impinge on the

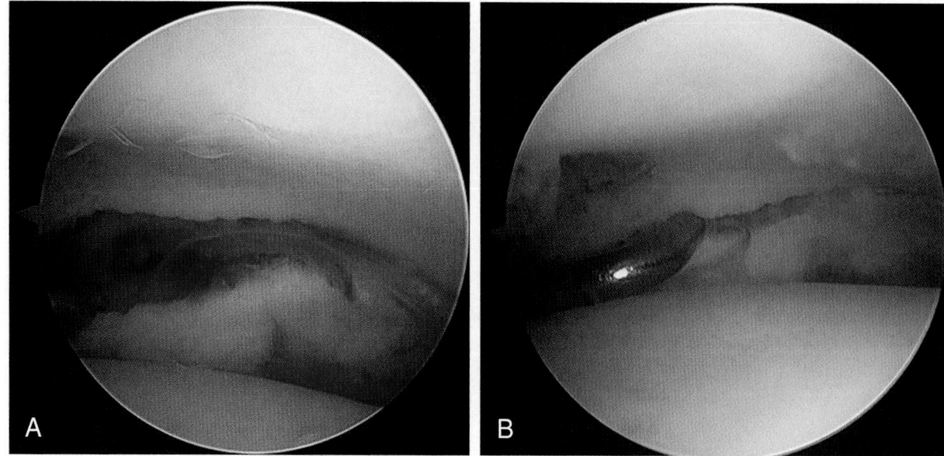

FIGURE 114-1 Arthroscopically assisted ankle fracture open reduction with internal fixation. **A,** The view of the medial malleolar fracture before reduction. **B,** The view of the medial malleolar fracture after reduction.

talus when it becomes thickened or scarred from an injury (Fig. 114-2).

Proposed causes for anteromedial impingement include injury to the deltoid ligament and capsule, resulting in scarring and hypertrophy of the synovium,[9] repetitive capsular traction resulting in "traction spurs,"[10] and repetitive dorsiflexion of the ankle.

With a syndesmotic injury, the anteroinferior tibiofibular ligament can become scarred and hypertrophied. Chronic synovitis can occur at the tibiofibular joint, resulting in a soft tissue lesion impinging on the talus.

Plicae have been well described in the knee. The origin of these lesions in the ankle is not well understood, but theories include congenital and traumatic causes. As with the knee, these fibrous cords typically can be found across the anterior ankle joint and have been implicated as a source of ankle pain, clicking, and occasional locking. *Plicae syndrome* refers to the painful impairment of joint function in which the only finding that helps explain the symptoms is the presence of thickened plicae. When encountered during an arthroscopic procedure, the thickened plicae are routinely excised.

Posterior ankle impingement can be caused by overuse or trauma. The overuse group comprises ballet dancers and athletes in sporting activities that involve forced plantar flexion of the foot. Repetitive plantar flexion results in swelling, partial rupture, and fibrosis of the posterior ankle capsule, synovium, and posterior ligamentous structures. A prominent posterior talar process or os trigonum can produce the syndrome.

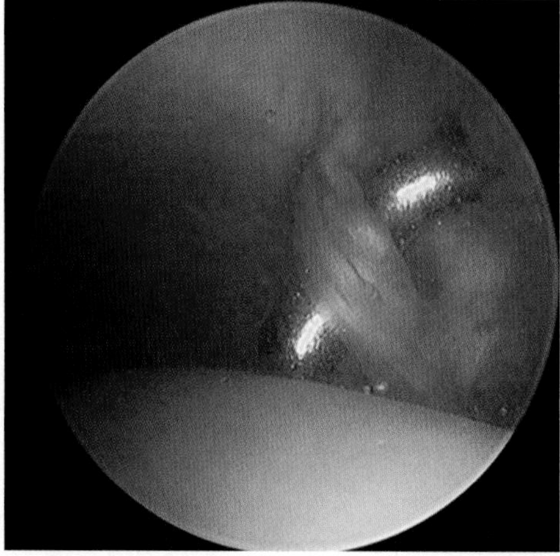

FIGURE 114-2 An anterolateral soft tissue impingement lesion.

The role of arthroscopy in the treatment of a patient with an inflammatory arthritic condition such as rheumatoid arthritis is limited. A patient with painful synovitis that is recalcitrant to conservative therapies may benefit from an arthroscopic complete synovectomy. The synovial lining is typically proliferative and thickened.

Pigmented villonodular synovitis (PVNS) is a benign neoplastic process of the synovium. It is most common in the knee but can be also seen in the ankle and hindfoot.[11,12] It is seen in two forms: generalized synovitis and a localized form. Localized lesions respond well to arthroscopy, but recurrence is common with the generalized form.

Septic arthritis of the ankle is amenable to treatment with arthroscopic lavage and debridement; however, only two case series have focused on arthroscopic treatment of ankle septic arthritis, and both included various joints in the study.[13] Despite the paucity of literature regarding the use of ankle arthroscopy in the management of septic arthritis, this practice is widely accepted.

Synovial chondromatosis is a benign condition in which the synovial lining of joints, bursae, or tendon sheaths undergoes metaplasia and ultimately forms cartilaginous loose bodies. Milgram[14] described three stages of the process. Stage I is the active synovial phase, without the presence of loose bodies. Stage II is the transitional phase, with both active synovial disease and chondral loose bodies. Stage III describes the burnout phase, with no further synovial activity and residual loose bodies.

Lateral ankle ligament injuries are the most common injuries that occur in sports and recreational activities (refer to Chapter 116 for full details regarding this pathology). Recently, arthroscopic and arthroscopically assisted reconstruction of the lateral ligament complex has been reported either by placation or anchor fixation techniques[15-17] and thermal shrinkage.[18-20]

Pain and disability from ankle arthritis may be treated with arthroscopy. In mild cases without significant loss of cartilage and in active patients for whom a fusion or replacement is not reasonable, arthroscopic debridement provides a low-risk alternative. In cases of end-stage arthritis, ankle arthrodesis may be indicated to relieve pain at the tibiotalar joint when prior conservative treatment has failed. Since the first description of arthroscopic ankle arthrodesis in 1983, this procedure has gained popularity. Contraindications include significant extensive bone loss, active infection, a neuropathic joint, and ankle fusion nonunion.

Arthroscopy of an acute ankle fracture can assist in the anatomic reduction of some fractures, diagnose syndesmotic instability, and assist in the treatment of concomitant osteochondral and chondral injuries. Direct visualization can confirm articular congruency and identify other fracture lines/fragments not seen on preoperative radiographs (see Fig. 114-1, *A* and *B*). Arthroscopy in the setting of chronic fractures can assist in the diagnosis and management of postfracture pathology. The indication for arthroscopy in the treatment of chronic ankle fractures (>3 months) is persistent joint pain that is unresponsive to conservative management.

History

Patients with anterolateral impingement typically report pain with weight-bearing activities after an inversion ankle injury that has not resolved. They can describe a feeling of instability, even without true mechanical instability, if the intermittent pain causes a feeling of giving way. Anteromedial impingement presents with anteromedial ankle pain with activities that place the ankle in a dorsiflexed position, such as running, kicking, or climbing stairs. The clinical presentation of syndesmotic impingement is similar to that of anterolateral impingement, with pain upon weight-bearing activities, variable swelling, and the feeling of locking or clicking of the ankle with range of motion.

Patient presentation can vary widely with synovial chondromatosis, with ankle pain, swelling, limited range of motion, and palpable nodules at the joint line.

Patients with posterior ankle impingement report pain toward the posterior aspect of the talus, mainly with plantar-flexion maneuvers.

Physical Examination

The diagnosis of anterolateral impingement is clinical, based on the physical examination. Molloy et al.[21] reported a sensitivity of 94.8% and specificity of 88% on special physical examination testing for impingement.[21] Patients exhibit palpable tenderness along the anterolateral corner of the ankle, along with anterior syndesmosis. Occasionally, asymmetric fullness along the anterolateral corner can represent scar tissue. Pain often can be elicited with passive dorsiflexion of the ankle, either while it is unloaded or with weight bearing. Tenderness at the sinus tarsi may be present but should be mild compared with the anterolateral ankle. An injection of a local anesthetic can confirm the diagnosis of soft tissue impingement when excellent pain relief is achieved.

Examination reveals anteromedial ankle joint tenderness and pain with dorsiflexion either while the ankle is loaded or with no weight bearing in patients with anteromedial impingement.

Patients with syndesmotic impingement have a more variable examination than do those with anterolateral or anteromedial impingement; findings can range from significant tenderness at the distal syndesmosis to no pain elicited on palpation. In chronic cases, examination of syndesmotic disruption (the squeeze test and external rotation test) may not be painful.

Patients with PVNS present with nonspecific findings such as a swollen, warm, diffusely tender ankle that is painful with activity. During the workup, aspiration of the joint can produce dark, serosanguineous fluid.

Palpation of the posterior talar process performed posterolaterally between the peroneal tendons and the Achilles tendon will reproduce the pain in patients with posterior impingement. The passive forced plantar-flexion test is executed with repetitive quick passive hyper–plantar-flexion movements with the patient sitting and his or her knee flexed at 90 degrees. van Dijk described application of a rotational movement at the point of maximal plantar flexion and stated that a negative test rules out posterior impingement.[6] The diagnosis is supported by relief of the pain with plantar flexion upon infiltration of an anesthetic.

Imaging

In the setting of anterolateral impingement, radiographs are often normal but can demonstrate anterior tibial and talar neck spurring. Standard anteroposterior and lateral radiographs may not detect the presence of all osteophytes, specifically off the medial aspect of the tibia and talus. van Dijk et al.[22] described an oblique anteromedial impingement view (a 45-degree craniocaudal radiograph with 30-degree external rotation of the leg and the foot in plantar flexion). The anteromedial impingement view improves diagnosis of both talar and tibial anteromedial osteophytes.[23] Radiographs may reveal ossification along the syndesmosis in the setting of syndesmotic impingement, and in cases in which instability is a concern, fluoroscopic external stress imaging is necessary to determine the presence of laxity. Radiographs can appear normal in stage I and early stage II cases in patients with synovial chondromatosis, whereas multiple calcific nodules within the anterior and posterior aspects of the ankle clearly indicates the diagnosis.

Plain radiographs may reveal an os trigonum or Stieda process in the setting of posterior impingement.

Magnetic resonance imaging (MRI) is the most valuable modality for evaluating soft tissue pathology. The reported sensitivity for an MRI scan in the diagnosis of anterolateral impingement varies from 39% to 100%, and its specificity varies from 50% to 100%.[24,25] MR arthrography with diluted gadolinium solution increases the sensitivity in diagnosing ankle impingement.[26] Although not required for the diagnosis of impingement, it is helpful in excluding other ankle pathologies, such as osteochondral defects. MRI can also identify soft tissue edema, bone edema involving an os trigonum/Stieda process, tenosynovitis of the flexor hallucis longus (FHL), and loose bodies when evaluating patients with posterior impingement. In the setting of PVNS, MRI scans typically reveal swollen synovial tissue and hemosiderin deposits. Computed tomography and MRI have been useful tools in the diagnosis of synovial chondromatosis. Depending on the extent of calcification and synovial proliferation, the appearance may vary.

Decision-Making Principles

A wide variety of pathologic conditions can be treated by means of routine anterior ankle arthroscopy. Diagnostic ankle arthroscopy without a preoperative diagnosis has limited value.[27] Relative contraindications for ankle arthroscopy include moderate degenerative joint disease and joint disease with severely reduced joint space, vascular disease, and severe edema. Absolute contraindications include severe degenerative joint disease not amendable to arthroscopic arthrodesis and a localized soft tissue infection.

Although septic arthritis can be treated effectively with arthroscopy, infection involving the soft tissue envelope around the ankle is best treated with an open debridement. In the early phases of synovial chondromatosis, with active synovial disease, a synovectomy with loose body removal is indicated. For patients with stage III disease, only removal of loose bodies is indicated.

When considering whether to perform an arthroscopy ankle arthrodesis, the surgeon should understand that this technique is an in situ fusion and that significant deformity in any plane is considered a contraindication. Coronal plane deformities greater than 15 degrees are not appropriate for an arthroscopic approach. Additionally, in the setting of osteoporosis or loss of bone stock of the talar body, an open approach with plate fixation should be considered to ensure adequate fixation.

Nonoperative Management

Initial management involves rest, activity modification, use of oral antiinflammatory medications, ice, corticosteroid injections, orthoses, and heel lifts, and physical therapy. Patients with chronic symptoms who fail to respond to conservative treatment after 3 to 6 months are appropriate surgical candidates. Surgery may be considered more urgently if the patient notes mechanical symptoms, such as catching or locking, which may suggest a loose body or cartilaginous flap tear.

General Surgical Technique: Ankle Arthroscopy

Arthroscopic Equipment

A range of arthroscope sizes are available, with the 2.7-mm size being the most versatile for the ankle and allowing visualization in the reduced space available in the medial and lateral gutters. The smaller sized arthroscopes are designed for smaller joints and include a shorter lever arm, which affords increased control over the instrument in a small joint and is preferred to prevent articular cartilage injury during the procedure. A 30-degree arthroscope is recommended for most ankle arthroscopic procedures because it increases the field of view (compared with a 0-degree scope) without the disadvantage of a central blind spot (as with the 70-degree scope). Occasionally a 70-degree arthroscope can be helpful, particularly when it is necessary to see around a corner, such as into the posterior ankle, but its use is accompanied by a learning curve. When performing hindfoot endoscopy, a 4.0-mm arthroscope is commonly used because the size and anatomic constraints are not as limiting as in anterior ankle arthroscopy.

As is the case with the arthroscope itself, a line of small joint instruments has also been developed; these instruments are smaller in diameter and have shorter lever arms. Availability of a probe, graspers, punches, curettes, and baskets is important. Other instruments now available include osteotomes designed for arthroscopic ankle arthrodesis, awls for microfracture, small joint drill guides and targeting devices, and small radiofrequency probes. A range of options are available for disposable arthroscopic shavers and burrs as well, ranging in aggressiveness and sizes from 2.0, 2.9, and 3.5 mm. Generally a 3.5-mm shaver is recommended; the smaller options can be quite useful in certain circumstances such as in tighter joints or in the gutters, although they do tend to reduce efficiency.

Inflow/Outflow

A two-portal or three-portal system (usually with use of the posterolateral portal for inflow) with gravity or a pump system can be used. A two-portal system is most commonly used for both anterior ankle arthroscopy and hindfoot endoscopy, along with a pump to improve flow and visualization. Frequently, if a soft tissue procedure such as a lateral ligament reconstruction is planned, a pump system is not used to minimize the amount of soft tissue fluid extravasation.

Positioning

For anterior ankle arthroscopy, the patient is positioned supine on the operating table. A beanbag can be used underneath the patient and positioned so that the ipsilateral hip is slightly elevated, and the remaining part of the beanbag is gathered under the thigh to hold the patient in position if distraction is applied. This area needs to be well padded. Alternatively, a padded leg holder or thigh support can be used and serves to position the limb and provide support to keep the patient in position when distraction is used. A nonsterile tourniquet can be placed on the thigh and inflated if necessary or according to the surgeon's preference. The patient should be positioned toward the end of the table to ease access and surgeon comfort while allowing enough room for the distraction setup to effectively apply a force.

For hindfoot endoscopic procedures, the patient is positioned prone. A small bolster or support under the operative leg will allow for adequate ankle motion. Again, a thigh tourniquet should be applied; it may be used more often in these procedures than during anterior ankle arthroscopy.

Distraction

Initially, distraction was described using the placement of pins in the calcaneus and distal tibia to allow the application of a distractive force.[28] Although this technique provides excellent distraction, disadvantages include risk of fracture, pin site infection, and neurovascular injury. Therefore noninvasive distraction has become the more favored option. Noninvasive distraction is performed using a disposable strap that passes over the dorsal foot and around the posterior aspect of the heel. This strap is attached to a sterile distractor that connects to the table rail (Fig. 114-3). To minimize the risk of neurovascular injury for either method of distraction, it is

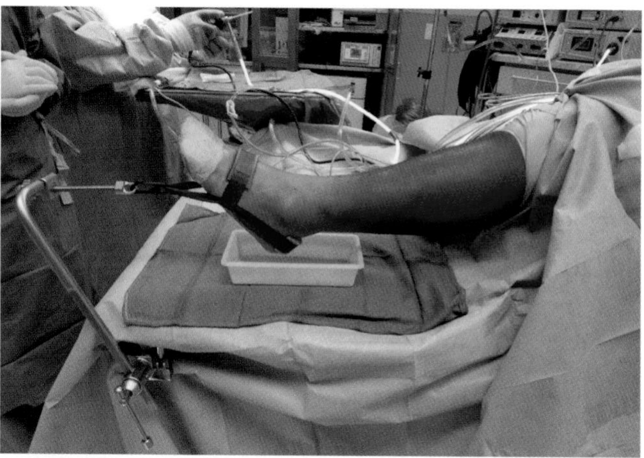

FIGURE 114-3 Noninvasive distraction. The foot is attached to a disposable harness that is attached to the distractor along the side of the operating table.

recommended that the distractive force be applied for a maximum of 90 minutes.

Anesthesia

Inducement of regional anesthesia with use of a popliteal nerve block can be very effective in managing postoperative pain and minimizing the need for general anesthetics. Administration of a popliteal nerve block can be performed with use of a nerve stimulator or ultrasound guidance. We recommend use of a popliteal nerve block in conjunction with general anesthesia to facilitate distraction and the use of a tourniquet if needed.

Tourniquet

A well-padded thigh tourniquet should be applied prior to patient positioning at the start of the case. Depending on the surgeon's preference and anticipated bleeding, the use of the tourniquet may or may not be necessary. Commonly the case can be performed without a tourniquet, but if bleeding becomes problematic, it can be inflated.

Arthroscopic Examination

The ankle can be divided into the anterior, central, and posterior compartments. Ferkel[4] has described the 21-point examination, including 8 points in the anterior compartment, 6 in the central compartment, and 7 in the posterior compartment. The anterior compartment examination includes the deltoid ligament, medial gutter, medial talus, central talus, lateral talus, talofibular articulation, lateral gutter, and anterior recess (see Fig. 114-3). The central compartment focuses on the tibiotalar articulation, examining the medial, central, and lateral aspects of this articulation, as well as slightly posteriorly looking at the posteroinferior and transverse tibiofibular ligaments and the reflection of the FHL tendon. The posterior compartment examination is performed while viewing from the posterolateral portal and includes the deltoid ligament, medial gutter, posteromedial talus and tibial plafond, central and lateral talus, posterior talofibular articulation, lateral gutter, and posterior recess.

AUTHORS' PREFERRED TECHNIQUE

Anterior Arthroscopic Debridement

Patients are placed in the supine position with a thigh tourniquet (inflation is optional). The patient's leg is secured on a nonsterile thigh holder. Before preparing the area, the course of the superficial peroneal nerve is identified by plantar flexing and inverting the foot. The path of the nerve is marked with a surgical marking pen. For use of noninvasive distraction, the foot strap harness is placed and distraction is applied to the foot. It is important to avoid excessive use of distraction. With longer procedures (more than 90 minutes) consideration should be given to relaxing some of the tension on the distraction device. Palpation of the joint line, anterior tibialis tendon, and peroneus tertius is performed. As previously described, the anteromedial and anterolateral portals are marked. At the marked anteromedial portal, sterile normal saline solution is infused through a 22-gauge needle. A knife with a No. 11 blade is then used to make a small vertical incision through the skin only. Blunt dissection through the subcutaneous tissue is made with use of a mosquito clamp. The blunt trocar with the attached arthroscope cannula (a 4.0-mm or 2.7-mm scope) is carefully introduced through the ankle capsule into the joint. The arthroscope (typically 30 degrees) is exchanged for the blunt trocar, and the inflow side post is opened to infuse normal saline solution. For most procedures, the inflow is set up to gravity pressure only or a pressure pump set to small joints. A 22-gauge needle is inserted at the anterolateral portal into the ankle joint and visualized with the scope. The position of this portal can be adjusted on the basis of the location of the ankle lesion. Using the same technique as with the anteromedial portal, the anterolateral portal is established. Sequential examination of the ankle is performed as previously described. A posterolateral portal can be established for inflow or visualization if necessary. For many anterior impingement lesions, visualization of the anterior compartment is maximized with minimal distraction and dorsiflexion of the ankle.

After the diagnostic examination, debridement with use of various arthroscopic tools and shavers is performed. Debridement includes removal of inflamed synovium, thickened adhesive bands and ligamentous tissue, osteophytes, and loose bodies. Typically the postfracture ankle and arthritic ankle is contracted and challenging to navigate. Iatrogenic injury to the already traumatized articular surface should be avoided. Osteophytes are first debrided of soft tissue, capsule, or adhesions. An arthroscopic burr, pituitary rongeur, and small osteotome can be introduced through both anterior portals to completely remove the spurs. The goal for adequate resection is to establish

Continued

an angle of 60 degrees with lines tangential to the talar neck and anterior tibia. Chondral lesions are debrided of loose fragments with a motorized shaver. Full-thickness lesions are debrided, and the subchondral base is drilled, similar to the technique described for microfracture/abrasion arthroplasty for talar osteochondral defect.

For anterolateral lesions, the diseased tissue may extend superiorly to the syndesmotic ligaments. For medial lesions, the arthroscope is placed in the anterolateral portal with instruments passed through the anteromedial portal. Care is taken to preserve the deep deltoid ligament. For cases of syndesmotic impingement, before preparing the limb, the stability of the syndesmosis is evaluated with stress radiographs obtained with use of an anesthetic.

Gravity inflow should be used in the setting of an acute ankle fracture to avoid excessive fluid extravasation into the soft tissues. Hemarthrosis, fibrinous debris, and chondral/osteochondral fragments are removed or repaired. Fracture reduction is performed with a Freer elevator, arthroscopic probe, or reduction tenaculum. Fracture fixation is performed based on the pattern of injury, and the arthroscope is used to confirm an anatomic reduction.

The portals are closed with use of nylon suture in a vertical mattress pattern.

AUTHORS' PREFERRED TECHNIQUE

Posterior Impingement

Patients are placed in a prone position, with placement of a thigh tourniquet. With the ankle in a neutral position, the posterolateral portal is made at the level of the tip of the lateral malleolus, just lateral to the Achilles tendon (Fig. 114-4). A vertical incision is made using a No. 11 blade through skin only. A mosquito clamp spreads the subcutaneous layer and is directed anteriorly in the direction of the interdigital web space between the first and second toe. Once the clamp touches bone, it is exchanged for a 2.7- or 4.0-mm 30-degree arthroscope. The camera is directed laterally. The posteromedial portal is made at the same level. Once the skin incision is made, a mosquito clamp is directed to the arthroscope shaft.

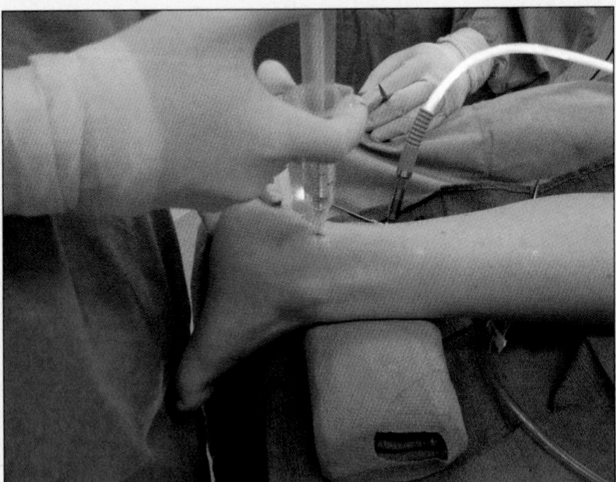

FIGURE 114-4 The setup for posterior ankle endoscopic procedures. The needle is placed at the posterolateral portal, directed to the first web space, and placed parallel to the weight-bearing axis of the foot.

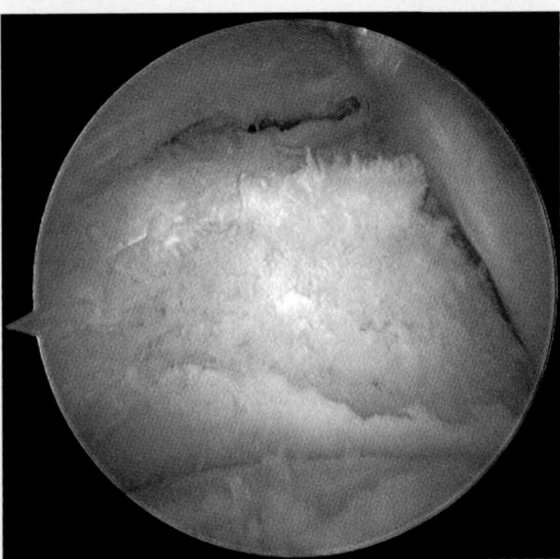

FIGURE 114-5 The view of the posterior ankle/subtalar joint after excision of an os trigonum.

When the mosquito clamp touches the arthroscope shaft, the clamp moves anteriorly toward the ankle joint, touching the arthroscope the entire way. The arthroscope is slightly pulled back, visualizing the tip of the clamp. An arthroscopic shaver is exchanged for the clamp, and the fatty tissue and synovium overlying the posterior ankle and subtalar joint are debrided. The posterior tibiofibular and talofibular ligament are identified. The posterior talar process, os trigonum, and FHL are identified. Care is taken to stay lateral to the FHL to prevent injury to the medial neurovascular bundle. Excision of an os trigonum or hypertrophic posterior talar process requires partial detachment of the posterior talofibular ligament, flexor retinaculum, and posterior talocalcaneal ligament (Fig. 114-5). After debridement, the skin portals are closed with nylon suture in a vertical mattress pattern.

AUTHORS' PREFERRED TECHNIQUE

Lateral Ankle Ligament Reconstruction

Position, equipment, distraction, and portal placement were outlined previously for a standard anterior ankle arthroscopy approach. After a complete diagnostic arthroscopy of the ankle and treatment of accompanying lesions, lateral ankle instability can be visually confirmed with talar tilt and anterior drawer maneuvers. The lateral gutter is debrided of all scar tissue, and the periosteum is removed off the anterior aspect of the fibula (immediately distal from the anterior-inferior tibiofibular ligament). With the suture-anchor technique, a suture anchor is delivered through the anterolateral portal and placed into the prepared surface of the fibula. An accessory anterolateral portal is made 1 to 2 cm in front of the tip of the distal fibula. The sutures are pulled through the accessory anterolateral portal, and deep stitches with the sutures are made in the lateral ligament complex. The knot is tightened with the foot held in eversion and with a slight posterior drawer force. With the thermal energy technique, the thermal electrode is passed through the anterolateral portal and serially swept across the area of the anterior talofibular ligament (and calcaneofibular ligament posteriorly) with the foot placed in an everted position.

Postoperative Management

We prefer use of a well-padded below-knee splint as the initial surgical dressing. This splint protects the limb, diminishes pain, and helps control swelling. The splint is removed around 10 to 14 days after surgery, and sutures are removed. For most conditions, a removable fracture boot is used to permit early motion exercises. The patient also increases weight bearing as allowed by pain and swelling of the limb. Formal physical therapy may also assist in facilitating the patient's rehabilitation and recovery. Patients typically perform therapeutic exercises without restrictions except if a lateral ligament reconstruction is performed; in that instance, limitation of inversion for the first 4 to 6 weeks can assist in early ligament healing. Discontinuation of the boot brace occurs around 4 to 6 weeks, followed by use of a lace-up ankle brace for patients with ligament reconstruction.

An exception to this general protocol is in cases of arthroscopic ankle arthrodesis; patients who have undergone this procedure are typically immobilized in a below-knee cast and restricted from weight bearing for approximately 6 to 8 weeks followed by progression of partial weight bearing to full weight bearing in a boot over another 4 to 6 weeks. Final discontinuation of the boot immobilization occurs once clinical and radiographic healing is confirmed.

Return to play in cases of loose body removal, synovectomy, and debridement of anterior or posterior impingement lesions is variable but in most cases is permissible 10 to 12 weeks after surgery. This time frame allows resolution of pain and edema along with advancement of the patient's rehabilitation and conditioning. Later phases of recovery focus on return to running, cutting and lateral movements, jumping, agility training, and sport-specific drills. Return to aggressive sports is, of course, very limited in cases of ankle arthrodesis, with many patients able to participate in light sporting activities but not sports that entail heavy running or cutting.

AUTHORS' PREFERRED TECHNIQUE

Arthroscopic Ankle Arthrodesis

As previously described, two- or three-portal arthroscopy is performed. Noninvasive or invasive distraction facilitates exposure. Good visualization may require removal of anterior scar tissue and osteophytes. The joint often has a large distal tibial and talar neck osteophyte that must be debrided not only for exposure but to achieve adequate apposition of the joint surfaces. All remaining articular cartilage is removed with use of an arthroscopic shaver, straight and angle curettes, and osteotomes. The posterior talus and posterior malleolus are best approached from the posterolateral portal. After removal of all residual cartilage, the subchondral surface is prepared with a motorized abrader, removing a 1- to 2-mm layer of bone to the level of viable bleeding bone (Fig. 114-6). After debridement, the distractor is removed and the foot is positioned. The ideal position for fusion is 0 to 5 degrees of valgus, neutral dorsiflexion, and external rotation matching the contralateral ankle (typically 0 to 5 degrees). Internal fixation is performed with 6.5- or 7.0-mm cannulated, partially threaded screws. Two-screw fixation includes one placed from the medial malleolus toward the lateral process of the talus and a second screw placed lateral traversing the fibula into the talus. Three-screw fixation includes a final screw placed laterally, either anterior or posterior to the fibula. Final fluoroscopic views of the ankle are taken to confirm screw length and placement, as well as reduction and compression of the joint.

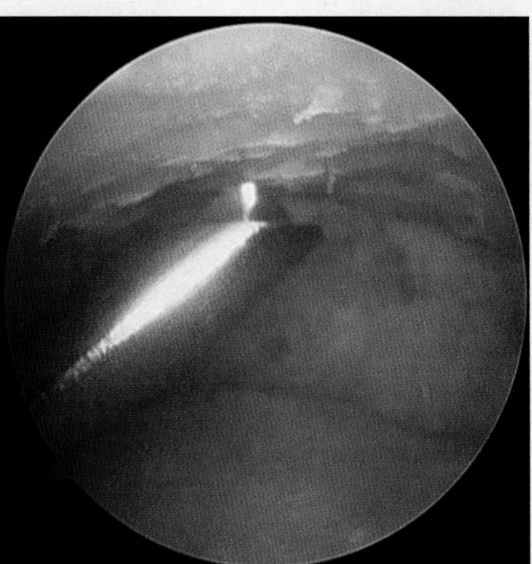

FIGURE 114-6 Arthroscopic preparation of the tibiotalar joint; the subchondral surface is debrided with use of a motorized burr.

Results

Most studies on ankle impingement are level IV case series, and rates of good to excellent patient outcomes are reported in more than 80% of cases.[13] Scranton and McDermott[29] compared open resection and arthroscopic resection of osteophytes in a retrospective study (level III). Length of stay and time to recovery were shorter in the arthroscopic group. In several prospective studies (level II), the success of arthroscopic debridement was reported as being between 73% and 96%.[30-32] One prospective, randomized (level I) study compared arthroscopic treatment of patients with a chronic syndesmotic injury both with or without medial instability.[33] The authors found no significant outcome difference between the two groups and reported an overall satisfaction rate of 90%.

Most studies involving the benefits of posterior ankle endoscopy involve level IV research.[34-37] Morag et al.[34] and Ogut et al.[35] reported on the results of endoscopic treatment of several pathologies in their patients, including Haglund's deformity, peroneal tendonitis, and Achilles pathologies. Another series reviewed the outcomes of 55 patients treated for posterior ankle impingement with hindfoot endoscopy.[36] Symptoms were caused by trauma in 65% of patients and by overuse in 35% of patients. Postoperative American Orthopaedic Foot and Ankle scores (AOFAS) improved, with patients in the overuse group more satisfied than those in the posttraumatic group.[36] Willits et al.[37] reported their results for 23 patients treated for posterior ankle impingement. All patients showed satisfactory scores on all outcome measures and a high rate of return to sports.

Only level IV studies for both plication and anchor fixation techniques are available at the time of the writing of this chapter.[15-20] Despite the debate over the effects of thermal energy on ligamentous tissue, the existing studies have demonstrated good results. Nery et al.[17] reviewed 38 patients treated with arthroscopic Broström-Gould repairs who were followed up an average of 9.8 years. Postoperative AOFAS scores were graded as excellent and good in 94.7% of patients. Prospective randomized controlled trials are needed to compare this approach with the standard open procedure.

Outcomes of degenerative ankles with arthroscopy have paralleled the experience of arthroscopic debridement of other joints. Treatment of specific degenerative pathology, such as impinging osteophytes, loose bodies, and limited chondral lesions, improves the chance of a good result.[38] Ogilvie-Harris and Sekyi-Out[39] reported on the arthroscopic debridement of 27 arthritic ankles and found that two thirds of patients had symptomatic relief (level IV). Amendola et al.,[40] in a level IV study, found uniformly poor results with arthroscopic debridement in 11 arthritic ankles. Patients with anterior tibiotalar osteophytes and loose bodies have demonstrated better outcomes after arthroscopic debridements.[41] The consensus in the literature is that arthroscopic ankle debridement for degenerative joint disease is only appropriate in select cases and should be reserved for persons with early-stage disease.

Arthroscopic ankle arthrodesis has demonstrated faster rates of union, decreased complications, reduced postoperative pain, and shorter hospital stays.[42-46] Myerson and Quill[42] compared patients who underwent open and arthroscopic arthrodesis in comparative studies (level III). Both groups demonstrated similar fusion rates, with a shorter time to union in the arthroscopic group. O'Brien et al.,[45] in another retrospective study (level III), noted that both the open and arthroscopic groups had a similar fusion rate; however, the arthrodesis group demonstrated shorter operating room times, tourniquet time, and hospital stays. In the study with the longest term of follow-up, Glick et al.[43] followed up 34 patients for an average of 7.7 years after arthroscopic ankle fusions. A 97% rate of fusion success was reported, with clinical results reported as excellent and good in 86% of patients.[43]

Two level I studies were conducted to compare ankle fracture treatment with ORIF with and without arthroscopy.[47,48] In the smaller study with 19 patients, Thordarson et al.[47] showed similar outcomes at 21-month follow-up. Takao et al.[48] compared 72 patients and found that the arthroscopic group had statistically higher AOFAS scores.

van Dijk et al.[27] compared the results of arthroscopic debridement in postfracture patients who had impingement symptoms with the results of those who had more diffuse ankle complaints (level II). At 2-year follow-up, the impingement group reported better pain relief with 86% satisfaction compared with the patients with grade II osteoarthritis, who had a satisfaction rate of 70%.[27] Utsugi et al.,[49] in a prospective case series (level IV), performed an arthroscopic debridement in 33 ankles at the time of removal of their ankle fracture hardware. These investigators recognized a negative correlation between the presence of arthrofibrosis and joint function. They stated that arthroscopic debridement resulted in functional improvement in 89% of the patients.[49]

Complications

The average complication rate of ankle arthroscopy in the literature ranges from 3.5% to 10.3%.[50-52] Neurologic injury is the most common complication reported, comprising almost half of all complications. Neurovascular injury can be contributed to incorrect portal placement, prolonged or inappropriate use of distraction, or use of a tourniquet. Anterolateral portal nerve injury can result in hypersensitivity or paresthesia over the intermediate branch of the superficial peroneal nerve. During noninvasive distraction, the foot strap has been implicated in the development of midfoot dysesthesias.[51] Overly aggressive anterior debridement can potentially result in hemarthrosis or deep peroneal nerve injury, although these complications are rare. Nonneurologic complications included wound complications, deep venous thrombosis, tourniquet complications, articular cartilage damage, compartment syndrome, and complex regional pain syndrome.[50]

Future Considerations

Given the small number of evidence-based studies that are available, it is difficult to determine the role of arthroscopic reduction internal fixation or arthroscopy-assisted ORIF in the management of ankle fractures. The incidence of cartilaginous injury associated with these fractures has been documented to be from 20% to 88% and may support routine arthroscopic techniques with future studies.[53-56]

Subtalar Arthroscopy

Arthroscopy of the subtalar joint was described by Parisien[57] in 1986 with the advent of improved arthroscopic technology and techniques, along with experience in ankle arthroscopy. Arthroscopy of the subtalar joint offered the ability to diagnose and treat intraarticular pathology that previously could only be addressed with open arthrotomy.[57,58] Early reports focused on portals located to allow access to the posterior facet of the subtalar joint, while acknowledging that visualization of the anterior and middle facets is prevented by the contents of the sinus tarsi and tarsal canal.[57,58] These descriptions included anterolateral and posterolateral portals for use with small-diameter arthroscopes. An anatomic study investigated the proximity of these portals to nearby neurovascular structures and found relative safety, with the sural nerve and its branches roughly 4 to 8 mm away from these sites.[59] These portals also allowed access to more than 90% of the posterior facet.[59]

History

Pathologic conditions of the subtalar joint produces pain, swelling, and stiffness that can present medially and laterally in the hindfoot. Patients particularly note difficulty ambulating on uneven ground. Symptoms are usually proportionate to the individual's level of activity.

Physical Examination

Careful physical examination can localize tenderness to the sinus tarsi and subtalar joint rather than the ankle joint. Inversion-eversion motion of the joint should be determined along with any obvious findings of crepitus. Examination of nearby structures may also help rule out other potential sources of pain, including the peroneal tendons. A diagnostic injection with a local anesthetic can prove useful but may require inclusion of radiopaque dye to allow radiographic confirmation that the injection is intraarticular and does not extrude into the ankle joint or peroneal tendon sheath, which may confound the test.[60]

Imaging

Standard weight-bearing radiographs of the foot and ankle are obtained to identify the presence of subtalar arthritis and assess overall alignment of the foot. Computed tomography and MRI can be obtained to identify occult pathology such as a focal cartilage abnormality or osteochondral defect, soft tissue inflammation, and the early presentation of arthritis.[61] However, these modalities may not fully evaluate the joint, and arthroscopy may ultimately provide so-called "gold standard" diagnostic assessment.[61]

Decision-Making Principles

Regardless of etiology, initial treatment focuses on nonoperative modalities. Use of antiinflammatory medications may relieve pain and swelling. Custom orthotic insoles can assist in improving hindfoot alignment and relieving impingement of the joint, and a lace-up ankle brace limits painful inversion and eversion. The benefit of physical therapy for subtalar conditions remains unclear but may be attempted for a short period. Corticosteroid injection of the subtalar joint can be performed to relieve inflammation and pain, although the duration may be temporary in most cases. Surgery is typically recommended when symptoms fail to respond to these measures after 4 to 6 months.

AUTHORS' PREFERRED TECHNIQUE

Arthroscopic Subtalar Debridement

For standard subtalar arthroscopy, the patient is placed in a lateral[61,62] or semilateral decubitus[63,64] position on the operating table. Noninvasive distraction may facilitate visualization of the joint, although in some cases simply positioning the limb on a bump may allow the joint to fall into varus.[62] Standard portals for subtalar arthroscopy include anterolateral, anterior or middle accessory, and posterolateral portals (Fig. 114-7).[58,59] The anterolateral portal is established 1 cm inferior and 2 cm distal to the tip of the lateral malleolus[58,59,61-64] in the palpable soft spot at the angle of Gissane. The portal can be localized by a needle inserted roughly 40 degrees in the semicoronal plane and aimed slightly cephalad, with insufflation of the joint capsule with normal saline solution. The anterior accessory portal is placed immediately anterior to the tip of the lateral malleolus and aiming horizontally in a medial direction,[58,59,62-64] with intraarticular confirmation performed with the arthroscope in the anterolateral portal. The posterolateral portal is located 1 cm above the level of the tip of the lateral malleolus and immediately lateral to the Achilles tendon.[58,59,62-64] A spinal needle can be placed to visually confirm the position again from the anterolateral portal prior to incision of the posterolateral skin. All portals are carefully created by incising only the skin with a scalpel blade

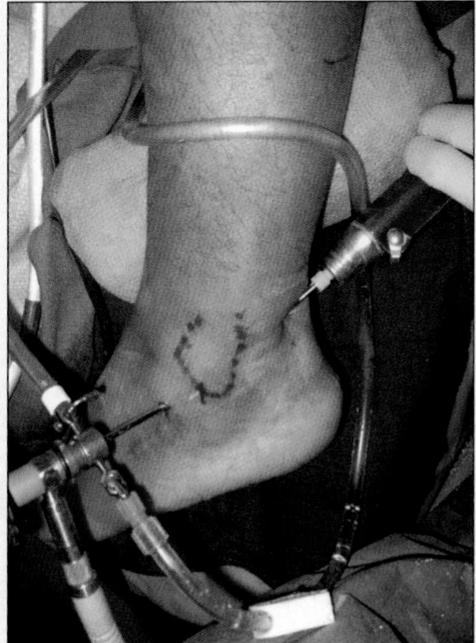

FIGURE 114-7 Subtalar arthroscopy portals. The arthroscope is in the anterolateral portal and the shaver is in the posterolateral portal.

Continued

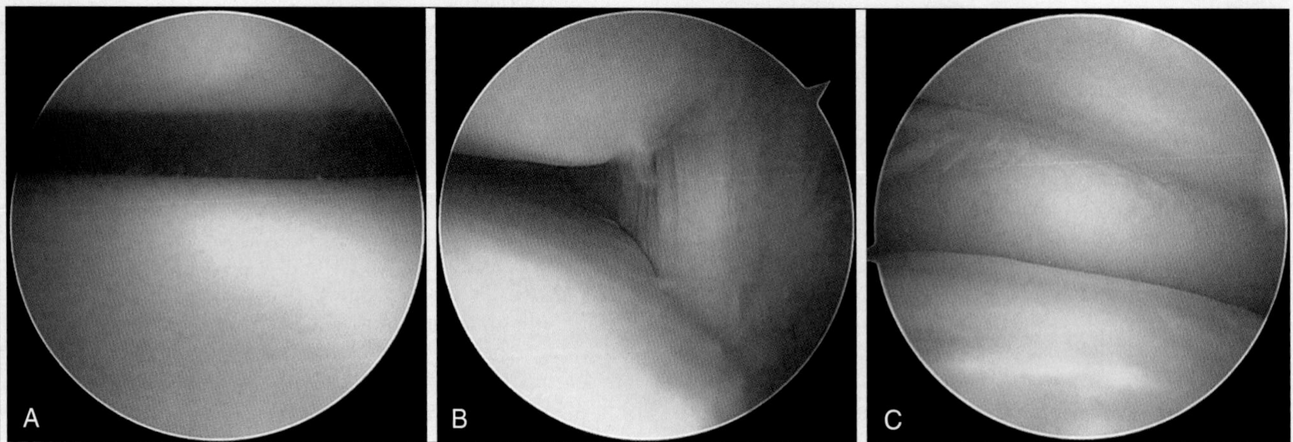

FIGURE 114-8 Views of subtalar arthroscopy. **A,** The posterior facet joint surface is visualized from the anterolateral portal. **B,** The view of the lateral recess beneath the lateral malleolus. **C,** The view of the posterior joint surface from the posterolateral portal.

to avoid injury to nearby nerves, followed by spreading of the subcutaneous tissues with a hemostat clamp and entry into the joint with a blunt trocar and cannula.

The use of small joint arthroscopes and instruments is necessary for subtalar arthroscopy. A 2.5- or 2.7-mm 30-degree arthroscope[58,59,61-63] is used along with 2.5- or 3.5-mm power shaver blades. A 2.7-mm 70-degree arthroscope may be useful in some instances to improve visibility. Use of specialized small joint basket forceps, probes, and grabber devices is appropriate. Soft tissue pathology such as synovitis, fibrosis, and chondral lesions are addressed with basket forceps and both fine and aggressive power shaver blades; bony lesions are debrided with small joint arthroscopic chisels and motorized burrs.

Visualization of the joint is performed by alternating placement of the arthroscope in the different portals, with instruments placed in the remaining portals. Inspection of the subtalar joint includes the interosseous ligaments anteriorly, the lateral recess inferior to the lateral malleolus, the chondral surfaces of the calcaneus and talus, and the posterior joint space (or pouch)[57] (Fig. 114-8).

Arthroscopy of the subtalar joint was initially described for debridement of soft tissue lesions or impingement (Fig. 114-9). Indications include the removal of loose bodies[61,62,64] along with the treatment of joint synovitis,[61,62,64] sinus tarsi syndrome,[62,63] cartilage flap tears,[61,62,64] and subtalar adhesions.[62,64] Indications have expanded to include the removal of osteophytes[64] and the treatment of arthritis.[62,64]

Subtalar arthroscopy has also been used to treat sequela of calcaneal fractures. Patients often have subtalar adhesions, contracture, and joint stiffness after an intraarticular calcaneal fracture,[65,66] manifesting as pain, stiffness, and difficulty walking on uneven ground.[65,66] Subtalar arthroscopy has been used to debride the sinus tarsi, intraarticular adhesions, and inflammation and fibrosis in the lateral recess and posterior joint space.[65,66]

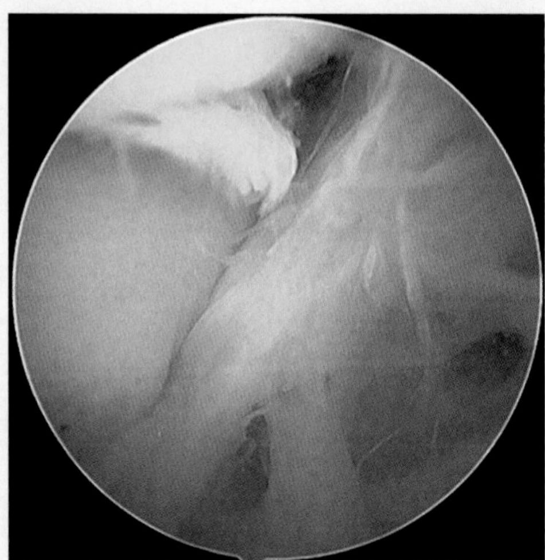

FIGURE 114-9 A view of torn subtalar interosseous ligaments before debridement.

AUTHORS' PREFERRED TECHNIQUE

Arthroscopic Subtalar Arthrodesis

Arthroscopic subtalar arthrodesis is indicated in the same instances as open arthrodesis, namely the treatment of end-stage posttraumatic arthritis, osteoarthritis, inflammatory arthritis, hindfoot deformity, or tarsal coalition.[67-69] Arthroscopic subtalar arthrodesis may result in less pain and morbidity than open arthrodesis[67,68]; older studies also suggested a shorter postoperative hospitalization,[67] although in contemporary practice subtalar fusion is commonly performed on an outpatient basis. Arthroscopic fusion may also result in less disruption of the osseous blood supply, which may facilitate bony healing.[68,70] Contraindications to arthroscopic subtalar fusion include hindfoot deformity of greater than 5 degrees of varus or 15 degrees of varus,[68,70] which may preclude effective arthroscopy and joint preparation. Significant bone loss, collapse, or osteonecrosis may also be contraindications.[70]

Early descriptions of arthroscopic subtalar arthrodesis used a supine position with a bump under the ipsilateral hip.[67,68] An anterolateral portal is created 1 cm distal and 1 to 2 cm anterior to the lateral malleolus, with an accessory portal placed immediately anterior to the malleolus.[67,68] A posterolateral portal is localized just adjacent to the Achilles tendon at the level of the posterior facet, which can be identified under fluoroscopy.[67,68] More recently, case series have discussed the advantages of prone positioning to allow better visualization of the posterior facet with little risk to the neurovascular bundle.[69,70] Initially, the prone approach was performed with three portals, but newer reports suggest excellent exposure with two portals.[69,70] The posterolateral portal is created as previously described. A posteromedial portal is made just medial to the Achilles tendon, and the blunt trocar is aimed laterally to touch the arthroscope.[69,70] The instrument is then carefully directed toward the posterior joint, staying lateral to the FHL tendon to avoid iatrogenic injury to the neurovascular structures.[69,70] Distraction of the joint can be performed with a soft tissue strap and clamp system similar to ankle arthroscopy.[68] Use of invasive pin fixation with an AO distractor is of historical interest only.[67] A blunt trocar can also be inserted into the joint via an anterolateral accessory portal to separate the joint surfaces and help exposure.[70]

Debridement of the sinus tarsi soft tissues and the interosseous ligaments is carried out with a motorized shaver from an anterior or posterior portal.[67] This debridement allows access to the anterior and middle facets, which can be debrided with a curette, although some authors believe that this procedure is not necessary.[69,70] The remaining cartilage of the posterior facet is then removed with curettes, motorized shavers, and power burrs, working through the various portals to access the joint.[69,70] Fixation is readily performed, especially when the patient is positioned prone. The use of one or two 6.5-, 7.0-, or 7.3-mm screws has been described.[68-70] The authors prefer use of two cannulated 6.5-mm compression screws directed from the calcaneal tuberosity across the fusion into the talar dome and neck, respectively. To augment biologic healing of the fusion, the use of demineralized bone matrix,[67] autologous tibial or iliac crest bone graft,[68] allograft cancellous bone,[70] or synthetic bone substitute[70] can be considered based on the surgeon's preference and patient risk factors. Postoperatively, the limb is immobilized for 2 weeks in a padded splint followed by use of a below-knee cast for 4 weeks while the patient is non–weight bearing.[67,69,70] After 6 weeks, the patient can begin partial weight bearing in a walking cast or removable boot brace and is typically able to resume wearing shoes by 10 to 12 weeks if radiographic healing has been achieved.[67,69,70]

AUTHORS' PREFERRED TECHNIQUE

Arthroscopically Assisted Treatment of Calcaneal Fractures

Treatment of comminuted intraarticular calcaneal fractures with ORIF has a high rate of soft tissue complications, including wound necrosis, dehiscence, and infection.[71,72] Extensile exposure can also cause significant soft tissue contracture and stiffness, compromising clinical outcomes. Recently, a trend has emerged favoring minimal incision or percutaneous fixation techniques when permitted by the fracture pattern to minimize such complications. Several authors have recommended concomitant use of subtalar arthroscopy to assist in removal of joint debris and confirm appropriate fracture reduction intraoperatively.[71,72] This technique is appropriate in two-part calcaneal fractures (type II Sanders classification), particularly tongue-type patterns; it is contraindicated in more severely comminuted fracture patterns (types III and IV).[71-73] The patient is placed in a lateral decubitus position on the operating table, and a tourniquet is applied to the thigh.[71-73] A combination of anterolateral, middle lateral accessory, and posterolateral portals is used.[71-73] A 2.0-mm or 2.7-mm arthroscope is used along with small joint instruments.[71-73] A partially threaded Schanz screw is inserted percutaneously into the displaced tongue fracture fragment or tuberosity to allow manipulation and reduction of the joint surface.[71-73] This maneuver can also be facilitated by a percutaneous elevator to disimpact and elevate the joint fragment along with Kirschner wires to act as a joystick.[71,73] Fine tuning of the reduction can be carried out based on the appearance of the congruity of the joint surface, which often appears reduced on fluoroscopy but still malreduced arthroscopically.[71-73] Provisional fixation is carried out with Kirschner wires followed by percutaneous lag or cannulated screw fixation.[71-73]

Postoperative Management

The patient is initially managed in a well-padded below-knee splint for 10 to 14 days, at which point the dressing is removed and sutures are withdrawn. In debridement procedures, the goal is to commence early range of motion and progressive weight bearing in a fracture boot orthosis. The patient then weans out of the boot as tolerated once pain and swelling subside. Formalized physical therapy can assist in the individual's transition toward functional recovery.

In patients treated for calcaneal fractures, non–weight bearing is maintained for roughly 8 to 10 weeks depending on the surgeon's confidence in the quality of fixation and the patient's bone stock. Early motion exercises, muscle stimulation, and strengthening are critical to prevent stiffness and atrophy after these types of fractures. As radiographic healing becomes apparent, weight bearing advances in a boot brace and then the patient progresses to wearing shoes.

Patients undergoing subtalar arthrodesis are non–weight bearing in a below-knee cast for a period of 6 to 8 weeks, again depending on fixation strength, bone quality, and progressive healing demonstrated on radiographs. This period is followed by progressive weight bearing in a removable boot orthosis until radiographic fusion is demonstrated. The patient then resumes use of comfort shoe wear, often by 12 to 14 weeks.

Results

Debridement procedures performed arthroscopically have been described in numerous level IV series. One report of 12 patients treated with subtalar arthroscopy indicated its utility in providing an accurate diagnosis, often more effectively than with radiographs or MRI scanning.[61] These authors indicated better results in patients treated for loose bodies or chondral tears, with worse results noted for patients with synovitis or arthritis.[61] A second series of 45 patients who underwent subtalar arthroscopy yielded 94% excellent or good results, even though 54% of the patients had Workers' Compensation claims.[62] The authors described a low complication rate, with three neurapraxias, one infection, and one portal fistula. They also found various pathologies during arthroscopy for so-called *sinus tarsi syndrome,* including interosseous ligament tears, arthrofibrosis, and subtalar arthritis; the authors recommended that this term be dropped in favor of more accurate diagnoses discovered during arthroscopy.[62] The authors of another series of 33 cases reached the same conclusion about the term *sinus tarsi syndrome* being vague and diagnostically inadequate.[63] These patients demonstrated interosseous ligament tears (88%), synovitis (55%), cervical ligament tears (33%), fibrosis (24%), and soft tissue impingement lesions (21%) upon arthroscopic evaluation. After debridement, patients had improvement in the Pain Visual Analogue Scale of 7.3 to 2.7 points, and 88% had excellent or good outcomes.[63] A comprehensive study of 115 patients treated with subtalar arthroscopy for debridement of soft tissue lesions, subtalar arthritis, calcaneal or talar fractures, and talocalcaneal coalitions produced overall 59% excellent, 38% good, and 3% poor results with use of the AOFAS Ankle-Hindfoot Scoring instrument.[64] Of the subgroup of patients with a preoperative diagnosis of "sinus tarsi syndrome," the authors found interosseous ligament tears, arthritis, loose bodies, osteochondral lesions, and fibrosis due to tarsal coalition.[64]

One level IV report demonstrated 82% pain relief in 17 patients treated for posttraumatic stiffness, with the remaining patients ultimately requiring subtalar arthrodesis for continued symptoms.[66] The authors noted that better results with arthroscopy occurred within a year of the initial fracture and with lower grades of cartilage damage or arthritis.[66] Surgeons have also reported successful arthroscopic treatment of subfibular impingement due to lateral calcaneal abutment after a calcaneal fracture.[74-76] Arthroscopy was performed after patients failed to respond to nonsurgical treatment with medications and injections.[74] The authors also believed that arthroscopic treatment allowed improved visualization and assessment of the joint cartilage compared with open arthrotomy.[74] These reports describe debridement of the lateral calcaneal exostosis due to the fracture with use of anterolateral, posterolateral, and middle accessory portals.[74-76] Initially, fibrosis is resected with use of a motorized shaver followed by removal of the calcaneal prominence with use of a burr to decompress the subfibular space.[74-76] In a retrospective series with limited numbers of patients, it was reported that pain relief was achieved in roughly 80% of cases, with the remainder needing subtalar fusion.[74,75] Clearly this technique warrants further study, but it may offer a less invasive option for these posttraumatic conditions.

Outcomes of arthroscopic subtalar arthrodesis are generally excellent. Scranton[67] retrospectively compared 12 patients who underwent open fusion versus five patients who underwent arthroscopic fusion. He noted a slightly longer operative time in the arthroscopic group but a 100% union rate compared with a 92% union rate in the open group. A prospective series of 41 arthroscopic fusions in 37 patients had a mean follow-up of 55 months.[68] Mean surgical time was 75 minutes. The authors noted delayed unions in the first three cases but subsequently had a 100% union rate by 11 weeks after initiating cast immobilization postoperatively. Amendola et al.[70] reported on 11 fusions in 10 patients treated with prone arthroscopic subtalar arthrodesis. Nine patients were very satisfied, one was satisfied, and one was dissatisfied because of a nonunion. The fusion rate was 91% by 10 weeks. No infections or nerve injuries occurred; one patient required hardware removal. Another series of 16 patients treated with prone arthroscopic subtalar arthrodesis had a follow-up of 72 months.[69] The operative time averaged 72 minutes. The authors realized a 94% union rate by 11 weeks with one nonunion; 81% had a good result, with 13% having a fair result and 6% having a poor result. Complications included one infection but no nerve injuries or deep vein thromboses. Arthroscopic subtalar arthrodesis appears to offer excellent clinical outcomes with few complications and a high union rate. Because of the technical difficulty, however, most authors agree that this procedure should be performed by experienced arthroscopists to minimize complications and optimize outcomes.

The management of calcaneal fractures by arthroscopically assisted reduction and fixation has been studied. Level IV case series have described outcomes with this technique in small numbers of patients. An early report discussed the utility of subtalar arthroscopy in calcaneal fractures in three ways.[72] A cohort of 28 patients who had previously undergone ORIF subsequently returned for hardware removal. At the time of that procedure, they underwent subtalar arthroscopy to assess the intraarticular reduction. The authors found that 23% had greater than a 2-mm step-off or Outerbridge grade III chondral damage, whereas another 23% had greater than a 1-mm step-off or grade II chondral changes. Only 53% had a congruent reduction.[72] A second cohort of 55 patients underwent ORIF with arthroscopic assessment of the quality of joint reduction; 22% of these patients still had residual step-off despite fluoroscopic evaluation that suggested good reduction.[72] A final group of 18 patients underwent arthroscopically guided percutaneous reduction and fixation of type II calcaneal fractures. Fifteen patients had a follow-up of 15 months, with 80% of patients pain free. Patients returned to work an average of 11 weeks after surgery.[72] Another study detailed results with arthroscopically assisted percutaneous reduction of type II calcaneal fractures.[73] The authors treated 22 patients with a follow-up of 33 months. They found correction of Bohler's angle postoperatively, which held up over time.[73]

Further, patients showed clinical improvement as measured by a Visual Analogue Pain Scale, the AOFAS Ankle-Hindfoot score, and the Short-Form 36 instrument; these results continued to improve up to 2 years after surgery.[73] In a similar study of 33 patients, improvements were found in AOFAS scores, with low rates of residual pain and maintained correction of Bohler's angle, reinforcing the results of prior reports.[71] Although this technique is indicated for a small subset of persons with calcaneal fractures and evidence-based studies are limited, the technique appears promising and will likely prove useful with additional study.

Complications

Complications after subtalar arthroscopy are uncommon. Most series report a low incidence of complications, although the retrospective nature of the vast majority of these reports potentially affects the reported incidence. Infection rates after subtalar arthroscopy have been reported to be from 0% to 1.1%.[62,64,70,77] A persistent sinus tract or fistula is rare, with reports of this phenomenon occurring in 0% to 2% of patients.[62,69] Nerve injuries including transient numbness or neurapraxia are the most frequent complication, ranging from 0% to 6%.[62-64,69,70] Authors of one large series of 186 patients treated with posterior ankle, subtalar, and hindfoot arthroscopy discovered an overall complication rate of 8.5%.[77] They did not find a correlation between complications and the surgeon's experience or the use or type of distraction used.[77] Neurologic complications were most common with a 3.7% incidence, including transient tibial neurapraxia, sural neurapraxia, and complex regional pain syndrome.[77] These complications were treated with oral gabapentin and subsequent neurolysis when necessary, whereas complex regional pain syndrome was addressed with gabapentin, physical therapy, and anesthetic injections. Emphasizing prevention, the authors recommended meticulous surgical technique, including careful portal placement, incision of the skin, and spreading of the subcutaneous tissues and minimizing the frequency of withdrawal and reinsertion of instruments through the portal sites to avoid nerve injury.[77] They also commented specifically on posterior subtalar and ankle arthroscopy, emphasizing the need to remain lateral to the FHL tendon to avoid iatrogenic nerve injury to the medial neurovascular structures.[77]

Endoscopic Haglund's Resection/ Calcaneoplasty

Pain in the posterior superior aspect of the calcaneus can be related to several factors that can be present in isolation or more commonly in combination. Retrocalcaneal bursitis, prominence of an enlarged superior calcaneal tuberosity (Haglund's deformity), insertional Achilles tendinosis, or inflammation of an adventitial bursa between the Achilles tendon and posterior skin can all cause pain in this area. A difference in outcomes between Achilles tendinosis and retrocalcaneal bursitis with Haglund's deformity has been noted, though the two often coexist.

Anatomically, the Achilles tendon inserts on the calcaneus between 10 to 13 mm distal to the superior aspect of the tuberosity with a crescent-shaped insertion that extends 3.5 mm anterior medially and 1.0 mm laterally on average from the most posterior point of the tuberosity.[78,79] The retrocalcaneal bursa is located between the Achilles tendon and the calcaneal tuberosity. It is a disk-shaped bursa that covers the posterosuperior angle of the calcaneus.[80] Mechanical irritation can lead to inflammation of the bursa, as well as hypertrophy of the tissue.

The sural nerve runs lateral to the Achilles tendon, and the plantaris tendon runs medially. The blood supply to the posterior calcaneus is from the medial and lateral branches of the posterior tibial artery and the peroneal artery.

History

Patients report posterior heel pain that is exacerbated by walking and climbing stairs. Often they note stiffness and pain upon arising from bed or after prolonged sitting. Some patients note swelling or enlargement of the posterior heel as well. These symptoms may wax and wane over time but generally worsen.

Physical Examination

On examination the posterior heel may appear swollen, or an enlargement of the posterior calcaneus may be present. The Achilles tendon is palpated for tenderness and any nodularity, which may signify tendinosis. The retrocalcaneal bursa is immediately anterior to the tendon and may be tender or boggy if inflamed. Direct pressure over the insertion point on the calcaneus may reveal tenderness along with painful spur formation.

Imaging

Calcification of the Achilles tendon noted on lateral radiographs as extensive calcification (>50%) in the tendon is a contraindication to endoscopic resection, and open resection should be recommended in that case. An MRI scan is frequently recommended to assess the tendon itself and also to confirm the presence of retrocalcaneal bursitis. Extensive tendinosis, splitting, or tearing seen on an MRI scan may be a contraindication to endoscopic debridement because open tendon debridement and repair will be necessary to fully address the pathology.

Decision-Making Principles

Most patients respond to nonoperative management including rest, activity modification (cross-training with low-impact activities), use of antiinflammatory medication and ice, and possible injection into the retrocalcaneal bursa, although a diagnostic injection with lidocaine is preferred to cortisone with lidocaine even in the bursa given the risk of tendon weakening and rupture. Use of heel lifts, open-backed shoes, and Achilles pads can also be helpful. Occasionally a fracture boot or short leg cast may be used in patients with very active symptoms. Surgical intervention is considered when nonoperative treatment has failed after a recommended minimum of 6 months. Endoscopic and open techniques have both been described and have been demonstrated to be effective, although less morbidity is associated with endoscopic debridement.[81,82]

AUTHORS' PREFERRED TECHNIQUE

Endoscopic Haglund's Resection

Positioning

The patient can be positioned either supine or prone with the foot and ankle free at the distal end of the operating table. This positioning allows for dorsiflexion and plantar flexion at the ankle with use of pressure from the surgeon's chest, leaving both hands free for manipulation of the instruments. In the supine position, a bump or well leg holder should be used to allow adequate working space. We prefer to use a prone position, with the ankle located just at the edge of the operating table. The procedure can be performed with use of a regional or general anesthetic. A well-padded thigh tourniquet should be placed because the bony resection can result in bleeding.

Portal Locations

Two portals are generally used, one medial and one lateral, although single medial portal use has been described as well.[81] The portals are located just medial or lateral to the Achilles tendon at the level of the superior aspect of the calcaneus. The lateral portal is often established first by making a vertical skin incision followed by blunt dissection to minimize the risk of injury to the sural nerve. A blunt trocar is then introduced, followed by the 4.0-mm 30-degree arthroscope (a 2.7-mm arthroscope can also be used in smaller patients). A needle is then used to localize the medial portal and is advanced in a lateral direction until it is visible. A vertical skin incision is then created followed by blunt dissection with a hemostat clamp. A 3.5- or 4-mm motorized shaver is then inserted, and resection of inflamed bursa and soft tissue will allow adequate visualization.

Retrocalcaneal Bursectomy

Resection of the retrocalcaneal bursa is performed once the portals have been established, allowing adequate visualization of the posterior calcaneus and anterior surface of the Achilles tendon. A 4-mm power shaver can be used to resect the inflamed bursal tissue. The use of an electrocautery device can also be helpful to remove the soft tissue and periosteum on the calcaneus.

Haglund's Resection

The goal of debridement of Haglund's deformity is to resect enough bone to eliminate the mechanical irritation of the tendon and bursal tissues. The resection needs to be carried down to the insertion of the Achilles both medially and laterally, which can be performed with the aid of intraoperative fluoroscopy to confirm adequate bony resection. A combination of a shaver, a burr, and a reciprocating rasp can be used (Fig. 114-10). The Achilles tendon is protected by maintaining the closed portion of the instrument against the Achilles while working on the resection. The edges can then be smoothed using a curette and bone rasp.

Achilles Tendon Debridement

The Achilles tendon is then visualized and inspected for diseased tissue. Diseased tendon can be resected with the shaver. An anatomic study had shown that as much as 50% of the tendon can be debrided safely if necessary.[83] However, actual repair of the tendon in the presence of partial tearing is difficult and likely requires an open procedure.

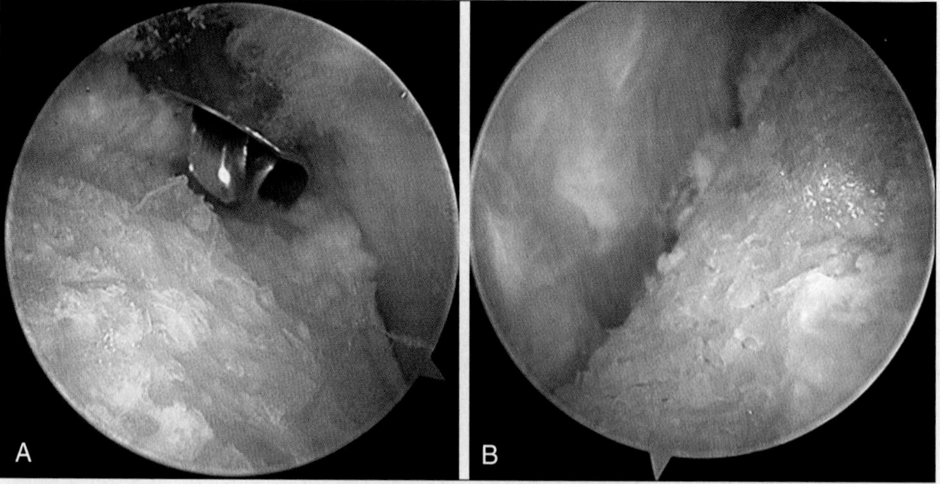

FIGURE 114-10 **A,** Endoscopic resection of Haglund's process with motorized burr. **B,** A view of the superior calcaneus after debridement.

Postoperative Management

Initially the patient is non–weight bearing and wears a padded below-knee splint to provide compression and minimize soft tissue tension that may affect wound healing. After 7 to 10 days, the splint is removed and the sutures are discontinued. The patient then advances to a removable fracture boot orthosis and can commence weight bearing. Physical therapy can assist in regaining range of motion and ankle strength and proprioception. Return to running and other sports typically occurs at 3 months after the procedure.

Results

Endoscopic treatment of Haglund's deformity and retrocalcaneal bursitis has been shown to be safe and effective.[82,84,85] van Dijk et al.[84] reported excellent or good results in 19 of 20 patients treated with endoscopic debridement. A retrospective study of 81 patients demonstrated excellent or good results in 75 patients (93%).[82] The authors did note a learning curve, with improved operative times after gaining more experience with the procedure.[82] In another retrospective series, excellent or good results were reported in 29 of 30 patients after 35 months of follow-up.[85] One patient did sustain a complete rupture of the Achilles tendon that required open repair.[85] A prospective study comparing open and endoscopic treatment in 17 and 33 patients, respectively, demonstrated similar outcomes with AOFAS Ankle-Hindfoot scores, a similar recovery time, and a faster operative time in the endoscopic group.[81] The endoscopic group also had fewer complications than did the open group, including fewer instances of wound infection, nerve injury, and scar tenderness.[81]

Complications

Potential complications include wound infection, delayed portal healing, incisional tenderness, sural nerve injury, heel numbness, incomplete pain relief, and Achilles tendon rupture. Most of these complications can be prevented with careful surgical technique, as previously detailed. Incomplete relief of symptoms may be due to improper patient selection in the setting of insertional calcification or extensive tendinosis; these patients may have better results with open procedures.

For a complete list of references, go to expertconsult.com.

Suggested Readings

Citation: Beimers L, Frey C, van Dijk CN: Arthroscopy of the posterior subtalar joint. *Foot Ankle Clin* 11:369–390, 2006.
Level of Evidence: V
Summary: The authors provide an excellent overview regarding the diagnostic and therapeutic indications for this technique. Additionally, the anatomy and technique of the procedure are explained in detail.

Citation: van Dijk CN: Hindfoot endoscopy. *Foot Ankle Clin* 11:391–414, 2006.
Level of Evidence: V
Summary: The author provides a review of hindfoot endoscopy and its relevance in posterior tibial tenosynovectomy, diagnosis of a peroneus brevis length rupture, peroneal tendon adhesiolysis, flexor hallucis longus release, os trigonum removal, endoscopic treatment for retrocalcaneal bursitis, endoscopic treatment for Achilles (peri)tendinopathy, and treatment of ankle joint or subtalar joint pathology.

Citation: van Dijk CN: Anterior and posterior ankle impingement. *Foot Ankle Clin* 11:663–683, 2006.
Level of Evidence: V
Summary: The author provides a review of the etiology and clinical features of ankle impingement. Additionally, a detailed explanation of the surgical technique and results are presented.

Citation: van Dijk CN, Scholten PE, Krips R: A 2-portal endoscopic approach for diagnosis and treatment of posterior ankle pathology. *Arthroscopy* 16:871–876, 2000.
Level of Evidence: IV
Summary: The authors describe a two-portal endoscopic approach of the hindfoot with the patient in the prone position. They describe a case of a professional ballet dancer with chronic flexor hallucis longus tendinitis and a posterior ankle impingement syndrome caused by an os trigonum of both ankles.

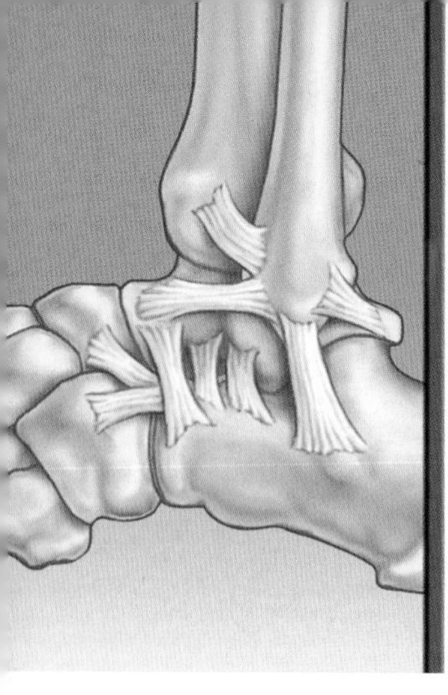

115

Sports Shoes and Orthoses

NICHOLAS LeCURSI

Sports Orthoses

Efficacy of Orthotic Treatment

Foot orthoses, also commonly called orthotics, arch supports, and inserts, have been applied to the treatment of pathologic musculoskeletal conditions for more than a century.[1] Orthoses in general are named according to the joints of the body that they cross or the body segments they encompass. The term *foot orthosis* refers to any orthotic device that is distal to the ankle. This naming convention was introduced in the early 1970s by the Committee on Prosthetic-Orthotic Education.[2]

A foot orthosis may be as simple as a prefabricated arch support available over the counter at the local pharmacy or as complex as a custom-designed device incorporating multiple elements of support. Whatever the type, the beneficial effects of a foot orthosis derive from its relative shape and stiffness with respect to the weight-bearing foot.

Although research suggests that foot orthoses are efficacious in the treatment of pathologic conditions, considerable variation exists in the reported reliability and effectiveness of orthotic treatment in outcome studies.[3] Clinical methodologies have been developed in an attempt to standardize treatment and improve the predictability of the clinical outcome.[4] Still, the results achieved by clinicians often differ, and interpractitioner variability appears to play a major role in the biomechanical response to orthotic intervention.[5,6] A paucity of objective evidence remains concerning *how* foot orthoses achieve favorable therapeutic results.[7] In spite of these variations, a growing body of objective evidence suggests that foot orthoses often produce positive clinical outcomes.[8-17] The potential benefits of a conservative, cost-effective treatment modality for some pathologic musculoskeletal conditions arguably justifies the continued prescription of foot orthoses and interest in orthotic-related research. However, an improved understanding of their mechanisms of action is necessary to enhance clinical methodologies and better inform their prescription.

Research

Historically, the primary focus of orthotic research has been the mechanical response of the lower extremity to orthotic action. Many studies have attempted to isolate the passive response of the limb by studying patients with neuropathy or by using cadaveric specimens.[18-20]

Studies have been performed to investigate the influence of discrete elements of orthotic support, such as base materials, interface materials, pads, and prefabricated and custom arch supports. Study results suggest that foot orthoses are capable of altering plantar pressure distribution, foot and ankle kinetics, and kinematics, as well as knee kinetics.[14,21-28]

Brodtkorb et al.[23] found that the thickness of a metatarsal pad was more significant than its positioning in load shielding the metatarsal heads and that the maximum load shielding effect occurred distal to the apex of the pad.

Kogler et al.[18,29,30] isolated the mechanical effects of arch supports and full-foot and forefoot wedges on plantar fascia strain. In these cadaveric studies they demonstrated the load-sharing effect of arch supports with the plantar fascia. The medial column of the foot approximated the arch support boundaries (Fig. 115-1).

Tsung et al.[28] investigated the effect of arch supports on plantar pressure distribution in patients with sensory neuropathy. In this study, the method of casting determined the shape of the arch support for patients with neuropathy and strongly influenced the plantar pressure distribution. Foot shape was captured with the subjects in non–weight-bearing, semi–weight-bearing, and full weight-bearing positions. The authors found that casting the foot in what they termed semi–weight bearing, with the subject standing with equal body weight on both feet, resulted in an orthotic shape with the least mean plantar pressure. The control of orthotic shape by the magnitude of the physiologic load produced orthoses with predictable plantar pressure distributions.

Guldemond et al.[20] investigated the effects of metatarsal pads, arch supports, and full-foot wedges on plantar pressure distribution in patients with neuropathy. The orthotic elements were added to a basic insole to alter its relative shape at the medial longitudinal arch and transverse arch.[20] This study revealed that the plantar pressure distribution could be altered in a predictable fashion and that the load shielding effects of the various elements were additive (Fig. 115-2).

Recent studies suggest that in addition to their direct mechanical influence, foot orthoses can also evoke a neuromotor response that may play a significant role in their function.[31,32] Evidence suggests that tactile stimuli may, under certain conditions, affect foot and ankle posture.[25,26] Several

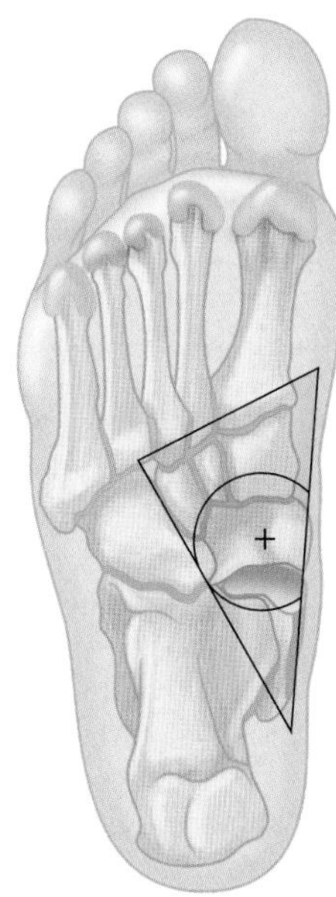

FIGURE 115-1 The plantar aspect of the bones of the right foot showing the primary support region for the longitudinal arch support mechanism of a foot orthosis. The partial circle indicates the position of the vertices of the orthotic support. *(From Kogler GF, Solomonidis SE, Paul JP: Biomechanics of longitudinal arch support mechanisms in foot orthoses and their effect on plantar aponeurosis strain.* Clin Biomech [Bristol, Avon] *11[5]:243–252, 1996.)*

authors have investigated the influence of comfort and surface texture on the biomechanical effectiveness of foot orthoses.[31,33,34]

Ritchie et al.[35] found that plantar sensory feedback influenced midfoot pronation. The addition of mild, nonmechanically supportive surface features plantar to the medial arch elicited active arch elevation in subjects while they were walking.[35]

Mundermann et al.[31] found that foot and ankle kinematics were related to orthotic comfort. In these studies, orthotic use also significantly changed muscle activity.[31,36]

These findings and other evidence suggest that the neuromotor response to orthotic stimuli may play a significant role in the orthotic influence on biomechanical function.[32,33,37] At this writing, the orthotic action upon a sensate, volitional foot appears to be some complex combination of direct mechanical action and the neuromotor response to the orthotic stimulus.[6,31,33,35]

Further exploration of the tactile response to orthotic mechanical action and the individual and combined mechanisms of action of functional elements in foot orthoses may help enrich our understanding of the complex nature of foot orthosis design. An improved understanding of these functional elements ultimately may also enhance communication for clinical collaboration and research.

Clinical Applications

Lower extremity injuries are extremely prevalent in runners.[38] Most running injuries are associated with overuse.[39] Although training distance and history of a previous injury are primary risk factors, a significant contributing factor in these injuries is lower extremity biomechanical abnormality.[14,38] When a biomechanical etiology can be identified, it is reasonable to assume that a mechanical treatment modality may be efficacious. At this writing, evidence suggests that foot orthoses may be efficacious in the treatment of metatarsalgia, plantar fasciitis, tendinopathies, stress fractures, compartment syndrome, and shin splints.[12-14,21,22,39-43] Foot orthoses may also be efficacious in the treatment of posterior tibial syndrome and foot pain resulting from postural pes planus and pes cavus.[9,10,44,45]

The complexity of foot orthosis action in treating foot pathology undoubtedly derives from the complexity of foot and ankle biomechanics and the neuromotor response to orthotic action. The clinician's initial approach to orthotic design is mechanically focused. The process typically begins with identification of the nature and severity of the biomechanical deficits associated with the pathology. Elements of orthotic support are selected with the intent to provide a beneficial mechanical influence that will address the biomechanical deficits.

The delivery of orthotic care is an iterative process of optimization of the orthotic design based on both subjective and objective clinical indicators. Patient comfort is an important clinical indicator used by most clinicians during orthotic fitting and optimization. Comfort in this sense implies not just the tactile feel of the orthosis but the beneficial change in biomechanical variables associated with orthotic treatment of the pathologic condition.[31] It is difficult to predict the response of a specific foot to orthotic support, which may account for some of the variability in patient satisfaction that occurs when treating the same condition with a similar orthotic design. Despite receiving an appropriate prescription, many patients require multiple adjustments to achieve pain relief, and imparting this information to the patient is critical to decrease rates of dissatisfaction. Some basic guidelines that may serve as a starting point for the prescription of orthoses to treat some sports-related injuries are shown in Table 115-1. Note that these guidelines are intended to serve only as a starting point.

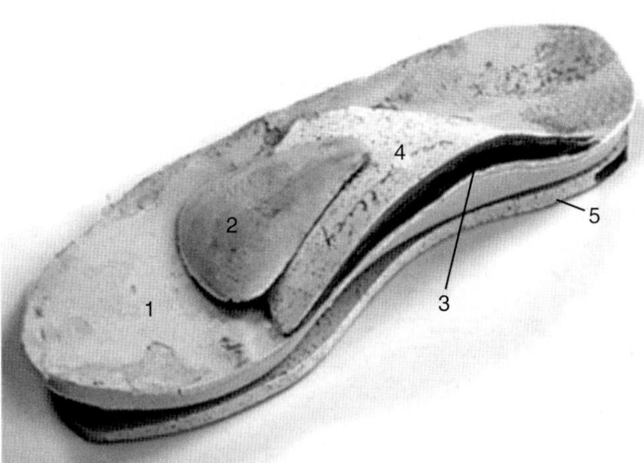

FIGURE 115-2 The right angular front view of a basic insole with components. *1,* Basic insole; *2,* metatarsal dome; *3,* "normal" arch support; *4,* "extra" arch support; and *5,* wedge (medial). *(From Guldemond NA, Leffers P, Schaper NC, et al: The effects of insole configurations on forefoot plantar pressure and walking convenience in diabetic patients with neuropathic feet,* Clin Biomech [Bristol, Avon] *22(1):81–87, 2007.)*

TABLE 115-1

GUIDELINE FOR THE ORTHOTIC TREATMENT OF SPORTS-RELATED PATHOLOGIES

Pathology	Elements of Orthotic Support in Foot Orthoses
Sesamoiditis with no other postural abnormality	Dancer pad—well out for the sesamoids
	P-cell foam insole with relief over first metatarsal head
	Addition of a reverse Morton's extension may sometimes provide additional symptomatic relief; this stiffens the forefoot while minimizing the pressure over the sesamoids
Metatarsalgia	Metatarsal pad with the distal aspect of the pad just proximal to the metatarsal heads
	Having the pad placed immediately plantar to the metatarsal head may actually increase pain
	Additional use of a Morton extension may decrease pain as a result of the elimination of metatarsophalangeal extension
Morton's neuroma with no other postural abnormality	A metatarsal pad is added to the native shoe insole with the apex of the pad at the neuroma
	A metatarsal pad is added to prefabricated orthosis with the apex of the pad at the neuroma
Plantar fasciitis with mild pes planus	A prefabricated orthosis if minimal depression of the medial longitudinal arch is present
	The addition of pressure relief with a cushioned heel for calcaneal pain may provide symptomatic relief
Mild pes planus	¾ length or full-length prefabricated insole with a supportive arch
Moderate to severe pes planus	Full-length orthotic with hindfoot inversion and medial arch support
	If forefoot varus/supination is present, additional medial forefoot support (i.e., additional material under the distal medial column) is required
Pes cavus	A soft custom orthosis may provide symptomatic relief by reducing plantar fascia strain
	A full-length custom orthosis with a lateral heel wedge and decreased arch in addition to a well out for the first metatarsal to accommodate the plantar-flexed first ray
Diabetic	A full-length accommodative orthotic fabricated from Plastazote

Elements of Orthotic Support

A simple flat insole added to a shoe may alter the comfort, pressure distribution, friction, or resistance to bacterial growth of the shoe.[24,46-49] Polyurethanes and elastomers such as Poron and Spenco, respectively, are examples of resilient insole materials that may enhance a shoe's comfort. Although cushioned insoles influence pressure distribution, it should be noted that evidence suggests that they appear to have little effect on shock attenuation.[50] Leather, vinyl, and silver-impregnated fabrics such as X-Static are examples of interface layers that may influence friction and discourage bacterial growth.

The addition of discrete pads to the native shoe insole may enhance the support or comfort of a shoe. Metatarsal pads and bars, arch pads, lifts, and wedges are support elements that are available in various materials including felt, elastomers, and polyurethanes. Felt is typically supportive, whereas elastomers and polyurethanes are typically more resilient and conformable. Several examples of orthotic materials, pads, and their applications are provided in Table 115-2.

Foot orthoses may be prefabricated or customized. The decision about whether to prescribe prefabricated or customized foot orthoses involves consideration of the posture of the weight-bearing foot. Also considered is the inclusion of elements of support in the foot orthosis design that are intended to treat the biomechanical deficits associated with the pathologic condition.

The primary application of prefabricated foot orthoses is the enhancement of medial longitudinal arch support. The shape of these orthoses is not typically customized to a specific foot; therefore, their application is usually limited to feet with normal arch height.

Customized foot orthoses fall into two primary categories: accommodative and corrective. The basis for the orthotic design is an anatomic model produced by casting, foam impression, contact, or optical scanning of the patient's foot.

The shape of the patient's foot while weight bearing determines the shape of an accommodative foot orthosis. Most commonly, these orthoses are designed to redistribute focal pressure or minimize the mean plantar pressure. Rigid deformities of the foot such as posttraumatic pes planus and arthrosis from a Lisfranc injury are best treated with an accommodative orthotic because any attempt to realign the foot will create increased focal pressure and pain. Foot orthoses for patients with diabetes are another example of an accommodative type.[51]

The shape of corrective foot orthoses is also anatomic, but with the inclusion of intentionally incongruous contours termed *modifications*. Examples of anatomic mold modifications are enhanced or reduced medial longitudinal arch support; metatarsal pad, medial, or lateral heel wedges; and medial or lateral forefoot wedges. The intent of these modifications is the incorporation of elements of support into the anatomic contour. These elements are often intended to influence foot and ankle kinetics and kinematics via redistribution of plantar pressure. The Functional Foot Orthosis and the University of California Biomechanics Laboratory orthosis are two examples of corrective types.

Selection of materials is an important aspect of foot orthosis design. Most foot orthoses are composed of multiple layers

TABLE 115-2

COMMON FOOT ORTHOSES, PADS, AND MATERIALS

Component	Example	Intended Application	References
Foam cushioned insole	Polyurethane: Poron* Ethylene vinyl acetate: P-cell* Polyethylene: Plastazote*	Decrease impulse Enhance comfort Decrease focal plantar pressure	Mills et al.[46] Paton et al.[49] Chiu and Shiang[24]
Antifriction insole	Leather interface	Decrease shear Reduce callus formation (diabetic applications)	Yavuz et al.[65] Lu[48]
Antibacterial insole	Silver impregnated fabric: X-Static*	Discourage bacterial/fungal growth	Sedov et al.[47]
Metatarsal pad		Decrease metatarsal head plantar pressure	Brodtkorb et al.[23] Guldemond et al.[20]
Cushioned heel cup		Decrease focal plantar heel pressure	Perhamre et al.[25]
Medial/lateral heel wedge		Influence center of pressure at heel Influence varus/valgus moment at heel Influence rate of change of inversion/eversion at heel Influence varus/valgus moment at knee	Huerta et al.[26,27] Leitch et al.[66] Bonanno et al.[67]
Full foot medial/lateral wedge		Influence varus/valgus moment at the knee Influence plantar fascia strain	Shelburne et al.[68] Kogler et al.[30]
Arch support (scaphoid pad)		Influence plantar fascia strain Influence plantar pressure distribution Influence joint angles of the weight-bearing foot	Kogler et al.[18,29] Tsung et al.[28] Kitaoka et al.[19]

*Acore Orthopaedics, Inc., Cleveland, Ohio.

including a base, intermediate layer, and interface layer. The use of multiple layers offers the combined benefits of their individual properties (Fig. 115-3). Firm base materials such as ethylene vinyl acetate with compressibility similar to that of shoe outsoles are typically used for the base layer of what are termed soft foot orthoses. Rigid base layers use materials such as polypropylene, copolymer, and fiberglass or carbon lamination. Laminated foot orthoses typically offer the highest stiffness while taking up the least room in the shoe.

Soft, resilient, and conformable intermediate layer materials include polyurethane foams, polyethylene foams, and elastomers. The intermediate layer helps to disperse plantar pressure and improve comfort.

The interface layer of a foot orthosis is typically leather, vinyl, or foam and may enhance the durability and hygiene of the orthosis or alter the friction between the foot and the orthosis. Polyethylene foam such as Plastazote may enhance the moisture control, friction, or pressure distribution of the interface layer. Fabrics may enhance the comfort, moisture control, or odor control of the orthosis.

One or more of the aforementioned elements of support may be incorporated into the orthotic design by virtue of the

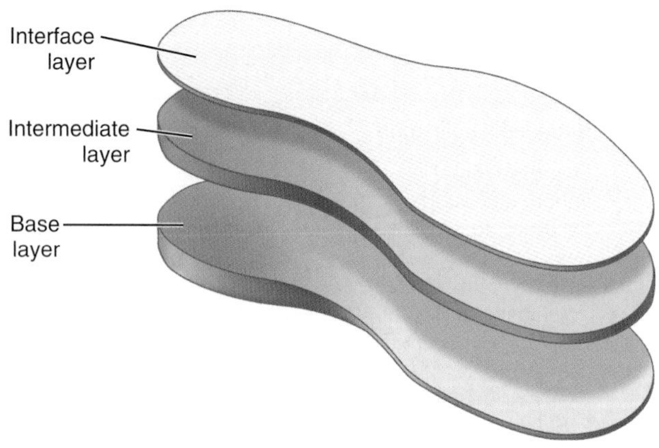

FIGURE 115-3 Foot orthosis construction.

method of casting or scanning, modification of the anatomic model, and the selection of materials for fabrication. The function of the orthosis is evaluated during the orthotic fitting and optimized for the comfort of the patient.

Sports Shoes

History of Sports Shoes

Because early humans were largely dependent on hunting, one can postulate that the earliest footwear was used in running. Upon the advancement and socialization of civilization, shoes took on symbolic functions.[52] Papyrus sandals for religious ceremonies and jeweled sandals for high-fashion gatherings have been discovered in the burial holdings of Egyptian pharaohs.[53] Although these examples have little to do with sports shoes, they foreshadow the current specialization, trendy colors, and designs incorporated into the construction of athletic shoe wear. Competitors in the early Greek games competed barefoot according to early drawings found on vases of that period (Fig. 115-4).[54]

Inasmuch as shoemaking was a well-developed trade by this time, it appears that early athletes eschewed comfort for the presumed benefits of barefoot performance—that is, less weight, a better feel for the surface, and improved traction.

Robbins and Waked[55] revived interest in barefoot running with their hypothesis that the excessive cushioning found in modern shoe wear prevents appropriate sensory feedback and results in a "pseudoneurotrophic" effect.

The sensibility of the plantar foot is a key reason that gymnasts and dancers perform with bare or minimally shod feet. While a person is running, plantar tactile reflexes and the intrinsic shock absorption system of the body complement one another and result in behavior modification to control load magnitude. Specifically, humans dramatically reduce impact force by altering knee and hip flexion at ground contact.[55] A series of studies by Robbins and coworkers[55] have proposed that cushioned shoes lead to negligible decreases in load because subjects decrease flexion to accommodate the instability produced by softer surfaces. A recent study demonstrated that subjects presented with a "deceptive" advertisement of the ability of a surface to cushion impact led them to increase the ground reaction force of a barefoot footfall when compared with a "warning" and "neutral" message, even though the surface was covered with an identical thickness of ethyl-vinyl acetate surfacing material.[56]

Although it is clear that Western-style shoes have contributed to many of the foot ills of modern society such as bunions, corns, calluses, and neuromas,[57,58] circumstantial evidence suggests that improvements in running shoe construction have reduced the prevalence of Achilles tendinitis and allowed greater numbers of average citizens to participate in the sport of distance running.[54]

A shoe designed for sports alone did not come into existence until the latter half of the nineteenth century. Croquet was a popular recreation during the Victorian period, and a croquet sandal appeared during this time.[52] Known as the *sneaker,* it was in use by the 1860s and had a fabric upper, a rubber sole, and laces.[52,54,59] Further sports development in the late 1800s spawned the need for durable but lightweight shoes with variable traction requirements depending on the playing surface. From these developments, we can trace the roots of the multibillion-dollar sports shoe industry and can conclude that the protection of our feet and fashionable design have always been important concerns of humankind. From this foundation, an explosion occurred in sports-specific footwear that has provided us with today's shoes for basketball, rock climbing, tennis, snowboarding, soccer, gymnastics, fishing, rollerblading, skating, jumping, sprinting, and so forth.

Anatomy of the Sports Shoe

For the sake of simplicity, the shoe can be broken down into two basic components: the upper and the bottom. The upper covers the foot, whereas the bottom cushions it and provides the interface between the foot and the surface. These two basic components are then subdivided into their various parts. The upper is composed of the toe box, toe cap, vamp, quarter, saddle or arch bandage, eyelet stay, eyelets, throat, tongue,

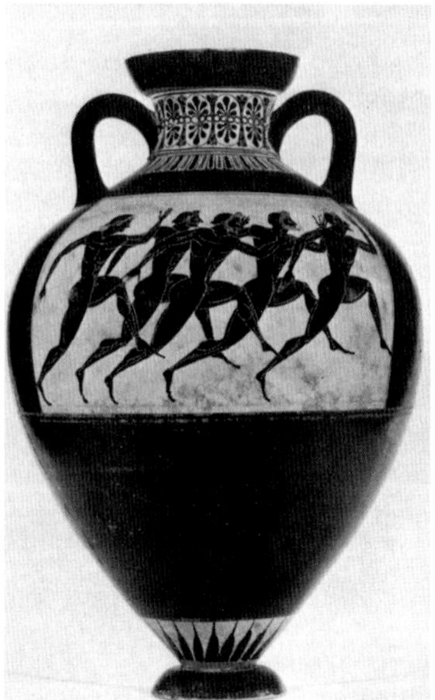

FIGURE 115-4 Competitors in the early Greek games competed barefoot, according to early drawings found on vases from that period. *(Courtesy Metropolitan Museum of Art, Rogers Fund, 1914.)*

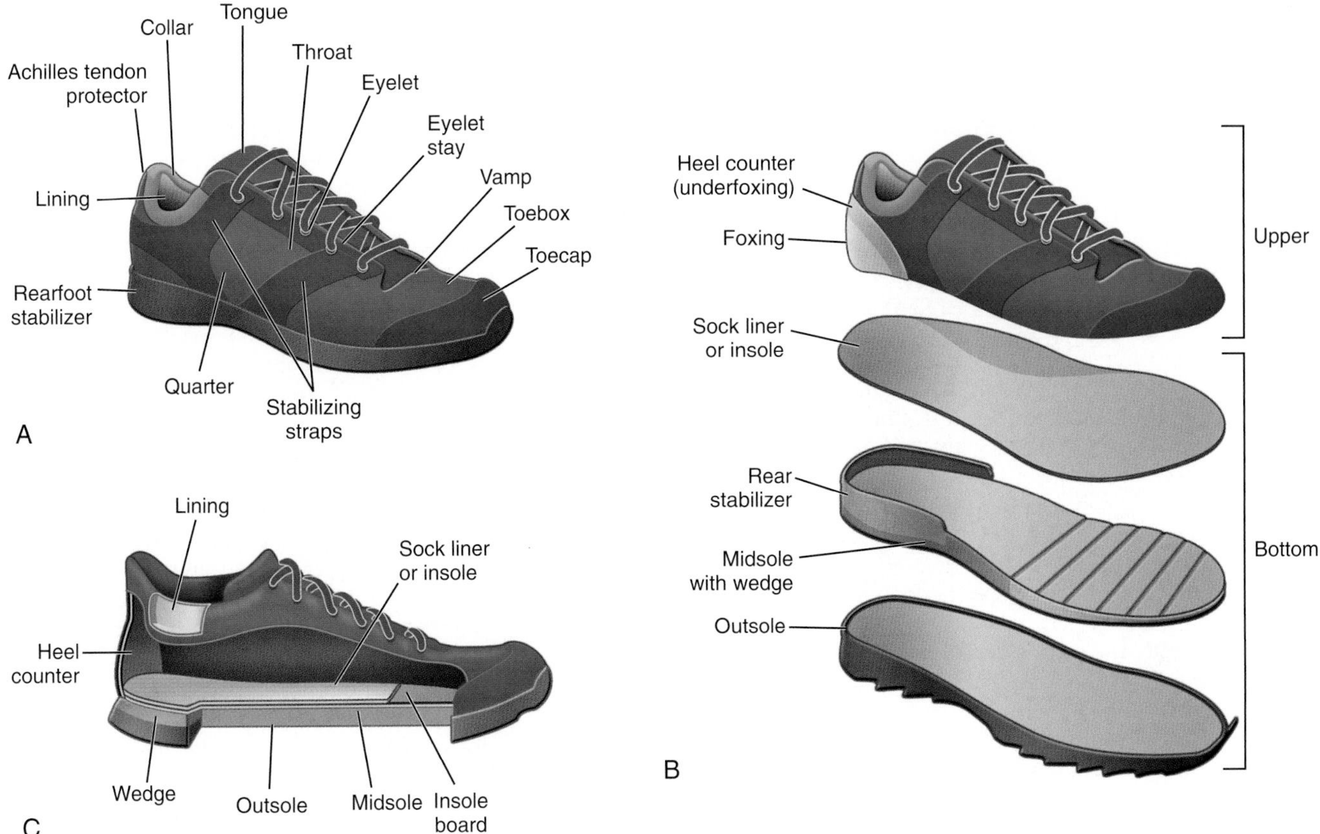

FIGURE 115-5 Illustrations of athletic shoes. **A,** An overview of the external appearance. **B,** Separation of shoe into its component parts. **C,** A sectional view of the interior of a shoe.

collar, Achilles tendon protector, heel counter, foxing, forefoot and rearfoot stabilizers, and lining. The bottom consists of a sock liner or insole, insole board, midsole, wedge, and outer sole. Although some of these names differ from those used in traditional shoemaking, the actual construction of a sports shoe does not vary remarkably from the traditional shoe manufacturing process (Fig. 115-5).

Midsole

Known as the *heart* of the running shoe, the midsole is sandwiched between the upper and the outsole of the shoe and provides the bulk of shock absorption. With the wedge, this component also produces the desired heel lift, rocker action, and toe spring. Through the use of canting and variable hardness, the midsole can control foot motion. With the use of anatomic contouring, even greater stability and comfort can be achieved. Variations in the materials used add another dimension to what the midsole can do for the foot.

Many of the more significant and recent design advances have occurred through alteration of the midsole.[60] These modifications are seen as significant enough by the manufacturers that they are frequently incorporated in the name or advertising campaigns of the various shoe products.

Outsole

The outsole is the bottom layer of the shoe that makes contact with the ground. The outsole can be constructed with different materials, patterns, colors, and densities. These factors, excluding color variations, can be used to modify the shoe's stability, flexibility, comfort, and shock absorption.

Proper Fit and Shoe Purchase Decisions

Although biomechanical abnormalities have caught the attention of both the athlete and the sports medicine practitioner in recent years, these problems are much less likely to be the source of day-in and day-out problems compared with the difficulties created by poorly fitting shoes. It is the poorly fitted shoe that creates such commonplace annoyances as blisters, ingrown toenails, certain forms of calluses, metatarsalgia, nerve compression syndromes, "black toes," corns, and a variety of other unnecessary ills. Most of these conditions are preventable with a working knowledge of shoe-fitting techniques.

The most classic case of a footwear-related problem is the bunion. Although some persons certainly have an anatomic predisposition to develop this condition, it has become evident from accumulated scientific research that the improperly fitted shoe is of major significance in the causes of bunions, or hallux valgus. Hoffman's study of barefooted peoples demonstrated "progressive characteristic deformation and inhibition of function" in people who wore shoes compared with those who remained shoeless.[61] Kato and Watanabe[58] pointed out the relationship between the development of hallux valgus as a clinical entity in Japan and the introduction of the Western-style shoe to replace the traditional geta sandal. Other studies have reached similar conclusions, but this evidence has had little effect on the shoe manufacturing industry or the consuming public, who continue to believe that the dainty foot is the most attractive foot.

Because fit and comfort are so critical, it would seem that the popular shoe surveys would try to determine how to achieve proper fit for the benefit of their readership. Evidently, proper fit is a matter of individual preference and is not quantifiable in the same sense that shock absorption and pronation control can be analyzed. Too many variables exist among persons, and major differences even exist between the right and left foot of the same person. Comfort and fit are a matter of individual preference—some people like a snug fit, whereas others prefer a more loosely fitting shoe; some people like the feel that a soft insole provides, whereas others do not like this sensation; and some people like the feel of a higher heel, whereas others cannot tolerate such a heel. In our own dealings with patients, it has become evident that although we can make suggestions based on reasonable empiric considerations, it is impossible for us to predict with accuracy which shoe a specific patient with a specific foot type will select as the most comfortable.

In determining the proper fit of a pair of shoes, it is commonly believed that the shoe may be somewhat uncomfortable on the first fitting but can then be "broken in" over time. Conversely, it is often thought that the shoe that feels comfortable in the store the first time will then fit comfortably for the rest of its natural life. Unfortunately, both of these concepts are subject to error. For these reasons, it is important to approach the purchase or fitting of a pair of athletic shoes thoughtfully. The decision to purchase a particular shoe should be based on the quality of construction (brand name may or may not be a factor in this consideration). One should avoid buying a shoe simply because it is made by a specific company or endorsed by a certain athlete. Many universities and professional sports teams receive shoes at considerable discounts or even have them donated for the publicity derived by the shoe company. In this situation, it is not uncommon to encounter fitting problems in certain athletes who simply do not have a foot that fits well into the selected shoe. Also, some athletes' feet require shoes with greater stiffness or other specific characteristics that are not available in the offered shoes. Rather than forcing athletes to adjust to the shoe for the sake of conformity, it is preferable to let them participate in the selection of a shoe that they know will fit well and that will allow them to perform to the best of their ability. Although this scenario is seldom possible in intercollegiate or professional sports, the sports medicine specialist should be sensitive to the relationship between poorly fitting shoes and certain complaints of the athlete, as well as the need to switch to a more supportive shoe when appropriate.

Three basic determinations need to be made when fitting shoes. One must first ascertain that the length is correct, which can be guided by the rule of thumb test that is performed by pressing on the end of the shoe while the wearer is applying full weight. Between half and a full width of the examiner's thumb should be present between the end of the longest toe and the end of the shoe. It is essential to note that for many people, the second toe is longer than the great toe. Another important test for length is to have the athlete kick the plantar forefoot into the ground as he or she would in a sudden stop. If the toes jam uncomfortably into the end of the shoe, the shoe will not last long, the toes will suffer, or the shoe will be shelved. It is wise to perform this test before the shoe is purchased. The next step in the fitting process is to determine proper width. The pinch test helps with this determination. The person stands in the shoe while the examiner tries to pinch a small amount of material in the upper between the thumb and index finger across the forefoot of the shoe.

The final test is a determination of the flex point of the shoe in relation to the metatarsal break of the foot. If the shoe does not have the proper degree of flexibility in the appropriate location, one can expect problems. In the past, the flexibility test was one of the common tests used by *Runner's World* in their annual shoe survey.[54] The shoe was bent through a 40-degree range, and the force required was measured with a strain gauge. It has been assumed that the less force required, the better, because this is the force that must be generated by the runner. This assumption includes a fallacy, however. It has become evident in shoes designed for artificial surfaces that the overly flexible shoe can predispose the wearer to sprains of the metatarsophalangeal joints, such as turf toe.[61] Furthermore, certain athletes may have underlying problems such as hallux rigidus or plantar fasciitis that are aggravated by an overly flexible shoe. Joseph,[62] in a study from the 1930s, found that the average male needs only 30 degrees of flexibility in the first metatarsophalangeal joint for normal walking and that the shoe with a stiffer sole provided better support for the foot. One can quickly realize that all the answers are not available on this aspect of comfort and fit. This area is one of many in which a great deal of individual variability exists in both objective and subjective factors.

A number of other considerations should be taken into account in the shoe selection process and are mentioned only briefly here. As noted earlier, the shape of the shoe is determined by the last, and this shape can be divided into either straight or curved forms. The straight last provides greater support along the medial aspect of the foot and is better suited to the athlete who has a lower arch or who tends to overpronate. Cheskin[63] also recommends the straight-lasted shoe for the athlete who participates in activities demanding slower and more controlled movements, whereas the curved last is better for faster movements. The curved last is generally better for the person who has an adducted foot or a cavus foot.

In purchasing shoes, one should try to mimic the conditions under which they will be worn as much as possible. Because feet tend to swell at the end of the day or after vigorous activity, this factor should be taken into consideration. In most persons, one foot is larger than the other or has certain anatomic features that mandate greater emphasis in the fitting process. One generally uses a specific sock in specific shoes, and it is important to remember this factor in the fitting process. Also, one's shoe size does not remain static over the years. Furthermore, even in the same manufacturer, variations can exist within the same labeled size for different shoes. It is estimated that nearly three fourths of Americans wear shoes that fit improperly, with the leading offenders being shoes that are too narrow or too short.[64]

The quality of production is not always the same for every shoe, even within the same product line. The purchaser should pay close attention to the construction of the shoe in the fitting process; a bad seam or an improperly applied layer will affect fit and comfort. The type of material used in the construction of the shoe upper is also of interest because it affects the conformability of the shoe, as well as its breathability. The temperature and humidity perceived by the foot are related to this latter property and are a factor in the shoe's comfort. One should appreciate the knowledge required of the athletic equipment manager or skilled salesperson in selecting the correct shoe for persons who have markedly varying feet and participate in numerous athletic endeavors.

It is quite common for persons involved in the care of athletes, particularly runners, to be asked for suggestions about the best running shoe, tennis shoe, skating boot, and so on. From the foregoing discussion, it should be obvious that no one shoe can fulfill all the criteria necessary to be the ideal shoe for all persons.

For a complete list of references, go to expertconsult.com.

Suggested Readings

Citation: Guldemond NA, Leffers P, Schaper NC, et al: The effects of insole configurations on forefoot plantar pressure and walking convenience in diabetic patients with neuropathic feet. *Clin Biomech* 22(1):81–87, 2007.

Level of Evidence: II

Summary: The effect of medial longitudinal arch pads, metatarsal pads, and full foot wedges on the plantar pressure distribution of a foot orthosis were investigated in patients with neuropathy. The effect of medial longitudinal and metatarsal pads appeared to be additive in decreasing pressure at the central and medial forefoot, with less pressure relief at the lateral forefoot.

Citation: Kogler GF, Solomonidis SE, Paul JP: Biomechanics of longitudinal arch support mechanisms in foot orthoses and their effect on plantar aponeurosis strain. *Clin Biomech (Bristol, Avon)*. 11:243–252, 1996.

Level of Evidence: II

Summary: The effect of medial longitudinal arch supports on plantar fascia strain was investigated in cadaveric specimens. Foot orthoses fabricated using foot molds created by elevating the medial longitudinal arch decreased plantar fascia strain more than did prefabricated and functional foot orthoses.

Citation: Mundermann A, Nigg BM, Humble RN, et al: Orthotic comfort is related to kinematics, kinetics, and EMG in recreational runners. *Med Sci Sports Exerc* 35(10):1710–1719, 2003.

Level of Evidence: II

Summary: The effects of foot orthosis posting and moulding on lower extremity kinematics, kinetics, electromyography, and perceived comfort were investigated in recreational runners. A significant correlation appeared to exist between the perceived comfort of foot orthoses and measured biomechanical variables.

Citation: Mills K, Blanch P, Chapman AR, et al: Foot orthoses and gait: A systematic review and meta-analysis of literature pertaining to potential mechanisms. *Br J Sports Med* 44(14):1035–1046, 2010.

Level of Evidence: II

Summary: The authors provide a systematic review of the effects of foot orthosis posting and molding on lower extremity kinetics and kinematics in normals. Foot orthosis posting reduced peak hindfoot eversion and tibial internal rotation, moulding attenuated shock, and the neuromotor influence of foot orthoses was inconclusive.

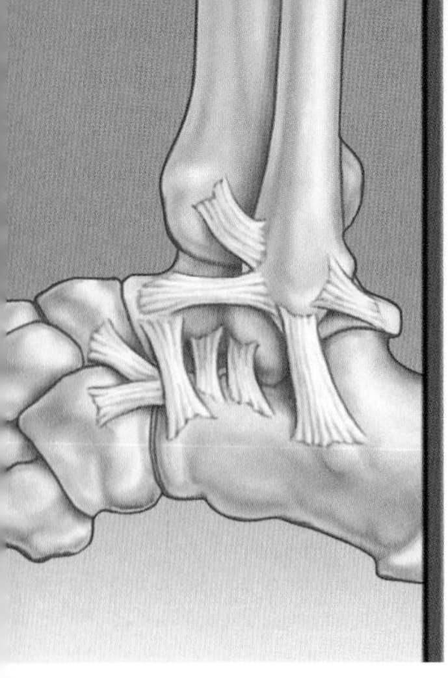

116

Ligamentous Injuries of the Foot and Ankle

ANDREW MOLLOY • DAVID SELVAN

The ankle is a highly specialized mortise joint that allows us to propel ourselves in an efficient manner. Anatomically it is a complicated joint that transmits 1.5 times the body weight when walking and up to 4 times the body weight when running.[1] Standing, walking, and all athletic ability requires stable, strong foot and ankle function to provide a stable platform for propulsion and yet allow adaptation for uneven surfaces and changes in speed and direction. This chapter covers the pathology, history and examination, investigation, treatment, and rehabilitation of ligament injuries of the foot and ankle.

Lateral Ankle Sprain

Ankle sprains are one of the most common soft tissue injuries affecting athletes of all sporting levels and account for nearly 40% of sports injuries.[1-7] Athletes in some sports such as basketball, football/soccer, running, and volleyball have a higher incidence of ankle injuries.[8-12]

The lateral ligament complex is most commonly involved, and the injury is caused by an inverted, plantar-flexed foot with an internally rotated hindfoot and an externally rotated leg.[2,3,8,13,14] The medial side is rarely injured.[15] These injuries can lead to chronic instability, which can cause significant public health issues in persons who do not participate in sports and can have a profound effect with regard to the time it takes to return to sports in athletes. The incidence of chronic ankle instability after an acute ankle sprain has been reported to be between 5% and 70%.[4,16-19]

Lateral ankle sprains comprise 85% of all ankle sprains.[12] The most common injured structure is the anterior talofibular ligament (ATFL; Fig. 116-1). The strain in the ATFL increases as the ankle moves from dorsiflexion into plantar flexion. The ATFL demonstrates lower maximal load and energy to failure values under tensile stress compared with the posterior talofibular ligament, calcaneofibular ligament (CFL), and anterior inferior tibiofibular ligament (AITFL),[20,21] which may explain why the ATFL is the most frequently injured lateral ligament.[22] The CFL is the second most common ligament to be injured, followed by the posterior talofibular ligament.[23] Injury of the ATFL causes increased internal rotation of the hindfoot and stress on the remaining ligaments.

Risk factors for lateral ankle sprains include a previous sprain, greater height and weight, limb dominance, pes cavus, a larger foot size, use of inappropriate footwear, generalized joint laxity, and reduced muscle reaction time due to neuromuscular control.[2-4,24-29]

History and Physical Examination

The mechanism of injury is usually an inverted, plantar-flexed foot with an internally rotated hindfoot and an externally rotated leg.[2,3,8,13,14] Persons with acute injuries have a preceding traumatic event that involves an inversion mechanism of injury with associated swelling, ecchymosis, and difficulty with weight bearing.

The findings frequently are the same in persons with acute and chronic injuries. However, persons with chronic injuries have a history of recurrent instability, which frequently occurs with less severe trauma. One must be careful to inquire about whether the patient has adapted his or her lifestyle to minimize injury, such as via cessation of regular sporting activities, avoidance of uneven ground, and not wearing high-heeled shoes. In persons with chronic instability, the overall severity of the injury is less and therefore patients tend to have less swelling and bruising, together with a diminished effect on the ability to fully bear weight after each episode.

Palpation should be specific with regard to tenderness over the course of the ligamentous structures, namely the ATFL, CFL, and AITFL, to aid in the diagnosis. Bony structures including the distal fibula, anterior process of the calcaneus, lateral process of the talus, and base of the fifth metatarsal should be palpated specifically to assess for possible fractures. One should also specify if tenderness of the peronei muscles is present from just superior to the metaphyseal flare of the distal fibula to the insertion point at the base of the fifth metatarsal. Tenderness to palpation within the ankle joint itself may suggest the presence of an osteochondral lesion. Although rare, dislocation of the hindfoot may occur, and limited passive motion should raise suspicion of this injury.

The anterior drawer test should be performed, along with talar tilt stress testing. The anterior drawer test assesses the integrity of the ATFL, whereas the talar stress test assesses the CFL, although it is sometimes difficult to identify specific ligaments from examination of an acute injury and the stress test is not very accurate.[3,30]

The anterior drawer test is performed with the patient seated and the distal tibia stabilized with one hand of the examiner while the other hand grasps the heel and the foot

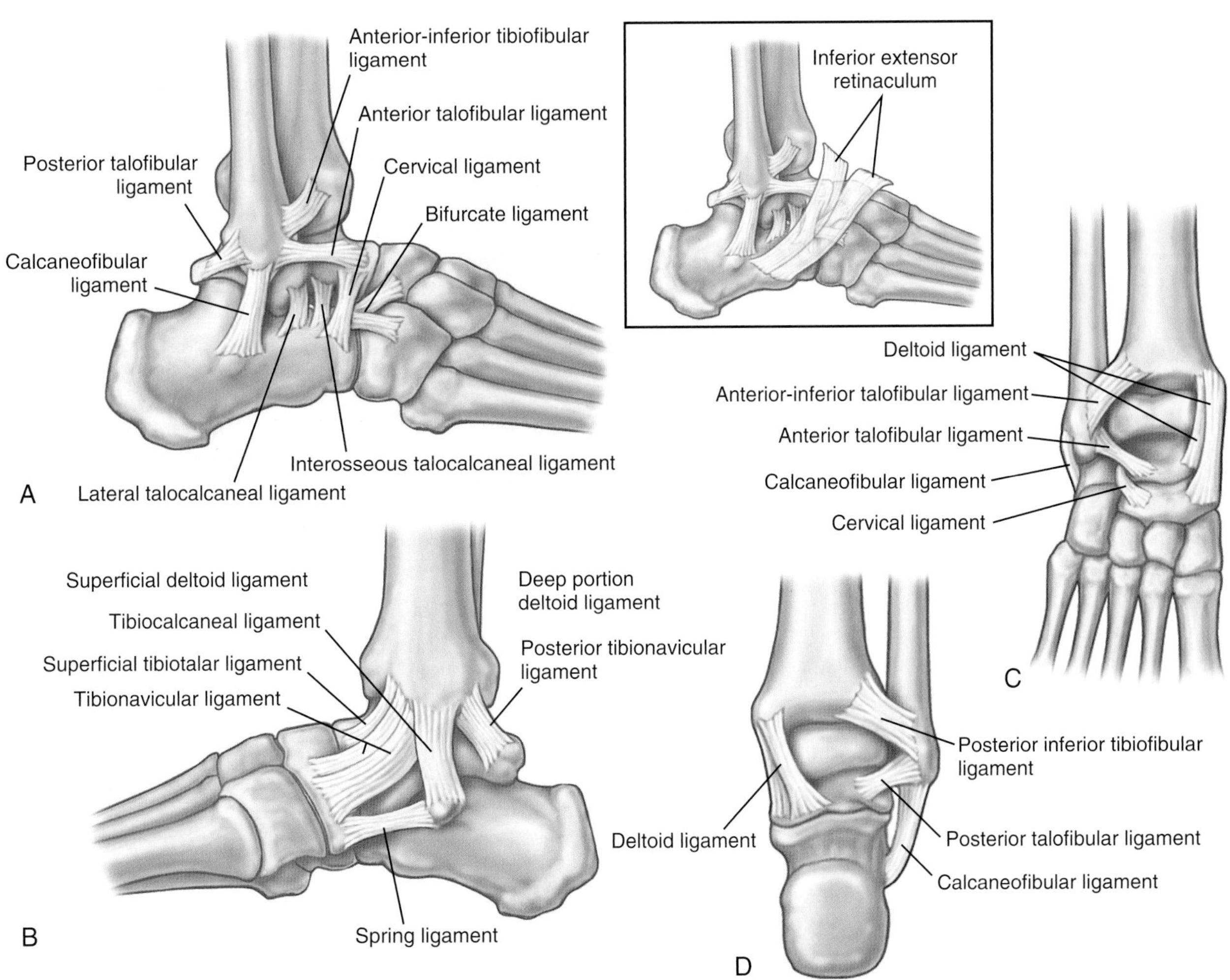

FIGURE 116-1 Compendium of the foot and ankle ligaments. **A,** The lateral view of the foot and ankle demonstrating the anterior talofibular ligament, calcaneofibular ligament, posterior talofibular ligament, anterior-inferior tibiofibular ligament, lateral talocalcaneal ligament, inferior extensor retinaculum, interosseous talocalcaneal ligament, cervical ligament, and bifurcate ligament. **B,** The medial view of the foot and ankle demonstrating the superficial deltoid ligament, including the tibionavicular, spring ligament, tibiocalcaneal, and superficial tibiotalar components. **C,** The anterior view of the ankle and hindfoot demonstrating the deltoid ligament with its superficial and deep components, the anterior-inferior tibiofibular ligament, the cervical ligament, the anterior talofibular ligament, and the calcaneofibular ligament. **D,** The posterior view of the ankle and hindfoot demonstrating the deltoid ligament with its superficial and deep components, the posterior-inferior tibiofibular ligament, the posterior talofibular ligament, and the calcaneofibular ligament.

is anteriorly translated. The ankle is initially in the neutral position, and the test is repeated with the ankle in plantar flexion. The test should be repeated on the other limb for comparison. In persons with a complete ATFL tear, the talus subluxates anteriorly and a dimple forms on the anterolateral joint area (the "sulcus sign"). Use of an ankle arthrometer can improve accuracy (Fig. 116-2).[31]

In the acute setting, if it is difficult to examine the patient because of pain, infiltration of a local anesthetic and reexamination of the patient provides a more accurate test result for the anterior drawer test.[32] However, it is more common in our practice to reexamine the patient a few days after the injury to avoid use of this invasive maneuver.

The talar tilt test is performed with the patient seated and the leg secured with the examiner's hand while the heel is grasped with the opposite hand and an inversion force is administered to cause talar tilt (Fig. 116-3). Results are compared with those of the other side to assess difference in the tilt. The test is performed with the ankle in both neutral and plantar flexion. The CFL is tested in neutral, whereas the ATFL is tested in plantar flexion, but once again this testing can be difficult to perform because the contribution of the subtalar joint sometimes can cause false-positive results.[33,34]

The examination is completed with checking of proprioception and joint hyperlaxity by calculating the Beighton score as shown in Table 116-1. A score of 4 or higher is indicative of hyperlaxity.

Imaging

Radiographs to assess ligamentous injuries include standard weight-bearing anteroposterior, lateral, and mortise views, as well as anterior drawer and talar tilt stress views, which can be obtained either manually or mechanically. The anterior drawer should measure less than 10 mm or within 3 to 5 mm of the opposite side. The talar tilt can range from 5 to 23

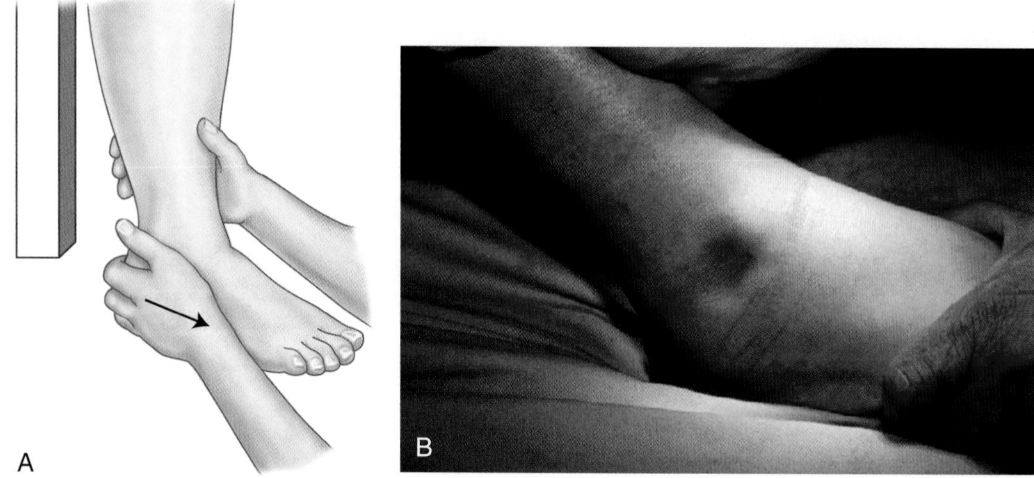

FIGURE 116-2 **A** and **B,** The anterior drawer test of the ankle. Note the skin dimple consistent with a positive test.

degrees, although the literature suggests that an absolute value of more than 10 degrees or more than 5 degrees when compared with the other side could be diagnostic.[3,34-36] The degree of tilt is calculated by measuring the difference in angle between the distal tibial articular surface and the dome of the talus (Fig. 116-4).

Magnetic resonance imaging (MRI) is the most accurate noninvasive modality and should be the test of choice to diagnose soft tissue injuries, although such testing is not routinely required in the setting of a routine ankle sprain. Upon clinical suspicion of a syndesmotic injury, osteochondral defect, or peroneal tendon injury, the use of MRI in the acute setting may be appropriate.

Multiple classifications and grading of ankle sprains exist, although none is superior. Maffulli classified them as grades I to III, but for sports injuries, Malliaropoulus further subdivided these grades to take into account the anterior drawer radiographs.[10,37] The classification is shown in Table 116-2. This grading is performed after 48 hours of rest and treatment with ice, compression, and elevation (RICE), together with gentle early range-of-motion exercises.

Associated injuries can include fractures of the lateral malleolus, lateral talar process, os trigonum, cuboid, and fifth metatarsal, as well as peroneal tendon tears/subluxations, intraarticular osteochondral lesions of the talus or tibia, medial ankle sprains, and syndesmotic injuries.[38]

Decision-Making Principles

Prevention is better than cure, but evidence supporting the use of proprioception exercises to prevent first-time sprains is limited, and no evidence exists to support the use of braces

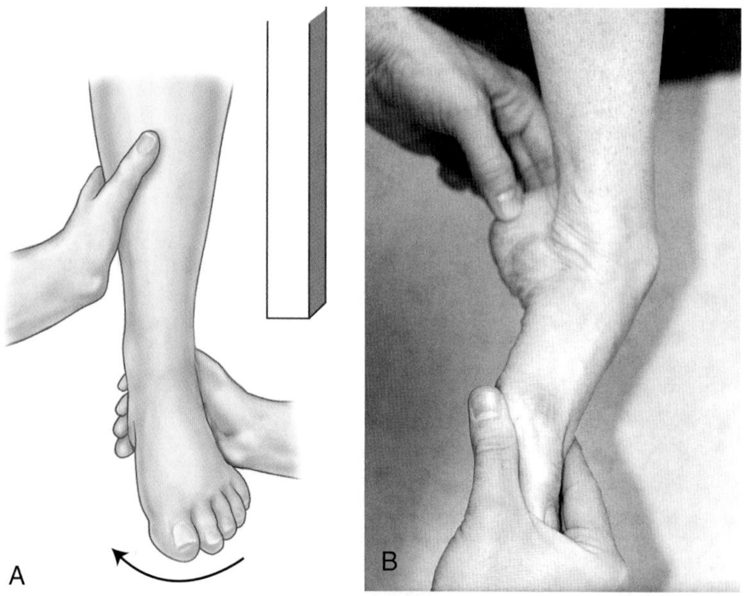

FIGURE 116-3 **A** and **B,** The talar tilt (inversion stress) test of the ankle.

TABLE 116-1

BEIGHTON SCORING METHOD

Testing	Points
Able to extend the little finger beyond 90 degrees	1 point for each side (maximum: 2)
Able to bend the thumb and touch the volar forearm	1 point for each side (maximum: 2)
Able to hyperextend the elbow beyond 10 degrees	1 point for each side (maximum: 2)
Able to hyperextend the knee beyond 10 degrees	1 point for each side (maximum: 2)
Able to lean forward and touch the ground with the knee straight	1 point

A score of ≥4 indicates hyperlaxity.

for prevention of first-time sprains.[10,39] The natural history of ankle sprains is that by 2 weeks after the injury, most patients experience rapid improvement of their pain, followed by a further 2 weeks when the pain subsides much more slowly. Rates of reinjury have been reported to be as low as 3% and as high as 54%, whereas in athletes it can range from 0 to 29% depending on the grade.[17,40]

At 1 year, most patients have been noted to still have some residual symptoms with pain and instability. Long-term follow-up at 3 years has revealed that as many as 34% of patients have had a repeat sprain and 36% to 85% have had a full recovery. The appropriate treatment of sprains therefore is imperative to aid early recovery and prevention of future sprains.

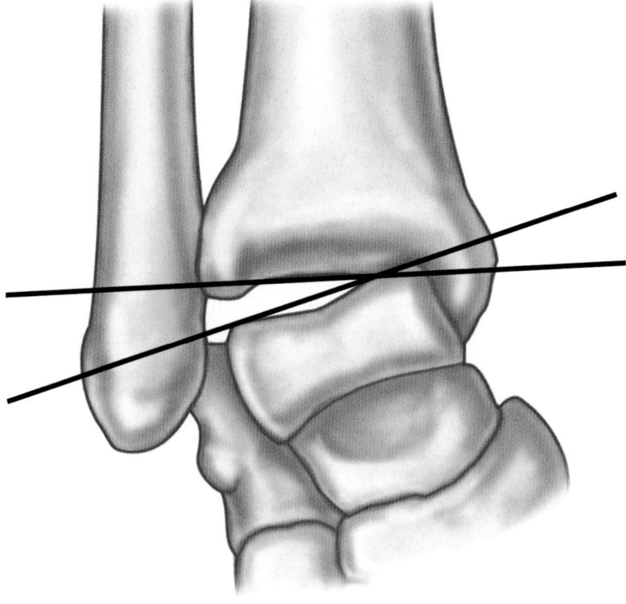

FIGURE 116-4 The talar tilt (inversion) as it would be seen on a stress radiograph. The talar tilt angle refers to the angle between two lines drawn to the tibial plafond and the talar dome.

TABLE 116-2

CLASSIFICATION OF ANKLE SPRAINS

Grade	I	II	III
Injured structures	Partial	ATFL	ATFL and CFL
Decrease in range of movement	<5	5-10	>10
Edema	≤0.5 cm	0.5-2 cm	>2 cm
Stress radiographs	Normal	Normal	>3 mm laxity

ATFL, Anterior talofibular ligament; *CFL,* calcaneofibular ligament.

Treatment

Conservative

The initial treatment of any acute sprain includes RICE, early range of motion, progressive weight bearing, and physiotherapy. The definitive treatment options available are casting or bracing, early functional rehabilitation, and surgery. The treatments depend on the severity of the injury and the patient's choice. Studies have shown that nonoperative treatment is as successful as operative treatment in the acute setting, and no evidence currently exists to support one treatment regimen over another.[3,41-43]

The CAST trial showed that casting relieves pain in the initial period and is as effective as an Aircast splint (DJO Incorporated, Vista, CA) but is better than Tubigrip (i.e., an elastic bandage) alone.[44] Casting is usually implemented for 3 weeks followed by 12 weeks of proprioceptive rehabilitation. Complications such as deep vein thrombosis have been reported, and most studies have shown that functional management is the nonsurgical treatment of choice and that casting is not routinely used.[8,45]

Functional management is classified as an early mobilization program with use of bracing and early rehabilitation. In the literature, functional management of these injuries is recommended as opposed to any other treatment such as immobilization. Authors of multiple articles and reviews have all come to the same conclusion.[4,8,16,45-47]

The purpose of rehabilitation exercise is to improve muscle strength, range of movement, and sensorimotor control, which are commonly impaired after an ankle sprain.

In most studies, functional treatment involved RICE for 48 hours followed by early supervised mobilization under the guidance of a physical therapist and progression to full weight bearing. Early isometric muscle strengthening is initiated within a week, progressing to isokinetic strengthening after 1 week, with proprioception and peroneal strengthening begun as soon as they can be tolerated. Gradually, as pain subsides, the therapy should be expanded to include muscle strength and endurance exercises. Some series include adjuvants such as cryotherapy, although no definite evidence has been found to show their effectiveness. The use of braces or aids to support the ankle is recommended in functional treatment and has been proved to decrease the rate of reinjury.[3,39,42,45,46,48-50] Numerous ankle braces are available; we recommend using braces that lace up and have a strap that "locks" the ankle to prevent inversion. Functional treatment should be performed for a minimum of 6 weeks.

Surgical Treatment

Operative treatment is reserved for persons for whom conservative treatment has failed, and it is not indicated in the acute setting. Persistent instability should be the primary complaint. Patients may have concomitant ankle pain; however, ankle pain without instability requires further investigation because repair of the lateral ligaments does not solve that problem. Inquiry should be made regarding the rehabilitation program carried out by the patient. If it is deemed to be insufficiently robust or if the patient has had issues with compliance, he or she should be referred for physical therapy. The aim of the program is to improve strength and speed of firing of the peronei, as well as proprioception. We have found it helpful to refer patients to physical therapists who specialize in the treatment of foot and ankle disorders. The incidence of patients who have residual functional instability ranges between 5% and 70%.[4,16-19]

Two forms of surgical treatment can be performed: anatomic and nonanatomic reconstructions. Anatomic repairs are more commonly performed in primary surgery. The seminal work on these repairs was carried out by Broström.[51] He described an end-to-end repair or an advancement of the torn end of the ATFL into the distal anterior fibula (Fig. 116-5). A total of 72% of patients were asymptomatic at 2.9 years, with 82% of those examined having a normal examination.

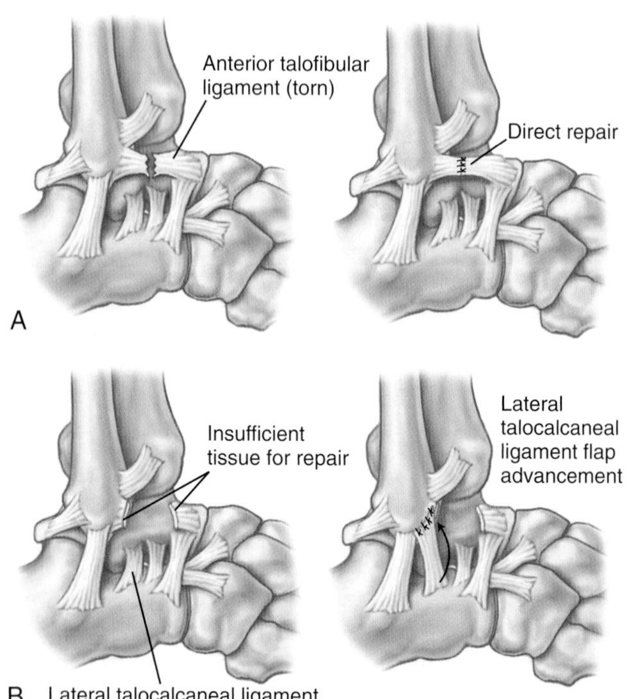

FIGURE 116-5 The repair of a chronic lateral ankle ligament rupture as described by Broström. **A,** A chronic anterior talofibular ligament (ATFL) rupture and direct repair. **B,** A chronic ATFL rupture with insufficient tissue for simple direct repair and reconstruction with advancement of the flap of the lateral talocalcaneal ligament into the fibula. *(Modified from Broström L: Sprained ankles. VI. Surgical treatment of "chronic" ligament ruptures.* Acta Chir Scand *132:551–565, 1966.)*

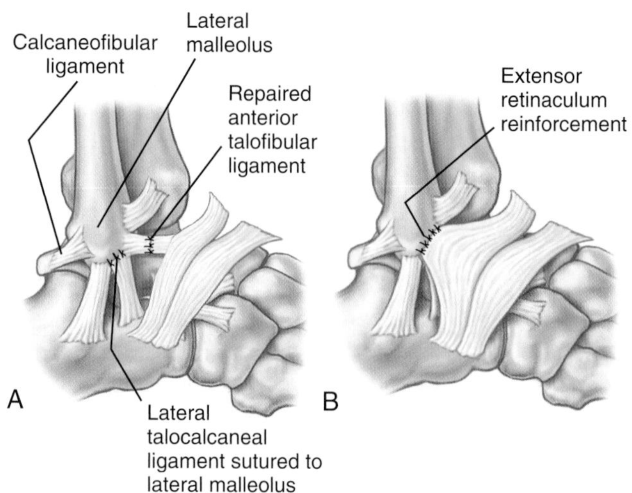

FIGURE 116-6 Gould modification of the Broström technique. After repair of the anterior talofibular or calcaneofibular ligament, reinforcements with the lateral talocalcaneal ligament (**A**) and extensor retinaculum (**B**) are made.

Gould et al.[52] described a modification of this technique, with excision of part of the scarred ATFL, ligament repair, and reinforcement with a ligamentous flap and the inferior extensor retinaculum (Fig. 116-6). Excellent results were again achieved. Karlsson et al.[53] described a further modification in which both the ATFL and CFL were advanced into a bony trough in the fibula together with reinforcement from a periosteal flap.

Some authors have advocated the simultaneous use of arthroscopy, which allows full evaluation of the ankle joint and treatment of any other pathologic conditions that are found, such as loose bodies, soft tissue or bony impingement, and osteochondral defects.[54,55] Although proponents of routine arthroscopy have demonstrated the presence of intraarticular pathologic features in a high percentage of patients, no clear evidence is available to indicate that routine arthroscopy affords a superior clinical result. The best indication for arthroscopy is the presence of ankle pain in addition to instability, or the presence of radiographic intraarticular pathologic conditions. Other authors have advocated performing the ligamentous repair arthroscopically as well, although this technique is presently in its infancy.[56,57]

Nonanatomic repairs include the Evans procedure and the Watson-Jones procedure, in which the peroneus brevis tendon is transferred to act as a lateral tie bar to prevent instability and inversion. Chrisman and Snook[58] described using a split peroneus brevis transfer along a more anatomic course to recreate the ATFL and CFL. Although good results were achieved, even at 10 years, moderate restriction in subtalar movement was still present.[59] Ligamentous reconstructions should be reserved for revision cases given the restriction of physiologic movement and are not recommended for use as the index procedure. Many authors have described free tendon grafts with use of the fascia lata, semitendinosus, and gracilis; however, these grafts are best used in cases of revision or ligamentous laxity given the excellent results achieved with primary repair.[60-63]

AUTHORS' PREFERRED TECHNIQUE

Lateral Ankle Sprain

1. The patient is positioned supine with the leg placed in an ankle distractor. Arthroscopy is performed with use of standard anteromedial and anterolateral portals. Any incidental pathology is then treated arthroscopically.
2. The patient is then placed in a lateral position. A longitudinal incision is performed over the distal fibula and the soft tissues distal to it. The subcutaneous tissues are dissected from the lateral ligament complex. Careful inspection for any branches of the superficial peroneal nerve should be performed.
3. A U-shaped incision is made in the lateral ligament complex 0.5 cm distal to the fibula. The incision extends from just superior to the origin of ATFL to just posterior to the origin of the CFL.
4. A subperiosteal flap is raised off the fibula for approximately 1.5 cm. Rongeurs are used to remove the lateral and distal cortex (Fig. 116-7). A suture anchor is placed at each of the positions of the origin of the ATFL and CFL.
5. The sutures are then used to draw the distal flap onto the distal fibula, and they are tied off. The edge of this distal flap is then sutured to the base of the subperiosteal flap.

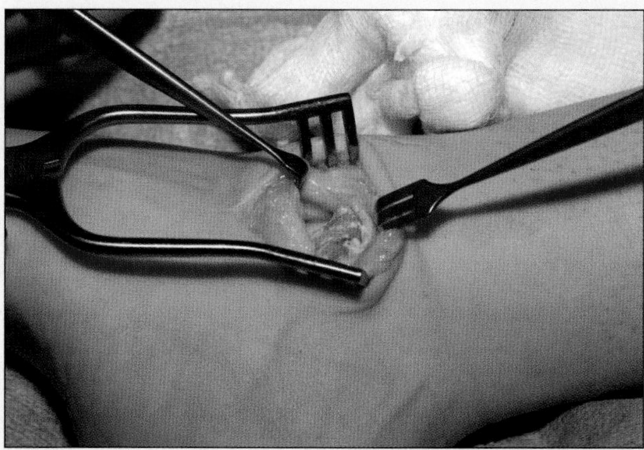

FIGURE 116-7 Intraoperative image showing cortical debridement of the fibula after a subperiosteal flap has been raised.

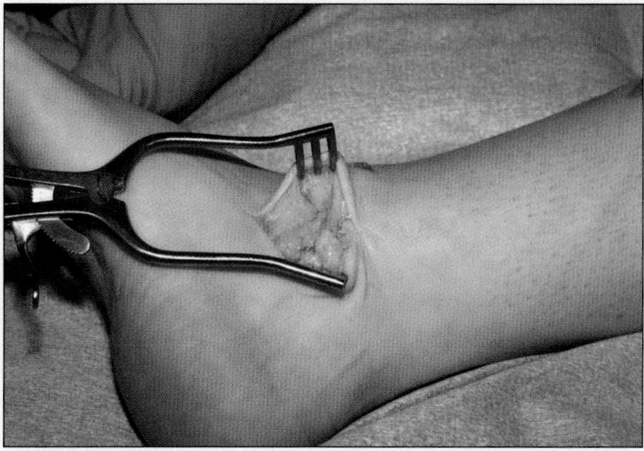

FIGURE 116-8 Intraoperative image showing the completed anatomic imbrication of the lateral ligament complex.

The subperiosteal flap is then sutured distally to lateral soft tissues to act as a double-breasted reinforcement (Fig. 116-8).

6. As an alternative to the use of suture anchors, a pants-over-vest technique is also very effective. The ATFL and CFL are transected 1 mm distal to the tip of the fibula. Bleeding of the cancellous bone of the distal cortex of the fibula is created with a rongeur. In this case, no subperiosteal proximal flap is created. The distal flap is then secured to the proximal soft tissue in a pants-over-vest fashion, taking care to perform an adequate imbrication to decrease the laxity; typically, two or three knots are required. The suture is begun on the distal flap, which allows the knot to be placed distally and away from the skin, and is then reinforced with figure of 8, number 0 absorbable suture after completion of the pants-over-vest imbrication.
7. The extensor retinaculum is then identified and sutured to the reconstruction and the periosteum of the fibula, with the hindfoot and ankle held in a neutral position and dorsiflexion.
8. The wound is closed in layers. The leg is placed into a below-knee backslab cast in dorsiflexion and eversion.

Postoperative Management

The patient wears a splint and is non–weight bearing for 2 weeks. At this stage the sutures are removed and the patient is allowed to bear weight in a locked range of motion walker boot.

At 4 weeks the range of motion walker is unlocked and physical therapy is begun. For the next 2 weeks this therapy consists of ankle range of motion exercises that are isolated to dorsiflexion and plantar flexion only and swelling management.

At 6 weeks the patient is weaned into a semirigid functional brace. The intensity of physical therapy can be increased, with more robust range of motion exercises (except forced inversion), early cardiovascular work, ankle-strengthening exercises, and proprioception exercises. Usually by 9 weeks the patient is being weaned out of the brace and is starting more sport-specific exercises, with progression to return to activity. The rehabilitation regime is obviously altered if other significant pathologic conditions were present in the ankle and addressed arthroscopically (e.g., an osteochondral defect).

Results

We studied a group of 18 consecutive patients prospectively with an average follow-up of 25 months.[5] Clinically, all ankles were objectively and subjectively stable, and the mean American Orthopaedic Foot and Ankle Score (AOFAS) was 89. All patients who played sports had returned to their sporting activities.

Complications

Patients can have persistent pain. In most cases, pathologic conditions explaining the pain will have been reviewed. With persistent long-term significant instability, the risk of posttraumatic osteoarthritis is undoubtedly increased. Most studies have shown that a small chance of recurrent instability exists in the long term. Our preferred method for dealing with cases of long-term instability is a Chrisman-Snook procedure.

Medial Ankle Sprains

Medial sprains are quite uncommon and represent 4% to 5% of all ankle sprains.[64-67]

The deltoid ligament is made up of the superficial and deep layers. The superficial layer originates from the superficial margin of the anterior part of the medial malleolus and attaches to the dorsal talus, navicular, and sustentaculum. The deep deltoid layer is made up of two parts, the deep anterior and deep posterior tibiotalar ligaments, which arise from the deep margin of the posterior colliculus and attach to the medial talus while blending with the medial capsule of the ankle joint.[68-70] The deep deltoid resists posterior and lateral translation in addition to valgus angulation of the talus. The superficial structures of the deltoid complex resist external rotation of the talus relative to the tibia and valgus stress. The flexor retinaculum and the posterior tibial tendon sheath also contribute to the medial ligament complex stability.

Medial sprains are graded I for a ligament stretch injury, II for a partial tear, and III for a complete tear.

History and Physical Examination

The deltoid ligament injury occurs when the hindfoot is in valgus and the forefoot is everted. The main risk factor for this type of injury is being a male athlete, with a possible link to pes planus deformity.[64,71] These injuries tend to be relatively high-impact injuries as opposed to simple "giving way" because of the relative strength and surface area of this ligament, as well as the higher inherent osseous stability of the ankle joint on the medial side.

A patient with an acute injury presents with medial-sided pain and swelling with ecchymosis. The patient may report hearing a "pop" on the medial part of the ankle before the onset of pain and usually has difficulty with weight bearing. Repeated episodes of giving way are uncommon with chronic injuries. Patients with chronic injuries tend to have residual pain together with a lack of trust in the ankle or a sense that "it just doesn't feel right."

After an appropriate focused physical examination is performed, the patient should be asked to lower himself or herself to a squatting position with the feet flat on the floor. In some more significant cases of deltoid insufficiency (usually chronic cases), the medial malleolus becomes overtly prominent compared with the other ankle (a positive medial malleolar pointing sign). It should also be noted whether pes planovalgus is present.

Examination of the superficial deltoid is performed with the patient seated with mild ankle plantar flexion. The heel is cupped in the examiner's hand and brought forward while the tibia is stabilized with the opposite hand. In the case of superficial deltoid insufficiency, enhanced external rotation of the talus is observed in comparison with the contralateral side. In acute superficial deltoid ligament injuries, the anterior portion of the medial malleolus is normally painful to palpation, but this sign may be absent in athletes with chronic instability.[68]

The deep deltoid ligament is assessed by examining the posterior translation of the talus from the tibia, which is best done with the patient prone with the legs hanging off the table. The degree of translation is compared with the other side.

Muscle function should be assessed. The main muscle to be tested is the tibialis posterior muscle. Patients should be asked to perform the double-heel raise test. The heel should smoothly swing from a valgus position to around 10 degrees of varus. The patient also should be asked to perform the single-leg raise test (except in the most acute settings). The patient should be able to perform this test with equal numbers and to an equal height on both legs.

If a valgus, pronated deformity of the foot corrects with single-heel raising, this finding indicates that the patient has a purely ligamentous injury (deltoid and spring ligament) with sparing of the tibialis posterior.[65]

Imaging

Radiographs to assess ligamental injuries include standard weight-bearing anteroposterior (AP), lateral, and mortise views. An AP hindfoot alignment view (Salzmann or Cobey view) is also indicated. Translational deformities can be assessed from the radiographs (Figs. 116-9 and 116-10).

Stress radiographs have some uses, particularly with the valgus stress test on an AP film bilaterally. A finding of more than 2 to 3 degrees of valgus is considered positive. Widening of the medial clear space by 6 mm is also suggestive of a medial injury.[68,72]

MRI can help assess the deltoid ligaments in detail and should be the investigation of choice.[73] However, the position

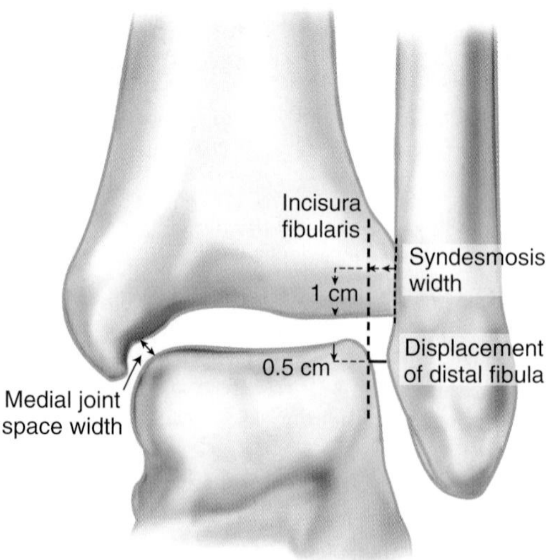

FIGURE 116-9 Techniques of measuring the lateral displacement of the lateral malleolus (mortise view) and the width of the syndesmosis (mortise view) and medial joint space (anteroposterior view). *(Modified from Harper MC: The deltoid ligament: an evaluation of need for surgical repair.* Clin Orthop *226:156–168, 1988.)*

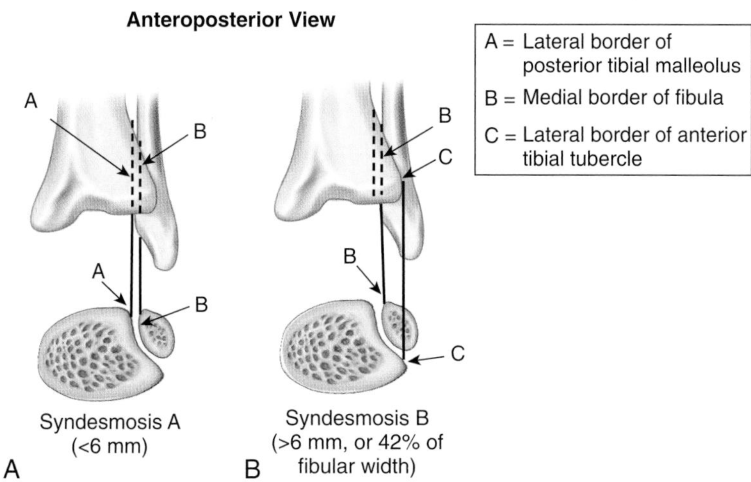

FIGURE 116-10 Syndesmotic radiographic criteria. **A,** The syndesmosis clear space as depicted on the anteroposterior view and by coronal section. The tibiofibular clear space is the distance between the lateral border of the posterior tibial malleolus (point *A*) and the medial border of the fibula (point *B*) on the anteroposterior radiograph. This space is normally less than 6 mm. **B,** The syndesmosis overlap as seen on the anteroposterior view and by coronal section. The tibiofibular overlap is the distance between the medial border of the fibula (point *B*) and the lateral border of the anterior tibial prominence (point *C*) on the anteroposterior radiograph. This space is normally greater than 6 mm, or 42% of the fibular width. *(Modified from Stiehl JB: Complex ankle fracture dislocations with syndesmosis diastasis.* Orthop Rev *14:499–507, 1990.)*

of the foot may influence the visualization of the relevant anatomy because the tibionavicular and anterior tibiotalar parts are best seen with the foot in plantar flexion, whereas the tibiocalcaneal and posterior tibiotalar parts are best seen in dorsiflexion.[74]

Decision-Making Principles

The primary decision is whether the ligaments have discontinuity, because this factor has the largest influence on potential treatments. One must ensure that the syndesmosis, spring ligament, and tibialis posterior are intact. Although clinical acumen is pivotal in this decision, further imaging is essential when a partial or complete tear of the deltoid ligament is suspected. Normally, operative treatment is indicated only with failure of conservative treatment unless additional pathologic conditions need to be addressed.

Treatment

Grade I (Strain)

Strains can be treated with a semirigid brace that allows ankle plantar flexion and dorsiflexion but prevents inversion and eversion. Elevation and cold therapy are also indicated for the first week. A structural rehabilitation program is indicated and should initially focus on proprioception and maintenance of range of motion. Return to sport is achieved in a graduated fashion as dictated by symptoms but normally occurs within 3 weeks, with use of a laced ankle brace for another 3 weeks.

Grades II (Partial Tear) and III (Complete Tear)

An MRI scan should be performed to see if any evidence exists of an avulsion or complete intrasubstance tear of the deltoid, as well as any of the other aforementioned pathologic conditions. If complete insufficiency of the deltoid is suspected, an examination with use of an anesthetic should be performed. Surgical repair is appropriate in the setting of documented instability.

If conservative treatment is indicated, initial immobilization is used to promote anatomic healing followed by physical therapy. Our preference is to treat patients initially in a locked range of motion walker with an orthotic to support the medial longitudinal arch. The patient can bear weight as tolerated but must keep the boot on at all times except for purposes of hygiene. At 4 weeks the boot can be unlocked from 5 degrees dorsiflexion to 30 degrees plantar flexion to commence early mobilization. At 6 weeks the boot is completely unlocked and can be removed during physical therapy for range of motion, proprioception, and ankle and inversion strength exercises.

AUTHORS' PREFERRED TECHNIQUE

Medial Ankle Sprain

If the ankle is unstable upon examination with use of an anesthetic, then surgical exploration can be indicated.

1. A medial longitudinal incision is performed from the medial malleolar metaphyseal flare down to the level of the talonavicular joint. The subcutaneous tissues are dissected off the deltoid ligament with careful inspection for any branches of the saphenous nerve in the superior margins of the wound.
2. If a superior avulsion is present, the torn ends of the ligament are dissected free. The cortex is removed with use of rongeurs. Two or three suture anchors are then used to reattach the ligament. Alternatively, bone tunnels can be used to anchor the ligament.
3. If an intrasubstance tear is present, the subperiosteal flap should be raised and suture anchors used as in the surgical technique for lateral ligament insufficiency.
4. The wound is closed in layers. The patient's ankle is placed in a backslab in dorsiflexion and inversion. The postoperative regimen is similar to that for conservative treatment once the patient progresses to a locked range of motion walker with an orthotic at 2 weeks.

The patient is gradually weaned out of the boot into a functional ankle brace and undergoes a graduated return to sport-specific exercises with return to play in a brace for a further 6 weeks.

Results

Evidence supporting acute surgical treatment of deltoid injuries is sparse. Some surgeons perform this procedure in conjunction with ankle fracture open reduction internal fixation, but no evidence exists to support this practice.

In a prospective series of 52 patients with chronic anterior deltoid incompetence, pain in the medial gutter was found in all ankles (100%), pain along the posterior tibial tendon was found in 14 ankles (27%), and pain along the anterior border of the lateral malleolus was found in 13 ankles (25%). Repair of the deltoid ligament was performed in all 52 patients, repair of the spring ligament was performed in 13 patients (24%), repair of the lateral ligaments was performed in 40 patients (77%), and an additional calcaneal-lengthening osteotomy was performed in 14 patients (27%). At a mean follow-up of 4.4 years (range: 2.0 to 6.6 years), the AOFAS hindfoot score had improved from 42.9 points preoperatively to 91.6 points. The clinical result was considered good to excellent in 46 cases (90%), fair in four cases (8%), and poor in one case (2%).[75]

Complications

Two possible local complications can arise from isolated deltoid injuries. Nonunited avulsion fragments or heterotropic ossification can produce localized osseous impingement at the medial gutter. They can also produce a local prominence that can rub against footwear. It is prudent to obtain a preoperative MRI scan to check for a medial osteochondral defect, the symptoms of which can be masked by the presence of these fragments. These fragments can be removed either through a deltoid-splitting incision or, for larger areas of ossification, by detaching the deltoid and reattaching it with suture anchors or bone tunnels (Figs. 116-11 and 116-12).

Chronic instability is the second complication and is most commonly due to insufficiency of the superficial deltoid. Hintermann et al.[76] described three types of this instability. Type I is due to a chronic avulsion from the medial malleolus, and type II is a chronic intrasubstance tear. They are treated as outlined in the section on acute injuries. Type III lesions are from the distal insertion of the deltoid. These lesions are repaired with nonabsorbable sutures into the spring ligament, as well as a suture anchor into the superior edge of the navicular tuberosity if additional insufficiency of the tibionavicular part of the superficial deltoid is present. With use of this treatment algorithm, the authors managed to achieve a 90% rate of excellent results at 4 years.

Chronic instability of the deep deltoid ligament is an extremely challenging condition. Many different choices of graft and graft fixation have been attempted with equivocal results.

Syndesmosis Sprain

The incidence of ankle syndesmosis injuries, or high ankle sprains, is around 15 per 100,000 in the general population and is much higher in the athletic population. These injuries can represent between 1% and 11% of all ankle injuries.[77,78]

The distal tibiofibular syndesmosis is composed of the anterior inferior and posterior inferior tibiofibular ligaments (AITFL and PITFL) and the interosseous membrane with its corresponding ligament.

The interosseous tibiofibular ligament is the strongest connection between the tibia and fibula and runs from the lateral distal tibia to the medial distal fibula. It is in continuation with the interosseous membrane proximally.[79]

The AITFL provides 35% of the resistance to diastasis stress of the syndesmosis, whereas the PITFL contributes 40% to 45%, and the remainder comes from the interosseous ligament.

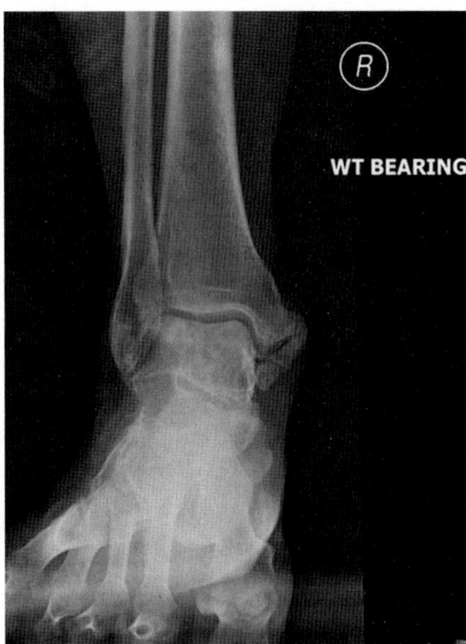

FIGURE 116-11 Radiograph showing a chronic heterotropic ossification after a deltoid ligament avulsion injury.

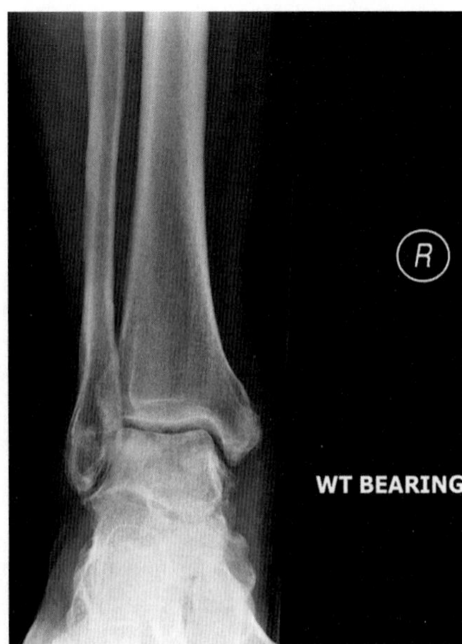

FIGURE 116-12 Postoperative radiograph 6 weeks after debridement of heterotropic ossification and reattachment of the deltoid ligament.

The AITFL is the first and most commonly injured ligament in a syndesmosis sprain, and the PITFL is the last ligament injured.

The syndesmosis, along with the deltoid ligament, prevents diastasis of the joint and maintains function. During non–weight-bearing plantar flexion, the distal fibula moves anteriorly and inferiorly and medially rotates after the internal rotation of the talus, whereas in dorsiflexion, the distal fibula glides in a posterosuperior direction and rotates laterally with the talus, which explains the mechanism of injury.[80]

History and Examination

The mechanism of injury is usually an externally rotated and dorsiflexed foot and axial loading,[81] which places stress on the ligaments. The AITFL fails first as noted, and the PITFL tries to stabilize the syndesmosis. With continued external rotation and/or abduction, the entire system fails and results in a diastasis.

Normally in most complete disruptions, associated injuries are found, such as Weber B or C fracture, Maisonneuve fracture, and also deltoid disruption and medial malleolar fracture, depending on the pattern of injury. Diastasis without fracture can occur but is extremely rare.

The clinical features that are in keeping with a syndesmosis injury classically are pain over the anterior and posterior tibiofibular ligaments. Often patients can point to this area where they have maximal tenderness. As the severity of the injury increases, the tenderness moves proximally to the anteromedial part of the fibula where the interosseous membrane is attached.

The combination of swelling, tenderness, laxity, weight-bearing reluctance, and radiographic findings allows the injury to be classified from grade I to III.

A grade I injury involves injury to the anterior deltoid ligament and the distal interosseous ligament but without tearing of the more proximal syndesmosis or the deep deltoid ligament. The AITFL often is very tender to palpation. Grade I injuries are stable because no diastasis is present.

A grade II injury involves disruption of the anterior and deep deltoid ligaments, as well as a tear in a significant portion of the syndesmosis, resulting in an unstable ankle.

Grade III injuries are unstable and involve complete disruption of the medial ligaments and extensive disruption of the syndesmosis and are often accompanied by a proximal fibula (Maisonneuve) fracture.

Many tests are available for diagnosis of a syndesmotic sprain, including the squeeze test, dorsiflexion compression test, external rotation test, manual stability test, cross-leg test, and heel thump test. All these tests are devised to stress the ligaments and thus reproduce the pain. The most reliable and most useful test is the external rotation test.[82]

The external rotation test is performed with the patient seated, the hip and knee flexed, and the foot and ankle in the neutral position. With the knee facing forward, a gentle external rotation is applied to the foot. The test is positive if the pain is reproduced at the anterior syndesmosis.

Imaging

Radiographs in these patients should include AP, mortise, and lateral views, including the entire tibia and fibula if a high fibular fracture is suspected. Ideally a weight-bearing view is preferred, but in a person with an acute injury, obtaining such a view may not always be possible. The three measurements that may help in diagnosing syndesmosis injuries are tibiofibular clear space, medial clear space, and tibiofibular overlap.

Recent data demonstrate that basing treatment of syndesmotic injuries on previously reported radiographic criteria can lead to unnecessary operative intervention or failure to treat.[83] The mean tibiofibular overlap is 8.3 mm on the AP and 3.5 mm on the mortise view, whereas the mean clear space is 4.6 mm on the AP and 4.3 mm on the mortise view. The least amount of overlap on the AP view was 1.8 mm. On the mortise view, a subset of patients had a complete lack of overlap (less than 0 mm), with the greatest gap noted to be 1.9 mm. The greatest clear space on the AP view was 8 mm, and on the mortise view it was 7.6 mm. The problem with relying on absolute values is that significant variations exist in the patient population, which may lead to misdiagnosis; therefore comparison with the contralateral lower extremity provides a more reliable "normal" measurement on which to base treatment. The clear space on the mortise view radiograph has been proved to be relatively independent of rotation, and 95% of patients have a less than 2-mm side-to-side difference.[82] If the initial radiographs are still not helpful, stress radiographs with the leg in external rotation may help assess for diastasis (Fig. 116-13).

If the diagnosis is still in doubt, three-dimensional imaging is warranted. Although computed tomography (CT) has been proved to show smaller diastases from 1 mm, MRI currently seems to be the more favored modality because of its high sensitivity and specificity and because it also helps show the injured anatomy and may aid in surgical planning (Fig. 116-14).

Decision-Making Principles

A chronic, unstable, untreated syndesmosis injury can predispose the patient to further injury, degenerative changes, chronic pain, and osteochondral lesions.[84] Therefore the key principle in the treatment of a syndesmotic injury is to maintain a high suspicion of the injury. Any evidence of widening of the syndesmosis, clear space, or fracture requires operative intervention.

Treatment

Grade I injuries are stable and can be treated nonoperatively. Rehabilitation with use of the RICE method with initial non–weight bearing in a boot and early mobilization is indicated. Serial radiographs may be indicated to ascertain that the injury has not progressed. The treatment is tailored to the athlete's progress. Once the swelling and pain have improved, early mobilization (between 3 and 6 weeks) is initiated. At this time, patients may still need some external support so they can start their rehabilitation program, starting with range of motion exercises and increasing to strengthening exercises as tolerated.

Grade II and III injuries are unstable and require surgical treatment. Many techniques have been described, including screw fixation, sutures with Endobutton, and tendon grafts.

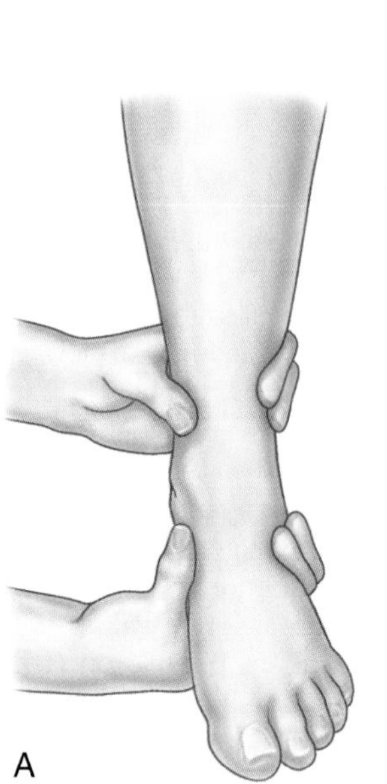
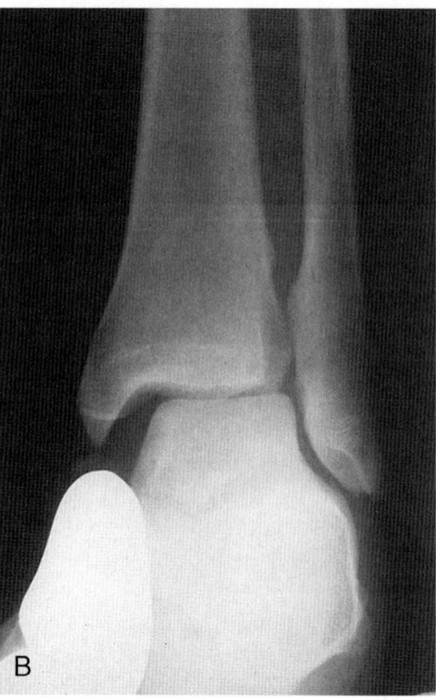

FIGURE 116-13 **A,** The direct eversion maneuver is accomplished with the patient in a seated and relaxed position. The examiner gently secures the leg and foot as a direct eversion or abduction force is applied across the ankle. Increased translation compared with the contralateral ankle is a positive result. **B,** A positive stress radiograph showing increased translation. *(**A,** Modified from Stiehl JB: Complex ankle fracture dislocations with syndesmotic diastasis.* Orthop Rev *19:499–507, 1990.)*

AUTHORS' PREFERRED TECHNIQUE

Syndesmosis Sprain

1. A longitudinal incision is made over the distal fibula. All branches of the superficial peroneal nerve are identified and protected.
2. The AITFL is carefully inspected. If an avulsion fragment is present, a decision is made about whether it can be fixed anatomically. Occasionally the ligament still has reasonable quality and a direct repair can be performed at the end of the procedure.
3. All extraneous fibrous tissue and any ossification is removed. The fibula is then reduced with a large reduction clamp. If it is irreducible or if significant force is required to achieve reduction, soft tissue may be interposed in the medial gutter. A separate medial incision is performed and the tissue is removed.
4. Fixation of the syndesmosis is performed with use of two tricortical 3.5-mm screws through a ⅓ tubular plate. These screws are inserted at 90 degrees to the joint line under fluoroscopic control.
5. The integrity of the deltoid ligament is then assessed both clinically and under fluoroscopic control. If it is found to be insufficient, a repair is performed as described in the deltoid ligament section. If possible, repair of the AITFL is then performed.

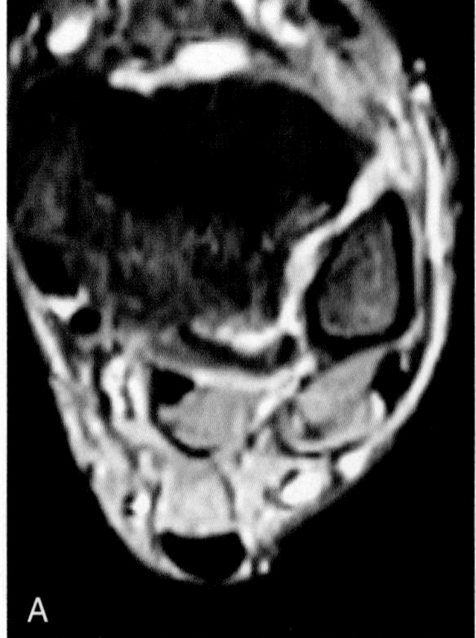
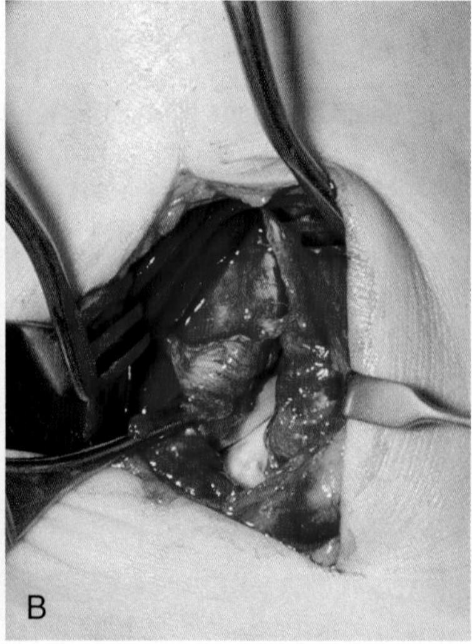

FIGURE 116-14 **A,** A magnetic resonance image demonstrating a complete tear of the anterior inferior tibiofibular ligament and a partial tear of the posterior inferior tibiofibular ligament. **B,** Open treatment of a syndesmotic rupture.

Postoperative Management

Patients are non–weight bearing in a cast or a removable controlled ankle motion walker for 6 weeks. Patients then graduate to using an unlocked range of motion walker boot or a semirigid brace for another 6 weeks. If screw removal is planned, patients are limited to nonimpact activity until removal of the hardware to minimize the risk of screw fracture. The rehabilitation program should then be carried out as for conservatively treated syndesmosis injuries.

Screws should be removed no earlier than 3 months after surgery. Removal between 4 and 5 months from the time of the injury allows increased time for the soft tissue healing to occur but increases the risk of hardware failure. One should consider later removal in patients with chronic injuries or in very heavy patients. Patients should be counseled that it will take at least 6 months for symptoms to resolve and that some patients will have a permanent decrease in function.

Results

Return to sport always takes longer in persons with syndesmotic injuries compared with persons with ankle sprains. Gerber et al.[66] studied a group of 96 military cadets, 16 of whom had a syndesmotic injury. At 6 months, their final outcome was worse than that of the subjects with lateral ligament injuries. Taylor et al.[85] showed that at 47 months, 23% of subjects had chronic ankle pain, 36% had ankle stiffness, and 18% had persistent swelling. Patients with longer recovery time frequently showed ossification of the interosseus membrane.

Wolf and Amendola[86] treated 14 patients who had a chronic syndesmotic injury but not diastasis with arthroscopic debridement and percutaneous screw fixation for 8 to 10 weeks in cases of latent instability. The short-term results were excellent in two patients, good in 10 patients, and fair in four patients.

Grass et al.[87] performed reconstruction of the AITFL and PITFL with the peroneus brevis tendon guided through bony channels in the distal tibia and fibula for patients with chronic syndesmotic instability. The first results in a series of 16 patients followed up for an average of 18 months were encouraging, with 15 of 16 having relief of pain and chronic instability.

Complications

Patients should be counseled that a significant minority (up to 20%) will have some degree of permanent symptoms. Patients with higher-grade injuries almost certainly have an increased chance of the development of posttraumatic osteoarthritis.

Patients should have regular weight-bearing radiographs after surgery and for some months after the removal of the metalwork because of the risk of recurrent diastasis. In the event of these complications, surgical strategies are available. Techniques of syndesmosis reconstruction have been described with use of autograft or allograft tendons, along with isolated syndesmosis fusion.

Bifurcate Ligament Sprain/Fracture of the Anterior Process of Calcaneum

The bifurcate ligament is commonly damaged by forceful inversion and plantar flexion of the foot, which can either cause a bifurcate ligament sprain or fracture of the anterior process of the calcaneum.[88,89]

The bifurcate ligament is a Y-shaped ligament composed of the calcaneonavicular and calcaneocuboid arms that originates from the anterior process of the calcaneum and attaches to the navicular and cuboid, respectively. It lies distal and anterior to the inferior lip of the fibula and superior and proximal to the base of the fifth metatarsal.

The anterior process of calcaneus fractures can be caused by tension, compression, or shear. Tension injuries cause avulsion fractures such as those seen with a plantarflexed inverted foot. Shear fractures are caused by forefoot abduction with the heel fixed to the ground and forced dorsiflexion. Compression fractures are caused by dorsiflexion eversion injuries, which tend to cause intraarticular fractures.

Degan classified these fractures into three types. Type I is an undisplaced fracture, type II is displaced fracture without intraarticular involvement, and type III is a displaced fracture involving the calcaneocuboid joint.[90,91]

History and Physical Examination

The history can be variable, but an inversion plantar flexion injury should lead one to look for this condition. However, this injury is not normally isolated, because ankle sprains, particularly on the lateral side, can be present along with the bifurcate sprain.[92]

The patient may have felt a pop or a snap with acute onset of pain followed by ecchymosis and swelling.

Examination confirms diffuse swelling over the lateral hindfoot and midfoot. The pain may be localized over the course of the ligament, which is normally separate from the ATFL, which is the other ligament that is often damaged with this mechanism of injury. Inversion and plantar flexion reproduces the pain. Broström suggested that the way to distinguish ATFL pain from bifurcate pain is to manipulate the heel to produce lateral-sided pain, whereas forced forefoot motion with the hindfoot stabilized will elicit bifurcate pain.[90]

Imaging

Routine AP, lateral, and oblique views of the foot and ankle are obtained. In persons with a bifurcate sprain, the radiographs are likely to be normal but may show an anterior process of a calcaneum fracture. The normal series may not always show the fracture, and therefore an oblique radiograph with the central ray directed 10 to 15 degrees superior and posterior to the middle of the foot is often useful because this technique projects over the process over the talus and makes visualization of the fracture much easier.[93]

CT is the preferred choice to assess fractures but is not useful for bifurcate sprains, for which MRI is superior.[88]

Decision-Making Principles

The treatment of bifurcate sprains is initially conservative. The only exception to this approach is the presence of a large or displaced anterior process fracture that may be amenable to surgical treatment. If such a fracture is suspected on plain radiographs, a CT scan should be performed to delineate the size of the fragment, whether it extends into the calcaneocuboid joint, and whether it is multifragmentary, which will determine the appropriateness of early surgery.

Treatment

Acute sprains are initially treated with RICE followed by range of motion and protected weight bearing. They can be initially supported with short removable boot, a walking cast, or a functional brace. Physical therapy emphasizes subtalar flexibility, motor function, and coordination.[93] The rehabilitation program starts with simple range of motion exercises, as well as isometric exercises. As the acute phase subsides, more aggressive therapies can be introduced, starting with closed-chain activities and graduating up to sport-specific exercises, followed by a graduated return to play. Søndergaard et al.[94] reported excellent results, with the time to return to sports averaging 21 days.

Chronic sprains can be treated similarly to acute sprains, but steroids can also be injected either intralesionally or intraarticularly at the calcaneocuboid level under fluoroscopic guidance. If symptoms do not diminish, operative treatment should be considered, which can be in the form of an open or arthroscopic procedure. However, operative treatment is rarely required.

AUTHORS' PREFERRED TECHNIQUE

Bifurcate Ligament Sprain

1. A lateral incision is made from just distal to the tip of the fibula toward the base of the fourth metatarsal. Care is taken not to damage any branches of the superficial peroneal nerve in the superior margins of the wound.
2. The extensor digitorum brevis is raised as a flap off the lateral border of the calcaneus, leaving a small cuff of tissue for later repair.
3. The sinus tarsi is identified as far distally as the superior aspect of the calcaneocuboid joint. Inflamed and fibrotic tissue is debrided with rongeurs. If a small malunited or nonunited fracture of the anterior process of the calcaneus is present, it is excised. If the procedure is acute and a large fracture is to be fixed, the fracture site is cleared, reduction is performed with a wire, and a headless compression screw is used for fixation.
4. Stress views of the hindfoot and ankle should then be performed to determine if any residual instability is present to help determine the postoperative regimen of mobilization.
5. The wound is closed in layers and a splint is applied.

Postoperative Management

The splint is kept in place for 2 weeks. A semirigid ankle brace is applied, and the patient is then allowed to bear weight. The same rehabilitation program is then used as outlined in the section on conservative treatment.

If any residual instability was present at the time of the operation, the patient's ankle is mobilized in a range of motion walker boot with the range of movement gradually increased over a period of 4 to 6 weeks. The patient then undergoes rehabilitation according to the more standard postoperative regimen. It should be noted that, unfortunately, symptoms can occasionally be protracted.

Results

No peer-reviewed articles are available that delineate the expected results from this injury.

Complications

The main complication is nonresolving pain with or without instability. Steroid injections with a further rehabilitation program can often be successful in relieving symptoms. In the rare cases in which pain persists, an arthrodesis may be required. Isolated calcaneocuboid fusion can be performed; however, union may be difficult to achieve. Arthrodesis of the triple-joint complex has a higher rate of union but imparts a significant loss of hindfoot motion.

Lisfranc Sprains

Lisfranc sprains or midfoot sprains occur at the Lisfranc joint, which is the second most common area in the foot to be injured in athletes after the metatarsophalangeal joint.[95,96] This area of the midfoot is named after Jacques Lisfranc, the French Napoleonic surgeon.

The incidence of midfoot sprains is around 4%. A Lisfranc sprain is a sprain of the midfoot due to a low-impact injury, whereas a Lisfranc fracture dislocation is the result of a high-impact injury.[97]

The midfoot is made up of five bones—the navicular, cuboid, and three cuneiform bones. The Lisfranc joint is the articulations between the three cuneiform bones and the cuboid bone with the five metatarsals. The shape of the articulating surfaces with the metatarsal bases provides primary stability, with the second tarsometatarsal joint acting as a keystone and providing stability in both the longitudinal and transverse arches.

These joints also classify the columns in the foot. The medial column is made up of the first ray and medial cuneiform bone, the middle column is made up of the second and third rays and middle and lateral cuneiform bones, and the lateral column is made up of the fourth and fifth rays with the cuboid bone. The rigidity of the medial and middle column is important to the function of the foot, and the Lisfranc ligament provides the rigid connection between the columns.[98]

Numerous ligaments in the Lisfranc joint provide the secondary stabilization. Dorsal and plantar ligaments are present, with the plantar ligaments being stronger than the dorsal ligaments.[99] The most important structure is the Lisfranc ligament, which is the plantar ligament running between the medial cuneiform and the base of the second metatarsal.[100]

History and Physical Examination

The mechanism of injury can be either direct or indirect.[101] Direct-force injuries as described by Myerson et al.[103] entail an axial-directed force acting on the dorsum of the foot, causing tension on the plantar surface and leading to injury. These injuries are usually higher-energy injuries in an industrial setting. Because of the mechanism of injury, open fractures and compartment syndrome are more common in this setting than in indirect injuries.

The more common indirect-force injuries are usually low-energy injuries and occur when a weight-bearing hyper–plantar-flexed foot with a rotational or bending force is applied to the foot or when the plantigrade foot is kept fixed to the floor (e.g., upon stamping in soccer) with the body rotating over the top of the foot. The severity of these injuries depends on the force and mechanism of injury.

In 2002 Nunley and Vertullo[102] classified Lisfranc injuries into three stages on the basis of radiographic and clinical findings and bone scan results. Stage I is a nondisplaced injury in which the patient may be able to bear weight but cannot return to sports. Stages II and III show displacement and require operative intervention. This classification has more relevance in low-energy injuries such as midfoot sprains.

Myerson and colleagues[103] classified Lisfranc injuries based on the classification performed by Hardcastle and colleagues.[104] Unfortunately, the classification systems do not significantly aid in determining treatment and outcome. A descriptive analysis of the involved joints, the presence of a fracture, and articular comminution is more useful than any particular classification scheme.

Associated injuries include a stress fracture of the base of the second metatarsal, particularly in female dancers with low-energy injuries, a nutcracker fracture of the cuboid, and compartment syndrome, particularly in high-energy injuries.

Clinical examination of the entire foot and ankle is performed to evaluate for other concomitant injuries. Patients usually present with pain and swelling and, depending on the extent of injury, may not be able to bear weight. Any ecchymosis present in the center of the plantar aspect of the foot is highly indicative of a Lisfranc injury.

Stability is tested in the sagittal plane if possible. With the midfoot secured with one hand and the other holding the first metatarsal, a dorsiflexion force is applied and abnormal translation and pain is noted compared with the normal foot on the other side. In the frontal plane, stability is tested with abduction and adduction forces. Myerson and colleagues described the pronation-abduction test, which is positive if it elicits pain and reproduces the patient's symptoms.[105] Pain with single-limb weight bearing is also suggestive of a Lisfranc injury and should be performed after obtaining appropriate imaging to ensure that no fractures have occurred.

Imaging

The best plain films are weight-bearing bilateral AP, lateral, and oblique views. Non–weight-bearing radiographs miss up to 50% of Lisfranc injuries and sprains.[97] Normal foot anatomy and congruency of the joints in all views should be assessed, and abnormal findings such as fracture and diastasis should be sought. Particular attention should be directed to looking for a "fleck sign," which is indicative of a cortical avulsion of the Lisfranc ligament (Fig. 116-15).

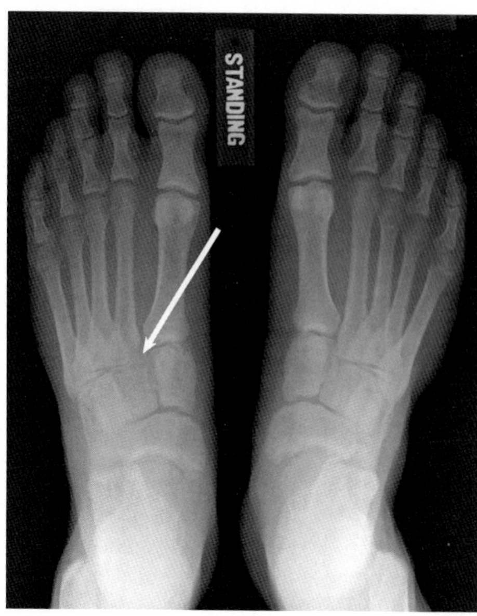

FIGURE 116-15 A patient with a Lisfranc injury identified by the "fleck sign" (*arrow*). In this case, the ligament itself remained intact and the injury occurs by avulsion of the ligament from the base of the second metatarsal. The function of the ligament is compromised, and operative intervention is indicated.

One should beware of normal appearances of non–weight-bearing radiographs when a high clinical index of suspicion exists. In this scenario, we recommend further imaging or conservative treatment until full weight-bearing films can be obtained. Single-limb weight-bearing views of the affected foot may also demonstrate subtle instability because patients shift weight to the unaffected extremity with a double-limb weight-bearing view.

The patient must be examined for Lisfranc variants with intercuneiform instability or disruption of the naviculocuneiform joint with an impaction fracture of the navicular. Stress radiographs are not routinely performed in the office because they cause extreme pain and patient guarding limits their utility. Examination with use of an anesthetic is typically required to determine the instability of the midfoot with manual stress testing. Pronation abduction and adduction stress testing is performed, and the joint is assessed with imaging.[97,106]

Bone scintigraphy has a very limited role. CT scanning can be helpful, particularly in demonstrating fracture patterns and the presence of any occult fractures. CT scans are particularly useful in assessing high-energy injuries.

MRI assessment of soft tissue is excellent and may be helpful, particularly with sprains and low-energy injuries; ligamentous anatomy and disruption can be examined when the diagnosis is in doubt.[106]

Decision-Making Principles

In cases with midfoot pain after an injury, the diagnosis of a Lisfranc injury is presumed. Nonoperative management is considered in cases with normal weight-bearing radiographs and/or corroborative MRI findings of an intact Lisfranc ligament. Biweekly weight-bearing radiographs for the first 6 weeks and a follow-up radiograph at 3 months are recommended to ensure that no displacement occurs. Any evidence of displacement or bony fracture requires operative reduction and stabilization.

Treatment

Stage 1 sprains can be treated conservatively with initial immobilization in a non–weight-bearing cast for 6 weeks. If the athlete is asymptomatic at this stage, a semirigid orthosis can be applied and the patient can be mobilized. If the patient still has symptoms, use of an ankle foot orthosis for an additional 4 weeks may be required.[96,100,102]

Range of movement can usually be initiated at around 8 weeks, but full weight bearing should not be initiated until 3 months after the injury. Supportive heel cushions may be needed once the athlete returns to training. Repeat imaging must be performed to ensure lack of displacement. Any diastasis or change in the alignment should be corrected with surgical intervention.

Patients with stages II and III are treated with surgery. The goal of surgery is to reduce the joints in an anatomic position and maintain this reduction until healing occurs. For this reason Kirschner wires should not be used because of the high incidence of recurrence of deformity. Usually the joints that need to be treated can be determined preoperatively, but fluoroscopic stress views should be carefully obtained intraoperatively to ensure that no residual instability is present.

The injuries can be addressed with screw or plate fixation. Reduction needs to be anatomic. Use of a bridging plate minimizes further articular injury because no screws cross the affected joints, and in cases of hardware failure, no intraarticular hardware will be present. However, during hardware removal, a large incision is required. In a prospective randomized study, Ly and Coetzee[107] noted their belief that better results could be achieved with use of primary fusion instead of fixation in all Lisfranc injuries except those with no or minimal displacement. However, Mulier et al.[108] demonstrated that fusion should be reserved for the more severely comminuted fracture dislocations.

AUTHORS' PREFERRED TECHNIQUE

Lisfranc Sprain

1. In minimally displaced injuries in patients with good bone stock, a percutaneous reduction may be attempted. Stab incisions are made over the lateral part of the base of the second metatarsal and the medial side of the medial cuneiform. A large reduction clamp is applied. Careful fluoroscopic examination is undertaken. If a perfect reduction is achieved, a 4.0-mm cannulated screw is inserted from the base of the second metatarsal into the medial cuneiform. The fluoroscopic examination is repeated along with stress views to see if any other joint requires stabilization. If so, they are addressed in a similar fashion. If this technique is to be used, it is essential that anatomic reduction be achieved. If any doubt exists about the possibility of anatomic reduction, conversion to an open operation should take place.
2. If a percutaneous reduction is not indicated or is unsuccessful, then an open procedure is performed. A longitudinal incision is made between the first and second metatarsals, extending proximally to the naviculocuneiform joint. The neurovascular structures are carefully retracted. Any interposed soft tissue or loose osseous fragments are removed. Reduction is performed from proximal to distal and medial to lateral. Therefore the intercuneiform should be stabilized, followed by the first tarsometatarsal, which creates a stable corner into which the second metatarsal can be reduced. In the setting of a naviculocuneiform variant, reduction of the intercuneiform joint allows for reduction of the impaction fracture of medial navicular. Fixation is then performed with the same cannulated screws or a bridging locking plate depending on bone quality and if associated fractures are present. If the third tarsometatarsal joint is involved, this condition is best addressed through a second incision based on the medial aspect of the fourth metatarsal, which also allows exposure of the cuboid if needed (Fig. 116-16).
3. Normally the fourth and fifth metatarsals reduce and remain stable. If this is not the case, Kirschner wires are used for 6 weeks because it is important to maintain high levels of flexibility in these joints.
4. Primary arthrodesis is reserved for the most severe injuries. This procedure is performed in a fashion similar to that performed for primary osteoarthritis. It is obviously complicated by the lack of bone stock, and bone grafting is often necessary.
5. The wounds are closed in layers. The foot is protected in a cast.

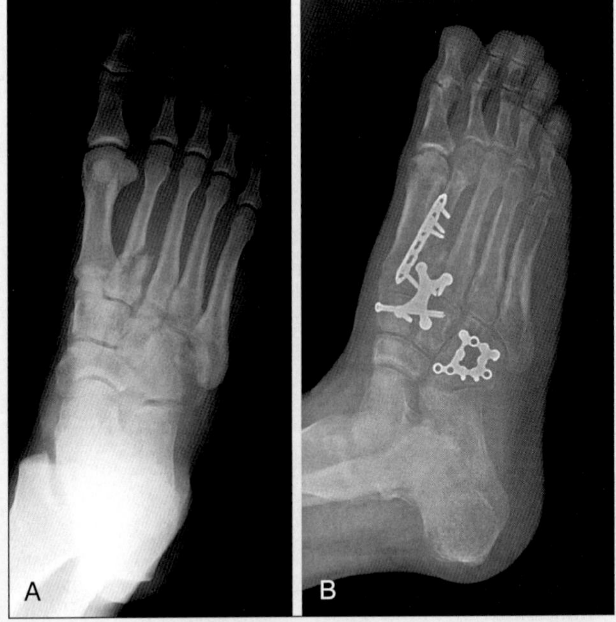

FIGURE 116-16 **A** and **B,** A combination of screw and plate fixation was used to maintain the reduction in a patient with a high-energy Lisfranc injury. Plate fixation is very useful in the setting of fractures of the base of the metatarsals that prevent adequate purchase for a screw. The patient also had a cuboid fracture that required plate fixation.

Postoperative Management

Patients are kept non–weight bearing for 6 weeks. This period is extended if high levels of comminution are present. The patient is then allowed to bear weight in a range of motion walker with an orthotic to support the medial longitudinal arch. Although no exact consensus exists with regard to the timing of hardware removal, it should be removed no earlier than 3 months after the procedure. Delaying hardware removal in obese patients and laborers may decrease the rate of late failure but increases the rate of hardware fracture. Removal of hardware from between 4 and 5 months offers a good compromise between ligamentous healing and hardware failure. The foot continues to be supported orthotically for a further 3 months. Physical therapy prior to hardware removal focuses on ankle and hindfoot movement, as well as low-impact cardiovascular work (e.g., use of an exercise bike). A graduated rehabilitation program can be undertaken after hardware removal.

Results

These injuries are significant. Average AOFASs are around 70 at medium-term follow-up for open reduction with internal fixation.[108,109] It should be noted that these scores included those of patients with the most severe injuries. The most significant factor for optimum results was the accuracy of reduction. Far better results are reported in athletes with more minor injuries that were able to be treated conservatively.[110,111]

Complications

The most significant complication is stiffness, residual pain, and posttraumatic arthritis. In this event, an arthrodesis is performed as a pain-relieving operation, although it may not improve the overall sporting function of the patient. If a primary arthrodesis is performed, then nonunion is also a reported complication in up to 33% of patients.[108] Complex regional pain syndrome is also widely reported. It is therefore necessary that soft tissues be handled as gently as possible during operative treatment.

For a complete list of references, go to expertconsult.com.

Suggested Readings

Lateral Ankle Sprains

Citation: Gould N, Seligson D, Gassman J: Early and late repair of lateral ligament of the ankle. *Foot Ankle* 1:84–89, 1980.
Level of Evidence: III
Summary: In this seminal article on operative treatment of chronic instability, the authors outline a description of a modification of the Broström technique.

Medial Ankle Sprains

Citation: Hintermann B, Knupp M, Geert IP: Deltoid ligament injuries: Diagnosis and management. *Foot Ankle Clin North Am* 11:625–637, 2006.
Level of Evidence: IV
Summary: The authors provide an overview of medial ligament injuries, a classification, an algorithm based on the classification, and the results of this algorithm.

Syndesmosis Sprains

Citation: Rammelt S, Zwipp H, Grass R: Injuries to the distal tibiofibular syndesmosis: An evidence-based approach to acute and chronic lesions. *Foot Ankle Clin* 13(4):611–633, 2008.
Level of Evidence: IV
Summary: In this article both acute and chronic injuries are reviewed and the authors' results for treatment of chronic injuries are detailed.

Bifurcate Ligament Injury/Fracture of Anterior Process of Calcaneum

Citation: Degan TJ, Morrey BF, Braun DP: Fractures of the anterior process of the calcaneus. *J Bone Joint Surg Am* 64A:519–524, 1982.
Level of Evidence: III
Summary: The authors classify fractures of the anterior process of the calcaneus, as well as treatment options and outcomes.

Lisfranc Sprains

Citation: Myerson MS, Fisher RT, Burgess AR, et al: Fracture dislocations of the tarsometatarsal joints: End results correlated with pathology and treatment. *Foot Ankle* 6:225–242, 1986.
Level of Evidence: III
Summary: In this seminal article the authors outline the etiology, classification, treatment algorithm, and outcomes of Lisfranc injuries.

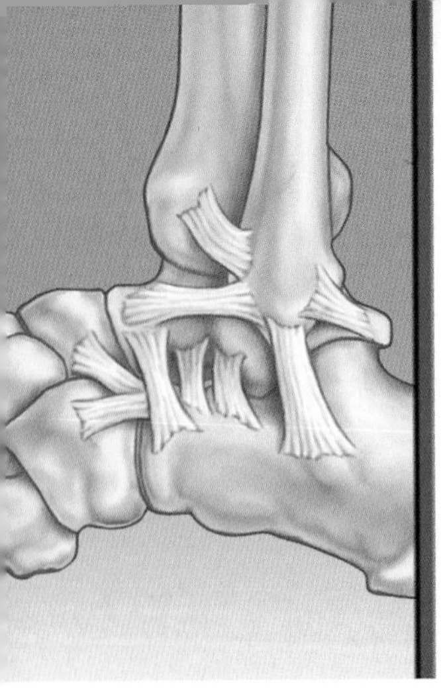

117

Tendon Injuries of the Foot and Ankle

TODD A. IRWIN

Anterior Tibial Tendon Injuries

Acute injuries to the anterior tibial tendon are uncommon and are often the result of open injuries or lacerations.[1] Chronic ruptures are decidedly more common, but they usually occur in an older population either as a result of minor trauma or with an insidious onset.

History

Open injuries or lacerations to the anterior ankle should elicit suspicion of an acute injury to the anterior tibial tendon. Often other structures may be injured concomitantly, including the extensor hallucis longus, extensor digitorum longus, and anterior neurovascular bundle.[2] Hockey players are at added risk because of the potential for boot-top lacerations from the hockey skate.[3]

Chronic ruptures are frequently missed initially because of the history of minor trauma that results in forced plantar flexion of the foot, sometimes with acute pain and the feeling of a "snap." Once the initial swelling and symptoms resolve, patients may notice a painless mass in the anterior ankle as a result of retraction of the proximal tendon. Often the diagnosis does not become apparent until the patient or a family member notices difficulty with walking or using stairs, a high-stepping gait, or weakness with dorsiflexion. Although chronic ruptures are not typically athletic injuries, several chronic ruptures have been reported after sporting activities such as cross-country skiing and fencing.[4,5] The differential diagnosis should include foot drop as a result of peroneal nerve palsy or L5 radiculopathy.

Physical Examination

In the chronic setting, swelling in the anterior ankle is a common finding. A mass (pseudotumor) may be palpable in the supramalleolar region as a result of retraction of the proximal tendon and is more commonly the presenting complaint in persons with chronic ruptures. Weakness to resisted dorsiflexion is expected but is isolated to the anterior tibialis with normal sensory findings, clearly differentiating this presentation from a radiculopathy or peroneal nerve palsy. High-stepping gait with recruitment of the toe extensors is likely (Fig. 117-1). If the patient has a chronic rupture, secondary claw toe formation may occur as a result of extensor recruitment. Walking on the heels demonstrates loss of dorsiflexion of the affected side.

Imaging

Magnetic resonance imaging (MRI) and dynamic ultrasound are the two most common imaging studies used to confirm the diagnosis. If the clinical situation is obvious based on the history and physical examination, further imaging is not necessary. However, if surgical intervention is planned, these studies may be useful for preoperative planning. Sagittal MRI scans provide the best view of the amount of retraction and subsequent gapping at the rupture site.

Decision-Making Principles

Surgical repair of an acute open injury should be performed. In the chronic setting, the patient's activity and lifestyle should be considered when determining whether operative or nonoperative treatment is appropriate. In a sedentary patient or a patient with multiple medical comorbidities who is a high surgical risk, nonoperative treatment is appropriate. In these patients the need for pain-free ambulation is easily resolved with the use of an ankle-foot orthosis. Patients who lead active lifestyles or refuse to use long-term bracing are best treated with surgical intervention in all cases. Use of age as a criterion is no longer appropriate because it has been clearly documented that older patients do very well with surgical intervention. The presence of a gastrocnemius contracture should be evaluated in all patients, and a gastrocnemius recession should be performed when such a contracture is present to increase range of motion and decrease strain on the repair.

Treatment Options

Acute ruptures should be treated with an end-to-end repair. When a laceration is the cause of the rupture, exploration of the wound is important to evaluate and repair concomitant tendon or neurovascular injuries. Timing, location of the rupture, and residual tendon quality are also important considerations. In the subacute setting (i.e., <6 to 8 weeks), primary repair may still be possible, but the surgeon should be prepared to use an autogenous or allogeneic graft if necessary. In the chronic setting, delayed reconstruction is often necessary and is usually achieved with either interpositional grafts or a tendon transfer. Interpositional autograft options include plantaris, extensor hallucis longus (EHL), extensor digitorum longus (EDL), peroneus tertius, and Achilles tendon.[6] The most common tendon transfer uses the EHL into the medial cuneiform, followed by the EDL.[7,8] Lengthening the anterior tibial tendon itself has also been described.[9] When the rupture occurs at the insertion of the tibialis anterior on the medial cuneiform, direct repair to the medial cuneiform can be achieved with use of suture anchors or an interference screw if the quality of the tendon is good. If the

AUTHORS' PREFERRED TECHNIQUE

Anterior Tibial Tendon Injury

The incision is centered over the course of the anterior tibial tendon; preoperative MRI or ultrasound may facilitate location of the proximal stump and guide incision length. The incision should be carried proximal to the site of the rupture to visualize the proximal stump. Distally the incision must be carried down to the proximal aspect of the distal stump. In cases of insertional rupture, this maneuver requires exposure of the medial cuneiform, which can be performed through a separate incision to minimize morbidity. Preservation of the superior extensor retinaculum should be attempted to minimize adhesions. Debridement of abnormal and diseased tendon should be performed prior to repair; this presentation is more likely to be seen in the older population. The amount of debridement may be significant enough to preclude end-to-end repair of the tendon, and the surgeon should be prepared to perform a graft reconstruction or tendon transfer in each case.

Intratendinous Rupture

In the setting of an acute intratendinous rupture, the proximal and distal stumps are prepared with a locking whipstitch. My preference is No. 0 nonabsorbable suture. Tension is placed on both the proximal and distal stumps, and the tendon should be apposed at neutral dorsiflexion of the ankle. In cases of late presentation, the proximal stump is contracted and direct apposition may not occur immediately. By placing traction on the proximal stump for 10 to 15 minutes, the muscle can be relaxed and end-to-end repair may be possible, mitigating the need for graft reconstruction. Placing additional suture crossing at the rupture site minimizes gapping of tendon under tension; this reinforcement can be performed with multiple figure of 8 sutures on the anterior and posterior aspects of the tendon. The tendon should not demonstrate any gapping with intraoperative plantar flexion of the ankle.

Chronic intratendinous ruptures or cases in which debridement has created a tendon gap cannot be repaired with end-to-end fixation. For the reconstruction to be successful, the proximal muscle belly of the anterior tibial tendon must be healthy and viable. Critical aspects of the procedure are exposure of the muscle with release of any scar tissue and ensuring that elasticity is present. If the muscle is fibrotic and nonviable, a tendon transfer should be performed as described later in this chapter. A hamstring autograft or allograft can be used to bridge the gap in this case. A doubled or quadrupled graft should be used given the cross-sectional diameter of the normal anterior tibial tendon. Side-to-side tenodesis or placement of the graft through a soft tissue tunnel within the proximal and distal stump of the tendon can be performed. Fixation to the proximal stump can be performed initially. Distal fixation can be performed either with a side-to-side tenodesis to the distal stump or through bone tunnel fixation into the medial cuneiform if the distal soft tissue is believed to be questionable. Use of fluoroscopy in conjunction with a guide wire facilitates placement of the bone tunnel. The ankle should be held in neutral dorsiflexion with maximal tension placed on the proximal limb. Fixation is then completed distally with multiple nonabsorbable sutures (my preference is No. 0) to the distal stump. In the setting of a bone tunnel through the medial cuneiform, a 5.5-mm interference screw can be used or the graft can be sewn upon itself. Use of a soft tissue button on the plantar aspect of the foot is a useful adjunct to fixation to further decrease the risk of pullout. After fixation, the sheath of the anterior tibial tendon is closed to prevent bowstringing of the reconstruction.

An alternative option to the use of a graft is an EHL transfer to reconstruct the anterior tibial tendon. An additional incision is made distally at the level of the first metatarsophalangeal joint, exposing both the EHL and extensor hallucis brevis. The EHL is affixed by tenodesis to the extensor hallucis brevis with the interphalangeal (IP) joint held in 20 degrees of dorsiflexion. The EHL is then sectioned immediately proximal to the tenodesis. The EHL is then passed through the medial cuneiform through a bone tunnel, and fixation can be performed with an interference screw or the tendon can be sewn back onto itself. The foot should be held in neutral with maximum tension placed on the tendon. Proximally, the stump of the anterior tibial tendon is secured to the EHL in a side-to-side fashion with moderate tension. Given the decreased power of the EHL relative to the Achilles tendon, an EHL transfer is more successful in the setting of a proximal tenodesis to increase the power that can be generated for dorsiflexion.

In the setting of a completely nonviable proximal anterior tibialis muscle belly, an isolated EHL transfer is unlikely to return full function. In this setting, transfer of the peroneus brevis or the posterior tibial tendon (PTT) may be required to provide sufficient dorsiflexion power.

Insertional Rupture

Insertional ruptures require a different approach relative to intratendinous ruptures. The lack of an adequate distal stump precludes tendon-to-tendon fixation. In these cases, fixation to the medial cuneiform with the aid of suture anchors is the most effective method. To maximize pullout, two suture anchors should be used and placed 45 degrees relative to the line of pull of the tendon, with the tip of the anchor angled proximally. Given the broad insertion of the tendon, one anchor can be placed within the medial cuneiform and the second anchor can be placed within the navicular or proximal aspect of the first metatarsal depending on the anatomy of the tendon and directed from plantar medial to dorsolateral. In the setting of a chronic rupture, use of a graft or an EHL transfer can be performed as previously described.

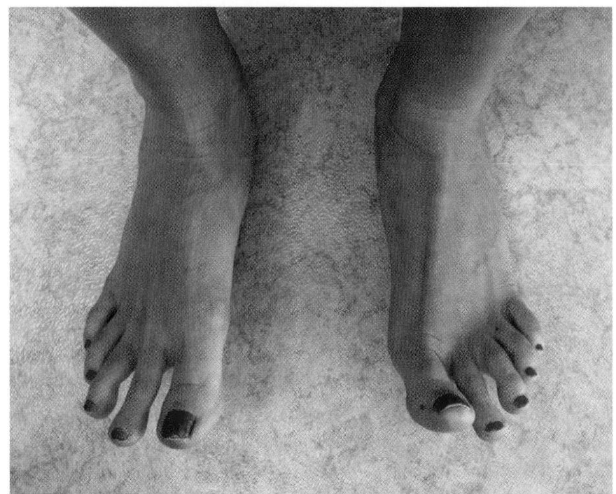

FIGURE 117-1 A patient with insertional rupture of the anterior tibial tendon. Note that with attempted dorsiflexion of the ankle, the extensor hallucis longus (EHL) and extensor digitorum longus (EDL) are recruited to allow for ankle dorsiflexion on the left side. The right side is normal and no EHL or EDL recruitment is needed. *(From Joos D, Kadakia AR: Extensor tendon disorders. In Miller MD, Sanders TG, editors:* Presentation, imaging and treatment of common musculoskeletal conditions: MRI-arthroscopy correlation, *Philadelphia, 2012, Elsevier.)*

quality of the tendon is poor, tendon transfer or allograft reconstruction is preferred.

Postoperative Management

The patient's ankle is typically immobilized with a cast and the patient is restricted from weight bearing for at least 4 weeks. For more complex or tenuous repairs, this period of non–weight bearing may be extended to a total of 6 to 12 weeks at the discretion of the surgeon. Patients are then transitioned to a removable boot, and weight bearing is started. Gentle range of motion may be initiated; however, passive plantar flexion is avoided until 12 weeks after surgery. At 12 weeks most patients can be weaned from the boot and strengthening can be started. Athletic activities and high-impact activities are avoided for 6 months.

Results

One study showed comparable outcome scores between patients treated operatively and nonoperatively. However, an age bias was present and recognized by the authors, as elderly patients were treated nonoperatively and younger active patients were treated operatively. The authors still recommended surgical repair or reconstruction in younger patients with an active lifestyle.[10] Three recent studies examined the results of surgical repair or reconstruction in both acute and chronic ruptures.[6-8] A total of 44 anterior tibial tendon ruptures were included in the three studies. Seventeen ruptures were repaired primarily and reconstruction was delayed for 27 ruptures, including 12 EHL tendon transfers, 3 EDL tendon transfers, and 12 interposition autogenous grafts. The three studies all showed improved outcome scores and high patient satisfaction. Although dorsiflexion strength was noted to be weaker compared with the nonoperative side, primary repair compared with delayed reconstruction showed no difference in dorsiflexion strength.

Complications

Complications of nonoperative treatment include a flat, pronated foot, decreased ankle motion, and Achilles contracture.[10] Operative complications were rare but included wound dehiscence, tendon adhesion to the extensor retinaculum, superficial peroneal nerve entrapment, and early failure requiring revision of interpositional autograft and tendon transfer operations.[6]

Posterior Tibial Tendon

Acute injuries to the PTT are relatively uncommon. The most common acute injury is a closed anterior dislocation of the tendon after disruption of the flexor retinaculum of the ankle; many of these injuries occur as a result of sporting activity. Most of the literature available regarding this injury is in the form of case reports, although a recent systematic review of the literature suggests that these injuries are more prevalent than originally thought.[11] Acute PTT ruptures are also relatively rare, although the majority occur in association with ankle fractures.[12] Posterior tibial tendinitis is relatively common in the athletic population and is usually associated with either a normal arch or pes planus. When this entity becomes chronic, it is termed *PTT dysfunction* (PTTD) and may ultimately lead to a progressive loss of arch. Johnson and Strom[13] developed the most used classification system for PTTD (also commonly referred to as *adult acquired flatfoot deformity*), and Myerson[14] added a fourth stage. Stage I is described as a tenosynovitis of the PTT without deformity. Stage II refers to tendon dysfunction leading to a flexible flatfoot deformity that is correctable. Stage III is a rigid flatfoot deformity, and stage IV refers to a stage III deformity with associated valgus ankle alignment. In the athletic population, stages I and II are by far the most common and are discussed later in this chapter.

History

Acute dislocations of the PTT usually occur after inversion of the ankle caused by a violent contraction of the posterior tibial muscle. The diagnosis is often missed initially, which leads the patient to report medial ankle pain or possibly a snapping sensation. Patients with tendinitis also report medial ankle pain and swelling that gets worse with activity. In athletes this pain may be debilitating because of the inability to run properly or perform any athletic activity that requires a strong push-off action.[15] The athlete may note worsening pain with elevating on the toes. In the chronic setting of any of the aforementioned entities, patients may report a progressive collapse of the arch with associated valgus position of the heel.

Physical Examination

Tenderness with or without swelling at the medial aspect of the ankle along the course of the PTT is a hallmark of any PTT disease. The tenderness may be primarily in the retromalleolar region, at the insertion of the tendon on the navicular, or along its entire course. In the setting of an acute or chronic

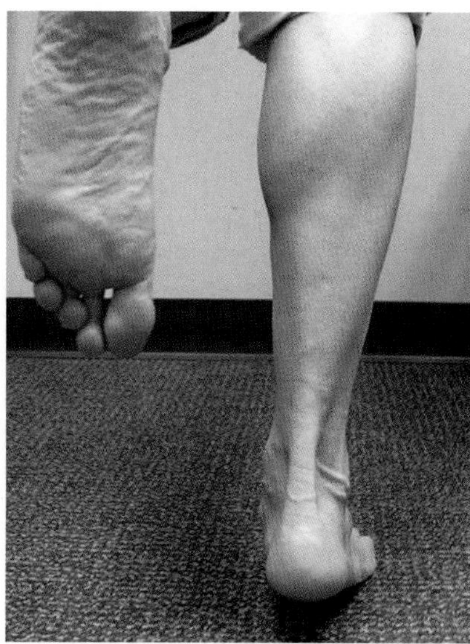

FIGURE 117-2 This patient is able to perform a single-limb heel rise, indicating the intact function of the posterior tibial tendon. Patients with stage I disease can perform this test, but it is very painful to do so. *(From Joos D, Kadakia AR: Flexor tendon disorders. In Miller MD, Sanders TG, editors:* Presentation, imaging and treatment of common musculoskeletal conditions: MRI-arthroscopy correlation, *Philadelphia, 2012, Elsevier.)*

dislocation, the tendon may be palpated as a cordlike structure anterior to the posteromedial ridge of the medial malleolus, although this finding is not always present. Resisted inversion of the foot with dorsiflexion or plantar flexion may elicit instability of the tendon, although again this finding is uncommon. A high degree of clinical suspicion is necessary to accurately diagnose acute or chronic PTT dislocation because these pathognomonic findings are variable. Resisted inversion of the foot while the ankle is plantar flexed should be tested. The ability to perform a single-limb heel raise should be tested because this maneuver isolates the PTT and is associated with inversion of the heel (Fig. 117-2). Patients who report medial ankle pain when attempting the single-limb heel raise or who are unable to perform this test should be suspected of having a pathologic condition of the PTT. The presence of an asymmetric pes planus deformity and hindfoot valgus is an indication that chronic PTT dysfunction is present. Range of motion of the hindfoot in inversion and eversion, as well as adduction and abduction of the transverse tarsal joints, should be tested to determine the flexibility of the deformity.

Imaging

Radiographs, MRI, and ultrasound are commonly used to confirm or diagnose pathologic conditions of the PTT. In the setting of dislocation, standard ankle radiographs may show a chip fracture of the medial aspect of the medial malleolus, representing disruption of the flexor retinaculum. Axial MRI scans may show the dislocated PTT sitting anterior to the disrupted flexor retinaculum, as well as the depth of the retromalleolar groove. However, if the tendon is appropriately located, bone edema present in the posteromedial aspect of the medial malleolus may be an indication that an injury occurred to the flexor retinaculum with associated tendon instability (Fig. 117-3). In these cases, dynamic ultrasound can be extremely useful to visualize the subluxation or dislocation of the PTT over the ridge of the medial malleolus. Associated tendon tears and excessive fluid in the tendon sheath can be visualized with either MRI or ultrasound. In the chronic setting, standing foot radiographs may demonstrate a pes planus deformity through an apex plantar lateral talo–first metatarsal angle, plantar gapping at the naviculocuneiform or first tarsometatarsal joint, or increased talonavicular uncoverage on the anteroposterior view. Hindfoot alignment views can also delineate the extent of hindfoot valgus that is present.[16] Debate exists about whether ultrasound or MRI provides a better evaluation of the extent of PTT disease in the chronic setting.[17,18]

Decision-Making Principles

Early diagnosis of PTT dislocation is difficult, which often leads to late presentation. If clinical suspicion is high and early diagnosis is achieved, it is reasonable to attempt conservative treatment with immobilization as long as the tendon is reliably located in the retromalleolar groove. However, because most cases have a delayed presentation, persistent symptoms are best treated with surgical intervention.

Acute PTT ruptures are most common in association with ankle fractures.[12] When an acute rupture is identified during fracture fixation, primary repair should be performed in the same setting.

PTT is almost exclusively treated conservatively initially because most patients, in particular younger patients and athletes, respond to nonoperative treatment. In the patient who does not respond to physical therapy, bracing modalities, and immobilization, surgical intervention is an option.[19]

PTT dysfunction is an often-discussed and sometimes controversial topic. Initially, stage I PTTD should be treated conservatively. Most cases abate or resolve, although rarely, surgical intervention is warranted despite no progressive loss of arch. With progressive degeneration and failure of the PTT, ligament failure occurs, leading to the flexible flatfoot deformity described in stage II. The spring (calcaneonavicular) ligament attenuates, leading to collapse of the talonavicular

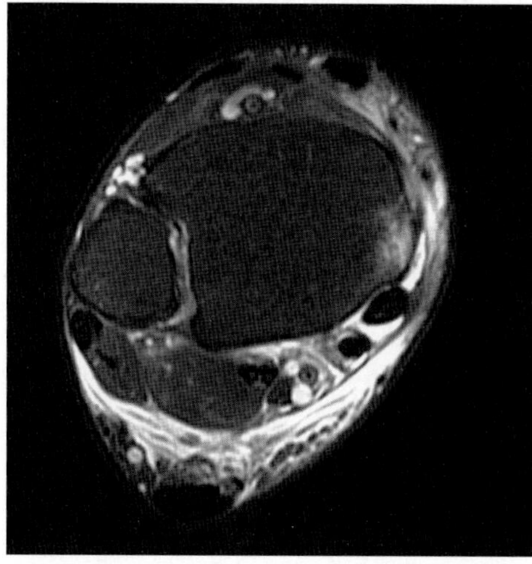

FIGURE 117-3 An axial T2-weighted magnetic resonance image of a subacute ankle injury. Note the posteromedial tibial bone edema, fluid within the posterior tibial tendon sheath, and the anterior false pouch where the posterior tibial tendon previously dislocated.

joint, and the interosseous ligament of the subtalar joint becomes involved, leading to a hindfoot valgus deformity.[30] Initially stage II PTTD should also be treated conservatively, because many patients subjectively and functionally improve.[20] However, if symptoms do not improve, surgical intervention should be considered prior to the development of a rigid deformity. This process can take many years; however, the surgical reconstruction of a rigid deformity (usually a triple arthrodesis) has significantly more morbidity than the joint-sparing procedures used to reconstruct a flexible flatfoot.

Treatment Options

Delayed presentation of a PTT dislocation commonly leads to surgical intervention based on persistent symptoms. The hallmark of surgery is retinaculum repair (if the tissue is amenable to repair) versus reconstruction. If advanced imaging shows evidence of a shallow retromalleolar groove, a groove-deepening procedure should be considered.[11,21] Evaluation for concomitant injuries such as a deltoid ligament tear, flexor digitorum longus (FDL) tear, or intraarticular ankle disease should also be conducted, and these injuries should be addressed if they are identified.

Conservative treatment for posterior tibial tendonitis first involves ankle bracing and physical therapy. If a pes planus deformity is present, orthotics with a longitudinal arch support with medial forefoot posting may provide some relief. If the pain is moderate to severe with even limited activity, immobilization in a walking boot is appropriate. When conservative treatment fails, surgical options include an open surgical release of the tendon sheath, tendoscopy, and/or possible FDL tendon transfer. Open release of the tendon sheath involves excision of scar tissue, a partial tenosynovectomy, and possibly intratendinous debridement if degenerative lesions are present (Fig. 117-4).[22] Tendoscopy is a less invasive option both for diagnostic purposes and to perform a tenosynovectomy.[23] If the tendon is excessively degenerated and is deemed to be insufficient, an FDL tendon transfer may be necessary and is the most commonly performed procedure for this problem.[24] In all surgical cases, evaluation for a possible gastrocnemius contracture should be undertaken and surgical release should be performed if such a contracture is present. Additionally, a concomitant medial slide calcaneal osteotomy can be considered in the setting of an FDL transfer despite lack of clinical deformity to prevent late recurrence.

The surgical options for stage II PTTD depend on the extent of the patient's dysfunction, as well as certain specific components of the developed deformity. Many patients with PTTD have a concomitant gastrocnemius contracture, and when such a contracture is present, a gastrocnemius recession should be performed. Second, the PTT itself should be evaluated and an FDL tendon transfer is performed to reconstruct the dynamic function of the tendon. The extent of PTT disease can vary from a mildly thickened tendon to severe degeneration with longitudinal and sometimes complete ruptures. In the case of moderate to severe degeneration of the tendon, the diseased tendon is resected, leaving the distal stump on the navicular. In the case of mild degeneration of the tendon, some surgeons opt to leave the PTT in place, whereas others choose to excise the tendon regardless of the extent of disease. Either way, an FDL tendon transfer is nearly always performed

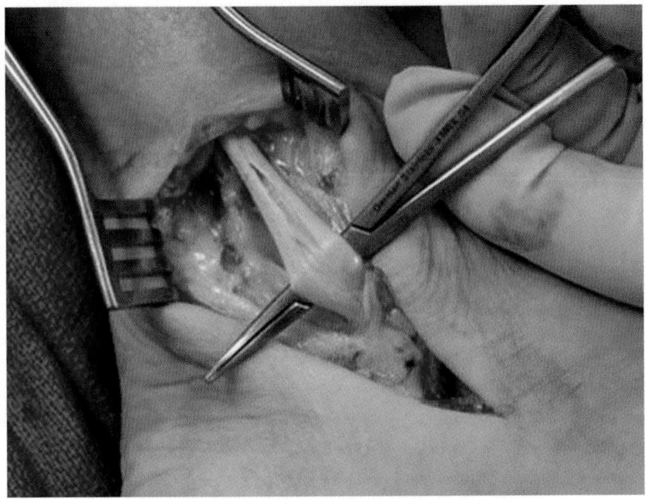

FIGURE 117-4 A longitudinal split tear in the posterior tibial tendon can be seen in stage I disease. This tear should be treated with debridement and tubularization of the tendon. If any evidence is seen of hindfoot valgus, excision and tendon transfer with the addition of a calcaneal osteotomy should be considered. *(From Joos D, Kadakia AR: Flexor tendon disorders. In Miller MD, Sanders TC, editors:* Presentation, imaging and treatment of common musculoskeletal conditions: MRI-arthroscopy correlation, *Philadelphia, 2012, Elsevier.)*

to augment the function of the damaged tendon. Third, because stage II PTTD implies a hindfoot valgus deformity, a medial displacement calcaneal osteotomy is usually performed to translate the weight-bearing portion of the heel back underneath the mechanical axis of the leg.[25,26] These three procedures account for a high proportion of the surgical treatment options in a patient with stage II PTTD. However, for a more advanced disease process that is not yet rigid, other options are available. The spring ligament should always be evaluated and either repaired or reconstructed if it is torn or insufficient. With significant forefoot abduction (evidenced by significant talonavicular uncoverage on the anteroposterior foot radiograph), a lateral column-lengthening procedure can be performed.[27] Options for lateral column lengthening are either through the neck of the calcaneus or through a calcaneocuboid distraction arthrodesis, although most surgeons today prefer to use the neck of the calcaneus. With midfoot collapse of either the first tarsometatarsal or naviculocuneiform joint, an associated arthrodesis of the involved joint helps to stabilize the medial column. This procedure also corrects a residual forefoot varus deformity, as does a plantar flexion osteotomy through the medial cuneiform.[28]

Postoperative Management

Patients who have undergone a flexor retinaculum reconstruction have a splint placed postoperatively and are instructed not to bear weight. After 2 weeks, a short leg cast or walking boot is applied and weight bearing is initiated. Six weeks after surgery an ankle lace-up brace is applied and range of motion is initiated and progresses over the next 6 weeks. Physical therapy can be started for range of motion and strengthening.

Patients who have undergone a tenosynovectomy for posterior tibial tendonitis are treated initially with a splint for the

AUTHORS' PREFERRED TECHNIQUE

Posterior Tibial Tendon Injury

Flexor Retinaculum Reconstruction

A curvilinear medial approach just posterior to the medial malleolus is made along the course of the PTT. The PTT and its sheath are evaluated for a possible false pouch anterior to the medial malleolus. A U-shaped flap consisting of retinaculum and medial malleolus periosteum is developed and cut anteriorly so that it is left attached to the posterior portion of the retinaculum. A trough is created at the anterior ridge of the retromalleolar groove using a small burr and is smoothed down with a rasp followed by bone wax. The retinaculum-periosteal flap is then passed into the trough from deep to superficial using intraosseous nonabsorbable sutures that lie posteriorly, minimizing soft tissue irritation. After imbrication of the retinaculum, the tendon should be stably located within the groove through all range of motion of the ankle.

Posterior Tibial Tenosynovectomy and Debridement

The tendon is approached as previously described, the PTT sheath is incised, and the tendon is evaluated. Diseased synovium is excised, with the incision extended as needed to ensure adequate debridement. Degenerative portions of the tendon are identified by the thickened and amorphous appearance (smooth with a lack of striations). The diseased portion is incised longitudinally, the nonviable portion is excised, and the longitudinal rent is repaired with running 3-0 Prolene sutures. Care is taken to avoid creating a full-thickness disruption of the tendon, resulting in discontinuity. The tendon sheath is then closed to prevent subluxation. If more than 50% of the tendon has been debrided, a concomitant FDL tendon transfer is indicated.

Flexor Digitorum Longus Tendon Transfer

The same approach to the PTT is used, extending it distal along the medial border of the foot. In these cases, the severity of tendon degeneration does not allow for repair and therefore it is resected, leaving a 1-cm stump on the navicular tuberosity for fixation. Securing the tendon to this distal stump theoretically allows the FDL to restore the stabilizing effect to the plantar midfoot through the multiple distal connections of the PTT. Isolated reconstruction to the navicular does not allow for restoration of this critical function of the PTT. The FDL tendon sheath is incised in the floor of the posterior tibial tendon sheath, inferior to the medial malleolus, and opened to a point 2 to 3 cm distal to the navicular tuberosity. The FDL tendon is dissected from its attachments to the flexor hallucis longus (FHL; master knot of Henry) and transversely cut as far distal as possible. Distal tenodesis can be performed at this point to help restore the function of the FDL; however, given the lack of gait disturbance, it is not required and is not routinely performed in my practice. A more proximal transection of the FDL, proximal to the knot of Henry, preserves the interconnections between the FDL and FHL but results in less tendon length for reconstruction. A 4.5-mm drill hole is created in the medial navicular tuberosity from dorsal to plantar, using fluoroscopy as a guide for placement of the hole. While holding the foot in 20 degrees of inversion and 20 degrees of plantar flexion, the FDL is delivered through the drill hole from plantar to dorsal, passed back onto itself if possible, and sutured to surrounding periosteum and the PTT stump using size 0 nonabsorbable suture. Tensioning is critical and the foot should not be able to evert past neutral after repair. Alternatively, especially in the setting of a short segment of FDL, the tendon can be sutured directly to the stump of the PTT or fixed to the navicular with dual suture anchors. No clinical superiority of fixation has been demonstrated.

Medial Displacement Calcaneal Osteotomy

To perform a medial displacement calcaneal osteotomy, make an incision posterior and inferior to the course of the peroneal tendons along the lateral hindfoot at 45 degrees to the plantar border of the foot. Dissect through subcutaneous tissues while avoiding sural nerve branches. Sharply incise through periosteum along the line of the incision and elevate 2 to 3 mm of periosteum dorsally and plantarly. Check the position of the planned osteotomy by inserting a small Kirschner (K) wire and assessing the position under fluoroscopy with a lateral and axial heel alignment view. Adjust as needed and perform the osteotomy using a larger saw blade, being careful to just perforate the far cortex to avoid injury to medial neurovascular structures; alternatively, the medial cortex can be perforated with an osteotome. Mobilize the posterior fragment using a wide osteotome or elevator, taking care not to crush the soft cancellous bone. Use of a wide elevator can minimize this complication. Translate the posterior tuberosity medially from 8 to 10 mm. Place one 6.5-mm partially threaded cannulated screw and check its position using lateral and axial fluoroscopy. Given the medial translation, the screw should be inserted relatively lateral on the tuberosity so that it remains with the distal calcaneus. Plates have also been developed for fixation, but given the low cost of the implant and high clinical success rate of screw fixation, they are not routinely used in my practice.

first 2 weeks, followed by use of a removable walking boot for 4 weeks. Early range of motion exercises are initiated and physical therapy can be considered, especially in athletes who are trying to return to play. At 6 weeks an ankle lace-up brace is worn, and full activity is allowed at between 6 and 8 weeks. For both of the aforementioned procedures, full return to sporting activity is variable but is expected at around 3 to 4 months after surgery. Use of an over-the-counter full-length arch support is encouraged to minimize recurrence.

Reconstructions for flatfoot deformity entail a longer recovery period. Patients wear a splint for the initial 2 weeks with the foot in an inverted and plantar-flexed position. A short-leg non–weight-bearing cast or controlled ankle motion boot is then used for 4 weeks, followed by weight bearing in a tall walking boot for 4 to 6 weeks. Physical therapy can be initiated about 8 to 10 weeks after surgery with an emphasis on inversion strengthening, with concomitant use of a lace-up ankle brace for a further 3 months. Sporting activity usually cannot be resumed until about 6 to 9 months postoperatively with the use of an over-the-counter orthotic to minimize stress on the reconstruction.

Results

Lohrer and Nauck[11] performed a systematic review of the literature regarding PTT dislocations and noted a higher prevalence than originally thought. Nearly 60% of the injuries were induced by sport. Of the 61 cases reported, only 10 were treated conservatively. Surgical treatment included a variety of retinaculum reconstruction techniques, direct suture repair, and retromalleolar groove deepening combined with reconstruction or repair. Results were rated as excellent in 80%, good in 13%, and fair in 7%. No comparison between surgical and conservative treatment could be performed.[11]

Tenosynovectomy for posterior tibial tendinitis has generally good results. McCormack et al.[19] published a series on tenosynovectomy in young competitive athletes. Twenty-two months after surgery, seven of eight patients had returned to full sports participation without difficulty. Teasdall and Johnson[29] reported results on 19 patients treated with synovectomy and debridement for stage I PTTD. Complete relief was reported by 74% of patients, whereas 16% had minor pain, 5% had moderate pain, and 5% had severe pain. Only 10% required conversion to a subtalar arthrodesis for progressive deformity and pain.

As the treatment of PTTD has evolved, so have the reported results in the literature. Alvarez et al.[20] reported the result of a structured nonoperative management protocol for stage I and stage II PTTD involving the use of a short-articulating ankle-foot orthotic and an aggressive physical therapy protocol including a home program.[20] Their patients had successful subjective and functional outcomes 83% of the time, whereas only 11% did not respond to conservative treatment and required surgery. Surgical intervention has also been shown to be beneficial in patients who do not respond to nonoperative treatment. Combining FDL transfer with a medial displacement calcaneal osteotomy has been shown to restore functional inversion and provide excellent pain relief and patient satisfaction, with variable radiographic and patient-perceived arch correction.[25,26]

Complications

The most common complication of PTTD is missed diagnosis leading to delayed presentation, because 53% of patients in a systematic review were initially misdiagnosed.[11] Tenosynovectomy for posterior tibial tendonitis is well tolerated with few reported complications, although if the tendon dysfunction is more chronic than originally thought, progression of the deformity may require further surgical intervention. Complications of PTTD correction include undercorrection with persistent pain, overcorrection resulting in varus hindfoot, and rarely, neurovascular injury either at the calcaneal osteotomy site or the FDL harvest site.[26]

Future Considerations

The treatment of PTT injuries and dysfunction will likely continue to evolve. The importance of the spring ligament in both acute injuries and chronic PTTD has been demonstrated.[30,31] Determining which patients will benefit from spring ligament repair or reconstruction and what effect this will have on the overall treatment algorithm is an area of current research. Novel rehabilitation protocols and early diagnosis may also lead to improved outcomes and more refined surgical protocols.

Flexor Hallucis Longus Injuries

Although lacerations to the FHL tendon have been reported, the most common pathology related to the FHL is tenosynovitis.[32,33] The FHL arises from the posterior aspect of the fibula and interosseous membrane. It then courses distally through a fibro-osseous tunnel posterior to the ankle joint, crosses deep to the FDL at the master knot of Henry in the midfoot and between the sesamoid bones in the forefoot, and inserts onto the base of the distal phalanx of the hallux. Symptoms can occur anywhere along this course, although the most common presenting complaint is posterior to the ankle. Both athletes and nonathletes may report symptoms consistent with FHL tenosynovitis, although the highest prevalence is seen in classical ballet dancers.[33-35] Stenosing tenosynovitis is a related clinical entity that is discussed. Posterior impingement of the ankle, often as a result of a large os trigonum, is commonly seen in association with FHL tenosynovitis and is often treated concurrently.[36]

History

The most common presenting complaint is pain in the posteromedial ankle that is worsened with activity. Chronic repetitive plantar-flexion activities such as en pointe dancing tend to exacerbate the symptoms. Triggering of the hallux may also be present in patients in whom a stenosing tenosynovitis has developed.[37,38] Triggering occurs as a result of a bulbous thickening of the FHL that causes the hallux to lock as the FHL attempts to pass through the fibro-osseous tunnel with plantar flexion or dorsiflexion of the ankle. Patients may also report limited dorsiflexion of the hallux, again as a result of stenosis at the proximal level of the fibro-osseous tunnel. Other less common complaints include pain medial and deep to the medial band of the plantar fascia in the midfoot and pain plantar to the first metatarsal.

Physical Examination

Pain associated with extreme plantar flexion of the ankle is the first indication that a pathologic condition is present posterior to the ankle. Although this pain may be an indication of posterior impingement, to isolate the FHL, further examination is required. Pain with resisted plantar flexion of the hallux is the hallmark of FHL tenosynovitis. Symptoms may worsen with dorsiflexion of the ankle as the musculotendinous junction is delivered into the fibro-osseous tunnel. Swelling may be present in the posteromedial ankle, and tenderness and crepitus may be present with palpation of the FHL while moving the hallux. The Tomassen sign is the finding of decreased passive dorsiflexion of the hallux with the ankle in neutral dorsiflexion that is improved with plantar flexion of the ankle. Upon forcible active contraction of the FHL, however, a snap or pop is noted in the posterior medial region of the ankle, and the patient is then unable to extend the IP or metatarsophalangeal joints of the great toe. Subsequent passive extension of the IP joint produces a painless snap or pop posterior to the medial malleolus with subsequent freeing of motion in the great toe.

The master knot of Henry is another potential area where the FHL can be symptomatic. Deep palpation just medial to the medial border of the plantar fascia that worsens with moving of the great toe can elicit pain. Pain with palpation of the plantar aspect of the first metatarsal, between the sesamoids and with motion of the great toe, can indicate distal entrapment of the FHL.

Imaging

Findings of standard foot and ankle radiographs are often normal, although lateral ankle radiographs may demonstrate an os trigonum or prominent posterior talar process. If suspicion of posterior impingement or FHL tenosynovitis is high or for confirmation of the diagnosis, an MRI scan is often performed. In one study, 82% of patients suspected of FHL tenosynovitis had positive MRI findings in the form of excessive fluid in the FHL tendon sheath posterior to the ankle[35] (Fig. 117-5). Ultrasound has also gained in popularity and can dynamically visualize the FHL, which may be helpful in confirming a stenosing tenosynovitis or in guiding an injection.[39]

Decision-Making Principles

Conservative treatment is the appropriate initial step in the management of both FHL tenosynovitis and stenosing tenosynovitis. If conservative treatment fails, symptoms have been present for longer than 3 months without relief, or the patient is a high-level athlete or performer who is unable to execute the desired activities, surgical intervention can be considered. It is important to determine the presence of posterior impingement, FHL tenosynovitis, or both because this information may help determine the appropriate approach and intervention. Some authors argue that the presence of triggering is an indication for earlier operative intervention.[40,41] Interestingly, Hamilton et al.[33] have reported the potential morbidity related to surgical intervention in the dancer population, both medically and professionally. They noted the competitive environment and stigma associated with having an injury as reasons professional dancers may elect to not have surgery, as well as reasons why amateur dancers may have been prevented from having a professional career. For this reason, understanding the patient's social situation is exceedingly important during a discussion of treatment options in this patient population.

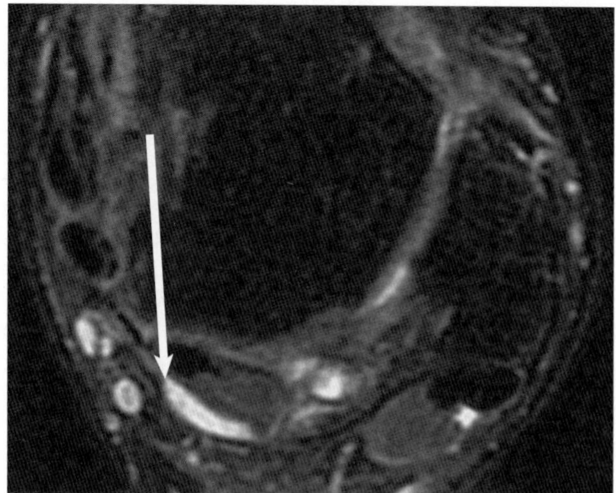

FIGURE 117-5 An axial T2-weighted image with high signal intensity (*white arrow*) adjacent to the flexor hallucis longus at the posterior aspect of the talus. *(From Joos D, Kadakia AR: Flexor tendon disorders. In Miller MD, Sanders TG, editors:* Presentation, imaging and treatment of common musculoskeletal conditions: MRI-arthroscopy correlation, *Philadelphia, 2012, Elsevier.)*

Treatment Options

Initial treatment for FHL tenosynovitis should include formal physical therapy including an FHL-specific stretching program, as well as use of antiinflammatory medication. Trial periods of bracing or boot immobilization are used if the pain is significant. Activity modification should also be instituted, in particular avoiding repetitive plantar-flexion activities such as dancing en pointe.

When conservative treatment fails, surgical intervention is an option. The great majority of patients who require surgical intervention have posterior ankle symptoms, although release of the FHL at the knot of Henry and between the sesamoids has been described.[35] Surgical techniques that have been described include addressing the FHL tenosynovitis alone or in combination with a suspected posterior impingement.[33,36] The treatment of choice for FHL tenosynovitis is release of the tendon sheath. In the case of stenosing tenosynovitis and triggering, the integrity of the tendon should be evaluated, and if tears or nodules are present, they are addressed with repair or debridement. The traditional surgical approach is through a medial approach to mobilize the neurovascular bundle, although posterolateral and posteromedial approaches have also been described.[33,35] If posterior impingement alone is being addressed, a straight posterolateral approach can be used to debride the impingement and remove the os trigonum if it is present. Access to the FHL fibro-osseous tunnel may be difficult, although by making the incision just lateral to the Achilles tendon and dissecting anterior to it, this difficulty may be minimized. Incising just medial to the Achilles tendon is another option to address both clinical problems and also minimizes manipulation and exposure of the tibial nerve.

Recently, posterior hindfoot arthroscopy has increased in popularity.[42,43] Most of these procedures have been performed for posterior ankle impingement, with or without clinical evidence of FHL tenosynovitis. If extensive debridement or repair of the FHL is required, conversion to an open procedure may be necessary.

Postoperative Management

After posterior hindfoot endoscopy, patients usually wear a splint postoperatively for 1 to 2 weeks, with subsequent transition to a boot or brace. Early ankle, subtalar, and great toe range of motion is initiated and encouraged. Some authors advocate a more functional postoperative course with early weight bearing and no immobilization.[42] For open procedures, it is reasonable to immobilize the ankle for 2 weeks to allow for wound healing, followed by a short course of boot

AUTHORS' PREFERRED TECHNIQUE

Posterior Hindfoot Arthroscopy

The patient is placed in the prone position, with the foot placed on two blankets slightly past the edge of the bed. A set of 4.5-mm arthroscopic equipment, including 5.0-mm shavers, curettes, and osteotomes, is required. Twenty milliliters of normal saline solution is injected into the posterior ankle starting just lateral to the Achilles tendon. A lateral portal is created just lateral to the Achilles tendon, slightly superior to the level of the tip of the fibula. Dissection is performed with a straight hemostat, being careful to direct the dissection straight anteriorly. A 4.5-mm arthroscope sleeve with trocar is introduced, followed by the arthroscope. The medial portal is made just medial to the Achilles tendon, at the same level, and dissecting slightly lateral toward the arthroscope tip. A 5.0-mm shaver is introduced and soft tissue debridement is performed. Be careful to stay lateral until visualization is improved with insufflation of the fluid to avoid iatrogenic damage to the neurovascular bundle. Continue debridement medially until the FHL tendon is visualized (Fig. 117-6). The neurovascular bundle should be protected as long as the dissection stays lateral to the FHL. Use a combination of the shaver, curette, grasper, and possibly the osteotome to remove the os trigonum or posterior talar process if it is deemed an inciting factor. Flex and extend the great toe to evaluate the FHL along its course. The arthroscope can be advanced relatively far distally into the fibro-osseous tunnel for further visualization. A shaver and biter can be used to debride the tendon and release the FHL tendon sheath. Conversion to an open posteromedial approach may be necessary if further debridement or repair of the FHL is necessary or if the sheath is unable to be adequately released.

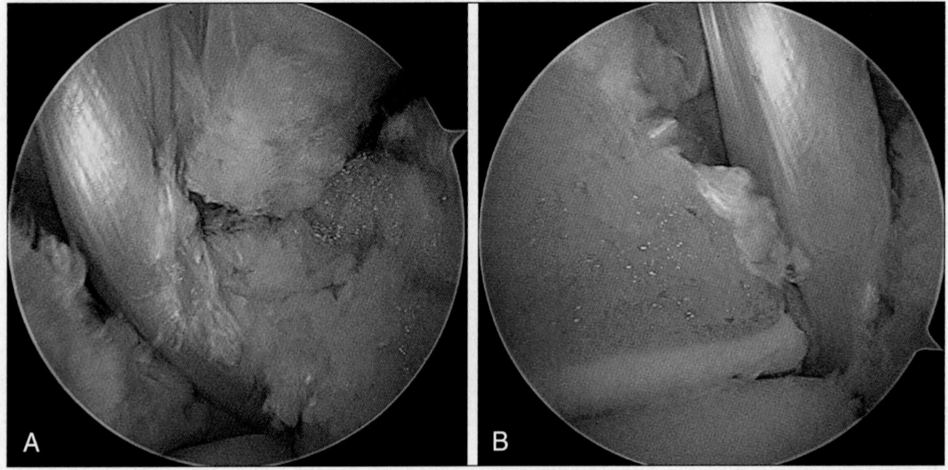

FIGURE 117-6 **A,** Posterior arthroscopic view of the flexor hallucis longus (FHL) tendon with incomplete longitudinal tear and surrounding synovitis. **B,** A view of the FHL after debridement of the surrounding synovitis and excision of impinging posterior talar process (note the fresh cancellous bone).

immobilization for 2 to 4 weeks. Early range of motion is initiated when the wounds have healed.

Return to sporting activities averages approximately 5 months. A formal physical therapy program may help shorten this time.[44] For dancers, achieving the en pointe position can be critical and may take a prolonged period depending on the severity of the preoperative condition. Although an endoscopic approach may shorten the time to return to play, studies are inconclusive.[42,43]

Results

Successful outcomes using nonoperative treatment alone have been reported to be as high as 64%.[35] The most common treatment used was an FHL-stretching regimen, in particular in patients with evidence of entrapment at the posteromedial ankle or limited dorsiflexion of the hallux.

Surgical outcomes have been promising in the more recent literature. In the series by Hamilton et al.,[33] 28 of 34 professional dancers had good or excellent results, whereas only 2 of 6 amateur dancers had equally successful outcomes. Kolettis et al.[40] reported that 11 of 13 ballet dancers were able to return to full dancing participation without restrictions after 5 months after an open medial release of the FHL. Marotta and Micheli[36] reported the results of 12 ballet dancers (15 ankles) who underwent excision of the os trigonum, through a lateral approach, for treatment of posterior impingement. At follow-up, 2 years after surgery, 8 (67%) still had occasional discomfort, but all 12 dancers returned to unrestricted dance activity.[36] In the review by Michelson and Dunn,[35] only 23 of the 81 patients with FHL tenosynovitis required surgical intervention, although each surgical outcome was deemed successful. Patients had significant subjective improvement after 6 weeks.[35] Similar good results have been seen after posterior hindfoot arthroscopy, although most of these cases were performed for posterior impingement, with or without FHL tendinitis. Scholten et al.[42] reported an increase in the American Orthopaedic Foot and Ankle

(AOFAS) hindfoot score from 75 to 90 at 3-year follow-up, although they did note that the patients with overuse injuries were more satisfied than were the patients with posttraumatic injuries. Willits et al.[43] reported similar high satisfaction rates in functional and clinical evaluations after posterior hindfoot arthroscopy in 24 ankles.

Complications

Typical postoperative complications such as wound healing problems and minor infections have been reported, although at low rates. Complications specific to an open approach for FHL tenosynovectomy include scar dysesthesias and rare transient nerve neuropraxias.[33,36] The largest review of posterior hindfoot arthroscopy procedures showed an 8.5% complication rate, including 2% with plantar numbness, 1.6% with sural nerve dysesthesias, and 2% with Achilles tendon tightness.[45]

Future Considerations

Higher clinical suspicion in the nondancer population should lead to increased awareness and earlier diagnosis. The development of more refined therapy protocols and further outcome studies may help decrease the need for surgical intervention. As arthroscopic techniques improve, a higher percentage of these cases may benefit from an arthroscopic technique that could potentially decrease rehabilitation time.

Peroneal Tendon Injuries

Peroneal tendon injuries are a common and increasingly recognized diagnosis, especially in the athletic population. Persistent lateral ankle symptoms after an ankle "sprain" should elicit suspicion of a peroneal tendon injury. Although most patients present with chronic injuries, acute tears of the peroneus brevis and less commonly the peroneus longus do occur. Peroneal subluxation or dislocation is another clinical entity that may be recognized acutely or chronically and is often associated with peroneal tendon tears. Disruption of the superior peroneal retinaculum (SPR), usually as a result of a forced contraction of the peroneals in a dorsiflexed position, can lead to peroneal instability. Chronic instability of the tendons can then lead to peroneal tendon tears, often of the peroneus brevis as it rubs over the posterolateral ridge of the fibula.[46] Finally, snapping of the tendons without evidence of subluxation or dislocation indicates an intrasheath peroneal subluxation.

History

Patients with acute tears of the peroneal tendons may report a sharp pain and acute "pop" at the lateral aspect of the ankle. However, most patients present several weeks or months after an acute injury and report lateral ankle pain or discomfort that worsens with activity. The pain may radiate proximally along the lateral aspect of the leg and may be associated with a snapping or popping sensation. Repeated episodes of ankle instability should raise suspicion of peroneal tendon involvement. Forced dorsiflexion of the ankle, such as when skiers quickly decelerate and stop, should alert the examiner to a subluxation or dislocation episode.[47,48] An accurate history can be extremely helpful in determining the true nature of the peroneal pathology.

Physical Examination

Swelling along the peroneal tendons in the posterolateral ankle, as well as distal and anterior to the tip of the fibula, is a consistent finding in persons with peroneal tendon disease. Tenderness to palpation along the retrofibular groove—or distally along the cuboid groove in the case of the peroneus longus—may indicate peroneal tendon tearing. Eversion and external rotation strength should be tested both from a contracted and lengthened position. Complete peroneal tendon ruptures are uncommon; most tearing occurs in a longitudinal fashion. Therefore peroneal tendon strength is often intact, although resisted contraction of either the peroneus brevis or longus may elicit pain. Pain with resisted eversion of the foot can indicate either peroneus brevis or longus involvement, although pain with resisted plantar flexion of the first ray (counterpressure at the plantar aspect of the first metatarsal head) indicates peroneus longus involvement. To evaluate for peroneal instability, resisted dorsiflexion and eversion should be tested while gently palpating the fibular ridge and feeling for tendon subluxation[49] (Fig. 117-7). Repeated circumduction of the foot can also elicit peroneal instability. If a palpable snapping or clicking of the tendons occurs with circumduction, but without evidence of subluxation or dislocation over the ridge of the fibula, intrasheath subluxation may be present. Finally, hindfoot and forefoot alignment should always be checked during examination while the patient is standing. The presence of cavovarus alignment increases the risk of peroneal tendinopathy and/or instability. A Coleman block test should be performed to determine if the varus hindfoot is the result of a plantar-flexed first ray alone or occurs in combination with a fixed varus heel deformity.[50]

Imaging

Standing foot and ankle radiographs should be performed as an initial assessment. Evidence of a hypertrophied peroneal tubercle may be a source of peroneal disease. The presence of an os peroneum, an accessory bone located just lateral to the cuboid and seen best on the oblique foot radiograph, is present in 10% to 20% of persons and is completely enveloped by the peroneus longus tendon.[51] An elongated or fractured os peroneum may indicate either chronic or acute disruption of the peroneus longus, respectively. A chip fracture identified just lateral to the lateral malleolus is an indication of an avulsion of the SPR and is likely associated with peroneal subluxation or dislocation.[52]

Advanced imaging most commonly involves either ultrasound or MRI. The advantages of ultrasound are not only that it is a noninvasive and inexpensive method, but that it allows dynamic evaluation of the peroneal tendons throughout their range of motion and with provocative maneuvers. Sensitivity, specificity, and accuracy of ultrasound in diagnosing peroneal tendon tears has been shown to be 100%, 85%, and 90%, respectively.[53] Comparison with the unaffected side is another advantage.

MRI is likely the most common modality ordered for suspected peroneal disease, especially considering the propensity for ordering MRIs in the primary care population. Axial

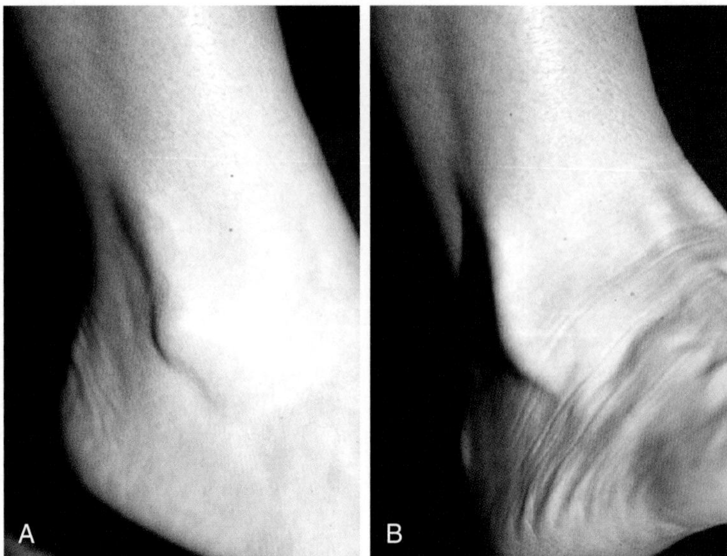

FIGURE 117-7 Dislocation of the peroneal tendons with dorsiflexion and eversion.

images provide the best cut for peroneal evaluation.[54] Torn tendons may appear thickened or nodular or they may have increased intrasubstance signaling, and excessive fluid within the tendon sheath usually indicates peroneal tendon disease (Fig. 117-8). The specificity of MRI to diagnose peroneus brevis tears, longus tears, or both has been shown to be 80%, 100%, and 60%, respectively.[55] However, both false-positive and false-negative results have been reported, and in my experience, false-positive results are relatively common.[56] Diagnosis and decisions about management should be made primarily by the history and physical examination, with advanced imaging used for confirmation or in unclear cases.

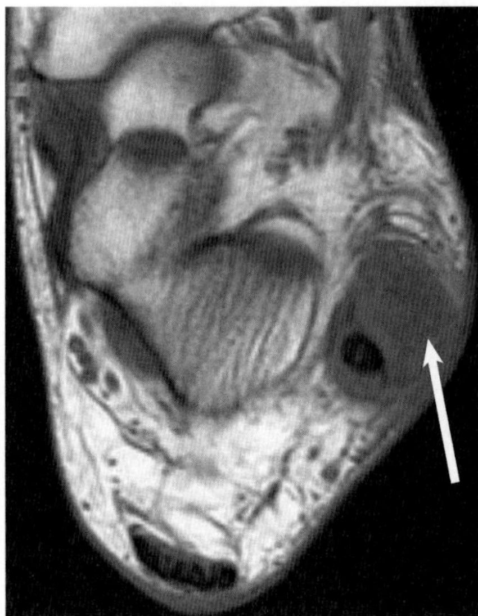

FIGURE 117-8 A T1-weighted axial magnetic resonance image with intermediate signal intensity in the location of the peroneus brevis (*arrow*). This was noted on multiple axial images, consistent with severe tendinosis of the peroneus brevis. Obvious thickening of the tendon is also noted. The normal peroneus longus is noted posterior to the pathologic brevis. *(From Joos D, Kadakia AR: Peroneal tendon disorders. In Miller MD, Sanders TG, editors:* Presentation, imaging and treatment of common musculoskeletal conditions: MRI-arthroscopy correlation, *Philadelphia, 2012, Elsevier.)*

Decision-Making Principles

Because acute peroneal tendon tears (or at least the recognition of them) are relatively uncommon, primary repair of the tendon tear is not always necessary unless it is diagnosed in a high-level athlete. Conservative treatment can almost always be tried initially, and decisions for surgical management can be made on the basis of the response to treatment. Peroneal tendinitis is almost always managed well with conservative treatment. Even mild degenerative tears of the peroneal tendons often respond to conservative treatment. Hindfoot alignment is important to consider because a simple orthotic may add significant benefit to the treatment protocol.

Peroneal tendon tears that are recalcitrant to conservative treatment likely benefit from surgical intervention. The extent and location of the tear are important determining factors with regard to the appropriate surgical option. Krause and Brodsky[46] based the method of surgical treatment on the cross-sectional area of tendon involvement. If 50% or more of the tendon remained after debridement of the damaged portion (grade I tear), they repaired the tendon. If less than 50% remained (grade II), proximal and distal tenodesis of the peroneus brevis tendon to the longus tendon was performed.[46] This rule is a good general guideline, although often multiple splits are present and the decision must be individualized. Peroneus brevis tears usually occur around the retrofibular groove. When a concomitant SPR disruption is present, reconstruction or repair of the SPR should be performed. Distal peroneus brevis tears are significantly less common. If the patient does not respond to conservative treatment, surgical debridement with reattachment to the base of the fifth metatarsal may be required.[57] Peroneus longus tendon tears occur less often than do brevis tears and are more likely distal to the tip of the fibula either at the peroneal tubercle or in the cuboid notch. In addition, in one study, 82% of peroneus longus tendon tears were associated with a cavovarus hindfoot position.[58] A similar approach to tendon debridement and/or repair can be used for the peroneus longus, although complete ruptures may be seen through the os peroneum or just distal or proximal to the os. In these cases, if direct repair is not possible, transfer into the cuboid is an option.[57] Tears seen in both the peroneus longus and peroneus brevis concomitantly are even less common, although they present a challenge when they are seen.[56]

Acute or chronic dislocating peroneal tendons, especially in the athletic population, should be treated surgically. Conservative treatment of dislocating tendons, either acute or chronic, has generally shown poor results.[51,59-62] The depth of the fibular groove has also been recognized as a contributing factor to peroneal tendon instability, and when it is recognized, the fibular groove should be deepened.[63] If chronic ankle instability is present, a lateral ankle ligament reconstruction should also be performed.[64] In the presence of a varus hindfoot or cavovarus deformity, cavovarus reconstruction should be considered.[50] Finally, when a low-lying peroneus brevis muscle belly or peroneus quartus is identified, appropriate debridement should be performed.[65,66]

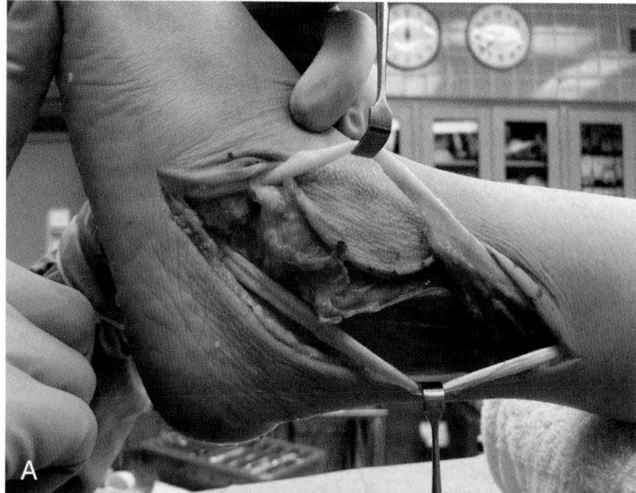

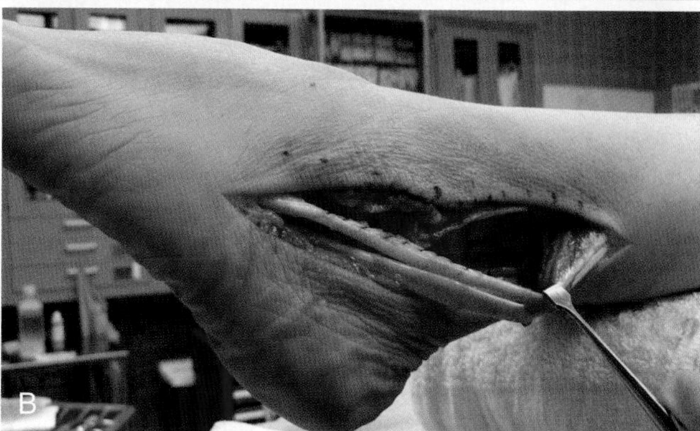

FIGURE 117-9 Intraoperative photographs of a patient who had a peroneus brevis tear in association with synovitis. **A,** Appearance of the tendons after excision of the synovitis. **B,** Tubularization of the peroneus brevis with a running nonabsorbable suture. *(From Joos D, Kadakia AR: Peroneal tendon disorders. In Miller MD, Sanders TC, editors:* Presentation, imaging and treatment of common musculoskeletal conditions: MRI-arthroscopy correlation, *Philadelphia, 2012, Elsevier.)*

Treatment Options

Conservative treatment includes use of nonsteroidal antiinflammatory drugs; physical therapy focusing on range of motion, peroneal strengthening, and proprioception; bracing with an ankle lace-up–type brace; or sometimes boot immobilization if symptoms are acute or severe.[57] In patients with a varus heel or cavovarus deformity, a simple lateral heel wedge or custom orthotic with lateral heel posting and a depressed first ray can be effective.

Surgical management of peroneal tendon tears first involves exploration of the tendon to determine the extent of tearing. When tenosynovitis is encountered, it should be debrided. As mentioned earlier, the tear can be debrided alone, debrided and repaired, or in severe cases, attached by tenodesis to the intact tendon (Fig. 117-9). In severe cases, the author has used the concept of "restoring at least one functioning tendon" via tenodesis of any remaining viable tendon. In the athlete, every attempt should be made to repair the tendons if possible.[57]

Peroneal tendon dislocation should be treated with reconstruction of the SPR. Eckert and Davis[52] came up with a classification system to define the injury to the SPR. In grade I injuries, the retinaculum and periosteum were elevated from the lateral malleolus, and the tendons lay between the periosteum and the bone. In grade II injuries (33% of their patients), the distal 1 to 2 cm of the fibrous ridge was elevated along with the retinaculum, and in grade III injuries (16% of their patients), a thin cortical rim of bone was avulsed along with the retinaculum, the fibrous lip, and the periosteum. Oden[48] described a similar classification scheme based on 100 cases but defined a type II injury as a tear rather than an elevation of the retinaculum from the fibula and added a type IV injury, an avulsion of bone from the posterior rather than anterior fibular insertion site. Several procedures have been described to treat the SPR insufficiency, including direct reattachment, reconstruction using either local or free grafts, rerouting the calcaneofibular ligament, and bone-block procedures.[52,61,67-69] When the peroneal tendons dislocate anteriorly to the fibula, a false pouch is often created that must be closed as part of the reconstruction. Multiple options for groove deepening have also been described. Direct groove deepening involves raising osteoperiosteal flaps with excavation of bone followed by laying back down the smooth osteoperiosteal surface.[70] Indirect groove deepening involves reaming out the posterior intramedullary fibula with use of a cannulated drill from the tip of the fibula and then tamping the intact periosteal surface to create a deeper groove.[71,72]

Associated pathologic conditions should also be addressed when present. Chronic lateral ankle instability can be treated with a modified Broström-Gould procedure, although in the presence of a peroneus brevis tendon tear, a modified Broström-Evans procedure is a useful alternative.[73] This procedure involves transferring the anterior one half to one third of the peroneus brevis into the distal fibula as an augmentation to the standard Broström procedure. If a varus heel is present, a lateralizing calcaneal osteotomy should be performed with use of either a standard oblique lateral-based wedge or a Z-shaped osteotomy.[74,75] When a hypertrophied peroneal tubercle is present, it should be excised.[51] In the case of intrasheath peroneal subluxation, groove deepening has been described as an effective treatment option.[76]

AUTHORS' PREFERRED TECHNIQUE

Peroneal Tendon Injury

Peroneal Tendon Repair

A curvilinear lateral approach is made over the peroneal tendons. If the SPR is intact, be careful to preserve a cuff lateral to the fibrocartilaginous ridge for later repair when incising through the retinaculum. Distal to the fibula, be sure to identify and release the separate sheaths in which the peroneus brevis and longus run, separated by the septa that attach to the peroneal tubercle. If the peroneal tubercle appears hypertrophied or is suspected of contributing to symptoms, have a low threshold to excise it. All tenosynovitis present is debrided. Evaluate the extent of the tendon tear and excise any degenerated tendon; if more than 50% of viable tendon remains, the tendon is repaired using a running, 4.0 absorbable suture. If the tendon is irreparable (i.e., generally <50% is viable, although this general rule can be modified), tenodesis to the intact tendon (longus or brevis) proximal and distal to the rupture site is performed with use of 2.0 or 3.0 nonabsorbable suture. Ensure that the tenodesis is performed both proximal and distal to the fibular groove to avoid fibular impingement.[77] In all cases, preservation of the function of the peroneus brevis is more critical than the function of the peroneus longus.

Chronic Peroneal Tendon Dislocation

In the setting of peroneal subluxation, the tendons are explored and synovectomy along with appropriate treatment of peroneal tendon tears are performed as previously described. The fibular groove should be deepened. A 3- to 5-cm-long cortical window of bone is carefully elevated from the posterior groove of the fibula, leaving the medial cortex intact. A burr is then used to deepen the groove by several millimeters. The cortical bone is then replaced and tamped down to provide a smooth surface for tendon gliding. Alternatively, the burr can be used directly on the posterior aspect of the fibula to deepen the groove. Use of a rasp to smooth the surface followed by bone wax creates a very smooth surface. This procedure negates problems with the cortical bone "popping" back into its original place. Indirect groove deepening can be performed with a large drill bit to ream out the posterior cancellous bone from the distal fibula. Bone tamping is used to collapse the retrofibular groove. Although this procedure preserves the gliding surface of the posterior fibula, the uncontrolled nature of this technique and the risk of fracture must be taken into consideration.

The tendons should lie within the groove without subluxation with gentle dorsiflexion and plantar flexion of the ankle. The SPR is then imbricated to the fibula through drill holes within the posterolateral border of the fibula (Fig. 117-10). The fibrocartilaginous ridge can also be used for fixation as an alternative to drill holes in the distal aspect of the fibula. Use of nonabsorbable No. 0 suture in a horizontal mattress fashion with the knot located on the SPR imbricates the tissue and prevents the knot from being placed in a subcutaneous location that can be irritating to the patient.

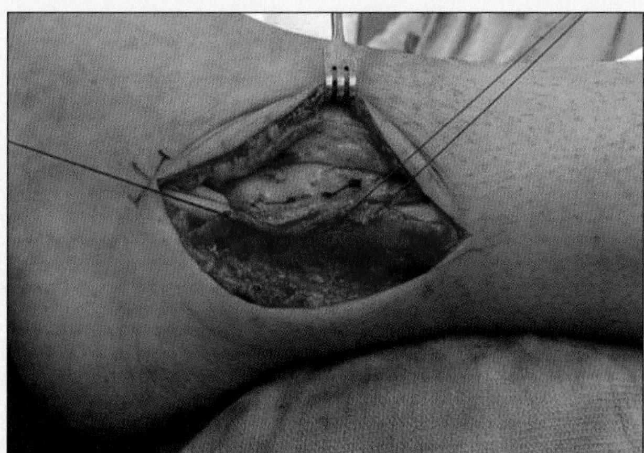

FIGURE 117-10 Repair of the superior peroneal retinaculum (SPR) is performed through drill holes in the fibula to imbricate the SPR to the deep aspect of the lateral fibula. It is critical to ensure that the SPR is placed to the underside of the lateral fibular ridge. *(From Joos D, Kadakia AR: Peroneal tendon disorders. In Miller MD, Sanders TG, editors:* Presentation, imaging and treatment of common musculoskeletal conditions: MRI-arthroscopy correlation, *Philadelphia, 2012, Elsevier.)*

Postoperative Management

Patients wear a short-leg, non–weight-bearing splint in the immediate postoperative period. After 2 weeks, a tall removable boot is worn and weight bearing is allowed. For most peroneal tendon procedures, it is important to initiate early ankle range of motion exercises to limit adhesion of the tendons. The patient can perform these exercises at home or with formal physical therapy. Inversion past 10 degrees from neutral is avoided until approximately 10 weeks after surgery to facilitate complete tendon healing. If concomitant osteotomies are performed to correct a cavovarus alignment, weight bearing is delayed until 6 weeks after surgery. At 6 weeks, most patients transition into an ankle lace-up–type brace, and activities progress. A realistic return to sporting activity is 4 to 6 months after surgery. Generally straight-ahead running is allowed at 3 months and cutting activities are allowed at 4 months, although this schedule is extremely variable.

Results

Outcomes of peroneal tendon repairs have mostly been reported in retrospective reviews and case reports. Bassett and Speer[78] reported that eight college-level athletes were able to return to full athletic activity after repair of five peroneus longus tendons and three peroneus brevis tendons, although the time frame was not discussed. AOFAS scores at medium-term follow-up after peroneal tendon repairs have been shown to be 82 to 85, with good to excellent patient-reported outcomes and normal to moderate peroneal strength in more than 90% of patients, although with prolonged time to maximum function.[56,79] In a recent study it was reported that the average return to activity was 3.2 months in an athletic population who underwent peroneal tendon repair and SPR reconstruction for symptomatic peroneal tendon subluxation.[80] However, Steel and DeOrio[55] reported that only 46% of 30 patients treated surgically for peroneal tendon tears were able to successfully return to sports.

Results of SPR reconstruction vary by the technique described. Eckert and Davis[52] reported only a 4% redislocation rate after SPR reattachment, although with only a 6-month follow-up. Maffulli and colleagues[81] performed anatomic repairs of the superior peroneal retinaculum on 14 patients with chronic, recurrent peroneal tendon subluxations. At follow-up of 38 months, none had experienced recurrent subluxations, and all had returned to their normal activities.[81] Poll and Duijfjes[69] reported on 10 patients in whom the insertion of the calcaneofibular ligament was mobilized and lifted with a cancellous bone block from the calcaneus. The peroneal tendons were then brought under the ligament, and the bone block was replaced and fixed with a small cancellous screw. They reported excellent results in all 10 patients and recommended the procedure because it precluded scarring and adhesions of the peroneal tendons to the surrounding structures.[69] Groove-deepening procedures have had similar good results. Zoellner and Clancy[70] reported on 10 patients using their technique and stated that the results were excellent at an average follow-up of 2 years. Porter et al.[82] modified their technique and accelerated the rehabilitation program and found no recurrent dislocations, minimal symptoms, and an average return to sports at 3 months after 3-year follow-up. Ogawa et al.[71] reported good clinical outcome scores and no recurrence of instability in 15 patients treated with the indirect groove-deepening method. Not surprisingly, the patients who had concomitant peroneal tendon tears had worse outcomes than those treated for instability alone.

Complications

Failure to diagnose the peroneal tendon tear or subluxation is likely the most common complication. Recurrent pain may be caused by inadequate debridement or failure to recognize and excise associated disease such as a low-lying muscle belly, peroneus quartus, or hypertrophied peroneal tubercle. Tendon adhesions and decreased mobility are another common cause of pain and dysfunction, especially after tenodesis is performed.[57] Recurrent tendon instability may be the result of persistent chronic lateral ankle instability and the subsequent strain on the SPR repair, as well as a failure to recognize and correct a subtle cavovarus alignment.

Future Considerations

Prospective studies are needed to determine the best and most appropriate SPR reconstruction method. Synthetic or specially processed allograft tissue may offer alternatives to local tissue when it is insufficient. The true benefit of groove-deepening procedures needs to be elucidated with higher level studies. As advanced imaging techniques improve, we may be able to better detect both peroneal tendon tears and subtle instability of the tendons and the fibulae that require groove deepening.

Achilles Tendon Injuries

The Achilles tendon is a common source of complaints in the orthopaedic surgeon's practice, especially in the athletic population. Acute Achilles tendon ruptures remain a very common injury and are prevalent in elite-level athletes, weekend warriors, and older patients. Surgical versus conservative treatment for acute Achilles tendon ruptures has followed a cyclical path in history and remains somewhat controversial. Chronic Achilles tendon dysfunction has been labeled many ways, including tendinitis, tendinosis, paratenonitis, and peritendinitis. Because these descriptions can be misleading, I agree with Maffulli and colleagues[83] that this entity should be termed *Achilles tendinopathy*. Most conditions are then further categorized into insertional versus noninsertional tendinopathy. Retrocalcaneal bursitis and Haglund's deformity (pump bump) are additional clinical entities that are associated with insertional disease.

History

Acute Achilles ruptures usually present after a traumatic event in which the patient feels as if he or she has been kicked or struck on the back of the ankle above the heel with subsequent weakness and difficulty with ambulation. This event is often the result of an explosive sporting maneuver, such as jumping for a rebound in basketball, but can be less significant and symptomatic if some intrinsic tearing was present. Although most patients seek immediate treatment, it is not uncommon for patients to disregard the initial event if the symptoms are mild and eventually seek treatment as a result of an altered gait, swelling, or heel walking.

Achilles tendinopathy causes chronic posterior ankle and heel pain that is worsened with activity. Runners show the highest incidence of noninsertional Achilles tendinopathy, which manifests as aching pain above the insertion of the Achilles, sometimes with associated swelling.[84] In early stages, the pain occurs only with prolonged running, but as the disease progresses, pain may occur even at rest. Insertional Achilles tendinopathy is seen in the athletic population but is more common as patients age and tendon degeneration occurs. Patients commonly localize their pain to the midline at the insertion of the Achilles on the calcaneus, although sometimes the pain is localized to the medial or lateral side. Exercise, stair climbing, and running on hard surfaces tend to exacerbate the pain. Symptoms may occur initially with strenuous activities alone but often progress to pain being present at rest.[85]

Physical Examination

Prone examination of both lower extremities provides all the information needed to determine the presence of an acute Achilles rupture. The resting tension of both Achilles tendons is evaluated by asking the patient to bend both knees and then inspecting the stance of the foot. Normal stance shows the foot plantar flexed about 20 degrees. Decreased stance (loss of plantar flexion) or asymmetry indicates a lengthened tendo-Achilles complex. A palpable gap and associated tenderness is often present at the rupture site, though these symptoms can be subtle if the injury is subacute. The most common site for rupture is 2 to 6 cm above the insertion on the calcaneus, thought to be secondary to an avascular zone.[86,87] The entire length of the gastrocsoleus complex should be palpated because ruptures can occur anywhere from the musculotendinous junction to the insertion on the calcaneus. The Thompson test is the classic and likely most sensitive way to determine a disruption in the Achilles tendon: with the knee flexed, squeeze the calf and inspect the motion of the foot.[88] If the foot plantar flexes, the Achilles is intact; if no motion occurs, discontinuity is present (Fig. 117-11).

Noninsertional Achilles tendinopathy classically presents with tenderness to palpation and swelling in the region proximal to the insertion of the Achilles tendon on the calcaneus. Similar to ruptures, this tendinopathy commonly occurs about 2 to 6 cm proximal to the calcaneal insertion (Fig. 117-12). Often a fusiform thickening of the tendon is palpated and tender. Assessment of lower extremity alignment is important, including limb-length inequality and the presence of cavus versus planus feet.

Insertional Achilles tendinopathy presents with the focus of tenderness on the posterior aspect of the insertional ridge of the calcaneus where the Achilles tendon inserts. Although not specific, midline tenderness tends to correlate with insertional tendinopathy, whereas lateral and less frequently medial tenderness tends to correlate with retrocalcaneal bursitis. Often a large prominence is noted on inspection either enveloping the entire posterior heel or predominantly laterally. When the bony prominence is isolated to the superolateral aspect of the calcaneal tuberosity, it is commonly referred to as a *Haglund deformity* (or pump bump). Testing for gastrocnemius tightness with the Silverskold examination should be performed for all patients suspected of having Achilles tendinopathy.

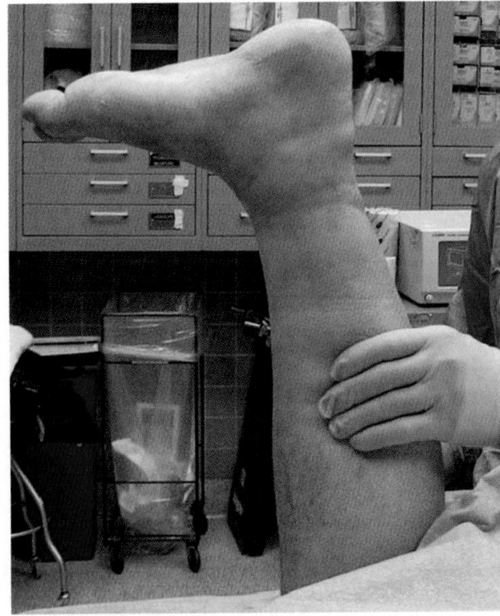

FIGURE 117-11 A positive Thompson test with a lack of plantar flexion with calf squeeze. *(From Joos D, Tran N, Kadakia AR: Achilles tendon disorders. In Miller MD, Sanders TG, editors:* Presentation, imaging and treatment of common musculoskeletal conditions: MRI-arthroscopy correlation, *Philadelphia, 2012, Elsevier.)*

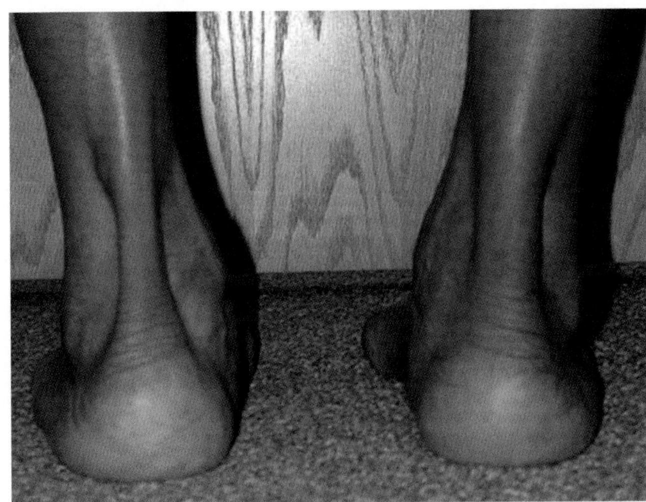

FIGURE 117-12 A patient with right Achilles tendinosis. Note the thickening of the tendon on the affected right leg compared with the normal left leg. *(From Joos D, Tran N, Kadakia AR: Achilles tendon disorders. In Miller MD, Sanders TG, editors:* Presentation, imaging and treatment of common musculoskeletal conditions: MRI-arthroscopy correlation, *Philadelphia, 2012, Elsevier.)*

Imaging

Standard ankle radiographs should be performed in most cases of Achilles tendon ruptures and all cases of Achilles tendinopathy. For ruptures it is important to evaluate whether a distal avulsion of the calcaneus is present, although this presentation is less common and suspicion should be raised on the examination. Soft tissue thickening or calcifications can be visualized in patients with noninsertional tendinopathy, whereas insertional disease may show a large bony spur at the insertional ridge, prominent Haglund deformity, or intratendinous calcifications. The width of the soft tissue shadow can also give an indication of tendon degeneration.

Ultrasound and MRI have become useful tools in identifying Achilles tendon disease, although neither is necessary to make the diagnosis in the great majority of cases. Ultrasound is the modality of choice to determine the proximity of the tendon edges in an acute Achilles rupture.[89] The dynamic nature of the test allows measurement of the gap present with the foot at neutral versus in 20 degrees of plantar flexion, which can have treatment implications. Although MRI can be useful in unclear cases or cases of chronic Achilles rupture, a recent study showed that physical examination findings were more sensitive in diagnosing acute Achilles ruptures than was MRI.[90]

For Achilles tendinopathy, ultrasound can be used to better delineate the presence of neovascularization in the tendon, which is a part of the degeneration process.[91] MRI can be used to better classify the degree of degeneration present in the tendon, as well as to distinguish intratendinous pathology from peritendinous pathology (Figs. 117-13 and 117-14). MRI has also been shown to help predict the response to nonoperative treatment in persons with insertional Achilles tendinopathy.[92] Both modalities can be used to assess response to treatment and for preoperative planning.

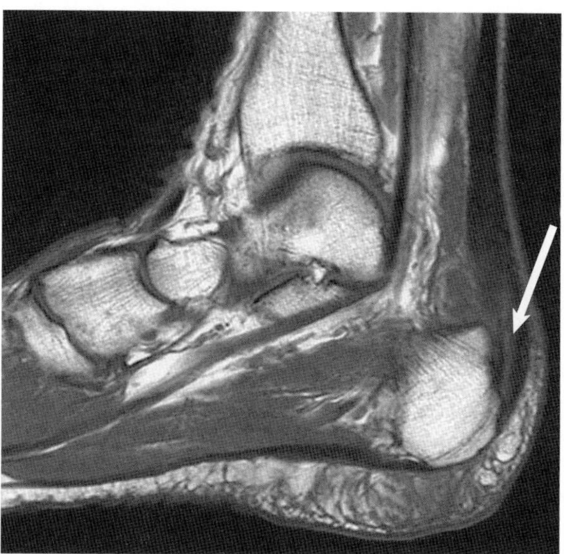

FIGURE 117-13 A T1-weighted magnetic resonance image of a patient with insertional Achilles tendinosis. Note the intermediate signal intensity and thickening of the tendon at the insertion of the Achilles tendon into the calcaneus (*arrow*). *(From Joos D, Tran N, Kadakia AR: Achilles tendon disorders. In Miller MD, Sanders TG, editors:* Presentation, imaging and treatment of common musculoskeletal conditions: MRI-arthroscopy correlation, *Philadelphia, 2012, Elsevier.)*

Decision-Making Principles

The debate between operative and nonoperative treatment for acute Achilles tendon ruptures has evolved with both improved surgical techniques and improved rehabilitation protocols. Multiple historical studies have compared the results of conservative versus surgical treatment.[93-99] However, rehabilitation protocols allowing motion and protected weight bearing earlier in the recovery period are now commonly used both during conservative treatment and after surgery with significant functional improvements.[100-104] The benefits and risks to both treatment options remain the same, although with these new rehabilitation protocols, the difference is not as stark. The advantage of nonoperative treatment is basically avoiding the risks (or disadvantages) of surgery: wound-healing problems, scar, and cost. The disadvantage of nonoperative treatment has historically been a higher repeat rupture rate and decreased strength and endurance compared with surgical treatment. Using a modern rehabilitation protocol, authors of two recent studies reexamined the question of operative versus nonoperative treatment. Willits et al.[103] showed equivalent repeat rupture rates and no clinically important difference in measured outcomes between operative and nonoperative groups, with increased complication rates in the operative group (18% vs. 8%). However, at the extreme plantar-flexion strength level measured (240 degrees/s), the surgical group showed a significant increase compared with the nonoperative group when measured as a ratio (affected/unaffected side). It was not stated how this measurement correlates clinically. Nilsson-Helander et al.[104] reported no difference in functional outcome scores between operative and nonoperative groups 12 months after surgery, with a 4% repeat rupture rate in the operative group and a 12% repeat rupture rate in the nonoperative group (the finding did not reach significance). Although a high rate of deep vein thrombosis (DVT) was found in the entire group (34%), all of the other complications reported were in the surgical group, mostly related to the scar. A systematic review of randomized controlled trials demonstrated a significantly reduced repeat rupture rate (3.6% operative vs. 8.8% nonoperative) and increased surgical complications with surgical treatment; however, no conclusion regarding return of strength could be made.[105] Although support has increased regarding the effectiveness of nonoperative treatment in Achilles tendon ruptures in the general population, most surgeons agree that in the athletic population, surgical repair is the most predictive method of restoring strength and ability to return to high-level sports. A frank discussion should be held with each patient to discuss the benefits and risks of both treatment options.

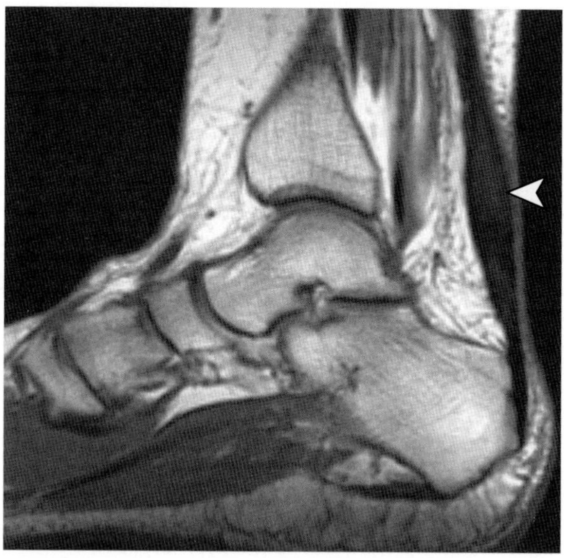

FIGURE 117-14 A T1-weighted magnetic resonance image of a patient with noninsertional Achilles tendinosis. Note the intermediate signal intensity and fusiform thickening of the tendon (*arrowhead*). *(From Joos D, Tran N, Kadakia AR: Achilles tendon disorders. In Miller MD, Sanders TG, editors:* Presentation, imaging and treatment of common musculoskeletal conditions: MRI-arthroscopy correlation, *Philadelphia, 2012, Elsevier.)*

Conservative treatment is always the first-line option in Achilles tendinopathy. If patients do not respond to the initial treatments such as rest, activity modification, footwear modification, and eccentric physical therapy, both invasive and noninvasive intermediate treatments are available and should be individualized to the patient. Noninvasive treatments for noninsertional tendinopathy include ultrasound, low-level laser therapy, shock-wave therapy, and glyceryl trinitrate patches.[84] Invasive treatments include platelet-rich plasma injections, prolotherapy, and aprotinin injections. Similar treatments have been described for insertional tendinopathy including shock-wave therapy and sclerosing injections.[85] Corticosteroid injections are not recommended based on the catabolic effect and subsequent risk of rupture.[106] Based on the limited literature available for most of these treatment options, insufficient evidence exists to support recommendation of these procedures, but the noninvasive treatments are relatively safe and may benefit some patients.

Surgical management can be considered for both insertional and noninsertional Achilles tendinopathy when nonoperative treatment fails. Because multiple surgical options exist, determining the appropriate procedure can be difficult. In general, for noninsertional tendinopathy, less invasive surgical treatments such as percutaneous longitudinal tenotomy and minimally invasive stripping procedures are appropriate for mild to moderate focal lesions, whereas open procedures including debridement, tenosynovectomy, and possibly FHL transfer are appropriate for moderate to severe tendinopathy.[107-110] Similarly, surgical management of insertional Achilles tendinopathy is dependent on the extent of degeneration of the Achilles tendon. Open retrocalcaneal decompression with Achilles tendon debridement and use of the Haglund excision have been used effectively for patients with persistent pain but minimal degeneration of the Achilles tendon, whereas an extensive debridement, reattachment of the Achilles tendon, and possible FHL transfer are more appropriate for patients with more extensive disease.[111-115]

Treatment Options

Conservative treatment of an acute Achilles tendon rupture should be managed with a modern rehabilitation program. As outlined by Willits et al.[103] and Tan et al.,[116] this protocol includes initial equinus immobilization for 2 weeks, followed by progressive weight bearing with heel lifts and range of motion with dorsiflexion blocks during the next 4 to 6 weeks. A physical therapy program is then initiated, including transition to footwear with a heel lift, open-chain exercises with a focus on eccentric strengthening, and eventual resistance exercises at about 10 weeks (Table 117-1).

Surgical options include primary open repair versus a "minimally invasive" or limited incision technique. The approach to primary open repair is usually performed just medial to the Achilles tendon, although central and lateral approaches can be used. Krackow, Bunnell, and Kessler suture configuration are all options, although one study showed that the Krackow technique was stronger than the others.[117] Two-strand versus four-strand repairs can be used, with four-strand repairs being biomechanically superior.[118] Limited incision techniques have increased in popularity since Ma and Griffith[119] reported their results in 1977. Assal et al.[120] and Amlang and colleagues[121] reported their results using specially designed devices to decrease risk of sural nerve injury and to ensure placement of the sutures within the paratenon. Currently neither treatment can be recommended over the other, although most surgeons would recommend an open repair in the elite-level athlete.

The conservative and surgical options for Achilles tendinopathy are listed in the Decision-Making Principles section. Endoscopic decompression of the retrocalcaneal space has also been described for insertional tendinopathy. Good clinical outcomes have been reported, although the ability to debride the tendon and remove any calcifications is limited.[122,123]

TABLE 117-1

PROTOCOL FOR NONOPERATIVE MANAGEMENT OF ACUTE ACHILLES TENDON RUPTURES

Timing	Treatment
Initial evaluation	Ultrasound or magnetic resonance imaging examination demonstrating less than 5 mm of gap with maximum plantar flexion or less than 10 mm of gapping with the foot in neutral position with greater than 75% of tendon apposition with the foot in 20 degrees of plantar flexion
Initial management	Cast with foot in full equinus with dorsiflexion block; non–weight bearing
2-week evaluation	Transition to a removable cast or cast boot with the foot in 20 degrees of plantar flexion with two 1-cm wedges in the cast boot; can bear weight as tolerated; the boot is to be worn 24 hours per day
4-week evaluation	Clinical examination: able to palpate continuity of the tendon; recommend repeat ultrasound or magnetic resonance imaging to verify that tendon edges are apposed without evidence of gapped ends; if tendon edges are not apposed, recommend surgical consideration; the boot is removed 5 minutes per hour when awake to perform active dorsiflexion to neutral with passive plantar flexion
6-week evaluation	Clinical examination to document continuity of the tendon; removal of one 1-cm wedge; continue active dorsiflexion to neutral with passive plantar flexion; initiate a physical therapy program to begin proprioception and non–weight-bearing muscle strengthening out of the boot
8-week evaluation	Clinical examination to ensure tendon continuity and evaluation with ultrasound or magnetic resonance imaging to document continued tendon apposition; if the patient has a lack of tendon healing or continuity, consider operative intervention; if the tendon is in continuity, recommend transition of boot to daytime wear only without use of a wedge; continue a formal physical therapy program
10-week evaluation	Discontinue use of the boot and use a 1-cm heel wedge for 3 more months; may start to ride a stationary bike and progress with the physical therapy program with weight bearing as tolerated with a lift in the shoe; no sprinting or running is allowed until use of the heel wedge is discontinued

Postoperative Management

Acute repair of Achilles tendon ruptures follow the same accelerated rehabilitation protocol as that used for nonoperative treatment (see the brief description in the Treatment Options section). Early motion and early weight bearing (after 2 weeks of immobilization) have been shown to significantly increase functional outcomes and health-related quality of life.[101,124] Patients are generally progressed into a shoe with

AUTHORS' PREFERRED TECHNIQUE

Achilles Tendon Rupture

I prefer to use an open repair technique for acute Achilles ruptures in the athletic population to ensure excellent tendon apposition and restoration of tension (Fig. 117-15). The patient is positioned prone, with the incision just medial to the Achilles tendon. Alternatively, the patient can be placed supine with the affected leg externally rotated using a medial approach to access the tendon. Although this technique can be used routinely, it is excellent for obese patients with respiratory compromise or patients with a compromised airway. One should sharply incise through skin, subcutaneous tissue, and paratenon to avoid devascularization of the skin edges. Identify the rupture and gently debride it of hematoma; do not debride frayed tendon edges. Place a Krackow locking stitch using No. 2 polydioxanone in the proximal and distal tendon stumps. Larger nonabsorbable No. 5 suture or newer No. 2 suture that has the strength of traditional No. 5 nonabsorbable suture is also frequently used. Four to five passes through both the medial and lateral column should suffice. If a four-strand repair is chosen, the second two strands should be passed orthogonal to the first (i.e., one in the coronal plane and one in the sagittal plane). Sutures are tied while holding the tendon edges apposed with the other suture limbs with the foot in about 20 to 30 degrees of plantar flexion. Epitendon suture is placed using 2-0 absorbable suture in cross-stitch fashion. The paratenon is carefully closed and a splint in 20 degrees of plantar flexion is applied to maximize perfusion to the posterior skin.

Noninsertional Achilles Tendinopathy: Tendon Debridement with Longitudinal Repair

For tendon debridement with longitudinal repair, a prone approach is used with a medial incision carried down through the paratenon. A longitudinal incision of the thickened, degenerative portion of tendon is performed. Sharp debridement of all degenerative-appearing tendon, essentially shelling out the inner core of the tendon, is carried out, taking care not to create a discontinuity (Fig. 117-16). Longitudinal repair is performed with tubularization of the healthy tendon edges and additional closure of the paratenon if possible.

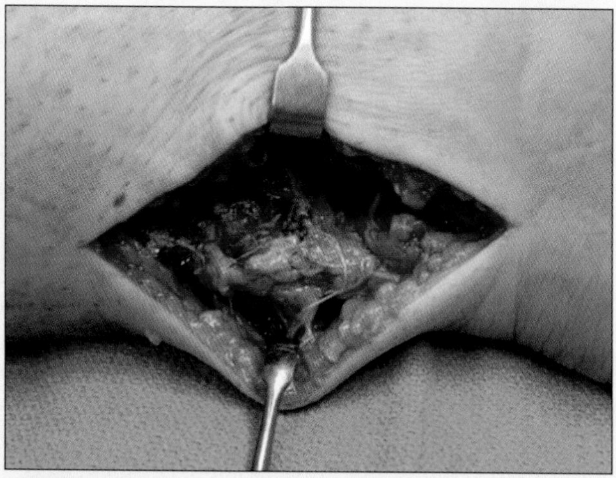

FIGURE 117-15 Intraoperative photograph of the Achilles tendon after repair. The tendon ends should be completely apposed without any gapping. *(From Joos D, Tran N, Kadakia AR: Achilles tendon disorders. In Miller MD, Sanders TG, editors:* Presentation, imaging and treatment of common musculoskeletal conditions: MRI-arthroscopy correlation, *Philadelphia, 2012, Elsevier.)*

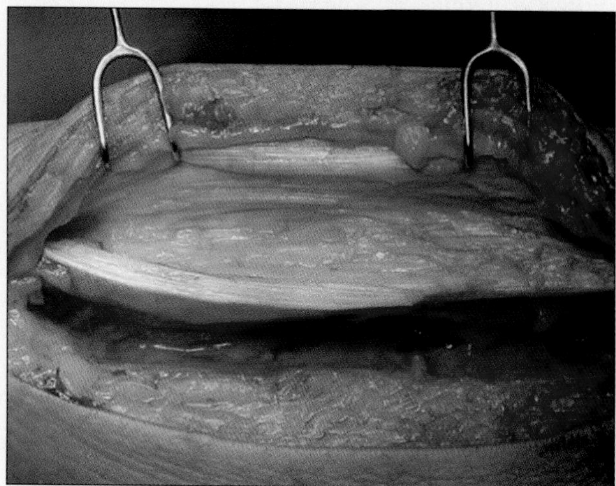

FIGURE 117-16 An intraoperative photograph demonstrating resection of the central diseased portion of the Achilles tendon. *(From Joos D, Tran N, Kadakia AR: Achilles tendon disorders. In Miller MD, Sanders TG, editors:* Presentation, imaging and treatment of common musculoskeletal conditions: MRI-arthroscopy correlation, *Philadelphia, 2012, Elsevier.)*

Insertional Achilles Tendinopathy: Achilles Debridement, Haglund Excision, FHL Transfer (If >50 Years Old), and Tendon Reattachment

The longitudinal midline approach is carried down through the paratenon, and the creation of paratenon flaps for later closure is undertaken. A longitudinal incision is made through the midline of the Achilles tendon, and detachment of the middle 75% of the Achilles insertion from the calcaneal ridge is performed. An attempt is made to preserve the far medial and lateral Achilles tendon attachments. Sharp debridement of all degenerative Achilles tissue is performed. Resection of the posterior superior prominence of the calcaneus (Haglund's deformity) is undertaken with a saw or osteotome from distal posterior to proximal anterior. Fluoroscopy is used to ensure that an adequate amount of bone has been resected to prevent further impingement. Excessive resection of the tuberosity is not required and may make reconstruction more difficult by minimizing the amount of bone for tendon fixation. Reattach the detached limbs of the Achilles tendon onto the calcaneus using two suture anchors placed distal to the FHL transfer, one medial and one lateral. Repair the midline tenotomy using size 0 or No. 1 nonabsorbable suture. Carefully close the paratenon, subcutaneous tissue, and skin and apply a splint in 20 degrees of plantar flexion.

FHL Transfer (If Necessary)

Divide the deep posterior fascia and identify the FHL muscle belly. Release the FHL tendon from its medial fibro-osseous tunnel and sharply divide as far distal as possible. Place tag suture using size 0 nonabsorbable suture. Note that the tibial nerve is located immediately medial to the tendon and must not be violated. Measure the diameter of the tendon and place a long Beath needle in the midline of the cut calcaneus through the plantar surface of the foot, again using fluoroscopy as a guide. Ream through the calcaneus using an appropriately sized reamer, slightly larger than the diameter of the measured tendon. Deliver the FHL through the reamed hole and place an interference screw in maximal tension with the foot held in 5 degrees of plantar flexion.

a heel lift at 8 to 10 weeks after surgery. Straight-ahead running is allowed at 3 months, and cutting exercises are allowed at 4 months. Return to full athletic activity is usually achieved by 9 months.

A similar postoperative course is followed in the patient undergoing debridement and repair of a noninsertional Achilles tendon lesion. For insertional Achilles tendon procedures, the postoperative course depends on the extent of surgery. If possible, the insertional attachment should be preserved in the athletic population. Weight bearing is delayed until 4 weeks after surgery in patients who undergo an FHL transfer. When Achilles reattachment is required, boot immobilization is maintained until 12 weeks to facilitate improved tendon to bone healing. Return to full sporting activities is generally delayed until about 12 months after surgery.

Results

Recent studies comparing nonoperative and operative treatment for acute Achilles tendon ruptures are discussed in the Decision-Making Principles section. In 1998, Speck and Klaue[125] prospectively evaluated the clinical outcomes of 20 patients who had 6 weeks of early full weight bearing in a removable ankle-foot orthosis after an open repair of a torn Achilles tendon. All 20 patients reached their preoperative level of sports activity and had no significant side-to-side difference in ankle mobility and isokinetic strength. No repeat ruptures occurred. In a larger prospective study, Mortensen and colleagues[102] randomly assigned 71 patients who had repairs of acute Achilles tendon ruptures to either conventional postoperative management (i.e., a cast for 8 weeks) or early restricted motion of the ankle in a below-the-knee brace for 6 weeks. They found that patients who engaged in early motion had a smaller initial loss in range of motion and returned to work and sports activities sooner than did patients managed with a cast. No repeat ruptures occurred in either group. In 2007, Twaddle and Poon[101] found that the common denominator between operative and nonoperative treatment was early motion. They found no differences in the outcomes of operative and nonoperative treatment in patients who were treated with early motion controlled with a removable orthosis. It is clear from these studies that early motion or an accelerated functional rehabilitation protocol, as well as early weight bearing, leads to improved functional results in both operative and nonoperative cases. The controversy regarding difference in strength and repeat rupture rate between operative and nonoperative treatment remains, although most investigators would agree the elite-level athlete should undergo surgical treatment. The definition of "elite," however, is debatable.

Limited incision techniques have also shown good results. In separate studies using a device designed to enhance the limited open repair, Assal et al.[120] and Calder and Saxby[126] reported no cases of repeat rupture, an average AOFAS score of 96 to 98, and return to previous sporting level in all patients. No wound healing difficulties were encountered in either study. The proposed benefit to the limited open repair procedure is a significant decrease in the wound healing and scar complications seen with the standard open repair procedure.

Eccentric exercises have demonstrated improved results in the nonoperative treatment of noninsertional Achilles tendinopathy compared with other therapies, primarily because of decreased pain.[127-129] Platelet-rich plasma injections have gained notoriety in recent years, but no comparison studies have been able to prove their efficacy in treating noninsertional Achilles tendinopathy.[130,131] Longitudinal tenotomies have shown good results in the running population.[107] Success rates greater than 80% have been obtained from open procedures with tenosynovectomy and tendon debridement.[109,132] Improved rates of pain, functional outcomes, and patient satisfaction have also been reported with use of FHL tendon transfers in severe cases of chronic Achilles tendinopathy.[110,133]

Surgical interventions for insertional Achilles tendinopathy have elicited similar patient satisfaction and good functional outcomes. Yodlowski et al.[112] reported that 90% of patients had complete or significant relief of symptoms after open retrocalcaneal decompression. Maffulli et al.[134] and McGarvey et al.[135] displayed good clinical results through a medial approach and a central tendon-splitting approach, respectively. Some factors that negatively affected outcomes included presence of intratendinous calcifications and age greater than 55 years.[111,135] When adding an FHL transfer, Den Hartog[114] reported significant improvement in AOFAS scores and an 88% rate of patient satisfaction. Similarly, Elias et al.[115] showed 95% patient satisfaction and no loss of plantar-flexion strength or power with use of a similar technique.[115]

Complications

Nonoperative treatment of Achilles tendon ruptures may lead to weakness and an elevated repeat rupture rate that has been shown to be 8.8% versus 3.6% in the operative group in a systematic review of randomized controlled trials.[105] However, this treatment avoids the surgical complications associated with open repair. The deep infection rate was found to be 2.36%, whereas noncosmetic scar complaints were reported in 13.1% in the surgical group. The most significant reported complication from limited open approaches for Achilles tendon repair is sural nerve injury, which was present in 13% of cases in one early study.[136] Improved designs using a jig to ensure placement of the suture within the paratenon have significantly decreased rates of sural nerve injury.[120,126] Rates of DVT after Achilles tendon ruptures have been reported to be as high as 34%, although a recent large review of a health care management database revealed DVT rates of 0.43% and pulmonary embolism rates of 0.34%.[104,137]

Postoperative complications were reported in 11% of patients in one large retrospective series of patients undergoing surgery for chronic Achilles overuse injuries.[138] These complications included skin edge necrosis, infections, sural neuritis, DVT, and sensitive or hypertrophic scars. Achilles tendon ruptures or avulsions have also been reported, albeit rarely.[111,139,140] Cock-up deformity and medial plantar nerve transection have been reported after FHL transfers.[141,142]

Future Considerations

Further prospective studies are needed to determine the efficacy of limited open approaches for acute Achilles tendon ruptures. Improved designs may permit stronger repairs, with the added benefit of decreased wound healing complications. The advancement of invasive, nonsurgical techniques for Achilles tendinopathy, with utilization of orthobiologics or autologous products such as platelet-rich plasma, may allow for improved results with less morbidity.

For a complete list of references, go to expertconsult.com.

Suggested Readings

Citation: Sammarco VJ, Sammarco GJ, Henning C, et al: Surgical repair of acute and chronic tibialis anterior tendon ruptures. *J Bone Joint Surg Am* 91(2):325–332, 2009.

Level of Evidence: IV (therapeutic)

Summary: Nineteen surgically repaired tibialis anterior tendon ruptures were evaluated, including eight early repairs and 11 delayed reconstructions. Functional dorsiflexion, improved gait, and good strength were achieved in most patients.

Citation: Lohrer H, Nauck T: Posterior tibial tendon dislocation: a systematic review of the literature and presentation of a case. *Br J Sports Med* 44:398–406, 2010.

Level of Evidence: III (therapeutic)

Summary: The authors performed a systematic review of the literature and evaluated 61 cases of posterior tibial tendon dislocations, including clinical presentation, treatment, and outcomes. More than half of the cases were missed initially and 83% were fixed surgically, of which 80% were judged to have excellent results.

Citation: Michelson J, Dunn L: Tenosynovitis of the flexor hallucis longus: A clinical study of the spectrum of presentation and treatment. *Foot Ankle Int* 26:291–303, 2005.

Level of Evidence: IV (therapeutic)

Summary: The clinical presentation and results of treatment in 81 patients with symptomatic flexor hallucis longus tenosynovitis were retrospectively evaluated. Nonoperative treatment was successful in 64% of patients, whereas successful outcomes were reported for all 23 patients treated surgically (the majority with FHL decompression and synovectomy at the posterior ankle).

Citation: Scholten PE, Sierevelt IN, van Dijk CN: Hindfoot endoscopy for posterior ankle impingement. *J Bone Joint Surg Am* 90(12):2665–2672, 2008.

Level of Evidence: IV (therapeutic)

Summary: The authors provide a retrospective review of 55 patients treated for posterior ankle impingement with posterior hindfoot endoscopy for both traumatic and overuse injuries. Outcome scores significantly improved and return to sports occurred at an average of 8 weeks, although patients in the overuse group fared slightly better than did those in the traumatic group.

Citation: Krause JO, Brodsky JW: Peroneus brevis tendon tears: Pathophysiology, surgical reconstruction, and clinical results. *Foot Ankle Int* 19:271–279, 1998.

Level of Evidence: IV (therapeutic)

Summary: Twenty patients with peroneus brevis tendon tears were evaluated and a new classification system was determined that defined tears as greater than or less than 50% of the cross-sectional area. Grade 1 tears were treated with debridement and repair, grade 2 tears were treated with tenodesis to the peroneus longus, and good to excellent results were achieved in the majority of patients, although with a prolonged return to maximum function.

Citation: Eckert WR, Davis EA Jr: Acute rupture of the peroneal retinaculum. *J Bone Joint Surg Am* 58:670–672, 1976.

Level of Evidence: IV (therapeutic)

Summary: Seventy-three skiers with acute peroneal tendon dislocations were evaluated and three grades of injury to the superior peroneal retinaculum were identified based on the location of disruption of the SPR on the posterolateral fibula. Surgical repair was deemed very successful, with only three cases of recurrent dislocation.

Citation: Willits K, Amendola A, Bryant D, et al: Operative versus nonoperative treatment of acute Achilles tendon ruptures: A multicenter randomized trial using accelerated functional rehabilitation. *J Bone Joint Surg Am* 92A:2767–2775, 2010.

Level of Evidence: I (therapeutic)

Summary: The authors report a randomized, controlled trial comparing operative versus nonoperative treatment of acute Achilles tendon ruptures in 144 patients with use of an accelerated functional rehabilitation protocol in both treatment groups. Outcome scores and clinical findings showed no clinically important differences between the groups and repeat rupture rates were equivalent, but complications were slightly higher in the operative group.

Citation: Suchak AA, Bostick GP, Beaupre LA, et al: The influence of early weight-bearing compared with non-weight-bearing after surgical repair of the Achilles tendon. *J Bone Joint Surg Am* 90A:1876–1883, 2008.

Level of Evidence: I (therapeutic)

Summary: Ninety-eight patients with surgically repaired Achilles tendons were randomized into either a weight-bearing group or a non–weight-bearing group at the 2-week postoperative visit. Health-related quality of life measures were significantly improved in the early weight-bearing group at 6 weeks, although no difference in outcomes was seen at 6 months.

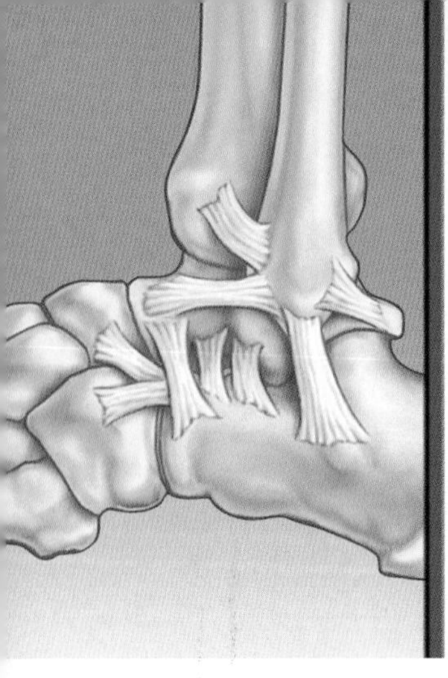

118

Articular Cartilage Injuries

DAVID R. RICHARDSON • KELLY R. McCORMICK

Osteochondral Lesions in the Foot and Ankle Region

Although a number of osteochondritic conditions in the foot and ankle have been described, most are rare and usually asymptomatic. The most common osteochondroses in the foot and ankle that cause symptoms and require treatment affect the talus, calcaneus, navicular, cuneiforms, metatarsals, and sesamoids.

The cause of osteochondrosis is complex and has been described as traumatic, constitutional, idiopathic, and hereditary. Most investigators now believe that numerous factors are responsible for these changes. For example, excessive physical demands during athletic activity may incite osteochondral changes in growing bone made vulnerable by constitutional factors. Once the process has begun, repetitive trauma or pressure may prolong recovery or contribute to deformity. All osteochondroses heal, but treatment may be required to relieve pain or prevent residual deformity, especially in osteochondroses around the foot and ankle in athletes. Treatment of any osteochondritic condition must be individualized to facilitate a rapid, safe return to activity and minimize sequelae of the condition.

Osteochondral Lesions of the Talus

History

The incidence of osteochondral lesions of the talus (OLT), at least in military recruits, has been steadily rising during the past 10 years and is 56 per 100,000 person-years.[1] Most lesions are unilateral, but 10% of patients may have bilateral OLTs.[2] Patients with acute injuries usually present with swollen and painful ankles or feet, limiting the specificity of physical examination. Patients with chronic injuries generally report mechanical symptoms, such as locking or giving way, or a feeling of instability of the ankle joint, in addition to pain and persistent swelling. Pain may occur only with certain ankle movements during sport or strenuous activity.

An OLT should be considered in any patient who presents with a history of a "persistent ankle sprain." Eighty percent of patients with traumatic OLT have a history of a seemingly benign ankle sprain. Taga and associates[3] found cartilage lesions in 89% of acutely injured ankles and in 95% of ankles with chronic injuries. They concluded that the longer the time from the initial injury, the more severe the associated cartilage lesions. Studies have found cartilage damage in up to 66% of ankles with lateral ligament injuries and 98% of ankles with deltoid ligament injuries.[4,5] In contrast, Komenda and Ferkel[6] found chondral injuries in only 25% of 55 unstable ankles. No correlation has been found between the amount of cartilage damage and the severity of the lateral ligament injury.[4]

Physical Examination

Visual inspection of the foot and ankle should be performed to identify areas of swelling and ecchymosis, which are critically important in the acute setting. Hindfoot alignment should be inspected from both the anterior and posterior aspects with the patient standing to determine if the patient has hindfoot varus or valgus, which may need to be addressed to improve the long-term outcome. The ankle and foot should be palpated to identify locations of tenderness; the medial and lateral corners of the talar dome should be palpated with the ankle maximally plantar flexed. A careful neurovascular examination is essential. Range of motion in the involved foot and ankle should be compared with that of the contralateral extremity. Stability of the ankle should be evaluated with an anterior drawer test with the ankle plantar flexed and dorsiflexed and with inversion and eversion stress testing. Other soft tissue or bony causes should be ruled out.

Imaging

Oblique and plantar flexed radiographic views that avoid tibial overlap generally show the lesion more clearly than plain films. If radiographs are suggestive but not diagnostic of OLT, technetium-99m bone scanning can help identify localized bony pathologic conditions. If an OLT is suggested by either radiography or bone scan, three-dimensional imaging such as computed tomography (CT) or magnetic resonance imaging (MRI) can provide more definitive information. The debate between modalities continues, but a study comparing the sensitivity and specificity of MRI demonstrated 96% for both, whereas the sensitivity and specificity of CT was 81% and 99%, respectively, although the differences were not statistically significant.[7] Axial and sagittal cuts can help determine the location of the lesion (anterior, medial, or posterior), as well as its depth and size (Fig. 118-1). MRI is useful for both preoperative evaluation and postoperative follow-up and has become the standard in noninvasive diagnostics. Anderson and colleagues[8] demonstrated that low

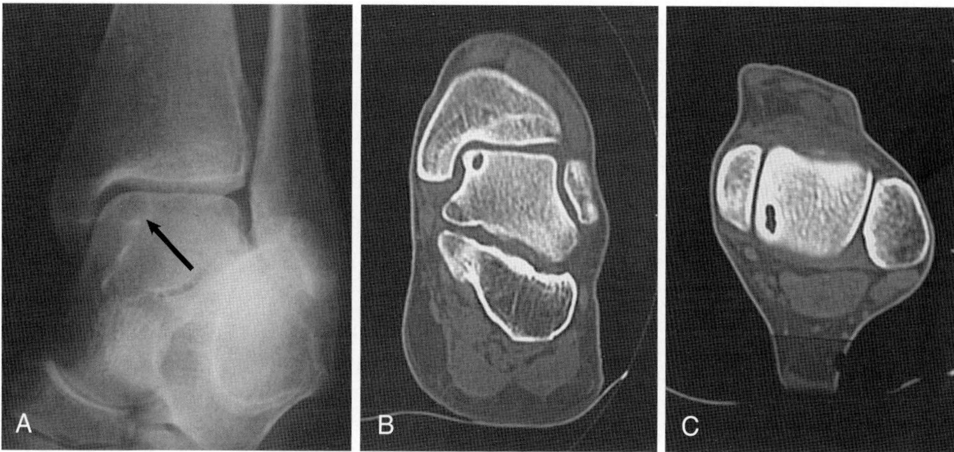

FIGURE 118-1 **A,** A posteromedial osteochondral lesion of the talus *(arrow)*. **B,** A coronal plane computed tomography (CT) image. **C,** An axial plane CT image. *(From Richardson DR: Ankle injuries. In Canale ST, Beaty JH, editors:* Campbell's operative orthopaedics, *ed 11, Philadelphia, 2008, Elsevier.)*

signal intensity in T1-weighted images is an early and definitive sign of even stage I lesions. A high signal rim between the osteochondral fragment and the talar bed is considered indicative of instability of the fragment, and joint fluid or fibrous granulation tissue is present as a result of the mobility of these fragments. It has been noted that the diameter of the lesion measured on MRI was significantly larger than that indicated on radiographs,[9] which is an important factor in preoperative planning. We recommend MRI evaluation to detect changes that provide information about the detachment and viability of the fragment and help make a decision about whether to preserve or excise the fragment (Fig. 118-2). MRI also may allow more appropriate treatment because it delineates the lesion more accurately than either plain radiography or CT.[10] OLTs that have a high signal rim on T2-weighted images are most likely unstable.[10] In a study of 22 ankles with OLT, Higashiyama and associates[11] found that the low and high signal rims present before surgery disappeared in 100% and 77% of ankles, respectively. A decrease in or disappearance of the signal rim correlated well with clinical results: no patient in whom the signal rim persisted had a good result. It has been suggested that helical CT, MRI, and diagnostic arthroscopy are significantly better than history, physical examination, and standard radiography for detecting or excluding OLT. Diagnostic arthroscopy does not perform better than helical CT and MRI.[10] In general, arthroscopy should not be used as the initial method for diagnosing OLT. In a recent study, MRI was used in combination with single photon emission CT to evaluate OLT to help determine if the OLT was incidental or truly symptomatic. Based on these images, three independent, blinded orthopaedic surgeons changed their treatment plan in 52% of the 25 cases.[12] By providing information on the subchondral plate and lesion depth, single photon emission CT may have additional diagnostic value.[13]

Decision-Making Principles

The choice of surgical or nonsurgical treatment depends largely on the patient's symptoms, age, and level of dysfunction and the size of the lesion. Uncontained lesions and lesions larger than 1.5 cm^2 have been associated with poor clinical outcomes and may need to be treated with a more extensive initial procedure.[14] Increasing age also was shown to correlate with poorer outcomes; however, after the age of 33 years, no difference in outcomes occurred.[14] Some patients may not have any functional deficits or complaints despite the presence of a lesion. An OLT discovered incidentally on diagnostic imaging does not always require surgery. Diagnostic injections into the ankle joint to delineate true ankle pain from other causes in the differential diagnosis can be helpful. However, mechanical symptoms such as locking, clicking, catching, or functional instability often require operative intervention. Chronic lateral instability in an ankle with an OLT can be successfully treated at the time of surgery.[15]

Treatment Options

Nonoperative

Although it is reported to be successful in only about half of patients,[16-19] nonoperative treatment generally should be attempted first in patients with cystic lesions (determined by CT) with or without communication to the ankle joint and acute nondisplaced lesions. In skeletally immature patients, nonoperative treatment may be tried for chronic nondisplaced

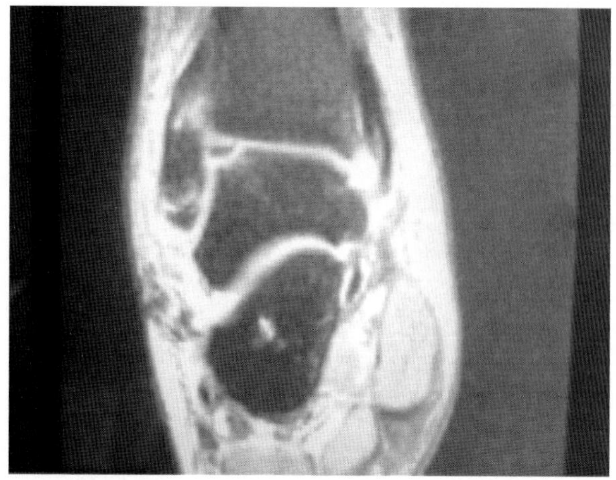

FIGURE 118-2 Magnetic resonance imaging appearance of a stage IV osteochondral lesion of the talus.

surface lesions as well. Nonoperative treatment is not recommended in adult patients with chronic symptomatic nondisplaced OLTs or in any patient with a displaced lesion.

Nonoperative treatment of acute OLT generally involves an initial period of non–weight bearing with cast immobilization, followed by progressive weight bearing and mobilization to full ambulation by 12 to 16 weeks. The recommended duration of nonoperative treatment is varied, with some authors recommending 6 months[18] and others up to 12 months[19] before operative treatment is chosen.

Based on the results of nonoperative treatment of 35 cases of chronic cystic OLT, Shearer and colleagues[20] concluded that (1) nonoperative management of chronic cystic OLT is a viable option with little or no risk for the development of significant osteoarthritis; (2) most lesions remain radiographically stable; (3) poor correlation exists between changes in lesion size and clinical outcome, although the few patients with lesions that decrease significantly in size tend to do well, and those with lesions that increase significantly in size tend to do poorly; (4) the development of mild radiographic changes of osteoarthritis does not correlate with clinical outcome; (5) the general course of chronic cystic OLT is benign, with more than half of patients improving to good or excellent results with nonoperative management; (6) lateral lesions tend to do better than medial ones; and (7) adult-onset lesions tend to do better than juvenile-onset lesions. Contrary to earlier reports, however, more recent investigations have determined that patient age is not an independent predictor of surgical results.[21] Alexander and Lichtman[22] suggested that a delay in treatment does not affect outcome, but more recent studies have questioned this suggestion.[23-25] Lesions presenting more than 1 year after injury or the onset of symptoms may have a poorer prognosis.[23] Also, radiographic results are improved when the interval between injury and operative treatment is reduced[23]; however, a correlation between radiographic appearance and clinical outcome has not been proven.

Operative

Options for open or arthroscopic treatment of OLT generally are based on one of three specific goals: (1) stimulating the bone marrow by debridement or drilling, with or without loose body removal; (2) securing the lesion to the talar dome so that it will heal in place; or (3) stimulating the development of hyaline cartilage (Box 118-1). Techniques include excision, drilling, and curettage, alone or in combination; internal fixation for acute lesions and cancellous bone grafting; osteochondral autograft or allograft procedures; and autologous chondrocyte implantation or transplantation.

BOX 118-1 Surgical Treatment of Osteochondral Lesions of the Talus

Abrasion chondroplasty
Marrow stimulation
- Debridement or microfracture
- Drilling: antegrade or retrograde

Internal fixation
- Headless screws, bioabsorbable devices, or Kirschner wires

Stimulation of hyaline cartilage
- Osteochondral autograft or allograft

Single plug
Mosaicplasty (multiple plugs)
- Autologous chondrocyte implantation (or matrix or membrane autologous chondrocyte implantation)

Lavage, Debridement, and Excision

Small, chronic, symptomatic lesions may benefit from arthroscopic lavage and debridement by removing catabolic cytokines and loose bodies from the ankle, which can be the source of mechanical symptoms. However, adding curettage and drilling has been associated with better results, and therefore arthroscopy and debridement alone is not recommended.[16,26]

Marrow Stimulation: Curettage, Drilling, and Microfracture

Marrow-inducing reparative techniques, such as abrasion, drilling, and microfracture, aim to stimulate chondroprogenitor cells within the underlying marrow. Penetration of the subchondral plate allows release of these cells into the defect. These stem cells populate the fibrin clot in the talar defect and produce a fibrocartilaginous matrix composed of chondroblasts, chondrocytes, fibrocytes, and an unorganized matrix that protects the surface from excessive loading. The disadvantage of these reparative techniques is the weaker mechanical properties of the type I collagen fibrocartilage matrix, which lacks the normal biomechanical and viscoelastic characteristics of type II hyaline cartilage.

Marrow stimulation generally is used as a first-line treatment for chondral lesions, and fair evidence (grade B recommendation) supports marrow stimulation as the index procedure or as a repeat procedure after failed arthroscopic management.[27] Arthroscopic results appear to be superior to those of open procedures.[27] In a metaanalysis that included 18 studies (388 patients), successful treatment was reported with bone marrow stimulation in 85% of patients (range, 46% to 100%).[17] OLTs associated with cyst formation have been successfully treated with marrow stimulation alone, achieving good to excellent results in 74% of patients.[28] When the overlying cartilage is intact, antegrade or retrograde drilling can effectively stimulate a response. Fair (level IV) evidence with consistently positive results is available to warrant a grade B recommendation for antegrade or retrograde drilling of OLTs with intact overlying cartilage.[27] Although antegrade (transtibial) and retrograde (transtalar) drilling are technically easy, both can result in cartilage damage and tibial necrosis.

Internal Fixation

Fixation devices include permanent or bioabsorbable low-profile pins, nails, or headless screws (Fig. 118-3). Acute OLTs do markedly better after fixation than do chronic lesions. Lesions need to be larger than 8 mm to allow secure internal fixation.

Restoration of Articular Hyaline Cartilage

Restorative techniques usually are recommended for defects larger than 1.5 cm^2. These techniques can include autologous chondrocyte implantation (ACI), matrix or membrane ACI, collagen-covered autologous chondrocyte implantation, arthroscopic allograft or autograft with platelet-rich plasma (PRP) implantation, osteochondral autograft, osteochondral autologous transfer system (OATS) and mosaicplasty, fresh

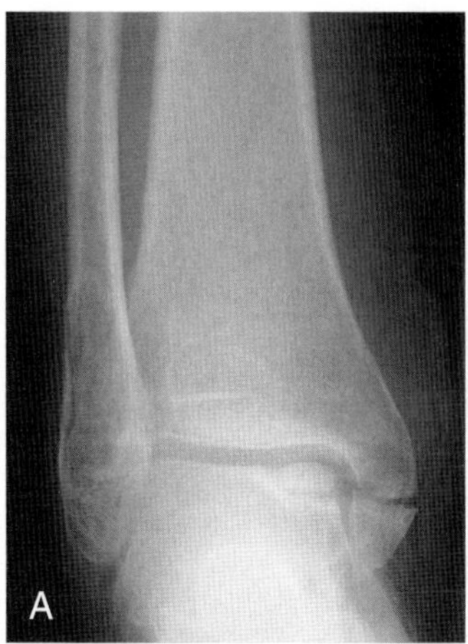

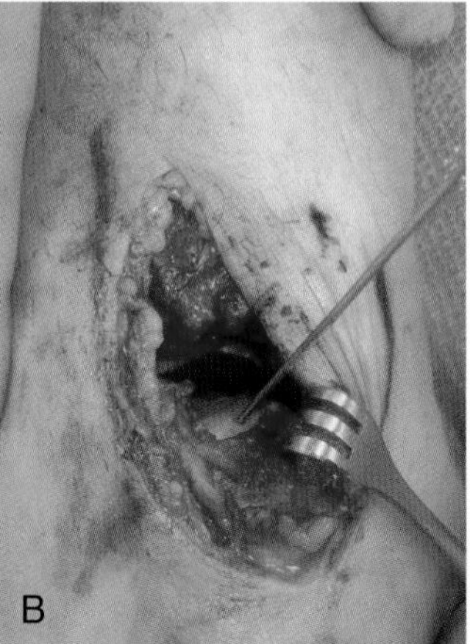

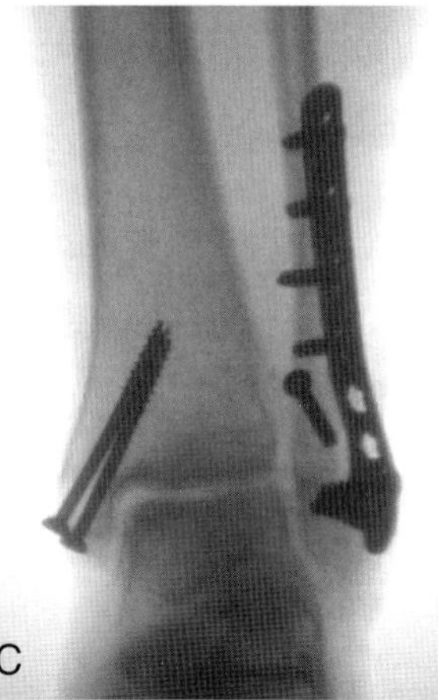

FIGURE 118-3 **A,** An acute osteochondral lesion of the talus associated with an ankle fracture. **B,** Kirschner wire was used to predrill for placement of an absorbable pin. **C,** Completed fixation.

osteochondral graft, stem cell–mediated implants, and scaffolds. These procedures generally are contraindicated in bipolar (kissing) lesions that involve both the tibia and the talus, as well as in patients with advanced generalized arthritis.[29,30]

Osteochondral autografting procedures such as OATS and mosaicplasty require the harvest of grafts from a donor site, such as the lateral supracondylar ridge or intercondylar notch of the femur, for insertion into the OLT. These techniques generally are used for moderate to large grade III or IV lesions. Concerns about donor site morbidity have prompted graft harvest from sites other than the distal femur, including the anterior talar dome, and the use of allografts.

Fresh-frozen allografts (the mega-OATS procedure) have been used for large osteochondral lesions in the knee but less commonly in the talus. Gross and colleagues[31] listed as their indication for this procedure a lesion at least 1 cm in diameter and 5 mm deep that could not be internally fixed. Chondrocyte viability is a primary concern, and it is essential that the graft be harvested within 24 hours of the donor's death and be stored at 4°C. One study found a minimal decrease in viability after 14 days of storage in a serum-free modified culture medium, but after 28 days, viability was significantly decreased.[32] Because most tissue banks require a 21-day screening process to minimize the risk of disease transmission and the grafts are not released for 3 days after screening is complete, the minimal time to implantation is 24 days. Other considerations, such as scheduling, can delay implantation even longer. Fortunately, the biomechanical properties of these allografts do not appear to deteriorate even after 28 days from procurement. Recent studies have suggested that, compared with current protocols, storage of osteochondral allografts at higher temperatures (25°C and 37°C) can increase the window of opportunity for implantation of optimal tissue from 14 to 42 days after disease-testing clearance.[33-35] A benefit of using an ipsilateral talar allograft is the ability to harvest from a similar area as the defect and thus have a closely matched graft.

Autologous Chondrocyte Implantation or Transplantation

ACI involves harvesting 200 to 300 mg of autologous chondrocytes from the distal femur, growing the cells in vitro for 2 to 5 weeks, and then implanting them into the defect. An autologous periosteal flap is harvested and sewn over the implanted cells and sealed with fibrin glue. A "sandwich" procedure has been described for lesions with concomitant bone loss.[36] The bony defect is grafted and covered with a periosteal patch with its cambium side facing the cartilage. A second periosteal patch with its cambium side facing the bone is sewn over the first patch to create a space for the cells. ACI is best suited for large and well-contained stage III or IV defects, large lesions with extensive subchondral cystic changes, and lesions in which previous operative treatment has failed. According to Ferkel and Hommen,[29] the ideal patient for ACI is between 15 and 55 years old and has no malalignment, degenerative joint disease, or instability of the joint. Because of concerns about donor-site morbidity after harvest from the distal femur,[37,38] other donor sites have been suggested. Giannini and associates[39] used detached osteochondral fragments as a source of cells.

Postoperative Management/Return to Play

After arthroscopic excision, curettage, and drilling, the patient is non–weight bearing in a boot for 4 weeks and then progresses to weight bearing in the boot during physical therapy. Active motion is begun at 12 days after surgery. After internal fixation or OATS, the patient is non–weight bearing in a cast for 8 weeks and then progresses to weight bearing in a boot for 4 weeks during physical therapy. A brace is then worn during a gradual return to activities as dictated by symptoms.

An athlete may return to play when he or she (1) has minimal or no symptoms and minimal swelling and (2) is participating in physical therapy without wearing the boot. After internal fixation, OATS, or cartilage replacement, a brace must be worn while participating in sports for 6 months after the procedure.

Results

Most of the literature about OLT consists of case series (level IV evidence) or case reports (level V evidence). For some of the newer techniques, numbers are too small and follow-up is too short to make definitive recommendations.

Text continued on p. 1437

AUTHORS' PREFERRED TECHNIQUE

Osteochondral Lesions of the Talus

For a stage I or II OLT, non–weight bearing in a cast or boot is first tried for 6 to 10 weeks, depending on the size of the lesion. If this strategy fails to relieve symptoms, arthroscopic excision, curettage, and microfracture or drilling is performed as follows:

- View anterolateral lesions through an anteromedial portal, with instrumentation for drilling, excision, or pinning inserted through an anterolateral portal, changing portals as necessary for optimal viewing and fixation.
- Posteromedial lesions can be more difficult to view and treat. With noninvasive distraction and use of a small, 2.7-mm scope in the anterolateral portal, most posteromedial lesions can be treated through anteromedial and posterolateral portals.
- Use a small, curved curette or curved microfracture awl to make perforations in the subchondral bone.
- If needed, make a small bony trough on the anteromedial tibia to improve access to posterior lesions.
- If the lesion still is not accessible, use a guide to place a Kirschner wire through the medial malleolus for drilling of the lesion (Fig. 118-4).
- A malleolar osteotomy may be required for pinning of larger lesions.
- Other helpful instruments are an open-end curette, a small 2.7-mm full-radius resector, and a small 2.7-mm burr.
- For lesions with intact overlying cartilage, use a retrograde drilling technique. This technique can be used for lesions of both the talus and the tibial plafond.
- Identify the lesion arthroscopically and with the use of fluoroscopy.
- Through a separate portal, insert a targeting drill guide similar to those used in ACL reconstructions but smaller and made specifically for ankle arthroscopy and direct it at the lesion. This procedure allows precise placement of the guide wire up to, but not through, the intact cartilage of the lesion.
- Place a drill over the guide wire with the use of fluoroscopy and pass it through the sclerotic zone, using a "loss-of-resistance" technique. Take care not to perforate the chondral surface.
- If the lesion is associated with a cyst, use a bone graft to fill the void (Fig. 118-5).

In a skeletally immature patient with a stage III OLT, a trial of conservative treatment is warranted before surgical treatment. For stage III or IV OLTs in skeletally mature patients, arthroscopic microfracture or drilling is the first choice, and good results have been obtained in about 90% of our patients (Fig. 118-6). The use of a noninvasive ankle distractor will help with visualization of posterior lesions. If this option fails to relieve symptoms, an osteochondral autograft (for lesions <1.5 cm^2; Table 118-1) or allograft (for lesions >1.5 cm^2) is used, as follows[40-43]:

- With the patient in a state of general anesthesia, prepare the affected lower extremity from the ankle to the knee. Examine the ankle arthroscopically to further delineate the chondral lesion.

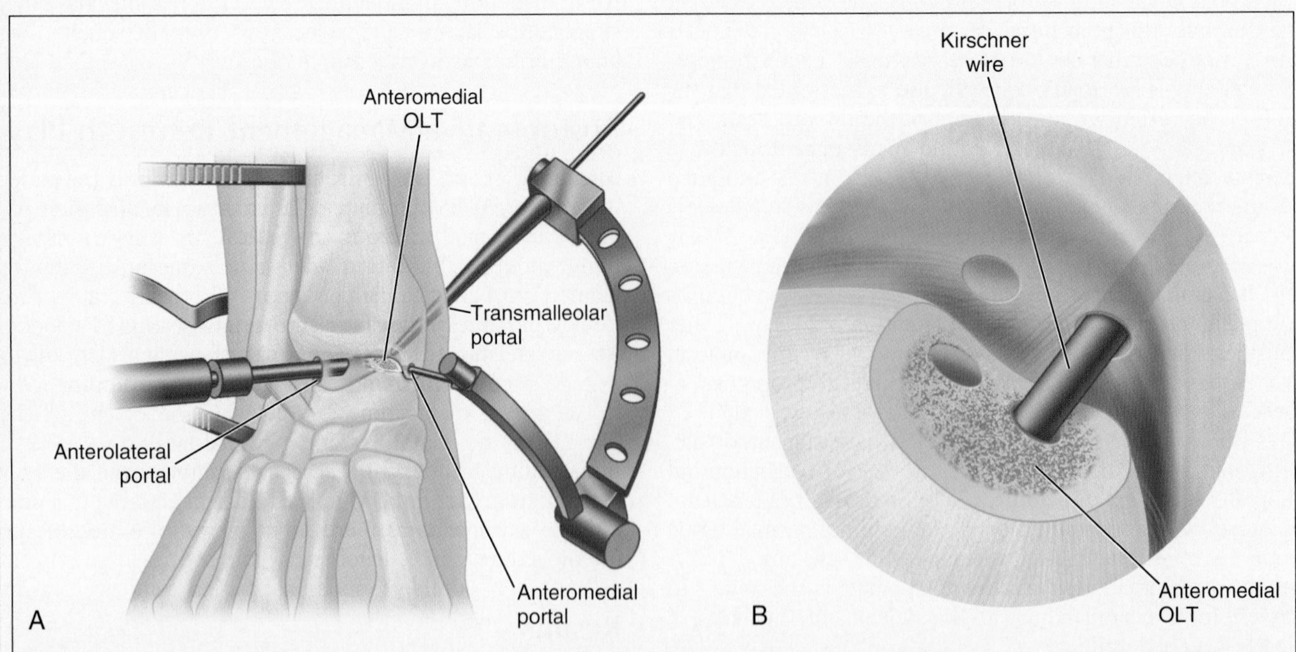

FIGURE 118-4 **A,** Transmalleolar drilling of an osteochondral lesion of the talus (*OLT*) using a guide. The scope is in the anterolateral portal, and inflow is through the posterolateral portal. **B,** Holes are drilled through the medial malleolus into the talus down to areas of bleeding bone. *(From Ferkel RD: Arthroscopy of the ankle and foot. In Mann RA, Coughlin MJ, editors:* Surgery of the foot and ankle, *ed 8, Philadelphia, 2006, Elsevier.)*

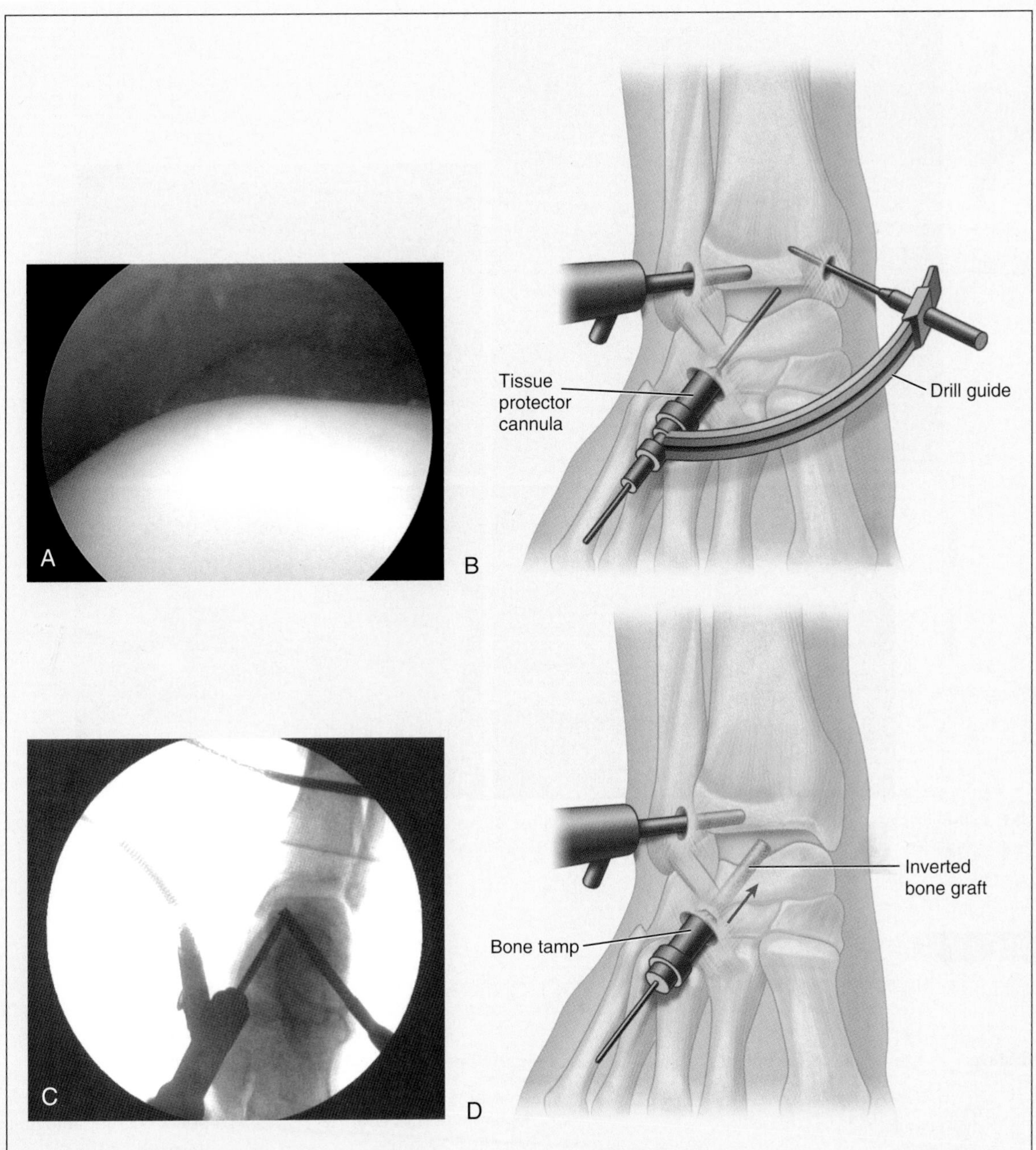

FIGURE 118-5 Retrograde drilling of an osteochondral lesion. **A,** Intact articular cartilage is confirmed arthroscopically. **B,** A guide pin is placed through the sinus tarsi with use of modified ligament guide. **C,** A subchondral lesion is drilled in a retrograde fashion. **D,** A graft is placed into the channel and gently compressed into position with a tamp and mallet. *(**B** and **D** from Richardson DR: Sports injuries of the foot and ankle. In Canale ST, Beaty JH, editors:* Campbell's operative orthopaedics, *ed 12, Philadelphia, 2013, Elsevier.)*

- Harvesters are made for lesions 5 to 11 mm (larger sizes also are available).
- The approach for osteochondral grafting is determined by the size and location of the lesion. Lesions in the anterior third of the talus may be reached through a standard anterior approach with a plafondplasty and maximal plantar flexion of the ankle. An anterior approach avoids osteotomy of the medial malleolus or fibula; however, an approach through a malleolar osteotomy allows more direct access to central and posterior lesions.[40]
- Approach lateral lesions through an anterolateral incision and perform a medial malleolar osteotomy for medial lesions. Rarely, a lateral malleolar osteotomy will be needed to access posterolateral lesions.
- Use a commercially available recipient sizer and harvester to create a recipient hole for the donor osteochondral

Continued

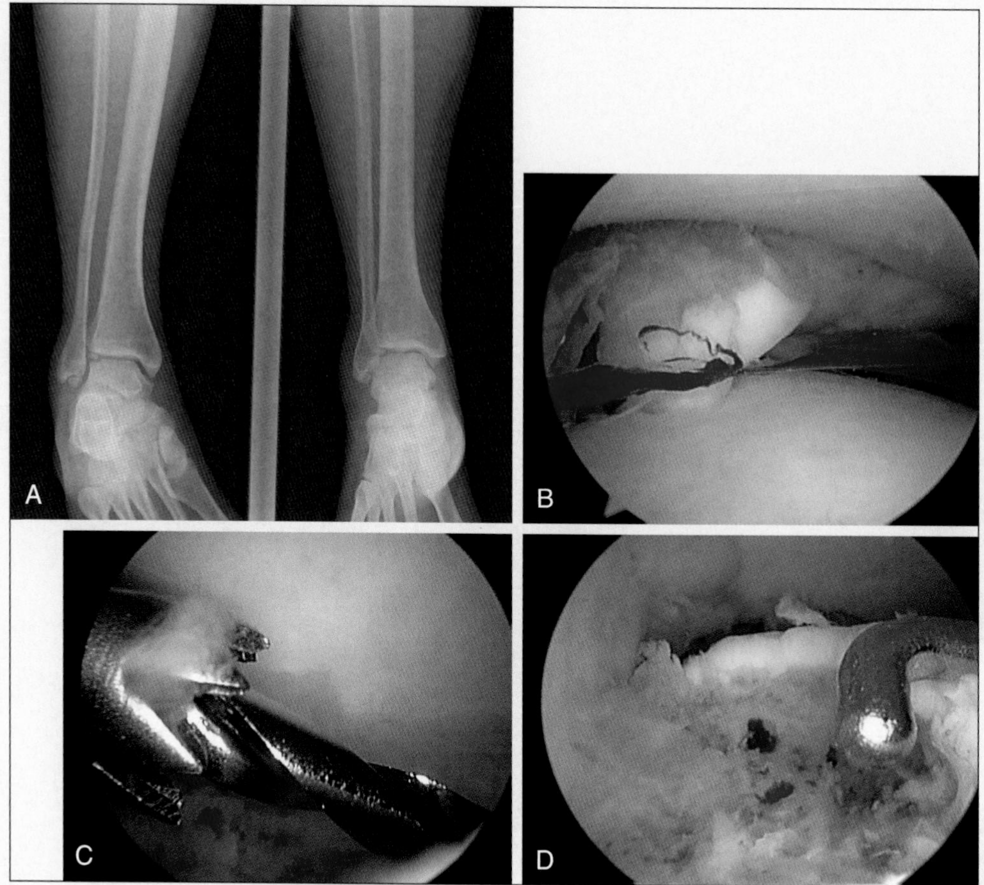

FIGURE 118-6 **A,** A stage IV osteochondral lesion of the talus. **B,** An arthroscopic view of a displaced osteochondral fragment. **C,** Arthroscopic excision and drilling. **D,** Note vascular channels created in the defect.

TABLE 118-1

AUTHORS' PREFERRED TREATMENT OF OSTEOCHONDRAL LESIONS OF THE TALUS

MRI Stage	Conservative Treatment	Primary Operative Treatment	After a Failed Primary Procedure
I or II	Cast or boot: non–weight bearing for 6-10 weeks	Arthroscopic excision, curettage, depending on size; ankle brace for 3 months	Damaged surface <1.5 cm^2, osteochondral autograft transport; >1.5 cm^2, osteochondral allograft microfracture/drilling
III	Cast or boot: Acute injury (<10 weeks) skeletally immature: non–weight bearing for 6-10 weeks Skeletally mature or chronic injury: proceed to operative treatment	Minimally damaged surface: arthroscopic transtalar drilling Damaged surface: microfracture/drilling	As above
IV	No role for conservative treatment	Minimally damaged surface: If <1 cm^2, arthroscopic transtalar drilling; if >1 cm^2, internal fixation Damaged surface: microfracture or drilling	As above
V	Cast or boot: weight bearing as tolerated for 6-10 weeks; ankle brace for 6 months	Cyst <1.5 cm: as above + bone graft Cyst >1.5 cm: bulk allograft	Minimally damaged surface: arthroscopic transtalar drilling + bone graft Damaged surface: microfracture or drilling

plug. Extract the plug to a depth of 10 mm (Fig. 118-7, *A* and *B*). Place the harvester perpendicular for dome lesions (Fig. 118-7, *C*) and at 45 degrees for talar shoulder lesions.

- Drill multiple holes into the subchondral bone of the recipient hole (Fig. 118-7, *D*).
- Obtain a graft from the ipsilateral knee, arthroscopically from the medial femoral condyle, or from the lateral femoral condyle through a small incision (Fig. 118-7, *E* and *F*). For talar shoulder lesions, obtain a graft from the lateral trochlea.
- Use the specially designed donor harvester to obtain osteochondral grafts that measure 5 to 11 mm in diameter and

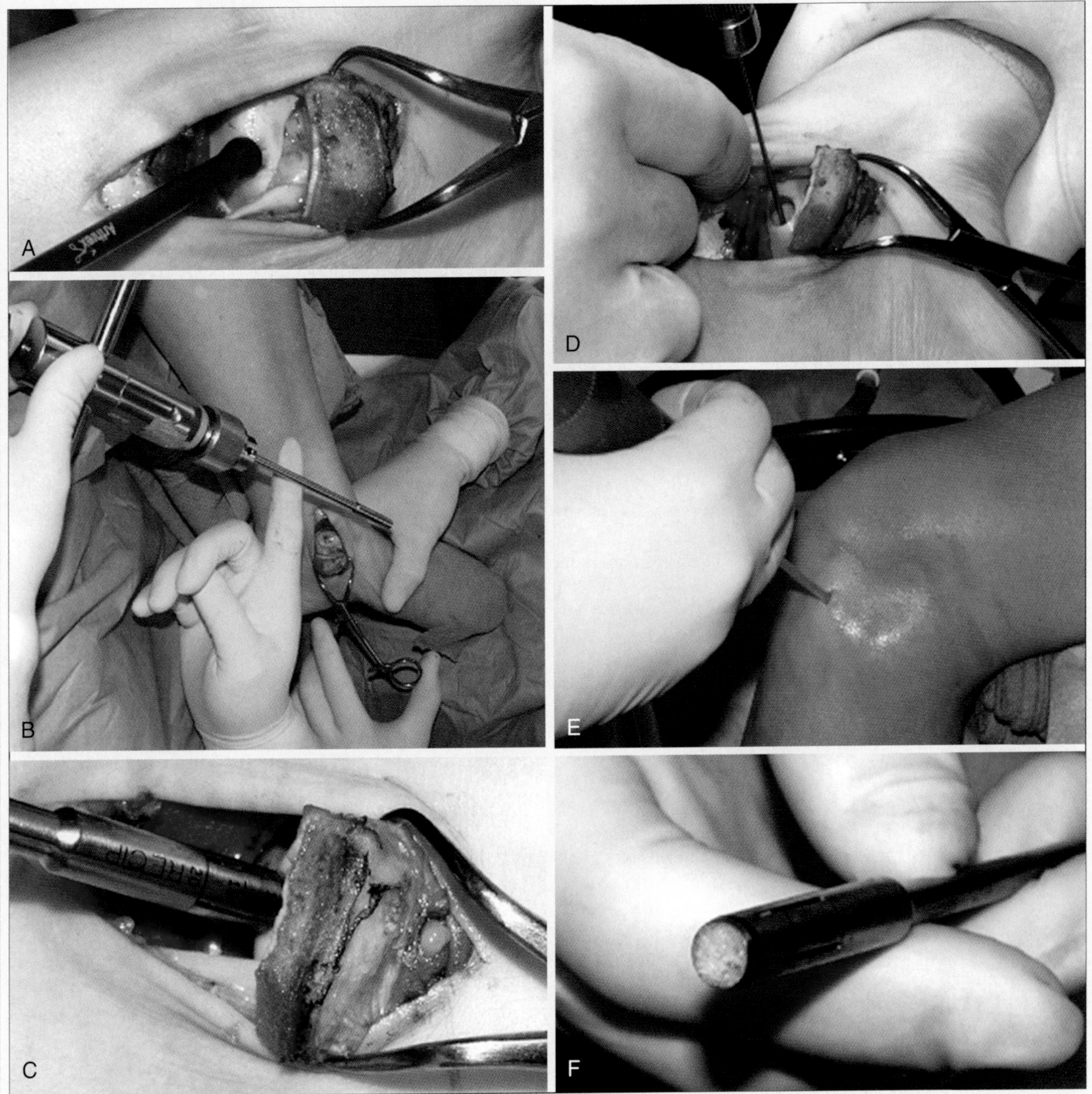

FIGURE 118-7 Osteochondral autograft and allograft transplantation. **A,** A trial sizer for the harvester. **B,** The recipient harvester. **C,** A plug 10 to 12 mm deep is removed from the recipient site. **D,** Multiple holes are drilled at the base of the lesion. **E,** An autograft is obtained from the femoral condyle with a donor harvester (for talar shoulder lesions, a graft is obtained from the corner of the trochlea). **F,** Donor graft in the harvester.

Continued

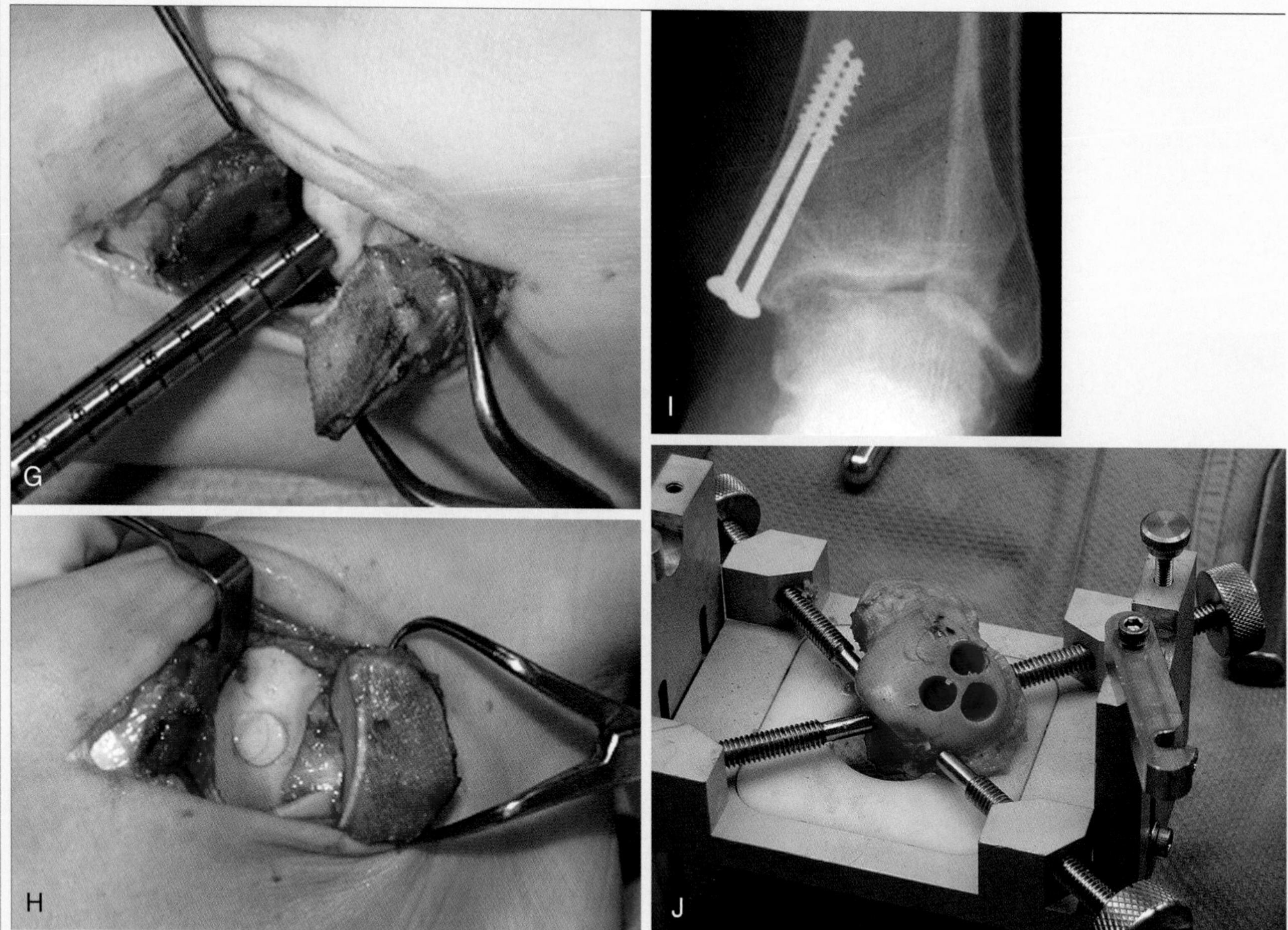

FIGURE 118-7, cont'd G and **H,** The graft is placed in the recipient hole. **I,** The malleolar osteotomy is secured with two partially threaded cancellous screws (holes are predrilled before the osteotomy). **J,** For large defects, allografts can be taken from the donor talus. *(From Richardson DR: Ankle injuries. In Canale ST, Beaty JH, editors:* Campbell's operative orthopaedics, *ed 12, Philadelphia, 2008, Elsevier.)*

10 to 12 mm in depth (slightly deeper than the recipient hole).

- Insert the cylindrical grafts carefully into the recipient hole using the designed extruder or collared pin through the donor harvester (Fig. 118-7, *G* and *H*).
- Do not remove the osteochondral autograft transfer harvester before completion of full graft extrusion, and do not allow the harvester to deviate from the insertion angle; either maneuver may cause fracture of the donor core.
- Use the sizer-tamp to gently tamp the core flush with the surrounding cartilage. Flush graft placement is important to restore near-normal joint contact pressure. An elevated graft significantly increases contact pressure at the graft site, and a recessed graft transfers excess pressure from the graft to the native cartilage rim.[41]
- Test range of motion of the ankle to ensure that the graft is well seated and secured.
- Close the incision and secure the osteotomy in the usual fashion (Fig. 118-7, *I*). Place one drain in the knee and apply a compressive dressing to the ankle. Apply a posterior splint with strips.
- For very large lesions (more than 3 cm^3), allografts can be harvested from an ipsilateral donor talus (Fig. 118-7, *J*). After direct access is obtained, resect, measure, and template the defect to allow a matched resection from the talar allograft. Graft any remaining cystic lesions with cancellous bone chips before allograft placement. Insert the allograft into the resected area to recreate the native morphology. Fixation of the allograft with screws[42] or bioabsorbable pins[43] is required for these bulk osteochondral allografts.

Shearer and colleagues[20] reviewed the results of nonsurgical management of 35 OLTs and concluded that nonsurgical management of chronic cystic (stage 5) OLT is a viable option with little or no risk for the development of osteoarthritis. Their clinical results were good or excellent in 54%, fair in 17%, and poor in 29%. A systematic review of 14 studies with a total of 201 patients showed only a 45% success rate of nonsurgical treatment of grades I and II and medial grade III OLTs, and nonoperative treatment of chronic lesions had a success rate of 56%.[16] The highest success rate was obtained with excision, curettage, and drilling (85%), followed by excision and curettage (78%) and curettage alone (38%). Shelton and Pedowitz[44] reported just 25% satisfactory results after nonoperative treatment of grade II and III lesions.

Gobbi and coworkers,[45] in a randomized trial comparing chondroplasty, microfracture, and OATS in 33 patients, found no significant differences in clinical results among the three methods. However, each treatment group contained a small number of patients, and three different surgeons were involved in the surgeries.

Noninvasive follow-up after cartilage repair techniques such as ACI or microfracture has become more common. To avoid the use of ambiguous terms, postoperative cartilage changes have been described in the literature with use of the magnetic resonance observation of cartilage repair tissue (MOCART) scoring system.[46] This scoring system describes the hyaline and fibrocartilage structure, degree of defect filling, and native border integration, as well as characteristics of the subchondral lamina and bone.

Authors of individual studies of various treatment methods have reported good results.

Lavage, Debridement, and Excision

In a systematic review by Verhagen and coworkers,[16] excision alone had an overall success rate of 38%, with a range of 30% to 100% in individual studies. Excision and curettage had a success rate of 76% (range, 53% to 100%). Arthroscopic procedures had a higher success rate (84%) than did open procedures (63%). Savva and associates[47] described repeat arthroscopic debridement in 12 of 215 patients who had arthroscopic treatment of OLT; at an average 6-year follow-up, results were good in all 12 patients, and eight had returned to their preinjury levels of sports.

Curettage and Drilling or Microfracture and Bone Grafting

Good to excellent results after drilling have been reported in 28% to 93% of patients. Ferkel and colleagues[29] reported 72% excellent or good results in 64 patients, Taranow and coworkers[48] reported an 81% success rate in 16 patients with retrograde drilling, and Becher and Thermann[49] reported 83% excellent and good results and 17% satisfactory results in 30 patients at an average follow-up of 2 years after microfracture. A recent prospective, randomized, level I study suggested that improved pain and function scores were obtained if the microfracture was supplemented with a postoperative hyaluronan injection.[50] To determine whether the presence of a subchondral cyst affected the results of arthroscopic microfracture or abrasion arthroplasty, Han and colleagues[51] compared the results in 20 defects that included cysts with those in 18 defects that did not include cysts and found no differences in the clinical results. They concluded that small cystic lesions can be successfully treated by arthroscopic microfracture or abrasion arthroplasty.

Lesion size may play a role in microfracture outcomes. Lesions larger than 150 mm, as calculated on MRI, have been reported to have a statistically significant increased risk of clinical failure (80% failure rate vs. 10.5% failure of lesions smaller than 150 mm).[52]

Autogenous Cancellous Bone Grafting

Saxena and Eakin[53] compared the results of microfracture procedures in 26 patients with the results after bone grafting in 20 patients. Overall, 96% of patients had excellent or good results, and no difference was found between the groups with regard to the percentages of those who returned to sports. However, bone grafting required a longer time to return to activity than did microfracture in patients participating in high-demand sports, but the two groups had similar postoperative American Orthopaedic Foot and Ankle Society (AOFAS) scores. Regardless of treatment type, patients with anterolateral lesions had the fastest return to activity and the highest AOFAS scores. Draper and Fallat[54] compared the results of 14 patients treated with bone grafting with those of 17 patients treated with curettage and drilling. At almost 5-year follow-up, patients who underwent bone grafting had better range of motion and less pain. However, Kolker and colleagues[55] reported that 6 of 13 patients required further surgery after open antegrade autologous bone grafting and concluded that autologous bone grafting alone should not be used as primary treatment for patients with symptomatic advanced OLT and deficient or absent overlying cartilage.

Few studies have been performed on retrograde drilling of OLTs. Techniques vary widely from fluoroscopy-controlled to computer-guided systems with fixed bony referencing. Gras et al.[56] showed an 86% decrease in surgical time using a Fluoro-Free navigation procedure. Anders et al.[57] demonstrated increased AOFAS and decreased VAS scores after retrograde drilling with a mean follow-up of 29 months; however, disrupted surface integrity resulted in poorer outcomes.

Osteochondral Autografts (Osteochondral Autologous Transfer System, Mosaicplasty)

Scranton and associates[58] reported 90% good to excellent results in 50 patients with type V OLT at an average 3-year follow-up after osteochondral autograft transplantation using a single, arthroscopically harvested graft from the distal femur. Thirty-two of their 50 patients (64%) had at least one previous operation that failed to relieve symptoms. Hangody and colleagues[59] described good to excellent results in 34 of 36 patients 2 to 7 years after mosaicplasty. Kreuz and coworkers[60] used mosaicplasty procedures for the treatment of 35 OLTs after failure of arthroscopic excision, curettage, and drilling. The osteochondral graft was harvested from the ipsilateral talar facet, and a malleolar or tibial wedge osteotomy was used to access central or posterior lesions. Although no nonunions of the osteotomies occurred, patients with small osteochondral lesions accessible through an anterior approach without additional osteotomy had the best results. Improved results also have been correlated with normal integration or minor incongruity of the transplant on follow-up MRI.[61]

Osteochondral Allografts

Although several studies have reported good results with osteochondral allografts in the knee, the literature includes few reports of its use in the ankle. Gross and associates[31] reported that six of nine allografts remained in situ with a mean survival rate of 11 years; three patients required arthrodesis because of graft resorption and fragmentation. Kim and colleagues[62] used tibiotalar osteochondral shell autografts in seven patients; at 10-year average follow-up, only four had excellent or good results. Complications included graft fragmentation, poor graft fit, graft subluxation, and nonunion.

Lesions on the talar shoulder have their own unique problems because of cartilage geometry and loss of articular buttress. Allografts may be considered in these situations when traditional treatment options would be difficult. Adams et al.[63] reported on eight patients who, at 4-year follow-up, had decreased pain and increased function after undergoing an osteochondral allograft. Half required an additional procedure, but none required arthrodesis or arthroplasty even though five had radiographic lucencies at the graft-host interface. Raikin[42] reported good or excellent results in 11 of 15 patients treated with allografts for large-volume cysts (a mean of 6059 mm) in the talar dome.

Autogenous Chondrocyte Implantation or Transplantation

Koulalis and colleagues[64] reported excellent to good results at 17 months' follow-up in all eight of their patients treated with ACI, and Whittaker and associates[65] described ACI in 10 patients, 9 of whom were "pleased" or "extremely pleased" with their results at 4-year follow-up; however, 1 year after surgery, Lysholm knee scores had returned to preoperative levels in only three patients, suggesting donor-site morbidity in the other seven patients. Baums and coworkers[30] reported 12 patients with ACI of the talus for defects that averaged 2.3 cm^2. At about 5-year follow-up, seven had excellent results, four had good results, and one had a satisfactory result. The AOFAS mean score improved from 43.5 before surgery to 85.5 after surgery. Patients who had been involved in competitive sports were able to return to their full activity levels. A recent large retrospective case series, however, suggests that patients tend to modify their return to play by decreasing their participation in contact and high-impact sports.[66]

A metaanalysis of 16 studies reporting the use of ACI for OLTs led to inconclusive results. All studies were level IV case studies and failed to show a superiority or inferiority of ACI compared with microfracture or other surgical techniques.[67]

Complications

The treatment of OLTs can have the same complications as any surgery: bleeding, infection, damage to anatomic structures, the need for further surgery, and the risk of continued pain or dysfunction. OLTs, however, have their own inherent risks, which depend on the procedure performed. For example, although it occurs rarely, the use of an allograft has the risk of disease transmission or immune response, and graft resorption or nonincorporation is always possible. The specific risks and benefits of each procedure must be discussed with the patient before any course is taken.

Future Considerations

New orthobiologic techniques are being developed to aid the body in healing itself. After reports of its successful use in other parts of the body, PRP is one orthobiologic technique that has been used for OLT treatment. In a recent level II study, Mei-Dan et al.[68] showed short-term pain reduction (6 months) and increased function after PRP injection into the ankle for nonoperative treatment of OLTs. The exact indications for the use of PRP, as well as its many different proprietary concentrations and configurations, have not yet been well established. Chondrogenesis[69] and marrow-derived cell transplant[70,71] currently are in the experimental stage of development, but they are promising new techniques that may drastically change the treatment of OLTs.

The evolution of novel surgical techniques, such as computer-assisted retrograde drilling,[72,73] and the advent of new biomaterials and orthobiologic techniques will further advance the treatment of OLTs.

Osteochondral Lesions of the Distal Tibial Plafond

Osteochondral lesions of the distal tibial plafond are much less common than those of the talus, and the literature includes little information about their cause, natural history, or treatment. It appears that they, like talar lesions, are primarily caused by trauma. Unlike OLTs, however, no preference to location is expressed within the articular surface of the plafond.[74] "Mirror image" or "kissing" lesions of the talus and distal tibia also have been described.[75] In one of the largest series of osteochondral lesions of the distal tibia,[76] 11 of 17 patients recalled an inversion injury to the ankle. Symptoms may include pain, stiffness, swelling, locking, and instability. Radiographs usually are not helpful, but MRI and CT can identify the lesion (Fig. 118-8). Treatment is similar to that of osteochondral lesions of the talus: debridement and curettage of the lesion, abrasion of the defect to subchondral bone, and drilling or microfracture of the subchondral bone. Mologne and Ferkel[76] reported excellent or good results in 14 of 17 patients an average of 44 months after debridement, curettage, abrasion, and drilling or microfracture. If this approach is unsuccessful, a retrograde osteochondral autograft or allograft transfer procedure can be performed[77,78]; instrumentation has been developed to make this process easier.

Osteochondrosis of the Metatarsal Head (Freiberg Disease)

History

First described by Freiberg[79] in 1914, osteochondrosis or osteonecrosis of the metatarsal head is most common in adolescent athletes who perform on their toes in either sprinting or jumping activities. It is more common in girls than in boys, making it the only osteochondrosis with a female predilection.

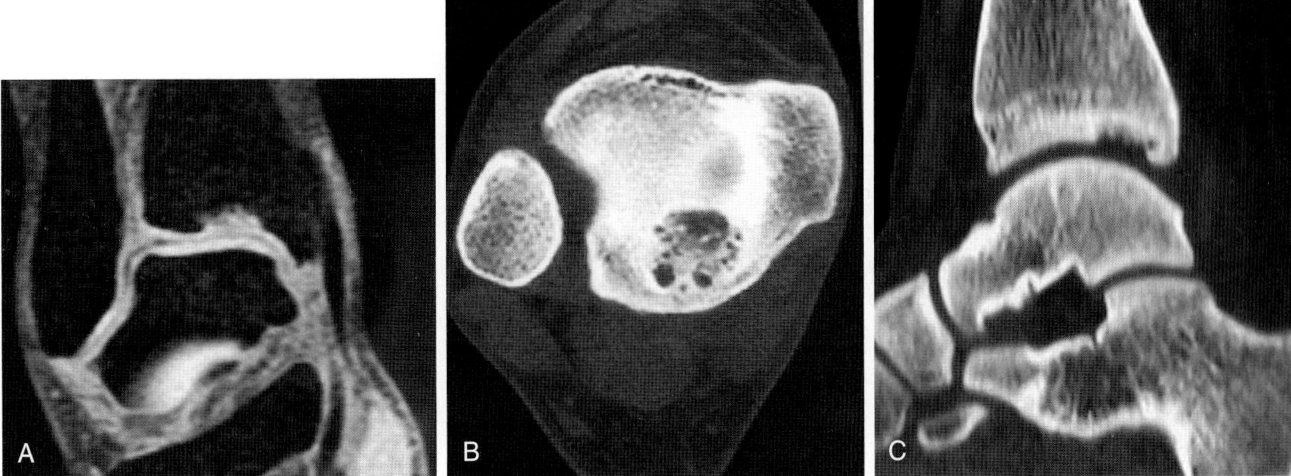

FIGURE 118-8 An osteochondral lesion of the distal tibia in a female collegiate basketball player. **A,** Coronal fat-suppressed magnetic resonance imaging. **B,** Axial computed tomography (CT) shows a posterior-central lesion and small subchondral cysts. **C,** A sagittal CT scan shows the depth of the defect. *(From Mologne TS, Ferkel RD: Arthroscopic treatment of osteochondral lesions of the distal tibia.* Foot Ankle Int *28:865–872, 2007.)*

The second metatarsal head, followed by the third metatarsal head, are most commonly involved. Fewer than 10% of patients have bilateral involvement. The pathogenesis is unknown, but Gauthier and Elbaz[80] found that patients with longer second metatarsals and excessive plantar pressure under the second metatarsal head had no significantly higher risk. These findings would appear to call into question mechanical stress as the sole or even the primary cause of Freiberg disease. The cause is likely multifactoral.[81]

Physical Examination

The initial presentation often is a vague forefoot pain that worsens with activity and weight bearing and is relieved with rest. The pain usually is worse at extremes of motion, with pain under and around the involved metatarsophalangeal joint. Palpation may identify swelling and a slightly increased temperature.

Imaging

The initial process of pain and synovitis is followed by radiographic findings of sclerosis, resorption of the subchondral plate, fracture, collapse, and fragmentation. Secondary degenerative changes and remodeling then occur in the flattened metatarsal head (Fig. 118-9).

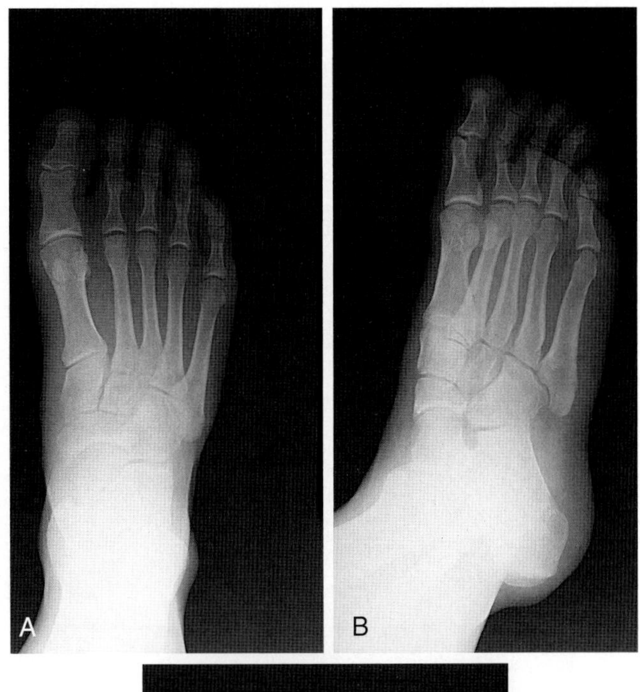

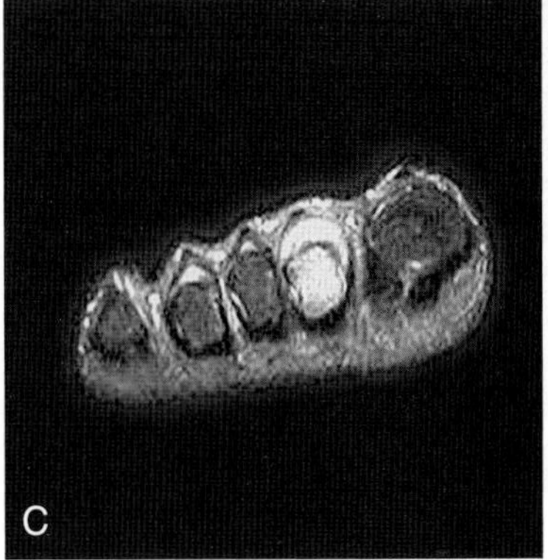

FIGURE 118-9 A Freiberg infarction. **A** and **B,** Note flattening of the second metatarsal head. **C,** Note marrow edema of the second metatarsal.

Treatment Options

Initial treatment is nonoperative, including metatarsal relief pads, restriction of running and jumping activities, and occasionally a short-leg walking cast worn for 6 to 12 weeks until acute symptoms are resolved. A number of operative procedures have been described for persistent symptoms, including debridement, synovectomy, drilling, osteotomy, interpositional arthroplasty, and joint replacement. Dorsal wedge or dorsiflexion osteotomy has been used successfully for all stages of the disease,[80,82-85] although the range of motion of the MTP joint is decreased. More recent innovations include the use of absorbable pins for fixation of the osteotomy, which obviates the need for a second operation for implant removal; arthroscopic techniques for synovectomy and drilling[86,87]; and osteochondral plug transplantation.[86,88,89] We have had good results with joint debridement and metatarsal head remodeling, as described by Freiberg and Mann, and use it most often.

Decision-Making Principles

Carro and coworkers[88] recommended an age-based approach to the treatment of Freiberg disease, beginning with arthroscopic synovectomy and debridement, followed by open or arthroscopic osteochondral transplantation in late adolescence and adulthood and an arthroscopic Keller procedure (with or without interpositional arthroplasty) for more severe involvement in late adulthood. However, in our experience, resection of the base of the proximal phalanx or the metatarsal head should be avoided to avoid transfer metatarsalgia or hallux valgus caused by instability of the second digit.

AUTHORS' PREFERRED TECHNIQUE

Osteochondrosis of the Metatarsal Head

Initial treatment is nonoperative, including restriction of sports activities and short-term cast-with-toe-plate immobilization. After acute symptoms resolve, metatarsal pads inserted proximal to the metatarsophalangeal (MTP) joint are used during running and sports. Operative treatment is indicated for persistent symptoms. For adolescents and young adults, joint debridement and removal of loose bodies usually are sufficient, and return to sports generally is possible in 6 to 8 weeks. More extensive surgery (e.g., dorsiflexion or a metatarsal-shortening osteotomy) is reserved for older patients with late-stage involvement.

Intraarticular Dorsiflexion Osteotomy

- Through a dorsal incision centered over the MTP joint, retract the extensor tendons and incise the capsule.
- Remove loose fragments from the MTP joint, taking care to preserve the soft tissue attachments to the capital fragment.
- Use a microsagittal saw to create a 5-mm intraarticular dorsally based closing wedge osteotomy, usually involving most of the arthritic portion of the metatarsal head.
- Place the apex of the osteotomy as proximal as possible to avoid shortening the metatarsal.
- Rotate the metatarsal head dorsally so that normal cartilage is articulating with the base of the proximal phalanx (Fig. 118-10).
- Fix the metatarsal head with a counter-sunk small compression screw or absorbable pin.

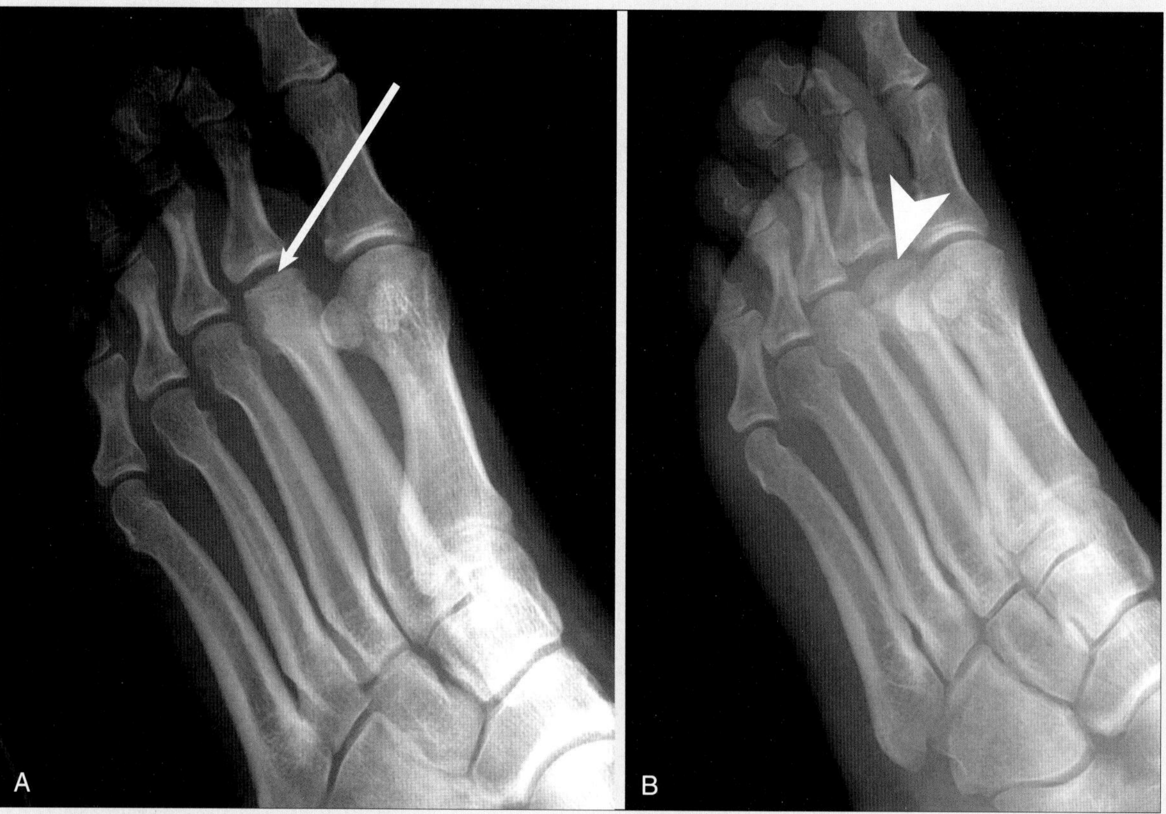

FIGURE 118-10 Oblique radiographs of a patient with Freiberg disease (**A**) with the characteristic flattening of the metatarsal head (*arrow*) treated with a dorsal closing wedge osteotomy (**B**). Note how the contour of the metatarsal head has been recreated (*arrowhead*). *(From Joos D, Sabb B, Kadakia AR: Osteochondral lesions. In Miller M, Sanders T, editors:* Presentation, imaging and treatment of common musculoskeletal conditions, *Philadelphia, 2011, Elsevier.)*

Postoperative Management

A light compressive dressing is applied, and the foot is immobilized in a short-leg walking cast for 4 weeks. After removal of the cast (and pin removal if pins are used), weight bearing as tolerated is allowed, but running and strenuous physical activity (sports) are not allowed for 4 more weeks.

Results

Gauthier and Elbaz[80] reported persistent symptoms in only 1 of 53 patients treated with dorsiflexion osteotomy. All 15 patients described by Kinnard and Lirette[83] had complete pain relief, and Capar et al.[90] reported good-to-excellent results in 16 of 19 patients (84%).

Complications

Reported complications of dorsiflexion osteotomy include osteonecrosis of the metatarsal head, transfer metatarsalgia, metatarsal shortening, nonunion of the osteotomy, loss of motion, and the development of arthritis.

For a complete list of references, go to expertconsult.com.

Suggested Readings

Citation: Baums MH, Heidrich G, Schultz W, et al: Autologous chondrocyte transplantation for treating cartilage defects of the talus. *J Bone Joint Surg Am* 88A:303–308, 2006.

Level of Evidence: IV

Summary: In 12 patients with deep focal lesions (average, 2.3 cm^2), seven had excellent results, four had good results, and one had a poor result at an average of 63 months after autologous chondrocyte transplantation. The mean American Orthopaedic Foot and Ankle Society score improved 45 points, and all patients involved in competitive sports were able to result to full activity levels.

Citation: Gobbi A, Francisco RA, Lubowitz JH, et al: Osteochondral lesions of the talus: Randomized controlled trial comparing chondroplasty, microfracture, and osteochondral autograft transplantation. *Arthroscopy* 22:1085–1092, 2006.

Level of Evidence: I

Summary: No differences were found in American Orthopaedic Foot and Ankle Society scores or subjective ratings among patients treated with chondroplasty (11), microfracture (10), or osteochondral autologous transfer (OAT) (12) at 12 and 24 months after surgery. At 24 hours after surgery, pain intensity was significantly higher in persons who had undergone OAT procedures.

Citation: Hassan AH: Treatment of anterolateral impingements of the ankle joint by arthroscopy. *Knee Surg Sports Traumatol Arthrosc* 15:1150–1154, 2007.

Level of Evidence: IV

Summary: Of 23 patients treated with arthroscopic debridement for ankle impingement after an ankle sprain, 21 had excellent or good results and 1 had a fair result at an average 2-year follow-up.

Citation: Kreuz PC, Steinwachs M, Erggelet C, et al: Mosaicplasty with autogenous talar autograft for osteochondral lesions of the talus after failed primary arthroscopic management: A prospective study with a 4-year follow-up. *Am J Sports Med* 34:55–63, 2006.

Level of Evidence: IV

Summary: American Orthopaedic Foot and Ankle Society scores improved by an average of 35.5 points in 35 patients treated with mosaicplasty after failed arthroscopic treatment. Subjective ratings were excellent in 17 patients, good in 15 patients, and fair in 3 patients.

Citation: McGahan PJ, Pinney SJ: Current concepts review: Osteochondral lesions of the talus. *Foot Ankle Int* 31: 90–101, 2010.

Level of Evidence: V

Summary: The authors provide an extensive review of the cause, diagnosis, and treatment of osteochondral lesions of the talus, with an emphasis on the outcomes of operative treatment.

Citation: Perumal V, Wall E, Babekir N: Juvenile osteochondritis of the talus. *J Pediatr Orthop* 27:821–825, 2007.

Level of Evidence: IV

Summary: After 6 months of nonoperative treatment of juvenile osteochondritis dissecans of the talus in 31 skeletally immature patients (mean age 12 years), 77% had persistent lesions as seen on radiographs; 42% of these patients required surgery for unhealed lesions and pain, even after an additional 6 months of nonoperative treatment. Despite persistent lesions viewed on radiographs, 46% had no symptoms.

Citation: Verhagen RA, Struijs PA, Bossuyt PM, et al: Systematic review of treatment strategies for osteochondral defects of the talar dome. *Foot Ankle Clin* 8:233–242, 2003.

Level of Evidence: III

Summary: The authors of this systematic review of the literature found that the average success rate was highest with excision, curettage, and drilling (86%), followed by excision and curettage (78%), and excision alone (38%).

Citation: Watson AD: Ankle instability and impingement. *Foot Ankle Clin* 12:177–195, 2007.

Level of Evidence: V

Summary: The author provides a review of the diagnosis and treatment of ankle instability and impingement.

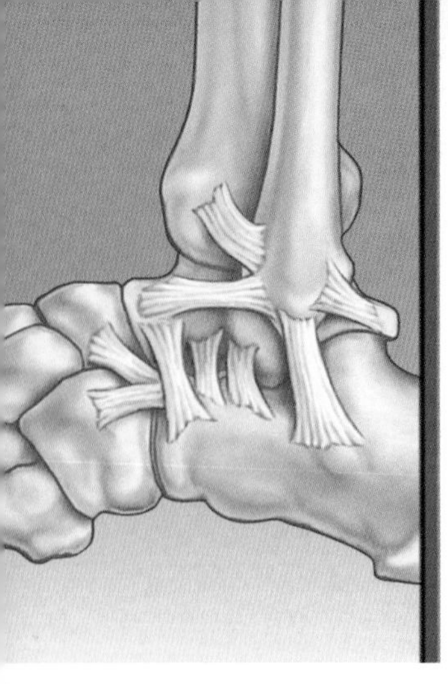

119

Heel Pain and Plantar Fasciitis: Hindfoot Conditions

ANISH R. KADAKIA

Posterior Heel Pain

Pain in the posterior, superior portion of the calcaneus may be multifactorial, ranging from retrocalcaneal bursitis, enlargement of the superior bursal prominence of the calcaneus, insertional Achilles tendinosis, or inflammation of an adventitious bursa between the Achilles tendon and the skin (Fig. 119-1).[1-6] Each of these entities may exist as an isolated condition or may be part of a symptom complex. Careful analysis of the patient's subjective complaints and objective findings are required to arrive at the correct diagnosis. Disorders of the Achilles tendon are covered in Chapter 117 and are not reviewed in detail here.

Retrocalcaneal bursitis may occur as an isolated entity but is more commonly associated with the prominent posterior superior bursal portion of the calcaneus, or Haglund's deformity. When Achilles tendinosis occurs concomitantly with this condition, it is generally located in the area of the Achilles tendon just at or above the insertion of the Achilles tendon at the posterior portion of the os calcis. Retrocalcaneal pain syndrome is commonly associated with a high-arched cavus foot and a varus heel.[1] The combination of these factors tends to produce a foot that does not dorsiflex as readily as a normal foot. The heel is prominent and is more susceptible to increased pressure from the tendons and the counter of the shoe.

History

The history is generally that of slow onset of dull aching pain in the retrocalcaneal area aggravated by activity and certain footwear. Footwear with a narrow heel counter is most commonly associated with this condition. Pain that starts after sitting or when arising from bed in the morning is commonly reported. At times the patient may have a history of the acute onset of pain, which is sometimes associated with a traumatic incident. When this history is reported, a rupture of the Achilles tendon or disruption of calcific tendinosis must be considered.

Physical Examination

Physical examination reveals swelling in the area of the retrocalcaneal bursa between the Achilles tendon and the calcaneus.[3,4] A prominence is generally present in the area of the superior portion of the heel. The swelling in the retrocalcaneal bursa will be found just anterior to the Achilles tendon. By palpating medially and laterally at the same time and with the aid of ballottement, one can sometimes feel fluid within the bursa (Fig. 119-2). With careful and discrete palpation, one can generally differentiate between swelling in the Achilles tendon and swelling in the retrocalcaneal bursa. The swelling of the Achilles tendon associated with retrocalcaneal bursitis is usually at the level of the tendon at or just proximal to the insertion. Dorsiflexion of the foot usually increases the pain in the area. A great deal of swelling and inflammation on examination may indicate involvement of both the retrocalcaneal bursa and the Achilles tendon. Redness and swelling may be present between the Achilles tendon and the skin, usually as a result of an adventitious bursitis produced by pressure of the shoe counter against the Achilles tendon. Periostitis may be present, which is a discrete localized area of tenderness of the os calcis, usually on the lateral side of the posterior portion of the os calcis and produced by pressure of the shoe counter. A "squeeze test" in which the palms of both hands apply moderate compression to the tuberosity should be performed to rule out the presence of a stress fracture. If the patient reports pain with this examination, a high suspicion for a stress fracture should be noted.

Imaging

A lateral view of the foot is taken with the patient standing, which allows biomechanical evaluation of the foot and evaluation of the specific points of the os calcis. The points of the os calcis are identified as the posterior margin of the posterior facet, the superior bursal projection, the tuberosity indicating the site of the Achilles tendon insertion, the medial tubercle, and the anterior tubercle.[7] The shape and appearance of the superior bursal prominence are noted. Evaluation of the lateral radiograph may be performed using the method described by Fowler and Philip, which measures the posterior calcaneal angle (Fig. 119-3).[8] Fowler and Philip consider the bursal projection prominent if the angle is greater than 75 degrees. Some authors have concluded that a combination of the Fowler angle and the angle of calcaneal inclination is more effective in correlating the radiographic appearance with symptomatology than the Fowler and Philip angle alone, with the combined angle being greater than 90 degrees in patients with symptomatic Haglund disease.[9,10]

Parallel pitch lines have been used by Heneghan and Pavlov[3] to determine the prominence of the bursal projection (Fig. 119-4). The base line is constructed by placing a line

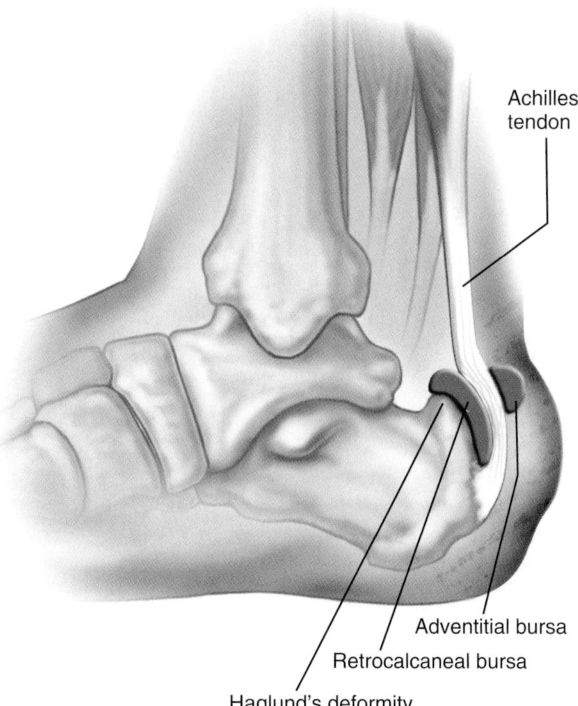

FIGURE 119-1 Haglund's deformity with a retrocalcaneal bursa between the Achilles tendon and the superior bursal prominence and an adventitious bursa between the Achilles tendon and the skin.

along the medial tuberosity and the anterior tubercle and a parallel line from the posterior lip of the talar articular facet. The bursal prominence is considered abnormal if it extends above this line.

Magnetic resonance imaging (MRI) has provided clearer insight into the anatomic abnormalities associated with posterior heel pain.[11-14] The imaging allows visualization of the Achilles tendon and the bursa, as well as demonstrating any bony abnormalities in the posterior superior calcaneus. In patients with a suspected stress fracture of the calcaneus, an MRI scan can be ordered to delineate the diagnosis in an expeditious manner so that the most appropriate treatment

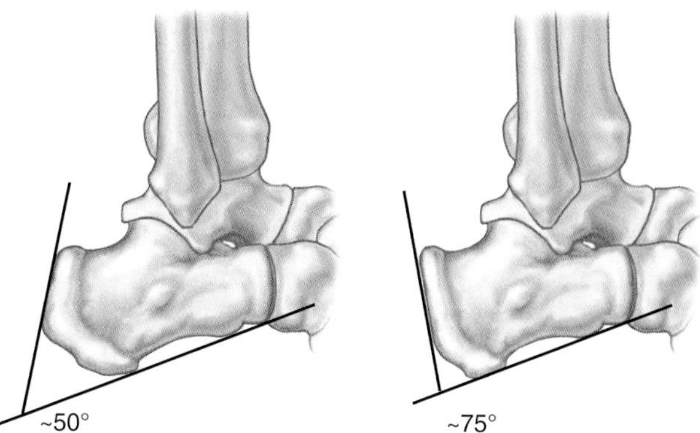

FIGURE 119-3 Measurement of the Fowler and Philip angle. The normal angle is shown on the left and an abnormal angle is shown on the right. The upper level of normal is considered to be 69 degrees. The drawing at the right indicates an abnormal angle of 75 degrees.

may be initiated. In patients refractory to nonoperative treatment, a preoperative MRI will define which anatomic structures need to be addressed (Fig. 119-5). The degree of tendinosis present in the Achilles tendon is easily visualized and distinguished from isolated bursitis.

Decision-Making Principles

Nonoperative treatment is successful at alleviating posterior heel pain regardless of cause in most patients. Adventitious bursitis is generally treated conservatively by softening the heel counter with use of a small U-shaped pad to relieve the pressure of the shoe or counter against the inflamed area; in addition, antiinflammatory medications are used. Surgical intervention performed solely for adventitious bursitis is unusual and carries a risk of wound slough, and thus it should be avoided if possible.

Retrocalcaneal bursitis and Haglund's deformity are generally managed by conservative measures consisting of antiinflammatory medication, decreased activity, padding to prevent

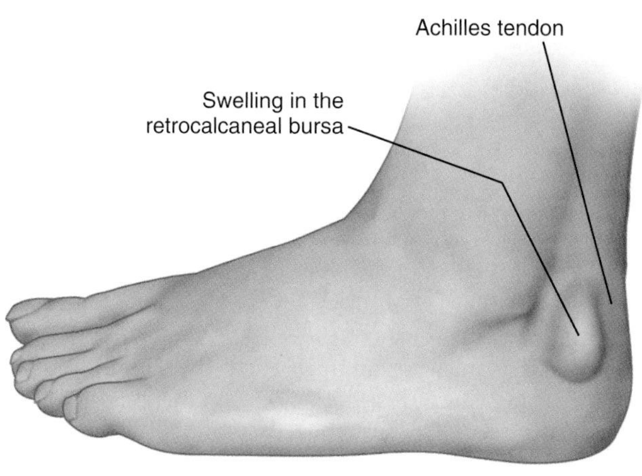

FIGURE 119-2 The area of the swelling; retrocalcaneal bursitis with swelling is anterior to the Achilles tendon.

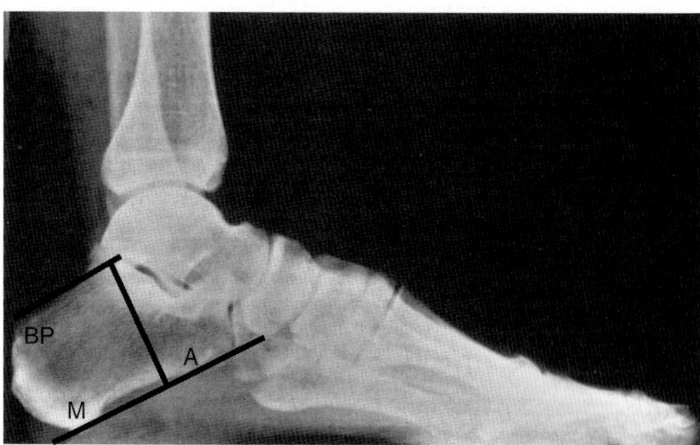

FIGURE 119-4 Parallel pitch lines used to determine the prominence of the bursal projection. A line is drawn along the medial tuberosity (*M*) and the anterior tuberosity (*A*). A parallel is constructed from the superior prominence of the posterior facet. If the bursal projection (*BP*) is above the superior line, the projection is considered abnormally large. *(From Pavlov H, Heneghan MA, Hersh A, et al: The Haglund syndrome: initial and differential diagnosis.* Radiology *144[1]:83–88, 1982.)*

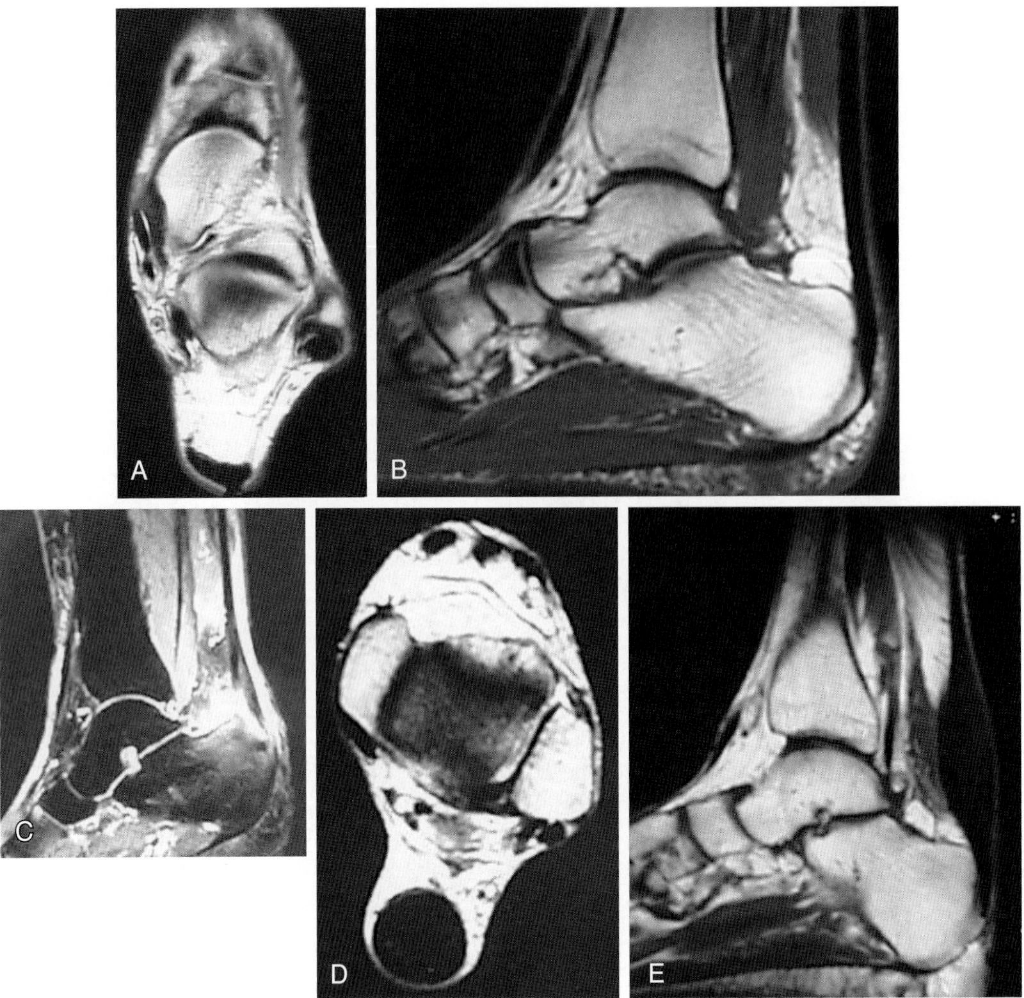

FIGURE 119-5 **A,** Axial magnetic resonance imaging (MRI) of a normal Achilles tendon showing the normal shape of the Achilles tendon. **B,** A sagittal MRI scan of a normal Achilles tendon showing the normal shape of the Achilles tendon. **C,** A sagittal MRI scan showing increased signal in the insertion of the Achilles tendon consistent with tendinosis. Increased fluid is present, demonstrating an inflamed bursa surrounding Haglund's deformity. **D** and **E,** Axial and sagittal MRI scans demonstrating chronic tendinosis of the Achilles with marked fusiform swelling of the tendon.

pressure on the affected area, orthoses or heel lifts, and strengthening and stretching exercises. If the condition does not respond to these modalities, then surgical intervention may be considered. Surgery generally consists of excision of the exostosis and the retrocalcaneal bursa and, at times, the adventitious bursa, if present, along with correction of the Achilles tendon disease with tendon transfer if necessary. Although good results after surgery are reported in most series, in the athlete, this condition may present a serious threat to continued full activity even after surgical intervention.

Treatment Options

Nonoperative Therapy

Initial goals of the treatment of patients with retrocalcaneal bursitis are to control pain and attempt to allow the patient to return to normal function and activity. Rest, particularly soon after the onset of symptoms, can be helpful. The duration of rest may be prolonged, depending on the increasing duration of symptoms.[15,16] Cross-training with low-impact exercises, such as an elliptical machine, swimming, or biking, may prevent deconditioning in the athlete. Modified regimens may be suggested for an athlete who is unwilling to cross-train.[16-18] In patients with exquisite tenderness, immobilization in a controlled ankle motion (CAM) boot or short-leg walking cast may be helpful.[17,19] Immobilization should be used cautiously in athletes because patients can have resultant tendon and muscle atrophy, degeneration, and decreased blood supply.[18,20]

Nonsteroidal drugs that are administered orally or delivered locally in the form of a patch may decrease local inflammation.[20-22] Cryotherapy and ice can decrease pain, swelling, and inflammation as well.[20-22] Corticosteroids that are taken orally, injected locally, or applied topically have been used.[23] Injections must be used cautiously because they can lead to a higher incidence of tendon ruptures and tendinopathy.[24,25] Animal model studies with intratendinous injections have been shown to result in localized tendon necrosis and decreased mechanical strength. If used, the steroid injection must be placed anterior to the tendon, in the area of the retrocalcaneal bursa.[20,21] The patient is immobilized in a CAM walker for 3 to 4 weeks to minimize the risk of tendon rupture after injection into the retrocalcaneal bursa.

Orthoses may help these patients by providing a heel lift function, correcting hyperpronation, or minimizing leg length discrepancies.[20,21] Care must be exercised when correcting hindfoot pronation deformities, because overcorrection can result in inflexibility of the hindfoot with decreased shock absorption.[21] Heel cups can decrease the strain on an Achilles tendon and elevate a prominent superior calcaneal tuberosity away from the tendon. High heels, clogs, open-back shoes, gel braces, and horseshoe pads can also provide symptomatic relief for the patient.[19,26]

If retrocalcaneal bursitis is present with a normal Achilles tendon, conservative therapy is implemented until the patient has been asymptomatic for 4 to 6 weeks. The patient may then return to sports participation starting with limited activity and working up to full activity within 4 to 12 weeks, assuming that they have recovered full strength and mobility without pain. If retrocalcaneal bursitis is associated with degeneration of the Achilles tendon, nonoperative treatment should be used until the patient is asymptomatic; a gradual increase in activity is then allowed over a 6- to 12-week period.

Operative Therapy

If the patient does not respond to these modalities, then surgical intervention may be considered. Surgery generally consists

AUTHOR'S PREFERRED TECHNIQUE

Posterior Heel Pain

Surgical procedures are usually performed for retrocalcaneal bursitis associated with the superior bony prominence. The retrocalcaneal bursa and the superior bursal prominence are excised. The adventitious bursa is excised if it is prominent. If the adventitious bursa is excised, the surgeon must take care to excise it carefully and meticulously to avoid adversely affecting the blood supply or the skin overlying this area because a skin slough can result in significant morbidity for the patient.

A medial or lateral incision or a combination of incisions 1.5 cm anterior to the Achilles tendon is made as determined by the location and width of the bony prominence (Fig. 119-6). Alternatively, a central posterior Achilles splitting approach can be used. Prone positioning can be used with all of the aforementioned incisions. A medial incision may be carried out with the patient supine and minimizes risk of damage to the sural nerve, but the superior calcaneal exostosis is typically lateral, which may make excision slightly more difficult. Given the elimination of sural nerve injury and simplified positioning, this is the author's preferred technique in these cases. If the patient has concomitant tendinosis of the Achilles tendon, the central posterior tendon splitting approach is used.

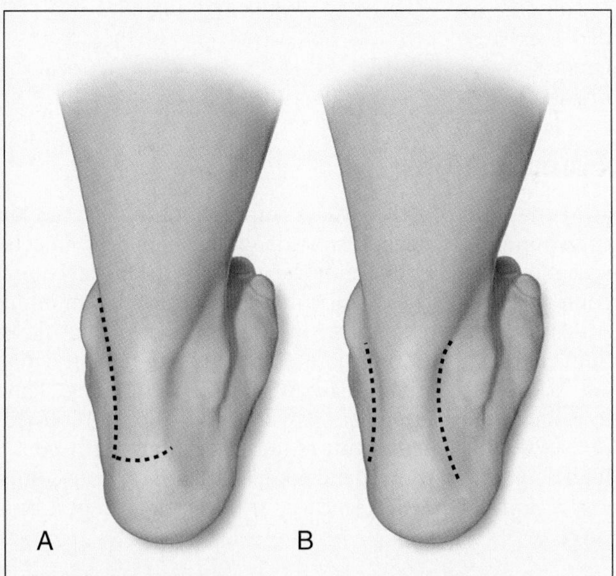

FIGURE 119-6 Surgical incisions for retrocalcaneal bursitis. **A,** The medial approach with J extension as described by Schepsis and Leach.[28] **B,** Medial and lateral approach incisions as described by Jones and James.[4]

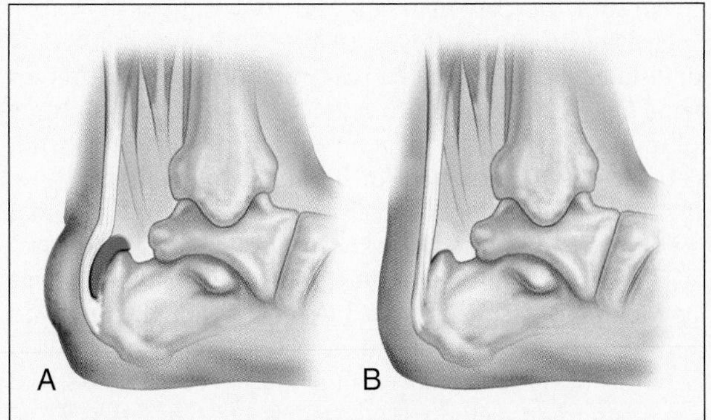

FIGURE 119-7 **A,** Haglund's deformity with prominence of the posterior superior portion of the os calcis. **B,** The appearance of os calcis after surgical resection of a posterior superior prominence for symptomatic Haglund's deformity.

After incision of the central aspect of the posterior skin, the incision is carried directly to the level of the paratenon and dissection is performed at this level to maintain full-thickness skin flaps to avoid skin loss. Attention should be given to the calcaneal branch of the sural nerve on the lateral side and the medial calcaneal nerve on the medial side. The Achilles tendon is inspected to confirm the presence and degree of tendinosis. Regardless of the surgical approach, the retrocalcaneal bursa is now excised. An exostosectomy is performed, removing the bone from the area of insertion of the Achilles tendon to the superior portion of the posterior facet of the os calcis (Fig. 119-7). Adequate bone is removed, and the edges are smoothed with a rasp. If greater than 50% of the insertion of the Achilles tendon is elevated from the calcaneus, repair with suture anchors is recommended to avoid rupture. In the case of a concomitant tendinosis, a flexor hallucis longus transfer may be required if a significant portion (>50%) of the Achilles tendon is excised as described in Chapter 117. The split in the Achilles tendon is repaired with an absorbable monofilament number 0 suture. The subcutaneous tissue and skin are closed after the procedure. Compressive dressings and plaster splints are applied to maintain 15 degrees of ankle plantar flexion to maximize perfusion to the posterior skin.

of excision of the exostosis and the retrocalcaneal bursa and at times the adventitious bursa, if present, along with correction of the Achilles tendon disease with tendon transfer if necessary. Although most authors report good results after surgery, in the athlete this condition may present a serious threat to continued full activity even after surgical intervention.

Postoperative Management

In cases in which the Achilles tendon is not involved, the patient is seen at 2 weeks for stitch removal and the lower extremity is placed into a removable CAM walker with the ankle at neutral position for an additional 4 weeks, and weight bearing is begun. A rehabilitation program for non–weight-bearing strengthening and range of motion is begun at this initial visit. Six weeks after surgery, the walking boot is removed and the patient is allowed to weight bear with a 7/16-inch heel lift during this time for 4 to 6 weeks. Therapy is continued and graduated to weight-bearing exercises. Patients are then advanced to regular footwear and continue to follow a strengthening program at home with a Theraband. Athletic activity is restricted for 3 months after surgery.

If surgery has been performed on the tendon in combination with excision of the retrocalcaneal bursa and exostosectomy, immobilization is continued for 8 weeks but active range of motion is begun at 3 weeks. Strengthening and stretching exercises are started at 6 to 9 weeks. Increased activity according to tolerance can be started at 12 weeks, and return to strenuous activity is allowed at 4 to 6 months if local symptoms have resolved.

Results

Ippolito and Ricciardi-Pollini[27] described three patients with invasive retrocalcaneal bursitis who had a large bursa and invasion of the os calcis. Pathologic examination revealed lymphoplasma cellular infiltrates containing proportionately more plasma cells than lymphocytes. Removal of the bursa provided clinical relief, and systemic rheumatic disease did not develop in later years.

Keck and Kelly[5] reported on 13 patients with 20 symptomatic heels that were treated surgically. In 17 heels the superior bursa was excised, and in three heels a dorsally based closing wedge osteotomy was performed. Good results were reported for 15 of the heels treated. The initial results were good in all but two patients, whose pain recurred as a manifestation of generalized rheumatoid arthritis. An osteotomy was used to reduce the posterior prominence, and results were rated good in two heels, fair in one heel, and poor in two heels. The authors believed that too few osteotomies were performed in this series to evaluate this method. A disadvantage of the osteotomy was that a longer convalescence was required.[5]

A series of 65 patients with Haglund disease was reported by Ruch[9]; 17 underwent resection of the posterior superior portion of the os calcis, with resection of the posterior superior aspect both medially and laterally and removal of sufficient bone to render the previous palpable prominence entirely absent.[9] The patients were evaluated 6 months to 5 years after undergoing surgery. Fifteen demonstrated good to excellent results with elimination of symptoms. Three of the patients required a second procedure to obtain the desired result.

Schepsis and Leach[28] reported that the majority of athletes, particularly runners, who presented with acute or chronic posterior heel pain were successfully managed nonoperatively using a combination of (1) a decrease in or cessation of the usual weekly mileage, (2) temporary termination of interval training and workouts on hills, (3) a change from a harder bank surface to a softer surface, (4) a 0.25- to 0.50-inch lift inside the shoe or added to the shoe, and (5) a program designed to stretch and strengthen the gastrocnemius-soleus complex.[28] These measures were combined with use of oral antiinflammatory medications and an occasional injection of corticosteroid into the retrocalcaneal bursa. Postural abnormalities were treated with orthotics. The authors retrospectively studied 45 cases of chronic posterior heel pain that were treated surgically in 37 patients. All but two of these patients were competitive long-distance runners who ran an average of 40 to 120 miles per week prior to the onset of symptoms. Their ages ranged from 19 to 56 years.

The surgical approach used by Schepsis and Leach[28] was a longitudinal incision 1 cm medial to the Achilles tendon that was continued transversely to form a J-shaped incision if necessary. A cast was applied and worn for 2 to 3 weeks, with weight bearing permitted after 1 week. When disease within the tendon required excision and repair, immobilization was continued for 1 to 2 weeks longer. Range-of-motion exercises were emphasized. A graduated program of swimming and stationary bicycling combined with isometric, isotonic, and isokinetic strengthening of the calf muscles was prescribed. Jogging was permitted after 8 to 12 weeks, but rarely sooner. Full return to a competitive level of sports activity usually required 5 to 6 months.

The patients were divided into three groups—those with Achilles tenosynovitis-tendinitis, those with retrocalcaneal bursitis, and those with a combination of both. In the 14 patients with retrocalcaneal bursitis, seven (50%) had excellent results, three (21%) had good results, and four (29%) had fair results. In the group with a combination of both conditions, five (71%) had excellent results and two (29%) had good results. It was noted that four of the six unsatisfactory results occurred in the group with retrocalcaneal bursitis.

Complications

More than half of all reported complications involve the surgical wound. Skin edge necrosis, superficial or deep infection, and seroma or hematoma formation are the most common complications. These complications can be minimized with postoperative splinting in 20 degrees of plantar flexion. Sural neuritis, tendon rupture, or disruption of the repair and deep vein thrombosis have also been reported. Failure to achieve complete relief of symptoms has been reported in up to 29% of patients with retrocalcaneal bursitis. Given the high demands of the athletic population, appropriate counseling regarding the outcomes is critical prior to performing surgery.

Future Considerations

Endoscopic techniques for the debridement of the retrocalcaneal space and the posterosuperior tuberosity of the calcaneus have been reported in the literature. Ortmann and McBryde[29] reported on 28 patients and 30 heels that were treated with endoscopic surgery; 86.67% of patients reported excellent results, with one major complication of an Achilles tendon rupture.[29] The medial column of the Achilles tendon, the sural nerve, and the plantaris tendons are at risk with use of this technique.[30] Despite these risks, the purported benefits of lower morbidity and recovery time make this procedure an excellent option for surgeons familiar with endoscopy.

Plantar Fasciitis

In reviewing the literature, it is apparent that many different theories exist about the cause of subcalcaneal pain, and hence many different methods of treatment have been suggested.[31-43] It has been said that although this condition is familiar to all orthopaedic surgeons, it is probably fully understood by none.[36]

Snook and Chrisman[44] noted that conflicting literature exists on this subject with regard to two salient points: that there is no accepted explanation of the cause of the condition and that no generally approved method of treatment exists. These investigators thought that the basic cause might lie in the subcalcaneal pad, which in some unknown manner lost its compressibility, either by local loss of fat with thinning or by rupture of the fibrous tissue septa. Ali[45] stated that "the painful heel is due to a fibrotic response, similar to plantar fibromatosis and not to the spur of bone which is the end result of recurrent strain on the plantar fascia." Tanz[46] thought that "inferior heel pain is often due to irritation of a branch of the medial calcaneal nerve." Similarly, Baxter and Thigpen[31] and Przylucki and Jones[47] advanced the thought that the heel pain is due to an entrapment neuropathy that involves the branch of the lateral plantar nerve to the abductor digiti quinti. It has been noted that this branch passes more proximally than is shown in most anatomic studies and is in the area of the heel spur.[31,48]

Heel spurs may be present or absent and may or may not be the primary pathologic entity in persons with heel pain. However, they must be considered in the context of the entire syndrome. Laboratory studies in most patients with subcalcaneal pain syndrome are normal. When the subcalcaneal pain syndrome is present, and especially if it is persistent and severe, consideration must be given to the diagnosis of a systemic disorder such as seronegative arthropathy. In patients with the subcalcaneal pain syndrome, it has been reported that the incidence of the subsequent development of a systemic arthritic disorder may be as high as 16%.[36]

History

The history usually reveals a slow but gradual onset of pain along the inside of the heel.[35-37] Occasionally the pain may be associated with a twisting injury of the foot, producing an abrupt onset of pain.[48] However, the clinical course is generally similar regardless of the onset. The location of the pain is generally described as along the medial side of the foot at the bottom of the heel. The pain is worse upon first arising in the morning and then decreases with increased activity. However, it may increase after prolonged activity. Periods of inactivity are generally followed by an increase in pain as activity is started again. Numbness of the foot is not present. When severe pain is present, the patient is unable to bear weight on the heel and will bear weight on the forepart of the foot.

Physical Examination

Specific examination of the foot reveals acute tenderness along the medial tuberosity of the os calcis along its plantar aspect. This tenderness may be at the origin of the central slip of the plantar fascia, or it may be deep, in which case it probably represents a deep inflammation, perhaps with involvement of the nerve to the abductor digiti quinti. The plantar fascia is palpated to determine whether the plantar fascia is tender just at its origin or throughout its course. The plantar fascia is also palpated for nodules, the presence of which suggests plantar fibromatosis. The plantar fascia is palpated both with the toes flexed so that it is supple and with the toes extended, which places tension on the plantar fascia. Careful examination of ankle range of motion is essential to identify any concurrent gastrocnemius or soleus contractures.

Common conditions in the differential diagnosis of heel pain should be ruled out. Tarsal tunnel syndrome may generate pain in the distribution of the calcaneal branch and first branch of the lateral plantar nerve and is typically elicited with palpation on the plantar medial aspect of the hindfoot, not directly under the foot. The associated sensory and motor changes are likewise not seen with plantar fasciitis (PF). Fat pad atrophy will often cause pain more posterior to the plantar tuberosity, directly under the calcaneus. Applying a squeeze around the calcaneus will elicit pain in patients with calcaneal stress fractures.

Imaging

Standing, full weight-bearing roentgenograms of the heel, including the foot, are taken in the anteroposterior and lateral standing projections. Roentgenograms taken in this manner will provide information about the osseous structures of the foot and specific details of the os calcis. Such radiographs will also help classify the foot as normal, flat, or cavus. The presence of a spur or calcification along the medial tuberosity will also be shown (Fig. 119-8). Axial non–weight-bearing views of the os calcis may be taken to provide information about the os calcis in a second plane.

Although much discussion has occurred about the relationship of the calcaneal heel spur to subcalcaneal pain, the relationship has not been definitely established. Tanz[46] stated that a heel spur is located in the origin of the short toe flexors and not in the plantar fascia. He noted that 15% of normal asymptomatic adult feet have subcalcaneal plantar spurs,

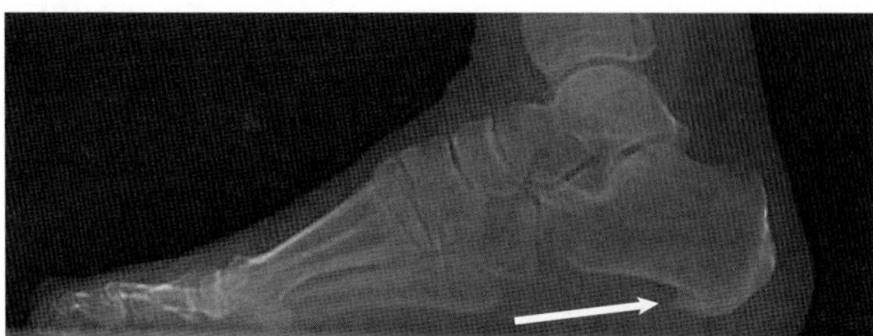

FIGURE 119-8 An inferior plantar spur (*arrow*) commonly seen in patients with plantar fasciitis.

whereas about 50% of adult feet with plantar heel pain have spurs. Tanz thought that heel spurs contributed to the plantar heel pain, although many patients with plantar heel pain did not have spurs. Snook and Chrisman[44] agreed with this supposition. In their report on 27 patients with subcalcaneal pain, they noted that 13 had a calcaneal spur and 11 did not have such a spur. Mann[49] stated that "over a long period of time, proliferative bony changes at the origin of the fascia may lead to the formation of a spur."

Shmokler and colleagues[50] reviewed 1000 patients at random with radiographs of the foot. They found a 13.2% incidence of heel spurs. Only 39% of those with heel spurs (5.2% of the total sample) reported any history of subcalcaneal heel pain. Shmokler and coworkers[50] believed that these statistics tended to support the premise that the presence of a heel spur did not mandate pain.

Intenzo and colleagues[51] studied 15 patients reporting chronic heel pain who underwent three-phase technetium-99m methylene diphosphonate bone scintigraphy. Ten patients demonstrated abnormal scan findings consistent with PF with uptake only in the early soft tissue phase, and they had responded to conventional therapy. Two patients were found to have calcaneal stress fractures, and one patient demonstrated a calcaneal spur that required no treatment. The remaining two patients had normal scans and did not appear to have PF clinically. These investigators found the three-phase bone scan useful in diagnosing PF and in distinguishing it from other causes of the painful heel syndrome.

Grasel et al.[52] evaluated various MRI signs of PF to determine if a difference exists in these findings between clinically typical and atypical patients with chronic symptoms resistant to conservative treatment.[52] These investigators found signs on MRI that included occult marrow edema and fascial tears. Patients with these manifestations seemed to respond to treatment in a manner similar to that of patients in whom MRI revealed more benign findings. MRI is not required to make the diagnosis of either PF or fibromatosis. The primary use is to rule out other conditions such as calcaneal stress fracture, plantar fascia rupture, neoplasm, and Baxter's neuritis.

Decision-Making Principles

Operative treatment for PF is reserved for patients with moderate to severe symptoms who have not responded to at least 6 months (or more conservatively 12 months) of nonoperative management. Currently, no prospective, randomized controlled trials exist that support any specific operative intervention for treatment of PF. Open techniques for plantar fascia release provide complete visualization of the fascia and allow the fascia to be incised in a controlled fashion. In addition, the first branch of the lateral plantar nerve can be decompressed with an open technique. Opponents of an open technique note a higher incidence of wound complications, infection, and postoperative pain and a longer return to work. Endoscopic plantar fascia release for treatment of PF has been suggested to reduce complications and provide an earlier return to work and activity. However, endoscopic techniques are limited by a small field of view and may result in inadequate resection of the plantar fascia. In addition, the lateral plantar artery and first branch of the lateral plantar nerve is not exposed during this technique, and injury may occur.

In a patient with a tight gastrocnemius with a positive Silverskold test, a gastrocnemius recession may relax the tension on the plantar fascia, relieving the pain. Successful relief of plantar foot pain after gastrocnemius recession has recently been demonstrated. Further research is required to validate these results.

Treatment Options

Nonoperative Therapy

Management of subcalcaneal heel pain should initially begin with nonoperative treatment. Although consensus does not exist on the efficacy of any particular conservative treatment regimen, it is agreed that nonsurgical treatment is ultimately effective in approximately 90% of patients. Because the natural history of PF has not been established, it is unclear how much of symptom resolution is in fact due to the wide variety of commonly used treatments. Activities are restricted according to the patient's symptomatic tolerance.

The mainstay of treatment is to stretch both the Achilles and plantar fascia. Simple plantar fascia stretching exercises are certainly the least expensive and easiest modality for patients to initiate. Plantar fascia–specific stretching has demonstrated superior success compared with isolated Achilles stretching (Fig. 119-9).

Nighttime dorsiflexion splints have demonstrated fair success in multiple randomized studies and are especially useful for relieving "start-up" pain in the morning. Resolution of symptoms has been reported as early as 12 weeks and may improve significantly even after 1 month of splint use.

Orthotics have demonstrated similar results to nighttime splints with better patient compliance. No conclusive evidence exists to support the use of a prefabricated versus a custom-molded orthotic. The use of a silicone heel pad is a simple and cost-effective method in patients without deformity.

Oral nonsteroidal antiinflammatory drugs have demonstrated trends toward improved patient pain and function but no statistically significant difference from placebo when used with other conservative modalities.

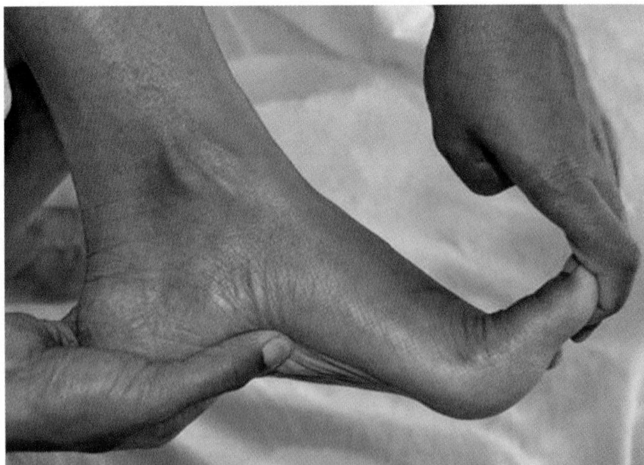

FIGURE 119-9 A plantar fascia–specific stretch is performed with the leg in a figure four position. The contralateral hand is used to dorsiflex the hallux and ankle. The ipsilateral hand is used to palpate the plantar fascia to ensure that it is taut.

Localized administration of corticosteroids, either through injection or iontophoresis, has demonstrated reliable short-term relief but no significant long-term benefit. The risk of plantar fascia rupture or fat pad atrophy must be weighed against the limited short-term benefit of corticosteroid injections, and repeat injections should be avoided. Iontophoresis may be a safer option but requires an increased time commitment and may be impractical in the typical clinic setting.

Cross-training activity is important. The patient should avoid repetitive impact activities such as running or use of a treadmill and instead cross-train with a bicycle or elliptical trainer. These options assist in maintaining conditioning and increasing flexibility while avoiding cyclic loading.

Once the patient has become asymptomatic without tenderness and has maintained this status for 4 to 6 weeks, a gradual increase in activity may be allowed. Use of the orthotic is continued for several months. After several months, use of the orthotic is discontinued unless the patient has a biomechanical abnormality of the foot such as a flatfoot or cavus deformity. If the patient has a flatfoot deformity, a device designed to correct the biomechanical abnormality, support the foot, and prevent the abnormal biomechanical stresses along the plantar fascia and the medial side of the heel is used. If the patient has a cavus deformity, a soft orthotic designed to decrease the shock and increase the weight-bearing area may be used indefinitely depending on the patient's symptoms. When a patient has a deformity and has had a significant episode of subcalcaneal pain requiring treatment, use of the orthotic can be continued permanently. Although the over-the-counter type of heel cup can be used initially to try to provide some symptomatic relief, in a patient with a true biomechanical abnormality, a specific orthosis should be used.

Postoperative Management

The patient is kept non–weight bearing for 2 weeks and then can bear weight in a short-leg cast for 2 more weeks; increased activity is started at 12 weeks. This operation is used only for patients with recalcitrant conditions. It carries with it the expectation that the patient will probably, but not certainly, be able to return to his or her preinjury status.

Results

In 1986 Lutter[43] outlined the decision-making process in athletes with subcalcaneal pain. He described 182 patients with heel complaints related to sports injuries; most of the patients were runners (76%). Approximately 20% of these patients required 3 to 4 months of conservative treatment before returning to sports activity. Five percent had chronic heel pain and did not recover within 9 to 12 months. For these patients, a surgical approach was considered. The procedure used in these patients depended on the preoperative

AUTHOR'S PREFERRED TECHNIQUE

Plantar Fasciitis

In the athlete, the least amount of surgery commensurate with high likelihood of a good result should be performed. In the athlete with recalcitrant subcalcaneal pain syndrome who desires to continue athletic activity, the exact site of the abnormality is evaluated carefully by means of differential blocks using a long-acting anesthetic such as bupivacaine hydrochloride. This evaluation allows more precise localization of the exact area of the pathologic condition. If clear evidence exists of an isolated gastrocnemius contracture without evidence of tarsal tunnel or Baxter's neuritis, an isolated gastrocnemius recession is considered.

Prior to surgery, nerve conduction and electromyographic studies are considered in patients in whom a tarsal tunnel syndrome is possible. Laboratory studies are performed to exclude systemic arthritis or spondyloarthropathies. Bone scans with technetium-99m may be considered if one suspects a fatigue fracture or if the exact location of the pain is not clear.

For partial release of the plantar fascia, the patient is positioned supine with a small bump placed under the contralateral hip to increase the external rotation of the affected limb. A tourniquet should be used to minimize the bleeding to ensure appropriate identification of the neurovascular structures. In all cases, the tourniquet is released and appropriate hemostasis is obtained prior to closure to minimize the risk of a hematoma and irritation of the nerves that may compromise the end result. A medial oblique incision along the heel is made as described by Schon (Fig. 119-10).[52a] Loop magnification may be used. The sensory branch of the medial calcaneal nerve is located, inspected, and preserved. If entrapment of the medial calcaneal nerve occurs as it comes through the fascia, this entrapment is explored and released. Subcutaneous fat is carefully dissected and retracted to expose the superficial fascia of the abductor hallucis, which is then incised. The abductor hallucis muscle is then retracted inferiorly and the deep fascia of the muscle is released to decompress the first branch of the lateral plantar nerve. The abductor is then retracted superiorly to visualize the plantar fascia. The medial one third of the plantar fascia is released under direct visualization and a 1-cm square segment is excised.

Any prominent calcaneal spur may be identified deep in the wound and carefully debrided back to a smooth, low-profile base. Removal of the spur is not required and may increase the risk of plantar fascia rupture and injury to the lateral plantar nerve. No specific criteria exist on which to base excision of the spur, only that "large" spurs should be excised.

After copious irrigation and hemostasis, the incision is closed with a nylon mattress suture and a short-leg cast is applied. The patient should not bear weight for 4 to 7 days. Weight bearing in a cast or an over-the-counter brace is maintained for 14 more days. At 3 weeks, weight bearing with a shoe is permitted. Running is started at 6 to 12 weeks, and activity is then allowed as tolerated. If the patient has a biomechanical foot abnormality, an orthotic device is used after the operation.

Continued

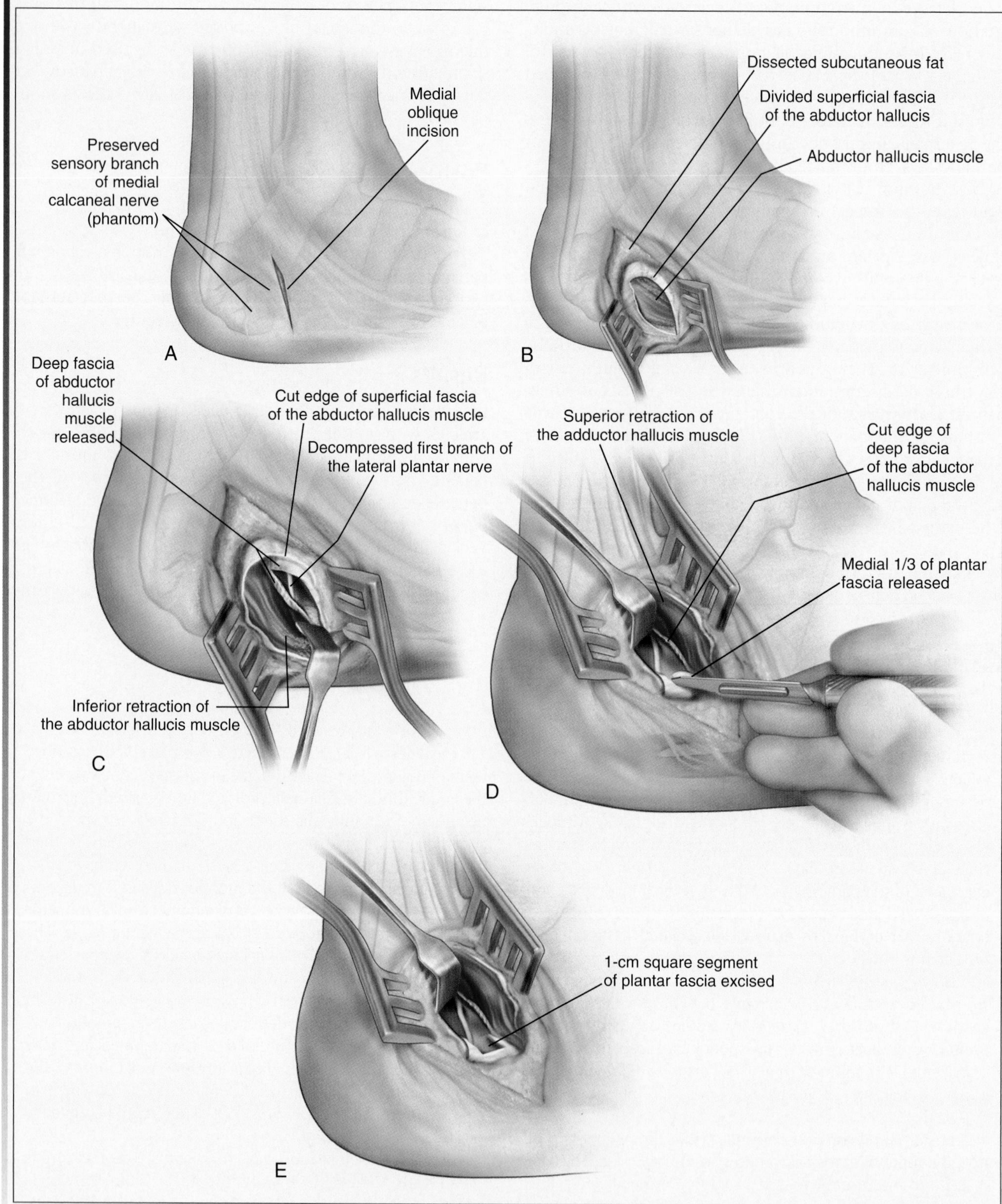

FIGURE 119-10 Plantar fascia and nerve release. **A,** Incision. **B,** Release of the abductor hallucis muscle. **C,** The abductor hallucis muscle is reflected proximally. **D,** The abductor hallucis is retracted distally. **E,** Resection of a small medial portion of the plantar fascia.

diagnosis and varied from release of the nerves to release of the fascia to complete exploration of the posterior tibial nerve and its branches and release of the plantar fascia. Cycling or swimming was begun 2 weeks after the operation. Gentle walk-dash run training and a gradual escalation up to running was allowed approximately 6 weeks after surgery. Patients were asked to refrain from walking until they were pain free and had no tenderness. If pain occurred with increasing activity, the workup was cut by 50% until the patient could tolerate the workup without pain.

Shock wave therapy has been examined in the treatment of chronic PF in athletes who run. Rompe et al.[53] demonstrated that after 6 months of treatments three times a week with shock wave therapy, the treatment group experienced greater relief than did the sham treatment group.

Baxter and Thigpen[31] performed 34 operative procedures in 26 patients with recalcitrant heel pain. The procedure consisted of isolated neurolysis of the nerves supplying the abductor digiti quinti muscle as it passed beneath the abductor with release of the deep fascia of the abductor hallucis longus and removal of the heel spur if it impinged on or produced entrapment of the nerve.[31] Among the 34 heels operated on, 32 had good results and 2 had poor results.

Clancy[39] treated patients with a medial heel wedge and flexible leather support, heel cord stretching, and rest for 6 to 12 weeks with a gradual return to running while wearing the orthotic and the medial heel wedge for 10 weeks. In patients who failed to respond to this treatment, surgery consisting of release of the plantar fascia and the fascia over the abductor hallucis longus was recommended. The 15 patients in whom surgery was performed returned to running within 8 to 10 weeks.

Henricson and Westlin[54] described 11 heels in 10 athletes who had chronic heel pain for which conservative therapy did not provide relief. The pain was due to compression of the calcaneal branches of the tibial nerve. Entrapment of the anterior calcaneal branch occurred where the nerve passed between the tight and rigid edges of the deep fascia of the abductor hallucis and the medial edge of the os calcis. Surgery consisted of identifying and releasing the tibial nerve and both calcaneal branches and releasing the deep fascia of the abductor hallucis. Follow-up for 58 months after surgery revealed that 10 of the 11 heels were asymptomatic. The patients had resumed athletic participation after an average of 5 weeks.

Leach and coworkers[55] described 15 competitive athletes in whom 16 operations were performed. Surgery consisted of release of the plantar fascia at the insertion of the os calcis, making the incision along the medial aspect of the heel. In one instance, the medial calcaneal nerve was involved in the inflammatory process. One patient returned to running at 6 weeks; the majority returned to running 9 weeks after surgery. Most patients continued to improve up to 6 months after the surgical procedure. Of the 15 operations, 14 were entirely successful in that the athletes returned to their previous level of activity. One failure occurred in a marathon runner who improved but was unable to train at the level he desired. No complications were reported.

In 1984 McBryde[56] reported that in his running clinic, PF comprised 9% of the total running disorders seen. The conservative (nonoperative) approach of McBryde and his group consisted of (1) ice massage for 2 minutes four to six times daily, including before and after runs, (2) heel cord stretching for 3 to 5 minutes three to four times daily, (3) posterior tibial and peroneal strengthening, (4) heel cushioning and control, and (5) use of antiinflammatory medication. This regimen was usually successful in treating runners with PF who were seen within the first 8 weeks. In runners with symptoms lasting longer than 6 weeks, a period of absolute rest with use of a cast was usually required. Orthoses were used. Five percent of the patients in the series underwent surgery, consisting of plantar fascial release through a short 1-inch longitudinal incision in the medial arch. All returned to a successful running program 6 to 12 weeks after surgery. Overall, among the 100 patients with PF, 82 recovered with a conservative approach, 11 stopped running, 5 underwent surgery (all of whom returned to running), and two refused surgery and continued to be symptomatic.

Snider and colleagues[57] reported 11 operations for plantar fascial release for chronic fasciitis in nine distance runners who had had symptoms for an average of 20 months and had not responded to nonsurgical treatment. The results of the operations were excellent in 10 feet and good in one foot with an average follow-up time of 25 months. Eight of nine patients returned to their desired level of full training at an average time of 4.5 months.

Rask[58] reported a medial plantar neurapraxia that he termed *jogger's foot*. Three cases were reported in which there was probable entrapment of the medial plantar nerve behind the navicular tuberosity in the fibromuscular tunnel formed by the abductor hallucis; the inciting factor was eversion of the foot. All three patients were treated successfully with conservative measures including a change in the running posture of the foot, antiinflammatory medication, and proper footwear.

In 2004, Saxena[59] reported on 16 athletes with intractable heel pain for whom conservative care had failed. Most of these athletes were runners. These patients were treated surgically with a uniportal endoscopic plantar fasciotomy. Saxena found that runners were able to return to athletic activity on average 2.6 months after surgery. Five poor results were found in patients with a body mass index greater than 27.

Complications

Acute complications after plantar fascia surgery are rare. Although few case series exist to determine reliable complication rates, the most commonly reported include wound dehiscence or infection. The most common complications reported after operative treatment for PF include further tearing or injury to the plantar fascia, collapse of the medial longitudinal arch, iatrogenic injury to the first branch of the lateral plantar nerve or neuroma formation, complex regional pain syndrome, and persistent pain. Complete excision of the plantar fascia has been associated with lateral column syndrome that presents a pain with weight bearing focused at the lateral border of the foot along the calcaneocuboid joint and fourth/fifth tarsometatarsal joints. In addition, recurrence rates after subtotal plantar fasciectomy have been reported as being approximately 10% in multiple studies.

Future Considerations

Increased focus on the role of a tight gastrocnemius complex and the effect on the function of the foot have begun to alter the surgical treatment for PF. With further research on biomechanical and clinical effect of a gastrocnemius release in patients with PF, the need for direct release of the plantar fascia may decrease. Although neither operation can be considered benign, patients with lateral column syndrome or injury to the lateral plantar nerve are severely limited without a good surgical recourse. Although injury of the sural nerve may occur, resection and burial can be performed, yielding an adequate result that does not preclude sporting activity.

For a complete list of references, go to expertconsult.com.

Suggested Readings

Citation: Yu J, Park D, Lee G: Effect of eccentric strengthening on pain, muscle strength, endurance, and functional fitness factors in male patients with Achilles tendinopathy. *Am J Phys Med Rehabil* 92(1):68–76, 2013.

Level of Evidence: II

Summary: The authors describe a prospective comparative study of 32 patients with Achilles tendinopathy who were placed into two treatment groups. One group underwent concentric strengthening and one underwent eccentric strengthening for an 8-week period. The authors were able to demonstrate a significant improvement in pain, balance, agility, and endurance in the patients who underwent eccentric strengthening. This article reinforces the critical nature of ensuring that therapy instructions are appropriately written for this disease process to focus on eccentric strengthening.

Citation: Kearney R, Costa ML: Insertional Achilles tendinopathy management: A systematic review. *Foot Ankle Int* 31(8):689–694, 2010.

Level of Evidence: III

Summary: The authors provide a systematic review of the literature regarding both operative and nonoperative management of insertional Achilles tendinopathy. Significant evidence favored conservative management, including both eccentric strengthening and shock wave therapy. The paucity of quality literature regarding operative intervention resulted in an inconclusive decision on the efficacy of surgery.

Citation: Digiovanni BF, Nawoczenski DA, Malay DP, et al: Plantar fascia-specific stretching exercise improves outcomes in patients with chronic plantar fasciitis. A prospective clinical trial with two-year follow-up. *J Bone Joint Surg Am* 88(8):1775–1781, 2006.

Level of Evidence: II

Summary: The authors of this very significant article definitively demonstrate that plantar fascia–specific stretching is the critical component in the nonoperative treatment of plantar fasciitis. Efficacy was noted 2 years after the initiation of treatment with a 92% satisfaction rate.

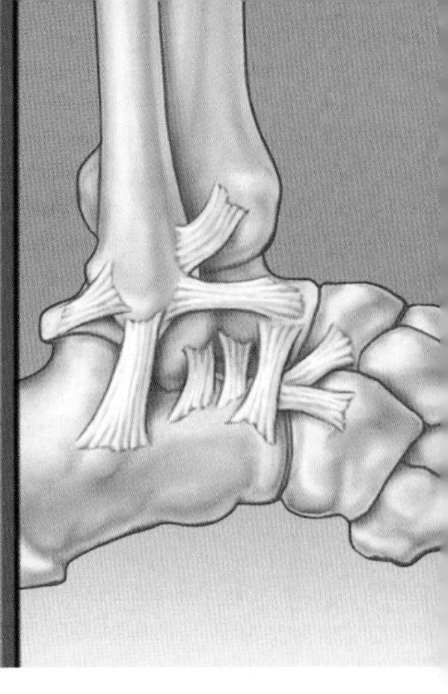

120

Forefoot Problems in Sport

ANTHONY PERERA • LYNDON MASON

Great caution must be taken in dealing with forefoot problems in athletes in particular. Although the outcomes are the same as in nonathletes, even a small decrease in performance may prove to be very significant for an athlete. Therefore, with certain exceptions, forefoot surgery should only be considered when conservative management has failed and the athlete is no longer able to play through the pain/dysfunction.

Turf Toe

Metatarsophalangeal (MTP) joint injuries are commonly the result of hyperextension. They are increasingly common[1-4] and can be characterized by a significant delay in return to sporting activities.[1]

History

Players may report localized pain, swelling, and pain with range of motion and ambulation; in addition, periarticular swelling and ecchymosis are typically present. Push-off is impaired with running, and it may be difficult to crouch with the MTP joint extended.[5]

Physical Examination

Clinical evaluation should include evaluation of hallux alignment, including clinical MTP joint reduction, or the presence of an intrinsic-minus posture (i.e., MTP extension and interphalangeal flexion), suggesting disruption of flexor hallucis brevis (FHB) tendon insertion. Palpation of plantar (including the individual sesamoids), medial, lateral, and dorsal structures for focal tenderness should be performed. Assessment of joint stability with respect to dorsoplantar stress and varus/valgus stress is critical. Weakness in plantar-flexion strength of the hallux may indicate loss of integrity of the plantar plate or the FHB. Point tenderness over the plantar aspect of the first MTP joint that worsens with passive extension of the toe is indicative of injury.

Imaging

Bilateral weight-bearing anteroposterior views can identify proximal migration of the sesamoids. A forced dorsiflexion lateral view assists in the diagnosis of failure of distal sesamoid migration and diastasis of a bipartite or fractured sesamoid. Magnetic resonance imaging (MRI) can be used to evaluate the presence and extent of capsular or plantar plate disruption[6] and also osseous or articular damage in the presence of normal radiographs.[7] Rodeo and coworkers[8] proposed a classification of first MTP joint injury (Box 120-1).

Decision-Making Principles

Operative intervention is rarely necessary in acute grade I and II injuries. Management is usually centered on conservative methods because surgery can be associated with a restricted range of motion. However, up to 25% to 50% of patients will have residual pain and limited dorsiflexion despite 6 months of rehabilitation[9]; some authors have therefore recommended surgical treatment of type III injuries.[10]

Treatment Options

Nonoperative

Ice, compression, and nonsteroidal antiinflammatory drugs may be used.[1,5,11,12] However, activity should be restricted in athletes with more severe injuries and significant discomfort. The patient can continue to participate in athletics if pain is minimal. A rigid forefoot insole[1,5,11] to stiffen the shoe and taping of the toe to compress the joint and limit dorsiflexion motion all help reduce the pain. For grade III injuries, immobilization and a period of restricted weight bearing is usually required for up to 8 weeks.

Return to sport depends on the severity of the injury, resolution of symptoms, and an athlete's sport or position. Ideally, painless 60-degree dorsiflexion will be achieved in the first MTP joint before running or explosive activities are attempted.[12] Serial examinations are important because deformity can progress with athletic activity.[12]

Operative

Operative treatment is necessary in more severe injuries with joint instability, retraction of the sesamoids, diastasis of a bipartite sesamoid or sesamoid fracture, traumatic hallux valgus, or the presence of a loose body or chondral injury. Arthroscopy is helpful in evaluating the injury, but an open approach (plantar medial with extension across the MTP joint if required) is most helpful; however, care must be taken with the plantar-medial nerve. Repair of the plate distal to the sesamoid can be achieved with suture anchors into the base of the proximal phalanx. Care must be taken to avoid overtightening this repair. Similar techniques can be used for diastasis of a bipartite sesamoid.

AUTHORS' PREFERRED TECHNIQUE

Turf Toe

To approach the sesamoids, the patient is positioned supine with the heel positioned as distal as possible on the bed. Dual incisions are recommended to repair a grade III turf toe (Fig. 120-1). A longitudinal medial incision is centered at the first MTP joint to access the medial sesamoid. Care is taken during dissection to leave a cuff of joint capsule for closure at the conclusion of the case. The medial plantar digital nerve lies adjacent to the sesamoid and should be protected. A longitudinal plantar incision is commonly used for the lateral sesamoid. The lateral plantar digital nerve is at risk during this approach and must be identified and protected to prevent neuroma formation.

The plantar plate is then repaired from lateral to medial with use of nonabsorbable or slow-absorbing suture. Care must be taken to avoid damage to the flexor hallucis longus. In the absence of tissue along the proximal phalanx, use of a suture anchor to secure the plantar plate has been described. Fracture of both sesamoids should be treated with cerclage of the sesamoids to restore continuity of the FHB and avoid a cock-up toe deformity. If one of the two sesamoids has severe articular damage, excision can be performed. However, in no case should both sesamoids be excised. Standard closure should be performed.

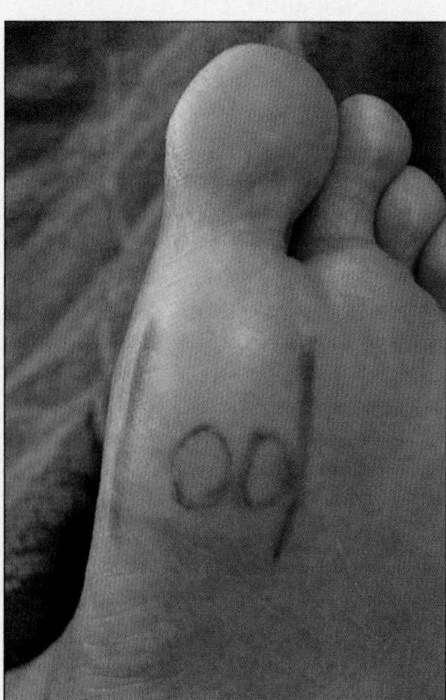

FIGURE 120-1 Dual incisions are required to repair a turf toe. Each individual incision can also be used for an isolated sesamoidectomy. Care must be taken to protect the plantar digital nerve during dissection. *(From Kadakia AR: Disorders of the hallucal sesamoids. In Miller MD, Sanders TC, editors:* Presentation, imaging and treatment of common musculoskeletal conditions, *Philadelphia, 2011, Elsevier.)*

Postoperative Management

Postoperative management must balance soft tissue healing with early range of motion of the MTP joint.[10] Immobilization in a removable splint (a toe spica splint in 5 to 10 degrees of plantar flexion with slight varus)[12] with restricted weight bearing continues for 4 weeks. Seven to 10 days after surgery, passive range of motion is begun. At 4 weeks, weight bearing and active range of motion are initiated in a walking boot. Wearing of modified footwear (i.e., a shoe with a stiff sole modified with a turf toe plate) is allowed at 8 weeks, with return to full sport at 3 to 4 months.

BOX 120-1 Classification of First Metatarsophalangeal Joint Injuries

GRADE 1: ACUTE SPRAIN OF THE FIRST MTP JOINT PLANTAR CAPSULE

Localized tenderness, swelling, and pain with dorsiflexion
Normal radiographs
Conservative treatment

GRADE 2: ACUTE SPRAIN OF THE FIRST MTP JOINT WITH SIGNIFICANT PLANTAR CAPSULE DISRUPTION

Ecchymosis, painful dorsiflexion, and loss of motion
Diastasis of a partite sesamoid or joint instability on radiographs
No degenerative first MTP joint changes
Conservative or surgical treatment

GRADE 3: CHRONIC SYMPTOMS INVOLVING THE FIRST MTP JOINT RESULTING FROM PREVIOUS INJURY

Loss of motion
Degenerative joint disease, hallux rigidus, or malalignment on radiograph
Treatment is often surgical

MTP, Metatarsophalangeal.

Results

Contrary to the common perception, evidence points to good outcomes when appropriate treatment is instigated. Most athletes with grade I and II injuries (53 of 56 in a series by Clanton et al.[1]) returned to sport within 3 weeks with careful conservative management. Even with grade III injuries, Anderson[10] found that seven of nine players returned to sport; two failed to resume playing because of pain and degeneration.

Complications

After a turf toe injury, athletes can experience persistent pain with toe-off and stiffness of the first MTP joint (Table 120-1). Instability, deformity, and degeneration can occur if the injury fails to heal well.

Sesamoid Dysfunction

The sesamoid complex of the first MTP joint plays a significant role in the function of the great toe (Box 120-2). Sesamoid dysfunction is uncommon; however, it can occur with arthritis,[13-17] trauma,[13,15,18-27] osteochondritis,[20,28-30] infection,[31-35] or sesamoiditis.[14,29,30,36] Abnormalities and complaints regarding the sesamoids of the hallux are much more common in professional athletes because of the stresses the first MTP joint is subjected to during athletic activities.[37,38] The medial sesamoid is more commonly injured than is the lateral sesamoid, because it bears greater force during normal gait.[39] The plantar lateral and plantar medial digital nerves are

TABLE 120-1

ANATOMIC CLASSIFICATION OF TURF TOE

ANDERSON CLASSIFICATION[92,93]		
Type of Injury	**Grade**	**Description**
Hyperextension (turf toe)	I	Stretching of plantar capsular ligamentous complex Localized tenderness, minimal swelling, minimal ecchymosis
	II	Partial tear of plantar capsular ligamentous complex Diffuse tenderness, moderate swelling, ecchymosis Restricted movement with pain
	III	Frank tear of the plantar capsular ligamentous complex Severe tenderness, marked swelling and ecchymosis Limited movement with pain, plus vertical Lachman test Possible associated injuries: Medial/lateral injury Sesamoid fracture/bipartite diastasis Articular cartilage/subchondral bone bruise
Hyperflexion (sand toe)		Hyperflexion injury to hallux MTP or IP joint May involve injury to lesser MTP joints as well
Dislocation	I	Dislocation of the hallux with the sesamoids No disruption of the intersesamoid ligament Frequently irreducible
	IIA	Associated disruption of the intersesamoid ligament Usually reducible
	IIB	Associated transverse fracture of one or both sesamoids Usually reducible
	IIC	Complete disruption of intersesamoid ligament with fracture of one of the sesamoids Usually reducible

IP, Interphalangeal; *MTP,* metatarsophalangeal.

located adjacent to the lateral and medial sesamoids. Impingement of either one of these branches may be a source of pain in the area of the sesamoids. Osteoarthritis of the sesamoids has been reported[13,14,16,17,28,40] in association with hallux valgus, hallux rigidus, and rheumatoid arthritis and as an isolated occurrence. When associated with a high-arched or cavus type of foot, a plantar-flexed first ray may be the cause of the callus formation. When a sesamoid is involved, a more localized or concentric lesion is usually present.

History

The most frequent subjective symptoms are pain and discomfort in the toe-off phase of gait located directly plantar to the sesamoids.

Physical Examination

A cavus foot or gastrocnemius contracture increase forefoot loading and therefore should be specifically assessed. A plantar keratosis beneath either the tibial or fibular sesamoid occasionally may accompany a symptomatic sesamoid. Another method to support the diagnosis of sesamoiditis is the use of the passive axial compression test.[41] The test is performed with the patient supine. After the sesamoids have been isolated, the hallux is maximally dorsiflexed at the MTP joint, which will cause distal migration of the sesamoids. The examiner's index finger is used to apply compression just proximal to the sesamoids. The patient's symptoms are reproduced with passive plantar flexion of the MTP joint, as the sesamoids are compressed against the metatarsal head and phalanx.

BOX 120-2 Sesamoid Function

- Protect the tendon of the flexor hallucis longus
- Absorb most of the weight bearing on the medial aspect of the forefoot
- Increase the mechanical advantage of intrinsic musculature of the hallux
- Elevate the first metatarsal head

Imaging

Often the most useful radiograph is the axial sesamoid view (Fig. 120-2). Fragmentation of a sesamoid in persons with osteochondritis may be seen on the axial radiograph. Radiographs are frequently normal despite subjective symptoms (sesamoiditis). MRI is one of the best methods for diagnosing disease of the sesamoids. Osteochondritis can be visualized very early, usually before any abnormality is seen on plain radiography. It is also useful in visualizing soft tissue abnormalities of the sesamoid mechanism.[42,43]

Decision-Making Principles

Most sesamoid problems in the athlete can be treated effectively without surgery. If conservative treatment has been unsuccessful, several surgical options are available depending on the pathologic condition. When considering surgical intervention, a concomitant deformity such as a gastrocnemius contractor or cavus foot alignment must be addressed.

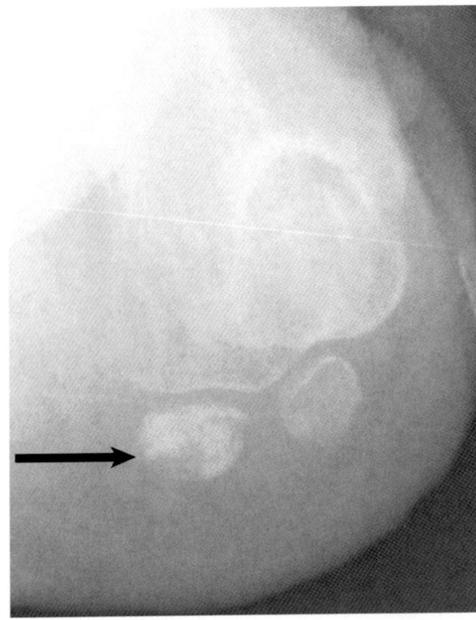

FIGURE 120-2 Sesamoid views allow visualization of the metatarsal-sesamoid articulation. This view clearly demonstrates sclerosis (*arrow*), flattening, arthritis, and fracture. *(From Kadakia AR: Disorders of the hallucal sesamoids. In Miller MD, Sanders TG, editors:* Presentation, imaging and treatment of common musculoskeletal conditions, *Philadelphia, 2011, Elsevier.)*

Treatment Options

Nonoperative

Activity and footwear modification, use of insoles, and treatment of the callosities are all helpful. In patients with sesamoid pain, a stiff insole or a rocker-bottom sole reduces metatarsal joint motion and can relieve pain with ambulation. The use of a dancer's pad, which is designed with a concavity for the sesamoids, is extremely useful in nearly all cases.

Operative

Surgical treatment includes a tibial or fibular sesamoidectomy, as well as sesamoid shaving. Excision of a single sesamoid does not usually lead to deformity as long as careful operative technique is used.[43] Removal of both tibial and fibular sesamoids is rarely indicated, because it predictably results in the development of a cock-up and intrinsic-minus deformity of the hallux. Arthrodesis of the MTP joint with excision of the sesamoid may alleviate arthritic symptoms and provides a stable medial buttress to the first ray, but it will severely compromise the function of an athlete. Although a sesamoidectomy is occasionally necessary for cases of intractable plantar keratosis (IPK), surgical shaving of the involved sesamoid may preserve function in the athlete and facilitate a more rapid recovery (Fig. 120-3).[42,43] Sesamoid shaving or resection in the presence of a plantar-flexed first ray is associated with a high rate of recurrence of the keratotic lesion.[44,45]

AUTHORS' PREFERRED TECHNIQUE

Sesamoid Dysfunction

Excision of the affected sesamoid with use of the previously described incisions is the treatment of choice, except in the case of an IPK. Care must be taken to avoid damage to the FHB and flexor hallucis longus. The soft tissue defect must be repaired to avoid iatrogenic deformity.

Postoperative Management

After sesamoid excision, a soft compression dressing is used, and the patient is allowed to ambulate in a postoperative shoe. Weight bearing on the heel is recommended to minimize soft tissue trauma to the forefoot and promote healing of the incision. Return to play after surgical intervention for sesamoid dysfunction is typically between 2 and 4 months after surgery. When shaving of the tibial sesamoid is performed, the athlete is allowed to resume running about 6 weeks after surgery.

Results

Sesamoidectomy has not been described as a treatment for acute fractures or nonfragmented nonunions of the sesamoids. However, it has been described for sesamoiditis. Saxena and Krisdakumtorn[46] reported a mean average return to activity between 7.5 to 12 weeks in 26 patients. Eleven professional/varsity athletes returned to sports at a mean of 7.5 weeks, whereas 13 "active" patients returned to sporting activity at a mean of 12 weeks.

Complications

Saxena and Krisdakumtorn[46] reported two cases of hallux valgus, one case of hallux varus, and two cases of postoperative scarring with neuroma-type symptoms in their series, representing a 19% complication rate. Transfer metatarsalgia may also occur.

Metatarsalgia

The term *metatarsalgia* is defined as pain of the plantar forefoot beneath the second, third, and fourth metatarsal heads.[47,48] It is an umbrella diagnosis incorporating many etiologic origins. Metatarsalgia can be subdivided into primary, secondary, and functional categories, along with pathologic conditions that arise during the stance and propulsive phases of gait.[48,49] The first ray bears 40% of the weight distribution of the forefoot, with the lesser four rays sharing the remaining 60%.[50] Bearing in mind that the first, fourth, and fifth metatarsal-tarsal articulations allow considerable flexibility compared with the more rigid second and third metatarsal-tarsal articulations,[51] any factor that lessens the ground force of the first metatarsal can increase the pressure applied to the lesser metatarsal heads. Metatarsal length discrepancy can similarly cause overload of one or more of the metatarsal heads. The most common pathology is the presence of an excessively long second metatarsal.[52] Hyperextension of the lesser toe MTP joint during gait can produce a dynamic plantar protrusion of the metatarsal head, as the toe is extending and the metatarsal head is forced plantarward.[48]

An IPK is a localized callosity occurring on the plantar aspect of the foot.[53] A generalized callus can develop in the forefoot of an athlete as a result of increased pressure, and it is normal for a moderate amount of callus to form; in contrast, an IPK is a well-localized keratotic lesion.

DiGiovanni et al.[54] studied a population of patients presenting with forefoot pain and found the incidence of

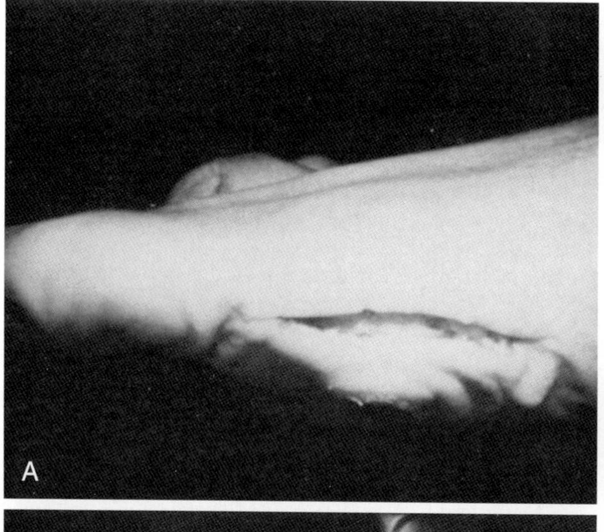

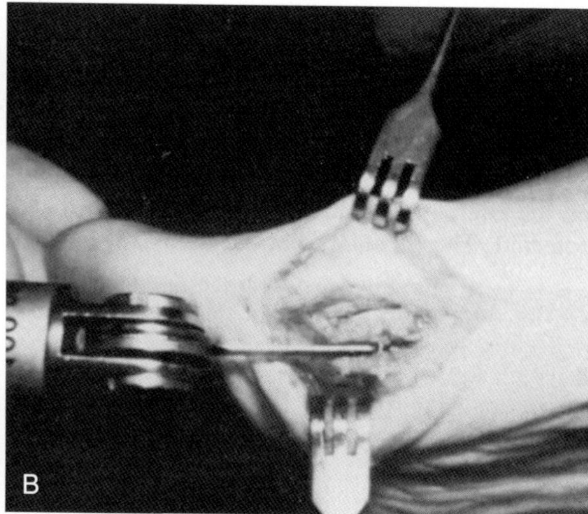

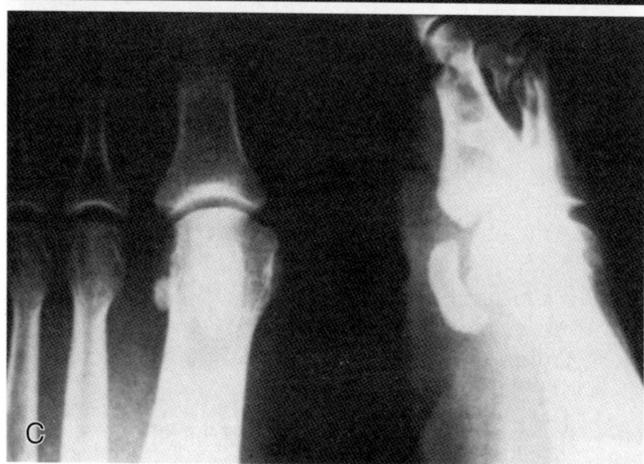

FIGURE 120-3 **A,** A plantar medial incision is used to expose the medial sesamoid for shaving. **B,** Half of the tibial sesamoid is shaved to treat an intractable plantar keratosis. Care is taken to protect the flexor halluces longus tendon. **C,** A radiograph after tibial shaving. *(Copyright M.J. Coughlin. Used with permission.)*

gastrocnemius contracture to be 65% (out of 34 patients). Many authors have emphasized the importance of gastrocnemius tightness in producing forefoot symptoms and the positive effect on the gait pattern when such tightness has been overcome.[55,56]

History

Barouk[57] emphasized the distinction between stance and propulsive metatarsalgia and advocated different treatments for these conditions. It is thus important to obtain a thorough history of the aggravating and relieving factors of the pain to try to discern between the two conditions. Athletes often report increased symptoms with specific activities or footwear. In persons with IPK, pain is usually directly under the callus.

Physical Examination

Physical examination first entails careful evaluation of the alignment of the foot when standing. The position of the hindfoot, the arch, and any great toe or lesser toe deformity should be noted. When a pes cavus deformity is suspected, a Coleman block test should be performed to determine if a fixed flexion deformity of the first metatarsal is present.[58]

The plantar aspect of the foot should be carefully evaluated, because the location of callosities can indicate the underlying problem. Stance-phase metatarsalgia generates proximal localized callosities or pain, whereas propulsive-phase metatarsalgia generates distal pain and a linear-type callosity.[57] Trimming of the callosity usually reveals a well-circumscribed keratotic lesion. Solitary keratotic lesions are sometimes difficult to distinguish from a wart; however, keratotic lesions occur directly under a bony prominence, and unlike warts, they are avascular.

A discrete IPK caused by a prominent metatarsal head lateral condyle can be seen on the lateral side of the metatarsal head, typically under the fourth metatarsal. Identification of this IPK is important because it is amenable to simpler surgical correction with a quicker rehabilitation and recovery and is a more predictable procedure than is a metatarsal osteotomy.

With suspected stance-phase metatarsalgia, the foot should be evaluated for abnormal plantar flexion of the lesser metatarsals. Elevation of the first metatarsal pushes the entire load of the second rocker onto the second metatarsal, resulting in isolated keratosis underneath the second metatarsal head.[48] Propulsive keratosis, however, occurs during the third rocker of the gait cycle when external rotation of the lower limb results in a shearing force. This produces a more rounded appearance of the callosity, which extends distally toward the toe.[48] Hypermobility of the first ray should be evaluated[59] along with midfoot mobility, because an unstable first ray can overload the lesser metatarsals.

Each MTP joint should be palpated to assess for position, synovitis, and joint stability. Each intermetatarsal web space should be palpated to assess for tenderness of the interdigital nerves. The Silfverskiöld test[60] is performed to evaluate for contracture of the gastrocnemius and the gastrocnemius-soleus complex; the foot is maintained in an inverted position to avoid dorsiflexion movements at the midtarsal joints.[48]

Imaging

Evaluation includes weight-bearing dorsoplantar and lateral views of the foot. Sesamoid views are included, depending on the location of the pain. The length of each metatarsal (MT) is assessed. Maestro et al.[52] described the "harmonic parabola" where in gait analysis studies they considered the lateral sesamoid of the first MTP joint as a pivot. They also emphasized the longitudinal axis of the second metatarsal, and the line passing through the center of the lateral sesamoid and bisecting a line perpendicular to the M2 longitudinal axis is termed the Maestro line.[49] This line must pass in through the center of the fourth metatarsal head to provide metatarsal harmony.

The slope of each MT and the difference in diaphyseal inclination between the first and second MT are assessed on the lateral view. Radiographic evaluation may contribute to the diagnosis of a subluxated or dislocated MTP joint. Careful attention is given to bony abnormalities that may be responsible for areas of increased pressure. If the IPK is large, then ultrasonography can be helpful, because dermoid inclusion cysts have been reported.[61]

An extended sesamoid view of the metatarsal heads end-on with the toes dorsiflexed out of the way is useful in identifying a prominent metatarsal head lateral condyle and abnormalities in the transverse arch.

Decision-Making Principles

If a keratotic lesion continues to be symptomatic and significantly impairs athletic function, surgical intervention is considered. Because of the lengthy postoperative recovery time and the possibility of restricted MTP motion, recurrence, or the development of a transfer lesion, a rigorous trial of trimming, padding, and orthotic management should be carried out before surgery is performed. Surgical release of a gastrocnemius contracture must be considered with great caution in athletes because a gastrocnemius recession may result in weakening of push-off. However, more recently, interest in performing a proximal medial gastrocnemius recession has increased. Abbassian et al.[62] have demonstrated that medial head release at the knee can be performed safely with use of a local anesthetic followed by immediate loading, and most importantly, the power loss is minimal. If all conservative efforts to treat metatarsalgia fail, then surgery is necessary. The goal of surgery is to distribute pressure evenly along the forefoot, thus reducing high-pressure areas. It is therefore essential to consider the clinical examination, pressure distribution, and x-ray evaluation to carefully plan a metatarsal osteotomy if this procedure is required. One should plan to correct metatarsal length to harmonize the parabola and elevate prominent heads to offload them.

Treatment Options

Nonoperative

The initial treatment of an IPK of any cause involves trimming the lesion to reduce the keratotic buildup. Trimming a callus also helps in differentiating it from a wart.

When the callus has been trimmed, a soft metatarsal pad is placed proximal to the keratosis to redistribute the pressure more uniformly. The use of a soft insole can alleviate the pressure further in athletes.[63] Athletic footwear should provide a wide toe box and a soft sole to lessen impact when running. A Plastazote orthosis can be fabricated to relieve pressure beneath the IPK and provide correction for a postural deformity.

Patients with tightness of the calf, be it gastrocnemius or the gastrocnemius-soleus complex, are taught stretching exercises to lengthen the muscles and thereby decrease pressure at the forefoot.

Operative

In all cases, the presence of a gastrocnemius contracture is treated with surgical release if the patient has persistent pain after engaging in a regimented nonoperative program (Fig. 120-4).

Mann and DuVries[64] proposed that a small, discrete, intractable plantar keratosis is caused by a prominent fibular condyle on the plantar aspect of the metatarsal head. DuVries[65] described a plantar condylectomy to correct this deformity. Mann and Mann recommend removal of 20% to 30% of the condyle through a dorsal incision.[66] This procedure was later modified by Mann and DuVries,[64] who performed an MTP arthroplasty, removing about 2 mm of the articular surface along with the plantar condylectomy. After MTP joint arthroplasty, MTP joint motion is diminished by 25% to 50%. Although stiffness does not always affect the function of a sedentary person, a competitive athlete typically requires more normal motion, and if so, an MTP arthroplasty is contraindicated.

Elevation of the metatarsal head can be achieved with use of a vertical chevron procedure.[64,67,68] A distal oblique osteotomy,[69-74] capital oblique (Weil) osteotomy,[48,49,75,76] and three-step (Maceira) osteotomy[48,77] are designed to both shorten the metatarsal and elevate the metatarsal head (Fig. 120-5). These procedures are best used in the treatment of propulsive-phase metatarsalgia. It is believed that elevation of about 3 mm is necessary for adequate decrease of pressure beneath the symptomatic metatarsal head.[78] Hansen[79] described midshaft segmental osteotomy in which two parallel cuts are made in the bone, which is subsequently fixed with a four-hole plate.

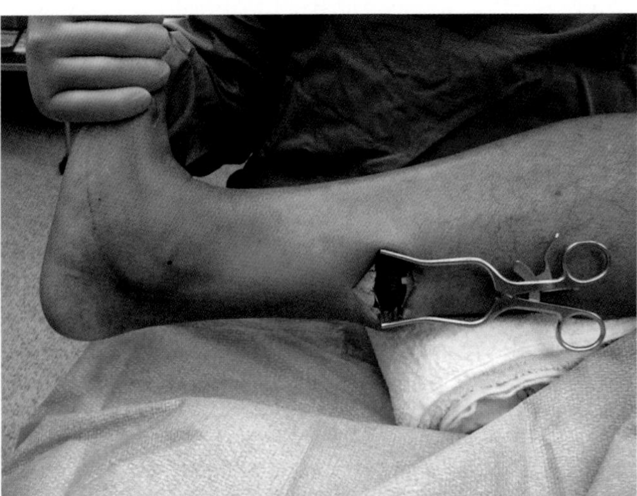

FIGURE 120-4 After release of the gastrocnemius fascia, improvement is noted in the dorsiflexion range of motion of the ankle with the knee extended.

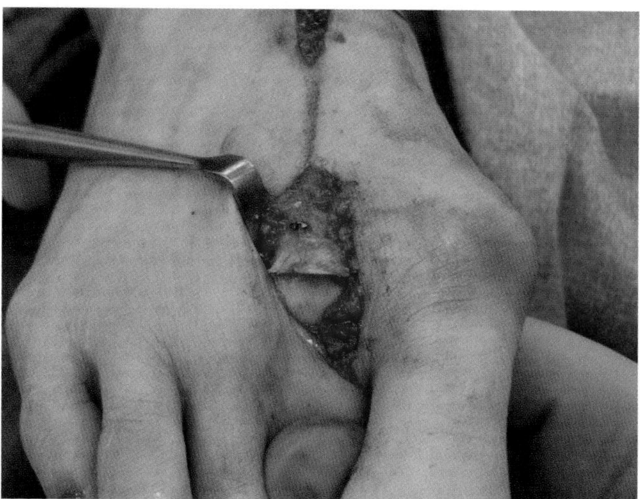

FIGURE 120-5 Intraoperative appearance of the metatarsal head after fixation with a 2.4-mm screw. Note the dorsal overhanging bone that must be removed to allow for appropriate articulation. *(From Seybold J, Kadakia AR: Claw and hammer toes. In Miller MD, Sanders TC, editors:* Presentation, imaging and treatment of common musculoskeletal conditions, *Philadelphia, 2011, Elsevier.)*

Galluch et al.[80] reported good results with this osteotomy in 95 patients. A 99.2% union rate was reported, and transfer lesions developed in five patients.

Postoperative Management

A compressive dressing is applied at the time of surgery, and the patient is allowed to bear weight in a postoperative shoe. After a metatarsal osteotomy, adequate time must be allowed for healing. Premature athletic activity may lead to failure of fixation, displacement of an osteotomy, or nonunion. In general, proximal metatarsal osteotomies require 6 to 12 weeks for osseous union to occur. A vertical chevron osteotomy, if performed with a thin oscillating saw blade, heals in about 6 weeks. After an MTP joint arthroplasty and condylectomy, about 6 weeks is necessary for adequate healing to occur at the MTP joint.

Once adequate healing has occurred (generally in 4 to 6 weeks), gentle range of motion is initiated at the MTP joint to diminish postoperative stiffness. When radiographs demonstrate bony union, aggressive walking activity is initiated. Taping of the forefoot or the use of soft metatarsal pads helps to alleviate symptoms with athletic activity during recovery from surgery. About 4 weeks after the initiation of walking, jogging is initiated, followed by running activities as pain permits.

Decreased range of motion is a significant risk after MTP arthroplasty, as well as after a distal metatarsal osteotomy. In the postoperative follow-up, one should pay close attention to any impending deformity or stiffness; it will be easier to start passive stretching or manipulation with use of a block or anesthetic earlier rather than later. In athletes, plantar flexion is very important. Full return to athletic activity is expected when bony healing occurs. Usually between 6 and 12 weeks after surgery, aggressive walking is initiated. Walking is advanced to jogging after 4 weeks as permitted by pain and swelling. The athlete then increases running activities as tolerated, gradually returning to sport between 3 and 6 months after surgery.

AUTHORS' PREFERRED METHOD

Metatarsalgia

When a competitive athlete requires a more normal motion, a distal metatarsal osteotomy is generally considered the osteotomy of choice. A number of osteotomies have been described in both treatment of stance-phase and propulsive-phase metatarsalgia, although distal osteotomies are generally used to treat propulsive metatarsalgia.

The distal metatarsal is approached dorsally, between the metatarsals if two are to be operated on. The collateral ligaments are released in order to release the plantar tissues in case of a hammer-toe deformity; if the toe is subluxed/dislocated, the plantar plate is likely to be torn and will require repair. The collateral ligaments may require reefing in case of coronal plane deformity. The most important step in a distal metatarsal osteotomy is to make the cut as parallel to the weight-bearing axis of the foot as possible to ensure that shortening does result in plantar flexion of the metatarsal head. Next, a parallel slice of the metatarsal is removed according to the amount of shortening/elevation that is required. This osteotomy is fixed with a screw and is performed under Image Intensifier control, assessing the metatarsal parabola (Fig. 120-6).

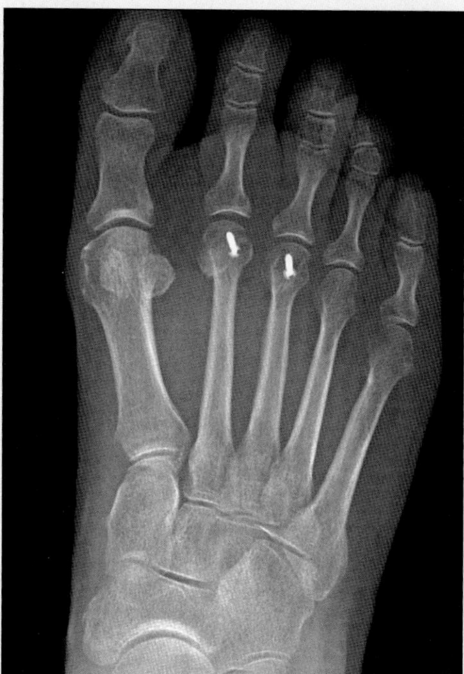

FIGURE 120-6 An anteroposterior radiograph of a patient after Weil osteotomy of the second and third toe. The normal cascade of the foot is preserved with the third toe slightly shorter than the second toe. Maintaining this cascade is critical to prevent iatrogenic metatarsalgia. *(From Seybold J, Kadakia AR: Claw and hammer toes. In Miller MD, Sanders TC, editors:* Presentation, imaging and treatment of common musculoskeletal conditions, *Philadelphia, 2011, Elsevier.)*

Results

In the treatment of an IPK, Winson and coworkers[74] found that 53% of the patients had significant postoperative symptoms, including transfer lesions in 32%, nonunion in 13%, and an overall recurrence of an IPK in 50% of patients. In 66 of the 124 feet, major postoperative complaints were noted. The authors stressed that in either a cavus or a rigid foot, a distal oblique sliding osteotomy was contraindicated.

In the treatment of propulsive stance metatarsalgia, the Weil-type or triple-step osteotomy is becoming the most accepted practice. Good to excellent long-term results have been noted in 70% to 100% of patients treated with a Weil-type osteotomy.[81-83] The three-step osteotomy was introduced to try to reduce complications observed with a Weil osteotomy. Espinosa et al.[48] reported that joint stiffness and floating toe deformities were rarely seen with this type of osteotomy. Pérez-Muñoz et al.[84] reported on 82 patients treated with a Weil or three-step osteotomy. They found recurrence of metatarsalgia in 4.3%, moderate joint stiffness in 60.2%, floating toes in 4.3%, and delays in bone healing in 7.5% of patients. All delayed unions occurred in the triple osteotomy group and were presumed to be a result of the decreased stability of the osteotomy.

Mann and DuVries[64] evaluated 100 patients with discrete IPKs and noted a recurrence rate of 17.6% after MTP arthroplasty. Of these recurrences, 5% were found under the symptomatic metatarsal. A transfer lesion developed in 13% of cases. Despite these results, 93% of the patients were satisfied with their outcome.

Complications

Complications reported with a Weil-type osteotomy include joint stiffness, floating-toe deformity, and transfer metatarsalgia. Stiffness may be caused by morphologic alterations of the MTP joint postoperatively, fibrosis, reaction to osteosynthesis material, or biomechanical alterations of the intrinsic musculature.[48,81,85] Beech et al.[76] noted that postoperative joint range of motion was reduced in most cases. Floating-toe deformity has been reported in up to 30% of cases.[86]

A 5% rate of complications was found after condylectomy and MTP arthroplasty for discrete IPK, which included fracture of the metatarsal head, avascular necrosis, drift of the involved toe, and cock-up of the involved toe.[86a]

Future Considerations

With further study of the effect of a gastrocnemius contracture on the incidence of forefoot pain, a shift away from bony correction of the foot pathology may occur if the outcomes are favorable. The morbidity from forefoot surgery as described is a major detriment to performing these operations in the athlete, and the possibility of a soft tissue correction without subsequent loss of athletic function would be very desirable.

Hallux Rigidus

History

Typical presenting symptoms of hallux rigidus are pain overlying the MTP joint from cartilage degeneration, possibly combined with mechanical shoe pain as a result of a dorsal bony prominence. The pain worsens over time with activity and typically improves with rest and elimination of restrictive footwear. Athletes will report a reduction in motion when crouching or during push-off. Once pain at night or at rest is noticed, the degeneration within the joint is generally widespread.

Examination

Hallux rigidus is a restriction of motion due to degenerative changes in the first MTP joint. The MTP joint may demonstrate a plantar-flexed position with a dorsal prominence (Fig. 120-7). Tenderness typically starts dorsolaterally on the joint line and is worse at the extremes of motion. With increased severity, the patient may have pain with the "grind test" in which the examiner impacts the phalanx on the first metatarsal head in the central range of motion. A positive test is consistent with end-stage arthritis, denoting that a simple cheilectomy will not be effective.

Imaging

Radiologic classification systems have been proposed but do not correlate well with clinical features. Narrowing of the joint, dorsal spurs from the metatarsal and phalanx, and loose body formation are common findings.

Decision-Making Principles

No reliable clinical classification systems have been developed for hallux rigidus. However, conservative measures must always be tried in the first instance for all athletes, and thus the real decision making lies in the choice between joint-sparing and joint-loss procedures. Clearly sporting requirements need to be considered, but some key clinical features will aid in the decision making. For instance, pain at night or at rest, crepitation upon passive motion, or a positive grind

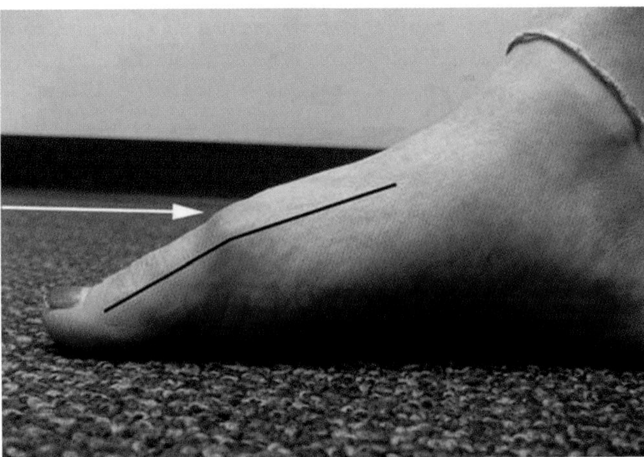

FIGURE 120-7 A patient with hallux rigidus with a fixed flexion deformity of the hallux. Note the large dorsal prominence (*arrow*). *(From Seybold J, Sabb B, Kadakia AR: Arthritides of the foot and ankle. In Miller MD, Sanders TG, editors:* Presentation, imaging and treatment of common musculoskeletal conditions, *Philadelphia, 2011, Elsevier.)*

test suggests a widespread problem that will not respond to a joint-sparing option and instead requires either fusion or a motion-sparing salvage procedure. Similarly, sesamoid pain will not be alleviated by an MTP cheilectomy. On the other hand, a smooth arc of motion (albeit reduced) and pain at end of range suggest that a cheilectomy is feasible.

The issue becomes difficult in cases of a failed cheilectomy or when the choice between cheilectomy and fusion is not clear-cut; in these cases, radiograph findings and visualization of the joint (arthroscopy is better than MRI) is helpful in determining whether the joint is salvageable.

Treatment Options

Nonoperative

Certain activities such as dancing or sprinting demand a high degree of dorsiflexion. These cases are difficult to manage conservatively other than to treat the patient with intraarticular corticosteroid injections and nonsteroidal antiinflammatory drugs. Because injections are likely to accelerate the wear within the joint, they must be used judiciously. The mainstay of conservative treatment is stabilization of the first MTP. Taping and orthotics can be very useful in pain control but, of course, reduces its motion.

Operative

Joint-sparing procedures should be performed for athletes if at all possible. If such procedures are not appropriate, joint-destructive but motion-sparing procedures (e.g., an osteotomy or interposition arthroplasty) should be considered; however, metallic or Silastic joint replacement has no role in the athlete. Ultimately, fusion surgery is a durable and long-term solution that allows robust activity.

Cheilectomy

A cheilectomy is the first line in surgical management. Impingement always starts dorsally and spreads downward, except in traumatic lesions, which start centrally; thus a cheilectomy is not appropriate for this group. Removal of the dorsal 25% of the joint and the osteophyte is very successful at removing the footwear irritation and the end-of-range impingement pain. It does not usually improve the range of motion, but it prolongs the athlete's career, even though it does not slow down the rate of progression (Fig. 120-8).

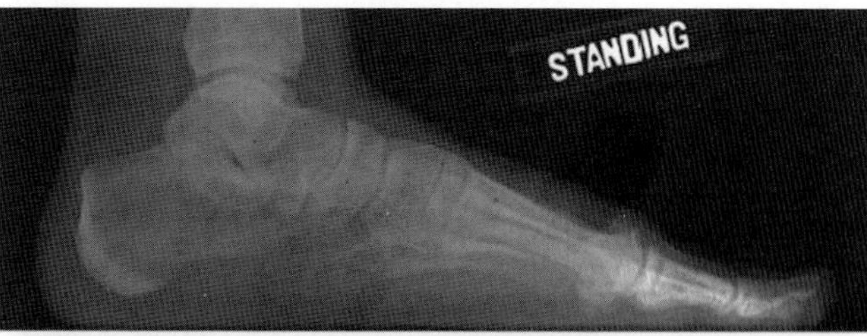

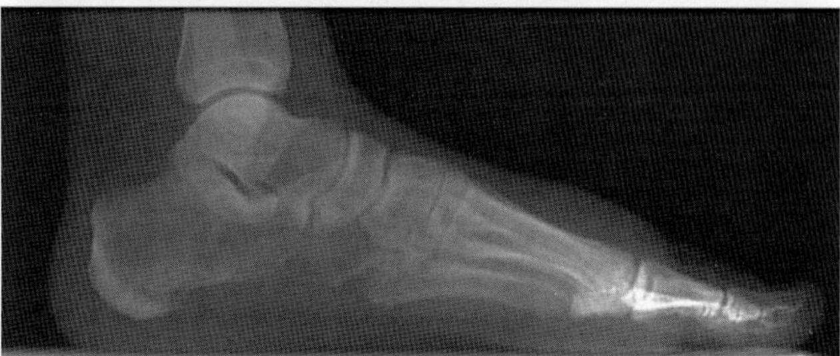

FIGURE 120-8 Preoperative and postoperative radiographs of a patient with grade II hallux rigidus who underwent a cheilectomy. The postoperative radiograph demonstrates removal of the dorsal osteophytes from both the metatarsal and the phalanx. The final appearance of the metatarsal reveals colinearity, with the metatarsal shaft indicating adequate bony resection. *(From Seybold J, Sabb B, Kadakia AR: Arthritides of the foot and ankle. In Miller MD, Sanders TG, editors:* Presentation, imaging and treatment of common musculoskeletal conditions*, Philadelphia, 2011, Elsevier.)*

Osteotomy

The Moberg procedure dorsiflexes the proximal phalanx, enabling greater movement through the third rocker before the MTP joint must engage, and thus it results in a functional increase in the dorsiflexion of the joint and can also decompress the joint.[87] A dorsal closing wedge is performed in combination with a cheilectomy; it is very stable and heals rapidly. If the joint has poor plantar flexion, then the toe may be too elevated, causing problems with footwear in stance. Rehabilitation is similar to that for a cheilectomy.

Two metatarsal osteotomies can be considered, especially in the athlete with advanced degeneration who runs. In the long or elevated metatarsal, a shortening/plantar-flexing osteotomy (the chevron type is the most stable) can be performed and is straightforward to plan, execute, and fix. If the metatarsal length is normal, then a dorsally rotating distal oblique osteotomy can be performed.

Motion-Sparing Procedures in Advanced Degeneration

Resection or interposition arthroplasty, although not joint sparing, can provide excellent pain relief while maintaining motion and may be preferable to arthrodesis in certain athletes for whom dorsiflexion is important, such as dancers or runners. Cosmesis may be poor with a short, elevated toe, but the range of movement may be excellent. A resection or Keller arthroplasty is not recommended in a young, active population, although the Valenti procedure, which resects the dorsal metatarsal head and dorsal phalangeal base and maintains length and plantar loading, can obviate some of these issues.[88]

MTP Arthrodesis

MTP arthrodesis remains the gold standard of pain relief and function[89]; although it comes at the cost of sacrificing any remaining movement, generally very little movement is left in persons with late-stage disease anyway. However, in athletes who require dorsiflexion or who have a short great toe, it should be used with caution. Care should also be taken in the person who has significant motion of the interphalangeal joint with uncovering of the phalangeal head and loading of the head. Loss of motion at the MTP joint will increase the loading on the phalangeal head in these cases, and this situation can be very difficult to manage.

The joint should be fused in 10 to 15 degrees of dorsiflexion to maximize the third rocker without setting the toe too high, in which case it may rub on the toe box (Fig. 120-9). Use of normal footwear can be resumed at 6 weeks after weight bearing on the heel in a protective shoe from the time of surgery. Participation in sports can generally be resumed 3 to 4 months after surgery. Nonunion mandates further surgery, but the rates with current implant techniques are very low.

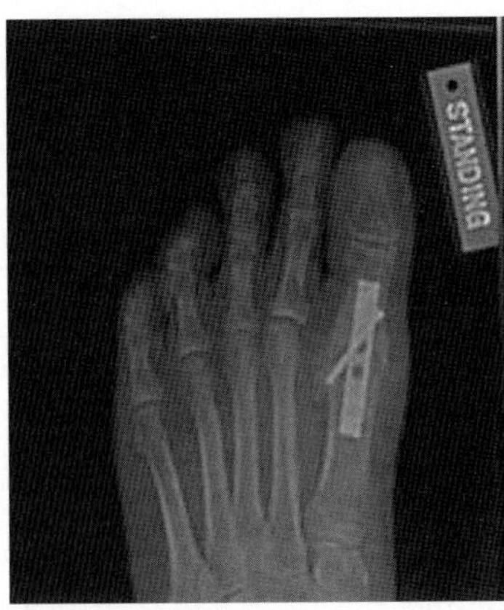

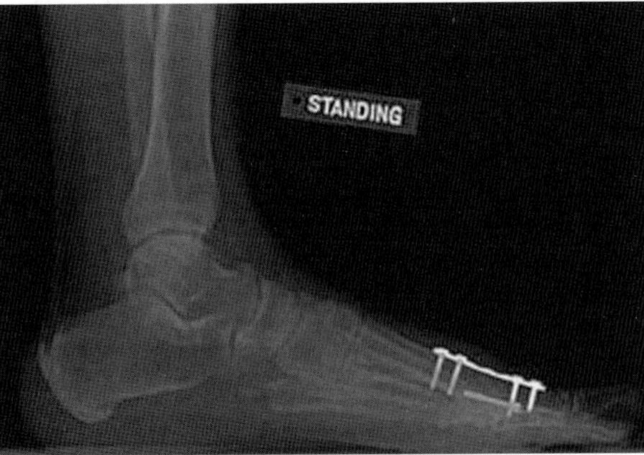

FIGURE 120-9 First metatarsophalangeal arthrodesis using a dorsal plate and lag screw for fixation. *(From Seybold J, Sabb B, Kadakia AR: Arthritides of the foot and ankle. In Miller MD, Sanders TC, editors:* Presentation, imaging and treatment of common musculoskeletal conditions, *Philadelphia, 2011, Elsevier.)*

AUTHORS' PREFERRED TECHNIQUE

Hallux Rigidus

Cheilectomy is the mainstay of treatment of the athlete. The joint is approached dorsally and the collaterals are released to allow full visualization; it is important to free up the sesamoids and plantar plate because they are frequently adherent to the underside and can restrict movement. After removal of the dorsal 25% of the head, it is refashioned to make it rounder and more congruent. One should attempt to achieve at least 80 degrees of dorsiflexion; if this degree of dorsiflexion is not achieved, consider a dorsiflexing osteotomy of the proximal phalanx (a Moberg osteotomy). Patients are able to bear weight and start gentle active motion immediately and can begin full rehabilitation once the wound has healed.

MTP fusion remains the gold standard in terms of pain relief and longevity, but if movement is important, our preferred motion-sparing option is the interposition arthroplasty.[90] A cushion of soft tissue is made from periosteum, attached fat, and tendon and stabilized by suturing to the plantar capsule. Alternatively, regenerative tissue matrix may be used as the interposition material. Implant arthroplasty has no role in the athletic population.

Results

In appropriate cases, cheilectomy has excellent outcomes, and rehabilitation is rapid. Approximately 70% of patients obtain excellent relief, 10% obtain modest relief, and 20% get no relief.[91] Microfracture of lesions below the level of the osteotomy or of isolated central lesions has an unreliable outcome.

Percutaneous and arthroscopic techniques appear to improve the rate of rehabilitation, but few data are as yet available on this subject. Arthroscopy allows visualization of the joint and therefore may be preferable. It is generally at least 8 weeks before running sports can be commenced, although cycling and swimming can be commenced earlier. It takes 3 to 4 months to achieve maximum outcome.

Complications

A cheilectomy can work very well, even in persons with radiologically advanced disease. However, a significant number of patients will have ongoing pain and stiffness that can limit participation in sports, and a small number may have significant arthrofibrosis that can prevent return to sport. This group is best served with revision to a fusion, although a course of intraarticular steroids may be of some benefit.

Outcomes from fusion are reliable with modern fixation techniques. Shortening of the big toe can cause rubbing on the end of the second toe, but this problem can be readily treated. A more difficult issue is the case with painful loading on the proximal phalangeal head, which occasionally requires conversion of a fused MTP joint into an interposition arthroplasty.

For a complete list of references, go to expertconsult.com.

Suggested Readings

Citation: Anderson RB: Turf toe injuries of the hallux metatarsophalangeal joint. *Tech Foot Ankle Surg* 1(2):102–111, 2002.
Level of Evidence: III
Summary: The author provides an excellent review of turf toe injuries combined with an algorithm of treatment from the surgeon's extensive experience.

Citation: Kadakia AR, Molloy A: Current concepts review: Traumatic disorders of the first metatarsophalangeal joint and sesamoid complex. *Foot Ankle Int* 32(8):834–839, 2011.
Level of Evidence: II
Summary: The authors provide a comprehensive review regarding the diagnosis and treatment of injuries to the metatarsophalangeal (MTP) joint and sesamoids. The review covers the current level of evidence and grades of recommendation for the treatment of first MTP capsuloligamentous injury and sesamoid pathology.

Citation: Barske HL, DiGiovanni BF, Douglass M, et al: Current concepts review: Isolated gastrocnemius contracture and gastrocnemius recession. *Foot Ankle Int* 33(10):915–921, 2012.
Level of Evidence: III
Summary: In this topical review, the authors define a gastrocnemius contracture, outline its impact on foot and ankle pathology, and review the potential role of an isolated gastrocnemius recession as treatment for select disorders.

Citation: Mann RA, Mann JA: Keratotic disorders of the plantar skin. *J Bone Joint Surg Am* 85(5):938–955, 2003.
Level of Evidence: III
Summary: The authors of this excellent review cover the possible etiologies and how to address the specific pathologic condition accordingly.

Citation: Seibert NR, Kadakia AR: Surgical management of hallux rigidus: Cheilectomy and osteotomy (phalanx and metatarsal). *Foot Ankle Clin* 14(1):9–22, 2009.
Level of Evidence: III
Summary: The authors provide a comprehensive review regarding hallux rigidus with a focus on joint-sparing procedures. The technique and results of multiple operations are discussed.

SECTION 9

Spine and Head

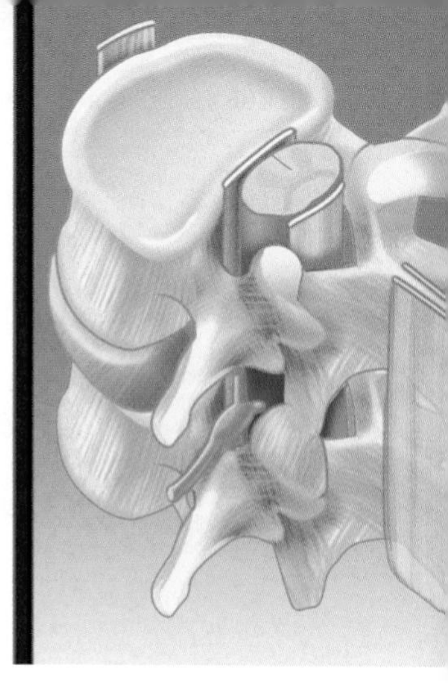

121

Head and Spine Anatomy and Biomechanics

NICOLAS V. JAUMARD • PETER P. SYRÉ • WILLIAM C. WELCH • BETH A. WINKELSTEIN

Despite technical advancements in protective gear and advocacy and enforcement of safety measures, sports and recreational activities still present risks for spinal and head injuries, particularly at the elite level of competition. Accidents that result in trauma of the spine or head can have dire physical, intellectual, and mental consequences because these structures consist of hard and soft tissues, including the central nervous system, with very complex interconnections at the macroscopic to cellular scales. A brief review of the relevant anatomy of the head and spine is presented in this chapter, highlighting important hard and soft tissues in the context of injury. The normal and pathologic biomechanics are then reviewed to provide a context for injury and treatment. A summary section integrates all these concepts.

Anatomy

The head and spine are both supportive anatomic structures that protect the brain, spinal cord, and nerve roots. Despite being adapted to human activities, these two complex anatomic bony structures remain susceptible to injury or trauma. Particularly during physical activities, spinal and head injuries present potentially debilitating consequences because of the intimate relationship of these hard tissues with the softer neural tissues they protect. Nonetheless, the hard tissues (i.e., the skull and vertebrae) and the soft tissues (i.e., the brain, ligaments, intervertebral disks, facet joint cartilage, muscles, and neural elements) can be damaged by nonphysiologic or repeated physiologic loading during athletic activities. Here we provide a brief overview of the relevant anatomic features of each tissue type to lay the foundation for a later discussion of the biomechanics of injury of these tissue types and considerations regarding their diagnosis, treatment, and management.

Skull (Cranium)

The skull is composed of 22 bones, including eight that surround and protect the brain; the other 14 bones make up the facial structures of the head. In adults, the skull bones are fused together by sutures that form a rigid structure. One exception is the mandible, which permits the opening and closing of the mouth via the temporomandibular joints. The eight bones that form the cranium include the frontal, parietal, temporal, and occipital (occiput) bones. The parietal bones join in the midsagittal plane to form the sides and roof of the cranium. The temporal bones make up the lower sides of the cranium, and the occipital bone completes the dorsal and posterior sides of the head (Fig. 121-1).

Spine

The cranium is connected to and supported by the spine, which is composed of 33 vertebrae. The spine contains five similar but distinct regions: (1) cervical, (2) thoracic, (3) lumbar, (4) sacral, and (5) coccygeal (Fig. 121-1, *A*). In the cervical, thoracic, and lumbar regions, adjacent vertebrae are connected by the intervertebral disc anteriorly and the facet joints ligaments and other connective tissues laterally and posteriorly (Fig. 121-1, *B*). The vertebrae in these spinal regions exhibit the same general structure with only slight variations in anatomy and size (see Fig. 121-1, *A*). Each of the sacral and coccygeal regions contains three to five fused vertebrae (see Fig. 121-1, *A*). Here we specifically focus on the cervical spine anatomy because it is the most flexible and thus the most prone to injury, and these injuries present potentially life-threatening consequences.

The cervical spine contains seven vertebrae that together create a lordotic curve (see Fig. 121-1, *A*). Each vertebra consists of an anterior vertebral body, transverse processes, and laminae that constitute the posterior neural arch (see Fig. 121-1, *B*). In the upper cervical spine, the first vertebra (C1; atlas) has only a bony ring with no vertebral body; the atlas encircles the dens of the second cervical vertebra as it protrudes rostrally from the vertebral body of C2 (axis). The atlas articulates with the occiput via a pair of bilateral synovial condylar joints. In the subaxial spine, intervertebral discs connect the vertebral bodies of adjacent vertebrae and provide support for axially directed loads.[1,2] The superior and inferior faces of the vertebral bodies articulate posterolaterally via the saddle-shaped joints of Luschka. The transverse processes are bony prominences that protrude laterally from the vertebral body. At each cervical level the bilateral facet (zygapophyseal) joints are positioned symmetrically in the posterolateral region of the vertebra and provide additional axial support for the transfer of loads applied to the spine; because of their oblique orientation, these joints also couple lateral bending and torsional motions (see Fig. 121-1, *B*). The facet joints are diarthrodial synovial joints with cartilage covering the surfaces of the opposing articular pillars, a synovial membrane that lines

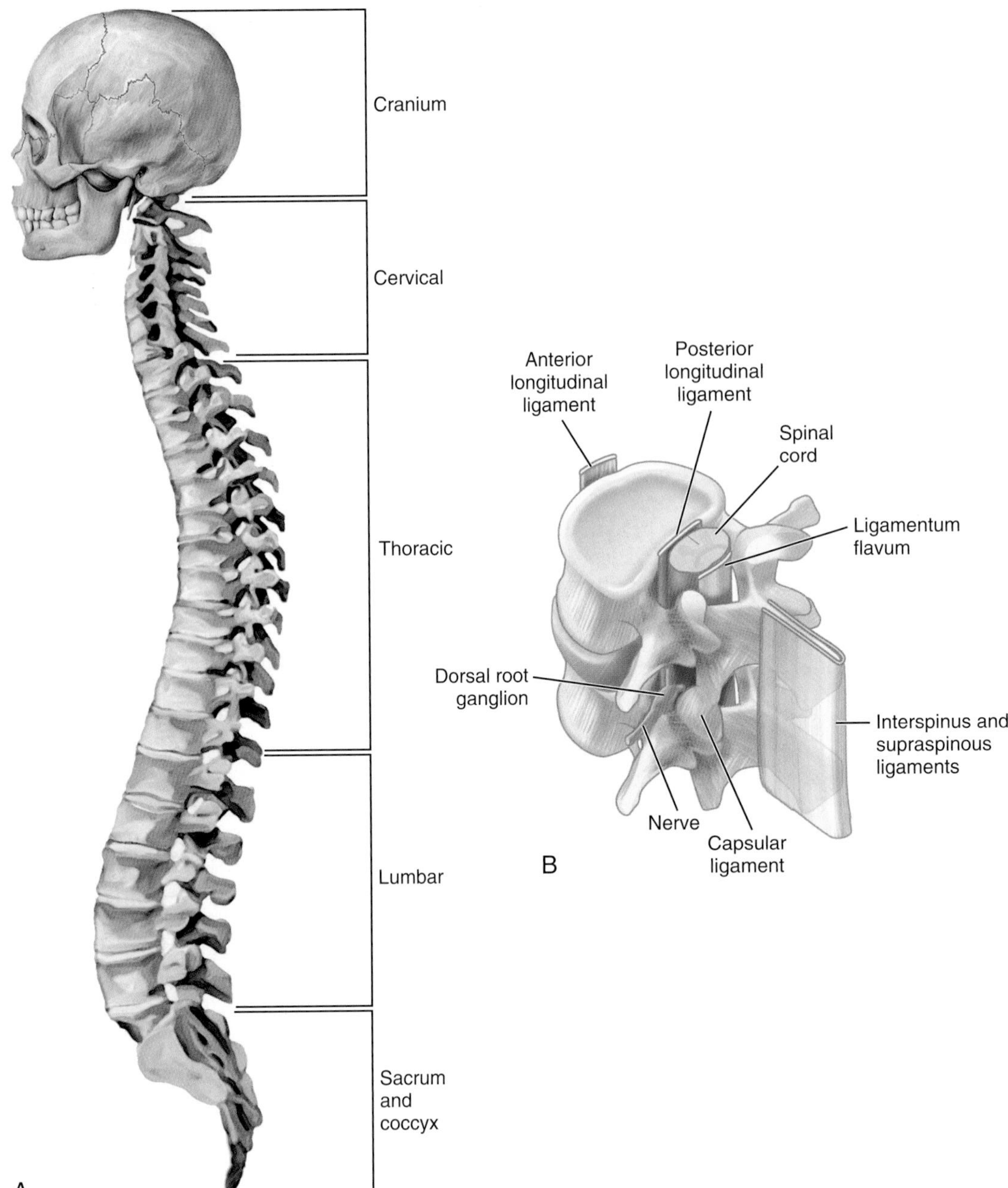

FIGURE 121-1 **A,** The left lateral view of the skull and spine. **B,** A detailed view of a spinal segment consisting of two vertebrae and their intervertebral disk, ligaments, and neural tissues.

the inside of the joint and maintains lubrication, and a ligamentous capsule that loosely envelops the entire joint.[3-6] Collectively, the facet joints and intervertebral disk provide mechanical stability across each segment and between vertebrae and guide spinal motions. In the lower cervical spine, the vertebral artery enters the transverse foramen at the C6 level and travels in the transverse processes to supply blood to the head, brain, and cervical tissues.

The thoracic spine is kyphotic, with 12 vertebrae; the lumbar spine is lordotic, with only five vertebrae (see Fig. 121-1, *A*). In these spinal regions the inferior and superior faces of the vertebral body are flatter and the transverse processes are more posterior and elongated than in the cervical spine. Ribs articulate with the lateral processes in the thoracic spine. In the lumbar region, the lateral processes are the longest and are positioned at the junction between the lamina and the vertebral body. The articular pillars are more posterior than in the cervical spine and are integrated within the laminae in the thoracic and lumbar spine regions. Also, the facet joints present a less coronal orientation and have a sagittal inclination that increases caudally to orientate the facet almost vertically in the lumbar region. It is important to note that anatomic variations will be found in approximately 10% of otherwise "normal" lumbar spines. These variations include segmentation abnormalities (lumbarized S1 or sacralized L5 vertebral bodies), spina bifida occulta (congenital partial or complete absence of lamina), pars interarticularis defects, and others.

Brain

Protected by the cranium, the brain contains 80 to 120 billion neurons that have connections limited to the brain itself and that also connect with neurons that extend caudally to become the spinal cord.[7-9] Collectively the brain, spinal cord, and nerve roots comprise the central nervous system. The brain is suspended in cerebrospinal fluid and has nearly symmetrical right and left hemispheres organized in four lobes (frontal, parietal, occipital, and temporal). The cerebellum lies in the posterior-central region of the brain and is connected to the brainstem along with the two hemispheres. Although the brain is mechanically protected by the thick bones of the skull, it is susceptible to physical damage from direct impact to and inertial loading of the head. Blows to the head can lead to brain tissue degeneration and long-term brain dysfunctions associated with psychiatric conditions.[10-13] Certainly, concussion is a common sports-related injury receiving increasing attention with its rising incidence in football, hockey, and other contact sports.[14-16] For instance, traumatic brain injury (TBI) comprised 5.1% of all the reported sports- and recreation-related injuries between 2001 and 2005, although estimates suggest that mild cases of TBI, which often are unreported, are 10 times more common than are severe cases of TBI.[14,15] Concussions are induced by contact and/or inertial forces exerted onto the human body. Such biomechanical forces produce linear and/or rotational accelerations of the head and cervical spine that are transmitted to the brain, where the resulting strains can produce damage in different zones. For instance, acceleration/deceleration in the anteroposterior direction and dynamic rotation in the sagittal plane are associated with frontal/occipital hemorrhage.[17] Although lateral rotations are associated with temporal lobe hemorrhages, they may also produce axonal shearing.[17] The strains induced by pressure gradients and shear forces in brain tissue can lead to a host of complex neuropathologic processes. Although 80% to 90% of the short-term neurologic impairment caused by concussion, such as loss of consciousness, resolves within the first 7 to 10 days, some athletes experience long-term physical, behavioral, neuropsychological, and personality changes.[16,18] The mechanical etiology of concussion and brain injury, as well as their neurologic consequences, are complex, and some aspects remain to be elucidated as discussed in a later chapter.

Intervertebral Disk

The intervertebral disk is the largest avascular and aneural structure in the body and connects with its adjacent vertebral bodies via a cartilaginous endplate through which it receives nutrients by diffusion. The normal disk is an ellipse-shaped tissue composed of water and proteins such as collagen, proteoglycans, and glycosaminoglycans.[19-24] Macroscopically it has two substructures, the anulus fibrosus and the nucleus pulposus. The anulus is a ring of concentric layers of crimped type I collagen fibers oriented 30 to 70 degrees from horizontal in an alternating pattern between adjacent layers.[19-22,25-29] Free nociceptive nerve terminals innervate in the outer third of the cervical anulus fibrosus, which supports its potential for pain generation under certain conditions when the outer layers of the disk become strained. The nucleus is an incompressible mucopolysaccharide gel rich in type II collagen fibers and proteoglycans that permit its hydration of up to 90%.[20,28] The gelatinous nucleus is surrounded by the anulus to confer upon the intervertebral disk the ability to absorb shock and to distribute and transfer compressive loads when applied to the spine.[30-34] As the disk degenerates, the water content is lost and annular fissuring occurs.[35,36] Generally these degenerative changes occur initially in the lower cervical and lumbar areas.

Ligaments

In addition to the disk, adjacent vertebrae are also connected by several ligaments. The seven main spinal ligaments are the anterior and posterior longitudinal, flaval, interspinous, supraspinous, and the two bilateral capsular ligaments (see Fig. 121-1, *B*). In the upper cervical spine, the transverse, apical, alar, and accessory ligaments also provide connectivity between the occiput, atlas, and axis. All of these ligaments are richly innervated and provide proprioceptive feedback about the head and neck position, as well as stabilize the neck during normal head and neck motions.[37,38] Because of the mechanical demands on the spinal ligaments, their importance for stability, and their innervation, these tissues are very important in sports medicine applications. However, a comprehensive review of the anatomy and biomechanics of the individual ligaments of the spine is beyond the scope of this chapter, and ligamentous injury and strain are covered elsewhere in this edition.

Muscles

The muscles of the spine are incredibly complicated, and a relevant review spans several length scales, from muscle to fiber to sarcomere. Again, a complete review is provided elsewhere, with a particular focus on injury. Several layers of muscles surround the bony spine, with anterior and posterior contributors to maintain head stability and facilitate coordinated motions. Eighteen, five, and eight major muscles are associated with the cervical, thoracic, and lumbar regions, respectively. Depending on their bony attachments and their length, these muscles activate to rotate, extend, and flex the spine forward or laterally.[39,40] They have relevance to biomechanics and injury in that their responses in the injury scenario can present extenuating factors for the clinician, both on the field and in the hospital setting.

Neurologic Tissues

The spine supports and protects the spinal cord and its exiting/entering spinal nerve roots. The spinal cord contains the neurons and associated supporting cells.[41] The spinal canal is formed anteriorly by the vertebral bodies and posteriorly by the laminae, from the lower half of the brainstem (medulla oblongata) to the first lumbar vertebra. In the lumbar spinal canal, nerve roots extend caudally within the canal from the end of the spinal cord between T12 and L2, forming the cauda equina, which extends caudally to the S5 level. Three membranes surround the spinal cord; these meninges are the pia mater, arachnoid, and dura mater, and they enclose the cerebrospinal fluid that bathes the spinal cord. Anterior and posterior nerve roots extend bilaterally from the spinal cord at each vertebral level. These roots exit the spinal canal through lateral neural foramina anterior to the facet joints (see Fig. 121-1, *B*). The cell bodies of the dorsal nerve root are contained in a dorsal root ganglion (DRG). This anatomic structure is usually located within, and protected by, the neural foramen. In the sacral area, the DRGs may lie completely outside of the neural foramen. The DRGs are vulnerable to trauma and are quite sensitive to mechanical loading.[42] Spinal nerves innervate both spinal and peripheral tissues. For instance, medial branches of the dorsal primary ramus from both the superior and inferior adjacent levels innervate the facet joint.[43]

Biomechanics

The relative motions of the various articulating structures of the spine relate to the loads experienced by the entire spine; in addition, the loads experienced by the individual spinal tissues vary with the spinal motions. Because of the interindividual variability in head and spine structures, the biomechanics of these structures depend on several factors, including the magnitude and direction of the applied loads, the rate of loading, the duration and location of the loads, the position of the head and spine at the time of loading, and the material and constitutive properties of the individual tissues.[39] Nevertheless, many biomechanical studies have been performed in vivo and with use of cadaveric spines from humans and other species and computational studies using computer models. Collectively, these investigations have provided a detailed understanding of spine biomechanics in both the normal and injured conditions. Here we review both conditions to provide a context for physiologic function and how it is altered during and after injury. We conclude this section with a discussion integrating both of these perspectives to provide a context for the following chapter.

Normal/Physiologic Biomechanics

The upper cervical spine exhibits unique biomechanics that distinguish it from the remainder of the cervical spine. Furthermore, because of differences in the anatomy between the spinal regions, differences also exist in the biomechanical responses between spinal regions, both at the segmental level and across the spinal region as a structure.[44,45] The occipital-axial complex can rotate up to 50 degrees in flexion-extension and up to 90 degrees in axial torsion, which corresponds to 50% of the motion of the entire cervical spine in each of these directions.[46-48] However, lateral bending in the upper cervical spine is limited to ±10 degrees,[49] whereas it ranges from 20 to 45 degrees for the cervical spine as a whole.[46,47]

Despite anatomic differences, the general biomechanical responses of the subaxial (C2-C7) cervical, thoracic, and lumbar regions are similar. The intervertebral disk, ligaments, and bilateral facet joints limit and guide the relative motions of adjacent vertebrae, which leads to highly nonlinear load-displacement relationships (Fig. 121-2).[50] These relationships are characterized by curves featuring two main zones, the neutral zone and the elastic zone. These two zones together constitute the range of motion (ROM) of a vertebral segment (see Fig. 121-2).[50] In the neutral zone, the vertebral motion segment is highly flexible, permitting a great amount of motion for very small applied loads. In the elastic zone, the spinal tissues begin to individually engage and undergo

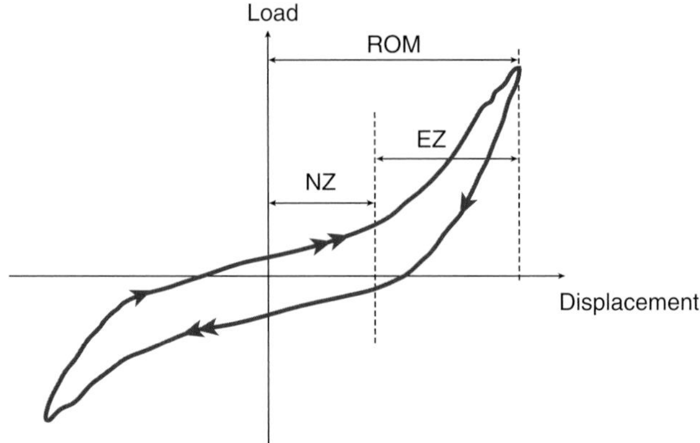

FIGURE 121-2 A representative load-displacement curve for a motion segment showing the nonlinear relationship between the segmental displacement (translation or rotation) and load (force or moment) generated. The difference between the loading (*double arrow*) and unloading (*single arrow*) indicates hysteresis. The elastic (*EZ*) and neutral (*NZ*) zones are defined and together comprise the total range of motion (*ROM*).

loading, with increasing stiffness as load increases. Such a stiffening behavior results from the viscoelastic properties of the intervertebral disk and of the ligaments as they deform inhomogeneously and nonlinearly with an applied load. The disk absorbs and distributes a compressive load and is mechanically comparable to a spring in parallel with a viscous damper (Fig. 121-3). Ligaments are like cables and can only resist tensile loading; as such, the posterior spinal ligaments tighten during spinal flexion and the anterior ligaments tighten during extension. These tissues are mechanically analogous to springs (see Fig. 121-3). The cervical neural arch and the facet joints also transfer and support 3% to 25% of a compressive load and limit the motion between adjacent vertebrae, especially in the extremes of extension and anterior translation.[1,51,52] Although the orientation of the cervical facet joints with respect to both the coronal and sagittal planes increase moving caudally,[49] the ROM in the subaxial cervical spine is similar at each level, ranging from 4 to 23 degrees in human voluntary and cadaveric studies of sagittal bending.[53,54]

In addition, vertebral rotations and motions about certain axes of the spine also induce simultaneous rotations and motions about another axis; this "coupling" is most extreme in the cervical spine.[51,55] Coupling occurs at all cervical levels but is particularly significant at the atlantoaxial junction.[47] For instance, extension is coupled with axial rotation in the C1-C2 joint,[56] and the ratios of lateral-to-axial and axial-to-lateral rotations range from 0.225 to 0.565 in the cervical spine.[53]

Injury

The hard and soft tissues of the spine are particularly susceptible to local damage and more widespread spinal injury when the tissue material and mechanical properties are reduced because of age, degeneration, or prior trauma. The vertebral bodies can bear compressive forces of up to 1700 N, 4000 N, and 8000 N in the cervical, thoracic, and lumbar regions, respectively.[47] Not surprisingly, the lumbar vertebrae, which are required to sustain more of the body's weight, can support a greater axial load. Because of the different loading patterns

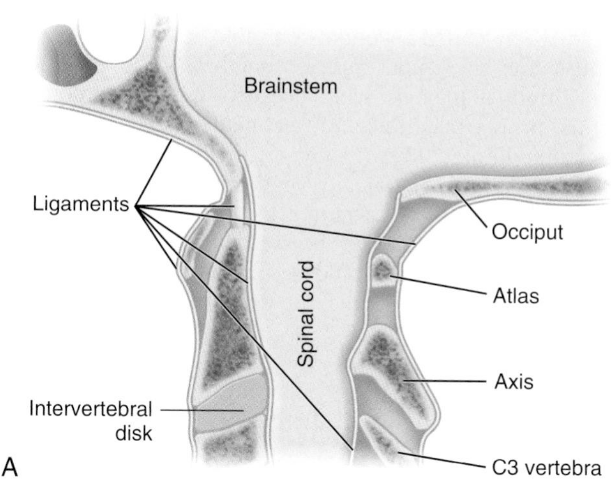

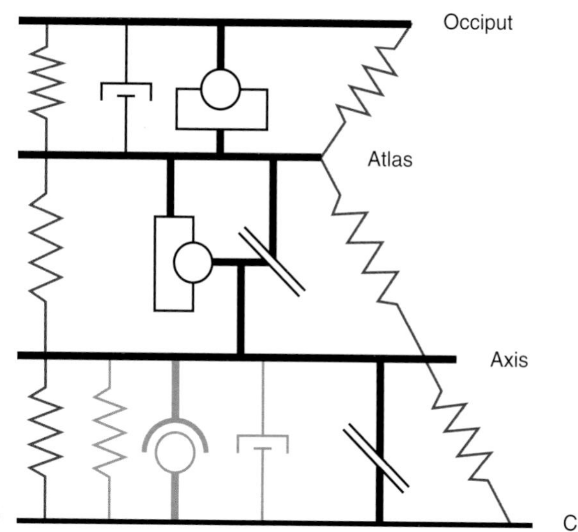

FIGURE 121-3 The major anatomic tissues of the upper cervical spine (**A**) and the matching mechanical analogues for biomechanical modeling using a free-body diagram (**B**). A ligament can be modeled by a spring and a disk by a spring and dashpot.

and vertebral structures, the spinal ligaments also exhibit a wide range of failure strengths that range from 76 to 436 N in the upper cervical spine, with the cruciate, alar, and anterior longitudinal ligaments being the strongest.[47] In the subaxial cervical spine, the capsular ligament and ligamentum flavum are the strongest, with failure strengths ranging between 47 to 264 N.[47] The anterior and posterior longitudinal ligaments in the lumbar spine are the strongest, with failure strengths reported from 100 to 510 N.[47] Similarly, the maximum compressive load that the intervertebral disk can withstand also increases from the cervical to lumbar spines: 74 N, 1800 N, and 5300 N in the cervical, thoracic, and lumbar regions, respectively.[47] Intervertebral disks are weaker in shear and can only resist shear loads of 20 N in the cervical spine and 150 N in the thoracic region.[47] Without protection from the facet joints, the intervertebral disks can only resist 1.8 Nm and 31 Nm of torsion in the cervical and lumbar spines, respectively.[47] Loading beyond any of these limits exceeds the tissue's tolerance and has the potential to produce injury and/or tissue damage. Moreover, it is important to recognize that muscle activation stabilizes the spine and helps protect it from excessive motion but can also produce loading to individual ligaments beyond their threshold for injury.[57,58] Also, the rib cage may afford the thoracic spine increased resistance to pathologic loading by providing increased biomechanical stability.[47]

Despite having the ability to adapt their mechanical properties, the anatomic structures of the spine can fail when mechanical loading becomes nonphysiologic. Injurious loads can result from a variety of scenarios: the combination of different loads, the application of physiologic loads in extreme spinal positions, and/or even from repetitive loading (fatigue) within the normal range.[55,59-61] The ensuing structural failures of the vertebrae, disk, and/or ligaments depends on the magnitude of the loads, their direction, and the rate of loading. For instance, the normally lordotic cervical spine dissipates axial compressive load through bending, but a straightened cervical spine, which can occur with a wide variety of head positions during athletic activities, can buckle and place individual vertebral segments in hyperflexion or hyperextension.[62,63] These extreme spinal deformations (i.e., hyperflexion and hyperextension) increase the risk of ligament tearing, facet joint subluxation, and/or fracture, even though the head and neck may not appear to be moving.[44,51] Other examples of this phenomenon are the injuries sustained by quarterbacks or rugby players when they are sacked from behind. At a high rate of loading, the instantaneous axis of rotation of a vertebra relative to its subadjacent vertebra moves upward into the top moving vertebra from its normal location during physiologic motions under the intervertebral disk. As a consequence, the inferior facets of the superior vertebra have an impact on the superior facets of the inferior vertebra instead of gliding posteriorly on them.[44,64] Such an extreme compression can produce facet joint hemarthrosis, cartilage fissures, and even facet fracture.[65,66]

Generally, disk and ligamentous injuries are not all fatal and do not completely destabilize the spine. For instance, in a cadaveric study, both the ROM and neutral zone have been shown to significantly increase by 50% to 60% in flexion after transection of the spinal ligaments (except the posterior longitudinal ligament) at the C5-C6 level.[67] In contrast, an annular cut of the C5-C6 intervertebral disc does not destabilize the segment until after facet capsule transection.[67] Similarly, a unilateral locked C5-C6 facet joint reduces segmental ROM by up to 3.6 degrees in all directions except ipsilateral torsion.[68]

Major damage and failure of the osseous and ligamentous spinal tissues can result in serious neurologic pathologies.[69,70] Because the spinal cord and neural elements are no longer protected in such cases, they can be subjected to injurious loading (e.g., pinching and shearing) by the surrounding tissues. However, undetectable and undetected structural failures of tissue can also occur and can lead to acute and chronic neurologic pathologies. Minor tissue damage can render the spine unstable and lead to nonphysiologic loading of the neurologic tissues in particular locations. For instance, subfailure stretching of the cervical capsular ligament in experimental in-vivo animal studies has been shown to produce microstructural collagen fiber realignment and laxity that can lead to central sensitization.[71,72] In addition, neurologic and vascular tissues can be loaded under nonphysiologic conditions even when the soft tissues of the spine only sustain minor damage. For instance, a transient reduction of the spinal canal diameter is induced by altered vertebral kinematics during high loading rates and can lead to spinal cord contusion.[44]

Integration of Biomechanical Considerations for Treatment

Despite decades of research, the biomechanics of the spine are still not fully understood, particularly in the context of sports injury. Although the mechanisms of spine injury might be similar for various loading scenarios, the injuries themselves are likely specific to the particular sport environment and the individual athlete because of the individual complexity of spinal anatomy, prior exposures, tissue tolerances, and changes with development, degeneration, and aging. However, with use of the principles and data already available, further investigations could be designed to fill in the gaps.

The human spine is elegant in its design, and when it is healthy, it functions well to protect the neural elements, support the body's weight, and maintain an upright posture during normal function. The spine has complex biomechanics that can be dramatically altered under traumatic loading such as can occur during athletic activities. Certain portions of the spine have a greater susceptibility to biomechanical failure and hence injury, particularly the regions where the anatomy transitions and the boundary conditions of the loading environment are modified. Although sports activities do not a priori subject the spine to the extraordinary loads that can occur with other traumas, such as motor vehicle collisions, the spine will behave in a similar biomechanical manner under similar force vectors.

Summary

The biomechanics of the spine are very complex and easily modified by trauma, with potential life-changing consequences, particularly for athletes. The small size and exposure of the cervical spine make it the most prone to injury of all of the spinal regions during athletic activities, despite the use of protective equipment. Disruption of cervical spine mechanics ranges from muscular deficit or dysfunction to ligament damage to disk injury to vertebral fracture. Because the head and spine protect the central nervous system and support the skeleton, spinal injuries and the subsequent altered spine mechanics lead to a host of pathologic spinal conditions. The pathologic mechanisms associated with spinal injuries are complex and not well elucidated, mainly because of confounding factors. In the most severe cases, the spinal cord has already been loaded beyond its physiologic limit either during or just after the spinal injury; nonetheless, no evidence of spinal trauma may be seen. Because of such confounding factors, proper diagnosis and treatment of spinal injuries are sometimes limited. In particular, on-site diagnosis of a cervical spine injury for high-velocity, high-impact sports (e.g., football and hockey) is not accurate and should not be based on the head and body motions observed during the injury. Therefore the medical team should be trained for, and equipment should be adapted to handle, the worst-case scenario.

Acknowledgment

We are grateful to the Catherine Sharpe Foundation for funding support.

For a complete list of references, go to expertconsult.com.

Suggested Readings

Citation: Panjabi MM: The stabilizing system of the spine. Part II. Neutral zone and instability hypothesis. *J Spinal Disord* 5(4):390–397, 1992.
Level of Evidence: Basic science article
Summary: In this basic science research article, the author defines the nonlinear relationship of the spine's load-displacement response in the context of instability. The author introduces the concept of the "neutral zone," how it is affected by injury and surgical instrumentation, and how it is altered in persons with spinal instability.

Citation: Myers BS, Winkelstein BA: Epidemiology, classification, mechanism, and tolerance of human cervical spine injuries. *Crit Rev Biomed Eng* 23(5-6):307–409, 1995.
Level of Evidence: Review
Summary: The authors provide a literature review of both adult and pediatric cervical spine injuries, synthesizing biomechanical tolerances and clinical classification to define injury mechanisms. The epidemiology also covers spinal cord injuries and is completed by a classification of injuries based on spinal loading.

Citation: Hubbard RD, Winkelstein BA: Dorsal root compression produces myelinated axonal degeneration near the biomechanical thresholds for mechanical behavioral hypersensitivity. *Exp Neurol* 212(2):482–489, 2008.
Level of Evidence: Basic science article
Summary: In this basic research article, the authors describe a pathomechanism by which transient nerve root trauma induces axonal degeneration and pain. Long-term behavioral symptoms are linked with the development of axonal degeneration and dysfunction, and the role of the magnitude (i.e., severity) of the compression in modulating such physiologic and injury outcomes is detailed.

Citation: Jaumard NV, Welch WC, Winkelstein BA: Spinal facet joint biomechanics and mechanotransduction in normal, injury and degenerative conditions. *J Biomech Eng* 133(7):071010, 2011.
Level of Evidence: Review
Summary: The authors provide a literature review of facet joint mechanics and adaptation to mechanical loading at various length scales in the context of different tissue health, based on both experimental and computational investigations. Mechanotransduction mechanisms are presented to provide an understanding of the physiologic implications of facet joint loading in healthy, injured, and degenerated spines.

122

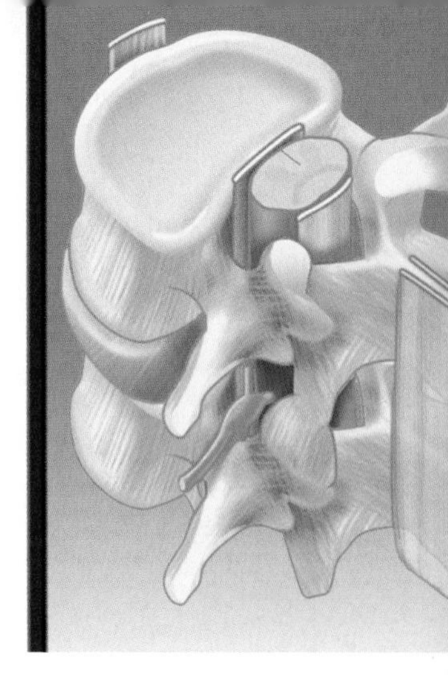

Emergency and Field-Side Management of the Spine-Injured Athlete

PETER P. SYRÉ • NICOLAS V. JAUMARD • BETH A. WINKELSTEIN • WILLIAM C. WELCH

Spinal injuries in sports are some of the more uncommon injuries encountered, with only 8.2% of spinal cord injuries being related to sports injuries.[1] However, when such injuries occur they can be among the most devastating. Although injuries can occur in all regions of the spine, most acute, debilitating, and devastating spinal injuries occur in the cervical spine.[2,3] Of all athletes in the United States, American football players sustain the greatest number of catastrophic spinal injuries, averaging approximately 7.8 catastrophic cervical spine injuries with incomplete recovery[4] and six quadriplegic events annually.[5] However, catastrophic injuries are not isolated to American football. Ice hockey is also associated with a high incidence of catastrophic spinal injuries.[3] Authors of one study found that of the 214 spinal fracture dislocations sustained by hockey players in Canada, 90% occurred in the cervical spine, where they can lead to more devastating and debilitating injuries.[6] Participation in sports such as gymnastics, rugby, and cheerleading also places players at risk for spinal injuries.[7]

Thoracolumbar injuries in sports are usually of the degenerative type and occur from repeated flexion or extension and slow degeneration of the soft tissue components of the spine. Fractures in that region of the spine occur as a result of severe trauma that is extremely uncommon in athletic activity, except in skiing and snowboarding accidents.[8,9] Accordingly, this chapter focuses primarily on the cervical spine, with mention of the thoracic and lumbar spines where appropriate.

A recent and growing trend has been to identify and quantify sports-related injuries. Although gross new neurologic and orthopaedic deficits obviously related to the witnessed traumatic event lend themselves to straightforward identification and prognostication, repetitive, less severe injuries may not do so. An excellent example of this phenomenon is concussion. In an effort to identify and limit these injuries, various pre- and postevent scoring systems, such as the IMPACT scoring system, have been developed.[10] Furthermore, ongoing development has occurred in the areas of restraint systems (such as the HANS system used in automotive sports), padding, and protective gear. Coaches and participants are receiving training in prevention, identification, and event-side management of sports-related injuries as well. The following sections review these efforts in more detail. With all of these points in mind, the emergency and field-side management of the athlete with a spine injury is reviewed and imaging, diagnostics, and surgical management are then briefly discussed as they follow from on-site management.

Field-Side Management

Preparation Before the Event

The diagnosis of spinal injuries in the athlete should begin off the field in the pre-event setting. As with all trauma, prevention is the foundation of the trauma ideology. To this end, pre-event preparation includes ensuring that the participant is outfitted with appropriately fitted equipment and that a pre-event program is dedicated to the awareness of spinal and neurologic injuries. Pre-event teaching should include appropriate playing techniques and, in the case of collision sports, appropriate collision maneuvers such as tackling in football.[6] For example, "spear tackling" in football places the cervical spine in a straightened position with an orientation that is more of an axial column without the protective benefit of its natural lordosis.[11] This maneuver was banned in 1976 by the National Collegiate Athletic Association under rule 912n because it was recognized then, and later demonstrated by Torg et al.,[12] that this type of play resulted in significant spinal injuries. This rule change was extremely successful in achieving what it set out to do. In the first year after the rule change, a significant reduction in the number of paralyzed players in football was noted, and since that time the numbers of catastrophic spinal injuries in football have remained in the single digits.[13-15] Further, rules that have been applied to prevent spinal injuries, such as the prohibition of cross-checking a player from behind in ice hockey, should be reviewed because they typically occur when the player is not expecting the check and has the neck in a flexed position. In this position the player lacks protective lordosis and often collides with the boards head first, placing an axial load on the cervical spine.

Athletes participating in motor sports are quite different from their on-field counterparts in that they are at a high risk for injury from high-velocity trauma. The injuries seen in these sports are similar to those in civilian motor vehicle accidents. The roadside management of motor sports is also much different from that of field sports because motor sports are usually staffed by trained emergency medical personnel who are accustomed to handling high-velocity trauma; these personnel are the same first responders who respond to other road collisions. Therefore motor sport athletes are rarely treated by a single roadside physician. They are rapidly assessed and transferred to dedicated trauma centers and undergo treatment according to advanced trauma life support (ATLS) guidelines, similar to the protocol used for persons with injuries that occur on highways on a daily basis.

Planning also means the appropriate designation of health care practitioners who can deal with an athlete with a spine injury. In the pre-event setting, a chain of command should be established and a team leader should be assigned who will take control of the care of the player who has a suspected spine injury on the field or track.[16] The team leader or medical personnel who is tasked with the care of the patient should be familiar with the basic biomechanics of the spine and the common injuries and injury mechanisms that may be encountered. Ideally, the event can be visualized by this team member and, armed with biomechanical knowledge and knowledge of classic injury patterns, he or she can predict the type and severity of a spinal injury.

Communication and prearrangements with a hospital system that has the capacity to handle a patient with a spinal cord and/or neurologic injury must also be made for transfer of care after acute on-site stabilization. If possible, a member of the medical team should accompany the injured athlete, thus providing excellent continuity of care and ensuring that accurate clinical information regarding the injury is communicated.

As with injuries to other parts of the body, a special tool kit will be required when a suspected spinal injury occurs, and it must be put together before the players take to the field.[17] This tool kit should include tools to properly remove protective equipment as necessary, such as a screwdriver, a set of wire cutters, and an 18-gauge needle to insert into air bladder padding systems to deflate them for easy removal. Removal of a face mask to gain access to an airway is often necessary in an athlete with a spine injury, and studies have been performed to show the best way of removing a face mask while maintaining spinal alignment.[18,19] A power drill is faster and easier to use and produces less head movement than does a manual screwdriver or the Trainer's Angel tool[18,19]; the power screwdriver applies the smallest anteroposterior forces (95 ± 138 N) and the smallest sagittal moment (12 ± 16 Nm) to the head during helmet removal.[19] Tools that stabilize the spine, such a hard cervical collar and spine board, are also a requirement. Noninvasive methods to secure the airway while maintaining stabilization of the spine should also be included in the tool kit, such as an oral or nasal airway. To perform an accurate and focused spine-oriented physical examination, the clinician must have a reflex hammer and a needle to perform an investigation of sensation. Motor sports require more specialized equipment. For example, extraction equipment is required for motor sports and marine rescue equipment is required for water-based sports.

Pregame radiologic screening of athletes remains a controversial subject because it has been shown that imaging modalities are poor at predicting which athletes are at risk for injury.[20,21] In addition to the poor predictive value, computed tomography (CT) and radiographs place the athlete at risk for unnecessary radiation exposure and magnetic resonance imaging (MRI) has a low yield, making it prohibitively expensive. Although athletes with either developmental or acquired cervical stenosis are predisposed to cervical spine injuries, such as transient quadriplegia, during play,[15,20] the rate of long-term consequences was extremely low in patients with transient quadriplegia who showed evidence of congenital stenosis.[14] Torg et al.[20] reported that "developmental narrowing of the cervical canal in a stable spine does not appear to predispose an individual to permanent catastrophic neurological injury and therefore should not preclude an athlete from participation in contact sports." Given all of these factors, and with evidence that even in the presence of abnormalities found on pregame screening examinations, athletes will not experience long-term consequences, screening has not been widely adopted and likely will not be adopted unless advances in technology occur or new data are found to lend support to screening.

Preparticipation physical examinations are excellent in screening out cardiac contraindications to athletic activity,[22] but in general these "sports" physical examinations are meant to screen out common general medical ailments and seldom are able to identify players who may be at risk for a spine injury. Screening is routinely performed in the special case of athletes who have achondroplasia or Down syndrome, in whom spinal anomalies are very common.[23] The Special Olympics established radiographic cervical spine screening in patients with Down syndrome in 1983 and may prevent athletes with Down syndrome from participating in specific sports in which the possibility of a spinal injury exists, such as diving, gymnastics, and weight lifting, among other activities.[24] Typical abnormalities in this population, however, are rather simple to identify on plain radiographs, making screening more feasible and having a higher yield. Additionally, persons with achondroplasia have a high incidence of spinal stenosis at all levels of the spinal canal and craniovertebral junction abnormalities with cervicomedullary compression and hydrocephalus.[25] Many medical centers use more intensive screening with MRI and patients undergo decompressive surgery if abnormalities are identified, even in patients who are not athletes.[26] Clinical symptoms typically drive the decision to undergo decompression and usually consist of pain, radiculopathy, and respiratory symptoms such as apnea due to brainstem compression. Cerebrospinal fluid diversion can also be undertaken if compression at the level of the foramen magnum is significant enough to cause hydrocephalus.[26]

On-Site Assessment

In the initial assessment in the field, clinical evaluation of an athlete with a potential spine injury should follow the classic ATLS protocol and begin with the "ABCDEs" (airway, breathing and circulation, disability, and exposure) used in any trauma evaluation. The first responder to the injury may encounter several scenarios. Banerjee et al.[11] divided these situations into three scenarios based on altered or normal level of consciousness and a compromised or normal cardiorespiratory status (Table 122-1). When approaching and evaluating the athlete, some cues indicate that a spine injury is present, including an altered level of consciousness, bilateral neurologic symptoms, or midline spinal pain or deformity.[8,27] When these signs and symptoms are present, the spinal injury protocol should be initiated as planned in the pre-event setting.

After manual spinal stabilization is performed, priority should be given to the airway, and if the athlete is wearing a face mask or helmet, it should be removed with the proper tools by an experienced member of the team. A jaw thrust can

TABLE 122-1

POTENTIAL CLINICAL SCENARIOS ENCOUNTERED IN CATASTROPHIC CERVICAL SPINAL TRAUMA

Scenario	Level of Consciousness	Cardiorespiratory Status
1	Abnormal	Compromised
2	Abnormal	Normal
3	Normal	Normal

Modified from Banerjee R, Palumbo MA, Fadale PD: Catastrophic cervical spine injuries in the collision sport athlete, Part 1: epidemiology, functional anatomy, and diagnosis. *Am J Sports Med* 32(4):1077–1087, 2004.

be performed or an oral airway can be placed to maintain patency of the airway. These maneuvers have less effect on the cervical spinal alignment than does the head tilt technique, which places the cervical spine in extension.[28,29] Ventilation also must be maintained, and for this purpose, bag-mask ventilation may be adequate. The cervical spine should be maintained during evaluation with use of manual stabilization to minimize secondary injury to the spinal cord during the evaluation procedures. However, traction must not be applied because it may further sublux the spinal column if significant ligamentous damage is present, and this subluxation can worsen a spinal injury.[30,31] Returning the spine to the neutral position will also minimize secondary injury but should not be performed if, during realignment, the athlete reports further pain or neurologic symptoms, if the athlete resists the movement, or if mechanical resistance is encountered, because these reactions can all indicate a worsening injury.[32,33] After stabilization of the ABCs, ATLS protocol can further guide the care of a patient, including obtaining a Glasgow Coma Scale (GCS) score to evaluate the ability to adequately assess the extent of injuries on the field. Mental status deterioration from baseline further dictates on-field management and concern because it has been shown that an inverse relationship exists between the GCS score and the risk of spinal injury, with patients who have a lower GCS score being at higher risk for a spinal injury.[34] Given this situation, athletes with altered mental status who are unable to completely communicate their extent of injuries are considered to have a spine injury until proven otherwise; the worst-case scenario is always assumed.

Should an athlete have a normal mental status, then initial evaluation on the field will include a brief spine-oriented history from the patient and a focused spine-oriented physical examination. Athletes at all levels generally minimize their complaints in favor of returning to play, so the clinician must be especially vigilant in obtaining an accurate history. Pain or a neurologic deficit is the usual complaint. It should be determined if the symptoms were acute in onset or if long-standing complaints became acutely worse with the injury. Localization of the symptom is also integral to understanding the diagnosis. Any prior spinal injury or deformity should be elicited, along with any family history of spinal problems. On the field, a brief history usually can be obtained, but if indicated the clinician should return to the patient later and obtain a more complete history. Several on-field assessment algorithms have been proposed and can aid in rapid triage for a player with a possible cervical spine injury (Fig. 122-1).[11,35]

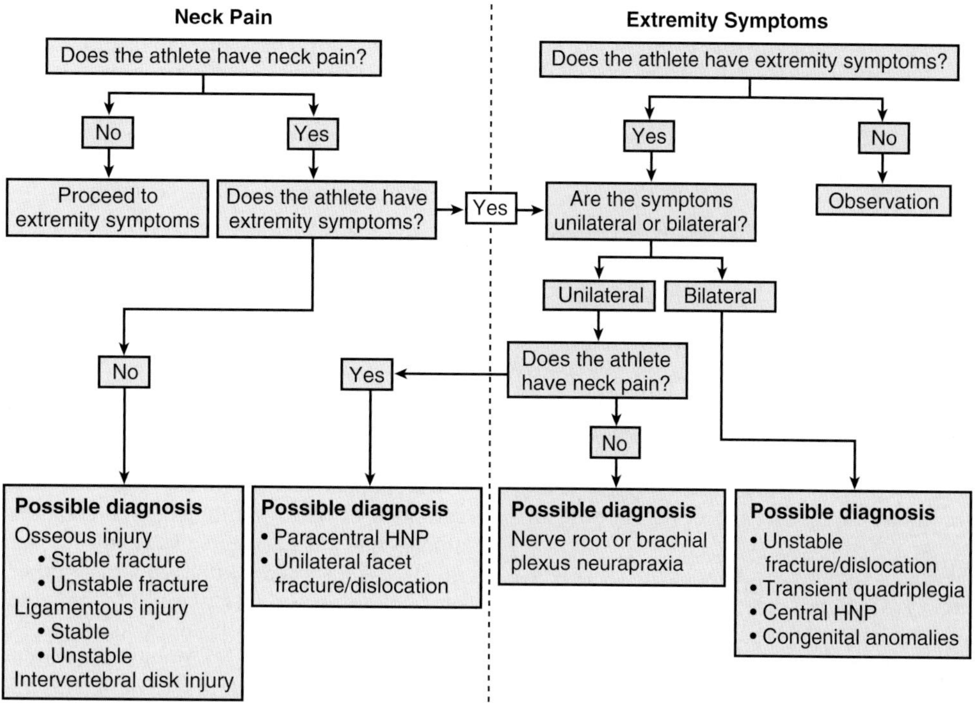

FIGURE 122-1 An algorithm for on-field evaluation of the cervical spine. *HNP*, Herniated nucleus pulposus. *(Modified from Banerjee R, Palumbo MA, Fadale PD: Catastrophic cervical spine injuries in the collision sport athlete, Part 1: epidemiology, functional anatomy, and diagnosis.* Am J Sports Med *32[4]:1077–1087, 2004, and Zahir U, Ludwig SC: Sports-related cervical spine injuries: on-field assessment and management.* Semin Spine Surg *22:173–180, 2010.)*

The Injured Athlete in a Prone Position

An injured athlete who is in a prone position presents special challenges. Again, one must initially assume that the player has a spinal injury until proven otherwise. Movement of the athlete must be undertaken by trained personnel to avoid further injury to the spine. Also, the mental status of the injured athlete will guide further management, and the airway remains the first priority. A conscious face-down athlete who is breathing should not be moved until a spine board and trained personnel are available, avoiding a possible second move onto a board.[8,36] In this case, if the athlete is not wearing protective equipment, the neck is stabilized with a rigid cervical collar in the prone position until the patient can be log-rolled into a supine position for further evaluation.[8,36] However, if an athlete is face down and is not breathing, the athlete must be log-rolled into a supine position so the airway can be accessed and a full evaluation can be performed. Ideally, the athlete will be log-rolled onto a spine board initially, but if one is not immediately available, the rescuers should not wait for one to arrive; the athlete can be rolled onto the playing surface and then moved onto a back board when it becomes available.

The proper log-roll technique should be performed with at least four rescuers if possible.[8] The team leader is positioned at the head and manually stabilizes the neck by holding the head with the fingertips on the mastoid processes bilaterally, the occiput cupped in the hands, and the thumbs pointed toward the face.[37] To prepare for the log-roll, the team leader holds the head with crossed arms so that when the athlete becomes supine the arms are no longer crossed. The remaining rescuers position themselves at the shoulders, hips, and legs of the athlete. The athlete's legs are placed straight and the arms are placed at the sides. The athlete can then be log-rolled using a push or pull technique. With use of either technique, the assistants all follow the command of the team leader and on command all rescuers roll the athlete so that the head, neck, shoulders, torso, and legs maintain alignment during the entire rolling maneuver. Once the athlete is supine, evaluation can continue.

On-Site Stabilization and Transfer

Concurrent with assessment of the injured athlete, rescuers must prevent any secondary injury to the spinal cord that can occur with excessive movement of the injured spine and must stabilize the spinal column. This procedure is most necessary in the area of the cervical spine where ligamentous laxity and possible fractures from injuries can disrupt the normal spinal architecture and biomechanics that protect the spinal cord. However, stabilizing the thoracic and lumbar spine is also of value because a secondary injury can also occur in these sections of the spine.

A hard cervical collar should be included in all sideline tool kits as previously discussed and should be applied as soon as possible if a spinal injury is suspected.[17] However, if the athlete is wearing protective equipment, it is sometimes not possible, and in fact can be dangerous, to apply a cervical collar.[38] Additionally, protective equipment, especially that worn by American football and ice hockey players, places the spine in a neutral alignment[11] and should not be removed, excluding the face mask, until reaching the hospital setting. Prior to the arrival of the collar, and in all athletes with protective equipment, rescuers need not wait to stabilize the spine and should do so manually if they suspect a spinal injury. Stabilization is performed by the team leader who manually stabilizes the neck by holding the head with the fingertips on the mastoid processes bilaterally, the occiput cupped in the hands, and the thumbs pointed toward the face[37] or holding the helmet in two hands similarly. The athlete's arms should not be crossed unless the athlete is prone and the stabilizer is preparing for a log-roll maneuver. In a situation in which a rigid cervical collar cannot be placed, more permanent stabilization can be provided once the athlete has been transferred to a back board. This stabilization can consist of sandbags or foam blocks attached to the spine board and can be implemented while protective equipment is still in place. Once again, traction should not be applied.[30,31] Similarly, loading of the neck in any other direction should be minimized to reduce the risk of secondary spinal cord injury during removal of the athlete's protective gear or his or her transfer and transportation to the hospital. Particularly, extension and compression of the cervical spine after a burst fracture or a bilateral facet dislocation have been shown to almost double the spinal canal occlusion.[39,40] This factor is important to consider because axial compression of 89 J applied to the cadaveric cervical spine already results in burst fractures that occlude the spinal canal up to 55% and produce a permanent height loss of 35%.[41] Therefore it is important to limit the loads imparted by the manipulation of an injured spine to reduce the risk of worsening neurologic injuries.

As mentioned, acute catastrophic injuries to the thoracolumbar spine in athletics are uncommon.[8] However, this spinal region is still at risk during movement induced by removal of protective equipment because the thoracolumbar junction can serve as a transition point of increased motion.[42] The same principles of stabilization and minimization of movement that are used with the cervical spine must also be used when caring for athletes with injuries of the thoracic and lumbar spines. Stabilization of the lumbar and thoracic spines can be accomplished with use of a rigid spine backboard, which also should be included in the sideline tool kit. If available, a full-body vacuum splint is an option for spinal stabilization and provides greater comfort for the athlete.[43] Stabilization of the spine should be maintained until a spinal injury has been ruled out with the appropriate diagnostic tools.[7]

Proper transfer of the athlete is as important as the initial stabilization of the spinal column because movement of the athlete can induce secondary injury to the spinal column if alignment is disrupted during movement. Movement of the prone patient has previously been discussed, but situations can arise in which an athlete is already supine or the prone athlete has already been placed in the supine position and must be transferred to a backboard or other spinal stabilizing piece of equipment. To place the athlete onto a spine board, the National Athletic Trainers' Association recommends use of the lift-and-slide technique rather than a log-roll technique,[7] because the lift-and-slide technique has been shown to produce less motion in the head and cervical spine.[44] However, compared with other techniques, more rescuers are required to correctly perform the lift-and-slide technique, and thus using it may not always be feasible.

Management of Protective Equipment

Care of an athlete with a spine injury in a collision sport is somewhat different than care provided to an athlete with other injuries, such as extremity injuries, in that same sport and in noncollision sports. In this case, the protective equipment can interfere with the treatment of the athlete, and when not dealt with properly, it can actually do more harm than good. Managing protective equipment correctly is paramount in the treatment of the athlete with a spine injury. Several guidelines have been established about when and how the removal of the equipment should be performed. In particular, the National Athletic Trainers' Association has developed guidelines on equipment removal (Table 122-2). Helmets, face masks, and shoulder pads are the most important and most studied pieces of equipment when considering an athlete with a spinal injury.

It is recommended that the face mask be removed as soon as the decision is made to mobilize and transfer the athlete and not to wait until respiratory compromise occurs to remove the mask.[7] Face mask removal can be complicated by the large variety of mechanisms used to secure the face mask to the helmet and the possibility of rusted fasteners. A powered cordless screwdriver is generally the fastest method of removal and produces the least amount of associated head movement.[18,45] Frequently the face mask is also attached via loops and thus a combined tool approach, in which a cutting tool is used in conjunction with a screwdriver, is the optimal approach for face mask removal.[46]

In American football and ice hockey, the helmet and shoulder pads work in conjunction to place the cervical spine in neutral alignment in the supine position. Thus they should not be removed individually because it has been shown that when one piece of equipment is removed in isolation, a significant change occurs in cervical spinal alignment.[47,48] Additionally, other studies have shown that it is possible to provide adequate immobilization of athletes on spinal backboards with protective equipment still in place.[49] To this end, the National Collegiate Athletic Association guidelines for football helmet management state that the helmet is not to be removed on the field in the case of a possible spine or head-injured player except in special circumstances, such as when an athlete has respiratory compromise and the airway cannot be properly accessed.[50] Furthermore, several studies have shown that removal of protective equipment leads to excessive motion of the spine and can lead to worsening of the injury.[51] The helmet and shoulder pads may be removed in special situations (see Table 122-2), but generally, sports medicine professionals recommend against removal of the helmet and shoulder pads until the athlete is in a hospital setting or until a spinal injury has been ruled out with use of adequate diagnostic tools.

Protective equipment in sports is usually used for head and upper body protection, and removal of protective equipment rarely interferes with thoracic or lumbar spine injuries. However, the thoracolumbar junction can act as a fulcrum for increased motion, putting neural elements at risk; thus, as with the cervical spine, minimizing excess motion and maintaining neutral alignment in the lower segments of the spine is also important when considering the removal of equipment.

Outpatient Setting

In the elective, ambulatory outpatient setting, the clinician has much more time and many more resources for evaluation of the athlete, although the principles remain the same. Overuse injuries are common in athletes and a discussion of these injuries is beyond the scope of this chapter, but they can present in similar ways as in the general population. Disk herniations, muscle strains, and sprains and chronic fractures are all possible. A thorough history can help discriminate between these injuries and can further guide follow-up care, imaging, and return to play. Localization and characterization of the pain and the temporal relationship of the symptoms should be ascertained, along with aggravating and alleviating factors. Any prior spinal injuries are of special interest to the clinician because a repeat injury can occur. The history is

TABLE 122-2

GUIDELINES REGARDING CIRCUMSTANCES UNDER WHICH EQUIPMENT SHOULD BE REMOVED

Helmet Removal Should Occur in Any of the Following Circumstances	Shoulder Pad Removal Should Occur in Any of the Following Circumstances
1. If, after a reasonable period of time, the face mask cannot be removed to gain access to the airway	1. Multiple injuries requiring full access to the shoulder
2. If the design of the helmet and chin strap is such that even after removal of the face mask, the airway cannot be controlled or ventilation cannot be provided	2. Ill-fitting shoulder pads resulting in the inability to maintain spinal immobilization
3. If the helmet and chin straps do not hold the head securely such that immobilization of the helmet does not also immobilize the head	3. Cardiopulmonary resuscitation requiring access to the thorax that is inhibited by the shoulder pads
4. If the helmet prevents immobilization for transport in an appropriate position	4. Any time the helmet is removed
5. Any time the shoulder pads are removed	

Modified from Kleiner DM, Almquist JL, Bailes J, et al: Prehospital care of the spine-injured athlete: a document from the Inter-Association Task Force for Appropriate Care of the Spine-Injured Athlete. Dallas, 2001, National Athletic Trainers' Association and Banerjee R, Palumbo MA, Fadale PD: Catastrophic cervical spine injuries in the collision sport athlete, Part 1: epidemiology, functional anatomy, and diagnosis. *Am J Sports Med* 32(4):1077–1087, 2004.

essential and can help the clinician develop an effective differential diagnosis to further investigate the problem with use of radiographic modalities as adjuncts to the physical examination.

Diagnostic Imaging

After stabilization and upon reaching a health care center, injured athletes undergo diagnostic imaging to characterize the extent of injury. Indications for imaging in persons who have sustained a trauma are typically defined as pain, neurologic deficit, distracting injury, altered mental status, and a high-risk mechanism of injury.[52] Standard diagnostic imaging in the case of the cervical spine classically consists of anteroposterior, lateral, and odontoid views and include the occiput-C1 and C7-T1 junctions. Protective equipment has been shown to interfere with sufficient imaging of the spine with plain radiographs[53,54] and must be removed with use of the established methods previously discussed to adequately image the spine. More health care centers are moving toward CT scanning as a first-line modality in persons with spinal trauma because CT is more time efficient[52] and has a higher sensitivity, specificity, and positive and negative predictive values compared with plain radiographs in the cervical spine[55] and the thoracic and lumbar spines.[56] Additionally, trauma centers routinely use CT to image the abdomen and pelvis so that reformatted images of the thoracic and lumbar spine can be obtained without further exposure to radiation.

Although CT scanning can be performed quickly and enables viewing anatomy in multiple planes and detailed bony architecture, patients are exposed to more radiation with CT scanning than with simple radiograph sequences. However, with newer advances in imaging, this exposure is becoming less of an issue. Some injured athletes may not require imaging when they reach a health care setting based on their clinical picture. The Canadian C-Spine Rule Study identifies low-risk patients (i.e., those who are ambulatory, do not have midline tenderness or the immediate onset of pain, are able to maintain a sitting position, and are able to turn their head 45 degrees without the onset of pain) who do not require imaging with a sensitivity of 100%.[57] Other criteria have been developed for the lumbar and thoracic spine as well,[58] although these criteria are not as widely accepted and can be used as an adjunct to the history and physical examination to guide further diagnostic testing. As such, in athletes who meet these criteria, diagnostic imaging may still be necessary.

Osseous disease is best viewed using CT scanning, but MRI is superior when viewing soft tissue injuries and is the only modality that can be used to image spinal cord disease directly. Ligamentous and disk pathology can be identified easily with use of this modality. MRI can also be used to further characterize the acuity of osseous injury by identifying edema within the osseous structures. Because MRI is more expensive and time consuming to perform compared with other imaging modalities, obtaining an MRI scan for all trauma victims is not practical. Therefore certain indications such as neurologic deficit or a suspicion of nerve root avulsion or vascular injury are used.[52] Athletes with chronic injuries also usually undergo MRI because the processes that cause these symptoms are similar to those of the general population, such as spondylitic disease.[59-61]

Spinal cord injury without radiographic abnormality (SCIWORA) was first defined as spinal injuries, typically in the cervical spine, without evidence of bony or ligamentous injury on complete, technically adequate plain radiographs or CT scans.[62,63] This condition has been seen in athletes, but in the era of MRI, with which soft tissues can be adequately imaged, it is no longer common, and cases of SCIWORA have since been found to have radiographically identifiable pathology. The term SCIWORA is still used, however; currently it usually describes a patient with a neurologic injury pattern suspicious for spinal cord injury but with normal alignment and no bony abnormalities seen on plain radiographs and CT imaging. In the case of an athlete who has a neurologic deficit and yet findings of adequate CT imaging are normal, an MRI is the next step, because early identification and treatment of spinal injuries is key to improving outcomes.[64]

Common Spinal Injuries

Although injuries to the spine are rather uncommon in athletics, when they do occur, they occur in a fairly consistent and stereotyped manner. Catastrophic thoracolumbar trauma typically requires high velocities or a significant force to produce injury and is rarely seen in athletic activity,[65] with the exception of some extreme sports such as airborne sports, skiing, and snowboarding.[66-68] Most thoracolumbar injuries in athletics result from chronic repetitive forces. Therefore injuries to the spine occur in the most vulnerable portion of the spine to athletic injuries, the cervical spine. Injuries to the cervical spine usually fall into one of the following categories: transient quadriplegia, stingers or burners, disk herniations (both acute and chronic) and fracture dislocations.

Transient quadriplegia, also known as spinal cord neurapraxia or cervical cord neurapraxia, refers to a spectrum of injuries ranging from complete self-limiting paralysis to simple weakness. First described by Torg et al.[20] in 1986, this condition is self-limiting and usually has minimal to no signs of radiographic abnormality, including on MRI.[35] The patient is frequently pain free with a full range of motion and no bony abnormalities. This injury pattern usually follows an axial load to the cervical spine while it is in a slightly flexed position. Treatment consists of expectant management. Return to play after transient quadriplegia is determined on a case-by-case basis, and no standard guideline exists.[69] However, athletes with abnormal imaging findings or congenital anomalies require special counseling and have a relative contraindication to returning to play.[70]

Stingers, also known as burners, are another common spine-related injury seen in athletes and consist of transient dysesthesias and numbness in the effected limb. Weakness can also be a component. More than half of all college football players have experienced this type of injury annually.[71] These injuries are unilateral and transient and affect the cervical nerve roots or brachial plexus. Neck pain is absent and range of motion is unhindered, and the hallmark of these injuries is their unilateral nature. Burners are usually described as stretch injuries to the brachial plexus or cervical roots, or alternatively foraminal compression injuries to the cervical roots when the head is placed in mild extension and lateral bending.[71] These injuries are self-limiting and typically resolve in 24 to 48 hours; they are treated expectantly with nonsteroidal antiinflammatory drugs and short-term immobilization. However, any symptoms lasting longer than 24 hours should be investigated with imaging and additional diagnostic studies.[72] Additionally, a single episode of a burner, once fully resolved, is not a contraindication to return to play.

Disk herniations can be acutely traumatic or chronic and can involve a variety of severities. The symptoms of axial pain with variable pain or tingling in a dermatomal distribution may signify the presence of nerve root compression from a disk rupture or neuroforaminal stenosis. Diagnostic imaging is typically obtained, with MRI as the modality of choice. Nonsurgical management (i.e., physical therapy and use of antiinflammatory medicines and epidural steroid injections) is attempted first, although surgery may be required if the symptoms increase in severity or if a worsening neurologic deficit is noted.[35]

Fracture dislocations are among the most common catastrophic cervical spine injuries[11] and can lead to neurologic disasters; they are manifested in a diversity of patterns. Within these injuries, concomitant ligamentous and other soft tissue damage can be present as well. Bilateral jumped facets are the most likely flexion-distraction injury,[39] require application of a great deal of force,[73] and can lead to significant neurologic injury in many cases.[74] Bilateral jumped facets can occur when an athlete assumes a flexed neck position and then receives an axial load to the head/spine, as in a diving injury. Patients with severe spinal injury are at risk for hypotension as a result of neurogenic shock and should be transferred to a center experienced in spinal injury as soon as possible for further evaluation and treatment. These types of injuries may be difficult to identify on plain radiographs, especially if they occur at the C7-T1 level. CT scanning is helpful if this type of injury is suspected.

Surgical Management

After appropriate diagnostic studies have been conducted, some athletes may require surgical intervention for their injury. The decision to pursue surgery should not be undertaken lightly. Although several strong indications exist for surgical intervention, such as a worsening neurologic deficit and incomplete neurologic injuries, few hard and fast guidelines are available that one can turn to when deciding on operative intervention in a patient with spinal trauma. In an attempt to better formalize the surgical decision-making process, the Spine Trauma Study Group has created the Thoracolumbar Injury Classification and Severity Score and the Sub-Axial Cervical Spine Injury Classification system.[75,76] With use of injury morphology (e.g., burst or compression, distraction or rotation/translation), the integrity of the discoligamentous complex, and neurologic status, a score is created that can aid the surgeon in deciding whether to proceed with surgery. These scores are meant only to guide surgeons and are not mandates on whether a patient does or does not require surgical intervention.

Summary

The goals in managing an injured athlete are to minimize the consequences of spinal trauma and avoid any secondary injury during removal of the protective gear, transfer, and transport to the hospital. Also, the team personnel should give the utmost attention to injuries that appear minor, such as concussions and neck sprains. Although some injured athletes might present symptoms of spinal injury without measurable changes in their spine biomechanics, they should be treated conservatively (i.e., with rest), because the spinal tissues may have sustained microstructural damage that can worsen their condition over time and/or put the athletes at a higher risk for a more severe spinal trauma. Finally, surgeons can use guidelines to decide the most appropriate medical treatment of a spinal injury. However, they should also consider and assess the biomechanics of the athlete's spine prior to and after medical treatment. Such consideration will help guide and educate the athlete regarding the most appropriate physical activities he or she can perform in both the short- and long-term.

For a complete list of references, go to expertconsult.com.

Suggested Readings

Citation: Stiell IG, Wells GA, Vandemheen KL, et al: The Canadian C-spine rule for radiography in alert and stable trauma patients. *JAMA* 286(15):1841–1848, 2001.

Level of Evidence: II (North American Spine Society Criteria)

Summary: The authors describe the creation and use of a decision rule regarding when to obtain C-spine radiography for alert and stable trauma patients based on a prospective cohort study.

Citation: National Collegiate Athletic Association: Guideline 4-F: guidelines for helmet fitting and removal in athletes. In Schluep C, editor: *2003–2004 NCAA Sports Medicine Handbook*, ed 16, Indianapolis, 2003, National Collegiate Athletic Association.

Level of Evidence: V (North American Spine Society Criteria)

Summary: The *Handbook* includes guidelines created by the National Collegiate Athletic Association on how to correctly fit athletic protective helmets and when to remove them in the case of a suspected spinal injury.

Citation: Kleiner DM, Almquist JL, Bailes J, et al: *Prehospital Care of the Spine-Injured Athlete: A Document from the Inter-Association Task Force for Appropriate Care of the Spine-Injured Athlete*, Dallas, 2001, National Athletic Trainers' Association.

Level of Evidence: V (North American Spine Society Criteria)

Summary: This document includes a uniform set of guidelines and recommendations created by the Inter-Association Task Force for Appropriate Care of the Spine-Injured Athlete regarding the prehospital management of athletes with suspected spinal injuries.

Citation: Andersen J, Courson RW, Kleiner DM, et al: National Athletic Trainers' Association position statement: Emergency planning in athletics. *J Athl Train* 37(1):99–104, 2002.

Level of Evidence: V (North American Spine Society Criteria)

Summary: This position statement created by the National Athletic Trainers' Association provides guidelines on the creation of preevent emergency planning, including the identification of personnel to be involved, the specification of necessary equipment to manage injured athletes, and communication and transportation arrangements.

Citation: Swartz EE, Boden BP, Courson RW, et al: National Athletic Trainers' Association position statement: Acute management of the cervical spine-injured athlete. *J Athletic Training* 44(3):306–331, 2009.

Level of Evidence: V (North American Spine Society Criteria)

Summary: This position statement created by the National Athletic Trainers' Association provides recommendations for how to best manage a catastrophic cervical spinal injury in an athlete, including emergency planning, stabilization, and airway management.

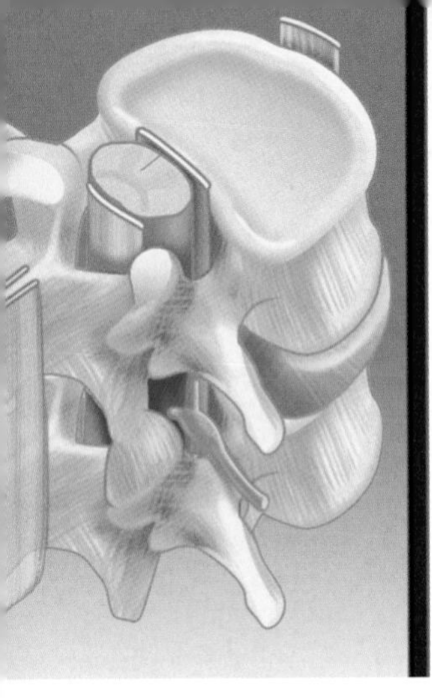

123

Head and Spine Diagnosis and Decision Making

RORY J. PETTEYS • NATHAN M. NAIR

Head

Overview of Pathologic Conditions

Head injuries can occur in a wide variety of contact and noncontact sports. Injuries include concussion, mild and severe traumatic brain injury, skull fractures, intracranial hematomas, cerebrospinal fluid leaks, cranial nerve injuries, and craniofacial injuries. Many of these injuries are serious and are associated with acute loss of consciousness, rapid neurologic decline, severe neurologic deficits, or disabling focal neurologic complications, usually leading to early evaluation by medical personnel, hospitalization, and sometimes surgical intervention. However, these symptoms occur in a minority of cases. Concussion and minor traumatic brain injury occur much more frequently and are far more likely to be seen by practitioners who specialize in sports medicine and by allied professionals involved in the care of athletes. This chapter focuses primarily on concussion and minor head injuries, with special attention directed to the pathologic basis and mechanisms of the disease process, as well as the pertinent components of the history and physical examination of the patient with a head injury.

Concussion

Head injury in athletics is a topic that has garnered much attention in medical and popular literature in recent years. Several tragic deaths and injuries in high-school football players, suicides in ex-National Football League players, and new evidence of the effects of repeated head injury have all brought this issue into the spotlight. The most common head injury among athletes is concussion. Although no universally agreed upon definition of "concussion" exists, the term should not be used interchangeably with "mild traumatic brain injury,"[1-3] because concussion can actually be a serious injury with longer term neuropsychological consequences. It is also important to distinguish concussion from postconcussion syndrome (PCS).

Concussion is characterized as a sudden and transient alteration in consciousness induced by traumatic forces applied directly or indirectly to the brain.[1,4,5] The latest (2009) Consensus Statement on Concussion in Sport[1] states that concussion may be caused by a direct impact to the head or by an impact to another part of the body that transmits impulse forces to the head. In adults, this impact most commonly occurs in falls and motor vehicle collisions, but in children, bicycle accidents and sports are the leading culprit.[4] In contradistinction to motor vehicle collisions and bicycle accidents, sports concussions are generally the result of lower velocity mechanisms and usually lead to disorientation and impaired consciousness rather than frank loss of consciousness.[3,6] Although the initial injury may or may not be associated with a loss of consciousness, some transient amnesia is usually present.[4] This amnesia is often typified by an inability to retain new information (antegrade amnesia) and less frequently involves a loss of autobiographical information.[4] However, patients often have some inability to recall the circumstances immediately preceding the injury, or even events that occurred hours or days prior to the impact (retrograde amnesia). The retrograde amnesia usually resolves, with affected persons eventually being able to recall preinjury events, but some period of antegrade amnesia can be permanent.[7] Injury to the brain is usually not apparent on macroscopic examination with computed tomography (CT) or magnetic resonance imaging (MRI),[1,8,9] but microscopic changes may exist, which will be further discussed.

Concussion is a common malady in athletes, especially participants in contact and field sports such as football, rugby, lacrosse, wrestling, boxing, basketball, field hockey, and soccer.[10,11] Despite the relative frequency of concussion, it seems likely that it is grossly underreported.[3,10,12] Efforts in the past two decades by sporting organizations, medical and professional associations, and other concerned groups have probably improved reporting of concussions, but underreporting remains a problem. The reasons for this underreporting are multifactorial, including the athlete's desire to continue playing, perceived negative consequences for the individual or team of reporting a concussion, and a lack of awareness of the symptoms and consequences of concussion.[3,12] The Centers for Disease Control and Prevention estimated a yearly rate of 1.5 million sports-related concussions in the United States,[3,13,14] but a more recent study puts that number as high as 1.6 to 3.8 million annually,[15] with many of these concussions not reported. Among high school football players, concussion rates are estimated at 15% per season, but several studies in which participants confidentially reported symptoms after a blow to the head put the rate as high as 35% to 40%.[3,12,16,17]

Pathophysiology of Concussion

Concussion is thought to be caused by rotational or angular acceleration forces that lead to neuronal shearing, whereas higher velocity linear acceleration-deceleration forces frequently cause macroscopic brain injuries.[3,18,19] The amnesia and brief loss of consciousness are possibly due to forces centered around the midbrain and thalamus, which lead to temporary disturbance of the reticular activation system.[4] At the cellular level, the stretching of axons leads to increased membrane permeability,[14,20,21] release of many neurotransmitters, including glutamate,[22] and an overall excitatory phase with increased metabolism and energy demands.[20,23] This phenomenon is followed by a period of neuronal suppression known as "spreading depression." Together, these metabolic changes can ultimately lead to permanent neuronal damage from axonal swelling and impaired neurotransmission, or even cell death.[20,21]

In addition to the derangements in cellular metabolism, animal models of concussion have also demonstrated a global uncoupling of cerebral metabolism and cerebral blood flow, so that metabolism increases while, paradoxically, blood flow decreases.[20,24] The mismatch of energy supply and demand is thought to increase the vulnerability of the brain to subsequent injury with potentially more severe and longer lasting effects and is the basis for the second impact syndrome.[20] Although this syndrome is rare, it is thought to occur in younger persons when two relatively minor injuries are sustained in short succession, before autoregulatory mechanisms in the brain have reset.[10,25] In some cases the subsequent injury has led to severe cerebral edema and death.[25]

The cellular and metabolic derangements induced by concussion and head injury are thought to produce short- and long-term neuronal dysfunction. Some, and perhaps many, of these changes are completely reversible. However, a growing body of evidence is demonstrating permanent irreversible changes at the cellular and structural level in athletes who have sustained repeated and frequent concussions and head trauma.[26] The exact causes and effects of these changes are not known, but many of the persons whose brains have been examined experienced depression, suicidal behaviors, and early dementia and had sustained repeated head trauma in their careers.[14,26] As the study of concussion and head trauma continues to advance, the body of knowledge will certainly increase, and our ability to treat athletes with sports-related concussions will improve.

Other intracranial components can be damaged in sporting collisions, including the dura and meninges, the bones of the calvarium, the cranial nerves, and the cranial vasculature. When involved, these structures can produce focal neurologic deficits or deformities or even life-threatening intracranial hematomas. Therefore these pathologic entities are more likely to be encountered in an acute setting and addressed promptly by emergency personnel or the appropriate specialists. That being said, any athlete with a head injury who has more than a brief loss of consciousness or has focal neurologic deficits, neurologic decline, subsequent loss of consciousness, or a seizure should receive urgent evaluation in an emergency care setting with appropriate neuroimaging, such as a CT or MRI scan of the head. It is unlikely that injuries of this type would be evaluated in an outpatient setting, but one must still be aware of possible pathologic conditions in persons with more severe injuries.

History

Obtaining a history for the patient with a suspected head injury is perhaps the most important element of the patient encounter. Concussion symptoms are frequently subtle and insidious and may not be present at the time of the interview. Therefore it is imperative to ask detailed questions about possible concussion symptoms in the time since the initial injury. The initial presentation of concussion ranges from an athlete being dazed with no loss of consciousness, to an unconscious athlete who has had a seizure. Symptoms from the time of impact and in the first 4 weeks are considered to be part of the initial concussion, whereas symptoms that persist after 4 weeks or new symptoms that occur are part of the PCS. This syndrome is highly variable and can last anywhere from weeks to several months.[1,3,4] Although a good deal of overlap exists between concussion and PCS, some important distinctions can be made.

The symptoms and signs of concussion are highly variable and can occur at different points after the initial impact. Somatic symptoms can include headache, nausea, vomiting, dizziness, vertigo, vision or hearing changes, tinnitus, photophobia, and fatigue. Cognitive symptoms can include unclear thinking, difficulty with memory or concentration, and hallucinations, and emotional symptoms can include sadness.[1-3] In most cases, some combination of these symptoms will be present immediately after the impact and can persist for varying periods. However, occasionally symptoms will emerge in the hours to days after an impact.

When obtaining the patient history, it is important to gain as much information as possible about the circumstances surrounding the initial impact, especially with regard to loss of consciousness and initial symptoms. This information can provide an indication of the severity of the initial concussion and help inform the decision of when to return to activity. Although the initial symptoms can be informative, it is imperative to determine symptoms that the athlete has experienced since the initial event and to what degree these symptoms have occurred. These symptoms may include subtle difficulties with concentration at school or work, emotional changes, or unclear thinking or may involve more overt symptoms such as headache, nausea, vision changes, imbalance, or photophobia. It is also important to know whether symptoms occur at rest or with activity. If any symptoms persist beyond 4 weeks after the injury, the diagnosis of PCS can be made. This diagnosis should prompt referral to a head injury specialist or clinical psychologist for further evaluation. If the athlete manifests any symptoms in the postinjury period, whether at rest or with activity, he or she should continue to rest and should not be allowed to return to activity. A detailed rehabilitation plan is discussed later in this chapter.

Physical Examination

Physical signs of concussion include loss of consciousness, drowsiness, disorientation or confusion, a dazed physical appearance, delayed motor and verbal responses, impaired neuropsychological abilities, amnesia, seizure, impaired balance, coordination, or gait, and emotional lability or irritability.[1-3] As previously stated, these signs often occur at the point of impact but can occasionally develop some time thereafter. Unlike the history, the initial assessment at the time of injury is important in the physical examination.

The initial assessment of an athlete with suspected concussion is usually carried out by a team physician, athletic trainer, or other trained individual in organized sport. Recreational athletes often are not evaluated at the point of injury and may present to an emergency or urgent care setting or a physician's office hours to days after the initial impact. The first priority is to evaluate the patient using standard emergency medical principles, ensuring adequate airway, breathing, and circulation. Consideration must also be given to the possibility of a coincident cervical spine injury, and immobilization is necessary if the patient reports neck pain or changes in strength or sensation in the extremities, or if the neurologic status is not able to be assessed (because the patient is unconscious or obtunded). If the patient is conscious and can be moved off the field of play, he or she should be brought to the sideline, where a detailed assessment can begin. A detailed neurologic examination should be performed to assess cranial nerve function, peripheral motor and sensory function, coordination, balance, and gait. Any focal neurologic deficits, prolonged unconsciousness, obtundation, or declining level of consciousness should prompt emergent transfer to a higher level of care.

With the initial medical assessment complete, a standardized symptom-based assessment tool should be used by the physician or qualified professional attending to the patient. Several of these tools are available, such as the Post-Concussion Symptom Scale, a component of the Sport Concussion Assessment Tool,[13] the Graded Symptom Checklist,[10] or the Head Injury Scale.[13] These comprehensive batteries have largely replaced concussion grading systems, which rely heavily on the presence of loss of consciousness and self-reported symptoms.[2,3] As previously mentioned, athletes commonly underreport or attempt to hide symptoms for a number of reasons, highlighting the importance of systematic testing.[3,6] Additionally, standard orientation questions to person, place, and time are unreliable tests of cognition compared with event-specific questions concerning the score, opponent, game rules, and play assignments, all of which are components of the Sport Concussion Assessment Tool assessment.[3]

Although these assessments can help systematize the evaluation of the potentially concussed athlete, they are best used as tools, not stand-alone diagnostic instruments. Concussion remains a clinical diagnosis that should be made by qualified personnel. Once the diagnosis of concussion is made, the athlete should not return to play on the date of injury and should be subject to further evaluation.[1,10,13] Some experts have advocated subsequent testing with the initial assessment tool at intervals of 2 to 3, 24, 48, and 72 hours after the injury.[10,27] Additional testing such as electroencephalography and medical imaging is usually not necessary and, when performed, it is frequently unrevealing. However, some recent studies have demonstrated subtle differences in electrophysiological testing[28-30] and advanced MRI.[30]

Although symptom-based evaluation is currently the most widely used assessment for concussion, recently several efforts have been made to develop objective neuropsychological testing batteries for the initial and follow-up evaluation of the concussed athlete. These assessments consist of computer-based programs that assess the athlete's attention, working memory, and speed of information processing. By conducting pre- and postinjury assessments, it is possible to make objective comparisons and determine the degree to which cognitive function is impaired. When paired with symptom-based assessment, the sensitivity of diagnosis[31] and ability to predict the length of recovery[32] are enhanced with computer-based testing. The overall sensitivity and specificity of computer-based testing alone has been demonstrated to be 80% to 90%.[32] However, as previously mentioned, these tests should be used in conjunction with other assessment tools and help inform the clinical diagnosis.

Ultimately, once an athlete is diagnosed with concussion, the responsible medical professional, coaching staff, the athlete, and the athlete's family are faced with the decision of when to return to physical and sport-related activity. Because no definitive medical treatments exist for concussion, the only effective therapy is physical and cognitive rest. A graduated return to play plan was recommended in the Consensus Statement on Concussion in Sport[1] and should be followed for a 1-week period at minimum as long as the athlete is asymptomatic at rest. This plan includes six rehabilitation stages and progresses from no activity through light activity and ultimately full-contact game play (Table 123-1). The plan should be tailored based on the severity of the initial injury and the individual athlete's history, especially if previous concussions are reported.[4,6] At each stage of the rehabilitation program, the athlete must be monitored for progression or return of symptoms, which, if present, would necessitate rest and deescalation of the activity level.

In conclusion, concussion is a common and likely underreported condition among athletes and is associated with potentially serious implications.

Spine

Overview of Pathologies

Neck and back pain in the athlete population are relatively common and can result from injuries to musculoligamentous, bony, neural, vascular, and disk structures.[33] These injuries are frequently minor injuries that cause discomfort and pain, but they can occasionally result in devastating neurologic injuries. Most serious injuries are recognized early and are handled by on-site emergency personnel, first responders, and emergency department staff. Therefore this section will focus on common outpatient complaints and diagnoses.

Spine Anatomy

The spine is divided into four functional segments; two are relatively mobile, and two are mostly rigid. The bony anatomy of the spine is characterized by 29 vertebrae that articulate with the vertebrae above and below to form functional spinal units. Each vertebra is composed of a vertebral body anteriorly connected to the posterior laminae, spinous process, and articulating facets by the pedicles. Between each vertebral body is an intervertebral disk. The spinal cord and nerve roots are transmitted through the spinal canal, which is surrounded by the vertebral body and posterior elements. Several ligaments connect the bony elements, providing additional support; these ligaments include the anterior longitudinal ligament, posterior longitudinal ligament, interlaminar

TABLE 123-1

GRADUATED RETURN-TO-PLAY PROTOCOL

Rehabilitation Stage	Function Exercise	Objective
No activity	Complete physical and cognitive rest	Recovery
Light aerobic exercise	Walking, swimming, stationary cycling <70% maximal heart rate; no resistance training	Increase heart rate intensity
Sport-specific	Sport-specific movements such as skating or running drills; no head impact drills	Add movement
Noncontact drills	Progression to more complex game-specific drills such as passing drills; may start resistance training	Exercise, coordination, and cognitive load
Full-contact practice	After medical clearance, participate in normal training	Restore confidence and assess functional skill by coaches
Return to play	Normal game play	

Data from McRory P, Meeuwisse W, Johnston K, et al: Consensus Statement on Concussion in Sport: the 3rd International Conference on Concussion in Sport held in Zurich, November 2008. *Br J Sports Med* 43(suppl 1): i76–i90, 2009.

Each stage lasts for approximately 24 hours, with the program taking approximately 1 week. If any symptoms recur during any stage, the player should immediately rest for 24 hours and, once asymptomatic, resume at the *preceding* stage. Concerns should be discussed with the athlete's physician.

ligaments, interspinous ligaments, facet joint capsules, and intertransverse ligaments. Several other specialized ligaments are found at each end of the spine in the craniovertebral junction and sacroiliac joints. The spinal musculature is mainly composed of longitudinally oriented muscles including the rectus, semispinalis, and splenius capitus muscles in the cervical spine and the erector spinae muscles in the thoracolumbar spine. The trapezius and rhomboid muscles also attach to the spine among other muscles. Also worth mentioning is that the course of the vertebral artery is intimately related to the cervical spine and can be affected in persons with cervical spine injuries.

Cervical Spine

The cervical spine is composed of seven vertebrae and permits most of the motion of the head with relation to the body. Each segment is therefore relatively mobile, with increasing motion occurring at the rostral end of the cervical spine. A gentle lordotic curve is characteristic of the cervical spine; straightening or reversal of this curve is indicative of an abnormality. Cervical spine injuries can occur in several different scenarios, including axial loading, translation, compression or distraction from impact, acceleration-deceleration, or excessive rotation.[34] Adolescent and pediatric athletes are more prone to ligamentous cervical injury for two reasons: (1) increased laxity of ligamentous structures and (2) increased head size relative to the remainder of the body.[35] Adults are more prone to bony fractures and disk herniations. However, the most common injury in both groups is muscular strain, also known as whiplash. Occasionally the vertebral arteries can be injured, especially in instances of excessive neck rotation, either accidental or intentional (e.g., chiropractic manipulation).

Thoracolumbar Spine

The thoracic spine is relatively rigid and therefore less prone to musculoligamentous injuries. However, high-impact collisions in some contact sports and among equestrians can result in a thoracic injury—frequently fracture or occasionally disk herniation. The lumbar spine, on the other hand, is much more mobile and prone to musculoligamentous injury; it is also a significant weight-bearing segment of the spine, supporting the upper body against the sacrum and pelvis caudally. Indeed, one of the most common outpatient complaints in adults is low back pain, frequently exacerbated by athletic activity.[36] Young athletes may also experience low back pain, which is also frequently due to musculoligamentous strain.[36] Less frequent causes of back pain in young athletes include ligamentous disruption, bony fracture, discogenic pain, and disk herniation. Spondylolysis, either congenital or acquired, is also a relatively common cause of chronic back pain in young athletes.[37,38] This condition is characterized by a defect in the pars interarticularis, usually of L5, that results in excessive motion between L5 and S1 and can cause nerve root compression and lower extremity radiculopathy.

Sacral Spine

The sacrum is composed of five fused vertebrae that articulate bilaterally with the pelvis and make up the posterior portion of the pelvic ring. The sacroiliac joint is one of the largest joints in the body and can be affected by a number of conditions. Athletic overuse injuries can result in sacroiliac joint inflammation or fractures and pain. Inflammatory and neoplastic diseases can also cause sacroiliac joint pain, but these diseases are not specific to athletes.

History

Obtaining the history in a patient with neck or back pain can help illuminate potential causes of the pain. It is important to attempt to define whether an inciting event led to the pain, such as a fall, collision, impact, or sudden increase in athletic activity. High-impact events, such as falls or collisions, should raise the suspicion for potential bony injury or ligamentous disruption.[34] Lower impact events and overuse are more likely to result in musculoligamentous strain or muscular spasm and pain during normal range of motion.

The nature of the patient's symptoms can also help determine the nature of the pathology. As with any history of pain, one should inquire about the onset of symptoms, whether the onset was abrupt or insidious, the duration of symptoms, whether symptoms are persistent or intermittent, worsening, inciting, and ameliorating factors, and whether the pain radiates. The presence or absence of neurologic symptoms should also be addressed, including headache, blurry or double vision, vertigo or imbalance, numbness or tingling of the extremities, impaired fine motor control (e.g., writing, buttoning shirts, tying shoes, opening doors, or handling keys and other small objects), impaired gait, and recent trips or falls.[39]

Musculoligamentous injury is usually associated with pain in the normal range of motion and is relieved by rest.[40] Icing and nonsteroidal antiinflammatory agents can also be helpful. Bony injury from fracture dislocation and acquired spinal deformity is usually more persistent and can be exacerbated by axial loading (weight bearing), as well as range of motion.[40] Nonsteroidal antiinflammatory drugs (NSAIDs) can be somewhat helpful but are frequently inadequate. Nerve root compression from disk herniation or another mechanism will frequently lead to radicular pain in the affected dermatome that is often described as a burning or tingling pain.[41] Radicular pain is also frequently more persistent than musculoligamentous pain and may also be refractory to NSAIDs. It is also common to have muscular weakness and paresthesias when nerve roots are involved. Injuries that result in compression of the spinal cord or cauda equina often have sudden dramatic implications, such as paralysis or severe paresis and sensory loss, but occasionally will have a more insidious or subtle presentation that may include imbalance, loss of fine motor control, bowel and bladder abnormalities, and subtle sensory changes. It is imperative to perform a detailed history and examination to identify any of these signs and symptoms and obtain the proper diagnostic studies.

Physical Examination

The physical examination of an athlete with suspected spinal injury should include a gross inspection of the area in question and palpation of the spinous processes in an attempt to elicit any point tenderness and detect any "step-off" or other deformity. Point tenderness over the spinous processes may indicate bony fracture and should prompt further evaluation. An obvious deformity should likewise prompt further investigation, and the patient should be immobilized until diagnostic studies can be obtained to ascertain the stability of the spine. It is also important to inspect global alignment, posture, and gait.

A thorough neurologic examination should also be performed if any spinal injury is suspected. In the case of collisions or falls, one should assess cognition, awareness, and attention because occult concussion may occur in these mechanisms as well. Examination of vision, oculomotor function, and balance can pick up subtle findings that may indicate vertebral artery injury in the case of some cervical injuries. Otherwise, it is important to perform a detailed and thorough examination of muscular strength, sensation, coordination, and fine motor control of the extremities. In the upper extremities, the intrinsic muscles of the hand, grip strength, wrist flexion and extension, biceps, triceps, and deltoid strength should all be assessed, as well as biceps, triceps, and brachioradialis reflexes and dermatomal sensation. Subtle signs of cervical myelopathy, including the Hoffman sign and impaired fine motor control, should also be assessed.

In the lower extremities, strength and power should be assessed in the quadriceps, tibialis anterior, extensor hallicis longus, soleus and gastrocnemius, and hamstrings, in addition to patellar, Achilles, and medial hamstring reflexes and dermatomal sensation. Upper motor neuron signs, including the Babinski sign, spasticity, and hyperreflexivity, should also be assessed. If bowel and/or bladder irregularities have been reported, it is prudent to examine perianal and genital sensation as well. Additionally, the straight leg raise and cross straight leg raise tests are useful in persons with lumbar radiculopathy.[42]

Most athletes with neck and back complaints have a self-limited musculoligamentous injury that will improve with rest and treatment with ice and NSAIDs. However, some more serious spinal pathologic conditions should be considered. A detailed history and physical examination, along with a working knowledge of spinal anatomy and disease, are imperative in the evaluation of these patients. An undiagnosed injury and return to activity could lead to potentially devastating neurologic injuries.

For a complete list of references, go to expertconsult.com.

Suggested Readings

Citation: McCrory P, Meeuwisse W, Johnston K, et al: Consensus statement on concussion in sport: The 3rd international conference on concussion in sport held in Zurich, November 2008. *Br J Sports Med* 43(Suppl 1):i76–90, 2009.

Level of Evidence: IV

Summary: This document is a revision and upgrade of the recommendations formed during the first and second International Symposia on Concussion in Sport. The document is intended for use by physicians, therapists, trainers, and other professionals involved in the care of injured athletes, either elite or recreational. The authors acknowledge that the science of concussion and concussion management are evolving fields, and therefore return-to-play decisions remain within the realm of clinical judgment on a case-by-case basis. The authors developed the Sports Concussion Assessment Tool (SCAT2) for use by persons evaluating concussed athletes.

Citation: Koh JO, Cassidy JD, Watkinson EJ: Incidence of concussion in contact sports: A systematic review of the evidence. *Brain Inj* 17:901–917, 2003.

Level of Evidence: III

Summary: The authors conducted a systematic review of the literature to estimate the incidence of concussion in contact sports. They found a relative paucity of good studies and several methodologic problems in reporting concussion incidence, especially for female athletes. That situation notwithstanding, the authors report that ice hockey and rugby have the highest incidence of concussion, with soccer having the lowest incidence. Male boxers and female taekwondo participants had the highest frequency of concussion among recreational athletes.

Citation: Guskiewicz KM, Bruce SL, Cantu RC, et al: Recommendations on management of sport-related concussion: Summary of the National Athletic Trainers' Association position statement. *Neurosurgery* 55:891–895, 2004.

Level of Evidence: IV

Summary: This article is an earlier—but one of the most comprehensive—reviews on the subject of concussion and concussion management in athletes. The effort stems from an effort by the National Athletic Trainers' Association to form a committee charged with developing a research-based position statement derived from the most recent scientific literature. The authors describe the recent literature and provide recommendations regarding concussion diagnosis, assessment, tools that can be used, and when to disqualify or refer an athlete to a physician, as well as special considerations for subpopulations, postconcussion care, and protective equipment.

Citation: McCrea M, Prichep L, Powell MR, et al: Acute effects and recovery after sport-related concussion: A neurocognitive and quantitative brain electrical activity study. *J Head Trauma Rehabil* 25:283–292, 2010.

Level of Evidence: IIa

Summary: The authors conducted a prospective study of 396 college and high school football players, including cohorts of 28 athletes with concussion and 28 matched control subjects. Concussed athletes and control subjects were evaluated at baseline during the preseason on measures of postconcussive symptoms, postural stability, and cognitive function, as well as quantitative electroencephalography (QEEG). These measures were repeated on the day of injury and at 8 and 45 days after injury. Injured athletes had more significant postconcussive symptoms in the first 3 days after injury, which resolved by days 5 to 8. However, QEEG demonstrated significant abnormalities in electrical brain activity on day 8 but not on day 45. The authors concluded that physiological brain recovery after concussion may continue after symptom resolution.

Citation: Lau BC, Collins MW, Lovell MR: Sensitivity and specificity of subacute computerized neurocognitive testing and symptom evaluation in predicting outcomes after sports-related concussion. *Am J Sports Med* 39:1209–1216, 2010.

Level of Evidence: IIb

Summary: The authors conducted a cohort study of 108 male high school football athletes who were diagnosed with concussion. Each athlete underwent computerized neurocognitive testing within 2.23 days of injury and separate discriminant function analyses (Post-Concussion Symptom Scale, symptom clusters, and Immediate Postconcussion Assessment and Cognitive Testing). The athletes were then followed up until return to play was permitted as established by international guidelines. The authors found that computerized neurocognitive testing increased the specificity and sensitivity of predicting a protracted recovery period (>14 days) when used alongside standard questionnaires.

Citation: Cantu RC, Li YM, Abdulhamid M, et al: Return to play after cervical spine injury in sports. *Curr Sports Med Rep* 12:14–17, 2013.

Level of Evidence: III

Summary: The authors review the history and salient features of cervical spine injury in athletes. Included is a description of a burner/stinger injury, musculoligamentous injury, cervical fracture, and acquired deformities, including cervical stenosis. The authors provide recommendations for return to play guidelines for various cervical spine injuries.

Citation: Mautner KR, Huggins MJ: The young adult spine in sports. *Clin Sports Med* 31(3):453–472, 2012.

Level of Evidence: III

Summary: The authors provide a description of sports-related spine injuries in young athletes. A detailed explanation of anatomic causes of back pain is included, as well as a list of red flags that should prompt further investigation. Recommendations are made for the evaluation and treatment of various commonly encountered spinal conditions in athletes.

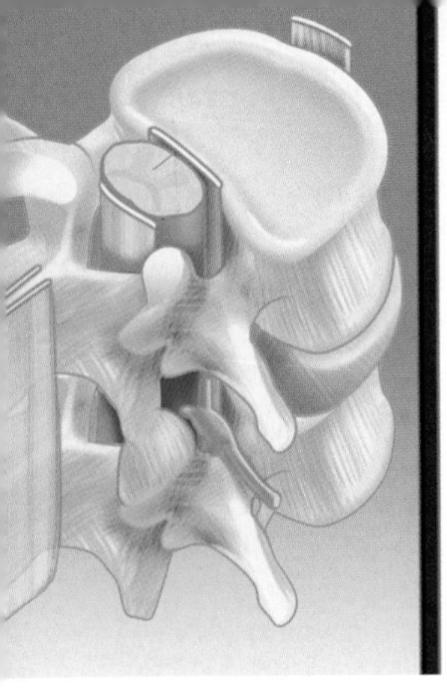

124

Head and Spine Imaging

ANOUSHEH SAYAH • FRANK BERKOWITZ

Head Imaging

After initial clinical evaluation and management, imaging can be a crucial step in the prompt workup and treatment of athletes with head trauma. An estimated 1.7 million people sustain traumatic brain injury (TBI) annually, and these injuries result in a third of all injury-related deaths in the United States.[1] The traumatic event is typically a one-time event, but the damage that follows is often a continuous and progressive process that can require multimodal and advanced imaging techniques for evaluation. Imaging can demonstrate the extent of primary pathologic conditions, including soft tissue injury, fractures, subdural and epidural hematomas, contusions, and diffuse axonal injury. Secondary injuries, such as cerebral swelling, herniation, hydrocephalus, infection, and ischemia/infarction, occur in a delayed fashion and warrant follow-up imaging. Long-term imaging may be used to determine the prognosis and rehabilitation options. The following sections review plain radiography, computed tomography (CT), and magnetic resonance imaging (MRI) modalities used in the evaluation of head trauma. The role of nuclear medicine is discussed briefly.

Indications for Head Imaging

Various criteria for use of CT after TBI have been recommended, although controversy remains regarding the timing of the imaging. Two of the more established guidelines are the New Orleans criteria and the Canadian Head CT rules. The New Orleans criteria limit the use of CT in patients with a minor head injury to patients with short-term memory deficit, drug or alcohol intoxication, evidence of trauma above the clavicles, age greater than 60 years, seizure, headache, or vomiting.[2] The Canadian Head CT guidelines similarly provide an imaging decision tool for adults with minor head trauma. These guidelines consist of a Glasgow Coma Scale score below 15 within first 2 hours, suspected open skull fracture, skull base fracture, vomiting, age greater than 65 years, retrograde amnesia, or a dangerous mechanism of injury.[3] Altered mental status, a focal neurologic deficit, and penetrating head injuries are other findings that should trigger an imaging evaluation.

In most cases diagnostic imaging of cerebral trauma should precede that of other concomitant injuries in the chest, abdomen, or pelvis. Additionally, one must consider whether primary cerebral disease, such as a ruptured aneurysm, caused the traumatic event. Suspicion of a head injury in an intoxicated patient warrants imaging, because up to 8% of intoxicated patients with minor head trauma are reported to have an intracerebral injury.[4,5] Increased rates of cerebral injury in children and the elderly also lower the imaging threshold in these populations because they may not show the typical warning signs or symptoms.[6] Patients with a history of coagulopathy or anticoagulant therapy have increased rates of delayed brain injury and merit early consideration for continued imaging.[7]

Imaging surveillance can help evaluate for new or worsening pathology. Bee et al.[8] report that 28% of patients with minimal brain injury show deterioration on repeat CT studies. Repeat imaging can assess for delayed or chronic traumatic sequelae (e.g., a reaccumulation hematoma, subdural empyema, brain abscess, brainstem bleeding, edema, tension pneumocephalus, and intraparenchymal hemorrhage), as well as guide rehabilitation and determine underlying functional abnormalities.

Imaging in Patients with a Sports-Related Concussion

Special consideration is given to concussion in this section because of the increasing attention given to this condition by the media and medical community. Concussion is generally accepted to be more of a functional/physiologic cerebral derangement than a structural abnormality. As such, CT and MRI do not have routine roles in the evaluation of concussion. Indeed, findings of CT and conventional MRI examinations are negative for most postconcussive athletes.[9] However, if the patient has posttraumatic signs and symptoms that raise suspicion for an intracranial lesion (e.g., loss of consciousness, altered mental status, amnesia, or a neurologic deficit), then CT imaging should be performed.[10]

Various modern, nonconventional imaging techniques investigated in the postconcussive setting consistently reveal brain abnormalities that are not detected with conventional examinations.[11] Cubon et al.[12] demonstrated subtle changes on diffusion tensor imaging (DTI) in postconcussive athletes and suggest this sequence as a tool to evaluate injury severity and determine management options. Functional MRI (fMRI) has shown an inverse relationship between brain activation and symptom severity immediately after a head injury in athletes.[13] Compared with neuropsychological testing, postconcussive fMRI is reported to have increased sensitivity to brain abnormalities in football players.[14] fMRI has also been used to document functional recovery after athletic concussion long after symptoms have resolved.[15] These techniques show potential in the investigative setting of concussion but are not yet in routine clinical use.

Plain Radiography

Historically, plain radiography or a "skull series" was the first, and often only, imaging study performed after head trauma. Because of the increasing availability of CT and MRI and the relatively lower sensitivities of radiography, radiographic imaging has markedly fallen out of favor.[16] Typical radiographic views include anteroposterior (AP) and lateral projections, with Caldwell, Townes, and/or Waters views available for further sinus and skull base evaluation. Skull fractures, pneumocephalus, foreign bodies, and penetrating injuries can be diagnosed with plain film. Visualization of foreign bodies is limited to radiopaque objects; wood and certain glass materials are not visible on radiographs. The paranasal sinuses may reveal fractures and/or hemorrhagic fluid levels. Mass effect may be determined by displacement of midline pineal gland calcifications or choroid calcifications. At present, however, radiographs are seldom used for evaluation of head trauma in adults and have almost completely been replaced by CT.

Computed Tomography

CT is generally considered the appropriate initial imaging examination in the acute posttraumatic setting because of ease of performance, availability, cost-effectiveness, and the ability to assess for acute pathologic conditions such as blood, mass effect, and fracture. Compared with other imaging modalities, CT is easier to obtain in patients who are connected to a ventilator, are in traction, or are agitated. The rapidity of CT imaging allows quick repeat imaging in studies with motion artifacts. CT data can be reconstructed into thin images for detailed evaluation and reformatted into various imaging planes and three-dimensional (3D) series.

Disadvantages of CT include the radiation dose delivered and artifacts from motion and beam hardening (notably in the posterior fossa). Small amounts of intracranial blood and linear skull fractures in the plane of section may be missed because of volume averaging.

CT findings can lag behind actual intracranial damage and thus early imaging (i.e., within 3 hours) may underestimate the degree of disease present.[17] Follow-up studies can assess for new or worsening pathologic conditions, such as delayed traumatic intracerebral hematomas and/or enlarging contusions.[18,19] Epidural hematomas have a lower threshold for repeat scanning; up to 65% can show enlargement on subsequent imaging.[20,21] Some authors argue that repeat studies should be performed 24 to 48 hours after all normal TBI head CT studies.[22,23]

Head CT scanning protocols are best performed with a slice thickness of 2.5 to 5 mm. Thinner axial images through the posterior fossa can be performed as needed. Scanning should include the foramen magnum and craniocervical junction. Noncontrast imaging is ideal in trauma situations because the presence of contrast material can mask intracranial hemorrhage.

Noncontrast CT scanning is excellent for subdural and epidural hematomas, although very small collections may be missed. Additionally, acute subdural hematomas in patients with anemia, coagulopathies, or associated arachnoid tears can be isodense to the adjacent brain parenchyma, making them difficult to detect. Low-density areas within acute hematomas suggest active bleeding, with hypodense regions reflecting active hemorrhage mixing with denser, clotted blood.[24] Subarachnoid hemorrhage (SAH) is well identified on CT and is typically seen over the cerebral convexities and in the basilar cisterns. Trace amounts of SAH may be missed on CT. The potential complications of SAH, including hydrocephalus and vasospasm, warrant follow-up imaging in the first days to weeks after trauma is sustained.

CT is also helpful for the detection of parenchymal contusions, with higher sensitivities for hemorrhagic contusions. Contusions are often coup-contrecoup in distribution and are mostly seen along the rough edges of the anterior cranial fossa, sphenoid wings, and petrous ridges (Fig. 124-1). CT is relatively insensitive for detection of diffuse axonal injury (DAI; also called *traumatic axonal* or *shear injury*).[25] Head CT findings are abnormal in fewer than half of all patients with DAI, with one third of patients with normal scans later demonstrating evidence of DAI on MRI.[26,27] This is likely because 80% of shear injuries are nonhemorrhagic and therefore are detected with less frequency on CT.[28] Delayed CT scanning may increase sensitivity for DAI because hemorrhagic foci increase and evolve over time. Long-term imaging may show associated encephalomalacia or Wallerian degeneration.

Secondary findings of head trauma include cerebral swelling, herniation, ischemia/infarction, and subdural hygromas. Loss of the gray/white matter differentiation and effacement of the cortical sulci and ventricles are notable CT findings of cerebral edema. Posttraumatic infarcts, which typically are hypodense regions following vascular distributions, have been reported in 8% of patients with a severe TBI.[29] Subdural hygromas or subdural cerebrospinal fluid (CSF) collections from tears in the arachnoid meninges can be seen up to several weeks after a head injury.

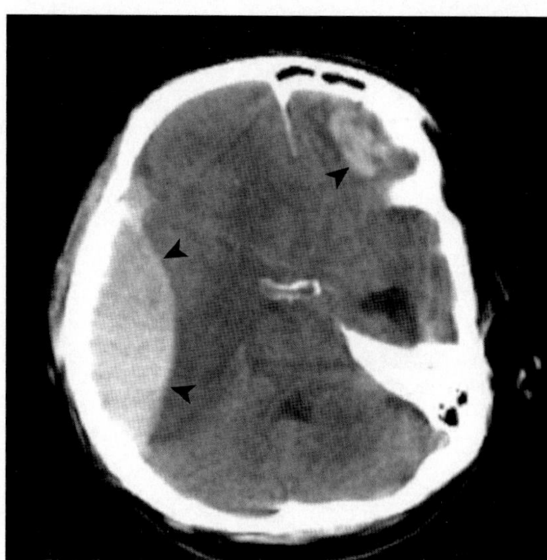

FIGURE 124-1 An axial computed tomography scan of the head in a soft tissue window demonstrates a right convexity epidural hematoma (*arrowheads*) and hemorrhagic anterior left frontal lobe parenchymal contusion (*arrow*) in a coup-contrecoup distribution. Also evident is parenchymal edema and loss of the basilar cerebrospinal fluid cisterns from parenchymal herniation.

Calvarial fractures are best evaluated with CT bone windows because they provide increased contrast between the calvarial cortices and the diploic space. Scout tomographic views may demonstrate fractures and should be evaluated in all studies. 3D projections are also helpful for delineation of fractures and their extent (Fig. 124-2).[30] Depressed or comminuted fractures should prompt evaluation for further intracranial damage. Skull fractures depressed more than the full thickness of the skull are of most concern and are typically surgical in nature. Pneumocephalus and/or fluid in the temporal bone (e.g., mastoid fluid) may herald the presence of a skull base fracture.

Persistent pneumocephalus should suggest the presence of a CSF leak. Nuclear medicine indium-111 or technetium-99 diethylene triamine pentaacetic acid cisternography can detect a leak but is not specific for determining the location of the defect. CT cisternography, with myelographic contrast, is excellent for detecting small osseous defects and provides the localization needed for surgical repair. Newer, high-resolution, heavily T2-weighted MRI sequences (e.g., 3D constructive interference in steady-state T2-weighted sequences) are also sensitive for skull base leaks and can aid in the detection of brain tissue herniated in association with the leak.[31]

The use of advanced CT techniques in persons with TBI is increasing, although they are mostly performed in the chronic setting for prognostication purposes. For example, CT perfusion is used to evaluate cerebral blood perfusion and can be more sensitive for small contusions compared with noncontrast CT. It is also reported to correlate well with functional outcomes. Normal or increased cerebral perfusion is seen in

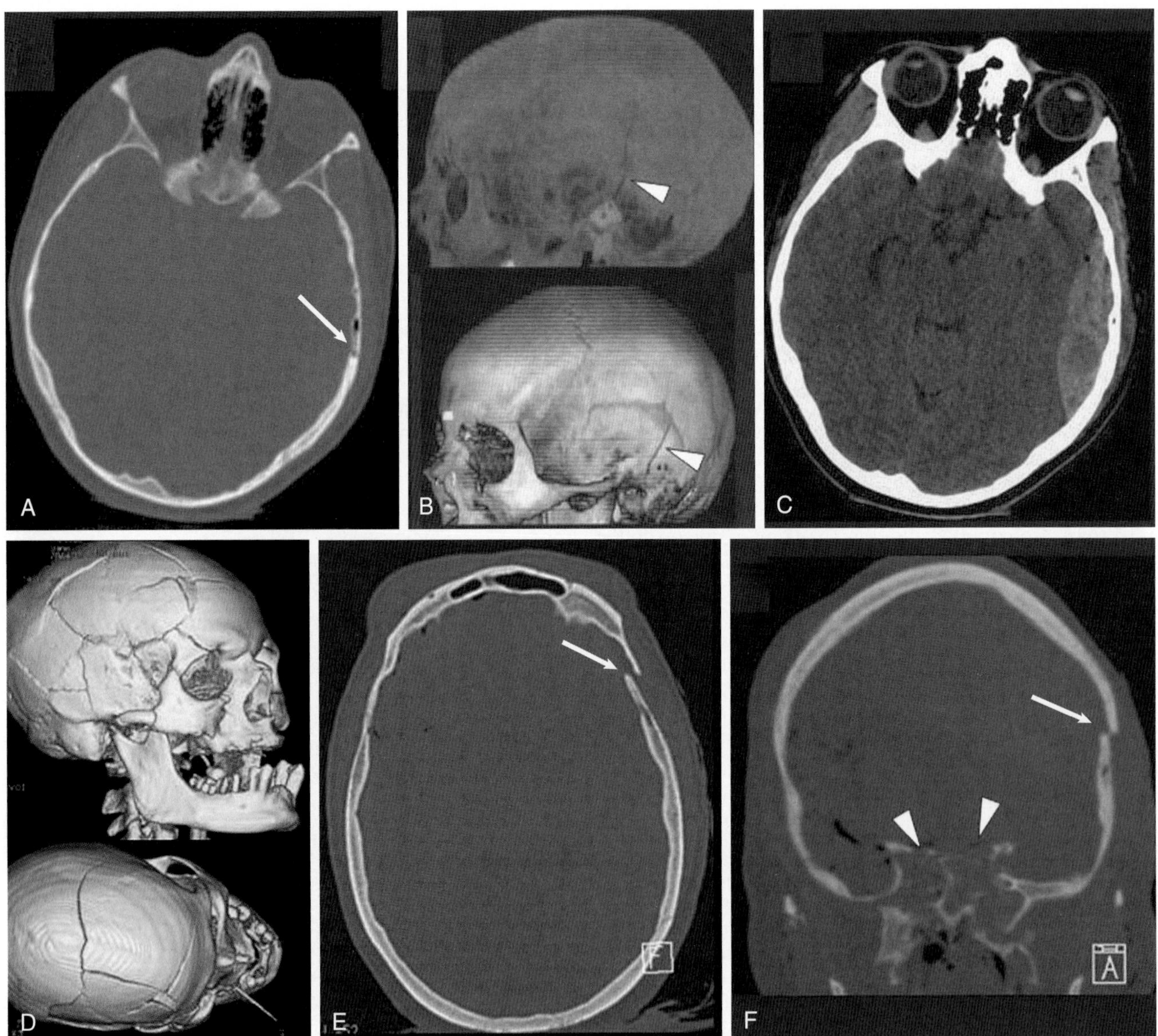

FIGURE 124-2 A left temporal calvarial fracture. An axial computed tomography head image in a bone window (**A**) reveals a linear calvarial fracture (*arrow*), which is better visualized in its entire course on three-dimensional volume-rendered reformatted images (**B** and **D**) (*arrowheads*). Soft tissue windows (**C**) demonstrate an underlying epidural hematoma. Axial (**E**) and coronal (**F**) bone window reformats demonstrate the degree of fracture displacement (*arrows*) as well as fractures at the skull base (*arrowheads*). *(From Law M, Som PM, Naidich TP:* Problem solving in neuroradiology, *Philadelphia, 2011, Elsevier.)*

patients with good clinical outcomes after head trauma, whereas oligemia is often found in patients with less favorable outcomes.[32]

Magnetic Resonance Imaging

MRI is more sensitive than CT for most posttraumatic pathologic conditions, including diffuse axonal injury, subdural hematomas, contusions, and brainstem lesions. In fact, CT has been reported to miss up to 30% of DAI lesions diagnosed with MRI.[26] Despite this situation, MRI is typically not the modality of choice for persons with an acute head injury and may not significantly change overall management of the patients with a TBI.[33,34] Instead, MRI is typically performed in the subacute and chronic settings to document the full extent of primary damage, secondary complications such as ischemia, and postoperative sequelae. MRI also aids with prognostication and often serves as a postinjury or posttherapy baseline examination.

MRI may help in the acute setting if CT findings do not fit with the clinical picture or if small hematomas or mild shear injury are suspected. The dural venous sinus and arterial systems can also be well evaluated with MRI for thrombosis, occlusion, or other vascular damage. Advantages of MRI include high contrast and spatial resolution, multiplanar acquisition capability, lack of ionizing radiation, the ability to characterize and date hemorrhage, little need for contrast material, and sensitivity for brainstem and posterior fossa injuries.

Disadvantages of MRI evaluation include significantly longer scan times, discomfort and claustrophobia (often requiring sedation or anesthesia), artifacts from implants, and poor sensitivity for pneumocephalus and skull base fractures. Various objects, implants, and medical devices can be contraindications for MRI. Each patient should be considered on an individual basis for compatibility issues. Studies are best performed on hemodynamic and neurologically stable patients because resuscitation efforts are difficult once the patient is in the machine.

Applicable MRI sequences for TBI imaging are fairly standard for current imaging practice. Sagittal T1-weighted imaging provides an overview of the midline structures. Axial T1- and T2-weighted sequences delineate anatomy and most intracranial pathologic conditions, including blood collections, mass effect, midline shift, hydrocephalus, and edema. Fluid-attenuated inversion recovery (FLAIR) imaging has increased sensitivity for detecting traumatic lesions and hematomas.[35] FLAIR imaging can detect small amounts of subarachnoid hemorrhage. Diffusion-weighted imaging (DWI) is optimal for diagnosing ischemia and sensitive for detecting many post-TBI lesions.[36] T2* gradient echo (GRE) and susceptibility-weighted imaging (SWI) are highly sensitive for hemorrhage, especially punctate foci of DAI that would be readily missed by other conventional sequences.[37,38]

DAI lesions on MRI are often diffuse and bilateral and most often located at the gray/white matter junction. Other common locations include the corpus callosum, basal ganglia, and brainstem. GRE and SWI sequences easily depict hemorrhagic foci, whereas FLAIR or T2-weighted images can pick up nonhemorrhagic lesions. DWI, and more specifically DTI, can be highly sensitive in detecting DAI lesions in the first hours after injury (Fig. 124-3).[39]

Specialized MRI techniques can aid in the long-term management and prognostication of patients with TBI. DTI and SWI sequences may correlate with cognitive impairment and functional outcomes,[40,41] and fMRI studies show changes in patients with varying degrees of TBI who demonstrate persistent changes in memory tasks.[42,43] MR spectroscopy can demonstrate decreased levels of the neuronal marker N-acetylaspartate in patients with a head injury, suggesting neuronal loss, notably in the corpus callosum.[44,45]

Nuclear Medicine

Radionuclide imaging of the patient with TBI consists mainly of cisternography for the evaluation of CSF leaks (as previously described) and positron emission tomography (PET) and single photon emission computed tomography (SPECT) imaging for long-term therapy and prognosis. Brain SPECT and PET imaging evaluates cerebral perfusion and metabolic activity. Cerebral hypoperfusion on SPECT and decreases in regional metabolism on PET are often seen in persons with acute and chronic brain injuries, even in patients without structural lesions on CT or MRI.[46,47] Normal or hyperemic results of initial SPECT examinations may predict favorable clinical outcomes in patients who have experienced head trauma.[48] Decreased regional metabolism on PET has been found to correlate with cognitive and behavioral disorders after TBI.[49]

Angiography

Angiography can be used to identify posttraumatic vascular injuries such as dissection, occlusion, and pseudoaneurysm and to determine lesion extent, location, type, and collateral supply. Abnormal findings include luminal narrowing from stenosis, abrupt cutoff from occlusion, irregular outpouchings from pseudoaneurysm, linear filling defects and flame-shaped luminal tapering in traumatic dissection, or extravasation from wall injury. Catheter angiography remains the gold standard but harbors a neurologic complication rate of 2.6%; the vast majority of these complications are transient or reversible.[50] The noninvasiveness, ease, and accessibility of computed tomographic angiography (CTA) and magnetic resonance angiography (MRA) have made these modalities increasingly popular. Unlike catheter studies, which evaluate only the lumen, MRA and CTA can also provide information about the arterial wall. CTA has higher spatial resolution and fewer flow-related artifacts than does MRA, although at the cost of ionizing radiation. The presence of brain ischemia after a head injury should prompt the clinician to exclude vascular injury. CT and MR venography can be used to evaluate for venous thrombosis and occlusion as a complication of a basilar skull fracture.

Pediatric Considerations

Skull fractures and intracranial injury from minor trauma are more common in children than in adults, especially in children younger than 2 years.[6] Subdural hematomas are more common in infants and young children than in teens and are usually bilateral. The prominent subarachnoid spaces of benign external hydrocephalus can mimic chronic subdural hematoma or hygroma in children younger than 2 years but can be distinguished by the presence of vessels traveling through the subarachnoid space. Epidural hematomas are less

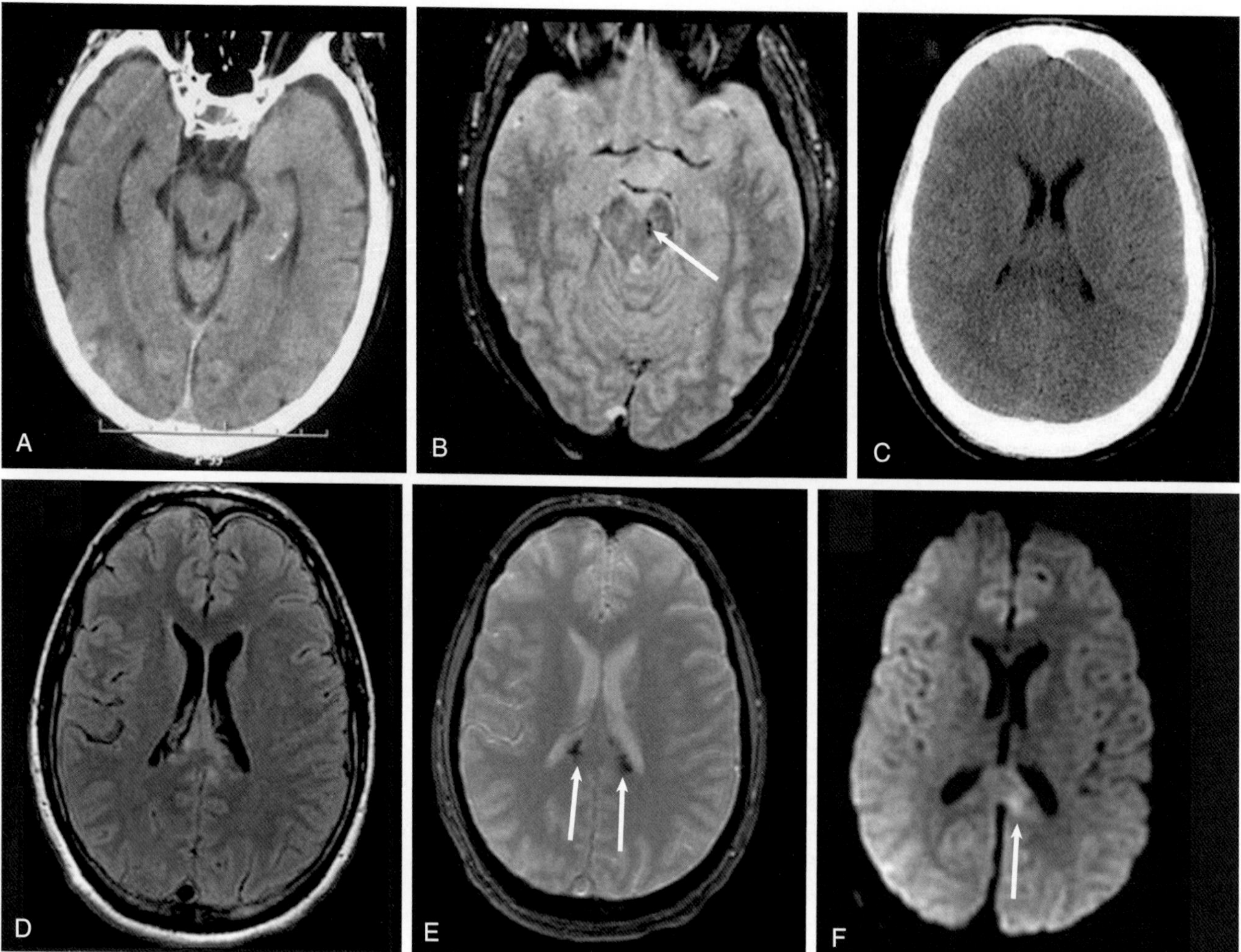

FIGURE 124-3 Diffuse axonal injury. Axial computed tomography of the head in soft tissue windows (**A** and **C**) does not show significant injury. However, magnetic resonance imaging gradient echo sequences at the same levels, respectively (**B** and **E**), reveal hemorrhagic axonal shear injury lesions along the splenium of the corpus callosum (*arrows*). The callosal lesions demonstrate hyperintensity on fluid-attenuated inversion recovery imaging (**D**) and restricted diffusion on diffusion-weighted imaging (**F**). *(From Law M, Som PM, Naidich TP:* Problem solving in neuroradiology, *Philadelphia, 2011, Elsevier.)*

common in infants, but if present the clinical presentation may be less dramatic than that seen in adults. Aggressive early CT imaging should be performed if an epidural hematoma is suspected.

Awareness of the risks of radiation related to radiography and CT imaging in the pediatric population is increasing. Theoretically, radiation exposure at a young age may predispose the patient to radiation-related neoplasms later in life. Children with a head injury are typically monitored closely for worsening symptoms before a CT scan is performed. Altered mentation, vomiting, or evidence of a skull fracture are strong indications for head CT scanning. Use of nonionizing imaging modalities (MRI or ultrasound) may be considered in certain cases. Further guidelines regarding pediatric imaging can be found at www.imagegently.org or via the American College of Radiology Appropriateness Criteria (www.acr.org/ac).

Spine Imaging

Athletics results in 8% of all new spinal cord injuries (SCIs) and is the main cause of spine injuries in persons younger than 30 years.[51] The highest incidence of SCI is seen in the late teens and early 20s, with a second peak likely in elderly persons; the lowest incidence is seen in young children.[52] Sports-related etiologies of SCI have declined from 14% of SCIs in the 1970s to 10% in 2000,[52] largely because of improvements in protective equipment, on-field management, and sporting rules (e.g., a spear tackling ban in football). Sports-related spine trauma is associated with a wide range of sports from football to gymnastics to diving, with mechanisms and severities of injury that are just as varied. Football accounts for the highest number of severe cervical spine injuries among high school and collegiate sports.[53] Furthermore, the cervical spine is the most injured spinal location among National Football League players.[54] In the following discussion we review the indications for spine imaging in the injured athlete and the various modalities available.

Cervical Spine

Indications for Imaging

Specific criteria regarding when and how to perform imaging for a patient with a posttraumatic cervical spine injury have been widely debated. The Canadian C-spine Rules (CCR) and the National Emergency X-Radiography Utilization Study (NEXUS) Low-risk Criteria are two guidelines that are now well established in clinical practice. Based on CCR, imaging should be performed in patients with a dangerous mechanism of injury, who are older than 65 years, and/or who have paresthesias. Conversely, patients with low risk factors who have at least 45 degrees of range of neck motion to the left and to the right do not require imaging.[55] Patients who are alert and lack any midline tenderness, have no focal neurologic deficits, are not intoxicated, or lack distracting injuries meet the NEXUS Low-risk Criteria and also do not need imaging evaluation.[56,57]

Plain Radiography

Despite the increasing availability of CT and MRI, radiographs are performed for most athletes with spine trauma before any other imaging evaluation. Plain radiography is quick, inexpensive, widely available, and can be performed at the bedside. However, radiographic imaging is highly technique dependent. The NEXUS study showed a near 100% negative predictive value for a three-view cervical spine series (lateral, AP, and odontoid), but only in studies that were deemed technically adequate. A good-quality film needs to be properly exposed and positioned, without motion or other artifacts. Specialized views may be needed for patients with limited range of motion, large body habitus, or bulky sports gear. Helmets and shoulder pads are usually not removed prior to imaging to avoid further cervical spine injury, although they often limit cross-table lateral studies and render only 20% to 35% of additional cervical spine views acceptable.[58] Findings missed on radiographs are often due to nondisplaced fractures, spontaneously reduced injuries, overlapping osseous structures, and studies with poor exposure, positioning, or motion.

The lateral cervical spine view should include all cervical vertebrae and the cervico-occipital and cervicothoracic junctions, without rotation (i.e., facet joints should overlap). Approximately 3% of injuries at the cervicothoracic junction are missed on plain radiography, mainly because of inadequate visualization at that level.[59] As such, if the top of T1 is not properly viewed, the wrists may be pulled toward the feet to remove the shoulders from the field of view. Additionally, higher exposure images centered on the lower cervical spine or swimmer's views can be performed. Swimmer's views are obtained by lifting one arm up to move the shoulder joint away from the lower cervical and upper thoracic spine. This view is not performed in patients with shoulder or arm injuries, unreliable examinations, or cord injuries (Fig. 124-4).

Evaluation for a cervical spine injury on the lateral view involves assessment of various anatomic lines and measurements. The prevertebral soft tissues should be less than 7 mm at the C2 level and less than 22 mm in adults (<14 mm in children) at C6. These measurements may be unreliable if the patient is intubated or has a nasogastric tube.[60] A normal prevertebral soft tissue width does not exclude fracture. Any disruption of the anterior spinal, posterior spinal, posterior pillar, or spinolaminar lines should raise suspicion for injury (Fig. 124-5). Although a small amount of physiologic subluxation (2 to 3 mm) can be seen involving several levels,[61] any amount of cervical anterolisthesis is worrisome.[62] Any positive or equivocal findings at radiography should be followed up with CT. Even if radiographs are normal, CT should be performed if the mechanism of injury is suspicious.

Various measurements are used to evaluate the cervical spine by radiography. Harris' rule of 12 states that the normal basion-dens interval, as well as the interval between the basion and posterior axial line, should not exceed 12 mm (Fig. 124-6).[63] The tip of the dens should not extend more than 5 mm above the line connecting the posterior hard palate to the opisthion, also known as *Chamberlain's line*. An atlantodental interval greater than 3 mm in adults or 5 mm in children is abnormal and likely reflects a transverse ligament injury.[64-66] The Powers ratio (the distance from the basion to the midportion of the C1 posterior laminar line divided by the distance from the opisthion to the midportion of the posterior surface of the C1 anterior ring) is used to assess for atlantooccipital dislocation; a ratio greater than 1.0 is abnormal.[67] Subluxation of the vertebral bodies may

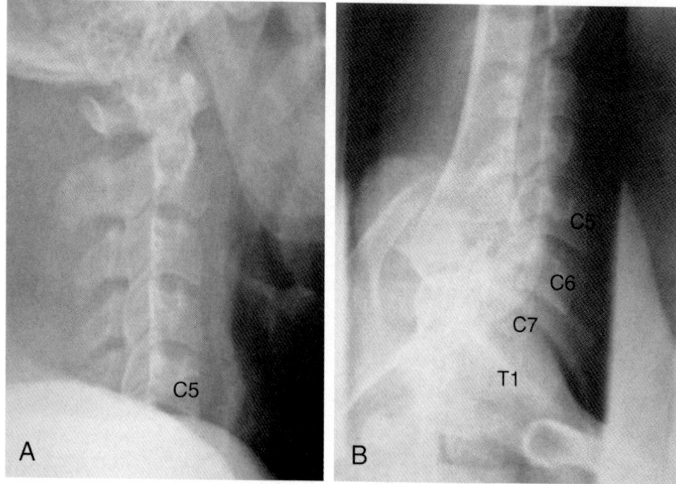

FIGURE 124-4 The initial lateral view (**A**) of the cervical spine is suboptimal for evaluation of the C6, C7, and T1 vertebral bodies. A subsequent swimmer's view (**B**) demonstrates bilateral jumped facet and greater than 50% translation of C6 on C7 not seen on the initial view.

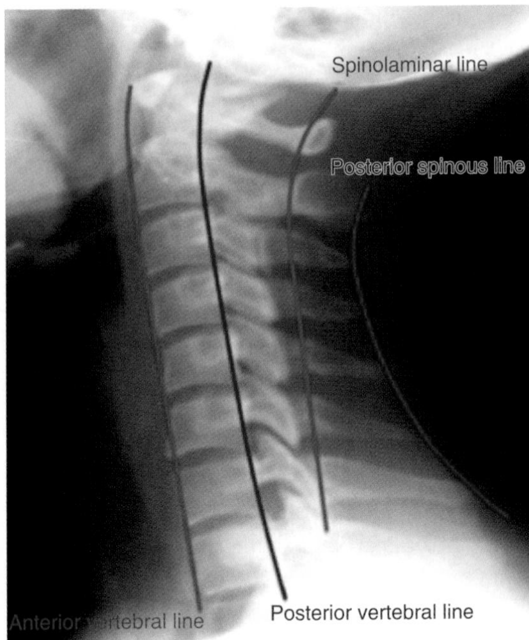

FIGURE 124-5 Lines of the cervical spine. Disruptions in any of these lines may herald an injury.

indicate facet dislocation: 25% subluxation is seen with unilateral dislocation, whereas 50% subluxation is seen with bilateral dislocation.

On AP views, the disk spaces should be uniform at each level and the articular masses should be superimposed. The tips of the spinous processes are vertically aligned; any malalignment may reflect rotational injury (e.g., facet dislocation). Disruptions in the lateral masses may indicate fracture.

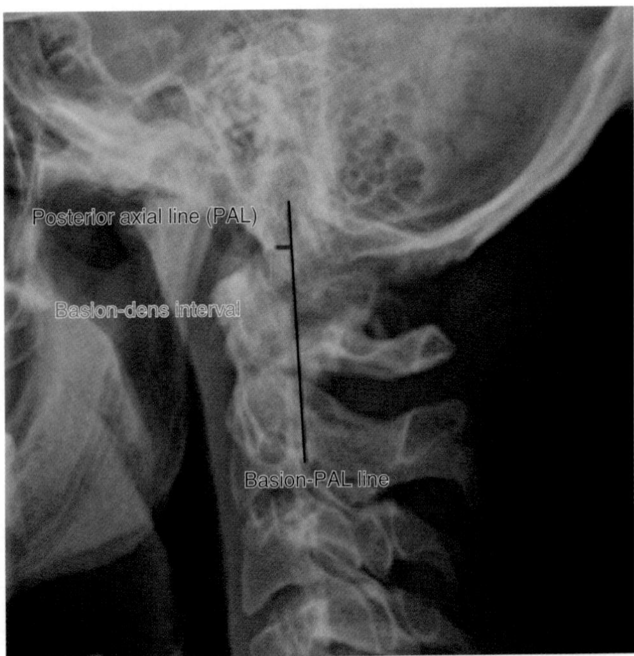

FIGURE 124-6 Harris' rule of 12. The basion-dens interval and posterior axial lines (*PAL*) should be <12 mm in length.

The open-mouth odontoid view requires patient cooperation and allows improved visualization of the occiput and C1 and C2 vertebral bodies for diagnosis of lesions such as Jefferson and dens fractures. The lateral margins of C1 normally lie within 1 to 2 mm of the C2 lateral mass margins. Any further overhang suggests a C1 fracture. Combined displacement of the bilateral lateral masses greater than 7 or 8 mm suggests a Jefferson fracture with an associated transverse ligament injury.[68,69]

Historically, flexion-extension views were used to assess for occult fracture or ligamentous injury and to rule out instability. Often this imaging was performed several weeks after injury in cases of persistent weakness despite negative radiographic or CT examination. However, various studies have consistently shown that flexion-extension views and dynamic fluoroscopic examinations are highly insensitive, with a reported 28% to 57% inaccuracy rate.[70,71] Bolinger et al.[72] report that only 4% of their dynamic studies visualized the C7-T1 level properly. As a result, the American College of Radiology recommends these examinations only in the occasional instances when MRI findings are equivocal and the patient has continued symptomatology.[73]

Computed Tomography

CT is the primary modality used in current trauma imaging because of its ease of use, speed, wide availability, ability to reconstruct in multiple planes, and increased sensitivity compared with radiography. In fact, 57% of diving-related fractures diagnosed with CT were initially missed on radiographs.[74] The NEXUS criteria study demonstrated that only 62% of cervical spine injuries were diagnosed with radiographs. Accordingly, the American College of Radiology recommends thin-section CT with sagittal and coronal reconstructions as the primary study of choice for patients with evidence of a cervical spine injury. If CT is unavailable, a three-view radiographic series should be performed until CT can be obtained.[73] CT should be performed using collimation of 1 mm or less so that good-quality sagittal and coronal reformations can be obtained. Axial images should be viewed with a slice thickness of 3 mm or less. It is important to look at both soft tissue and bone windows.

Evaluation usually begins with the reformatted images. On sagittal reformatted images, it is important to assess alignment of the anterior vertebral bodies, posterior vertebral bodies, spinolaminar line, and facet joints. On CT, the atlas-dens interval (predental space), facet joint spaces, and atlantooccipital joint spaces should all be no more than 2 mm in the adult and 2.5 mm in the child. Sagittal reformats are also good for evaluating the prevertebral soft tissues. Separation of the prevertebral fat stripe from the bone may indicate edema or hemorrhage related to a fracture or ligamentous injury. This is best evaluated in the upper cervical spine.

CT is optimal for osseous structures, aiding in fracture diagnosis and evaluation of fracture fragments within the spinal canal. CT can demonstrate ligamentous injury in a high proportion of cases, although MRI is far superior for this purpose.[75] Disadvantages of CT include the radiation dose, motion artifacts, and streak artifacts through the lower cervical spine due to attenuation from the shoulders. Patient motion during the CT acquisition can falsely suggest malalignment. Careful review of the axial images shows slices with motion artifact at the level of apparent step-off (Fig. 124-7).

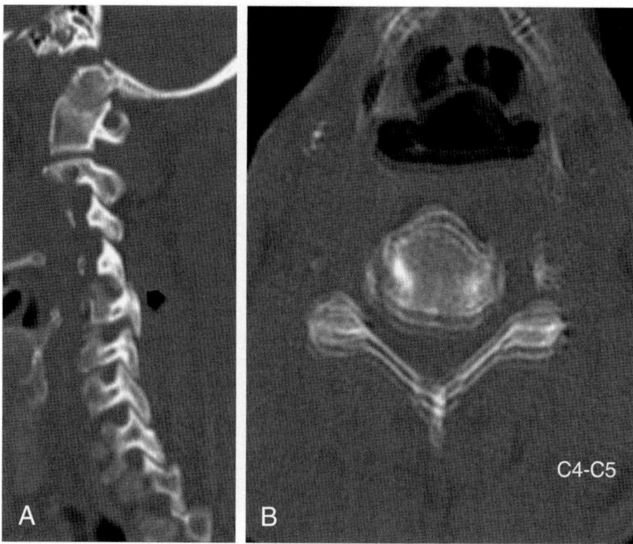

FIGURE 124-7 Sagittal reconstruction (**A**) demonstrates possible C4-C5 facet dislocation (*arrowhead*). Further evaluation of the source axial data at the C4-C5 level (**B**) shows significant motion artifact creating the apparent facet dislocation.

CTA provides an excellent depiction of the cervical arteries and should be performed when a vascular injury is suspected. Most spinal vascular injuries are located in the cervical spine. The vertebral arteries are injured more often than the carotid arteries, mainly because of their fixed location within the osseous transverse foramina. Fractures suspicious for concomitant vascular injury include transverse foramen fractures and complex subluxated/dislocated vertebral fractures (Fig. 124-8). CTA and MRA are both appropriate techniques for the investigation of suspected vascular injury. CTA is performed with an injection of iodinated contrast material, whereas MRA may be obtained with or without use of gadolinium contrast material. Catheter angiography is typically reserved for further evaluation or intervention (e.g., embolization) of a known lesion.

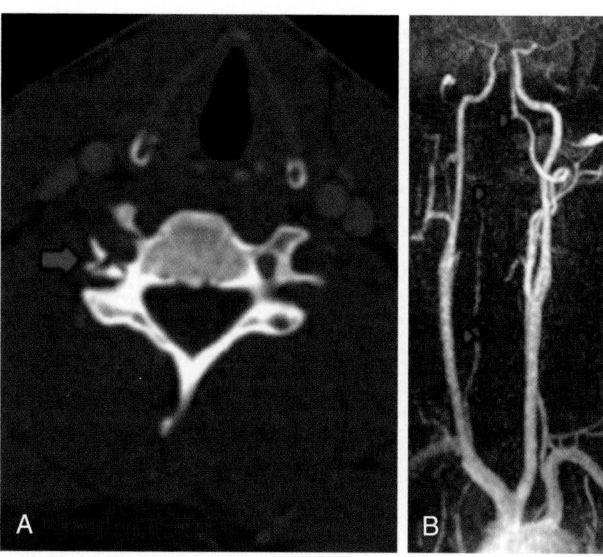

FIGURE 124-8 A transverse foraminal fracture with resulting vertebral artery dissection. **A,** An axial computed tomography cervical spine image shows a right transverse foramen fracture (*arrow*). **B,** Maximum intensity projection from magnetic resonance angiography reveals irregular narrowing and occlusion of the right vertebral artery (*arrowheads*).

CT myelography has mostly been replaced by high-resolution MRI sequences, although contraindication to MRI, MRI unavailability, significant spinal hardware, or physician preference may dictate its use. Myelography can demonstrate canal stenosis, foraminal stenosis, nerve root compression or avulsion, and cord compression. Nonionic water-soluble iodinated contrast is instilled into the spinal subarachnoid space, which is accessed via lumbar puncture. The C1-C2 level can also be accessed if necessary. Spot fluoroscopic images are generally obtained prior to CT myelographic imaging.

Magnetic Resonance Imaging

MRI is typically reserved for patients with spinal trauma who have a neurologic deficit, worsening neurologic status, or a neurologic examination that does not fit with CT or radiographic findings or require preoperative evaluation. It is the modality of choice for cord disease and can help identify causes of cord contusion or compression. Levitz et al.[76] demonstrated that 87% of athletes with recurrent stinger symptoms have MRI evidence of disk bulge, protrusion, or herniation. As a result, symptoms persisting beyond 24 to 36 hours should raise suspicion for cord injury and be evaluated with MRI.[77]

Advantages of MRI include high contrast resolution (with excellent soft tissue, spinal cord, and ligamentous delineation), lack of ionizing radiation, no need for contrast material in most cases, and the ability to image in multiple planes. High-resolution sequences can be used to evaluate the spinal canal and its contents in a myelographic fashion, without requiring intrathecal contrast material.

Typical MRI sequences include sagittal T1-weighted sequences for anatomy; sagittal T2-weighted sequences for spinal cord disease and ligamentous structures; sagittal short tau inversion recovery (STIR) for marrow or soft tissue edema, ligamentous injury, and cord lesions[78]; axial T2-weighted sequences for the cord, foramina, and epidural space; and axial GRE for cord hemorrhage and neural foramina. Optional sequences include sagittal proton density to confirm ligamentous disruption and to better visualize epidural collections/blood; sagittal GRE for cord hemorrhage; and DWI for cord ischemia. MRA along with fat-saturated T1-weighted axial sequences can be performed to evaluate the cervical vasculature for traumatic lesions such as dissection or vertebral artery injury (Fig. 124-8).

Disadvantages of MRI include increased time, increased cost, limited availability, presence of MRI-incompatible devices and implants, smaller gantry sizes, artifacts from metallic hardware, and claustrophobia or the need for sedation. Regions of the spine of the most clinical interest should be imaged first in case the patient moves or becomes uncomfortable later in the study. Quick, limited surveys of the spine can be performed as necessary. MRI also has an overall high false-positive rate (25% to 50%) and a low sensitivity for osseous injury (55%).[79,80] Consequently, MRI is not used for first-line imaging, and abnormalities should always be correlated with the clinical examination, as well as with findings from other radiologic studies.

MRI is the best tool available for evaluation of cord pathology. Findings of interest include the extent of hemorrhage, length of edema, and evidence of parenchymal disruption such as compression or transection. Follow-up imaging may reveal subacute to chronic posttraumatic changes such as a syrinx, cyst formation, and chronic atrophy. SCI without radiographic abnormality (SCIWORA) syndrome was coined by Pang and Pollack[81] in 1989 to describe cord injury without findings on radiographs or CT. SCIWORA was initially described and most commonly occurs in the pediatric population, likely because of inherent cervical spine elasticity. SCIWORA is also seen in adults with a cervical spine injury, often from acute trauma superimposed on preexisting spondylosis, and involves up to 12% of adult cord injuries.[82]

MRI is sensitive for a range of other pathologies that can be seen after spine trauma. MRI is ideal for posttraumatic disk injury, which may be indicated by asymmetric narrowing or widening of the disk space or increased T2 signal intensity in the disk itself. Ligamentous disruption is well identified on MRI as a focal gap in the ligament often with adjacent soft tissue edema, with or without an associated hematoma. Soft tissue injury or edema is best imaged in the first 3 days after injury before it begins to resolve (Fig. 124-9). The exclusion of epidural hematoma is a common indication for MRI after spinal injury, especially in cases of suspected cord or cauda equina impingement. Epidural hematomas can be seen in up to 41% of spine injuries,[83] although most are not clinically significant.[84] Although MRI can assess for spinal canal stenosis, currently only athletes with prior cervical cord neurapraxia undergo MRI screening for stenosis. In patients with nerve root avulsion, MR is reported to be as sensitive and even more accurate than CT myelography for detecting pseudomeningoceles.[85] The pseudomeningocele often appears as an epidural or soft tissue mass or CSF collection within the neural foramen (Fig. 124-10).

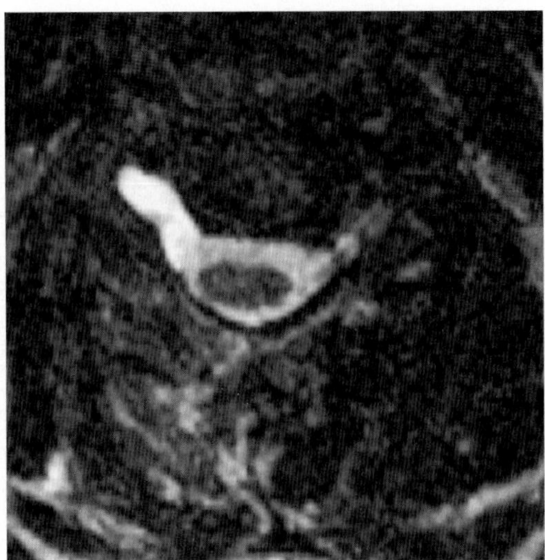

FIGURE 124-10 Nerve root avulsion with a pseudomeningocele. An axial gradient echo magnetic resonance imaging sequence through the C6 vertebral body shows masslike hyperintensity in the right transverse foramen, representing a pseudomeningocele from nerve root avulsion. The right-sided roots are less conspicuous compared with the left-sided roots.

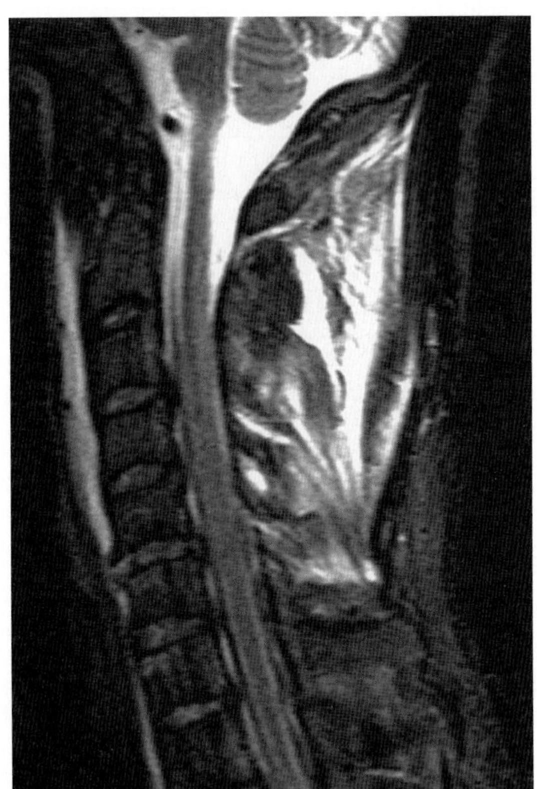

FIGURE 124-9 An anterior and posterior ligamentous and soft tissue injury. A magnetic resonance imaging short tau inversion recovery sequence through the cervical spine reveals diffuse signal abnormality in the posterior soft tissues indicative of soft tissue edema and posterior ligamentous injury. The presence of prevertebral edema and anterior longitudinal ligament tear with disk injury at the C4-C5 level classifies this injury as a three-column injury. *(From Naidich TP, Castillo M, Cha S et al:* Imaging of the spine: expert radiology series, *Philadelphia, 2010, Elsevier.)*

Pediatric Considerations

Spine injuries are less common in the pediatric population compared with adults. Fewer than 1% of children evaluated after blunt trauma show radiographic evidence of cervical spine injury.[86] The aforementioned CCR and NEXUS criteria can be applied to children older than 14 years because their spines are typically developed by this age.[73] Guidelines for performing imaging in patients younger than 14 years are less well defined. Younger children frequently have upper cervical spine lesions, whereas teens have lower cervical, adult-type injuries. Radiography is usually first-line imaging, with high sensitivity for cervical spine trauma, in the pediatric population.[87] Head stabilization can improve visualization of the cervicothoracic junction on lateral cervical spine radiographs and can reduce radiation dose by decreasing need for additional views.[88] It is important to note that lateral views in children may reveal up to 2 mm of physiologic pseudosubluxation at the C2-C3 level, which can cause disruption of anterior and posterior cervical lines, although the spinolaminar line should remain intact.

Early CT evaluation of children at high risk for cervical spine injury may result in more effective cervical spine clearance.[89] CT must be used judiciously in children, however, given the relative low risk of spine injury in children and the need to minimize their exposure to radiation. Hernandez et al.[90] report that multidetector CT in patients younger than 5 years may be of little clinical benefit and results in substantial increases in the radiation dose.[90] As such, the use of CT in children can be limited to the specific levels of concern based on clinical examination and findings of preceding studies.

Thoracolumbar Spine

The thoracic and lumbar (T/L) spines differ from the cervical spine in that the thoracolumbar spine has more support from surrounding musculature, the rib cage, and soft tissues. Khan et al.[91] summarized the specific mechanisms of T/L spine injury in a variety of sports. Most injuries are sprains and are usually not imaged unless pain persists over several weeks. A recent study of National Football League players over 11 seasons revealed that lumbar injuries made up 31% of all spine injuries, 7% of which were fractures. Thoracic spine injuries resulted in only 4% of injuries (12% of which were fractures) but resulted in the most days missed from play.[54]

Indications

Indications for imaging of the thoracolumbar spine include back pain, midline tenderness, neurologic deficit, cervical spine fracture, a Glasgow Coma Scale score less than 15, a major distracting injury, or intoxication.[92] Imaging assessment typically begins with radiographic examination, with CT to follow. MRI can be obtained to evaluate disease involving the spinal cord or canal. Up to 16% of patients with T/L fractures have a concomitant noncontiguous fracture elsewhere in the spine and therefore should undergo complete spine imaging.[93]

Plain Radiography

Plain radiography of the T/L spine begins with AP and lateral views. The combined AP and lateral T/L spine radiographs can show up to 90% of bony fractures.[91] In severely injured patients, a cross-table lateral view supplants the standard lateral view. The upper thoracic spine is obscured on the lateral view by the shoulders and is best evaluated on the AP view. The AP view is used to assess osseous alignment and evaluate interpedicular distances, which should gradually increase in a craniocaudal direction. The lateral view provides good visualization of the vertebral body heights, disk space heights, and sagittal alignment and is thus ideal for compression fractures and pathologic listhesis. Acute changes in disk space height can be seen with posttraumatic herniations.

Oblique views of the lumbar spine can be obtained to better visualize the lamina and posterior elements for fractures and spondylolysis. Flexion-extension views of the lumbar spine can evaluate for instability, often signaled by greater than 3 mm of change from flexion to extension. Other potential radiographic signs of T/L spinal instability include widened facet joints, interspinous widening, a sudden increase in interpedicular space, facet dislocations, and loss of more than 50% of vertebral body height. Vertebral displacement/translation or increased interpedicular distance is worrisome for three-column injury.

Computed Tomography

Indications for CT imaging of the thoracolumbar spine include abnormality on a preceding radiograph, clinical discrepancy between the clinical examination and radiography, or suspicion of spondylolysis in an athlete with chronic low back pain. CT is also used in obtunded or unreliable patients to look for occult injuries. Noncontrast CT is viewed in bone and soft tissue windows and sagittal and coronal reformats, as in the cervical spine. Reformats from CT chest, abdomen, and pelvis examinations are more sensitive for disease than is plain radiography in the T/L spine,[94] which is especially helpful in the pediatric population, for whom radiation dose is an increasing concern. CT myelography is used to detect cord, cauda equina, or canal pathology in cases in which MRI is unavailable or contraindicated.

Magnetic Resonance Imaging

Thoracic and lumbar MRI is often performed to evaluate for cord lesions (i.e., compression, edema, or hemorrhage) and cauda equina syndrome. Paraspinal soft tissue, ligamentous, and disk injury is also well evaluated with MRI. Indications for MRI of the T/L spine mainly involve neurologic deficits or deficits that are not explained by radiographic imaging. Emergent MRI is performed in cases of cauda equina syndrome or progressive neurologic deficit. MRI is often not performed if CT and radiographs are normal, unless neurologic symptoms persist. MRI does have a high false-positive rate, with abnormalities in up to 64% of asymptomatic lumbar spines,[95,96] and therefore findings need to correlate with the clinical examination.

Sequences include sagittal T1, sagittal T2, sagittal STIR, axial T1, and axial T2. GRE and DWI sequences, as well as coronal plane imaging, can be performed as clinically necessary. Kinematic flexion-extension MRI studies to evaluate unstable injuries and subluxations are available, although they are not part of common clinical practice.[97] Follow-up MRI studies are obtained for new or progressive symptoms to evaluate for residual/recurrent cord compression, arachnoid adhesions, syringomyelia, or myelomalacia.

Nuclear Medicine

Nuclear medicine imaging is not regularly performed in the acute evaluation of athletic spine injury. The most common sports-related spine indication is the use of technetium-99m bone scans for suspected spondylolysis in the athlete with chronic low back pain and negative radiography. SPECT imaging is often added to increase spatial resolution. A bone scan is highly sensitive but relatively nonspecific for pars defects compared with CT,[98] although CT can be normal with chronic fractures.[99] A positive bone scan often indicates that the defect is in an active phase in which immobilization may be of greatest benefit and may also demonstrate impending pars fractures.[100]

For a complete list of references, go to expertconsult.com.

Suggested Readings

Citation: Haydel MJ, Preston CA, Mills TJ, et al: Indications for computed tomography in patients with minor head injury. *N Engl J Med* 343(2):100–105, 2000.

Level of Evidence: II

Summary: The authors of this prospective study evaluated 520 consecutive patients for the purpose of establishing a set of clinical criteria that can identify patients with minor head trauma who do not require computed tomography scanning of the head.

Citation: Stiell IG, Wells GA, Vandemheen K, et al: The Canadian CT head rule for patients with minor head injury. *Lancet* 357(9266):1391–1396, 2001.

Level of Evidence: II

Summary: The authors of this prospective study evaluated 3121 consecutive patients to derive a clinical decision rule regarding the use of computed tomography of the head in patients with a minor head injury.

Citation: Stiell IG, Wells GA, Vandemheen KL, et al: The Canadian C-spine rule for radiography in alert and stable trauma patients. *JAMA* 286(15):1841–1848, 2001.

Level of Evidence: II

Summary: The authors of this prospective study investigated 8924 consecutive patients with the aim of creating a clinical decision guideline that is sensitive for detecting acute cervical spine injury and for deciding when to use cervical spine radiography.

Citation: Hoffman JR, Wolfson AB, Todd K, et al: Selective cervical spine radiography in blunt trauma: Methodology of the national emergency X-radiography utilization study (NEXUS). *Ann Emerg Med* 32(4):461–469, 1998.

Level of Evidence: I

Summary: The authors of this multicenter prospective study evaluate the validity of a previously developed set of criteria used to rule out cervical spine injury and determine which patients benefit from cervical spine radiography.

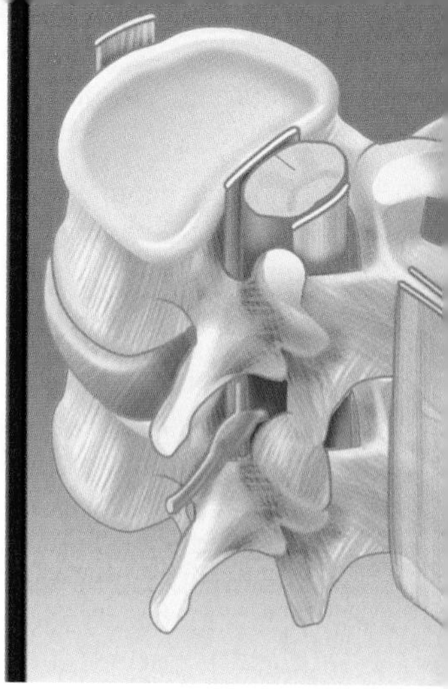

125

Concussion and Brain Injury

HEIDI C. ROSSETTI • JEFFREY T. BARTH •
DONNA K. BROSHEK • JASON R. FREEMAN

Among the wide range of injuries that occur in the sports arena, traumatic brain injury (TBI) is a health problem that has garnered increasing public awareness during recent years. This heightened interest has been largely driven by intense media exposure, as well as the retirement of prominent professional athletes with cognitive and behavioral dysfunction purportedly representing lingering sequelae of brain injury. Player safety concerns have become an area of special focus for professional leagues, such as the National Football League (NFL) and National Hockey League, as well as organizations such as the International Olympic Committee and the National Collegiate Athletic Association, with a resulting impact on collegiate, high school, and recreational sports.

Key to a discussion of sports brain injury is an understanding of the terminology applied to the topic. TBI is an umbrella term that encompasses a range of clinical labels that vary based on severity. Mild traumatic brain injury (mTBI) involves an impact to or acceleration/deceleration of the head resulting in at least a temporary alteration in consciousness or loss of consciousness (LOC) of less than 20 minutes, a Glasgow Coma Scale score of 13 to 15, and no findings on neuroimaging.[1] mTBI is alternately referred to as *mild head injury, minor head injury,* and *concussion*. The vast majority of brain injuries sustained by athletes are mild events that would be considered concussions[2]; moderate, severe, and penetrating traumatic brain injuries are less common. For practical purposes, in this chapter mTBI, mild head injury, and concussion are considered synonymous and the term *concussion* is used throughout this chapter.

The intent of this chapter is to provide a resource for the clinician on the diagnosis and management of sports concussion. A brief historical context for the issue of sports concussion, relevant definitions, and epidemiology are presented; the clinical presentations that can occur after a concussive blow are also reviewed, and a clear concussion management and return-to-play (RTP) decision-making process is given.

Background

Concussion is not a modern phenomenon. Numerous references to cranial injury can be found in ancient medical reports and mythological literature by such figures as Hippocrates and Homer. The recognition of concussion as a separate entity from more severe head injuries was made as far back as the first century AD by Rhazes, an Arabian physician who described concussion as an abnormal physiologic state lacking gross traumatic brain lesions. Modern-day literature, however, has predominately focused on moderate to severe brain injuries, with relatively little attention given to mild brain injuries, whether sports-related or not.

The topic of concussion began to be taken seriously by medical science in the 1980s, when clinical and epidemiologic studies received media attention in a *Wall Street Journal* article, "Silent Epidemic: Head Injuries Often Difficult to Diagnose, Get Rising Attention." The growing consensus that mild head injury was in fact not innocuous was based on the identification of neuropsychological deficits in problem solving, attention, and memory lasting up to 3 months after a trauma was sustained.[3] Additionally, primate studies documented histologic evidence of axonal shear and strain during experimentally induced acceleration-deceleration mild head injury.[4,5]

Because the study of concussion does not lend itself to randomized controlled trials, significant strides were made when Barth and colleagues[6] turned to the collegiate sports arena to address the problem of finding adequate control subjects and accounting for the effects of premorbid functioning in the study of concussion. The sporting venue provided a large number of potential participants who were likely to experience mild acceleration-deceleration head trauma. Data from 10 universities showed that athletes who sustained a concussion had neurocognitive deficits at 24 hours and 5 days after concussion but recovered by the tenth day, a recovery curve that has been replicated by other studies.[7,8] This seminal study set the methodologic standard for baseline and serial neuropsychological testing as the best way to determine the effect of concussion, and this approach of using individual athletes as their own controls and as a model for understanding brain injury in general was termed the Sports as a Laboratory Assessment Model (SLAM).[9] The SLAM approach helped establish concussion as a sports medicine issue with broader implications for mTBI in other areas (e.g., motor vehicle accidents).

Definition of Concussion

As noted at the outset of this chapter, a widely varying set of terms and defining parameters exist for the topic of concussion, and this lack of clarity and consistency has hampered the study of concussion to a significant degree. The two most common definitions used in sports concussion research are from the American Academy of Neurology (AAN) Practice Parameters and the International Symposia on Concussion in Sport (ISCS) group (commonly referred to as the Vienna, Prague, and Zurich Conferences). In 1997, the AAN defined concussion as an altered mental state that may or may not include LOC.[10] Four years later, the ISCS group proposed that concussion is a "complex pathophysiological process affecting the brain, induced by traumatic biomechanical forces," and included five common features of concussion that incorporate clinical, pathological, and biomechanical constructs to supplement the definition: "1. Concussion can be caused by direct impacts to the head, face, neck, or elsewhere on the body with an 'impulsive' force transmitted toward the head; 2. Concussion typically results in the rapid onset of short-lived impairment of neurological function that resolves spontaneously; 3. Concussion may result in neuropathological changes, but the acute clinical symptoms largely reflect a functional disturbance rather than a structural injury; 4. Concussion results in a graded set of clinical syndromes that may or may not involve LOC; and 5. Concussion is typically associated with grossly normal structural neuroimaging studies."[11]

This definition was reaffirmed by the 2008 and 2013 Consensus Conference in Zurich[12,13] and reflects the current trend toward emphasizing the biomechanical force, time course of symptoms, and the functional nature of the injury, as opposed to the structural emphasis used in more severe forms of TBI.

Epidemiology

The Centers for Disease Control and Prevention estimates that approximately 1.6 to 3.0 million sports-related concussions among high school students will be reported each year in the United States, and during the past decade, emergency department visits for sports concussions among children and adolescents increased by 60%.[14,15] Such estimates likely underestimate the actual occurrence, given that many leagues lack the medical oversight to identify concussions.[16] Recent studies suggest that 8.9% of all high school athletic injuries were concussions,[17] and estimates for collegiate sports range from 5% to 18%.[18] The incidence of sports concussion is expected to continue to rise in part because of the increase in sports participation by both male and female athletes at the collegiate and high school levels, but also because of increased knowledge and detection of the injury.

Pathophysiology

A full discussion of the pathophysiology underlying concussion is beyond the scope of this chapter. The interested reader is referred to the work of Giza and Hovda for a thorough understanding of the topic. In brief, concussion occurs as a result of linear and rotational accelerations and decelerations to the brain and is thought to cause a multifactorial neurometabolic cascade of physiologic changes. This process begins with cell body expulsion of sodium and potassium into the intracellular space and an influx of calcium, as well as mild edema and a resultant decrease in cerebral blood flow in the setting of initial hyperglycolysis. As glucose is consumed and blood flow is limited, a state of hypoglycolysis ensues, which slows the neurochemical return to homeostasis. This dysautoregulation explains how clinical signs of brain dysfunction can be observed in the absence of prominent physical damage. This cascade begins within minutes of the injury and can be active for several weeks.[19]

Clinical Presentation

When the question is raised as to why concussion in sports represents an important problem that must be identified, the answer lies in the known consequences demonstrated by concussed athletes, who may present with acute, catastrophic, lingering, or long-term sequelae.

Although it is controversial and rare, a potentially catastrophic outcome from concussion termed *second impact syndrome* (SIS) is sometimes manifested. This most severe consequence of concussion was part of the initial impetus for a formalized approach to concussion management and RTP criteria. First described in 1973,[20] the syndrome is said to occur when a second concussion is sustained before the symptoms of the first have fully resolved. The second impact may appear minor and may not occur on the same day. The athlete may not initially appear injured but may collapse and lose consciousness shortly after the event, with respiratory failure, coma, and even death possibly ensuing. Underlying the SIS phenomena is the notion that the brain appears to have a decreased threshold for sustaining a concussion of any severity with each subsequent trauma.[21] The pathophysiology behind SIS is not fully understood, but it has been suggested that the subclinical edema and increased intracranial pressure from the first concussive impact make the brain successively more vulnerable to the second impact through autodysregulation and subsequent vascular engorgement. This condition manifests as malignant cerebral edema and herniation of the uncus or the cerebellar tonsils through the foramen magnum, resulting in brainstem failure.[22]

Postconcussive syndrome (PCS) is another possible clinical presentation after a sports concussion is sustained. Most concussed athletes demonstrate gradual, spontaneous recovery, generally within 2 to 10 days after injury,[6,7,12,23] consistent with laboratory animal studies showing short-lived effects of concussion,[19] and with metaanalytic studies demonstrating no evidence of impairment beyond 3 months.[24,25] However, the fact that some persons experience persistent sequelae has been recognized for quite some time. For example, at 3-month follow-up, 34% of an mTBI clinical (nonsports) sample had not yet returned to work, and 24% demonstrated measurable neurocognitive deficits.[3] Prolonged recovery (>3 months) with no obvious underlying neurophysiologic cause fits the criteria for PCS. This phenomenon is relatively new to the field of sports concussion, and no widely accepted standard exists for making the diagnosis. Also unknown is the actual incidence of PCS, although it is assumed to occur in a very small percentage of athletes.

The clinical presentation of PCS is characterized by neurologic symptoms, such as headache, dizziness, and nausea; cognitive deficits, such as impaired attention, slowed mental processing, and memory dysfunction; and emotional disruption, including depression or irritability. It is important to note that the presence of one or more of these symptoms 3 months after a concussion is sustained in an athlete is not diagnostic of PCS, given that such symptoms are extremely common in a host of other conditions. For example, PCS symptomatology has been demonstrated in 81% of subjects in a chronic pain sample with no history of concussion.[26] As such, the clinician may find the identification of PCS difficult. One challenge is that the athlete may present with vague, subjective symptoms that are nonspecific. Issues of effort and secondary gain may also be a contributing factor in some cases. Furthermore, the differential diagnosis often includes mood and anxiety disorders, as well as sleep disruption, which can lead to or mimic PCS symptoms. Neuropsychological assessment can be quite useful in this situation, because objective evaluation can help parse out the factors contributing to the athlete's atypical presentation.

In addition to the clinical presentations of SIS and PCS, a third potential clinical presentation known as chronic traumatic encephalopathy (CTE) can occur after multiple concussions.[27] This outcome appears to be the possible long-term result of repeated concussions and subconcussive blows and has been studied in groups of retired football, rugby, and boxing athletes.[28-30] The combination of repetitive sports head injury–related damage with that of age-related neuronal loss[31] may result in the development of clinical signs of CTE, often appearing years after the end of the athlete's career.[32] CTE is characterized by long-term deficits in executive functioning, processing speed, verbal learning, and visual memory; motor impairments, including impaired coordination, spasticity, and parkinsonism; as well as behavioral problems such as emotional dysregulation and disinhibition.[30,33] Referred to as "dementia pugilistica" in early literature,[34] CTE in its advanced stage can be clinically indistinguishable from other advanced dementias. Neuropathologically, CTE is a progressive tauopathy with gliosis and neurofibrillary tangles, as well as common gross elements of reduced brain weight, enlarged ventricles, volume loss in the corpus callosum, cavum septum pellucidum, and scarring and neuronal loss of the cerebellar tonsils.[35] The pathology of CTE has been most frequently demonstrated in the brains of professional athletes[36] and can be widespread throughout the brain given the nonfocal nature of repeated head trauma.

Although long-term deficits in the form of PCS can manifest after a single concussive blow, it is generally assumed that a concussed athlete can expect a favorable prognosis if the injury is safely managed. The risk of outcomes such as SIS, PCS, and CTE can be significantly reduced with proper concussion identification, examination, and intervention.

Examination

The goal of sports concussion examination is to identify the concussion, assess the injury, determine its effects, and devise appropriate interventions. The traditional approach to this task involved simply gauging the signs and symptoms of the concussion and their resolution over time. Many different classification schemes for concussion exist, and definitions and criteria continue to evolve. Until the wide dissemination of the ISCS (also known as Zurich) Conference guidelines, the two most widely used systems for grading concussion were those proposed by the AAN in 1997 and Cantu in 2001. These systems used three grades to represent mild, moderate, and severe concussion based on the clinical presentation of the athlete and placed considerable emphasis on LOC (AAN) or posttraumatic amnesia (PTA; Cantu) as severity indicators. Despite early TBI literature showing that coma duration is an important predictor of outcome,[37] authors of more recent studies have found that the relationship between LOC and injury outcome in the realm of mTBI and sports concussion is less certain.[38] Concussion grading systems are now considered obsolete, and an individualized approach to concussion diagnosis and management is favored, consistent with the ISCS guidelines.

Although monitoring subjective symptoms is an important aspect of concussion management, it cannot be the sole means of gauging effect and recovery. It is now understood that fewer than half of concussed athletes spontaneously report their symptoms,[39] citing doubt that the injury was severe, not wanting to leave the game, or general lack of awareness about concussion as reasons for not reporting. For these and other reasons, the modern model for concussion examination, outlined by the Zurich Conferences, emphasizes an individualized approach that incorporates neurocognitive evaluation. Several computer-administered measures (outlined later) are validated for the assessment of concussion sequelae. The standard practice has evolved to include such standardized tools in both preseason and postinjury assessment. The Zurich guidelines recommend that athletes not resume a gradual progression of activity until their concussion symptoms have remitted. Thus neurocognitive testing has become a valuable tool in identifying subtle cognitive symptoms and their resolution.

Baseline (Preseason) Assessment

The true beginning of the evaluation and subsequent management of sports concussion begins prospectively with baseline neurocognitive testing. To refer again to the SLAM approach, a widely used model for understanding and addressing the multifactorial nature of sports-related concussion, the process should involve the collection of preseason baseline data for all athletes engaged in sports with a high risk for concussion, retesting injured athletes, and performing serial testing throughout the process of recovery. The importance of obtaining baseline information for an athlete cannot be overstated. The results of any evaluation vary based on many factors other than the actual injury, including intelligence and cultural background, learning disabilities, and previous concussion history.[40] This situation applies to neurologic findings as well; for example, up to 20% of athletes normally experience a headache while in the midst of competition,[41] and approximately 3% of the healthy population exhibit pupillary asymmetry.[42] Erroneous conclusions about the cognitive and neurologic state of an athlete may be drawn without an awareness of these baseline characteristics.

Neurocognitive baselines may be obtained for athletes with use of computerized methods in an individual or group setting with a trained examiner. Several tools are available for the specific purpose of assessing concussion severity and resolution. These tools include the Automated Neuropsychological Assessment Metrics[43]; the Immediate Post-concussion Assessment and Cognitive Testing (ImPACT Applications Inc., Pittsburgh, PA)[8,44]; the Concussion Resolution Index (HeadMinder Inc., New York, NY)[45]; and the Computerized Cognitive Assessment Tool (Axon Sports [formerly CogSport], Wausau, WI).[46] The Automated Neuropsychological Assessment Metrics measures processing speed, resistance to interference, and working memory. The Immediate Post-concussion Assessment and Cognitive Testing tool was developed specifically for athletes and assesses reaction time and a range of attentional and memory skills, accompanied by a self-report postconcussion scale. The Concussion Resolution Index is a Web-based set of cognitive tasks that measure simple and complex reaction time, attention, memory, and cognitive processing speed. Axon is also a Internet-based system and includes eight tasks designed to sample a range of cognitive functions.

Sideline Assessment

Once baseline data have been obtained, the focus shifts to the evaluation of injuries sustained on the field of play. The first step in the assessment of concussion is to recognize that a concussion may have occurred. It is important to remember that most injured athletes exhibit no obvious indications that they are concussed. Therefore sideline assessment is warranted for any athlete who has received a significant blow to the head or an athlete who does not appear to "be him or herself" in response to a lesser degree of contact.[47] This assessment involves evaluation of the athlete on the field, or more commonly on the sideline, and usually is conducted by a physician or a certified athletic trainer with expertise in concussion evaluation and management.

An obvious goal of the sideline assessment is to determine if the athlete has signs that signal the presence of severe intracranial or spinal cord injury and whether transport to a medical facility is required.[48] After that determination, the athlete is examined for signs of alteration in consciousness. Over time, less emphasis has been placed on LOC, PTA, and retrograde amnesia as indicators for diagnosis and classification of the severity of concussion. These classic signs remain helpful but nonessential in the venue of sports concussion given that they appear in a minority of injured athletes.[49]

In general, the sideline evaluation should assess for signs of confusion, loss of balance, headache, dizziness, and slowed responding, in addition to informal cranial nerve, motor, sensory, and reflex testing[50] and cognitive screening. For athletes with no obvious acute symptoms, physical maneuvers such as push-ups or jumping jacks can help determine whether concussive signs or symptoms develop with exertion and resultant increased intracranial pressure.[48] Sideline assessment should also incorporate a mental status examination that targets orientation, concentration, and memory. Assessment of level of orientation can consist of standard questions pertaining to person, place, and time. Concentration may be gauged by tasks such as repeating strings of three to five digits both forward and backward, serial subtraction of numbers, or repeating a well-known verbal sequence such as months of the year or days of the week backward. Memory can be informally and qualitatively assessed by recall of three items at different intervals after the injury or repeating assignments of a number of previous plays.[38,50]

Although these informal methods of sideline assessment are helpful, a standardized approach is preferable.[51] A number of standardized methods for determining the severity of a concussion and the initial symptoms have been developed for use in the sideline evaluation of athletes. The Post-Concussive Symptom Scale—Revised is a 21-item self-report scale consisting of terms and descriptors commonly used by athletes.[52] Each symptom is rated on a 7-point Likert scale ranging from 0 to 6, with a total score ranging from 0 to 126. Many of the items refer to symptoms that emerge after the acute stage and are not appropriate for sideline use (e.g., "trouble falling asleep"), and no guidelines for determining a symptomatic or asymptomatic score have been published. The Standardized Assessment of Concussion (SAC) is a 5-minute measure administered by a trained physician or athletic trainer and includes five orientation questions, a five-word learning test, reciting digits backward, reciting the months of the year in reverse, and delayed word recall.[53] The SAC provides a 30-point composite score to gauge neurocognitive function and also includes a standard neurologic screening, exertional maneuvers, and means of assessing LOC and PTA. Normative data for comparison are also available.[54] The SAC is available in paper form and a pocket-card format and has been adapted for use with smartphone technology. The Balance Error Scoring System is an objective measure of postural stability for use on the sideline.[55] The 5-minute procedure requires the injured athlete to maintain three stances (double, single, and tandem) for 20 seconds with the eyes closed and both hands on his or her hips. Scoring is based on six types of errors over six test trials. The Standardized Concussion Assessment Tool (SCAT-2) is another standardized tool that incorporates the aforementioned SAC and a modified version of the Balance Error Scoring System, in addition to the Glasgow Coma Scale and a rating of common physical signs and concussive symptoms, with a total possible score of 100. The Zurich Conference recommended use of the SCAT-2 for concussion assessment.[12] The SCAT-2 is our preferred method of sideline concussion assessment. The tool is easily accessible online and may be freely copied for distribution to individuals, teams, groups, and organizations.

After a sideline evaluation, any athlete considered to have sustained a concussion should undergo a medical evaluation with a more detailed neurologic consultation to determine the need for neuroimaging and/or electrophysiologic testing. Finally, to provide an objective basis for detecting the effects of the concussion, the athlete should undergo postinjury neurocognitive assessment. This brief repeat evaluation can occur within 24 to 48 hours after the suspected concussion if the athlete appears to be symptom free. This aspect of concussion management may provide increased sensitivity for identifying cognitive impairment resulting from concussion when physical symptoms are limited or resolved.[56] However, conducting the brief repeat evaluation 7 days after the injury has been found to provide more unique information regarding impairment than routine assessment conducted relatively close in time to the sideline assessment.[57]

Comprehensive Assessment

In the case of a single uncomplicated concussion or subconcussive event, it is generally anticipated that the athlete will experience full resolution of symptoms within the 2- to 10-day natural recovery curve. In cases with an atypical presentation, a more comprehensive evaluation may be necessary. Athletes with preexisting or comorbid conditions (e.g., learning or attention disorders, depression, or substance abuse), athletes who report or demonstrate a slower than expected recovery or who have sustained multiple previous concussions should be considered for expanded assessment. In these situations, a referral for comprehensive outpatient neuropsychological evaluation is indicated, which includes a clinical interview, record review, and objective testing of aptitude and cognitive functioning and provides individualized recommendations for the athlete and relevant treatment providers. In addition, further medical assessment may be warranted for atypical concussion cases (e.g., neuroophthalmology).

Imaging

Acute evaluation of concussion may incorporate at least one form of brain imaging. Computed tomography is an appropriate choice to rule out the presence of intracranial hemorrhage and skull fracture and is the imaging option of choice for concussion evaluation in most emergency departments. Magnetic resonance imaging (MRI) with an angiogram can be obtained if carotid dissection or stroke is suspected, and MRI studies may also identify a diffuse injury such as axonal shearing.

It is important to emphasize that most concussions are unlikely to produce observable signs upon testing with these traditional radiologic techniques. This phenomenon is explained by the notion that the neurophysiologic changes that occur after concussion involve low levels of axonal strain and a temporary disruption of cellular and vascular function,[19] which would not likely manifest as an identifiable form of structural brain damage upon imaging. However, it is possible that more sophisticated imaging may have potential utility. For example, it has been proposed that diffusion tensor imaging may have relevance because of its ability to detect axonal damage.[58] Functional MRI, positron emission tomography, and single photon emission computed tomography techniques are the subject of ongoing investigations into the identification of a functional correlate for the neurophysiologic disruption involved in mTBI. However, as yet these techniques are not well validated in the field of sports concussion and are not always readily accessible in a clinical setting. For this reason, although structural neuroimaging continues to rule out the presence of serious pathology that would be beyond that of a mild concussive injury, brain imaging is less relevant in the context of typical concussion management.

Management

An athlete who experiences one concussive event is three times more likely to sustain another concussion in the same season, usually within 10 days of the first injury.[59] As previously outlined, the athlete is at heightened risk for consequences such as SIS, PCS, and CTE with repeated concussions, particularly during the acute stage when the brain is more susceptible to subsequent insult. The prolonged recovery of multiply concussed athletes has been demonstrated with lingering cognitive and gait stability deficits.[21,60] Players who sustain a concussion are more likely to experience LOC with the next injury.[21,61] Furthermore, the force threshold for concussive injury may be far less for a second impact[59]; therefore subconcussive events must be considered as possible risk factors when discussing concussion outcome and management. A subconcussive blow is an apparent brain insult with insufficient force to cause the hallmark symptoms of concussion.[62] These more minor events conceivably occur at a high rate during both competitive play and practice. Investigation with use of the Head Impact Telemetry System to record the frequency, magnitude, and location of head impacts found that a group of college football players sustained on average 1000 subconcussive impacts over the course of a single season.[63] The notion that repetitive blows may cause equivalent, if not greater, damage than a single mild concussion has been suggested previously.[64]

It is possible that the number of concussions sustained plays a more important role in long-term outcomes than does the severity of the concussions. The animal experimental literature has shown that two or more concussive blows produce greater deficits than predicted by single blows and that repeated blows can accelerate the deposition of β-amyloid.[65] The heightened risks of repeat concussive injury have also been extended to human studies.[59,66] What is unknown is "how many is too many," and this number will vary for individual athletes.

Different groups and individuals are more susceptible than others, and the nature of their symptoms and deficits may vary. For example, younger athletes appear to be particularly vulnerable to negative outcomes, with greater susceptibility to SIS and longer recoveries.[67] Compared with their college counterparts, high school athletes may be more vulnerable to concussion, exhibit a more protracted recovery, and have longer lasting cognitive deficits.[8,68] Differences by gender may also exist, with some evidence that females experience a higher incidence of PCS compared with their male counterparts, although this literature is still equivocal.[69,70]

Given the well-documented risks involved in returning an athlete to play, the potential for delayed onset of symptoms; variable symptom reporting; the nonlinear, individualized nature of recovery; and the known long-term risks for such consequences as CTE, the accepted standard for concussion management is that concussed athletes are held from competition until they are completely asymptomatic at rest and during exertion (which involves either physical or cognitive activities). When the previously outlined examination process is followed, the clinician is equipped with appropriate data with which to approach an RTP determination.

Return to Play

The primary focus of concussion management revolves around the appropriate implementation of RTP guidelines. Historically many different classification systems have been used to guide RTP decisions. The AAN published multiple guidelines and classification systems for concussion management from 1990 to 2005, all of which were based on clinical experience and expert opinion. The Cantu system of concussion grading was also revised to guide RTP decisions, and the Colorado Medical Society is another frequently referenced model for RTP.[71,72] These models added much to the field of sports concussion but were criticized for lack of empirical basis and standardization and for being overly restrictive.

Newer approaches have replaced the use of grading systems of acute symptoms with more emphasis on the individual's path of symptom resolution rather than preconceived timelines. This process has been guided by recommendations of the ISCS, which produced a series of consensus documents that evolved from the first summary statement in 2001 (Vienna Conference) to a second statement in 2004 (Prague Conference), and the third and forth iterations following the Zurich Conferences in 2009[12] and 2013.[13]

The Zurich consensus models and the most recent AAN evidence-based guidelines (published in 2013) provide the

TABLE 125-1

ZURICH GRADUATED RETURN-TO-PLAY PROTOCOL

Rehabilitation Stage	Functional Exercise at Each Stage of Rehabilitation	Objective of Each Stage
1. No activity	Complete physical and cognitive rest	Recovery
2. Light aerobic exercise	Walking, swimming, or stationary cycling, keeping intensity <70% of maximum predicted heart rate No resistance training	Increase heart rate
3. Sport-specific exercise	Skating drills in ice hockey, running drills in soccer; no head impact activities	Add movement
4. Noncontact training drills	Progression to more complex training drills, such as passing drills in football and ice hockey May start progressive resistance training	Exercise, coordination, and cognitive load
5. Full contact practice	After medical clearance, participate in normal training activities	Restore confidence and assess functional skills by coaching staff
6. Return to play	Normal game play	

From McCrory P, Meeuwisse W, Johnston K, et al: Consensus Statement on Concussion in Sport: The 3rd International Conference on Concussion in Sport held in Zurich, November, 2008. *South Afr J Sports Med* 21(2), 36–46, 2009.

most current and thorough models with which to approach RTP. The protocols call for immediate removal from practice or play after a suspected concussion, standardized sideline assessment, and no RTP on the day of injury. The Zurich RTP protocol (Table 125-1) follows a stepwise process that progresses through six graduated steps that take 24 hours each. If any postconcussion symptoms occur within a step, the athlete is returned to the previous asymptomatic level for another 24 hours until resuming the graded process. It should be noted that cognitive rest and restriction from cognitive exertion (e.g., schoolwork, video gaming, and texting) is equally important to physical rest and restriction from physical exertion during the course of recovery. Clinicians involved in the care of athletes should be well versed in the Zurich guidelines and should engage in a dynamic approach to RTP that takes into account the individual's history with careful attention paid to age, number of previous concussions, severity of concussion, and comorbidities such as other health issues, mood disturbance, and substance use. The 2013 Zurich consensus statement recommends that children and adolescents not return to sports until they have successfully returned to academics.[13] The 2013 AAN guidelines suggest a conservative approach to RTP for children and further recommend no RTP for any concussed athlete until he or she is assessed by a licensed health care professional trained in concussion management.[73]

Retiring an Athlete

One of the most challenging aspects of sports concussion management is the issue of when to retire an athlete from play. In the face of limited empirical data on the topic and the great variability in both immediate symptoms and long-term effects that individual athletes demonstrate after sustaining single or multiple concussions, no clearly defined method exists to guide the clinician or team. However, several important factors clearly must be taken into consideration to make a reasoned decision. When an athlete begins to demonstrate a longer period of recovery from symptoms, experiences concussive symptoms from forces that are increasingly mild, or does not return to baseline neurocognitive functioning, then it may be time for the athlete to stop playing.[74] In addition, the athlete's functioning in multiple settings should be considered; for example, problems at school or home or behavioral problems can signal the need to consider retirement from play.

Interventions

Sport concussion interventions are targeted in three main areas. The most critical means of intervention is education. Concerted efforts must be made to improve concussion awareness for athletes, their parents, coaches, and athletic trainers, and school and league administrators. A basic understanding of what constitutes a concussion, the signs to look for, the importance of removing the athlete from further concussion risk, and the need to obtain an appropriate examination will go a long way toward improving outcomes. The need for education is highlighted by actions such as the passage of the Lystedt Law, named for Zackery Lystedt, who sustained a TBI when he returned to a middle school football game after experiencing a concussion. The legislation, passed in 2009, aims to protect athletes by mandating that athletes, parents, and coaches be educated about the dangers of concussions each year, that a player suspected of having a concussion be removed from play, and that a licensed health care professional clear the athlete for RTP.[75] "Lystedt Laws" are being enacted nationwide to outline educational requirements and the need for clearance by a qualified professional any time a concussion is suspected.

A second area of intervention is, of course, prevention. The data on protective equipment are somewhat mixed with regard to whether headgear and helmets actually reduce concussion incidence. It has been suggested that such equipment has little ability to stop concussion, because helmets are not able to prevent deceleration and rotation forces on the brain. However, it is established that they absorb some of the impact forces on the brain and prevent other forms of injury, such as skull fracture.

The most powerful means of prevention may be rule changes within the sport, and a clear precedent exists for organizational changes. For example, the NFL made the tackling method of using one's head or helmet to hit another player ("spearing") an illegal technique in an effort to curb serious injury. Attention should be directed to both game time and practice activity; for example, part of the recent NFL collective bargaining agreement between owners and players resulted in a limit to the number of contact drills in practice. Rules such as limiting helmet-to-helmet contact by enacting penalties or other consequences would have beneficial effects for athlete protection and brain health. Furthermore, fair play and the distinction between aggressive play and violence should be emphasized within sporting organizations.

Conclusion

The neuroscience and clinical study of sports concussion remains a developing area that has increasingly become the focus of both laypeople and researchers alike in light of the knowledge that concussions can exert meaningful effects on the athlete both in the short and long term. Given the number of variables that can influence concussion symptoms and length of recovery, individualized clinical management of concussed athletes guided by a clearly defined concussion evaluation process is paramount. The challenge for the future is to delineate factors that contribute to individual susceptibility to concussive blows, the variables that influence prognosis, and methods of preventing catastrophic, prolonged, and long-term outcomes, as well as to increase the awareness of sport concussion in players, their families, sporting organizations, treatment providers, and the general public.

For a complete list of references, go to expertconsult.com.

Suggested Readings

Citation: Belanger HG, Vanderploeg RD: The neuropsychological impact of sports-related concussion: A meta-analysis. *J Int Neuropsychol Soc* 11(4):345–357, 2005.
Level of Evidence: II
Summary: This metaanalysis of 21 studies involving 790 cases of concussion and 2014 control cases was conducted to determine the impact of sports-related concussion across six cognitive domains. Results provide compelling evidence that sports-related concussion has no significant effect on neuropsychological function by 7 to 10 days after injury in the athletic population at large, although long-term participation in sports involving head contact may be associated with small, adverse sequelae.

Citation: Echemendia RJ, Cantu RC: Return to play following brain injury. In Lovell M, Echemendia R, Collins M, et al, editors: *Traumatic brain injury in sports: An international neuropsychological perspective*, Lisse, The Netherlands, 2004, Swets and Zeitlinger.
Level of Evidence: V
Summary: The authors propose a model for return-to-play decision making that takes into account the complexity of multiple factors and variables. Informed decision making involves consideration of data from many different sources.

Citation: Giza CC, Hovda DA: The neurometabolic cascade of concussion. *J Athl Train* 36(3):228–235, 2001.
Level of Evidence: II
Summary: The authors use more than 100 articles from both basic science and clinical literature to review the underlying pathophysiologic processes of concussive brain injury and relate these neurometabolic changes to clinical sports-related issues such as injury to the developing brain, overuse injury, and repeated concussion.

Citation: Gysland SM, Mihalik JP, Register-Mihalik JK, et al: The relationship between subconcussive impacts and concussion history on clinical measures of neurologic function in collegiate football players. *Ann Biomed Eng* 40(1):14–22, 2011.
Level of Evidence: II
Summary: This study is the first to investigate the relationship between repetitive subconcussive head impacts and clinical measures of neurologic impairment while monitoring sustained impacts throughout the course of a single collegiate football season. The methodologies presented could help establish a foundation for future longitudinal study aimed at answering questions about the possible relationship of recurrent subclinical blows and later depression, early-onset dementia, and chronic traumatic encephalopathy.

Citation: McCrory P, Meeuwisse W, Aubrey M, et al: Consensus statement on concussion in sport—the 4th International Conference on Concussion in Sport held in Zurich, November 2012. *Br J Sports Med* 47:250–258, 2013.
Level of Evidence: V
Summary: These guidelines improved on those previously presented by the same conference in Vienna and Prague and constitute the most widely used protocol for our current understanding of and approach to sport concussion.

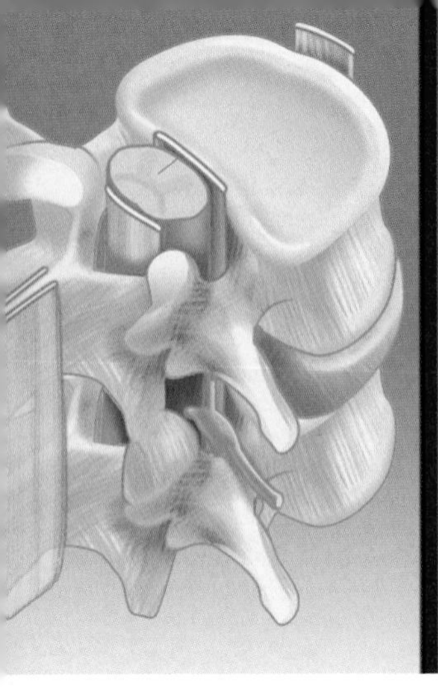

126

Cervical Spine Injuries

JESSE L. EVEN • MARK S. ESKANDER • WILLIAM F. DONALDSON III

This chapter describes the history, physical evaluation, imaging, diagnoses, treatment, and return-to-play recommendations of common cervical spine injuries encountered by the team physician or trainer using the most up-to-date and highest level of clinical evidence (level III to V). Because a cervical spine injury can lead to permanent neurologic damage, the margin for error is low. Medical providers should therefore always maintain a high index of suspicion for a potential cervical injury. Although severe neurologic injuries are infrequent in most sports settings, it is imperative that the medical staff be educated in basic spine precautions, triage, and cervical spine immobilization techniques.

History

Every year more than 10,000 cases of cervical spine injuries occur in the United States, of which 10% are associated with athletic events, making contact sports second only to motor vehicle accidents as the cause of cervical spine injury.[1,2] More than 11,000 cases of spinal cord injuries occur each year in the United States, and again, approximately 10% are sports-related injuries, with these injuries ranking as the fourth most common mechanism of spinal cord injury.[3] The injuries are most commonly associated with high-risk sports, including football, gymnastics, Olympic diving, equestrian sports, surfing, rugby, wrestling, soccer, ice hockey, skiing, and snowboarding.[4-6] The most extensively studied sport is American football, and one of the largest databases of football-related injuries that has been assembled is from the Annual Survey of Football Injury Research (ASFIR), which has completed data from 1931 to 2007. The ASFIR is supported by many institutions, including the National Collegiate Athletic Association and the American Football Coaches Association, with the goal of tracking injuries to make football safer through equipment improvement, rule changes, and improved coaching techniques. According to the ASFIR, 1006 direct football-related deaths have occurred, with 12% of these deaths resulting from cervical spine injuries. The research has led to rule changes that have had a significant impact on cervical spine injuries, with the most important rule change coming in 1976 when spear tackling was outlawed. In 1976 the incidence of permanent quadriplegia in college football players was 10.66 per 100,000 participants. The incidence was reduced to 1.33 per 100,000 participants after spear tackling was outlawed and helmets were modified.[7] Although these major neurologic conditions are a rare occurrence, it is important that the training staff, team physicians, and emergency medical technicians be aware of these types of injuries so that all persons can be prepared when they do occur.

A frequently encountered injury is a temporary neurologic disability such as a cervical neurapraxia, also known as a *stinger* or *burner*. Cervical neurapraxia can be seen in up to 50% of collegiate football players throughout the season.[8] These injuries, although not as devastating, can be a cause of great concern to the athlete, coaching staff, and family members. Treatment, along with return to play, are important decisions that must be made by the training staff in consultation with the team physician.

Physical Examination/ On-Field Evaluation

The key to dealing with any catastrophic situation is planning and preparation. A cervical spine injury on the playing field should be approached in an organized manner. Any team physician or trainer should have a plan, and the necessary equipment should be in place before a spinal injury occurs on the field. The plan includes having a chain of command in place that designates who will direct the immobilization and transportation of the injured athlete. This team leader can be the head trainer or team physician, but a clear leader must be defined to protect the injured player from a disorganized and dangerous situation. Equipment should also be available on site, including a spine board, stretcher, cervical collar, helmet removal set, and access to telecommunications, to facilitate immobilization of the patient with a spinal cord injury to a hospital or trauma center equipped to handle such an injury. Proactive planning is paramount to optimize the outcome for the injured athlete.

As with any trauma, the ABCs (airway, breathing, and circulation) should be addressed in a person with a cervical spine injury. Rapid immobilization of the cervical spine by manual traction or cervical orthosis immobilization should be performed while the ABCs are being assessed. The cervical spine of an injured athlete should be immobilized and he or she should be placed onto a spine board; the ABCs can then be evaluated after the spine is protected (Fig. 126-1). Extreme care must be used when placing the injured athlete on the spine board. A recent cadaveric model showed statistically

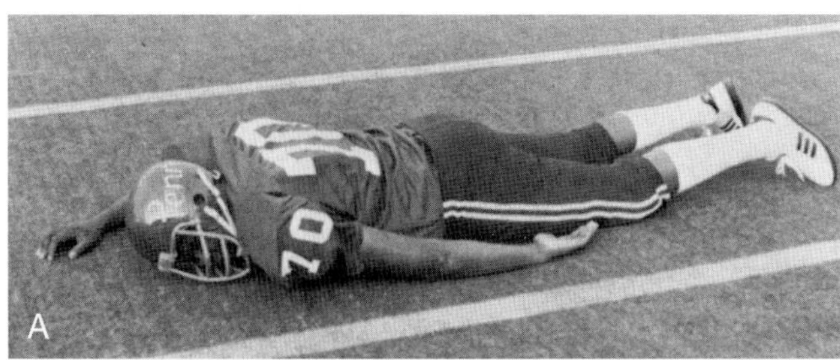
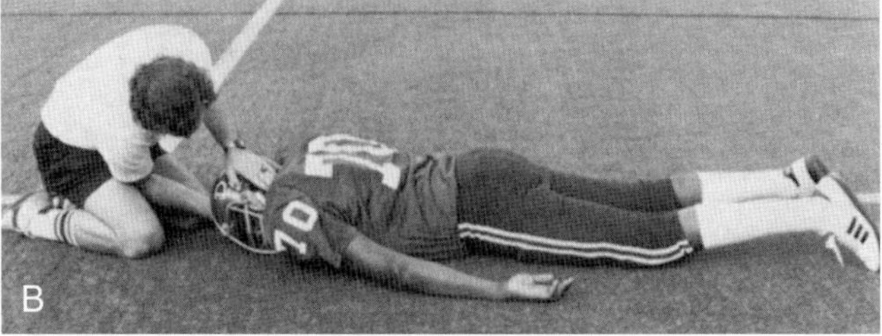

FIGURE 126-1 **A,** Athletes with a suspected cervical spine injury may or may not be unconscious. All athletes who are unconscious should be managed as though they have a significant neck injury. **B,** Immediate manual immobilization of the head and neck unit. One should first check for breathing. *(From Torg JS, editor:* Athletic injuries to the head, neck and face*, Philadelphia, 1982, Lea & Febiger.)*

significant movement even with use of spine board precautions.[9] Multiple studies have been performed to evaluate the removal of shoulder pads and helmets in football players during the past 20 years. The consensus of these studies is to leave shoulder pads and the helmet in place for transport to minimize movement of the cervical spine.[10-15] If a player who is wearing a helmet is not breathing, the face mask alone should be removed. The chin strap should be left in place to keep the helmet on to maintain the cervical spine in line with the shoulders. If the airway is compromised after the face mask is removed (Figs. 126-2 and 126-3), a jaw thrust or head tilt can be performed (Figs. 126-4 and 126-5). If the player's cardiopulmonary status is intact and he or she is alert and following commands, a baseline neurologic examination should be performed to assess the injury. The player should be transferred in full uniform to the nearest hospital that is equipped to handle spine trauma.

Fortunately, most cervical spine injuries do not result in catastrophic injury; most patients will be ambulatory, and examination will reveal that the neurologic system is intact. It is important to understand when more advanced imaging is indicated. The National Emergency X-ray Utilization Study (NEXUS) is a multicenter, prospective observational study designed to determine the clinical criteria indicating the need for radiographic imaging of the spine in patients who have sustained a blunt cervical spine trauma. The study included more than 34,000 patients with blunt trauma to the head and neck, and they were evaluated for the presence or absence of five clinical criteria, including midline cervical tenderness, focal neurologic deficits, normal cognition, level of intoxication, and painful and distracting injuries (Fig. 126-6). The authors reported that of the 34,000 patients included in the study, 818 had cervical spine injuries. All but 8 of the 818 were identified with use of their criteria, which equates to a negative predictive value of 99.8% and 99% sensitivity. The criteria led to a 12.9% reduction in the use of radiographs that were not indicated. The study authors concluded that a patient has an extremely low probability of having a cervical spine injury if none of the five criteria is present.[16,17] Although this study was designed to address imaging indications for emergency medicine doctors, it also applies to the team physician/trainer. In a fully conscious athlete with cervical trauma, the spine can be cleared with very high confidence using the same five clinical criteria. If any of the criteria are not met, then radiographs should be obtained.

Imaging

Plain films should be obtained when the possibility of a cervical spine injury is a concern, the NEXUS criteria are not met, and the patient has a neurologic deficit. A three-view cervical spine film (at a minimum) should be obtained, which includes an anteroposterior, lateral, and open-mouth odontoid view. It is important to obtain full visualization of the entire cervical

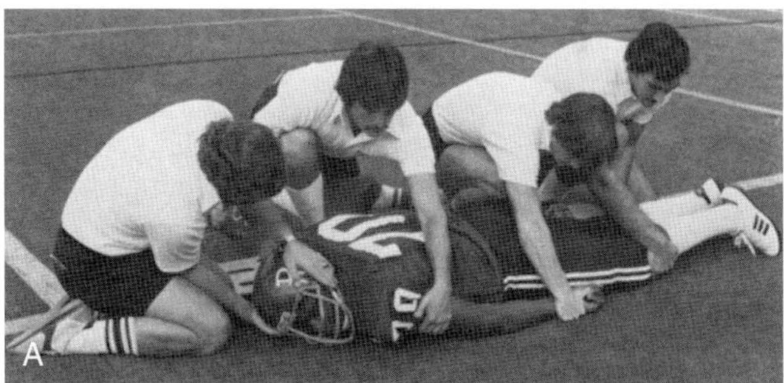
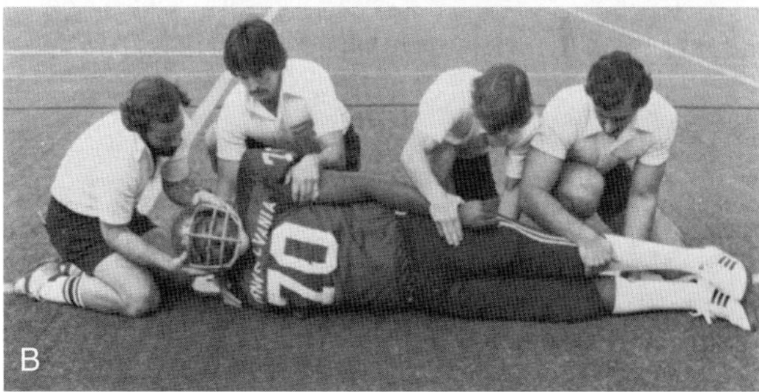
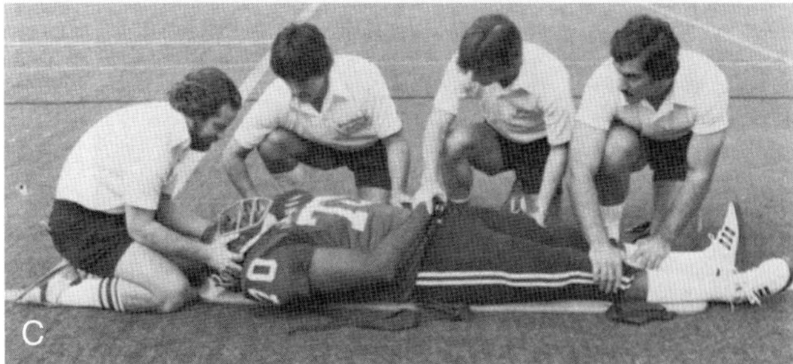

FIGURE 126-2 **A,** Logrolling an athlete onto a spine board requires four persons: the leader, who immobilizes the head and neck and commands the medical support team, and the remaining three persons, who are positioned at the shoulders, hips, and lower legs. **B,** The leader uses the crossed-arm technique to immobilize the head. This technique allows the leader's arms to unwind as the three assistants roll the athlete onto the spine board. **C,** The three assistants maintain body alignment during the roll. *(From Torg JS, editor:* Athletic injuries to the head, neck and face*, Philadelphia, 1982, Lea & Febiger.)*

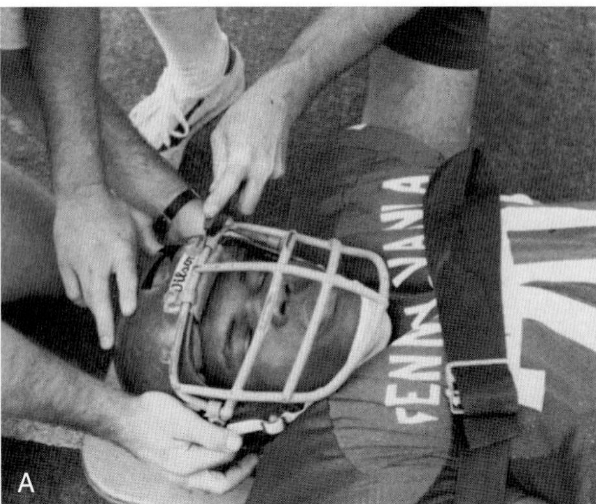

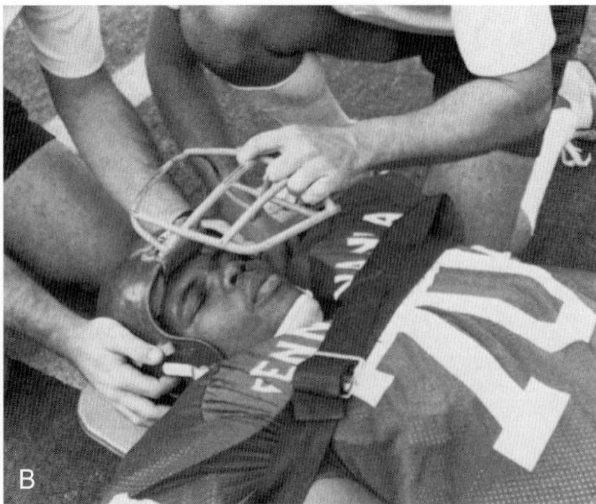

FIGURE 126-3 The head and helmet must be securely immobilized. **A,** Remove cage-type masks by cutting the plastic loops with Dura shears, EMT scissors, or a Trainer's Angel. Make the cut on the side of the loop away from the face. **B,** Remove the entire mask from the helmet so that it does not interfere with further resuscitation efforts. *(From Torg JS, editor:* Athletic injuries to the head, neck and face, *Philadelphia, 1982, Lea & Febiger.)*

spine, including the C7-T1 junction. A swimmer's view lateral may be required to assess the lower cervical spine, especially in athletes, because of their robust shoulder and neck musculature. If no fracture or dislocation is noted on the three-view series, a flexion and extension view can be added to evaluate for any dynamic instability. If a fracture is not identified and the player is tender to palpation on physical examination, advanced imaging is recommended.

Computerized tomography (CT) scans should be obtained for any patient who presents with any neurologic deficit, especially partial or complete paralysis. A full traumagram should be obtained if the athlete has partial or complete paralysis. CT scans have been shown to be extremely sensitive to fractures and/or dislocations of the spine.[18] They have the ability to evaluate the cervicothoracic junction, which is often difficult to visualize and typically cannot be seen on plain radiographs, especially in large patients. CT reconstruction in the sagittal, coronal, and axial plane allows identification of subtle injuries that otherwise would be missed on plain films. The downside of CT is that it does not show soft tissue injury to the ligamentous structures or detailed views of the intervertebral disks.

Magnetic resonance imaging (MRI) is a useful diagnostic tool to evaluate the soft tissue of an athlete's cervical spine when concern exists about the possibility of injury to the spinal cord, posterior ligamentous complex, and intervertebral disks. MRI should be obtained for any athlete who presents with a persistent neurologic deficit, the potential for herniated disks, or traumatic injury to the posterior ligamentous complex. Multiple articles have been written about the sensitivity of MRI for evaluating the posterior ligamentous complex in traumatic situations.[19]

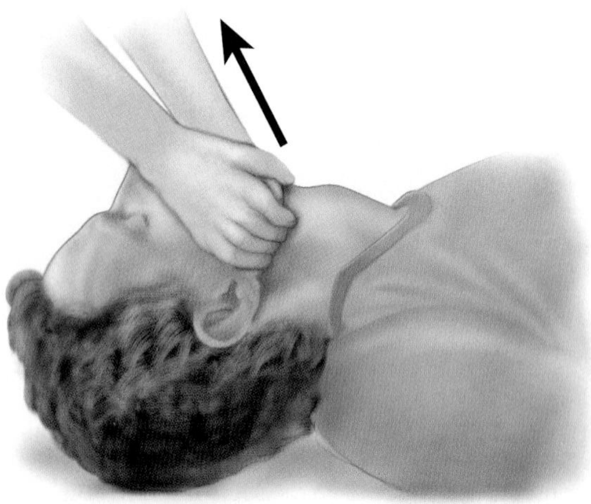

FIGURE 126-4 The jaw-thrust maneuver for opening the airway of a person with a suspected cervical spine injury.

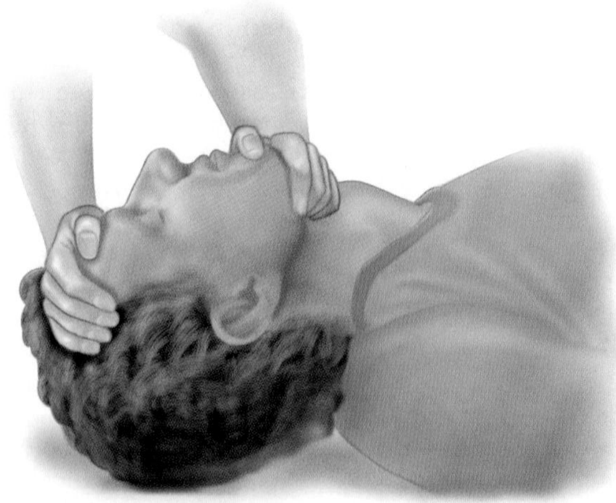

FIGURE 126-5 The head tilt–jaw lift maneuver for opening the airway. This maneuver is used if the jaw-thrust maneuver is inadequate or if the athlete is wearing a helmet.

NEXUS Clinical Criteria

Five components to clear cervical spine

- No midline cervical tenderness
- No focal neurologic deficit
- Normal alertness
- No intoxication
- No painful, distracting injury

FIGURE 126-6 National Emergency X-Radiography Utilization Study (NEXUS) clinical criteria.

Electromyographic examinations may be helpful in evaluating patients with persistent symptoms of neurapraxic injury, such as stingers or burners. These studies should be delayed 3 to 4 weeks after the injury to help with baseline values, and they can help predict recovery with subsequent serial examinations. Electromyographic examinations are also helpful in distinguishing between preganglionic and postganglionic injuries. Patients with preganglionic injuries show an absence of motor innervations and have a very poor prognosis for recovery. Brachial plexus injuries, which demonstrate loss of motor and sensory potentials, are postganglionic injuries, and they have a much better prognosis compared with preganglionic injuries.[20]

Decision-Making Principles/Diagnoses

Strain/Sprain

Cervical strain and sprain are frequent injuries seen in most sports. The patient usually has localized pain in the cervical spine area after an injury with diminished range of motion and tenderness to palpation. By definition no paresthesias or weakness should be identified on examination. When tenderness to palpation is present, and depending on the mechanism of injury, a plain film radiograph may be warranted. Physical examination is paramount to determine if radiographs are needed and if the neurologic status is intact. The range of motion of the athlete should be examined, including flexion, extension, lateral bending, and rotation. If these motions are intact and painless, then no further imaging is needed, and the athlete is allowed to resume activity. If the patient has less than full range of motion, pain, motor weakness, or paresthesias with examination, then at a minimum flexion/extension/anteroposterior films are required. If persistent pain continues or pain out of proportion with range of motion is present, advanced imaging may be warranted to rule out an acute intervertebral disk herniation or ligamentous injury.

Neurapraxic Injuries

Stinger/Burner

A stinger or burner usually presents as a burning pain that radiates from the shoulder down the deltoid into the arm and hand. It can also present with numbness and motor weakness in the most common C5 and C6 distributions (deltoid and biceps weakness).[8,21] These symptoms may last several minutes to several days but by definition do not leave any permanent neurologic deficits and result in negative imaging evaluations. Once a participant has had one episode of a neurapraxic injury, he or she has a 49% to 65% chance of recurrence.[22]

The mechanism of injury that causes neurapraxic injuries has been debated in the literature, and numerous theories have been postulated regarding the cause of these injuries. The most common theory is that the neurapraxic symptoms are caused by a traction injury to the brachial plexus/nerve roots. The anatomic location of the injury is also debated in the literature. Some investigators believe that the injury is caused by nerve root trauma from a traction injury.[23,24] Other authors have postulated that the injury is from a brachial plexus/peripheral nerve injury[8,25] and thus should be treated and classified as a peripheral nerve injury according to the Seddon classification.[26]

Burning Hands Syndrome

As described by Maroon,[27] burning hands syndrome presents with a burning and dysesthesia and associated hand and arm weakness. It is thought to be a variant of central cord syndrome, with cord compression of the spinothalamic and corticospinal tracts. As with stingers and burners, most of these episodes resolve on their own within minutes to days.

Transient Quadriplegia

Transient quadriplegia is temporary and usually resolves within minutes, but in some cases it can last up to 36 to 48 hours. It has also been named *spinal cord concussion*[28] and *cervical cord neurapraxia*. The incidence in football is 7 per 10,000 participants. The pathophysiologic mechanism is not understood; a number of mechanisms have been suggested, including hyperflexion, hyperextension, and axial loading with the prior two mechanisms. A pincer mechanism described by Penning[29] involves narrowing of the anteroposterior diameter of the cord with flexion and extension because of the infolding of the posterior longitudinal ligament and ligamentum flavum. Multiple retrospective studies have shown that patients who experience transient quadriplegia usually have no significant spinal abnormalities that would predispose them to a spinal cord insult, nor are these patients predisposed to have a permanent spinal cord injury.[30]

Herniated Disks

Herniated disks can be a chronic issue or may develop acutely. They usually present with axial neck pain and radicular pain in the upper extremities. They can present with numbness and weakness. Most can be treated conservatively, but in cases of persistent radiculopathy, neurologic weakness, or numbness, a decompression procedure may be indicated. An extremely rare presentation is of an athlete with an acute onset of paraplegia or quadriplegia with negative plain film or CT scan findings. In this presentation an emergent MRI is warranted to rule out an acute herniation with spinal cord compression.[31,32]

Fractures

Fractures of the cervical spine can be defined as stable or unstable and with associated neurologic deficits. Stable fractures include spinous process fractures, lamina fractures, and vertebral body fractures that show no instability on flexion/extension radiographs. Historically, the radiographic criteria for an unstable fracture have been defined in the literature as more than 3.5 mm of horizontal movement or 11 degrees of angular displacement between two adjacent vertebrae (Figs. 126-7 and 126-8).[33] Compromise of the anterior ligament and posterior ligamentous complex can also lead to instability and must be assessed with MRI scanning to evaluate these structures.

Fractures of the cervical spine are delineated by the levels where they are located. The upper spine consists of the C1 and C2 vertebrae. The subaxial spine consists of vertebral bodies C3-C7. The unique anatomy of the C1 and C2 vertebral bodies leads to different types of fractures compared with vertebral bodies of the subaxial spine, which all have similar anatomic features.

Upper Cervical Fractures

The C1 and C2 complex is a combination of bony and ligamentous attachments and articulations. Any disruption of these articulations can cause instability and possible neurologic damage. Instability of the C1/C2 articulation is usually defined by the atlantodens interval, which is measured on a lateral radiograph or sagittal CT reconstruction. The space between the posterior aspect of the anterior C1 ring and the anterior aspect of the C2 dens in adults should be less than 3 mm. If the transverse alar ligament (TAL) is compromised, this interval is greater than 3 mm. The TAL functions as a checkrein to keep the dens from protruding into the spinal canal posteriorly and subsequently compressing the spinal cord. However, this injury rarely causes neurologic damage because of the large amount of space available for the cord in the upper cervical spine. If the condition is not treated, the patient may become myelopathic as the spinal cord undergoes impingement from the dens (Fig. 126-9). These patients most likely need a C1/C2 fusion.[34]

The C1 vertebra is shaped like a ring and thus is susceptible to axial loads. A ring must usually break in two places because of its geometry. Jefferson first described the fracture of the C1 ring in 1920.[35] These fractures are typically noted on axial CT scans or on open-mouth odontoid views. The stability of a C1 fracture is defined by measuring the lateral overhang of the lateral masses of C1 over the lateral masses of C2 on odontoid views or coronal CT reconstructions. If the combined overhang is greater than 7 mm, then the TAL is most likely injured, resulting in instability, and likely requires surgical intervention (Fig. 126-10).

The most common fracture of the C2 vertebra is the fracture of the dens. These fractures were organized into three major types by Anderson and D'Alonzo (Fig. 126-11).[36] Type I fractures are an avulsion of the tip of the odontoid from the

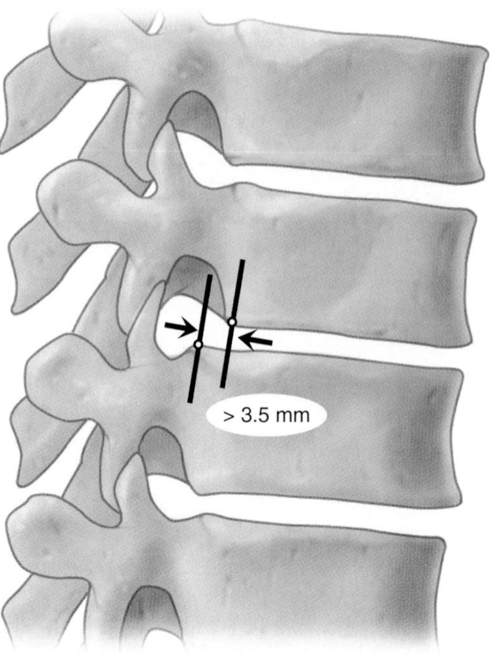

FIGURE 126-8 The method for determining translatory displacement, as described by White and colleagues. Using the posteroinferior angle of the superior vertebral body as one point of reference and the posterosuperior angle of the vertebral body below, the distance between the two in the sagittal plane is measured. A distance of 3.5 mm or greater suggests clinical instability. *(From White AA, Johnson RM, Punjabi MM, et al: Biomechanical analysis of clinical stability in the cervical spine.* Clin Orthop *109:85, 1975.)*

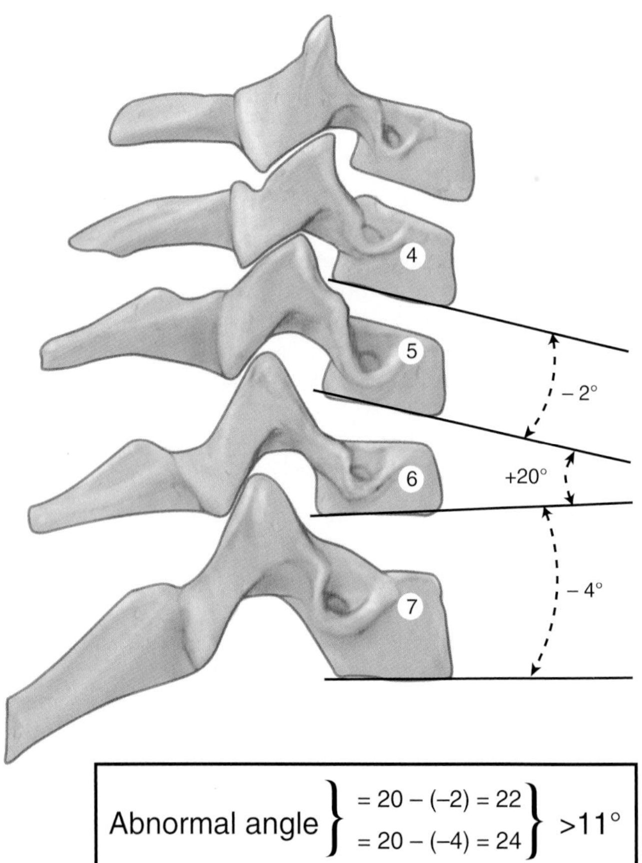

FIGURE 126-7 Abnormal angulation between two vertebrae at any one interspace is determined by comparing the angle formed by the projection of the inferior vertebral body that borders with that of either the vertebral body above or the vertebral body below. If the angle at the interspace in question is 11 degrees or greater than that of either adjacent interspace, it is considered to be clinical instability by White and associates. *(From White AA, Johnson RM, Punjabi MM, et al: Biomechanical analysis of clinical stability in the cervical spine.* Clin Orthop *109:85, 1975.)*

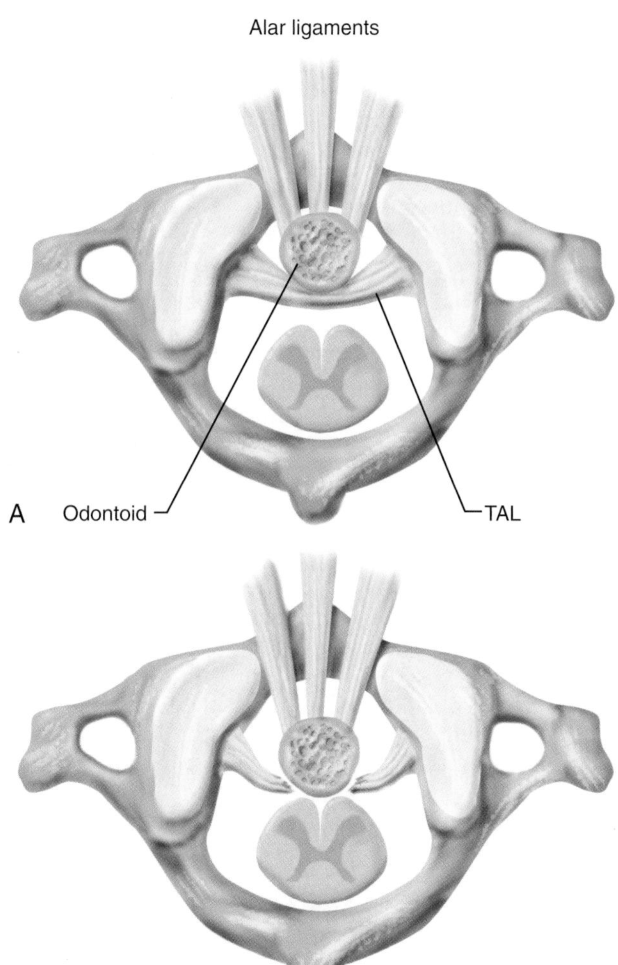

FIGURE 126-9 **A,** The atlantoaxial complex as seen from above. **B,** The disruption of the transverse ligament (*TAL*) with intact alar ligaments results in C1-C2 instability without cord compression. *(Modified from Hensinger RN: Congenital anomalies of the atlanto-axial joint. In The Cervical Spine Research Society Editorial Committee:* The Cervical Spine, *ed 2, Philadelphia, 1989, JB Lippincott.)*

alar ligament. These fractures are rarely seen and usually require immobilization for comfort only. Type II injures are fractures through the base of the den/body interface of C2. These injuries have a nonunion rate of 36% to 50% with nonrigid immobilization. They are usually treated with cervical immobilization with use of a rigid collar or halo device or possible C1/C2 surgical fixation or C2 dens screw fixation. Up to 85% unite with halo immobilization.[37] Type III fractures are fractures through the body of dens in the vascular cancellous bone of C2. These fractures usually heal without complication with use of a rigid cervical orthosis for 4 to 6 weeks and have a very low nonunion rate.

Another common C2 fracture is the so-called hangman's fracture or traumatic spondylolisthesis of the C2 posterior arch. This fracture is an unstable injury and must be treated with a rigid orthosis such as a rigid cervical collar or halo immobilization device. These injuries are rarely associated with neurologic injuries when they are isolated because they enlarge the spinal canal diameter as a result of the fracture pattern.

Subaxial Fractures/Dislocations

One of the most common types of fractures in the subaxial spine is the compression fracture. This injury consists of compression of the anterior aspect of the vertebral body and is only a one-column injury as described by Denis (Fig. 126-12).[38] Most of these fractures are stable and can be treated in a rigid cervical collar for 4 to 6 weeks.

A burst fracture consists of a two-column injury to the vertebral body and is inherently more unstable. These fractures are defined as unstable if they have more than 11 degrees of cervical kyphosis or 3.5 mm of spondylolisthesis (slippage) of the vertebral body compared with the rostral vertebral body (Fig. 126-13).[33] Unstable fractures are typically treated surgically, usually with a posterior spinal fusion or anterior corpectomy and fusion.

A more serious variant of the burst fracture is the so-called teardrop fracture. It received this name because the anterior-inferior fragment of the vertebral body, as noted on the cervical spine lateral view, looks like a teardrop. A high incidence of quadriplegia occurs with this type of injury. Two planes of

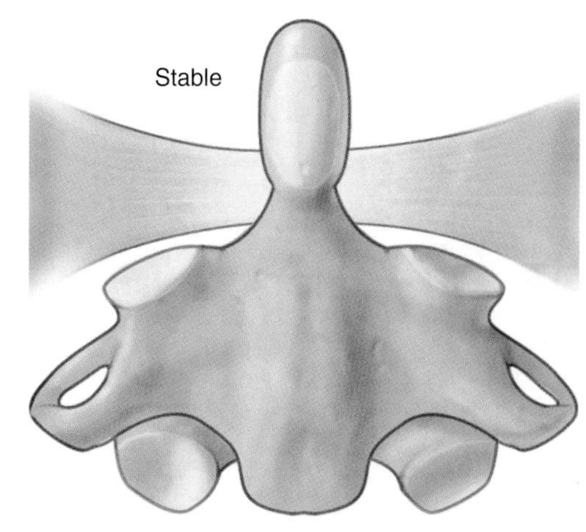

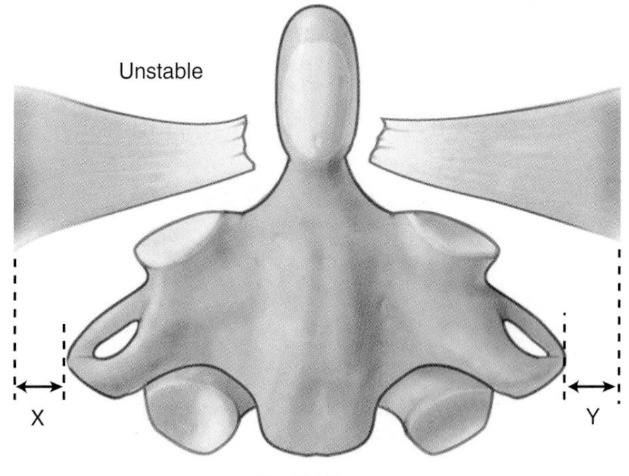

FIGURE 126-10 A comminuted Jefferson fracture with both the transverse ligament intact (stable configuration) and a transverse ligament rupture (unstable configuration). *(Modified from White AA, Punjabi MM:* Clinical biomechanics of the spine, *Philadelphia, 1978, JB Lippincott.)*

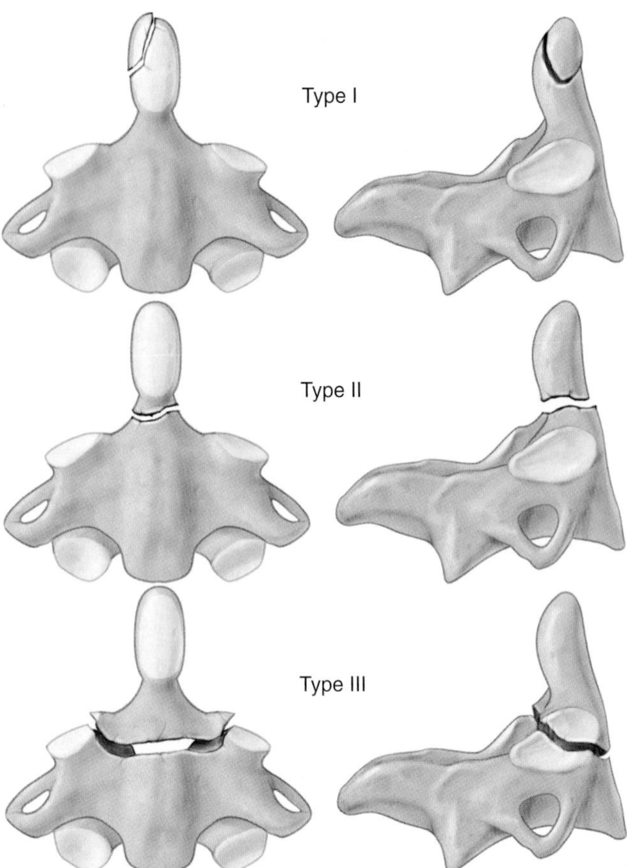

FIGURE 126-11 The three types of odontoid fractures in both the anteroposterior and lateral planes. Type I is an oblique avulsion fracture from the upper portion of the odontoid. Type II is a fracture of the odontoid process at its base. Type III is an odontoid fracture through the body of C2. *(Modified from Anderson LD, D'Alonzo RT: Fractures of the odontoid process of the axis.* J Bone Joint Surg Am *56:1663–1674, 1974.)*

injury have actually been described with this fracture. The first plane is the coronal plane injury that causes the pathognomonic teardrop fragment seen on the lateral radiograph. The other fracture is in the sagittal plane through the midbody of the vertebra.[39-42] This plane can be seen only on CT coronal reconstruction, and any patient with the classic teardrop anterior-inferior injury should have a CT scan to rule out the more serious sagittal plane injury (Fig. 126-14). The posterior elements and the posterior ligamentous complex are usually also injured. These fractures are not stable and require surgical treatment, usually with an anterior corpectomy and fusion along with posterior stabilization and fusion.

Facet dislocations are extremely rare in athletes. They are usually associated with high-energy motor vehicle accidents. However, the health care professional must be able to recognize this dislocation pattern on plain radiographs, along with the clinical signs associated with the dislocations. Two pairs of facet joints are present for every vertebra in the cervical spine from C3 to C7. These joints are overlapped like shingles on a roof, and with severe flexion they can distract enough to translate over each other, causing a facet dislocation on one side or both. Unilateral facet dislocations are associated with torticollis and severe axial neck pain with possible isolated nerve root injury. Radiographs show between 10% and 25% subluxation of the superior vertebral body over the caudal body below (Fig. 126-15). These injuries must be anatomically reduced. Reduction can be performed in the emergency department with cervical tongs and weight in an awake and alert patient. If reduction is not possible, the patient is taken to the operating room for open reduction and internal fixation after an emergent MRI is obtained to evaluate for a concomitant herniated disk.[43] Bilateral facet dislocation has a much more grave prognosis and a higher incidence of neurologic compromise, including quadriplegia. On radiographs the vertebral body is subluxated 50% or greater on the caudal vertebra below (Fig. 126-16). An emergent reduction and

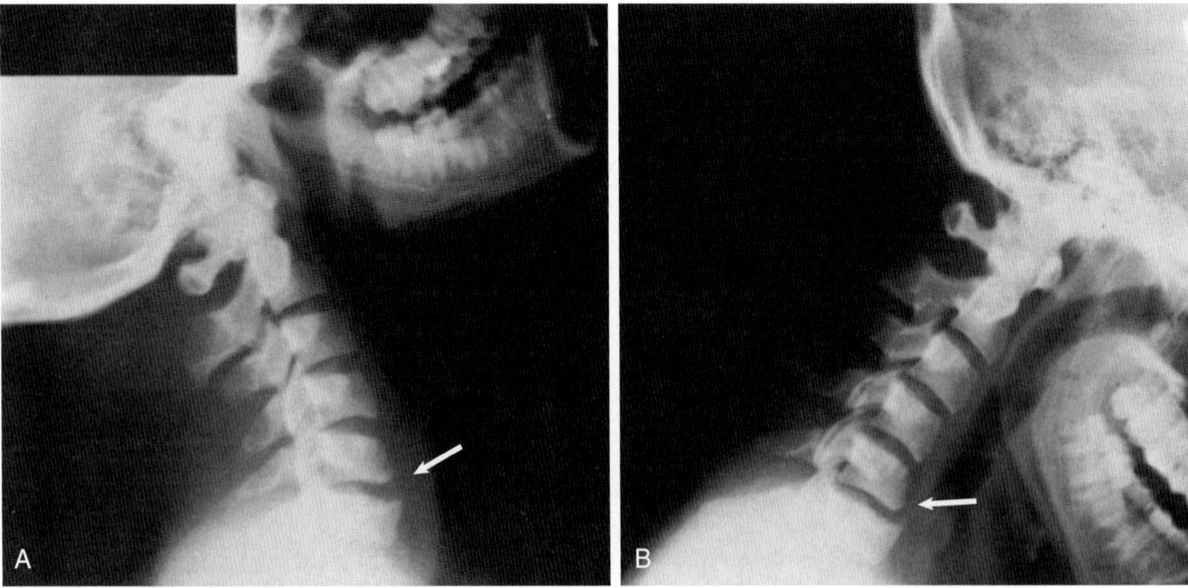

FIGURE 126-12 **A** and **B,** A type I vertebral body end plate compression fracture involving the superior aspect of C6 (*arrows*). Extension and flexion views demonstrate absence of evidence of instability. *(From Torg JS, editor:* Athletic injuries to the head, neck and face, *Philadelphia, 1982, Lea & Febiger.)*

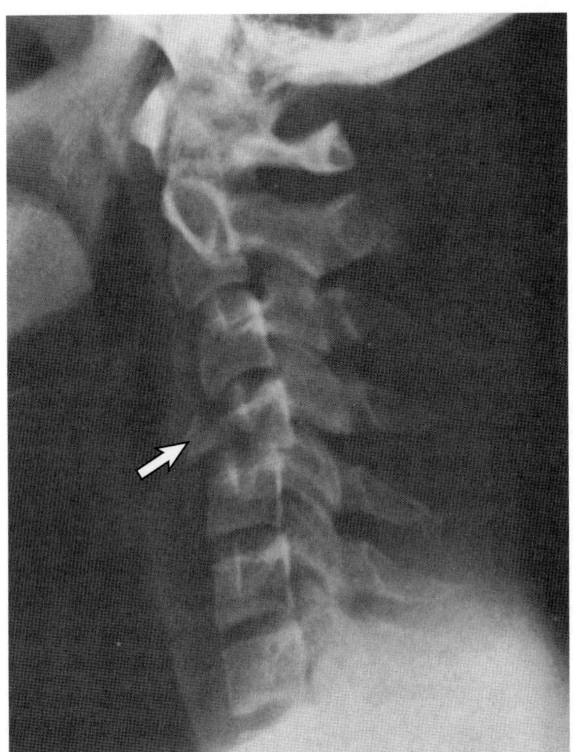

FIGURE 126-13 A type III comminuted burst fracture of C4 with displacement of fragments into the vertebral canal (*arrow*). *(From Torg JS, editor:* Athletic injuries to the head, neck and face, *Philadelphia, 1982, Lea & Febiger.)*

operative stabilization is performed. Bilateral facet dislocations usually result in the disruption of the posterior ligamentous complex and therefore are usually operated on posteriorly to address this injury and allow for facet reduction.

Spinal Stenosis

Spinal stenosis has historically been defined as a subaxial (C3-C7) spinal canal of less than 14 mm on a lateral plain film.[30] According to Torg et al.,[46] any ratio of less than 0.8 of the spinal canal to the vertebral body would be considered spinal stenosis. However, they have noted that this ratio of 0.8 does not predispose football players to spinal cord injury and should not be a contraindication to participation in sports. Athletes have been shown to have large vertebral bodies compared with control subjects, thus skewing the denominator in the ratio and causing an overdiagnosis of spinal stenosis in athletes with use of the Torg method.[44]

Spinal cord injuries are catastrophic consequences that can occur in contact sports such as American football and high-energy sports such as equestrian sports. Complete spinal cord injuries are life-changing injuries that have a huge impact on society and the families of patients with spinal cord injuries. The cost to society is estimated to be $9.7 billion.[45] Approximately 11,000 new spinal cord injuries occur each year.[45] The incidence of permanent cervical quadriplegia is 0.33 per 100,000 in high school athletes and 1.33 per 100,000 in college athletes.[7,46] Cantu and Mueller[47] describe the most likely scenarios of cervical spinal cord injuries in American football. Most of the injuries occur during a game and not during practice. More than 71% of the players injured were playing defense and were making a tackle at the time of the injury. Almost 80% sustained a fracture dislocation of the cervical spine. The quadriplegia risk went up substantially as the level of football increased from high school to professional football. The spinal precautions described earlier in this chapter should be implemented for any player with a suspected spinal cord injury, along with the trauma protocol for assessing the airway, breathing, and circulation. Complete spinal cord injury has a very poor prognosis and is rarely reversible, and usually function is recovered at only one spinal root level.

Incomplete spinal cord injuries have a much better prognosis than complete injuries but are also life-changing events for patients with these injuries. The four classically described types of incomplete spinal cord injury syndromes are the central cord, Brown-Séquard, anterior cord, and posterior cord syndromes.

Central cord syndrome is the most common type of incomplete spinal cord injury. It is usually associated with a hyperextension injury in patients who have congenitally narrowed spinal canals. The hyperextension injury leads to injury to the central gray matter and to the central corticospinal tracts. The distribution of the gray matter in the corticospinal tract consists of upper extremity neurons more centrally and lower extremity neurons more laterally, and thus the upper extremities are more affected than the lower extremities in persons with a central cord injury (Fig. 126-17). The typical presentation is upper extremity motor weakness that is much more pronounced than the lower extremity weakness. Patients also have more weakness distally in the extremity than proximally. A nonspecific loss of sensory patterns and commonly bladder and sexual dysfunction are associated with this injury. Persons who have this injury have a relatively good prognosis, with a majority of patients regaining the ability to walk, along with bowel and bladder control and the use of their upper extremities. The most common residual effect is decreased strength in the intrinsic muscles of the hand.[48,49] Factors associated with good to excellent recovery include young age, absence of spinal cord signal abnormality on MRI, level of education, absence of spasticity, and early motor recovery.[50] A large variability exists in the literature regarding treatment for central cord injuries, with most historical studies recommending nonsurgical management and immobilization in a rigid cervical orthosis and possible decompression procedures several weeks to months after the initial injury. No prospective surgical versus nonsurgical studies have been performed, and thus an unbiased recommendation is not possible at this time.

Brown-Séquard syndrome is an incomplete spinal cord injury that results in a hemisection of the cord from penetrating trauma, vascular insult, or unilateral facet fracture/dislocation (Fig. 126-18). It includes ipsilateral loss of motor function below the injury, along with loss of proprioception. It also results in disruption of contralateral spinothalamic pathways (pain and temperature), usually two levels below the lesion. Patients with this injury have an overall good prognosis, with most persons regaining the ability to ambulate and control bowel and bladder function.

Anterior cord syndrome is a variant of incomplete spinal cord injury that causes injury to the anterior two thirds of the spinal cord and results in loss of all motor function below the injury, with the weakness being equivalent in the upper and

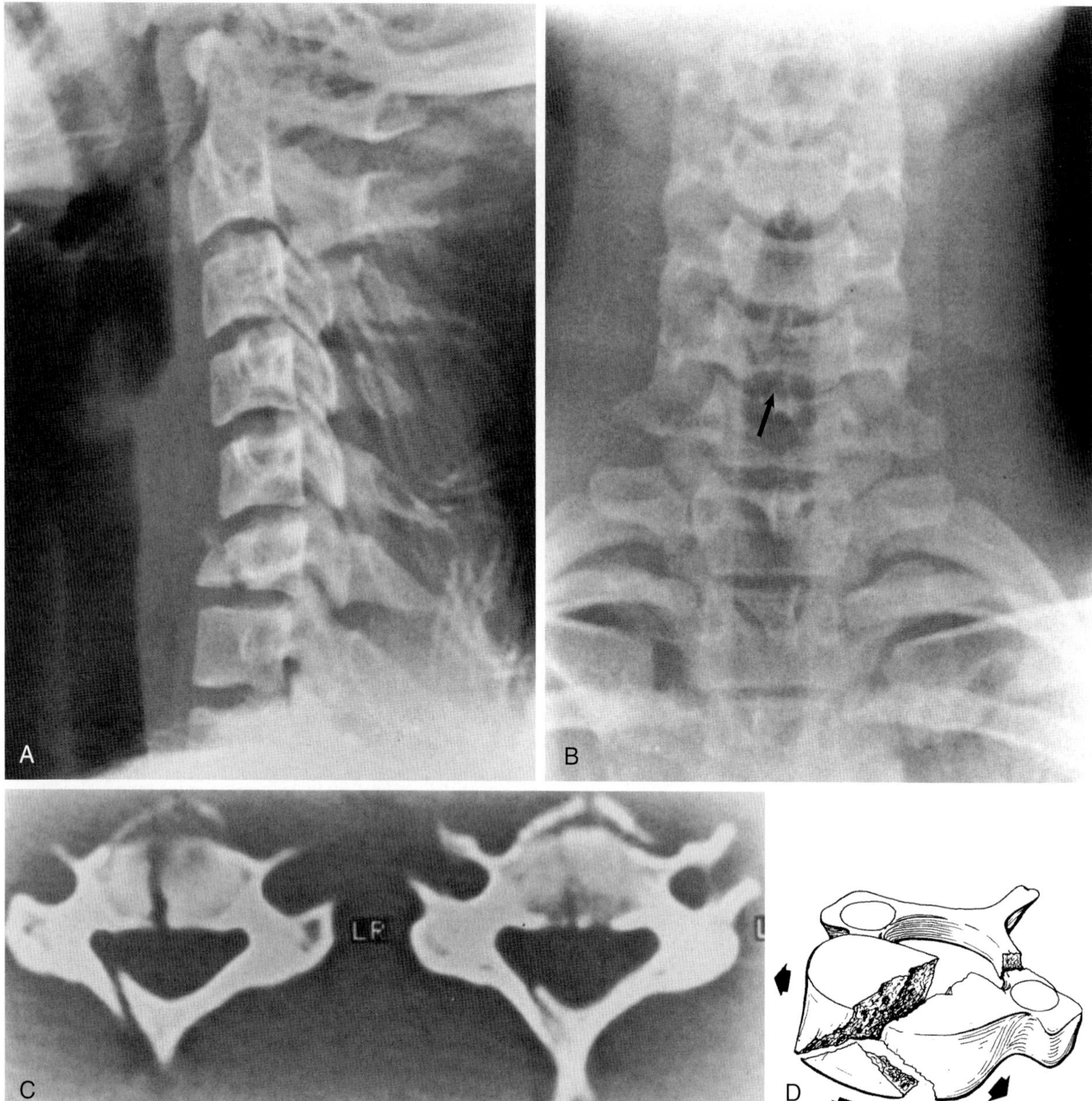

FIGURE 126-14 **A,** A three-part, two-plane fracture of C6. The lateral view demonstrates prevertebral soft tissue swelling and an anteroinferior fracture fragment of C6 involving the entire vertebral body height and one third of the vertebral body width. Approximately 1 mm of posterior displacement of the inferior aspect of the posterior vertebral body is present. The C6-C7 intervertebral disk space is minimally narrowed posteriorly with associated capsular disruption and fanning. **B,** The frontal view demonstrates a faint, linear radiolucency through the C6 vertebral body indicating a sagittal vertebral body fracture (*arrow*). Mild lateral mass displacement is present. **C,** Computed tomographic examination demonstrates the sagittal fracture extending completely through the vertebral body with disruption of the lamina on the right. **D,** A diagrammatic representation of the three-part, two-plane vertebral body compression fracture demonstrates the anteroinferior teardrop as well as the sagittal vertebral body fractures and associated fracture through the lamina. *(**A,** From Torg JS, Pavlov H, O'Neill MJ, et al: The axial load teardrop fracture.* Am J Sports Med *19:355–364, 1991.)*

lower extremities (Fig. 126-19). The injury is typically caused by a hyperflexion injury with bony instability, acute disk herniation, or formation of an anterior spinal canal hematoma. It can also be caused by direct injury to the anterior spinal artery, resulting in a spinal cord stroke of the anterior two thirds of the spinal cord. The dorsal columns are spared in the injury, so patients have preservation of vibration and proprioception. Patients with this injury overall have a very poor prognosis for a return of motor function and control of bowel and bladder functions.

Posterior cord syndrome is the rarest of the incomplete spinal cord syndromes. It is usually caused by an insult to the posterior spinal artery, resulting in ischemia of the dorsal columns of the spinal cord, which leads to loss of deep touch, proprioception, and vibratory sense. Patients have no loss of motor function or pain or temperature sensation, but they

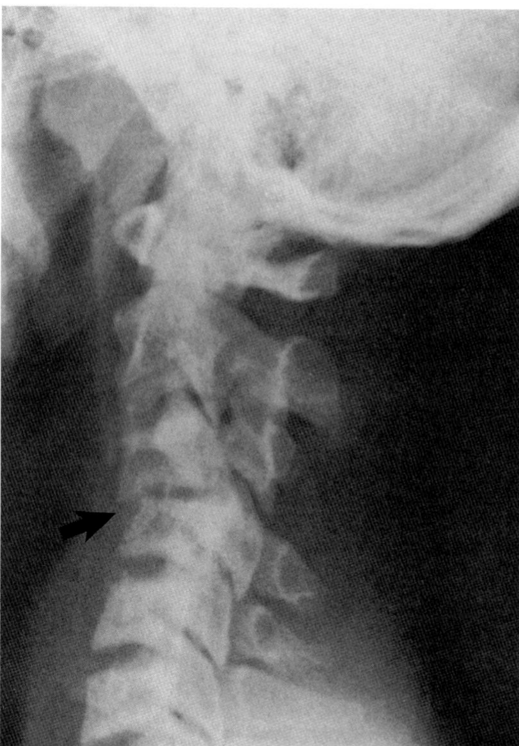

FIGURE 126-15 A unilateral C3-C4 facet dislocation resulting in a complete motor and sensory deficit distal to the lesion. Fanning of the spinous processes of C3 and C4 and more than 20% anterior displacement of the body of C3 on C4 is present (*arrow*). *(From Torg JS, Sennett B, Vegso JJ, et al: Axial loading injuries to the middle cervical spine: analysis and classification.* Am J Sports Med *19:17–25, 1991.)*

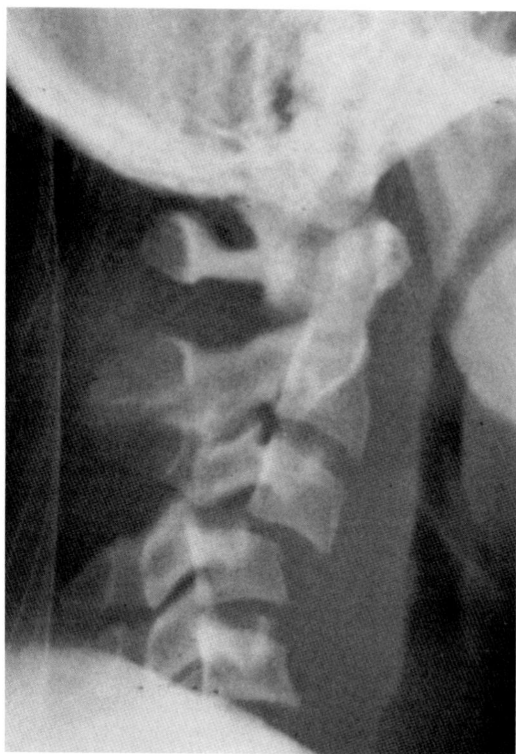

FIGURE 126-16 A bilateral facet dislocation at the C3-C4 level demonstrates anterior angulation, as well as translation greater than 50% of the width of the vertebral body associated with spinous fanning. The lesion resulted in quadriplegia. *(From Torg JS, Sennett B, Vegso JJ, et al: Axial loading injuries to the middle cervical spine: analysis and classification.* Am J Sports Med *19:17–25, 1991.)*

have significant trouble coordinating the movement of limbs because of the lack of proprioception.

Treatment Options/Return to Play

Sprain/Strain

Most sprains and strains of the cervical spine resolve over a few days to weeks. Usually treatment is activity modification and possible suspension of participation in sports, depending on the pain of the athlete while playing. The athlete may resume full participation once the full painless range of motion is reestablished and no tenderness to palpation is noted on examination.

Neurapraxic Injuries

The main treatment for any neurapraxic injury includes cessation of participation in sports until all of the symptoms have resolved. Criteria for return to play consist of full strength on physical examination, no pain with range of motion of the cervical spine or extremities, and no numbness or tingling that radiates into the upper extremities. As described earlier, after an athlete has one episode of a neurapraxic injury, he or she has a 50% chance of a recurrent episode if participation in the same sport continues. The patient and family must be informed of this risk. If a recurrent injury occurs, steps must be taken to protect the patient, which may include equipment modification such as use of a "cowboy collar" in football or physical therapy that focuses on shoulder and neck strengthening, which has been shown to aid in the prevention of some neurapraxic injuries (Figs. 126-20 and 126-21).[24] Vaccaro et al.[22] outlined some return-to-play criteria for patients with transient quadriplegia, stingers, and burners (see Table 126-1).

Most herniated disks can be treated nonoperatively, especially in the absence of any motor weakness or sensory changes. However, if the patient has neurologic deficits or persistent radicular symptoms for up to 6 months, surgical intervention may be warranted. Recent studies have shown

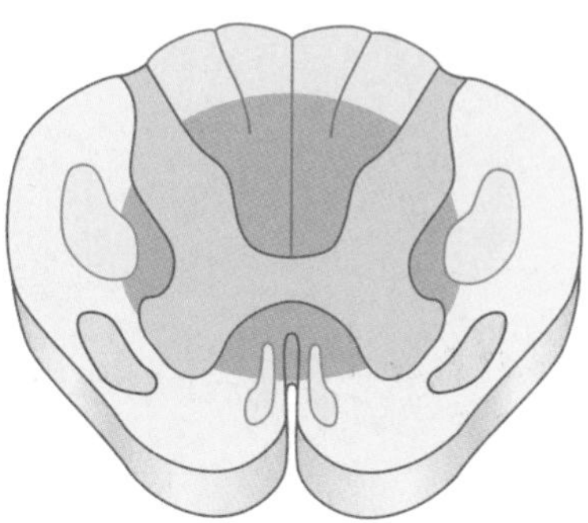

FIGURE 126-17 Central cord syndrome.

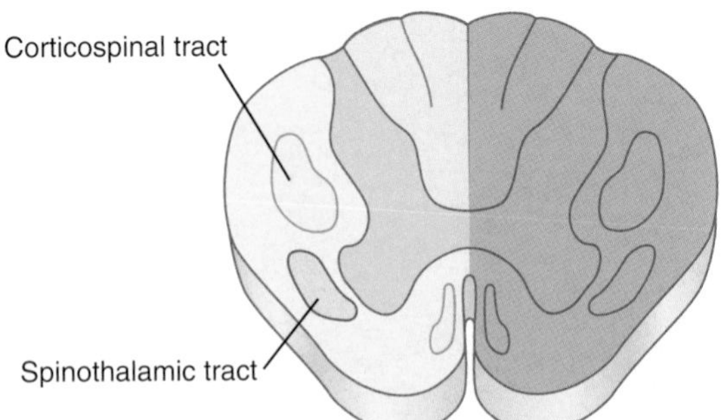

FIGURE 126-18 Brown-Séquard syndrome.

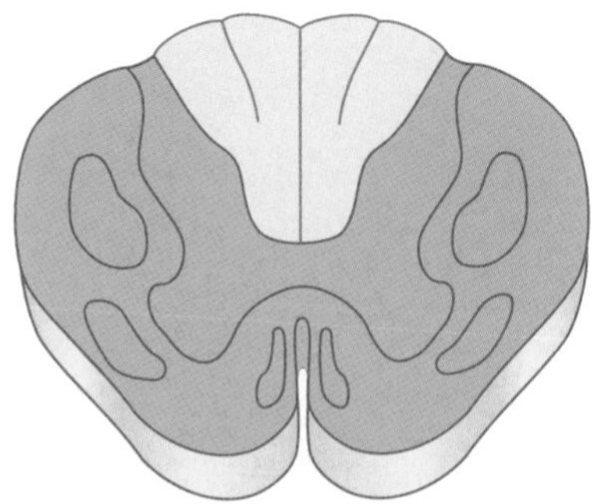

FIGURE 126-19 Anterior cord syndrome.

that surgical and nonsurgical outcomes are worse if radicular pain is treated after the 6-month range.[51] Depending on where the herniation is located anatomically, it can be treated with an anterior cervical diskectomy and fusion in the cervical spine or a microdiskectomy if it is located in the lumbar spine. Studies have shown that a healed anterior cervical diskectomy and fusion preserves the strength and integrity of the cervical spine and should not be an exclusion for return to sports.[2]

Fractures of the cervical spine can be incidental injuries, such as spinous process, transverse process, or avulsion fractures. These injuries are usually treated conservatively with use of a hard or soft cervical orthosis for 4 to 6 weeks or until full range of motion and pain have resolved, and they usually do not require any permanent restrictions regarding return to play. Other fractures of the cervical spine that require reduction or surgical stabilization may preclude return to play, but because of the large variability in fracture pattern and injury, the final decision must be made by the spinal surgeon in conjunction with the team physician.

Recurrent injury and return to play in patients with spinal stenosis and cervical cord neurapraxia have been addressed by Torg et al.[52,53] in several articles. In 1997 they reported on 110 patients with spinal stenosis who had a cervical cord neurapraxia. Of those 110 patients, 63 returned to play, with 56% (35 of 63) sustaining a recurrent episode of neurapraxia. None of the recurrent episodes led to any permanent injury or sequela. The conclusion of these investigators was that persons with stenosis and an uncomplicated episode of cervical cord neurapraxia could return to play without increased risks of permanent neurologic deficits.[52] In 2002 they published guidelines for return to play for athletes with spinal stenosis and a previous history of cervical cord neurapraxia[53] (see Table 126-2 for a summary of these guidelines).

Any complete or incomplete spinal cord injury prevents return to play in the sport in which the injury was sustained, but patients can participate in many noncontact and Paralympic sports after such an injury. Studies have shown that return to an adaptive sport is important for self-perception and quality of life for disabled athletes.[54]

Conclusion

Cervical spine injuries are the most serious injuries that can occur during sporting events and can lead to permanent paralysis and death. Prevention is the most important step that can be taken to deter the injury. When an injury does occur, it is paramount for the health care provider to be well educated regarding spine immobilization, airway protection,

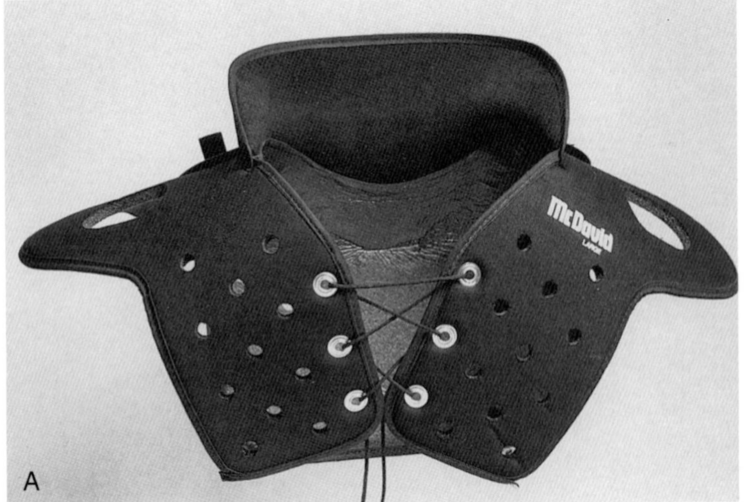

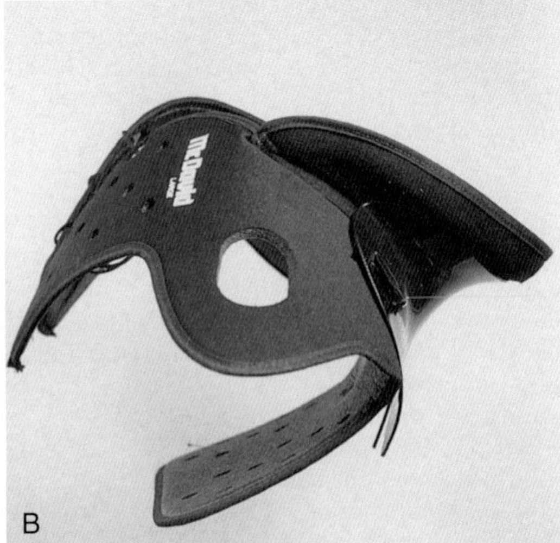

FIGURE 126-20 Frontal (**A**) and lateral (**B**) views of the cowboy collar. This device, which is worn under the shoulder pads, effectively limits the extremes of extension and lateral bending of the cervical spine.

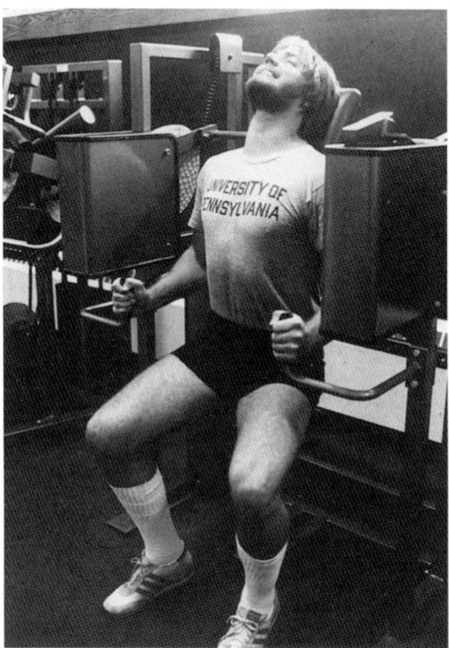

FIGURE 126-21 Crucial in the effective management of the athlete with recurrent burners is the implementation of an aggressive, year-round neck and shoulder muscle strengthening program. Use of variable-resistance isotonic "neck machines" is effective.

and pertinent radiologic and medical workup. As a first responder, the trainer, team physician, or paramedic should have the appropriate training before handling such serious injuries. A violation of protocol has potentially dire consequences for the injured athlete. A spine board, equipment to remove face masks and other items that could potentially hamper airway and spine management, and on-site electronic communication to allow immediate contact with the local trauma center should be available at any contact sporting event. Athletes can recover from most sporting injuries, but a cervical spine injury can be a life-changing event for the athlete. The first responder must have the knowledge, equipment, and protocols in place to reduce the chance of further injury.

TABLE 126-1

CERVICAL SPINE INJURIES IN ATHLETES: CURRENT RETURN-TO-PLAY CRITERIA

No contraindication	1. <3 episodes of burners lasting <24 h
	2. 1 episode of TQ with no residual deficit
Relative contraindication	1. Prolonged burner or TQ >24 h
	2. >3 episodes of burners or >2 episodes of TQ
Absolute contraindication	1. >2 episodes of TQ
	2. Cervical myelopathy on imaging/hx
	3. Cervical pain/neurologic deficit

hx, History; *TQ,* transient quadriplegia.

TABLE 126-2

GUIDELINES FOR RETURN TO PLAY FOR AN ATHLETE WHO PREVIOUSLY SUSTAINED CERVICAL CORD NEURAPRAXIA

No contraindication	1. Torg ratio <0.8 in an asymptomatic patient
Relative contraindication	1. Torg ratio <0.8 with one episode CCN
	2. An episode of CCN with intervertebral disk and/or degenerative changes
	3. An episode of CCN with MRI evidence of cord deformation
Absolute contraindication	1. An episode of CCN with MRI evidence of a cord defect or edema
	2. An episode of CCN with ligamentous instability, symptoms >36 h, and/or multiple episodes

CCN, Cervical cord neurapraxia; *MRI,* magnetic resonance imaging.

For a complete list of references, go to expertconsult.com.

Suggested Readings

Citation: Hoffman JR, Mower WR, Wolfson AB, et al: Validity of a set of clinical criteria to rule out injury to the cervical spine in patients with blunt trauma. National Emergency X-Radiography Utilization Study Group. *N Engl J Med* 343(2):94–99, 2000.

Level of Evidence: I

Summary: The authors of this landmark article discuss the criteria that should be used to determine if radiographic evaluation should be obtained after blunt trauma to the cervical spine. More than 34,000 patients were studied in 21 different centers across North America to determine the validity of the criteria.

Citation: Maroon JC, Bailes JE: Athletes with cervical spine injury. *Spine (Phila Pa 1976)* 21(19):2294–2299, 1996.

Level of Evidence: III

Summary: The authors of this article provide an excellent overview of the most common types of cervical spine injuries seen in sports. On- and off-field management strategies are also discussed.

Citation: Rihn JA, Hilibrand AS, Radcliff K, et al: Duration of symptoms resulting from lumbar disc herniation: effect on treatment outcomes: analysis of the Spine Patient Outcomes Research Trial (SPORT). *J Bone Joint Surg Am* 93(20):1906–1914, 2011.

Level of Evidence: I

Summary: Although this article does not specifically address cervical disk herniations, it has been instrumental in advising patients about their prognosis as it relates to the length of the delay in undergoing decompression for disk herniations. Patients who underwent decompression prior to having symptoms for 6 months had better results than did patients who waited longer than 6 months. This article is one of the many excellent reports from the Spine Patients Outcome Research Trial (SPORT) study group.

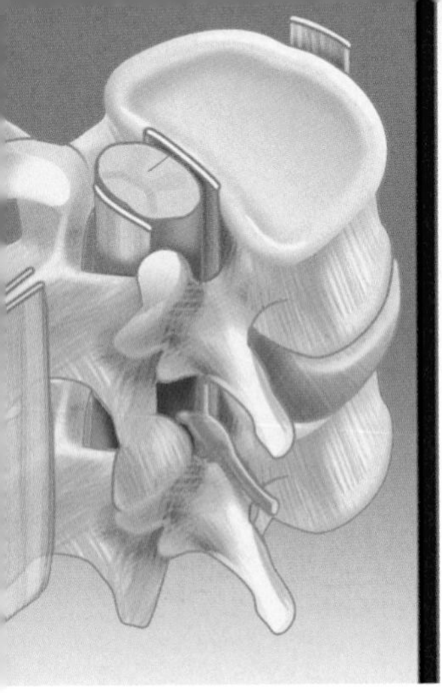

127

Stingers

DAVID GOODWIN • S. BABAK KALANTAR

Brachial plexus injuries are among the most common neurologic injuries sustained by athletes in contact sports. Brachial plexopathies, more commonly referred to as *stingers,* are reversible unilateral upper extremity injuries that can present with pain, numbness, tingling, and/or occasional weakness. Stingers can represent a broad spectrum of injuries that include brachial plexus and cervical nerve root injuries. Stingers were first described by Chrisman et al.[1] in 1965 after a lateral neck sprain that caused transient paresthesias and paralysis to the involved upper extremity. Since its initial description, the pathophysiology, management, and potential complications of stingers have become much better understood.

Stingers most commonly occur in collision sports such as football, rugby, and wrestling. Fifty percent of athletes in these contact sports report sustaining a stinger during their athletic careers.[2] Sallis et al.[3] found that 65% of football players sustained a stinger during their careers. Authors of another study estimated that the incidence of stingers among football players is 7.7% per year.[4] Football players have the highest risk of sustaining a stinger at the cornerback position, with the offensive linemen being the second most affected position.[3]

Stingers are purely peripheral nerve injuries that do not affect the spinal cord. Symptoms are not typically bilateral and do not affect the lower extremity. Stingers most commonly affect the C5 and C6 motor and sensory distributions.[5-7] Although stingers are usually temporary, lasting seconds in most cases, effects of some stingers may last weeks or may even result in permanent disability and loss of function. In this chapter we review the natural history, diagnosis, and management of stinger injuries.

History

On the field, the mechanism of injury is typically a consistent identifier of a stinger injury. The symptoms of a stinger occur immediately after contact of the head, neck, or shoulder. The injured athlete may be seen either supporting the affected extremity or "shaking out" the affected extremity.

Athletes frequently describe a painful sensation that radiates from their neck to their fingers after an impact to the shoulder or neck. Some athletes may describe a "dead arm" sensation with transient paralysis and a burning paresthesia from the shoulder to the fingertips. Over the course of seconds to minutes, motor and sensory function typically normalizes, with full recovery within 10 minutes in most athletes.[5] In 5% to 10% of athletes, effects of a stinger may last several hours or longer and may last as long as a few weeks.[8]

Physical Examination

After an athlete with a suspected injury is removed from competition, a mental status examination is performed to rule out a possible head injury. The physical examination begins at the neck, with assessment for tenderness along the cervical spine. If tenderness is identified, a cervical collar is applied until further examination and imaging can rule out a cervical spine injury. If no tenderness is present, then active range of motion of the player's cervical spine is assessed. Loss of neck range of motion is rare with stingers and is associated with more severe cervical spine injuries.

Next, a focused screening examination for upper extremity motor and sensory deficits is conducted by testing the C5 (deltoid strength and lateral upper arm sensation), C6 (wrist extensors and lateral forearm sensation), C7 (triceps or wrist flexion strength and middle fingertip sensation), C8 (finger flexion strength and medial forearm sensation), and T1 (hand intrinsic strength and medial arm sensation) neurologic levels (Fig. 127-1 and Table 127-1). Any deficits upon examination should alert the physician to suspect a neurologic injury and warrant further investigation.

In persons with brachial plexus injuries, unilateral weakness and loss of sensation persist while pain is present[7]; however, neurologic deficits quickly subside after the pain resolves.[7] The most common areas of weakness include the deltoid, biceps, supraspinatus, and infraspinatus muscle groups.[5-7] Injuries of the upper trunk of the brachial plexus can be distinguished from nerve root injuries involving C5 and C6 levels because the long thoracic and dorsal scapula nerve functions are preserved in persons with brachial plexus injuries. The long thoracic nerve may be tested by performing the serratus wall test (i.e., asking the patient to face a wall, and while standing 2 feet from the wall, pushing into the wall with open palms). If a long thoracic nerve palsy is present, the examiner will observe scapular winging medially. The dorsal scapular nerve may be assessed by testing the strength of the levator scapulae and rhomboid major and minor muscles. Persons with rhomboid weakness may have mild scapular winging at rest, with the scapula displaced laterally and upwardly rotated.[9] The rhomboids may be

TABLE 127-1

EVALUATION OF MOTOR FUNCTION IN BURNERS AND OTHER BRACHIAL PLEXUS INJURIES

Muscle	Innervation	Clinical Test
Deltoid	Axillary (C5, C6)	Shoulder abduction
Supraspinatus	Suprascapular (C5, C6)	"Full can" abduction
Infraspinatus	Suprascapular (C5, C6)	External rotation
Biceps brachii	Musculocutaneous (C5, C6)	Elbow flexion
Pronator teres	Median (C6, C7)	Forearm pronation
Triceps brachii	Radial (C7, C8)	Elbow extension
Abductor digiti minimi	Ulnar (C8, T1)	Fifth digit abduction

From Kuhlman G, McKeag D: The "burner": a common nerve injury in contact sports. *Am Fam Physician* 60(7):2, 1999.

tested by having the patient place his or her palm on the lower back facing outward and then pushing the palm away from the lower back against resistance provided by the examiner.[9] The rhomboids should be observed and palpated by the examiner throughout this examination.

Additional tests may yield further clues to diagnosis. Performing the Tinel test at Erb's point may elicit paresthesias in the affected extremity, suggesting an injury distal to the cervical nerve roots. Erb's point is located on the neck 2 to 3 cm superior to the clavicle in line with the C6 vertebra. At Erb's point, the upper trunk of the brachial plexus is immediately subcutaneous, making it vulnerable to injury.

The Spurling test may also be performed by having the athlete extend the neck while tilting the head to the side of

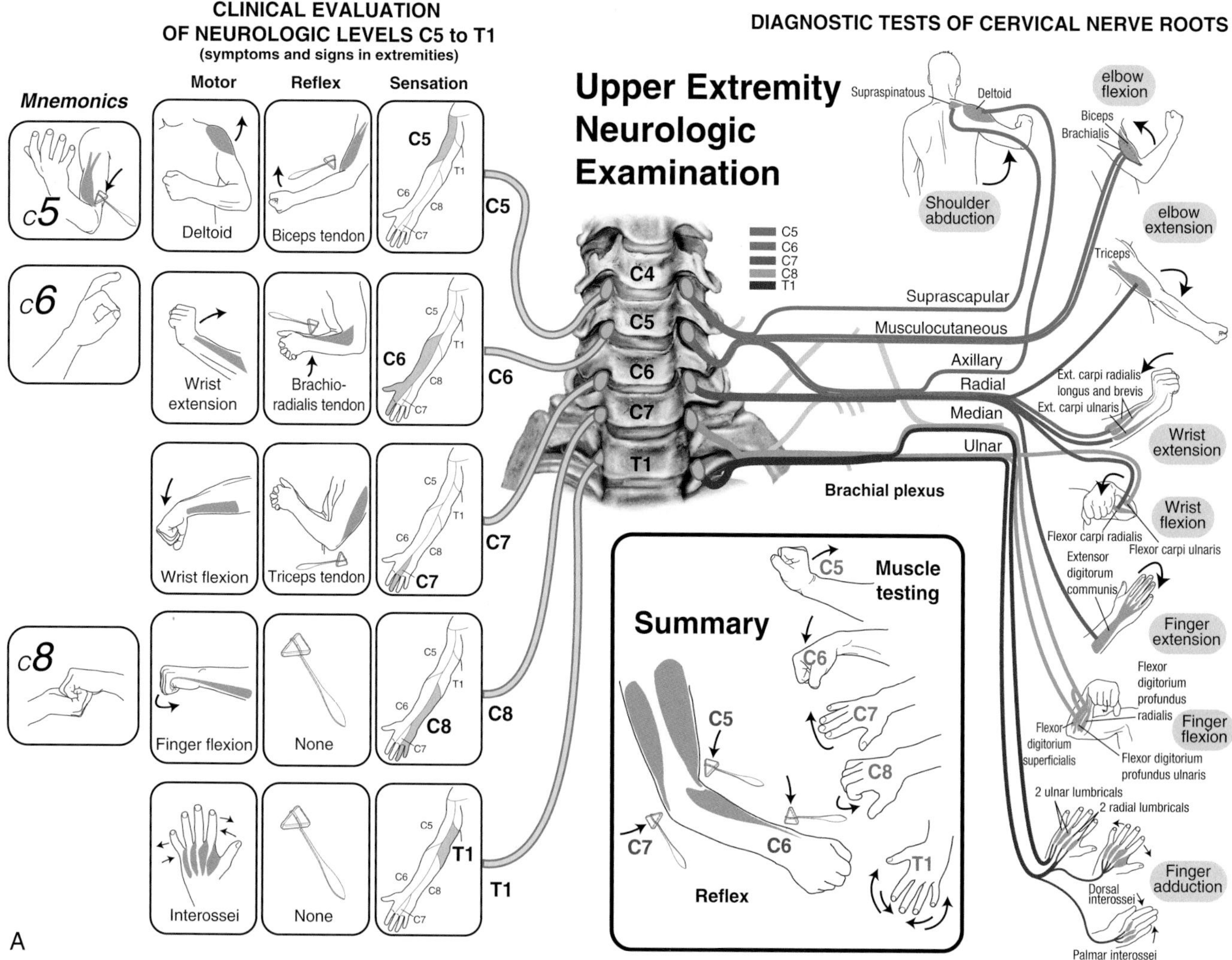

FIGURE 127-1 **A** and **B,** Examination of the upper extremity for strength, sensation, and reflexes. *(From Miller MD, Thompson SR, Hart JA:* Review of orthopaedics, *Philadelphia, 2012, Elsevier.)*

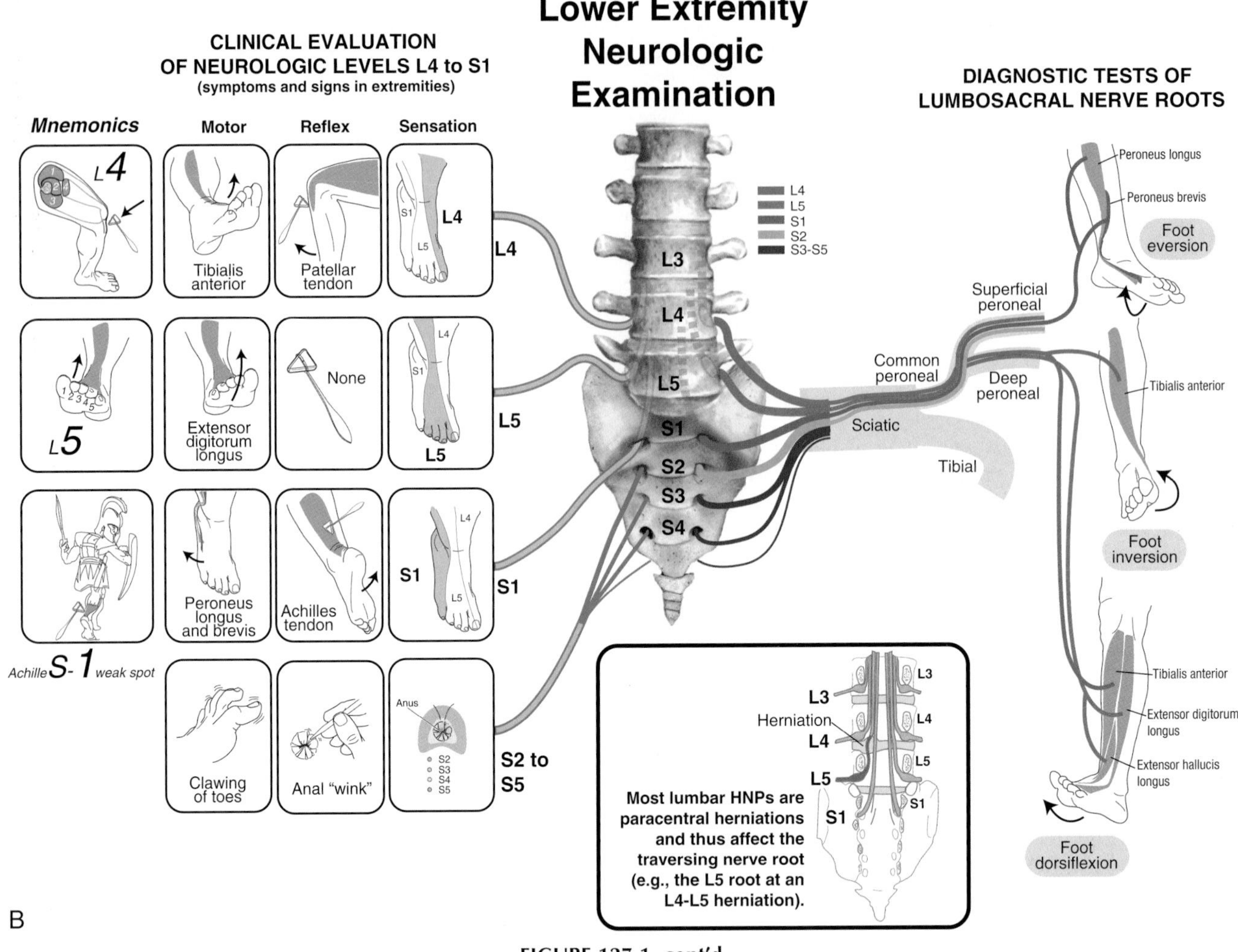

FIGURE 127-1, cont'd

the injury as the examiner applies axial traction. A positive test reproduces pain down the affected extremity, indicating cervical radiculopathy.

Bilateral upper extremity symptoms, restricted neck range of motion, cervical spine tenderness, and symptoms in the lower extremities are rarely associated with stingers and should alert the physician to a more significant cervical spine injury.

Imaging

Imaging should be considered in any athlete with persistent upper extremity pain or weakness or pain with cervical spine range of motion. Initial imaging typically begins with cervical spine radiographs with flexion and extension views to evaluate for fracture or instability. However, recent investigators have questioned the validity of radiographs because of concerns about whether they are sensitive enough to rule out cervical fracture. Computed tomography (CT) has been shown to be more sensitive than radiographs in assessing cervical fractures, and some authors advocate the use of CT if a high level of suspicion exists or the mechanism of injury suggests a possible fracture.[10-12] Acheson et al.[10] retrospectively reviewed cervical spine CT scans and radiographs in 49 patients who were found to have cervical fractures with CT. In this group, 135 fractures were identified with CT, whereas 64 (47%) were seen or suspected on screening radiographs. The authors concluded that conventional radiographs fail to detect a large number of fractures, with potentially significant ramifications.[10] Similarly, Nunez et al.[11] conducted a retrospective review of 88 patients with cervical spine fractures. Radiographs and helical CT images were then reviewed by emergency radiologists. In this study, cervical spine fractures not detectable with radiographs were detected with CT for 32 patients.[11] Without CT imaging, a cervical spine fracture would have been missed in 36% of the patients in this study.

A prospective study by Bailitz et al.[12] compared the diagnostic accuracy of cervical spine radiographs with cervical CT in consecutive patients at a level I trauma center. All patients meeting one or more of the National Emergency X-Radiography Utilization Study criteria underwent cervical spine radiographs and cervical spine CT scans. A total of 1505 patients were included in the study, and 78 (4.9%) were found to have cervical spine fractures on radiographs or CT, with 50 of the injuries found to be clinically significant. A fracture was defined as clinically significant if it required operative treatment, halo application, and/or rigid cervical collar application. CT was 100% sensitive and radiographs were 36% sensitive in detecting clinically significant injuries.[12] Patients were further subdivided into low-, medium-, and high-risk groups for cervical spine injury based on the mechanism of injury, the presence of focal neurologic deficits, age, and associated injuries as defined by Blakemore et al.[13] Radiograph sensitivity among the low-, medium-, and high-risk groups was 25%, 37%, and 46%, respectively, with the lowest sensitivity for low-risk patients. The authors concluded that CT should replace radiographs for the detection of clinically significant cervical spine injuries in all patients with a low, medium, or high risk for cervical spine trauma.[12]

The role of magnetic resonance imaging (MRI) in the evaluation of a stinger is limited. MRI may be useful when it is suspected that disk herniation or foraminal stenosis is contributing to the injury. However, MRI is more helpful when nerve root or nerve transection injury is a concern.

Radiographs, MRI, and CT may also be used to evaluate an athlete's Torg ratio. The Torg ratio is the sagittal spinal canal diameter divided by the sagittal vertebral body diameter. The Torg ratio was first described by Torg et al.[14] in 1986. These investigators retrospectively reviewed 32 athletes who had reported transient neurologic symptoms sustained during play in contact sports. Twenty-nine of the athletes were injured playing football, and 23 were National Football League athletes. All patients in this series were male. Clinical records and postinjury radiographs were reviewed in all patients. More specifically, Torg et al.[14] reviewed lateral cervical spine radiographs to assess evidence of congenital anomalies, instability, disk disease, and spinal stenosis. The authors presented the "ratio method," defined as the sagittal diameter of the spinal cord divided by the anteroposterior width of the vertebral body, as a measure to predict stinger injuries (Fig. 127-2). Torg et al.[14] compared the 32 athletes who had transient neurologic injury with 49 healthy male subjects of comparable age using the ratio method and concluded that a ratio of less than 0.80 indicated significant spinal stenosis and increased risk of sustaining a transient neurologic injury in contact sports.

In a later study, Torg et al.[15] reviewed 110 cases of stingers; 109 of the athletes were male, with an average age of 21 years, and 87% of the injuries occurred while they were playing football. The patients were followed up for an average of 3.3 years. All patients underwent radiographs of the cervical spine, and 53 patients underwent MRI. Torg et al.[15] found the average ratio in affected patients to be 0.68. They concluded that a smaller Torg ratio is a significant predictor of sustaining a stinger and that radiographs and MRI should be obtained in all patients who report a history of transient neurologic injury sustained during contact sports.[15] Fifty-six percent of patients in this study also reported a second stinger injury sustained during the study. The patient's age, level of sports participation, and MRI findings of disk herniation or degenerative disk disease were not found to be significant predictors of recurrent injury.

Although Torg et al.[15] associated a smaller Torg ratio with a higher risk of transient neurologic injury, routine screening of asymptomatic football players has been a controversial topic in collegiate and professional competition. Meyer et al.[16] followed up 266 collegiate football players and identified 40 athletes who had sustained a stinger. Among the 40 collegiate

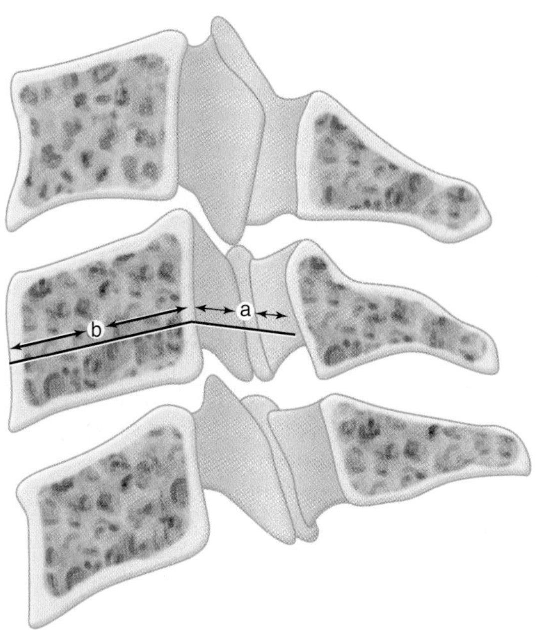

FIGURE 127-2 The ratio method defined by Torg and colleagues uses a cervical spine lateral radiograph to predict an athlete's risk of sustaining a stinger. The Torg ratio is defined as the canal diameter (*a*) divided by the vertebral body diameter (*b*). *(Modified from Torg J, Pavlov H, Genuario S, et al: Neurapraxia of the cervical spinal cord with transient quadriplegia.* J Bone Joint Surg *68:1354–1370, 1986.)*

football players who had sustained stingers, the average Torg ratio was significantly smaller than in those who had not sustained such an injury. Meyer et al.[16] concluded that athletes with a Torg ratio of less than 0.8 had a three times greater risk of sustaining a stinger than did players with a Torg ratio greater than 0.8.

Not all investigators have confirmed the predictive value of the Torg ratio. Castro et al.[4] prospectively followed up 165 collegiate freshman football players at Tulane University. Athletes underwent cervical spine radiographs before their freshman season and were followed up throughout their collegiate football career (range, one to five seasons); 7.7% of athletes reported sustaining a stinger during collegiate competition. Images from the stinger population were compared with those of asymptomatic football players. The authors concluded that the Torg ratio was not predictive of sustaining a stinger.[4] However, among athletes who had previously sustained a stinger, Castro et al.[4] did find an association between the Torg ratio and the risk of recurrence. The authors concluded that a Torg ratio less than 0.70 may be an independent risk factor for repetitive brachial plexus injuries but not for sustaining a first-time stinger. This finding led the authors to recommend that a more appropriate threshold for significant stenosis to be defined as a Torg ratio less than 0.7, instead of the 0.8 previously advocated by Torg et al.[15] and Meyer et al.[4,16]

Page and Guy[17] used screening lateral cervical spine radiographs to measure the Torg ratio in 125 football players at the University of South Carolina. Athletes were followed up for 3 years, and during that period 11% reported sustaining a stinger that resulted in time lost from practice or competition. Among the 11% who sustained stingers, 37% had a Torg ratio less than 0.8. Page and Guy[17] found that players with a Torg ratio of less than 0.8 were four times more likely to experience a stinger than athletes with a Torg ratio greater than 0.8. However, the positive predictive value of using a Torg ratio of 0.8 was 22%. Based on these results, Page and Guy[17] concluded that the Torg ratio was not accurate in predicting stinger injuries and therefore is not useful as a screening tool in asymptomatic athletes.

Herzog et al.[18] evaluated radiographs, CT scans, and MRI scans in asymptomatic professional football players. The two goals of this study were to assess for variances in spinal structure and to determine if an accurate screening method exists for cervical stenosis. Herzog et al.[18] concluded that although the Torg ratio was sensitive in detecting congenital spinal stenosis, the Torg ratio had a poor positive predictive value and therefore was not useful as a screening tool for cervical stenosis and for an increased risk of stingers in this population.

Levitz et al.[19] examined cervical spine radiographs and MRI scans in 55 athletes with recurrent brachial plexopathies; 93% of athletes in this study had either cervical disk disease or narrowing of the neural foramen on MRI. A 53% rate of cervical stenosis also was identified. Levitz et al.[19] concluded that the combination of disk disease and foraminal stenosis may predispose these athletes to recurrent stingers. Similarly, Kelly et al.[20] also found that adult athletes with cervical disk degeneration and foraminal stenosis from facet arthrosis have a significantly higher risk of sustaining a stinger.

Unfortunately, no consistent answer has been found regarding whether cervical stenosis is a risk factor for sustaining a stinger. Prospective and retrospective studies have both shown that cervical stenosis is a risk factor; however, many athletes with cervical stenosis in contact sports never sustain a stinger. Limited data support the use of cervical spine imaging as a screening tool for stingers prior to sustaining an injury.

Electromyography (EMG) has also been used in the evaluation of athletes with persistent weakness or pain after a stinger is sustained. EMG is helpful in determining the location and severity of injury. This information is useful in prognosis and management of a stinger. Timing of an EMG examination is important to accurately obtain the degree of injury sustained. EMG evidence of denervation is maximal at 21 to 35 days after injury when Wallerian degeneration distal to the injured nerve has occurred.[21] Denervation is shown in an EMG report in the form of fibrillation potentials. In an athlete with transient symptoms lasting less than 48 hours, EMG is not recommended. One study showed that athletes with stinger symptoms lasting longer than 72 hours correlated best with positive EMG findings, suggesting that a shorter duration of symptoms is unlikely to be the result of a grade 2 or 3 injury.[8]

Diagnosis and Mechanism of Injury

Stingers can be categorized as occurring either proximal or distal to the clavicle. In proximal injuries, the cervical nerve roots are affected. These injuries involve both flexor and extensor musculature.[6] Injuries distal to the clavicle affect the division level of the brachial plexus and involve either flexor or extensor musculature.[6]

Stingers are also classified as grades 1, 2, or 3 based on the severity and duration of symptoms, as well as EMG findings (Table 127-2). Grade 1 brachial plexopathies are the most common. Grade 1 injuries represent neurapraxias. In this injury, all of the structures of the nerve affected remain intact. Focal demyelination resulting in a conduction block but no axonal loss is found on EMG. Grade 1 injuries consist of mild, moderate, or severe neurapraxias. In mild neurapraxias, symptoms of mild paresthesias last seconds, and physical examination results are normal. Moderate neurapraxias may last minutes to hours. Physical examination findings are typically abnormal in motor or sensory strength in at least one muscle group or dermatome. In severe neurapraxias, symptoms remain unresolved 12 hours after injury and may last longer. Most grade 1 injuries resolve within minutes but may last as long as 6 weeks.[6]

Grade 2 brachial plexopathies are less common and more severe than grade 1 injuries. Grade 2 injuries represent neurapraxia with axonotmesis in which the axon is disrupted but the epineurium remains intact. As a result, Wallerian degeneration occurs distal to the injury site. Because the epineurium remains intact, the nerve regenerates at approximately 1 to 2 mm per day. EMG evaluation shows positive waves and fibrillation potentials 2 to 3 weeks after the injury, after Wallerian degeneration has occurred. Neurapraxia with axonotmesis is characterized by significant motor and sensory deficits lasting more than 3 weeks because of axonal disruption. Athletes with grade 2 injuries typically have a complete recovery, but achieving a complete recovery may take 12 to 18 months.

Grade 3 brachial plexopathies are the most severe of all stingers but fortunately are rare. Grade 3 injuries represent neurotmesis in which the axon and all components of the nerve itself are disrupted. As in grade 2 injuries, Wallerian degeneration occurs distal to the injury site, but in grade 3 injuries, the epineurium is no longer intact and the nerve is not able to regenerate. Recovery requires operative repair and prognosis is highly variable, ranging from complete recovery

TABLE 127-2

CLASSIFICATION OF STINGER INJURY DEFINED BY NERVE INJURY, ELECTROMYOGRAPHIC FINDINGS, AND PROGNOSIS FOR RECOVERY

Grade	Nerve Injury	Electromyographic Findings	Prognosis
1	Neurapraxia	Normal	Most resolve within minutes
2	Axonotmesis	Positive waves with fibrillation	Recovery in 12-18 months
3	Neurotmesis	Acute denervation	Variable; possible complete loss of function

to complete loss of function of the nerves involved. EMG studies show acute denervation 2 to 3 weeks after the injury.

The degree of nerve damage sustained in a stinger is the result of several variables, including pressure intensity, duration, and the mechanism of injury. One area particularly susceptible to injury is Erb's point. At Erb's point, the upper trunk of the brachial plexus is immediately subcutaneous and is particularly vulnerable to injury.[22] A direct blow to this area for even a short duration may have more severe consequences than an injury sustained elsewhere.

Three mechanisms of injury have been proposed as the cause of stingers: compression, traction, and hyperextension (Fig. 127-3).[3,16,23] Compression injuries occur when the fixed brachial plexus undergoes compression between the shoulder pad and the superomedial scapula.[22] In football players, this injury occurs when the shoulder pads are pushed into Erb's point where the brachial plexus is most superficial. Compression injuries also result from foraminal stenosis of the cervical spine. In this scenario, cervical spine extension decreases the diameter of the foramen. Rotation of the head further decreases foraminal diameter and places the nerve root at risk for injury.

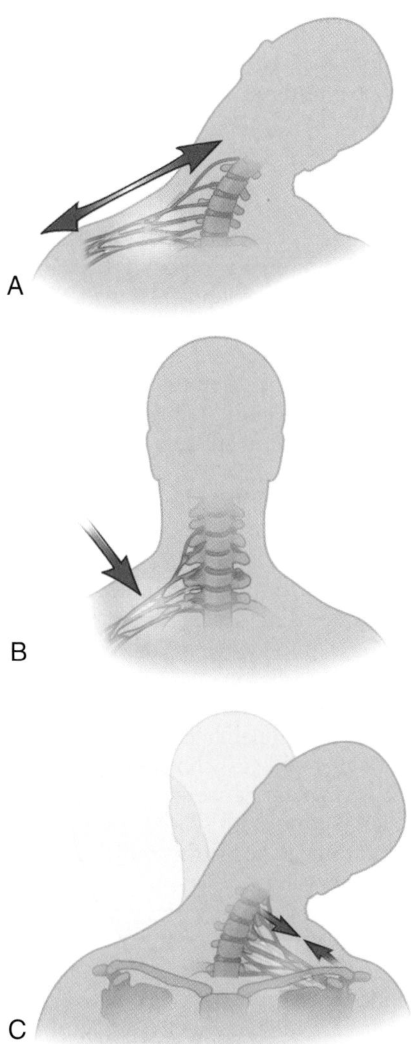

FIGURE 127-3 Mechanisms of stingers. **A,** Traction to the brachial plexus from ipsilateral shoulder depression and contralateral lateral neck flexion. **B,** A direct blow to the supraclavicular fossa at Erb's point. **C,** Compression of the cervical roots or brachial plexus from ipsilateral lateral flexion and hyperextension. *(From Kuhlman G, McKeag D: The "burner": a common nerve injury in contact sports.* Am Fam Physician *60[7]:2035–2040, 1999.)*

Traction injuries are the result of lateral flexion away from the side of injury with ipsilateral shoulder depression,[1] which places tension on the brachial plexus. This mechanism of injury is common in football and is typically seen during a block or tackle.[4] It is less common in athletes with a short, thick neck.[1] It may also occur after a fall from a bike when the shoulder hits the ground.

The third mechanism, hyperextension, occurs when cervical spine hyperextension compresses the nerve root at the intervertebral foramen.[19,24] Hyperextension elevating the affected side briefly narrows the cervical foramina and results in transient nerve root compression with associated motor and sensory findings.[20] This injury is more common in athletes with foraminal stenosis or degenerative disk disease.

In young athletes, the most common mechanism of injury is believed to be compression injuries to Erb's point.[6] In one review of the stinger mechanism of injury, Meyer et al.[16] prospectively followed up 266 collegiate football players. All athletes had cervical spine radiographs completed upon entering the study. Meyer et al.[16] analyzed the players' injury mechanism, radiographs, and time lost from competition. Forty (15%) of players had reported a symptomatic stinger, with 31 (11.6%) reporting associated neck pain with the stinger. Of the 40 symptomatic athletes, 85% reported compression-type injuries and 15% reported a traction etiology. No cases of hyperextension-type injuries were reported. The amount of time lost as a result of the injury also varied based on the mechanism of injury. In hyperextension injuries, the average time lost from competition is 12.3 days, versus 1.5 days for traction injuries.[16]

Treatment Options

The treatment of brachial plexus injuries begins on the field. Withholding an athlete from competition while evaluating him or her and performing a physical examination may allow the clinician to differentiate between a stinger and a potentially more serious cervical spine injury. Many stingers resolve so quickly, with symptoms lasting only seconds, that the athlete may return to play without alerting a physician or trainer.[25] Initial management of stingers includes rest and pain control.

Players with grade 1 stingers are permitted to return to competition when symptoms resolve and physical examination results, including motor, sensory, and cervical spine range of motion, are normal. According to this guideline, athletes with mild neurapraxias are permitted to return to sports immediately. Athletes with moderate neurapraxias are withdrawn from competition and undergo serial examination at the time of injury, at the end of the game, and 24 hours after the injury, including radiographs of the cervical spine (anteroposterior, lateral, flexion/extension, and open-mouth odontoid views). Players with severe neurapraxias are reexamined repeatedly over a 2-week period and permitted to return to sports when physical examination findings return to normal.

In addition to cervical spine radiographs, MRI or CT may also be considered, but no guidelines have been developed for the use of MRI, CT, or EMG in the evaluation and management of grade 1 stingers.[26]

Patients with grade 2 injuries should undergo cervical spine radiographs and serial examination over the course of 2 weeks after the injury. If symptoms remain at 2 weeks, EMG may be warranted to assess for nerve injury and to identify the site of the injury. EMG is not helpful immediately after the injury because Wallerian degeneration of the distal axon has not yet occurred. MRI scanning should be performed if nerve root or spinal cord injury is a concern. Players with grade 2 injuries may return to sports when full restoration of strength and sensation is demonstrated on examination with full painless range of motion of the cervical spine. These athletes should use protective equipment when returning to play. EMG should not be used to gauge when to return to play because electrical abnormalities in this study may persist for months after the injury and after symptoms have resolved.

Athletes with grade 3 stingers are prohibited from returning to sports because of persistent weakness. An EMG or MRI should be obtained and surgery may be considered based on the possibility of return of nerve function.

Athletes who sustain a stinger are likely to benefit from physical therapy. The first step in physical therapy is restoration of cervical spine range of motion,[27] which may be achieved with active and passive flexion, extension, and rotation exercises. After restoring range of motion, cervical spine strengthening begins. Cervical spine strengthening should be accompanied by range of motion and strengthening of the affected upper extremity.[27]

Return to Play

In severe cases in which nerve function does not return to baseline within 48 hours, the athlete may benefit from a period of rest and aggressive physical therapy focusing on cervical and upper extremity strengthening.

Athletes who have multiple stingers may continue to participate in sports as long as their strength remains normal. However, athletes with multiple episodes of stingers may warrant further imaging investigation while withholding from competition.

Weinstein[28] recommended that the decision to permit an athlete to return to contact sports be based on clinical and electrodiagnostic studies. Athletes with demonstrable weakness beyond 2 weeks' duration should undergo EMG evaluation. Based on these EMG studies, athletes with clinical weakness and moderate fibrillation potentials are withdrawn from play, whereas those with sequential EMG studies revealing no spontaneous potentials or only mild positive waves may return to the preinjury level of activity, as long as clinical improvement occurs with full pain-free cervical motion and return of full strength.

In cases of upper extremity weakness and moderate positive waves on EMG, Olson et al.[6] recommend withholding an athlete from competition. However, no guidelines are currently available with regard to how often to repeat studies or when an athlete can return to competition when no clinical weakness is evident but EMG studies remain abnormal.

In some cases, EMG studies may never normalize. Bergfeld et al.[29] found that 5 years after sustaining a stinger, the EMG findings of 80% of athletes with previously abnormal EMG findings remained abnormal even after restoration of full strength at 5 years from the time of injury. Bergfeld et al.[29] concluded that although EMG findings may remain abnormal, athletes may be able to return to competition after motor and sensory examinations have returned to baseline.

Weinstein[28] suggests that chronic EMG abnormalities after sustaining a stinger are likely related to changes in the motor unit and are not signs of axonal denervation. Weinstein[28] recommended using both clinical weakness and EMG abnormalities when deciding when an athlete may safely return to competition.

Evidence pertaining to the management of stingers in athletes remains limited. Most treatment guidelines are based on expert opinion without randomized controlled evidence to support one modality over another.

Complications

A common complication of stingers is recurrence. Also known as chronic burner syndrome, recurrent stingers are estimated to occur in as many as 57% of athletes who have sustained a previous stinger.[3] Levitz et al.[19] followed up a subset of 55 athletes with recurrent stingers to identify physical and radiographic similarities among this population. In 83% of patients with recurrent stingers, the mechanism of injury was hyperextension. The Spurling sign was positive in 70% of patients, 53% had foraminal stenosis, and 93% had disk disease on MRI. This study identified persons most at risk for recurrent stingers as a subpopulation of athletes with degenerative spine disease in the cervical spine. Levitz et al.[19] also concluded that degenerative disk disease and foraminal stenosis may be contributing factors to recurrent stingers.

The more concerning sequelae of sustaining a stinger is permanent neurologic injury. Although only 5% to 10% of athletes with stingers have symptoms longer than several hours, this percentage represents a large population of athletes at risk for a potentially disabling neurologic deficit.[8] Permanent neurologic injury is most common in persons with grade 3 injuries in whom complete nerve transection has occurred. Without surgical intervention, complete nerve recovery is unlikely, and depending on the nerve involved, the injury may result in significant functional deficit and disability. It has also been found that some athletes who sustain repetitive stingers may experience permanent nerve root dysfunction.[5] However, because of the large population of athletes who sustain recurrent stingers, it is difficult to predict which athletes are most at risk for this complication.

Future Considerations

Future research into stinger injuries is focused on prevention. Several studies have explored the screening of athletes who may be at risk for sustaining stingers with use of radiographs, MRI, or CT. Although such screening remains a controversial topic, other considerations include the use of protective equipment. In football players, properly fitting shoulder pads may offer some degree of protection to the athlete.[30] Other enhancements such as use of a neck roll, a custom-fit orthosis, and a cowboy collar may play a role in preventing stingers. A biomechanical study by Hovis and Limbird[30] evaluated the ability of a neck roll, a cowboy collar, and a custom-fit

AUTHORS' PREFERRED TECHNIQUE

Stingers

Any case of neurologic deficit sustained during competition warrants investigation to rule out fracture or cord injury. If symptoms are transient and the level of suspicion for such injuries is low, the athlete is examined on the sideline. If the athlete demonstrates paresthesias or a focal neurologic deficit on examination, he or she is removed from competition and reexamined after the game. If symptoms are present upon examination the following day, the athlete undergoes cervical spine radiographs and is reevaluated within 2 to 4 days. If concern about a potential cervical fracture is significant, CT is considered. Any athlete with symptoms present at that time undergoes MRI of the cervical spine. If symptoms fail to resolve after 2 weeks, EMG studies are obtained. Throughout this time, the athlete continues to undergo weekly examination to monitor neurologic recovery.

We do not routinely recommend physical therapy in athletes who have sustained stingers unless the patient demonstrates severe muscle spasm in the absence of neurologic deficits on examination.

If at any time the athlete is able to demonstrate full active range of motion of the cervical spine with no deficits on motor or sensory examination, that athlete is permitted to return to competition (Fig. 127-4).

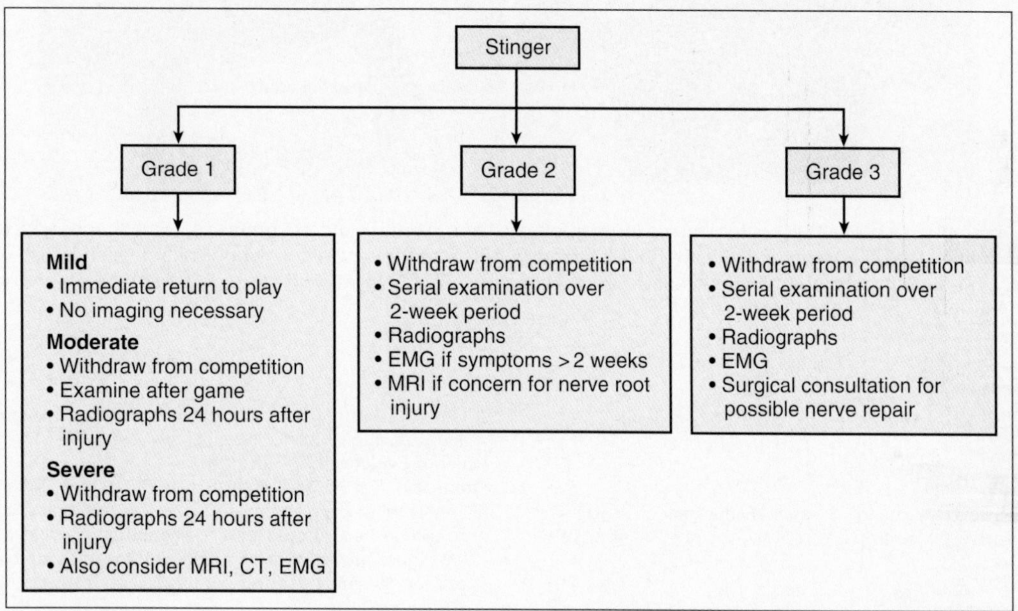

FIGURE 127-4 Management of stingers based on grade of injury. *CT,* Computed tomography; *EMG,* electromyography; *MRI,* magnetic resonance imaging.

orthosis to restrict cervical spine motion (Fig. 127-5). The authors concluded that all three braces limited hyperextension, with the custom-fit orthosis restricting motion the most.[30] However, none of these devices significantly reduced lateral motion. As a result, the equipment used in this study may have limited efficacy in preventing traction-type injuries of the brachial plexus. In addition, limiting cervical spine motion may have deleterious effects on an athlete's performance. Further exploration in the area of prevention is needed.

Controversy remains about how to manage the patient with abnormal EMG studies who is otherwise asymptomatic after sustaining a stinger. Does the abnormal EMG represent an ongoing neurologic injury that is best managed by continuing to hold the athlete from competition, or is it safe to return to sports when symptoms have resolved? Future research correlating EMG findings to return to play and risk assessment for recurrent injury would be beneficial.

A limited number of studies have investigated the management of stinger injuries sustained by athletes. Most of what we know is based on expert opinion and has not been substantiated by randomized controlled trials. Future research into risk factor assessment, as well as how to manage the athlete with a neurologic deficit after a stinger, would help elucidate the best management of this injury.

Summary

Stingers are brachial plexus injuries commonly encountered in athletes who participate in contact sports. Most cases present with transient neurologic findings, such as weakness or paresthesias, that last seconds to minutes. In cases with longer sustained neurologic symptoms, further workup is warranted to rule out more serious nerve or spinal cord injury. An athlete should not return to competition until neurologic symptoms have resolved.

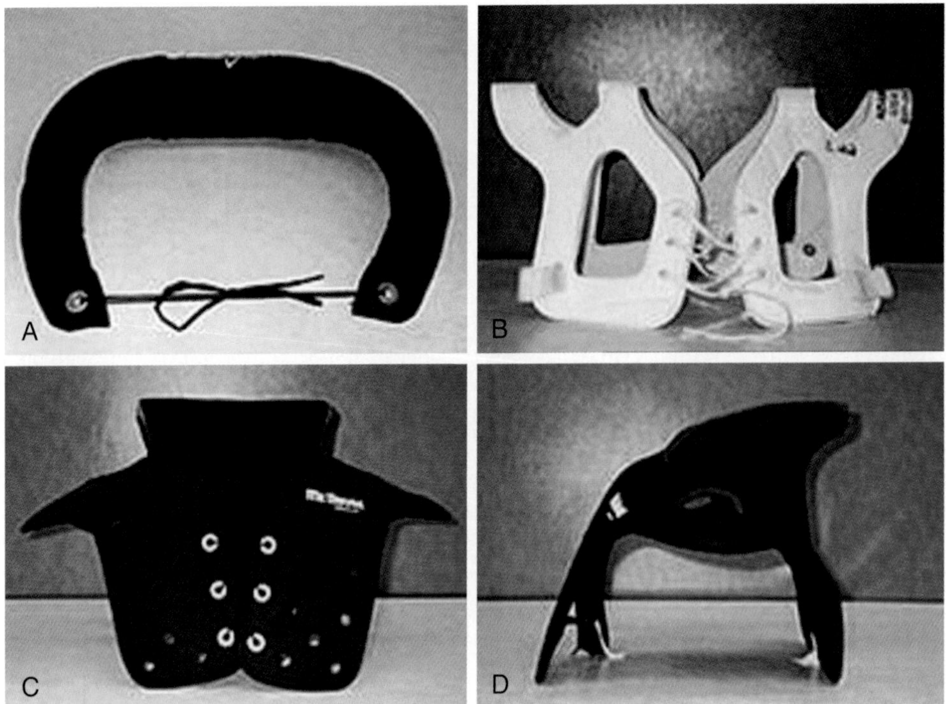

FIGURE 127-5 Examples of protective equipment for football players who have sustained burners. **A,** A neck roll, which attaches to the shoulder pads. **B,** A lifter, which is worn underneath shoulder pads. **C,** The anterior view of a cowboy collar, which is also worn underneath shoulder pads. **D,** The lateral view of a cowboy collar. *(From Kuhlman G, McKeag D: The "burner": a common nerve injury in contact sports.* Am Fam Physician *60[7]:2035–2040, 1999.)*

For a complete list of references, go to expertconsult.com.

Suggested Readings

Citation: Torg J, Pavlov H, Genuario S, et al: Neurapraxia of the cervical spinal cord with transient quadriplegia. *J Bone Joint Surg Am* 68A:1354–1370, 1986.
Level of Evidence: IV
Summary: The authors conducted a retrospective review of 32 athletes who sustained cervical neurapraxias. This article introduced the ratio method (later described as the Torg ratio) as a tool to predict the risk of sustaining a stinger with use of cervical spine radiographs. The authors also investigated the incidence of stingers and the risk of permanent neurologic injury after sustaining a stinger.

Citation: Vaccaro A, Klein G, Ciccoti M, et al: Return to play criteria for the athlete with cervical spine injuries resulting in stinger and transient quadriplegia/paresis. *Spine* 2:351–356, 2002.
Level of Evidence: IV
Summary: The authors conducted a literature review to evaluate guidelines for return-to-play criteria after cervical spine injuries in the athlete. In a section of this article the authors evaluated stingers and introduced guidelines for when it may be appropriate for an athlete to return to competition after sustaining a stinger.

Citation: Herzog R, Wiens J, Dillingham M, et al: Normal cervical spine morphometry and cervical spinal stenosis in asymptomatic professional football players: plane radiography, multiplanar computed tomography, and magnetic resonance imaging. *Spine* 16:S178–S186, 1991.
Level of Evidence: II
Summary: The authors evaluated cervical spine radiographs, computed tomography scans, and magnetic resonance imaging scans in asymptomatic professional football players. The authors concluded that the Torg ratio has a poor predictive value with regard to which athletes are at increased risk for sustaining a stinger but that it is a sensitive tool in detecting congenital spinal stenosis.

Citation: Herman M: Cervical spine injuries in the pediatric adolescent athlete. *Instr Course Lect* 55:641–646, 2006.
Level of Evidence: IV
Summary: Herman discusses common cervical spine injuries in the pediatric adolescent athlete along with the diagnosis, natural history, and management of stingers, as well as other cervical spine injuries commonly encountered in this population.

Citation: Levitz C, Reilly P, Torg J: The pathomechanics of chronic, recurrent cervical nerve root neurapraxia: The chronic burner syndrome. *Am J Sports Med* 25(1):73–76, 1997.
Level of Evidence: IV
Summary: The authors evaluated the mechanism of injury and magnetic resonance imaging scans in 55 athletes who sustained more than one stinger. The authors concluded that cervical spine stenosis and disk disease may lead to an alteration in normal spine mechanics, placing this subset of patients at higher risk for recurrent stingers.

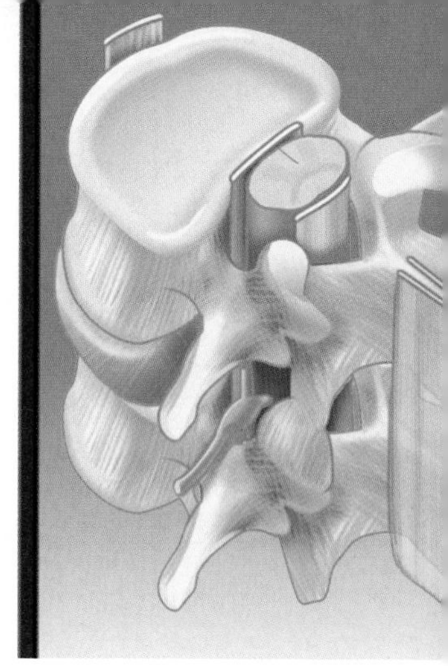

128

Thoracolumbar Spine Disorders in the Adult

WILLIAM LAUERMAN[†] • MATTHEW RUSSO

Athletes comprise a unique subset of the general population and are exposed to unusual forces that may predispose them to specific injury patterns. Spine injuries account for up to 15% of all athletic injuries,[1] most of which tend to be of soft tissue origin. With higher levels of training, increased physical demands on the body, and decreased time to rest, low back pain has become an important limitation for training and continuing to compete at a high level.

This chapter reviews basic concepts of thoracolumbar spine anatomy, mechanics, and associated disorders with specific attention to the athletic population. As always, the key aspects of a complete history and physical examination are essential, with appropriate imaging studies to confirm the diagnosis and guide treatment. Particular focus is aimed at nonoperative treatment algorithms with the goal of allowing the athlete to return safely to competition and training as quickly as possible.

Relevant Anatomy and Biomechanics

Bony

The majority of the vertebral column is composed of the thoracolumbar spine, with its contrast of the relatively rigid thoracic spine and the increased mobility of the lumbar spine. The thoracic vertebral column provides the origin for the ribs, with 12 thoracic vertebrae separated by intervertebral disks that articulate through diarthrodial facet joints. Because of the stability and rigidity of the rib cage and the frontal plane orientation of the facet joints, the thoracic spine is the least mobile segment of the spine.

The lumbar vertebrae are larger and wider than their thoracic counterparts and make up the last five vertebrae. Compared with the thoracic three-joint complex, the lumbar articulations are oriented in a more sagittal plane, allowing for increased flexion and extension but with significantly less rotation.

The thoracic spinal cord is protected by a small, round spinal canal. The spinal cord typically ends at the L1-L2 level, and the resultant collection of individual spinal nerve roots caudal to this point is referred to as the *cauda equina*. This distinction is important during injury because the nerve roots in the cauda equina are generally able to respond as peripheral nerves, whereas injury to the spinal cord may be irreversible.

Intervertebral Disk

Together with the facet joints, the intervertebral disk provides the third articulation of the three-joint complex of spinal articulation. Each disk is composed of an outer fibrous layer designed to resist torsional stress (anulus fibrosus) and an inner gelatinous shock-absorbing mass (nucleus pulposus; Fig. 128-1).[2]

Ligaments

The anterior and posterior longitudinal ligaments mark the ventral and dorsal borders of the vertebral bodies and are the two major spinal ligaments that support the thoracolumbar spine. Moving further dorsally, the ligamentum flavum provides the posterior wall of the vertebral canal and becomes much thicker in the lumbar spine in an attempt to replace the loss of bony overlap between adjacent lumbar laminae. The supraspinous and infraspinous ligaments are also enlarged in the lumbar spine and run between the spinous processes throughout the spine.

Muscular

Whereas the thoracic rib cage serves as an inherent stabilizer of the thoracic spine, it is the spinal musculature and ligaments that provide most of the support in the lumbar spine. The erector spinae muscles run longitudinally and function bilaterally to produce back extension and unilaterally to produce lateral bending throughout the thoracolumbar spine. Assisting with spine extension and rotation are the splenius muscles, which arise from the midline and run laterally. Deep to the erector spinae is the transversospinal musculature, which contributes to extension, lateral bending, and rotation of the vertebral column. Muscular strains involving the erector spinae and transversospinalis muscles are common in the athletic population.

Biomechanics

The range of motion of the thoracolumbar spine is composed of the individual intervertebral movements producing flexion, extension, lateral flexion, and rotation of the vertebral

[†]Deceased.

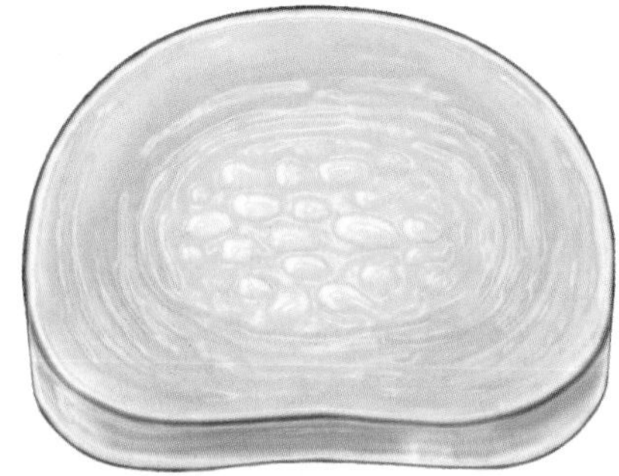

FIGURE 128-1 Anatomy of the thoracic disk.

column.[3] As the spinal curvature changes from thoracic kyphosis to lumbar lordosis, the relationship of the vertebrae to the center of gravity shifts from posterior to anterior, resulting in a vulnerable transition point at the thoracolumbar junction for fracture and dislocation.

It has been demonstrated that the lumbosacral articulation is exposed to the highest forces in the thoracolumbar spine. The oblique inclination of the sacrum subjects the neural arch to both anterior compressive and shear forces. The erector spinae also place increased stress on the neural arch in the erect stance.

Risk Factors for Injury

Athletes have multiple risk factors for the development of thoracolumbar injury, including prior back injury, poor conditioning, repetitive loading, improper technique, and abrupt increases in training.[4] In a prospective cohort study of 679 varsity athletes, the most significant risk factor for lumbar injury was a history of injury in this area. Athletes who had a history of a spine injury sustained a recurrent spine injury at three times the rate of control subjects who did not have a prior injury.[5] It is likely that the next most significant risk factor can be seen with activities that involve repetitive loading of the spine, such as occurs in gymnastics. In a cross-sectional study by Goldstein et al.,[6] female gymnasts had a markedly increased prevalence of lumbar spine abnormalities seen on magnetic resonance imaging (MRI) when compared with swimmers, whose sport generally does not place an axial load on the spine.

Clinical Evaluation

History

Based on the initial history, thoracolumbar spine disorders in athletes generally can be divided into those related to acute trauma and those involving a slow progression of symptoms, usually as a result of chronic repetitive trauma (Table 128-1). In cases involving acute trauma, it is important to determine whether the athlete was truly asymptomatic before the more significant symptoms began. Diagnosis of thoracolumbar disorders must follow the same format as any clinical evaluation, starting with an accurate and thorough history, a complete physical examination including lower extremity evaluation, and specific diagnostic studies based on the findings of the history and physical examination.

Although it is helpful to try to identify a single traumatic episode, often no sudden event led to the acute onset of symptoms. It is important to ask the patient about the onset of pain (acute vs. insidious) and the presence of preexisting pain before the event or the day on which it was noticed. In many patients with thoracolumbar disorders, a relatively long history of gradually worsening pain, culminating in a single day or event when more significant pain was noticed, can be elicited. When a single traumatic event can be identified, it is important to inquire about the presence of any transient neurologic signs or symptoms at the time of onset (e.g., the inability to move an extremity, any degree of numbness, or loss of bowel or bladder function). Although these symptoms are extremely rare with sports injuries to the thoracolumbar spine, their occurrence, if present, should be elicited.

A helpful mnemonic when obtaining a history of pain is to obtain a CLEAR picture of the patient's pain. ***C*** represents the *character* of the pain complaint (e.g., burning or stabbing). ***L*** represents the *location* of the pain. Clinical terms such as back, buttocks, hips, or spine frequently mean different things to different people, and it is essential to have the patient accurately define where he or she experiences the pain. ***E*** represents *exacerbation*: What makes the pain worse? It is usually activity that makes the pain worse, but certain activities and positions may be particularly painful and should be determined. ***A*** stands for *amelioration*: What can the patient do to lessen the pain? In general, rest reduces or relieves most musculoskeletal back pain. Finally, ***R*** stands for *radiation*: Where does the pain go? Pain that radiates below the knee (true radicular pain) is important to elucidate because it may have an impact on diagnosis and management decisions.

"Red flags" are important questions that must be asked of all persons with spine injuries or acute low back pain and may indicate serious pathology. These red flags include the presence or absence of neurologic symptoms, including the presence of leg pain or paresthesias that may signify nerve root compression or irritation. Although bowel or bladder dysfunction is unusual, it is important to inquire about its presence to avoid missing cauda equina syndrome. Pain occurring with rest or at night may signify a mass lesion of the spine or spinal cord and must be ruled out.

TABLE 128-1

INJURY CLASSIFICATION OF THORACOLUMBAR INJURIES

Acute	Chronic
Fracture-dislocation	Isthmic spondylolysis and spondylolisthesis (type IIA and IIB)
Acute pars fracture (type IIC)	Lumbar disk injury, diskogenic pain
Acute traumatic disk herniation	Disk herniation
Infection	Apophyseal injury
	Disk degeneration
	Overuse syndrome
	Spinal deformity
	Spinal tumor
	Infection

A thorough medical history must also include any history of cancer or previous orthopaedic injuries, including childhood spine problems. Because activity restriction with or without physical therapy is often the initial treatment, it is important to note if these therapies have already been prescribed—specifically which physical modalities were used, whether the patient was compliant, and the response to treatment. Any history of medication usage and the response to it should also be sought. Finally, the previous use of bracing or casting should be explored. Identifying the type of brace, the regimen prescribed, patient compliance, and whether any sports participation was attempted while wearing the brace provides a foundation for further treatment options. A social history should also be obtained, including occupational activities (e.g., heavy lifting) and other risk factors for spine disorders.

A review of systems should be conducted, with the presence of any constitutional symptoms such as fever, chills, or weight loss noted. Finally, the presence of any psychosocial factors such as depression should be identified. It cannot be overemphasized that a thorough history provides the groundwork for an appropriate yet focused physical examination and is essential for an accurate diagnosis.

Physical Examination

Examination of the patient with a low back complaint begins with inspection, which cannot be performed adequately unless the patient wears an examination gown that opens in the back, is disrobed down to his or her underwear, and has removed his or her shoes and socks. The skin is inspected and the presence of any skin lesions, such as café-au lait spots or striae, is noted. Asymmetry of the shoulders, pelvis, scapulae, and skin creases is noted. The Adam forward-bend test should be performed to note any asymmetry of the ribs or flank, suggesting scoliosis. The patient's gait is then observed, including toe and heel walking. A broad-based gait may suggest an underlying disorder such as myelopathy that may be further evaluated by having the patient walk with a tandem gait (i.e., having the patient heel-toe walk as in a sobriety test). Palpation of the back is then performed at the level of each spinous process to help define where the most pain is experienced. The exact site of tenderness is noted, whether in the midline, in the paraspinal region, in the buttocks, or over the trochanteric bursae. Palpation may also identify a step-off in the lower lumbar spine, suggesting a high-grade spondylolisthesis.

Range of motion of the spine should then be tested. Forward flexion is a complex motion of the lumbar spine, sacroiliac joints, and hip joints with an average range of 40 to 60 degrees. Limitation of forward flexion may represent disk disease, although hamstring tightness or spasm, commonly seen in persons with spondylolysis and spondylolisthesis, may also limit forward flexion. Pain on extension of the lumbar spine, particularly with a painful catch, is commonly seen in persons with spondylolysis or spondylolisthesis, with average extension of 20 to 35 degrees. The major motion of the thoracic spine is rotation, measured with the feet in place and rotation at the shoulders to average 90 degrees. The inability to bend or rotate because of inhibition by a protective muscle spasm may be an indication of injury of one of the functional units of the spine.

TABLE 128-2

MUSCLE TESTING OF THE LOWER EXTREMITIES

Nerve Root	Muscle Group	Reflex
L1	Hip flexion	
L2	Hip flexion	
L3	Knee extension	
L4	Foot dorsiflexion–knee extension	Knee jerk
L5	Big toe extension–foot eversion	Posterior tibial
S1	Foot plantar flexors–knee flexion	Ankle jerk

A neurologic examination should also be performed, with the presence of leg atrophy or asymmetry noted. Light-touch sensory testing, motor strength assessment, and testing of the reflexes should be performed. Evaluation of the thoracic spine is essentially limited to sensory light-touch examination of the thorax. An initial rough examination of lower extremity strength testing can be performed by asking the patient to squat down, raise up, and perform both toe and heel walking. The patient is then seated on the edge of the table with the feet dangling off the side for strength testing of the major muscle groups according to the standard nomenclature on a 0 to 5 scale, including the hip flexors, adductors, quadriceps, hamstrings, tibialis anterior, foot everters, extensor hallucis longus, and foot plantar flexors (Table 128-2). A sensory examination of the lower extremities is then carried out by light-touch testing (Fig. 128-2). If cord compression is suspected, sensory pin-prick testing may be performed.

The presence of upper motor neuron findings such as spasticity, hyperreflexia, clonus, extensor plantar response (the Babinski sign), or asymmetry of the superficial abdominal reflexes should also be noted. Tension signs, such as the straight-leg–raising sign, the bowstring sign, and the femoral nerve stretch test, should also be assessed because they are sensitive for disk herniation. The most common test of sciatic nerve irritation is the straight-leg–raising test,[7] which is intended to reproduce radicular symptoms of pain along the anatomic course of the sciatic nerve by stretching the dura and nerve roots. It is important to note that it is not back pain alone but rather recreation of the patient's radicular pain that constitutes a positive test. Symptoms usually begin at about 30 to 35 degrees of hip flexion (Fig. 128-3). Similarly, the bowstring sign[8] is performed by having the patient flex the knee to 90 degrees and bend forward while the examiner presses a finger into the popliteal space. Again, radicular pain in sciatic nerve distribution indicates a positive test.

The femoral nerve tension sign is a similar test to examine femoral nerve distribution radiculopathy. With the patient in prone position, the knee is flexed to 90 degrees and the hip is extended. Radicular pain in the femoral nerve distribution (anterior thigh) indicates a positive test.

Physical examination of acute spine injuries on the field is unique and requires careful examination and immobilization because of potential neurologic injury. If the clinician suspects a possible spinal column injury of any type, the patient must be immobilized in the same position as he or she was found without any attempt to remove equipment, such as a helmet,

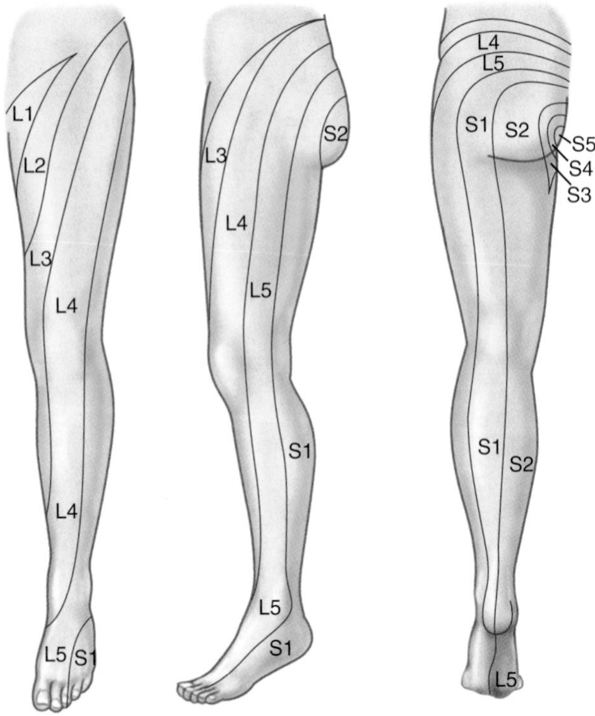

FIGURE 128-2 Dermatomal innervation of the lower extremities.

and transported with the aid of a spine board. Adequate spinal immobilization on a spine board is the only method for preventing catastrophic neurologic injury in a patient with spinal instability or injury. Examination of associated nonspinal areas is also important because back pain may be due to nonspinal causes, including the abdomen, the hips, and, when indicated, the sacroiliac area.

An accurate and working differential diagnosis is possible only after a careful history and physical examination is complete and is essential to help guide appropriate diagnostic testing to further narrow the differential.

Imaging

Radiographic imaging studies are costly, time-consuming, and sometimes inaccurate in identifying the source of back pain. Furthermore, it is relatively uncommon for a radiographic abnormality to alter treatment in the early phase of most cases of back pain. It is essential to bear in mind that a radiographic diagnosis does not need to be made in most cases, including conditions such as spondylolisthesis and disk herniation, at the time of initial assessment. The decision for imaging in the athlete with back pain is thus determined by several factors, including the severity and duration of symptoms and the response to previous treatment.

Plain radiographs are the usual initial imaging test.[9] They are indicated in an athlete with a history of acute trauma in whom fracture is suspected or in the presence of neurologic symptoms. We more typically obtain plain radiographs in patients with significant symptoms lasting more than 3 to 4 weeks. The standard lumbar radiographic series includes standing anteroposterior and lateral views of the lumbar spine, as well as a spot lateral (coned down) view of L5-S1 (Figs. 128-4 through 128-7). Plain lateral radiographs can identify 80% of pars defects (Fig. 128-8) and essentially all cases of spondylolisthesis.[10] These views also identify virtually all significant fractures, such as compression fracture of the vertebral body. If a pars defect is suspected but not identified on the plain anteroposterior and lateral views, oblique views of the lumbar spine can be ordered (Figs. 128-9 and 128-10).[11] The pars interarticularis is well visualized on an oblique view in the form of the neck of a Scotty dog; the presence of a collar, or disruption of the neck, is suggestive of spondylolysis (Fig. 128-11).

Standing posteroanterior and lateral scoliosis radiographs are ordered if truncal asymmetry or hyperkyphosis is present on physical examination (Fig. 128-12). It is important to recognize that hyperkyphosis, with or without mild secondary scoliosis, is frequently misinterpreted by primary care practitioners as scoliosis; therefore the initial scoliosis evaluation should include a lateral radiograph.

When spinal instability is suspected outside the acute setting, specialized lateral flexion-extension views may also be performed. The limitations of plain radiographs to visualize only the space occupied by the disk and the spinal canal rather than the contents themselves must be understood. Furthermore, plain radiographs are unable to accurately visualize significant bony destruction, with up to 50% of medullary vertebral body bone destruction not visualized on plain radiographs.[11]

Nuclear imaging with a technetium-99m bone scan can be helpful in identifying occult lesions of the spine not seen on plain radiographs. Increased osteoblastic (bone production) activity produces an increased intensity on bone scan, whereas disruption of metabolic activities of bone or bony absorption results in a decreased amount of visible tracer. Bone scans are commonly indicated early in the evaluation of stress fractures or stress reactions of the pars interarticularis.

The sensitivity of technetium is enhanced with single photon emission computed tomography (SPECT), which provides tomographic images of the radiotracer in the lumbar spine (Fig. 128-13). SPECT scanning is the preferred imaging modality for identifying occult pars interarticularis lesions.[12] It is also sensitive, although nonspecific, for identifying other bony lesions such as tumors of the posterior elements and diskitis. Some of these lesions may be missed on MRI. Although technetium scanning is sensitive in identifying occult cases of spondylolysis, it is less useful in determining the acuity of an injury because a bone scan may be abnormal for up to 18 months after fracture.

Computed tomography (CT) allows the clinician to visualize a complex three-dimensional image of the thoracolumbar spine, creating cross-sectional images in all three planes that may be used for reconstruction but at the cost of high doses of radiation.[13] This imaging modality is useful in certain conditions, particularly in the evaluation of spondylolysis.[14] Although not as sensitive as SPECT scanning, CT using 3-mm parallel cuts is a very sensitive modality for identifying pars defects. It is also very specific for differentiating pars defects from sclerosis of the pars or the pedicle and from tumors such as osteoid osteoma or osteoblastoma. In addition, CT is useful for monitoring healing of a pars defect. CT provides the best definition of the bony anatomy of the posterior elements of the lumbar spine, but multiple studies have shown that it is

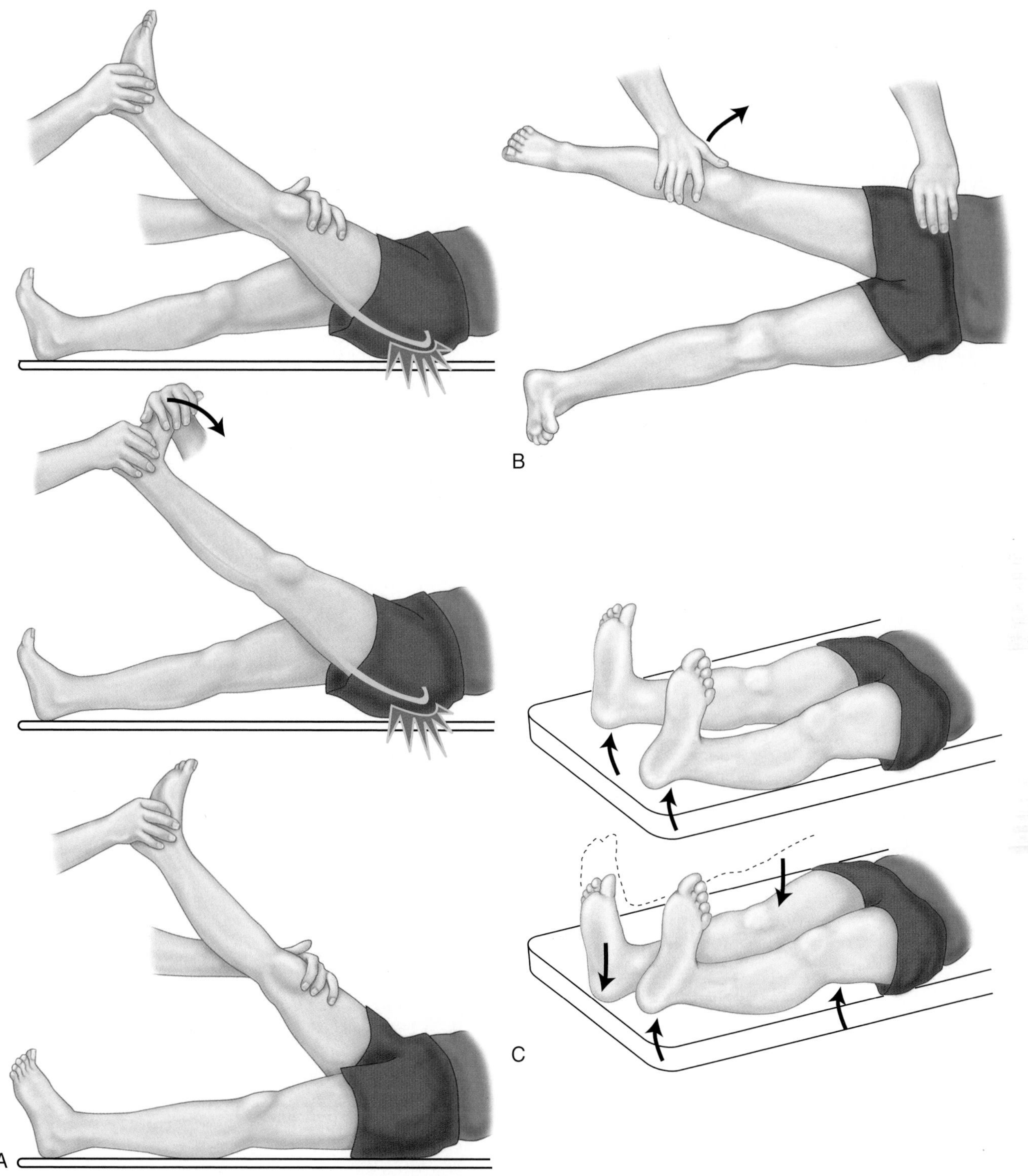

FIGURE 128-3 A, Straight-leg–raising test. **B,** Femoral stretch test. **C,** The Milgram test.

not be useful or cost-effective in routine scanning for thoracolumbar pain.[15,16]

MRI is commonly used for patients with clear-cut neurologic signs or symptoms and for patients who are clinically deteriorating. Similarly, a history of constitutional symptoms merits early evaluation with MRI. We also typically use MRI in the athlete with functionally disabling pain for longer than 3 months. Although 3 months may still be relatively early in the disease process, patient expectations generally mandate its use (Fig. 128-14).

The obvious advantages of MRI are that it is noninvasive, does not deliver any ionizing radiation, and provides orthogonal imaging of the entire lumbar spine. It is the test of choice for herniated nucleus pulposus, disk degeneration, or

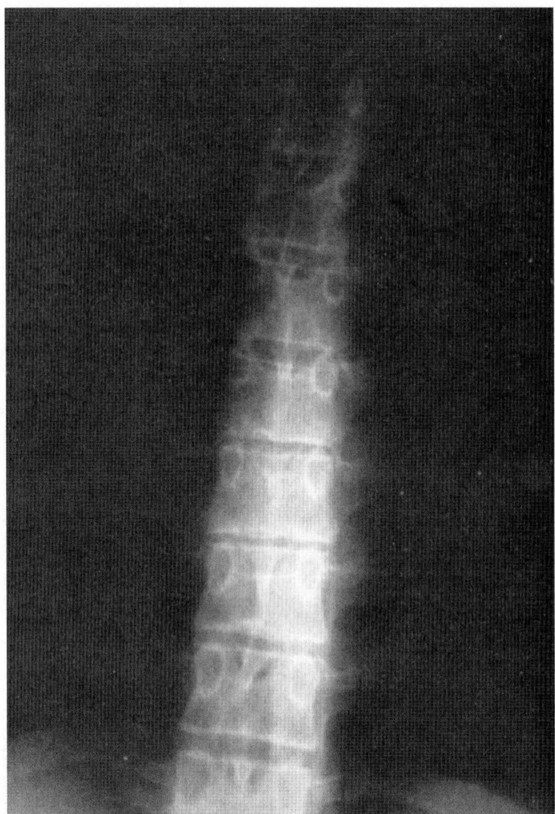

FIGURE 128-4 Normal anteroposterior anatomy of the thoracic spine.

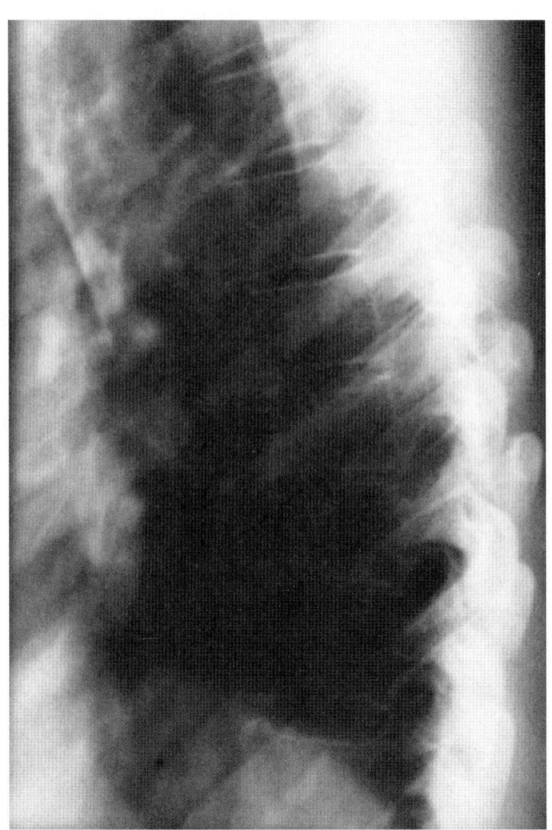

FIGURE 128-5 Normal lateral anatomy of the thoracic spine.

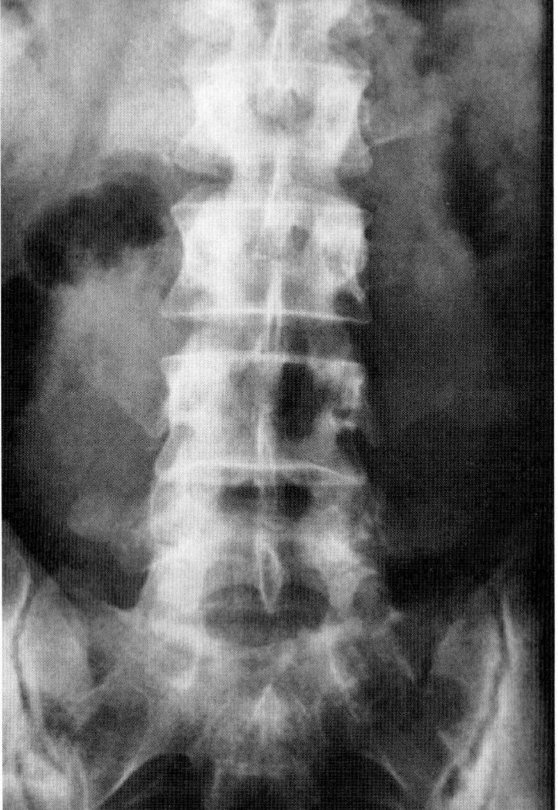

FIGURE 128-6 Normal anteroposterior anatomy of the lumbar spine.

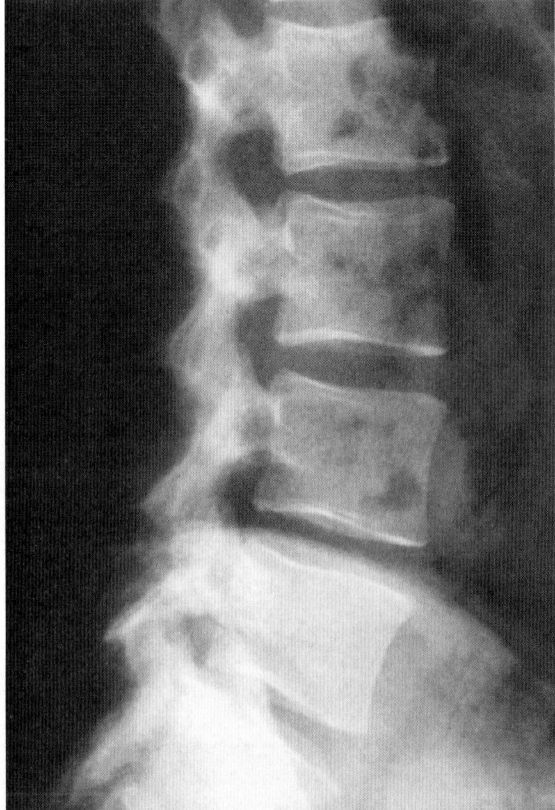

FIGURE 128-7 Normal lateral anatomy of the lumbar spine.

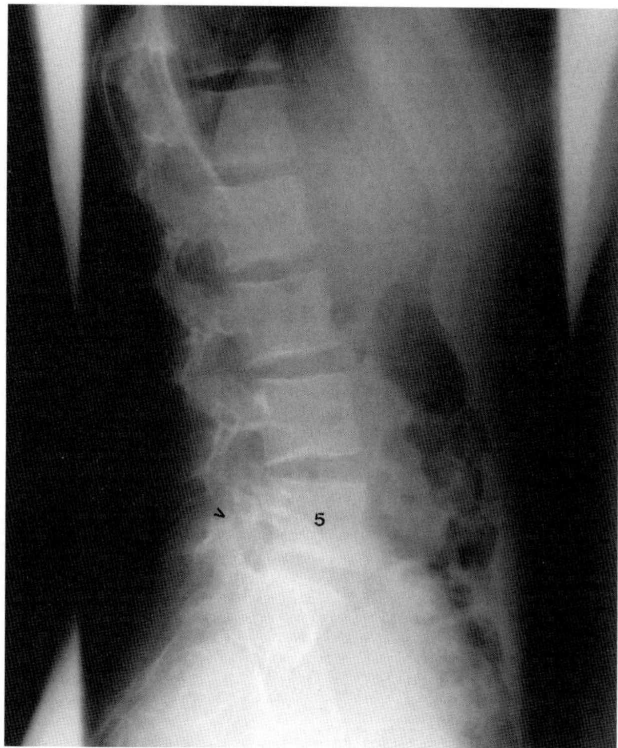

FIGURE 128-8 A plain lateral radiograph of the lumbar spine from a 15-year-old soccer player with low back pain for 8 months demonstrates lysis of the pars interarticularis at L5 (*arrowhead*) without spondylolisthesis.

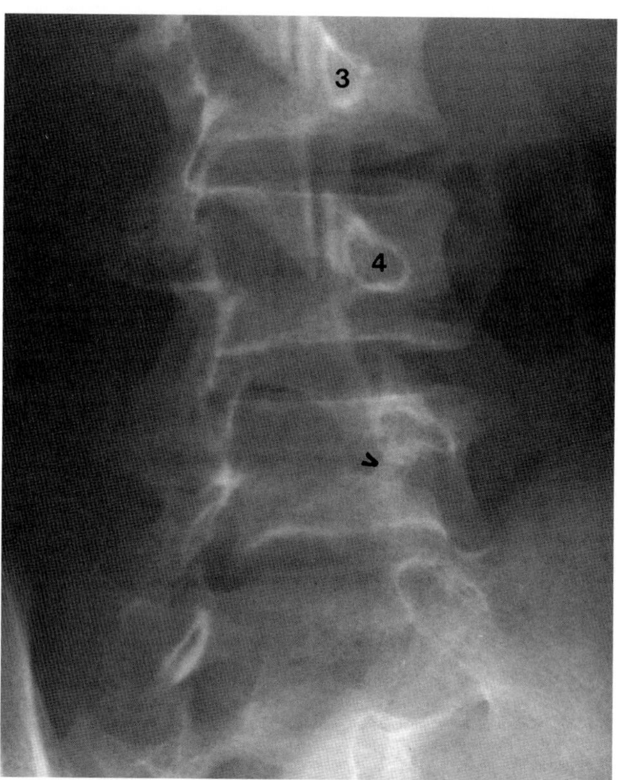

FIGURE 128-9 A defect in the pars interarticularis of L5 (*arrowhead*) is seen on this oblique radiograph. The normal bony continuity of the pars (the "neck of the Scotty dog") of L3 and L4 can also be appreciated.

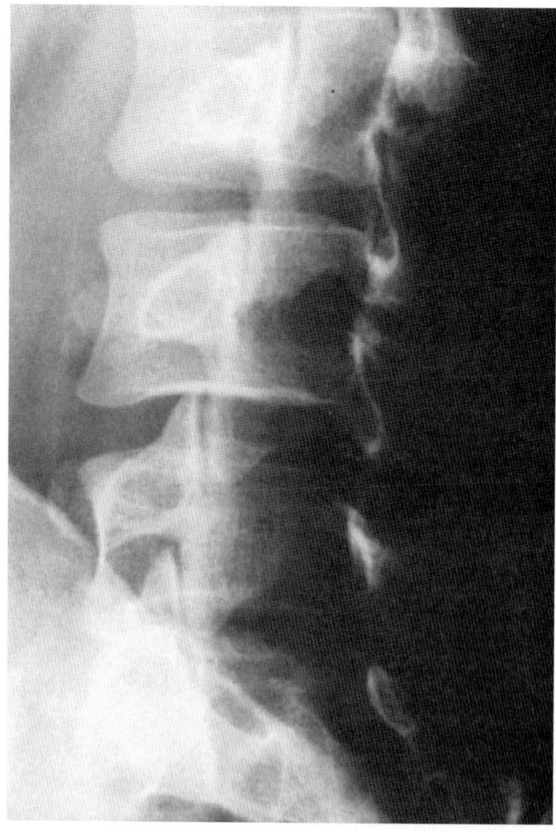

FIGURE 128-10 Oblique projection of the lumbar spine.

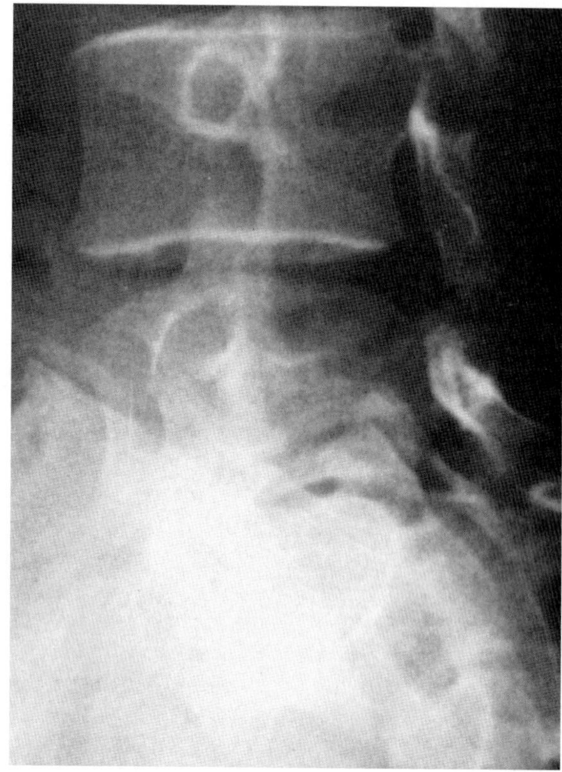

FIGURE 128-11 Spondylolysis of the lumbar spine.

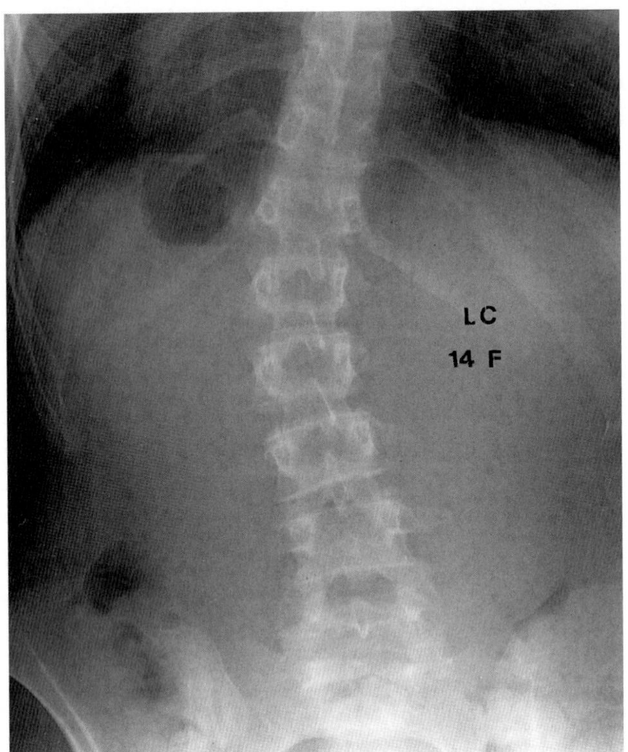

FIGURE 128-12 A 16-year-old football player was struck in the back during a game and experienced acute onset of low back pain. Plain lateral radiography demonstrates isthmic spondylolisthesis at L5-S1. By the time of his orthopaedic evaluation, he was asymptomatic, and he has been symptom free for more than 2 years.

infection.[17] The clinician should be aware that disk abnormalities are common in asymptomatic persons. By the age of 50 years, autopsies of 95% of adult subjects show evidence of disk space narrowing, calcification, or marginal sclerosis.[18] Results are similar in living patients, with degenerative changes present in 87%.[19] Pars defects, on the other hand, may not be best identified with MRI. The usefulness of MRI in diagnosing spondylolisthesis is its ability to identify the presence or absence of foraminal stenosis and nerve root compression on the parasagittal images.[20-22] Such foraminal stenosis is a common cause of radicular leg pain in patients with spondylolisthesis, particularly in patients with high-grade slips.

In cases in which surgery is elected in the patient with spondylolysis or spondylolisthesis, we routinely perform MRI to help exclude other sources of pain. MRI is also helpful in identifying and defining rare but ominous causes of back pain, including intraspinal diseases such as tumors, intraspinal lipomas, and a tethered cord, which usually present with neurologic findings. Tumors of the anterior column, although rare, and infections of the spine are also optimally imaged with MRI. On the other hand, MRI is inferior to CT for defining bony lesions of the posterior elements.

Specific Sport Injuries

Throughout training and competition, athletes place high demands on the thoracolumbar spine that serve to increase the rate of injury and vary with the specific sport played. Football players are at high risk for thoracolumbar injury

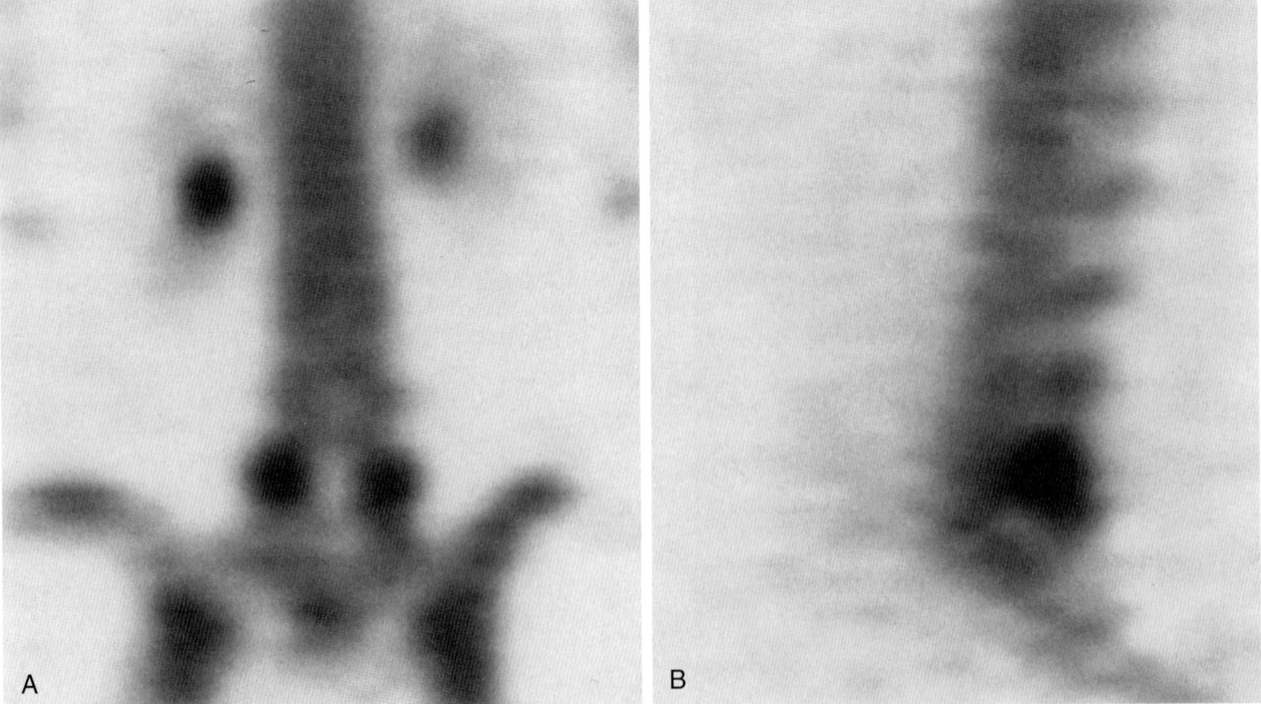

FIGURE 128-13 Coronal (A) and sagittal (B) single-photon emission computed tomographic images from a 15-year-old boy with uptake in the region of the L5 pars interarticularis, consistent with spondylolysis.

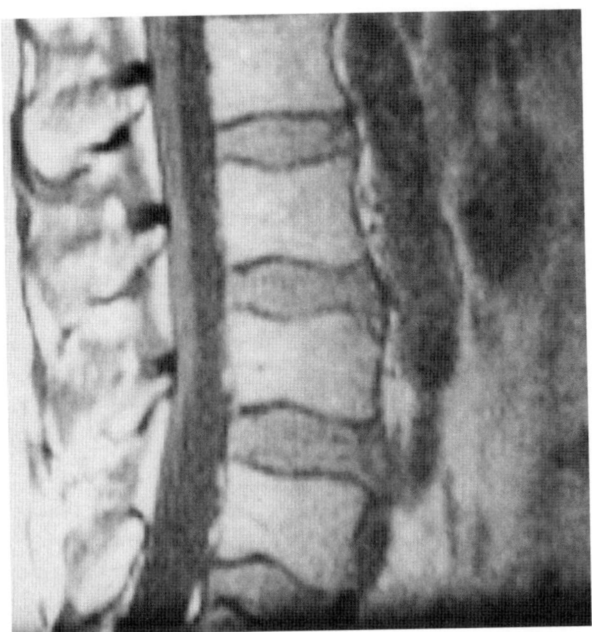

FIGURE 128-14 A normal magnetic resonance imaging scan of the lumbar spine.

because of high-force axial loading and hyperextension experienced by the spine during blocking.[23] These forces, as well as torsional strain, can lead to the development of spondylolysis, acute spine injury, and chronic back pain.[24] Gymnasts also undergo axial loading and hyperextension of the spine, thus increasing the rate of lumbar spondylolysis. One study comparing gymnasts with a general age-matched population found that 11% of gymnasts had injury to the pars interarticularis compared with fewer than 3% of the general population.[25] Weight lifters often experience paraspinal sprains and strains, spondylolysis, spondylolisthesis, and herniated nucleus pulposus, with rare serious flexion-distraction injuries occurring when the athlete attempts to squat with too heavy a weight while using improper technique.[26] Gerbino and d'Hemecourt[27] demonstrated that herniated lumbar disks are more common in football players and weight lifters, whereas traumatic injuries to the lumbar spine are more common in wrestlers and hockey players.

Paraspinal Soft Tissue Injury

Sprains and Strains

The most common cause of chronic low back pain in the athlete can be attributed to injury of the paraspinal soft tissue musculature.[28] If the physical examination is benign and findings of imaging studies, including MRI and bone scanning, are normal, a chronic strain or overuse syndrome can be assumed. Typically, these patients present with a prolonged history of backache and exhibit a high level of frustration because of the ongoing pain and the absence of a clear diagnosis.

Evaluation of these patients begins with a thorough history and physical examination, with careful identification as to whether the injury was caused by a direct blow versus a twisting movement and elucidation of any previous back complaints before the injury. The physical examination should also note any observation of protective muscle spasm, restrictive motion, and tenderness to palpation. In most cases, symptoms resolve over a period of several weeks. However, some cases of recalcitrant low back pain may persist for a year or longer.

A sprain is defined as a ligamentous injury that occurs as a result of stretching the ligament beyond its capacity but without resulting in discontinuity.[29] Similarly, a strain is defined as a similar process involving muscle fibers either at the muscle tendon junction or within the muscle belly. Both processes are treated similarly, with most patients responding well to a regimen of activity restriction, nonsteroidal antiinflammatory drugs (NSAIDs), moist heat, and a program of stretching and strengthening exercises followed by gradual resumption of activity. Antispasmodic agents may be used to control muscle spasms, because they are often the most debilitating part of any musculoligamentous injury. Bracing rarely has a role in persons with nonspecific chronic low back pain. Trigger point injections with a local anesthetic and a corticosteroid are occasionally useful, but epidural steroid injections are reserved for patients with radicular pain from a disk herniation. Continued stretching theoretically reduces the risk of repeat injury by allowing full range of motion and muscle strengthening.

Piriformis Syndrome

Piriformis syndrome, which is often confused with radicular pain, is a diagnosis of exclusion that presents with signs and symptoms of sciatic nerve irritation, usually as a result of a traumatic blow to the buttock. The result is an acute neuritis of the proximal sciatic nerve just under the piriformis. Patients with this syndrome may be unable to sit and have tenderness at the greater sciatic notch and deep palpation over the piriformis. Provocative testing includes the Pace test (resisted abduction/external rotation) and the Beatty maneuver (abduction against gravity). MRI shows the absence of other causes for radicular pain, such as spinal stenosis or herniated disk disease. Most patients are best treated nonoperatively with NSAIDs and physical therapy.[30]

Posterior Facet and Sacroiliac Joint Dysfunction

Lumbar facet joint pain is often the result of a rotational injury that disrupts the joint capsule and leads to hypermobility, inflammation, and articular injury. Pain is often reproduced with extension, direct palpation, and rotation of the lumbar spine and is usually treated nonoperatively with a focus on lumbar stabilization and physical therapy.

Sacroiliac joint dysfunction is a rare but important cause of chronic low back pain that is increased in specific athletic populations such as rowers and cross-country skiers.[31,32] Sacroiliac joint dysfunction is also known to affect patients with seronegative spondyloarthropathies, such as ankylosis spondylitis, Reiter syndrome, and psoriatic arthritis. It usually presents as unilateral pain just inferior to the posterior superior iliac spine.[33] Bone scans are useful to confirm the diagnosis, with treatment consisting of conservative measures and/or CT-guided steroid injections to the affected sacroiliac joint.

BOX 128-1 Typical History and Physical Examination Findings

Spondylolysis and Spondylolisthesis
- Back pain with back extension maneuvers
- Usually acute exacerbation of chronic low-grade pain
- Limited forward flexion due to hamstring tightness
- Palpable step-off of lumbar spinous processes (for high-grade slip)
- Tenderness with pressure on and movement of the affected spinous process

Lumbar Disk Herniation
- Pain with sitting or any maneuver that increases intraabdominal pressure (e.g., coughing or sneezing)
- Often of sudden onset
- Significant back pain and stiffness with postural abnormality (sciatic list)
- Neurologic abnormalities are often absent, but the patient may have weakness or reflex change
- A high incidence of a positive tension sign (e.g., a straight-leg–raising sign, bowstring sign, or femoral nerve stretch test)

BOX 128-2 Wiltse-Newman Classification of Spondylolysis

I. Dysplastic
II. Isthmic
  A. Lytic-fatigue fracture of pars
  B. Elongated pars
  C. Acute pars fracture
III. Degenerative
IV. Traumatic
V. Pathologic

From Wiltse LL, Newman PH, Macnab I: Classification of spondylolysis and spondylolisthesis. *Clin Orthop* 117:23–29, 1976.

Spondylolysis and Spondylolisthesis

Spondylolysis and associated spondylolisthesis are common causes of low back pain in the athlete. The term spondylolysis refers to a chronic fatigue fracture of the pars interarticularis, whereas spondylolisthesis refers to a pars fracture with associated anterior subluxation of the involved vertebra on the subjacent vertebra.[34] The condition results from both hereditary and environmental factors.[35] The athlete with spondylolysis or spondylolisthesis typically presents with a history of chronic low-grade back pain, sometimes with an acute exacerbation. Box 128-1 helps to differentiate key aspects of the clinical history compared with disk herniation.

The degree of slippage is based on Meyerding's classification, whereby the superior aspect of the sacrum is divided into quarters and the slip is described as the relationship of the L5 vertebral body to the sacrum (S1) (Fig. 128-15).[36] Spondyloptosis occurs when the body of L5 sits anterior to the sacrum—a slip of more than 100%. Associated physical findings seen with high-grade slips include flattening of the buttocks, a transverse abdominal crease, and gait alterations. In the thin patient, a palpable step-off of the lower lumbar spinous processes may be appreciated, and painful limitation of extension is frequently associated with a painful catch on back extension. A hamstring spasm is frequently present, and forward flexion may be limited because of the tight hamstrings.

It is helpful to be familiar with the classification system of Wiltse-Newman based on the causative factor for slippage (Box 128-2).[37] Type I is a dysplastic slip due to congenital abnormality of the facet. Type II is an isthmic slip as a result of a pars interarticularis defect. Type III is a degenerative slip resulting from degenerative changes at the facet joint, and types IV and V result from traumatic and pathologic causes, respectively.[38]

The most common form of spondylolisthesis in athletes is type II (isthmic), with type III (degenerative) being the next most common. It is important to recognize that unlike type II, degenerative (type III) spondylolisthesis has an intact neural arch, often resulting in central canal narrowing, and typically presents as lumbar spinal stenosis in older adults, rarely before 40 years of age.[39] Isthmic spondylolisthesis does not result in central canal narrowing because the posterior elements remain in place as the vertebral body moves anteriorly, and it commonly presents in adolescents (Table 128-3). In addition to disk degeneration and facet arthrosis, the translation involved in degenerative spondylolisthesis occurs as a result of intersegmental instability,[40] with usually less than 30% anterolisthesis.[41] The level of translation also differs between degenerative and isthmic-type spondylolisthesis,

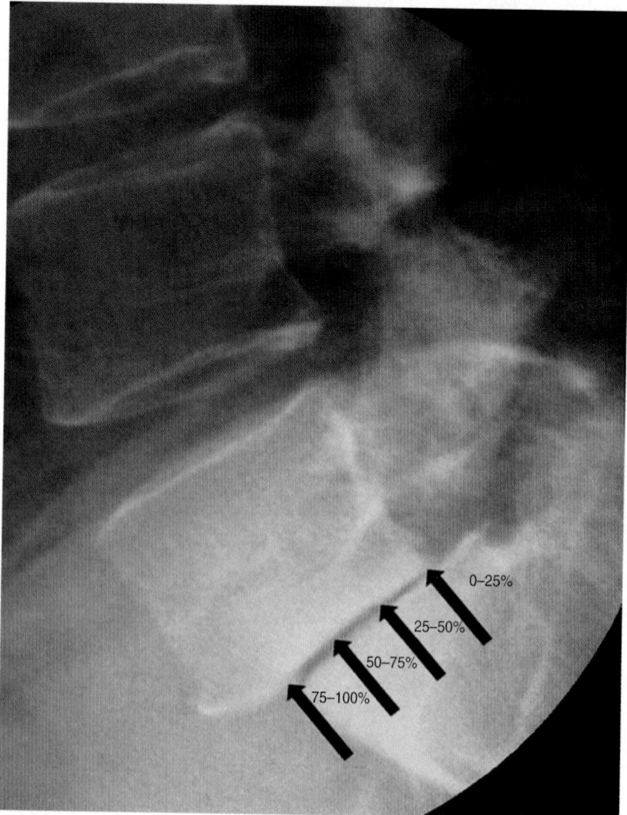

FIGURE 128-15 Classification of spondylolisthesis: grade I, 0% to 25% slip; grade II, 50% to 75% slip; grade IV, 75% to 100% slip; and grade V, spondyloptosis (complete displacement of upper vertebra in front of lower vertebra). *(From Wiltse LL, Winter RB: Terminology and measurement of spondylolisthesis.* Clin Orthop *117:23–29, 1976.)*

TABLE 128-3

DEGENERATIVE VERSUS ISTHMIC SPONDYLOLISTHESIS

	Degenerative Spondylolisthesis	Isthmic Spondylolisthesis
Age of onset	>40 yr	~10 yr
Level	Any level; most commonly at L4-L5	Any level; most commonly L5-S1
Pars interarticularis	Intact	Lysis
Central canal	Narrowed	Patent
Foraminal canal	Narrowed	Narrowed
Degree of slip	<30% of inferior vertebral body	No limit

with L4-L5 being the most common location for degenerative spondylolisthesis and L5-S1 the most common location for isthmic spondylolisthesis.

Multiple types of pars defects may be seen, including, most commonly, fatigue fracture of the pars (type IIA), elongation of the pars (type IIB), and acute fracture of the pars (type IIC), which in our experience is extremely rare. The concept of fatigue fracture of the pars interarticularis as the underlying disorder in spondylolysis was first popularized by Wiltse.[42] It is believed that in certain persons, the pars is susceptible to repetitive hyperextension stresses and that a hereditary predisposition to this susceptibility exists. Elongation of the pars interarticularis (type IIB) may be seen without frank fracture and may permit the development of anterolisthesis. Most low-grade isthmic spondylolistheses does not progress after 18 years of age.[43] However, progression of anterolisthesis may occur because of associated degenerative changes in the disk at that level and may present as leg pain due to foraminal narrowing, nerve root compression, and disk collapse.[44] Other factors that increase risk for progression are high-grade slips with high slip angles.[45]

Diagnostic studies start with plain radiographs. A standing spot lateral view identifies 80% of pars defects but may be supplemented with oblique views if needed. SPECT is the most sensitive study for identifying occult pars defects not seen on plain radiographs (Fig. 128-16). CT can also be helpful to more clearly define the pars fracture and help differentiate the rare acute fracture of the pars from the much more common chronic lesion (Fig. 128-17). Degenerative spondylolisthesis can often be diagnosed with standing lateral radiographs, noting that flexion views often exacerbate the slippage and extension views tend to reduce it.[46]

Nonoperative Treatment

The primary goal of treatment is relief of back pain and the resumption of full activities, including sports. The goal is not to heal a pars fracture or to reduce a slippage but to render the patient asymptomatic or minimally symptomatic. It is important to stress this point to the athlete from the onset. Most patients with symptomatic spondylolysis or spondylolisthesis are prescribed an initial trial of nonsteroidal NSAIDs, moist heat, and activity limitation. Depending on the severity and duration of the patient's symptoms, athletic participation may be either restricted or eliminated, with some studies suggesting removal from athletic participation for a minimum of 3 months.[47] As the symptoms resolve, athletic participation is gradually resumed, the patient is weaned off medication, and a lumbar stabilization program is usually started. The athlete is encouraged to continue these exercises, even if he or she is asymptomatic, for at least one season and frequently longer. Patients with spondylolysis who strictly adhere to a conservative treatment protocol can expect good-to-excellent long-term outcomes of greater than 90%.[48]

Unfortunately, some patients either fail to respond to treatment or experience a recurrence of pain. In these

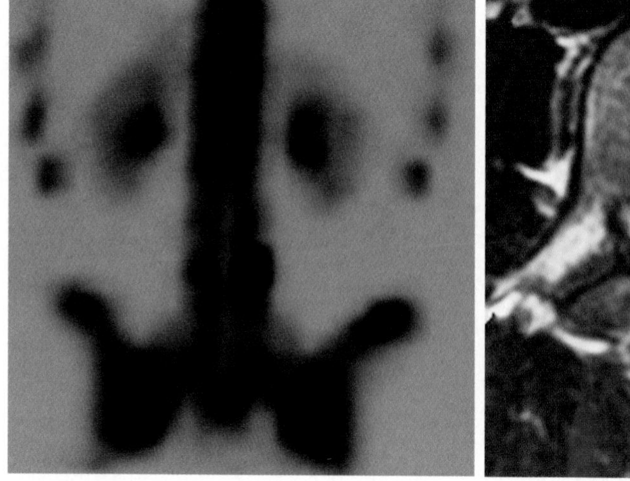
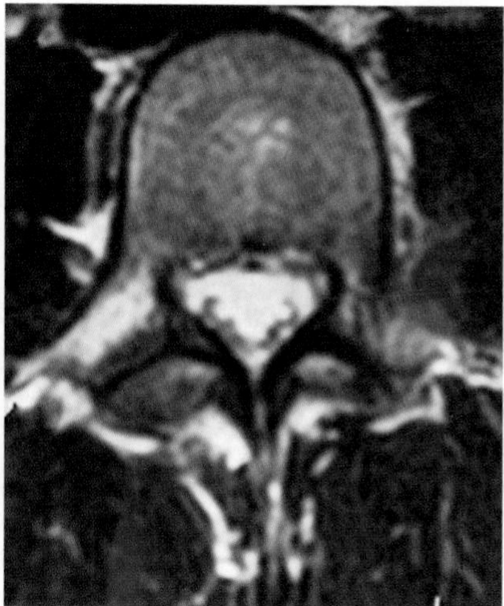

FIGURE 128-16 Single photon emission computed tomography imaging with increased tracer uptake and matching magnetic resonance imaging with edema in pars area.

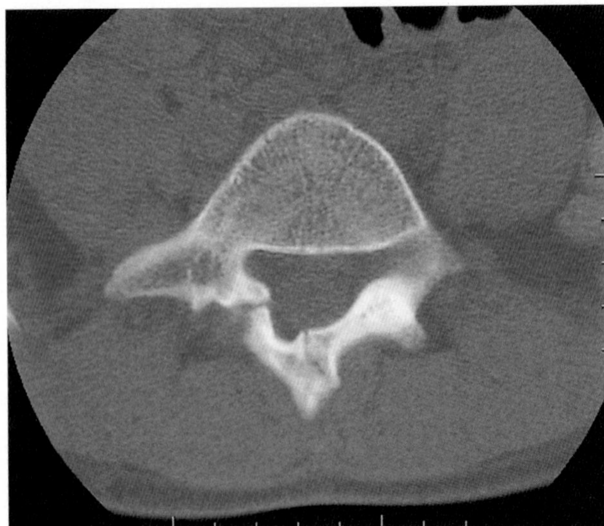

FIGURE 128-17 An axial computed tomographic image of a 17-year-old football player demonstrating unilateral spondylolysis with sclerosis of the contralateral pars.

circumstances, we typically repeat the course of treatment and try to ensure that compliance has been adequate. Another option in this setting is the use of bracing, which is most applicable in the skeletally immature athlete.[49] The most common regimen is to wear a Boston antilordotic brace on a full-time basis initially, with gradual weaning over a 6- to 12-week period. In the adult athletic population, bracing is of limited use, with the goal to render the patient asymptomatic rather than to promote healing of a pars fracture. In high-level athletes concerned about returning to competition quickly, bracing may result in further loss of core strength and deconditioning and therefore is often not the best treatment in this population. Acute fracture of the pars interarticularis is unusual, but when a fracture is identified early, healing can sometimes be achieved. The most reliable method of immobilizing the lumbosacral junction is with a pantaloon spica cast, although some authors report an acceptable healing rate with other types of bracing.[50] Serial CT can be useful in following the progression of the defect to healing. However, the physician must always keep in mind the significant radiation exposure inherent in CT scanning.

Thoracolumbar Fractures

A review of the literature tells us that specific anatomic zones of the spine are more prone to injury than others, with the incidence of thoracic and lumbar injuries as follows: T1-T10, 16%; T11-L1, 52%; and L1-L5, 32%.[51] Fracture or dislocation of the anterior column of the thoracolumbar spine is unusual, although any suspicion of high-speed axial loading mechanism warrants the use of a spinal board (Fig. 128-18). Of utmost importance in terms of workup and management options is the presence of any neurologic deficits. If radiographs are inconclusive or if a neurologic deficit is present, even if transiently, CT or MRI should be performed. Potential surgical management decisions are based on three critical factors that must be elucidated at presentation: injury mechanism and pathology, neurologic status, and posterior ligamentous integrity.[52] These three factors are also the basis of the Thoracolumbar Injury Classification and Severity Score, which uses specific point values assigned to each category based on the injury severity and is used to guide treatment.[53] Ligamentous injury to the posterior column should be suspected when increased space between adjacent spinous processes is seen on lateral radiographs or when physical examination demonstrates ecchymosis, interspinous tenderness, or the presence of a gap between the spinous processes. CT is most useful in cases in which a fracture is suspected to evaluate bony anatomy, perform fracture classification, and provide information about the spinal canal.

The three-column classification first described by Denis is also one of the most commonly used systems to assess spinal stability and further guide treatment decisions (Fig. 128-19).[54-56] In this classification, the spine is divided into three columns: (1) anterior column: anterior longitudinal ligament and anterior vertebral body; (2) middle column: posterior vertebral body and posterior longitudinal ligament bordered by the origin of the pedicles; and (3) posterior column: the remaining posterior elements, including pedicles, facet joint, lamina, and spinous process.[57] Although it is useful for assessment of bony stability, Denis' three-column classification fails to account for the patient's neurologic status, nor does it provide accurate prognostic information. The Thoracolumbar Injury Classification and Severity Score system as previously described accounts for these limitations and has become a useful and widely accepted classification system for thoracolumbar fractures.[58]

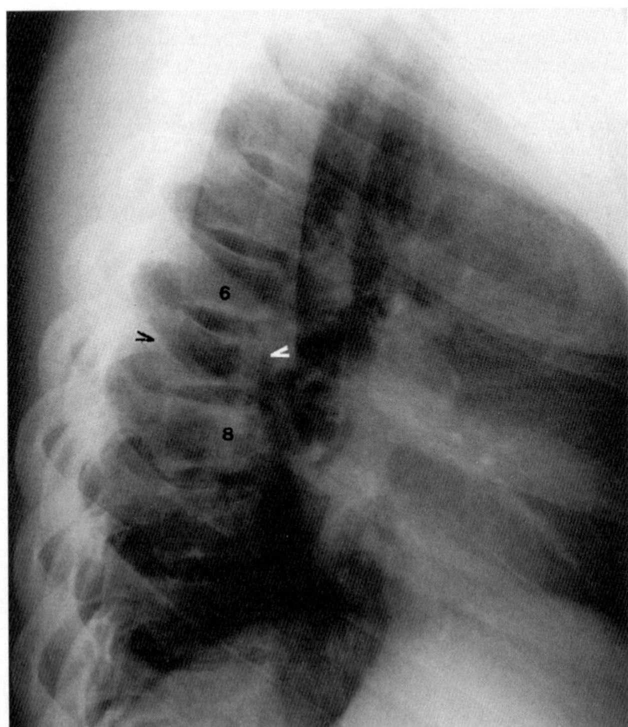

FIGURE 128-18 A 14-year-old boy was thrown from his bike during a competition, landed on his head and neck, and experienced the sudden onset of midthoracic pain. Findings of neurologic tests were normal. Plain lateral radiography demonstrated mild wedging at T6 and T8 and a more significant wedge compression fracture of T7 (*arrowheads*). The absence of end-plate irregularity or Schmorl node formation differentiates this case from Scheuermann kyphosis, which would also involve multilevel wedging.

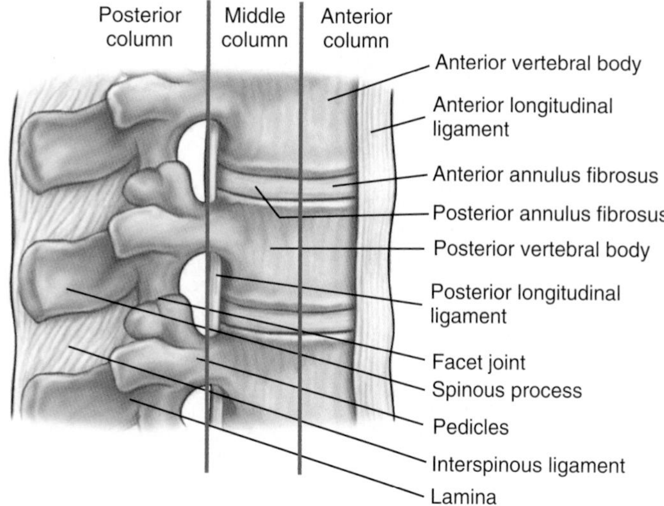

FIGURE 128-19 The commonly used three-column classification system to assess mechanism of injury and inherent spinal stability.

Compression Fractures

The most common thoracic spine fracture is the compression fracture (Fig. 128-20), which often occurs in the lower thoracic spine or at the thoracolumbar junction. This type of fracture occurs as a result of failure of the anterior column in flexion with preservation of the middle column, and thus it results in rare neurologic sequelae. It usually is seen after a history of significant trauma in the younger athlete or after prior osteopenia in the older athlete. Some compression fractures at the thoracolumbar junction are not easily seen on plain radiographs and must be carefully scrutinized at the level of pain or tenderness. Diagnosis on lateral radiographs is made by comparing the anterior versus posterior aspects of the vertebral body in question. Less than 25% compression of the anterior vertebral body is usually treated with conservative management and possible bracing in the form of a molded thoracolumbar spine orthosis for prevention of further flexion of the thoracic spine.

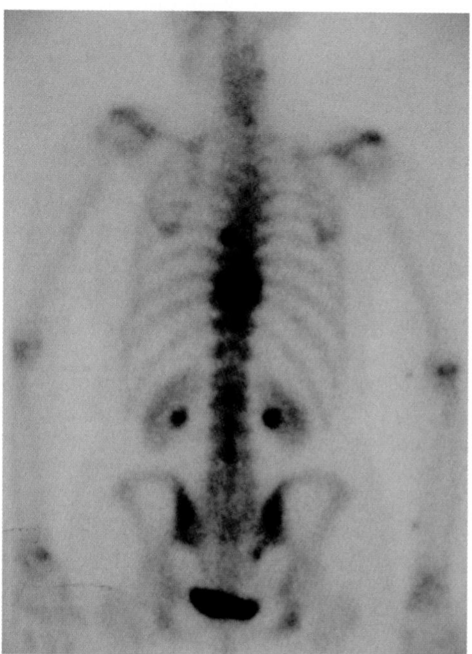

FIGURE 128-20 A thoracic compression fracture not visualized on a lateral radiograph in a mature recreational walker but identified on a bone scan.

Thoracolumbar Burst Fractures

Similar to compression fractures, the mechanism of a burst fracture may result from flexion and axial loading of the spine. Burst fractures, however, involve both the anterior and middle columns with frequent neurologic compromise due to bony retropulsion of the posterior aspect of the vertebral body into the spinal canal (Fig. 128-21).[59,60] Most burst fractures without neurologic injury are treated conservatively; however, some investigators have suggested that indications for more aggressive treatment include collapse of more than 50% of the vertebral body height, compromise of more than 50% of the spinal canal, or more than 20 degrees of kyphosis at the level of injury.[61]

Transverse Process Fractures

A direct blow to the lumbar spine is capable of producing a fracture of the transverse process. In most cases, this type of fracture is stable without any type of neurologic injury, although the suspicion must remain high for abdominal or retroperitoneal injury, especially involving the kidney.[62,63] The clinician should have a low threshold for abdominal imaging with a CT in any patient who has abdominal pain or hematuria with an associated lumbar transverse process fracture. Because of the stability of isolated transverse process fractures, these injuries are treated conservatively, allowing adequate time for fracture healing, which is often prolonged because of distraction of the fragments from the paraspinal musculature.

Thoracolumbar Disk Herniation

Half of all symptomatic disk herniations present with the insidious onset of back pain, leg pain, or both, with a small

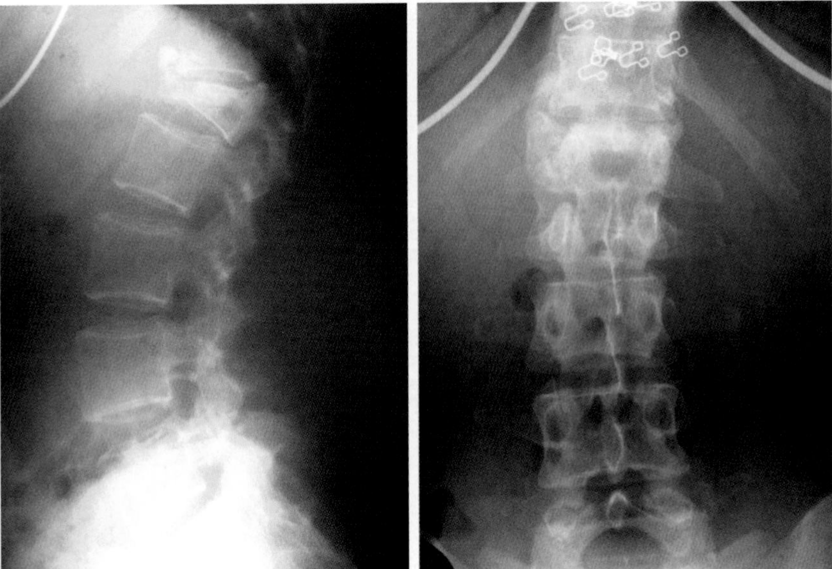

FIGURE 128-21 A 38-year-old woman involved in a dune buggy "hard landing" sustained a burst fracture of L1 without neurologic deficit and was treated with a thoracolumbar spine orthosis. She is asymptomatic and has returned to normal sports activities but not dune buggy riding.

number occurring as a result of acute trauma. Disk herniation occurs when the gelatinous inner material of the nucleus pulposus pushes through the outer anulus fibrosus layer of the disk and protrudes into the spinal canal. If the amount of herniation is large enough, it may produce mechanical compression of the neurologic structures within the canal.[64]

Thoracic Disk Herniation

The thoracic spine accounts for approximately 1% of clinically relevant disk herniations. The most common locations in the thoracic spine involve levels T9 to T12.[66] In a recent review study, the authors conclude that in patients with thoracic disk herniation, pain was present in 57% of patients, sensory changes in 24%, motor deficits in 17%, and bowel or bladder incontinence in 2%.[67,68] Intercostal nerve root impingement as a result of posterolateral thoracic disk herniation may produce chest wall pain or numbness along the dermatomal distribution, whereas central disk herniation may exhibit no pain symptoms but rather bilateral lower extremity weakness or paralysis.[68,69] Central disk herniation may also produce other long tract findings such as hyperreflexia, clonus, and upgoing plantar response (the Babinski sign).[70,71]

Lumbar Disk Herniation

Almost 90% of all symptomatic disk herniations occur in the lumbar spine. The initial presentation varies greatly among athletes, with many unable to relate the pain to a specific event or activity. On the other hand, other athletes may recall sudden radicular pain with preceding back pain.[72] Most lumbar herniations involve L4-L5 and/or L5-S1 levels and thus produce calf pain with compression of the L5 or S1 nerve roots. Other presentations depend on the location of disk herniation, with anterior thigh pain and positive findings of a femoral nerve stretch test being the most common presentation in patients with impingement of L2, L3, or L4 nerve roots. A positive tension sign (i.e., the straight leg raising test or bowstring sign) is present in most patients with a clinically significant disk herniation at L5 or S1 with radicular shooting pain traveling below the knee.

Cauda equina syndrome, including bowel and bladder incontinence, is a rare but serious complication of lumbar disk herniation resulting from sacral nerve root impingement. This condition should always be ruled out because of the need for urgent surgical decompression to attempt to preserve bowel and bladder function.[73-75] Another urgent consideration in patients with lumbar disk herniation is the presence of a progressive neurologic deficit, which may indicate a need for surgical intervention.[76]

Appropriate diagnostic studies to evaluate disk herniation include MRI and CT-myelography. Treatment for all thoracolumbar disk herniations depends on the clinical presentation, the presence of neurologic symptoms, and the location of the disk herniation. Isolated nerve root compression is often due to posterolateral disk herniation and may be treated nonoperatively initially, with surgical intervention considered only after the patient fails to respond to conservative management for at least 4 to 6 weeks. Rarely, a large central disk herniation may present with significant neurologic signs and symptoms and thus require early surgery.

Nonoperative measures generally include activity restriction, physical therapy, pain medication, and use of epidural steroid or nerve root block injections. Once the patient is able to walk without a limp and has a near-normal range of back motion, physical therapy is initiated. We generally prescribe a McKenzie back exercise program under the supervision of a physical therapist and allow the patient to resume normal activities gradually, including sports, as the symptoms subside. In a retrospective review of 342 professional athletes diagnosed with lumbar disk herniations, Hsu et al.[77] demonstrated that no difference in outcome occurred between operative and nonoperative cohorts, specifically regarding ultimate return to play (average 82%) and career length (average 3.4 years after diagnosis). In fact, Major League Baseball players who underwent lumbar diskectomy had a shorter career compared with the nonoperative cohort (256 vs. 471 games played, respectively).[77] Another retrospective review shows that in patients with lumbar disk herniation treated with conservative management, 38% improved within 1 month, 52% improved by 2 months, and 73% improved by 3 months.[78] Furthermore, several studies suggest that about 80% of patients with radicular pain due to lumbar disk herniation significantly improve without surgery within 6 weeks.[79-81]

Lumbar Spinal Stenosis

As discussed previously, the spinal cord tapers in the lumbar spine to produce spinal nerve roots that emerge as the cauda equina, located in the central spinal canal, and exiting bilaterally through the neural foramen between each lumbar vertebrae. Each nerve root is named after the superior pedicle at that level (e.g., the L4 nerve root exits below the L4 pedicle). Lumbar spinal stenosis occurs when either the central spinal canal, the lateral recesses (subarticular groove), or the foraminal canal becomes narrowed, resulting in compression of the thecal sac or individual nerve roots. This phenomenon typically occurs in persons with a developmentally narrowed canal with superimposed degenerative changes of the disk and facet joints.

A few causes of neural compression include disk herniation and protrusion, hypertrophic laminae or ligamentum flavum, degenerative changes of the facet joints, and spondylolisthesis. Typical central canal lumbar stenosis is often a result of degenerative changes at the facet joint, where the minimum cross-sectional area often occurs at the interfacet level (Box 128-3).[82] Lateral stenosis can be further broken down into three specific anatomic zones based on the course of the nerve root exiting the canal: the entrance, mid, and exit zones.[83] Whatever the cause of stenosis, many studies have attempted but ultimately failed to define a threshold cross-sectional area that produces symptoms of clinical stenosis.[84] No statistically significant correlation seems to exist between the severity of spinal stenosis as measured by dural cross-sectional area and the severity of clinical symptoms,[85] and therefore imaging alone cannot predict symptomatic lumbar stenosis.[86] MRI of the lumbar spine is the diagnostic imaging study of choice for confirmation of clinically suspected lumbar spinal stenosis, although CT is often used in patients with previously implanted hardware or who are unable to tolerate MRI (e.g., because of a pacemaker).

In the athletic population, clinically significant stenosis is rising as a cause of radicular symptoms in active, older adults because of degenerative changes and hypertrophy of the facet joints. The presentation is often gradual back and leg pain, although acute worsening may occur within the setting of a degenerative process with sudden concomitant disk herniation. Straight-leg testing may not be positive with isolated lateral stenosis and is often negative with central stenosis.[87] The term "neurogenic claudication" is used to describe the clinical syndrome of leg pain, weakness, or numbness exacerbated by walking/standing and relieved by sitting or bending forward as caused by lumbar stenosis.[88,89] It is important to rule out vascular claudication, which is capable of producing similar complaints, with the exception of worse symptoms while bending forward and, often, abnormal findings of arterial Doppler studies (Table 128-4).[90] Neurogenic claudication is relieved by bending forward because this position allows the spinal canal to expand and release nerve compression.[91]

BOX 128-3 Spinal Stenosis

Anatomic Zones for Stenosis

Central canal stenosis
Lateral recess stenosis
Foraminal stenosis
Extraforaminal stenosis

Spinal Alignment

Normal
Spondylolisthesis
Scoliosis
Kyphosis
Multidirectional malalignment

TABLE 128-4 VASCULAR VERSUS NEUROGENIC CLAUDICATION

Evaluation	Vascular	Neurogenic
Walking distance	Fixed	Variable
Palliative factors	Standing	Sitting, bending
Provocative factors	Walking	Walking, standing
Walking uphill	Painful	Painless
Bicycle test	Positive (painful)	Negative (painless)
Pulses	Absent	Present
Skin	Loss of hair, shiny	Normal
Weakness	Rarely	Occasionally
Back pain	Occasionally	Commonly
Back motion	Normal	Limited
Pain character	Cramping, distal to proximal	Numbness, aching, proximal to distal
Atrophy	Uncommon	Occasionally

Degenerative Disk Disease

All patients who live long enough eventually experience degenerative disk disease of the lumbar spine, which is usually present by middle age.[92] Athletes have an increased risk of the development of degenerative changes of the spine because of repetitive loading and intense training over many years that varies with the sport being played. One retrospective study examining Olympic athletes found an increased rate of lumbar disk degeneration compared with healthy control subjects.[93] Another cross-sectional study comparing university athletes with students who were not athletes also confirmed increased disk degeneration in the athletic group as seen on MRI.[94] Activities involving increased mechanical loading of the spine seem to increase a person's risk of back

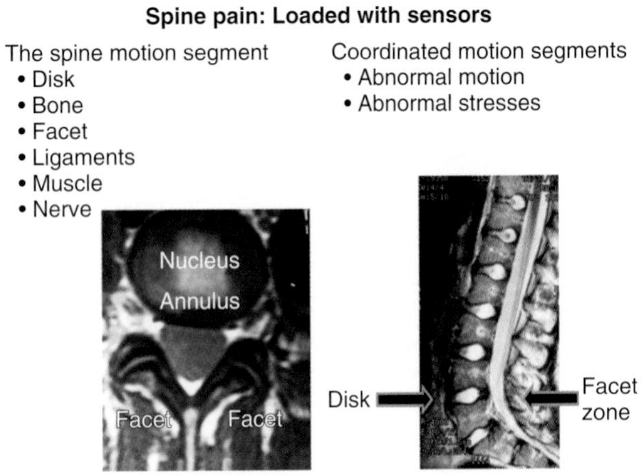

Spine pain: Loaded with sensors

The spine motion segment
- Disk
- Bone
- Facet
- Ligaments
- Muscle
- Nerve

Coordinated motion segments
- Abnormal motion
- Abnormal stresses

Nucleus
Annulus
Facet
Facet
Disk
Facet zone

FIGURE 128-22 Spine pain.

pain and degenerative changes, whereas endurance exercise seems to be protective.[95]

Degeneration of the lumbar disk may include disk protrusions or anular tears, ultimately leading to marginal osteophyte formation and remodeling of the facet joints. These changes may or may not be associated with symptoms of low back pain or radicular pathology. It is therefore important to remember that not all common degenerative changes seen on imaging are the source of the patient's pain.[96,97]

Kirkaldy-Willis and colleagues[98] developed the degenerative disk cascade model to further examine the natural progression of degenerative changes of the spine. Assuming a three-joint spine complex consisting of the disk and each posterior facet joint, the degenerative cascade explains periods of mechanical dysfunction, instability, and restabilization (Fig. 128-22). Degenerative disk disease may be evaluated by MRI as described by Pfirrmann, demonstrating progressive loss of signal and disk height seen on T2-weighted images and graded I to V in severity.[99]

Anular tears are caused by radial tears of the disk through the anulus fibrosus and may become painful because of its sensory innervation to the outer layers.[100-102] T2-weighted MRI is often used for diagnosis of an annular tear, but controversy remains about whether any correlation exists with the patient's symptoms.[103,104] Less popular, controversial, and invasive lumbar diskography may also be used to assess the integrity of the disk by injecting dye into the disk and assessing the patient's pain, as well as viewing the radiographic image. Similarly, pressure-controlled manometric diskography may be more effective in distinguishing between symptomatic and asymptomatic anular tears.[105] Similar to diskography, diagnosis of facet joint pain may also be made by injection of the joints under fluoroscopic control with resultant pain relief.[106]

Nonoperative Treatment

Initial Treatment

Most athletes presenting with new-onset back pain respond quickly to a series of general measures (Box 128-4), and thus it is rarely essential to make a specific diagnosis early in the course of the patient's complaints. Furthermore, it is rarely cost-effective to order sophisticated imaging of recent-onset back pain except in unusual circumstances.

Many athletes present with a more chronic pain of insidious onset. The presence of incapacitating pain causing the patient to stay home or be bedridden should lead to a more aggressive evaluation. Similarly, a history of constitutional symptoms such as unexplained weight loss, fever, night pain, or the presence of significant neurologic signs or symptoms suggests the need for prompt imaging.

Unless one or more red flags are present, activity is restricted for most patients and generic treatments are begun, such as moist heat, stretching, and use of over-the-counter medications such as acetaminophen or ibuprofen. The goal of this approach is to rule out more serious underlying disease and help the patient return to full activity with minimal or no pain, which may require relatively frequent reevaluation.

In most cases, improvement will occur. Depending on the duration and severity of the patient's symptoms and the rapidity of improvement, the athlete is allowed to gradually return to his or her daily activities, and a program of back and core strengthening exercises is then begun under the guidance of a physical therapist. We usually recommend lumbar stabilization exercises and typically insist that an actual physical therapist rather than an athletic trainer or personal trainer teach and supervise the initiation of the program; a self-taught approach should not be used. Once the exercise program has

BOX 128-4 Treatment Options

ACUTE LUMBAR STRAIN

Limited period of activity restriction
Moist heat and tissue massage
NSAIDs
Stretching and strengthening program
Gradual return to play

SPONDYLOLYSIS AND SPONDYLOLISTHESIS

Activity restriction with or without bracing
NSAIDs
Physical therapy with core strengthening (stabilization program) and stretching
Surgical stabilization if pain >1 year or high-grade (grade III or IV) spondylolisthesis

LUMBAR DISK HERNIATION

Initial period of restricted activity
NSAIDs and moist heat
McKenzie back program (generally an extension program)
Surgical treatment if unacceptable pain for 6 to 12 weeks (physical and radiographic findings must correlate) or progressive weakness or cauda equina syndrome

OVERUSE SYNDROME

Plain radiography, magnetic resonance imaging, and bone scan correlate (must rule out other conditions)
Activity restriction, NSAIDs, moist heat, and physical therapy program
Alternative treatments may be considered (e.g., chiropractic or acupuncture)
Gradual resumption of activities
If symptoms recur, change to a less competitive level of athletic participation or change sport

NSAIDs, Nonsteroidal antiinflammatory drugs.

been mastered without recurrence of pain, gradual resumption of athletic activities is allowed. Because pain is a strictly subjective complaint, it is difficult to define objective guidelines for when the patient can resume specific activities. We find that the most useful guideline is the presence of minimal or no pain, full range of motion, and a normal neurologic examination.

Another aspect of the management of the athlete with ongoing back pain is counseling. The athlete often may not understand that back pain is a relatively common occurrence. It is imperative that the physician reinforce the fact that this condition may occasionally involve a prolonged recovery. It also needs to be emphasized that the exact cause of the pain may not always be determined.

Because the appropriate role of imaging studies is to guide treatment, imaging should be conducted only when it can reasonably be expected to have a significant impact on therapeutic decision making. In general, imaging is rarely helpful and therefore not indicated in the first 2 to 4 weeks that a patient has symptoms. We typically wait 2 to 4 weeks before obtaining plain radiographs for persons whose back pain fails to improve significantly. If plain radiographic findings are negative and the pain persists, we consider ordering an MRI scan after the patient has symptoms for 6 to 12 weeks. When the presence of a spondylolysis is a particular concern, we often proceed to SPECT before ordering MRI. If the MRI results are normal and symptoms persist for 6 months or longer, we often recommend technetium bone scanning.

Spinal Stabilization and Core Strengthening

Core strengthening is an important part of the support mechanism of the spine and can be achieved with tensioning of the thoracolumbar fascia and strengthening of the deep lumbar stabilizer muscles.[107] A recent review article describes the core as "a muscular box with the abdominals in the front, the paraspinals and gluteals in the back, the diaphragm as the roof, and the pelvic floor and hip girdle musculature as the bottom."[108] This core strength ensures a solid support for body movement and allows for the distribution of forces to and from the remainder of the body. For the competitive athlete, core strength is necessary for biomechanical efficiency and decreases the risk of injury.[109]

The lumbar spine is particularly vulnerable to injury from lack of stabilization and therefore has the most to gain from core strengthening. The deep lumbar musculature originates directly on the lumbar vertebrae to control each motion segment and is mostly responsible for the relationship of one vertebrae to another.[110] Several studies have identified a beneficial relationship between specific thoracolumbar pathologies, core strengthening, and improved overall outcome. It is well documented that poor core stability is often present in patients with back pain,[111] and deep lumbar exercises have been shown to improve symptoms in radiographically proven spondylolisthesis and spondylolysis.[112] One study was able to show that patients with a first episode of back pain treated with lumbar strengthening had a reduced risk of recurrence of pain (35% at 3 years) compared with an age-matched control group without strengthening (75% at 3 years).[113]

Specific exercises that have been shown to be important in spinal stabilization include deep lumbar musculature providing intersegmental control, superficial muscles (transverse abdominis and pelvic floor) that increase intraabdominal pressure, global muscles (latissimus dorsi and quadratus lumborum) that control trunk movement, and neural control.[114]

Medications

A recent review summarizing 50 randomized controlled clinical trials on the therapeutic effect of medications on low back pain identified several effective medications for acute and chronic low back pain.[115] NSAIDs were identified as being effective for both acute and chronic low back pain, whereas muscle relaxants were effective only for acute low back pain and antidepressants were effective in persons with chronic low back pain. If NSAIDs are administered, it is recommended that administration of a proton-pump inhibitor also be considered to reduce complications of acid reflux and erosion.[116-118] Lastly, corticosteroids are useful in the setting of back pain with the presence of radicular symptoms to reduce nerve compression and inflammation.[119]

Trigger Point Injections

Trigger point injections may be used in the management of acute and chronic low back pain and are often incorporated into a physical therapy regimen.[120] Patients who receive the most benefit from trigger point injections have suspected myofascial syndrome due to increased muscle spasm with localized injection of myofascial trigger points.[121] The ideal chemical to be injected is debated among clinicians, with most using either botulinum toxin or bupivacaine. Graboski et al.[122] compared these two agents for the treatment of myofascial pain syndrome and found no difference in the outcomes measured and thus recommend use of bupivacaine, which is less expensive.[122] To date, data are insufficient to support the judicious use of trigger-point injections.[123]

Operative Treatment

Indications

Few indications for operative management are generally accepted. A therapeutic dilemma arises in the patient who achieves acceptable symptomatic relief with activity restriction but is unable to resume athletic activity without recurrence of symptoms. Surgery may be considered under such circumstances, but return to high-level sports competition after surgery is unpredictable. Other less common indications for surgery include a significant or worsening neurologic deficit or the presence of cauda equina syndrome.

A patient with symptomatic disk herniation should have a chief complaint of radicular pain and a positive straight-leg–raising sign to be considered a good surgical candidate. MRI is the preferred confirmatory diagnostic test to identify a disk herniation and must correlate with the patient's symptoms, neurologic examination, and tension sign (i.e., the straight-leg–raising test or bowstring test).

Decompression

Typical decompressive surgery for disk herniation involves hemilaminotomy and partial diskectomy to relieve mechanical compression of the involved nerve root(s).[124,125] The goal of decompression surgery is to reduce radicular leg pain symptoms. Relief of back pain is not predictable and should not be the primary goal of surgery. More than 90% of appropriately selected adults experience significant long-term relief of their sciatica after an uncomplicated diskectomy, and a recent Cochrane update suggests that a diskectomy provides faster relief of sciatica compared with traditional nonoperative treatment.[126]

Fusion

The traditional gold standard surgical treatment for lumbar spondylolisthesis and instability in the athlete is posterior spinal fusion.[127] For an L5 spondylolysis or low-grade L5-S1 slip, fusion from L5 to the sacrum is typically performed. Instrumented posterolateral fusion with an autogenous iliac crest bone graft has a very high success rate with minimal morbidity and is our preferred approach.[128] Some authors have shown varying benefits of fusion surgery compared with a thorough physical therapy regimen, with one study demonstrating no advantage[129] but others showing superior outcomes in the fusion group.[130-132] The risks and benefits of surgery and a candid discussion of recovery time and expectations must be discussed individually with the athlete and vary depending on the pathology.

Return-to-Play Criteria

Much controversy exists in the orthopaedic and sports medicine community regarding decisions about returning to sports participation after thoracolumbar spine injury. Each case is considered independently and reviewed according to the nature of the injury, current signs and symptoms, response to treatment, and physical demands of the sport. However, a general consensus exists regarding criteria that most clinicians believe should be met prior to resumption of sport activity, including minimal current symptoms and near-baseline active range of motion, strength, and endurance.[133] Once these parameters are met, gradual resumption of drills and conditioning allow a period of transition before full play is allowed.

Return to collision sports after an injury is much more difficult. Although successful conservative or surgical treatment of lumbar disk herniation is generally well accepted for return to full contact sports, this does not apply to spondylolisthesis or spondylolysis, which remains case dependent.[134] Burnett and Sonntag[135] have published an excellent summary of their recommendations for return to contact sports after spinal surgery (Table 128-5).

TABLE 128-5

RECOMMENDATIONS FOR RETURN TO CONTACT SPORTS AFTER SPINAL SURGERY*

Operative Location/Procedure	Return to Contact Sports
Cervical	
Occiput–C2 region	No
Subaxial region	
Posterior foraminotomy	
Single-level	Yes
Multilevel	Yes
Posterior laminectomy (with or without fusion)/laminoplasty	
Single level	Yes
2 levels	Yes
>2 levels	No
Anterior diskectomy fusion/arthroplasty	
Single level	Yes
2 levels	Yes
>2 levels	No
Anterior foraminotomy	
Single level	Yes
Multilevel	Yes
Anterior corpectomy	
Single level	Yes
Multilevel	No
Thoracic	
Cervicothoracic junction zone	No
Midthoracic	
With deformity	Yes
Without deformity	Yes
Thoracolumbar junction zone	No
Lumbar	
Diskectomy/laminectomy/laminoplasty	
Single level	Yes
Multilevel	Yes
Anterior or posterior fusion/arthroplasty	
Single level	Yes
Multilevel	Yes

From Burnett MG, Sonntag VKH: Return to contact sports after spinal surgery. *Neurosurg Focus* 21(4):E5, 2006.

*To be considered eligible for a full return to activity, patients must be pain free, neurologically intact, and have completed an uneventful rehabilitative course.

Conclusion

Today's athletes have enormous pressure to succeed with unprecedented training regimens that place their bodies at high risk for thoracolumbar injury. As physicians, health care professionals, coaches, and trainers, we have an obligation to provide our athletes with the correct diagnostic and therapeutic approaches that will minimize time spent away from training and allow them to compete at their preinjury level.

Athletes depend on a healthy body, relying on their speed, strength, and agility to succeed. The spine remains at the core of all movement, providing a foundation of support when it is healthy and a constant source of pain and disability when it is injured. Knute Rockne has proven he knows how to succeed in athletics, agreeing that success is built on many aspects, including discipline, strength, training, and respect for your opponents, topped with prayer, although he admitted that "prayers work best when you have big players."

For a complete list of references, go to expertconsult.com.

Suggested Readings

Citation: Lawrence JP, Greene HS, Grauer JN: Back pain in athletes. *J Am Acad Orthop Surg* 14:726–735, 2006.
Level of Evidence: V
Summary: The authors of this excellent review article provide a clear systematic approach to diagnosis and management of back pain with a specific focus on the athlete.
Citation: Tallarico RA, Madom IA, Palumbo MA: Spondylolysis and spondylolisthesis in the athlete. *Sports Med Arthrosc Rev* 16:32–38, 2008.

Level of Evidence: V

Summary: The authors provide a brief, well-organized review of a topic for which both diagnosis and treatment are difficult. In six pages, the authors answer most of the challenging clinical questions that arise in the treatment of spondylolysis and spondylolisthesis in the athlete.

Citation: Tokuhashi Y, Matsuzaki H, Uematsu Y, et al: Symptoms of thoracolumbar junction disc herniation. *Spine* 26(22):E512–E518, 2001.

Level of Evidence: IV

Summary: In this retrospective case series, the authors analyze patients with thoracolumbar junction disk herniation, specifically with regard to presenting signs and symptoms. The authors brilliantly correlate the affected spinal level as diagnosed with imaging and confirmed with operative findings to clinical motor and sensory deficits.

Citation: Jonsson B, Stromqvist B: Symptoms and signs in degeneration of the lumbar spine: A prospective, consecutive study of 300 operated patients. *J Bone Joint Surg Br* 75B(3):381–385, 1993.

Level of Evidence: II

Summary: In this well-structured study, the authors compare presenting signs and symptoms of lumbar disk herniation, lateral spinal stenosis, and central spinal stenosis with diagnosis confirmed intraoperatively.

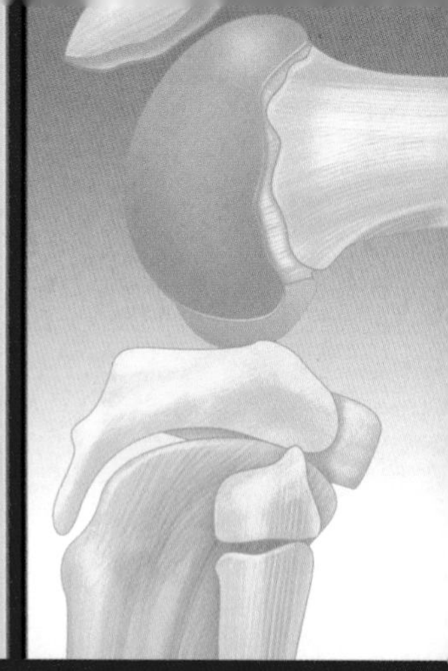

SECTION 10

Pediatric Sports Medicine

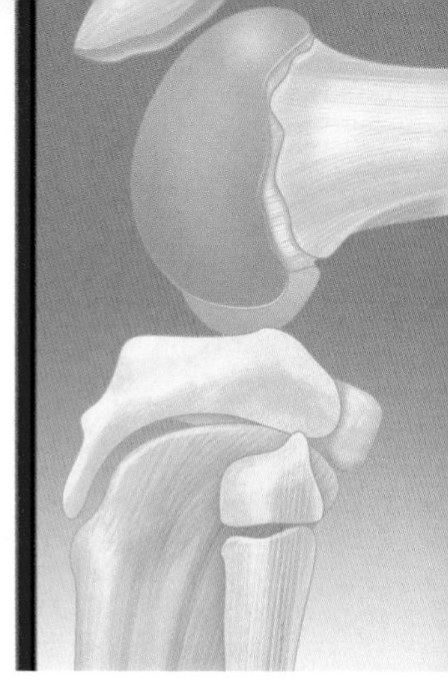

129

The Young Athlete

MININDER S. KOCHER

Sports injuries in pediatric and adolescent athletes are being seen with increasing frequency because of increased participation in higher competitive levels at younger ages, increased recognition of injuries in this age group, and the advent of arthroscopy and magnetic resonance imaging (MRI). The pediatric athlete differs from the adult athlete in terms of physiology, growth, psychology, and skills. Injury patterns are specific to the age of the athlete and the sport he or she plays. An understanding of the special considerations of pediatric athletes and common injury patterns in this population is necessary for the successful management of their sports injuries.

Epidemiology

Pediatric Sports Participation

During the past 30 years, the number of children and adolescents participating in physical activity and team sports has significantly increased, with the largest increase among female adolescents.[1] The overall trend has shifted from the largely unstructured, unsupervised "free play" of the early twentieth century to the evolution of organized and highly structured youth sports activities.[2] It is estimated that at present up to 30 million children and adolescents participate in an organized sport in the United States. In 1995, reports indicated that 15 million 5- to 14-year-olds played baseball in the United States.[3]

The Youth Risk Behavior Survey (YRBS) was a large population-based study performed throughout the 1990s that enabled accurate assessment of emerging trends in youth sports participation. Results from the 1997 survey indicated that 62% of U.S. high school students participated in one or more sports teams, with the majority playing in a combination of both school and nonschool teams.[4]

The YRBS study highlighted a number of significant demographic differences when results were compared for age, gender, and ethnicity. Although the number of girls participating in sports teams has increased fivefold during the past 30 years, a disparity continues to exist between genders according to the 1997 YRBS study.[1] Whereas almost 70% of male high school students participate in sports, only 53% of similarly aged female high school students exhibit the same level of sporting interest.[1,4] This gender disparity was even more dramatic among ethnic minorities, with only 40% of Hispanic and African American girls participating compared with 62% and 71% for boys, respectively.[4]

Furthermore, progression into adolescence was also associated with a reduction in the involvement of both boys and girls in vigorous sporting activities.[1,4] In boys, participation in vigorous exercise (defined as activity causing shortness of breath, lasting at least 20 minutes, 3 days a week) reduced from 81% in grade 9 to only 67% by grade 12.[1] As expected, this trend was even more pronounced in girls, with 61% of female ninth graders participating in vigorous exercise compared with only 41% by twelfth grade.[1]

The growth and increasing popularity of school and community youth sports programs have become an integral part of American youth culture and have the potential to enhance the long-term physical and psychosocial health of children and adolescents who participate in these programs.[4]

Pediatric Sports Injury

Increased youth participation in sports and physical activities and specialization in particular sports (and positions) at an earlier age have resulted in an increase in sports-related injuries as a result of trauma and overuse.[2] The annual incidence of sports injuries within the United States is estimated to be around 3 million, with up to 70% of those injuries resulting from youth sports activities.[3] High school athletics account for more than 2 million injuries annually, including 500,000 doctor visits and 30,000 hospitalizations.[5] More than 3.5 million children younger than the age of 14 years are treated annually for sports injuries.[5] The financial costs of managing these injuries in 1996 was well in excess of $1 billion.[3]

Pediatric sports injuries are often unique not only in terms of the underlying pathologic findings but also with regard to the challenges in managing these injuries. Many patients participate in several teams during a given season, the rest periods between seasons are short if not nonexistent, and the demand for sporting success from parents, schools, and sporting establishments is increasing.[6]

Pediatric sports injuries can be classified according to the age of the athlete, the type of injury, and the type of sport/activity being played when the injury occurred.[7] From an epidemiologic standpoint, these classifications assist in identifying potential risk factors for injury and implementing prevention strategies and rehabilitation plans that are appropriate for the age of the patient and the sport being played.

Several studies have identified a correlation between an increased risk of sports-related injury and the increased age of the pediatric athlete.[7] A number of explanations for these findings have been postulated, including a greater opportunity for injury in the adolescent athlete because of longer game times, along with more frequent and intense practices.[7] The provision of medical assistance at many high school and college games allows increased reporting of injuries.[7] It appears that anatomic factors such as the increased size of the athletes and the resultant increased force and speed of collisions play an insignificant role, because the same trend was noted for both contact and noncontact sports.[7]

Sports injuries can be broadly divided into acute traumatic and overuse-type injuries according to their pathophysiologic characteristics.[7] Whereas many acute traumatic injuries are the result of random events, overuse injuries are often the result of entrenched training errors and therefore have greater potential for prevention.[7] The difficulty lies in identifying these overuse injuries because initially they can be only subtly disabling when compared with an immediate fall to the ground after a sprain, for example.

It is important that an injury be viewed in the context of the sport in which it occurred because an injury that may be functionally disabling for one sport may have no relevance in another sport.[7] Furthermore, it is important for physicians to recognize that time lost from sports participation is often more of a concern to athletes and their coaches than the nature of the injury itself.[7] These perceived differences in injury severity inevitably affect management programs.

Among school athletes, football has the highest rate of injury, with wrestling not far behind.[3] The rate of injury in both males and females at the high school and college levels is comparable, with the exception of knee injuries, which occur at a slightly greater rate in females at the college level.[8] Fortunately, fatal sports injuries are rare. Mueller and Cantu[9] reported 160 nontraumatic deaths in high school and college athletes in the United States between 1983 and 1993, with the primary cause being heart related; only a small number of the injuries were heat related. These investigators also reported 53 traumatic deaths from 1982 to 1992 in football players, resulting primarily from head and neck trauma.[9]

Exercise Physiology

Endurance Training

The increased popularity of endurance sports such as swimming, running, rowing, and cycling among children and adolescents has heightened awareness of aerobic training as a means of maximizing performance.[10,11] The beneficial effect of aerobic training in adults is now well established, with increases in maximal oxygen uptake (VO_2max) of up to 15% to 20% reported in the literature.[11] The ability to enhance the aerobic capacity of children and adolescents through endurance training remains controversial, however, because many of the studies to date have been methodologically flawed and largely neglected adolescents.[10-14]

Although several physiologic parameters may be used to measure aerobic fitness, VO_2max is the most commonly used in studies involving adult endurance.[10,11] The usefulness of this parameter in children has been questioned because most children fail to ever reach the plateau consistent with VO_2max.[10,11] As a result, VO_2max has been replaced with peak VO_2 in pediatric endurance studies, which instead measures the highest VO_2 level achieved prior to the point of voluntary exhaustion.[10,11]

Despite the traditional view that prepubescent children are incapable of improving their aerobic capacity through endurance training, evidence to the contrary is now emerging in the literature.[10,11] A review of 22 studies by Baquet et al.[10] demonstrated that a 5% to 6% increase in peak VO_2 among both children and adolescents is possible with appropriate aerobic training. The ability to achieve these increases is influenced by several factors, including baseline peak VO_2 levels, program design, maturity level, and genetics.[10,11]

The role of pubertal status on a child's ability to enhance aerobic capacity through endurance training remains unclear because of a lack of quality longitudinal data.[10,11] Early research indicated that for the same relative training intensity, greater gains in peak VO_2 were demonstrated for circumpubertal relative to prepubertal subjects.[10,11] Two theories have been used to explain this finding: first, the existence of a so-called *maturational threshold* below which training-induced adaptations in aerobic fitness were physiologically limited, and second, the fact that the greater level of habitual activity among children maintained their VO_2 closer to its maximum potential, making additional increases in peak VO_2 more difficult to achieve.[10,11] Although data are limited, evidence is slowly emerging to contradict these theories as a better understanding is gained of the role of genetic, environmental, and endocrine influences.[10,11,14] High-quality longitudinal studies that document not only chronologic age but also maturity status are essential.[11]

Designing a program that incorporates appropriate levels of training duration, frequency, and intensity is essential to achieving the desired increase in aerobic capacity.[10,11,14] In their literature review, Baquet et al.[10] found that three to four 30- to 60-minute sessions per week was optimal. Interestingly, no clear relationship was found between the length of training program and peak VO_2 improvement.[10] Training intensity is generally defined in terms of the percentage of maximal heart rate.[10,11] Several studies have confirmed that a heart rate that exceeds 80% of maximum is required to obtain significant increases in peak VO_2.[10]

Comparison between continuous and interval training and the effect on peak VO_2 is limited to prepubertal children.[10,14] Nine of the 16 studies reviewed by Baquet et al.[10] demonstrated a significant increase in peak VO_2 after continuous training. However, only 3 of the 16 studies showed improvement when the heart rate was less than or equal to 80% of the maximum.[10] The implementation of continuous training among children poses difficulties with regard to compliance and motivation.[14] Interval training is not only easier to put into practice but has more consistently positive results. Programs that combine continuous and intermittent exercises make interpretation of results difficult.[10]

The increasingly competitive nature of sports has resulted in reluctance by athletes to take adequate breaks from training and performing.[15] The damaging effects of prolonged endurance training on skeletal muscle and function are well documented in the literature, as is the huge capacity of human skeletal muscle for repair and adaptation, given adequate recovery time.[15] A study by Grobler et al.[15] demonstrated that whereas minor exercise-induced muscle damage is a precursor for adaptation, the reparative capacity of skeletal muscle is limited and the cumulative effects of repetitive trauma and injury to skeletal muscle may lead to reduced performance, especially in long-distance runners. Further research is needed to investigate the limits of skeletal muscle regenerative capacity after a chronic injury.[15]

Flexibility

Extremes of joint and ligament laxity have important implications for the pediatric athlete because of the increased risk of both acute traumatic and overuse-type sporting injuries, in addition to a number of degenerative orthopaedic conditions, many of which have long-term implications for sports participation and performance.[16,17]

Childhood is associated with a gradual reduction in flexibility, with the greatest loss occurring around puberty as a result of a growth-induced muscle-tendon imbalance.[18] This loss of flexibility is less pronounced in females.[18] Excessive tightness during this time of rapid growth is thought to play a major role in both acute and overuse-type injuries affecting in particular the lower back, pelvis, and knee.[17] Slight improvements in flexibility are observed after the pubertal growth spurt in both males and females until early adulthood, at which point it plateaus and then starts to decline once again.[18]

Although only 4% to 7% of the general population meets all the criteria for generalized ligament laxity, evaluation of flexibility remains an essential component of the clinical assessment of a young athlete because it enables identification of the persons at increased risk, in addition to providing invaluable information for injury prevention and rehabilitation programs.[17,19] Studies performed by Marshall and colleagues in 1980 demonstrated that increased flexibility was associated with a greater risk of sports-related injuries, particularly in sports requiring rapid change of direction or acceleration.[17]

Although several instrumented tests are available to test the flexibility of individual joints, it is the use of simple screening tests such as the modified Marshall test devised in 1978 that are more commonly used as a routine part of the clinical assessment of the young athlete.[17] By measuring thumb to forearm apposition, the modified Marshall test can quickly identify extremes of flexibility that warrant further, more in-depth investigation and assessment that is relevant to the athlete's given sporting interest.[17]

Strength Training

Traditionally, strength training was discouraged among the pediatric population because of the perceived risk of growth disturbances and other injuries.[16] However, research during the past 20 years has demonstrated that not only can strength training be a safe and effective component of any comprehensive fitness program, but it can also provide clear health benefits to the pediatric age group.[20-23] These benefits include improved athletic performance as a result of increased coordination, muscle strength, and power, in addition to enhancement of long-term health as a result of increased cardiorespiratory fitness, reduced risk of injury, and improved bone mineral density and blood lipid profile.[21,22,24]

Research shows that expertly tailored strength-training programs in children and adolescents are associated with increased muscle strength and performance advantages in sports such as football and weight lifting.[24] Increases in strength of 50% to 65% above baseline have been reported in the prepubescent athlete over a 2- to 3-month training period.[25] In the preadolescent child, however, this increased strength occurs in the absence of muscle hypertrophy, highlighting the role of neurogenic adaptation as the likely cause. Neurogenic adaptation refers to the recruitment of increased motor neurons that can fire with each muscle contraction.[24] Moreover, the loss of benefits after the program is discontinued for 6 weeks provides further evidence for this hypothesis.[22] In contrast, strength training during and after puberty is further enhanced by the hormonally induced increase in muscle growth that occurs in both males and females.[24]

Although the risk of injury associated with strength training is real, research shows that it is no greater than in any other sport when adult supervision is available to ensure use of proper technique and implementation of safety precautions.[22,24] Data obtained by the National Electronic Injury Surveillance System between 1991 and 1996 were used to estimate that strength training was responsible for more than 20,000 injuries annually in the group of athletes who were younger than 21 years.[26] However, the usefulness of these results is limited by the lack of distinction between competitive and recreational injuries or comments regarding the quality of the equipment being used or the presence of adult supervision.[24] Of note, 40% to 70% of the injuries were attributable to muscle strains, primarily within the lumbar area.[24] Case reports indicate that children and adolescents participating in strength training may be at risk of specific lumbar injuries, including herniated intervertebral disks, paraspinous muscle sprains, spondylolisthesis, and pars interarticularis stress fractures.[22]

Thermoregulation and Heat-Related Injuries

Even though heat-related illnesses are preventable,[27] heat stroke remains the third most common cause of exercise-related death among high school athletes in the United States after head injuries and cardiac disorders.[28]

Several physiologic characteristics unique to the pediatric population contribute to the thermoregulatory disadvantage they face in extreme climatic conditions, including increased surface area to body mass ratio, reduced sweating capacity, greater generation of metabolic heat per mass unit, and a slower rate of heat acclimatization.[27,29] A large surface area to body mass ratio is advantageous in mild to moderate climates because of the increased convective surface it provides.[28] In hot, humid weather, however, this large ratio provides a larger area for heat influx, thereby raising the core temperature and increasing the risk of heat-induced illnesses.[28] Conversely, in cold climates, enhanced metabolic heat production and cutaneous vasoconstriction are often insufficient to overcome the heat lost from their vast surface area, particularly in cold water.[30]

Sweat glands play a central role in the pediatric athlete's ability to thermoregulate. By 3 years of age, the number of sweat glands a person shall possess is fixed.[28] Despite having a greater density of sweat glands per skin area than adults, the sweating capacity in children is restricted because of a lower sweating rate and a higher sweating threshold.[31] As a result, the ability of children to dissipate body heat by evaporation is reduced until the transition is made to an adult sweating pattern in late puberty.[27,29]

The reluctance of children to drink while engaging in prolonged exercise further exacerbates this thermoregulatory disadvantage.[32] The American Academy of Pediatrics recommends prehydration in addition to enforced periodic drinking during the course of prolonged exercise.[27,33] Although water is readily available, flavored drinks are often easier for children to tolerate.[27] Moreover, because the risk of dehydration is even greater in children with certain diseases or conditions such as cystic fibrosis, diabetes, and anorexia, the need for optimal fluid intake during exercise is essential.[27]

Psychosocial Aspects of Sports Participation

Psychosocial Development

Participation in sports activity is associated with a large number of health benefits that can influence both physical and psychosocial well-being. The social interaction associated with sports participation is instrumental in a child's psychosocial development, including character development, self-discipline, emotion control, cooperation, empathy, and leadership skills.[31] The acquisition of new skills aids in building confidence and self-esteem.[31] It also allows children to experiment with success and failure in a low-risk environment.[34]

The YRBS study mentioned earlier in this chapter was a nationally representative study conducted throughout the 1990s by the Centers for Disease Control and Prevention. It evaluated the new trends in sports participation with a particular focus on health behaviors.[4] The study revealed a strong positive trend between sports participation and several types of positive health behaviors in white males and females, including consumption of fruit and vegetables as part of a healthy diet, reduced levels of smoking or illegal drug use, and a reduced risk of suicide.[4] This trend was not found among ethnic minorities, however, and among Hispanics and African Americans, the risk of negative health behaviors actually increased with sports participation.[4]

Readiness for Sport

Knowledge of cognitive and motor developmental milestones and the factors that motivate children and adolescents to participate in sports is essential when designing sports activities that are both rewarding and beneficial.[31,34] Motor development is a sequential process like any other developmental milestone, and the rate of progression varies among children.[35] Participation in most sports requires fundamental motor skills such as kicking, throwing, running, jumping, and catching.[35] Most children acquire these skills through informal "play," but mastery often requires more formal instruction and repetition.[35] Although this process of acquisition and mastery can potentially be accelerated through intensive instruction and practice, research shows that it rarely speeds up motor development or leads to enhanced athletic performance.[35]

The principal motivating factors for young children to participate in sports activities are fun and enjoyment.[31] For an activity to be viewed as enjoyable, it must include a certain level of excitement but ultimately a sense of personal achievement associated with the improvement or mastery of specific skills.[31] We must acknowledge that whereas virtually all children have the ability to acquire new motor skills, the ease of acquisition and degree of mastery may vary among children.[34] Research has shown that children who feel less competent with one particular skill are less likely to continue with that sport in the long term.[34] Therefore it is important that young children be exposed to a range of sports that challenge and enable them to acquire a variety of fundamental motor skills.[34]

Progression into adolescence is not only associated with a number of physical changes resulting from the pubertal growth spurt but also a shift in the motivational factors influencing sports participation.[31,34] Cognitive and motor development is now sufficient to allow for the incorporation of strategy into sports such as football or basketball.[35] The need for fun and excitement is overtaken by social factors such as interaction with friends and physical appearance, although mastery of skills remains important.[31,35] Differing rates of progression through puberty can result in inequality within and between genders.[35] Persons who experience earlier growth spurts may be temporarily taller, heavier, and stronger, which often leads to unrealistic expectations because of the erroneous conclusion that they are destined to become better athletes than their less mature peers.[35]

Adult Involvement

The level of adult involvement has increased significantly with the evolution of organized youth sports. Although the traditional role of "supervisor" still exists, the nature of adult involvement in youth sports has also evolved. An increased level of sophistication has developed as a result of the advent of specialized coaches, sports psychologists, nutritionists, and personal trainers, all of which undoubtedly affect the psychosocial development of the young athlete.

Adults are vital for the enforcement of rules and the creation of a safe, controlled environment in which to impart their knowledge and assist children and adolescents in the acquisition of new skills and the development of appropriate attitudes regarding sports.[27,28] However, the involvement of adults in sports activities can also have a detrimental impact on psychosocial development through the expression of negative and unsportsmanlike behavior, negative reinforcement, and the enforcement of demands and expectations that exceed the child's abilities.[31,34]

In the early years of life, parental influence is instrumental in the development of lifelong core values and attitudes.[31] By 12 years of age, a child's attitudes to winning are already well established and often directly reflect the values held by their parents.[31] These values and attitudes are often acquired through observation of parental behavior, and although extreme parental behavior is rare, the use of negative comments or reinforcements is frequent.[31] Variation was found between sporting codes, with the greatest incidence of extreme parental behavior occurring in soccer and rugby.[31] Children of relaxed and supportive parents who positively reinforce their child's performance are not only more self-confident but are more likely to be successful athletes.[31,34]

As the child progresses to adolescence, the role of parents starts to diminish as the role of the coach increases.[31] Through the provision of feedback and reinforcement, coaches have a large impact on the confidence and self-perception of the young athlete.[31]

The increasingly competitive nature of sports has led to a shift in goals that are largely adult-oriented and focus on winning at any cost.[3] Competitive behaviors start to emerge at 3 to 4 years of age, and the potential exists to either enhance or exploit this trait through the use of sports.[31] The danger arises when the demands and expectations placed on young athletes by their parents or coaches exceed their abilities.[31] This phenomenon can result in the development of unhealthy competitive behavior with serious antisocial interpersonal consequences or even problems such as burnout and chronic stress.[31,36]

Nutrition

The nutritional concerns of the pediatric athlete are complex and unique compared with those of their adult counterparts because they involve the interaction between normal growth and development and the optimization of athletic performance.[37,38]

During the 1980s it was erroneously believed that leanness correlated with enhanced athletic performance as a result of studies that demonstrated a positive correlation between running performance and percentage of body fat.[39] Not only is scientific evidence lacking to prove that weight reduction alone improves athletic performance, but in fact deliberate caloric restriction in children and adolescents is likely to have detrimental implications, not only for their athletic performance but also for their growth and development and general health.[39] Unfortunately, these erroneous beliefs are often perpetuated today by coaches who have little or usually no training in nutrition for athletes.[39] The employment of school-based coaches is often dependent on the success of their teams, and controlling an athlete's weight is often the easiest parameter by which a coach can try to ensure athletic success.[39] In fact, by reducing fat in the diet, it is possible that essential sources of protein and minerals and vitamins such as calcium, magnesium iron, zinc, B12, and other fat-soluble vitamins that are critical for growth also may be eliminated from the diet.[38]

Diet should play an integral role in any comprehensive training program, with specific attention to energy requirements, including appropriate combinations of protein, carbohydrates, fat, vitamins, and minerals.[38] These requirements are often subject to large interindividual variation not only between sporting codes but often within a given sport.[38]

Results of the YRBS study in the 1990s confirmed that children and adolescents involved in regular sporting activities not only maintain healthier diets including greater amounts of fruit and vegetables but are often less concerned with caloric intake and energy balance.[4] For young athletes, the energy requirements must be sufficient to ensure normal growth and development but must also provide the additional calories to account for physical training.[38] The recommendations for estimated energy requirements in young athletes set by the Food and Nutrition Board are based on age, height, weight, and physical activity classification.[38]

Protein is an essential part of a young athlete's diet because it is required to build amino acids necessary for the growth and development of lean body mass and healthy bones but also as an alternative to carbohydrates as a source of energy.[38] Research is lacking regarding the recommended daily protein intake for young athletes.[38] Twelve percent to 15% of the dietary energy of adults should come from protein; however, the energy demands of children are greater, especially when they are involved in competitive, intensive training during periods of rapid growth.[38]

Research shows that children and adolescents up to the age of 13 to 15 years have restricted glycolytic capacity, which calls into question the role of high-carbohydrate diets for younger children.[38] Regardless, nutritionists recommend that at least 50% of a young athlete's diet consist of carbohydrate because of the importance of this energy source during high-intensity training.[39] A significant amount of research is needed with regard to the optimal nutrition of the pediatric athlete.

Performance-Enhancing Substances

The use of performance-enhancing substances is increasing among children and adolescents as a result of media exposure, the availability of so-called *natural supplements*, the absence of formal drug testing in schools, and the increasingly competitive nature of youth sports.[40] Pediatric athletes are at high risk because of increased susceptibility to societal pressures at a time where they are often dealing with complex developmental and psychosocial changes.

The term *ergogenic* is derived from the Greek "to make work" and refers to the inherent ability of many substances to enhance athletic power and/or endurance.[40] In many cases, the ergogenic effects of a substance are actually secondary to their intended use.[40] It is therefore essential that physicians dealing with athletes, especially those competing in high-level sports, have a working knowledge of substances that contain ergogenic properties, because inappropriate prescribing/counseling may result in the disqualification of an athlete from a competition.[41]

Anabolic-Androgenic Steroids

Although a wide range of performance-enhancing substances are available in the United States, anabolic-androgenic steroids are by far the most publicized and intensely studied. Anabolic-androgenic steroids are a synthetic analog of the male hormone testosterone, and their use in the pediatric athlete for both performance and enhancement of the physique has been documented in the medical literature for well over 20 years.[40] The use of androgenic steroids is widespread; an estimated 4% to 12% of male adolescents and 0.5% to 2% of female adolescents used anabolic-androgenic steroids in the 1990s even though they were banned by almost every major athletic governing body.[41]

As the name suggests, anabolic-androgenic steroids have both masculinizing and tissue-building effects, and thus when they are used in conjunction with adequate strength training and proper diet, they have the ability to increase muscle size and strength, enabling high-intensity workouts and possibly even a reduced recovery time after workouts.[40] As a result, athletes who are attracted to the substance tend to be those whose sport requires strength (such as weight lifters, throwers, and football players) or frequent, high-intensity workouts (such as swimmers and runners).[40]

Research conducted by Kindlundh et al.[41] in 1999 demonstrated a significant correlation between the use of anabolic-androgenic steroids in adolescents and the abuse of other common drugs such as alcohol, tobacco, cannabis, and opioids.

Although the perceived performance-enhancing benefits appear high, the adverse effects of using anabolic-androgenic steroids are extensive and often irreversible.[40] In addition to the personality changes and psychological problems that are associated with steroid use, premature closure of epiphyseal plates with subsequent linear growth arrest, irreversible alopecia, gynecomastia, and acne and irreversible masculinization of secondary sexual characteristics in females are just a few of the more dramatic and often psychologically devastating adverse effects of anabolic-androgenic steroids.[40,42]

Regulation of Performance-Enhancing Substances

Drug testing is both time consuming and expensive, making the widespread testing of young athletes virtually impossible.[32] Nonetheless, many schools and youth organizations have implemented voluntary drug testing, which has a dual benefit of identifying and providing assistance for athletes with abuse problems and reducing the peer pressure to use drugs.[30]

With the introduction of the Dietary Supplement Health and Education Act in 1994, the role of the Food and Drug Administration in regulating "natural supplements" was eliminated.[15] Since that time, "natural agents" such as creatinine, androstenedione, and dehydroepiandrosterone (DHEA) have been widely accessible via health stores and the Internet.[15] This accessibility results in an erroneous perception that these substances are "safe," even though the absence of regulatory control eliminates any legal requirement of manufacturers to declare all active ingredients and potential interactions and fully test their products for short- and long-term effects.[30]

The use of performance-enhancing drugs among athletes of any age is unethical, unhealthy, and potentially life-threatening.[32] As physicians we have a responsibility to acquire and impart factual knowledge to young athletes who are contemplating the use of these substances. Although the effectiveness of using scare tactics that emphasize the negative effects of substance use has been questioned, a clear role exists for positive counseling with regard to healthy alternatives such as strength training and conditioning, nutrition, and skill acquisition through coaching and camps.[32]

Arthroscopy in Children

The use of arthroscopy in the pediatric and adolescent population has dramatically expanded during the past decade as a result of increased youth participation in sport and the subsequent rise in sports-related injuries.[6] With the advent of smaller, more sophisticated arthroscopic instruments during the past decade, the major obstacle to the application of arthroscopy in children was overcome.[6] In fact, after extensive experience, Gross[43] noted that despite the difference in joint size, basic techniques of arthroscopy are largely the same in both children and adults. At present, arthroscopy is indicated in the management of several shoulder, elbow, wrist, hip, knee, and ankle injuries within the pediatric population.[6] Advantages of arthroscopy in this population include reduced postoperative morbidity, smaller incisions, more rapid return to activities, decreased inflammatory response, and improved visualization of joint structures.[6]

Shoulder injuries in the pediatric athlete include acute fractures, overuse injuries such as Little League shoulder (Fig. 129-1), and shoulder instability (Fig. 129-2). Most major shoulder injuries requiring arthroscopy are related to instability and can be divided into two descriptive groups: traumatic anterior instability and multidirectional instability.[4,6,38-41,43-51]

The incidence of elbow injuries continues to increase as a result of the growing popularity of youth sports. Many of the elbow injuries are repetitive, overuse-type injuries, such as osteochondritis dissecans (OCD), which is prevalent in athletes who participate in baseball, racket sports, and gymnastics.[52] In fact, "Little League elbow" is now an accepted term for a common overuse injury in young throwing athletes, with etiologies including a fragmented medial epicondyle (Fig. 129-3), OCD (Figs. 129-4 and 129-5), ulnar hypertrophy, and medial epicondylitis.[49,52-54]

Wrist arthroscopy is not a commonly practiced treatment modality among pediatric and adolescent patients because many injuries achieve successful healing nonoperatively and because of the restricted size of the joint space.[54] Kocher et al.[55] noted an increasing incidence of repetitive use–type injuries such as triangular fibrocartilage injuries (Fig. 129-6), and they believe that arthroscopy is indicated for debridement or determination of the extent of ligamentous injury in patients who fail to respond to nonoperative therapies.[55,56]

Although hip arthroscopy is a commonly used diagnostic and treatment modality for pathologic conditions of the hip

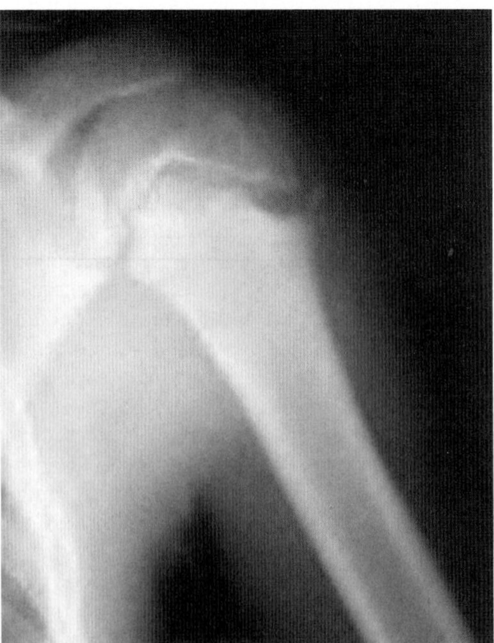

FIGURE 129-1 An example of "Little League shoulder," which is associated with widening of the proximal humeral physis as a result of repetitive overuse.

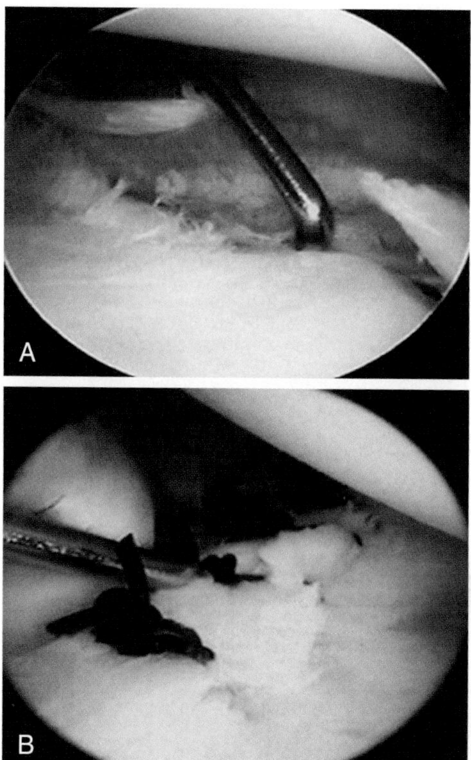

FIGURE 129-2 Traumatic anterior shoulder instability. A, Bankart lesion. B, Repair of a Bankart lesion.

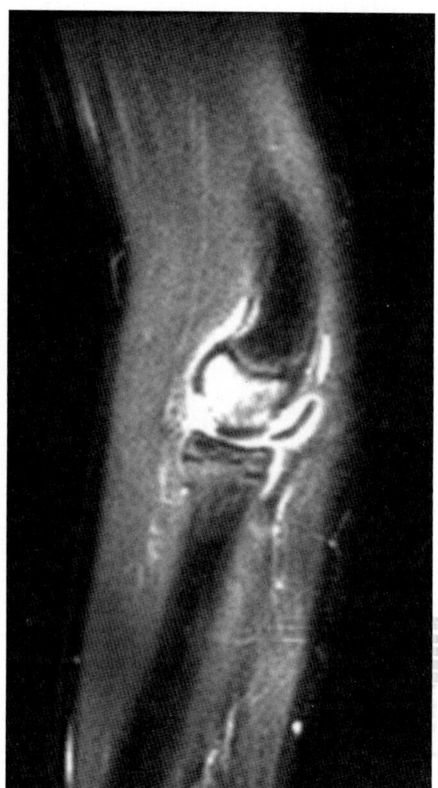

FIGURE 129-4 A sagittal magnetic resonance imaging scan of the elbow demonstrating a chondral defect of the capitellum associated with osteochondritis dissecans.

in the adult population, its application in the pediatric population is just beginning to increase. Indications in the pediatric population include isolated labral tears (Fig. 129-7), loose bodies, chondral injuries, and internal derangement associated with Perthes disease and epiphyseal dysplasias.[57-60] The risk of complications, although small, does exist and includes pudendal nerve irritation and recurrent injury.[6]

Currently the largest application of arthroscopy in the pediatric and adolescent population is in the treatment of knee disease and is directly attributable to increased athletic activity.[43] Key indications for knee arthroscopy include OCD (Figs. 129-8 and 129-9), discoid meniscus, tibial spine fractures (Figs. 129-10 and 129-11), and partial and complete anterior cruciate ligament tears.[61-69]

At present, the use of ankle arthroscopy in the pediatric population is restricted to a small number of

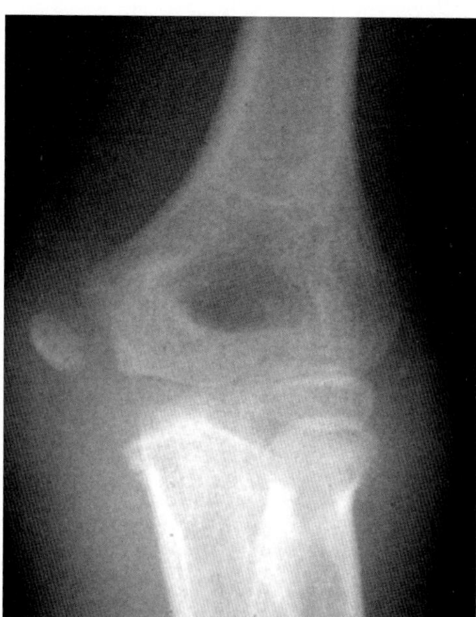

FIGURE 129-3 Medial epicondyle widening associated with "Little League elbow."

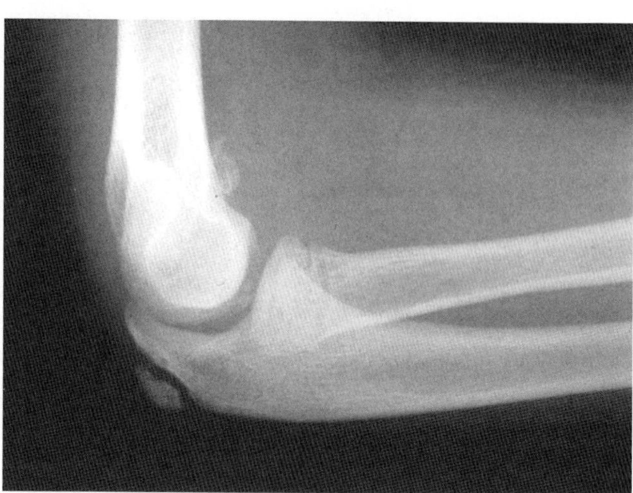

FIGURE 129-5 A lateral radiograph of the elbow demonstrating a loose body in the anterior elbow.

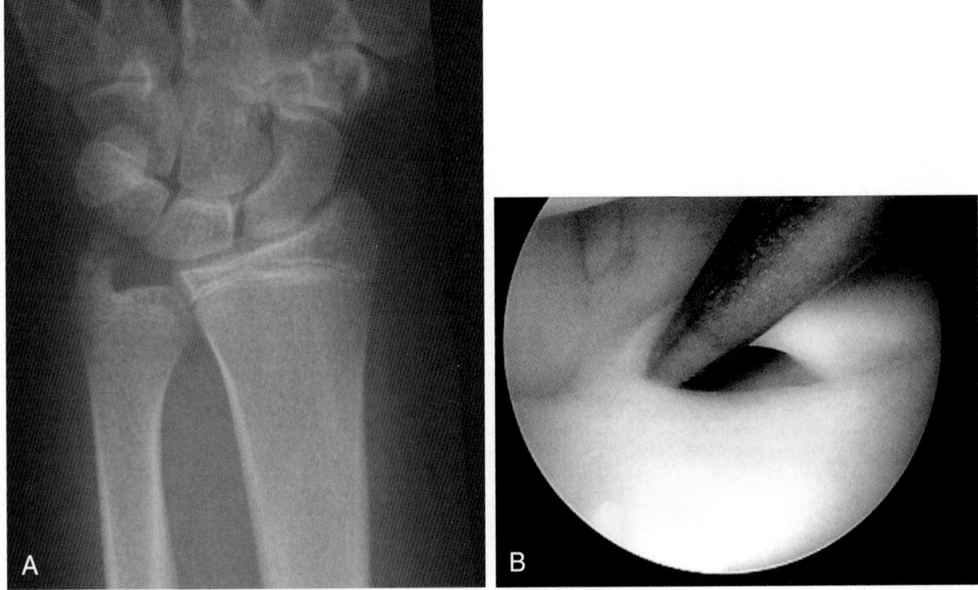

FIGURE 129-6 An ulnar styloid fracture (**A**) associated with a triangular fibrocartilage tear (**B**).

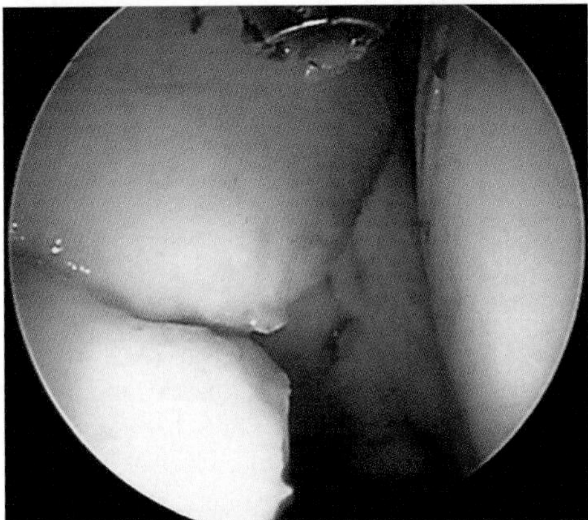

FIGURE 129-7 A radial labral tear of the hip.

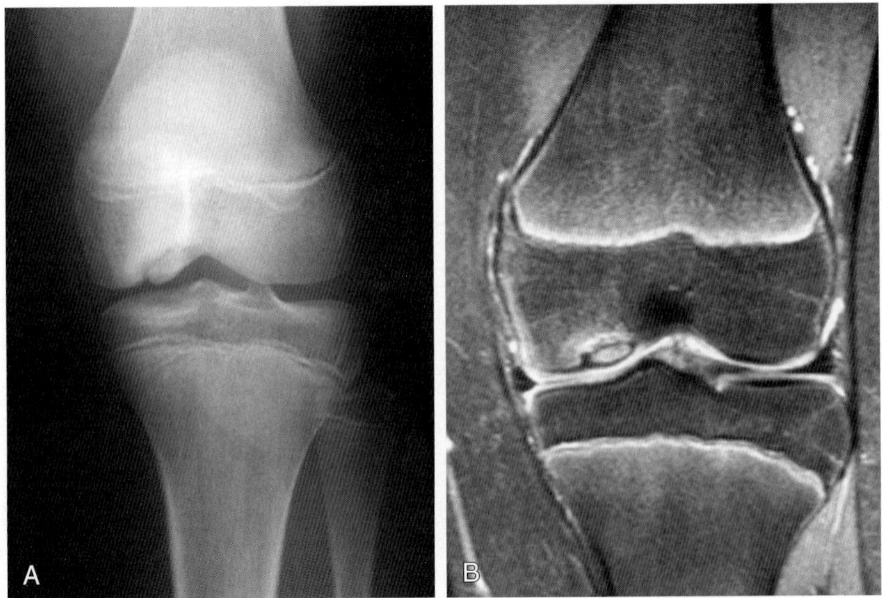

FIGURE 129-8 Osteochondritis dissecans of the knee. **A,** An anteroposterior radiograph. **B,** A corresponding coronal magnetic resonance image.

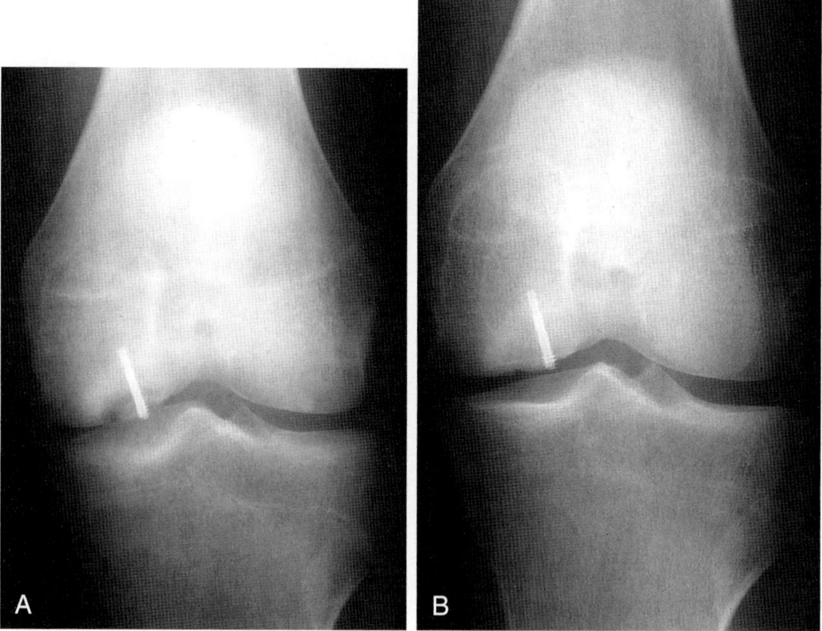

FIGURE 129-9 Fixation of an unstable osteochondritis dissecans lesion of the knee. **A,** An anteroposterior radiograph obtained immediately after the operation. **B,** A radiograph obtained 3 months after the operation demonstrating healing of the lesion.

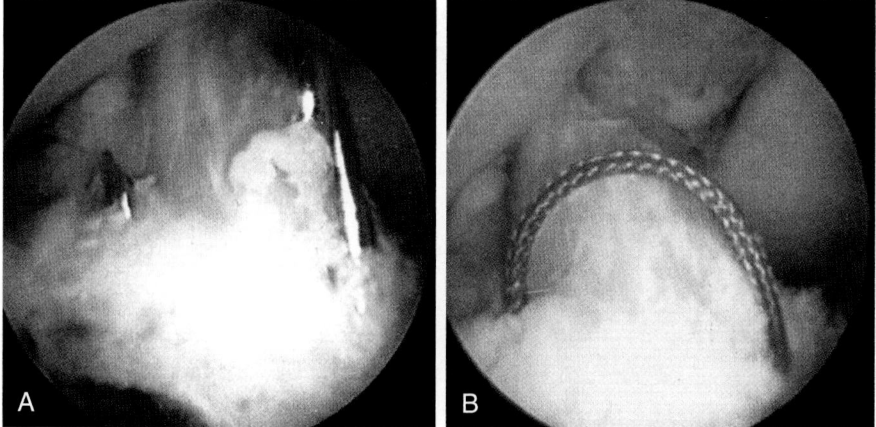

FIGURE 129-10 Suture fixation of a tibial spine fracture. **A,** Guide wires brought through the tibial spine fragment. **B,** Suture fixation.

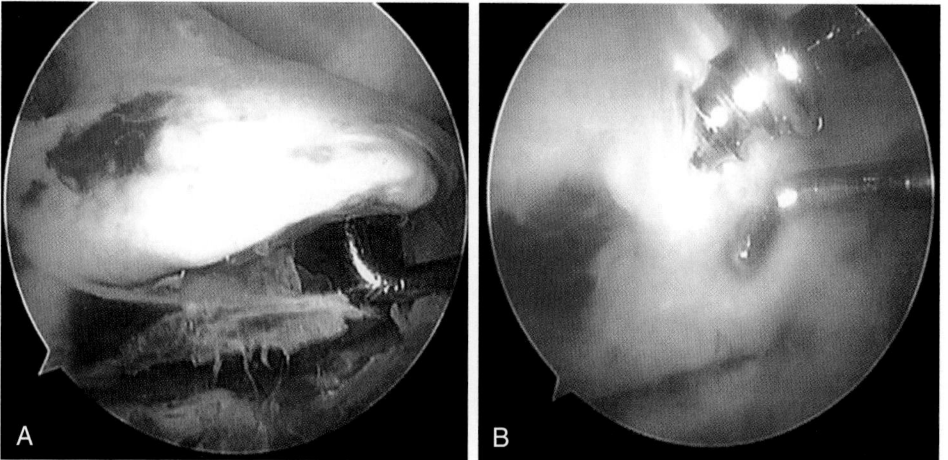

FIGURE 129-11 Epiphyseal cannulated screw fixation of a tibial spine fracture. **A,** A displaced fracture. **B,** Screw fixation.

conditions including OCD, loose body removal, and triplane fracture repair because of technical challenges resulting from the size of the joint and the risk of neurovascular damage.[43,70-73]

Conclusions

Pediatric sports injuries are being seen with increased frequency. Just as the child is not a "little adult," the pediatric athlete is not a "little adult athlete." An understanding of the unique considerations of the pediatric athlete with respect to epidemiologic factors, endurance, flexibility, strength, thermoregulation, psychology, and nutrition is important background knowledge. Recognition of common injury patterns of the shoulder, elbow, wrist, hip, knee, and ankle is essential to effective management.

For a complete list of references, go to expertconsult.com.

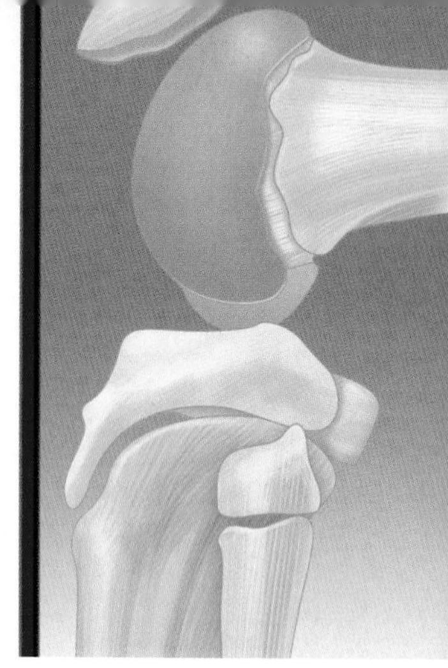

130

Imaging Considerations in the Skeletally Immature Patient

JOHN P. CLEMENT

Sports-related injuries in the pediatric population have increased in incidence during the past decade as a result of both an increasing number of children engaged in sports and the intensity of their activity. Traumatic injuries remain common, and overuse and stress-related injuries have become more frequent, even appearing in toddlers. Although many of these conditions mimic their adult counterparts, several considerations unique to immature skeletons influence both imaging diagnoses and subsequent therapies. Nontraumatic entities such as tumors, infections, and developmental variations may also be a source of symptoms. This chapter discusses various imaging modalities and their implementation in imaging the skeletally immature athlete. Several common normal skeletal variations are also presented, as well as traumatic and pathologic processes particular to the pediatric patient.

Skeletal Maturation

Bone develops by either intramembranous mesenchymal ossification or by endochondral ossification. Intramembranous ossification is a process by which primitive mesenchymal cells directly differentiate into membranous bone, and it is responsible for the development of such bones as the skull, clavicle, and facial bones. Endochondral ossification reflects a process by which the bones are first cartilaginous and then are transformed into bone. The long bones, vertebrae, and skull base are formed by the process of endochondral ossification. Skeletal maturation proceeds in a fairly predictable manner, with ossification centers appearing in their cartilaginous precursors in a relatively defined sequence.[1] The process may be delayed or accelerated in some children. Radiographs of the hand and wrist are often used to evaluate the bone age of a patient through comparison of the ossification centers with compiled female and male standards.[2] Epiphyseal and apophyseal ossification centers have variable appearances depending on the particular bone and the degree of ossification. Ossification centers may appear fragmented or sclerotic and may be mistaken for pathologic processes (Fig. 130-1). Comparison with atlases of normal developmental variants or the opposite extremity often resolves confusion.

Developing long bones have four discrete parts defined by their location with respect to the physis, or growth plate. The epiphysis and metaphysis flank the growth plate, whereas the diaphysis comprises the shaft of the bone, merging into the metaphysis in a region termed the metadiaphysis. Short tubular bones have a physis on only one side of the bone, at the site of greatest joint motion. Apophyses are ossification centers protruding from a bone; they do not articulate with a movable joint and therefore do not contribute to linear bone growth. They often comprise ligament and tendon attachment sites to bone (Fig. 130-2). The primary ossification center is the first to form, usually in the diaphysis of the chondral precursor. Early diaphyseal ossification occurs around the main diaphyseal nutrient vessel, which splits and extends toward the metaphyses. The secondary ossification centers form in the epiphyses and appear in a predictable pattern. Their formation is triggered by the invasion of juxtaarticular blood vessels. During the first 18 months of life, an anastomotic communication of vessels occurs across the physis, allowing processes such as infection or tumor to readily cross. From 18 months until physeal closure, these anastomoses do not exist, and the physis serves as a relative barrier to further extension of metaphyseal or epiphyseal pathologic processes.[3]

The physis is the growth center of long bones and is responsible for bone lengthening. It is composed of parallel columns of chondrocytes in various stages of differentiation into bone. The chondrocytes divide in the germinal zone, along the epiphyseal side of the physis. They continue to grow in the adjacent proliferative zone and further swell in size in the hypertrophic zone. These cells give rise to the cartilage matrix that eventually ossifies by the process of endochondral ossification within the zone of provisional calcification. Ossification subsequently occurs along the metaphyseal portion of the physis. As skeletal maturity evolves, the physis become thinner with a mild degree of irregularity, finally closing as the bone reaches maturity. Bone widening occurs through osteogenic activity of the surface periosteum.

The physis, specifically the junction of the metaphyseal bone with the physeal cartilage, is the weakest element of growing bone. Additionally, the diaphyseal cortex is relatively thick and strong, whereas the metaphyseal cortex is comparably weaker. Fractures therefore often occur at the metaphyseal-physeal junction. The perichondrium is a ring of tissue that is tightly attached to the bone at this location. In contrast, the periosteum enveloping the diaphyseal cortex is loosely attached. Subperiosteal processes (e.g., infection, hematoma, or tumor) may extend up the diaphysis by elevating this loosely attached periosteum (Fig. 130-3). However,

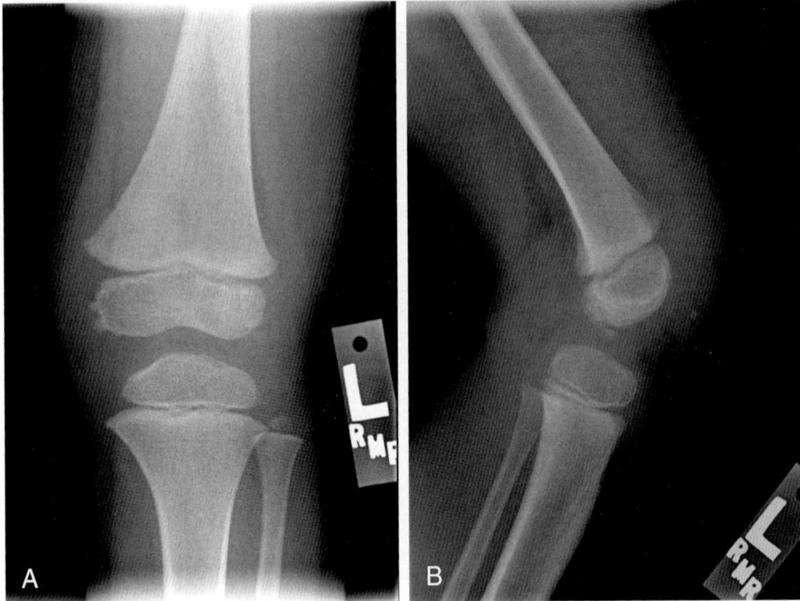

FIGURE 130-1 Normal knee epiphyseal ossification. Radiographs of the left knee in the anteroposterior (**A**) and lateral (**B**) projections demonstrate a fragmented and irregular appearance to the medial aspect of the distal femoral epiphyseal ossification center. This variation is normal and should not be mistaken for a fracture or reactive bone formation.

the perichondrium provides a relative barrier to further extension into the joint.

Imaging Considerations

Imaging in the pediatric patient presents challenges that are infrequently encountered in the adult patient. The foremost challenge is that patients often are not cooperative, which manifests as motion that not only degrades image quality but also may lead to a completely nondiagnostic examination. In the worst-case scenario, motion artifact may result in an erroneous diagnosis. Additionally, some examinations require injection of contrast material that may introduce discomfort, leading to motion. Sedation is often required in younger patients to obtain images of an adequate quality, usually in the setting of examinations of a longer duration, such as magnetic resonance imaging (MRI). Radiographs and computed tomographic (CT) examinations can usually be performed without sedation, although some views may need to be repeated. The rapidity of image acquisition afforded by multidetector CT scanners has diminished the need for sedation during CT examinations.[4]

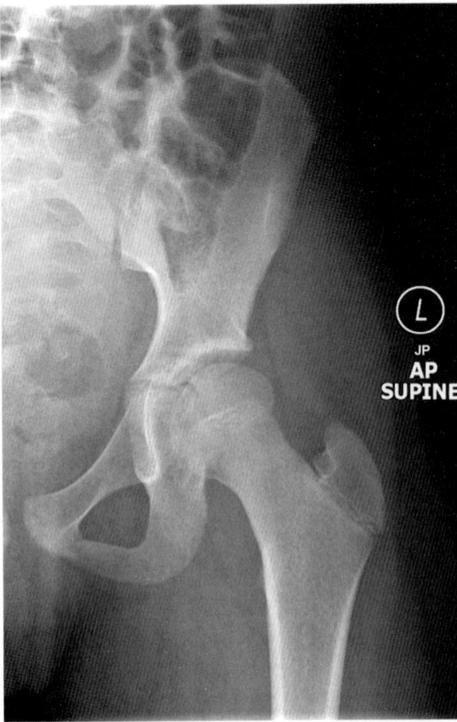

FIGURE 130-2 A supine anteroposterior radiograph of the left hip demonstrates the normal greater trochanteric apophysis with physeal radiolucent cartilage separating it from the subjacent intertrochanteric femur.

A second feature of pediatric imaging that is often overlooked is the size of the anatomy being imaged. For example, a child's knee is much smaller than the knee of an adult. Spatial resolution in radiography, CT, nuclear medicine, and MRI is relatively maximized and cannot be increased further when applied to smaller pediatric anatomy. Therefore, by definition, the detail of a particular anatomic structure is less well visualized in the pediatric patient compared with the adult patient. Magnification makes anatomy look bigger but does not add any increase in the underlying spatial resolution. This phenomenon is especially relevant in MRI, in which motion combined with the small size of the underlying anatomy often leads to interpretative challenges.

A final consideration in pediatric imaging is radiation dose. Adequate genital shielding should be provided for all patients undergoing radiographic and CT examinations. With radiography in children, dosages are decreased as dictated by the parameters used to obtain the radiographic images. With CT, however, incorrect imaging parameters generate examinations that are perfectly diagnostic but may impose substantial patient radiation dosages. Imaging facilities should be familiar with pediatric CT protocols designed to minimize patient

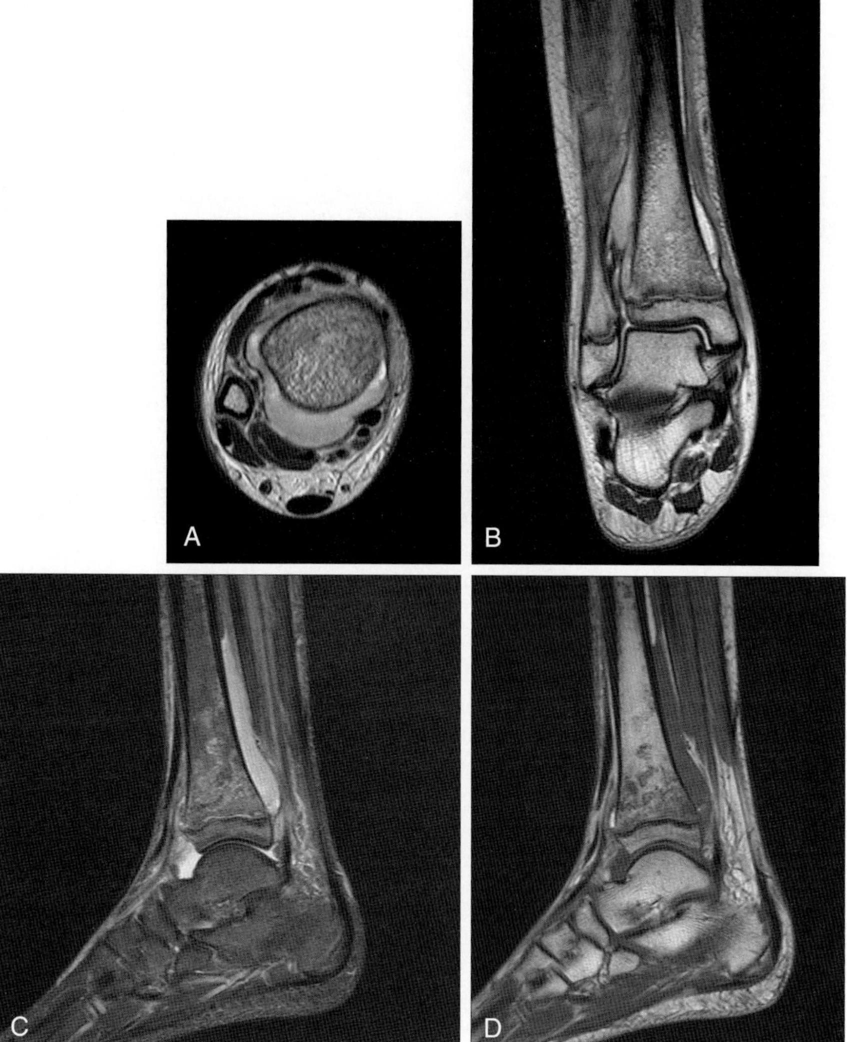

FIGURE 130-3 A subperiosteal abscess. Axial (**A**) and coronal (**B**) T2-weighted magnetic resonance images of the ankle demonstrate a T2-weighted bright subperiosteal fluid collection extending nearly circumferentially about the metadiaphyseal region of the distal tibia. The fluid collection extends to the physis but not beyond it, which is also seen in the T2-weighted fat-saturated sagittal magnetic resonance image (**C**). The abscess is the result of distal tibial metaphyseal osteomyelitis as evidenced by an abnormal signal in the marrow, a high signal on the T2-weighted fat-saturated image, and heterogeneously low signal on the T1-weighted sagittal magnetic resonance image (**D**).

dosage yet provide adequate diagnostic images.[5] As an ordering physician, it is imperative to consider as many diagnostic scenarios as possible so that the appropriate imaging procedure may be performed, decreasing the need for further imaging and an additive radiation dose. The radiologist is at your service in this regard.

Imaging Techniques

Radiography

Conventional radiography remains the mainstay for the initial evaluation of musculoskeletal processes in the pediatric patient. As with adult radiography, two orthogonal views of any anatomic location are required for adequate assessment. Occasionally, comparison views of the opposite extremity are obtained to differentiate a suspected abnormality from a normal or developmental variation.[6] In some cases this comparison may be achieved with a single view. Motion may occasionally interfere with image quality either by blurring the image or by leading to suboptimal positioning for assessment of a particular anatomic structure. The technologist should review all images for adequacy and perform repeat scans as necessary. Optimally, this review is performed in conjunction with the interpreting physician so that repeat or comparison views may be obtained expeditiously.

Computed Tomography

CT is performed to provide a more detailed anatomic assessment of soft tissue and osseous injuries. It is often used in preoperative and postoperative fracture assessment to evaluate intraarticular extension, alignment, and healing. Two-dimensional reformations and three-dimensional reconstructions often provide superior visualization of injuries (Fig. 130-4). With current-generation multidetector scanners,

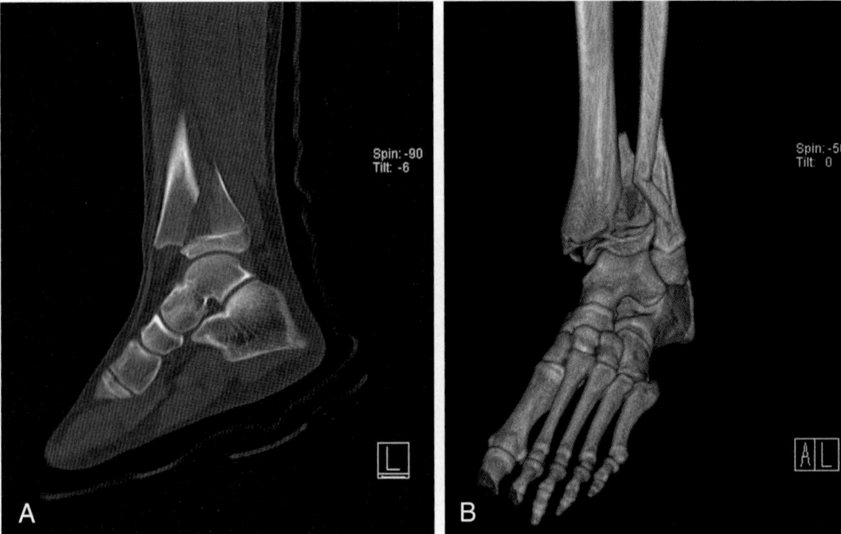

FIGURE 130-4 A triplane fracture with three-dimensional reconstructions. **A,** A sagittal reformatted computed tomographic image of the left ankle demonstrates a displaced triplane fracture. **B,** A three-dimensional reconstruction of the same ankle allows better visualization of fragment relationships. An angulated elongated fracture to the left distal fibula is also evident.

sedation is rarely needed. CT is also commonly used in the assessment of bone lesions because it permits visualization of the internal architecture of the lesion, often leading to a definitive diagnosis.[7] CT may also be used to guide a biopsy of such lesions.

Magnetic Resonance Imaging

As in adults, MRI provides superb soft tissue contrast resolution in children. It is an excellent modality for imaging bone marrow, joints, cartilage, tendons, and soft tissues. Unfortunately, MRI requires a relatively long period for image acquisition. Cooperative patients can often undergo imaging without intravenous sedation, but younger patients may require medicinal assistance to remain still for adequate imaging.

Ultrasonography

Musculoskeletal ultrasonography is used for select purposes in the pediatric patient. It is an excellent modality for visualizing nonmineralized structures. It is most commonly used in the assessment of the neonatal hip (Fig. 130-5). Other uses include the assessment of large tendons and soft tissue masses, as well as determining the presence or absence of joint effusions. As in adult patients, ultrasound may be used to guide aspiration, injection, or biopsy of soft tissue pathologic entities in children.

Scintigraphy

Bone scintigraphy is performed with technicium-99m methylene diphosphonate. Pediatric scans are performed in a similar fashion as adult scans. Immediate flow, blood pool, and delayed-phase images may be obtained. Additionally, single photon emission CT images may also be acquired. Single photon emission CT images are especially useful in the evaluation of the pediatric spine for the presence of occult pars stress fractures.[8] Compared with adult bone scans, pediatric bone scans are typically more difficult to interpret. First, spatial resolution is diminished because of the smaller size of the imaged structures, although this diminishment does not usually produce significant difficulties with diagnosis. Second, the physeal growth centers are quite metabolically active and take up a tremendous amount of radiotracer (Fig. 130-6), and thus pathologic processes (e.g., fractures, tumors, and infection) in close proximity to an active physis may be obscured. Spot images may be acquired in select cases to distinguish periphyseal pathologic processes from activity in the adjacent physis.

Imaging of Specific Structures

Bone

Cortical bone appears similar on both pediatric and adult imaging studies, including radiography, CT, and MRI, with the only difference being the relatively thinner appearance of

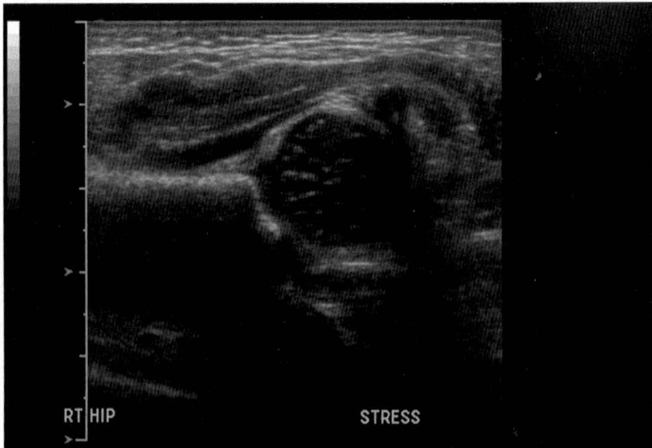

FIGURE 130-5 An ultrasound image of a neonatal hip. A coronal ultrasound view of the left hip demonstrates the cartilaginous femoral head that appears stippled and lies within the acetabulum with normal coverage of the femoral head.

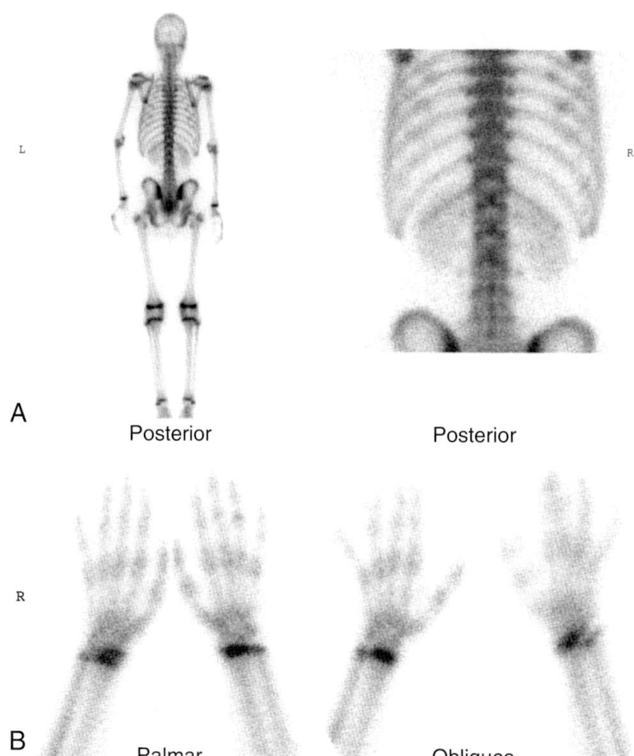

FIGURE 130-6 A normal pediatric bone scan. **A,** A whole-body bone scan in a 13-year-old boy shows physiologic uptake throughout the skeleton. Normal physeal uptake is present, seen particularly in the areas of the knees, ankles, and wrists. **B,** Bone scintigraphic spot images of the hands in the same patient show normal uptake in the distal radial and ulnar growth plates.

pediatric bone. On the other hand, medullary bone has a different appearance in the pediatric skeleton compared with the adult skeleton. Although the medullary bone itself is quite similar, the bone marrow it contains is quite different. Pediatric patients have a pattern of red and white marrow distribution that evolves with age and is different than in the adult patient.[9] Although it is indistinguishable on radiography, CT and MRI are both capable of differentiating red and yellow marrow, with MRI proving far superior. On MRI, fatty marrow is bright on T1-weighted images with an intermediate signal on T2-weighted images. It has low signal on fat-suppressed images. Red marrow is of intermediate to low in signal intensity on T1- and T2-weighted images.

At birth, nearly the entire osseous skeleton is composed of red marrow. When epiphyses and apophyses ossify, they contain red marrow only transiently before converting to yellow marrow. Conversion from red to yellow marrow proceeds from the extremities to the axial skeleton, beginning in the distal bones of the hands and feet and proceeding proximally in a relatively symmetric manner. Within a long bone itself, epiphyses and apophyses initially convert, followed by the center of the diaphysis, distal metaphysis, and finally the proximal metaphysis. If the patient has an increased demand for hematopoiesis (e.g., in persons with chronic anemia and leukemia), reconversion may also occur. Reconversion generally proceeds in the reverse pattern of conversion. Natural variations in red and yellow marrow distribution occur from patient to patient. Small differences are normal, but significant asymmetries are worrisome for an underlying marrow infiltrative process.

The appearance of the physis varies depending on the age of the patient, the specific bone imaged, and the imaging modality used. With radiography, the physis appears as an area of transverse lucency at the junction of the metaphysis and epiphysis. If the epiphysis has not yet ossified, it is not defined as a discrete linear structure, but rather merges with the epiphyseal cartilage. The physis may be wide, narrow, smooth, or irregular, depending on the specific bone imaged (Fig. 130-7). Comparison views may be helpful in difficult cases. With age, the physis gradually narrows, finally disappearing in the mature skeleton. With CT, the physis has a similar appearance to that seen radiographically. Using two-dimensional reformations, CT affords a more detailed examination of the structure of the physis.

MRI demonstrates the cartilaginous physis, as well as the adjacent metaphysis and epiphysis. The physis typically has a high signal on fat-suppressed T2-weighted images and proton density images, reflecting the water content of the physeal cartilage. It is higher in signal than adjacent epiphyseal cartilage (Fig. 130-8). As the physis matures, the high signal thins as the thickness of cartilage within the physis decreases. As described earlier, scintigraphy demonstrates intense radiotracer uptake at the physis proportional to its osteoblastic activity. Maturing physes demonstrate proportionately less activity, whereas the closed and fused growth plate is quiescent.

Cartilage

Normal cartilage has soft tissue attenuation on imaging in both the pediatric and adult patient. It is not readily visualized on either radiographs or CT scans. Loss of cartilage can be inferred by the assessment of relative joint space narrowing. Cartilage can be visualized on ultrasound. It is typically hypoechoic with through transmission of the ultrasound beam. In young pediatric patients who have large unossified cartilage structures such as the femoral or humeral heads, bright specular reflectors within the cartilage correspond to vascular channels. Ultrasound is often used in the evaluation of developmental dysplasia of the neonatal hip.[10]

As in the adult, cartilage is best visualized with use of MRI techniques in children. Cartilage is uniformly hypointense on T1-weighted images and intermediate in signal on T2-weighted fat-saturated images. T2-weighted images provide excellent contrast of cartilage with adjacent high-signal joint fluid and low-signal subchondral bone. High-field magnets permit greater spatial resolution and therefore better morphologic assessment of cartilage integrity. Growth plate cartilage typically has a higher signal on T2-weighted images compared with epiphyseal cartilage.[11]

Hyaline cartilage and epiphyseal unossified cartilage do not demonstrate increased uptake on radionuclide bone scans. However, the growth plates along epiphyseal and apophyseal growth centers demonstrate intense radiotracer uptake.

Soft Tissues

The appearance of soft tissues in the pediatric musculoskeletal system is similar to that of their adult counterparts across imaging modalities. These tissues include tendons, ligaments,

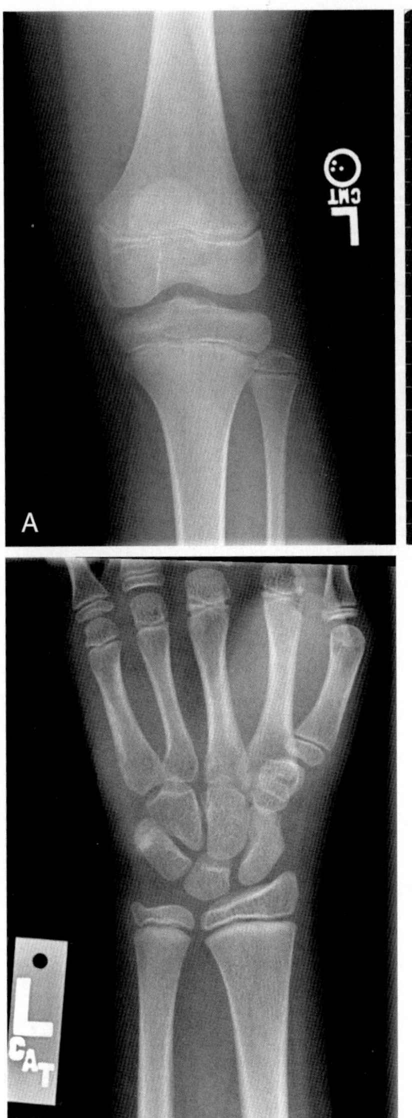

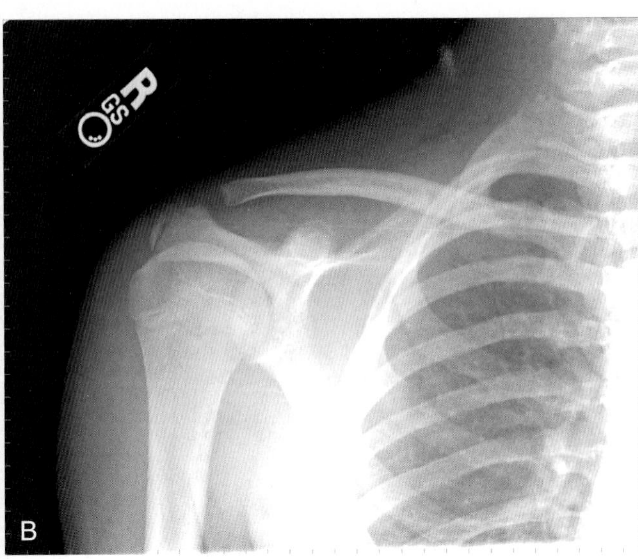

FIGURE 130-7 Normal growth plates. **A,** An anteroposterior radiograph of the knee shows a normal lucent appearance of the distal femoral, proximal tibial, and proximal fibular growth plates in a 12-year-old girl. **B,** An anteroposterior internal rotation view of the right shoulder shows a normal appearance of the growth plates of the tip of the acromion and the tip of the coracoid, as well as the proximal humerus. In internal rotation, the proximal humerus demonstrates a double lucency that should not be mistaken for fracture. **C,** An anteroposterior view of the left hand shows normal distal radial and ulnar physes. Additionally, growth plates along the distal aspect of the metacarpals are also well visualized. The lack of a growth plate along the proximal aspect of the second to fifth metacarpals is normal. The proximal aspect of the first metacarpal, adjacent to a quite mobile joint, has its own growth plate.

menisci, labra, bursae, and muscles. For the most part, all of these structures are best visualized using the multiplanar capabilities and excellent soft tissue contrast afforded by MRI techniques. Ultrasound is often useful in the differentiation of solid and cystic mass lesions and is occasionally used in the assessment of tendons of the extremities.

Imaging Musculoskeletal Processes

Trauma

In the pediatric patient, both soft tissue and osseous injuries are common. Diagnosis of fractures in the child is more difficult because of the smaller size of the bones, the presence of the radiolucent growth plate, and the variable amounts of epiphyseal ossification. MRI often provides significantly more information with respect to the extent of a childhood fracture compared with plain film radiography (Fig. 130-9). The pattern of fracture in the child depends on the stage of skeletal maturation. Compared with the adult skeleton, pediatric bone is more pliable and may actually bend without completely fracturing. This phenomenon is more commonly seen in infants and toddlers.

As a general rule, childhood fractures heal more quickly than their adult counterparts, and nonunions are infrequent. The periosteum and endosteum are capable of exuberant callus formation, much more so than in the adult patient. Fracture healing also occurs in the setting of the constantly remodeling and growing pediatric bone, which may lead to alterations of growth that eventually manifest as a bone deformity. Compared with fractures in adults, fractures in children are capable of greater bony remodeling after healing, leading to correction of significant angular deformities and fragment offset. Angular deformities are more readily remodeled and corrected in the plane of adjacent joints as opposed to perpendicular to those joints.

Incomplete fractures are common in young children, reflecting the pliable nature of their bone structure. A bowing fracture reflects a bend in the bone without a cortical break. A greenstick fracture is an incomplete fracture with a cortical

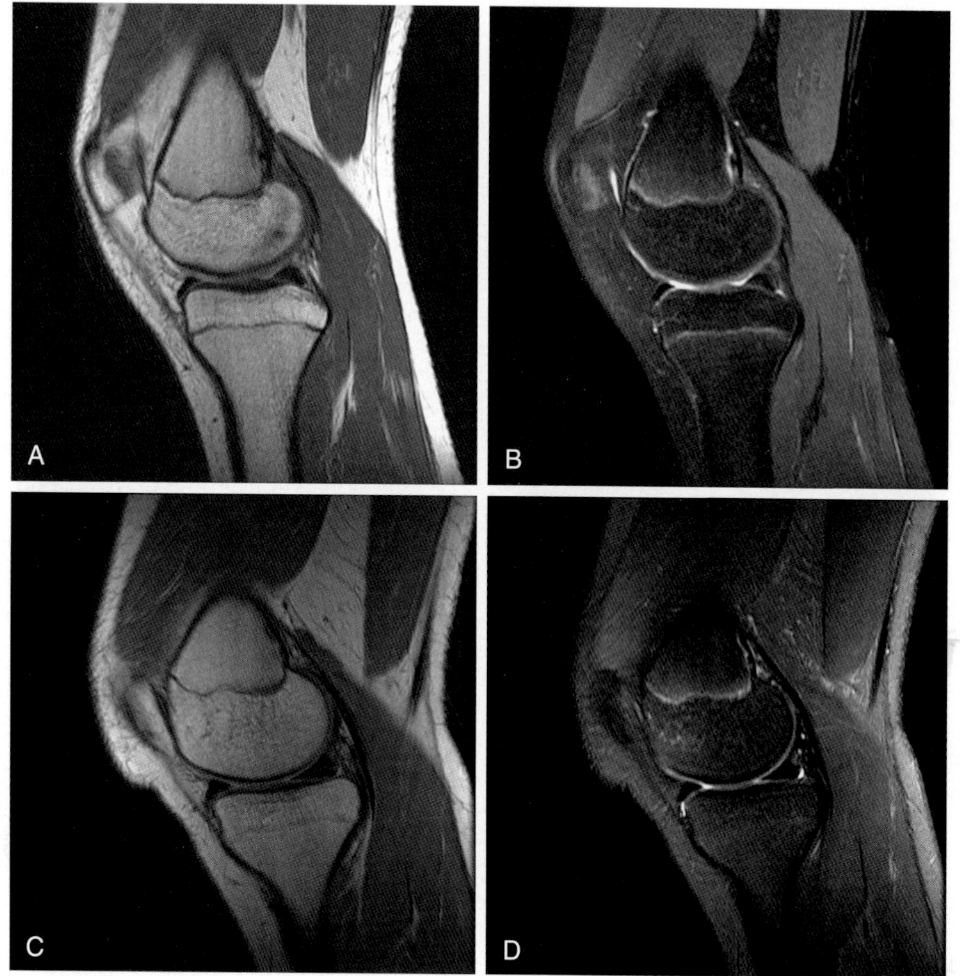

FIGURE 130-8 Magnetic resonance imaging of normal physis. **A** and **B,** Sagittal T1-weighted and fat-saturated T2-weighted magnetic resonance images of the knee in a 14-year-old girl demonstrate a normal appearance to the distal femoral and proximal tibial physeal cartilage. Nonossified cartilage has low signal on T1-weighted images and a high signal on the T2-weighted images. The tibial physis is slightly thinner than the femoral physis. **C** and **D,** Sagittal T1-weighted and fat-saturated T2-weighted magnetic resonance images of the same knee obtained 2 years later demonstrate progressive physeal closure. The tibial physis has completely closed, whereas the femoral physis remains open, although it is thinner than its appearance in **B**.

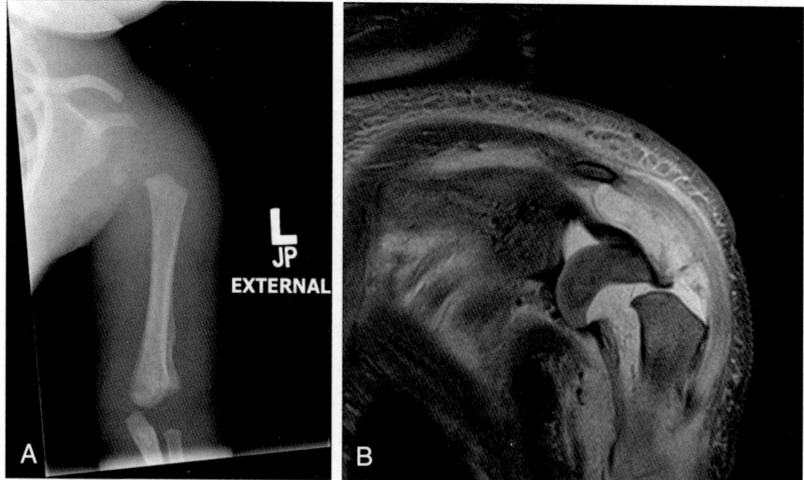

FIGURE 130-9 A displaced Salter-Harris type I fracture. **A,** An anteroposterior externally rotated image of the left shoulder demonstrates abnormal alignment of the proximal humeral ossification center with the humeral metaphysis without acute fracture. Diffuse soft tissue swelling is present. The periosteal reaction in the distal humerus is the result of a subacute healing fracture in this patient, who experienced recurrent episodes of child abuse. **B,** A coronal T2-weighted fat-saturated magnetic resonance image of the same shoulder demonstrates a medially displaced epiphysis consistent with a displaced Salter-Harris type I fracture. The periosteum is stripped from the medial aspect of the proximal humeral shaft, and a large joint effusion and soft tissue swelling are present.

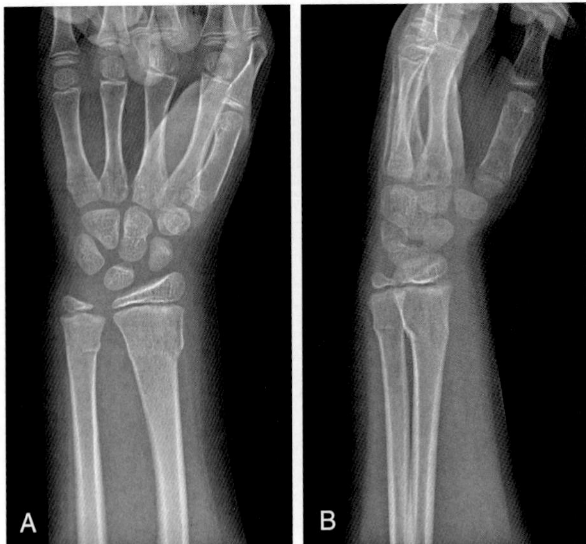

FIGURE 130-10 A buckle fracture of the radius and ulna. Anteroposterior (**A**) and lateral (**B**) radiographic images of the left wrist and distal forearm demonstrate buckle fractures to the distal radius and ulna with minimal angulation. Diffuse soft tissue swelling is present.

break along the tensile (convex) side of the cortex but not on the compressive (concave) side. If the site of cortical failure occurs along the compressive side of the bone, a buckle fracture occurs, with a protuberance of bone at the site of deformity. In the wrist, along the distal metaphysis of the radius, this type of fracture is commonly called a torus fracture (Fig. 130-10).

The physis often lies at the center of traumatic injuries to the immature skeleton. It is the weakest part of the developing bone. Childhood fractures are often characterized by their involvement of the physis according to the Salter-Harris classification system. A Salter-Harris type I fracture represents a separation of the physis. A Salter-Harris type II fracture has a fracture plane through the physis and metaphysis, whereas a Salter-Harris type III fracture involves the physis and epiphysis. A Salter-Harris type IV fracture involves the metaphysis, physis, and epiphysis (Fig. 130-11). Finally, a Salter-Harris type V fracture represents a crush injury to the physis. All of these injuries may result in growth abnormalities from physeal damage, with Salter-Harris type V injuries having the greatest likelihood of growth abnormalities.

The most important fracture not to be overlooked in the pediatric patient is the nonaccidental fracture. Nonaccidental trauma is a significant cause of morbidity and mortality in the pediatric population.[12] It is an entity that crosses all gender and socioeconomic boundaries. By law, the interpreting physician is required to report findings compatible with child abuse.

The diagnosis of child abuse depends on the evaluation of a particular fracture with respect to the expected activities of the child, the skeletal maturation of the child, and the fracture pattern. Children who have been subjected to nonaccidental trauma have several characteristic findings. Metaphyseal corner fractures, also called *bucket-handle fractures*, are commonly seen in the distal long bones, including the femur, humerus, radius, and tibia. They are considered pathognomonic of child abuse (Fig. 130-12). Spiral fractures in the long bones of infants and toddlers are also suspicious. Unusual fractures including fractures of the metacarpals, posterior rib fractures, skull fractures, scapular fractures, or spinous process fractures may be seen. Finally, fractures in various stages of healing are also highly suspicious for child abuse. To this end, a radiographic skeletal survey or a bone scan is often performed in young children to screen for further occult trauma.[13]

Extremity Fractures

In the upper extremities, the most common fractures in the pediatric patient occur in the radius, clavicle, and humerus. Greenstick fractures are common, and these fractures usually heal completely (Fig. 130-13). In the proximal humerus, the growth plate, corresponding to the anatomic neck of the humerus, will appear at two levels, and this appearance should not be mistaken for a proximal humeral fracture (see Fig. 130-7).

The elbow is a common sight of fracture. The presence of an elbow joint effusion, delineated by distention of the joint and displacement of adjacent anterior and posterior fat pads, indicates a high likelihood of fracture.[14] In younger children, a supracondylar distal humeral fracture is most common, whereas in adolescents, radial head fractures are more common (Fig. 130-14). Medial epicondyle avulsion fractures result from the action of the flexor carpi ulnaris. The avulsed fragment may become displaced, becoming trapped in the joint and leading to mechanical symptoms. Knowledge of the normal sequential appearance of the ossification centers of the elbow is important to distinguish a displaced medial epicondylar fragment from a normal trochlear ossification center. Elbow dislocations are uncommon in the child but more so in the adolescent population, and when they do occur, they are invariably posterior. Avulsion of the medial epicondyle is a common concomitant injury.

Distal radial and ulnar fractures are also common in the pediatric population. These fractures usually take the form of buckle or torus fractures to the distal radius and occasionally the ulna. Bowing deformities without fracture occur in the mid shaft of the radius and ulna. The "both bones forearm fracture" refers to fractures to the midshaft of the radius and ulna, usually transverse and nondisplaced. Physeal injuries to the distal radius also frequently occur. More distal carpal and metacarpal fractures are infrequent in the pediatric population; they increase in frequency in the teenage years and into adulthood.

In the lower extremities, fractures are most common in the area of the hip and ankle. In the hip, a slipped capital femoral epiphysis describes a displacement of the proximal femoral growth plate. It is more frequent in obese adolescents and is more common in males.[15] The femoral epiphysis usually slips posteriorly and inferomedially. The fracture differs slightly from a classic Salter-Harris type I fracture in that it occurs between the proliferative and hypertrophic zones of the physis as opposed to through only the hypertrophic zone. Both mechanical and endocrine conditions have been implicated as potential etiologies (Fig. 130-15). The workup of unexplained knee pain in an adolescent athlete should include both an anteroposterior and frog-leg lateral radiograph of the pelvis to evaluate for slipped capital femoral epiphysis.

Fractures in the area of the knee are relatively uncommon and typically take the form of Salter-Harris type II or III

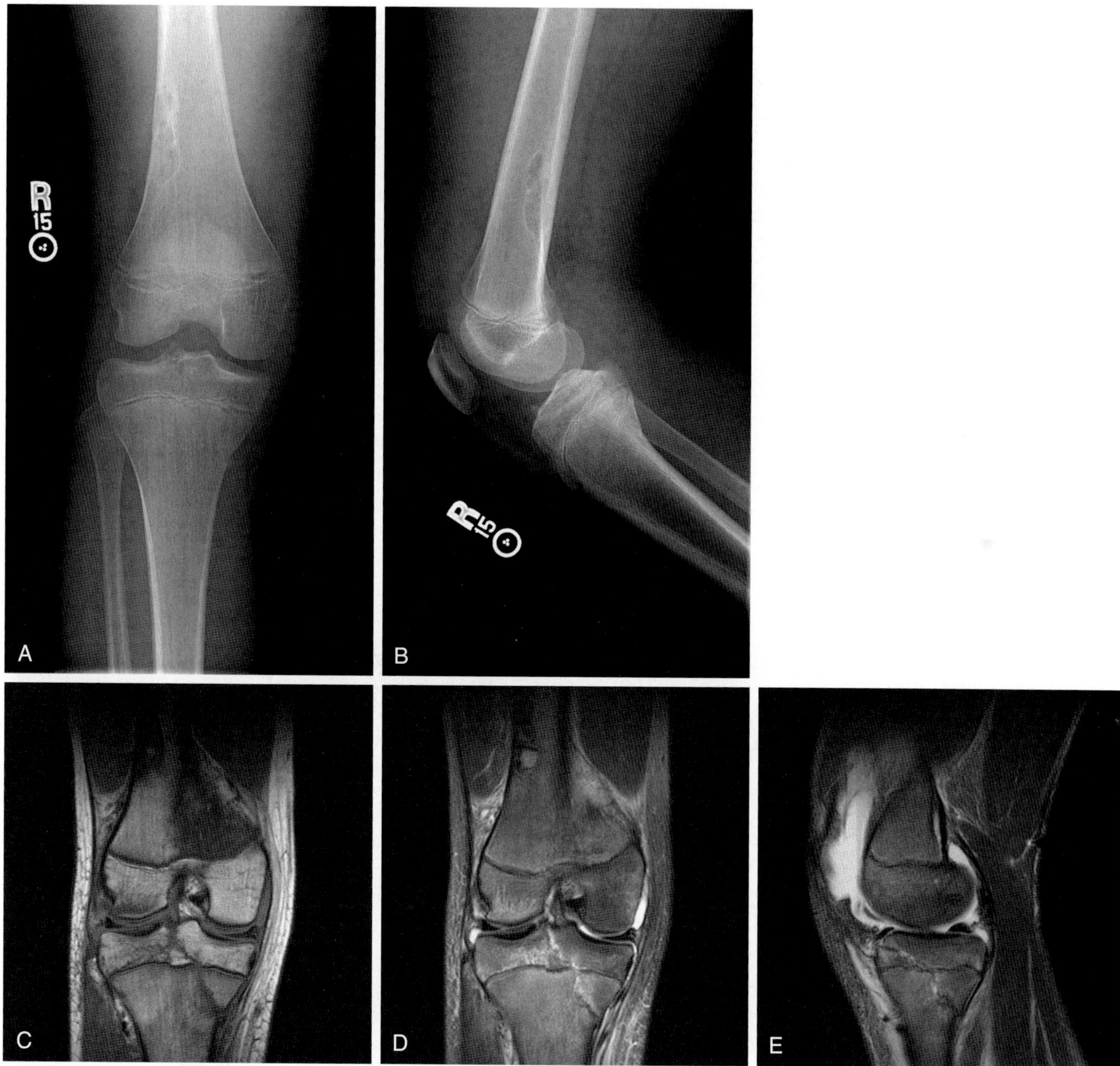

FIGURE 130-11 A Salter-Harris type IV fracture of the knee. Anteroposterior (**A**) and lateral (**B**) radiographic images of the right knee demonstrate a linear fracture line through the mid aspect of the epiphysis extending through the physis and exiting from the medial aspect of the metaphysis. The fracture is nondisplaced. A joint effusion is present on the lateral view. The fracture line is also well visualized on the coronal T1-weighted (**C**) and T2-weighted fat-saturated (**D**) magnetic resonance images. The sagittal T2-weighted fat-saturated magnetic resonance image (**E**) also demonstrates the fracture; it also shows a large joint effusion with a fluid-fluid level confirming an intraarticular fracture.

fractures to either the distal femur or proximal tibia. Fractures to the tibial tuberosity occur in male adolescents when the knee is forcibly flexed against a tightly contracted quadriceps. These fractures are typically diagnosed radiographically. However, if the fracture is nondisplaced, an MRI scan may be required to diagnose the fracture and determine the degree to which the fracture may extend into the proximal tibial physis. The proximal tibial physis is the most common site for Salter-Harris type V fractures, which occur in the setting of impaction injuries. Patella fractures are infrequent and are usually transverse in orientation. Developmental patellar variations such as a bipartite or tripartite patella should not be confused with patellar fractures, although these variations are occasionally a source of knee pain.

In the ankle, an 18-month window occurs during adolescence in which the distal tibial physis closes asymmetrically. This window occurs at about 12 years of age in girls and 15 years of age in boys. Generally, the physis closes from medial to lateral and posterior to anterior, leaving the anterolateral physis vulnerable to injury. Triplane fractures are Salter-Harris type IV fractures, named for their fracture extension in coronal, transverse, and sagittal planes. They occur as a result

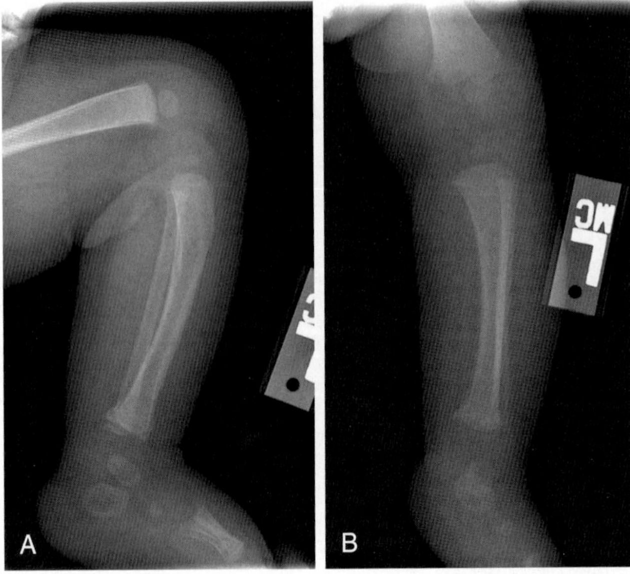

FIGURE 130-12 A metaphyseal corner fracture. Lateral (A) and oblique (B) images of the lower left leg in a toddler show a circumferential metaphyseal corner fracture of the distal tibia. When it is circumferential in the area of the metaphysis, it is termed a bucket-handle fracture. This fracture is nearly pathognomonic of child abuse.

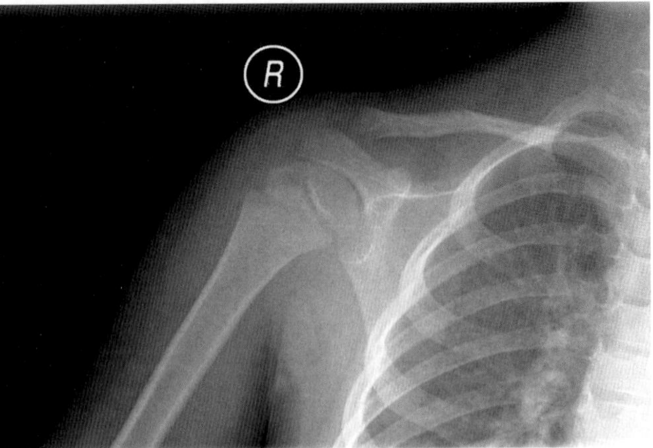

FIGURE 130-13 A clavicular greenstick fracture. The frontal view of the right clavicle and shoulder demonstrates a focal cortical break along the superior aspect of the middle third of the clavicle with minimal angulation. The inferior cortex is intact. Findings are consistent with a greenstick fracture of the clavicle.

of external rotation of the foot with respect to the distal tibia. The fracture extends through the epiphysis in the sagittal plane and travels horizontally through the unfused lateral aspect of the physis, finally exiting the metaphysis in the coronal plane. Juvenile Tillaux fractures are Salter-Harris type III fractures that are similar to triplane fractures, but without the metaphyseal component. The Tillaux fracture is a result of avulsion forces of the anterior talofibular ligament along the anterolateral aspect of the distal tibial epiphysis during external rotation of the foot (Fig. 130-16).[16]

Avulsion injuries are common in the adolescent athlete and often occur at apophyses, the attachments of tendons to bone.[17] Avulsion fractures usually present after a forceful muscle contraction with subsequent pain and limited motion. Abnormal forces across joints may lead to avulsion injuries along the attachments of ligamentous and capsular structures. These injuries may be quite subtle, with only a small fleck of cortical bone avulsed. Chronic microstress may also lead to avulsion fractures or stress changes in the underlying bone, termed apophysitis. In the adolescent population, the pelvis is the most common site for avulsion injuries. Typical locations include the rectus femoris attachment along the anterior inferior iliac spine, the sartorius attachment to the anterior superior iliac spine, and the hamstring insertion to the ischial tuberosity. Other sites include the knee, ankle, foot, shoulder,

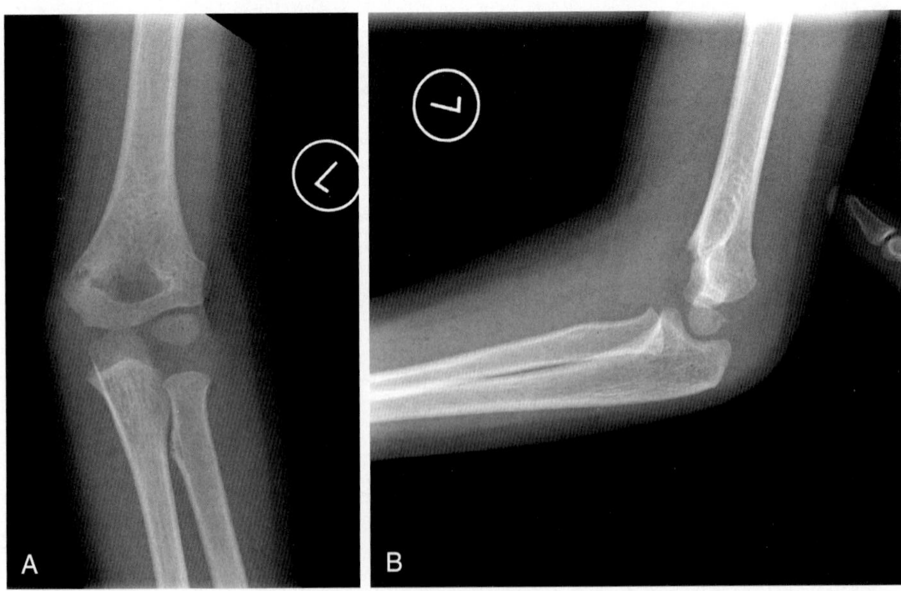

FIGURE 130-14 A supracondylar fracture. Anteroposterior (A) and lateral (B) radiographic images of the left elbow demonstrate a supracondylar fracture of the distal humerus with very minimal posterior angulation. A large elbow joint effusion is present that is well seen on the lateral view by displacement of the normal anterior and posterior fat pads.

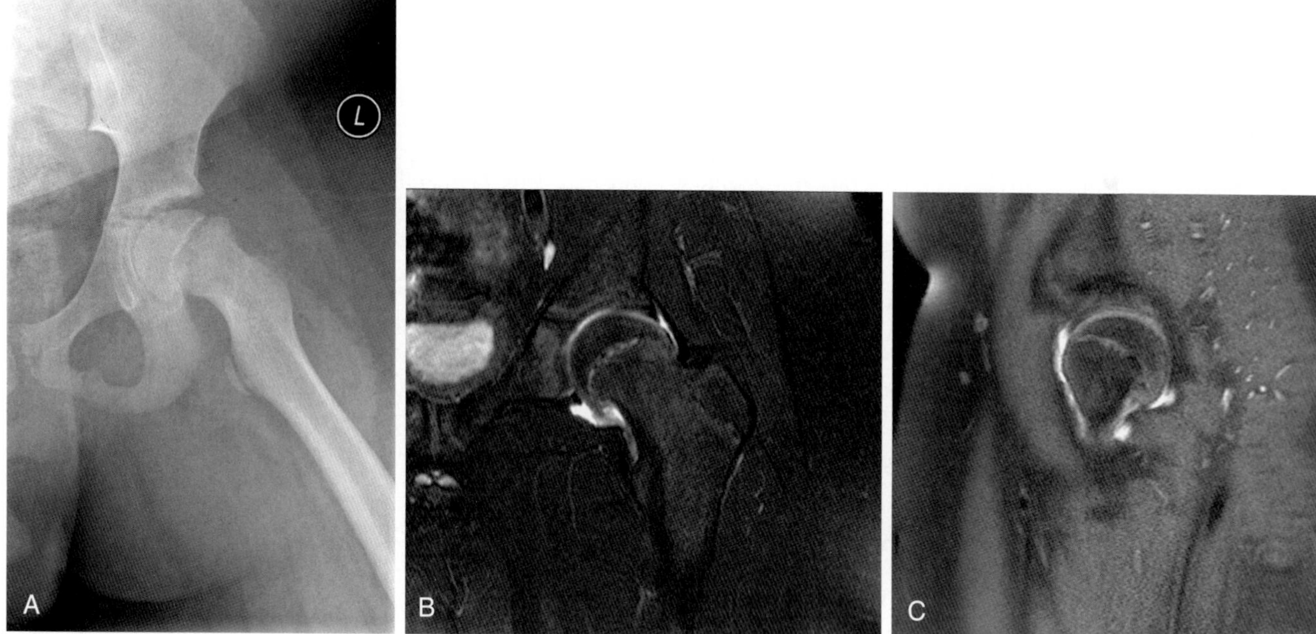

FIGURE 130-15 Slipped capital femoral epiphysis. **A,** An anteroposterior radiographic view of the left hip shows malalignment of the femoral epiphysis with the subjacent femoral metaphysis in an adolescent. The patient has a large body habitus as indicated by the generous soft tissues on the film. **B** and **C,** Coronal and sagittal T2-weighted fat-saturated magnetic resonance images of the same hip confirm malalignment of the femoral epiphysis with slippage posteriorly and inferomedially. Minimal edema in the physis and a small joint effusion are present.

and wrist. The presence of an avulsion fracture is associated to a large degree with other ligamentous injuries.

Radiography is usually diagnostic in the evaluation of avulsion fractures. CT images provide a more detailed cross-sectional view, allowing avulsed fragment size and displacement to be more accurately assessed. CT examination is especially valuable in detection of subtle avulsion injuries in complex structures such as the hand, wrist, or foot. MRI images actually are less sensitive to the detection of avulsion fractures compared with CT. Avulsion injuries generally produce far less marrow edema compared with linear fractures.[18] Additionally, tiny avulsed cortical bone fragments are devoid of signal on MRI and may be overlooked. Conversely, stress apophysitis as a result of chronic avulsive forces is well visualized using MRI, demonstrating prominent bone marrow edema.

Healing of avulsion injuries may produce a diagnostic dilemma. In the adolescent athlete, avulsion injuries often heal with exuberant hypertrophic bone formation, often mimicking a more sinister malignant lesion on radiographs. In these cases, CT or MRI can play a role in evaluation, allowing visualization of the healing avulsion fracture and excluding the presence of a destructive lesion.[19]

Osteochondroses

Osteochondroses are defined as noninflammatory and noninfectious derangements of bone growth that occur at bone growth centers during periods of activity. Disordered bone growth then results in morphologic alterations to the epiphysis or apophysis. Although the exact cause of osteochondroses is unknown, trauma is believed to play a significant role, with

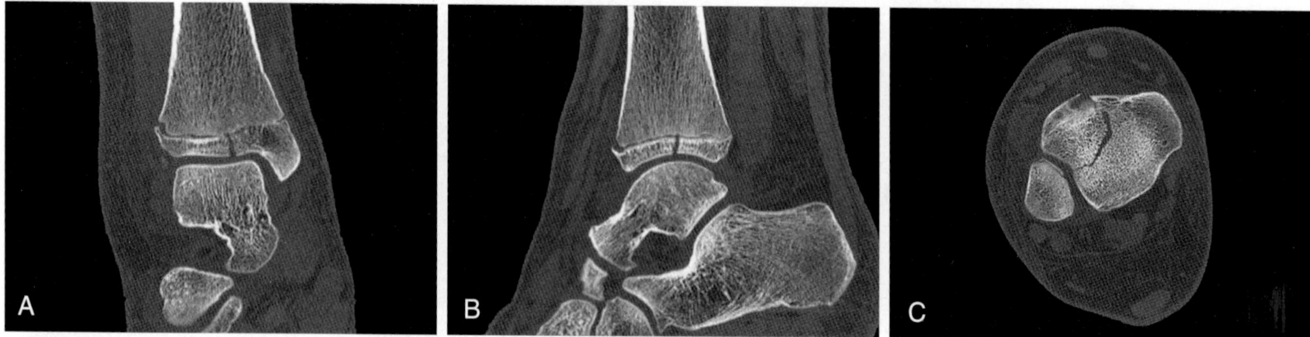

FIGURE 130-16 Juvenile Tillaux fracture. Coronal (**A**) and sagittal (**B**) computed tomographic reformations of the ankle demonstrate a minimally displaced fracture to the anterolateral tibial epiphysis. The medial aspect of the physis is fused, whereas the lateral aspect of the physis is widened. The minimally displaced anterolateral Tillaux fragment is well seen in the axial (**C**) computed tomographic image.

subsequent compromise of blood supply, bone necrosis, and finally bone regrowth.

Osteochondritis dissecans most commonly affects teenagers and young adults. It is possibly posttraumatic in origin as a result of impaction injuries.[20] The condition is most common in the lateral aspect of the medial femoral condyle followed by the medial talar dome. It is occasionally bilateral. Radiographs demonstrate a linear lucency in the subchondral bone (Fig. 130-17). If the fragment is free floating, the patient may have mechanical symptoms. MRI plays an important role in the assessment of the osteochondral fragment.[21] Magnetic resonance arthrography is often useful in the assessment of potentially loose osteochondral fragments.

Idiopathic avascular necrosis of the femoral capital epiphysis, termed Legg-Calvé-Perthes disease, is a common cause of hip pain with maximal incidence in the 5- to 10-year-old patient. It is more common in boys by a 5:1 margin and is usually unilateral. Patients present with slowly progressive joint pain and gait disturbances. Early diagnosis may be made with MRI that shows typical findings of bone necrosis.[22] Radiography demonstrates more progressive findings, including subchondral fractures, fragmentation, and flattening of the femoral head with mixed lucency and sclerosis and increased joint spacing as a result of swollen epiphyseal cartilage and joint effusion (Fig. 130-18).

Osgood-Schlatter disease is an osteochondrosis of the tibial tubercle. It is frequently bilateral and is commonly seen in teenagers, with boys outnumbering girls 3:1. Clinical findings most commonly involve pain over the tibial tubercle. This entity, also termed *tibial tubercle stress apophysitis,* results from chronic repetitive injury to the tibial attachment of the infrapatellar tendon, often as a result of sports that entail jumping,[23] and leads to a fragmented appearance to the tibial tubercle, with ossification in the distal infrapatellar tendon. Radiographs support the diagnosis. MRI may demonstrate bone marrow edema in the tibial tubercle, as well as edema in the attachment of the infrapatellar tendon. Sinding-Larsen-Johansson disease is an osteochondritis of the intrapatellar tendon attachment to the inferior patellar pole. It demonstrates changes similar to that seen in Osgood-Schlatter

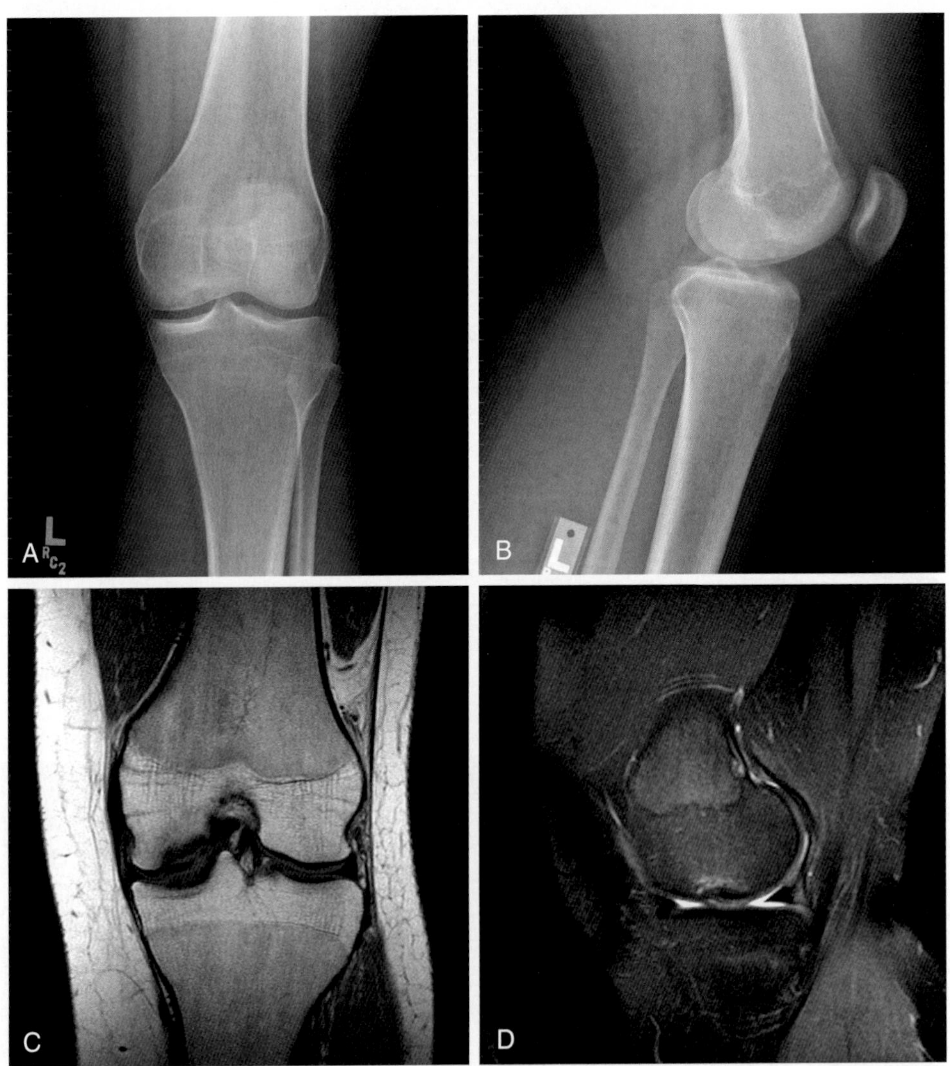

FIGURE 130-17 Osteochondritis dissecans. **A** and **B,** Anteroposterior and lateral views of the left knee demonstrate a subtle area of lucency in the lateral aspect of the anterior weight-bearing portion of the medial femoral condyle. **C** and **D,** Coronal T1-weighted and sagittal T2-weighted fat-saturated magnetic resonance images confirm the presence of an osteochondral lesion at this location. The fragment remains in situ, and the overlying cartilage is intact.

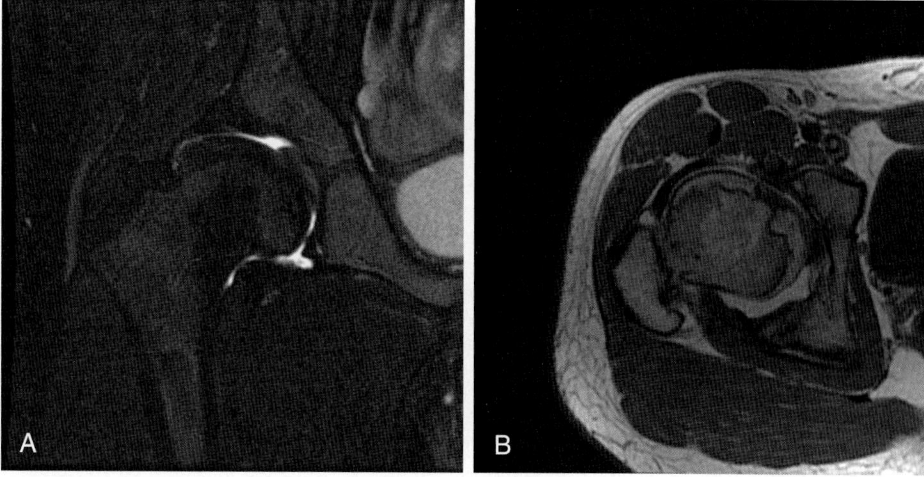

FIGURE 130-18 Legg-Calvé-Perthes disease. Coronal T2-weighted fat-saturated (**A**) and axial T1-weighted (**B**) magnetic resonance images of the right hip after intraarticular gadolinium injection demonstrate coxa magna with a flattened, widened femoral epiphysis. These findings are consistent with long-standing Legg-Calvé-Perthes disease.

disease, but along the inferior margin of the patella.[24] The superior pole of the patella can also be affected by a similar set of clinical symptoms and radiographic findings.

Kohler disease is a relatively rare osteochondrosis affecting the tarsal navicular. It affects children in the 3- to 5-year age range, typically boys. Patients report midfoot pain with gait disturbances. Radiographs demonstrate an irregular, sclerotic, and occasionally flattened navicular bone. The condition is usually self-limited, with the navicular resuming a normal shape 2 to 4 years after presentation.[25]

The Frieberg infraction usually affects the head of the second metatarsal. It most commonly presents in teenagers with foot pain. Radiographs demonstrate flattening of the head of the second metatarsal. Over time, degenerative arthritis of the second metatarsophalangeal joint ensues.

Blount disease, also termed *osteochondrosis deformans tibiae,* is a developmental deformity of the proximal tibia. Three forms have been described: infantile, juvenile, and adolescent.[26] In each of these forms, abnormal stress is placed on the posteromedial tibia, leading to growth suppression of the posteromedial physis. The decrease in longitudinal growth that ensues leads to further varus angulation and progressive worsening of the condition. Radiographic findings include sloping and fragmentation of the medial epiphyseal ossification center, widening of the growth plate, and beaking of the medial metaphysis. MRI is often helpful in the evaluation of the growth plate, especially in the case of adolescent Blount disease, which is often due to premature fusion of the medial portion of the proximal tibial growth plate.[27]

Infection/Inflammation

Osteomyelitis

In the pediatric patient, osteomyelitis is usually hematogenous in origin, either from transient asymptomatic bacteremia or sepsis. It most commonly occurs in the metaphyses, which contain slow-flowing venous sinusoids at the terminal segments of medullary vessels. The physis represents a relative barrier to epiphyseal spread. However, transphyseal spread may occur in infants younger than 18 months of age because of the presence of transphyseal vessels, which may allow the development of subsequent septic arthritis. Increased intramedullary pressures as a result of infection may lead to bone necrosis. Alternatively, increased pressure often results in transcortical extension of infection. The relatively loose attachment of the periosteum along the metaphysis and diaphyseal regions allows the longitudinal dissection of subperiosteal abscesses along the shaft of bone (see Fig. 130-3). Further extension through the periosteum may lead to soft tissue involvement. The firm attachment of the periosteum at the physis often prevents extension into the joint, except in the case of the proximal femur, proximal humerus, distal tibia and fibula, and the proximal radius where the metaphyses are intraarticular, thus permitting direct seeding of these joints.

The most common sites of osteomyelitis are the metaphyses of actively growing large bones, which includes the proximal and distal ends of the femur, proximal tibia and humerus, and distal radius. Flat bones, specifically the ilium, vertebrae, and calcaneus, are also commonly involved. The most common organism in the pediatric population is *Staphylococcus aureus*, which is most relevant when treating pediatric and adolescent athletes with osteomyelitis.

Radiographs are insensitive to the early changes of osteomyelitis. Bone destruction may take up to 10 days to become evident. Soft tissue changes such as soft tissue swelling and obliteration of normal fat planes, although subtle, are detected earlier than bone changes. The diagnosis of osteomyelitis can be made much earlier with the use of MRI, which shows changes of bone marrow edema in the involved metaphysis. MRI is also capable of showing complications of osteomyelitis such as intraosseous abscess formation, subperiosteal abscess formation, and soft tissue extension (Fig. 130-19).[28] Three-phase scintigraphy is also sensitive to the detection of osteomyelitis, although interpretation may be confounded by activity in the developing physis adjacent to an area of metaphyseal osteomyelitis (Fig. 130-20).

Septic Arthritis

Septic arthritis is a relatively common clinical emergency in the pediatric patient. It may develop hematogenously, either

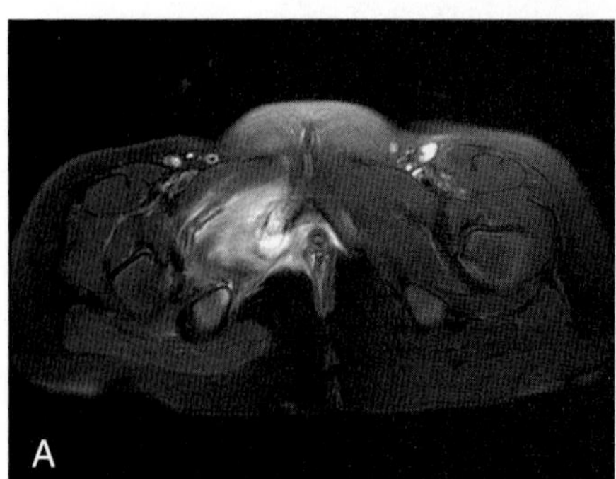
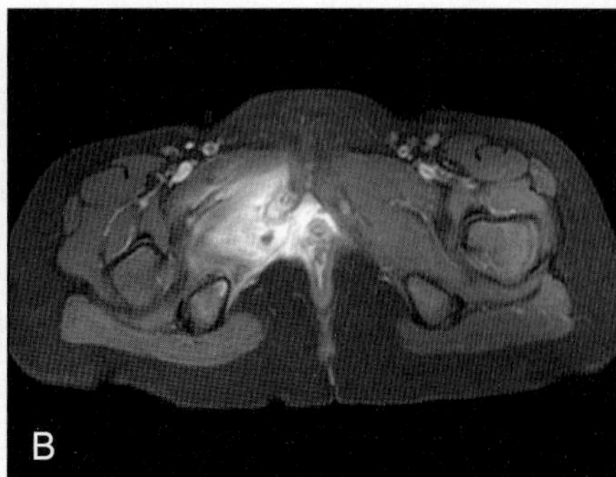
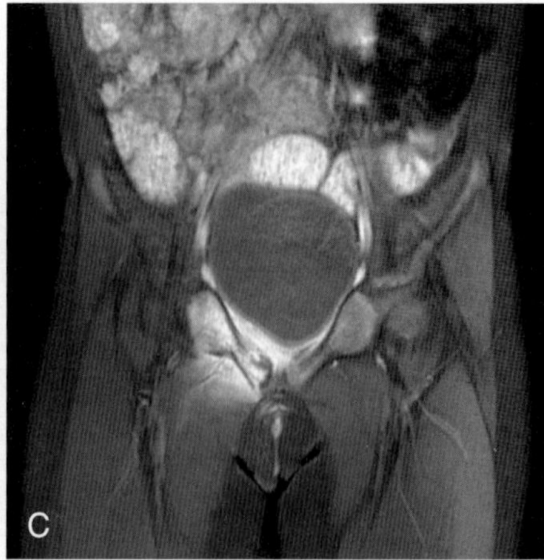

FIGURE 130-19 Pubic osteomyelitis. Axial T2-weighted fat-saturated (**A**) and T1-weighted fat-saturated gadolinium-enhanced magnetic resonance images in the axial (**B**) and coronal (**C**) projections demonstrate edema in the right pubis with prominent enhancement of the bone and adjacent soft tissues. Findings are consistent with pubic osteomyelitis. A small peripherally enhancing soft tissue abscess is present on the postgadolinium images.

by being directly seeded from synovial blood vessels, by contiguous extension from adjacent metaphyseal osteomyelitis or soft tissue cellulitis, or rarely from a direct puncture wound. Once the joint is infected, it effectively becomes an abscess. Increased pressure in the joint leads to compromised blood supply to the epiphysis. In combination with active infection, this process leads to rapid bone and cartilage destruction and dissolution.

Imaging findings in persons with septic arthritis are nonspecific. Joint effusions are common, although they may be absent in small joints in which the relatively thin joint capsule allows decompression into the adjacent tissues.[29] Imaging, especially MRI, allows for the detection of joint effusions and other potential etiologies such as osteomyelitis, soft tissue cellulitis, tumors, or even occult trauma. Ultrasound is an efficient modality that can also be used to detect joint effusions and to guide joint aspiration. Transient toxic synovitis is a self-limited condition that may mimic septic arthritis. It is thought to be viral in origin and usually involves the pediatric hip. It often produces a joint effusion, but patients are likely to have less pronounced symptoms compared with a truly septic joint. In general, however, a very low threshold should exist for arthrocentesis of a suspected infected joint.

Inflammatory Arthritis

Juvenile idiopathic arthritis, formerly known as juvenile rheumatoid arthritis, is the newest terminology for a group of poorly understood arthropathies that affect children.[30] It is a chronic inflammatory arthropathy in which the immune system targets the synovium, leading to synovial hypertrophy and hyperemia with joint effusions. In addition to the bone and cartilage destruction that results from chronic inflammation of the joints, the chronic hyperemic state also leads to growth disturbances, including epiphyseal overgrowth and thin gracile diaphyses. These processes may lead to significantly deformed joints, depending on the severity of the disease (Fig. 130-21).

Juvenile idiopathic arthritis has been subdivided into five subtypes depending on the symptoms and number of joints involved. Oligoarthritis affects fewer than five joints in the first few months of the disease. Extraarticular manifestations include uveitis, iritis, or iridocyclitis. Polyarthritis affects five or more joints and is often symmetric in distribution. It has more of a predisposition for small joints compared with oligoarthritis, which tends to affect larger joints. Systemic arthritis, also termed *Still disease,* is a systemic disease that affects

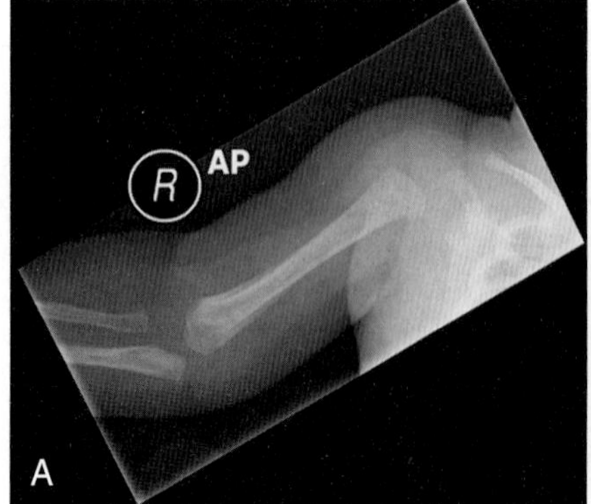

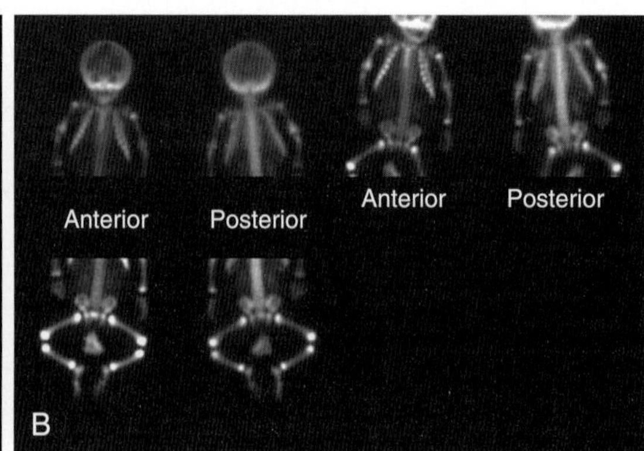

FIGURE 130-20 Humeral osteomyelitis. **A,** A frontal radiograph of the right humerus in a young child shows abnormal periosteal new bone formation along the distal diaphysis and metaphysis of the right humerus. **B,** A bone scan demonstrates asymmetrically increased uptake along the distal metaphysis of the right humerus compared with the left humerus. A biopsy revealed osteomyelitis.

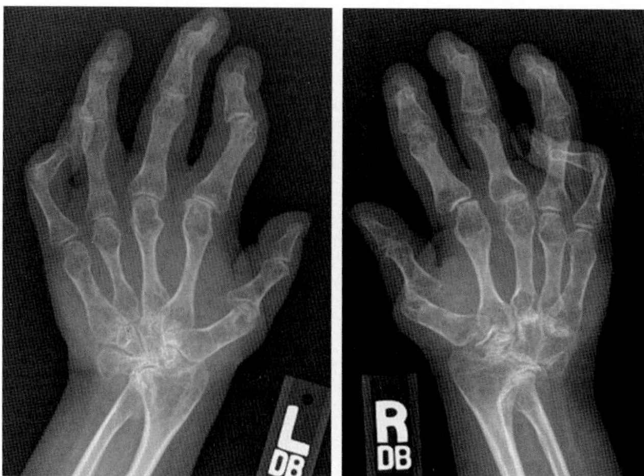

FIGURE 130-21 Juvenile idiopathic arthritis. Anteroposterior radiographs of the bilateral hands of a child show severe deformity as well as osteopenia, joint space narrowing, and carpal destruction with collapse. Growth disturbances manifest as ballooning epiphyses and shortened metacarpals.

joints and internal organs. Patients have high fever and a rash. Eye involvement is rare. A fourth category of juvenile idiopathic arthritis is the psoriatic variant, in which patients with an inflammatory arthropathy also have typical psoriatic skin and nail manifestations. Finally, enthesitis-related arthritis affects the spine, hips, and entheses (tendon attachments to bone). It is more common in males and in families with a history of spondyloarthropathies. Eye involvement is also common.

Making the diagnosis of juvenile idiopathic arthritis may be difficult. It is often a diagnosis of exclusion that is arrived on after other entities have been excluded. Imaging studies are nonspecific, demonstrating joint effusions and synovial proliferation. MRI may aid in demonstrating the condition of the joints, specifically the articular cartilage. Radiographs are also helpful in following the progression of the disease and assessing bone growth and deformity.[31]

Benign Lesions

Several benign bone conditions may affect pediatric patients. Some of these conditions are painful and require surgical intervention. They may mimic sports-related injuries such as stress fractures. Others are entirely incidental findings that may be seen on radiographs obtained for other reasons and should not be mistaken for malignant lesions. Finally, some lesions, although benign, may predispose the patient to pathologic fractures. Preventative intervention should be considered with respect to lesion morphology and the child's activity level.

Osteoid osteomas are benign bone-forming lesions that are often encountered in the pediatric and young adult patient. Patients classically report pain that is worse at night and relieved by aspirin. Lesions may be seen anywhere but are most common in the femur, tibia, and posterior elements of the spine. A central lucent nidus, usually less than 1 cm in size, may be intramedullary, cortical, or periosteal. The nidus often has a small focus of central mineralization. These lesions are extremely inflammatory. Often an exuberant, thick, benign-appearing periosteal reaction and sclerosis occur. If the lesion is intraarticular, a joint effusion may be present. MRI demonstrates both periosteal and soft tissue edema about the lesion, which is best seen on T2-weighted fat-suppressed or short tau inversion recovery sequences (Fig. 130-22). CT is the imaging modality of choice for demonstrating the nidus and the adjacent periosteal reaction. CT may also be used to guide a radiofrequency probe into the lesion to effect ablation, with a high percentage of therapeutic success.[32]

Chondroblastomas are infrequent benign cartilaginous epiphyseal or apophyseal lesions seen most commonly in teenagers. They are typically seen in the area of the knee and the distal humerus. Patients present with pain, tenderness, swelling, and occasionally a joint effusion. Plain film radiographs demonstrate a round or oval well-marginated lucent lesion eccentrically in the epiphysis. The majority of these lesions have a small amount of internal matrix, although a large percentage is uniformly lucent. Occasionally a benign periosteal reaction is present. MRI demonstrates the lesion well with low signal on T1-weighted images and heterogeneous signal on T2-weighted images as a result of the variable internal cartilage stroma and mineralization. Adjacent inflammatory changes are common; they manifest as bone marrow edema and are well out of proportion to the size of the actual tumor (Fig. 130-23).

Giant cell tumors are infrequent in young children and rarely appear in a bone before physeal closure. Most of these tumors occur in young adults and present with either low-grade pain or pathologic fracture. These tumors are usually eccentric, lytic, and located along the subarticular end of the bone. They typically lack a sclerotic rim. MRI readily displays

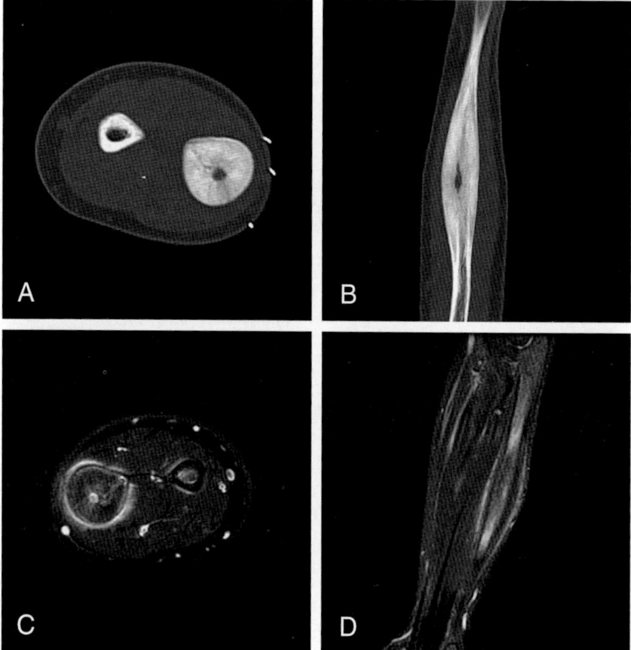

FIGURE 130-22 Osteoid osteoma. Axial (**A**) and coronal reformation (**B**) computed tomographic images of the left forearm demonstrate circumferential marked periosteal new bone formation along the shaft of the ulna with a central lucent nidus corresponding to an osteoid osteoma. Corresponding axial (**C**) and coronal (**D**) T2-weighted fat-saturated magnetic resonance images show both periosteal and cortical high-signal edema along the involved portion of the bone.

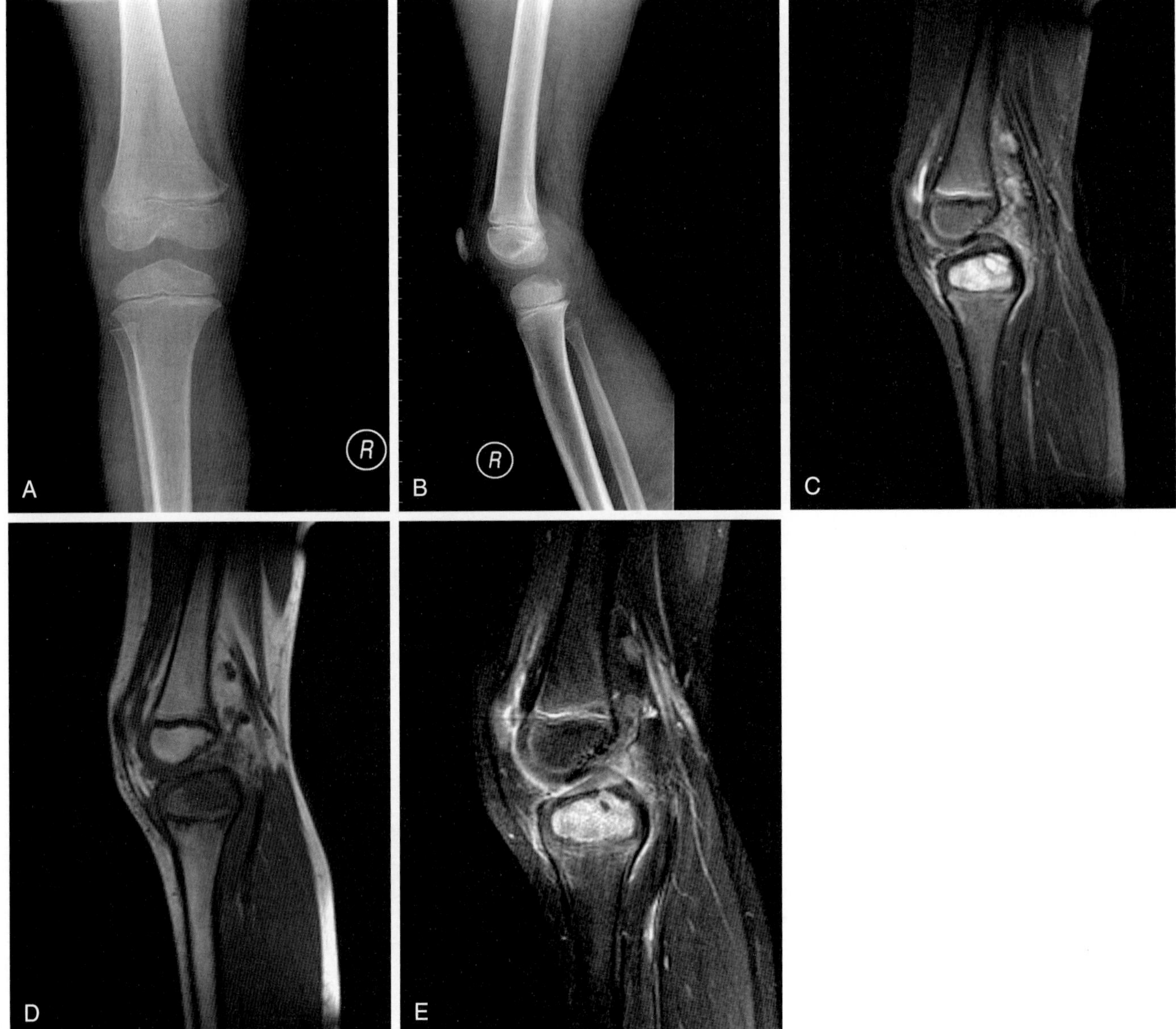

FIGURE 130-23 Chondroblastoma. **A** and **B,** Anteroposterior and lateral radiographs of the right knee demonstrate a subtle lytic lesion in the posteromedial aspect of the proximal tibial epiphysis in a young patient with knee pain and limp. Sagittal short tau inversion recovery (**C**), T1-weighted (**D**), and T1-weighted fat-saturated gadolinium-enhanced (**E**) magnetic resonance images of the same knee confirm the presence of a cartilaginous lesion and show extensive adjacent epiphyseal enhancement and edema consistent with the robust inflammatory response elicited by a chondroblastoma.

the tumor and allows assessment of cortical or subchondral breakthrough (Fig. 130-24).

Benign fibrous cortical defects, also termed *nonossifying fibromas,* are benign asymptomatic lesions of bone often seen incidentally. They are cortical lesions and often are seen eccentrically in the metadiaphyseal regions of the long bones, particularly in the area of the knee. Radiographically, they are well-marginated, lobular, and have a well-defined sclerotic margin (Fig. 130-25). Larger nonossifying fibromas may lead to pathologic fracture. Over time the lesions involute, with bone filling the fibrous lucent defect. On MRI, the lesions have low signal on both T1- and T2-weighted images, with a thick low-signal rim corresponding to peripheral sclerosis. MRI is not necessary in their evaluation because radiographs are usually diagnostic.

Intraosseous hemangiomas are commonly seen in the spine, skull, and facial bones. Typical radiographic and CT findings are prominent thickened vertical trabeculations. Mild bone expansion may be present. MRI often demonstrates macroscopic fat within the lesion. Rarely, these lesions may be symptomatic.

Solitary or unicameral bone cysts are common bone lesions usually found in the proximal metaphysis of the humerus or femur. Radiographically, they appear as expansile, well-marginated lucent lesions with internal bony septations. They are asymptomatic unless a pathologic fracture has occurred as a result of the weakened bone. A "fallen leaf," corresponding to a free osseous fragment in the dependent portion of the lesion, is seen in a fair number of cases of pathologic fracture (Fig. 130-26). MRI demonstrates the

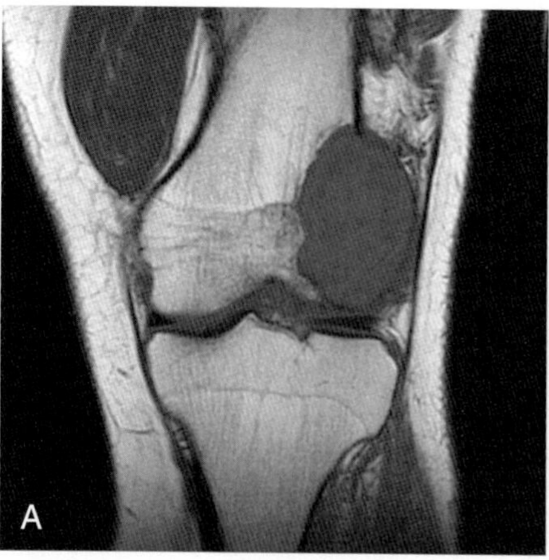

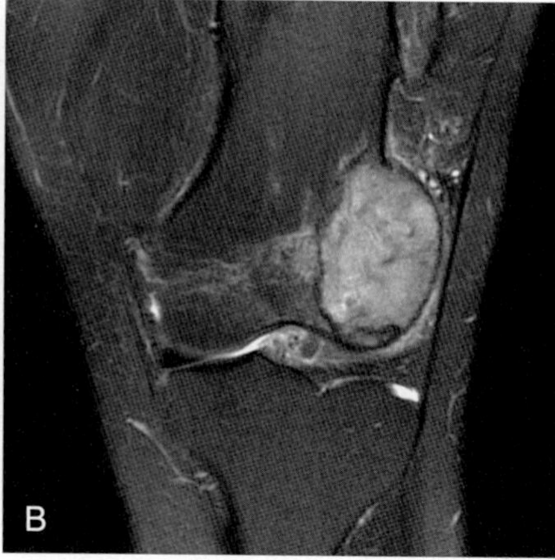

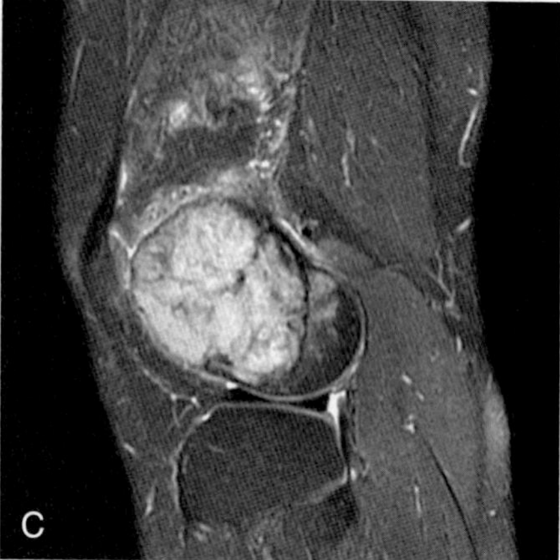

FIGURE 130-24 A giant cell tumor. Coronal T1-weighted (**A**) and coronal (**B**) and sagittal (**C**) T2-weighted fat-saturated magnetic resonance images of the knee demonstrate an eccentric low-signal lesion in the lateral femoral condyle extending to the subchondral cortex. A biopsy confirmed a giant cell tumor. Note that the physes are closed, as is typical with these lesions.

cystic nature of the lesion, which is uniformly quite bright on T2-weighted images. Solitary bone cysts differ from aneurysmal bone cysts (ABCs) in that the latter contain blood-filled cavernous spaces, are reactive in origin, and are often symptomatic. ABCs are often expansile and may break through the cortex. On MRI, they commonly demonstrate dependent fluid-fluid levels. ABCs can be found in association with other more aggressive or even malignant lesions.

Osteochondromas, also termed *exostoses,* are a very common form of bone dysplasia. The lesion forms from a metaphyseal outgrowth of cartilage, usually in a tubular bone such as the femur, tibia, or ribs. The exact etiology is unknown. The island of cartilage grows as an epiphysis grows, eventually ossifying. By definition, the marrow cavity of the lesion is contiguous with the marrow of the subjacent parent metaphysis, and a cartilage cap of variable thickness thins with age. The lesions may be sessile, with a broad base of attachment, or exophytic. The latter lesions may extend several centimeters into adjacent soft tissues and result in mechanical symptoms such as myositis, adventitial bursal formation, or nerve impingement (Fig. 130-27). They are also prone to fracture. These lesions are typically seen incidentally on imaging examinations. If they are painless, no further workup is required. If they are painful, MRI is indicated to assess soft tissue changes and the structure of the lesion, in particular the cartilage cap, which in rare cases may degenerate into chondrosarcoma.[33] Rarely patients may have numerous osteochondromas, termed *hereditary multiple exostoses.* These patients have a higher incidence of malignant degeneration compared with patients who have a solitary osteochondroma and should be monitored accordingly.

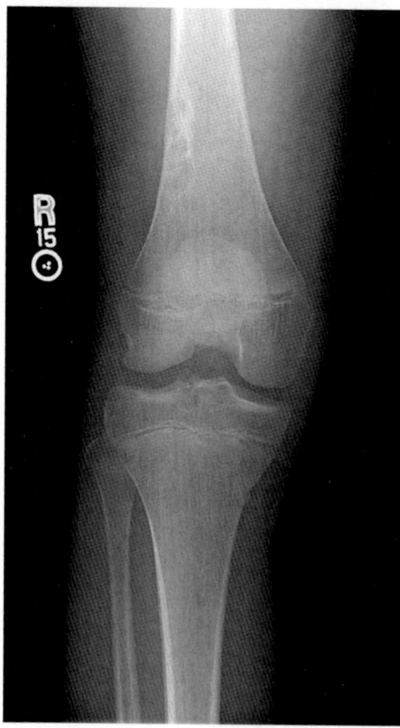

FIGURE 130-25 A nonossifying fibroma. An anteroposterior radiograph of the knee demonstrates an eccentric, lobular lesion along the lateral aspect of the distal femoral diaphysis with a well-marginated sclerotic border corresponding to a benign nonossifying fibroma.

Fibrous dysplasia is a common benign disorder in which bone is replaced by fibrous tissue. It is usually monostotic, although polyostotic forms exist, usually associated with a number of endocrine abnormalities. Fibrous dysplasia usually arises in growing bones of older children and adults. Common locations include the proximal femur, tibia, ribs, and craniofacial bones. Affected bone is predisposed to pathologic fracture, and chronic deformity may result. Lesions are usually asymptomatic. Radiographically, fibrous dysplasia is a well-circumscribed lytic lesion in a long bone, often with a hazy ground-glass appearance of the internal matrix. It is well marginated, often with a thick sclerotic border. It may be slightly expansile with scalloping of the endosteal cortex, but it does not demonstrate cortical breakthrough or a soft tissue mass (Fig. 130-28). Lesions usually demonstrate increased uptake on bone scintigraphy. This modality is used to assess for polyostotic disease.

Aggressive Lesions

Osteosarcoma is the most common primary malignancy of bone in the 10- to 25-year-old age group, comprising more than half the malignant bone lesions in the first two decades of life. The most common location is the metaphyses of long

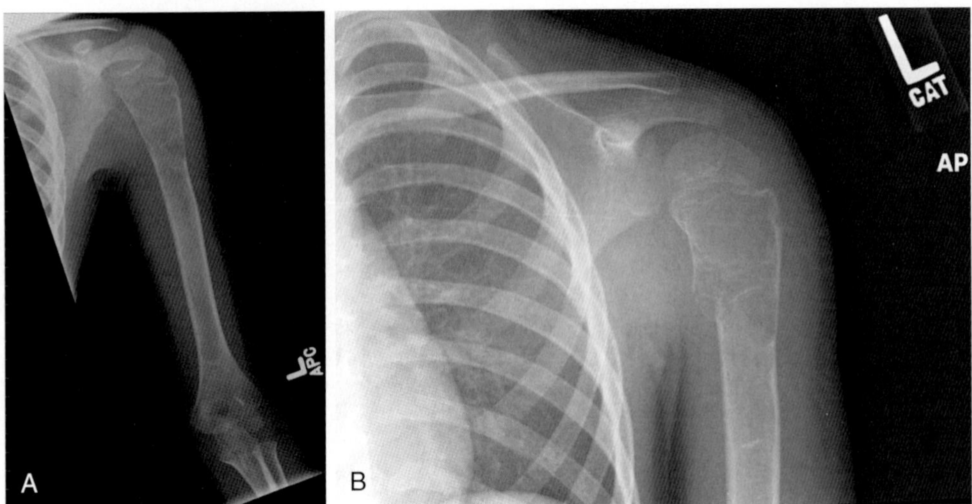

FIGURE 130-26 A unicameral bone cyst with a pathologic fracture. **A,** An anteroposterior view of the left humerus demonstrates an expansile, elongated, lytic lesion in the proximal metaphysis of the left humerus. A few thin internal bony septations are present. **B,** A frontal view of the left shoulder in the same patient 4 days later shows a pathologic fracture through the lesion with a fallen fragment of bone in the dependent aspect of the bone cyst.

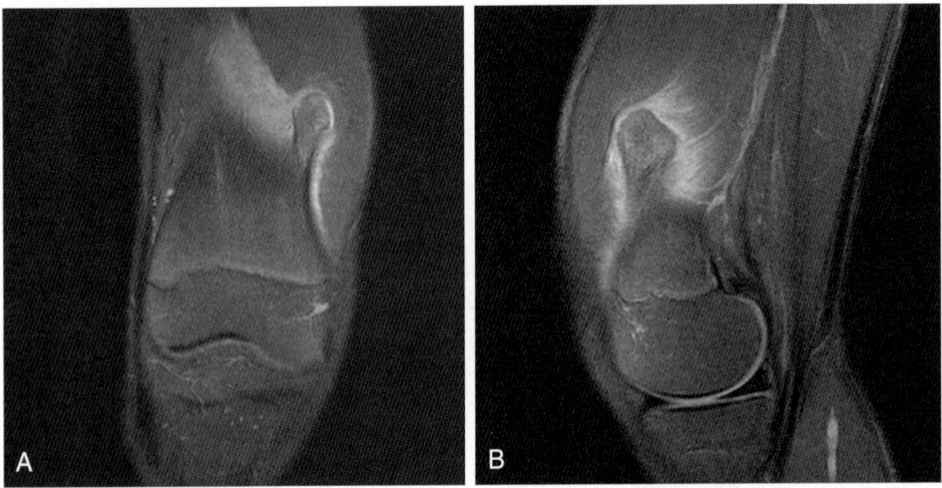

FIGURE 130-27 An exophytic osteochondroma. Coronal (**A**) and sagittal (**B**) T2-weighted fat-saturated magnetic resonance images of the knee are shown in an adolescent with medial knee pain and a palpable, painful mass. An exophytic osteochondroma is arising from the medial metaphysis of the distal femur. Its internal marrow is contiguous with the marrow of the distal femur. Inflammatory changes are present in the soft tissues surrounding the osteochondroma with formation of a tiny adventitial bursa.

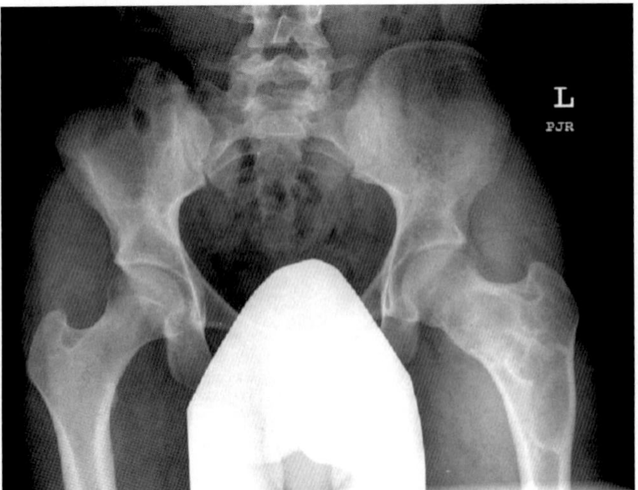

FIGURE 130-28 Fibrous dysplasia. An anteroposterior radiograph of the pelvis demonstrates an expansile, mixed lytic and sclerotic lesion in the proximal left femur corresponding to an area of fibrous dysplasia.

bones, with greater than 50% of lesions occurring in the area of the knee. However, tumors may arise in any bone. Males have a slightly higher incidence than do females. The appearance of the lesion varies with the degree of matrix produced by the lesion. Some types are quite osteoblastic with extensive new bone formation. Chondroblastic subtypes produce cartilaginous matrix, whereas others produce predominately fibroblastic stroma. Parosteal osteosarcoma originates from the periosteum and often wraps around the diaphysis, growing outside the bone. This subtype is infrequent in children, with a peak incidence in the third decade. Telangiectatic osteosarcoma can be entirely lytic, often appearing cystic. It occurs most commonly in the area of the knee.

On radiographs, a typical osteosarcoma appears as a destructive eccentric metaphyseal lesion with mixed lytic and sclerotic regions. The tumor often penetrates the cortex, leading to formation of malignant-appearing periosteal new bone in a sunburst configuration. Radiographs are usually diagnostic. MRI is quite useful in mapping the true extent of the tumor, both within the bone marrow and adjacent soft tissues (Fig. 130-29). Tumors typically have low signal on T1-weighted images, displacing normal fatty marrow. Osteosarcomas heterogeneously have a high signal on T2-weighted images and demonstrate heterogenous enhancement. Areas of mineralization appear as signal voids within the tumor mass. If a long bone such as the femur is involved, MRI should

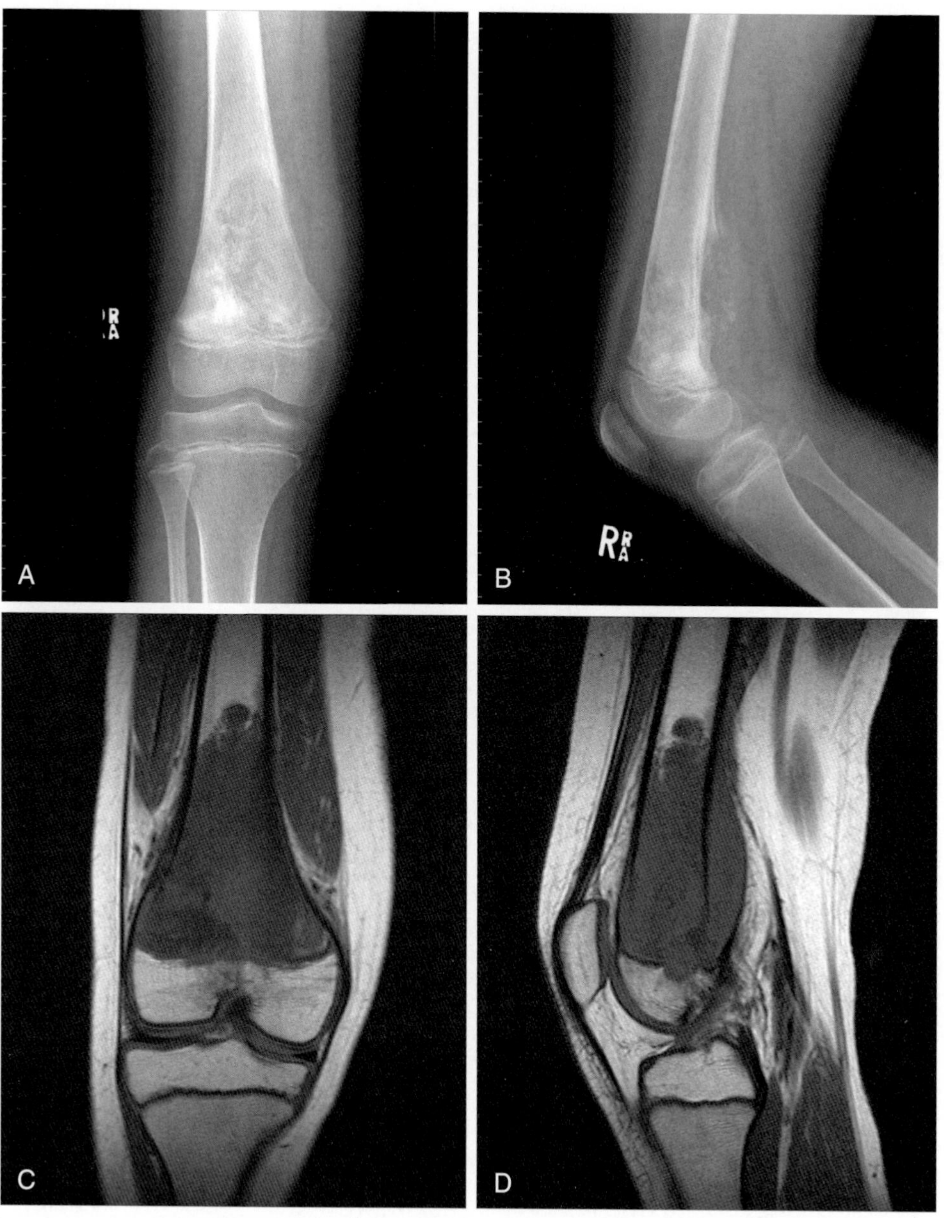

FIGURE 130-29 Osteosarcoma. Anteroposterior (**A**) and lateral (**B**) radiographs of the right knee demonstrate a lytic lesion in the right femoral metaphysis that shows areas of internal mineralized matrix. The lesion has eroded through the posterior cortex of the femur, extending into the adjacent soft tissues and lifting the periosteum to form a Codman triangle. Coronal (**C**) and sagittal (**D**) T1-weighted magnetic resonance images reflect the true extent of the tumor within the marrow cavity with low-signal tumor replacing the high-signal fatty marrow. Destroyed posterior femoral cortex with soft tissue extension can also be appreciated on the sagittal view.

include the entire length of the bone to evaluate for "skip lesions." Osteosarcomas typically avidly take up radiotracer on bone scintigraphic examination. CT of the chest is often used to detect metastatic lesions. Ossifying metastatic lesions may show uptake on bone scans.

Ewing's sarcoma is the most common malignant bone tumor in the first decade of life, usually occurring after 5 years of age. It is two times more common in males but is rare in Asians and African Americans. Children often present with systemic symptoms such as fever, pain, and an elevated white blood cell count. The most common location is the femoral diaphysis. However, lesions are also common in the flat bones of the pelvis, as well as the ribs and spine. Radiographically, Ewing's sarcoma appears as a predominantly lytic, permeative lesion in the diaphysis of a long bone. It has poorly defined margins. A periosteal reaction is common, often appearing either in a sunburst configuration or lamellated like an onion skin. Rarely, benign, thick, wavy periostitis may be seen. Ewing's sarcoma often has a large soft tissue component. CT and MRI are often helpful in demonstrating the entire osseous and soft tissue extent of the tumor (Fig. 130-30). Bone scintigraphy demonstrates both the primary lesion and bone metastatic lesions, which is a common presentation in Ewing's sarcoma.

Several other malignant tumors may affect bone. In children younger than 12 months, neuroblastomas are the most

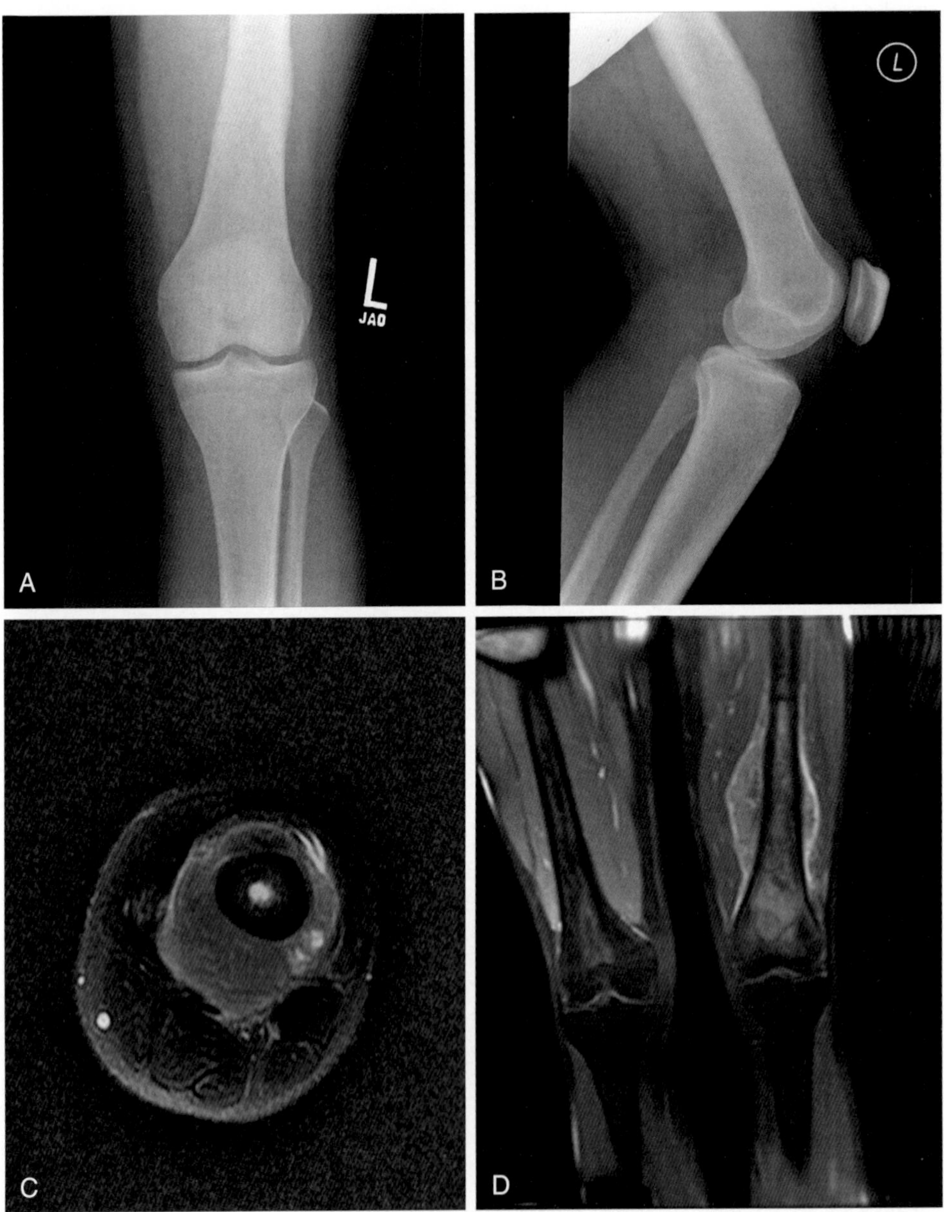

FIGURE 130-30 Ewing's sarcoma. **A** and **B,** Anteroposterior and lateral radiographs of the left knee demonstrate a subtle permeative lesion in the distal diaphysis of the femur with a mild periosteal reaction. Tissue planes are distorted, indicating a large soft tissue component. **C** and **D,** Axial T2-weighted fat-saturated and coronal T1-weighted fat-saturated gadolinium-enhanced magnetic resonance images of the femur confirm the presence of an elongated mass in the diaphysis of the femur extending into the distal metaphysis. A large soft tissue component is extending circumferentially around the femur. A biopsy revealed Ewing sarcoma.

common cause of bony destructive lesions. Like Ewing's sarcoma, they are small blue cell tumors that infiltrate marrow. They are most common in the chest, where they are termed *Askin tumors*. They are often associated with a pleural effusion and have a poor prognosis. Leukemia also commonly involves the skeleton, demonstrating osteopenia and focal osteolytic lesions on radiographs. MRI is sensitive to marrow infiltration from leukemia. Neither leukemia nor neuroblastomas produce tumor matrix.

Conclusion

Imaging of the pediatric skeleton, although similar to that of the adult skeleton in many respects, often presents unique technical and diagnostic challenges. At the center of these challenge lies the growth plate and epiphyseal ossification centers. Their continued evolution with age is reflected across their appearance on radiographic, CT, scintigraphic, and MRI examinations. Familiarity with normal variations is crucial to accurate diagnoses. Pediatric traumatic injuries differ from those of adults in both patterns of injury and healing. Additionally, the report of pain in the pediatric patient is often not secondary to a traumatic etiology but may reflect a host of conditions particular to the growing skeleton, including both benign and aggressive entities.

For a complete list of references, go to expertconsult.com.

Suggested Readings

Citation: Wootton-Gorges SL: MR imaging of primary bone tumors and tumor-like conditions in children. *Radiol Clin North Am* 47(6):957–975, 2009.

Level of Evidence: V (expert opinion)

Summary: The authors of this article provide a broad introduction to pediatric magnetic resonance imaging and address a wide spectrum of pathologic entities.

Citation: Kan JH, Kleinman PK: *Pediatric and Adolescent Musculoskeletal MRI: A Case-Based Approach*, Secaucus, NJ, 2007, Springer-Verlag.

Level of Evidence: IV (case based)

Summary: The authors describe a case-based approach to the magnetic resonance imaging presentation of pediatric musculoskeletal disorders including bone, joint, and soft tissue injuries.

Citation: Karantanas AH: *Sports Injuries in Children and Adolescents*, Secaucus, NJ, 2011, Springer.

Level of Evidence: IV (case based)

Summary: Karantanas provides a multimodality presentation of pediatric imaging, specifically focused on childhood sports injuries.

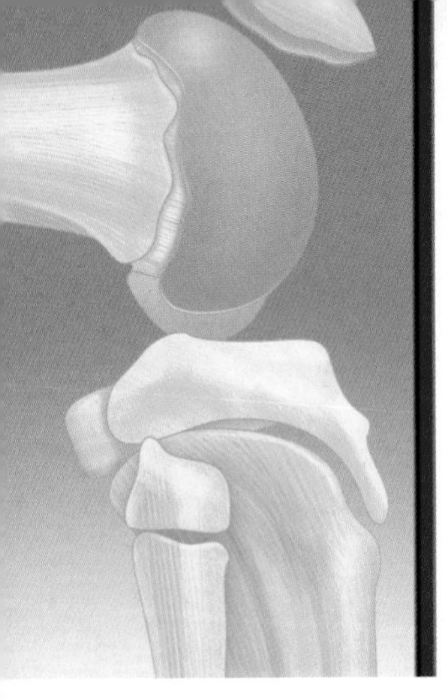

131

Shoulder Injuries in the Young Athlete

RALPH J. CURTIS

Shoulder injuries in the skeletally immature athlete are relatively uncommon but are significant in terms of interfering with sports participation.[1] Shoulder injuries in young athletes demonstrate both similarities and differences compared with injuries encountered in the adult. In younger patients the injury more often involves fracture through the open growth plates; in the adolescent patient with open physes, the injury tends to be more that in the adult, involving soft tissues, which may lead to instability.[2,3] Injury types tend to differ with age, as do injury rates. Injury rates increase steadily with age, with the highest rates seen in the high school age group.[4-6]

Sports injuries to the immature shoulder can be caused by both macrotrauma and microtrauma. Macrotrauma in the young shoulder usually results in an acute failure through the physis or, less frequently, from failure of the soft tissues. This injury pattern is the opposite of the pattern found in adults, who are more likely to have injuries from failure of ligament or tendon as opposed to bone. Failure as a result of repetitive stresses (microtrauma) is also more likely to result in a bony physeal injury in the young athlete and is much less likely to lead to stress injuries involving rotator cuff tears or labral injuries.

Anatomy

Injuries to the musculoskeletal system in the young athlete can be similar to those found in the adult but also can be uniquely different based on the anatomy of growing bone. In the skeletally immature athlete, all bone contains growth plates, or physes, that represent the primary site of longitudinal bone growth. This area of rapidly growing cartilage transitions to bone by a process called *endochondral ossification*. Due to the nature of this rapid development, physes have much less tensile strength than the surrounding bony epiphysis and metaphysis, thereby rendering the physis more vulnerable to injury as a result of compressive and shearing forces. Injuries to the growth plate are characterized by rapid healing and remodeling as well as the potential for growth arrest or disturbance.[7]

Clavicle

The clavicle is an S-shaped bone that occupies a subcutaneous position extending anteriorly from the sternoclavicular joint medially to the acromioclavicular (AC) joint laterally. It is more cylindrical in configuration medially and is somewhat flattened and narrow laterally. The clavicle provides attachment for many of the major shoulder girdle muscles, including the trapezius, deltoid, sternocleidomastoid, and pectoralis major muscles. It also provides a bony roof over the thoracic outlet, protecting the axillary vessels and brachial plexus.

The clavicle forms by intramembranous ossification during the fifth gestational week from two different areas in the diaphyseal portion of the bone. The medial physis of the clavicle is the most important, providing up to 80% of the remaining longitudinal growth of this bone. The medial epiphysis is one of the last in the body to ossify, appearing between 12 and 19 years of age and fusing to the shaft of the clavicle at age 22 to 25 years. The lateral clavicular epiphysis is rarely visualized radiographically, ossifying and fusing during a period of a few months at about 19 years of age.[7,8]

Scapula

The scapula is a large, flattened, triangular bone positioned at the posterolateral aspect of the bony thorax situated between the third and ninth ribs. It provides attachment for many of the major muscles about the shoulder and is a mobile base for the glenohumeral joint at the glenoid. It has five major components—the body, neck, spine, glenoid, and coracoid.

The body of the scapula is oriented at a 30- to 45-degree angle to the coronal plane of the body. It is concave on its costal surface with slight convexity on the dorsal surface. The dorsal surface of the body of the scapula is divided by a thin ridge of bone known as the *spine of the scapula* into the supraspinatus and infraspinatus fossae. At the lateral edge of the scapular spine, these two fossae communicate by the spinoglenoid notch. The acromion is an extension of the spine of the scapula laterally that rotates to form a flattened roof above the shoulder joint.[7]

The lateral portion of the scapular body narrows to form the scapular neck, which supports the glenoid fossa. The glenoid is a concave, pear-shaped structure covered with articular cartilage that is oriented laterally at approximate right angles to the long axis of the scapular body. The glenoid has an average of 5 degrees of superior tilt and retroversion of 3 to 9 degrees in relationship to the long axis of the scapula.[9,10]

The coracoid process is a bony projection off the anterior surface of the scapula just medial to the scapular neck. It projects anteriorly and laterally and serves as the origin of several muscles and ligaments that provide stability at the AC joint. Superiorly and medial to the coracoid is the suprascapular notch, which contains the suprascapular nerve.

The body of the scapula forms by intramembranous ossification through multiple ossification centers that are highly variable in terms of number and position. The base of the coracoid and upper glenoid have a common physis that is apparent by age 10 years. A variable ossification center can appear at puberty at the tip of the coracoid and may be mistaken as an avulsion fracture. The acromion ossifies by forming several ossification centers that appear by puberty and fuse by the age of 22 years. Failure of fusion of one of the acromial physes can result in an unfused os acromiale, which may have clinical implications in impingement.[8,11,12]

Proximal Humerus

The proximal humerus consists of four main components: humeral head, greater tuberosity, lesser tuberosity, and metaphyseal portion of the shaft. The humeral head has a large, convex, oval shape covered with a hyaline cartilage that articulates with the glenoid. The head forms an upward head shaft angle between 130 and 140 degrees and is in 25 to 30 degrees of retroversion as it relates to the humeral epicondyles.[13] Adjacent to the articular surface on the posterior and superior aspect is a prominent projection of bone known as the *greater tuberosity*. On the anterior surface is a smaller prominence of bone known as the *lesser tuberosity*. The tuberosities are separated by a shallow groove that allows passage of the long head of the biceps tendon into the glenohumeral joint. The anatomic neck is that space between the articular cartilage and the ligamentous and tendinous attachments on the tuberosities. The surgical neck is that portion of the proximal humerus that lies below the tuberosities and above the metaphysis.[7] The tuberosities serve as the attachment point for the tendons of the rotator cuff musculature.

The humerus is completely ossified throughout its diaphysis and metaphyseal portions at birth with the secondary ossification center for the head appearing in the first 6 months. The secondary ossification center for the greater tuberosity appears by age 3 years, followed by the secondary center for the lesser tuberosity about 2 years later. By age 5 to 7 years, the three proximal ossification centers of the humeral head, greater tuberosity, and lesser tuberosity coalesce to become a single proximal ossification center. The proximal humeral physis is predominately extracapsular along the surgical neck except medially, where it becomes intracapsular. The proximal humeral physis usually closes between 18 and 22 years of age and accounts for approximately 80% of longitudinal growth of the humerus.[8]

The classification of proximal humeral injuries in skeletally immature athletes is outlined in Box 131-1.

BOX 131-1 Classification of Proximal Humeral Injuries in Skeletally Immature Athletes by Location

I. Proximal humeral physeal fracture
   A. Salter-Harris I-II: common
   B. Salter-Harris III-IV: uncommon
II. Metaphyseal fracture
III. Lesser tuberosity fracture
IV. Stress injury
   A. Little Leaguer's shoulder

The Salter-Harris classification of physeal injuries is based on the orientation of the fracture line in relation to the physis and can be applied to proximal humeral physeal fractures. Proximal humeral physeal fractures from macrotrauma are commonly Salter-Harris type I or II injuries. Although Salter-Harris type III-IV fractures can occur, they are rare in sports and are more commonly a result of high-energy trauma, such as motocross.[88-90] Lesser tuberosity fractures are uncommon and represent avulsion injuries secondary to the force generated in the subscapularis tendon. Stress injuries to the proximal humeral physis are actually stress fractures caused by repetitive microtrauma.[91]

The Neer and Horowitz classification of displacement is also commonly used when describing proximal humerus fracture.[92]

Glenohumeral Instability

The glenohumeral joint of the shoulder in young athletes is susceptible to injury in high-demand sports activities as a result of both macrotrauma and repetitive microtrauma. The anatomy of the glenohumeral joint allows a high degree of functional mobility but with a sacrifice of inherent stability. Although the shoulder is susceptible to the development of pathologic instability, the same forces that result in soft tissue injury with instability in the adult commonly result in fracture through the proximal humeral physis in the skeletally immature young athlete.[14,15]

The incidence of shoulder instability in the young athlete is unknown. It has been reported that the adolescent athlete with open physes has an incidence of shoulder instability similar to that seen in adults, whereas in children younger than 12 years instability is less common. In the classic review by Rowe of 500 dislocated shoulders, only 8 patients were younger than 10 years old, whereas 99 patients were between 10 and 20 years of age.[16,17] Only 9 of 212 patients with traumatic glenohumeral dislocations had open physes in a series reported by Wagner and Lyne,[18] representing a 4.7% incidence rate.

Reports of glenohumeral dislocation due to trauma in children younger than 10 years of age are limited to very small numbers and case studies.[19,20] Many reports in the literature include patients between 11 and 20 years of age, but data for skeletal maturity are not included. Most of these studies involve traumatic instability treated by surgical reconstruction and do not address instability treated by nonoperative means.[21]

In addition to instability due to trauma, atraumatic shoulder instability as a result of underlying multidirectional laxity is commonly encountered in younger patients and must be recognized when treating athletes in these age groups. Studies describing multidirectional laxity with subluxation of the shoulder demonstrate this problem to be more common in younger age groups.[22] A classification of shoulder instability in young athletes is listed in Box 131-2.

BOX 131-2 Classification of Shoulder Instability in Young Athletes

Degree of Instability
1. Dislocation: complete, requiring reduction
2. Subluxation: incomplete, not requiring reduction

Direction of Instability
1. Anterior
2. Posterior
3. Multidirectional
4. Inferior (luxatio erecta)

Etiology of Instability
1. Traumatic instability
   a. Macrotraumatic: single event
2. Atraumatic instability
   a. Voluntary: volitional
   b. Involuntary: not controllable

Frequency of Instability
1. Acute instability: single episode
2. Recurrent instability: multiple episodes
3. Chronic instability: locked dislocation

Traumatic Anterior Instability

History

Anterior instability of the glenohumeral joint is the most common type of instability associated with macrotrauma. This direction of instability represents more than 90% of traumatic dislocations in all age groups and is frequently seen in collision and contact sports. To be categorized as a traumatic dislocation, the patient's history should include significant injury and an appropriate mechanism of forced abduction and external rotation at the shoulder applied to an outstretched arm. As a result of this force the humeral head is translated anteriorly, causing damage to the anterior-inferior glenohumeral ligaments and labrum, eventually subluxating or dislocating. The anterior soft tissue injury that includes stripping of the labrum and capsule from its insertion on the rim of the glenoid is termed a *Bankart* or *Perthes' lesion* (Fig. 131-1). During a dislocation the posterior-superior aspect of the humeral head impacts against the anterior rim and neck of the glenoid, often resulting in an impaction fracture called a *Hill-Sachs lesion*.

Recurrent instability of the shoulder is the most common complication associated with nonoperative treatment after an acute traumatic anterior dislocation. The age of the athlete at the time of the first dislocation is the single most important factor in assessing the risk for recurrent instability after an acute anterior dislocation. The risk for recurrence is inversely proportional to the patient's age. For patients younger than 20 years who want to continue to be athletically active, the risk for recurrent dislocation ranges between 48% and 100%. A 100% incidence of recurrence in children younger than 10 years and a 94% incidence of recurrence in adolescent and patients aged 11 to 20 years old have been reported by Rowe.[16] Many reports document a recurrence rate of 80% to 90% in traumatic dislocations for adolescent patients aged 12 to 18 years, but few distinguish the number of patients with open physes.[21,23] Wagner and Lyne[18] reported an 80% recurrence rate in 10 patients with clearly open proximal humeral physes. Marans and associates[24] reported on the natural history after anterior dislocation in 21 children between the ages of 4 and 15 years with open physes at the time of initial dislocation. They found a 100% recurrence rate no matter what postreduction treatment program was used. In a 10-year prospective study by Hovelius and colleagues,[25] a 48% recurrence rate after primary anterior dislocation was documented in young patients.

The evaluation of the young athlete with suspected recurrent anterior instability begins with a thorough history. Some patients have required multiple trips to the emergency department for reduction of anterior dislocation, whereas others with subluxation often relate a history of recurrent pain in the provocative position rather than feelings of instability. Many of these patients describe a feeling of a "dead arm" when an instability episode occurs. Careful consideration should be given to the initial injury to rule out the possibility of atraumatic instability, which should be treated much differently.

Physical Examination

Acute

Patients with an acute traumatic glenohumeral anterior dislocation present with pain and obvious deformity from the anteriorly displaced humeral head and relatively prominent acromion. The humeral head is located anteriorly and inferiorly and can sometimes be visualized or palpated in the axilla. The affected arm is usually supported by the opposite hand and held in a slightly abducted and externally rotated position. Motion is limited by pain. The athlete who presents after a subluxation episode or after dislocation with spontaneous reduction demonstrates tenderness with guarding but no deformity.

Careful examination of the neurologic and vascular status is mandatory. The axillary nerve is the most commonly injured neurologic structure after dislocation, but additional brachial

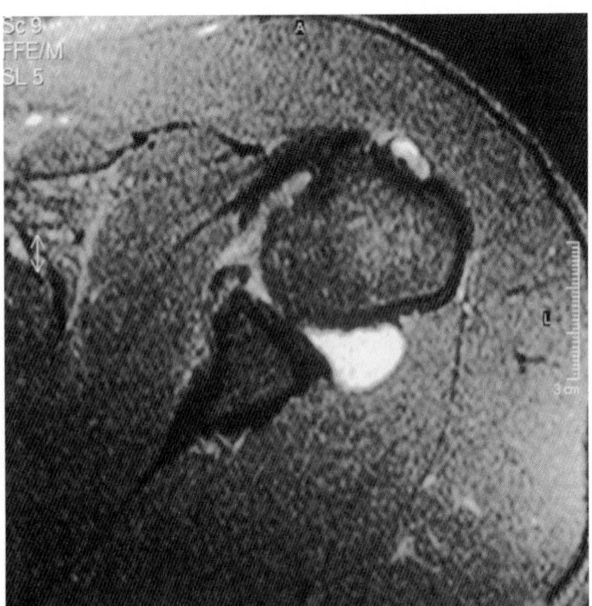

FIGURE 131-1 Magnetic resonance image of the shoulder demonstrating an anterior Bankart lesion in a case of recurrent anterior instability.

plexus involvement may be present. Axillary nerve injury has been reported in between 5% and 35% of first-time anterior shoulder dislocations.[14] Examination of the axillary nerve can be accomplished by first testing the sensory distribution of the axillary nerve along the upper lateral arm by light touch or pinprick. The motor innervation to the deltoid can be evaluated by having the patient abduct the dislocated shoulder as the examiner supports the affected elbow with one hand while palpating the deltoid for contraction with the opposite hand. This can be accomplished without causing the patient undue pain and confirms function of the axillary nerve (Fig. 131-2). The presence of both the radial and ulnar pulses should be noted. Absence of the pulses or swelling with a rapidly expanding hematoma suggests a rare vascular injury.[26]

Recurrent

Clinical examination in the athlete with recurrent instability usually reveals a full range of motion and normal physical appearance. Strength is generally equal to the opposite side with occasional mild weakness in external rotation against resistance. Provocative tests for anterior instability are usually positive.

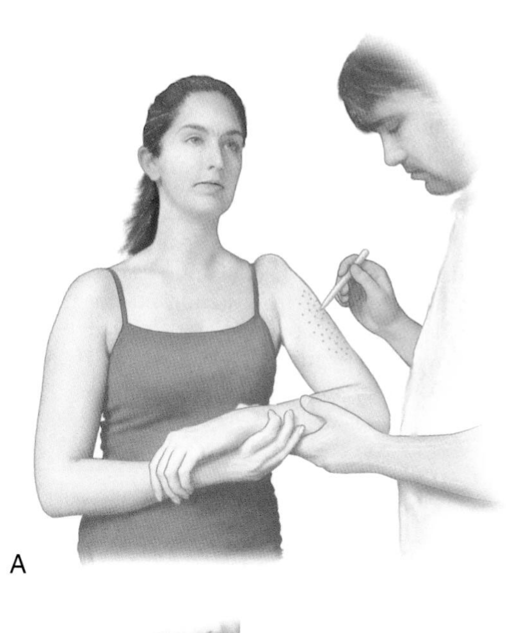

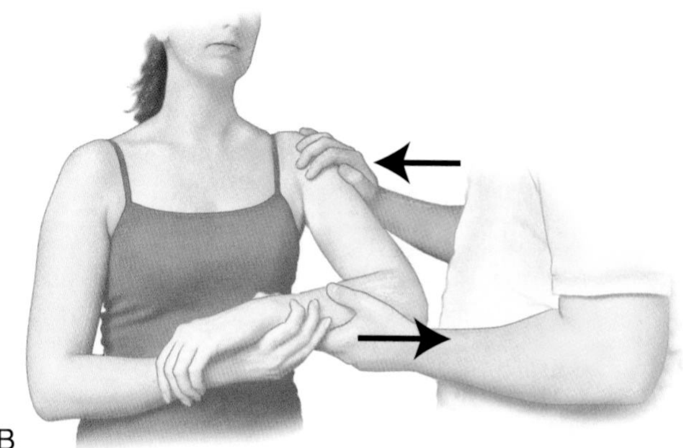

FIGURE 131-2 Clinical evaluation of the axillary nerve during initial assessment of a patient with anterior dislocation. **A,** Sensory distribution can be tested to light touch on the upper lateral arm. **B,** Motor testing is accomplished by palpating contraction of the deltoid muscle during resisted abduction.

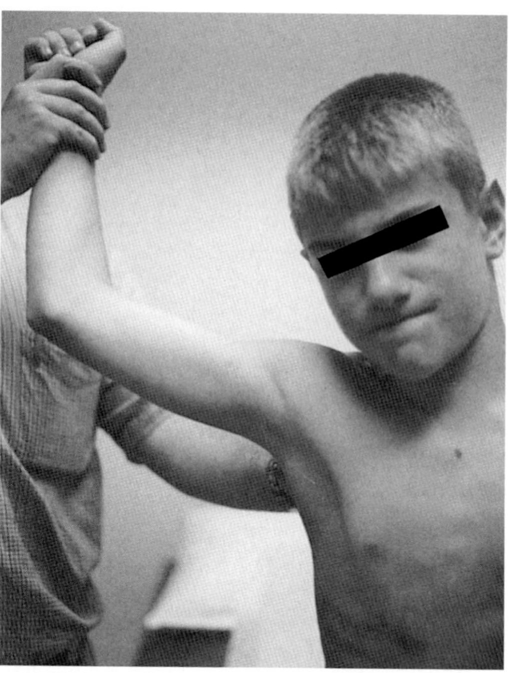

FIGURE 131-3 A positive anterior apprehension test in a young athlete with recurrent anterior instability.

Provocative tests for anterior instability include the anterior apprehension test and the relocation test.[27] The anterior apprehension test is performed with the patient standing or seated while the examiner is positioned at the side (Fig. 131-3). The examiner stabilizes the scapula with one hand, placing the thumb on the posterior aspect of the shoulder joint while the opposite hand is used to bring the patient's arm into abduction and external rotation. The result is positive when the test elicits a feeling of apprehension or instability with or without pain.

The relocation test is performed with the patient supine and the examiner standing at the side. The examiner performs the apprehension test in this supine position and then repeats the test with one hand applying a posteriorly directed force to the anterior shoulder. A resultant decrease in apprehension with this maneuver represents a positive test.

Imaging

Routine Radiography

Acute and recurrent traumatic instability of the shoulder is best evaluated initially with routine radiography. In the young athlete with open physes, fracture of the proximal humerus should always be suspected and ruled out with routine radiographs.[28,29] The trauma series for the shoulder includes three views: the anteroposterior (AP) view, an axillary lateral view, and a trans scapular Y view. It is important to image the shoulder in at least two planes oriented at right angles to the other to confirm the actual position of the humeral head in relation to the glenoid. In cases of anterior instability, the humeral head can be seen situated anterior and inferior to the normal position in the glenoid (Fig. 131-4). Postreduction films in both planes are important to confirm reduction and

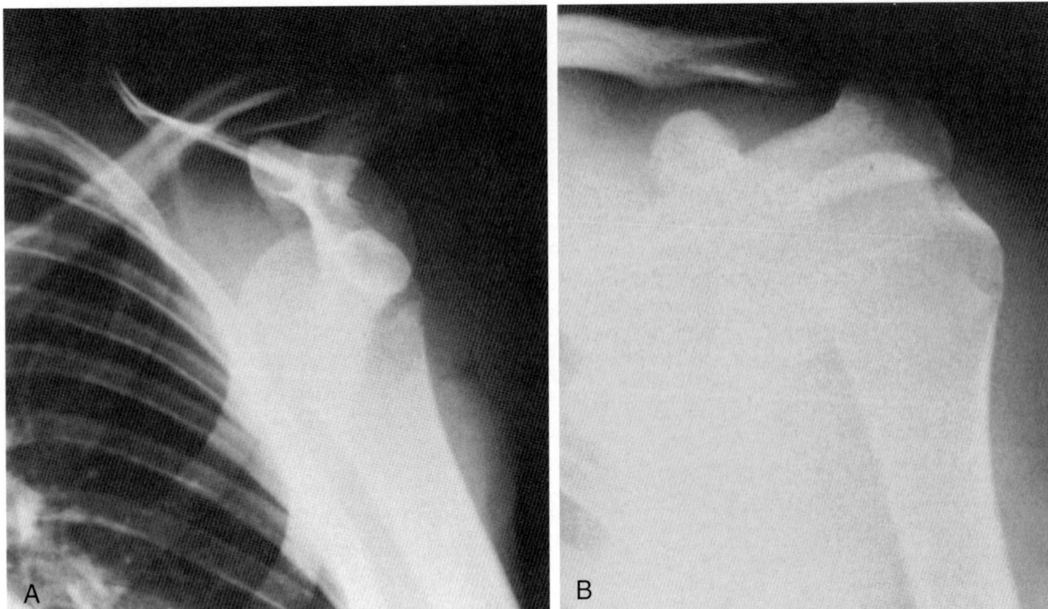

FIGURE 131-4 Anterior dislocation of the shoulder as demonstrated on anteroposterior plain radiographic view. **A,** Initial film shows an anteroinferior dislocation with the humeral head in the dislocated position. **B,** Postreduction film shows the humeral head in normal relation to the glenoid. Note the Hill-Sachs lesion (indentation fracture of the posterosuperior humeral head).

assess for fractures that are difficult to visualize in the dislocated shoulder. The postreduction films often reveal a posterolateral humeral head impaction fracture (Hill-Sachs lesion) but can also reveal fractures involving the anterior glenoid rim (boney Bankart lesion). The anterior glenoid rim is best evaluated for fracture or deficiency on an axillary lateral or modified axillary lateral view (West Point view).[30] The size and position of the glenoid rim fracture and, to a lesser degree, the Hill-Sachs fracture have been reported to affect the success of surgical treatment for recurrent anterior instability.

Magnetic Resonance Imaging

Magnetic resonance imaging (MRI) has become the standard to assess and evaluate shoulder instability. MRI is commonly combined with arthrography to evaluate injury to capsular and labral structures, articular surfaces, and tendons. Damage to these soft tissue structures can be successfully visualized in a high percentage of cases (see Fig. 131-1).[31]

Treatment Options

Nonoperative Treatment

The initial treatment for a dislocated shoulder, whether acute or recurrent, is accomplished by closed reduction. A careful assessment of the neurovascular status should be performed both before and after reduction, with particular attention to axillary nerve function. Early reduction can often be accomplished without anesthesia, but if significant pain and muscle spasm limit success then appropriate intraarticular anesthesia or intravenous analgesia and sedation are used.[32,33] Closed reduction of a suspected dislocation in the athlete younger than 14 years before radiographic confirmation is certainly more hazardous than in an adolescent or adult due to the higher frequency of proximal humeral physeal fracture in this age group. If possible, radiographs should be taken before reduction.

The traction/countertraction technique for reduction of anterior shoulder dislocation (Fig. 131-5) is performed with the patient in the supine position. Longitudinal traction is applied to the arm on a continuous basis while countertraction is applied to the thorax with a sheet passed around the patient's trunk through the axilla. Reduction is accomplished by loosening the humeral head from its locked position on the anterior glenoid rim by overcoming muscle spasm through the longitudinally applied traction. Once the head is disimpacted spontaneous reduction occurs.

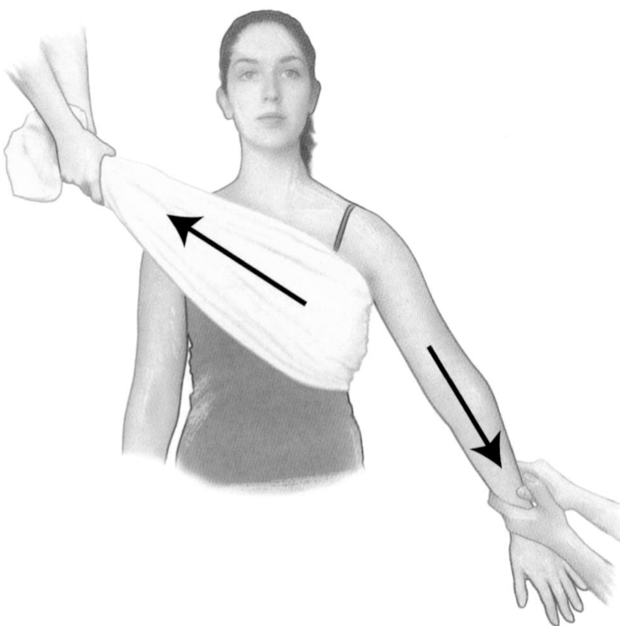

FIGURE 131-5 The traction/countertraction technique for reduction of anterior dislocation of the shoulder.

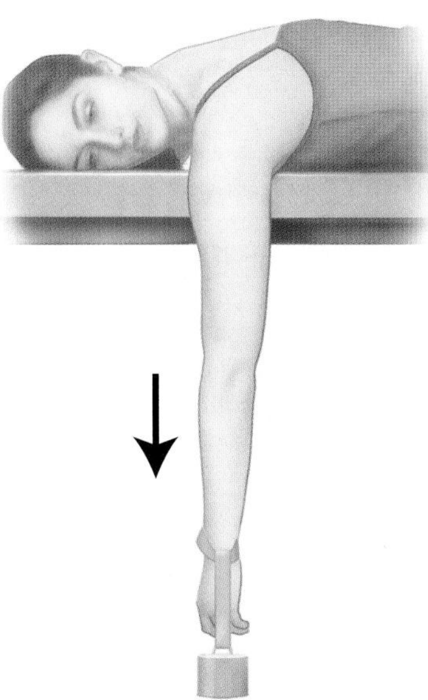

FIGURE 131-6 Stimson's maneuver for reduction of anterior dislocation of the shoulder.

In the Stimson's maneuver for closed reduction (Fig. 131-6), the patient is placed prone on an examination table. The dislocated arm is allowed to hang off the edge of the table while a weight of 10 to 15 pounds is suspended from the patient's wrist. Spontaneous reduction of the humeral head occurs as the shoulder musculature is relaxed by the gravity-assisted traction. This technique is particularly useful in situations of a single person attempting the reduction.

The abduction maneuver for reduction is performed with the patient in the supine position. The arm is supported by the examiner with the elbow flexed. The shoulder is gently abducted and externally rotated into the overhead position, thus reproducing the mechanism of injury. Reduction occurs as the arm is then brought to the side with extension, adduction, and gentle internal rotation.

After closed reduction, appropriate radiographs are obtained to confirm the position of the humeral head and to rule out associated fracture. The arm is immobilized in a sling for comfort and protection. A rehabilitation program is begun as soon as comfort allows in an attempt to prevent recurrent instability.

In the athlete with recurrent anterior instability of the shoulder, nonoperative treatment has had limited success in preventing further recurrence. Although aggressive rehabilitation programs and bracing have been used to decrease frequency, these methods are a temporizing measure before definitive surgical treatment is performed.

Operative Treatment

Rarely is acute surgical treatment for open reduction of an uncomplicated traumatic anterior dislocation necessary. Closed reduction is usually successful when the necessary muscular relaxation is obtained.

On occasion, after initial closed reduction, surgical stabilization as the definitive treatment for initial traumatic anterior dislocation in the young, at-risk athlete has been reported.[34-38] If the athletic demand or seasonal timing dictates, consideration for primary repair seems to be a reasonable option when compared to the 48% to 100% recurrence rates found in patients with skeletal immaturity after conservative treatment.[15,39] Less invasive arthroscopic procedures have been documented to be successful, resulting in up to 88% success rate.[38] One recent prospective study in treating acute dislocations reported a 75% recurrence rate after immobilization and rehabilitation compared with an 11% recurrence rate after arthroscopic stabilization.[40] Jones and associates[41] compared the results of primary arthroscopic Bankart repair to late reconstruction after failed conservative treatment in skeletally immature adolescent patients aged 11 to 18 years. They found a similar satisfaction rating and a lower recurrence rate (12.5% vs. 18.75%) for the acute surgical group.

Surgical reconstruction is the treatment of choice for recurrent traumatic anterior instability of the shoulder and has resulted in good success rates. Historically, many types of procedures have been successfully used in the treatment of recurrent dislocation. The most common types of anterior reconstruction of the shoulder are bone block–type procedures (Bristow, Latarjet), subscapularis shortening procedures (Putti-Platt, Magnuson-Stack), and capsular procedures (Bankart, capsulolabral reconstruction). Although these procedures have all been successful at limiting recurrent dislocation, many long-term studies demonstrate less success at eliminating subluxation and complications such as pain, limited motion, hardware failure, and premature arthritis.[42-54]

Today, anterior reconstruction procedures are directed toward restoring normal anatomy with direct repair of the capsulolabral structures. These procedures have been reported to have a high success rate combined with a low complication rate and are the most commonly used.[55] Repair to bone is accomplished with a variety of suture anchors. Metallic fixation devices are avoided, particularly in the athlete with open physes.

There are limited data available regarding specific results for surgical treatment of recurrent anterior instability in skeletally immature patients. Most studies of anterior reconstruction include both patients who are skeletally mature and immature, but results are not specifically subcategorized by age or radiographic criteria. Reports of surgical reconstruction by a variety of techniques in skeletally immature patients by Wagner and Lyne[18] and Marans[24] identified good short-term results. Postacchini[56] reported a 100% success rate in a group of adolescent patients treated with surgical reconstruction. Both the open and arthroscopic capsulolabral repairs have been successful.[55] Recent reports by Cole,[57] Freedman,[58] and Karlsson[59] demonstrated good results of both open and arthroscopic treatment for recurrent anterior dislocation.

Postoperative Management

After closed reduction of an acute dislocation, immobilization in a sling is followed by a period of supervised rehabilitation. Aggressive rehabilitation focuses on strengthening the rotator cuff, deltoid, and periscapular muscles. Plyometric exercises are added in the later rehabilitation phase in an attempt to improve proprioceptive function for return to sports-specific activities. The length of immobilization and the type and length of rehabilitation are somewhat controversial. Recurrent dislocation is the single biggest problem in shoulder instability after an acute traumatic dislocation. At least two studies

AUTHORS' PREFERRED TECHNIQUE

Acute Traumatic Anterior Dislocation

Closed reduction is the initial treatment of choice after acute traumatic anterior dislocation. Physical examination with careful attention to the neurologic status of the axillary nerve is performed before and after closed reduction. In children younger than 14 years, I prefer radiographic evaluation with a trauma series to confirm the diagnosis and rule out associated fracture before reduction. In adolescents aged 14 years and older, on-the-field gentle closed reduction can be attempted before radiographic evaluation. I prefer traction/countertraction or Stimson's maneuver for closed reduction. A sling is adequate for postreduction immobilization. An aggressive rehabilitation program focusing on dynamic stabilization is used in an attempt to avoid recurrence.

Despite the high incidence of recurrence in young patients, nonoperative treatment is still my treatment of choice. On occasion, adolescent athletes with a documented traumatic lesion to the anterior labrum who participate in high-risk collision sports are considered for primary surgery. Successful results in treating young athletes with primary surgical repair have been obtained with arthroscopic capsulolabral repair techniques with suture anchors.[60,61]

In the skeletally immature patient who has documented recurrent traumatic anterior shoulder instability, surgical reconstruction is indicated. I prefer a modification of the open capsular procedure originally described by Rockwood and reported by Wirth and associates.[55] This procedure is performed with the patient under general anesthesia through a modified axillary incision. The procedure combines a direct repair of the Bankart lesion using bioresorbable suture anchors with a capsular shift as necessary to address capsular injury or laxity (Fig. 131-7). A sling is used postoperatively for 3 to 4 weeks, followed by a vigorous 6- to 9-month rehabilitation program before return to competitive sports.

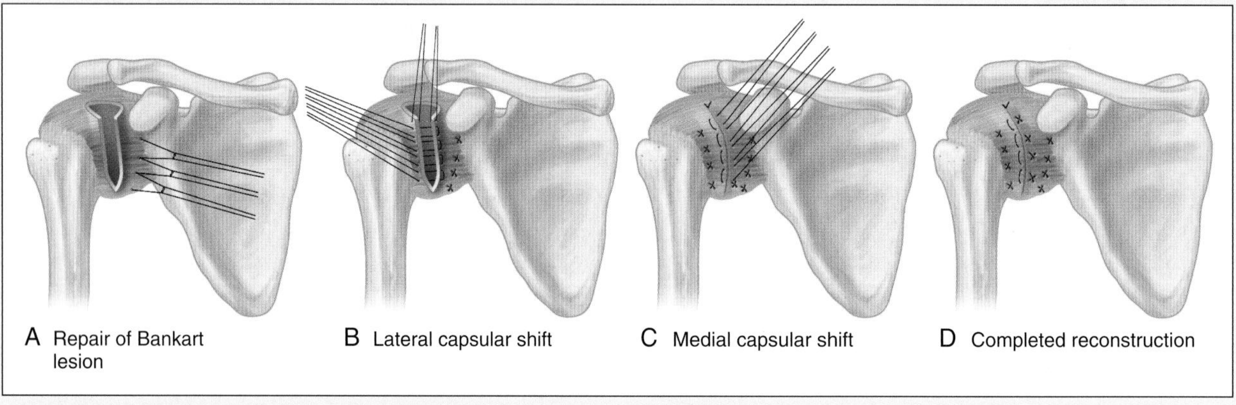

FIGURE 131-7 The author's preferred technique for anterior reconstruction of the shoulder. **A,** The Bankart lesion is repaired with suture anchors in the glenoid rim. **B,** A vertical split is made in the mid-capsule from the rotator interval to at least the 6 o'clock position. The lateral capsule is then shifted laterally and superiorly beneath the medial capsular flap. **C,** The lateral capsular flap is then closed over the medial flap. **D,** The completed repair after direct repair of the Bankart lesion and capsular shift as needed to provide stability.

have demonstrated lower recurrence rates in young, at-risk patients treated with 4 to 6 weeks of immobilization and a 3- to 6-month delay in return to athletic activities.[62,63] Other reports suggest that neither the length of immobilization nor the type or duration of rehabilitation alters the natural history of recurrence.[64] Hovelius[39] has published a 10-year prospective study that confirmed that neither the type nor the duration of the initial treatment had any effect on the rate of recurrence.

After surgical reconstruction for recurrent instability, the shoulder is protected in an immobilization device for 1 month while gentle range of motion is allowed. During the second month, range of motion is stressed while avoiding the extremes of abduction and external rotation. At 4 weeks, rotator cuff and scapular strengthening exercises are started. The athlete begins core strengthening and running at the 6-week stage. At 12 weeks, the athlete is started on general weightlifting activities and proprioception retraining. Contact sports are avoided for 6 months.

Return to Play

After closed treatment of an acute traumatic anterior shoulder instability episode, the athlete must regain full range of motion and protective strength as well as demonstrate stability in the overhead position without apprehension before return to play. If the athlete continues to demonstrate apprehension in the provocative position, a recurrent dislocation is more likely to occur. Therefore the decision about return to play must be made on an individual basis. Bracing to avoid the apprehension position may be useful, but there has been no documented evidence supporting the technique.

After surgery, the goal of reconstruction of the shoulder is to return the athlete to all activities without symptoms of instability. These goals usually require 6 to 9 months after surgical reconstruction to achieve. If the athlete has regained adequate range of motion and protective strength without signs of apprehension in the provocative position, the patient can return to contact and overhead sports.

Complications

The single most common complication of treatment for acute anterior shoulder instability is recurrent instability. As previously mentioned, the recurrence rate in the skeletally immature athlete is documented to be in the range of 48% to 100%. Other complications include axillary nerve injury, which may be present in up to 35% of cases but is usually transient.[27]

Complications associated with surgical treatment include recurrence of instability, loss of range of motion, and neurologic injury.

Traumatic Posterior Instability

Historically, traumatic posterior instability of the shoulder is reported to be much less common than anterior instability in all age groups, representing only 4% of traumatic dislocations. However, many recent studies of shoulder instability reported over the past decade seem to indicate that posterior instability is actually more common than once recognized. These study results were likely attributable to improved imaging techniques and greater awareness of the problem.

Many studies of posterior instability include adolescent patients, but little data are available regarding whether these patients have completed skeletal maturity.[64-67] Few reports of preadolescent patients with posterior instability exist in the literature. Foster and associates[68] described a case of an isolated traumatic posterior shoulder dislocation in a 10-year-old child. Most cases of posterior instability in young patients are associated with multidirectional atraumatic instability rather than as a result of trauma.

Posterior instability of the shoulder, whether dislocation or subluxation, often results in stripping of the posterior-inferior labrum and capsular ligaments from their attachment on the posterior glenoid, which is termed a *reverse Bankart lesion*. When the anterior aspect of the humeral head dislocates and makes contact with the posterior rim of the glenoid, the result often is an impaction fracture called a *reverse Hill-Sachs lesion*.

History

The mechanism of injury can be either direct or indirect. Commonly in contact sports, a force directed along an outstretched arm with the shoulder adducted, internally rotated, and flexed can drive the shoulder posterior. This would appear to be the most common mechanism in football offensive linemen during blocking. A direct mechanism of injury can result from a blow to the anterior aspect of the shoulder that can result in posterior shoulder instability. Either of these mechanisms can occur in the course of contact sports. In addition, posterior instability can occur indirectly as a result of a seizure or electrical shock. During seizure activity, violent contraction of the strong shoulder internal rotators forces the humeral head posterior. Any report of shoulder pain in an athlete who has had a seizure should be taken seriously, and a posterior dislocation should be suspected.[27]

Clinically, patients with posterior instability of the shoulder report pain and limited ability to move the arm. In cases with complete dislocation, patients are usually aware that the shoulder is out of place but may not be able to describe the direction of the dislocation. Subluxation is much more common than dislocation in athletes. When subluxation occurs, the prominent report is pain with a transient sensation of instability. Remember that in the skeletally immature athlete, fracture through the proximal humeral physis is more common than dislocation and may mimic instability clinically.[14]

For athletes involved in contact sports, recurrent posterior instability after an acute episode is not uncommon. These episodes usually represent recurrent subluxation rather than dislocation. These patients are more likely to report pain or a dead-arm sensation associated with specific activities rather than instability. Approximately half of patients with recurrent posterior subluxation have a sensation of instability but can rarely identify the direction.

Physical Examination

Acute

Posterior dislocation of the shoulder is less apparent on clinical examination when compared with the more common anterior dislocation and can easily be overlooked. The arm is usually held across the abdomen with the shoulder internally rotated and adducted. The shoulder is tender to palpation and the patient avoids motion. Only on close inspection by visualizing the shoulder from above can the clinician visualize flattening of the anterior aspect of the shoulder with prominence of the coracoid and a fullness posteriorly created by the dislocated humeral head. The hallmark of the diagnosis is a lack of shoulder external rotation and inability to supinate the forearm.[27] These examination findings are subtle and sometimes difficult to elicit in the acute situation because of swelling and pain. The lack of clinical findings can lead the examiner to a delay in diagnosis.

Examination of the athlete after a posterior subluxation episode is usually relatively normal on clinical inspection. The shoulder may demonstrate tenderness at the joint line, mild swelling, and decreased range of motion. Pain is usually elicited with cross-arm adduction and the posterior apprehension maneuver. The posterior apprehension test is performed with the patient upright, either standing or seated, with the examiner positioned on the symptomatic side. The arm is taken into horizontal adduction with the shoulder flexed 90 degrees while the examiner applies a posteriorly directed force across the flexed elbow. A feeling of apprehension or instability is a positive test.[27]

The jerk test is similar to the posterior apprehension test in terms of position. The examiner puts the arm into the horizontally adducted position and attempts to subluxate the shoulder posteriorly.[27] When the arm is then moved rapidly into a horizontally abducted position, the shoulder is reduced with a palpable and often visible jerk. The jerk test may be positive for crepitus and a catch when the arm is taken from the adducted to the abducted position.

Recurrent

In recurrent posterior instability, examination of the athlete is characterized by normal appearance, range of motion, and strength on manual muscle testing. Positive provocative tests include the posterior apprehension test and jerk test. The O'Brien test classically described for SLAP (**s**uperior **l**abrum, **a**nterior to **p**osterior) lesions is often positive.[27]

Imaging

Radiographs

The radiographic evaluation of posterior instability of the shoulder includes the three-view trauma series: the AP view, the axillary lateral view, and the transscapular Y view. These radiographs should include at least two views in planes at 90 degrees to each other. Radiographic findings on the AP view are very subtle even when the humeral head is completely posteriorly dislocated. The diagnosis is confirmed with a lateral radiograph, either axillary or transscapular Y view, demonstrating the posterior dislocation of the humeral head. On the axillary view, the empty glenoid is apparent with the humeral head lodged on the glenoid posteriorly. Postreduction films are important in both the AP and lateral planes to confirm the position of reduction and evaluate for associated fracture. Common radiographic findings include a reversed Hill-Sachs impaction fracture on the anterior surface of the humeral head and marginal fractures of the posterior glenoid rim, called a *reverse boney Bankart lesion*.

Magnetic Resonance Imaging

MRI has become the standard in evaluating posterior instability of the shoulder in all situations except acute dislocation. Combined with arthrography, MRI provides detail about the soft tissue injuries associated with posterior instability including labral, chondral, and tendinous pathology. Both the size of the reverse Hill-Sachs lesion and posterior Bankart lesion can be assessed (Fig. 131-8).

Treatment Options

Nonoperative Treatment

Initial treatment of posterior dislocation of the shoulder in the young athlete includes adequate workup to confirm the diagnosis and exclude fracture. When the diagnosis is confirmed, closed reduction is usually successful. Appropriate analgesia and sedation should be used to obtain adequate muscular relaxation during reduction. With the patient in the supine position, traction is applied to the adducted arm in line with the deformity. Countertraction is accomplished by stabilizing the chest while exerting lateral pressure on the upper arm, lifting the humeral head back into the glenoid fossa. The arm is usually stable at the side and can be immobilized in a sling. If instability is present after reduction, an external rotation splint or spica cast can be applied.

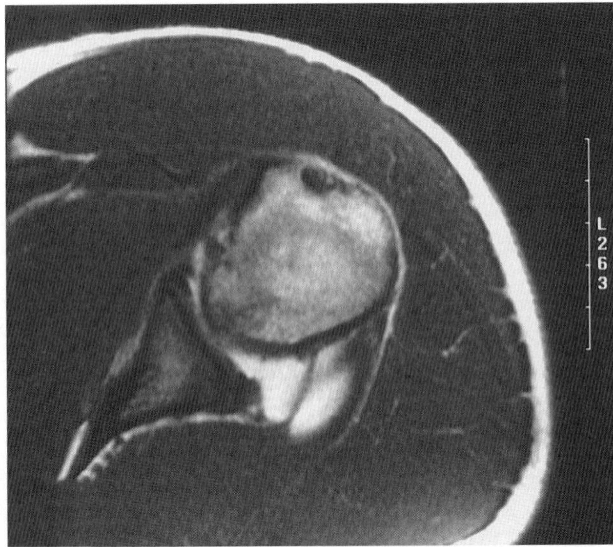

FIGURE 131-8 Magnetic resonance image of the shoulder depicting a posterior (reverse) Bankart lesion, including stripping of the capsulolabral complex from the posterior rim of the glenoid.

Operative Treatment

Surgical treatment is rarely required for initial treatment of a posterior dislocation. Open reduction of a locked posterior dislocation has been described in adults. Surgery may become necessary after an acute traumatic posterior dislocation associated with fracture of the lesser tuberosity, proximal humeral physis, or with a major fracture of the posterior glenoid rim, resulting in uncontrollable instability despite external rotation bracing. Open reduction and internal fixation of the fracture is usually sufficient to provide stability.

Surgical repair has been successful in the treatment of recurrent posterior shoulder instability. Both open and arthroscopic techniques that address the posterior capsulolabral injury (reverse Bankart lesion) often combined with capsular repair have been described. Results of both open and arthroscopic techniques have been similarly successful. Recent studies by Kim and colleagues,[69] Bradley and colleagues,[70] and Mair and associates[67] have described greater than 90% success with arthroscopic posterior capsulolabral reconstructions in athletic populations. Wolf and colleagues[71] and Misamore and Facibene[72] have documented 81% to 92% good results with traditional open capsular techniques. Although all these reports include young athletes there are few data documenting skeletal maturity.

Postoperative Management

The goal of postreduction treatment is to regain full range of motion and strength without apprehension. After the prescribed immobilization period of 3 to 6 weeks, an aggressive rehabilitation program is begun. Active and assisted range of motion avoiding cross-body adduction is started when appropriate. This is followed by focused strengthening of the rotator cuff and scapular rotators. As strength progresses, additional chest, shoulder, and back exercises are started in the weight room. Complete rehabilitation for return to overhead and contact sports may require 4 to 6 months after acute instability.

Rehabilitation and bracing are rarely effective in eliminating symptoms in patients with recurrent posterior instability of the shoulder. By improving protective strength and limiting range of motion in the provocative position, nonsurgical treatment may decrease the symptoms of instability, allowing the athlete an opportunity to complete a season before obtaining definitive treatment.

After surgery the operative shoulder is immobilized for 1 month in an external rotation brace. At the 4- to 6-week stage, rotator cuff strengthening and scapular strengthening are instituted, along with range of motion exercises. Avoidance of provocative cross-arm adduction maneuvers and pressing activities is continued for 12 weeks. At 12 weeks, a full weight room strength program and proprioception retraining are

AUTHORS' PREFERRED TECHNIQUE

Acute Posterior Dislocation

For the pediatric and adolescent athlete with an acute posterior dislocation of the shoulder, radiographic confirmation is required to exclude proximal humerus fracture before attempted reduction. Closed reduction is accomplished by applying longitudinal traction to the arm with countertraction to the torso. Stability is assessed after reduction, and immobilization in a brace is tailored to the most stable position. Radiographs after reduction should confirm position and exclude fracture.

In cases of suspected posterior shoulder subluxation, workup with magnetic resonance arthrography is obtained to confirm the diagnosis. Most cases are treated with a short period of immobilization followed by an intensive rehabilitation program. Primary surgery can be considered for a high-performance athlete in whom a significant reverse Bankart lesion is identified. Arthroscopic posterior capsulolabral reconstruction has been successful in allowing athletes to return to their preinjury level of participation.

Athletes with well-documented recurrent posterior instability of the shoulder who demonstrate a reverse or posterior Bankart lesion on magnetic resonance arthrography should be treated surgically. I prefer arthroscopic posterior capsulolabral reconstruction performed in the lateral position (Fig. 131-9). After careful assessment of the pathology, repair of the posterior Bankart lesion is accomplished. The glenoid in the area of the defect is debrided, followed by insertion of biocomposite suture anchors placed along the posterior rim of the glenoid. The sutures are then passed deep to the labrum and capsule to advance these structures back to their anatomic position, thus restoring the labral buttress. Additional repair of capsular injury, rotator cuff pathology, and removal of loose bodies can be performed as well. Postoperative immobilization is in an external rotation brace.

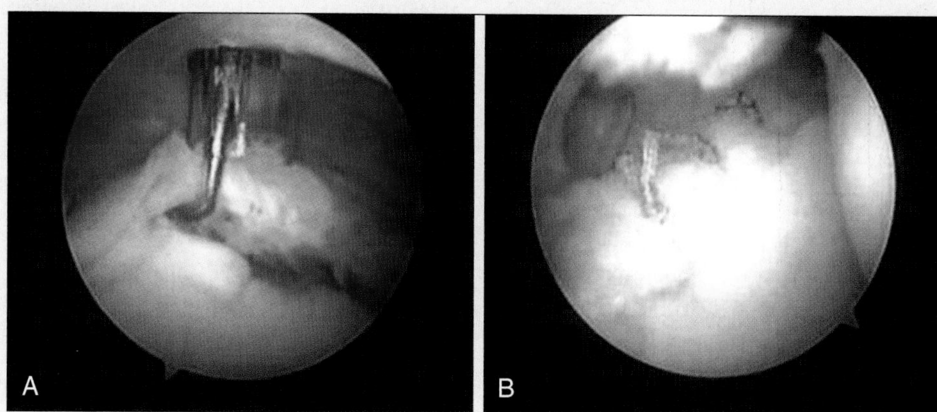

FIGURE 131-9 Arthroscopic images during a posterior capsulolabral repair. **A,** The probe is on the posterior labrum, which has detached from the posterior inferior glenoid as a reverse Bankart lesion. **B,** After repair of the posterior capsulolabral injury.

begun. Sports-specific noncontact activities can begin at 4 months, with anticipated return to contact at 6 months.

Return to Play

As for most injuries to the shoulder, return to play after posterior instability treated with nonoperative or operative techniques requires relatively normal function before return. Full range of motion and strength in the injured arm must be present without apprehension in the provocative position. Sports-specific activities should return to normal before return to contact sports.

Atraumatic Instability

Atraumatic instability of the glenohumeral joint in the skeletally immature athlete is common, but the actual incidence of this subset of instability has not been reported in the literature.[73] Atraumatic instability is usually characterized by redundancy and hyperelasticity of the capsule with increased intraarticular volume, resulting in multidirectional laxity of the shoulder. This multidirectional laxity is not always symptomatic but is a prerequisite for pathologic atraumatic instability. Multidirectional laxity may be associated with a true syndrome of collagen deficiency, such as Marfan or Ehlers-Danlos syndrome. Emery and Mullaji[74] have reported signs of instability in 57% of shoulders in boys and 48% in girls in a study of normal school-aged children.

History

Atraumatic instability can be categorized as voluntary or involuntary depending on the degree of conscious control the patient exerts on the shoulder during the instability episode. A shoulder "dislocation" in a child or adolescent without a clear, significant history of trauma suggests an instance of atraumatic instability. These patients have inherent joint laxity, and the glenohumeral joint can be dislocated voluntarily or involuntarily as a result of minimal trauma. Episodes of instability may occur with activities such as throwing, hitting an overhead serve in tennis and volleyball, or swimming. These episodes do not constitute significant trauma, and a high index of suspicion for atraumatic instability should be maintained in these cases.

Atraumatic instability associated with secondary impingement symptoms is a common cause of shoulder pain in the young athlete involved in sports that require repetitive overhand motion, such as swimming, baseball, and volleyball. These patients rarely report instability, but instead report pain exacerbated by high-demand sports activity. Most of these individuals do not recognize their own inherent multidirectional laxity; it is therefore difficult from the patient's history to determine that instability is truly the primary underlying pathology.

Voluntary instability is accomplished by patients with multidirectional laxity through conscious firing of certain muscle groups and inhibition of their antagonists while combining these muscle manipulations with certain arm positions that lead to subluxation of the glenohumeral joint (see Fig. 131-7). The most notable finding in cases of voluntary instability is the lack of pain associated with the subluxation or dislocation episode. Pathologic voluntary instability is never recognized as such by the individual and is often associated with psychological or emotional instability.[75-77]

Physical Examination

On examination the shoulder, range of motion is normal and specific tenderness is usually absent. Signs of multidirectional laxity at the shoulder are always present. A positive sulcus sign (Fig. 131-10) is recognized as a dimpling of the skin or sulcus noted below the acromion when manual longitudinal traction is applied to the arm. This is a result of inferior subluxation of the humeral head within the glenohumeral joint.

Significant humeral head translation can also be elicited with the drawer test, as described by Gerber and Ganz (Fig. 131-11).[78] The drawer test is performed with the examiner seated at the patient's side, stabilizing the scapula with one hand while the opposite hand manually translates the humeral head anteriorly and posteriorly. Most of these patients demonstrate evidence of ligamentous hyperlaxity in multiple other joints, including hyperextension at the elbows, knees, and metacarpophalangeal joints. Skin hyperelasticity with striae may also be present and may suggest the presence of an underlying collagen abnormality.

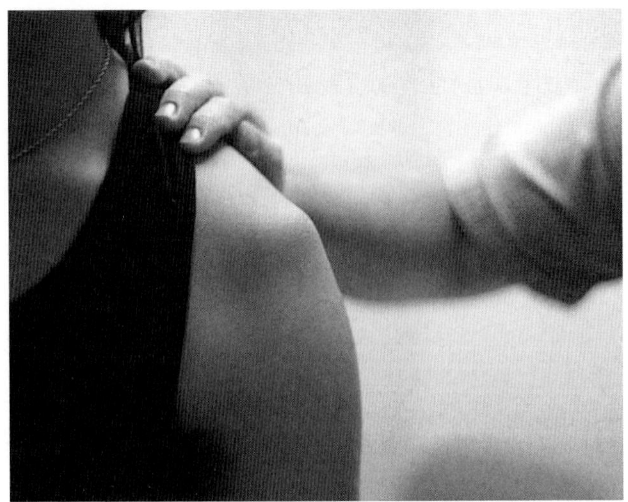

FIGURE 131-10 The Sulcus sign commonly associated with multidirectional laxity of the shoulder.

Some athletes present with secondary impingement findings, and the multidirectional laxity at the shoulder may be difficult to detect. Restricted motion from pain, impingement findings, and painful resisted external rotation are common.

Imaging

The radiographic examination in athletes with atraumatic instability is normal. Stress radiographs can be used to supplement the clinical examination to demonstrate instability in the anterior, posterior, and inferior directions but is usually unnecessary. Findings such as the Hill-Sachs lesion of the humeral head or glenoid rim fracture are not characteristic of atraumatic instability and may suggest a traumatic etiology.

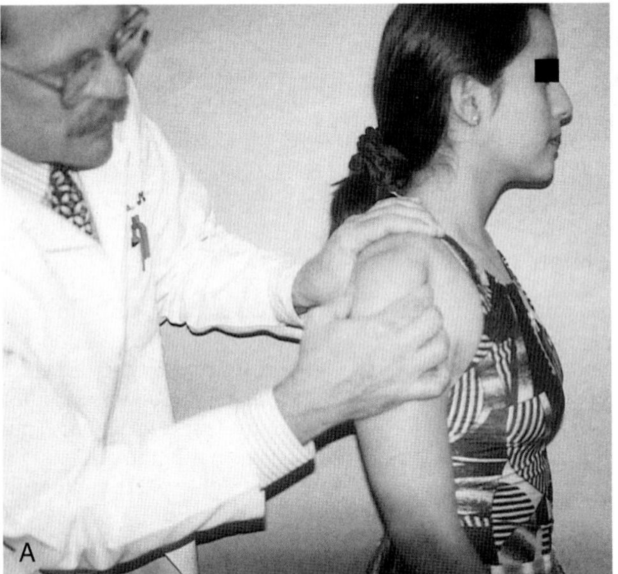

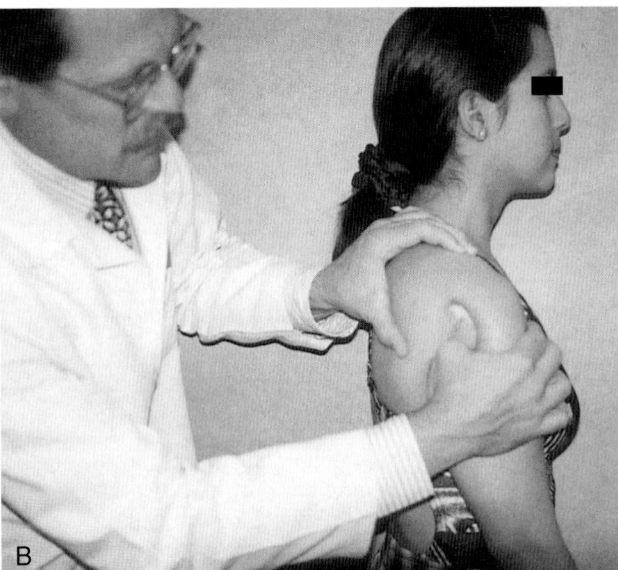

FIGURE 131-11 The load and shift, or anteroposterior drawer test.

Magnetic resonance arthrography commonly demonstrates an abnormally patulous, redundant capsule with a large intraarticular volume and occasional inflammation without structural damage.

Treatment Options

Nonoperative Treatment

Treatment of patients with atraumatic instability begins with a thorough history and physical examination to confirm the diagnosis. A nonoperative approach is indicated as the initial treatment in every case of atraumatic instability. This nonoperative treatment emphasizes a vigorous rehabilitation program involving strengthening of the dynamic stabilizers, improvement of proprioception, and avoidance of provocative activities. Most patients with atraumatic instability improve their symptomatic shoulder instability with this program. Burkhead and Rockwood[63] reported an 80% success rate in the treatment of atraumatic instability with a vigorous rehabilitation program (Fig. 131-12). Neer and Foster,[79] in the classic description of multidirectional laxity, restricted surgical intervention to patients who did not respond to a 12-month rehabilitation program.

For athletes who demonstrate voluntary atraumatic instability, the same conservative program is indicated but the prognosis is more guarded. Huber and Gerber[80] have reported a series of 25 children with voluntary subluxation of the shoulder followed up for an average of 12 years. They found that 16 of 18 children managed by "skillful neglect" had successful outcomes compared with only 3 of 7 who underwent stabilizing operations.[80] Postacchini and associates[56] demonstrated 100% failure in adolescent patients with voluntary atraumatic instability treated surgically. It is therefore extremely important for the clinician to recognize the young athlete with a voluntary component to instability and treat the patient with nonsurgical methods.

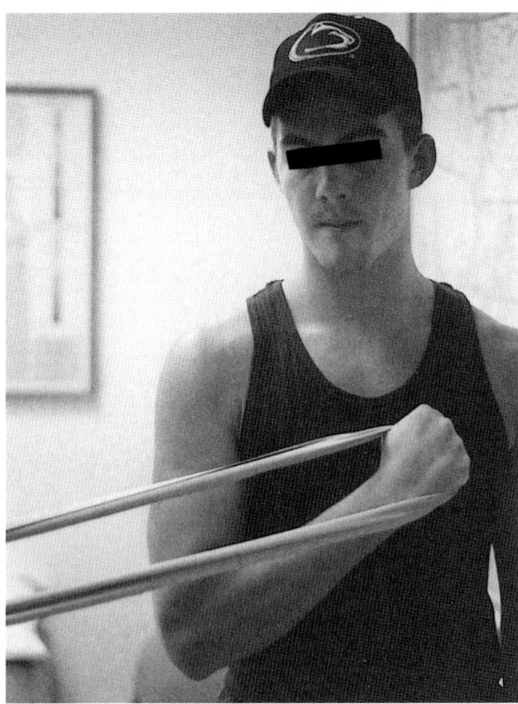

FIGURE 131-12 Rehabilitation of the rotator cuff to improve dynamic stability of the shoulder.

Operative Treatment

Patients with a voluntary component to shoulder instability should never be considered for shoulder reconstruction. Neer and Foster[79] reported success in patients with multidirectional atraumatic instability who did not improve after a thorough rehabilitation program using the inferior capsular shift procedure.[79] Mizuno and associates[81] reported two cases of surgical treatment in young children with disabling multidirectional instability who were treated successfully with the inferior capsular shift. Many adolescent patients have been included in other large studies on surgical treatment of this difficult problem and appear to have successful results proportional to those reported for adults.[82]

AUTHORS' PREFERRED TECHNIQUE

Atraumatic Instability

A careful history and physical examination should be used to confirm the diagnosis of atraumatic instability with underlying multidirectional laxity. Voluntary instability should be ruled out. In all cases of atraumatic instability, initial treatment should be conservative. Many of these patients present with impingement-type symptoms from sports overuse. Treatment begins with avoiding the provocative activity, gentle stretching, and administering nonsteroidal antiinflammatory medications. After symptoms have improved, a rehabilitation program focusing on improving dynamic stability through rotator cuff strengthening, scapular control, and proprioceptive retraining is instituted. Only after completion of a supervised rehabilitation program for 9 to 12 months would additional aggressive intervention be considered. Surgery includes an inferior capsular shift reconstruction to address the redundant capsule. I prefer an open capsular shift through an anterior deltopectoral approach. The rehabilitation program should be highly regimented and proceed more slowly than after a standard shoulder reconstruction. Care must always be taken to exclude the athlete with voluntary dislocation, who will be at greater risk for a poor outcome after surgical treatment.

Postoperative Management

Patients who undergo a capsular shift reconstruction are treated with a very slow and controlled postoperative program. Immobilization in a sling continues for 6 weeks after surgery. At that time, a gentle range of motion program is begun along with a rotator cuff and scapular muscle strengthening program. Ballistic training and heavier weightlifting activities are deferred for at least 4 months. Return to full activities requires 6 to 9 months.

Return to Play

Patients treated for atraumatic instability must have little or no pain with rehabilitation activities before consideration for return to athletics. They should also demonstrate full range of motion and adequate dynamic strength to provide stability. This level of improvement may be difficult to confirm on examination; a progressive trial of sports activity may therefore be necessary in the decision for return to play.

Physeal Injuries

Proximal Humeral Physis

Although fractures involving the upper extremities are the most common injuries in athletes with open physes, the incidence of proximal humeral physeal injuries has been reported to range between 2% and 6.7%.[83-85] Despite this relatively low incidence, these injuries can be serious in terms of time lost from participation.[86]

Injuries to the proximal humeral physis in sports can occur as a result of either macrotrauma or microtrauma.[87] Macrotrauma usually results in an acute failure of the osseous structures due to a single event in high-energy sports such as football, soccer, and hockey. Microtraumatic injury occurs as the result of repetitive subthreshold stresses that result in failure over time in activities such as throwing or volleyball.

Fractures of the proximal humeral physis can be classified by location and the degree of displacement (Box 131-3). In addition, fracture stability is important in the treatment algorithm and depends on the degree of initial displacement and the degree of initial trauma.

BOX 131-3 Proximal Humeral Physeal Fracture Grades of Displacement

Grade I: <5 mm
Grade II: up to one third the width of the shaft
Grade III: up to two thirds the width of the shaft
Grade IV: greater than two thirds the width of the shaft, including total displacement

History

Fractures through the proximal humeral physis are more common in adolescents as they near skeletal maturity than in younger children. Type I fractures are less common and tend to occur in athletes younger than 12 years. In adolescent athletes 12 years and older, most fractures are Salter-Harris type II lesions (Fig. 131-13).[93]

The exact mechanism of proximal humeral physeal injuries is not completely clear, but direct and indirect mechanisms of injury have been described.[94] Anatomically, the proximal humerus is surrounded by a periosteal sleeve that is thicker posteromedially and weaker on the anterolateral aspect of the

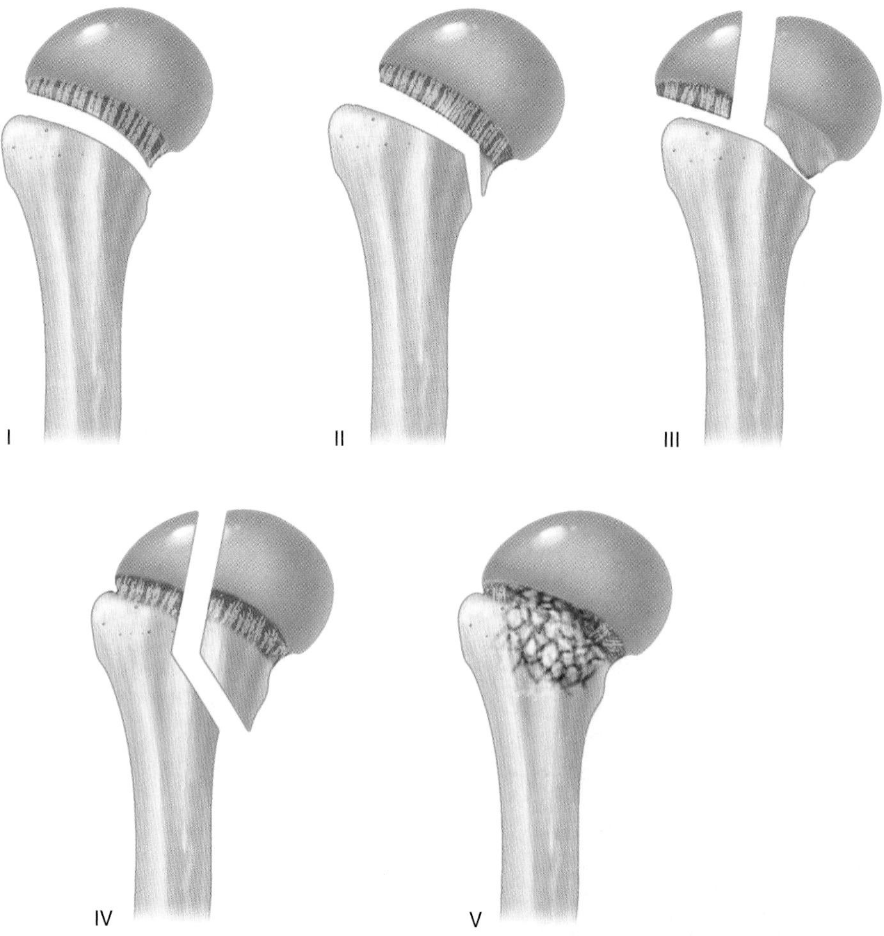

FIGURE 131-13 The Salter-Harris classification in proximal humerus fractures. Type I: transverse fracture involving the physis. Type II: transverse fracture involving the physis with a metaphyseal fragment. Type III: transverse fracture involving the physis and an epiphyseal fragment. Type IV: longitudinal fracture across the physis from epiphysis to metaphysis. Type V: a crushing injury to the physis.

proximal humerus. In fractures involving the humeral physis, the proximal metaphyseal fragment is usually displaced anteriorly and laterally through this weakened area. This injury may be the result of a direct blow to the shoulder by a posterolateral force that adducts the humeral shaft and forces it anteriorly. This direct mechanism may occur in any contact sport but is most common in football. Fracture of the proximal humeral physis may also result from an indirect force from a fall backward on an outstretched hand. The resultant force is transmitted proximally through the humeral shaft with the shoulder extended and adducted, driving the metaphyseal fragment anteriorly and laterally. This mechanism of a fall would be possible in almost any sport.

Physical Examination

Athletes with nondisplaced fractures often present with only minimal swelling and tenderness localized over the proximal humerus. Motion and resisted rotation are limited because of pain. When greater degrees of physeal displacement are present, considerable bleeding into the soft tissues can produce marked swelling. The athlete reports pain with any motion and usually holds the extremity adducted to the chest, supported at the elbow and forearm with the opposite hand. There is more diffuse tenderness that is poorly localized on palpation. The neurologic and vascular status of the upper extremity must be assessed to rule out injury to any peripheral nerves, the brachial plexus, or vascular structures.[95] Because of the nature of the indirect force transmitted up the extremity longitudinally, a thorough evaluation for ipsilateral fractures should be performed.

Imaging

Routine radiographs of the shoulder, including the AP view, axillary lateral view, and scapular lateral view, are adequate in most cases to demonstrate the presence of a proximal humeral physeal fracture.[96] The common proximal and lateral displacement of the metaphyseal fragment is best visualized on routine AP view of the shoulder, whereas the scapular lateral view is often best to demonstrate the degree of apex anterior angulation often present. A computed tomographic scan (CT) is occasionally helpful to determine the fracture patterns and degree of displacement in comminuted fractures or lesser tuberosity fractures.[96]

Treatment

The proximal humeral physis contributes approximately 80% of the longitudinal growth of the humerus, thus allowing great potential for remodeling after fracture. The younger the athlete, the greater the potential for remodeling, and the need for anatomic alignment is less important. However, in the adolescent athlete with only 12 to 18 months of growth remaining in the proximal humeral physis, adequate remodeling time to correct functional deformity may not remain. The dilemma for the treating physician then becomes when to use aggressive treatment for these fractures. Malunion with residual deformity from varus or shortening is well tolerated functionally due to the wide range of motion of the glenohumeral joint and the independent function and non–weight-bearing status of the upper extremity.[96] However, several authors have reported cases of older adolescent athletes with difficulty in overhand throwing sports due to loss of shoulder motion as a result of a less than anatomic reduction after treatment of proximal humeral physeal fractures.[97,98]

Nonoperative Treatment

Many reports in the literature have demonstrated that for most individuals with proximal humeral physeal fracture, despite initial displacement simple immobilization often produces satisfactory results for return to athletic activities.[87,97,99-101] Other series, however, have reported both subjective complaints of pain and objective findings of decreased shoulder motion in the adolescent athlete involved in overhand sports treated without reduction.[98]

In cases of nondisplaced to mildly displaced or angulated proximal humeral physeal fractures, treatment is usually successful without attempting reduction of the fracture. Initial protection in a sling followed by rehabilitation is usually all that is necessary to obtain a good result.

Most authors reserve attempts at closed reduction for displaced fractures.[102] The argument for reduction of the fragments is that it decreases the degree of shortening and varus deformity that develops if the malalignment is allowed to persist. Various closed methods have been advocated to realign the fracture fragments into a more anatomic position. Closed reduction can be performed under anesthesia by bringing the distal shaft fragment into flexion with some abduction and external rotation to align it with the flexed, abducted, and externally rotated proximal epiphyseal fragment.[96] After closed reduction, options to maintain position without internal fixation include a sling, brace, cast, or olecranon pin skeletal traction. Today, most authors would not use a cast or traction to maintain reduction but would perform percutaneous fixation in cases of an unstable fracture.[103]

Operative Treatment

The literature offers mixed results when reviewing operative treatment of proximal humeral physeal fractures.[87,98,104-106] Indications for operative treatment include inability to gain an adequate closed reduction or inability to maintain anatomic closed reduction. Unfortunately, closed reduction alone does not always result in a stable fracture in which reduction can be maintained. Closed reduction followed by percutaneous pin fixation under fluoroscopic control is a highly effective method of maintaining an unstable reduction. The percutaneous technique uses two smooth or threaded tip pins passed from the metaphysis retrograde across the fracture into the humeral head. This technique has the advantage of maintaining fracture alignment with the arm in the normal position, supported only with a sling or brace. The pins can be removed within 2 to 3 weeks due to the rapid healing of the physeal fracture. Retrograde nailing with elastic nails has gained popularity, particularly in fractures involving the metaphysis.[107-109]

On occasion, an open reduction is necessary when a satisfactory reduction cannot be obtained by a closed manipulation or in cases of open fractures or vascular injuries. Failure to obtain adequate closed reduction is more common in Salter-Harris type III and IV injuries and occasionally in cases of Salter-Harris I and II fractures in which the periosteum or the biceps tendon has become interposed in the fracture site. Fixation after open reduction can include smooth or threaded tip pins, screws, retrograde nails, or contoured plate fixation. Screws and plate fixation would only be used in athletes very near skeletal maturity. Many reports have cited the success of open reduction and fixation in these difficult cases, with most patients returning to sports without limitations.[108,109]

AUTHORS' PREFERRED TECHNIQUE

Proximal Humeral Physis

Nondisplaced or mildly displaced fractures can usually be treated with a sling. Early active motion is allowed when the pain and swelling have subsided. Rapid callus formation provides stability for progressive motion and strength.

In displaced physeal fractures, the age of the injured athlete dictates to what degree an anatomic reduction will be required. In patients younger than 12 years, the proximal humeral physis has tremendous remodelling potential; anatomic reduction is therefore unnecessary. However, as the athlete nears maturity, much less displacement can be tolerated without interfering with shoulder motion. This is particularly relevant for athletes who require a full range of glenohumeral motion for throwing and overhand sports activities. If indicated, closed reduction is accomplished with the patient under general anesthesia. If the reduction is stable, an abduction sling is used for comfort and protection. If the fracture proves to be unstable, reduction is maintained with percutaneous insertion of threaded tip pins passed from the metaphysis proximally into the epiphyseal fragment. These pins can be removed 3 to 4 weeks after surgery, followed by rehabilitation.

On occasion, closed reduction is inadequate and open reduction is accomplished through a deltopectoral incision. Percutaneous threaded tip pins are again inserted to temporarily secure the reduction. In these cases, interposition of the periosteum or the long head of biceps is usually interposed in the fracture, which blocks reduction, and must be removed to facilitate adequate reduction.

Postoperative Management

If the patient is treated nonoperatively, a sling is used for comfort and shoulder motion is started as early as tolerated. When early callus is noted on radiographs, the athlete can begin active and assisted shoulder motion. Strengthening of the rotator cuff and deltoid and scapular muscles is added when pain has decreased and range of motion has progressed.

After operative intervention, a sling and pendulum exercises are used until percutaneous pins are removed at 3 to 4 weeks. After pin removal, sufficient callus is usually present so that rehabilitation can advance as tolerated.

Return to Play

Return to sports participation can resume only after radiologic healing of the fracture and complete rehabilitation. This would require full range of motion of the shoulder and strength appropriate for the specific sport. Return to contact sports and overhand throwing may require up to 10 to 12 weeks.

Complications

Acute complications associated with proximal humeral fractures in young athletes are rare but include neurologic and vascular injuries that occasionally require intervention.[95,96]

Major skeletal complications include growth arrest, malunion, and avascular necrosis of the humeral head. Growth arrest after fracture is very unusual, although varus deformity and shortening from malunion are common but well tolerated. In the adolescent nearing skeletal maturity, fracture deformity can occasionally produce a disabling loss of motion for an overhead athlete.[97]

Avascular necrosis of the humeral head is rare in the skeletally immature athlete. Most case reports describe transient symptoms with little long-term disability.[97,110]

Lesser Tuberosity Fractures

Fracture of the lesser tuberosity portion of the proximal humeral physis is uncommon as an isolated injury.[111-115] This injury represents an avulsion of the tuberosity by a violent contraction involving the subscapularis tendon. The most commonly reported mechanism is one of a forced external rotation against an internal rotation resisting force, which may occur in upper extremity–dominated contact sports such as football and wrestling.[96]

These fractures are difficult to diagnose in the acute situation, possibly because of difficulty in radiographic visualization of the fracture and a lack of specific clinical findings. Up to 50% of cases of lesser tuberosity fracture in the skeletally immature athlete have been reported to be missed on initial presentation.[116,117]

History

The athlete usually gives a history of a traumatic injury in a contact sport involving an external rotation force applied to the arm in a leveraged position. Acutely the patient has mild swelling, limited range of motion, and pain. Weakness of internal rotation may be noted by the patient. Many of these patients present several weeks after injury with persistent shoulder pain and weakness after a previous injury.

Physical Examination

If the athlete presents after acute injury, the shoulder is diffusely tender and guarded. Mild swelling may be present. Motion is limited by pain and strength testing is limited. If the presentation is delayed, the range of motion has usually improved but weakness and pain are noted with resisted internal rotation. The lift-off test and the belly press test may be positive.

Imaging

Standard radiographs, including AP, axillary lateral, and transscapular lateral views, should be performed to evaluate all shoulder injuries possibly caused by trauma. Fracture of the lesser tuberosity physis may be difficult to visualize on the AP and scapular lateral views because of overlap with the humerus and scapular neck. The axillary view may provide the best visualization of the fracture fragment but may be difficult to obtain in the acute setting.[96] CT scans will demonstrate the fracture if needed and MRI may be used to assess the shoulder for other soft tissue injuries.

Treatment Options

If the fracture is nondisplaced it can be successfully treated with nonoperative management. A sling is used for protection for 4 to 6 weeks followed by rehabilitation. Displaced fractures and nondisplaced fractures with a delay in treatment are commonly treated surgically.[118,119] Some authors recommend surgical treatment for all lesser tuberosity avulsion fractures

in throwing athletes because malunion may lead to decreased overhead sports function.[96,116] Surgical repair of the lesser tuberosity fracture can be accomplished with heavy suture through drill holes, suture anchors, or screw fixation. Surgical repair should avoid iatrogenic damage to the remaining portion of the proximal humeral physis. Results with surgical treatment have been reported as good in terms of full return to athletic function.[118-121]

AUTHORS' PREFERRED TECHNIQUE

Lesser Tuberosity Fractures

I prefer surgical treatment for repair of lesser tuberosity fractures unless the fracture is completely nondisplaced. In most cases the fracture is easily reduced and can be fixed with nonmetallic, biocomposite suture anchors without risk to the remaining proximal humeral physis. Postoperative immobilization in a sling is used for comfort during the initial 3 to 4 weeks of rehabilitation.

Postoperative Management

The literature provides very few guidelines concerning postoperative management. The patient is initially placed in a sling for the first 4 to 6 weeks. Range of motion and strength are then gradually increased with physical therapy until the athlete is fully rehabilitated.[96]

Return to Play

After treatment the patient must regain full range of motion and strength before returning to competitive sports activity. This usually requires 4 to 6 months.

Complications

Both nonunion and malunion of fractures of the lesser tuberosity have been reported.[116,118] Nonunited fractures are usually painful, and malunited fragments often lead to bony impingement anteriorly, which can limit motion. This can be disabling for the athlete who uses his shoulder for overhand sports activities.

Stress Injuries: Little Leaguer's Shoulder

Little Leaguer's shoulder represents failure or stress fracture through the proximal humeral physeal plate as a result of repetitive microtrauma. The most common cause is the application of repetitive rotational forces applied to the proximal humerus in the immature athlete during the throwing motion. Numerous cases have been described in the literature; in fact, stress fracture of the proximal humeral growth plate may be the most common stress injury in athletes aged 11 to 14 years.[122-126] This injury is the corollary to internal impingement seen in adults and older adolescents.

The forces generated in the upper extremity during the throwing motion and overhand sports motion are considerable both in rotation and compression at the shoulder. When these types of repetitive forces are applied to the physis over time, it is easy to understand how injury could occur. Today, more and more skeletally immature athletes are participating in year-round overhand sports with substantial increased exposure. As would be expected, the increased exposure has led to an increase in the incidence of proximal humeral stress injury. For this reason, strict pitching limits have been developed by many organizations governing youth baseball.[126]

In addition to increased volume of forces across the shoulder, other factors may create microtrauma in young, skeletally immature pitchers. Several investigators have observed that the incidence of shoulder symptoms in young pitchers also relates to form, with those who had poor pitching skills being more likely to have symptoms.[127-129]

History

Most patients with a proximal humeral stress fracture are between the ages of 11 and 14 years and are involved in throwing or repetitive overhand sports. The majority of these athletes are boys who participate in baseball, but athletes involved in volleyball and softball can also be affected. Pain is usually gradual in onset over weeks to months, with a superimposed subacute episode that brings the problem to attention. Often a short trial of rest has been tried, with improvement followed by recurrent symptoms upon return to throwing.

Physical Examination

Physical examination is normal, without swelling, deformity, or discoloration. There is localized tenderness to palpation over the proximal humerus. Restricted range of motion can be present secondary to pain. Pain can usually be elicited with resisted external rotation and abduction.

Imaging

On plain radiographs, widening of the proximal humeral physeal plate is the hallmark finding. This widening usually begins laterally and extends across the physis as the stress lesion progresses. Comparison views are helpful in early cases to distinguish subtle physeal changes. MRI and bone scan studies are unnecessary for diagnosis in most cases and do not add information that would alter treatment protocols.

Treatment

Rest is the primary treatment for this stress injury. The athlete should refrain from throwing and all other activities, including lifting, hitting, or contact, until there are no symptoms with daily activity. At that stage rehabilitation is started, including shoulder stretching and strengthening of cuff and scapular stabilizers. Return to overhead athletics is allowed when radiographs are normal, the athlete is asymptomatic, and rehabilitation is completed. This usually requires 8 to 12 weeks. A throwing protocol is often used, focusing on gradually increasing the amount of pitching along with frequency and velocity, with a special focus on core and lower extremity strengthening and stability. The athlete's pitching technique and frequency should be addressed before return to pitching is considered.[126]

Complications

Although rare, displacement of the proximal humeral physis with continued throwing in the clinical setting of stress

fracture has been documented.[126] Treatment after displacement may require reduction and internal fixation. Avascular necrosis of the epiphysis has also been reported.[110] All these cases occurred in high-performance male pitchers who were 11 to 13 years old.

Lateral Clavicle Physeal Fractures

Although injuries to the distal clavicle in children are similar in many ways to the adult AC joint injury, the distinct differences are a reflection of the developmental anatomy of the distal clavicle. The distal clavicle is surrounded by a thick periosteal sleeve that is continuous laterally with the AC joint capsule and inferiorly with the coracoclavicular ligaments. The physis of the distal clavicle lies within the periosteal sleeve medial to the attachment of the AC joint capsule. The epiphysis, which is rarely apparent radiographically, is tightly bound to the AC joint; failure in the skeletally immature athlete therefore usually occurs through the physis as opposed to an adultlike dislocation through the AC joint. Classification of distal clavicle injuries is based on the degree of disruption of the periosteal sleeve and the direction and degree of displacement of the shaft fragment (Box 131-4).[130]

History

Typically, the athlete has a history of a fall on the point of the shoulder. The blow directed to the scapula can lead to disruption of the periosteal sleeve and fracture through the physis. There is immediate pain, and the athlete may relate a feeling of instability. Transient symptoms of numbness or dysesthesia are occasionally experienced, similar to that of a brachial plexus burner.[131,132] The injury may occur with an indirect mechanism, such as a fall on an outstretched, adducted arm that drives the humeral head into the acromion.[131,132]

Physical Examination

On inspection, the amount of deformity relates to the degree of injury. Mild type I and type II injuries may demonstrate only localized swelling, whereas type III and type V injuries are characterized by clinically significant deformity caused by the displaced distal clavicle shaft. Type II injuries may appear fairly benign when visualized from the front, but when inspected from above the deformity of the displaced clavicle posterior into the trapezius can be recognized. The athlete often supports the affected arm with the opposite hand and resists shoulder range of motion. Tenderness to palpation over the distal clavicle is uniformly present. Muscle strength testing is limited by pain. Neurologic testing should be performed to rule out brachial plexus involvement. In less severe cases, the cross-arm adduction test is usually positive. This test is performed by positioning the shoulder into flexion of 90 degrees followed by bringing the arm across the chest into adduction. Pain referable to the AC joint region is a positive test finding.[131-133]

BOX 131-4 Classification of Distal Clavicle Physeal Injuries

- **Type I injury:** sprain of AC ligaments with the periosteal sleeve intact
- **Type II injury:** sprain of AC ligaments with partial disruption of the periosteal sleeve and slight widening of the AC joint
- **Type III injury:** disruption of the periosteal sleeve with instability and superior displacement of the distal clavicle by 25%-100% on the AP radiograph
- **Type IV injury:** disruption of the periosteal sleeve, posterior displacement of the clavicle into the trapezius muscle
- **Type V injury:** disruption of the periosteal sleeve, deltoid and trapezius muscle detachment, clavicle displaced into subcutaneous position, greater than 100% displacement on the AP radiograph
- **Type VI injury:** periosteal sleeve disrupted with inferior displacement of the clavicle beneath coracoid process

AC, Acromioclavicular; *AP,* anteroposterior.

Imaging

In suspected trauma the shoulder should be examined with plain radiographic views in at least two planes taken at right angles to the other, including the AP and axillary lateral views. However, in the case of injury to the distal clavicular physis, routine AP views may be overpenetrated for this area; a special Zanca view may therefore be indicated.[134] This view is performed by angling the beam 10 to 15 degrees toward the head and using only 50% of the standard AP shoulder penetration. The distal clavicular epiphysis is rarely visualized on plain films because it appears and fuses over a short period at approximately age 19 years. Distal physeal injury is therefore inferred by the degree of shaft displacement in relation to the acromion and coracoid in an athlete in the appropriate age range.

Comparison views of the opposite shoulder can often be useful particularly when trying to determine the normal coracoclavicular distance. This distance from the superior aspect of the coracoid to the undersurface of the clavicle is used to determine the degree of clavicular shaft displacement, which relates to classification of this injury. The axillary lateral view is important to differentiate a type IV injury from a type II injury by demonstrating the posterior position of the shaft fragment in relation to the acromion. Stress views of the shoulder are not necessary in assessing distal clavicular physeal injury.[131]

Treatment Options

Nonoperative Treatment

Injuries to the distal clavicular physis represent Salter-Harris type I injuries, and healing is virtually always the rule. The periosteal sleeve remains in continuity with the AC joint capsule and the coracoclavicular ligaments; stability is achieved when the periosteal sleeve fills with healing new bone. Even in cases with large degrees of displacement, remodeling potential in this injury is significant and residual deformity is unusual. Nonoperative treatment is therefore acceptable in most type I, II, and III cases of distal clavicular physeal fracture.[131,132,135-138] In younger patients with greater degrees of remodeling potential, even cases of type V injury should be considered for nonoperative treatment. Nonoperative treatment includes a short period of immobilization and supportive care with ice and analgesics followed by a progressive rehabilitation and return to play program.

Surgical Treatment

Surgical treatment for fractures of the distal clavicular physis is reserved for type IV injuries, type VI injuries, and type V injuries in adolescents who have less remodeling capability. The procedure includes reduction of the displaced shaft fragment and repair of the periosteal sleeve supplemented with temporary transacromial or coracoclavicular fixation.[131,132,137,139-141]

AUTHORS' PREFERRED TECHNIQUE

Distal Clavicle Physeal Injuries

For all type I, type II, and type III injuries and type V injuries in athletes younger than 12 years, I prefer nonoperative treatment. A sling is used for comfort, with active range of motion beginning as fast as tolerated. Ice and oral analgesics are often needed for approximately 1 week. As soon as tolerated by the patient, range of motion exercise is started followed by light strengthening. Typically, strength and stability are achieved in 6 to 8 weeks with remodeling progressing for up to 1 year.

For athletes with type IV or VI injury, and type V injury in patients older than 12 years, I prefer operative repair. This includes reduction of the shaft fragment into the periosteal tube with suture repair and temporary fixation with a lag screw and washer from clavicle to coracoid. The screw and washer can typically be removed at 6 weeks. Rehabilitation follows screw removal and includes range of motion and strengthening.

Postoperative Management

After surgery a sling is used for 2 weeks, allowing early hand and elbow motion and shoulder pendulum exercises. Between 2 and 6 weeks gentle shoulder motion progresses, but lifting is not allowed. After screw removal rehabilitation for strength is achieved.

Return to Play

As with most shoulder injuries in the skeletally immature athlete, return to play requires that the patient has completed treatment and rehabilitation. The athlete should have no pain, full range of motion, and good strength. After treatment for type I or type II injury this may only take 1 to 2 weeks; type III and type V injuries treated nonoperatively will take 4 to 6 weeks.

After surgical treatment, return to play follows implant removal and rehabilitation, which may require 10 to 12 weeks.

Results

Because of the great potential for healing and remodeling of this fracture in this age group, results for treatment of an injury to the distal clavicular physis are uniformly good. Several reports in the literature for both surgical and nonoperative treatment demonstrate good results.[137,138,141,142]

Complications

Although malunion and the common complications of any surgery are possible, there have been no reports of problems during treatment of this injury.

Medial Clavicle Physeal Fractures

The epiphysis of the medial clavicle is the last epiphysis in the body to appear radiographically, at approximately 18 years of age, and the physis does not close until age 23 to 25 years.[143,144] Physeal injuries to the medial clavicular physis are therefore much more common in the skeletally immature athlete compared with dislocation of the sternoclavicular joint. This is an important distinction because these physeal injuries have a much higher likelihood of healing and remodeling compared with sternoclavicular dislocation.

The incidence of injuries to the medial end of the clavicle in children is not well documented. Many case reports and small series have described this injury with estimates that medial injuries represent between 1% and 6% of all clavicular injuries in skeletally immature patients.[145-150]

Medial physeal injury of the clavicle is classified according to the anatomic position of the shaft fragment in relation to the epiphysis and sternum. The shaft can be displaced either anteriorly or posteriorly as it penetrates the periosteal sleeve that remains attached medially to the epiphysis and joint capsule.

Although anterior displacement is the most common type of injury, posterior displacement is the most important to recognize because of potential impingement of structures within the mediastinum by the shaft fragment. Most of these physeal fractures are characterized as Salter-Harris type I and II injuries (Fig. 131-14).[151]

History

Injury to the medial clavicle can occur as a result of either direct or indirect forces. Although uncommon, a force may be applied directly to the anteromedial aspect of the clavicle during contact sports, resulting in a fracture through the physis. If displacement results, the shaft fragment would penetrate the periosteal tube posteriorly and potentially become retrosternal, with possible injury to structures within the mediastinum.

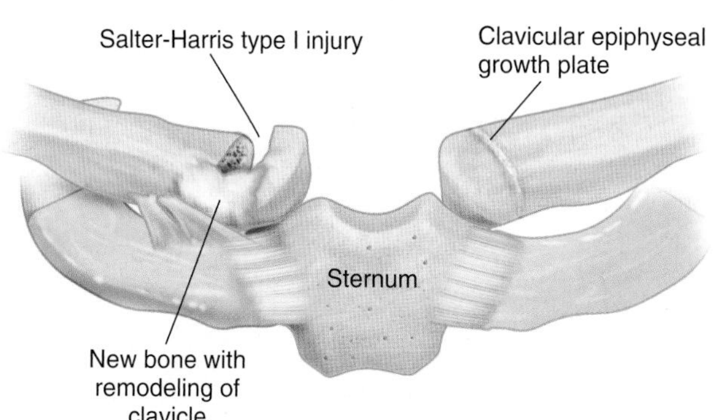

FIGURE 131-14 Salter-Harris type I injury to the medial clavicle with anterior displacement.

Many investigators have reported that the indirect mechanism is the most common.[144] A typical history given by the athlete includes a fall with the athlete's opposite shoulder on the ground while several other players pile on top of the shoulder, applying significant compressive force directly to the medial clavicle. When the shoulder is compressed with a posterolateral force and rolled forward, an ipsilateral posterior displacement of the shaft fragment can result. In contrast, a compression force to the anterolateral aspect of the shoulder results in anterior displacement of the shaft.

Most athletes with medial clavicular physeal fracture have immediate pain with a specific traumatic episode. It is important to elicit any symptoms of impingement on mediastinal structures if a posterior displacement is suspected. Symptoms of shortness of breath, choking or difficulty swallowing, or any neurologic or vascular symptoms should be of concern to the examiner.

Physical Examination

In a nondisplaced injury to the medial physis, the ligaments of the joint and periosteal tube are intact. The patient reports pain with range of motion of the upper extremity. The area is typically swollen and tender to palpation, but instability and crepitus are absent.

In a more severe injury to the physis with displacement of the shaft fragment, swelling and severe pain with any movement of the arm are common. The injured arm is often supported with the normal arm, and the head may be tilted toward the side of the dislocated joint because of spasm of the surrounding musculature. Swelling may be substantial, disguising the position of the displaced shaft fragment. Careful palpation of the shaft in relation to the epiphysis and sternum should be performed in an attempt to discern anterior versus posterior displacement. In suspected posterior displacement, careful examination of the upper extremity should document neurologic status and adequacy of pulses or any venous congestion that may be present. Breathing difficulties, voice changes, or a choking sensation should be noted. If the patient demonstrates some or all of these signs and symptoms of mediastinal impingement, treatment becomes a relative emergency and should be promptly instituted.

Imaging

Radiography

Plain radiographs of the medial clavicle, including the AP and lateral views, can be very difficult to interpret for fracture or displacement of the medial clavicle because of overlap with other structures, including sternum, ribs, and spine. A special oblique view, known as the *serendipity view,* has proved to be the most valuable plain radiographic technique. With the patient supine in the center of the x-ray table, the tube is tilted at a 40-degree angle off the vertical, centered directly on the sternum. The cassette is placed squarely on the table under the patient's upper shoulders and neck so that the beam aimed at the sternum projects both medial clavicles onto the film. This oblique view demonstrates a side-to-side comparison of the medial clavicle and sternoclavicular joint and allows evaluation of potential displacement or fracture.[144,152]

Computed Tomography

The CT scan is the best technique to study all injuries of the medial clavicle and sternoclavicular joint (Fig. 131-15). A CT scan demonstrate fracture, dislocation, and displacement with more consistency and accuracy than plain radiographs and should be used in all cases of suspected medial clavicle injury.

Treatment Options

As is the case of all fractures involving physes, the expectation for rapid healing and significant remodeling in fractures of the medial clavicle is the rule. With this in mind, treatment of these fractures will be generally more conservative than in cases of sternoclavicular joint dislocation. Conclusive data regarding recognition, treatment, and specific outcomes are limited to case reports and small series, but results of treatment for this injury are generally good by whatever means.[145-149,153]

Treatment is based on both the degree and direction of displacement of the shaft fragment, with special attention to cases with posterior position of the shaft fragment that may result in impingement of mediastinal structures.[154-158]

In physeal fractures with mild to moderate displacement in either direction, treatment is always by observation and

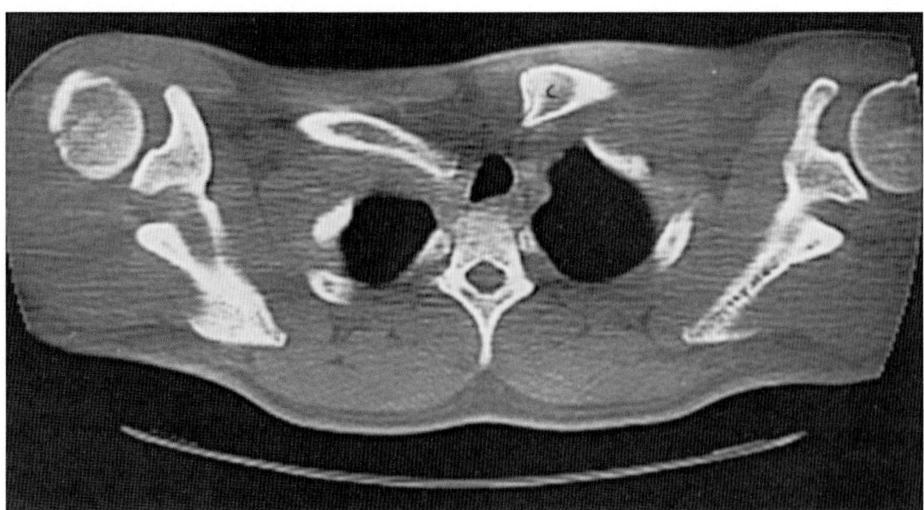

FIGURE 131-15 Computed tomographic scan demonstrating posterior displacement of a medial clavicle fracture.

supportive care. These fractures are stable with any type of immobilization, and remodeling of any deformity is the expectation.

If significant anterior displacement of the medial physeal injury is recognized, closed reduction can be considered. If attempted, closed reduction should be performed with the patient under general anesthesia and positioned supine with a pad between the shoulders. While applying lateral traction on the arm, direct pressure is applied to the anteriorly displaced clavicle while the shoulder is pushed posteriorly. The reduction is maintained by placing the patient in a figure-of-eight splint. If the clavicle fracture is unstable, the deformity is accepted, and healing and remodeling of the fracture will usually correct any residual deformity. Some clinicians suggest that benign neglect can be successful for all fractures with anterior displacement.[159]

In athletes who demonstrate posterior displacement of the medial physeal fracture, closed reduction should be performed with the patient under general anesthesia (Fig. 131-16). With the patient in the supine position and a pad placed between the shoulders, traction is applied to the abducted arm, which is then slowly brought into extension. It may be necessary to apply lateral and anterior traction to the medial clavicle either manually or with a percutaneous towel clip to accomplish reduction. The reduction is usually stable, with the shoulders held back in a figure-of-eight dressing or strap. If the posterior physeal injury cannot be easily reduced closed, and if the patient has no symptoms of impingement of the mediastinal structures, the injury can be treated expectantly. Healing and remodeling commonly result in a stable clavicle with no long-term sequelae.[160]

Open reduction of a medial clavicular physeal injury is indicated for cases of irreducible posterior displacement in a patient with signs and symptoms of compression of the mediastinal structures. Reduction performed open is usually accomplished without difficulty. Reduction is maintained by

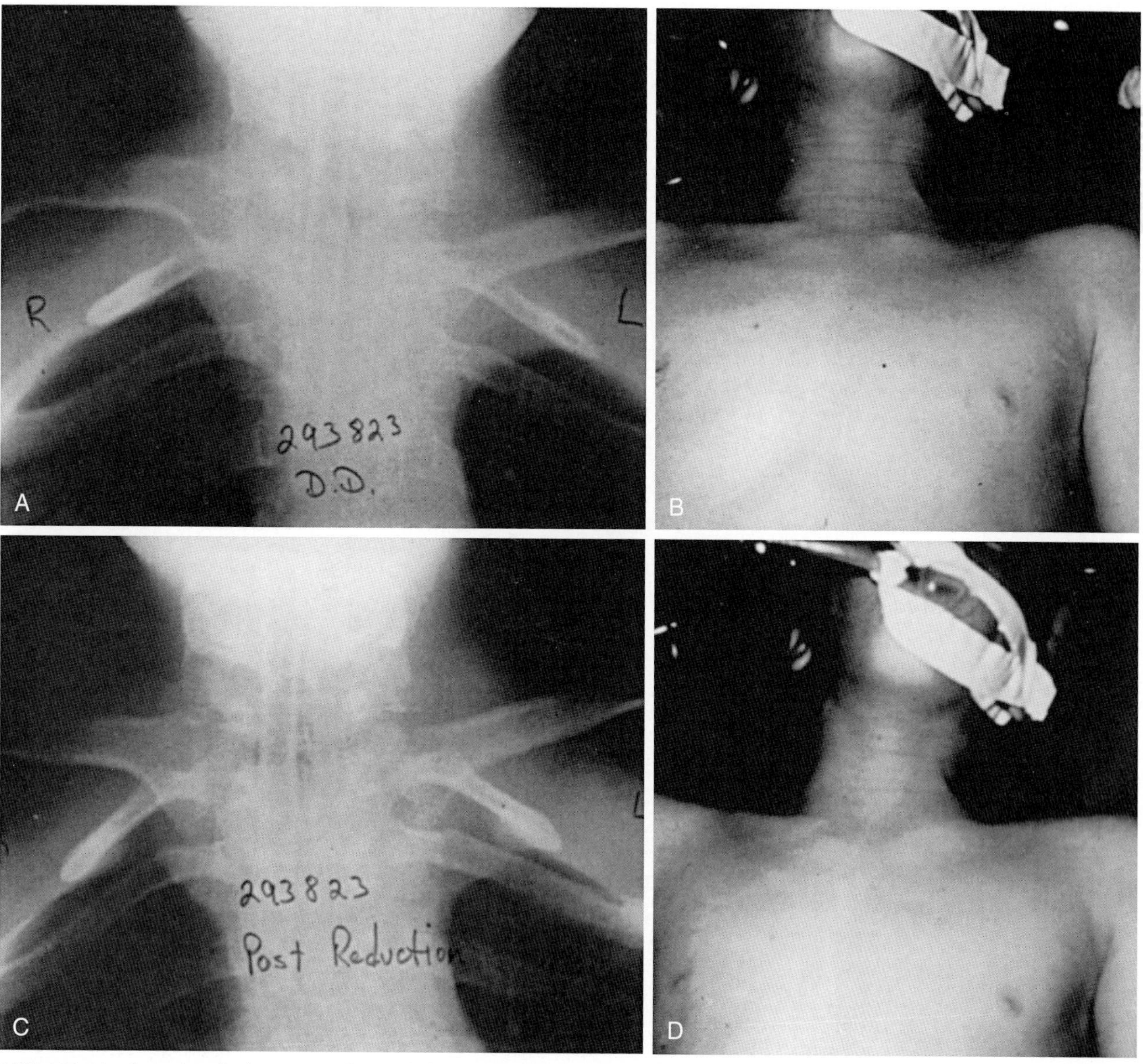

FIGURE 131-16 Posterior displacement of a medial clavicle physeal fracture. **A,** Serendipity view demonstrating posterior displacement of the left side. **B,** The patient before reduction. **C,** Serendipity view after closed reduction. **D,** Clinical appearance after reduction. *(From Rockwood CA, Matsen FA, editors:* The shoulder, *ed 2, Philadelphia, 1998, WB Saunders.)*

repairing the thick periosteal tube and maintaining the patient in a figure-of-eight brace as for closed reduction. Successful results for the open treatment of posteriorly displaced medial clavicular physeal fractures in young athletes has been reported.[161-163] The literature has documented many cases of complications with metallic internal fixation to maintain reduction of these fractures and is therefore not recommended.[152,164-167]

AUTHORS' PREFERRED TECHNIQUE

Medial Clavicular Physeal Fractures

Treatment of mild to moderately displaced medial clavicular physeal fractures is nonoperative. The great potential for healing and remodeling improves even fairly substantial deformities. A sling is used for comfort, and rapid active motion is encouraged followed by rehabilitation as the athlete progresses to healing.

In the treatment of completely displaced anterior physeal fractures, closed reduction with the patient under general anesthesia is completed in an attempt to minimize deformity. Immobilization is accomplished with a figure-of-eight splint or sling. Incomplete or unstable reduction is accepted with the expectation that significant remodeling will take place.

Closed reduction of posteriorly displaced fractures of the medial clavicular physis is the treatment of choice. Open reduction is reserved for patients in whom closed reduction is unsuccessful and those with signs and symptoms of mediastinal impingement. Repair of the periosteal sleeve around the fracture maintains reduction; metallic fixation is always avoided. In a posteriorly displaced fracture without impingement symptoms or unstable fractures without symptoms, the fracture is treated with benign neglect.

Postoperative Management

For all medial clavicle fractures treated nonoperatively and fractures after closed or open reduction, the patient is initially placed in a sling or figure-of-eight brace. Upper extremity motion is encouraged as soon as possible, with active assisted stretching exercise starting at approximately 2 to 4 weeks. Full active motion and light strengthening exercise begin in the fourth week; heavier weightlifting, particularly in the press position, is delayed for 8 weeks.

Return to Play

Most young athletes can return to noncontact sports by 8 to 10 weeks when full motion and adequate strength are present. Contact sports require complete protective strength and should be delayed for an additional 2 to 4 weeks to allow remodeling of the medial clavicle.

Complications

Acute complications associated with medial clavicular physeal fracture are primarily limited to impingement of mediastinal structures because of posterior displacement of the shaft fragment. When symptoms and signs are present, prompt reduction, either closed or open, should be performed to prevent short- and long-term sequelae. Long-term issues related to malunion are unusual in the skeletally immature patient because of the great propensity for remodeling of the physeal fracture with time.

Many complications have been previously reported with the use of metallic implants for fixation of fractures and dislocations in this area. Pin breakage and migration have lead most authors to recommend that metal not be used in the medial clavicle and sternoclavicular joint.[152,164-167]

For a complete list of references, go to expertconsult.com.

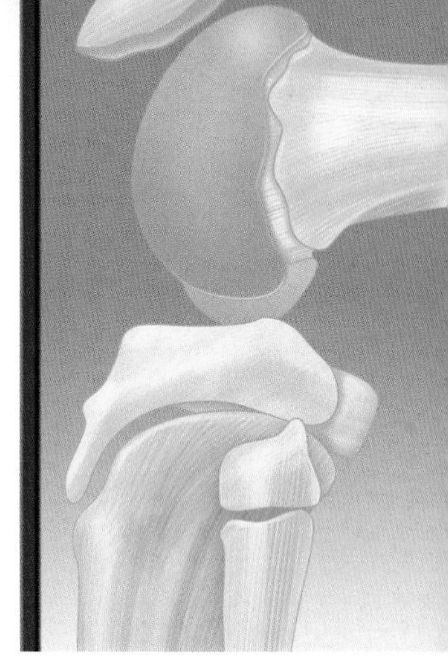

132

Elbow Injuries in Pediatric and Adolescent Athletes

JAMES P. BRADLEY • LUKE S. AUSTIN • FOTIOS P. TJOUMAKARIS

Elbow injuries in athletic children and adolescents are a distinct clinical entity when compared with the adult population. The presence of the distal humeral physis, multiple ossification centers, developing muscular and ligamentous attachments, and articulating cartilage can contribute to characteristic pathologic conditions in vulnerable patient populations. Based on the age of the patient, the duration and location of symptoms, and the specific sport, the clinician can arrive at the diagnosis and develop a clear treatment strategy. Nonoperative treatment often can result in a high degree of success when treating this patient population; however, several conditions may require surgical intervention.

Relevant Anatomy and Biomechanics

Osteology

Skeletal growth around the elbow typically follows a characteristic development process. The elbow joint consists of the articulation of the distal humerus with the ulna (the ulnohumeral joint), the articulation of the distal humerus with the radial head (the radiocapitellar joint), and the proximal articulation of the radius and ulna (the proximal radioulnar joint). Skeletal maturation occurs from the primary ossification centers of the humerus, radius, and ulna, along with six secondary ossification centers. The sequence of ossification is the capitellum, proximal radius, medial epicondyle, trochlea, olecranon, and lateral epicondyle.[1-3] When evaluating radiographs, variation can occur in the appearance of the ossification centers as distinct structures, and correlation with the contralateral extremity can help determine disease in questionable cases.

The ossification of the distal humerus extends to the condyles at birth and progresses through the secondary centers at various stages of development. The lateral condyle and capitellum appear in the second year of life.[4] On a normal lateral radiograph of the elbow, the anterior humeral line intersects the anterior third of the capitellar ossific nucleus (Fig. 132-1). This line is helpful in characterizing supracondylar fracture displacement in children. In the third year of life, the proximal radius ossific nucleus begins to ossify and is typically present in most children by age 4 years. Notches or clefts in the proximal radius metaphysis can sometimes be seen and are considered part of the normal variability of maturation.[5,6] The medial epicondylar ossific nucleus begins to ossify between the ages of 5 and 6 years; however, fusion of the epiphysis does not occur until 15 to 16 years of age, placing this physis under stress during the throwing motion well into adolescence.[7] The secondary ossification center of the olecranon process appears around age 7 to 9 years, whereas the trochlear ossific nucleus appears around age 9 to 10 years.[8] The last center to appear is the lateral epicondyle, usually after age 10 years, and this center rapidly fuses to the lateral condyle shortly after being visible on radiographs. A thorough understanding of the stages of ossification and the appearance of the centers of ossification is critical for clinicians who treat pediatric elbow injuries (Fig. 132-2). Any heterogeneous appearance to the nuclei or differences relative to the contralateral extremity in terms of size, density, position, or fragmentation could indicate abnormal development and may be the result of repetitive stress to the elbow, inducing vascular changes with resultant alterations in the maturation process. A failure to appreciate the normal progression of growth at the elbow could result in misdiagnosis, improper treatment, and progressive developmental abnormality.

The osseous anatomy surrounding the elbow contributes significantly to stability of the elbow joint. Approximately 50% of elbow stability arises from the congruity of the ulnohumeral articulation.[9] In serial olecranon excision studies, progressive loss of the proximal olecranon resulted in linear decreases in elbow stability at 0 and 90 degrees of elbow motion.[10] The radial head provides 15% to 30% of valgus stability to the elbow joint and may be more important in the throwing athlete to providing valgus stability through the midrange of motion.[9] Studies evaluating the load transmission across the elbow joint have shown that forces of up to three times body weight can be seen, and forces that are generated during throwing may be even higher.[11,12] Thus it is not surprising that a small deficiency in the elaborate stability-controlling mechanisms of the elbow may have a significant and cumulative effect on elbow function.

Ligaments and Soft Tissue

Whereas 50% of the stability of the elbow joint arises from the osseous anatomy, the remaining 50% is derived from the ligamentous and soft tissue attachments (e.g., the anterior capsule, the medial or ulnar collateral ligament [UCL], and the lateral radial collateral ligament).[9] With regard to the muscular attachment sites around the elbow, laterally the

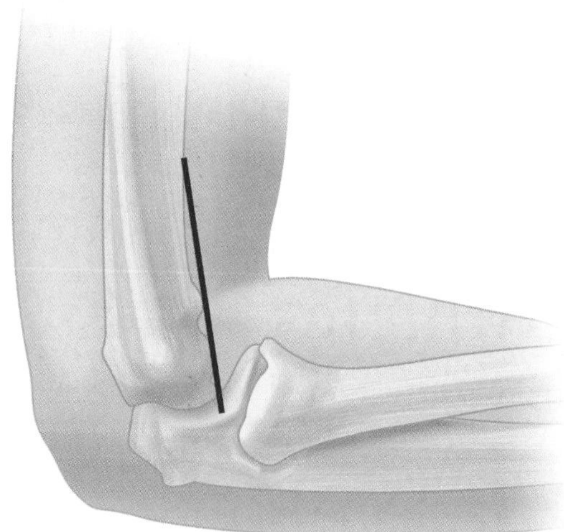

FIGURE 132-1 On a normal lateral radiograph of the pediatric elbow, the anterior humeral line intersects the anterior third of the capitellum and is helpful in characterizing displacement in supracondylar humerus fractures.

common extensor origin is located at the lateral epicondyle and can be a common source of pathologic findings in persons who participate in racquet sport and repetitive motion activities. This source is perhaps more prominent in the adult population, with abnormalities classically located within the extensor carpi radialis brevis (lateral epicondylitis). Anteriorly, the brachialis and biceps serve as a powerful flexor and supinator of the elbow, respectively. Posteriorly, the triceps attachment on the proximal aspect of the olecranon serves as the main extensor to the elbow and can be injured in young athletes who have an eccentric contractile injury. Although injury or strain of these muscle groups can occur, this pathologic condition is less often seen in the pediatric population.

Medially, the flexor and pronator attachment sites serve as powerful medial stabilizers to the elbow, particularly in the athlete whose sport entails throwing. Repetitive strain at this site can be seen in the throwing population or, alternatively, in golfers, in whom it can manifest as medial epicondylitis.

The UCL complex of the elbow is a broad ligament on the medial side of the elbow that provides restraint to valgus stress (Fig. 132-3).[13] The ligament consists of three portions: the anterior oblique bundle, the posterior oblique bundle, and the transverse ligament or intermediate bundle. The anterior oblique bundle is the main medial stabilizer to the elbow and arises from the medial epicondyle with an insertion to the medial aspect of the coronoid process. This ligament becomes more important during high-velocity throwing, when a large valgus force is placed on the medial elbow structures. Both the anterior and posterior bundles of the ligament provide stability during the full arc of motion, with the anterior band having a larger burden in extension and the posterior band having a more important role in flexion. The lateral collateral ligament provides varus stability to the elbow and in recent years its role as a major contributor to posterolateral rotatory elbow stability has been more extensively studied.[14] The lateral collateral (or radial collateral) ligament complex is composed of three main parts: the lateral UCL, the radial collateral ligament, and the accessory lateral collateral ligament (Fig. 132-4). The radial collateral ligament courses from the lateral epicondyle to the annular ligament of the proximal radioulnar joint. The lateral UCL courses from the posterior lateral epicondyle, travels across the annular ligament, and attaches on the crista supinatoris of the ulna. This ligament is the primary restraint to posterolateral elbow stability. The accessory lateral collateral ligament originates from the inferior aspect of the annular ligament and attaches to the tubercle of the supinator. The lateral ligamentous complex is classically injured or disrupted during an elbow dislocation or iatrogenically during surgery around the posterolateral aspect of the

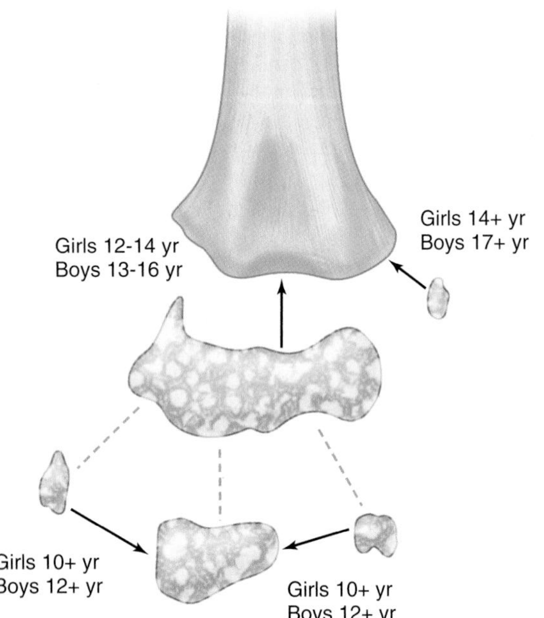

FIGURE 132-2 The usual ages at which the ossific centers fuse to each other and to the distal humerus in boys and girls.

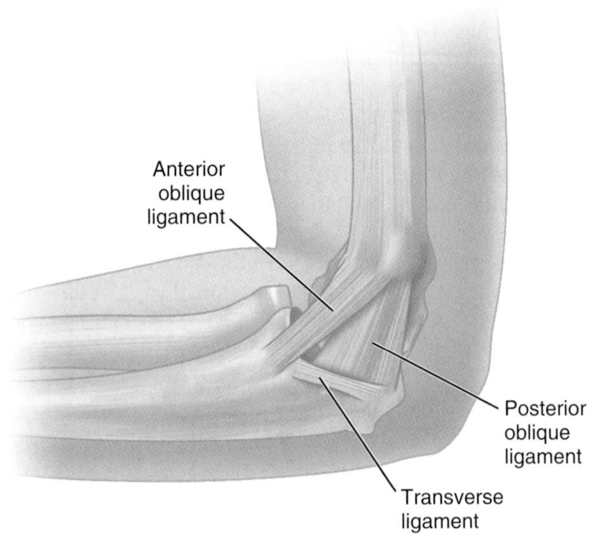

FIGURE 132-3 The ulnar collateral ligament of the elbow consists of the anterior oblique bundle, the intermediate bundle, and the posterior oblique bundle.

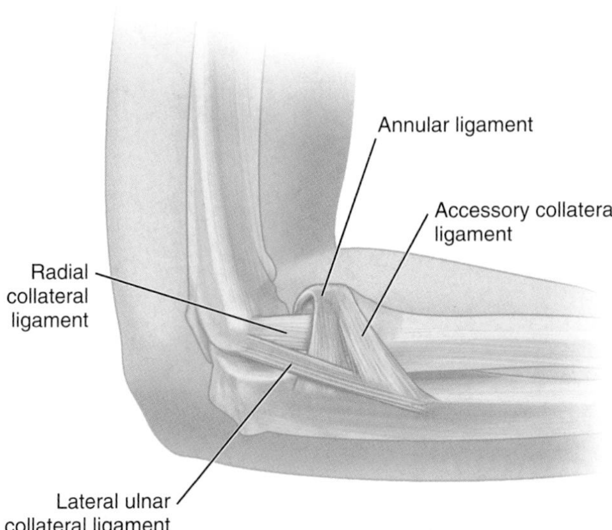

FIGURE 132-4 The lateral collateral ligament complex of the elbow is demonstrated, including the lateral ulnar collateral ligament, the radial collateral ligament, and the accessory collateral ligament.

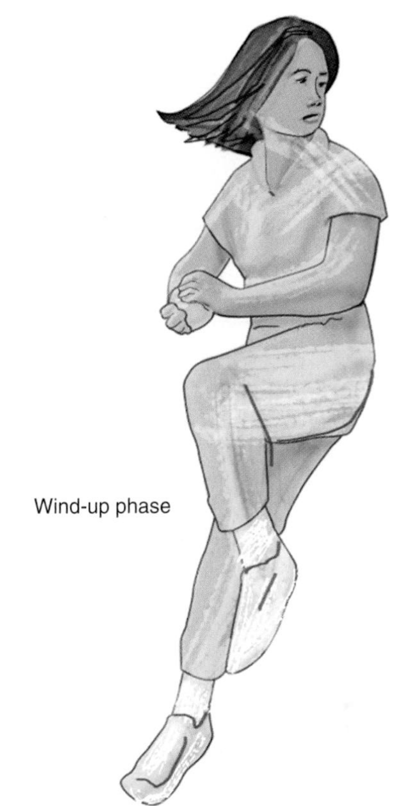

FIGURE 132-5 The wind-up phase of throwing.

elbow. These ligaments, combined with the anconeus muscle, form a lateral elbow complex that provides both dynamic and static restraint to elbow instability in both varus and rotation. The lateral ligament complex is rarely injured in children as a result of repetitive use or microtrauma; however, the medical literature includes case reports that describe reconstruction or repair of this complex when persistent instability exists.[15,16] The diagnosis is often challenging because children may describe vague pain and soreness with certain activities but without the characteristic instability that is the hallmark of this clinical entity in adults.

Biomechanics in Throwing Sports

Throwing Motion

The throwing motion is common in many sports played by children and adolescents. Football, baseball, and overhead racquet sports such as tennis are the characteristic activities that demonstrate the biomechanics of the elbow during throwing and are most common in this age group. The pitching motion has been analyzed extensively in the adult and pediatric sports medicine literature. Repetitive valgus and distraction forces of the medial pediatric elbow have been observed during pitching and are thought to be the etiology in the development of medial UCL disease, medial epicondylitis, and epicondyle avulsions. The pitch has been divided into five stages[17-19]:

1. Wind-up (ends when the ball leaves the nonthrowing hand; Fig. 132-5)
2. Early cocking (shoulder abduction and rotation; ends when the forward foot hits the ground; Fig. 132-6)
3. Late cocking (maximum shoulder external rotation is achieved; Fig. 132-7)
4. Acceleration (begins with internal rotation of the humerus and ends with ball release; Fig. 132-8)
5. Follow-through (ends when all motion is complete; Fig. 132-9)

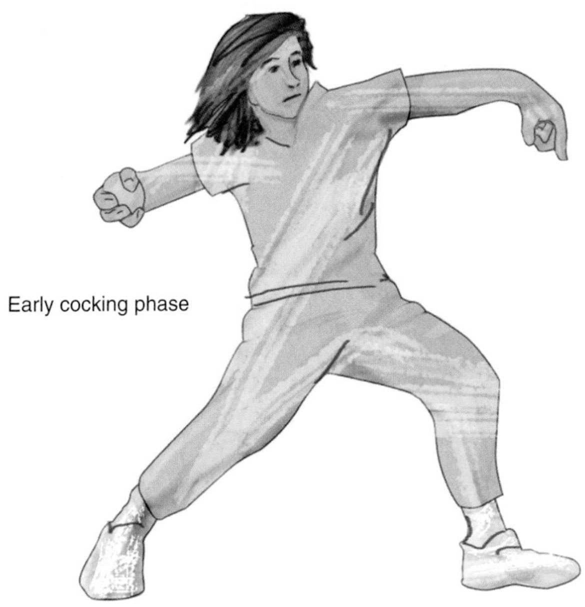

FIGURE 132-6 The early cocking phase of throwing.

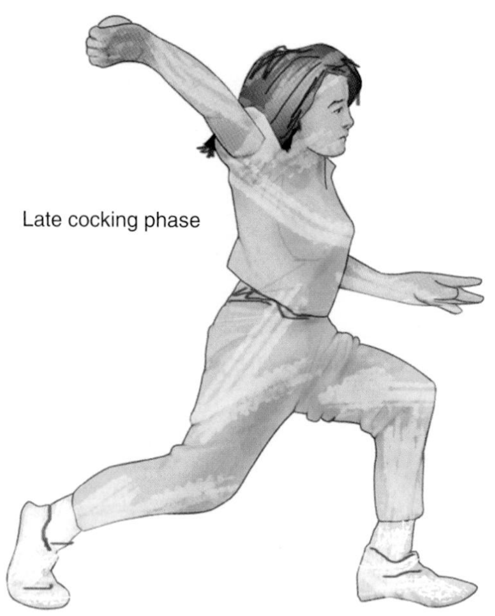

FIGURE 132-7 The late cocking phase of throwing.

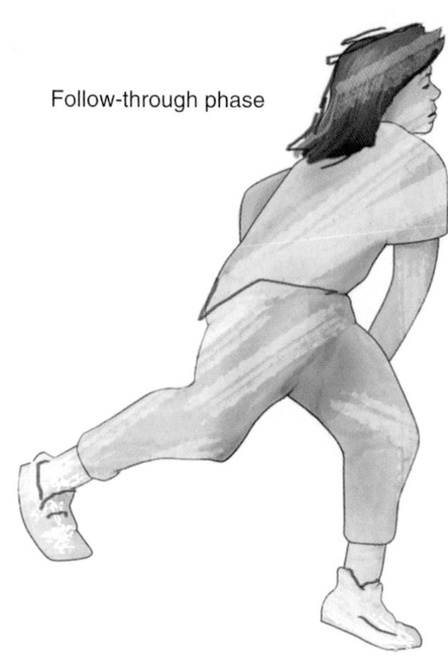

FIGURE 132-9 The follow-through phase of throwing.

One of the fundamental concepts in understanding the throwing motion as it relates to pitching is the "kinetic chain."[20] The kinetic chain of throwing refers to the role that core and proximal musculature play into the development of force required for throwing. Proximal muscle activation results in postural adjustments that allow the body to balance the forces that are required for throwing.[21] These muscle activations create force moments, which are a product of adjacent segment motion and position. The moments occur at proximal segments and are important for generating force delivered to distal motion segments such as the elbow.[22] One investigation demonstrated that younger pitchers may not produce as much force generation from their lower core segments, which may place larger demands on the upper extremities of youths who pitch and can ultimately cause pain and disability.[23] Other investigations have documented that youths who pitch and adults who pitch have similar kinematics, while also demonstrating that youth pitchers who are deficient in their mechanics on key parameters are less efficient, place higher valgus loads across their elbows, and demonstrate higher humeral internal rotation torque.[24,25] Lack of proximal force production may cause the elbow to be lower than the shoulder during the acceleration phase of throwing (as a result of a lack of elbow elevation and extension prior to shoulder rotation), which places increased tensile forces on the medial elbow.[20] In the ideal motion, maximal elbow extension occurs prior to maximum shoulder rotation, which couples internal rotation of the shoulder to pronation about the elbow, preventing medial tensile or valgus overload. Teaching proper throwing mechanics in youth sports and limiting the opportunities of young throwers to "overuse" their arms is critical in preventing pathologic conditions of the elbow.

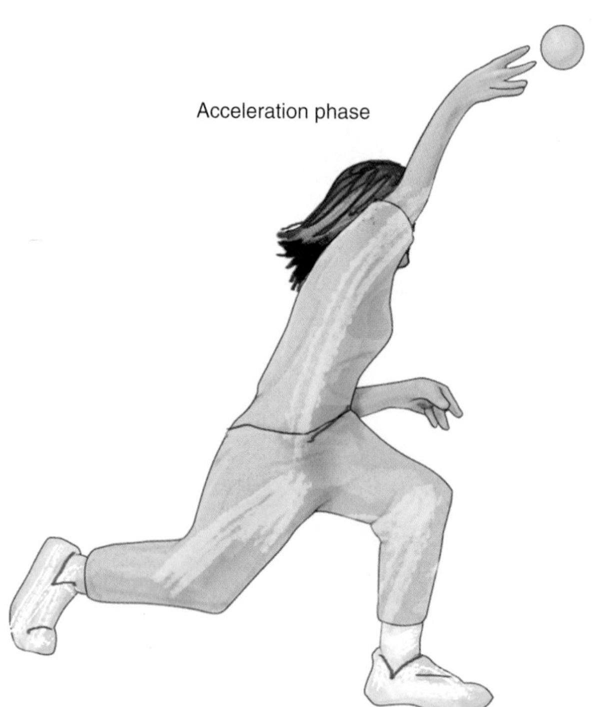

FIGURE 132-8 The acceleration phase of throwing.

Forces Around the Elbow During Throwing

During the early and late cocking phases of throwing, significant distraction forces are placed on the medial elbow structures. This tensile force is transmitted to the medial UCL and medial epicondyle. In the pediatric population, the most vulnerable area of injury is the medial epicondylar physis, which can be avulsed with repetitive injury. In addition, the UCL can become stretched or incompetent, the flexor pronator mass can become strained, and the ulnar nerve can be stretched, resulting in neurologic symptoms. Whereas distraction forces are applied on the medial elbow, compressive forces are encountered on the lateral elbow structures during the early and late cocking phases.[17-19] Sequelae of this repetitive compression of the radial head against the capitellum can result in growth disturbances, osteochondral fractures and loose bodies, and altered growth of the radial head.[17,18]

During the acceleration phase of throwing, extreme pronation of the forearm results in a tension force on the lateral and posterolateral elbow structures. Lateral epicondylitis may result from repetitive overuse and strain of these muscles during this phase of throwing. During follow-through, hyperextension of the elbow places strain on the olecranon process and the anterior capsule. In late adolescence and into young adulthood, this stress can manifest as posteromedial elbow spurs, posterior/triceps spurs, and traction spurs of the coronoid process. Classic overload symptoms of the elbow result from forces generated during the throwing motion and are helpful in determining pathologic findings: tensile overload of the medial restraints, compression overload of the lateral elbow, shear forces of the posteromedial elbow, and extension overload of the lateral restraints.[18,26]

Overview of Pathologies

Little Leaguer's Elbow

Little Leaguer's elbow, or medial apophysitis, is a broad term used to describe a spectrum of pathologic conditions that can occur in the young baseball player or thrower. Although we typically associate this spectrum of injury with baseball, a wide range of throwing or overhead sports including javelin, tennis, and football can present in a similar fashion. The throwing motion in the developing athlete is associated with significant force across the medial elbow.[18] During the throwing motion, and particularly in the late cocking phase of throwing, a valgus traction force is created on the medial elbow structures (i.e., the medial epicondyle, epicondylar apophysis, and medial ligament complex), whereas a compressive force is transmitted to the lateral side of the elbow (radial head and capitellum). With repetitive stress to the medial elbow, microtrauma and potentially degeneration of these structures may occur.[27] The subsequent tissue breakdown can cause the characteristic spectrum of disease: delayed or accelerated growth of the medial epicondyle, traction apophysitis and fragmentation of the medial epicondyle, medial epicondylitis, osteochondritis of the capitellum, hypertrophy of the ulna, osteochondral injury to the radial head, and olecranon apophysitis with delayed physeal closure.

Aside from overuse and repetitive stress to the medial elbow, young pitchers are believed to have altered mechanics relative to older athletes. Younger pitchers may initiate trunk rotation earlier in the throwing motion, which causes hyperangulation at the shoulder and increased torque along the longitudinal axis of the humerus during late cocking, predisposing them to elbow and shoulder pathology.[27] Early trunk rotation occurs before the scapula and humerus are properly positioned in space. The resultant increase in horizontal abduction of the shoulder during stride results in excessive angulation of the shoulder throughout the cocking phase, which can predispose the athlete to anterior shoulder instability and an elevation in the horizontal adduction force applied to the humerus. When obtaining the history, a focus on the athlete's prior education regarding proper throwing mechanics, initiation of pitch counts with rest periods, and supervision for manifesting symptoms are all helpful in determining the prevention strategies that were in place for the athlete prior to the development of symptoms and can help guide treatment. Young athletes may not present in a typical fashion, and the symptoms may range from medial elbow pain and decreased throwing effectiveness to decreased throwing distance.

History

Obtaining a thorough history in pediatric and adolescent patients can often be challenging. The clinician must assess the overall affect of the child, as well as the importance of the sport in his or her daily life. Some children may underreport their symptoms so they may continue playing, whereas other children may overreport their symptoms in situations in which they feel pressured to compete by family or friends or pressured by the requirements of the daily routine. The age of the patient is important because it may provide a clue to the potential diagnosis. Patients in their early childhood and in whom the secondary ossification centers have yet to appear are more likely to report pain originating from the medial elbow as a result of repetitive injury to the ossification center and apophysis.[18] Throwing forces may impede the characteristic appearance and growth of these ossification centers. In adolescence (which terminates with the fusion of the secondary centers of ossification with their respective long bones), muscle mass and force generation during throwing dramatically increase. In this age group, avulsion of the medial epicondyle can occur with resulting fracture displacement (Fig. 132-10). Incomplete avulsions are more common near the

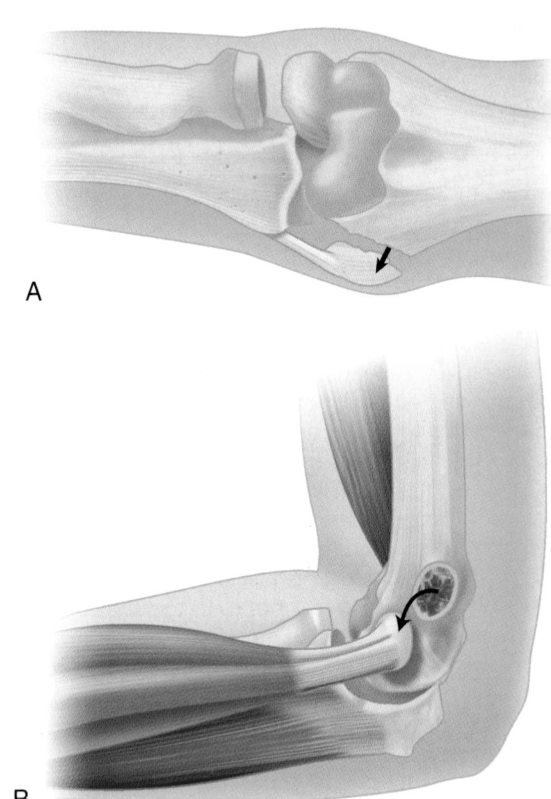

FIGURE 132-10 **A** and **B,** An avulsion fracture through the medial epicondyle, with attached ulnar collateral ligament and flexor/pronator mass.

end of adolescence as fusion of the medial epicondyle occurs. With repetitive stress to the medial epicondyle, nonunions and delayed unions may occur and cause continued pain into young adulthood. When the patient enters young adulthood (after fusion of all the secondary ossification centers), injuries to the muscles and soft tissue attachments of the elbow are more common. Injury to the ulnar collateral ligament and strain of the flexor/pronator mass are characteristically seen as overuse syndromes in this patient cohort.

In addition to age, the position of the throwing athlete should be elicited. Pitchers and quarterbacks place the most strain on their arms within their respective sports relative to other position players. In baseball, the likelihood of injury is more prevalent in pitchers and less likely in infielders, catchers, and outfielders in decreasing order.[17] Athletes who engage in throwing often injure themselves as a result of repetitive overuse rather than direct trauma, making hand dominance an important factor in determining injury.

In addition to this demographic information, the clinician should inquire about pain, which is often the presenting complaint. The onset, character, duration, intensity, location, persistence, and temporal association (e.g., night, day, or with activity) of the pain are important in both diagnosis and formulating a treatment plan. The onset of the pain can be gradual with an overuse injury pattern or more sudden if an avulsion fracture of the medial epicondyle is encountered. The pain may be dull or aching in patients with chronic injuries or sharp and severe when a more identifiable, acute episode is the culprit.

The duration of the pain is important in determining prognosis. Short episodes of soreness are distinguished from pain that is present before, during, and after throwing, which is a more worrisome finding that could represent chronic overuse and portend a poorer prognosis. The location of the pain can help determine which structures are at risk. The temporal association of the pain is important in determining the most likely site of pathologic findings. Pain during the throwing motion in the late cocking phase typically implies medial overload or instability in a young adult or adolescent patient. Pain at rest or at night could indicate another underlying cause, and a neoplastic process should be ruled out in these instances.

In addition to pain, other symptoms may be present. Decreased range of motion, swelling, decrease in velocity or control, and paresthesias or dysesthesias into the upper extremity, particularly the ulnar nerve, can also occur and should be evaluated. After the symptoms have been elicited, a more detailed athletic history should also be obtained. The number of innings pitched, pitch count, type of pitches thrown, pitching rotation schedule, and training schedule can help determine if the athlete is placing his or her arm at risk for injury. Identifying a strain prior to ligament incompetence or growth plate disturbance is important to optimize treatment and prognosis. Associated injuries should also be evaluated, as well as any downstream (wrist/hand) or upstream (shoulder/neck) symptoms that could compromise successful treatment.

The surgical history of the elbow and shoulder should also be evaluated because altered biomechanics of both joints can place increased strain on the elbow during throwing. A thorough medical and family history should also be elicited for all patients with particular attention to any history of osteochondritis, Perthes disease, Kohler disease, and Osgood-Schlatter disease. When patients with any of these diseases participate in sports that increase the articular cartilage demand around the elbow, the likelihood of abnormal epiphyseal development is increased.[17] In addition, a history of delayed skeletal maturation could cause a young child to throw on an age-determined team beyond his or her physiologic tolerance, which could lead to elbow abnormalities.

Physical Examination

The physical examination is first focused on the overall demeanor and affect of the young athlete. The examination should proceed in a fairly systematic fashion to decrease the risk of missing associated injuries. A complete examination of the cervical neck for range of motion, tenderness, and associated provocative tests (e.g., the Spurling test) can help determine cervical spine pathology. Both shoulders should be examined for strength, range of motion, and stability. Abnormalities of the scapulothoracic joint, including scapular dyskinesia, should be sought, as should any evidence of internal rotation contracture of the glenohumeral joint, which can contribute to pathologic conditions of the elbow.[20] Both elbows should first be inspected and evaluated for any asymmetry, deformity, or hypertrophy. Throwers often have hypertrophy of the muscles of their dominant arm or an alteration of the carrying angle. Range of motion of the elbows is assessed in flexion and extension, along with pronation and supination. The medial, lateral, and posterior elbow structures are palpated to elicit any tenderness. Because of the relative subcutaneous position of the osseous structures around the elbow, the medial epicondyle, lateral epicondyle, radial head, olecranon process, and collateral ligaments are readily identified and palpated to specifically identify any areas of discomfort. Patients with medial apophysitis typically demonstrate a flexion contracture greater than 15 degrees with point tenderness over the medial epicondyle.[28]

Palpation of the ulnar nerve is also performed in flexion and extension to evaluate for tenderness and subluxation. With slight flexion, the olecranon fossa can be examined and gentle pressure can indicate pain over the posteromedial or posterolateral portion of the olecranon fossa. In slight flexion of 25 to 35 degrees, the olecranon is "unlocked" and the ligamentous stability of the elbow can be assessed. The lateral ligaments are assessed with slight varus and internal rotation stress applied to the arm, whereas the medial ligaments are assessed with valgus and external rotation stress applied to the arm.[29] With the elbow flexed 90 degrees and the patient actively supinating, the distal biceps tendon can also be palpated in the antecubital fossa. The insertion of the triceps muscle is also easily identified on the olecranon process, and both of these muscles can be actively tested with flexion/supination and extension, respectively. Comparison is made to the contralateral extremity for any subtle differences that could indicate elbow instability or weakness. The examination concludes with a detailed neurovascular examination of the distal extremity.

Imaging

Routine radiographs are an essential part of the evaluation of children and adolescents with elbow pain. Anteroposterior (AP), lateral, reverse axial, and comparison views are often obtained to rule out any osseous injury or irregularity of the growth centers. When injury to the ligaments is suspected, stress views can be obtained; however, a normal stress view does not rule out the presence of a significant ligamentous injury. Within the spectrum of Little Leaguer's elbow, a variety of pathologic conditions can be seen on radiographs. Fragmentation, enlargement, or fracture of the medial epicondyle can sometimes be appreciated.[30] Laterally, osteochondritis dissecans (OCD) can be appreciated as a lucency in the capitellum on oblique radiographs, or in advanced cases, degenerative arthritis and loose bodies may be visualized. Posteriorly, hypertrophy of the ulna may be present, which can impinge in the olecranon fossa of the distal humerus. With repetitive impingement, osteophytes and loose bodies may be visualized in the posterior compartment. Occasionally, stress fractures of the ulna or olecranon apophysis can occur, in addition to delayed union at these sites. Classic findings of medial apophysitis include fragmentation and widening of the medial epiphyseal lines relative to the contralateral elbow.

Although most diagnoses can be confirmed with a thorough history, physical examination, and review of radiographs, other imaging modalities have been shown to increase sensitivity and the specificity of diagnosis. Ultrasound has been investigated as a potential imaging modality for evaluating OCD lesions of the capitellum and fragmentation of the medial epicondyle.[31] Bone scans can help determine areas of increased activity in persons with overuse injuries, and computed tomography (CT) scans can help better identify osseous anatomy in instances of fractures and loose bodies with osteophyte formation. Perhaps the most sensitive imaging modality is magnetic resonance imaging (MRI). MRI is helpful in evaluating the soft tissue structures of the elbow (UCL, biceps, triceps, and extensor/flexor tendon attachment sites), the articular cartilage (OCD, loose bodies, and avascular necrosis), and epiphyseal development (apophysis and epiphysis).[32,33] In addition, in cases of OCD, MRI can help in decision making with regard to surgical intervention. MRI often demonstrates more positive findings in patients with Little Leaguer's elbow than do traditional radiographs; however, these findings rarely alter clinical management of these patients.[18]

Decision-Making Principles

No hallmark sign accompanies the diagnosis of Little Leaguer's elbow; often it is the constellation of symptoms, physical signs, and confirmatory findings on radiographs or MRI that leads to the diagnosis. A high index of suspicion is warranted when any child presents with elbow pain and is involved in competitive sports that entail throwing. With prompt diagnosis and treatment, patients can often avoid more serious and long-term sequelae that are associated with this spectrum of injury. Perhaps equally as important is recognizing the variability and normal findings that exist in this population. Hypertrophy of the throwing arm, valgus alignment of the extremity, and flexion contractures are fairly common in this patient population and by themselves rarely warrant treatment in asymptomatic patients.[34]

Treatment Options

Treatment of Little Leaguer's elbow is tailored toward the specific diagnosis that is causing the pain or disability. Because this diagnosis can present along a continuum of injury, from a strain of the medial epicondyle to fracture and incompetence of the UCL, treatment is dependent on a multitude of factors: the injury severity, acuity, level of disability, and age. In patients who do not require acute surgical intervention and who have the capacity to heal, a period of rest is often warranted. In most cases, abstinence from throwing for 4 to 6 weeks results in cessation of symptoms. Use of ice and nonsteroidal inflammatory medications has been shown to be beneficial in the acute stages. Currently no role exists for the use of injected corticosteroids in the management of medial apophysitis. In more severe cases, use of a removable posterior splint with immobilization may be warranted. After 6 weeks of rest, range of motion is restored with gentle exercises and strengthening is begun. After 8 weeks, a throwing program is generally begun. Beyond rest, proper instruction on throwing mechanics may reduce the incidence of elbow injuries in these patients. In a recent investigation, it was found that youth who pitched with better pitching mechanics produced lower humeral internal rotation torque, lower elbow valgus load, and more efficiency during throwing.[24] This study has implications for the prevention of injury through better instruction. With regard to the frequency of pitching and the types of pitches thrown, a prior report demonstrated that the slider was associated with an 86% risk of elbow pain in youth who pitch, and a strong association was found between shoulder and elbow injuries and the number of games played and pitches thrown.[35] Perhaps the best treatment strategy known is prevention. Preventing excessive pitching in youth sports, discouraging year-round play, and delaying the use of breaking pitches will likely have a positive impact on the young pitcher's medial elbow. Current guidelines from Little League recommend that young athletes not be allowed to pitch curveballs until the age of 14 years (±2 years). Current guidelines have been developed for pitch counts in youth baseball as well, with the recommendation that any athlete younger than 10 years should pitch fewer than 75 pitches per day, with 3 rest days for any days in which more than 60 pitches are thrown. This amount can be increased by intervals of 10 for every 2 years of chronologic age, with the pitch threshold for 3 days of rest increased to 75 pitches.[36]

Results

Most patients with medial apophysitis return to sports at their preinjury level of competition with conservative treatment. No large-scale results of conservative management of this entity have been published. Because this diagnosis encompasses such a wide range of pathologic conditions, each distinct clinical entity has a varying prognosis with treatment.

Complications

With repetitive injury, after return to sport, the athlete is at risk for the development of growth disturbances around the elbow, persistent pain, avulsion fractures, OCD, and valgus instability after physeal closure.

Osteochondritis Dissecans and Panner Disease (Osteochondrosis)

OCD is a focal lesion of the capitellum that typically occurs in adolescents between 13 and 16 years of age. Theories regarding the origination of this pathologic process vary, with some authors believing that the compressive forces from throwing result in valgus overload and contribute significantly to its development. Other investigations have pointed to the biomechanical mismatch between the capitellum and radial head as a causative mechanism. The etiology of this disease is multifactorial and likely results from microtrauma in the setting of cartilage mismatch and joint susceptibility.[37] Histology from patients who underwent surgery for OCD of the capitellum demonstrated damage to the articular cartilage surface as a result of repetitive stress after a degenerative and reparative process of articular and subchondral fracture.[38] Separation of the fragment occurs on the cartilage surface and may proceed to the subchondral bone in advanced stages.[38]

Panner disease is a clinical entity that is distinct from OCD and is more common in younger patients. This clinical entity is a reversible, degenerative process of the capitellum that begins earlier in childhood, typically between the ages of 7 and 10 years, and involves the secondary ossification center of the capitellum. The hallmark of Panner disease is a process of degeneration followed by regeneration and recalcification.[31,39] Potential causes of Panner disease have been attributed to endocrine disorders, fat embolism, congenital and hereditary factors, the tenuous blood supply of the capitellum, and repetitive trauma. In the child, the most common cause of lateral elbow pain is Panner disease; however, by adolescence OCD becomes the most common source of this pain. Panner disease has a rather acute onset, with fragmentation of the entire capitellar ossific nucleus.

History

Patients with OCD most commonly report elbow pain with decreased ability to throw and may localize their symptoms on the lateral side of the elbow. The onset is typically insidious, and as the process progresses, loose bodies may form, which can cause the sensation of a "locking elbow." Patients report joint stiffness and lack of range of motion and may report catching within the joint. Patients with Panner disease may have difficulty describing their symptoms; however, it is usually an aching lateral-sided elbow pain that may be accompanied by swelling. Patients may report an inability to throw a ball or achieve terminal extension of the elbow. Most patients with either condition do not report a traumatic injury or other inciting event. It is important to identify causative mechanisms such as repetitive throwing, endocrine disorders, or family history that could implicate the diagnosis.

Physical Examination

In persons with Panner disease, the dominant arm is typically affected. On physical examination, patients may report tenderness over the lateral elbow and capitellum with slight effusion and synovial thickening. Range of motion is typically affected, with a lack of terminal extension of 20 to 30 degrees.[40] Also noticeable may be a slight lack of pronation or supination with tenderness while attempting this movement.[37]

In patients with OCD, the elbow may not demonstrate significant swelling. Because this clinical entity is commonly associated with Little Leaguer's elbow, many of the clinical manifestations are similar. Tenderness and laxity of the medial elbow, tenderness over the lateral epicondyle and capitellum, and clicking of the joint may be evident. In most patients, the pain may be difficult to localize because of the spectrum of pathologic conditions that is characteristic in these patients. Patients typically have diminished range of motion, and in the setting of loose bodies, they may have acute, sharp pain with certain movements.

Imaging

In the setting of Panner disease, radiographs in the early stages of the disease demonstrate irregularity of the capitellum with areas of radiolucency and sclerosis, particularly near the physis. After several months, radiographs show enlarged areas of radiolucency with reconstitution of the bony epiphysis. After a period of 1 to 2 years, the epiphysis returns to a normal configuration without flattening. In some patients, the adjacent radial head may undergo early maturation compared with the contralateral elbow.

In the setting of OCD, supplemental radiographs such as oblique views or 45-degree flexed views can help better visualize the lesion in suspected cases. The classic finding in pediatric and adolescent OCD is a focal area in the anterolateral capitellum with rarefaction and irregularity of the articular surface. Sclerotic bone may surround the lesion and loose bodies may be seen when the articular lesion becomes detached.[31] Healing of the lesion can take months to years and is visualized on radiographs as ossification of this radiolucent lesion. CT with or without arthrography may help better delineate the osseous anatomy and articular surface. MRI is the most sensitive test and may detect lesions prior to their appearance on radiographs. In lesions that appear early in the disease process, T1-weighted sequences may detect decreased signal intensity within the lesion, with a normal appearance on T2-weighted sequences. In more advanced cases, high signal intensity and cyst formation around the lesion could indicate impending detachment and loose body formation (Fig. 132-11).[41] More advanced MRI techniques with gadolinium may help to define fragment stability and determine staging and prognosis.

Decision-Making Principles

In persons with Panner disease, the key to optimal management is proper diagnosis and recognition. When the clinician recognizes that Panner disease is usually a self-limited

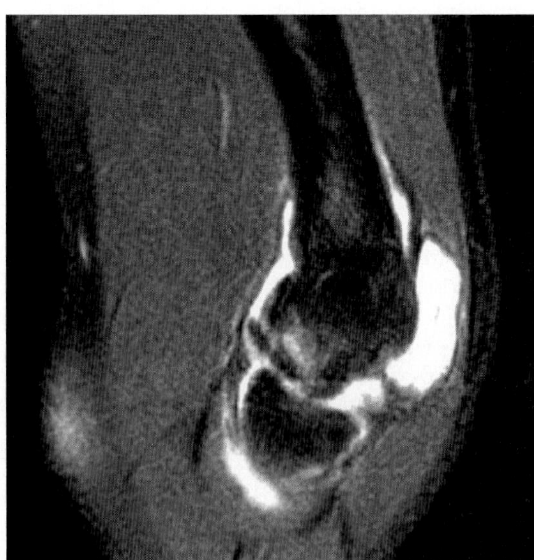

FIGURE 132-11 A T2-weighted sagittal magnetic resonance imaging scan of a detached or semidetached osteochondritis dissecans lesion in a 12-year-old male adolescent.

TABLE 132-1

CHARACTERISTICS OF OSTEOCHONDRITIS DISSECANS LESIONS BASED ON STABILITY

Classification	Capitellar Growth Plate	Range of Motion
Stable	Open	Normal
Unstable	Closed	Restricted

Data from Ruchelsman DE, Hall MP, Youm T: Osteochondritis of the capitellum: current concepts. *J Am Acad Orthop Surg* 18:557–567, 2010.

condition that disappears by adolescence, proper care and instruction can be provided to both the patient and family. With OCD, several factors determine proper management and treatment. Classification systems of OCD have been devised to help standardize reporting and define treatment. In one of the first classification systems based on AP radiographs, the authors outlined three grades of OCD.[42] In grade I, radiographs demonstrated a translucent cystic shadow in the middle or lateral capitellum. In grade II, a clear zone or split line between the lesion and the adjacent subchondral bone is evident. In grade III, loose bodies are present.[42] In another study, the authors correlated the arthroscopic findings with those found on MRI to devise a classification of elbow OCD. In this system, surgically defined lesions were those in which a lesion was found to be grade III or higher, indicating a high signal intensity rim around the lesion that implied instability of the lesion upon probing.[41] Further systems devised by the International Cartilage Repair Society have not shown a strong correlation to treatment or outcomes in the peer-reviewed literature.[43] A more recent classification has been proposed that classifies lesions as stable or unstable and is dependent on the ability of the lesion to heal based on the physiologic condition of the elbow (Table 132-1). Based on this classification system, unstable lesions demonstrate improved results with surgery.[43] As the characterization of capitellar lesions evolves, it will become increasingly important to use this information to predict prognosis and guide treatment. Management of OCD of the elbow is primarily determined by the integrity of the articular cartilage and the stability of the lesion. Unstable lesions are typically managed with surgical intervention, whereas stable lesions demonstrate more intrinsic ability for healing.

Treatment

In the early stages of OCD, treatment is largely nonoperative. Early-grade, stable lesions are typically managed with a period of rest and cessation of sports participation. The amount of time that the patient refrains from participating in sports is determined by the length of time that symptoms persist. The typical duration is 3 to 6 weeks, followed by a 3- to 6-month period of progressive strengthening and range of motion until full participation is achieved. Bracing and use of nonsteroidal antiinflammatory medication may have a role; however, these treatments are largely supportive and have not been shown to provide tremendous benefit in the literature.[43,44]

Surgery for OCD of the elbow is typically reserved for patients who have loose bodies, report mechanical symptoms, and have unstable lesions on radiographs or MRI or who have failed to respond to nonoperative management after 6 months and have a stable lesion. The best surgical procedure for patients with OCD of the elbow is a topic of considerable debate. Surgical options include open or arthroscopic fragment excision (with or without abrasion arthroplasty, drilling, or microfracture), fixation of the unstable or displaced lesion, bone grafting, osteotomy, and osteochondral autograft transplantation (the OAT procedure). Our preference is fixation of these fragments when they are larger and when adequate purchase can be obtained with a 3.0-mm minifragment cannulated screw. Screw removal is typically necessary 3 months after fixation and healing. When smaller lesions are present, loose body removal and microfracture of the defect is a good surgical option.

Results

The spontaneous healing rates of patients with OCD are varied, and the results in the literature vary from excellent to poor. In a recent investigation, the authors found that 25 of 30 early-stage lesions healed at final follow-up, whereas only 1 of 9 late-stage lesions had healed.[37] A significant correlation of healing with open physes was noted. In another study with longer follow-up, the authors found that more than 50% of the patients with stable lesions treated nonsurgically had mild discomfort at a mean follow-up of 13.6 years.[44] In a different study, 50% of patients treated nonsurgically had persistent elbow symptoms with activities of daily living and also demonstrated radiographic evidence of osteoarthritis at 12.6-year follow-up.[45] These results demonstrate the variability in the outcomes of these patients; however, proper assessment of the stability of the lesion may be the reason for the discrepancy in the data.

For surgical treatment, the results may depend on the technique used, the stage of the lesion, and the length of follow-up of the patients. For open excision of the fragment and debridement, Bauer et al.[46] demonstrated poor results at long-term follow-up, with 40% of patients reporting recurrence of symptoms and loss of elbow extension. These patients all had advanced lesions at the time of surgery. Other studies have demonstrated more encouraging results, with nearly 50% of patients returning to athletics.[43] Short- and midterm results of patients who have undergone arthroscopic debridement and marrow stimulation techniques such as drilling or microfracture are encouraging; however, long-term outcomes of these studies are currently lacking. In one report, the authors studied three elite gymnasts who underwent arthroscopic debridement and microfracture after failure of an initial trial of nonoperative management. They found full range of motion and return to sport in all three patients at 1-year follow-up with hyaline-like cartilage on postoperative MRI.[47] In a more recent report, the authors reported improvement in Disabilities of the Arm, Shoulder and Hand scores and symptoms; however, many of the patients demonstrated decreased ability to participate in some sports because of their elbow.[48] In a large retrospective review of fragment fixation versus excision, the authors compared 12 patients who underwent fixation with 55 patients who underwent excision of the unstable lesion. The authors found that fragment fixation performed better than removal, and they recommended bone grafting for higher grade lesions.[43] Osteotomy is a surgical option in the management of these patients, but it is rarely performed in the United States. In Japan, one study demonstrated good outcomes in baseball pitchers, with six of seven returning to sports and all seven demonstrated remodeling of the capitellum at 6 months with a mean increase in range of motion of 12 degrees.[49] In lesions that engage the radial head, are large in surface area, or are higher grade, the OAT procedure offers the ability to restore articular cartilage to the capitellum. The short-term results of the OAT procedure in the literature are promising, with more than 90% of patients in most series returning to their preinjury level of function without radiographic degenerative changes.[50-52]

Complications

Patients with Panner disease have relatively few complications. Most patients demonstrate the natural history of the condition with progression to healing. A few may experience worsening symptoms, loose body formation, and progression to an OCD clinical scenario. With OCD, most complications arise from incomplete healing of the lesion. Progression to loose body formation, osteoarthritis, limited range of motion, and disability can occur, and athletes should be counseled on the possibility of not returning to their preinjury level of sport. Surgical complications can include infection, stiffness, hardware failure, neurologic injury (affecting the ulnar nerve), and failure to restore normal congruity to the elbow.

Medial Epicondyle Avulsion Fractures

Medial epicondyle fractures are common fractures in children and adolescents, accounting for 11% to 20% of all elbow fractures in this patient population.[53] In many instances, this fracture pattern is associated with elbow dislocation; however, in the throwing athlete, this situation is rarely the case and it is more commonly associated with repetitive overuse and traction on the medial epicondyle from the flexor/pronator mass.[54] Alternatively, a valgus force on the elbow while falling on an outstretched hand can also cause this injury pattern. These fractures most commonly occur in boys, with a peak incidence in age of 11 to 12 years.[53-56]

History

Patients who sustain this injury likely report acute, sudden pain in their elbow localized over the medial epicondyle. Patients may have reported a subluxation event or feeling a pop in their elbow that precipitated the swelling and discomfort. The history of pain may include sudden elbow pain in the setting of chronic elbow symptoms. A thorough and detailed athletic history is warranted to associate the pathologic condition with the throwing motion, and the constellation of findings seen in Little Leaguer's elbow should be sought.

Physical Examination

Physical examination typically demonstrates swelling in the area of the elbow, loss of a normal elbow contour (in cases of dislocation), and crepitus with range of motion. Diminished range of motion is present, and associated neurologic symptoms may occur because the ulnar nerve lies in close proximity to the posterior aspect of the medial epicondyle. In patients who require surgery, elbow stability can be assessed with the gravity-assisted valgus stress test (Fig. 132-12).[57]

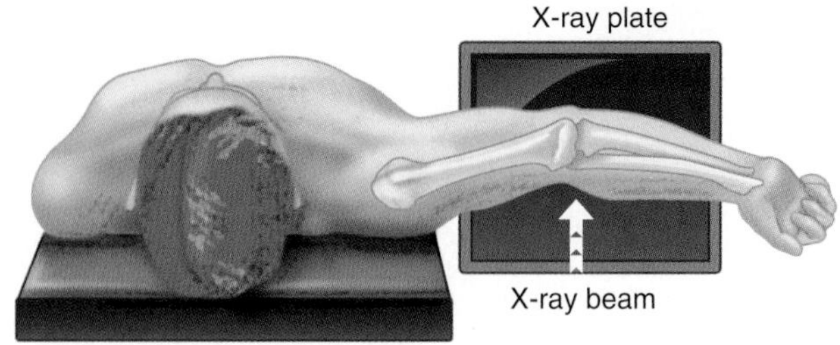

FIGURE 132-12 The gravity stress test is shown. The arm is placed in full external rotation, permitting the weight of the forearm to deliver a valgus stress to the elbow.

Imaging

The diagnosis is typically made with standard AP, lateral, and oblique radiographs of the elbow. Evaluating displacement on the AP radiograph may be the most accurate method of diagnosis; however, several studies have demonstrated the difficulty of and low interobserver agreement with assessment of displacement.[58] CT can be used to more accurately assess displacement in patients with these fractures; one study demonstrated that in cases in which the fracture was thought to be minimally displaced on radiographs, significant displacement was encountered on CT.[59]

Decision-Making Principles

The management of medial epicondyle fractures is controversial. Traditionally, this injury has been managed conservatively, and good results have been reported.[60-63] The decision to treat the fracture surgically is typically reserved for open fractures and injuries in which fracture fragments are incarcerated within the joint space. Surgical fixation may be indicated for severely displaced fragments, cases in which valgus instability is present in the athlete who places a high demand on the elbow, and when the ulnar nerve is compromised. With regard to fracture displacement as an indication for surgery, some authors advocate fixation for fragments with as little as 2 mm of displacement, whereas other authors recommend this treatment for fragments demonstrating greater than 15 mm of displacement.[61-63] Integrating the clinical history, examination, radiographs, and demands of the patient are all important in selecting the proper treatment for patients in this setting.

Treatment

Our preferred nonoperative treatment consists of immobilization in a long-arm cast with the elbow flexed to 90 degrees for 4 weeks. After removal of the cast, a splint can be applied with progressive range of motion and return to sports after union is achieved. Surgical techniques for fractures meeting surgical criteria include suture repair, Kirschner wire fixation, screw fixation, and excision of the fragment with suturing of the soft tissue to the medial periosteum.[64,65] Goals of surgery are to recreate the normal stability and mechanics of the elbow and to create an epiphysiodesis of the medial epicondyle. Rigid internal fixation with screws (3.0 or 3.5 mm, depending on the size of the epicondyle fragment) allows for earlier mobilization and may provide optimum stability.[60] Postoperatively, patients can be managed with a posterior splint, gentle exercises, and return to play once union is achieved and symptoms resolve.

Results

Reported results of nonoperative and operative management have generally been acceptable in the medical literature, even when fibrous union is achieved.[60-63] A shift toward operative treatment in recent years is likely due to the emerging concept of medial elbow stability in throwing athletes. If bony union is the primary outcome variable, surgical fixation provides better results in this regard, with a recent systematic review demonstrating 92% union in the surgically treated group and 50% union in the group managed without surgery.[66] Despite the higher union rates with screw or wire fixation, the patients managed without surgery achieved pain levels comparable with those of the surgical treatment group, with a trend toward less pain in the conservatively managed cohort. Functional outcome studies have demonstrated relative favorability for both treatment modalities, with some reports demonstrating improved functional results in patients managed without surgery. Although substantial valgus deformity occurs in fewer than 10% of patients, one study reported cubitus valgus as high as 35% after treatment.[67] Some studies have also demonstrated loss of range of motion after both surgical and nonsurgical treatment (37 degrees and 15 degrees, respectively).[54]

Complications

Complications from either treatment modality include loss of range of motion, nonunion, and cubitus valgus. Surgical complications include myositis ossificans, septic arthritis, pin tract or wound infections, and radial nerve injury.[68]

Medial Collateral Ligament Injury

Injuries to the UCL, although uncommon in children and adolescents, have an increasing incidence as muscle mass and force increase in young adults. UCL injuries occur more commonly in adults but have been seen and treated in young adults and adolescents. This spectrum of injury is closely associated with Little Leaguer's elbow and is part of the spectrum of injury that can be seen with valgus stress placed on the elbow during sports that entail throwing, particularly pitching.

History

Most patients have an insidious progression of discomfort and report pain over the medial elbow for months or even years before the ligament is definitively torn. Ruptures of the ligament occur as a sudden traumatic event, after which the elbow is painful enough to warrant cessation of throwing. Often patients report preexisting problems with elbow pain prior to this catastrophic event. Patients with overuse or attenuation of the ligament report medial elbow pain that is exacerbated by throwing, particularly in the late cocking and acceleration phases of throwing.[69]

Physical Examination

On physical examination, patients demonstrate tenderness along the course of the UCL, from the medial epicondyle to the sublime tubercle. Subtle findings of instability are often present, demonstrated by flexing the elbow to 25 degrees to unlock the olecranon from its fossa and gently stressing the medial side of the elbow. This test assesses the competency of the anterior band of the UCL, as does the moving valgus stress test.[69] The posterior band of the ligament is tested with the milking maneuver, which is performed by pulling the patient's thumb with the forearm supinated, shoulder extended, and elbow flexed more than 90 degrees. Typically, pain with these maneuvers can be indicative of subtle instability and is deemed a positive finding.

Imaging

Plain radiographs are typically normal, except in cases of chronic injuries where the findings of valgus extension overload are found, such as posterior spurring and osteophyte formation. In patients with chronic valgus instability, excessive forces are placed on the posteromedial elbow during terminal elbow extension, which can result in degenerative changes of the posteromedial compartment, manifesting as spurring and joint space narrowing on routine radiographs. Stress views can be obtained, and relative widening of greater than 2 mm (compared with the contralateral extremity) can be considered a positive finding and indicative of instability. Comparison views may be necessary to more accurately determine pathology. MRI is the most sensitive test to evaluate the UCL and also helps delineate concomitant pathologic conditions in the area of the elbow. MRI and MRI arthrography may demonstrate thickening of the ligament in many asymptomatic patients. In patients with instability, the ligament may demonstrate attenuation or a tear from either the medial epicondyle or the sublime tubercle. Chondromalacia of the posteromedial compartment could indicate chronic valgus instability and may also be detected on MRI.[70,71]

Decision-Making Principles

When considering surgical versus nonsurgical treatment, many factors go into determining the optimum strategy. Patients are likely surgical candidates when they have experienced an acute rupture, have signs of chronic instability, and have failed to respond to conservative treatment. Surgical treatment is best reserved for patients who wish to continue participating in sports that place a high demand on the medial elbow, including sports that entail throwing and gymnastics.[69,72]

Treatment

In most instances, conservative treatment is warranted, which consists of rest, immobilization, use of nonsteroidal antiinflammatory medication, and physical therapy to restore strength, flexibility, and stability. The flexor and pronator muscle groups should be targeted because they are important secondary dynamic stabilizers to valgus stress around the elbow.[73] Targeted evaluation of the throwing motion and biomechanics should be instituted by the coaching staff and trainers to identify any problems that could be contributing to the development of UCL abnormalities.

Surgical treatment for UCL insufficiency is offered after failure of a trial of 6 months of conservative management with persistent symptoms in the older athlete whose sport entails throwing. Complete tears of the ligament in young athletes typically require surgical intervention. In select cases, direct surgical repair of the ligament can be attempted when direct avulsions off the medial epicondyle occur and the native ligament appears to be of good quality. When a tenuous ligament repair is imminent, reconstruction of the ligament is a better

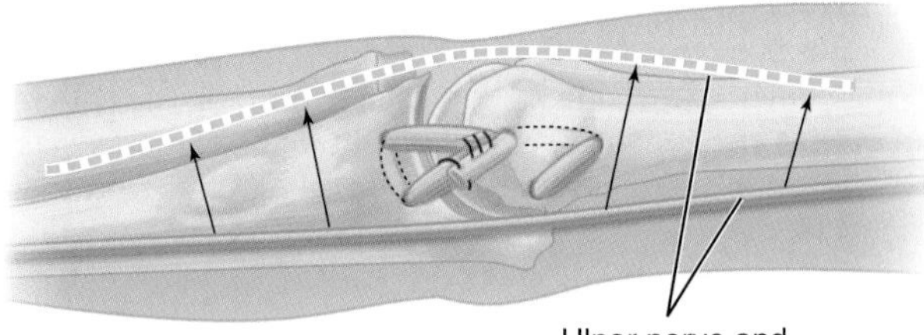

FIGURE 132-13 An example of a medial collateral ligament reconstruction with anterior submuscular transposition of the ulnar nerve.

option with a palmaris or gracilis tendon autograft.[74] Surgical reconstruction with a tendon graft is also indicated in the following circumstances: acute ruptures in throwers who lack enough remaining tissue ligament for a primary repair, the need to reestablish valgus stability in the presence of symptomatic chronic laxity, after debridement of calcific tendonitis in athletes if insufficient tissue is available to effect a primary repair, and when multiple episodes of recurring pain with throwing occur after periods of conservative care.[75-77] Figure of eight tendon reconstruction, as advocated by Jobe et al.,[72] or the docking technique, as advocated by Altcheck, are good options, and good results have been reported in the literature (Fig. 132-13).[72,78,79]

Results

Many young patients respond favorably to a trial of conservative treatment. In one study of athletes that outlined the treatment of UCL insufficiency with conservative treatment, 42% of patients returned to sport[80]; however, no randomized prospective studies have been performed to compare this treatment method with surgical reconstruction. Prospective and retrospective studies evaluating the outcome of UCL reconstruction have demonstrated favorable results, with the majority of athletes returning to their preinjury level of participation. In one study evaluating the results in high school baseball pitchers, 74% of athletes were able to return to high-level throwing, which is comparable with the results seen in more mature athletes.[81] In a systematic review of UCL reconstructions, the authors found favorable results overall with success rates improved with use of a muscle-splitting approach, less handling of the ulnar nerve, and use of the docking technique.[82] Overall, results range from a 70% to 90% successful return to sport at the preinjury level.[72,79,81-83]

Complications

Complications of surgical reconstruction include infection, fracture of the medial epicondyle and proximal ulna, ulnar nerve injury, and persistent pain and instability.

Posterior Elbow Pathologic Conditions (Posteromedial Impingement and Olecranon Osteochondrosis)

Injuries to the posterior compartment of the elbow are rare injuries in children and adolescents (Fig. 132-14). These injury patterns typically develop as late sequelae of chronic overuse syndromes (e.g., Little Leaguer's elbow and valgus extension overload). Pathologic conditions of the posterior elbow develop in response to chronic and repetitive extension overload from repetitive triceps contraction during the deceleration and follow-through phases of throwing. Posteromedial impingement is a term that denotes abutment of the medial aspect of the olecranon against the olecranon fossa as a result of valgus stress during terminal extension. Childhood injuries are more characteristically olecranon apophysitis and osteochondrosis with irregular ossification. In athletes approaching adolescence and young adulthood, these injuries are more commonly stress fractures or avulsion injuries of the olecranon apophysis with physeal widening, delayed fusion, or fragmentation.[84,85] In young adults and after skeletal maturity, this spectrum of injury presents as posteromedial elbow impingement as a result of valgus extension overload, with osteophytes, loose bodies, and persistent elbow pain.[69]

History

Patients with pathologic conditions of the posterior elbow typically report pain in the posterior compartment of the elbow. This pain may be most noticeable as the elbow is taken into extension or during the follow-through phase of throwing. Symptoms of locking or catching within the elbow joint could be a result of the presence of loose bodies.

Physical Examination

Physical examination shows pain in terminal extension, and patients may have tenderness to palpation over the posteromedial elbow and olecranon fossa. Because this injury can be the result of chronic valgus instability, assessment of the UCL should also be performed with stress testing as previously described. Tenderness over the proximal olecranon apophysis could indicate a stress fracture in this region, and distal triceps pain or pain with resisted elbow extension may indicate pathologic conditions within the extensor mechanism.

Imaging

Routine radiographs may demonstrate the presence of stress fractures or widening of the olecranon apophysis. These

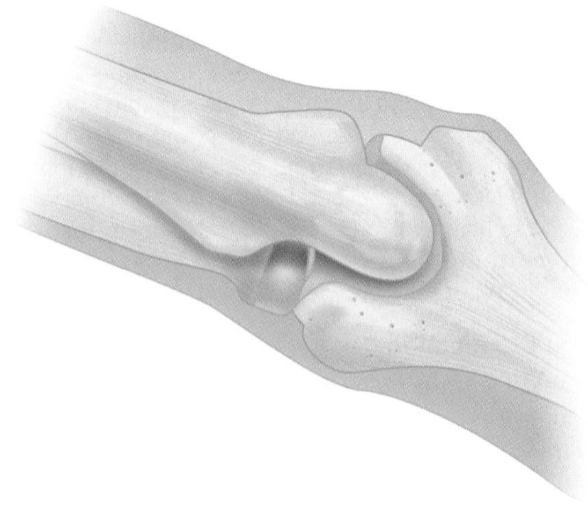

FIGURE 132-14 The posterior compartment of the elbow.

radiographs should be inspected for fragmentation, avulsions, or delayed fusion, which could indicate pathologic findings at this site. In cases in which injury is suspected, comparison views of the contralateral elbow can be obtained. With posteromedial impingement, osteophytes of the posteromedial olecranon may be visualized, along with loose bodies within the posterior compartment. Traction spurs of the proximal olecranon and triceps attachment are seen best on the lateral projection.[86-88] MRI can be used to evaluate for concomitant pathologic conditions such as UCL tears, osteochondral lesions, and stress reactions and can help locate loose bodies within the joint space.

Decision-Making Principles

Posterior elbow abnormalities are best managed on the basis of the presenting diagnosis. The age of the patient often determines the most likely diagnosis in this setting. Younger patients are more likely to respond to conservative treatment, particularly when chronic insufficiency of the UCL has yet to develop. In older patients, avulsions of the proximal olecranon and triceps attachment and other injuries that denote chronicity may require surgical management.

Treatment

Treatment is tailored to the individual according to the age of the patient and the diagnosis. Osteochondrosis and stress fractures in younger patients usually respond to a period of rest (with or without immobilization), with progression to range of motion and strengthening exercises after symptoms resolve. When returning to play, throwers are typically advanced with a rehabilitation program focusing on proper throwing mechanics and neuromuscular control, with progression to dynamic control and improvement of power. Avulsion[89] fractures with less than 2 mm of displacement can usually be treated conservatively with splint immobilization followed by functional range of motion and strengthening exercises. Small apophyseal fragments that do not compromise the extensor mechanism can be excised in patients who fail to respond to conservative treatment. Large avulsion fragments can be surgically treated with screw or suture fixation. In patients who have stress fracture nonunions or delayed union of the olecranon physis, open reduction and internal fixation with bone grafting is a viable option when a protracted period of conservative treatment fails.[86] Removal of loose bodies and posteromedial osteophytes can also be performed for more mature patients who have persistent posteromedial elbow symptoms. A minimally invasive arthroscopic approach should be instituted in these cases to possibly optimize function and decrease morbidity. Posterior olecranon spur resection should be performed with care, because increasing bone resection creates more strain in the UCL with valgus load.

Results

The results of nonsurgical treatment are generally favorable, with most patients returning to sports after a trial of conservative treatment. Results of stress fracture and delayed physeal closure with surgical fixation have been reported in the literature in small case series with favorable outcomes in nearly all patients.[86] Excision of spurs and loose bodies can provide symptomatic relief in most patients; however, addressing the underlying valgus instability through physical therapy or medial ligament reconstruction may be necessary to prevent further episodes. The pediatric literature has a paucity of data regarding this treatment because most reports focus on the adult athletes.

Complications

Complications can include nonunion, persistent pain, progression of posterior compartment osteoarthritis, and disability. Surgical complications include infection, wound complications, persistent nonunion, and progression of instability or iatrogenic instability as a result of surgical treatment.

Medial/Lateral Epicondylitis

A common anatomic location for pain in pediatric tennis players is the elbow, with 25% of 16- to 18-year-old boys and girls reporting previous or current elbow pain in survey data from the United States Tennis Association.[90] Medial epicondylitis, lateral epicondylitis, or apophysitis of either epicondyles can be seen in skeletally immature and developing tennis athletes. Racquet sports place significant demand on the developing elbow as a result of repetitive eccentric contraction of the wrist extensors.[91] This demand can also be seen in throwers during the follow-through phase of throwing.[92] Repetitive microtrauma in patients with open physes can lead to apophysitis during childhood and the early adolescent period, with transition to epicondylitis in the late adolescent and young adult patient populations. Lateral epicondylitis has been associated with equipment issues used in racquet sports, including grip size, metal racquets, tightly strung racquets, and racquets with increased vibration.[93,94] Poor mechanics related to the backhand technique have also been associated with lateral epicondylitis. Proper[95] equipment sizing and instruction on proper mechanics of play are paramount in preventing this injury from developing and becoming a persistent problem for the young athlete. Anatomic studies examining the extensor carpi radialis brevis, which is implicated in lateral epicondylitis, have shown a unique anatomic location that makes its undersurface vulnerable to abrasion against the lateral edge of the capitellum during elbow motion.[96] Medial epicondylitis, although not as common as lateral epicondylitis, can be seen more commonly in baseball pitchers, golfers, and athletes who create significant valgus force at the elbow.[97] Valgus force created at the elbow can place increased strain on secondary stabilizers such as the flexor and pronator muscles, which arise from the medial epicondyle.[98] Poor technique with improper warm-up and fatigue can lead to injury and inflammation of the flexor/pronator mass. Implicated muscles of this muscle group are the flexor carpi radialis and pronator teres. In a prior study, the authors found macroscopic tearing of the flexor/pronator group in all of the patients who underwent surgical treatment for medial epicondylitis.[99] Just as with lateral epicondylitis, medial epicondylitis can be treated and hopefully prevented with proper mechanics, warm-up, and stretching so that symptoms do not persist into adulthood.

History

Patients with lateral epicondylitis typically report a burning-like pain on the lateral side of the elbow. Initially the pain is primarily activity related, and activities involving wrist extension may precipitate the pain. This injury is common in

patients who play racquet sports, and this history should be elicited. Medial epicondylitis is similar in presentation to lateral epicondylitis, with symptoms arising from the medial elbow. Patients should be asked about exacerbating sports and activities for both conditions and if any associated neurologic symptoms are present, such as numbness and tingling, to rule out compression neuropathies.

Physical Examination

In persons with lateral epicondylitis, physical examination usually demonstrates pain and tenderness to palpation over the common extensor origin of the lateral epicondyle. Patients have pain with resisted wrist extension referred to the lateral side of the elbow. Range of motion is usually not affected. Persons with medial epicondylitis present with pain and tenderness to palpation over the medial elbow and may demonstrate increased pain with resisted wrist flexion. Pain may be associated with valgus stress testing of the elbow, which could indicate underlying valgus laxity as the cause of the pain.

Imaging

Routine radiographs are usually normal; however, in some cases, calcification may be present at the tendon origin. In younger patients, widening and fragmentation of the apophysis may be seen. MRI evaluation may prove useful in instances in which there is a question of diagnosis. MRI may demonstrate increased signal on T2-weighted imaging or partial tearing of the tendon attachment of the lateral epicondyle. The reliability of MRI in detecting pathologic conditions was demonstrated to be excellent in a recent study, with good interobserver agreement; however, no correlation of MRI findings with symptoms was found in the patients studied.[100]

Decision-Making Principles

Most young patients with medial and lateral epicondylitis are managed nonoperatively. Surgery is rarely indicated in this patient population. Most patients respond to conservative treatment measures and modification of activity with a short period of cessation of sports participation.

Treatment

Conservative treatment is mostly supportive for epicondylitis and apophysitis in the pediatric and adolescent patient populations. Cessation of sports participation and inciting activity is begun with or without a course of antiinflammatory medication and physical therapy. Therapy is aimed at restoring range of motion, stretching the offending muscle group, and strengthening the muscles surrounding the elbow. Counterforce straps and wrist braces may offer additional relief from symptoms in patients who are not responding to other conservative measures. Additional therapies such as shock wave treatment, ultrasound, and light wave therapy are investigational and have shown variable results in the literature.[101,102] Corticosteroid injections may be offered to young adults, although their utility in treating this condition has been questioned. A recent level I study in adults comparing autologous blood, corticosteroid therapy, and placebo saline solution injection for the treatment of lateral epicondylitis demonstrated no advantage of one treatment over the other.[103] The role of platelet-rich plasma is currently being intensely investigated, with some studies demonstrating improvement in patients with lateral epicondylitis.[104] Surgery is rarely indicated in this patient population but can consist of debridement of the extensor or flexor tendon in refractory cases. Surgery can be performed with a percutaneous, arthroscopic, or open technique.

Results

Results of conservative treatment are generally favorable with both lateral and medial epicondylitis. In a systematic review evaluating the different types of therapy for lateral epicondylitis, the authors found that all types of therapy substantially improved the outcomes of patients, with eccentric strengthening being the most exhaustively studied.[101] Eccentric strengthening exercises have demonstrated benefit in the literature; however, whether this treatment is better than stretching alone or stretching with concentric strengthening is not clear.[102,105] Nonsteroidal antiinflammatory medications (both topical and oral) are routinely prescribed for persons with epicondylitis; however, studies have shown both positive benefit and no benefit when compared with placebo.[106,107] Current use of this modality is based on physician preference and the ability of the patient to tolerate treatment. Corticosteroid injections are still routinely used in practice for alleviating the pain of lateral epicondylitis. Although studies have shown acute benefit, most investigations that report long-term outcomes demonstrate no advantage to the use of corticosteroid for this condition.[108-111] Surgical treatment, although rarely offered to young patients, has shown good results in the literature, regardless of the technique used, with one study showing improvement in outcomes in more than 90% of patients.[99,112-116] The treatment of medial epicondylitis mirrors the outcomes of lateral epicondylitis, with most patients responding favorably to nonsurgical management and good to excellent results in most patients who are ultimately candidates for surgical intervention.[117]

Complications

Complications from conservative treatment are rare. Antiinflammatory medications may cause impaired renal function and gastrointestinal adverse effects, although in younger patients these effects are usually self-limiting. Corticosteroids may cause pigmentation changes of the skin and fat atrophy with a low risk of tendon rupture.[118] Surgical treatment complications include infection, iatrogenic elbow instability from excessive release, nerve injury, and heterotopic ossification.[99,118-120]

Summary

The treatment of elbow maladies in children and adolescents requires a thorough understanding of developing skeletal anatomy, biomechanics of sport, and a multitude of pathologic conditions that are characteristic in this patient population. With thorough history-gathering techniques, a comprehensive physical examination, and judicious use of musculoskeletal imaging, the diagnosis is usually readily delineated. Treatment is largely nonoperative in this patient population; however, understanding the need for surgery in select cases can help optimize the outcome.

For a complete list of references, go to expertconsult.com.

Suggested Readings

Citation: An KN, Morrey BF: Biomechanics of the elbow. In Morrey, editor: *The Elbow and Its Disorders*, Philadelphia, 1985, WB Saunders.
Level of Evidence: Book chapter
Summary: This chapter focuses on the biomechanics of the elbow as it relates to anatomy, range of motion, and stability.

Citation: Jobe FW, Stark H, Lombardo SL: Reconstruction of the ulnar collateral ligament in athletes. *J Bone Joint Surg Am* 68A:1158–1163, 1986.
Level of Evidence: IV
Summary: The authors of this case series outline the results of ulnar collateral ligament reconstruction in 16 athletes (most of whom were in sports entailing throwing). After surgery, 10 of the 16 athletes returned to their previous level of competition.

Citation: Yadao MA, Field LD, Savoie FH 3rd: Osteochondritis dissecans of the elbow. *Instr Course Lec* 53:599–606, 2004.
Level of Evidence: Book chapter/instructional course lecture
Summary: The authors of this comprehensive review outline the pathophysiology, diagnosis, and treatment of osteochondritis dissecans of the elbow joint. The article is a very good review of current concepts regarding this topic.

Citation: Chen FS, Diaz V, Loebenberg M, et al: Shoulder and elbow injuries in the skeletally immature athlete. *J Am Acad Orthop Surg* 13:172–185, 2005.
Level of Evidence: Review article
Summary: The authors of this review article provide an overview of common shoulder and elbow maladies in pediatric and adolescent patients. Little Leaguer's elbow, osteochondritis dissecans, epicondylitis, and other pathologic conditions are comprehensively reviewed.

Citation: Nirschl RP, Pettrone FA: Tennis elbow: The surgical treatment of lateral epicondylitis. *J Bone Joint Surg Am* 61A:832–839, 1979.
Level of Evidence: IV
Summary: Tennis elbow surgery was performed for eight elbows in one of the first reports of this technique. An overall improvement rate of 97.7% was reported, with 85% of patients returning to rigorous activity.

the soft tissues can also provide valuable information, especially when considering tendonitis in the differential diagnosis. In younger patients, the clinician may encounter resistance to frank palpation of the area of interest because of the patient's discomfort. If this portion of the examination is attempted early in the encounter, the patient may be less willing to participate in further examination techniques. Therefore consideration should be given to delaying direct palpation of the injured site until the end of the encounter.

Forearm supination and pronation, measured from the neutral position, as well as wrist flexion and extension should be documented and compared with the contralateral limb. When one is interested in the digits or possible pathologic findings distal to the wrist, the resting posture of the hand should be noted, as well as flexion measurement and the presence of any extension lag or hyperextension at the metacarpophalangeal (MCP), proximal interphalangeal (PIP), and distal interphalangeal joints. Malrotation of a digit is often easiest to determine while observing active grip or passive tenodesis, observing for the presence or absence of digit scissoring (Fig. 133-1).

A basic strength examination should include resisted wrist extension and flexion, grip, and interosseous strength. In pediatric and adolescent patients, strength should always be compared with the contralateral limb because normal strength is often difficult to estimate in younger patients. As in adults, strength can be graded on a 0 to 5 scale, with a 5/5 grade corresponding to the patient's full strength of the contralateral, unaffected limb. Objective strength measurements using a dynometer or other device are usually not performed in young patients.

In general, sensation can be tested with use of the light-touch technique unless a nerve injury is suspected. In these cases, two-point discrimination or monofilament testing should be documented compared with the contralateral, unaffected limb. When a digital nerve injury is suspected, the area of sensation loss should be documented as radial or ulnar and compared with the unaffected side.

The radial and ulnar arteries should be palpated at their respective anatomic locations at the volar wrist. Capillary refill should be used to assess the perfusion of the digits distally. In general, refill after pressure is applied should occur in less than 1 second in a well-perfused hand.

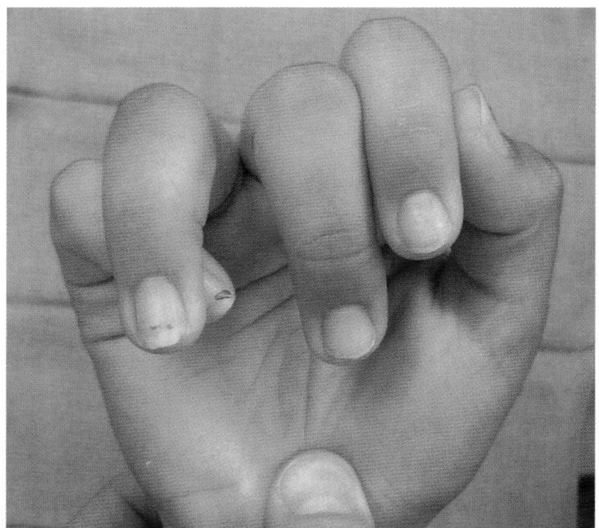

FIGURE 133-1 Digit scissoring that suggests a rotational deformity.

Provocative tests that can aid in diagnosis of certain pathologic conditions are covered in the following sections.

Imaging

Most radiographic evaluations begin with radiographs of the affected wrist or hand. The key to using radiographic evaluation effectively is to understand and order the appropriate views. Orthogonal views are necessary, but not always sufficient, in the pediatric wrist and hand. Specific views often may be necessary to perform a complete radiographic examination; these specific views are discussed in the following sections. In pediatric and adolescent patients, consideration should also be given to minimizing overall radiation exposure. Finally, when interpreting radiographs, if the clinician is unfamiliar with the pattern of ossification or normal development variants in the wrist and hand, a pediatric skeletal atlas, such as the classic text by Greulich and Pyle, should be consulted.

Computerized tomography (CT) scanning can be useful in definitively diagnosing occult fractures that are not seen on radiographs. In addition, we use CT with every pediatric and adolescent scaphoid fracture and fracture nonunion. Detailed imaging of these injuries can provide the clinician with an accurate diagnosis and assist with surgical planning as described in the following section. However, to minimize radiation exposure in growing children, it should be used judiciously. Its use in specific clinical scenarios is described in the following section.

Magnetic resonance imaging (MRI) is a powerful imaging tool and has been shown to be useful when evaluating a variety of injuries in pediatric and adolescent patients, including distal radial physeal injury, triangular fibrocartilage complex tears, and scaphoid fractures (described later). However, MRI is an expensive and time-intensive modality that may require sedation, especially in younger patients. Given these issues, it should be used judiciously in the pediatric and adolescent population.

A magnetic resonance (MR) arthrogram can be useful in the wrist for examining the condition of the triangular fibrocartilage complex (TFCC), as well as the integrity of the intercarpal ligaments. This modality is more widely used in adults but may not be as convenient or well tolerated in pediatric patients given its inherent invasiveness. In adolescent patients in whom history and physical examination suggest TFCC or intrinsic ligament injury and who can tolerate an injection and cooperate with the procedure, an MR arthrogram may be considered.

Ultrasound has been reported to be useful in pediatric and adolescent patients to help confirm diagnosis of extensor and flexor tenosynovitis[5] and to aid in the diagnosis of a thumb UCL injury.[6] In addition, ultrasound can also help differentiate soft tissue swelling from fluid-filled structures (i.e., ganglion cysts), which may narrow the differential diagnosis. Ultrasound is easy to perform in the office setting, provided that equipment is readily available and the clinician or clinician's staff is adept at performing the study and interpreting results. This modality also allows for dynamic imaging.

Decision-Making Principles

After thorough evaluation with a complete history, detailed physical examination, and appropriate imaging techniques, a diagnosis is made. The clinician now must weigh treatment options with the patient and parents and come to a decision regarding treatment. Additional considerations must be made in the pediatric and adolescent athlete before arriving at a treatment plan, including but not limited to the following considerations:

1. Will the patient be able to tolerate or cooperate with treatment?
2. Are the clinician's goals for treatment the same as those of the patient and/or family?
3. How will the injury and recommended treatment affect sports participation both now and in the future as the patient grows and matures?

In the following sections, selected injuries and conditions are reviewed in further detail, from evaluation to treatment and return to play. The sections emphasize diagnostic pearls, specific treatment options, and evidence-based results when available to provide the clinician with a practical guide to caring for pediatric and adolescent wrist and hand injuries.

Triangular Fibrocartilage Complex Injury

The TFCC is a confluence of soft tissue structures at the ulnar side of the wrist that provides stability, absorbs axial load, and ensures smooth articulation between the radius and the ulna.[7] In pediatric patients, the components of the TFCC, including the triangular fibrocartilage, meniscal homologue, radioulnar ligaments, ulnocarpal ligaments, and the subsheath of the extensor carpi ulnaris, are prone to injury as they are in adults. An increase in diagnosis of these injuries in pediatric and adolescent patients has followed the increase in other sports-related injuries in this population discussed previously.

History

Injuries to the TFCC in pediatric and adolescent patients can present either acutely after a recent traumatic event or chronically with a history of remote injury. In chronic cases, a history of injury is not necessarily recalled. If it is recalled, the mechanism is usually a fall on an outstretched, pronated extremity.[8,9] Injuries to the TFCC can occur in conjunction with fractures of the distal radius or ulnar styloid.[8] The patient's history of symptoms should include ulnar-sided wrist pain. In athletes, this symptom often is related to specific sports-related activity, such as gripping. In pediatric and adolescent patients particularly, it is important to note that the pain may not be debilitating enough to prevent sports participation.[8]

Physical Examination

Physical examination may reveal ulnar-sided tenderness, although tenderness at any one point does not specifically correlate with a TFCC injury. A provocative test called the TFCC compression test has been described but not evaluated in pediatric or adolescent patients. This test consists of axial loading, ulnar deviation, and rotation of the wrist. A similar test called the "press test," in which the patient is asked to use his or her affected wrist to push up from a chair from a seated position, was shown to have a 100% sensitivity for TFCC injury in adults.[10] It has not been evaluated in younger patients. When evaluating ulnar-sided wrist pain, it is also important to evaluate the stability of the distal radioulnar joint; passive laxity in volar and dorsal translation should be compared with the contralateral wrist.

Imaging

Radiographs centered at the wrist are obtained for patients with suspected TFCC pathology. Acute findings may include an ulnar styloid fracture. Ulnar styloid nonunions may be seen in patients who have a remote history of a traumatic event and chronic symptoms. Positive ulnar variance can be associated with TFCC pathology and should be measured with a posteroanterior view in neutral rotation (i.e., no supination and no pronation). A pronated view effectively increases and a supinated view decreases measured ulnar variance. In addition, radiographs allow evaluation of any coexisting bony pathology unique to pediatric and adolescent patients, such as physeal changes or a Madelung deformity (a volar and radial deformity of the distal radius caused by physeal growth disturbance) that may or may not require additional treatment.

Although newer high-resolution 3.0-Tesla MRI machines have shown greater sensitivity and specificity in diagnosing TFCC injury in adult patients,[11] false-positive and false-negative findings still occur. Positive results in particular must be evaluated in conjunction with the patient's history and findings of the clinical examination to prevent overtreatment, especially in younger patients. Although not specifically studied in pediatric or adolescent patients, MRI findings of a TFCC injury or a complete tear in asymptomatic adult patients is common in asymptomatic wrists, with one recent study showing a prevalence of greater than 50%.[12]

MR arthrography has been considered the gold-standard imaging modality for TFCC injury. This technique provides a high-intensity fluid signal at the location of perforations in the TFCC tissue. MR arthrography for this application has not been specifically evaluated in pediatric and adolescent patients. In our practice, MR arthrography is not used in young pediatric patients. We do recommend use of this modality in adolescent patients who are willing to cooperate with the examination because it adds diagnostic value. However, it is important to recognize that MR arthrography may occasionally provide false-negative results when compared with arthroscopic examination.[13]

Decision-Making Principles

In approaching a pediatric or adolescent patient with a suspected TFCC injury, the clinician must take into account the time course of the injury (i.e., acute vs. chronic), as well as the injury pattern. Chronic injuries have proven their instability and by definition lack a propensity to heal without intervention. On the other hand, acute injuries in the pediatric or adolescent patient may heal or may not become symptomatic.

TABLE 133-1

CLASSIFICATION OF TRAUMATIC INJURIES TO THE TRIANGULAR FIBROCARTILAGE COMPLEX IN PEDIATRIC AND ADOLESCENT PATIENTS AND SURGICAL TREATMENT RECOMMENDATIONS

Palmer Class	Location	Treatment Recommendation
1A	Central	Debridement
1B	Ulnar attachment	Repair
1C	Distal attachment	Repair
1D	Radial attachment	Repair

The pattern of the injury should be considered. Generally, injury to the TFCC is classified into Palmer class 1 (traumatic) and Palmer class 2 (degenerative).[14] Palmer class 1 lesions are further categorized depending on the location of the tear (Table 133-1), whereas Palmer class 2 lesions are categorized depending on the extent of degenerative changes. Because of inherent patient characteristics and the mechanism of injury, most TFCC injuries in pediatric and adolescent patients are Palmer class 1 (traumatic).[15] Few reports have focused on TFCC injuries in pediatric and adolescent patients, but several investigators have suggested that many injuries in these patients are most commonly avulsions of the TFCC from the insertion on the distal ulna (Palmer class 1B).[8,15,16] Other peripheral tears, which are more amenable to surgical repair, may be more common than central perforations in pediatric and adolescent patients (Fig. 133-2).

Treatment Options

After a traumatic event in which a TFCC injury without distal radioulnar injury is either diagnosed or suspected, our first-line treatment is full-time immobilization in either a wrist brace or short-arm cast. A cast avoids the parental challenge of ensuring compliance with a removable brace and therefore should be strongly considered. As described in the preceding section, many TFCC injuries occur in conjunction with a distal radius or ulnar styloid fracture. Although no data have been published regarding acute treatment of TFCC injuries in pediatric or adolescent patients with wrist fractures, our practice is to treat the fracture first, allow appropriate healing and rehabilitation, and address the TFCC injury if and when it becomes symptomatic.

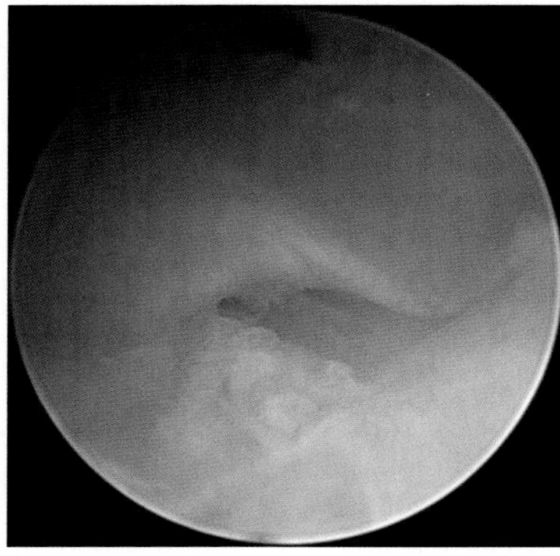

FIGURE 133-2 A tear of the triangular fibrocartilage complex at its peripheral radial-sided attachment in an adolescent athlete.

The mainstay of surgical treatment of Palmer class 2 (degenerative) TFCC injuries is arthroscopic debridement with or without ulnar shortening. Because pediatric patients generally present with Palmer class 1 (traumatic) injuries, arthroscopic debridement has less of a role in this population. We recommend arthroscopic debridement for younger patients with central tears that are not amenable to repair.

Repair of TFCC injuries in pediatric and adolescent patients should be restricted to patients for whom nonoperative management has failed and who have an injury pattern that is amenable to surgical repair.[15] Various techniques have been described for open and arthroscopic repair in adults,[16-19] and any of these techniques can be used in pediatric or adolescent patients. No single technique has been shown to be superior in pediatric or adolescent patients. Bae and Waters[15] have recommended an outside-in arthroscopically assisted repair technique for pediatric and adolescent patients with Palmer class 1B tears.[15]

AUTHORS' PREFERRED TECHNIQUE

Repair of TFCC Injuries

Arthroscopic repair in pediatric and adolescent patients begins with diagnostic arthroscopy. The typical 3-4 portal is used for introduction of the arthroscope, and a 4-5 or 6U portal is the working portal. We often use a separate 18- or 19-gauge needle as an outflow device in the 6U or 6R position. Through the working portal, debridement is performed arthroscopically to prepare the injured portion of the TFCC for repair. During this process it is important to leave enough tissue to repair as well as debride to bleeding tissue if possible to facilitate healing. An outside-in technique is then used to complete the repair. An incision is made longitudinally in line with the 6U portal, and blunt dissection is taken down to the wrist capsule. Care should be taken during this dissection to protect the dorsal sensory branch of the ulnar nerve. An 18- or 19-gauge needle preloaded with a 2-0 or 3-0 Vicryl or polydioxanone suture is then passed through the capsule, across the ulnar aspect of the TFCC tear, and into the fibrocartilage. A fine hemostat is used to puncture the capsule distal to the needle and grasp the suture intraarticularly. The suture is then brought out of the wrist joint and tied over the exposed capsule. Additional sutures should be added to the repair until the TFCC regains appropriate tension, which can be judged with use of an arthroscopic probe.

Patients with TFCC injuries can often have coexisting pathologic findings that should be addressed at the time of surgery, including positive ulnar variance and osteochondral injuries.

Postoperative Management

After arthroscopic debridement, the wrist is placed into a sugar-tong plaster splint for 2 weeks and then converted to a short-arm cast or removable wrist brace for 2 to 4 weeks depending on the severity of the injury. If repair is performed, a sugar-tong plaster splint is placed in neutral rotation for 2 weeks, followed by use of a long-arm plaster or fiberglass cast for 4 weeks. A removable wrist brace is used for the final 2 weeks of immobilization. Forearm rotation through the distal radioulnar joint can jeopardize the repair and should be avoided with use of long-arm immobilization for at least 6 weeks.

Rehabilitation in patients undergoing debridement should commence as soon as immobilization is discontinued. Wrist and hand therapy that focuses on strengthening with a gradual increase in resistance should continue for approximately 6 weeks. A recommendation regarding return to sports should be based on the patient's symptoms, activity level, and progress achieved with rehabilitation. Wrist and hand therapy for strengthening should commence after 6 weeks of immobilization and should continue for at least 6 weeks. Upon successful completion and abatement of symptoms, the patient may return to sports, usually at 3 months after the surgical procedure is performed.

Results

No level I data have been published on treatment results of TFCC injury in pediatric or adolescent patients. A single case series has been published on this topic. Terry and Waters[8] reviewed 29 pediatric patients (with a mean age of 13.4 years) who had surgically documented TFCC tears. Half of these patients had an associated distal radius fracture at the time of injury. All patients in this study presented with ulnar-sided wrist pain, and 12 presented with distal radioulnar joint (DRUJ) instability. Surgical treatment consisted of arthroscopic debridement, open repair, or arthroscopic repair depending on the pattern of TFCC injury and concurrent treatment of related pathologic conditions, including excision of the ulnar styloid or DRUJ stabilization. The procedures led to 89% excellent results at an average of 21 months based on a modified Mayo wrist score.

Complications

A complication that should be avoided during treatment is iatrogenic injury to the dorsal sensory branch of the ulnar nerve. This terminal sensory branch of the ulnar nerve runs subcutaneously along the ulnar border of the wrist and can be injured during placement of the 6U or 6R portals if dissection to the wrist capsule is not performed carefully. Additionally, if not treated appropriately, injuries to the TFCC can result in dysfunction of the DRUJ, leading to joint instability and eventual degeneration.

Future Considerations

An increased awareness of TFCC injuries in young patients raises many further questions. Research in this area should be directed not only toward decision making regarding operative treatment types, such as repair versus debridement, but also to defining which patients are most likely to benefit from operative intervention, which has yet to be determined in the pediatric and adolescent patient population. In addition, with the increased use of high-resolution MRI in this patient population, subtle TFCC irregularities will undoubtedly be diagnosed in many patients. It is still unclear which of these irregularities actually constitute clinically significant injury or change in the structure of the TFCC that warrants intervention.

Intercarpal Instability

Intercarpal instability can be divided into three major types: scapholunate, lunotriquetrial, and midcarpal instability. These conditions often differ in injury mechanism, presentation, and clinical significance. However, all three share a common pathologic pattern; an injury causes alteration in the normal functioning of the biomechanical link between the wrist and the hand. Intercarpal instability is rare in pediatric and adolescent patients. The literature consists mostly of case reports and one retrospective study of scapholunate ligament injury.[20-24] Lunotriquetral and midcarpal instability are essentially unreported in pediatric and adolescent patients. Often, when intercarpal instability is diagnosed, other pathology, such as TFCC or chondral injury, is present.[24]

History

Pediatric and adolescent patients with wrist instability caused by a scapholunate injury often present with nonspecific chronic wrist pain. They may have a history of traumatic injury with or without fracture of the distal radius or ulna. A history of previous unsuccessful treatments, especially in patients with chronic wrist pain, is possible.

Physical Examination

The physical examination should focus on the location of tenderness; the scapholunate interval can be found distal to Lister's tubercle on the dorsum of the wrist. Anatomic snuffbox tenderness may also be present. The sensitivity and specificity of these examinations in pediatric and adolescent patients has not been studied. The scaphoid shift test[25] can identify injury to the scapholunate ligament. In this test, the examiner places his or her thumb on the palmar tuberosity of the scaphoid. He or she then asks the patient to move the wrist from ulnar to radial deviation. In a normal wrist without scapholunate ligament injury, the pressure on the palmar tuberosity of the scaphoid prevents normal flexion of the scaphoid, which occurs when the wrist is moved from ulnar to radial deviation. With a torn scapholunate ligament, the scaphoid is forced to subluxate dorsally; when pressure is removed, the scaphoid "shifts" back into place, resulting in a clunk or snapping sensation characteristic of a positive result. This positive result can also occur in overall "lax" wrists, and thus a general assessment of ligamentous laxity should be performed, as well as comparison with the contralateral wrist. The scaphoid shift test has not been evaluated specifically in the pediatric and adolescent patient population, and it is important to remember that provocative tests for scapholunate ligament instability may be negative despite injury in this population, especially if the patient has a partial injury.[24]

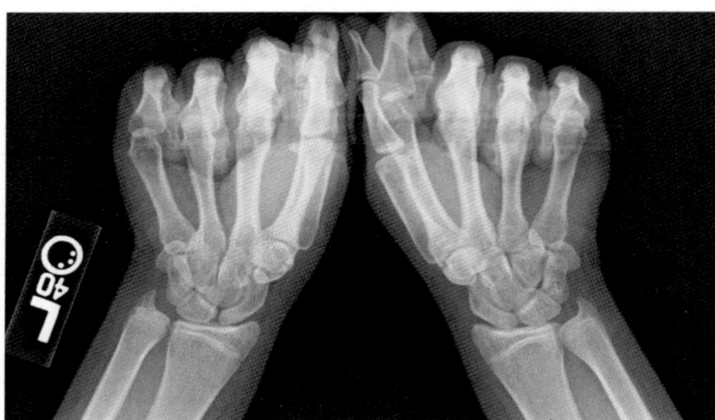

FIGURE 133-3 A bilateral grip stress view showing a widening of the scapholunate interval on the left wrist.

Imaging

Standard anteroposterior (AP), lateral, and oblique plain radiographs of the wrist should be obtained. A scapholunate interval asymmetry greater than 2 mm between the affected and unaffected wrists is abnormal in adults and may suggest an injury to the scapholunate ligament; greater than 5 mm of contralateral asymmetry in adults is diagnostic of a tear and is referred to as the "Terry Thomas" sign.[26] However, because of the ossification process of the carpal bones, the interval in pediatric and adolescent patients may be increased.[27] In addition, ossification of the carpal bones may be asymmetric from side to side, and therefore contralateral comparison can be unreliable.[28] Dynamic stress radiographs may be obtained to aid in the diagnosis. In pediatric and adolescent patients, obtaining these radiographs may be of significant benefit given the unreliability of static films as previously described. A useful technique for dynamic stress radiographs is to have the patient grip a round, cylindrical object and obtain an AP film of both wrists on the same plate. This technique allows for easy side-to-side comparison as well (Fig. 133-3).

MRI has shown usefulness in the diagnosis of scapholunate ligament and other intercarpal ligament injury in adults. The sensitivity and specificity of MRI for scapholunate ligament injury in pediatric and adolescent patients has not been reported. However, in a study of the arthroscopic treatment of partial scapholunate tears in pediatric and adolescent patients, only 11 of the 32 patients who were confirmed to have an injury with arthroscopy had MRI findings suggestive of injury.[24] We have used MR arthrograms to assist in making a diagnosis for adult patients, but this modality may be less useful in pediatric and adolescent patients because of its invasiveness. Arthroscopy remains the gold-standard imaging technique for detection of scapholunate ligament injuries in pediatric and adolescent patients, as well as in adults.[26]

Decision-Making Principles

Few data have been published to guide treatment decisions for intercarpal instability in pediatric and adolescent patients. In general, the injury can be classified as acute or chronic and partial or complete. After classification of the injury and consideration of the patient's symptoms and resulting disability, the clinician can begin to outline a treatment plan. All acute injuries should be considered for nonoperative management, whereas chronic injuries may be more amenable to surgical intervention. Partial injuries may only require immobilization, or in chronic cases, debridement. Complete injuries usually necessitate a surgical repair or reconstruction. Giessler et al.[29] have published a classification system for scapholunate tears that is based on their arthroscopic appearance, and it can also be helpful in guiding treatment.

Treatment Options

Pediatric and adolescent patients who present with acute or chronic wrist pain from suspected intercarpal instability or scapholunate injury should be treated initially with a course of nonoperative management. Immobilization with either a cast or a full-time brace for 4 to 6 weeks is appropriate. Hand therapy should be initiated upon discontinuation of immobilization with a focus on the intrinsic hand musculature, as well as the wrist flexors and extenders. After failure of this nonoperative management, surgical treatments may be considered. These injuries are rare in pediatric and adolescent patients, and generally management in this population is similar to that in adult patients.

Partial scapholunate ligament tears are amenable to arthroscopic debridement. Diagnostic wrist arthroscopy should be performed, including examination of the scapholunate ligament from both the radiocarpal and midcarpal joints (Fig. 133-4). The extent of the tear can be determined by probing the ligament with a right-angle arthroscopic probe. If the extent of the tear is significant, pinning the interval with Kirschner wires (K wires) is advisable. Surgical treatment of complete tears should also begin with diagnostic arthroscopy. In more acute presentations of complete tears, the scapholunate ligament can be reapproximated with suture anchors after an open dorsal capsulotomy. To protect this repair, the scapholunate and scaphocapitate intervals should be immobilized with K wires. In chronic, complete scapholunate tears, a reconstructive procedure should be considered. Perilunate dislocations represent the most severe type of scapholunate injury and can be reduced from an open dorsal approach. In these cases, acute repair of the scapholunate and lunotriquetral ligaments is performed, followed by pinning of scapholunate, lunotriquetral, and midcarpal intervals.

AUTHORS' PREFERRED TECHNIQUE

Intercarpal Instability

In pediatric and adolescent patients, we recommend nonoperative management if at all possible as previously described. In acute settings in which complete injury is apparent with evidence of static instability on radiographs, with perilunate dislocations, or in cases of chronic instability that have not responded to prior treatments, operative treatment should be performed as in adults.

Postoperative Management

Patients should be immobilized for at least 6 weeks to allow for adequate ligament healing. A brace can be used for 2 to 4 weeks after immobilization with a cast. No agreed-on postoperative management protocol exists, but we lean toward a

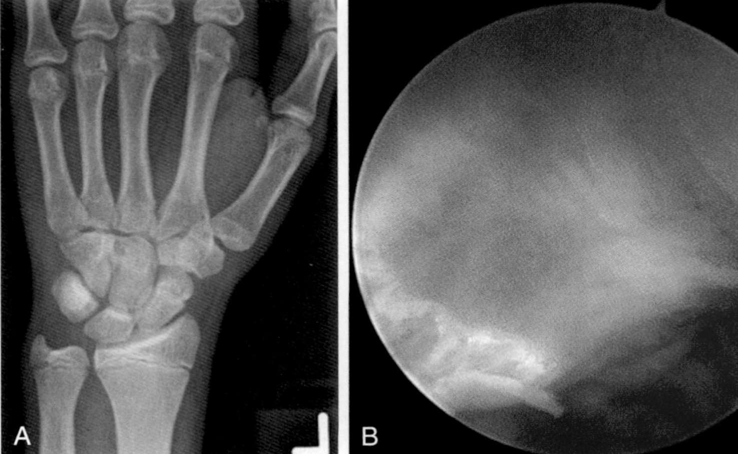

FIGURE 133-4 A partial scapholunate injury in an adolescent basketball player with a scaphoid fracture. **A,** A radiograph demonstrating a scaphoid fracture without significant scapholunate interval widening. **B,** An arthroscopic view from the radiocarpal joint of an inflamed scapholunate ligament without complete injury.

conservative progression toward activity because of the inherent difficulties with intraarticular ligament healing. Hand therapy and rehabilitation should begin after demonstration of clinical healing (i.e., the patient is pain free with no tenderness on examination), stability, and preserved reduction of the scapholunate interval on postoperative radiographs.

Return to Play

To safely return to play, the athlete must demonstrate pain-free motion and gripping activities, which usually does not occur until an adequate course of immobilization and hand therapy has been completed. We expect that the patient will not be able to return to sports for at least 3 months.

Results

A single retrospective study has reviewed the results of the arthroscopic treatment of partial scapholunate injuries in pediatric and adolescent patients.[24] All 32 patients in this study were treated with arthroscopic debridement and all concomitant injuries, including TFCC tears and chondral injuries, were addressed at the time of surgery. At the time of the last postoperative follow-up session (a mean of 43 months), the modified Mayo wrist score of the 28 patients examined had increased from 66.3 to 91.6. Eight patients required further surgery after their index procedure because of continued pain or a return of symptoms. Alt et al.[30] reported the results of three pediatric and adolescent patients with complete scapholunate tears. All three patients were treated with arthroscopy and open ligament repair. They were reported to be pain free and without noticeable scapholunate widening on AP radiographs at an average follow-up of 2.3 years.

Complications

After operative treatment, clinicians should be wary of pin-site infections and loss of scapholunate reduction or persistent scapholunate interval widening. In addition, delayed ossification of the proximal pole of the scaphoid can occur in younger patients.

Future Considerations

Given the limited number of cases of pediatric and adolescent intercarpal instability found in the literature, further reporting of these clinical entities would facilitate a better understanding of their effect on pediatric and adolescent patients. In adults, intercarpal instability can lead to debilitating degenerative conditions, such as scapholunate advanced collapse after chronic scapholunate ligament injuries. It is important for the sports clinician to have an understanding of these conditions to avoid such potential devastating outcomes in young athletes.

Distal Radial Physeal Stress Injury

Like all other growth centers of the immature skeleton, forces influence the biology of the physis of the distal radius. Repetitive compressive stress at the physis in particular can lead to injury, and therefore any pediatric or adolescent athlete who repetitively loads his or her wrist is prone to distal radial physeal stress injury. In particular, gymnasts are prone to these stress-related effects because of their reliance on the wrist as a weight-bearing joint during activity.[31-37] In male and female gymnasts as a group, the incidence of injury to the distal radial physis has been estimated at 1.9 and 2.7 per 100 seasons in two separate studies.[38,39]

In addition to causing pain and dysfunction during activity, stress injury to the physis of the distal radius may lead to growth disturbance.[33,34] This phenomenon can be explained through the application of the Hueter-Volkmann law, which asserts that increased compression at the physis leads to a reduced growth rate. Mechanistically, the injury may be secondary to blood supply compromise and the disruption of mineralization.[40] The threshold both for stress-related injury or growth disturbance has not been defined. In addition, previous basic science research has demonstrated the effects of the Hueter-Volkmann law on physes under static compressive loading.[41-44] In physes exposed to different levels of physiologic dynamic loading (simulating different levels of normal activity), Niehoff et al.[45] showed little difference in physeal growth.

History

The age of the patient is important. The physis is at greatest risk of injury during the periods of highest growth rate,[46-48] and therefore clinicians should be most suspicious for physeal injury in patients presenting during the adolescent growth spurt, usually between the ages of 10 and 14 years. Both female and male athletes are at risk. The patient usually reports pain on the dorsal aspect of the wrist that is exacerbated with activities requiring weight bearing through the wrist.[31,32,35] Patients with a high activity level may have an increased likelihood of developing symptoms, but athletes at any skill or activity level can experience a stress injury. A recent study of precompetitive and competitive young gymnasts with an average age of 9.3 years reported wrist pain in 56% of the patients, with 51% showing evidence of physeal stress injury on radiographs.[32] An increased number of training hours and length of training were correlated with pain symptoms; no significant difference in symptoms was found between males and females.

Physical Examination

Often, pain from a distal radial physeal stress injury cannot be reproduced on physical examination. The patient may have tenderness at the dorsal aspect of the wrist, but this finding is neither sensitive nor specific. No specific provocative tests exist for a distal radial physeal stress injury, but in select patients, axial loading through the wrist may provoke pain symptoms. Usually, the only reliable method to provoke symptoms is to reproduce the activity that elicits pain in the athlete. Loss of wrist extension is possible, especially in patients with long-standing symptoms.

Imaging

Plain radiographs may show physeal widening, sclerosis, beaking, haziness, or irregularity.[31,36,49] Alternatively, some patients with mild cases may show a normal physeal appearance, whereas in severe cases, premature physeal closure may be observed.[49] Premature physeal closure can lead to a shortened appearance of the radius or an abnormal radial inclination on radiographs. Positive ulnar variance appears as a radiographic finding in gymnasts in particular but has not been shown to be associated with wrist pain or radiographic findings of distal radial physeal injury in this population.[32,37] The clinician should also take into account that pediatric patients usually have negative ulnar variance until skeletal maturity.[50]

MRI has been shown to be useful in the diagnosis of physeal injury in the distal radius. Typical MR findings include edema on both the metaphyseal and epiphyseal ends of the physis, cartilage extension into the physis, and vertical fractures.[51-53] Late findings can include abnormal physeal closure in severe cases, although this finding is often observed on radiographs. If plain radiographs appear negative, MRI can detect these subtle changes if physeal injury is suspected.

Decision-Making Principles

The degree of physeal injury should help guide the clinician regarding treatment recommendations. As previously noted, a grading system for a stress injury to the distal radius physis has been proposed based on radiographic findings.[32] Although this radiographic grading system was correlated with patient symptoms, it was not used specifically to guide treatment. Any decision regarding treatment should take into account the severity of the patient's symptoms, as well as imaging findings. In addition, consideration should be given to the patient's current sports participation because treatment may influence his or her ability to continue to play.

Treatment Options

Prevention of this repetitive stress injury is the best cure, but no training regimen or protocol has been specifically shown to be preventative. Bracing has not been shown in the literature to prevent distal radial physeal injury. As a rule, the only method that allows physeal stress injury recovery once it has occurred is cessation of the offending activity. Immobilization may be required to decrease acute symptoms and prevent activity participation in certain patient populations, but prolonged immobilization is not advised. No studies have been performed to specifically define the length of avoidance of the offending activity. If cessation of activity does not lead to a recovery of the physis and premature closure ensues, surgical treatment of any resulting deformity may be indicated. As indicated by the small number of reported cases, these clinical scenarios are rare.

AUTHORS' PREFERRED TECHNIQUE

Distal Radial Physeal Stress Injury

We recommend cessation of activities that lead to compressive forces through the wrist until tenderness and pain at the distal radius have dissipated. To facilitate this restriction in a young active patient, we recommend application of a short-arm cast for 4 to 6 weeks. We have not found that radiographs are generally useful for judging healing.

Return to Play

After the resolution of symptoms, the patient can gradually resume training. We recommend at least 4 weeks without pain symptoms prior to returning to play. To begin, the athlete can start at 25% of the preinjury compressive loading activity level. After 1 to 2 weeks, this level may be gradually increased as tolerated by the patient. Full return to play should not be expected before 10 to 12 weeks after the diagnosis. Once a patient is fully recovered, the training regimen should be altered to include alternating compressive and tensile activity and cyclical increases in intensity.

Results

No studies have directly reported the outcomes of different treatment modalities for distal radius physeal injury. The existing literature consists of a number of retrospective case series of young gymnasts with this condition. A recent review of these case series reported that nearly all patients had symptomatic relief with cessation of the offending activity.[54] However, several cases of premature closure of the distal radial physis have been reported in this patient population.[37,55-57]

Complications

Failure to diagnose and treat distal radius physeal stress injury has the potential to lead to a progression of the underlying physeal biologic disturbance and a growth arrest. In younger athletes, this outcome can lead to abnormal development of radial height and inclination, as well as positive ulnar variance, which can alter the normal biomechanics of the wrist over time.

Future Considerations

As previously stated, the threshold for injury to the distal radius physis or any physis of the immature skeleton has not been precisely defined. Although it is generally agreed that repetitive compressive stress at the distal radial physis leads to injury, a better understanding of specific risk factors, including biomechanical analysis of stress patterns within the distal radial physis during different activities, might be helpful to prevent injury.

Scaphoid Fractures

The most commonly fractured carpal bone in pediatric athletes is the scaphoid,[58] and yet the incidence of this injury in pediatric and adolescent patients is low; it is estimated to be 0.6 per 10,000 in one study.[59] Previous literature has suggested that fractures of the distal pole are more common in the pediatric population.[60,61] However, a recent review of pediatric scaphoid fractures over a 15-year period showed that most fractures occurred at the scaphoid waist, likely in part because of the pediatric population's increased participation in adult-type athletic activities.[62]

History

Scaphoid fractures usually occur after a fall on an outstretched extremity, often with the wrist in radial deviation. Patients usually report immediate pain and swelling after the inciting event. Specifically, pain is located at the dorsum of the wrist, at the scaphoid tubercle, or at the anatomic snuffbox. However, pediatric and adolescent patients may continue activity, causing a delay in presentation. Pain is often reported with wrist motion or weight bearing through the wrist.

Physical Examination

The classic teaching is that pain from a scaphoid fracture is present at the anatomic snuffbox, the area of the dorsal radial aspect of the wrist between the extensor pollicis longus and the tendons of the first dorsal compartment, the extensor pollicis brevis and abductor pollicis longus. In adult patients, tenderness in this location has been shown to be highly sensitive (up to 100%) but not specific for a scaphoid fracture.[63,64] Tenderness at the scaphoid tubercle and pain with the scaphoid compression test have also been reported in the literature as positive in patients with scaphoid fractures.[63] In this report, Grover[63] showed that the scaphoid compression test had a sensitivity of 100% and a specificity of 80% in patients with a mean age of 36 years. No studies have specifically addressed the sensitivity and specificity of these examination tests in pediatric or adolescent patients.

Imaging

Patients with history and physical examination findings suggestive of scaphoid fracture should have AP, lateral, oblique, and scaphoid radiographic views of the wrist. The scaphoid view consists of a posterioanterior view of the wrist in ulnar deviation with the x-ray beam angled 20 to 30 degrees proximally. Nondisplaced and minimally displaced scaphoid fractures can be missed on initial radiographs in up to 37% in the pediatric and adolescent population.[59,65] When clinical suspicion for fracture is high, the wrist should be immobilized and radiographs repeated at 2 weeks to help prevent delayed treatment.[66]

MRI can be useful in the diagnosis of scaphoid fractures in pediatric and adolescent patients. The use of MRI in younger patients is attractive because of the lack of radiation exposure. In pediatric and adolescent patients, its use has been shown to help avoid unnecessary immobilization if performed within 10 days of the injury.[67] In addition, Cook et al.[68] reported a 100% negative predictive value if MRI is performed within 6 days of injury in patients aged 8 to 15 years. Ultrasound has also been proposed as an imaging technique to diagnose scaphoid fractures when initial radiographs are negative in adults.[69] This modality holds promise for use in pediatric and adolescent patients but has yet to be studied in younger patients.

In our experience, radiographs are usually adequate. If displacement is suspected, we obtain a CT scan for further evaluation and preoperative planning. If any suggestion of avascular necrosis is noted, an MRI is ordered. CT should be used to follow up on fracture healing. In our experience, radiographs are not adequate to determine the extent of bone bridging across a scaphoid fracture, which is the hallmark of healing. For patients interested in returning to weight-bearing or contact sports, a CT scan should be obtained to confirm scaphoid fracture healing. Typically, this scan should be performed at the 2- to 3-month time frame depending on the radiographic appearance and clinical examination.

Decision-Making Principles

Displacement of the fracture, chronicity of the fracture, location of the fracture, and age of the patient at presentation should help guide the clinician in selecting treatment. Nondisplaced and minimally displaced fractures should all be considered for cast immobilization. Displaced fractures, whether presenting acutely or delayed, may require internal fixation. Scaphoid waist and proximal pole fractures, which are the most prone to progress to nonunion because of the pattern of blood supply, may benefit from early internal fixation. Finally, patients who are closer to skeletal maturity may also benefit from internal fixation compared with younger patients.

As summarized by Trumble et al.,[70] early internal fixation should be considered in scaphoid fractures with displacement greater than 1.0 mm, the presence of comminution, location at the proximal pole, a delay in diagnosis or presentation, angulation in the sagittal plane greater than 45 degrees, or in patients with poor perceived compliance to avoid nonunion. Although meant for adult patients, these guidelines can be applied to adolescent patients who are nearing skeletal maturity and many younger patients as well.

Treatment Options

Nonoperative treatment consists of cast immobilization. No studies in pediatric and adolescent patients have defined the best method of immobilization for this population, but generally a thumb spica cast should be applied. The question of whether the cast should extend above the elbow has not been answered in pediatric and adolescent patients and is left to the clinical judgment of the treating physician.

Numerous operative techniques for internal fixation of the scaphoid have been described, including K wires, noncannulated headless compression screws,[71] and cannulated headless variable-pitch compression screws.[72] Specifically in pediatric and adolescent patients, a compression screw should be placed for fractures that require internal fixation.

Results

Traditionally, most pediatric and adolescent patients with scaphoid fractures have been treated with cast immobilization. Successful treatment with immobilization has been reported in several retrospective series.[59,75,76] More recently, Gholson et al.[62] published a retrospective review of 351 scaphoid fractures in pediatric and adolescent patients (ages 7 to 18 years) over a 15-year period. Their results showed a 90% healing rate in patients with acute, minimally displaced fractures treated with casting. In patients treated with screw fixation, the healing rate was 96.5%. No studies have prospectively studied the outcomes of cast immobilization versus internal fixation in pediatric and adolescent patients.

Return to Play

For scaphoid fractures treated either with casting or with operative fixation, patients should not return to sports until they are pain free and nontender on clinical examination at both the proximal snuffbox and the distal poles. In addition, a CT scan should be performed to confirm the presence of at least 50% bridging bone. For individual sports, Slade et al.[77] published guidelines for return to play and immobilization technique for individual sports after fixation of a scaphoid fracture with headless compression screws. For example, they recommended that gymnasts return to play without immobilization no sooner than 8 weeks from surgery, with CT scan evidence of 50% bridging bone.

Complications

Scaphoid fractures in the pediatric population can often be overlooked, leading to nonunion and complicating treatment. In pediatric and adolescent patients, up to one third of scaphoid fractures present as nonunions.[62] Because of the tenuous blood supply to the scaphoid, even fractures that were treated with immobilization or internal fixation initially may progress to nonunion. Gholson et al.[62] reported a 3.5% nonunion rate in patients treated with internal fixation. Treatment of scaphoid nonunion is challenging and requires internal fixation with nonvascularized or vascularized bone grafting.

Thumb Ulnar Collateral Ligament Injury

UCL injury in pediatric and adolescent patients is differentiated from the injury in adults by the presence of the physis of the proximal phalanx. The UCL normally inserts onto the ulnar base of the proximal phalanx, and in patients with open physes, injury to the UCL can be transferred to the weak physis and result in a Salter type I, II, or III injury. Alternatively, a "pseudo" UCL rupture can occur in which the physis fails but the UCL remains competent.[78]

History

A thumb UCL injury can be seen in skiers and is often referred to as "skier's thumb." The abducted thumb experiences a valgus stress as the skier's pole is planted during a fall. Alternatively, thumb UCL injuries can occur during contact sports, such as football. Injury to the thumb UCL ranges from a simple sprain of the ligament to an avulsion injury of the ligament off the epiphysis of the proximal phalanx, resulting in a Salter-Harris type III injury. If the diagnosis is missed after initial examination and treatment, chronic injury to the thumb UCL results in chronic ulnar-sided thumb pain and instability during pinching or gripping activity.

Physical Examination

The clinical presentation of a thumb UCL injury in pediatric and adolescent patients mirrors that in adults. In the acute setting, swelling and tenderness are present at the ulnar border of the thumb. Range of motion should be documented both at the thumb interphalangeal joint and at the MCP joint. A manual test of ligamentous laxity in the coronal plane at the MCP joint can be diagnostic. The thumb is grasped between the examiner's thumb and index finger and a valgus stress is applied to the MCP joint. Pain and laxity compared with the contralateral side suggest a UCL injury. An injection of lidocaine at the site of the injury decreases the pain associated with this examination technique while allowing evaluation of laxity, especially in patients with acute presentations.

Imaging

Radiographs of the thumb in at least two planes can reveal a fracture at the epiphyseal base of the proximal phalanx in a Salter type III pattern. Displacement of this fragment suggests a pediatric version of a Stener lesion, in which the avulsed fragment of the proximal phalanx and the intact UCL is blocked by the adductor aponeurosis.[79]

An ultrasonographic stress test has been described as a method to confirm diagnosis of a thumb UCL injury[80,81] and may be helpful in pediatric and adolescent patients who are

AUTHORS' PREFERRED TECHNIQUE

Scaphoid Fractures

In younger pediatric patients, we recommend nonoperative treatment with thumb spica casting extending above the elbow for 4 weeks followed by application of a short-arm cast until healing is complete. Although previous literature has suggested that nonoperative treatment can be successful in most nondisplaced or minimally displaced pediatric and adolescent scaphoid fractures,[62] our bias is to operatively treat all waist and proximal pole fractures in older pediatric and all adolescent patients (Fig. 133-5). Diligent fracture care can help prevent scaphoid nonunion, which is a problematic complication in young, active patients. In patients treated nonoperatively and in those with screw fixation, immobilization should continue until healing is complete. Our criteria for judging healing include the absence of tenderness to palpation at the anatomic snuffbox or the scaphoid tubercle and evidence of radiographic healing and radiographs taken at monthly intervals. However, radiographs can be unreliable indicators of healing, and we routinely obtain a CT scan at 3 months in all patients with a fracture pattern that is prone to nonunion, including scaphoid waist and proximal pole fractures or in patients who would like to return to weight-bearing or contact sports.

If operative treatment is selected on the basis of fracture and patient characteristics, we recommend that a long (but subchondral) headless compression screw be placed down the central axis of the scaphoid either through an open or percutaneous approach. No implant has been shown to be superior to another. However, improved biomechanical stability after a simulated fracture in cadaver specimens has been shown with long compression screws placed centrally down the axis of the scaphoid.[73,74] Preoperatively, a CT scan is obtained to confirm fracture location and displacement. Arthroscopy can be performed prior to screw placement to assess the condition of the soft tissues of the wrist (Fig. 133-5, *B*). Concurrent injuries to the TFCC and intercarpal ligaments are possible and may require treatment at the time of the procedure.

For screw placement, a K wire is used to locate the center of the proximal pole of the scaphoid under fluoroscopy, which can be performed either percutaneously or with direct visualization of the proximal pole through a dorsal capsulotomy. Once the appropriate location of the K wire down the central axis of the scaphoid is confirmed with use of fluoroscopy and the appropriate length is determined, the trajectory is hand drilled over the wire, and a compression screw is placed. A screw that is 4 mm shorter than the measure proximal to distal pole length has been shown to be biomechanically superior to shorter screws.[73]

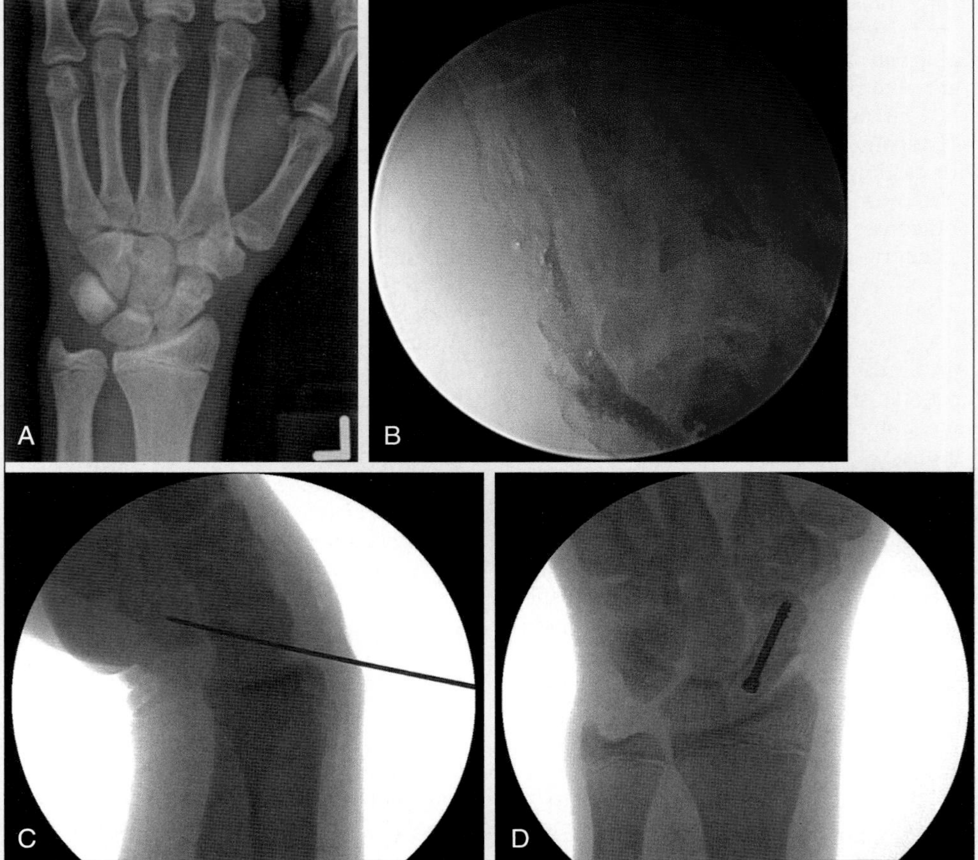

FIGURE 133-5 A scaphoid fracture in an adolescent basketball player treated with percutaneous compression screw fixation. **A,** A minimally displaced fracture is observed on a radiograph. **B,** An arthroscopic view of the fracture. **C,** Kirschner wire placement in the central axis of the scaphoid. **D,** The final position of a compression screw in the anteroposterior plane.

not ideal candidates for MRI. In addition, one recent study reported a sensitivity of 92% and a positive predictive value of 99% with ultrasound examination of UCL injuries in adolescent and adult patients; findings were confirmed after surgical treatment.[6]

MRI is the gold standard of imaging modalities for soft tissue injuries in the wrist and hand. For UCL injuries in pediatric and adolescent patients, MRI can be a helpful alternative to lidocaine injection and clinical examination, which can be a difficult procedure for pediatric and adolescent patients.

Decision-Making Principles

Sprains or stable ligamentous tears are treated nonoperatively. Avulsions of the UCL on its epiphyseal insertion can be treated nonoperatively if the fragment is minimally displaced or not displaced. Displaced avulsions should be reduced surgically and maintained with internal or percutaneous fixation. We recommend a threshold of 2 mm as measured on any radiographic view to consider surgical treatment in pediatric and adolescent patients. Partial UCL injuries without gross instability on examination should be considered for nonoperative treatment. Complete midsubstance ruptures are rare in pediatric and adolescent patients, but resulting instability should be treated with surgical repair. A UCL tear with a Stener lesion[82] should be repaired surgically because healing with use of conservative means is not reliable.

Treatment Options

UCL injuries that are amenable to nonoperative treatment should be immobilized in a short-arm thumb spica cast for 6 weeks. After removal of the cast, a removable thumb spica brace should be used. In patients who do not respond to nonoperative treatment, have a Stener lesion, or have chronic instability, operative treatment is indicated. An open approach to the ulnar base of the thumb proximal phalanx is performed and the injury is identified. Suture anchors or bone tunnels to avoid the physis are used to repair disrupted ligament. An avulsion fracture of the base of the proximal phalanx should be anatomically reduced and fixation applied. In chronic cases, reconstructive techniques may be required because primary repair can be difficult.

Results

Published data regarding the results of thumb UCL injuries in pediatric and adolescent patients are scarce. It is generally an uncommon injury. In healthy young patients with stable partial injuries, healing should be expected after appropriate immobilization. Acute ligamentous and bony repairs must be

AUTHORS' PREFERRED TREATMENT

Thumb Ulnar Ligament Injury

For injuries that involve an avulsion fracture at the base of the thumb proximal phalanx, we recommend using 1.0- or 1.2-mm screw fixation whenever possible (Fig. 133-6). Kirschner wires can also be used but may not provide sufficient stability. Screws also eliminate complications associated with K-wire fixation, such as pin-site infections. Care after surgery consists of immobilization for 4 to 6 weeks in a thumb spica cast followed by a return to motion. Earlier return to motion may be considered for stable bony repairs compared with ligamentous repairs or reconstructions.

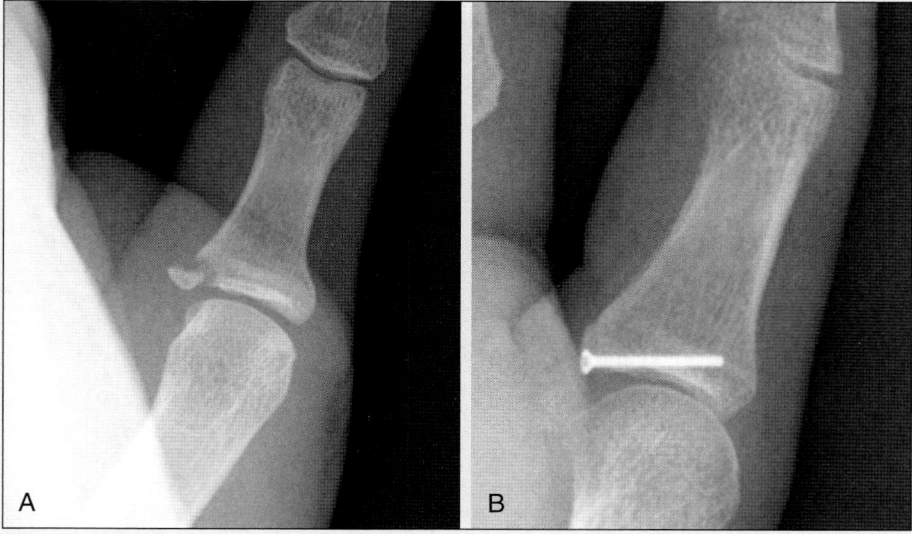

FIGURE 133-6 Avulsion of the insertion of the ulnar collateral ligament of the thumb in a nearly skeletally mature adolescent after a kickball injury. **A,** A typical pediatric and adolescent avulsion fracture pattern. **B,** Reduction of the fracture and fixation using a 1.0-mm cortex screw.

protected with immobilization to ensure adequate healing. Close clinical follow-up is recommended to ensure compliance and prevent failure of treatment in this population.

Return to Play

After nonoperative or operative management, immobilization should be provided with a thumb spica splint or cast for 6 weeks. Hand therapy should be initiated after this 6-week period, along with a gradual return to activity. In sports with high levels of hand contact, such as basketball, a full 2 to 3 months should be expected prior to return to sport. Clinical examination should reveal no tenderness or pain, and stress examination should be negative. In the case of UCL injuries with associated fractures, radiographs can be used to follow the progression of healing.

Complications

Authors of a recent retrospective study of 127 patients, including 15 adolescent patients, who were treated surgically for UCL injury in a single institution over a 10-year period reported that the most common complications included temporary neurapraxia of the radial sensory nerve in 6.5% of patients and temporary stiffness in 4% of patients.[6] Chronic regional pain syndrome developed in two patients. Additional complications include chronic instability from failed previous treatment or failed identification of a Stener lesion, pin-site infections if K wires are used for fracture fixation, and fracture nonunion in avulsions of the epiphysis of the proximal phalanx if stable fixation is not maintained.

"Jammed" Finger

The fingers are vulnerable to injury in almost every athletic endeavor. In fact, a recent epidemiologic study of 100 U.S. high schools showed that among fractures sustained during school-sponsored athletic activities, the most common location was the hand and fingers (28.3%).[3] The small finger was the most commonly affected digit, and the proximal phalanx was the most commonly fractured bone. Although most fractures and soft tissue injuries can be treated similarly to those in adult patients, several injuries that are more specific to pediatric and adolescent patients deserve attention. These injuries include the Seymour fracture, which is a displaced physeal fracture of the distal phalanx with nail bed laceration first described by Seymour[83] in 1966, proximal interphalangeal (PIP) joint injuries, and mallet finger.

History

Usually, the "jammed" finger involves a history of hyperextension or hyperflexion of the affected digit after contact with a ball, the ground, or another athlete. Immediate pain and swelling is common, and the patient often has to be removed from play. In some cases, however, the patient does not remember the event and may present subacutely with pain and swelling during activity. Seymour fractures occur with some associated crushing injury. PIP injuries, including problematic fracture-dislocations, often occur in athletes participating in contact sports (e.g., football and rugby) or sports that involve catching a ball (e.g., basketball, volleyball, and football).[84] Mallet finger involves the disruption of the extensor mechanism insertion on the distal phalanx and can occur with hyperflexion injuries. In young patients with open physes, these injuries can represent Salter-Harris type III injuries.

Physical Examination

Tenderness and swelling at the site of injury is encountered. In Seymour fractures, close examination of the nail bed should be documented, as well as the presence of any exposed distal phalangeal bone. Deformity in the sagittal, coronal, and rotational planes should be identified in PIP joint injuries, and range of motion should be tested. The initial extensor lag for mallet fingers is recorded.

Imaging

AP, lateral, and oblique films should be obtained at the affected site. Further advanced imaging studies are not needed in most cases. In general, it is prudent to obtain radiographs in all patients presenting after sustaining a "jammed" finger if there is any clinical concern for injury.

Decision-Making Principles

Most of the treatment of "jammed" finger injuries occurs in the emergency department without assistance from orthopaedic or hand surgeons, and these injuries can easily be treated closed as long as appropriate reduction and immobilization are performed. On follow-up with the sports clinician, evaluation should include repeat radiographs to assess the quality and maintenance of reduction, as well as an assessment of the type of immobilization used. If there is a question of poor reduction, alignment, or instability that is not being treated adequately in a closed manner, the clinician should be prepared to address these issues operatively in a timely manner. Hand fractures and soft tissue injuries in young patients heal quickly, and lasting dysfunction is risked if these injuries are inadequately treated.

Results

The treatment goal for any pediatric or adolescent patient who presents with a "jammed" finger after appropriate diagnosis is a painless, flexible, and functional digit. Although specific evidence-based results of treatment of the aforementioned injuries is limited for pediatric and adolescent patients, the healing potential in young, healthy athletes is high, and if appropriate treatment is initiated in a timely manner, in our experience the aforementioned goals of treatment can be expected to be achieved.

Complications

Failure to diagnose the previously described injuries appropriately can lead to a delay in treatment and permanent dysfunction of the affected digit. In particular, appropriate repair of nail bed lacerations in patients with Seymour fractures will help prevent abnormal nail plate growth or failure of nail plate growth. Achieving and maintaining appropriate reduction of PIP joint injuries will prevent future stiffness and malalignment detrimental to appropriate hand function.

AUTHORS' PREFERRED TECHNIQUE

"Jammed" Finger

Most treatments for the jammed finger, regardless of the underlying injury, can be performed in the emergency department with use of a local digital block with 1% or 2% lidocaine; we do not use epinephrine. In younger patients, a weight-based dosing check should be performed to prevent overuse of the local anesthetic. In very young patients, conscious sedation may be necessary to facilitate patient cooperation.

A Seymour fracture is an open fracture and should be thoroughly irrigated and appropriately debrided of any foreign or devitalized material. A tetanus booster and antibiotic coverage, usually a first-generation cephalosporin, is prescribed. Close attention should be directed to the nail complex. Usually, nail plate removal is required to facilitate examination and repair with 6.0 absorbable sutures of the nail bed. This step is vital in ensuring appropriate healing and restoration of the nail anatomy. Soft tissue can be interposed between the fracture fragments and should be removed at the time of debridement. The previously removed nail plate can be tucked under the eponychium. Stabilization can be achieved with use of a sterile dressing and a hand cast in younger patients.

Proximal interphalangeal joint injuries range from volar plate disruptions to simple dislocations to complex physeal fracture dislocations. In general, pediatric and adolescent patients with open physes and injury to the PIP joint can be treated with closed reduction and casting for 3 to 4 weeks, with exact timing dependent on the stability of the injury pattern. Buddy taping can be used to maintain rotational alignment. Radiographs should be obtained on a weekly basis to ensure a concentric PIP joint and that fractures remain within 5 to 10 degrees of angular deformity. The patient should have no rotational deformity, and intraarticular incongruity should be less than 1 to 2 mm. Fractures that are unable to be reduced to fit these parameters in a closed manner or that lose reduction over time should be treated operatively with K-wire or preferably screw fixation (Fig. 133-7). Isolated PIP joint dislocations can be treated with a brief course of splinting for 10 to 14 days, followed by a return to active range of motion.

Mallet finger in pediatric and adolescent patients presents either with bony involvement, which is usually a Salter-Harris type III injury to the dorsal epiphysis of the distal phalanx, or without fracture. Both of these types of injuries can be effectively treated without surgery. We recommend extension splinting of the distal interphalangeal joint only for 8 weeks, followed by another 4 weeks of nighttime splinting. K-wire pinning is rarely needed except for open injuries. In our experience, chronic presentations of mallet finger in pediatric patients can also be successfully treated with use of a trial of extension splinting. In severe cases that are not responsive to splinting, tenodermodesis, a resection and advancement of skin and tendon sutured together as a unit, can be considered.[85-87]

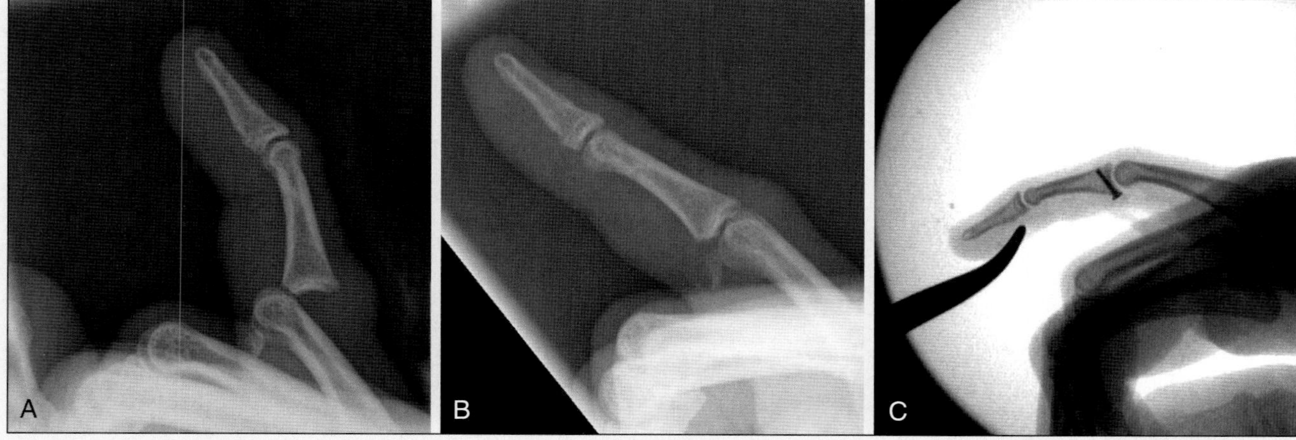

FIGURE 133-7 Unstable fracture-dislocation of the proximal interphalangeal (PIP) joint in an adolescent football player. **A,** A film of the injury shows dorsal dislocation of the PIP joint. **B,** A postreduction film from the emergency department. **C,** An intraoperative image showing placement of a 1.0-mm cortex screw.

Diligent monitoring of splint compliance during mallet finger treatment should prevent excessive distal phalanx extensor lag and its corresponding dysfunction. During closed treatment of mallet finger, the clinician and patient should carefully watch the skin beneath the splint to prevent the development of pressure-induced breakdown.

For a complete list of references, go to expertconsult.com.

Suggested Readings

Triangular Fibrocartilage Complex Injuries

Citation: Terry CL, Waters PM: Triangular fibrocartilage injuries in pediatric and adolescent patients. *J Hand Surg* 23(4):626–634, 1998.

Level of Evidence: IV

Summary: A retrospective review of 29 children and adolescents with traumatic tears of the triangular fibrocartilage complex who underwent operative treatment showed excellent results in 89% of patients. The authors also noted a high percentage of patients who had coexisting pathologic findings that required treatment.

Distal Radial Physeal Stress Injury (Gymnast's Wrist)

Citation: DiFiori JP, Caine DJ, Malina RM: Wrist pain, distal radial physeal injury, and ulnar variance in the young gymnast. *Am J Sports Med* 34(5):840–849, 2006.

Level of Evidence: Not applicable

Summary: A review of the literature describing the etiology, pathophysiology, treatment options, and preventative techniques for wrist pain in skeletally immature gymnasts led to the recommendation of early identification and treatment of pathologic findings in this at-risk population. The authors stress the importance of graduated training regimens and slow return to sport after a physeal injury.

Scaphoid Fractures

Citation: Gholson JJ, Bae DS, Zurakowski D, et al: Scaphoid fractures in children and adolescents: Contemporary injury patterns and factors influencing time to union. *J Bone Joint Surg Am* 93A(13):1210–1219, 2011.

Level of Evidence: III

Summary: The authors of a retrospective review of the treatment of 351 scaphoid fractures over 15 years in children and adolescents report an overall 90% healing rate with cast treatment and a 96.5% healing rate after surgical treatment. The most common fracture pattern in the series was a scaphoid waist fracture (71%), followed by distal pole (23%) and proximal pole (6%) fractures.

Hand Fractures

Citation: Kozin S, Waters P: Fractures and dislocations of the hand and carpus in children. In *Fractures in Children*, Philadelphia, 2010, Lippincott Williams & Wilkins.

Level of Evidence: Not applicable

Summary: The authors present current recommendations for nonoperative and operative management of hand fractures in skeletally immature patients.

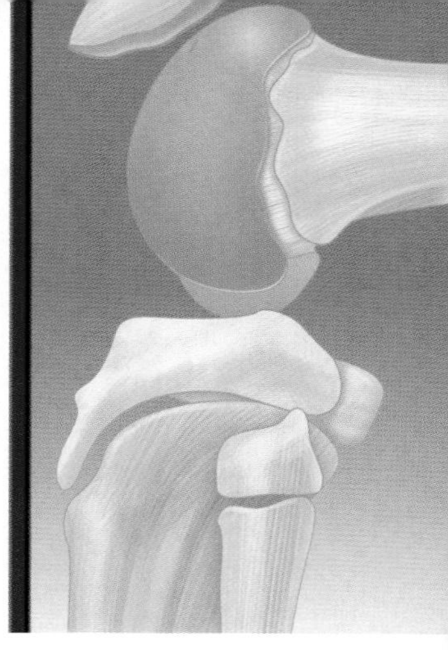

134

Pediatric and Adolescent Hip Injuries

YI-MENG YEN • MININDER S. KOCHER

Almost a decade ago, it was estimated that more than 30 million children in the United States participated in organized sports programs, with a third of them sustaining an injury that required evaluation by a nurse or physician.[1] Compared with adults, children and adolescents have physical and physiologic differences that may cause them to be more vulnerable to injury. Children may not have as much coordination and may experience musculoskeletal imbalance because limb mass increases faster than limb length.[2] Muscle tendon growth lags behind bone growth, and growing cartilage is more susceptible to stress and injury. The increased incidence of injury in children and adolescents is due in part to the increased participation in competitive sports and the propensity for children to focus on a single sport, leading to an increased risk of overuse injuries. More recently, it has been reported that up to 2.6 million youth athletes have injuries that warrant a visit to the emergency department, costing almost $2 billion per year.[3]

Injuries to the hip and pelvis in pediatric and adolescent patients have been reported in the past several decades[4-9] but are receiving an increased level of attention because of advances in arthroscopic treatment and magnetic resonance imaging (MRI). Injuries in the area of the hip can be caused by a single traumatic event or by repetitive microtrauma. Most injuries in the area of the hip in children are soft tissue, apophyseal, or bony injuries that require supportive management; only a significant minority of such injuries require surgical intervention. Several unique hip conditions are specific to the pediatric population, including slipped capital femoral epiphysis (SCFE), hip dysplasia, and Legg-Calvé-Perthes disease. In this chapter we focus on an overview of common hip injuries in pediatric and adolescent athletes.

Bony Injuries

Avulsion Fractures

Avulsion injuries are common among skeletally immature athletes and those approaching skeletal maturity because of the inherent weakness of the open apophysis. These injuries are commonly seen in the area of the knee, heel, and elbow. Avulsion fractures result from indirect trauma caused by sudden, violent, and unbalanced muscle contractions and are most common between the age at which the secondary ossification center appears and the age at which the ossification center fuses. Sports such as soccer, rugby, ice hockey, gymnastics, and sprinting that involve kicking, rapid acceleration and deceleration, and jumping are commonly associated with avulsion fractures. Intensive training exposes the epiphyseal plate to repeated tensile stress while overstrengthening the muscles around the joint. The inherent weakness of the epiphyseal plate, combined with the increased demand on the musculature, predisposes the adolescent athlete to an avulsion injury. Once the injury has occurred, the bony displacement is limited by the periosteum and the surrounding muscle fascia.

The sites for apophyseal injury in the area of the hip include the ischium (hamstring attachment), anterior inferior iliac spine (rectus femoris), anterior superior iliac spine (sartorius), iliac crest (abdominal musculature), lesser trochanter (iliopsoas; Fig. 134-1), or greater trochanter (abductors). In a study of 203 avulsion fractures, 54% of the fractures occurred at the ischial tuberosity, whereas 22% were anterior superior iliac spine fractures and 19% were anterior inferior iliac spine fractures.[10] Most injuries occurred in soccer and gymnastics. The clinical presentation typically follows a traumatic incident with an acute onset of localized pain and the description of a "pop." Palpation and passive stretching of the muscle is typically quite painful, and patients assume a position that places the least amount of tension on the involved muscle. Although clinical presentation is often diagnostic, radiographic imaging is useful to determine the location, size, and degree of bony displacement.

Initial management of most avulsion fractures is conservative, including rest and application of ice, followed by protected weight bearing with crutches until symptoms resolve.[11] Progression to light isometric stretching, full weight bearing, and strengthening exercises occurs when the patient is pain free. Return to sports occurs after full pain-free range of motion and full strength is achieved, which can take from 6 weeks to 6 months. The need for surgical intervention for avulsion fractures is rare and is indicated only in patients in whom the fragment has been displaced greater than 2 cm or who have loss of function or painful nonunion. In the case of an ischial tuberosity avulsion fracture, several investigators have advocated repair if the bony fragment if greater than 2 cm; otherwise the fibrous nonunion can lead to chronic buttock pain, decreased hamstring strength, or potentially symptoms of the sciatic nerve.[11-15] Although it is generally agreed that large displaced fragments greater than 2 cm may

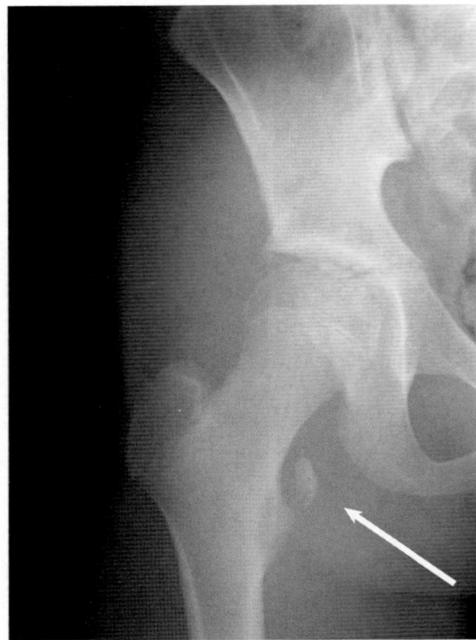

FIGURE 134-1 A lesser tuberosity avulsion fracture in a skeletally immature patient. The arrow denotes the site of avulsion.

require surgical fixation, the optimal timing of surgery remains unclear (Fig. 134-2).

Stress Fractures

Stress fractures of the femoral neck are most commonly seen in distance runners and young people enlisted in the military, with an incidence as high as 21% to 31% in these groups.[16-18] Similarly, the incidence of femoral neck stress fractures in young female athletes has been reported to be as high as 20%.[19] Stress fractures originate from either abnormal forces on normal bone (fatigue fractures) or normal forces on abnormal bone (insufficiency fractures).[20] These overuse injuries result from repetitive microtrauma on the bone and occur when the extent of damage exceeds the remodeling process. The most common sites of stress fractures in the hip occur in the femur, pubic rami, iliac crest, and sacroiliac joints.[21] Stress fractures of the femoral neck are particularly important because they often are untreated or unrecognized and can lead to the potentially devastating consequence of an acute femoral neck fracture.[22,23] Female athletes are more likely to experience stress fractures because of the classic female athlete triad: amenorrhea, eating disorders, and low bone density.[23-25] Additional risk factors include chronic use of glucocorticoids, smoking, hyperparathyroidism, hyperthyroidism, malabsorption syndromes, and calcium deficiencies.[26-37]

Stress fractures of the hip often present with only subtle clinical symptoms, making the diagnosis difficult. Hip pain associated with these stress fractures presents with an insidious onset of vague groin discomfort that is worse with activity and alleviated by rest. Patients often provide a history of a recent increase in the amount of time that they run or engage in other activity. As the fracture worsens, pain may occur earlier or even at rest. On physical examination, pain may be reproduced at the extremes of range of motion, particularly with internal rotation.[38] A positive Trendelenburg test, the inability to perform a straight-leg raise test against resistance, and the inability to hop on the affected side should raise suspicion of a stress fracture.[39] Plain radiographs are often negative in the acute setting, and therefore advanced imaging may be required. A bone scan or MRI can be more helpful for diagnosing a stress fracture and should be considered if plain films are not diagnostic (Fig. 134-3).

Management of hip stress fractures is based on the location, chronicity, and causative factors.[8] Femoral neck fractures occur in two patterns: tension and compression.[40] Tension-sided stress fractures are located on the superolateral femoral neck; they are more common in adults and may become displaced. These types of stress fractures should be managed with percutaneous cannulated screws placed up the femoral neck. Tension-sided compression fractures are at higher risk for nonunion, deformity, and avascular necrosis. Compression-sided fractures occur in the inferomedial neck, which is rarely displaced but can cause a mild varus deformity. Younger patients typically present with compression-sided femoral neck stress fractures, which can be managed conservatively.[41,42] In most adolescents, conservative treatment includes non–weight bearing on the affected leg until radiographic union is achieved and use of nonsteroidal antiinflammatory drugs; in addition, gentle range of motion and regional muscular

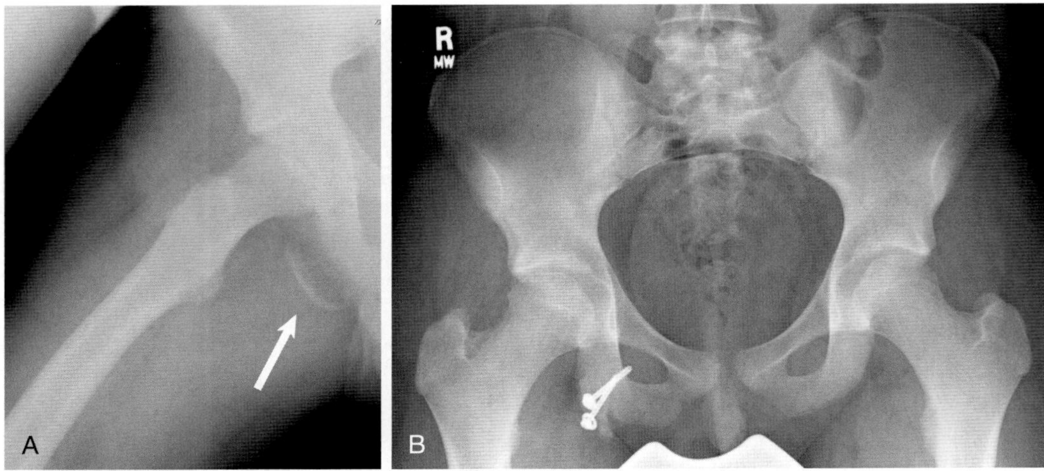

FIGURE 134-2 **A,** An ischial tuberosity avulsion fracture. The arrow denotes a large fragment of the ischium. **B,** The same patient after open reduction and internal fixation.

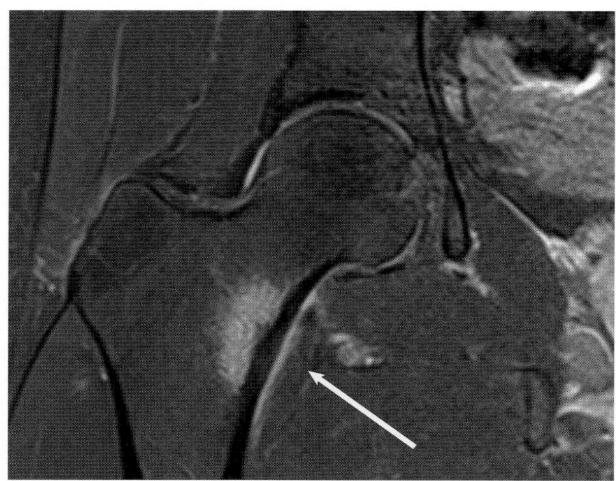

FIGURE 134-3 A magnetic resonance imaging scan depicting a stress fracture of the intertrochanteric region of the hip in a female adolescent. The arrow denotes an area of edema resulting from the stress fracture.

strengthening can be initiated. If healing does not occur within 6 to 8 weeks, use of a bone stimulator may be attempted. Return to play should be allowed only after complete fracture healing is demonstrated on clinical and radiographic examination. Treatment of any underlying endocrine disorder or other disorder is paramount to prevent recurrence.

Fractures

Fractures in the area of the hip are relatively rare in the adolescent and pediatric population and account for fewer than 1% of fractures. These fractures usually result from high-energy trauma or a fall from a height rather than from participation in sports. Fractures can occur in the femoral head and neck, the subtrochanteric region of the femur, and around the pelvic ring. Fractures in the area of the pelvis can occur as single breaks due to the elasticity of the child's pelvis and can injure the triradiate cartilage and lead to growth disturbances of the acetabulum.[43-45] Radiographs of the pelvis and orthogonal views of the hip are usually diagnostic, but CT scans can be useful in many cases.

Fractures of the acetabulum are generally treated nonoperatively in cases of minimal displacement, disruption of a small fragment, stable fracture patterns, or Salter-Harris type I or II fractures of the triradiate. Operative intervention has been recommended in comminuted, open, and unstable fracture patterns, but long-term results have not been encouraging.[43-46]

Fractures of the femoral head and neck are classified by the method of Delbet as type I (transphyseal), II (transcervical), III (cervicotrochanteric), and IV (intertrochanteric).[47] Type I fractures are the least common but have the highest rate of osteonecrosis (38% to 100% depending on the presence of femoral head dislocation).[8,48] Irreducible fractures require open reduction and internal fixation.[49] Type II and III fractures should be treated with anatomic reduction and internal fixation[49] and are the most commonly encountered femoral neck fractures in children. Type II fractures have approximately twice the risk of avascular necrosis compared with type III fractures.[8,48] Decompression of the capsular hematoma associated with femoral neck fractures may have a role in treatment because lower rates of avascular necrosis have been observed in patients who underwent capsular decompression.[50] Type IV fractures and subtrochanteric femur fractures are extracapsular and have the most favorable prognosis. These fractures should be treated with anatomic reduction and internal fixation with blade plate fixation or screw-side plate fixation.[51-54] In some cases, intramedullary nailing or a dynamic hip screw can be used for subtrochanteric fractures of the femur.[55] Postoperatively, these patients are generally instructed to ambulate with crutches, with protected weight bearing.

Dislocation

Hip dislocation is relatively uncommon in the adolescent population and accounts for less than 5% of all traumatic hip dislocations. Traumatic hip dislocation in children differs from dislocation in adults in that it is classified as a low-energy injury in most patients when it results from sports injuries or a fall from relatively low heights.[14,56-58] This difference is due to increased joint laxity in children, making dislocation possible with relatively minor trauma.

Although the femoral head in children may dislocate in any direction, posterior dislocations occur most frequently and account for more than 90% of all dislocations.[56,57,59,60] The hip is usually held in flexion, adduction, and internal rotation with a posterior dislocation. The neurovascular status must be documented thoroughly, and blunt trauma to the ipsilateral knee should be noted. Diagnosis can be made by history and physical examination. The femoral head can sometimes be palpated posteriorly. Radiographs, which should include a view of the entire pelvis and orthogonal views of the affected hip, are usually diagnostic. Radiographs should be examined carefully to evaluate for ipsilateral physeal injury or an associated femoral neck fracture. A CT scan can be useful to detect bony fragments within the joint, as well as concomitant injury.

The treatment for a traumatic hip dislocation is an emergent closed reduction within the first 6 hours of the time of injury to minimize the risk of avascular necrosis The incidence of avascular necrosis is about 5% to 15% in all patients but increases by as much as 20-fold if the reduction is performed more than 6 hours after the injury occurs.[56,59] Closed reduction can be performed in the emergency department, but we prefer to perform the reduction in the operating room with inducement of general anesthesia and use of imaging (Fig. 134-4). Open reduction is performed only if the hip is irreducible after two to three reduction attempts or if soft tissue or bony fragments are interposed between the head and acetabulum. The approach should be the same as the direction of the dislocation—for example, a posterior approach for a posterior dislocation. The acetabulum should be cleared of any debris, osteochondral fragments should be fixed if they are large enough, and the soft tissue should be repaired if possible.

The major complication after a dislocated hip is avascular necrosis of the femoral head.[56,57,61,62] When a traumatic dislocation is associated with femoral epiphysiolysis, the risk of avascular necrosis is almost 100%.[60,63,64] A patient who has had a delayed reduction should undergo MRI to assess for avascular necrosis 3 to 6 months after the injury. An alternative algorithm has been proposed that entails obtaining an

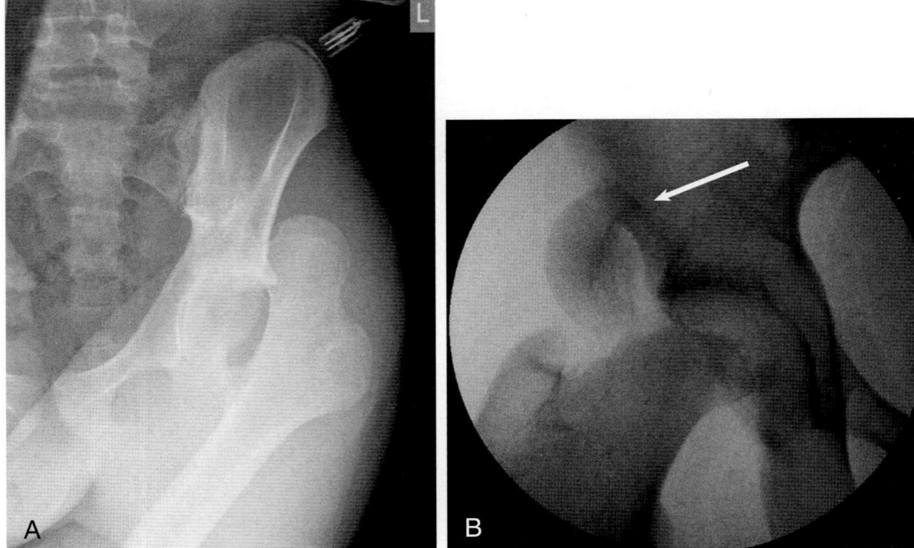

FIGURE 134-4 **A,** Posterior dislocation of the hip in skeletally immature patient. **B,** Epiphysiolysis (*arrow*) during reduction of a dislocated hip. Open reduction and internal fixation of the epiphysis was necessary.

MRI scan 6 weeks after the injury. If the marrow signal is normal, no further imaging is necessary, but if an abnormal signal is noted, a follow-up scan should be performed at 3 months.[65] Other complications include sciatic nerve injury, late posttraumatic osteoarthritis, coxa magna, heterotopic ossification, and recurrent dislocation.[58]

Recently, two studies have been performed regarding intraarticular pathologic evaluation by hip arthroscopy after hip dislocation.[66,67] In all patients, intraarticular disease was documented in all cases, including chondral damage, labral tears, and adhesions. Ligamentum teres tears have been documented as a cause of persistent hip pain.[68] However, hip arthroscopy in the acute setting may be difficult because of fluid extravasation and should only be considered by the most experienced surgeons.

Pathologic Lesions

Very rarely, both benign and malignant lesions may be found when evaluating a patient for hip pain. The most common benign lesions are simple bone cysts and osteoid osteomas, whereas the most common malignant tumors are osteosarcoma and Ewing's sarcoma.[69] Radiographs and advanced imaging (CT and/or MRI) should be obtained to evaluate the location and size of the lesion, the presence of a fracture, soft tissue extension, and metastatic manifestations. Some simple benign lesions heal or regress spontaneously and require only close observation, whereas others may require surgical intervention if they are quite large. If malignancy is suspected, referral to an orthopaedic oncologist is advisable because adjunctive and wide resection surgery may be indicated.

Soft Tissue Injuries

Muscle Injury

Muscle strains and contusions are common in young athletes.[70] Muscle strains are associated with improper warm-up, a previous injury, fatigue, weather conditions, and uneven surfaces, among other factors.[71,72] A muscle strain occurs in the hip area when muscle is functioning eccentrically, that is, the muscle is contracting while being lengthened. The most susceptible muscles involved are those that cross two joints, in particular the rectus femoris, hamstrings, and adductors.[72] A fall or a direct blow causes a muscle contusion that is commonly seen in athletes who participate in contact sports.

The diagnosis of a muscle strain or contusion is typically straightforward. For a muscle strain, a high-velocity activity is usually being performed, and the patient reports a sudden and intense pain in the affected muscle. The patient usually has localized pain and tenderness of the affected muscle with varying degrees of ecchymosis. The patient is usually unable to continue the activity and cannot immediately use the muscle. A contusion can be distinguished from a muscle rupture by the ability to continue using the muscle, and it can be distinguished from a strain by the mechanism of injury. Nonsurgical treatment varies, but all options involve the same principles. Early use of a compression wrap and icing helps control edema, bleeding, and swelling. Nonsteroidal antiinflammatory drugs are used for the first several days. Immobilization and partial weight bearing can help provide comfort and muscle protection in the early period. Early initiation of range of motion and gentle stretching with progression to strengthening can be implemented when muscle pain is absent. Functional activities can start once strength has returned. Surgical intervention is rarely indicated.

Myositis ossificans can occur after moderate or severe injuries.[71] The vastus intermedius of the quadriceps is most commonly affected in persons with this condition. It is usually diagnosed clinically by the presence of persistent soft tissue swelling, particularly with a muscle that is warm and tender. The diagnosis becomes evident with heterotopic bone formation seen on a radiograph around 2 to 4 weeks after the injury. The size of the myositis ossificans usually stabilizes by 6 months, but it can cause continued pain and can delay rehabilitation.[73] Surgery is usually not indicated.

Bursitis

Bursitis occurs at two major areas around the hip, the iliopsoas bursa and the greater trochanteric bursa. The iliopsoas bursa is the largest synovial bursa in the body and is located between the iliopsoas tendon and the lesser trochanter, extending upward into the iliac fossa beneath the iliacus muscle.[74] The greater trochanteric bursa is located on the lateral side of the greater trochanter and cushions the gluteal tendons, iliotibial band, and tensor fascia latae.[75] A smaller, less commonly affected bursa is the iliopectineal bursa, which is situated between the iliopsoas muscle belly and the femoral head. Causes of bursitis include chronic microtrauma, arthritis, regional muscle dysfunction, overuse, and acute injury.[75,76] Hip bursitis is commonly caused by repetitive motion of the hip during cycling or running or a direct injury to the hip such as a fall or a tackle onto the greater trochanter.

The clinical presentation depends on which bursa is affected. Iliopsoas bursitis causes pain in the anterior groin, tenderness over the lesser trochanter, and pain with resisted hip flexion (Stinchfield test).[77] Symptoms of trochanteric bursitis include pain on the lateral aspect of the hip and thigh and pain when moving from sitting to standing and when walking up stairs. Having the patient lie on his or her side and reproduce the motion of riding a bike can elicit tenderness. In both cases, erythema, swelling, and warmth may be present over the front or side of the hip. Diagnosis is usually clinical, and imaging is often unnecessary. Plain films can sometimes show round calcifications that are isolated around the greater trochanter in the case of trochanteric bursitis.[75] Ultrasound or MRI can be used to localize areas of inflammation.

Treatment of bursitis is almost always conservative and includes rest, use of ice and nonsteroidal antiinflammatory drugs, gentle stretching, and physical therapy. Ultrasound-guided steroid injections may help alleviate the painful symptoms of bursitis. In recalcitrant cases, a surgical bursectomy or tendon release may be helpful (performed in an open manner or arthroscopically).[78-81]

Athletic Pubalgia

Athletic pubalgia is a term used to refer to pain around the groin and can encompass osteitis pubis, adductor dysfunction, a sports hernia, or another pelvic/abdominal muscular injury. Most people refer to athletic pubalgia as a sports or sportsman hernia,[82-84] although no universally accepted definition exists. Adductor dysfunction causes tenderness localized to the adductor longus insertion, and on examination the patient has pain with adduction against resistance and with stretching in abduction. This condition is usually managed with nonoperative management, including rest and physical therapy. Occasionally the use of injected corticosteroids can provide relief,[85] whereas adductor tenotomy has been shown to provide long-term relief in recalcitrant cases.[86,87]

Osteitis pubis causes tenderness to palpation at the pubic symphysis. Chronic osteitis pubis can cause chronic changes that induce inappropriate osteoclastic activity and osseous resorption on plain radiographs[88,89] and the so-called secondary cleft sign on MRI,[90] whereas edema is seen around the pubis on MRI in acute cases.[91,92] Normally osteitis pubis is treated with rest and physical therapy,[93] with use of injections[94,95] and surgical intervention[96,97] in recalcitrant cases.

Athletic pubalgia is a syndrome that occurs as a result of weakness of the posterior wall of the inguinal canal and results in both nerve irritation and disruption and instability of the muscular attachments.[82,98-101] Athletic pubalgia can be thought of as an overuse injury[102,103] in which the muscular attachments of the pelvis are unbalanced, which leads to a loss of postural control and an increase in the shear forces across the pelvis. Most patients report insidious unilateral, dull, achy pain in their groin that is significantly exacerbated by activities such as running, cutting, or twisting. Coughing, sneezing, and Valsalva-type maneuvers usually worsen the pain. Physical examination can reveal tenderness over conjoined tendon, the adductor origin, the distal rectus insertion, and the inguinal canal. It is important to distinguish athletic pubalgia from an inguinal or femoral hernia. Newer types of MRI imaging can be useful in showing rectus abdominis tendon injury and subtle abnormalities of the myofascial layers of the abdominal wall.[104,105] Prevention with core and hip stability and flexibility is paramount in decreasing the incidence of athletic pubalgia.[106] Nonoperative measures include rest, use of antiinflammatory drugs, strengthening of core musculature, and postural control.[107,108] Surgical exploration should be considered if nonoperative treatment has failed after 3 to 6 months and other diagnoses have been excluded. Surgical repairs include primary pelvic floor repair without mesh,[109,110] open anterior mesh repair,[111,112] and laparoscopic mesh repair.[113] Surgical repairs should be referred to an appropriate general surgeon.

Snapping Hip (Coxa Saltans)

A snapping hip is characterized by an audible or visible popping or snapping when the hip is brought through a certain range of motion. The condition can be painful and is often exacerbated by sporting activities, particularly running uphill and downhill. Three types of snapping hip typically have been described: lateral or external (iliotibial band), internal or medial (psoas), and intraarticular.[114] The external type is the most common and involves the posterior border of the iliotibial band or the anterior border of the gluteus maximus tendon snapping over the greater trochanter when the hip is flexed from an extended position or with internal and external rotation while the hip is extended.[115] The external snapping is often visible as the iliotibial band clunks over the greater trochanter. The internal snapping hip is the iliopsoas tendon snapping over the iliopectineal eminence or the femoral head, and it is often painful and audible.[116] The intraarticular snapping can be caused by a loose body, a chondral flap, a labral tear, or synovial plica.[117,118]

The patient's history and physical examination are usually diagnostic for the location and cause of the snapping hip. Patients with an external snapping hip can often reproduce the symptoms voluntarily. Internal snapping hip occurs when moving the hip from a flexed and abducted position to an extended and adducted position; this snapping can often be seen on ultrasonography. MRI is indicated if an intraarticular pathologic condition is suspected. Initial management for coxa saltans externa or interna includes physical therapy for stretching of the iliotibial band or iliopsoas. Antiinflammatory medications, rest, and bursal injections also can be effective.

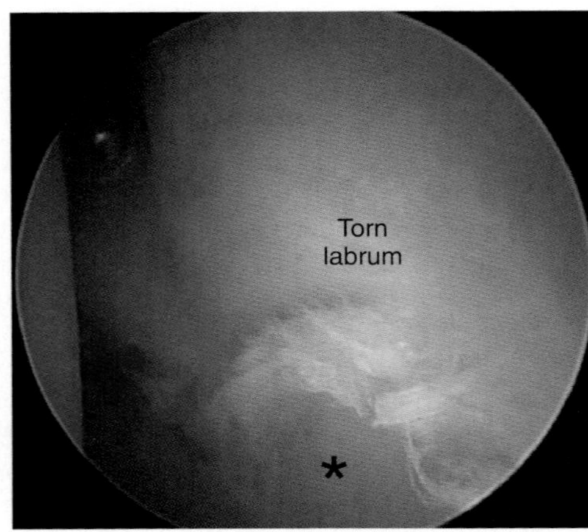

FIGURE 134-5 An arthroscopic view of a left hip depicting a large torn labrum. The asterisk denotes the articular surface of the acetabulum.

If conservative management does not relieve the symptoms, surgical intervention may be considered. Open surgical approaches that involve fractional lengthening or release have been performed,[119-121] although few reports have been described in adolescents.[116] Recently arthroscopic treatment has been described, with good short-term success for both coxa saltans interna and externa.[81,122-125]

Labral Tears

The acetabular labrum is a ring of fibrocartilage that almost encircles the acetabulum of the hip joint and is believed to deepen the acetabular, enhance joint stability, and provide a fluid seal for the articulating femoral head and acetabulum.[126-128] Injuries to the labrum occur during sports because of mechanical stresses or twisting in sports such as football, soccer, ballet, and ice hockey. The patient may report hip or groin pain and experience catching or locking of the hip during certain maneuvers. Disorders such as hip dysplasia and femoroacetabular impingement increase the risk of labral tears. Tears can occur in any part of the labrum but are more common in the anterosuperior portion of the acetabulum, perhaps because of the higher stresses in this region.[129] Radiographic imaging of the pelvis and hip can demonstrate a dysplasia, femoroacetabular impingement (FAI), or other abnormality, but an MR arthrogram is the most commonly used modality for diagnosing labral tears.[130,131]

The standard for diagnosing and treating acetabular labral tears has become arthroscopy. Conservative management may be able to alleviate pain, but surgical repair or debridement is the most definitive treatment (Fig. 134-5). Several studies have shown good long-term results and return to sports after labral treatment in both adults and adolescents.[132-135]

Acquired Disease

Femoroacetabular Impingement

FAI has been gaining increasing attention as a common etiology of hip pain in athletes.[136,137] Anatomically, the concept of FAI is that certain minor morphologic alterations to the hip joint occur that, when combined with repetitive abutment of the femoral head-neck junction against the anterior rim of the acetabulum, leads to chondrolabral dysfunction and eventual early degeneration of the hip joint. The morphologic alterations may be either on the acetabular side (pincer impingement) or the femoral head–neck side (cam impingement) or both.[138] FAI is now being recognized as a significant cause of hip pain in the adolescent population.[139]

Patients often present with an insidious onset of groin pain that is made worse with sporting activity. Patients can have an associated labral tear and often describe their pain with their hand cupped over the anterolateral hip with the thumb and forefinger in the shape of the letter C.[140] Impingement can be detected with decreased hip flexion and limited internal rotation and a positive impingement (flexion, adduction, and internal rotation) test. Radiographic imaging should include an anteroposterior view of the pelvis and orthogonal views of the hips.[141] A bony prominence on the head-neck junction is indicative of a cam lesion, whereas acetabular overcoverage or retroversion on the radiograph is termed a *pincer lesion*. Additional MRI scans can be helpful for evaluation of the soft tissues of the joint, including the cartilage and labrum.[142]

Treatment goals include improving hip muscle flexibility, pelvic tilt, strength, and posture. Progression of arthritic changes from impingement can be gradual but has the potential for severe permanent injury to the articular surfaces of the joint if left untreated. Refractory pain should be managed surgically by either open surgical dislocation or arthroscopic treatment.[136,143] Good results have been achieved in the adolescent population with arthroscopic intervention.[144]

Legg-Calvé-Perthes Disease

Legg-Calvé-Perthes disease is an idiopathic self-limiting condition involving avascular necrosis of the femoral epiphysis. The exact etiology of the disease is largely unknown, although a number of vascular causes have been proposed. In the past 100 years since it was first described, little insight has been gained into the cause and pathophysiologic features of this condition. It typically presents within the first decade of life, predominantly among boys aged 4 to 8 years.[145] Bilateral involvement is uncommon, occurring about 15% of the time, but is almost never simultaneous. The pathogenesis is complex and passes through multiple stages: the initial avascular necrosis, fragmentation, resorption, and collapse, followed by reossification. The Catterall[146] and Herring et al.[147] classifications are the two most common classification systems to provide a prognosis, depending on the necrosis location and percentage of femoral head involvement. The natural history of the disease is variable, being largely dependent on age at the time of diagnosis and the degree of involvement of the femoral head. Age younger than 9 years and less than 50% involvement of the femoral head are predictive factors for a good prognosis.[147] The younger the child is at the time of the onset of disease, the greater the time he or she has for subsequent growth and remodeling. Results of one study showed that 50% of patients who had childhood Perthes disease and did not receive treatment experienced osteoarthritis in the fifth decade of life.[148]

Perthes disease is specific to the hip joint and typically presents as an insidious, unilateral painless limp. If pain is present it is usually mild and is commonly referred to the knee. The most common physical examination findings

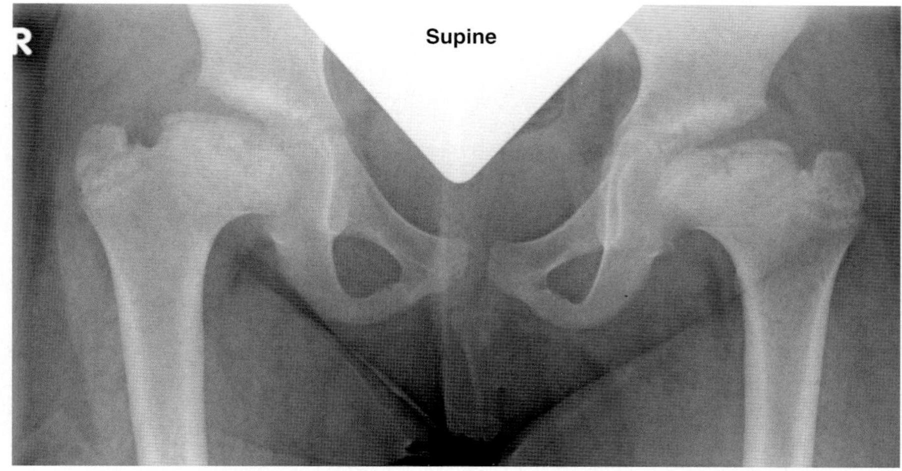

FIGURE 134-6 Bilateral Legg-Calvé-Perthes disease. The right side of the femoral head is in the reossification stage, whereas the left side is in the fragmentation stage.

include decreased internal rotation and abduction of the hip. Anteroposterior and lateral radiographs are diagnostic (Fig. 134-6). The goal of treatment is to try to contain the femoral head within the acetabulum, which can be performed by traction, casting, abduction bracing, tendon releases, or osteotomies of the femur or acetabulum. At present, conclusive data are lacking in the literature regarding the superiority of one treatment method over another. In patients with severe disease, surgical intervention appears to be preferable compared with nonoperative treatment. Patients older than 8 years with the classification of B or B/C according to Herring et al. have a better outcome with surgical intervention.[147] Adolescents with a history of Legg-Calvé-Perthes disease may present later in life with an abnormally shaped femoral head that predisposes them to FAI. A recent article on arthroscopic treat of residual cam deformity in four patients with Perthes disease showed restoration of hip geometry and good short-term results.[149]

Slipped Capital Femoral Epiphysis

SCFE involves the posterior displacement of the proximal femoral epiphysis with concomitant extension and external rotation of the femoral neck and shaft. It is a common hip disorder of adolescence, occurring most frequently in obese African American boys between 10 and 16 years of age.[150] SCFE is usually associated with pubertal growth but may be attributed to trauma, endocrine disorders, or inflammatory disorders. Increased body mass index is also a significant risk factor.[151] Bilateral involvement can occur in up to 60% of cases.[152] Classification of SCFE has been traditionally based on the acuity of symptoms and the severity of the slip; however, a greater emphasis is now being placed on the mechanical stability of the slip because it has a greater prognostic value. Patients with a mechanically stable slip can bear weight with or without crutches, whereas a patient with an unstable slip is unable to bear weight because of pain.[153] An unstable slip typically represents an acute physeal fracture with displacement.

Accurate, early diagnosis of SCFE is important to prevent short- and long-term complications, including chondrolysis of the joint and avascular necrosis of the femoral head. The average duration of symptoms is 5 months for stable slips; complaints are often insidious and ambiguous, with activity-related hip, thigh, or knee pain.[7] The delayed onset of significant pain and dysfunction may allow for progression of a stable to an unstable slip, which has major implications for long-term prognosis.[154] Physical examination shows obligate external rotation of the affected side, and anteroposterior and frog-leg lateral radiographs are diagnostic. If a slip is suspected but findings of plain films are negative, an MRI should be obtained (Fig. 134-7). Treatment is always operative, with the gold standard now involving in situ pinning with a single screw crossing the physis. Severe slips with significant deformity have recently been treated with a modified Dunn osteotomy with a surgical dislocation approach.[155-158] However, a clear relationship exists between stability and severity of the slip and the postoperative risk of avascular necrosis. Additionally, a cam lesion can develop at the time of the SCFE. Although remodeling can occur,[159,160] damage to the acetabular labrum and cartilage has been noted in both open and arthroscopic approaches.[161,162]

Conclusion

A multitude of injuries can occur in the area of the hip and pelvis; some occur as a result of a disease process, but most occur as the result of trauma. The prevention of such injuries in the adolescent and pediatric population is immensely important. Almost all sports involve the use of the lower extremity and core stability. A number of studies have linked the importance of core stability and the development of hip and pelvic injuries.[163-167] These studies underscore the importance of developing, strengthening, and maintaining the flexibility of the core muscle group. Improvement of the core muscle group can help decrease the likelihood and/or severity of hip and pelvic injury in adolescent athletes. Further research and programs to develop and improve strategies to prevent injury are warranted.

For a complete list of references, go to expertconsult.com.

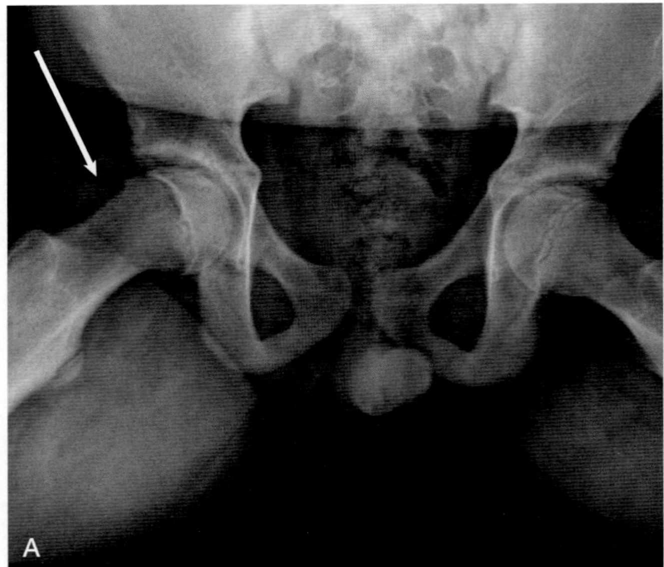

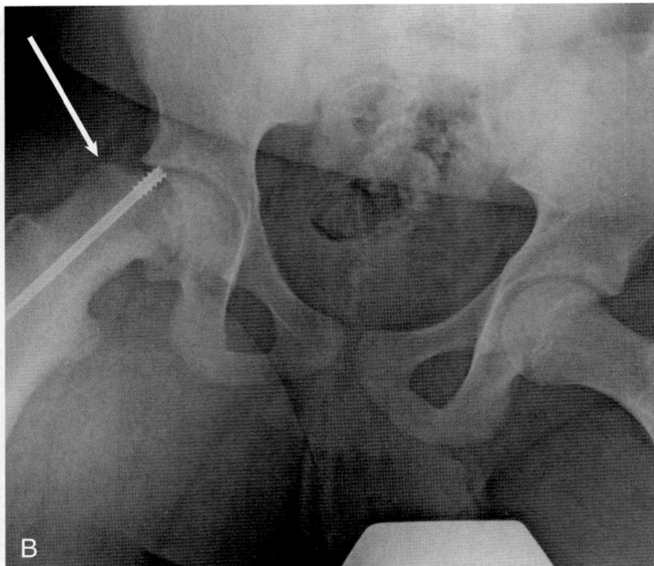

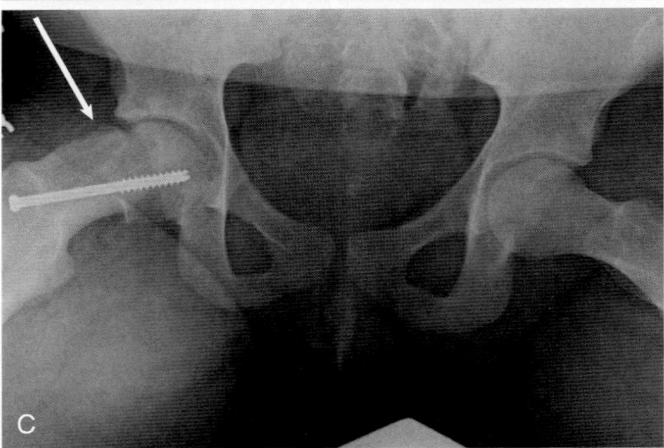

FIGURE 134-7 **A,** Mild slipped capital femoral epiphysis on the right hip that underwent in situ pinning with a single cannulated screw. The arrow depicts the slip. **B,** In the same patient, the epiphysis grew off the screw and continued to slip. The arrow shows the increase in the metaphyseal bump. **C,** After repinning of the slipped capital femoral epiphysis with fusion of the physis. The arrow shows the residual femoroacetabular impingement.

Suggested Readings

Citation: Rossi F, Dragoni S: Acute avulsion fractures of the pelvis in adolescent competitive athletes: Prevalence, location and sports distribution of 203 cases collected. *Skelet Radiol* 30(3):127–131, 2001.

Level of Evidence: IV

Summary: The authors provide a retrospective review of the prevalence, location, and sports distribution of pelvic avulsion fractures in adolescent patients. Soccer and gymnastics were the sports with the highest risk of these fractures, and the ischial tuberosity or attachment of the hamstring was the most common site of injury.

Citation: Wootton JR, Cross MJ, Holt KW: Avulsion of the ischial apophysis. The case for open reduction and internal fixation. *J Bone Joint Surg Br* 72B(4):625–627, 1990.

Level of Evidence: V

Summary: This small case series demonstrates that open reduction and internal fixation of ischial tuberosity fractures (the most common type of pelvic avulsion fractures) can lead to full function, including participation at the Olympics.

Citation: Milgrom C, Finestone A, Shlamkovitch N, et al: Youth is a risk factor for stress fracture. A study of 783 infantry recruits. *J Bone Joint Surg Br* 76(1):20–22, 1994.

Level of Evidence: IV

Summary: This study of a large prospective series of military recruits demonstrates that the risk of stress fracture was inversely proportional to age and that each year after about age 17 years reduced the stress fracture risk by 28%.

Citation: Mehlman CT, Hubbard GW, Crawford AH, et al: Traumatic hip dislocation in children. Long-term followup of 42 patients. *Clin Orthop Relat Res* (376):68–79, 2000.

Level of Evidence: IV

Summary: The authors report a long-term follow-up study of pediatric patients who underwent hip dislocation. A delay in reduction after 6 hours resulted in a 20-fold increase in avascular necrosis.

Citation: Minnich JM, Hanks JB, Muschaweck U, et al: Sports hernia: Diagnosis and treatment highlighting a minimal repair surgical technique. *Am J Sports Med* 39(6):1341–1349, 2011.

Level of Evidence: V

Summary: In this review of sports hernia diagnosis and treatment, good short-term results are shown using a newer minimally invasive surgical technique.

Citation: Dobbs MB, Gordon JE, Luhmann SJ, et al: Surgical correction of the snapping iliopsoas tendon in adolescents. *J Bone Joint Surg Am* 84A(3):420–424, 2002.

Level of Evidence: IV

Summary: The authors provide the first report of treatment of snapping iliopsoas tendon in adolescents with use of an open technique, with good results at 4 years with no subjective loss of strength.

Citation: Kocher MS, Kim YJ, Millis MB, et al: Hip arthroscopy in children and adolescents. *J Pediatr Orthop* 25(5):680–686, 2005.

Level of Evidence: IV

Summary: The authors provide the first published report on use of hip arthroscopy in the treatment of multiple pediatric disorders with good success.

Citation: Ganz R, Parvizi J, Beck M, et al: Femoroacetabular impingement: A cause for osteoarthritis of the hip. *Clin Orthop Relat Res* (417):112–120, 2003.
Level of Evidence: IV
Summary: The authors of this classic article describe the concept and possible etiology of femoroacetabular impingement.
Citation: Herring JA, Neustadt JB, Williams JJ, et al: The lateral pillar classification of Legg-Calve-Perthes disease. *J Pediatr Orthop* 12(2):143–150, 1992.
Level of Evidence: IV
Summary: The authors of this classic article describe the lateral pillar classification system in Legg-Calvé-Perthes disease. This classification system has a high correlation in asphericity of the femoral head at skeletal maturity.
Citation: Loder RT, Richards BS, Shapiro PS, et al: Acute slipped capital femoral epiphysis: The importance of physeal stability. *J Bone Joint Surg Am* 75A(8):1134–1140, 1993.
Level of Evidence: IV
Summary: The authors of this classic article describe the classification of slipped capital femoral epiphysis as stable or unstable.

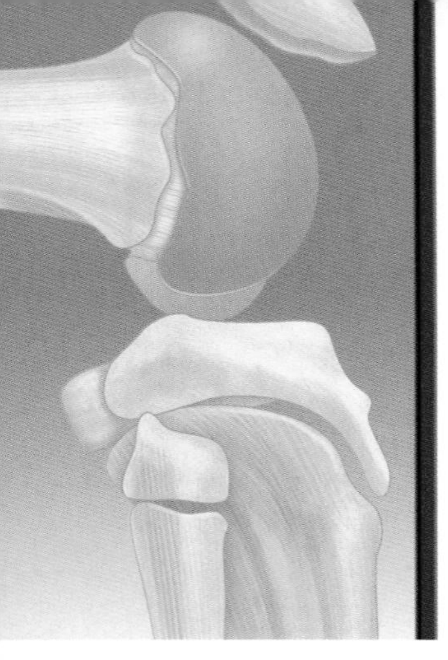

135

Knee Injuries in Skeletally Immature Athletes

MATTHEW D. MILEWSKI • STEPHAN J. SWEET • CARL W. NISSEN • TRICIA K. PROKOP

With the rapid increase in participation in youth athletics, the incidence of knee injuries among skeletally immature athletes has also risen dramatically. This increased participation in youth athletics has coincided with increased awareness of knee injuries among providers, including athletic trainers, physical therapists, and sports medicine physicians, along with improvements in diagnostic modalities such as ultrasound and magnetic resonance imaging (MRI), leading to a substantial increase in the incidence and prevalence of these injuries in young athletes. This chapter provides insight into the epidemiology, presentation, diagnosis, treatment, and rehabilitation of common sports-related knee injuries in skeletally immature athletes.

Anterior Cruciate Ligament Injuries

Injuries to the anterior cruciate ligament (ACL) in skeletally immature athletes were traditionally thought to be rare. Historically, the incidence of ACL rupture in this population was reported as 1% to 3.4%.[1-4] Avulsion of the tibial spine was reported to be more common than ACL rupture.[3] However, as awareness of these injuries has increased, and with improvements in diagnostic modalities, especially MRI, ACL rupture is increasingly recognized in skeletally immature athletes who present with a knee injury. Injuries to the ACL have been reported in children as young as 4 years of age.[5] In patients presenting with a hemathrosis, the incidence of ACL rupture has been reported to be between 26% and 65%.[6-9] It is now believed that the rate of ACL rupture in patients with open physes may exceed the rate of tibial spine fractures.[10] Whether a young athlete sustains an ACL rupture or a tibial spine fracture may depend on the loading rate at the time of injury and also the intercondylar notch.[11-13]

History and Physical Examination

Skeletally immature athletes who have sustained an ACL rupture present very similarly to more mature athletes with similar injuries. As stated previously, the rate of ACL injury in a patient presenting with a hemarthrosis approaches 70%.[14] Patients often state that during a pivoting or cutting activity they heard a "pop," felt immediate pain and swelling in the knee, and were unable to return to full activity. As with other populations, the skeletally immature athlete may sustain an ACL rupture after a contact injury, but noncontact injuries are more common. After such an injury, athletes may describe continued instability with cutting or pivoting activities or can often have symptoms even with activities of daily living.

On examination, skeletally immature athletes should be assessed for an effusion and range of motion (ROM); in addition, a neurovascular examination and standard knee ligament and hip and ankle assessments are required. Special attention should be directed to the Lachman, anterior drawer, and varus/valgus laxity tests both on the affected and contralateral knees because skeletally immature athletes can often have increased laxity globally, and asymmetry in their examinations is an important diagnostic criteria. Patients with a suspected ACL rupture should also be closely examined for pathologic meniscal findings, with an assessment of joint line tenderness, flexion pinch, and McMurray tests. An assessment of patellar instability is also crucial in this population of young athletes who present with a painful effusion because this diagnosis can often mimic an ACL injury.

Especially crucial to the examination of a skeletally immature patient with a potential ACL rupture is an assessment of physical maturity. Several methods may be used to assess physical maturity in adolescents. Tanner and Whitehouse[15] correlated physiologic development signs with height, weight, height velocity, and weight velocity. Tanner staging is the most common means of assessing physical maturity on physical examination. Although many pediatricians are familiar and comfortable with this staging assessment, many sports medicine physicians may be unfamiliar or uncomfortable with this process. Self-Tanner staging, intraoperative Tanner staging, and growth relative to family members can be used to supplement the physical examination.[16]

Imaging

Standard sports-oriented radiographs of the knee should be obtained for skeletally immature athletes presenting with a suspected ACL injury. These radiographs include a standing anteroposterior (AP), standing notch or tunnel view, and lateral and sunrise views to assess for associated injuries such as osteochondritis dissecans (OCD; seen best on the notch view), patellar subluxation (seen best on the Merchant view), tibial spine fracture (seen best on the lateral view), and physeal injuries. In cases in which surgical intervention is likely, a mechanical axis radiograph for limb length and a standardized posteroanterior radiograph of the left hand is recommended to determine bone age using the Greulich and Pyle atlas. Further mention of bone age in this chapter refers to this technique.[17] A simplified version of determining bone age has been recently developed.[17a] Often contralateral knee views are necessary to better assess any asymmetry in the physes if a distal femoral or proximal tibial physeal injury is suspected. A Segond fracture or lateral capsular avulsion adjacent to the proximal tibia can be seen and is highly correlated with an ACL injury.

MRI has increasingly become the modality of choice for imaging the ACL. Direct evidence of ACL injury on MRI includes discontinuity of ACL fibers in any three imaging planes and the "empty notch sign" in which fluid signal instead of ACL signal is seen at the proximal attachment site; this finding is best observed on T2-weighted images. In the acute setting, the injured or ruptured ACL can appear as an edematous mass with increased T2-weighted signal and abnormal morphologic features. In the subacute setting, it can appear discontinuous and less edematous with a more linear fragmented appearance, or it may even be completely absent in the chronic setting.[18,19] In some cases, a nearly normal ACL can be seen on the sagittal images when the ACL has sustained scarring down to the posterior cruciate ligament. This presentation also can be a point of confusion at the time of arthroscopy because the distal portion of the ACL can appear normal and can also create a pseudo end point on examination.

Indirect evidence on MRI of an ACL injury can include a hemarthrosis and a pivot-shift bone contusion, which is usually seen on the lateral femoral condyle and posterolateral tibial plateau. In addition, evidence of a deepened sulcus sign may be seen with an irregular-appearing lateral femoral condyle sulcus with a depth greater than 2 mm. Other indirect evidence of ACL injury on MRI includes a visible Segond fracture, the anterior drawer sign (i.e., increased anterior tibial translation), or buckling of the posterior cruciate ligament, which may be nonspecific.[20]

Decision-Making Principles

The decision to proceed with operative treatment of the ACL-deficient knee in a skeletally immature athlete is challenging and currently evolving for athletes, parents, and providers. The rationale for operative treatment of ACL injuries in skeletally immature patients is based on recent studies documenting the increased risk of meniscal damage, chondral damage, chronic instability, and inability to return to sports in these athletes.[21] These risks must be balanced against the potential complications associated with ACL reconstruction in this population, which include growth arrest with resulting angular deformity or leg-length discrepancy.

The risk of growth disturbance has been examined in numerous animals with use of a transphyseal reconstruction technique across open physes.[22-25] Guzzanti et al.[22] first demonstrated this risk in a rabbit model. Houle et al.[24] and Edwards and Grana[25] also showed significant risk of deformity with soft tissue grafts placed under tension across both canine and rabbit physes. Stadelmaier et al.[23] showed no evidence of physeal arrest when tension was not applied to soft tissue grafts.

Several clinical studies have reported growth disturbances associated with ACL reconstruction in the skeletally immature athlete.[3,26,27] Risk factors associated with growth disturbances and angular deformities include transphyseal hardware fixation or bone plugs and lateral extraarticular tenodesis. A recent metaanalysis reported a 1.8% overall risk of growth disturbance in skeletally immature athletes undergoing ACL reconstruction.[28]

Prevention

ACL injuries in all athletes can have serious short- and long-term consequences, especially in the youngest populations. Strategies to prevent these injuries have been developed and are becoming increasingly refined and important both on an individual and public health level.[29] These programs focus on education, stretching, proprioceptive training, plyometrics, sports-specific agility, jump and landing training, and progressive resistance weight training for the lower extremities.[30-34] Sports medicine providers may want to consider implementing these preventive training programs, especially for high school athletes. It is still unclear if pre–high school-aged patient populations are able to comply and take advantage of the benefits of these training programs.

Conservative Treatment

Traditional recommendations for the treatment of the ACL-deficient knee in the skeletally immature athlete included delayed surgical treatment until skeletal maturity with interim functional bracing, physical therapy, and activity modification.[4,35-38] Certain circumstances may dictate conservative treatment or a delay in surgical intervention, such as personal or medical reasons that would increase the risk of surgery or in the setting of an incomplete ACL tear without a secondary injury.

Treatment of Partial ACL Tears

Treatment of partial ACL tears in the skeletally immature athlete entails decision-making principles similar to those used in athletes with complete ACL tears. If the clinical examination and the patient's symptoms are consistent with instability with activities and the inability to return to sport, or if the patient has associated injuries such as meniscal tears or chondral damage indicative of an ACL-deficient knee or if recurrent effusions are present, a partial ACL tear should be considered functionally incompetent. If the young athlete's symptoms and examination findings are not indicative of instability, then conservative treatment with functional bracing, physical therapy, and activity modification could be considered.

Treatment Algorithm for ACL Reconstruction Based on Skeletal Maturity

Milewski et al.[16] have described an algorithm for deciding the operative surgical technique in skeletally immature athletes (Figs. 135-1 and 135-2). After appropriate decision making has been conducted and conservative treatment has been considered, skeletal age is determined by bone age using radiographs of the hand.

For prepubescent adolescents (i.e., those with a skeletal age <7 years), the physeal-sparing combined intraarticular and extraarticular reconstruction technique with an iliotibial band described by Kocher at al.[39] is recommended. Older

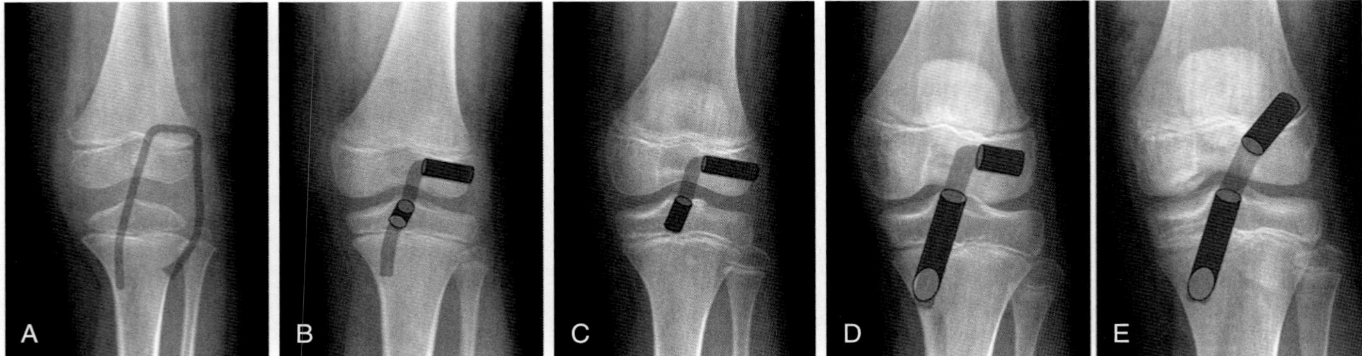

FIGURE 135-1 Radiographs revealing representative images of patients with bone ages of 6 to 14 years. **A,** Bone age of 6 years: Micheli-Kocher intraarticular extraarticular procedure. **B,** Bone age of 8 years: Anderson all-epiphyseal procedure, which has been modified. **C,** Bone age of 10 years: Ganley-Lawrence all-epiphyseal docking procedure. **D,** Bone age of 12 years: Hybrid all-epiphyseal femoral transphyseal tibial procedure. **E,** Bone age of 14 years: Transphyseal femoral and tibial reconstruction with soft tissue only at the level of the physis. *(From Milewski MD, Beck NA, Lawrence JT, et al: Anterior cruciate ligament reconstruction in the young athlete: a treatment algorithm for the skeletally immature.* Clin Sports Med *30[4]:801–810, 2011.)*

children with a small lateral femoral condyle may also be appropriate candidates for this technique.

For athletes with a skeletal age of 7 to 12 years, an all-epiphyseal reconstruction as described by Lawrence et al.[40] is advocated. Ganley has recommended a modification to this technique, and the technique is described by Anderson[41] for use in adolescents who have less than 20 mm of epiphyseal length. In these patients, cortical button fixation is used on both the femur and tibia for an all-epiphyseal tunnel procedure with a hamstring autograft.

For 13-year-old female athletes and 13- to 14-year-old male athletes, transphyseal reconstruction with a quadrupled hamstring autograft is recommended. This procedure can be modified using the hybrid anatomic technique with an all-epiphyseal femoral tunnel and a transphyseal tibial tunnel if a significant amount of growth is believed to remain and if the surgeon prefers to use the newer anatomic ACL techniques of centering the tunnels within the anatomic footprint.

Treatment

ACL Reconstruction Techniques

Once operative treatment of an ACL-deficient knee is elected, it must be decided whether to use a physeal-sparing or physeal-respecting technique or a traditional technique for

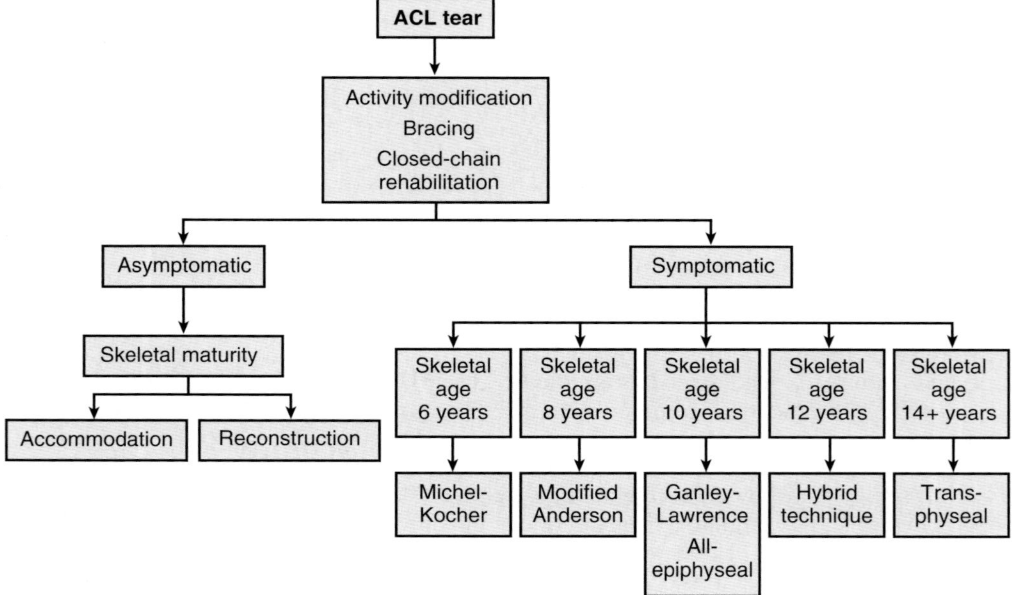

FIGURE 135-2 A treatment algorithm for patients with a ruptured anterior cruciate ligament (ACL). After a trial of activity modification, bracing, and closed-chain rehabilitation, symptomatic patients are candidates for surgical reconstruction. Prepubescent patients are at greatest risk for growth disturbances, and physeal-sparing techniques such as an all-epiphyseal or combined intraarticular and extraarticular reconstruction are used. Soft tissue transphyseal reconstruction is performed on older/postpubescent patients. *(From Milewski MD, Beck NA, Lawrence JT, et al: Anterior cruciate ligament reconstruction in the young athlete: a treatment algorithm for the skeletally immature.* Clin Sports Med *30[4]:801–810, 2011.)*

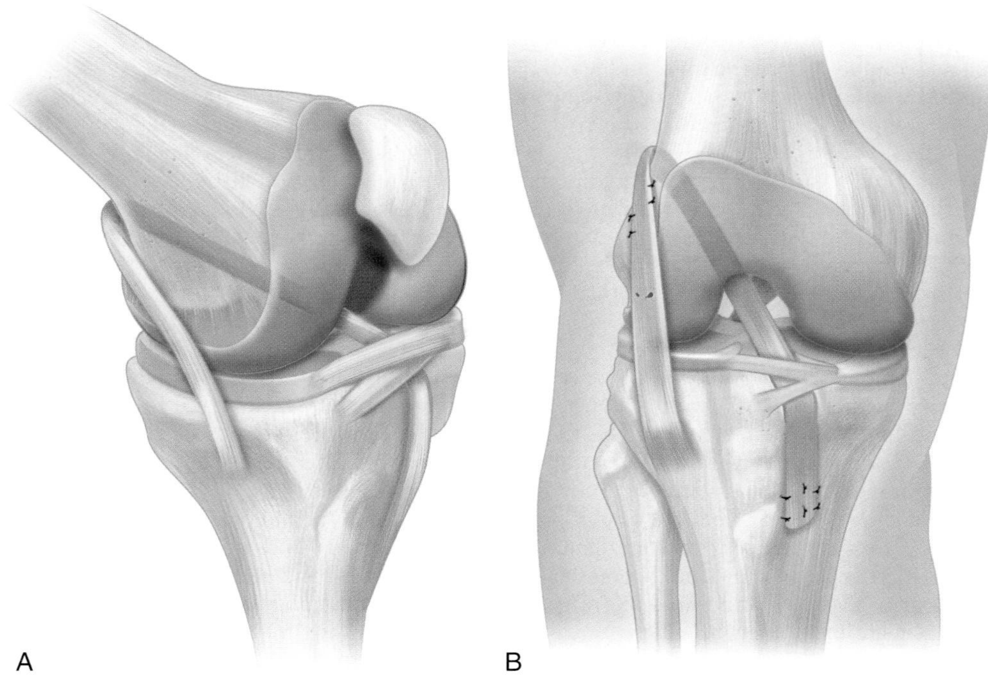

FIGURE 135-3 **A** and **B,** The iliotibial band graft is passed over the top of the lateral femoral condyle, through the knee, under the intermeniscal ligament, and into the groove in the proximal tibia. The graft is sutured to the lateral femoral condyle with the knee in 90 degrees of flexion and 15 degrees of external rotation. It is then sutured to the periosteum of the proximal tibia with the knee in 20 degrees of flexion. *(From Scott WN, editor:* Insall and Scott surgery of the knee, *ed 5, New York, 2012, Elsevier.)*

ACL reconstruction. Physeal-sparing techniques for ACL reconstruction were initially described with use of patellar tendon grafts without drill holes by DeLee and Curtis[2] and using hamstring tendon grafts by Brief[42] and Parker et al.[43]

Kocher et al.[39] have described and advocated use of a physeal-sparing combined intraarticular and extraarticular reconstruction with an autogenous iliotibial band in prepubescent children who are at Tanner stage 1 or 2. This reconstruction technique has no bone tunnels and incorporates a lateral extraarticular iliotibial band reconstruction to help control rotation as described by Losee et al.[44] (Fig. 135-3).

Anderson,[41] as well as Guzzanti et al.,[45] have described physeal-sparing hamstring graft reconstruction techniques. Both techniques require extraosseous tensioning of the graft across the tibial physis. Anderson's reconstruction technique uses a hamstring graft tensioned across epiphyseal tunnels in the femur and tibia with the graft extending out of the tibial tunnel and across the tibial physis and attached with a screw and post construct in the tibial metaphysis.

Lawrence and colleagues at Children's Hospital of Philadelphia have recently described an all-epiphyseal ACL technique using femoral and tibial epiphyseal tunnels confirmed with intraoperative computed tomography (CT).[40] Use of an intraoperative CT scan or fluoroscopy is necessary to avoid the physes (Fig. 135-4).

More traditional transphyseal reconstruction techniques have also been used in skeletally immature athletes.[46,47] These techniques become more appropriate as the patient approaches skeletal maturity. Aronowitz et al.[46] and Kocher et al.[48] have shown that Tanner stage 3 athletes have little risk of angular

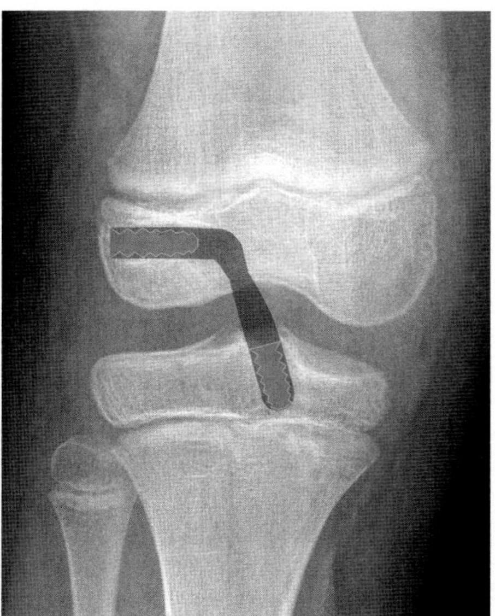

FIGURE 135-4 The Ganley/Lawrence all-epiphyseal anterior cruciate ligament reconstruction with tunnel placement, with fixation within the epiphyses. *(From Milewski MD, Beck NA, Lawrence JT, et al: Anterior cruciate ligament reconstruction in the young athlete: a treatment algorithm for the skeletally immature.* Clin Sports Med *30[4]:801–810, 2011.)*

deformity or leg-length discrepancy. Shea et al.[49] used MRI of children's knees to show that drill holes could ideally affect less than 5% of the total volume of both the tibial and femoral physes and was central in the tibia but more peripheral in the femur, which was hypothesized to increase the risk of growth arrest.

Investigators in many older series relied on traditional transtibial tunnel drilling for transphyseal reconstructions. The more vertical tunnels used in these techniques may minimize physeal damage by producing a hole of a smaller aperture in the physis. However, the vertical graft position may not fully restore the normal kinematics of the knee and may be less "anatomic" by centering less graft in the anatomic ACL footprint. Independent femoral drilling techniques such as those using an accessory medial portal, a two-incision technique, or a retrograde drilling outside-in technique have been advocated to place the femoral tunnel within the anatomic footprint.[50] In skeletally immature athletes with open physes, Nelson and Miller[51] have shown that the femoral tunnel produced by these drilling techniques crosses the lateral femoral physis obliquely and eccentrically and would potentially damage a much larger area of physis and perichondral ring than a more vertical, less anatomic tunnel. Given the increased risk of growth disturbance with these newer anatomic reconstruction techniques, an all-epiphyseal femoral tunnel combined with a traditional transphyseal tibial tunnel hybrid technique may be used (Fig. 135-5).[16,51]

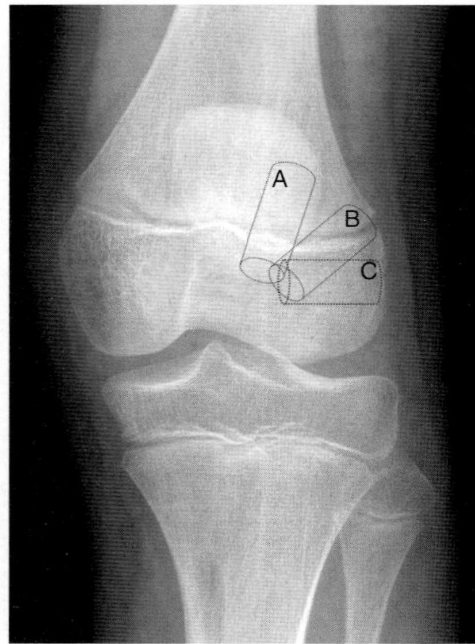

FIGURE 135-5 The amount and location of femoral physis affected using different operative techniques. **A,** The location of a vertically orientated tunnel, which affects less of the femoral physis but is typically outside the native anterior cruciate ligament (ACL) footprint. **B,** The location of a classic anatomic accessory medial portal, or outside-in technique, that places the tunnel anatomically in the ACL footprint but affects a large portion of the distal femoral physis. **C,** The location of a femoral tunnel, which is in the anatomic center of the ACL footprint within the epiphysis in a trajectory. It avoids the femoral physis. *(From Milewski MD, Beck NA, Lawrence JT, et al: Anterior cruciate ligament reconstruction in the young athlete: a treatment algorithm for the skeletally immature.* Clin Sports Med *30[4]:801–810, 2011.)*

Postoperative Management and Rehabilitation

Postoperative rehabilitation after ACL reconstruction in the skeletally immature athlete is similar to the approaches used in more mature athletes. It is generally recommended that postoperative rehabilitation be divided into phases with specific criteria for progression. Emphasis on attainment of these goals rather than a precise postoperative time frame allows adaptations to be made as needed for the skeletally immature athlete.

The focus of the first phase of rehabilitation is to decrease postoperative impairments while protecting the patient and the surgical intervention. Goals for this phase are to decrease pain and joint effusion, obtain full knee extension and 90 degrees of knee flexion, and restore patella mobility and volitional quadriceps activation.[53,54] The goals of the second postoperative phase are to eliminate pain and effusion, progress toward full knee flexion, restore normal ambulation, improve proprioception, and progress strengthening of quadriceps and hamstrings.[53,54] Postoperative rehabilitation should emphasize strengthening and neuromuscular control to allow the patient to initiate running and plyometric training during the third phase.[53,54]

To obtain significant improvements in knee strength and overall function, strengthening exercises should be performed both in the open and closed kinetic chain position.[55] It has been shown that open kinetic chain knee extension exercises performed isotonically between the ranges of 90 and 40 degrees of knee flexion and isometrically at 90, 60, or 0 degrees of knee flexion increase strength and minimize patellofemoral joint stress while allowing for protection of the graft.[56-61]

Additionally, closed kinetic chain strengthening exercises should be implemented as dictated by weight-bearing status, pain control, and range of motion. Closed kinetic chain exercises not only assist in strengthening but also are functional and emphasize co-contraction and neuromuscular control. Knee flexion ROM should be limited to between 0 and 60 degrees during closed chain strengthening to decrease stress placed on the ACL graft and patellofemoral joint.[58,60]

Additional emphasis should be placed on strengthening and neuromuscular training of the hip and core of athletes after ACL reconstruction. Impairments in transverse plane hip motions, frontal plane knee motions, and trunk displacement have been shown to increase risk of ACL injury, especially in female athletes.[62-65] Injury prevention training with a focus on strengthening and lower extremity alignment has demonstrated improvements in hip and knee kinematics in female athletes.[66]

Return to play is not based on one specific criterion but instead on a constellation of criteria including ROM, proprioception, functional strength, and knee/graft stability.[67] In general, most skeletally immature athletes are able to return to sports approximately 6 to 12 months after undergoing their reconstruction. Some authors have advocated bracing during participation in athletics after combined extraarticular and intraarticular iliotibial extraphyseal reconstruction has been performed.[68]

Complications

The most serious complications of ACL injuries and reconstructions in skeletally immature patients are those associated

AUTHORS' PREFERRED TECHNIQUE

ACL Reconstruction

- Given the increased incidence of secondary injuries and less optimal outcomes with conservative or delayed reconstructive procedures in skeletally immature athletes, we attempt to schedule ACL reconstruction within the first 3 to 5 weeks after the injury.
  - Elimination of effusion and regaining full ROM are preferred.
  - Inability to gain full, painless ROM often denotes displaced meniscal fragments. In this case, earlier intervention is appropriate.
  - Patients should be encouraged to use crutches until ambulation without a limp is achieved.
  - Crutch use after ambulation without a limp is preferred to prevent meniscal injury.
- Our graft choice is uniformly hamstring autografts in these primary ACL reconstructions.
  - Although grafts smaller than 8 mm have been shown to have an increased rate of failure,[52] we have not found this to be true in midterm follow-up and therefore continue to use these grafts even when grafts with a diameter of 6 mm are present.
- The determination of which physeal-respecting approach we use depends on the skeletal age of the patient and relative remaining growth as determined by a posteroanterior radiograph of the left hand.
- Our approach for prepubescent athletes is to perform an all-epiphyseal reconstruction with fixation performed within the physis. Combined intraarticular and extraarticular reconstruction that spares the physes can also be used in this population, especially if the patient's skeleton is very immature or the epiphysis is insufficient for adequate tunnel lengths.
  - Use of fluoroscopy or an intraoperative CT scan is essential to ensure that femoral and tibial tunnels appropriately respect the femoral and tibial physes.
  - Setting up the C-arm or intraoperative CT scanner before beginning the operation is helpful so that "real time" drilling with guidance can be performed.
  - The proximal tibial epiphyseal tunnel should generally be at least 20 mm to attempt an all-epiphyseal ACL reconstruction to ensure an adequate length of graft in the tunnel for fixation and incorporation.
  - Tibial and femoral drilling can be performed with a retrograde drill such as the FlipCutter (Arthrex, Naples, FL) using fluoroscopic guidance.
  - Placing a small-diameter Kirschner wire prior to drilling with the retrograde drill is useful to ensure that tunnel placement successfully avoids the physes. These drill systems are not cannulated, and thus the guide wire is removed prior to drilling.
  - Fixation can be performed with interference screws as initially described or with loop fixation for both the femoral and tibial portions.[40]
- In pubescent patients we perform a hybrid fixation with epiphyseal fixation on the femur and transphyseal drilling on the tibia and fixation distal to the tibial physis and apophysis.
  - Fluoroscopy is again key to successfully avoiding the femoral physis. It can also be used to measure the distance from the tibial aperture to the tibial physis for appropriate tibial screw length.
  - Tibial tunnel placement should be made as vertical as possible to minimize the aperture created in the physis.
- In late pubescent patients, fixation is performed with loop fixation on the femur and expansion devices on the tibia.
- Transphyseal femoral tunnels, when used, should attempt to cross the femoral physis as centrally as possible without jeopardizing the femoral tunnel footprint to lessen the possibility of differential physeal growth.

with growth disturbances. Findings of animal studies and anecdotal reports of human growth disturbances demonstrate that these concerns are valid. The possibility of growth disturbance needs to be fully disclosed and discussed with patients and their families. The appropriate approach then needs to chosen given the patient's skeletal age, and long-term follow-up is necessary to watch for the earliest signs of any growth disturbance, including useof long leg mechanical axis radiographs until skeletal maturity is achieved.

Future Direction

The increased incidence of ACL injuries in skeletally immature athletes has increased the need to look deeper into the issues surrounding this devastating injury. The most important questions that need to be studied and answered are the long-term outcome with regard to function and arthritic conditions of the different techniques.

Meniscal Injuries

The incidence of meniscal tears in skeletally immature athletes has been increasing,[69] likely because of improved awareness by sports medicine providers, increased youth sports participation, and increased use of advanced imaging such as MRI. Identifying and treating these meniscal injuries in young athletes is crucial to maintaining normal joint mechanics and preserving and protecting articular cartilage. Preserving as much of the meniscus as possible is crucial, especially in the adolescent athlete, because of the long-term consequences of aggressive debridement.[70]

Development

The meniscus forms by 8 weeks of embryologic development (Fig. 135-6). By week 14 it has a normal anatomic appearance.[71] The entire meniscus is vascularized during the fetal

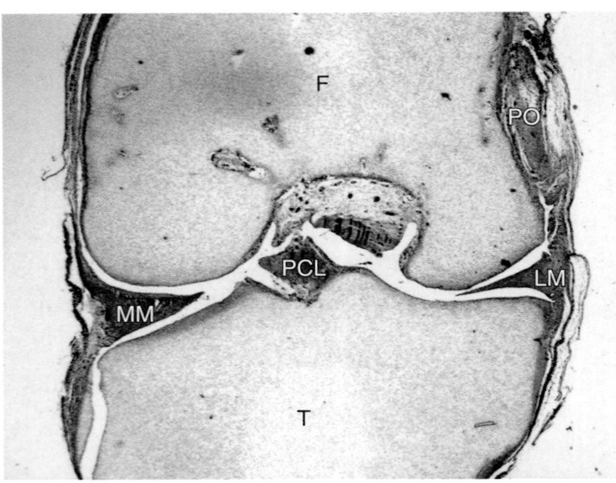

FIGURE 135-6 Fetus HK24F, 12.5 weeks old, frontal section (see text). *F,* Femur; *LM,* lateral meniscus; *MM,* medial meniscus; *PCL,* posterior cruciate ligament; *PO,* popliteus muscle; *T,* tibia (Goldner, ×20). *(From Scott WN, editor:* Insall and Scott surgery of the knee, *ed 5, New York, 2012, Elsevier.)*

period, but this vascularization gradually recedes by age 9 months, with the central third already avascular at this point in development.[72] By 10 years of age, the meniscus has developed its adult structure, with only the peripheral 10% to 30% of the medial meniscus and only the peripheral 10% to 25% of the lateral meniscus receiving a direct vascular supply.[73]

Anatomy

The meniscus consists of type I collagen fibers that are arranged in a circumferential pattern parallel to its long axis with radial, oblique, and vertical fibers that reduce hoop stresses.[74] Inferior meniscal surfaces are flat, whereas the superior surfaces are concave. This shape allows for conformity of the femoral condyles with the tibial plateau surfaces. The meniscus is thus able to increase contact area and congruency, thereby reducing contact stresses and aiding in shock absorption. The medial meniscus is C-shaped; it covers approximately 50% of the medial tibial plateau and attaches to the medial joint capsule by the meniscotibial and coronary ligaments. It is able to translate approximately 2.5 mm posteriorly with femoral rollback during knee flexion. The lateral meniscus is circular, covering approximately 70% of the lateral tibial plateau. There are no attachments to the capsule at the popliteal hiatus, and the lateral meniscus translates 9 to 11 mm with knee flexion.[74,75] The ligaments of Humphrey and Wrisberg are accessory meniscofemoral ligaments that are present in up to 84% of people.[76]

History and Physical Examination

In adolescents, nondiscoid meniscus injuries are usually a result of trauma during sports and typically involve a twisting injury or directional change. Pain is usually the chief complaint, but effusion, giving way, and mechanical symptoms such as snapping, catching, and locking also may be present. In one study, meniscal tears were found in 47% of preadolescents (aged 7 to 12 years) and 45% of adolescents (aged 13 to 18 years) with an acute traumatic knee hemathrosis.[8] In both age groups the authors found that the medial meniscus was most commonly injured (70% in preadolescents and 88% in adolescents). A possible ACL tear should always be suspected in this population because 36% of the adolescents in this series with meniscal injuries also had an ACL tear.

On examination, effusion is usually indicative of intraarticular pathologic conditions in this age group. Skeletally immature athletes with meniscal injuries often have joint line tenderness on palpation. It is sometimes difficult to examine children with a painful knee, and they might not tolerate full ROM. One option is to use a modified McMurray maneuver, which involves pain with rotational varus or valgus stress at 30 to 40 degrees of knee flexion. It is always important to check ACL integrity with a Lachman test and compare it with the contralateral side because a high correlation exists with meniscus disease. The Lachman test is a reliable indicator of ACL injury. KT-1000 measurements were found to be increased in younger patients when measuring anterior tibial translation.[77] When physical examination was performed by experienced examiners, Kocher et al.[78] found that it was 62% sensitive and 81% specific for medial meniscus tears and 50% sensitive and 89% specific for lateral meniscus tears.

Imaging

Initial workup should include standard AP, lateral, tunnel, and sunrise radiographic views. These views are helpful in detecting patellar dislocation, osteochondral fractures, physeal fractures, and loose bodies. The tunnel view is included to evaluate for osteochondritis desiccans. The sunrise view may show patellar subluxation.

When the history and physical examination are suggestive of a meniscal tear and radiographs are normal, an MRI is usually ordered. Compared with adults, MRI in children has lower sensitivity and specificity in assessing meniscus tears because of the higher vascularity of a child's meniscus, which appears as intrameniscal enhancement, resembling meniscal tears.[79] Children younger than 12 years were found to have 62% sensitivity and 78% specificity compared with 90% sensitivity and 96% specificity in children between the ages of 12 and 16 years.[78] When evaluating an MRI for a meniscal tear, one should look for the enhancement to extend to the superior or inferior surface of the meniscus.

Decision-Making Principles

The basic principle in the treatment of meniscal injuries in children and adolescents is to preserve as much meniscal tissue as possible to minimize subsequent articular cartilage degeneration. The developing meniscus has an increased potential for healing because of its increased vascularity. When the history, physical examination, and imaging are consistent with meniscal injury and appropriate conservative options have been tried or considered, then surgery can be recommended in the skeletally immature patient.

Treatment Options

Nonoperative

After a meniscal injury is confirmed, initial management with conservative treatment including rest, activity modification, physical therapy for strengthening, and possible bracing can be considered. This approach is usually recommended for patients without mechanical symptoms or with imaging findings that are inconclusive or indeterminate. If the patient remains asymptomatic, then initial nonsurgical management can be continued.

Operative

Symptomatic meniscal tears in children and adolescents that have failed to respond to conservative treatment are usually treated surgically. Longitudinal tears in the red-red zone that measure 10 mm or less and are manually displaceable less than 3 mm may heal without repair.[80] Arthroscopic partial meniscectomy is most commonly performed but does produce increased contact stresses. Cadaver studies showed a 65% increase in contact stress when removing small bucket-handle medial meniscus tears. Debridement of the posterior horn of the medial meniscus can increase contact stresses almost to the level of a total meniscectomy, which is 235% of normal.[81] Authors of one study with a 5.5-year follow-up in 20 patients with an average age of 15 years old who underwent partial or total meniscectomy found that 75% were still symptomatic, 80% had radiographic evidence of osteoarthritis, and 60% were dissatisfied with their results.[70] At 10- to 20-year follow-up, 50% of patients who underwent a total meniscectomy had evidence of osteoarthritis based on radiographic evidence, symptoms, and functional loss.[82] Current indications for a partial meniscectomy in the skeletally immature athlete include irreparable meniscal tears such as radial tears, horizontal cleavage tears, and a complex degenerative tear in the white-white zone. It is preferred that as limited a partial meniscectomy as possible be performed for a damaged, unstable meniscus. A total meniscectomy is contraindicated.

Many meniscus tears in skeletally immature patients can be repaired. The types of tears most amenable to repair include longitudinal tears in the red-red zone or red-white zone, bucket-handle tears without significant injury to the bucket-handle fragment, and lateral meniscus posterior horn tears, which have a good vascular supply. All techniques first require debridement of loose degenerative edges and rasping of the perimeniscal synovial edges or trephination into the peripheral zone to promote vascular inflow to the repair site. The inside-out vertical mattress suture technique is still considered the gold standard. It uses absorbable or nonabsorbable suture with flexible needles that are placed through the meniscus in vertical or horizontal fashion and are tied down over the capsule through a separate incision. When repairing posterior horn tears, a posterolateral or posteromedial approach must be made to protect the posterior neurovascular structures with retractors. An outside-in technique is often helpful for isolated anterior horn tears or anterior portions of bucket-handle tears. If needed, open repairs can be performed through either posterolateral or posteromedial incisions for peripheral tears and are useful for posterior horn medial meniscal tears in patients with tight medial compartments.[83] All-inside techniques have gained popularity again. Previously, these techniques included use of devices such as darts, arrows, and screws to anchor the meniscal tear to the capsule or peripheral meniscus. Unfortunately, they did not have the ability to compress across the tear site. Newer repair systems are suture based and provide the ability to compress at the tear site.

Postoperative Management

Postoperative management after meniscal surgery in skeletally immature patients is similar to management in adults, with the understanding that postoperative restrictions are often more difficult in this population. Before the surgery is performed, both the young athlete and his or her family must understand the expectations for activity restriction and rehabilitation after surgery. If bracing, weight-bearing restrictions, or specific rehabilitation protocols will need to be followed postoperatively, improved compliance will be achieved if the family is counseled appropriately before surgery.

Postoperative protocols are typically separated into meniscal repair and transplantation or meniscectomy. It is essential that the physical therapist be informed of the type of surgical intervention performed, because variations in postoperative protocols are made according to the type, location, and size of the meniscal injury.[84] Concomitant procedures such as ligamentous reconstructions or comorbidities such as articular cartilage damage also affect the potential for rehabilitation and the plan of care.[84]

Most surgeons allow patients who have had partial meniscectomies to begin weight bearing as tolerated immediately. Rehabilitation after a meniscectomy can progress as tolerated with the initial goals of eliminating pain and effusion, attaining knee ROM of 0 to 90 degrees with good patellar mobility, ambulating without an antalgic gait, and regaining volitional neuromuscular control of the lower extremity. Full and painless knee ROM should be obtained approximately 6 weeks after the operation.[84] Ongoing rehabilitation should emphasize strengthening of the lower extremities while progressing toward return to the previous level of function by the third postoperative month.

For isolated meniscal repairs, many surgeons restrict weight bearing for up to 6 weeks and restrict ROM in a hinged knee brace to minimize joint compressive forces and shear stresses, especially in the extreme range of flexion. The initial phases of rehabilitation emphasize decreasing pain and swelling, improving ROM, and regaining volitional quadriceps activation while protecting the surgical repair. Therapeutic exercises and neuromuscular training should progress in a manner consistent with postoperative ROM and weight-bearing guidelines. Return to sport after isolated meniscal repair is generally allowed 3 to 6 months after the operation if the young athlete has regained full ROM and adequate strength and remains asymptomatic. Regardless of the type of surgical intervention, patients should be monitored for pain in the tibiofemoral compartment, painful clicking at the knee, lack of progress with ROM, decreased patellar mobility, or persistent joint effusion.[84]

Results

The results of partial or total meniscectomies in children and adolescents are poor, with early onset of osteoarthritis.[70,81] Although increased success rates are associated with meniscal repairs in younger patients, few long-term outcome studies have been performed regarding meniscal repair in this age group. In one series of 29 arthroscopic meniscal repairs in 26 patients with a mean age of 15.3 years, no meniscal symptoms were noted at an average of 5 years of follow-up, and 24 of

26 patients returned to their preinjury level of sports activity. Of note, 15 of 26 patients had a simultaneous ACL reconstruction, all the tears were in the posterior horn of either the medial or lateral meniscus, and 22 of the 29 tears were in the red-red zone. The mean time between injury and surgery was 6.7 months. Twenty-five repairs were performed with the inside-out technique, and four were performed with an all-inside technique.[85] In another series of 71 meniscal repairs in adolescents with a mean age of 16 years, clinical healing was seen in 75% at a mean 51-month follow-up. All tears extended into the avascular white-white zone and were repaired with use of an inside-out technique. In patients undergoing a simultaneous ACL reconstruction, the success rate was even higher at 87%.

Complications

Complications from arthroscopic partial or total meniscectomy or meniscal repair are rare but may include painful neuroma, arthrofibrosis, complex regional pain syndrome, and iatrogenic chondral injury from the surgery or from a protruding implant.

Future Considerations

Although short-term and midterm results are encouraging for meniscal repair, especially in the setting of simultaneous ACL reconstruction, long-term results are needed to determine if newer techniques for meniscal preservation are successful in decreasing the risk of osteoarthritis in the future for these skeletally immature athletes.

Discoid Meniscus

The discoid meniscus was first described by Young in 1887 after cadaveric dissection. It is almost exclusively found in the lateral meniscus and in some studies has been shown to have a higher prevalence of approximately 15% in Asian populations; however, it has a prevalence of only 3% to 5% in the U.S. population.[86] Approximately 20% of patients with a discoid meniscus have bilateral discoid menisci. The true prevalence of discoid menisci is unknown because many discoid menisci are asymptomatic.

Discoid menisci generally occupy greater than normal coverage of the lateral tibial plateau and are uniformly thickened. They can represent a spectrum of meniscal morphologic features and stability. Discoid menisci are thought to be a congenital anomaly because menisci are not discoid-shaped during development. Increased meniscal thickness and width may also be due to compensatory changes for an unstable meniscus during development.[87]

Classification

The Watanabe classification system is most commonly used (Fig. 135-7).[88] This classification system describes three types of discoid meniscus based on arthroscopic appearance and stability of the meniscus. Type I (stable, complete) menisci are stable to probing and complete; the meniscus is block shaped and covers the entire lateral tibial plateau. Type II (stable, incomplete) menisci cover 80% of less of the tibial plateau. Type III menisci, also known as the Wrisberg variant (unstable), have a thickened posterior horn but otherwise appear normal. They lack posterior meniscal attachments with the exception of the meniscofemoral ligament of Wrisberg, which causes the lateral meniscus to have posterior horn hypermobility. When the knee goes into extension, the posterior horn can be pulled into the intercondylar notch and can result in snapping knee syndrome. Klingele et al.[89] examined peripheral rim instability patterns of 128 discoid menisci. They found that 62.1% were complete and 37.9% were incomplete. Peripheral rim instability was found in 28.1%, of which 47.2% occurred in the anterior horn, 38.9% in the posterior horn, and 11.1% in the middle third. Peripheral instability was more common in younger patients, with a mean age of 8.2 years, and in patients with complete discoid lateral menisci.

History and Physical Examination

The clinical presentation of a discoid meniscus may vary. Stable discoid menisci usually are first noticed in older children who present with mechanical knee symptoms similar to those of a meniscal tear. These stable menisci are prone to tearing because of increased thickness and abnormal vascularity.[72] Compared with normal menisci, discoid menisci

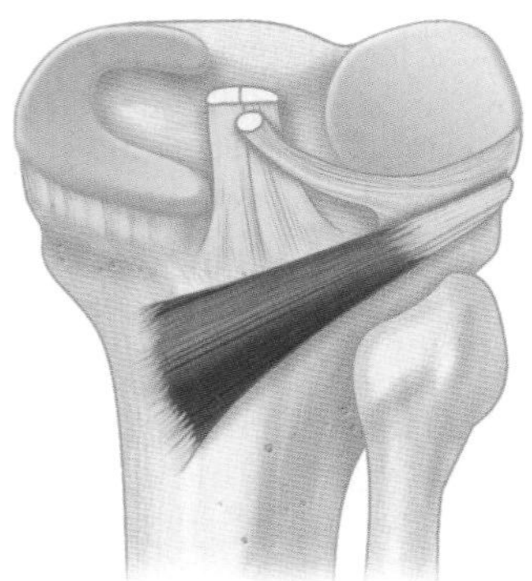

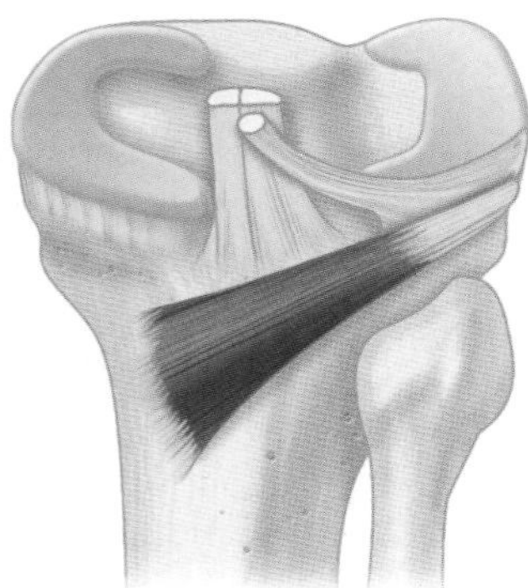

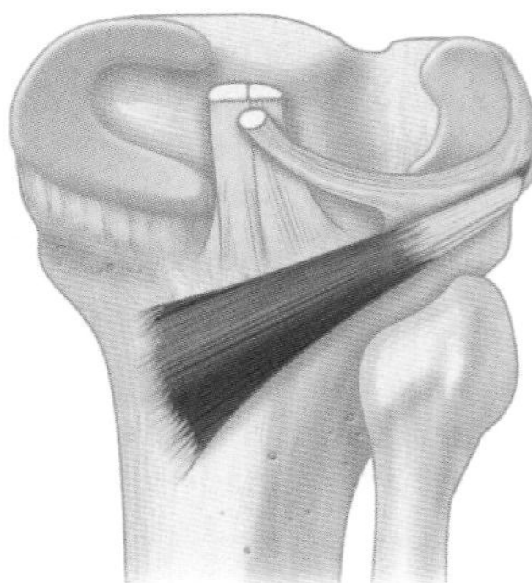

FIGURE 135-7 The Watanabe classification of discoid lateral meniscus. Type I is a complete variant, type II is a partial variant, and type III is a Wrisberg variant. *(From Scott WN, editor:* Insall and Scott surgery of the knee*, ed 5, New York, 2012, Elsevier.)*

have also been shown on transmission electron microscopy to have a decreased number of collagen fibers with a more disorganized pattern.[90] Discoid menisci without an associated tear are often asymptomatic and are often found incidentally on MRI or during knee arthroscopy.

Children with unstable discoid menisci often present with intermittent snapping and popping within the knee. This phenomenon is called "snapping knee syndrome" and usually occurs when the knee is brought from flexion to extension; it may cause pain and apprehension.[91] Unstable discoid menisci are usually found in younger patients with a Wrisberg type I discoid appearing morphology, in which the meniscus is a solid block covering the entire tibial plateau.[89]

Physical examination findings can include joint effusion, limited motion, terminal extension discomfort, a lateral joint line bulge, joint line tenderness to palpation, and pain or popping during the McMurray test. This popping during the McMurray test is a result of subluxation of the unstable lateral meniscus. Very often a lack of terminal extension mimicking a knee flexion contracture is present in children with discoid menisci. It is always important to examine and assess the symptom history of the contralateral knee as well because of the high rate of bilateral discoid menisci.

Imaging

Standard knee radiographs are normal in most children with discoid menisci, but some radiographs occasionally indicate subtle findings, such as squaring of the lateral femoral condyle, a widened lateral joint line, cupping of the lateral tibial plateau, and mild hypoplasia of the tibial spine.

MRI is the radiographic study of choice for diagnosing a discoid meniscus. The diagnosis is made if the transverse meniscal diameter is greater than 15 mm or 20% of the tibial width on coronal views, or if continuity of the anterior and posterior horns of the lateral meniscus is seen on three or more consecutive sagittal images of 5-mm thickness.[92,93] Types II (incomplete) and III (Wrisberg variant) discoid menisci may appear normal on MRI. However, type III discoid menisci may appear to have some minimal posterior horn anterior subluxation or have a high signal on T2-weighted images between the lateral meniscus and joint capsule, resembling a peripheral tear appearance.[94] MRI has been shown to have low sensitivity (38.9%) in diagnosing a discoid lateral meniscus in children compared with a 88.9% sensitivity of physical examination.[95]

Decision-Making Principles

If a discoid meniscus is asymptomatic and found incidentally, it should be treated with observation. The knee is functioning well and may have adapted to this abnormal anatomy. Surgery is indicated in patients with symptomatic discoid menisci for whom conservative management has failed, similar to the management of normal meniscal tears. This surgical indication includes discoid menisci with or without an associated tear as defined on MRI.

Treatment Options

After it has been decided that a symptomatic discoid meniscus will be managed arthroscopically, the first issue to address is the size. This issue is addressed with a partial meniscectomy, also called *saucerization*. Saucerization is performed to create a stable and functional remaining meniscus that will provide adequate shock absorption. A minimum of 6 to 8 mm of the peripheral rim is left intact. Larger peripheral rims have been shown to have higher repeat tear rates.[96] This remnant peripheral rim may be thicker than a normal meniscus and may require an undersurface debridement to recreate a more normal structure.

If peripheral instability occurs after saucerization, meniscal repair to the capsule is performed. Meniscal tears after saucerization are repaired in the same fashion as a nondiscoid meniscus tear. Remaining tears that cannot be repaired undergo debridement to a stable rim. If a horizontal cleavage tear remains, then the unstable leaflet is usually debrided.

A total meniscectomy is rarely performed in children and adolescents; it is generally reserved for only the most difficult of unsalvageable cases.

Postoperative Management

Postoperative management is similar to that of other pathologic meniscal conditions. Immediate weight bearing is usually allowed after saucerization alone. Physical therapy is often started immediately to work on ROM. It is crucial to work on extension exercises immediately because many of these patients have long-standing terminal extension limitations from their chronic discoid meniscus. Patients who undergo saucerization and meniscal repair are placed in a hinged knee brace with restricted ROM between 0 and 90 degrees for 6 weeks. They are allowed partial weight bearing up until this point. Return to sports is generally allowed around 3 or 4 months after the surgical procedure is performed.

Results

A total meniscectomy was traditionally used for the treatment of symptomatic discoid menisci, and although this approach is no longer recommended, the long-term results have been reported with mixed findings. Habata et al.[97] and Okazaki et al.[98] found excellent functional scores with minimal radiographic changes after a total meniscectomy at 14- to 16-year follow-up. It has been suggested that young patients adapt to increased articular cartilage stress after meniscectomy. Authors of another study examined 17 knees in children with a mean age of 9 years who were treated with a total meniscectomy.[99] They found that 10 knees had clinical symptoms and radiographic changes of lateral compartment arthritis at 19.8-year follow-up. Two of the knees had lateral femoral condyle OCD lesions. Authors of another study compared long-term clinical and radiographic outcomes in a series of 125 complete and incomplete discoid menisci managed with partial or total meniscectomy.[100] They found better radiographic results at 5-year follow-up with partial meniscectomy. The long-term prognosis was based on the volume of removed meniscus.

Saucerization has become more accepted as standard treatment for discoid menisci. Short- and midterm results of this treatment have been reported. In a retrospective review, authors looked at 11 knees in children with a mean age of 11.5 years who were treated with arthroscopic saucerization for their discoid menisci.[101] At 4.5-year follow-up, all patients had good to excellent clinical results with no radiographic degenerative changes. Authors of another study looked at 27 consecutive discoid menisci in children with a mean age of 10.1 years who were treated with saucerization and repair.[102] Prior to repair, they found that 77% of the discoid menisci were unstable, with anterior horn instability being most common. At 3.1-year follow-up, 21 patients had excellent clinical results and 3 patients reported residual knee pain. Although midterm results are encouraging, long-term results to demonstrate whether saucerization can prevent the development of clinical and radiographic osteoarthritis are still lacking.

Patients who have undergone a total meniscectomy may be candidates for meniscal transplantation. In a cadaveric study of nondiscoid knees, a total lateral meniscectomy was found to decrease the total contact area by 45% to 50% and increase peak local contact pressure by 235% to 335%.[103] Even though the discoid knee has some anatomic and biomechanical differences compared with the nondiscoid knee, these changes are quite significant and should be considered when contemplating meniscal transplantation after a total meniscectomy. A meniscal transplantation may increase the total contact area and decrease the peak local contact pressure. In a study of 14 patients who underwent meniscal allograft transplantation after a previous total meniscectomy for a torn discoid lateral meniscus, Lysholm knee scores improved from 71.4 to 91.4 at a mean 4.8-year follow-up.[104] Only one allograft tear was observed in six second-look arthroscopies. These midterm results are encouraging.

Complications

Complications related to arthroscopic treatment of discoid menisci are similar to those of normal menisci. Perhaps most concerning are the risks of late arthritis, especially in patients with total or subtotal meniscectomies. A higher rate of retearing of the abnormal discoid meniscus tissue may be expected compared with normal menisci. Also, an association of lateral femoral condyle OCD lesions has been reported with discoid menisci after meniscectomy.

Although it is not a complication, sports medicine providers should be aware of the high rate of bilateral discoid menisci. Patel et al.[105] recently reported on children with symptomatic bilateral discoid menisci compared with children who had bilateral discoid menisci, only one of which was symptomatic. They found that patients younger than 12 years and those with complete or Wrisberg-type menisci were more likely to have symptoms and require surgical treatment for their contralateral discoid menisci.

Future Considerations

The increasing understanding of the pathogenesis of the discoid meniscus has led to debate regarding the treatment of stable asymptomatic discoid menisci. Traditionally these menisci are managed with observation; however, prophylactic debridement may possibly prevent symptoms, instability, or future tears. Also, long-term results are needed to address the risks of arthritis in the lateral compartment when counseling patients who have undergone meniscal saucerization with or without repair.

Patellar Instability

Patellar instability affects approximately 43 of 100,000 children.[106] It has been generally accepted that it is easier to return to sport after a patellar instability episode compared with other knee ligamentous injuries or instability in other joints such as the glenohumeral joint. However, Atkin et al.[107] demonstrated that only 66% of athletes were able to return to sport after patellar instability and 50% had some degree of limitation at 6-month follow-up. The rate of redislocation is high in pediatric and adolescent populations. Buchner et al.[108] showed that patients younger than 15 years had a 52% redislocation rate versus a 25% rate for the entire cohort. Cash and Hughston[109] found a 60% redislocation rate in younger adolescents aged 11 to 14 years versus a 33% rate for older adolescents aged 15 to 18 years. Authors of one study found a higher dislocation rate in women, but subsequent metaanalysis has shown no real sex predilection.[110] A family history of patellar instability has been shown to be a major risk factor for repeat dislocation in patients with a previous dislocation.[107,111]

Embryology

The patella develops during the seventh week of gestation but does not begin to ossify until age 4 to 6 years.[112] The patellar facets and trochlear sulcus are well formed in neonates but become more evident as the cartilage thins with age on both the patella and trochlea. The cartilaginous sulcus has been shown to measure between 134 and 155 degrees and remain consistent through development, but the osseous sulcus angle is inversely proportional to age (Fig. 135-8).[106]

Pathoanatomy and Risk Factors

Multiple anatomic factors and potential genetic predilection can lead to the risk for recurrent patellar instability in young athletes. These factors include family history; patellar alta; trochlear dysplasia; increased anatomic Q angle; increased tibial tubercle–trochlear groove distance; medial patellofemoral ligament (MPFL) insufficiency; vastus medialis oblique (VMO) hypoplasia; contractures of the lateral knee structures, including the lateral retinaculum, iliotibial band, and rectus and vastus lateralis; femoral anteversion; tibial external torsion; genu valgum; and possibly excessive foot pronation.

History and Physical Examination

Young patients who have had an episode (or episodes) of patellar instability often provide a more vague description of their symptoms than do adult patients. Very often young patients report that "my knee dislocated" or provide a history very similar to that of an ACL injury, reporting that they twisted, heard or felt a "pop," and had immediate pain and swelling. If they report a true patellar dislocation on a field of play, it is important to ask if a reduction was required or performed on the field or at a local emergency department. It is also important to assess if they have a history of patellar subluxation or dislocation or if a family history of this entity exists. Mechanical symptoms after such an event including locking, popping, and catching can be indicative of a loose body. A history of prior knee pain is especially important to

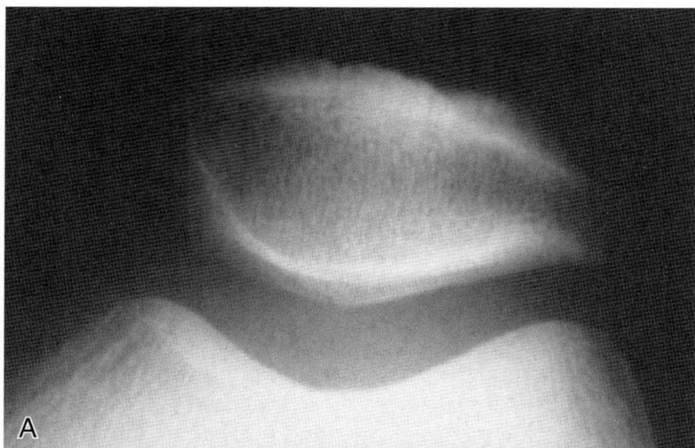

FIGURE 135-8 The sunrise view of the patellofemoral joint in an adult man (**A**) and an 8-year-old boy (**B**). *(From Hinton RY, Sharma KM: Acute and recurrent patellar instability in the young athlete.* Orthop Clin North Am *34:385–396, 2003.)*

consider, including anterior knee pain and pain when using stairs and squatting, for example. These young athletes should also be assessed for contralateral knee pain or instability symptoms. Awareness of a history of joint hyperlaxity can also be useful when assessing these patients.

When examining a young athlete either after a frank patellar dislocation or when chronic patellar instability is present, it is important to assess for signs of an effusion or hemarthrosis. Quadriceps girth or size should be assessed compared with the contralateral side, especially in the area of the VMO. A full knee examination as previously outlined should be performed to check for associated ligament injury, joint line tenderness, and meniscal signs. Specific to assessment of the patellofemoral joint, a patellar apprehension test should be performed to assess for subjective instability. Patellar glide and tilt tests should be performed to assess for increased lateral translation and increased lateral retinacular tightness, respectively. As knee ROM is assessed, patellar tracking should also be assessed. The presence of a J sign is indicative of patellar instability. The patient's overall lower extremity alignment should also be assessed specifically for the Q angle and for femoral anteversion, external tibial torsion, and pes planovalgus.

Imaging

Standard radiographs should be obtained, including standing AP, lateral, notch, and Merchant views. The lateral radiograph should be assessed for patellar alta, which is a risk factor for patellar instability. The Insall-Salvati ratio is difficult to use in pediatric patients because portions of the patella and tibial tubercle are still cartilaginous. Instead, the Blackburn-Peel method can be used, or the Koshino method can be used in pediatric patients to assess patellar height (Fig. 135-9).[113,114] AP, lateral, and Merchant views can be assessed for signs of patellar fracture, sleeve avulsions, or patellar or femoral osteochondral fracture. However, radiographs have been shown to detect only 23% of osteochondral injuries.[115]

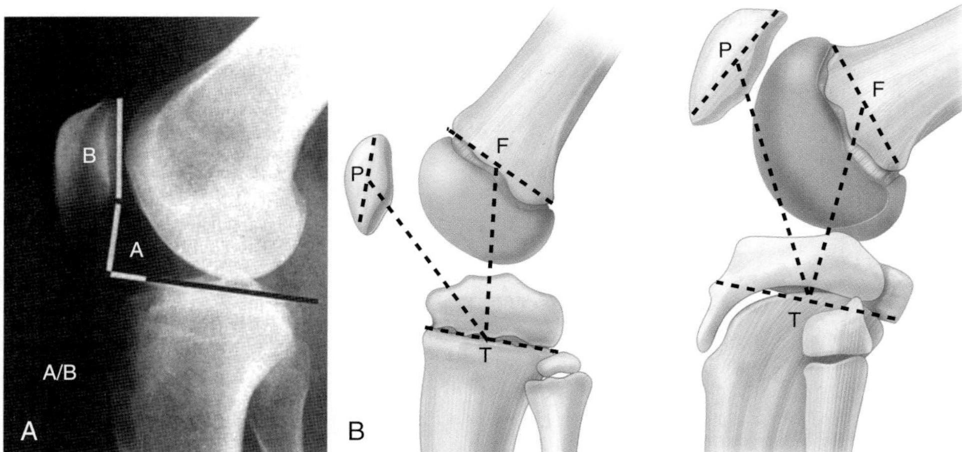

FIGURE 135-9 **A,** The Blackburne-Peel ratio (A/B) compares the perpendicular distance from the lower articular margin of the patella to the tibial plateau (A) and the length of the articular suface of the patella (B). **B,** The Koshino index (PT/FT) compares the patellar-tibial (PT) distance between the midpoint of the patella (P) and the midpoint of the proximal tibia at the physis (T) with the femoral-tibial (FT) distance between the midpoint of the femur at the physis and the midpoint of the proximal tibia at the physis (T). *(**A,** From Blackburne JS, Peel TE: A new method of measuring patellar height.* J Bone Joint Surg Br *59:241–242, 1977. and Scott WN, editor:* Insall and Scott surgery of the knee*, ed 5, New York, 2012, Elsevier. **B,** From Koshino T, Sigimoto K: New measurement of patellar height in the knees of children using the epiphyseal line midpoint.* J Pediatr Orthop *9:216–218, 1989.)*

MRI is useful in assessing patients after a patellar instability episode for several reasons. It has been shown to be 85% sensitive and 70% accurate in detecting an MPFL injury.[116,117] MRI can determine the location and extent of an osteochondral injury, along with the site of MPFL disruption. A typical bone bruise pattern can be seen after patellar dislocation with edema under the medial patellar facet and along the midportion of the lateral femoral condyle.

Decision-Making Principles

Patellar instability can be a tremendously challenging problem for skeletally immature athletes, parents, and sports medicine providers. First, the scope of the patient's patellar instability needs to be assessed, and it should be determined whether the instability is acute and traumatic or chronic and atraumatic. Second, the presence of an osteochondral fracture or cartilaginous loose body should be assessed both by the history of mechanical symptoms, physical examination, and potentially advanced imaging. The presence of a loose body might necessitate earlier surgical intervention. In addition to assessing the knee for signs of patellar instability, the entire patient needs to be considered in terms of risk factors for patellar instability, including patella alta, a shallow trochlear groove and trochlear dysplasia, MPFL injury, patellar tilt, valgus knee alignment, femoral anteversion, external tibial torsion, pes planovalgus, and hypoplastic tibial tubercles.

Treatment Options

Nonoperative Management

Conservative treatment of a first-time patellar dislocation without mechanical symptoms indicative of a loose body is standard. Some controversy exists regarding the issue of whether immobilization should be used immediately after a dislocation. Maenpaa and Lehto[118] reported a dislocation rate that was three times higher with immediate mobilization compared with initial immobilization. In general, most sports medicine providers immobilize the knee for several weeks followed by gradual mobilization. A hinged knee brace, often with a lateral buttress for patellar stabilization, can be used until full painless ROM is possible. Physical therapy is recommended to assist initially with regaining ROM, soft tissue swelling mobilization, quadriceps strengthening (especially focusing on the VMO), electrical stimulation for VMO activation, and patellar taping. McConnell taping has been shown to decrease pain and increase quadriceps activity during rehabilitation, despite perhaps not truly medializing the patella.[119,120] Later stages of rehabilitation focus on continued quadriceps strengthening, gait training, closed-chain exercises, proprioceptive training, and sports-specific training before allowing a full return to activities. Return to play is usually allowed after full ROM is restored without pain, swelling, or instability symptoms. Some providers may choose to allow return to play once strength is 80% to 85% compared with the contralateral side, along with a satisfactory single-leg hop test and two-legged hop test.

Operative Treatment

In first-time acute patellar dislocations in skeletally immature patients, immediate operative intervention is generally reserved for patients who have a displaced osteochondral fracture or lesion. Open reduction and fixation of osteochondral lesions is generally reserved for lesions greater than 1 cm in diameter with bone attached to the fragment. Smaller lesions or lesions without bone attached are generally treated with removal of the loose body. The osteochondral lesion can be treated with chondroplasty or microfracture initially. Larger lesions may require further treatment, which can include osteochondral autograft transfer (OATS), autologous chondrocyte implantation (ACI), or osteochondral allograft treatment.

The medial patellofemoral ligament is the primary ligamentous restraint to lateral dislocation. Once surgical treatment is determined to be necessary, reestablishing the integrity of the MPFL is crucial to restoring patellar stability. Acutely, the MPFL can be repaired, but such repair has shown mixed long-term results.[121-124] The MPFL can be reconstructed with either autograft or allograft in skeletally immature athletes. It is crucial for the graft to be of sufficient length, especially if a loop-type construct that is doubled back is used (Fig. 135-10). In skeletally immature patients with open distal femoral physes, the anatomic MPFL femoral attachment point, which is just posterior to the medial epicondyle, is very close to the physis. The graft fixation or graft tunneling procedures performed in more mature patients would risk a growth disturbance or arrest, and thus it is often necessary to place the femoral attachment point in a nonanatomic position to avoid the physis. This position is generally just anterior and proximal to the medial epicondyle and 4 to 5 mm distal to the growth plate.[125] This position is somewhat controversial, however, with other surgeons suggesting that the femoral tunnel or attachment point be placed just proximal to the physis. Patellar fixation can be performed with a single or double tunnel. Screw fixation can be used in the patella, or a loop can be used through the patella without hardware. The application of appropriate tension to the graft in MPFL reconstruction is always crucial, but especially in skeletally immature patients in whom the femoral fixation point also needs to avoid the physis. According to Wall and Romanowski, tension of between 30 and 60 degrees of flexion should be placed on the MPFL graft.[125] If the patella tracks medially in flexion, the pin is moved distally. If the patella tracks medially in extension, the pin is moved proximally. If the pin is too anterior, it tightens in terminal extension and flexion. If the pin is too posterior, it loosens in terminal extension and flexion.

Skeletally immature athletes, and in particular especially young children with patellar instability, present a unique challenge to sports medicine care providers. Surgical options such as tibial tubercle osteotomies are not possible in young patients who have open tibial physes. A number of "nonanatomic" reconstruction procedures have been used both historically and in patients with particularly difficult and challenging cases of patellar instability, such as athletes with congenital patellar dislocations, collagen disorders, neuromuscular and metabolic syndromes, and mechanical alignment issues.

The isolated lateral release is rarely used or indicated in patients with traumatic instability but often is needed in combination with other procedures in patients with long-standing chronic patellar dislocations or congenital dislocations.

The Galeazzi procedure involves use of the semitendinosus as a restraint to lateral subluxation. The semitendinosus is

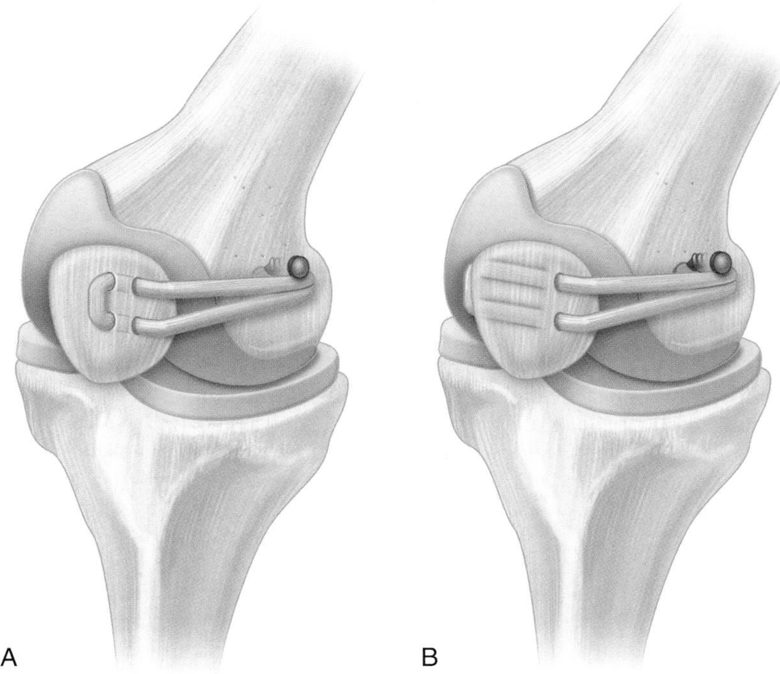

FIGURE 135-10 **A**, Medial patellofemoral ligament (MPFL) reconstruction using a gracilis tendon that is looped through two tunnels in the medial half of the patella. The tunnels exit in the midline of the patella, avoiding tunnels that pass across the full width of the bone. The femoral fixation at the adductor tubercle is by means of an interference screw. **B,** MPFL reconstruction using a free gracilis tendon that is passed through two transverse tunnels in the proximal part of the patella. The femoral fixation at the adductor tubercle is by means of an interference screw. *(**A,** From Scott WN, editor:* Insall and Scott surgery of the knee*, ed 5, New York, 2012, Elsevier, courtesy M. Lind. **B,** From Christiansen SE, Jacobsen BW, Lund B, et al: Reconstruction of the medial patellofemoral ligament with gracilis tendon autograft in transverse patellar drill holes.* Arthroscopy *24:82, 2008.)*

harvested proximally with an open-ended tendon harvester, leaving the distal portion attached. The patella is exposed, and often a lateral release is performed. A patellar tunnel is made from proximal lateral to distal medial. The semitendinosus tendon is passed retrograde and folded over the anterior surface of the patella and secured there with suture. Tension is applied to the graft at 45 to 60 degrees of flexion.

The Roux-Goldthwaite procedure is another nonanatomic reconstruction procedure that has been used in skeletally immature patients.[126-128] This procedure involves splitting the patellar tendon and detaching the distal end of the lateral half, which is then passed posterior to the medial half and reattached medially into the pes anserinus. Although tension is also applied at 45 to 60 degrees of flexion in this procedure, it is difficult to achieve appropriate tension in both limbs of the patellar tendon, which is one of the criticisms of this technique. This patellar tendon rerouting procedure is generally combined with a medial retinacular plication.

Multiple tibial tubercle osteotomies are available for realignment in the surgical treatment of patellar instability but require that the tibial tubercle physis be closed. Premature closure of the tibial tubercle portion of the tibial physis can result in an recurvatum deformity. Once the tibial tubercle physis has closed, the most popular option is currently the anteromedial tibial tuberosity transfer popularized by Fulkerson.[129,130] Earlier versions include the Hauser osteotomy, which included a distal medial transfer of the tibial tubercle combined with a lateral retinaculum release and medial imbrication along with the Elmslie-Trillat osteotomy, which involved only medialization, and the Maquet osteotomy, which involved only anterior elevation of the tubercle.

Postoperative Management

Rehabilitation after MPFL reconstruction should emphasize lower limb alignment in all phases of rehabilitation to avoid dynamic hip internal rotation and knee valgus, which can lead to stress on the healing reconstruction.[131] A skeletally immature athlete often wears a hinged patellar stabilizing brace for approximately 6 weeks. Full weight bearing is generally allowed unless a simultaneous microfracture or osteotomy was performed. Weight bearing may progress from ambulation with crutches and a knee brace locked in extension to ambulation with crutches and the brace unlocked. Use of crutches and the brace may be discontinued when the patient demonstrates sufficient strength and control of the limb to protect the knee from transverse and frontal plane stress.[131]

Initial phases of rehabilitation emphasize quadriceps activation and ROM with the goal of attaining 90 degrees of knee flexion by 6 weeks after the operation to prevent adhesions.[131] Younger patients undergoing more extensive patellar realignment procedures, especially nonanatomic reconstructions, may require a longer immobilization period and a slower rate of mobilization. Rehabilitation should continue to progress with strengthening, ROM, and proprioception training until the patient is ready to return to unrestricted sports at approximately 6 months after surgery, depending on the patient's function and symptoms.[131]

Results

MPFL reconstruction has been associated with excellent results in terms of preventing recurrent patellar instability. In two series combined, only 5 of 170 patients who had undergone MPFL reconstruction experienced repeat subluxation or dislocations.[132,133] Failed MPFL reconstruction may be associated with trochlear or patellar dysplasia.[134] Nonanatomic reconstruction techniques have good results in select patients but should be recommended with caution in skeletally immature athletes who do not have congenital patellar dislocations, collagen disorders, neuromuscular and metabolic syndromes, and mechanical alignment issues.

Complications

The surgical treatment of patellar instability has multiple potential pitfalls and complications. Potentially the most disheartening complication is recurrent instability. As previously mentioned, failure of MPFL reconstruction with recurrent instability is usually due to unrecognized trochlear or patellar dysplasia. Arthrofibrosis is another potential complication of any surgical treatment of the knee. In the skeletally immature athlete, potential growth arrest after a ligament reconstruction with or without an osteotomy is a particular concern, and careful preoperative planning and intraoperative attention should minimize this risk. Patellar fracture is a recognized complication after MPFL reconstruction.[135] Minimizing the size and number of tunnels and related hardware within the patella can help reduce this risk. Patellofemoral arthrosis is a particularly concerning complication after patellar instability surgery and is difficult to quantify in this population. It can certainly be part of the natural history of articular cartilage damage caused by recurrent patellar instability. It can also be a potential complication of overtension of an MPFL reconstruction, improper femoral tunnel placement, or overloading of the patellofemoral joint with improper translation of the tibial tubercle osteotomy.

Future Considerations

As the sports medicine community advances the ligament reconstruction of the medial patellofemoral ligament, techniques for skeletally immature athletes will need to focus on reconstructions that are anatomic, spare the physes, decrease the risk of patellar fracture, minimize the risk of dislocation, and reduce the risk of applying too much tension.

Osteochondritis Dissecans

OCD is an acquired potentially reversible lesion of subchondral bone that often results in delamination of the articular surface and sequestration of subchondral bone. The term was originally coined by Konig in 1887, who recognized at that time that it was a potential cause of loose bodies and degenerative changes.[136] The peak prevalence of OCD diagnosis is noted during the preteen years; OCD is thought to be rare among children younger than 10 years and less common after skeletal maturity. The estimated incidence of adolescent OCD is between 0.2% and 0.3% based on knee radiographs and 1.2% based on knee arthroscopy studies.[137] The male/female ratios have been quoted as being between 2 : 1 and 5 : 3, although the incidence of OCD diagnoses in females is on the rise.

Etiology

Several theories have been proposed regarding the etiology of juvenile OCD, including both single and repetitive trauma. Green[138] reported a 40% rate of trauma prior to diagnosis of OCD in 1966. Since then, authors have found an increased incidence in young, very active athletes, with a statistically significant association between OCD and increased involvement in sports. In Sweden it was found that 55% to 60% of patients with OCD participated in high-level sports.[137,139,140] In 1933 Fairbanks concluded that the OCD lesion on the medial femoral condyle was caused by repetitive contact on the tibial spine, a conclusion later supported by other authors.[141,142] However, Cahill has refuted some of these claims by showing no history of trauma in 204 cases of OCD; he postulated a stress reaction or fracture as the cause of the lesion.[143]

Inflammation has also been proposed as a possible causative factor in the formation of the OCD lesion and, in fact, was Konig's original hypothesis. Other investigators have postulated that a genetic predisposition exists for OCD lesions.[144-147] This theory was refuted by Petrie[148] but supported by the association of OCD with other diseases such as familial epiphyseal dysplasia, Legg-Calve-Perthes disease, and Stickler syndrome.[140]

Regardless of the etiology, ischemia or avascular necrosis has been proposed as the first event in the formation of juvenile OCD.[149,150] In 1978 Milgram showed that revascularization occurred in partially attached lesions. Limited uptake of radionuclide and labeled tetracycline has also been shown in these lesions.[151] However, in 1950 Rogers and Gladstone[152] disagreed with the idea of ischemia as a cause by showing vascular anastomoses in more than 200 specimens, and Yonetani et al.[153] showed no osseous necrosis in their samples of OCD.

History and Physical Examination

The skeletally immature athlete with an OCD lesion often presents with the insidious onset of knee pain that is worse with participation in high-energy sports. As the lesion progresses, symptoms occur with minimal activity and eventually at rest. At more advanced stages of disease, patients have pain, swelling, effusions, and mechanical symptoms such as locking, popping, and catching if a loose body is present. Ligamentous stability and a lack of meniscal disease are usually found. The Wilson maneuver or sign involves pain elicited by extension of the knee from 90 degrees of flexion to 30 degrees of flexion while internally rotating the tibia. Pain should be relieved by external rotation in the same arc, which is obviously specific for lesions involving the medial femoral condyle in the classic location and has been found to have poor reliability as a specific test for OCD lesions (Fig. 135-11).[154]

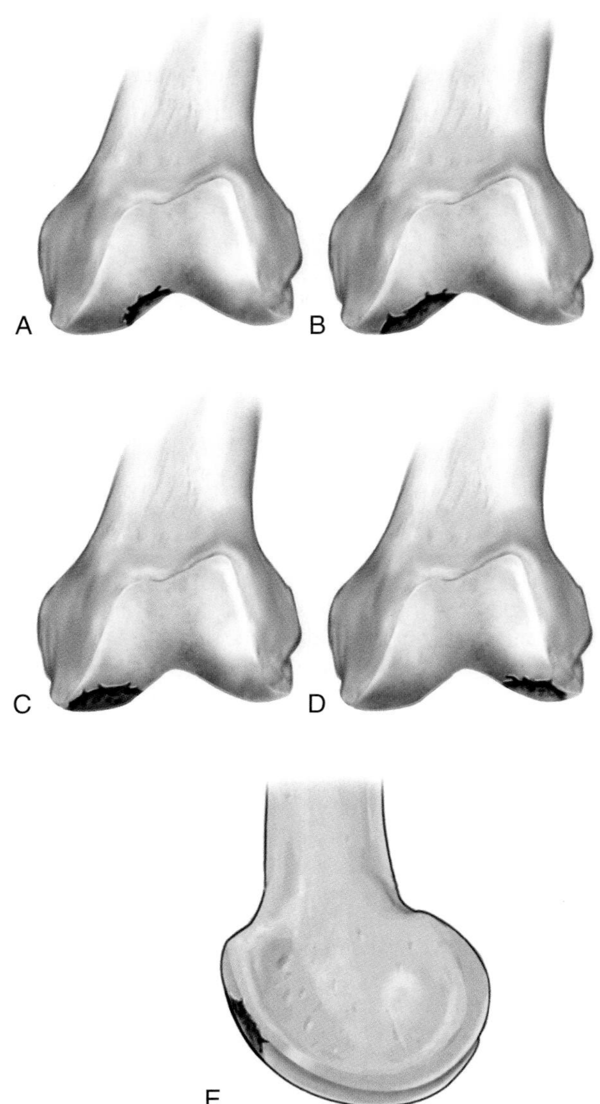

FIGURE 135-11 Location of osteochondritis dissecans of the femoral condyles. Medial condyle: classic, 69% (**A**); extended classic, 6% (**B**); inferocentral, 10% (**C**). Lateral condyle: inferocentral, 13% (**D**); anterior, 2% (**E**). *(Modified from Aichroth P: Osteochondritis dissecans of the knee.* J Bone Joint Surg Br *53:440–447, 1971.)*

Radiographs

Standard radiographic evaluation includes an AP, lateral, sunrise, and a notch or tunnel view for a patient with a suspected OCD lesion of the knee. Of these views, the notch view is often the most revealing and specific. Many medial femoral condyle OCD lesions can be missed on a standard AP view and are better seen on the notch view.

CT scans have been used in the past, but because of radiation concerns and improvements in technology, MRI has now largely replaced the use of CT scans for OCD evaluation. Bone scans were used in the past and were shown to be useful for classifying OCD lesions by Cahill and Berg when compared with radiographs.[155] This grading system had five stages based on radiograph and bone scan activity but was later reported to have limited correlation with lesion stability and the future need for surgery.[156] Paletta et al.[157] were able to show that in four of five patients with open physes and increased uptake on a bone scan, their OCD lesions healed without surgery.

MRI has become a standard higher level imaging modality to assess OCD lesions in skeletally immature patients. DeSmet et al.[158,159] defined the criteria on MRI for instability in adult OCD lesions. They found that a high signal line beneath the lesion was the most predictive. Other signs of instability included a focal defect or fracture in the articular cartilage along with the presence of subchondral cysts. Kijowski et al.[160] found that the criteria cited by DeSmet et al. was 100% sensitive and specific for adult OCD but not for juvenile OCD, for which it was only 11% specific for instability. They found that secondary criteria with a high signal rim could increase specificity to 100%. These secondary criteria were multiple breaks in the subchondral bone plate, outer rim of low T2-weighted signal intensity, and a rim of fluid signal intensity (Table 135-1 and Figs. 135-12 and 135-13).

Unfortunately, no valid or reliable criteria currently exist with which to grade or prognosticate juvenile OCD. This problem is being addressed by a multidisciplinary, multicentered national group referred to as ROCK (Research on Osteochondritis of the Knee). Currently the ROCK group has established radiographic and arthroscopic grading scales and shown them to be valid and reliable. An MRI system is being developed and will be evaluated soon to help providers not only in the diagnosis of juvenile OCD but also guide the treatment and future prognosis of these lesions.

Decision-Making Principles

In the treatment of juvenile OCD lesions, determining the stability of the lesion at presentation and trying to predict which lesions may become unstable over time is paramount.[161,162] Although deciding whether a lesion is stable is difficult, in this skeletally immature population, some authors have shown that conservative treatment works well for stable lesions and leads to good outcomes.[161,162] In an effort to better define stable lesions, Wall et al.[162] developed a nomogram to predict the potential for healing of an OCD lesion. This predictive tool took into account aspects of the lesion,

TABLE 135-1

MRI CLASSIFICATION OF KNEE OSTEOARTHRITIS DISSECANS

Stage	Description
1	Small change of signal without clear margins of fragment
2	Osteochondral fragment with clear margins but without fluid between fragment and underlying bone
3	Fluid partially visible between fragment and underlying bone
4	Fluid completely surrounding fragment but fragment still in situ
5	Fragment completely detached and displaced (loose body)

MRI, Magnetic resonance imaging.

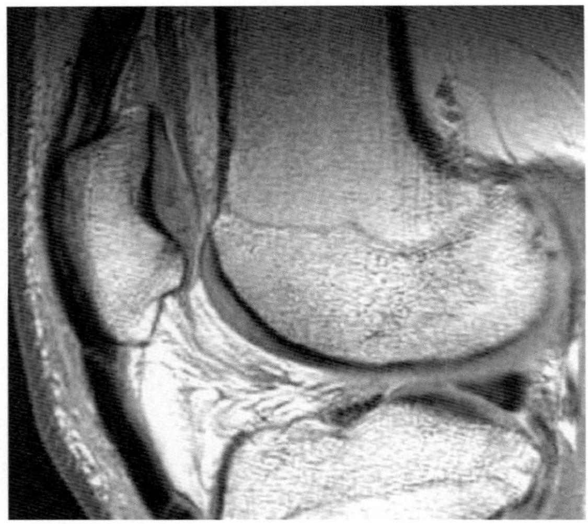

FIGURE 135-12 Osteochondritis dissecans of the patella.

including the relative size, location, and symptoms, and has been used effectively for stable lesions.

In a multicenter trial of the European Pediatric Orthopaedic Society it was also found that stability was associated with a good prognosis.[140] In this trial it was also found that smaller lesions, lesions in the most common location (i.e., the lateral edge of the medial femoral condyle), a lack of sclerosis on radiographs, and lesions in younger patients did better overall. Unfortunately, it was also shown that pain, swelling, radiographs, and CT scans were not good predictors for dissection of the lesion. However, when a separation between the native and progeny bone existed, surgical intervention led to improved results.

During the past several years, many medical organizations have begun to emphasize and produce clinical practice guidelines (CPGs). The American Association of Orthopaedic Surgeons (AAOS), as a part of this process, has recently put together a CPG for the treatment of OCD.[163,164] The AAOS was able to make only a few recommendations to help guide the diagnosis and care of OCD in adults or adolescents in this CPG but did describe and propose the research necessary to improve the care of persons with these lesions.

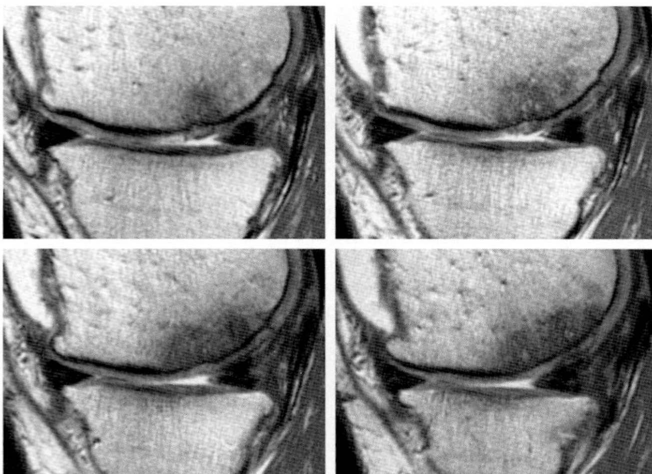

FIGURE 135-13 Osteochondritis dissecans of the femur.

The treatment of juvenile OCD is in a stage of evolution. The study and long-term evaluation of current treatment techniques is underway at many centers; the multi-centered ROCK group is part of this effort. As these centers and groups compile data to help direct care, the decision process will become more clear and evidence directed. To a great extent, however, only level IV and V evidence is available at this point.

A developing trend is the increasingly aggressive care that is being promoted. This trend is driven by two somewhat obvious but underappreciated issues. First, the chance for achieving an excellent outcome is better when the OCD is in the early stages of the continuum of its progression. The second issue is the significantly poor results that occur once the progeny bone/lesion becomes loose or free.

Treatment Options

The initial step in the algorithm of the treatment of juvenile OCD depends on the stability of the lesion. Nonoperative treatment focuses on off-loading the lesion.[161] Off-loading traditionally was achieved with a long leg cast but has now evolved to include the use of crutches, braces, unloader braces, and more permanent steps such as osteotomies. Although they are not standardized, most unloading protocols recommend at least 6 weeks of care, with some protocols extending to as long as 6 months.[162,165,166]

Preoperative examination and radiographic findings may suggest the extent of the lesion, but the final determination of the full extent of the lesion is assessed arthroscopically and occasionally by miniarthrotomy. As many investigators have shown, preoperative evaluations are often found to be incomplete at the time of arthroscopy, and thus equipment and time must be available for all potential treatment options.

In lesions that were determined to be stable at initial presentation but have failed to progress toward healing or are determined to be stable but have a risk for progression, care is directed toward stimulating healing of the lesion. This stimulation is often accomplished by drilling of the lesion to stimulate the reestablishment of a vascular supply, which is performed either in a transarticular or extraarticular fashion. This technique is generally reserved for lesions in situ, with the decision of which method of drilling to perform being dependent on the condition of the articular cartilage and the location of the lesion. Some investigators advocate transarticular drilling, which allows visualization of the lesion arthroscopically and treatment of the entire lesion. The drawback to this technique of drilling is that the articular cartilage surface is violated by the drilling.[167,168] Extraarticular drilling avoids the penetration of the articular cartilage but requires another means of determining complete treatment of the lesion. This determination can be achieved with the use of fluoroscopy intraoperatively.[169] Both methods have produced good results in appropriate patients.

The other branch of the algorithm in juvenile OCD involves the treatment of unstable lesions. The decision to attempt fixation of the lesion is dependent on several factors, including the age of the patient, the size and depth of the lesion, the presence or lack of bone on the progeny fragment, sclerosis of the bone, and the condition of the articular cartilage.

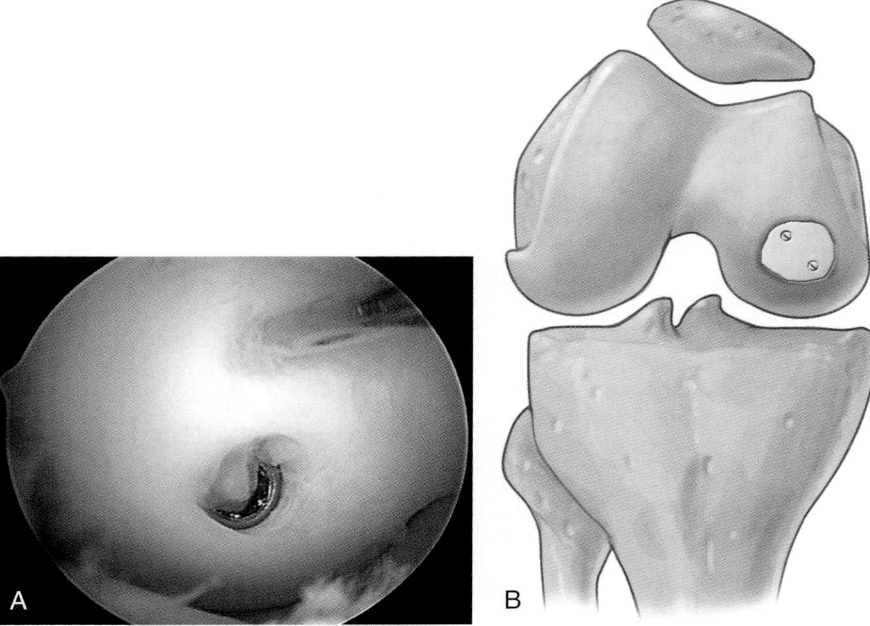

FIGURE 135-14 Screw fixation of an osteochondritis dissecans lesion. Note that the screw is seated below the articular cartilage surface to reduce injury to the tibial articular surface. *(From Miller MD, Cole BJ, Cosgarea A, et al, editors:* Operative techniques: sports knee surgery, *Philadelphia, 2008, Elsevier.)*

If the progeny fragment remains in situ or is partially attached with a bony fragment on it, then fixation of the lesion is generally recommended. Many fixation methods are available, including bioabsorbable screws,[170-172] metal screws,[168,173-176] pins or darts, and bone pegs (Fig. 135-14).[169,177-179] The bioabsorbable screws have the advantages of not interfering with MRI and not needing to be removed, but they are more fragile, and multiple reports have been made of hardware failure with use of these devices.[180] Other investigators have used biologic fixation for these lesions with use of OATS. This technique is technically demanding and requires a donor site with requisite donor site morbidity. However, it offers a biologic fixation method without the need for hardware or eventual hardware removal. Longer term studies along with comparison studies are needed to examine these fixation techniques.

More involved lesions including those that are completely loose or hinged, similar to a trap door, may require more extensive steps to improve the chance of healing. If the lesion is hinged, it is generally recommended that the sclerotic bone beneath the lesion be removed to allow better bleeding bone surfaces for healing. Some authors suggest bone grafting or use of bone graft substitutes during this process.[181,182] Once the lesion has been prepared and reduced either arthroscopically or through a mini open approach, the previously noted fixation devices can be used.

For lesions that are not salvageable at the time of arthroscopic examination, OCD treatment options are similar to those used for other articular cartilage salvage and reconstruction options. Removal of the loose fragments alone has resulted in poor outcomes in long-term follow-up.[183-185] Lesions in which the loose OCD lesion has fragmented into smaller pieces and lesions that no longer have bone stock on the articular cartilage lesion are not considered salvageable. In addition to providing biologic fixation, OATS plug transfers can provide autograft articular cartilage to fill a full-thickness defect. Other options for larger lesions include ACI and fresh osteochondral allograft transplantation.

Results

Results of OCD treatment vary greatly according to the qualities of the lesion at the time of treatment, as well as the associated co-morbidities that exist. Most authors, however, note that symptomatic stable lesions, when treated appropriately both technically and during their rehabilitation, do very well; this has been our experience as well. In these situations, once long-term healing has occurred, patients have normally functioning knees and often forget that their problem ever existed. Unstable lesions, although more variable, can also have excellent outcomes. The key to their prognosis is the recreation and reestablishment of a smooth cartilage surface with a solid subchondral bone foundation. Even larger, initially unsalvageable lesions can have excellent outcomes with the use of osteochondral allografts when the lesion is treated appropriately. A concern with the use of allografts includes reports of midterm failures when, for unknown reasons, the allograft fragment fails. This outcome has been reported by some investigators after 4 years of an otherwise excellent course.[186]

Complications

Few complications occur in the treatment of juvenile OCD. Intraoperative concerns include improper placement of fixation devices or breakage of drill pins and screws. Nontechnical complications revolve primarily around the failure of healing of the lesions and the cartilage degeneration that can result.

AUTHORS' PREFERRED TECHNIQUE

OCD Lesions

- It is our bias that symptomatic knee OCD lesions should undergo arthroscopic evaluation with treatment at an early stage.
  - This bias is based on the fact that less chance of progeny bone/lesion displacement exists earlier in treatment. This view is certainly controversial, because many surgeons have reported satisfactory healing of OCD lesions with extended periods of conservative treatment.
- Arthroscopic management should include:
  - Probing of the lesion helps determine stability. Probing is followed by drilling if the lesion is stable or fixation with bioabsorbable or metal screws, bone plugs, or dowels if any element of instability is noted.
  - Drilling can be performed transarticularly or extraarticularly using smooth, small-diameter (0.045 or 0.062) Kirschner wires.
  - Transarticular drilling should be performed with direct visualization arthroscopically.
  - Extraarticular drilling should be performed with fluoroscopic guidance to ensure that the pins are engaging the lesion in both the AP and lateral projections. We often use the Micro Vector drill guide system (Smith & Nephew, Andover. Massachusetts) to assist with placement of the initial pin.
    - It is also necessary to ensure that the articular cartilage is not violated with the pin.
    - Extraarticular drilling, to ensure adequate penetration of the lesion, is performed eight times per square centimeter.[169]
    - When or if the lesion has begun to fragment, we attempt to save the progeny fragment by debriding the base of the lesion either arthroscopically or via an open procedure. The base is then grafted with bone as needed and fixed with appropriate screws or bone plugs.
    - If the OCD fragment is not salvageable, we will debride the lesion to a stable cartilage rim and perform marrow stimulation at the base of the lesion.
    - If symptoms continue, we recommend that the lesion be treated with a cartilage reparative procedure (such as ACI) if the depth of bone loss is less than 4 mm or with OATS or a fresh osteochondral allograft if the patient has greater bone loss.

Future Considerations

The treatment of juvenile OCD is evolving. As the lesions become better recognized and evaluated, better care decisions and presumably better long-term outcomes will occur. As the AAOS pointed out in their CPG, a substantial need exists for better-designed studies that look at all of the issues surrounding OCD diagnosis and care. As mentioned, many of these studies are underway, and we hope they will be completed soon.

Osteochondroses of the Knee

Disordered endochondral ossification of a previously developing epiphysis results in osteochondrosis.[187] The stresses of repetitive activity can lead to changes within the apophysis, a primary area of development in the young athlete. As the skeleton matures, changes in the bone and cartilage of the apophysis can cause the symptoms that lead to the diagnosis of tendinopathy. Advanced radiographic findings are consistently found within the tendon in mature individuals; however, in young athletes, radiographic findings show changes only in the bone and cartilage. Classically, young athletes with osteochondrosis present with pain localized to the origin or insertion of a tendinous insertion.

Osgood-Schlatter Disease

In the early 1900s two separate clinicians, Osgood and Schlatter, first reported osteochondrosis of the tibial tubercle. They described pain over the tibial tubercle with running and jumping in active adolescents. The disease occurs in children who are undergoing rapid growth when stress is placed on the developing tubercle through patellar tendon force. Osgood and Schlatter stressed that this condition is due to repetitive loading in the area causing a traction apophysitis of the tibial tubercle, not an avulsion fracture.

Osgood-Schlatter disease is now one of the most well-known overuse syndromes. It was originally reported to be more common in boys than in girls.[188,189] The prevalence in girls is on the rise because of the increasing number of female athletes. Girls typically experience the condition between the ages of 10 and 13 years, and boys experience it between the ages of 12 and 14 years, coinciding with their growth spurts. Its incidence was found to be 21% in athletic adolescents compared with 4.5% of nonathletic adolescents.[188] Osgood-Schlatter disease is found bilaterally in 20% to 30% of affected persons.

This condition develops most commonly in boys who participate in the sports of running, basketball, and hockey, whereas it develops most commonly in girls who participate in the sports of gymnastics, volleyball, and figure skating. These sports involve running and jumping, which require repeated loading of the knee in flexion and forced extension of the knee by eccentric quadriceps contraction. The force of the quadriceps extensor mechanism is magnified by the patellar mechanism and transferred to the immature tibial tubercle.

The exact cause of Osgood-Schlatter disease has yet to be identified, but it is universally found in adolescents who undergo a rapid period of growth. During this time an imbalance occurs between bone and muscle growth, which may lead to susceptibility of the apophysis to overuse injury. Several studies have attempted to identify a relationship between patella alta, Osgood-Schlatter disease, and tibial tubercle avulsion fractures.[188,190,191] None of these studies has found a link between any of these three entities. Repetitive microtrauma appears to be an integral part of the development of Osgood-Schlatter disease because there is a much lower prevalence in nonactive persons.[188]

Patients usually present with pain and swelling over the tibial tubercle. These active adolescents may report increased pain with running, jumping, or kneeling. The pain is usually

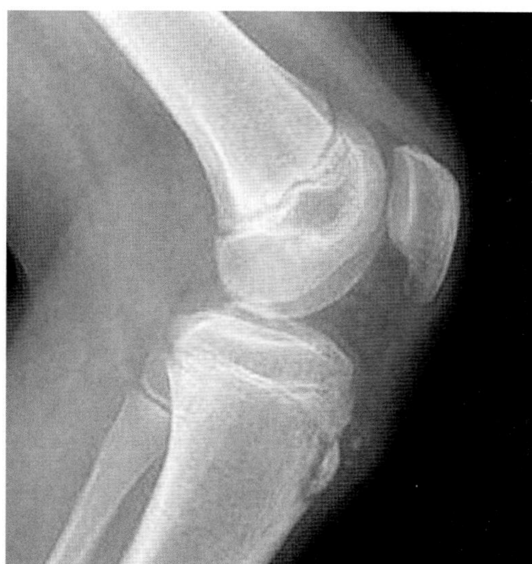

FIGURE 135-15 Osgood-Schlatter disease of the tibial apophysis.

gradual in onset. Parents often report that they notice an antalgic gait. Tenderness to palpation, swelling, and prominence of the tibial tubercle are often found on physical examination. The distal half of the patella tendon may be tender to palpation. Quadriceps and hamstring tightness may be appreciated. Pain can also be reproduced with resisted knee extension. Bone irregularities can often be palpated in chronic cases. The differential diagnosis of Osgood-Schlatter disease includes avulsion fracture of the tibial tuberosity, patellofemoral stress syndrome, pes anserinus bursitis, Sinding-Larsen-Johansson disease, and infection.

To further evaluate the tibial tuberosity, plain radiographs of the affected knee are ordered. The lateral radiograph is the most helpful in assessing the extensor mechanism (Fig. 135-15). Patients with Osgood-Schlatter disease may have separation or fragmentation of the tibial tubercle apophysis. The tibial tubercle may also be enlarged. Radiographs are also important for excluding other diagnoses such as cysts, tumors, or infection.

The natural history of Osgood-Schlatter disease has been evaluated.[188,192,193] Krause et al.[192] looked at 50 patients with Osgood-Schlatter disease. Half of the patients were treated with a form of nonoperative treatment, and half of the patients received no treatment. When followed up to adulthood, most patients in both groups had no residual symptoms. Treatment usually entails activity modification, ice, stretching, and strengthening exercises. Stretching should focus on the quadriceps, hamstrings, and iliotibial band. Occasionally immobilization in a splint or brace is needed to control pain. The splint or brace should be removed daily for exercises to maintain knee ROM. Whereas symptoms are usually self-limited, pain may persist until the apophysis closes. Some of these patients may continue to have pain as adults because of the formation of a separate ossicle. Surgical excision of the ossicle is required in the rare cases in which nonsurgical treatment fails to treat this pain.[194] Pihlajamaki et al.,[195] in a long-term follow-up study of military recruits who underwent surgery for the treatment of unresolved Osgood-Schlatter disease, reported that 87% had no restrictions of daily activity and 75% returned to their preoperative activity level.

Sinding-Larson-Johansson Disease

Sinding-Larson-Johansson disease is an osteochondrosis of the inferior pole of the patella. It is predominantly seen in active adolescent boys between the ages of 11 and 13 years. No reports have been made yet of an increased prevalence in females associated with increased young female athletic activity. Sinding-Larson-Johansson disease traditionally presents in slightly younger patients compared with those with Osgood-Schlatter disease because the maturation of the inferior pole of the patella occurs before that of the tibial tuberosity. Rarely, the diagnoses of both of these conditions at the same time have been reported.[196,197]

Patients with Sinding-Larson-Johansson disease report pain at the patella–patella tendon junction associated with running, jumping, and ascending or descending stairs. The pain improves with rest. On physical examination, patients have tenderness to palpation at the patella–patella tendon junction, and they occasionally have swelling. The examination should also look for other possible causes of activity-related anterior knee pain. A palpable defect at this junction and an extensor lag or inability to perform a straight-leg raise should raise concern for a patellar sleeve fracture.

Anteroposterior, lateral, and Merchant radiographic views of both knees should be obtained. At the inferior pole of the patella, calcification or ossification can often be identified (Fig. 135-16). These radiographs can also aid in the diagnoses of other entities, including patella sleeve fractures, Osgood-Schlatter disease, bipartite patella, patella alta, and patella baja.

Sinding-Larson-Johansson disease is a self-limited condition with resolution of symptoms after full maturation of the inferior pole of the patella, which is usually a 12- to 18-month period. Treatment is similar to the treatment for Osgood-Schlatter disease. The emphasis of treatment is on decreasing pain and inflammation with activity modification and use of ice and antiinflammatory medications. Physical therapy programs emphasize an eccentric quadriceps loading program and lower extremity stretching.[198] Sports participation should be limited until symptoms improve. Few late sequelae of the

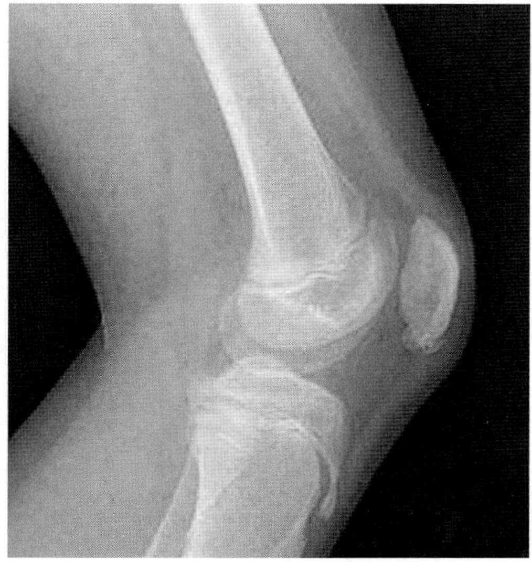

FIGURE 135-16 Sinding-Larsen-Johansson disease.

disease occur, with one report of a fracture through a previously united ossicle.[199] Remaining symptomatic separate ossicles are rare. Excision could be considered in adults who have pain when nonoperative management fails.

Superior Pole Osteochondrosis

Similar to Osgood-Schlatter and Sinding-Larson-Johansson diseases, superior pole osteochondrosis is a traction apophysitis. Very few reports of superior pole osteochondrosis have been made.[200-202] It can be distinguished from Osgood-Schlatter and Sinding-Larson-Johansson diseases by clinical examination and radiographic findings. It is most commonly found in active boys between the ages of 10 and 11 years. Patients report anterior knee pain that is poorly localized by the patient. Palpation of the superior patella-quadriceps junction reproduces pain. Radiographs show various stages of fragmentation and ossification based on chronicity of symptoms. Tyler and McCarthy[200] found osteonecrosis and reparative changes on histologic examination in patients with superior pole osteochondrosis. These findings are similar to those seen in persons with Osgood-Schlatter and Sinding-Larson-Johansson disease.[203] Like these other entities, superior pole osteochondrosis is a self-limited process. Treatment consists of activity modification, use of ice and antiinflammatory medication, and therapy.

Physeal Fractures in the Area of the Knee

Skeletally immature athletes are at risk for unique injuries in the area of the knee involving their open physes. These injuries usually require significant trauma but have been associated with a variety of sporting activities. Their diagnosis and treatment involve special consideration. Distal femoral physeal fractures represent fewer than 1% of all fractures in children and between 6% and 9% of physeal fractures.[204,205] However, they are associated with a 20% to 90% complication rate.[206-212] Most commonly, they are associated with a growth disturbance or angular deformity. The distal femoral physis produces approximately 70% of the growth of the femur or a length of approximately 9 to 10 mm per year. The physis is more undulating than other long bone physes and therefore fractures often extend through multiple layers of the physis. Tibial spine fracture is another unique injury in the skeletally immature athlete. It involves an avulsion of the ACL chondroepiphyseal attachment. It has a similar pattern of injury as ACL injury but in a younger population. These injuries have been associated with a variety of meniscal and chondral damage intraarticularly. Kocher et al.[213] found the incidence of meniscal tears with these fractures to be 3.8%. Other unique proximal tibial physeal injuries include tibial tubercle avulsions and proximal tibial physeal fractures. Because the proximal tibial physis is more stable than the distal femur, these injuries represent fewer than 1% of all physeal separations. However, these injuries require significant force and trauma and therefore associated injuries are common and need to be closely followed. Tethering of the popliteal artery to the posterior tibia occurs that places it and its branches at risk during these physeal injuries. Distal swelling and compartment syndrome can be associated with these injuries. The tibial tuberosity may avulse in adolescents, especially during jumping or eccentric loading landing patterns, which can cause contraction of the quadriceps against the fixed tibia or passive flexion of the knee against a contracted quadriceps.

History and Physical Examination

Distal femoral physeal fractures in skeletally immature athletes are most commonly the result of torsional or valgus stress against the knee. Bright et al.[214] have shown in an animal model that the prepubescent male is less resistant to physeal separation and that the physis is weakest in torsion. The mechanism of injury can also dictate the fracture and physeal injury pattern.[214] Bending causes physeal separation on the tension side of the fracture, whereas the Salter-Harris II metaphyseal fragment usually occurs on the compression side. This fragment, referred to as the *Thurston-Holland fragment,* represents a portion of the metaphysis that has fractured while the physis remaining attached to this segment is not separated. The Salter-Harris type II fracture pattern is the most common fracture pattern for displaced distal femoral physeal fractures. In addition, Salter-Harris type III fractures can occur when the medial condyle fractures off both through the physis medially and extending through the intracondylar notch with valgus stress. The medial collateral ligament (MCL) remains attached to the condylar fracture during valgus stress and can occur as the physis begins to close because this physis generally closes centrally first. Many of these physeal fractures in the area of the knee are present with a pronounced hemarthrosis, particularly the tibial spine fractures. Affected patients often report hearing a "pop" and having instability after an awkward landing or during a cutting activity. Patients with a tibial tubercle avulsion or proximal tibial physeal fracture often had a hyperextension injury. Because the metaphysis is often posteriorly displaced, the popliteal artery may stretch in the area of the trifurcation. A series of vascular examinations is needed if proximal tibial physeal injury is suspected.

On examination, patients with a distal femoral physeal fracture may exhibit abnormal laxity on varus or valgus stress that can mimic an MCL or lateral collateral ligament/posterolateral corner injury. They have been associated with residual ligamentous laxity after healing (8% in one series) that may represent stretch injury to the ligament in addition to the physeal fracture.[207] Salter-Harris type III fractures of the medial femoral condyle are highly associated with cruciate ligament injuries. In addition to a thorough examination of knee stability, it is crucial to document the neurovascular status distally. As mentioned previously, these fractures can be associated with vascular compromise in some cases. Also, varus stress injuries may result in peroneal nerve stretch and neurapraxia. Patellar height should also be measured and compared with the contralateral knee because patella alta can be seen in tibial tubercle avulsions along with patellar sleeve avulsion fractures. When examining the tibial tubercle, it is important to distinguish a chronic condition such as Osgood-Schlatter disease from an acute tibial tubercle fracture or avulsion. Both a history of symptoms and their severity, along with physical examination findings such as knee effusion, patellar height difference, and inability to perform a straight-leg raise, help distinguish these two entities.

Imaging

In addition to standard radiographs, stress views were traditionally recommended to evaluate a patient for a suspected distal femoral or tibial physeal fracture. However, given the risk of further damage to the physis and improvement in MRI, MRI may be a better means of evaluating potential physeal injuries that are not clear on radiographs or when compared with contralateral films. A CT scan can be used for evaluating intraarticular extension, especially in the cases of Salter-Harris type III and IV fractures of the distal femur, tibial spine, and tibial tubercle fractures.

Tibial spine fractures are often classified by the Meyers and McKeever classification system (Fig. 135-17).[215] Type I fractures are minimally displaced; type II fractures are hinged anteriorly with an intact posterior portion; and type III fractures are completely separated (Figs. 135-18 and 135-19). Type IV fractures were added to the classification system later and are also completely displaced and rotated.[216]

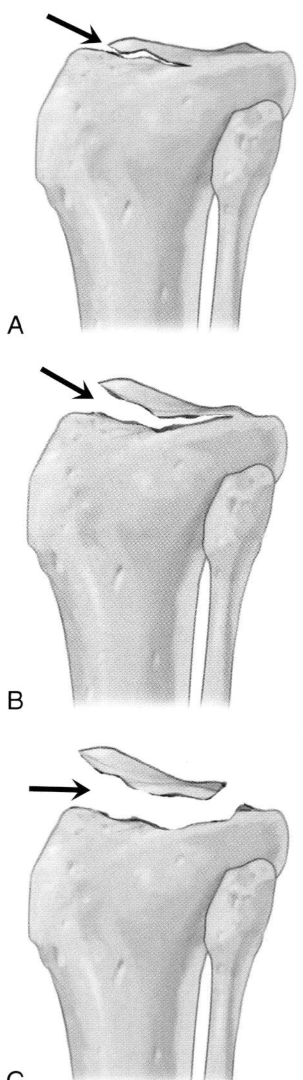

FIGURE 135-17 Meyers and McKeever classification of tibial eminence fractures in children. **A,** Type I is a nondisplaced fracture. **B,** Type II is a displaced fracture that is hinged posteriorly. **C,** Type III fractures are completely displaced.

Tibial tubercle and proximal tibial physeal fractures are also best evaluated on the lateral view or in the sagittal plane. A CT scan is sometimes needed to evaluate for intraarticular extension or displacement. A modified Watson-Jones classification system of tibial tubercle fractures has been developed. Type I fractures are a physeal separation through the tubercle apophysis but distal to the junction of the ossification centers of the tubercle and the epiphysis. Type II fractures are a physeal separation through the junction of the tubercle and epiphysis. Type III fractures extend through the proximal tibial epiphysis intraarticularly. Type IV fractures extend posteriorly through the physis. Type V fractures involve an avulsion of the periosteal attachment of the patellar tendon.

Decision-Making Principles

Treatment Options

Distal femoral physeal fractures can be treated both conservatively and operatively, with the amount of initial displacement generally dictating the treatment plan. Closed reduction and immobilization is best for a nondisplaced or minimally displaced fracture. Closed reduction and percutaneous pinning versus screw fixation is appropriate for displaced Salter-Harris type I and II fractures that reduce anatomically with closed reduction. If screw fixation is used, the Salter-Harris type II fragment must be large enough for adequate screw purchase (if the screw is placed proximal and parallel to the physis). In general, rigid immobilization or supplemental pin fixation is often needed in addition to fixation of the Thurston-Holland fragment, given the large lever arm distal to the fracture fixation. Open reduction and internal fixation are advocated for irreducible Salter-Harris type I and II fractures and all displaced Salter-Harris type III and IV fractures of the distal femur (Fig. 135-20).

Tibial spine fractures that are nondisplaced or reduce anatomically with closed reduction using hyperextension and casting can be treated in a closed fashion with immobilization. In general, the knee must be kept in full extension or slight hyperextension to maintain reduction, and casting or brace immobilization needs to continue for 4 to 6 weeks depending on the radiographic progression of healing. For tibial spine fractures that do not respond to closed reduction, multiple techniques are available for reduction and fixation. Traditionally, open reduction using a parapatellar arthrotomy approach and screw fixation was used. Screws are generally kept within the epiphysis to avoid damage to the physis. Arthroscopic reduction and internal fixation techniques are also available now. Lateral and medial meniscal tears have been described in conjunction with tibial spine fractures, and arthroscopic examination allows for diagnosis and treatment of these lesions. Meniscal tears and the intermeniscal ligament have been described as blocks to reduction and often need to be addressed to allow an anatomic reduction (Fig. 135-21). Once reduction is achieved arthroscopically, either percutaneous screw fixation or suture fixation can be performed. Suture fixation involves passing sutures through the chondroepiphyseal portion of the tibial spine avulsion and bringing these sutures down across the physis; tension can be applied, and they can be tied across a metaphyseal bone

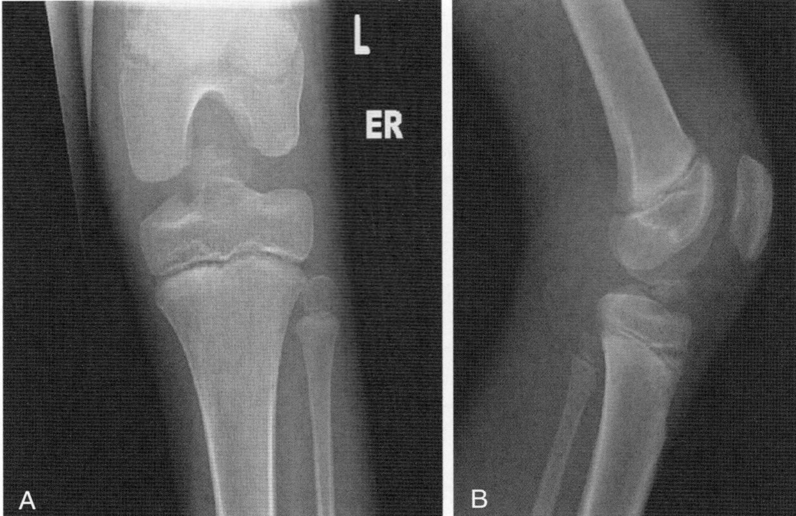

FIGURE 135-18 Anteroposterior (**A**) and lateral (**B**) radiographs of a type III tibial eminence fracture.

bridge. This technique is generally reserved for tibial spine avulsions that have insufficient bone stock for screw fixation (Fig. 135-22).

Nondisplaced proximal tibial physeal fractures can also be treated with immobilization with a cast and eventually a brace. Minimally displaced fractures can be treated with closed reduction and smooth pin or screw fixation. Depending on the age of the athlete, smooth pin fixation may be more appropriate for younger patients with wide-open physes. Open reduction and internal fixation is reserved for fractures that fail to respond to closed reduction, are widely displaced, have intraarticular step-off, or have associated neurovascular issues that need to be addressed simultaneously. Tibial tubercle fractures follow a similar decision-making algorithm. Some persons have advocated the use of arthroscopy to evaluate and assist in the treatment of intraarticular fractures. However, this technique should be undertaken with caution because these patients are already at risk for increased swelling distally given the risk of vascular injury, and the added fluid extravasation from arthroscopy can increase the risk of compartment syndrome.

Complications

Each physeal fracture pattern around the knee has been associated with complications. The major complications include nonunion, malunion, neurovascular compromise (particularly with proximal tibial physeal fractures), compartment syndrome, growth arrest and/or angular deformity (particularly with distal femoral physeal fractures), associated ligamentous injury or residual laxity (particularly with tibial spine fractures and intraarticular distal femoral physeal fractures), and stiffness/arthrofibrosis.[206-212,217-227] Particular attention should be given to the difficult situation of arthrofibrosis after physeal

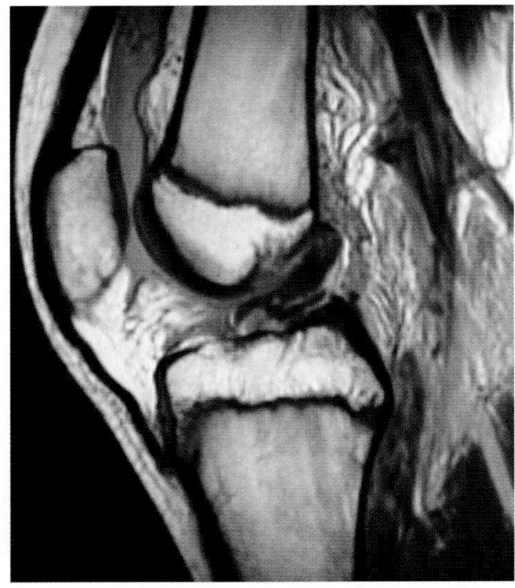

FIGURE 135-19 A sagittal magnetic resonance imaging section showing a type III tibial eminence fracture.

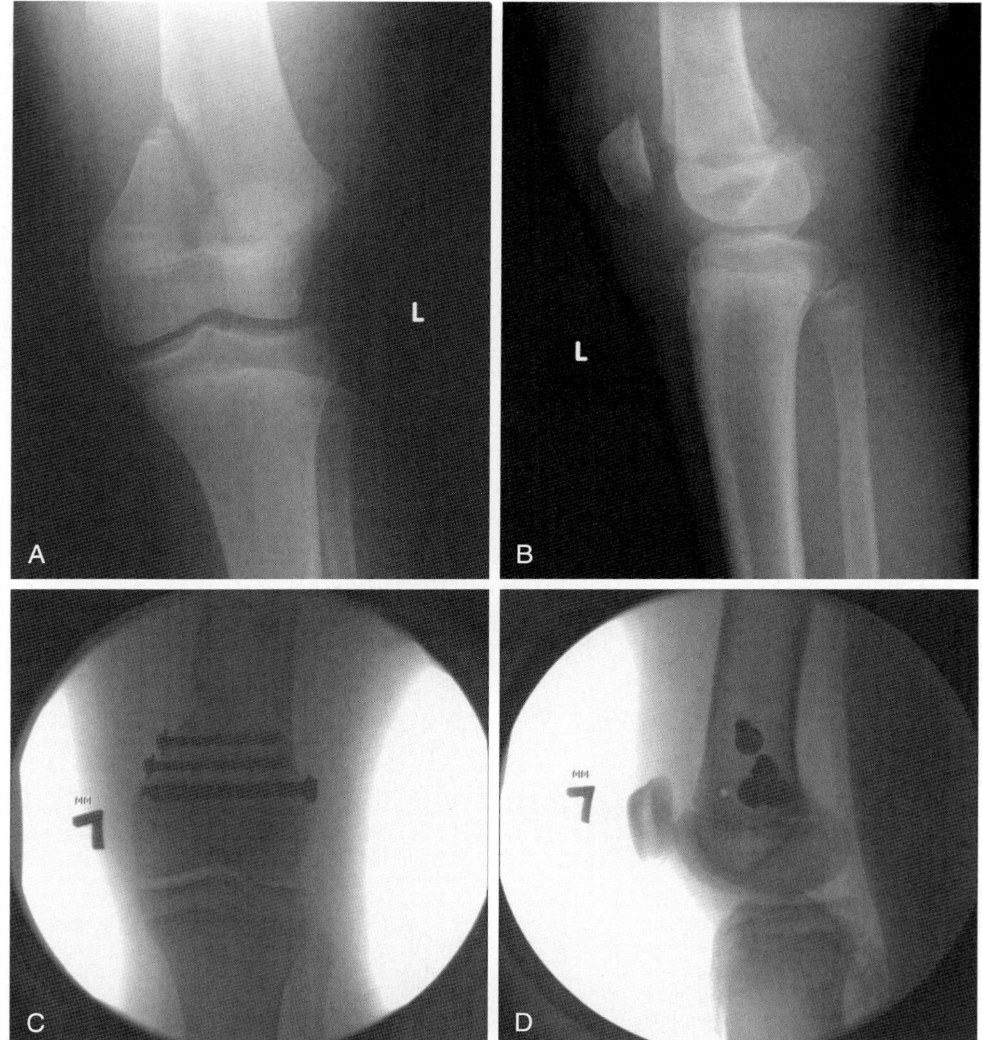

FIGURE 135-20 **A,** An anteroposterior (AP) radiograph of distal femoral physeal fracture. **B,** A lateral radiograph of a distal femoral physeal fracture. **C,** An AP radiograph after closed reduction internal fixation of a distal femur physeal fracture. **D,** A lateral radiograph after closed reduction internal fixation of a distal femoral physeal fracture. *(Courtesy Children's Orthopedic Center. From Scott WN, editor:* Insall and Scott surgery of the knee*, ed 5, New York, 2012, Elsevier.)*

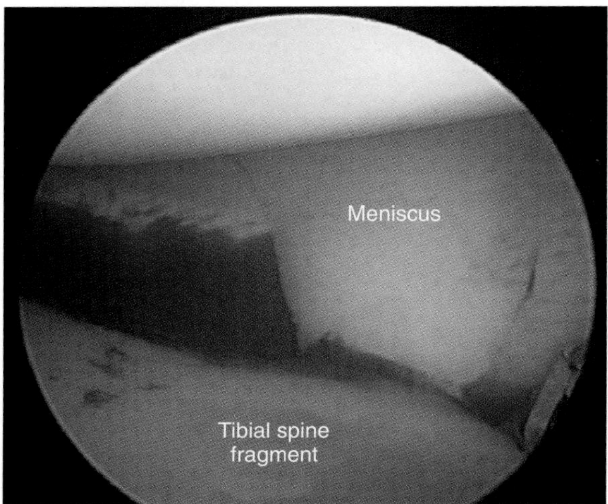

FIGURE 135-21 Anterior horn of the medial meniscus entrapped under the tibial spine fragment. *(From Scott WN, editor:* Insall and Scott surgery of the knee*, ed 5, New York, 2012, Elsevier.)*

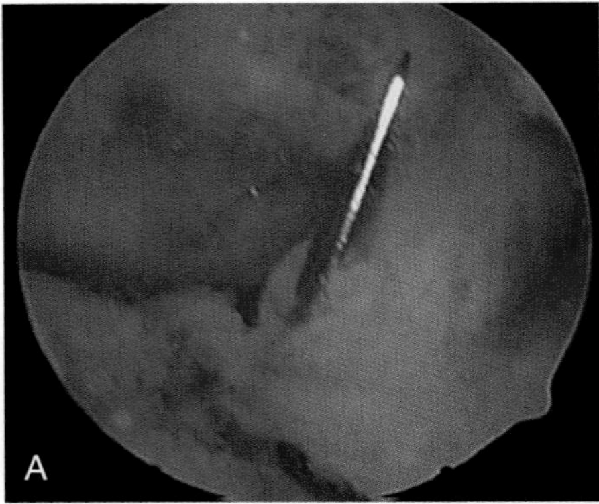

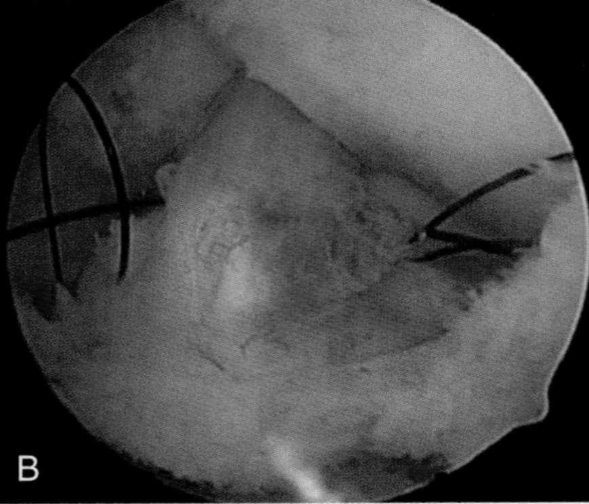

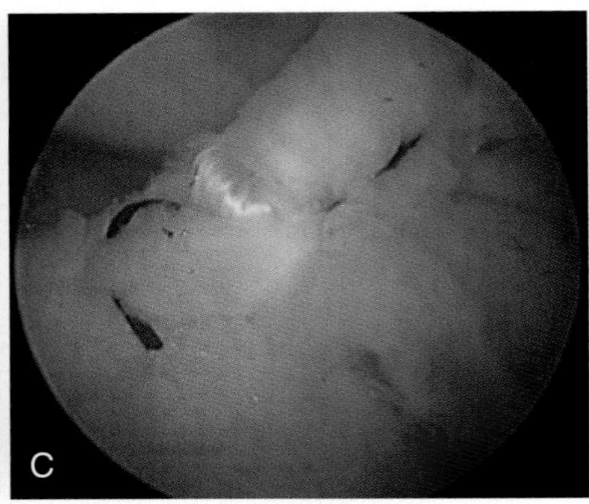

FIGURE 135-22 Treatment of a type II tibial spine fracture with arthroscopic reduction and suture fixation. **A,** Drilling of guide wire with an anterior cruciate ligament (ACL) guide system. **B,** Hewson suture passers on either side of the ACL and passage of absorbable sutures through the ACL. **C,** The final appearance after suture fixation. *(From Scott WN, editor:* Insall and Scott surgery of the knee*, ed 5, New York, 2012, Elsevier.)*

or tibial spine fractures. Vander Have et al.[228] recently reported a 12.5% risk of distal femoral physeal fracture and subsequent growth arrest after manipulation following tibial eminence fracture treatment complicated by arthrofibrosis.

For a complete list of references, go to expertconsult.com.

Suggested Readings

Citation: Anderson AF: Transepiphyseal replacement of the anterior cruciate ligament in skeletally immature patients. A preliminary report. *J Bone Joint Surg Am* 85A(7):1255–1263, 2003.

Level of Evidence: IV

Summary: Anderson reports one of the first case series of transepiphyseal anterior cruciate ligament reconstruction with use of quadruple hamstring autograft. This article includes an excellent technical description of the procedure along with relevant figures and fluoroscopic images.

Citation: Kocher MS, Garg S, Micheli LJ: Physeal sparing reconstruction of the anterior cruciate ligament in skeletally immature prepubescent children and adolescents. *J Bone Joint Surg Am* 87A(11):2371–2379, 2005.

Level of Evidence: IV

Summary: The authors of this classic article describe physeal-sparing, combined intraarticular and extraarticular reconstruction of the anterior cruciate ligament and provide a minimum of 2-year follow-up data. An excellent technical description of the procedure accompanies results that show a low revision rate and minimal risk of growth disturbance.

Citation: Lawrence JT, Argawal N, Ganley TJ: Degeneration of the knee joint in skeletally immature patients with a diagnosis of an anterior cruciate ligament tear: Is there harm in delay of treatment? *Am J Sports Med* 39(12):2582–2587, 2011.

Level of Evidence: III

Summary: The authors of this excellent cohort study show that increased time from injury to anterior cruciate ligament reconstruction in children younger than 14 years of age was associated with an increased risk of medial meniscal tears and lateral compartment chondral injury.

Citation: Lawrence JT, et al: All-epiphyseal anterior cruciate ligament reconstruction in skeletally immature patients. *Clin Orthop Relat Res* 468(7):1971–1977, 2010.

Level of Evidence: IV

Summary: The authors of this case series describe an anatomic all-epiphyseal anterior cruciate ligament reconstruction technique for skeletally immature patients. Fluoroscopic or intraoperative computed tomography scan image guidance is necessary for tunnel placement.

Citation: Kocher MS, Klingele K, Rassman SO: Meniscal disorders: Normal, discoid, and cysts. *Orthop Clin North Am* 34(3):329–340, 2003.

Level of Evidence: V

Summary: The authors provide an excellent review of meniscal disease in pediatric and adolescent patients. Topics include meniscal tears, discoid meniscus, and meniscal cysts.

Citation: Palmu S, et al: Acute patellar dislocation in children and adolescents: A randomized clinical trial. *J Bone Joint Surg Am* 90A(3):463–470, 2008.

Level of Evidence: II

Summary: In this prospective study, nonoperative and acute surgical repair is compared for first-time patellar dislocations in children younger than 16 years. Long-term follow-up showed a high rate of recurrent instability in both cohorts but similar subjective outcomes. Initial surgical treatment was not recommended in this population. A family history of patellar instability was shown to be a significant predictor for recurrence.

Citation: Chambers HG, et al: Diagnosis and treatment of osteochondritis dissecans. *J Am Acad Orthop Surg* 19(5):297–306, 2011.

Level of Evidence: IV

Summary: In this clinical practice guideline, recommendations are outlined based on a systematic review of the published literature on osteochondritis dissecans treatment. Although the recommendations are graded as mostly weak or inclusive, this review will help shape future research.

Citation: Wall EJ, et al: The healing potential of stable juvenile osteochondritis dissecans knee lesions. *J Bone Joint Surg Am* 90A(12):2655–2664, 2008.

Level of Evidence: II

Summary: In this excellent study of stable osteochondritis dissecans lesions in skeletally immature patients, lesions with an increased size, associated swelling, and/or mechanical symptoms are shown to be less likely to heal. A nomogram is produced from their data to predict healing based on normalized height/weight and symptoms.

Citation: Kocher MS, et al: Tibial eminence fractures in children: Prevalence of meniscal entrapment. *Am J Sports Med* 31(3):404–407, 2003.

Level of Evidence: IV

Summary: In this large case series of operatively treated type II and III tibial eminence fractures, a high rate of meniscal entrapment is shown under displaced fractures. The anterior horn of the medial meniscus was most commonly entrapped. Operative treatment was recommended for all type III eminence fractures and type II fractures that did not reduce in extension.

Citation: Vander Have KL, et al: Arthrofibrosis after surgical fixation of tibial eminence fractures in children and adolescents. *Am J Sports Med* 38(2):298–301, 2010.

Level of Evidence: IV

Summary: Case series from four institutions show a high rate of arthrofibrosis after operative treatment of tibial eminence fractures. The series also show an increased risk of iatrogenic physeal fracture from manipulation after inducement of anesthesia. Conclusions include focusing on sufficient stabilization at the time of the initial surgery to allow early postoperative rehabilitation and performing subseqent manipulation only upon inducement of anesthesia in conjunction with a lysis of adhesions.

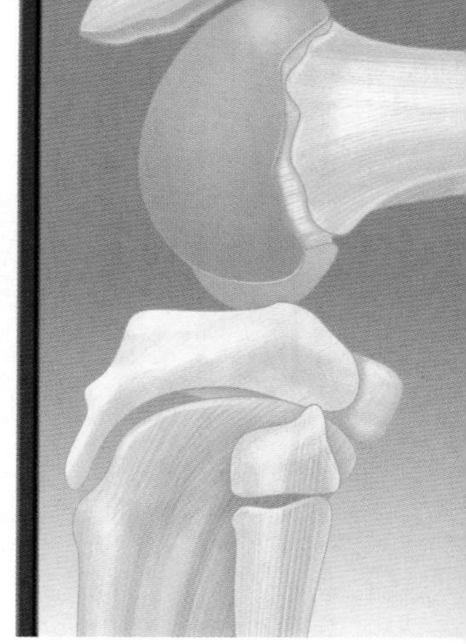

136

Foot and Ankle Injuries in the Adolescent Athlete

J. ANDY SULLIVAN • THOMAS R. LEWIS

Most of the injuries that occur in the ankle and foot of the pediatric athlete are not unique to athletic participation but occur normally during childhood. Some injuries, however, occur with greater frequency in the athlete. The conditions covered in this chapter occur in childhood and may present in the athlete, raising the question of whether the athlete should be allowed to participate in sports activities. As a general rule, in all of these conditions, if a patient has an injury or an operation, we allow return to play when he or she has no pain, full range of motion, and the strength and ability to perform all the activities involved in the sport.

Variations of Normal Anatomy

Tarsal Coalition

Tarsal coalition is a bony or fibrous or cartilaginous connection of two or more of the tarsal bones. The cause is unknown, but it has been established that the condition results from failure of differentiation and segmentation of the primitive mesenchyme.[1] The overall incidence is 1% to 3%.[1-3] The most common coalitions are the calcaneonavicular and talocalcaneal types, which are bilateral in about 60% and 50% of cases, respectively.[2-4] More than one type of coalition can exist in one foot. In a review of 60 cases of tarsal coalition, Clarke[5] found that 6 of 30 patients had multiple coalitions in the same foot. The exact mode of inheritance is unknown, but it is postulated to be autosomal dominant with variable penetrance.[2]

Most patients seek medical care during early adolescence, at a time when the coalition is ossifying. The pain is vague in nature and insidious in onset. The patient may have a history of precipitating trauma. Sports participation or running over uneven ground may accentuate the pain. The pain is thought to be due to microfractures in the coalition.[6] Physical findings include pain on palpation over the subtalar joint, limited subtalar motion, and at times pes planus and ankle valgus. The peroneal muscles may be tight and resist inversion, but true muscle spasm occurs rarely (Fig. 136-1). Any condition that injures the subtalar joint can produce similar symptoms.

The clinical diagnosis can be confirmed by radiographic imaging. Plain radiographs, especially the 45-degree oblique view (Fig. 136-2), usually demonstrate the calcaneonavicular coalition and other less common coalitions, such as the calcaneocuboid. The talocalcaneal coalition (TCC) is difficult to visualize on plain radiographs, but secondary changes, which may suggest the need for other studies (Fig. 136-3), include beaking and shortening of the talar neck, a middle subtalar facet that cannot be seen, elongation of the lateral process of the calcaneus, and a ball-and-socket ankle joint (see Fig. 136-3).

Crim and Kjeldsberg[7] studied two groups of 30 patients with tarsal coalition and 17 control subjects. A second group of patients with 150 weight-bearing radiographs for nontraumatic foot pain were reviewed for cases of undetected tarsal coalition. These investigators identified several previously undescribed plain radiographic signs for coalitions. For calcaneonavicular coalitions, these signs were altered navicular structure and visualization of the bar on the anteroposterior (AP) radiograph. For TCCs, the changes were a dysmorphic sustentaculum tali, nonvisualization of the middle subtalar facet, and shortening of the talar neck. When these criteria were used in the 150 prospective cases, three previously undetected coalitions were diagnosed and then confirmed by computed tomography (CT) with no false-positive results.

If a calcaneonavicular coalition is present on plain radiographs, a CT scan should be obtained to ensure that no other coalitions exist, which is necessary for surgical planning (see Fig. 136-2). A CT or magnetic resonance imaging (MRI) scan can also be performed if a coalition is suspected clinically but none is identified on plain films. CT is easily performed, delineates bone quite well, and can be formatted into a three-dimensional (3D) image that is useful when planning surgery. MRI has the advantage of demonstrating fibrous or cartilaginous lesions, as well as bony lesions. MRI has the advantage of the absence of radiation but at three times the cost of CT.

El Rassi and colleagues[8] reviewed 19 patients with symptoms and signs consistent with tarsal coalition and normal imaging studies. These investigators used technetium-99m scintigraphy and found slightly increased uptake in the middle facet. They obtained good or fair results in all patients after resection of hypervascular capsule and synovium, which had produced arthrofibrosis.

The initial treatment of these conditions should include conservative measures aimed at relieving the pain. These measures are empirical and include casting and the use of various shoe inserts and orthotics. The main indication for surgical resection is persistent pain. For calcaneonavicular coalition, resection of the bar with interposition of the extensor

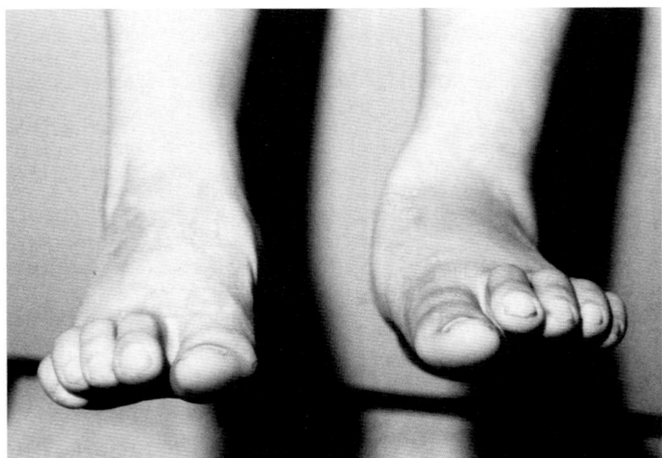

FIGURE 136-1 This patient had a tarsal coalition in the left foot. Note that the foot is held in an everted position. Attempted inversion caused pain and resistance.

digitorum brevis is usually associated with good results. Studies by Cowell[2] and Jayakumar and Cowell[4] indicated that 23 of 26 feet treated in this manner became symptom free.

TCC historically was more difficult to recognize, and its surgical management is less certain.[10] Before the advent of CT, the diagnosis was often confirmed at the time of surgery. Jayakumar and Cowell[4] reported that up to one third of their patients responded to conservative treatment, and they believed that few indications for resection exist. This conclusion was based on evidence from family studies indicating that many adults with tarsal coalition were asymptomatic. The surgical alternatives include resection of the bar with interposition of fat or tendon, calcaneal osteotomy, and triple arthrodesis.

Scranton[11] reviewed 14 patients with 23 symptomatic TCCs. Five feet (in three patients) were treated successfully with casts. Four feet were treated with triple arthrodesis. Eight patients with 13 coalitions that had been resected had a good result. The review was performed at a mean of 3.9 years after surgery. In Scranton's series, about half of the joint surface was removed in some patients.[11] In the series reported by Swiontkowski and associates,[12] 10 patients were treated for TCC—4 by resection of the bar, and the remainder with some type of arthrodesis. This article stressed that the talar beak is not a true degenerative sign and therefore is not a contraindication to resection of the bar. Olney and Asher[13] evaluated 9 patients with persistent pain from 10 middle-facet TCCs who were treated with resection of the bar and an autogenous fat graft. At an average follow-up of 42 months, the results were rated excellent in 5 patients, good in 3 patients, fair in 1 patient, and poor in 1 patient. In one patient who underwent a repeat operation, the fat graft was replaced by fibrous tissue.

Luhmann and Schoenecker[14] used CT to evaluate TCC in 25 feet. They quantified heel valgus and the size of the coalition relative to the posterior facet. The ratio of mean TCC cross-sectional area to the posterior facet was 53.4%. Mean hindfoot valgus was 17.8 degrees. Statistical analysis determined a significant association between TCC greater than 50% the size of the posterior facet and poor outcome ($P = .014$). Heel valgus greater than 21 degrees was also associated with poor outcome ($P = .014$). However, good results were obtained in some patients with a TCC greater than 50% and in patients with heel valgus greater than 21 degrees. These investigators advocate using the CT information for a preoperative discussion with patients and families.

Comfort and Johnson[15] reviewed resection of 20 TCCs at an average of 29 months of follow-up. They found good or excellent results with resections involving less than one third of the total joint surface. They did not find increasing age to be a contradiction to the procedure. Gantsoudes et al.[16] have provided an excellent review of outcomes with use of interpositional fat. In 49 feet with a minimum follow-up of 12 months (and an average follow-up of 42.6 months), an average score of 90/100 (excellent) was achieved with use of the American Orthopedic Foot and Ankle Society Hindfoot scale. Eleven patients (34%) required subsequent surgery to correct foot alignment. Good to excellent results were achieved in 85% of patients.[16]

The management of these coalitions is still controversial and awaits the results of larger series with longer follow-up.

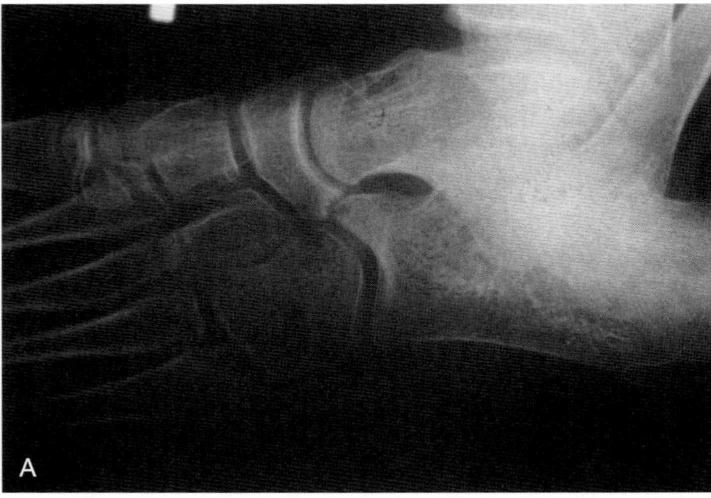

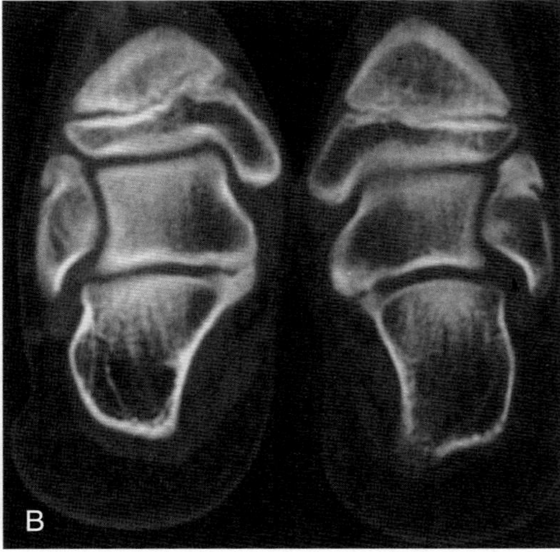

FIGURE 136-2 Plain radiography (**A**) and a computed tomographic scan (**B**) showing calcaneonavicular and talocalcaneal coalitions, which occurred bilaterally in this patient. The patient presented with a painful, rigid foot and was having difficulty playing tennis.

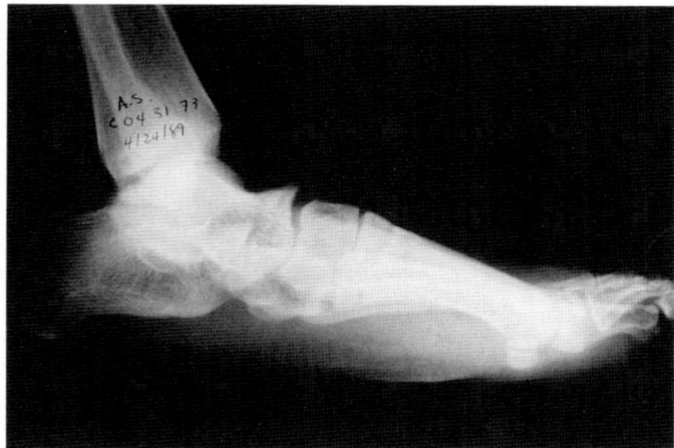

FIGURE 136-3 A lateral radiograph of the foot. Note the beaking of the talus and the widening of the talonavicular joint. The subtalar joint is narrowed.

Patients with persistent symptoms who do not have degenerative findings have the option of continued conservative care, resection of the coalition, or arthrodesis. Talar beaking is not necessarily a degenerative sign. Factors to consider are the size of the coalition and the age of the patient. Severe malalignment of the foot is a contraindication to resection alone. A sliding osteotomy or medial closing wedge as described by Cain and Hyman[17] can be used to realign the foot.

Adolescent Bunion

The cause of adolescent bunion is unknown. Fifty percent to 60% of patients have a positive family history.[18] Patients with this condition have an increased intermetatarsal angle (the angle between the first and second metatarsals, normally 10 degrees) and an increased first metatarsal–phalangeal angle (normally 20 degrees). Many patients also have a relaxed flatfoot and a long first metatarsal ray. None of these conditions is known to be the cause of adolescent bunion. Footwear has been implicated, but because bunions occur in cultures in which shoes are not worn, this theory seems unlikely.

Patients with adolescent bunion report pain, prominence, and difficulty associated with footwear. On examination, lateral deviation of the toe is found, along with a medial prominence and a wide forefoot. The bursa that is a prominent part of the adult deformity may be present but is usually less impressive. Arthritis and decreased range of motion are also less common. The patient should be evaluated with AP and lateral weight-bearing radiographs. The joint space is usually maintained. The sesamoids may be laterally displaced in advanced cases. The medial eminence of the metatarsal head is prominent, and a sagittal groove may be present medially.

Children should be treated nonsurgically whenever possible. Alteration or stretching of footwear may alleviate symptoms. Although some series have claimed a success rate of 80% to 95%, this high rate of success has not been the universal experience. Factors implicated in these complications included failure to correct the abnormal deviation of the first metatarsal, failure to correct the soft tissues, weight bearing that was begun too early, inadequate immobilization, and osteotomy performed distal to the open physis. Patients with a hypermobile flatfoot or a long first ray also seemed to be more prone to recurrence.

Indications for surgery include pain that is not responsive to conservative measures and severe deformity. The goals of surgery should include realignment of the first ray and of the metatarsophalangeal joint, cosmesis, and prevention of arthritis. Arthrodesis and resection have no place in the normal child. In general, the most common procedures are distal soft tissue realignment, a distal osteotomy such as the Mitchell or chevron technique, or a proximal realignment or Scarf osteotomy combined with soft tissue procedures. In the senior author's experience, it is not unusual for a female athlete to present with a bunion, usually bilateral. Often these athletes are basketball or soccer players and have increased intermetatarsal and metatarsophalangeal angles. In these patients the most common procedure the senior author now performs is a bunionectomy, release of the abductor hallucis, a Scarf osteotomy, and capsular imbrication. Most patients have returned to sport in 3 to 6 months. Postoperatively the senior author has the patient wear a cast for 6 weeks, and then the wearing of regular shoes is gradually resumed.

Accessory Navicular

Numerous accessory ossicles can occur in the foot, and awareness of these accessory ossicles is necessary to avoid confusing them with an acute fracture. The most common accessory ossicles are the os trigonum posterior to the talus and the os vesalianum at the base of the fifth metatarsal. The accessory navicular is a separate ossification center of the navicular. It may be completely separate or joined by a synchondrosis. It may also present as a large or cornuate (horn-shaped) prominence on the medial side of the navicular (Fig. 136-4). We

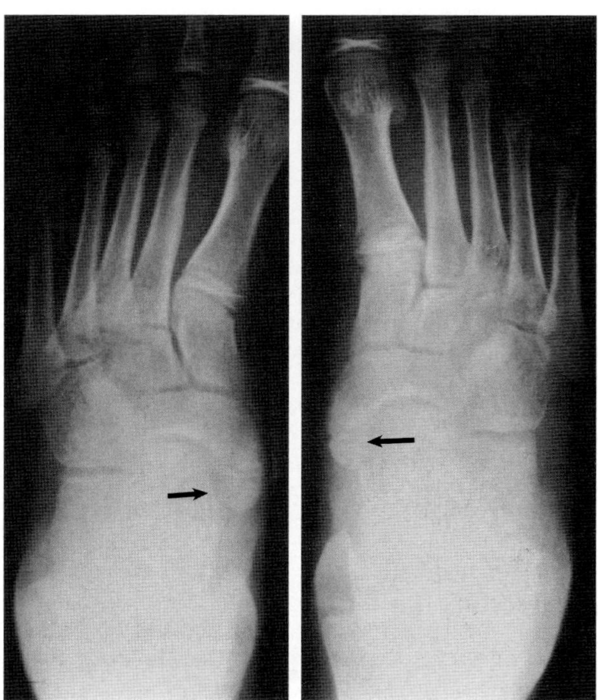

FIGURE 136-4 Large bilateral cornuate prominent accessory naviculars (*arrows*). They are joined by a synchondrosis to the navicular.

now know that only a small slip of the tendon inserts into this ossicle and that these patients are no more likely to have flatfoot than are those with a normal navicular.[19]

Many of these patients are asymptomatic. Symptomatic patients experience pain directly over the prominence, usually from footwear over the prominence. If the shoes are stretched or altered over this prominence, symptoms may be relieved. Other patients experience pain when the posterior tibial tendon is stretched or placed under tension. In persons with persistent pain, simple excision of the ossicle without rerouting of the tendon is usually successful.[19,20]

Cavus Foot

Cavus is defined as an increase in the height of the longitudinal arch of the foot. A variety of other modifiers, such as cavovarus and calcaneocavus, are used to further describe the position of the heel. Often the patient has claw toes or hammer toes and metatarsal head calluses. The presenting complaint can be pain or abnormal wear of the shoe. A cavus foot is usually the result of muscle imbalance that is caused by an underlying neurologic disorder. The patient should undergo a meticulous neurologic examination so that evidence of disorders such as Charcot-Marie-Tooth disease, spinal dysraphism, or a spinal tumor can be detected. Initial radiographic evaluation should include weight-bearing views of the feet and at least an AP view of the entire spine in search of an occult spinal anomaly. An MRI of the entire spine and a neurologic consult are indicted if any question exists of an underlying neurologic disorder.

Soft Tissue Injuries

The ligaments of the ankle insert on the epiphyses distal to the physeal line (Fig. 136-5). Because the physis is the weakest link in this bone-tendon-bone interface, it is usually the part that gives way when significant force is applied to the ankle. Serious ankle sprains are unusual in the skeletally immature athlete. Physeal fractures that do occur are discussed in the next section. Minor ankle sprains occur and are diagnosed by a history of inversion or eversion strain with findings of tenderness over the anterior talofibular or deltoid ligament. Treatment consists of the usual conservative means of rest, ice, compression, elevation, and immobilization. Formal rehabilitation is rarely necessary but may be beneficial for the competitive athlete. Continued pain or disability should provoke a search for other more serious injury.

Recurrent subluxation of peroneal tendons can occur in the adolescent athlete. Usually, a history of injury is followed by recurrent episodes of a snapping sensation and pain. The subluxation can be provoked by forceful dorsiflexion with the foot everted. In patients whose symptoms are sufficiently severe, surgical correction may be indicated. Surgical alternatives include deepening the groove on the fibula, creating a bony block, and reconstructing the superior peroneal retinaculum. The first two are rarely useful in treatment of the pediatric athlete because the physis is still open. Poll and Duijfjes[21] reviewed 9 patients aged 15 to 45 years (average age, 25 years) who underwent reconstruction with the posterior calcaneofibular ligament attached to a bone block. Results were said to be good.

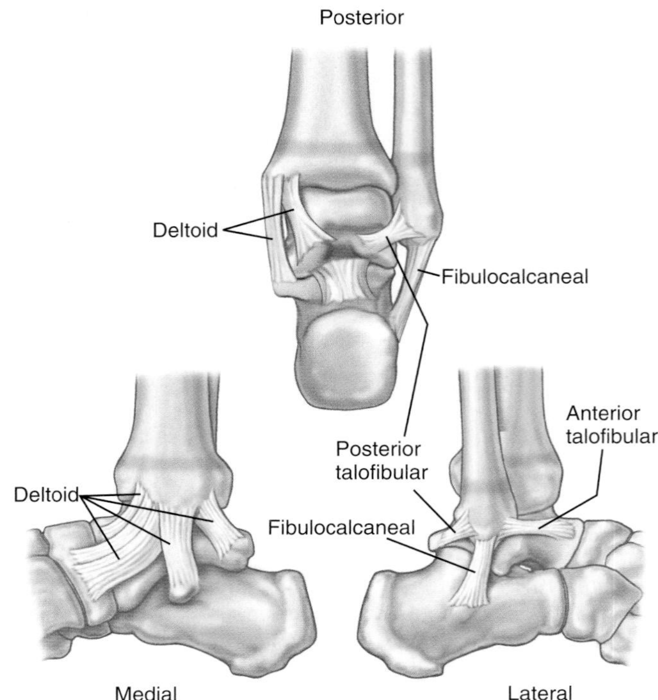

FIGURE 136-5 Posterior, medial, and lateral views of the ligaments of the ankle.

Contusions on the foot are treated in the same way as those on any other area. Blisters are a frequent problem and require alleviation of the stress, which is usually provided by a new shoe and protection until healing occurs. Tinea pedis (athlete's foot) usually responds to a regimen of antifungal medication, along with education about the need to change socks frequently and to use antifungal powders.

Fractures Around the Ankle

Numerous systems have been proposed to classify ankle injuries. All of these classification systems take into account the position of the foot at the time of injury and the force applied. The Salter-Harris classification[22] is based on the mechanism of injury and the pathoanatomy of the fracture pattern through the physis, as interpreted on plain radiographs. The authors described types I through V. Type V, a crush injury to the physis, is difficult to recognize on plain radiographs at the time of injury and is not discussed in this chapter (Fig. 136-6). Podeszwa has an excellent review of this topic and points out that these physeal fractures are second only to fracture of the radius in frequency.[23]

In the skeletally immature patient, the tibiotalar joint surface is rarely disturbed. The injury pattern changes in adolescence as the physis begins to close. The outcome of the injury depends on the type of physeal injury and its management. Tension injuries usually produce Salter-Harris type I and II injuries of the physis. Compression forces can produce Salter-Harris type III and IV injuries. Podeszwa and Mubarak[23] state that the incidence of accessory centers of ossification is 20% in the medial malleolus and 1% in the lateral malleolus.

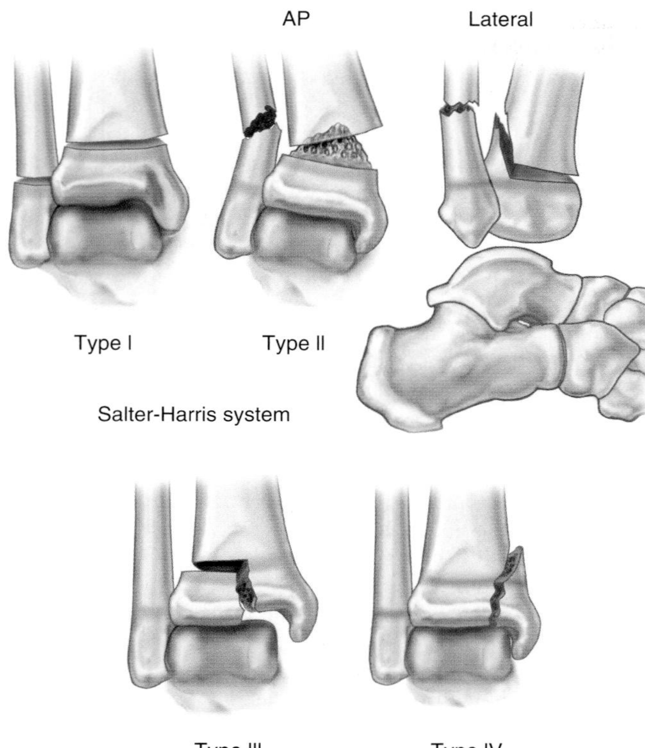

FIGURE 136-6 Fracture patterns of the distal tibial and fibular physes classified by the Salter-Harris system. *AP*, Anteroposterior.

CT and MRI are valuable techniques in assessing and classifying some fractures, especially those that are intraarticular, because they allow more accurate evaluation of the fragments. Carey and associates[24] performed a study of plain films and MRI in 14 patients with acute injuries. The direct visualization of cartilage afforded by MRI improved evaluation of growth plate injury in each case. MRI changed Salter-Harris classification or staging in 2 of 9 patients for whom fractures were visualized on conventional radiographs, allowed the detection of radiographically occult fractures in 5 of 14 cases, and resulted in a physical change in management for 5 of the 14 patients studied. MRI has an important role in the evaluation of acute pediatric growth plate injury, particularly when diagnostic uncertainty persists after the evaluation of conventional radiographs. MRI allows detection of occult fractures, may alter Salter-Harris staging, and may lead to a change in patient management.

Rohmiller and colleagues[25] have recently used the Lauge-Hansen system to look at the mechanism of injury in Salter-Harris type II distal tibial fractures. This topic is discussed later in this chapter.

Clinical Evaluation

The mechanism of injury and the time elapsed since the accident should be noted. The neurovascular status of the foot should be carefully documented. The amount of swelling and the status of the skin are important. Gentle examination should be carried out to seek areas of point tenderness, especially over the physis. This examination may be more useful than radiographs in the diagnosis of Salter-Harris type I injuries of the fibula.

Radiographs should always include three views of the ankle, which are required so the physician is able to see some fractures and determine whether the ankle mortise is disrupted. Plain tomography and CT may be indicated in the juvenile fracture of Tillaux and in triplane fractures, which are discussed later in this chapter. Because treatment and prognosis depend on the Salter-Harris classification, the fractures are discussed according to fracture type. Charlton and colleagues[26] recommended open reduction in physeal fractures with a gap of 3 mm or more. They found entrapped periosteum as the main offender in causing the gap. Trapped periosteum has been implicated in an increased incidence of premature physeal closure. These authors also recommended removal of epiphyseal metallic implants used in Salter type III and IV fractures of the tibia because the contact pressures as measured in cadavers are increased by the presence of epiphyseal screws. They mention the alternative use of bioabsorbable screws to obviate the need for removal.[26] As a general rule, any metallic fixation crossing the physis should be removed to lessen the risk of physeal closure.

Salter-Harris Type I

Rohmiller and colleagues[25] combined Salter-Harris type I and II fractures of the distal tibia and found an incidence of premature physeal closure (PPC) of 38%. No distinction was made between types I and II. Salter-Harris type I fractures of the fibula are common and may be missed entirely or misdiagnosed as a sprain. The characteristic history of an external rotation force in a patient who presents with localized tenderness and swelling directly over the distal fibular physis is diagnostic. The radiograph shows only localized swelling and widening of the fibular physis. Many of these injuries are probably unrecognized and untreated.

Salter-Harris Type II

The Salter-Harris type II injury is uncommon or is infrequently recognized in the fibula. Salter-Harris type II injury of the distal tibia combined with a fracture of the distal fibula is one of the most common injuries of the ankle, accounting for 47.3% of cases in the series compiled by Peterson and Cass.[27]

Rohmiller and colleagues[25] studied 91 Salter-Harris type I and II fractures. Treatment options include no reduction and use of a cast, closed reduction and use of a cast, closed reduction and use of percutaneous pins and a cast, and open reduction with internal fixation. They found a 39.6% incidence of PPC. With use of the Lauge-Hansen classification system, they found a significant increased incidence of PPC in pronation-abduction injuries (54%) compared with supination–external rotation injuries (35%). The most important determinant of PPC was the amount of fracture displacement after reduction. In some cases, periosteum is trapped in the fracture site medially, blocking reduction. These investigators thought that operative treatment may decrease the incidence of PPC. They recommended less than 2 mm of displacement in a child with 2 years of growth remaining to decrease the risk for PPC.

Traditional treatment consists of wearing a long-leg bent-knee cast for 2 to 3 weeks followed by a short-leg walking cast for 4 weeks. Dugan and coworkers[28] reviewed 56 patients with this injury who were treated with a long-leg weight-bearing cast for 4 weeks. The patients had no nonunions and no angular deformities, with one case of clinically insignificant premature closure of the growth plate. Use of a long-leg weight-bearing cast for 4 weeks appears to be the treatment of choice because it allows early healing, low morbidity, and rapid rehabilitation.

Salter-Harris Type III

In adolescents, a Salter-Harris type III injury is also known as the *juvenile fracture of Tillaux*. The distal tibial physis closes first in the central region and then from the medial side toward the fibula. An external rotation force applied to the partially closed physis applies traction on the physis through the anterior talofibular ligament. This process avulses a fragment of the lateral physis, which remains attached to the ligament (Fig. 136-7). Closed reduction with use of an anesthetic should be attempted. The injury can be treated in a closed manner if the fragment is not displaced more than 2 mm or if it can be reduced in a closed manner and percutaneously fixed. Most of these injuries require open reduction and fixation of the fragment with a pin or cancellous screw. Fractures of the medial malleolus can be either type III or IV injuries. If displaced less than 2 mm, they may be treated in a closed manner. Initially this treatment should consist of wearing a long-leg non–weight-bearing cast for 3 weeks, followed by wearing a short-leg walking cast for 3 weeks. These injuries are the most unpredictable of ankle epiphyseal injuries. Near-anatomic reduction must be obtained.[29]

Salter-Harris Type IV

The Salter-Harris type IV group includes some of the medial malleolar fractures and the triplane fractures. The triplane fracture, first described by Marmor, is so named because the fracture lines extend from the physis into the transverse, sagittal, and coronal planes (see Fig. 136-7).[30-33] This type of fracture may be mistaken for a Salter-Harris type II injury if the radiographs are not carefully scrutinized.

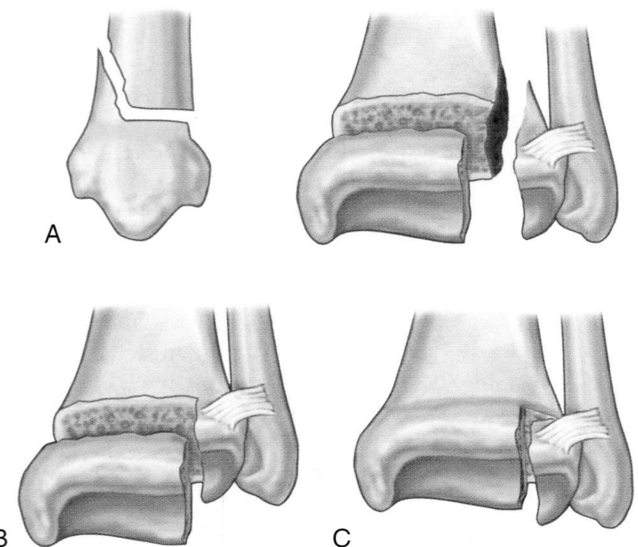

FIGURE 136-7 **A** and **B,** The triplane fracture can consist of two or more fragments. **C,** The juvenile fracture of Tillaux.

Many authors have described this fracture and have argued about the number of fragments involved.[30,32,33] Most of these studies were based on plain radiography. Figure 136-7 illustrates the possibilities. In the two-part fracture, the main fragment is the tibial shaft, including the medial malleolus and a portion of the medial epiphysis. The second fragment is the remaining epiphysis, which is attached to the fibula. In the three-part injury, the third fragment is usually an anterior free epiphyseal fragment. Brown and colleagues[34] studied 51 children with tibial triplane fractures. By evaluating them with CT with multiplanar reconstructions, these authors have used the best radiographic evaluation possible to define the number of fragments. The classic two-fragment type with medial epiphyseal extension was most frequent (occurring in 33 of 51 children). All three-fragment types (occurring in 8 of 51 children) had a separate anterolateral fragment. Extension to the medial malleolus was common (occurring in 12 of 51 children). None of the four reported fracture types involving anteromedial extension was seen.

Karrholm[35] reviewed the literature on this injury. Triplane fracture made up 7% of physeal injuries in girls and 15% in boys. Of the injuries, 35% were treated closed without manipulation, 30% by manipulation and casting, and 35% by open reduction and internal fixation.

If this injury can be reduced to within 2 mm, it may be treated in a closed manner. In the series reported by Cooperman and associates,[30] 13 of 15 fractures were treated in a closed manner, and in the series reported by Dias and Giergerich,[31] 5 of 8 were treated in this way. In the series by Ertl and colleagues,[32] residual displacement of more than 2 mm was associated with a high incidence of late symptoms. Obtaining a reduction of less than 2 mm by either closed or open means did not ensure an excellent result. Poor results may be related to damage done to the articular surface or to the amount of displacement. Fractures outside the weight-bearing area did not show this tendency toward poor results.

Evaluation of the adequacy of reduction in this injury is difficult, and because most authors recommend manipulation after inducement of general anesthesia, the only radiographic means of diagnosis available is plain radiography. Our preferred method is manipulation by internal rotation of the foot after the patient is sedated; this manipulation is usually performed in the emergency department. If any question exists about the adequacy of reduction on plain radiographs, CT or plain tomography is used to evaluate the articular surface and the reduction (Fig. 136-8). If displacement is greater than 2 mm, open reduction with internal fixation is performed, which may require two incisions. The first is an anterolateral incision, which permits identification of the anterolateral fragment. Usually, it is first necessary to reduce and fix the posterior fragment. If this procedure cannot be performed in a closed manner, a second posteromedial approach is used to reduce the fragment under direct vision. Fixation is achieved with cannulated screws, cancellous screws, or pins. These injuries require the patient to wear a cast for 6 weeks.

Prediction of Outcome

The prognosis for an ankle fracture in a skeletally immature patient depends on the following factors:

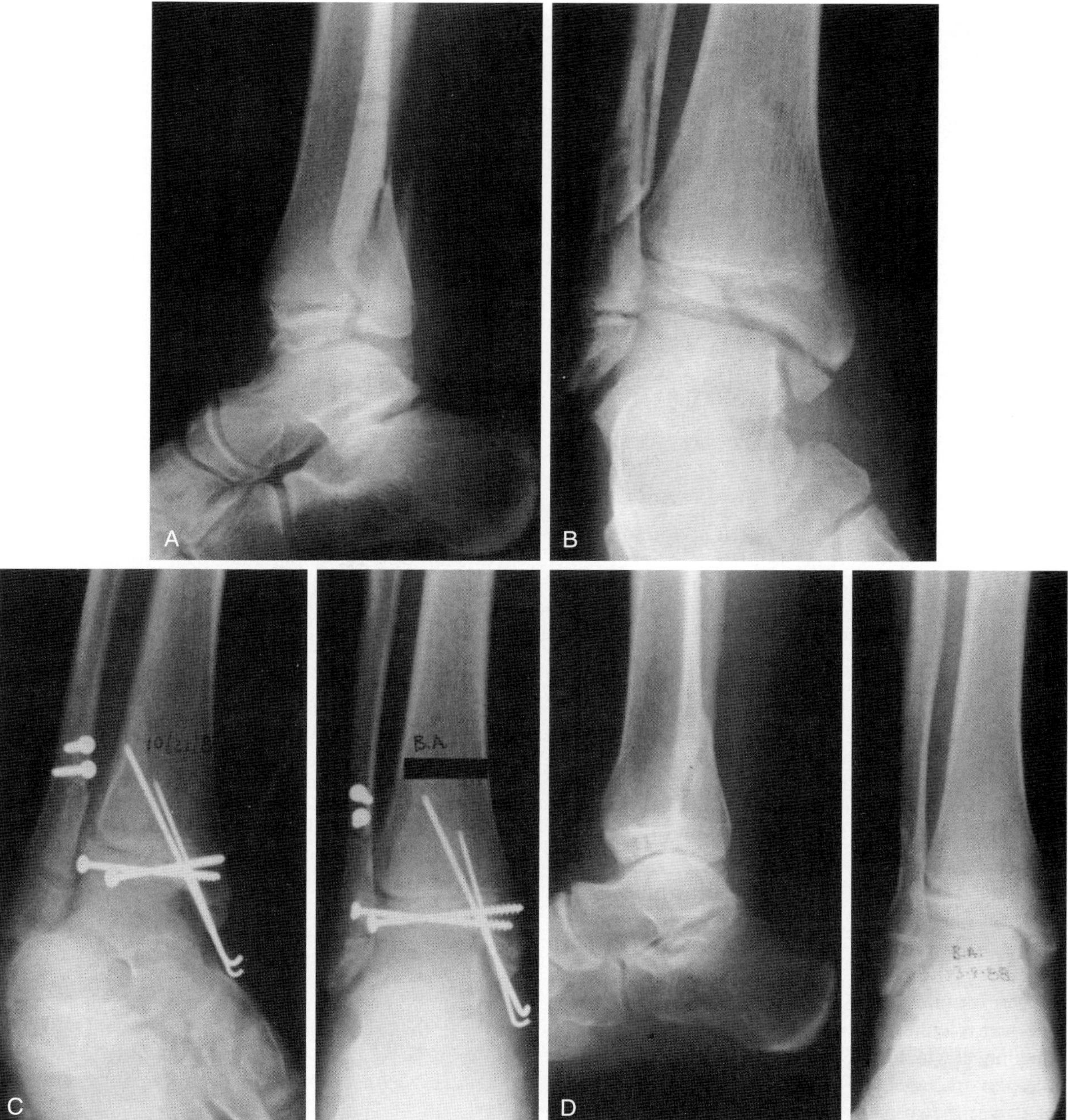

FIGURE 136-8 **A** and **B,** The position attained after manipulation of a severely displaced triplane fracture. The position was not acceptable, and thus further imaging was not necessary. **C,** The position achieved by open reduction. **D,** The position retained after hardware removal.

1. Mechanism of injury
2. Salter-Harris classification
3. Quality of the reduction
4. State of skeletal maturity
5. Amount of displacement
6. Miscellaneous modifiers (e.g., open fracture, vascular injury, infection, systemic illness, and interposed periosteum)

Spiegel and colleagues[33] retrospectively studied a series of closed distal tibial physeal injuries. One hundred eighty-four patients (of 237) were followed up for an average of 28 months. The authors looked specifically at the complications of angular deformity of greater than 5 degrees and shortening of more than 1 cm, joint incongruity, or asymmetric closure of the physis. These complications appeared to correlate with the Salter-Harris type, the amount of displacement or comminution, and the adequacy of reduction. The patients were divided into the groups shown in Table 136-1.

The overall complication rate was 14.1% for 184 patients. Salter-Harris II injuries of the tibia appeared to be the least predictable because the incidence of complications remained about the same, regardless of the amount of displacement.

TABLE 136-1

COMPLICATIONS OF ANKLE FRACTURES

Group	Complication Rate (%)	Salter-Harris Group and Bone Involved
Low risk (89 patients)	6.7	Types I and II of the fibula, type I of the tibia, types III and IV with displacement of less than 2 mm, epiphyseal avulsion injuries
High risk (28 patients)	32	Types III, IV, and V of the tibia Tillaux and triplane
Unpredictable (66 patients)	16.7	Type II of the tibia

Data from Spiegel PG, Cooperman DR, Laros GS: Epiphyseal fractures of the distal end of the tibia and fibula. *J Bone Joint Surg Am* 60: 1046, 1978.

Displacement is not always mentioned as one of the factors involved in prediction of outcome, but it is intuitive that greater displacement implies greater force, with damage more likely to the articular cartilage, the circulation, and the soft tissues important in healing. Karrholm[35] thought the good results were based on the adequacy of the reduction.

Near-anatomic reduction of type II injuries of the tibia is desirable. Gruber and associates[36] have shown in an animal model that interposed periosteum in an intact physis produces a spectrum of changes at the tissue level and a small but statistically significant leg-length discrepancy compared with fracture alone. Because this is a spectrum, it may explain the unpredictable nature of these injuries and support the need to remove interposed periosteum (Fig. 136-9). Residual displacement after attempted closed reduction may be a result of this interposition.

The patient in Figure 136-10, *A*, was treated by closed manipulation and casting. He had residual medial displacement (see Fig. 136-10, *B* and *C*). Follow-up radiographs show the development of a defect in the medial cortex. A valgus ankle deformity subsequently developed (see Fig. 136-10, *D*), which would indicate that the medial physis and suspected interposed periosteum grew more than the lateral side. He required a varus tibial osteotomy and physeal closure. Although some patients experience normal growth despite the medial cortical defect, the unpredictability and high frequency in the article by Rohmiller and colleagues[25] support a near-anatomic reduction with less than 2 mm of displacement in a child with more than 2 years of growth remaining. These injuries must be followed up until the patient attains skeletal maturity or a normal growth pattern is ensured because some patients will experience premature closure and an angular deformity.[29]

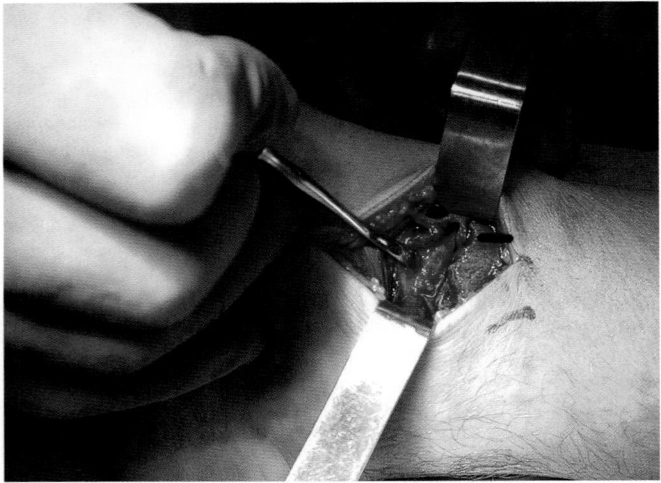

FIGURE 136-9 The Freer elevator is on the metaphyseal periosteum that is inverted into the physeal fracture site. The black mark is on the epiphyseal fragment.

The juvenile fracture of Tillaux and the triplane fracture result from incomplete closure of the physis. Because growth is nearing an end, angular deformity and shortening are uncommon. In these patients, the tibiotalar joint surface is disturbed and must be restored to as near normal as possible to prevent incongruity and subsequent traumatic arthritis. In the series by Cooperman and colleagues,[30] triplane fractures were reduced by internally rotating the foot while the patient was in a state of general anesthesia. The adequacy of reduction was determined by plain tomography. Dias and Giergerich[31] reported on 9 Tillaux and triplane fractures that were followed up for an average of 18 months, and all patients did well.

Peterson and Cass[27] reviewed all Salter-Harris type IV distal tibial injuries seen at the Mayo Clinic, with particular attention given to injuries of the medial malleolus. Nine of 18 patients with these injuries experienced premature physeal closure of a sufficient degree to require additional surgery for physeal bar resection, angular deformity, or leg-length discrepancy. Thirteen of these patients received their care at the Mayo Clinic, and of these, 11 had closed injuries. Six patients were treated with closed reduction and a short-leg cast. Five patients underwent open reduction and internal fixation. Five additional patients in the study had been referred to the clinic because of complications of a closed injury that had been treated in a closed manner. The investigators concluded that oblique radiographs are necessary to ensure an accurate diagnosis and to confirm the adequacy of the reduction. Some injuries that resemble type III injuries are actually type IV injuries. The authors also found that partial arrest that results in angular deformity was more common than complete arrest. They concluded that three patterns of medial malleolar injury exist and that type IV injuries constitute the most common and most dangerous pattern because they usually occur in a patient who has remaining growth potential (Fig. 136-11). The authors also concluded that the medial malleolus requires anatomic reduction, which often necessitates open reduction and internal fixation.

In any patient with an open physis, it is preferable to avoid crossing the physis with a fixation device. This goal can usually be achieved by placing smooth pins from metaphysis to metaphysis or from epiphysis to epiphysis. At times, crossing the physis cannot be avoided. Smooth pins can be used, and care should be taken that they do not cross within the physis. Patients need to be followed up until skeletal maturity is achieved or until one is certain that a normal growth pattern is occurring. An asymmetric Harris growth arrest line may be the earliest clue to an abnormal growth pattern (see Fig. 136-11).

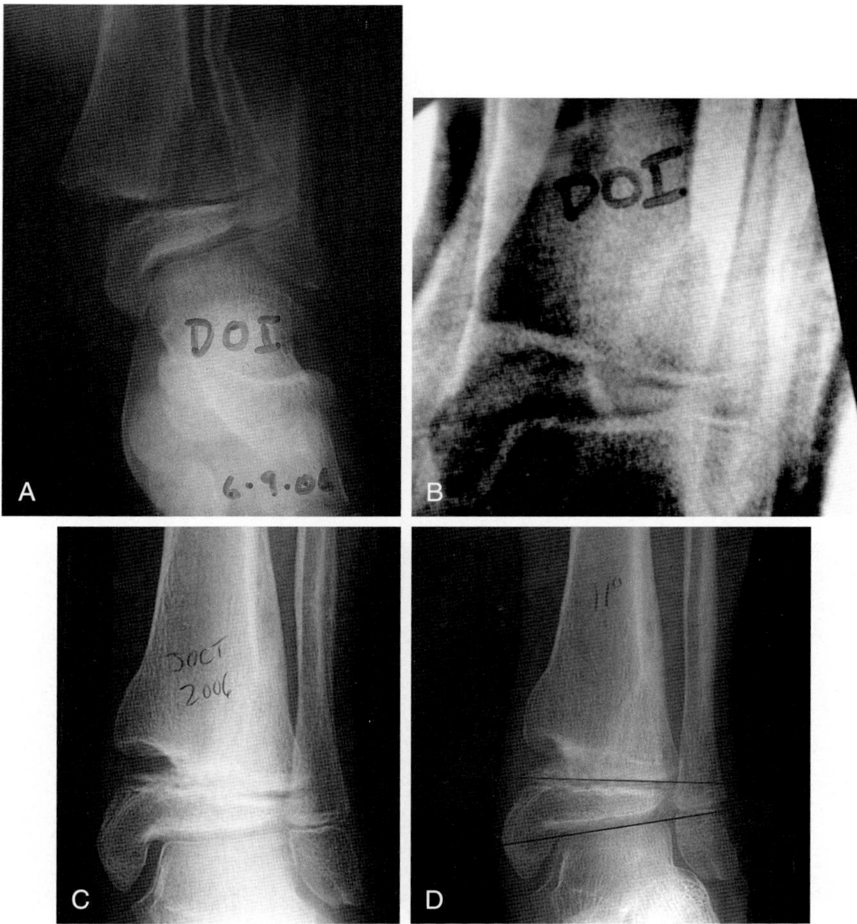

FIGURE 136-10 **A,** An anteroposterior (AP) radiograph on the day of injury of this Salter-Harris type II tibial fracture. **B,** A postreduction AP radiograph. **C,** An AP radiograph at 4 months. **D,** An AP radiograph at 2 years.

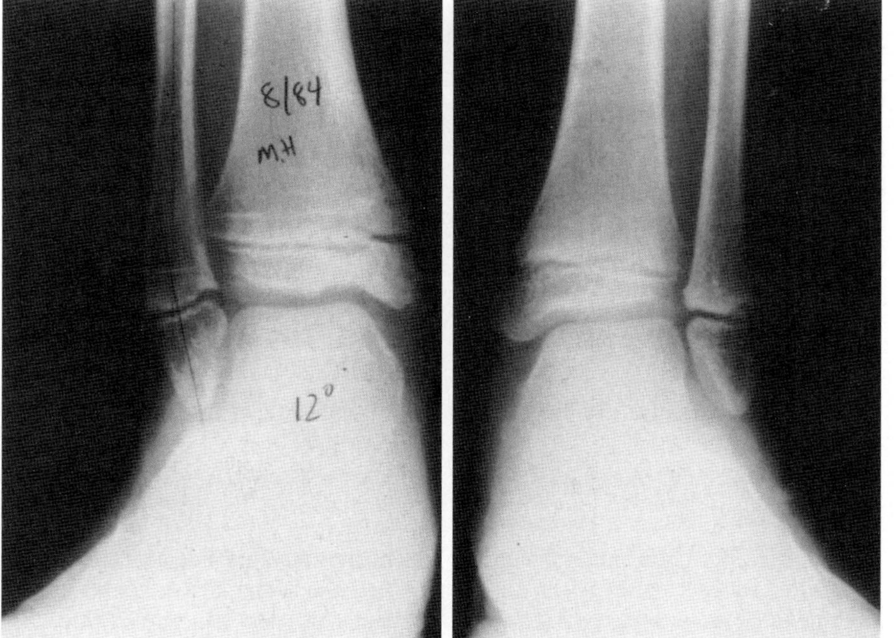

FIGURE 136-11 This patient sustained a Salter-Harris type IV medial malleolar fracture, which was treated in a closed manner. The patient was referred 6 months after injury, at which time she had trouble remembering which ankle had been injured. These radiographs were taken 18 months after the injury. Resection of a bony bridge and interposition were required. She resumed growth, and the fibular angular deformity had been corrected. Note the irregular Harris growth arrest lines.

Fractures in the Foot

Fractures of the foot resulting from participation in sports are unusual in children. Fractures of the metatarsals can result from direct trauma (Fig. 136-12) and can be treated by immobilization in a short-leg walking cast. The most controversial fracture in the foot may be an avulsion injury at the base of the fifth metatarsal.

Fractures of the fifth metatarsal in children can be divided into distal physeal fractures, fractures of the proximal diaphysis, and avulsion fractures of the apophysis. The fifth metatarsal has its epiphysis distally and an apophysis proximally. The tendon of the peroneus brevis is inserted into the apophysis. With inversion stress, the apophysis can be avulsed. Findings include tenderness at the base of the fifth metatarsal and radiographic confirmation of widening of the apophysis. Treatment should be symptomatic with compression and partial weight bearing until the pain subsides. Use of crutches and an elastic bandage may be sufficient. Two to three weeks in a short-leg cast or boot also yields good results.

Fracture of the proximal diaphysis of the fifth metatarsal (Jones fracture) is less common in skeletally immature patients and usually occurs in the 15- to 20-year age range.[37] When such fractures occur, a trial of immobilization in a short-leg walking cast is indicated because many acute fractures heal. Even fractures with delayed union may heal if they are treated conservatively.[38] Early operative intervention in highly competitive athletes has been advocated by some investigators, but others have shown that each patient needs to be treated individually because some of these fractures will heal if treated conservatively, allowing early return to athletics.[37-39] Early

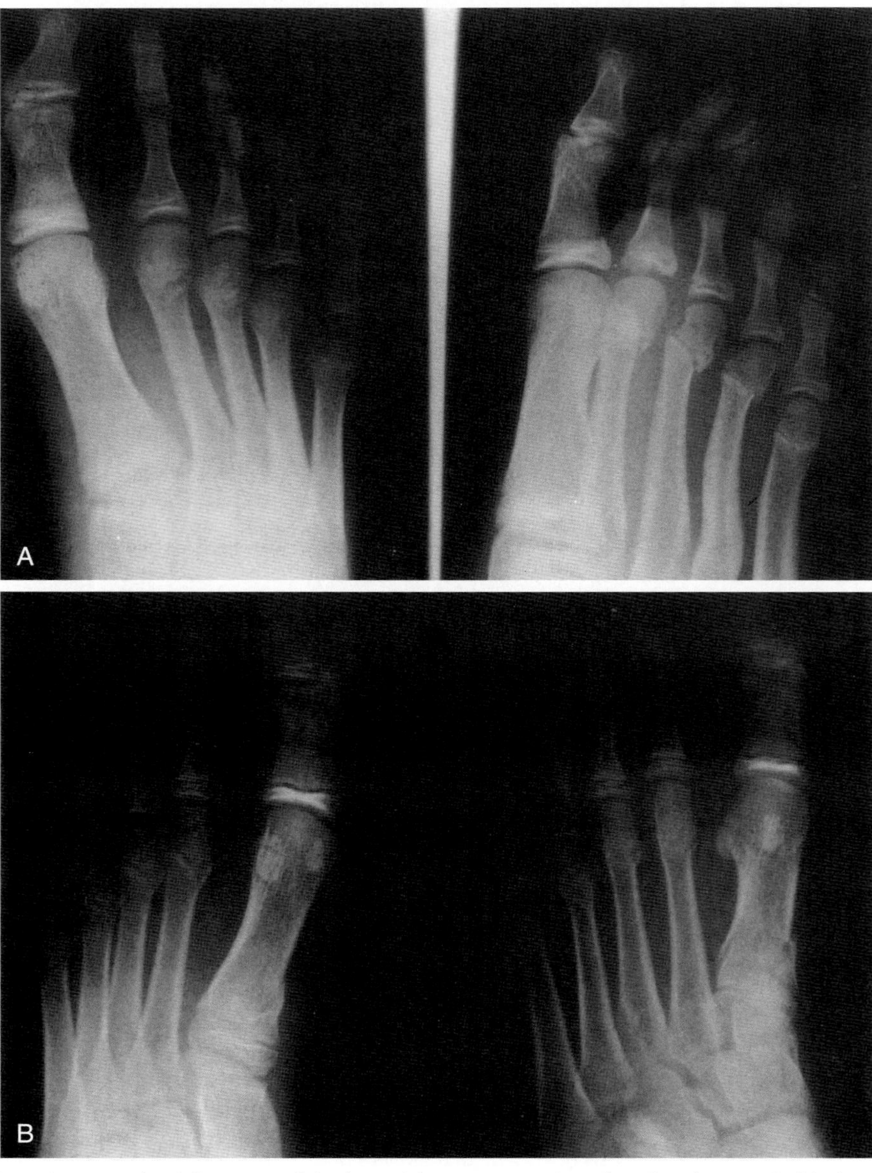

FIGURE 136-12 **A,** This patient sustained fractures of the lateral four metatarsal necks when he caught his foot on a base while sliding. **B,** This patient sustained a fracture of his first metatarsal when he was stepped on during a football game.

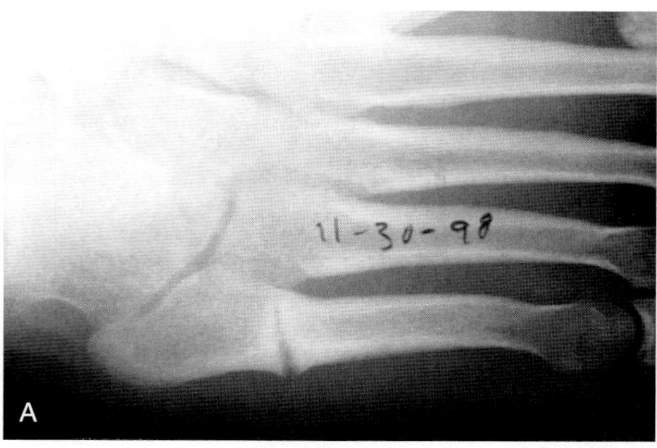

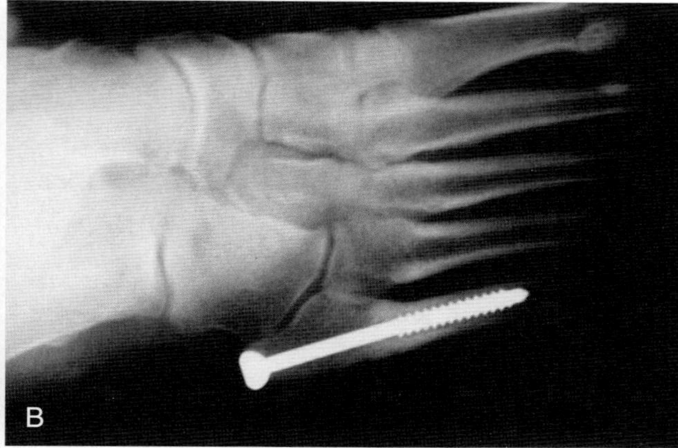

FIGURE 136-13 **A,** This patient sustained a fracture of the diaphysis of the fifth metatarsal. This radiograph was obtained 2 months after treatment with a cast. The metatarsal was tender to palpation, and the patient walked with a limp. **B,** This radiograph was obtained after treatment with internal fixation and a local bone graft from the calcaneus.

operative intervention in the pediatric athlete is rarely if ever indicated. Patients with established nonunion require operative treatment that includes reopening of the medullary canal, bone grafting, and internal fixation (Fig. 136-13).

Fractures of the toes are unusual in athletes. Buddy taping a fractured toe to the adjacent toe or wearing appropriate shoes for a few weeks and avoiding participation in sports until the toe is asymptomatic is the approach used to treat most phalangeal fractures. Articular fractures are even more rare. The only one that may merit consideration of operative management is an intraarticular physeal fracture of the great toe. These fractures should be reduced to as near-anatomic alignment as possible by whatever means necessary (Fig. 136-14).

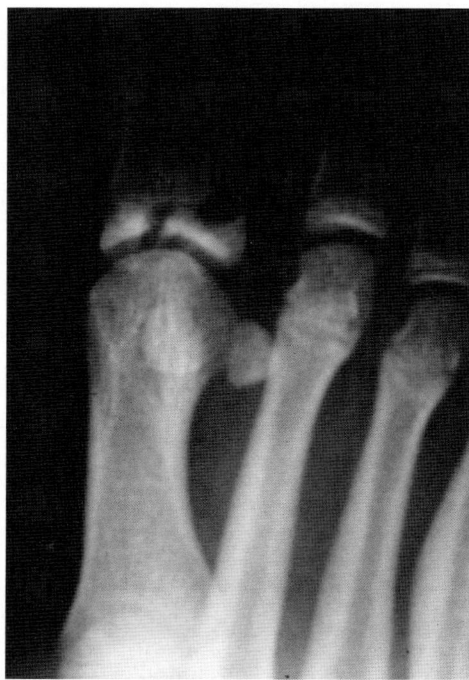

FIGURE 136-14 This intraarticular fracture was treated with closed reduction and percutaneous pinning.

Stress fractures are less common among children than adults but cannot be entirely dismissed. Some children participate in marathons and other sporting events that can result in stress fractures. Basketball, soccer, and other team sports have tournaments that may require considerable running. The stress fracture shown in Figure 136-15 resulted from a tournament and was thought to be a sprain. Stress fractures are also common in high school cross-country athletes. Given that it is a stress reaction and requires rest and/or immobilization before resumption of activity, a stress fracture is often a season-ending event for runners.

Yngve[40] found 131 pediatric stress fractures in 23 references in the literature. Two of the 131 reports documented metatarsal fractures—two of the tarsal navicular and one of the medial sesamoid. The primary training error was "too much too soon." Other factors that should be considered are a change in training surface or equipment (shoes) and a sudden change in intensity of training (tournaments). Diagnosis depends on an appropriate history, a high index of suspicion, and the presence of localized tenderness. The differential diagnosis includes contusion, tendinitis, and sprains.

The initial radiograph may be normal but should be diagnostic in half of cases. One should look for cortical thickening or a translucent fracture line. A bone scan may be diagnostic at this stage and may be particularly helpful if the diagnosis is in question and one wishes to avoid immobilization. A bone scan may be indicated when the diagnosis is in doubt and the athlete wishes to return to play. MRI has also been used to identify occult stress fractures. Conversely, immobilization for 2 weeks in a cast is usually diagnostic in that pain is relieved; repeat radiographs are then positive, making a bone scan unnecessary. Although some of these fractures heal without use of a cast, the athlete should be immobilized for protection from himself or herself, as well as from well-meaning parents and coaches.

Osteochondral Lesions of the Talus

The term osteochondritis dissecans (OCD) has been used to describe lesions in the dome of the talus. These lesions have been attributed to a vascular insult, but trauma has been implicated, especially in anterolateral lesions.[41-44] Berndt and

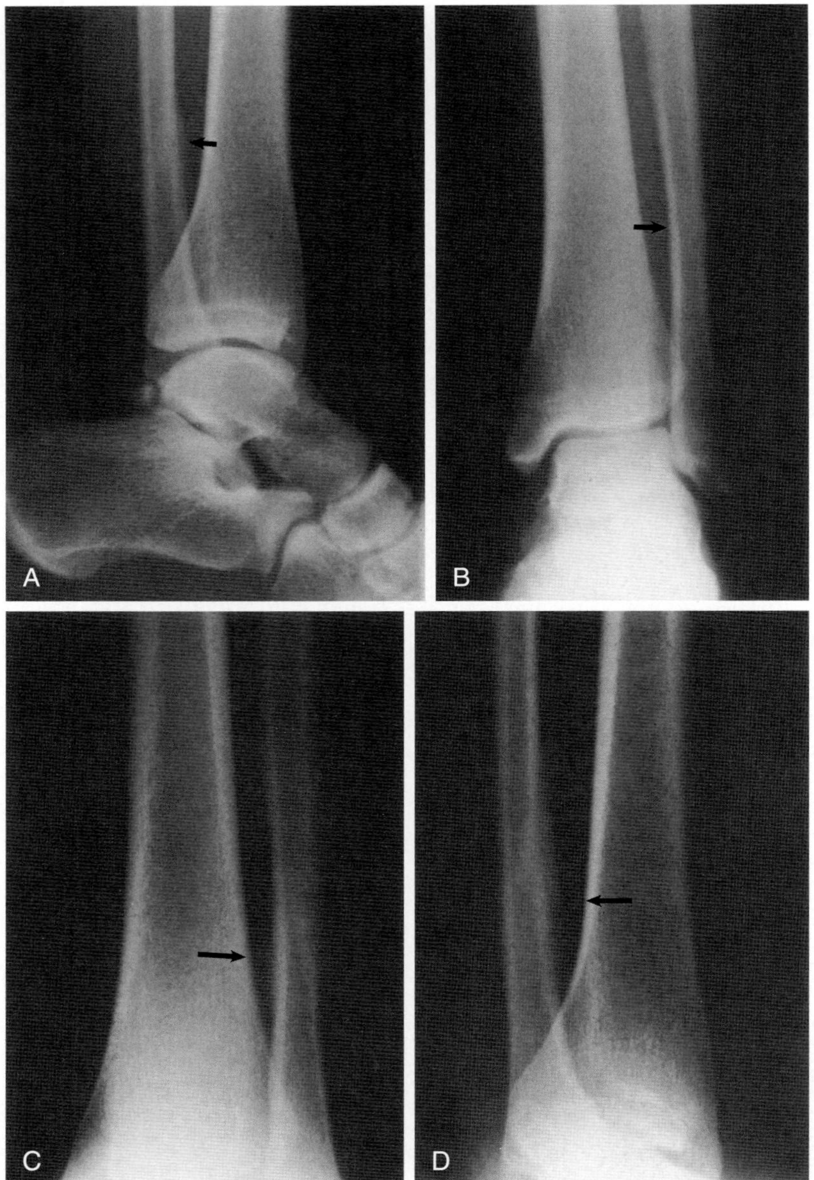

FIGURE 136-15 This patient presented with localized tenderness just above the ankle. After being injured in a basketball tournament, she continued to play with a presumptive diagnosis of a sprained ankle. The initial radiographs (**A** and **B**) showed periosteal elevation (*arrows*). Follow-up radiographs (**C** and **D**) taken after 2 weeks of treatment with a short-leg walking cast illustrate new bone formation (*arrows*).

Harty[41] developed a classification system based on the amount of damage and the degree of displacement involved. This system, in a slightly modified form, is still in use:

Stage I: Localized trabecular compression
Stage II: Incompletely separated fragment
Stage IIA: Formation of a subchondral cyst
Stage III: Undetached, undisplaced fragment
Stage IV: Displaced or inverted fragment

Most series consist predominantly of adults; however, 21 of 29 patients studied by Canale and Belding[42] experienced onset of symptoms during the second decade. CT and MRI can reveal lesions not seen on plain films and also make staging more accurate. These techniques may reveal that this disorder is more common among adolescents than was previously suspected. Hao et al.[43] compared conventional MRI with 3D MRI (fast spoiled gradient recalled acquisition in the steady state; FSPGR) in a group of 21 patients with suspected cartilage lesions. All lesions were confirmed by arthroscopy. The investigators concluded that T1-weighted 3D fat-suppressed FSPGR MRI is more sensitive than is conventional MRI in detecting defects of articular cartilage covering osteochondral lesions of the talus.[43] Proper treatment depends on identification of the lesion and accurate staging.

Canale and Belding[42] suggested that nonoperative treatment by immobilization of all stage I, stage II, and medial stage III (Berndt and Harty classification) lesions would result in a high percentage of good clinical results and delayed development of arthrosis. Persistent symptoms after conservative treatment were an indication for operative treatment by excision and curettage. These investigators further recommended that all stage III lateral lesions and all stage IV lesions be treated by immediate excision and curettage of the lesion. Anderson and associates[43a] recommended immobilization for 6 weeks for patients with stage I and II fractures, but they cautioned that these patients need to be followed up for a prolonged time so that delayed development of arthrosis can be detected. Operative treatment was recommended for patients with stage IIA, III, and IV lesions.

Letts and colleagues[44] reviewed 24 children treated since 1983 for OCD of either the medial or lateral dome of the talus (two were bilateral). The average age at presentation was 13 years, 4 months. Nonoperative treatment included activity restriction, physiotherapy, and immobilization. Surgical intervention was required in 15 ankles (58%). Surgical treatment included arthroscopy (1), arthrotomy and drilling of the defect (9), drilling with excision of the lesion (3), excision of the lesion (2), and pinning of the fragment (1). Most recent follow-up revealed resolution or decreased symptoms in 25 patients (96%) and no change in one patient. MRI was useful in preoperative assessment in six cases. In this series, a slight female preponderance was noted (58%). Higuera and coworkers[44a] reported good to excellent results in 94.8% of children. Cuttica et al.[45] reported favorable results with marrow stimulation techniques such as drilling or microfracture in contained lesions measuring less than 1.5 cm^2. For larger uncontained lesions, they recommend consideration of a more extensive initial procedure.[45]

Osteochondroses in the Foot

The osteochondroses are a group of conditions of unknown origin. Suggested causes have included endocrinopathies, vascular phenomena, infection, and trauma.[46] Many of these conditions are now known to represent radiographic variations of normal ossification of the epiphysis. Most are named for the person or persons who originally described them. They all include a pattern of clinical symptoms coupled with a radiograph that suggests that the epiphysis or apophysis is undergoing necrosis. In the foot, the most commonly described conditions are Kohler syndrome and Freiberg infarction.

Kohler syndrome is a clinical syndrome consisting of pain in the midfoot coupled with a finding of localized tenderness over the navicular. Radiographs demonstrate increased density and narrowing of the tarsal navicular. Irregular ossification in this bone may be the rule rather than the exception, and thus the existence of this condition is in question (Fig. 136-16). Williams and Cowell[47] reviewed a series of patients with the following findings. Thirty percent of males and 20% of females demonstrated irregular ossification in the tarsal navicular. Most patients appeared to respond to 6 weeks of immobilization in a cast. All 23 patients eventually became asymptomatic, and the navicular became normal. The authors believed that patients treated in a cast became asymptomatic sooner than did those treated with shoe inserts. Regardless of treatment, no long-term problems were associated with this condition, again raising the question of whether it is a distinct pathologic condition.

Freiberg infarction is a condition of condensation and collapse of the metatarsal head and articular surface. It commonly occurs during the second decade of life while the epiphysis is still present.[48] It is of unknown cause and is more common among females. Many causes have been proposed, but repetitive trauma probably plays a role. The lesion occurs most commonly in the second or third metatarsal (Fig. 136-17),[46] which are the longest and least mobile of the metatarsals. The patient presents with pain on weight bearing and has localized tenderness over the metatarsal head. Radiographs reveal collapse of the articular surface (see Fig. 136-17). Conservative treatment with a cast or orthotic device that minimizes weight bearing over the involved head is often successful in relieving the pain. Surgical treatment consisting of removal of loose bodies or bone grafting has been reported for persistent symptoms. A dorsiflexion osteotomy to relieve weight bearing has also been reported to work well. Removal of the metatarsal head should be avoided because this procedure results in transfer of weight bearing to the adjacent

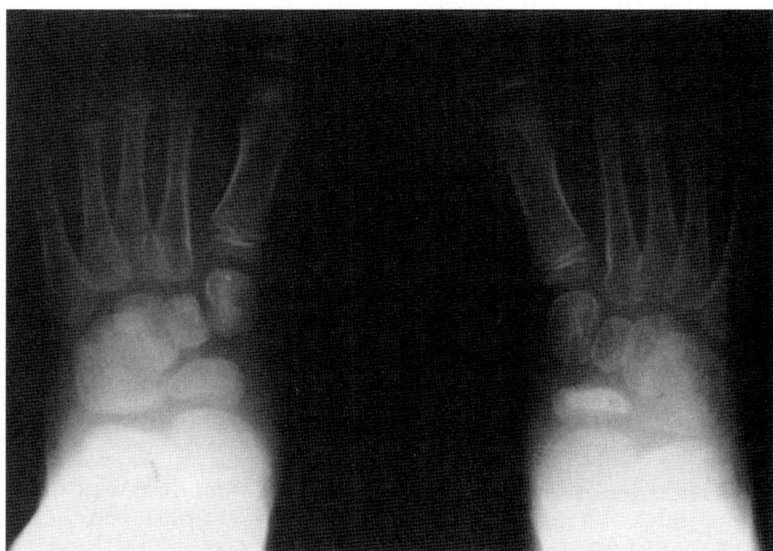

FIGURE 136-16 This patient presented with undisplaced fractures of the metatarsals. The condensed, narrowed appearance of the navicular is the same as that seen in patients with Kohler syndrome, but it was an incidental finding in this patient.

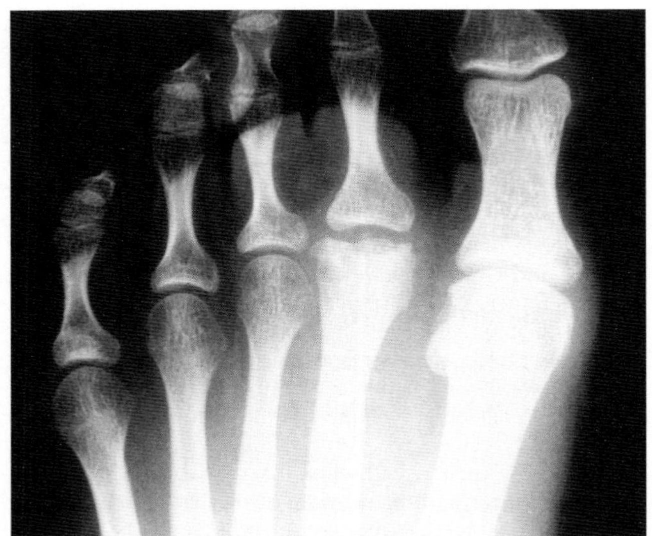

FIGURE 136-17 This anteroposterior radiograph of the foot shows irregularity and collapse of the second metatarsal head.

metatarsal heads. Prosthetic replacement has also been tried but is not indicated in children. In most instances, the disease runs its course, and the head reossifies within 2 to 3 years.

Sever disease is a term used to refer to a nonarticular osteochondrosis or a traction apophysitis (Fig. 136-18). The real question is whether a distinct syndrome exists and, if it does, whether the apophysis has anything to do with it. The calcaneal apophysis appears and develops in the 5- to 12-year age range and is typically irregular. Often, a child with heel pain and an irregular apophysis has the same radiographic finding in the opposite asymptomatic heel. Rachel et al.[49] recently reported a 5% rate of diagnosis of another lesion on lateral radiographic images of children with heel pain and presumed calcaneal apophysitis. In response, they recommend routine lateral radiographs of children presenting with insidious onset of heel pain to rule out other potentially more aggressive diagnoses.[49] These children are usually in the 9- to 12-year age range and are active in sports. They may have a tight heel cord. The calcaneus serves as the insertion of the powerful gastrocnemius-soleus muscle and the origin of the plantar fascia. Traction or overuse can strain these structures, producing pain. Stretching may be beneficial. Symptomatic treatment by avoidance of the offending exercise is usually curative. Shock-absorbing inserts or a heel cup may be advantageous. A heel lift to relieve some of the pull of the gastrocnemius-soleus, or at times an arch support for a child with a high arch, may provide symptomatic relief as well. Heel cord stretching exercises may be tried. Additionally, splinting at night and/or short-term immobilization in a controlled ankle movement walker boot or weight-bearing cast may provide symptom relief. One must carefully search for the point of maximal tenderness and seek its cause rather than implicating an irregular apophysis, which is probably not the source of the pain. The exact time frame for resolution of symptoms in children with heel pain is unknown and at times can be vexing. If we believe that the child has complied with the previous conservative measures and is no better after 2 to 3 months, we proceed with further workup, such as a bone scan and other studies, to seek more occult sources of the pain.

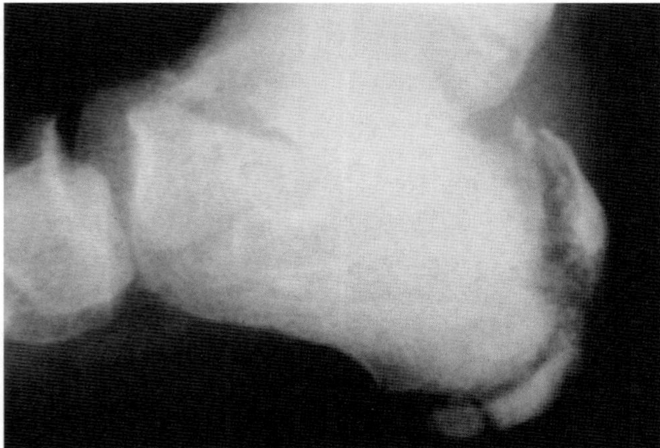

FIGURE 136-18 A lateral radiograph of the calcaneus. Note the irregularity, especially in the superior part of the apophysis. Fragmentation and increased density are common occurrences in the calcaneal apophysis.

Systemic Illness

Systemic illness can present with foot pain and must be considered in the pediatric and adolescent athlete. Rheumatoid arthritis or hemophilia can involve the subtalar joint. Osteomyelitis can involve the foot but is unusual unless the patient has a history of a puncture wound. Acute lymphocytic leukemia is a great masquerader and can infiltrate the bones of the foot. Although they are rare, these types of diseases must be considered. One cannot develop tunnel vision and believe that all pain in an athlete is of a traumatic origin.

Shoes and Orthotics

The athletic shoe business is lucrative, as is shown by the intense marketing, endorsement, and competition for the introduction of new technology and an edge in the marketplace. Little scientific evidence supports the hype associated with shoe sales. Most often, the advertisements depict current sports heroes wearing shoes from the high end of the price scale, and they tell us little about the shoes themselves. Athletic shoes should fit adequately in both width and length. The models and range of widths available are more limited for children. The material should be reasonably soft. Too often, children's athletic shoes are made of stiff, unyielding, synthetic material and are poorly padded around the heel counter. Multisport shoes with small-diameter, evenly spaced cleats that distribute weight bearing more evenly are preferable to cleated or studded shoes. Padding over the heel counter and ankle may increase comfort. Most shoes now come with a built-in arch support that has little scientific basis but may give some support to children with a well-developed arch. Children with flatter feet may actually find it necessary to remove the pad. Barefoot running or running in toe shoes is a hot, controversial topic for which no literature relating to children is available, and the senior author certainly would not recommend it.

Orthotics is another area of controversy. An asymptomatic flexible flatfoot should be left alone. No evidence exists to support the idea that an orthotic will bring about any structural change in such a foot. A painful flatfoot should prompt a thorough search for its cause, such as a tarsal coalition. Orthotics may be tried in a patient with aching feet or shins and a flexible flatfoot. Heel cups may be beneficial in the symptomatic treatment of heel pain. Little if any scientific information is available about the use of sports orthotics in children.

For a complete list of references, go to expertconsult.com.

Suggested Readings

Citation: Vincent KA: Tarsal coalition and painful flatfoot. *J Am Acad Orthop Surg* 6(5):274–281, 1998.

Level of Evidence: V

Summary: Vincent provides a comprehensive review of the types of tarsal coalition and their diagnosis and management.

Citation: Letts M, Davidson D, Ahmer A: Osteochondritis dissecans of the talus in children. *J Pediatr Orthop* 23(5):617–625, 2003.

Level of Evidence: IV

Summary: Since 1983, 24 children treated for osteochondritis dissecans of the talus at a major Canadian pediatric referral center were followed up. Two children had bilateral involvement, for a total of 26 lesions. The patients included 10 boys and 14 girls. The lesion involved the medial aspect of the talus in 19 patients, the lateral aspect in 5 patients, and the central talar dome in 3 patients. Magnetic resonance imaging was very useful in preoperative assessment in six cases. Surgical intervention was required in 15 ankles (58%). Results at the most recent follow-up revealed resolution or decreased symptoms in 25 patients (96%) and no change in 1 patient (4%).

Citation: Podeszwa DA, Mubarak SJ: Physeal fractures of the distal tibia and fibula (Salter-Harris Type I, II, III, and IV fractures). *J Pediatr Orthop* 32(Suppl 1):S62–S68, 2012.

Level of Evidence: V

Summary: The authors provide an excellent up-to-date review of physeal fractures of the distal tibia and fibula.

Citation: Gantsoudes GD, Roocroft JH, Mubarak SJ: Treatment of talocalcaneal coalitions. *J Pediatr Orthop* 32(3):301–307, 2012.

Level of Evidence: IV

Summary: A retrospective review was performed for all patients who underwent surgical treatment for a symptomatic talocalcaneal coalition over a 13-year period. Ninety-three feet were treated with excision and fat graft interposition by six surgeons. The authors concluded that a symptomatic talocalcaneal coalition can be treated with excision and fat graft interposition and that good to excellent results can be achieved in 85% of patients. Patients should be counseled that a subset may require further surgery to correct malalignment.

Citation: Cuttica DJ, Smith WB, Hyer CF, et al: Osteochondral lesions of the talus: Predictors of clinical outcome. *Foot Ankle Int* 32(11):1045–1051, 2011.

Level of Evidence: IV

Summary: A retrospective review of a group of patients treated operatively for osteochondral lesions of the talus was performed to determine factors that may have affected outcome. The treatment of osteochondral lesions of the talus remains a challenge for the foot and ankle surgeon. Arthroscopic debridement and drilling often provide satisfactory results. However, larger lesions and uncontained lesions are often associated with inferior functional outcomes and may require a more extensive initial procedure.

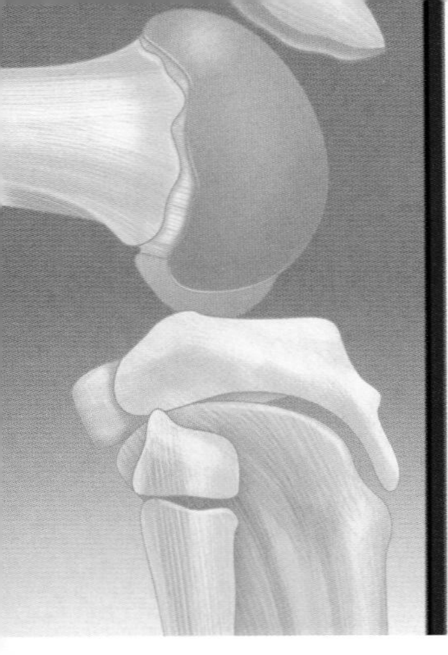

137

Head Injuries in Skeletally Immature Athletes

TRACY ZASLOW • DAVID L. SKAGGS

The incidence of sports and recreation-related traumatic brain injuries (TBIs) has increased during the past decade.[1] The two most common athletic activities associated with emergency department treatment for TBI are bicycling and football.[1] Risk for TBI is inherent to participation in sports and recreation activities, and compared with adults, children and adolescents have an increased risk for TBIs, with increased severity and prolonged recovery.[2] TBI is a term that encompasses a broad range of head injuries and includes concussion, skull fracture, epidural hematoma, subdural hematoma, intracerebral hematoma, and subarachnoid hemorrhage.

Concussion

Concussion is defined as a complex, transient, pathophysiologic process that affects the brain and is induced by traumatic biomechanical forces.[3] Concussions occur with rapid onset and involve short-lived neurologic impairment that typically resolves spontaneously. *Acute clinical presentation reflects a functional disturbance rather than structural injury.* Injury occurs on a biochemical level without significant detectable gross anatomic changes, which supports the understanding that the changes are based on temporary neuronal dysfunction, not cell death.[4] Biochemical neuronal dysfunction occurs as a result of a combination of shifts in ion balance, altered glucose metabolism, impaired connectivity, and changes in neurotransmission. This biochemical dysfunction presents clinically in patients with a constellation of symptoms that may include any combination of one of more of the following: headache, dizziness, confusion, disorientation, hearing/visual disturbances, and/or loss of consciousness. It is important to understand that this range of clinical symptoms may or may not involve loss of consciousness. Historically, athletes referred to concussive episodes as a "ding" or "getting your bell rung"; these terms may describe the disorientation experienced by the athletes and are suspicious, if not defining, for a concussive injury. Results of neuroimaging studies (i.e., skull radiographs and head computed tomography [CT] or magnetic resonance imaging [MRI]) are typically normal, further supporting the understanding that concussion is a functional disturbance without true gross structural abnormality.

Biomechanics and Pathophysiology

When rotational or angular acceleration forces are applied to the brain, a shear strain occurs on the neural elements, leading to a neurometabolic cascade and the clinical features of concussion. The biomechanical injury to the brain causes an immediate release of excitatory neurotransmitters (Fig. 137-1).

The binding of the excitatory neurotransmitters, such as glutamate, lead to further neuronal depolarization with further destabilization of the ionic equilibrium, including influx of calcium and efflux of potassium (Fig. 137-2).[5]

To restore the ionic homeostasis, neuronal membrane potential energy (adenosine triphosphate) is required to enable operation of the sodium-potassium pump. This increased glucose demand ("hypermetabolism") occurs in the face of decreased cerebral blood flow. Metabolic supply/demand mismatch leads to cell dysfunction and increased vulnerability of the cell to a second insult (Fig. 137-3).

After the initial period of "hypermetabolism," a period of decreased metabolism occurs in the concussed brain. Calcium levels may remain elevated and impair mitochondrial oxidative metabolism, further worsening the energy deficits. Additionally, neurofilament and microtubule function is disrupted by intraaxonal calcium flux, impairing posttraumatic neural connectivity.

On average, these biochemical changes take 7 to 10 days to normalize in adults (see Fig. 137-2), but normalization can take longer in the growing brain of a child and adolescent. Interestingly, the clinical recovery parallels this biochemical normalization. Changes in cerebral blood flow may also occur with concomitant impairment of vascular autoregulation, which can result in cerebral edema and may persist beyond the acute phase.

Epidemiology

Twenty-one percent of all traumatic brain injuries among children in the United States are associated with sports participation.[6] Although death from a sports injury is rare, the leading cause of death from a sports-related injury is a brain injury. Football, gymnastics, and ice hockey reported the highest number of sports-related fatalities from 1982 to 2010 according to the 28th annual report of the National Center for Catastrophic Sport Injury Research.[7]

Concussions occur commonly in sports in which helmets are and are not worn. Three hundred thousand sports-related concussions associated with loss of consciousness occur annually. However, only 8% to 19% of concussions are associated with a loss of consciousness,[8,9] and thus rates of

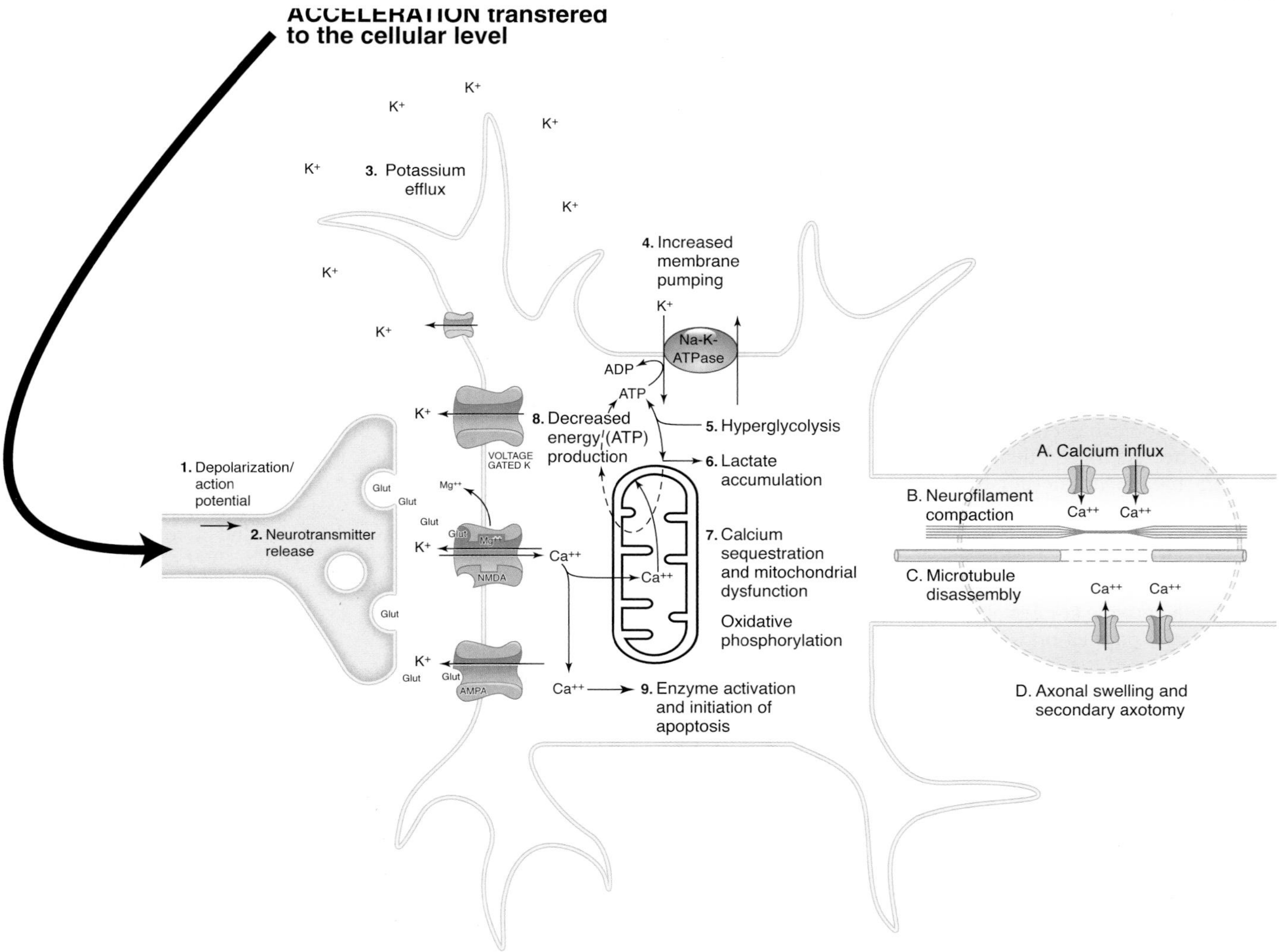

FIGURE 137-1 The biochemical changes that occur in the neuron with concussion. *ADP,* Adenosine diphosphate; *ATP,* adenosine triphosphate; *ATPase,* adenosine triphosphatase. *(Modified from Giza CC, Hovda DA: Ionic and metabolic consequences of concussion. In Cantu RC, Cantu RI, editors:* Neurologic Athletic and Spine Injuries, *Philadelphia, 2000, WB Saunders.)*

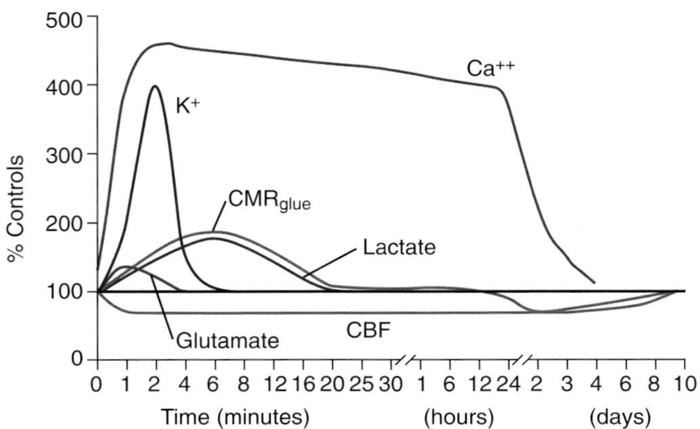

FIGURE 137-2 Ionic and metabolic consequences of concussion. *CBF,* Cerebral blood flow; *CMR,* cerebral metabolic rate. *(From Giza CC, Hovda DA: Ionic and metabolic consequences of concussion. In Cantu RC, Cantu RI, editors:* Neurologic Athletic and Spine Injuries, *Philadelphia, 2000, WB Saunders.)*

sports-related concussion are estimated at 1.6 to 3.8 million sports-related concussions per year.[10] The rate in high school athletes is 0.14 to 3.66 injuries per 100 player seasons at the high school level, accounting for 3% to 5% of injuries in all sports.[11,12] At the collegiate level, the exposure rate is 0.5 to 3.0 injuries per 1000 athlete exposures.[12] Trends have shown a significant (60%) increase in concussion rates in young athletes (<19 years old) during the past decade.

Although sports participation overall is increased, this increase is likely related to better reporting, recognition, and

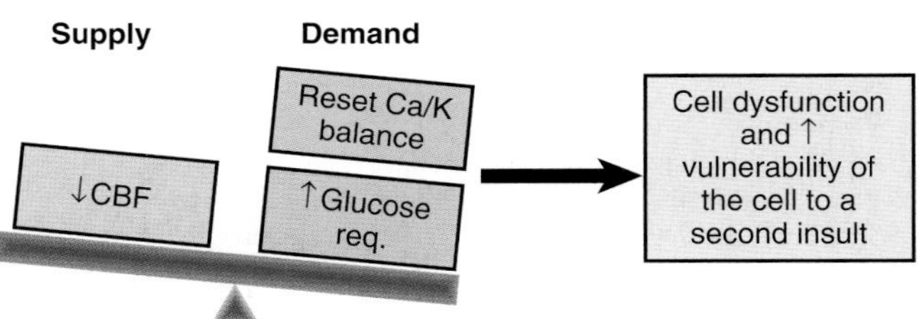

FIGURE 137-3 Metabolic supply/demand mismatch in the neuron after concussion. *CBF,* Cerebral blood flow.

diagnosis of concussion. Historically, concussion reporting rates have been poor. In a survey of 1532 varsity football athletes, 47% of players who sustained concussions continued to play without reporting their injuries to anyone. The most common reason athletes did not share the presence of symptoms was that the athletes did not believe the concussion was serious enough to report. Other reasons for underreporting were that athletes did not want to leave the game, did not realize a concussion was sustained, and did not want to let their teammates down.[13] Another study reported that 70.4% of football players and 62.7% of soccer players experienced symptoms of concussion within one season,[14] further supporting the understanding that the current reported concussion rates are likely much lower than actual rates because of unrecognized concussions.

Concussion can occur in any sport from football to basketball to cheerleading; different studies have shown different incident rates. One metaanalysis of 23 articles indicated the highest incident rates for tae kwon do (8.77 per 1000 athlete exposures), rugby (9.05 per 1000 player games), amateur boxing (7.9 per 1000 athlete exposures), and boys' high school ice hockey (3.6 per 1000 athlete exposures).[11] When specifically looking at rates of sports-related concussion in the high school population, another study showed that boys' sports accounted for 53% of athlete exposures and 75% of all concussions. Football had the highest incident rate and accounted for the majority of concussions (53.1%), followed by boys' lacrosse (9.2%). Among girls' sports, soccer had the highest rate of concussions and was the second-highest of the 12 high school sports studied.[15]

History

Concussions can present seconds, minutes, hours, or days after an indirect or direct force to the head. The signs and symptoms of concussion fall into four main categories: physical, cognitive, emotional, and sleep (Table 137-1).[16,17]

The self-reported Postconcussion Symptom Scale is a useful tool for initial assessment and serves to facilitate follow-up as well. The scale is a 7-point Likert scale graded from 0 (no symptoms) to 6 (severe symptoms); multiple scales are available with a range of symptoms included. Although no specific scale has been assessed for reliability, self-reported postconcussive symptoms are associated with ongoing cerebral hemodynamic abnormalities and mild cognitive impairments.[18] Headache is the most frequently reported symptom.[19] Loss of consciousness occurs in 8% to 19% of concussions[8,9] and is not a defining feature of concussion; however, when prolonged loss of consciousness (>30 seconds) occurs, further evaluation may be necessary.

Understanding the presence of preexisting medical and mental health disorders, including migraine headaches, depression, anxiety, learning disabilities, cognitive delays, and attention-deficit disorders, is important because concussion may cause an exacerbation of underlying symptoms; additionally, athletes with preexisting conditions may have a more complicated and prolonged recovery course. Athletes with preinjury depression, sleep disturbances, and/or attention-deficit/hyperactivity disorder may not have a baseline (preinjury) symptom score of zero and thus are not expected to have a symptom score of zero prior to considering return to play.

Recognizing concussion may be difficult in athletes for a number of reasons. Athletes may not recognize symptoms as serious and thus not report them. Symptoms may be delayed and not appear until several hours after a concussive event occurs.[20] Also, athletes may not volunteer their symptoms to avoid restriction from play and because they fear they will let down their teammates.[13]

Physical Examination

Initial assessment on the sidelines follows the protocol of all acute head and neck injuries and begins with assessment of the airway, breathing, and circulation (ABCs) and stabilization of the cervical spine. If an athlete is unconscious after head or neck trauma, a cervical spine injury is assumed until neurologic function in all four limbs is determined to be intact and the athlete reports no neck pain or cervical spine tenderness on palpation. Immediate emergency transport with cervical precautions is essential if this evaluation is unable to be completed; if the athlete is wearing a helmet and pads, the gear should not be removed for transport, but the face mask should be removed to provide access to the airway. For athletes in whom cervical spine injuries are not suspected, evaluation can be performed on the sidelines.

Sideline assessment includes review of the athlete's symptoms, neurologic evaluation, and cognitive and balance testing. Initial neurologic testing should begin with evaluation of eye response, verbal response, and motor response as per the Glasgow Coma Scale. The next steps included further

TABLE 137-1

SIGNS AND SYMPTOMS OF CONCUSSION

Physical	Cognitive	Emotional	Sleep
Headache	Feeling "foggy"	Irritability	Drowsiness
Nausea	Feeling slowed down	Sadness	Sleeping more or less than usual
Vomiting	Difficulty concentrating	Anxiety	Difficulty falling asleep
Balance problems	Amnesia	Emotional lability	
Visual problems	Confusion	Depression	
Sensitivity to light	Slow response to questions		
Sensitivity to noise	Repeating questions		
Fatigue	Difficulty with schoolwork		
Dazed/stunned affect	Loss of consciousness		
Seizure			

evaluation of neurologic status with examination of pupil size and symmetry, vision, reflexes, sensation, and strength. When the athlete appears stable, testing of memory, coordination, concentration, and gait/balance can ensue. Numerous sideline assessment tools are available to facilitate expedient and standardized assessments, both as printable forms and smartphone applications, including Maddocks questions,[21] Standardized Assessment of Concussion,[22] Balance Error Scoring System (BESS),[23] and the Sport Concussion Assessment Tool 3 (SCAT3).[3] The SCAT3 was released as part of the Consensus Statement on Concussion in Sport: The Fourth International Conference on Concussion in Sport held in Zurich in November 2012 and is also available as a free smartphone application that enables test results to be sent via e-mail after completion.[20] In all of these tests, individualized baseline information is useful.

The Maddocks questions are a set of sport-specific questions designed to evaluate orientation, short-term memory, and long-term memory; these questions may provide more accurate responses then the usual orientation to time, day, date, and location. Examples of Maddocks questions are "Who scored last in the match?" and "Did your team win the last game?" These questions are useful only on the sidelines (not in a clinic setting) and are included in the comprehensive SCAT3.

Balance is an important part of the assessment after head trauma. Historically, the Romberg test has been used to assess balance subjectively. However, the BESS provides a quantifiable balance test that is straightforward to perform and objectively assesses postural stability. The BESS may be performed on the sidelines or in a clinic setting.[24-26] The BESS test has been shown to be a valid and reliable tool.[27,28] The BESS test is performed with the patient in three positions, first on a firm surface and then on a less-stable surface, a 10-cm-thick piece of foam. The three positions, which are well described in the SCAT3, include (1) standing flat on both feet with the hands placed on the iliac crest; (2) standing on a single leg on the nondominant foot; and (3) standing in tandem stance, heel-to-toe, with the nondominant foot in back of the other. The athlete is instructed to hold each position, to the best of his or her ability, for 20 seconds while the examiner observes the athlete for errors (Box 137-1). The examiner scores the test by adding the number of errors (one error point for each error during each 20-second test). Because fatigue and setting have an effect on the test, it is recommended that the test be completed 15 minutes after cessation of exercise and in the same setting where the follow-up testing will be performed.[29,30] Ideally, athletes will have a baseline evaluation that includes the BESS test prior to the start of the season so that comparison of postinjury and baseline testing may be incorporated to most reliably incorporate balance testing results into the return-to-play plan.

Although basic neurocognitive assessments are included as part of the Standardized Assessment of Concussion/SCAT3, more in-depth testing may be helpful to determine a player's readiness for safe return to play, especially in cases with chronic symptoms and questions of the athlete's truthfulness. Neuropsychological testing can be performed in one of two ways—with pencil-and-paper testing administered by a neuropsychologist or with computerized neuropsychological testing. Accessibility, time, and cost often limit the practical implication of the pencil-and-paper testing, but it can be extremely useful in cases complicated by prolonged symptoms and difficulty returning to school. Computerized testing is currently used more widely because of the ease of use and short testing times (30 to 45 minutes). Ideally, baseline neuropsychological testing is performed prior to injury to enable it to be used most effectively. Schools and teams have begun to offer and administer tests proctored by school personnel, usually athletic trainers.

BOX 137-1 Balance Testing Errors

Hands lifted off the iliac crest
Opening eyes
Step, stumble, or fall
Moving the hip to >30 degrees of abduction
Lifting the forefoot or heel
Remaining out of the test position for >5 seconds

Imaging

Results of conventional neuroimaging (i.e., skull radiographs and head CT/MRI scans) are usually normal in persons who have had a concussion; however, prudent utilization of neuroimaging must be considered if an intracranial structural injury is suspected. The signs and symptoms that increase concern for a more serious injury include a worsening severe headache, seizures, focal neurologic signs, and circulatory changes (Box 137-2).

Other considerations to help determine when neuroimaging is appropriate are prolonged loss of consciousness (>30 seconds) and persistently worsening symptoms. A CT scan is the first-line testing modality recommended to evaluate for intracranial hemorrhage and skull fractures during the first 24 to 48 hours after injury.[31] Performing a CT scan is absolutely not recommended for all concussed athletes, especially children, because of a small increased risk of brain cancer and leukemia as a result of radiation exposure.[32] MRI is most effectively used in cases of prolonged symptoms (>3 weeks) and is primarily performed to rule out underlying structural pathology such as Arnold-Chiari malformation or arteriovenous malformation, which may cause a prolonged recovery from a concussive injury. Emerging MRI and functional

BOX 137-2 Red Flags for Intracranial Structural Injury

Severe, worsening headache
Seizures
Focal neurologic findings
Repeated emesis
Significant drowsiness/difficulty awakening
Slurred speech
Poor orientation/significant confusion
Significant irritability
Slowed pulse
Increased systolic blood pressure with decreased diastolic blood pressure
Pupil irregularity

imaging modalities including diffusion tensor imaging, magnetic resonance spectroscopy, singlephoton emission CT, and cerebral angiography may facilitate the diagnosis of concussion and assist in making return-to-play decisions.

Decision-Making Principles

The differential diagnosis of concussion includes epidural hematoma, subdural hematoma, intracerebral hematoma, and subarachnoid hemorrhage.

Epidural hematoma is a rapidly progressing intracranial hematoma that occurs from a tear of the middle meningeal artery that normally supplies the dura (the outermost covering of the brain). A fracture of the temporal bone often precipitates this hematoma. Blood accumulates between the skull and the dura and can rapidly reach a fatal size within 30 to 60 minutes. The classic clinical presentation is an athlete who sustains a blow to the head with immediate loss of consciousness followed by a lucid interval. However, the presentation can vary; sometimes the athlete may not lose consciousness, or he or she may regain consciousness with symptoms of severe, progressing headache followed by a decline in the level of consciousness. These worsening symptoms occur because the clot accumulation is causing increased intracranial pressure. If the diagnosis is an epidural hematoma, it is often obvious within the first 1 to 2 hours after injury. Treatment is emergent evacuation of the hematoma because if the pressure is removed and no further bleeding occurs, a significant recovery can be made. However, if it is not treated expediently, an epidural hematoma can rapidly lead to death. All athletes who sustain a head injury must be monitored closely and frequently for the first 24 to 48 hours with direct access to full neurosurgical services in the event of emergency.

A *subdural hematoma* occurs as a result of bleeding between the brain surface and the dura; it is considered the most common fatal head injury in athletes.[33] A subdural hematoma may occur as a result of one of a few different mechanisms, including a tear in a vein(s) running from the surface of the brain to the dura; diffuse injury to the surface of the brain; a torn venous sinus; or, less commonly, a torn small artery on the surface of the brain. Subdural hematomas are associated with brain tissue injury and thus are associated with a greater morbidity because even if the clot is evacuated early, underlying brain tissue injury has already occurred.

An *intracerebral hematoma* occurs from intracranial hemorrhage from bleeding into the brain substance itself, usually from a torn artery or congenital vascular lesion such as an aneurysm or arteriovenous malformation. Clinically, athletes present with rapidly progressive neurologic deterioration after a head trauma. Immediate medical attention is essential, but death occasionally occurs before the athlete is even transported to a medical facility. A full autopsy is recommended in these cases to establish the potential underlying anatomic malformation and to clarify the causative factors.

A *subarachnoid hemorrhage* is intracranial bleeding within the cerebrospinal fluid space along the surface of the brain. Bleeding occurs most commonly after head trauma from disruption of the tiny surface brain blood vessels. However, it can also result from a ruptured cerebral aneurysm or arteriovenous malformation. Brain swelling may be associated and may require a decompressive craniectomy, but surgery is not required for the hemorrhage itself.

Treatment Options

Treatment of concussion is entirely nonoperative. The goal of managing an athlete with concussion is to facilitate expedient resolution of symptoms and safe return to play. Initial treatment involves physical and cognitive rest and requires comprehensive education of the patient and his or her caregivers so they understand the management plan. Management practices are based on the Third International Conference on Concussion in Sports,[3] which is the current standard of care. Previously many grading systems were used for concussions; however, all of the recent guidelines now focus on symptoms and returning to play. Regardless of the severity of the injury, an athlete is not allowed to return to play as long as symptoms are present.

Physical rest involves broadly withholding an athlete from all physical exertion. This restriction is based on the pathophysiologic principle that in the setting of a metabolic imbalance and energy crisis within the brain, any increased energy demand in the brain from physical activity may worsen symptoms and delay recovery.[39] Physicians must be clear with athletes that restriction from physical activity includes all weight training, cardiovascular training, physical education classes, and leisure activities and not just restriction from competition and organized team training.

Cognitive rest is also essential to minimize symptoms and maximize recovery. After sustaining a concussion, athletes often report difficulty attending school, taking tests, and keeping up with assignments. Cognition is "exercise" for the brain and requires increased energy demand in the face of the postconcussion energy crisis in the brain and thus should be avoided until symptoms subside. Cognitive rest may involve staying home from school, attending only a few classes, decreased schoolwork load, allowance of extra time to complete coursework and tests, avoiding standardized testing, and taking rest breaks during the day. Additionally, all activities that require concentration or offer stimulus to the brain must be avoided as part of cognitive rest, including playing video games, using the computer, watching television (especially intense, dramatic, violent programming), listening to loud music, and exposure to bright lights. Lastly, because of slowed reaction times, licensed drivers with a concussion should avoid driving until they are cleared for activity.

Return to Play

After a concussion, athletes should not return to play until all symptoms are resolved, and current recommendations are for no same-day return to play, especially for the pediatric or adolescent athlete. Legislation has been passed in many states requiring all athletes with a suspected concussion to be removed from any sports participation until they are given clearance to return to play from a licensed health care professional. Although most athletes display resolution of symptoms within 7 to 10 days, the recovery time frame may be longer in children and adolescents.[20]

For deciding when to return to play, asymptomatic athletes are directed to follow a medically supervised stepwise process, based on the summary and agreement statement of the Fourth International Conference on Concussion in Sports.[20] The patient should never return to play while symptomatic, and all return-to-play programs must be individualized because

TABLE 137-2

GRADUAL RETURN-TO-PLAY PROTOCOL

Level	Activity
1	No activity, complete rest until asymptomatic and cleared by physician
2	Light aerobic exercise (e.g., walking, stationary cycling)
3	Sport-specific training (e.g., skating for hockey, running for soccer)
4	Noncontact training drills
5	Full-contact training after medical clearance
6	Game play

every athlete recovers at a different pace. The following protocol is recommended by the Fourth International Conference on Concussion as a guideline to be completed with appropriate supervision (Table 137-2):

> *Each level requires at least 24 hours and a minimum of 5 days is required to progress through the protocol to be cleared for full participation. However, any return of symptoms at any stage of the protocol is indication that concussion recovery is inadequate. If any post-concussion symptoms occur the patient should drop back to the previous asymptomatic level and try to progress again after 24 hours. If an athlete completes all levels with minimum of 24 hours between levels, the athlete is considered cleared for all activities. Athletes with a history of multiple concussions or prolonged post-concussion syndrome may require longer intervals as they progress through each level of recovery.*

Athletes who have sustained traumatic intracranial bleeding may begin the gradual return-to-play protocol for noncontact sports after a minimum of 6 weeks to enable the bone flap to heal after a craniotomy; however, after traumatic intracranial bleeding, it is recommended that athletes not return to contact sports.

Complications

Although the large majority of concussions self-resolve within 7 to 10 days, complications may occur, including postconcussion syndrome, second-impact syndrome, long-term effects, and chronic traumatic encephalopathy.

Postconcussion syndrome refers to the presence of symptoms beyond the normal duration of recovery. Many variations exist in the specifics of the postconcussion syndrome definition, and no set of criteria is universally accepted. The two most commonly applied definitions are proposed by the World Health Organization International Statistical Classification of Diseases and Related Health Problems (ICD)-10 and the *Diagnostic and Statistical Manual of Mental Disorders*, fourth edition (DSM-IV) (Table 137-3).

Second-impact syndrome is a debated term that applies to the pathophysiology that occurs when an athlete sustains a second head trauma prior to complete symptom resolution after an initial head injury. Second-impact syndrome results in cerebral vascular congestion that progresses to diffuse cerebral swelling and is associated with a high mortality rate. This second hit occurs during the period of enhanced vulnerability characterized by an increased brain cell demand for glucose in the face of reduced cerebral blood flow and impaired cerebral vascular autoregulation. Because pediatric and adolescent athletes have demonstrated longer recovery times from the initial decreased cerebral blood flow,[2] these younger athletes are at higher risk of second-impact syndrome.

The long-term effects of one or multiple concussions are largely unknown because minimal large-scale scientific investigation of the long-term consequences of brain injury in athletes has been performed. A study of high school athletes showed that symptom-free athletes with a history of two or more concussions performed similarly on testing when compared with youth athletes who had experienced a recent concussion. Similarly, cumulative academic grade point averages were significantly lower for youth athletes with two or more previous concussions.[35] A metaanalysis reviewing eight current articles that evaluated high school and collegiate athletes also demonstrated that multiple concussions were associated with statistically significant deficits, but only on measures of executive and delayed memory.[36]

Studies of amateur boxers reveal similar chronic neurocognitive effects[37]; however, professional boxers show much more significant long-term neurocognitive effects, with older studies showing that 17% of retired boxers demonstrate chronic traumatic encephalopathy.[38] A genetic predisposition to chronic traumatic encephalopathy may exist. More recent studies accounting for the reduction in exposure to repetitive head trauma and increasing medical monitoring of boxers predicts a lower incidence in the future.[37-39]

Chronic traumatic encephalopathy is a progressive degenerative disease of the brain that occurs in persons with a history of repetitive head trauma, including symptomatic concussions and asymptomatic subconcussion threshold hits to the head. Trauma triggers the progressive brain cell degeneration,

TABLE 137-3

WHO AND DSM-IV POSTCONCUSSION SYNDROME DEFINITIONS

	WHO ICD-10	DSM-IV
Minimum duration of symptoms	NA	3 mo
Number of symptoms	3	3
Defining symptoms	Headache Dizziness/vertigo Easily fatigued/ easily tired Irritability Poor concentration Forgetfulness Sleep disturbance Depression Anxiety	Fatigue Disordered sleep Headache Vertigo/dizziness Anxiety Depression Personality changes Apathy

DSM-IV, Diagnostic and Statistical Manual of Mental Disorders, 4th edition; *ICD-10,* International Statistical Classification of Diseases and Related Health Problems; *WHO,* World Health Organization.

Modified from Kashluba S, Casey JE, Paniak C: Evaluating the utility of ICD-10 diagnostic criteria for postconcussion syndrome following traumatic brain injury. *J Int Neuropsychol Soc* 12:111–118, 2006; and *American Psychiatric Association: Diagnostic and Statistical Manual of Mental Disorders,* ed 4, Washington, DC, 2000, American Psychiatric Association.

leading to an accumulation of an abnormal protein called tau. Changes can occur months, years, and decades after the traumatic events. Chronic traumatic encephalopathy presents clinically with symptoms of headaches, memory loss, disorientation, impaired judgment, impulse control problems, aggression, depression, tremors, abnormal gait/speech, and ultimately dementia and sometimes suicide; often the diagnosis is made postmortem at autopsy.

National Football League retirees with a history of three or more concussions show a threefold increase in the risk of depression and memory problems and a fivefold increased prevalence of mild cognitive impairment (e.g., memory, concentration, and speech) when compared with retirees without a history of concussion.[40,41]

Future Considerations

Currently, concussion is a diagnosis made subjectively based on history and supported by neurocognitive and balance testing; however, no diagnostic test is available to facilitate an objective diagnosis. Future research and medical advances will likely further elucidate the underlying disease and improve the diagnosis and management of concussive injuries.

For a complete list of references, go to expertconsult.com.

Suggested Readings

Citation: McCrory P, Meeuwisse W, Aubry M, et al: Consensus statement on concussion in sport: The 4th International Conference on Concussion in Sport held in Zurich, November 2012. *Br J Sports Med* 47(5):250–258, 2013.

Level of Evidence: III

Summary: Although evidence-based recommendations are limited, the authors of this article review consensus based on a systemic review of current medical literature and expert opinion for diagnosis and management of concussion.

Citation: Halstead ME, Walter KD, The Council on Sports Medicine and Fitness: Clinical report: Sports-related concussion in children and adolescents. *Pediatrics* 126(3):597–615, 2010.

Level of Evidence: III

Summary: Although evidence-based recommendations are limited, the authors of this review provide a summary of current medical literature, which is a helpful tool for the management of concussion in children.

Citation: Giza CC: The neurometabolic cascade of concussion. *J Athl Train* 36(3):228–235, 2001.

Level of Evidence: III

Summary: This article is an excellent review of the underlying neuropathophysiologic processes of concussive brain injury and the associated neurometabolic changes in relation to clinical sports-related issues. Results from more than 100 articles of basic science and clinical medical literature are summarized.

Citation: Maugans TA, Farley C, Altaye M, et al: Pediatric sports-related concussion produces cerebral blood flow alterations. *Pediatrics* 129:28–37, 2012.

Level of Evidence: III

Summary: The authors report a small study in which 12 children who experienced sports-related concussion were evaluated with use of multiple modalities, including ImPACT neurocognitive testing, T1- and susceptibility-weighted magnetic resonance imaging, diffusion tensor imaging, proton magnetic resonance spectroscopy, and phase-contrast angiography.

Citation: Riemann BL, Guskiewicz KM, Riemann BL, et al: Effects of mild head injury on postural stability as measured through clinical balance testing. *J Athl Train* 35(1):19–25, 2000.

Level of Evidence: III

Summary: The authors of this study investigate the efficacy of a clinical balance testing procedure for the detection of acute postural stability disruptions after mild traumatic brain injury.

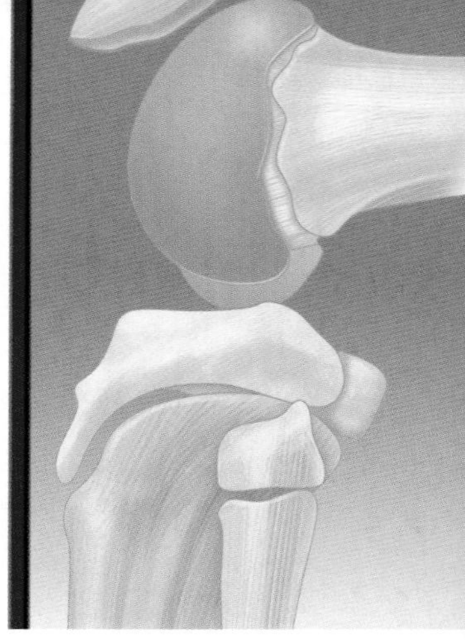

138

Spine Injuries in Skeletally Immature Athletes

LINDSAY ANDRAS • DAVID L. SKAGGS

Many aspects of the care of the spine in pediatric athletes are challenging. Sports physicians play several roles in this setting. First, they may be asked to evaluate a child or adolescent with a known condition and weigh in on whether he or she can safely participate in athletic activities. Second, when an acute traumatic event has occurred, sports physicians may be asked to evaluate and provide initial management for the injured athlete. Additionally, sports physicians manage and treat conditions that create chronic pain or deformity and may have an impact on sports participation.

These varied roles are complicated by the anatomic differences between the mature and growing spine. Thus in addition to injuries that are observed in both children and adults, the growing spine leads to injuries that are unique to the pediatric and adolescent populations. This chapter describes the relevant anatomy and related injuries observed in the young athlete as well as key components in the evaluation of these spine conditions and their management. In addition, guidelines for both restriction from sports and timing of return to athletic activities are provided.

Anatomy

Fracture patterns and biomechanics, particularly in the cervical spine, differ for children based on age. In younger children, the fulcrum is at C2-C3 because of their proportionally large skulls. Consequently, for children younger than 8 years, 87% of cervical spine injuries occur at or above C3 and 50% are associated with head injuries.[1] Older children have fracture patterns similar to those of adults, with the subaxial spine most commonly affected.

Diagnosis of cervical spine injuries in the child can be challenging, particularly in the younger age groups, because much of the cervical spine has not yet ossified. The anterior ring of C1 does not ossify until after the age of 1 year, making detection of injury in this region especially challenging (Fig. 138-1). Between the ages of 3 and 6 years, fusion of the dens to the neural arches and anterior body occurs, which can be mistaken for a fracture at the base of the odontoid. By age 6 years, the spinal canal of the cervical spine has reached adult dimensions. Lateral radiographs show a progressively increasing facet angle from birth to 8 years of age that allows motion through flexion and extension and contributes to the appearance of pseudosubluxation often seen at C2-C3 and C3-C4. Pseudosubluxation can be differentiated from true subluxation on plain radiographs by the maintenance of the Swischuk line, which is a straight line drawn along the spinolaminar line (the anterior edge of the posterior neural arch; Fig. 138-2). Additionally, incomplete ossification often gives the appearance of wedging of the cervical vertebral bodies on lateral radiographs until age 10 years. The atlantodens interval (ADI) may be increased in children. As opposed to adults, in whom a normal ADI is less than 3 mm, in young children the ADI may be up to 4.5 mm without signifying injury.

Additional considerations also exist in the thoracolumbar spine compared with the adult spine. The ring apophysis that extends peripherally around the vertebral body is adherent to the annulus of the intervertebral disk and can be at risk for injury. These injuries may be mistaken both clinically and radiographically for a pediatric disk herniation.

General History and Physical Examination for Evaluation of the Pediatric Spine

The sports physician can evaluate the spine of a pediatric patient in preparation for participation in athletic activities, after an acute event that occurs while participating in a sport, or when the patient has chronic pain. It is important to differentiate the more common generalized aches and pains that accompany both athletic training and adolescence from more serious causes of pain. Atypical pain may be indicative of a more serious injury, a tumor, infection, or another more severe clinical entity. Box 138-1 outlines key elements in the history that can guide the clinician in making this distinction.

In evaluating spinal injuries, the mechanism and impact can alert the clinician to more critical conditions. In acute scenarios in which a potentially unstable spine injury is suspected, proper immobilization of the spine is necessary to prevent worsening of the injury. For children younger than 7 years, a pediatric backboard with a recess should be used to accommodate their proportionally large head size and prevent additional injury from the acute flexion that can be caused by a traditional backboard.

The physical examination is critical but also challenging in the child with suspected spinal injury. In cases in which spinal instability is not suspected, the focused neurologic examination outlined (Box 138-2) provides an efficient assessment and can be performed even in young children.

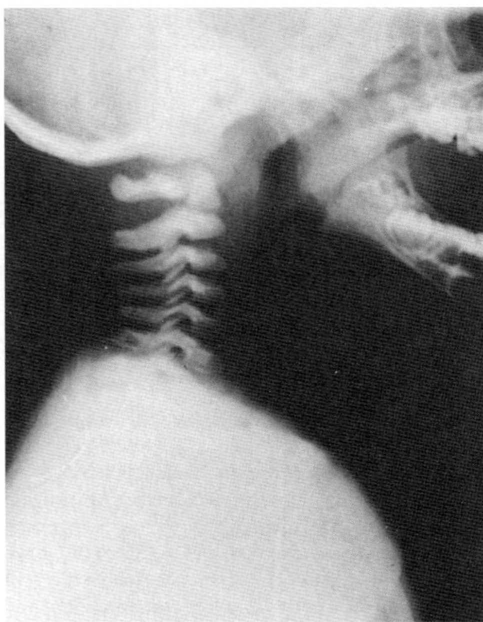

FIGURE 138-1 Detection of cervical spine injuries or abnormalities in the young child can be challenging, because much of the cervical spine has not yet ossified. The anterior ring of C1 does not ossify until after the age of 1 year and is not visible on plain radiographs at that age, as depicted here.

BOX 138-1 Pediatric Back Pain Red Flags

The following pain characteristics are not associated with typical muscular back pain and warrant further investigation.

- Night pain
- Pain in young children, especially if they stop playing
- Frequent pain at rest, not including sitting (pain with prolonged sitting in school is extremely common in teens with mechanical low back pain)
- Back pain associated with an abnormal gait, limp, unsteadiness on feet, etc.
- With associated constitutional symptoms (e.g,. fever, lethargy, weight loss, loss of appetite)
- Atypical location, especially thoracic rather than lumbar pain (although pain in the trapezius/periscapular muscles is often due to backpacks)
- History of worsening pain
- With neurologic symptoms or physical findings (cavus foot, etc.)
- Kyphosis
- With important cutaneous findings (e.g., high and deep dimple, hairy patch, café-au-lait spots suggestive of neurofibromatosis)
- Positive finger test (child localizes pain to area the size of a fingertip)
- Positive coin test (have child keep the back straight when picking something up)
- Listing to side on Adams forward bend
- Tight hamstrings (popliteal angle >50 degrees)

Atlantoaxial Instability

Atlantoaxial instability may be either acute, as a result of a traumatic event, or chronic. Acute atlantoaxial instability may occur as a result of severe flexion of the cervical spine. An ADI of 5 mm or more in children in the setting of an acute injury may signify that the transverse ligament has been injured and that instability is present. Magnetic resonance imaging (MRI) may further elucidate the extent of the injury. If the transverse ligament is injured, posterior spinal fusion of C1 and C2 is usually necessary to prevent further compromise to the spinal cord.

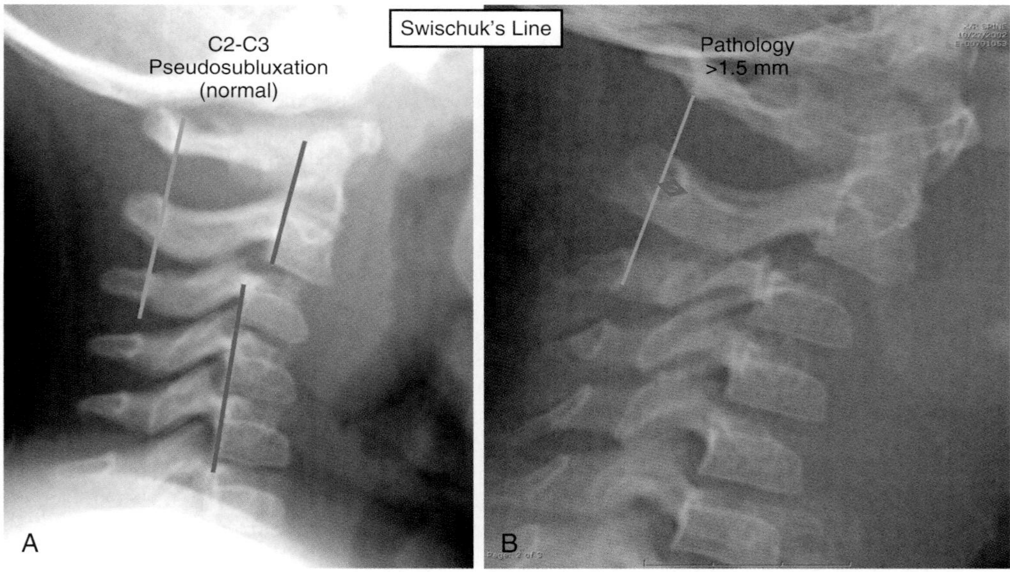

FIGURE 138-2 Pseudosubluxation can be differentiated from true subluxation on plain radiographs by the maintenance of the Swischuk line (green), which is a straight line drawn along the anterior edge of the posterior neural arch. **A,** The patient has no acute injury, which is confirmed by the maintenance of this line. **B,** The patient has a change in the relation of the posterior elements to this line, which represents true subluxation. *(Courtesy Children's Orthopedic Center, Los Angeles, CA.)*

BOX 138-2 60-Second Neurologic Examination

Hop on each foot, one at a time
Walk on heels
Reflexes
Foot inspection
Ankle dorsiflexion to assess muscle tone and clonus
Sensation
Popliteal angle

From Skaggs DL, Flynn JM: *Staying out of trouble in pediatric orthopaedics,* Philadelphia, 2005, Lippincott Williams & Wilkins.

Atlantoaxial Instability in Syndrome

More commonly the physician is faced with management of chronic atlantoaxial instability in patients with Down syndrome. This instability may be either symptomatic or asymptomatic. The estimated incidence of asymptomatic atlantoaxial instability in persons with Down syndrome is up to 22%, whereas only 2% to 3% of persons with Down syndrome have symptomatic atlantoaxial instability.[2] The literature currently does not include any reports of children with Down syndrome without preceding neurologic symptoms who have had a traumatic injury with sports participation that resulted in progression to symptomatic instability. The history and physical examination are especially important in the evaluation of these patients.

History and Physical Examination

The history is key in this patient population because the physical examination may be challenging. Symptoms to inquire about include neck pain, fatigability, difficulty walking, abnormal gait, and worsening coordination or clumsiness. Physical examination should include evaluation of neck range of motion, gait, strength, spasticity, hyperreflexia, and clonus.

Imaging

Both the screening and management of atlantoaxial instability in persons with Down syndrome have become extremely controversial. The American Academy of Pediatrics has retracted its recommendation for assessment of potential atlantoaxial instability and currently advises against imaging in asymptomatic persons.[3] Conversely, the Special Olympics have screening requirements for sports participation that typically consist of a lateral cervical spine radiograph in flexion, neutral position, and extension. In children, the guidelines established by Special Olympics state that an ADI of greater than 4.5 mm is considered to be atlantoaxial instability.[4] Other authors have suggested that measurement of the space available for the cord (spinal canal width) of less than 14 mm is a more relevant predictor of neurologic injury. If either an abnormal space available for the cord or an abnormal ADI is detected, further evaluation by a pediatric spine surgeon is warranted. In cases in which the ADI is greater than 10 mm or the child is symptomatic, an MRI scan may be helpful in the evaluation.

A similar issue for pediatric athletes with Down syndrome is the consideration of atlantooccipital hypermobility. Atlantooccipital instability has been underappreciated and should be considered when evaluating radiographs in this population.[5] A Power's ratio of greater than 1.0 signifies anterior instability.[6] In addition, posterior instability has also been described, but the clinical significance of this instability is as yet unclear.[7]

Decision-Making Principles

Activity restriction on the basis of asymptomatic atlantoaxial instability is a topic of great controversy. Opponents argue that no cases have been reported of patients with isolated radiographic atlantoaxial instability who sustained a neurologic injury as a result of sports participation.[8] In addition, no cases have been reported of asymptomatic atlantoaxial instability progressing to symptomatic atlantoaxial instability as a result of a sports-related injury.[9] Nevertheless, the present recommendations from the Special Olympics Committee are for restriction from the sports listed in Box 138-3 unless the participant has written certification by two physicians acknowledging the acceptance of risks by the parent or guardian. For patients with an ADI of greater than 10 mm, spinal fusion is generally recommended. Figure 138-3 shows our preferred treatment in the screening and management of asymptomatic persons with Down syndrome.

Currently no recommendations exist regarding atlantooccipital hypermobility in terms of clearance for the Special Olympics or other sporting activities in the young athlete with Down syndrome, but it should be considered when monitoring for the more common atlantoaxial instability.[5]

Treatment

Aside from activity restrictions, no other nonoperative treatments are available for atlantoaxial instability. Operative management consists of posterior arthrodesis. Prior to fusion, particular attention needs to be given to the occipitocervical articulation. If any evidence of instability is observed at this level, the occiput should be included in the fusion. Many techniques for atlantoaxial fusion have been described, including use of wires, plates, and transarticular screws with either a rib or iliac crest graft. For smaller children, two commonly used techniques are the Mah modified Gallie

BOX 138-3 Special Olympics Participant Restriction

The Special Olympics restricts participation in sports that involve hyperextension, radical flexion, or direct pressure on the neck or upper spine unless a radiograph demonstrates no evidence of cervical spine instability*:

- Butterfly stroke and diving starts (swimming)
- Diving
- Pentathlon
- High jump
- Equestrian sports
- Gymnastics
- Football (soccer)
- Skiing
- Warm-up exercises placing stress on the head and neck

*Or two documented discussions with a physician regarding risks.

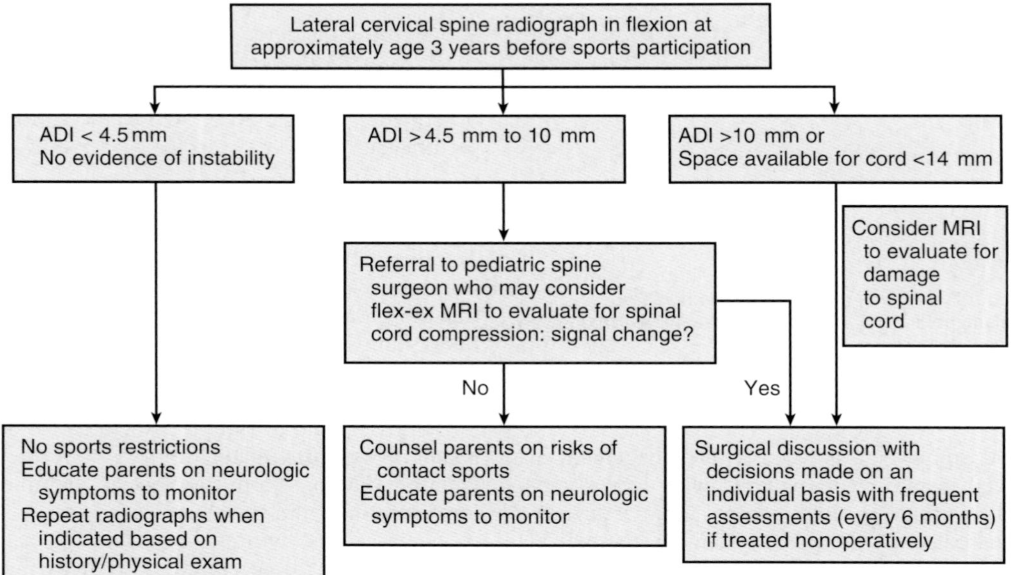

FIGURE 138-3 The authors' screening protocol for asymptomatic patients with Down syndrome. *ADI,* Atlantodens interval; *flex-ex,* flexion-extension; *MRI,* magnetic resonance imaging.

technique and the Brooks technique. In the Mah modified Gallie technique, a wire is passed under the posterior arch of C1, looped over a threaded Kirschner wire that is placed in the spinous process of C2, and then tightened to secure a rectangle of corticocancellous autograft in position.[10] In the Brooks technique, two sublaminar wires are passed under both C1 and C2 and used to secure two trapezoids of the iliac crest graft that are wedged between C1 and C2.[11] Halo vest immobilization is required until bony fusion has been achieved.

Results

Fusion rates in the setting of atlantoaxial instability in persons with Down syndrome have historically been poor and range from 40% to 80%.[12] An improvement in these results has been reported by Menezes and Ryken[13] by incorporating the occiput when indicated and implementing prolonged immobilization with a halo postoperatively, with recommendations of 4 months for C1-C2 fusion and 6 months when the occiput is included. Complication rates are high for this procedure. Segal et al.[14] have reported a 100% complication rate and an 18% mortality rate.

Rotatory Atlantoaxial Subluxation

A common cause of acute torticollis is rotatory atlantoaxial subluxation, which occurs when the lateral mass of the atlas locks behind the ipsilateral lateral mass of the axis. It is most often traumatic in nature in healthy children, although other possible causes exist, such as Grisel or Sandifer syndrome. Rotatory atlantoaxial subluxation may occur after even minor trauma during sports participation or even with coughing episodes. It also may be associated with conditions that feature ligamentous laxity in this region, including Down syndrome, Marfan syndrome, or rheumatoid arthritis.

History and Physical Examination

On presentation patients have a "cock robin" torticollis with their head tilted toward one shoulder and their chin rotated in the opposite direction. Patients may report neck pain and occasionally occipital neuralgia or symptoms of vertebrobasilar insufficiency. This condition is easily differentiated from muscular torticollis both by the acuity and by the absence of a palpable sternocleidomastoid on the shortened side. The lengthened sternocleidomastoid may feel tight from being stretched. Most affected children are neurologically intact, but a thorough neurologic examination should be performed.

Imaging

Radiographic evaluation should include an open-mouth anteroposterior and lateral radiograph of the cervical spine. The technician should take the image as a true lateral view of the skull, which results in images that are more easily interpreted and show a true lateral view of the axis and rotation of the remainder of the spine. For further evaluation or if the diagnosis is unclear, a computed tomographic (CT) scan can provide additional clarity (Fig. 138-4). Historically, dynamic CT scans have been recommended but may not be worth exposure to additional radiation on a routine basis.

Treatment

Treatment is time dependent because the subluxation becomes more difficult to reduce with the passage of time. Additionally, persistent subluxation may damage the transverse ligament and result in subsequent instability or recurrence if a reduction is obtained.[15] In general, if the diagnosis is made and treatment starts 1 month or less from the time of the injury, then nonoperative management with either a cervical collar or head halter traction is often sufficient. In patients in whom

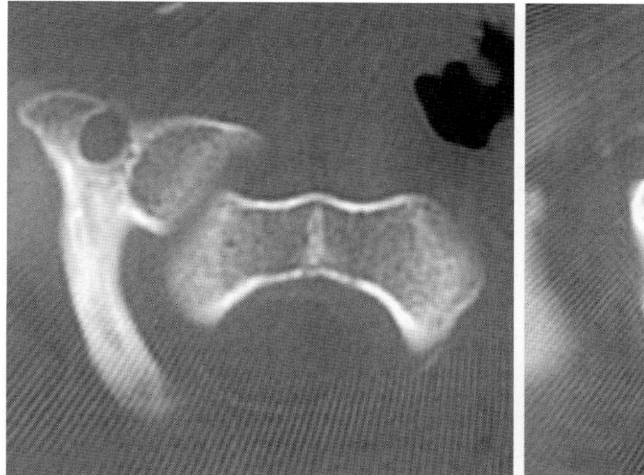

FIGURE 138-4 A computed tomography scan showing that C1 is subluxated on C2 with the lateral mass of the atlas locked behind the ipsilateral lateral mass of the axis. *(Courtesy Children's Orthopedic Center, Los Angeles, CA.)*

treatment is initiated less than 1 week after the onset of symptoms, immobilization in a soft collar for a few days is often sufficient to both obtain and maintain a reduction. For patients who begin treatment 1 to 4 weeks after the onset of symptoms, head halter traction can be used. If reduction is attempted with head halter traction, the position can be maintained with the use of a noninvasive halo. If these measures fail or if the injury occurred more than 4 weeks prior to the beginning of treatment, closed reduction with a noninvasive halo may be attempted, with reduction likely once the head is rotated past midline. A CT scan confirms the reduction. Use of the noninvasive halo may be continued for 4 to 6 weeks to allow scarring and maintenance of the reduction.[16] If instability or loss of reduction occurs, then repeat reduction with the noninvasive halo followed by surgical stabilization with posterior atlantoaxial fusion is indicated.

Odontoid Fractures

Odontoid fractures account for 10% of all cervical spine injuries in children and the majority of pediatric cervical spine fractures.[17] In children younger than 7 years, the fracture occurs through the synchondrosis at the base of the dens. This position can make the diagnosis more challenging because the synchondrosis may be mistaken for a fracture or, conversely, the fracture may be assumed to be the synchondrosis and overlooked (see Fig. 138-5).

Classification

Odontoid fractures in children are described with use of the adult classification system of Anderson and D'Alonzo. Type I is an avulsion fracture of the tip of the dens. Type II is the most common and is through the base of the dens. In type III, the fracture extends into the vertebral body.

History and Physical Examination

Odontoid fractures occur more commonly from flexion mechanisms but have also been described from forced hyperextension. Although most authors have reported that pediatric

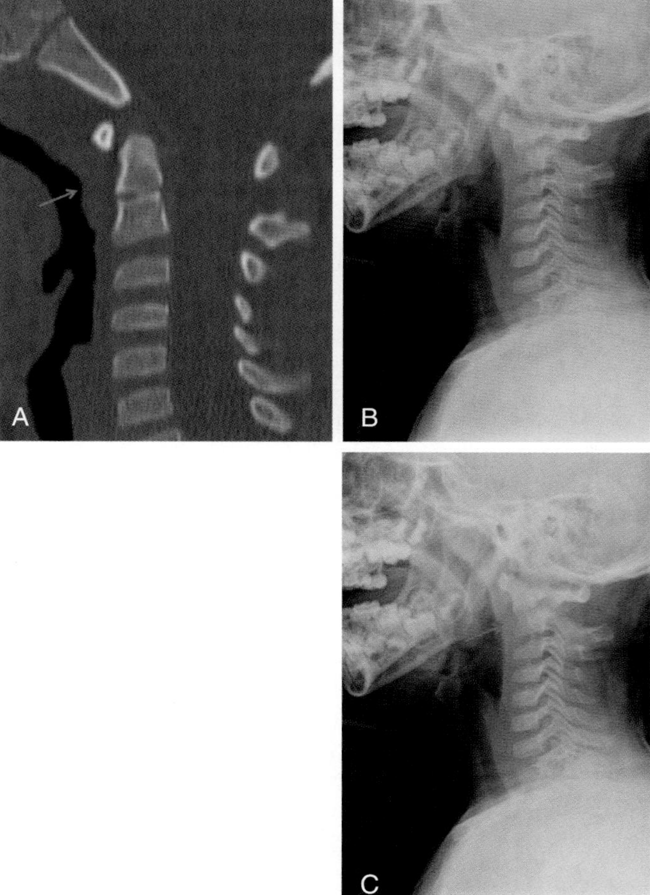

FIGURE 138-5 A 4-year-old boy who had sustained a fall on his head had an initial computed tomography scan (**A**) and radiograph (**B**) that were read as negative. The odontoid fracture (*arrow*) was missed because it was assumed to be just his normal physis despite the associated swelling. He presented 2 weeks later to his primary care physician with neck pain; a lateral radiograph taken at that time (**C**) shows significant displacement through the fracture site. Treatment consisted of closed reduction and halo placement. *(Courtesy Children's Orthopedic Center, Los Angeles, CA.)*

odontoid fractures are not associated with neurologic injury, one series reported neurologic injury in 8 of 15 children younger than 6 years who had odontoid fractures.[18] A thorough physical examination should be performed to evaluate for this possibility. Typically these children have neck pain and decreased range of motion. Direct point tenderness is not necessarily present.

Imaging

The synchondrosis at the base of the dens should be fused by age 6 years. After this age, any evidence of a radiographic abnormality in this region suggests a fracture. In children younger than 7 years, great care must be taken to not mistake normal anatomy for an acute injury or conversely to neglect a fracture by attributing it to normal development. Assessment for swelling in the retropharyngeal space can be helpful in this differentiation. Nevertheless, the clinician should keep in mind that if the patient is crying, the child will have an apparent increase in the width of the retropharyngeal space. In situations in which the diagnosis is unclear and clinical suspicion is high, an MRI may be obtained for further evaluation. Figure 136-5 shows the initial CT scan of a 4-year-old boy who fell on his head and whose odontoid fracture was missed because this fracture was assumed to be just his normal physis despite the associated swelling. He presented to his primary care physician with neck pain 2 weeks later, and a lateral radiograph showed significant displacement through the fracture site.

Treatment

Most of these injuries can be treated by stabilization in a halo vest. The alignment of the fracture is generally improved with the head positioned in slight extension. The amount of acceptable angulation and the potential for remodeling varies with age and remains controversial, although one report of patients younger than 3 years with angulation of greater than 30 degrees showed that remodeling led to a normal structure with no associated sequelae.[19] In children 7 years of age or older, the fractures behave more like adult fractures and are treated accordingly. Cases of nonunion of type II odontoid fractures in this group have been reported and can be treated with a screw placed via a direct anterior approach.[20] Consideration should also be given to the possibility of instability, which necessitates surgical fusion.

Congenital Anomalies of the Cervical Spine

Congenital anomalies may involve either failure of formation or segmentation of vertebrae. Numerous anomalies exist, and each case warrants evaluation for concomitant stenosis or instability. Evidence of instability may warrant surgical management and at the very least avoidance of sporting activities. One such clinical entity is os odontoideum. In this condition, the dens is not fused to the body of the C2 vertebrae. Another commonly encountered congenital anomaly is that of Klippel-Feil, the term given to a congenital fusion (or failure of segmentation) of two or more cervical vertebrae.

Classification

Klippel-Feil anomalies are divided into two types. Type I is a multilevel deformity in which a large fusion mass is present, and type II is a fusion of either one or two levels.

History and Physical Examination

Although os odontoideum was once believed to be exclusively a congenital condition, more recently a posttraumatic cause has also been proposed.[21] Evidence supports both posttraumatic and congenital causes, and in reality, two separate clinical entities may exist.[22] The clinician may be evaluating a patient because of an incidental radiographic finding or because pain or neurologic symptoms are present.

Patients with Klippel-Feil syndrome may have the classic triad of a low hairline, a short neck, and decreased cervical range of motion, but these findings are present in fewer than 50% of cases.[23] These patients may also have an associated Sprengel deformity due to failure of the scapula to descend. Evaluation of a person with Klippel-Feil syndrome also may be in response to an incidental radiographic finding. In all cases a thorough evaluation for any neurologic symptoms or physical findings must be performed.

Imaging

At a minimum, imaging consists of anteroposterior, lateral, and flexion extension radiographs of the cervical spine. In cases of odontoid abnormalities, improved visualization is obtained with an open-mouth odontoid view. If evidence of instability or concern about instability is present on the basis of neurologic abnormalities, an MRI of the spine is warranted. A flexion-extension MRI is preferred in many cases to evaluate for any signal changes indicative of dynamic cord compression.

An additional consideration in the patient with congenital anomalies of the spine is the increased incidence of genitourinary issues in this patient population, which should be evaluated by renal ultrasound prior to consideration of sports participation. The presence of renal abnormalities, such as a solitary kidney, may pose additional risks with sports participation.[24] Although recommendations vary, a diagnosis and discussion of the risks prior to sports participation are warranted.[25]

Treatment

In cases of os odontoideum in which the patient has neurologic symptoms and evidence of radiographic instability, a cervical fusion of the first and second cervical vertebrae is indicated. In cases of asymptomatic instability, the treatment is controversial, and both radiographic surveillance and surgical management have been recommended. Little evidence supports either decision over the other. In persons with os odontoideum, as well as odontoid agenesis or hypoplasia, participation in contact sports is usually contraindicated. The literature includes multiple reports of injury to patients with previously undiagnosed os odontoideum that resulted in a neurologic injury, including respiratory-dependent quadriplegia.[26]

In persons with Klippel-Feil syndrome, the potential for spinal cord injury is due to the abnormal motion of the unfused segments. Pizzutillo[27] has reported that more than 90 cases of neurologic injury have occurred in patients with Klippel-Feil syndrome because of associated occipitocervical anomalies, chronic instability, disk disease, or degenerative joint disease.[27] More than two thirds of these cases were associated with a single-level fusion of the upper cervical spine.[28] Although no consensus has been achieved on this topic, a congenital fusion at level C3 or higher is sometimes considered a relative contraindication to participation in collision sports and warrants evaluation by a pediatric spine surgeon. Conversely, patients with a one-level fusion below the level of C3, a normal neck range of motion, the absence of occipitocervical abnormalities, and the absence of instability do not have any contraindication to sports participation.[26]

Spinal Cord Injury Without Radiographic Abnormality

The acronym SCIWORA was coined by Pang and Wilberger[30] to describe a spinal cord injury with either motor, sensory, or combined deficits in the absence of any vertebral fracture or malalignment on plain radiographs or a CT scan. Although SCIWORA has been described in persons of all ages, it is most commonly observed in the pediatric population and accounts for an estimated 19% to 34% of all spinal cord injuries.[29-31] A great deal of controversy surrounds this condition, including its definition, diagnosis, and optimal management. In some cases the term is a misnomer because clear evidence of the neurologic injury is observed on MRI. In some series, such as the one reported by Bosch et al.,[32] 50 of the 60 MRI scans obtained were interpreted as normal.[32] Conversely, a recently published metaanalysis found that of the 392 cases identified, every patient with a diagnosis of SCIWORA with an MRI scan had evidence of either intraneural or extraneural injury.[33] In a series by Hamilton and Myles,[34] the onset of neurologic symptoms was delayed in 23% of cases (range, 6 to 72 hours).

History and Physical Examination

Patients with SCIWORA have sustained a traumatic event and have a subsequent neurologic deficit. Most cases of SCIWORA involve the cervical spine, but cases involving the thoracic and lumbar spine have also been described.[35] Sports injuries are the third most common mechanism, after motor vehicle accidents and falls. SCIWORA is most commonly associated with a flexion injury, but distraction and extension injuries have also been described with this diagnosis. The severity of the neurologic injury is highly variable, ranging from isolated nerve root involvement to complete quadriplegia. The spine is usually tender with the presence of significant local swelling or a hematoma.

Imaging

By definition, the absence of any vertebral fracture or malalignment on plain radiographs or a CT scan must be observed to assign the diagnosis of SCIWORA. MRI scans of the brain and spine are also obtained for persons with this condition to evaluate for evidence of spinal cord injury and any other central nervous system abnormality in the differential. Several anatomic explanations for the more frequent occurrence of SCIWORA in the pediatric cervical spine have been proposed, including a more horizontal orientation of the facet joints, anterior wedging of the vertebral bodies, and increased elasticity of the ligaments and joint capsules. A sentinel finding on MRI of a ligamentous Chance fracture that may be missed on plain films is significant as evidenced by a subcutaneous hematoma around the failed posterior elements and/or an increased T2-weighted signal at the interspinous ligament.

Treatment

A wide spectrum of severity is found in this condition, ranging from deficits localized to one nerve root to complete paralysis. Because of the variation in clinical presentations, the appropriate management is difficult to determine. Use of corticosteroids, mannitol, hyperbaric oxygen, and bracing have all been described.[32] The variable treatment protocols instituted from one institution to the next have further confounded this analysis and made it impossible with the currently available data to ascertain if steroids are of true benefit. Some authors have also argued against bracing or immobilization; they believe it is not indicated based on a lack of associated instability. Other authors, including Launay et al.,[33] have recommended treatment with immobilization. In their study, they compared a subgroup of 93 patients treated with immobilization only (with no use of steroids or other medications) and divided them into groups who were immobilized for 8 weeks and for 12 weeks. These investigators observed complete recovery in 42% of the patients immobilized for 12 weeks but in only 34% of the patients immobilized for 8 weeks.[33]

At our institution, the following protocol is used in the management of persons with SCIWORA: In cases in which evidence of spinal instability exists (including ligamentous Chance fractures), we believe that spinal fusion with instrumentation is the most reliable treatment to protect the patient from further injury and allow early rehabilitation. If no evidence exists of an occult injury that may be associated with instability, then we do not routinely immobilize these patients.

Scoliosis

Scoliosis is defined as curvature of the spine of greater than 10 degrees. Although most cases of scoliosis are idiopathic, idiopathic scoliosis is a diagnosis of exclusion. The clinician should be careful to consider other diagnosis such as neurofibromatosis, Marfan syndrome, or Ehlers-Danlos syndrome, with which the scoliosis may be associated. Many patients with adolescent idiopathic scoliosis—which has a prevalence of nearly 3%—participate in sports.[36] Once other potential concomitant conditions have been eliminated, idiopathic scoliosis is not a contraindication to participation in sports.

History and Physical Examination

At presentation, approximately 20% of patients with scoliosis have back pain, which is similar to the percentage of adolescents who have back pain in general.[37] For back pain that is localized, constant, progressive, predominantly occurs at night, or limits activities, further evaluation with MRI is warranted. The clinician should also ask about constitutional symptoms and any bowel or bladder issues. These atypical symptoms necessitate further evaluation for other causes and for spinal cord compression.

The risk of progression depends not only on the curve magnitude but also on genetic predisposition and the amount of growth remaining, which are important considerations in the history. When and how the curve was detected can provide insight into the severity and rate of progression. Family history is often positive, with approximately 10% of first-degree relatives affected and 8% of second-degree relatives affected.[38] Assessment of the amount of growth remaining is critical in the prognosis. Age at menarche and parental height can be helpful in this assessment.

Physical examination can be divided into three components: (1) assessment of the curve, (2) evaluation for any neurologic concerns, and (3) examination for any stigmata that suggest a cause that is not idiopathic. While the patient is standing upright, one should assess whether the shoulders and pelvis are level or if they are unbalanced. Also evaluated at this time are whether the shoulders are centered over the pelvis or if the patient has a truncal shift with the shoulders to one side or another. The Adams forward bend test then allows assessment of the rotation. Prominence should be noted on the same side as the convexity of the curve. In cases in which a lumbar prominence is noted on the concavity, a leg length discrepancy should be suspected, and the curve may be compensatory. With the patient bent forward, scoliometer readings can be obtained. A reading of 7 degrees on a scoliometer is considered abnormal and correlates to an approximately 20-degree curve,[39] which is an indication to order radiographs.

After assessment of the curve, a focused neurologic evaluation should be performed (see Box 138-2). Any change in sensation or strength, gait abnormality, foot deformity, unequal reflexes, or sustained clonus suggests a cause that is not idiopathic. Cutaneous findings of axillary freckles, more than three café-au-lait spots, or neurofibromas suggest neurofibromatosis. A high-arched palate, ligamentous laxity, and pectus deformities warrant consideration of Marfan syndrome.

Imaging

If the clinical examination suggests the possibility of scoliosis, then initial radiographic evaluation consists of a standing posteroanterior and lateral radiograph of the thoracolumbar spine. This radiograph ideally includes the pelvis and is not collimated to allow for evaluation of closure of the triradiate cartilage and the Risser sign, which are important components in assessing the growth remaining and the risk of progression. Care should be taken to evaluate for concomitant pathologic conditions on the lateral radiograph. In particular, in persons with symptomatic spondylolysis/spondylolisthesis, an associated scoliosis is present in 25% to 40% of cases, but it may be easily overlooked if the focus is entirely on the spinal curvature.[40]

Attention should also be directed to the sagittal contour of the patient with idiopathic scoliosis. Because scoliosis is a three-dimensional deformity, significant rotation and resultant hypokyphosis is generally observed through the thoracic region. If this area is instead kyphotic, one should suspect other etiologies. In cases in which a cause other than idiopathic scoliosis is suspected, an MRI should be obtained. Although recommendations vary, indications for an MRI include (1) neurologic abnormality (weakness/abnormal reflexes), (2) severe pain, (3) young patients (younger than 11 years) with curves greater than 20 degrees, (4) atypical patterns (i.e., a left-sided thoracic curve, congenital scoliosis, short angular curves, or a severe deformity >70 degrees), and (5) rapid progression (i.e., >1 degree per month).[41]

Treatment

Treatment is based on the risk of curve progression. The two major components in the evaluation are the curve magnitude and skeletal maturity (i.e., the amount of growth remaining). Lonstein and Carlson[42] have reported that if the condition is not treated, 68% of patients who are at Risser level 0-1 with a 20- to 29-degree curve will progress, whereas only 23% of patients who are at Risser level 2-4 with a curve of the same magnitude will show signs of progression.[42] Currently, none of the genetic testing available reliably allows identification of the curves that will progress as opposed to curves that will not progress.

Nonoperative treatment consists of bracing. Protocols and indications vary. Much of the debate centers around the contradictory evidence with regard to bracing. Much of the research that has been performed is complicated by compliance issues. In 2010, Katz et al.[43] published an article on bracing in persons with idiopathic scoliosis; brace monitors were used to measure the compliance. In this study, 82% of patients who wore a brace more than 12 hours a day did not have a progression of their curve, compared with 31% who did not progress with brace wear of fewer than 7 hours per day. Additionally, two brace treatment protocols were used. In one protocol, patients were instructed to wear the brace 23 hours per day, and in the second, they were instructed to wear the brace 16 hours per day. No difference was observed in either the number of hours the brace was worn or in the incidence of progression between these two groups. In this series, nighttime wear was not shown to be effective.[43] In general, bracing with a thoracolumbosacral orthosis (Boston brace) can be considered for curves of 25 to 40 degrees, with substantial growth remaining (Risser level 3 or less) and a curve apex below T7.

For curves that reach 50 degrees, surgical intervention is generally recommended. This recommendation is based on the high rate of progression of curves of that magnitude even after skeletal maturity and the ultimately significant cardiopulmonary effects.[44] Currently, posterior spinal fusion with pedicle screw fixation is the most common surgical treatment for idiopathic scoliosis. The selection of levels for posterior spinal fusion varies among surgeons but in general should include the Cobb angle and avoid ending the construct at any level of kyphosis (especially T6-T8). In general, a straight line drawn through the center of the sacrum should travel through the vertebrae at the distal end of the construct. If curves are compensatory, that is, less than 25 degrees on bending, then a selective fusion of the structural curve can be performed.[45] Complications include ileus (6%), early infection (1% to 2%), late infection (up to 5%), pseudarthrosis (3%), and neurologic deficit (0.4% to 0.7%).[41]

Scoliosis and Sports Participation

A curious finding has been the increased incidence of scoliosis detected in athletes who participate in some sports. For example, Becker[46] reported a 16% incidence of scoliosis in swimmers, and in all of these cases, the curves were toward the dominant hand. Similarly, Hellstrom et al.[47] reported a 13% incidence of scoliosis in tennis players. The significance and true validity of such reports is currently unclear. Numerous studies have demonstrated that exercise is not sufficient to inhibit the progression of idiopathic scoliosis. Although it may not alter the natural history, swimming has been shown to help maintain flexibility of the spine, as well as strength and endurance.[46]

Although it is widely recognized that scoliosis should not present a contraindication to sports participation, many questions remain about when it is appropriate for patients to return to sports in cases in which athletes have undergone surgical treatment. Survey responses from 261 pediatric spine surgeons indicate that the majority of these surgeons allow children to return to noncontact sports participation between 6 months and 1 year after spinal fusion for adolescent idiopathic scoliosis.[48] Even more variable was the timing for return to contact sports. In most cases of uncomplicated posterior spinal fusion for idiopathic scoliosis, we allow return to sports as tolerated, including contact sports, at around 3 months after the operation. However, this return is dependent on the understanding of both the patient and parent that some very small increase in the risk of a catastrophic spinal injury may exist, along with the agreement to undertake this shared risk.

Varying reports have been made regarding the long-term impact of surgical treatment for scoliosis on sports participation. In 2002, a survey of patients with scoliosis who were treated both operatively and nonoperatively reported no significant difference in sports participation, but both groups had decreased participation compared with control subjects.[49] More recently, Fabricant et al.[50] reported a correlation between the distal level of the fusion and return to sports after posterior spinal fusion. In their study, only 59% returned to their preoperative level of athletic activity at an average of 5.5 years of follow-up.[50] Their study did not include a nonoperatively treated group for comparison. Selective posterior spinal fusions, more stable constructs with pedicle screws, and postoperative protocols with earlier return to physical activity may help improve outcomes, but as of yet, data on this topic are limited.

Spondylolysis/Spondylolisthesis

Spondylolysis is a defect in the pars interarticularis and is most commonly found at the L5 level. It is by far the most common cause of back pain, accounting for up to 47% of cases in the adolescent population in some series.[51] The prevalence of spondylolysis is approximately 6% among whites and as high as 25% in the Inuit population.[52,53] Approximately 80% of cases are bilateral, whereas 20% of cases are unilateral. When a patient has an associated slippage of a vertebra in relation to the adjacent vertebra, the term "spondylolisthesis" is used.

Classification

Spondylolisthesis can be classified on the basis of either the type of the spondylolisthesis or the degree of displacement. The five types of spondylolisthesis are dysplastic, isthmic, degenerative, traumatic, and pathologic.[54,55] Of these, dysplastic (in which facet joints allow anterior translation) and isthmic (associated with a lesion of the pars interarticularis) types are most commonly encountered in children. Spondylolisthesis can also be classified by the degree of displacement in relation to the adjacent vertebra with use of the Meyerding grading system (shown in Fig. 138-6, with an example of a grade 3 spondylolisthesis), where 1% to 24% = 1, 25% to 49% = 2, 50% to 74% = 3, and 75% to 100% = 4. Cases in which the amount of displacement exceeds 100% are referred to as *spondyloptosis*.

History and Physical Examination

Spondylolysis is associated with sports such as gymnastics, volleyball, football, diving, and pole vaulting in which repetitive hyperextension occurs, but it is frequently seen in almost any sport. A typical history is one of activity-related back pain that is well localized to the lower spine, with radiating pain in the buttocks or legs in some cases. Approximately 40% of patients recall a traumatic event at the onset of pain.[56]

On physical examination, patients may have lumbar hyperlordosis. Conversely, they may have flattening through the lumbar region in cases of severe pain or a high-grade spondylolisthesis.[57] Patients with symptomatic spondylolysis/spondylolisthesis almost always have pain with standing spine hyperextension, especially during single-leg stance or with concomitant twisting. Hamstring contractures are commonly associated with spondylolysis/spondylolisthesis. In some severe cases, this condition leads to the abnormal gait pattern described by Phalen and Dickson[58] consisting of crouching, a short stride, and an incomplete swing phase.

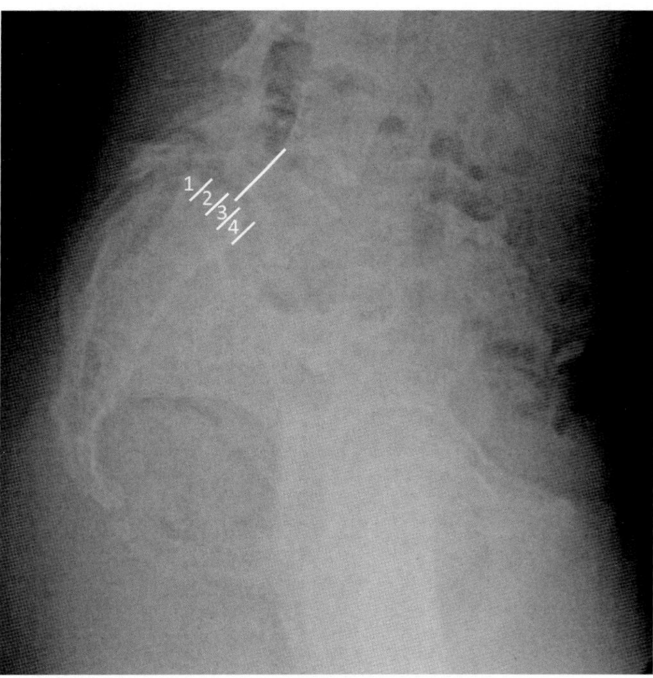

FIGURE 138-6 An example of grade 3 spondylolisthesis using the Meyerding grading system. This system describes the percentage of translation of the superior vertebral body relative to the inferior vertebral body. Grade 1 = 1% to 24%; grade 2 = 25% to 49%; grade 3 = 50% to 74%; and grade 4 = 75% to 100%. Cases in which the amount of displacement exceeds 100% are referred to as spondyloptosis. *(Courtesy Children's Orthopedic Center, Los Angeles, CA.)*

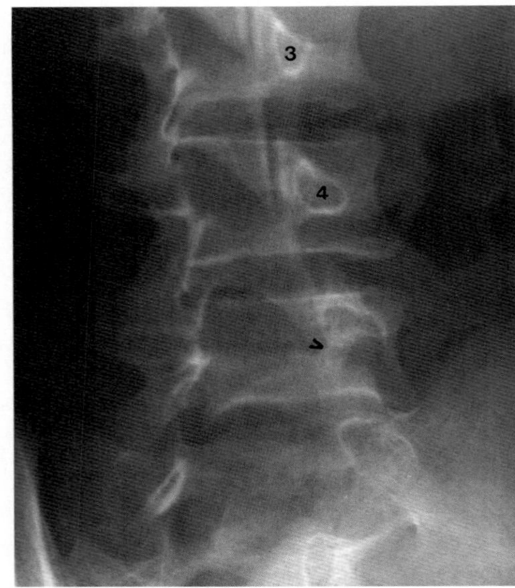

FIGURE 138-7 The characteristic "collar of the Scottie dog" observed on oblique radiographs. *(Courtesy Children's Orthopedic Center, Los Angeles, CA.)*

Imaging

A great deal of controversy exists regarding the optimal imaging modality for evaluation of spondylolysis. Although the characteristic "collar of the Scottie dog" observed on oblique radiographs is often difficult to appreciate, plain radiographs are commonly used as first-line imaging (Fig. 138-7). In some series, more than half of spondylolysis lesions (53%) can be missed on plain films alone.[59] A single photon emission CT bone scan is more sensitive for detecting defects of the pars but is nonspecific and thus is positive for other pathologic conditions, including infection, osteoid osteomas, and neoplasms.[60] Single photon emission CT also misses cold lesions. Consequently, our practice is to obtain a spot lateral of L5-S1 and then move directly to a limited CT if the signs and symptoms are consistent with a spondylolysis.

Since the advent and development of CT, many studies have verified that CT is more sensitive than plain radiographs in detecting early spondylolytic lesions.[61,62] Additionally, even in patients with radiographs that demonstrate spondylolysis, a CT scan may be helpful for treatment planning to assess the acuity of the spondylolytic lesion.[62] MRI has been suggested as another imaging modality for evaluation of spondylolysis, but the reported sensitivity ranges from 25% to 86%.[63-65] In our own series, we found that up to 64% of spondylolysis cases in symptomatic patients can be missed if MRI is the only diagnostic imaging study performed.[66] Consequently, it is standard protocol at our institution to obtain a limited CT scan when presented with a patient whose history and physical examination are suggestive of spondylolysis and an MRI scan that appears "normal."

Treatment

Most children have resolution of symptoms with conservative treatment consisting of activity modification and bracing. In acute cases, the goal is to achieve bony union. Rest and bracing should be continued for a minimum of 3 months. Although reports in the literature are variable, an estimated 75% to 100% of acute unilateral lesions and 50% of acute bilateral lesions heal (Fig. 138-8), whereas essentially no chronic defects heal.[57] Approximately 90% of athletes return to their prior level of sports participation at an average of 5 to 6 months,[67] which suggests that in many cases a fibrous union is sufficient for symptomatic improvement because the rates of returning to sport exceed those of bony union.[57]

No consensus has been reached regarding the type of bracing or protocol for wear. The Boston thoracolumbar sacral orthosis, an antilordotic brace, and braces with a thigh cuff have all been used. Some authors suggest that braces be worn for 23 hours a day for 4 to 6 months.[68] In general, when we are attempting to heal the fracture, our preferred treatment of patients with acute spondylolysis is to begin with an antilordotic brace worn any time the patient is weight bearing, including a thigh cuff if tolerated, for the first month. A lumbar sacral orthosis without a thigh cuff provides very little

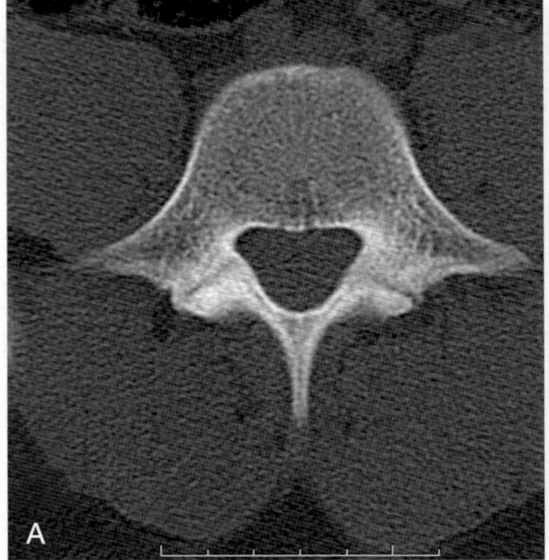

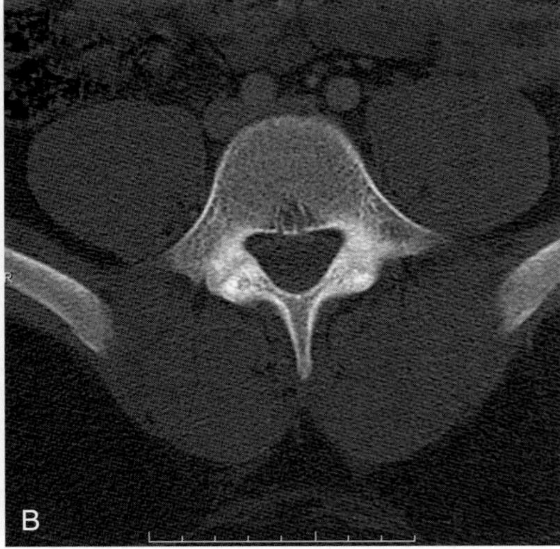

FIGURE 138-8 **A,** The presence of a bilateral pars defect on a noncontrast computed tomography (CT) scan consistent with a diagnosis of acute spondylolysis. **B,** A subsequent CT scan with contrast-confirmed healing of the defect after successful conservative treatment. *(Courtesy Children's Orthopedic Center, Los Angeles, CA.)*

immobilization to L5-S1. In acute cases, bracing is continued for 3 months and a limited CT scan is then performed to evaluate for bony healing prior to return to sport.

In chronic cases in which the bone does not heal, conservative treatment is based on symptoms. A variety of braces prevent excessive hyperextension of the lumbar spine. In some cases, patients can return to their prior level of activity while using such a brace. Core strengthening may play a role in long-term prevention of symptoms.

In cases in which the patient has unresolved pain after more than 6 months of conservative treatment, intolerance of conservative treatment, a greater than 50% slip of the spondylolisthesis, or severe neurologic symptoms, surgical intervention is considered. Numerous techniques have been described both for direct repair and for fusion of the involved segment. A direct repair should not be considered in cases of spondylolisthesis. Techniques for direct repair include Buck's technique of direct screw fixation across the pars defect, wiring between the transverse and spinous process, and pedicle screws with an attached sublaminar hook described by Kakiuchi.[69-71] Prior to consideration of a direct repair, an MRI scan should be obtained to evaluate the integrity of the intervertebral disk. If the intervertebral disk is abnormal, a fusion is preferred. Fusion may consist of a posterior only approach, with or without a transforaminal lumbar interbody fusion. A great deal of controversy continues to exist with regard to in situ fusion versus reduction of the spondylolisthesis. The increased neurologic risks of reduction must be weighed against the risks of implant failure, slip progression, and pseudarthrosis associated with in situ fusion.[72,73] See Figure 138-9 for our treatment algorithm for spondylolysis/spondylolisthesis.

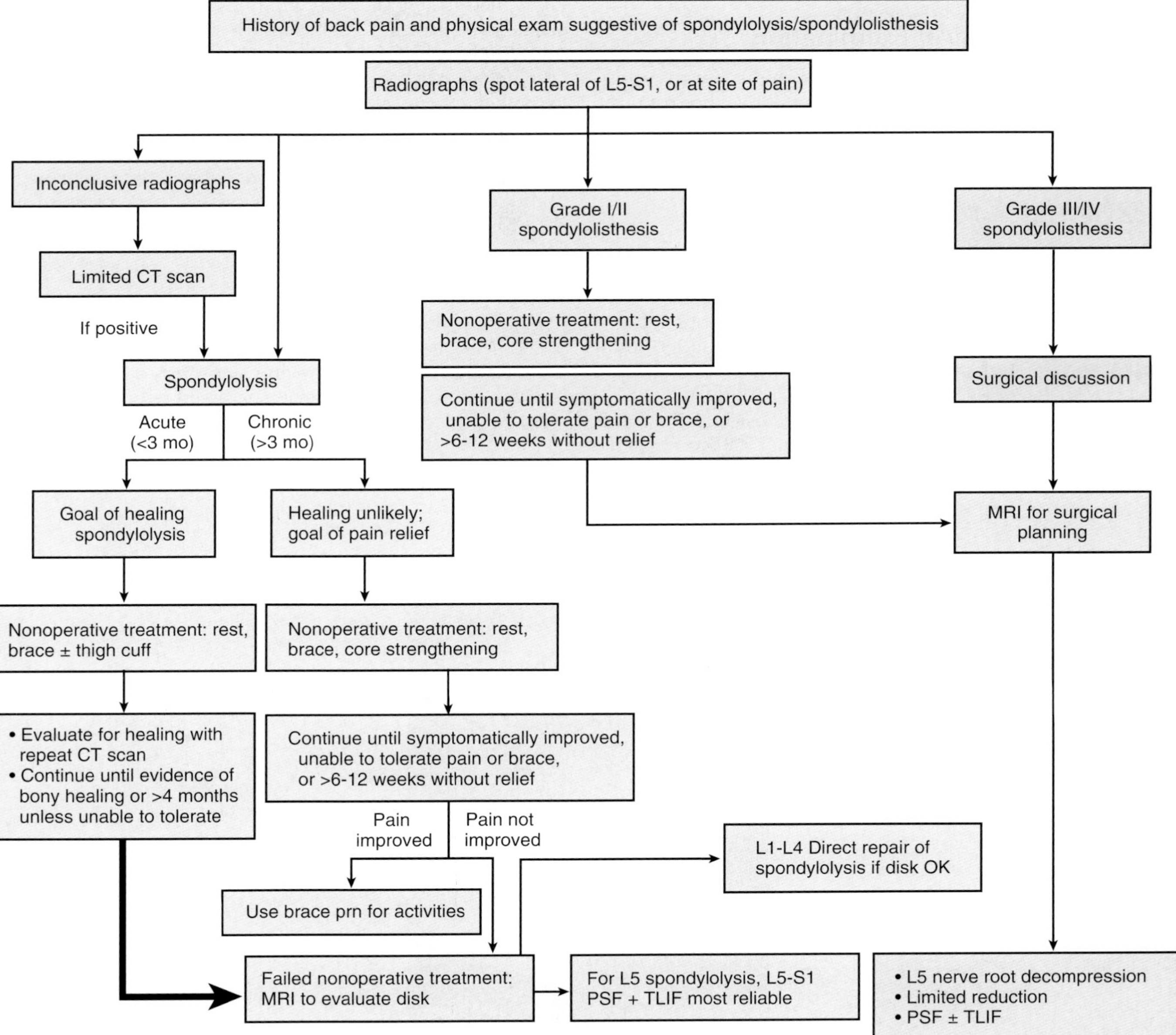

FIGURE 138-9 A treatment algorithm for spondylolysis/spondylolisthesis. *CT*, Computed tomography; *MRI*, magnetic resonance imaging; *prn*, as needed; *PSF*, posterior spinal fusion; *TLIF*, transforaminal lumbar interbody fusion.

Results

Rates of return to sports participation after surgical treatment are high, ranging from 80% to 100%.[74] Figure 138-10 shows an example of a patient treated with fusion who returned to a high level of sports participation.

Apophyseal Ring Fractures

The vertebral ring apophysis appears at the age of 6 years and fuses to the vertebral body at the age of 17 years.[75] Mechanical stress on the apophyseal ring can lead to a fracture of the vertebral growth plate, resulting in an apophyseal ring fracture. This clinical entity, unique to the immature pediatric spine, causes pain similar to that of a disk herniation.

History and Physical Examination

Pain is usually described as acute in onset and is often severe. Radicular pain is less common than in adult disk herniations because the injury is less likely to have a lateral component. A straight-leg raise test may be positive.

Imaging

This injury is often difficult to appreciate on plain radiographs, although such radiographs are generally obtained as an initial step in evaluating the patient with back pain. A CT scan allows accurate characterization of the osseous injury (see Fig. 138-11). MRI is generally obtained as well in these cases to allow for evaluation of the adjacent intervertebral disk and nerve roots. However, MRI scans frequently miss this injury or are misread as a disk herniation because the thin bony component of the apophysis may not be appreciated (see Fig. 138-11).

Treatment

In contrast to herniated disk material, the posterior endplate lesion is typically not absorbed. Although injuries with very small osseous fragments may be treated conservatively, such treatment usually results in severe pain for many months. The mainstay of treatment is surgical excision of the protruding fragment. A recent report by Higashino et al.[76] supports favorable long-term outcomes in patients with these injuries.

Sacral Facet Fractures

Sacral facet fractures are a rare injury but an important diagnosis to recognize. This diagnosis should be considered in the young athlete who has localized back pain with extension. This diagnosis may be easily missed on plain radiographs, bone scans, and MRI, which are frequently negative in these cases.[77,78] CT is the imaging modality of choice in cases in which this diagnosis is suspected. An example is shown in Figure 138-12. Authors of a recent case series of elite athletes reported that two of three patients had resolution of their back pain and return to sport after removal of the intraarticular fracture fragments by a minimally invasive muscle-sparing approach.[78] In the third patient, who had previously been a level 9 gymnast, the injury had occurred 2 years prior to diagnosis. This patient had a transient improvement in pain, but her back pain recurred and she was unable to return to competitive sports.

Conclusion

In addition to the injuries of the spine observed in adults, care of the pediatric spine includes consideration of these conditions. Evaluation of the growing spine may be challenging, but with appropriate treatment, successful return to sport can often be achieved in pediatric and adolescent athletes.

For a complete list of references, go to expertconsult.com.

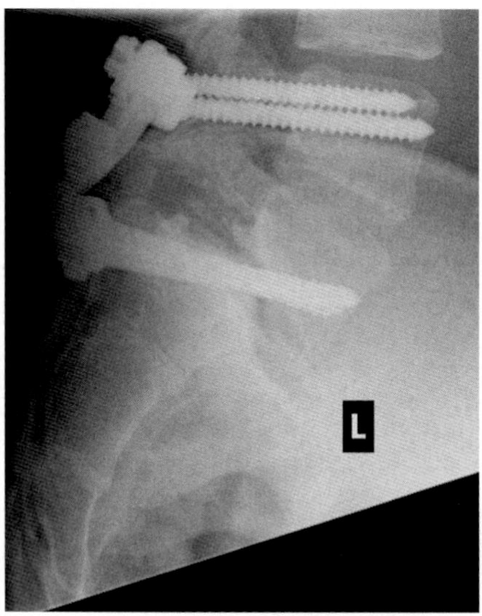

FIGURE 138-10 A postoperative radiograph of a 15-year-old boy who underwent an L4-S1 posterior spinal fusion and returned to basketball to receive a scholarship to play Division I basketball. *(Courtesy Children's Orthopedic Center, Los Angeles, CA.)*

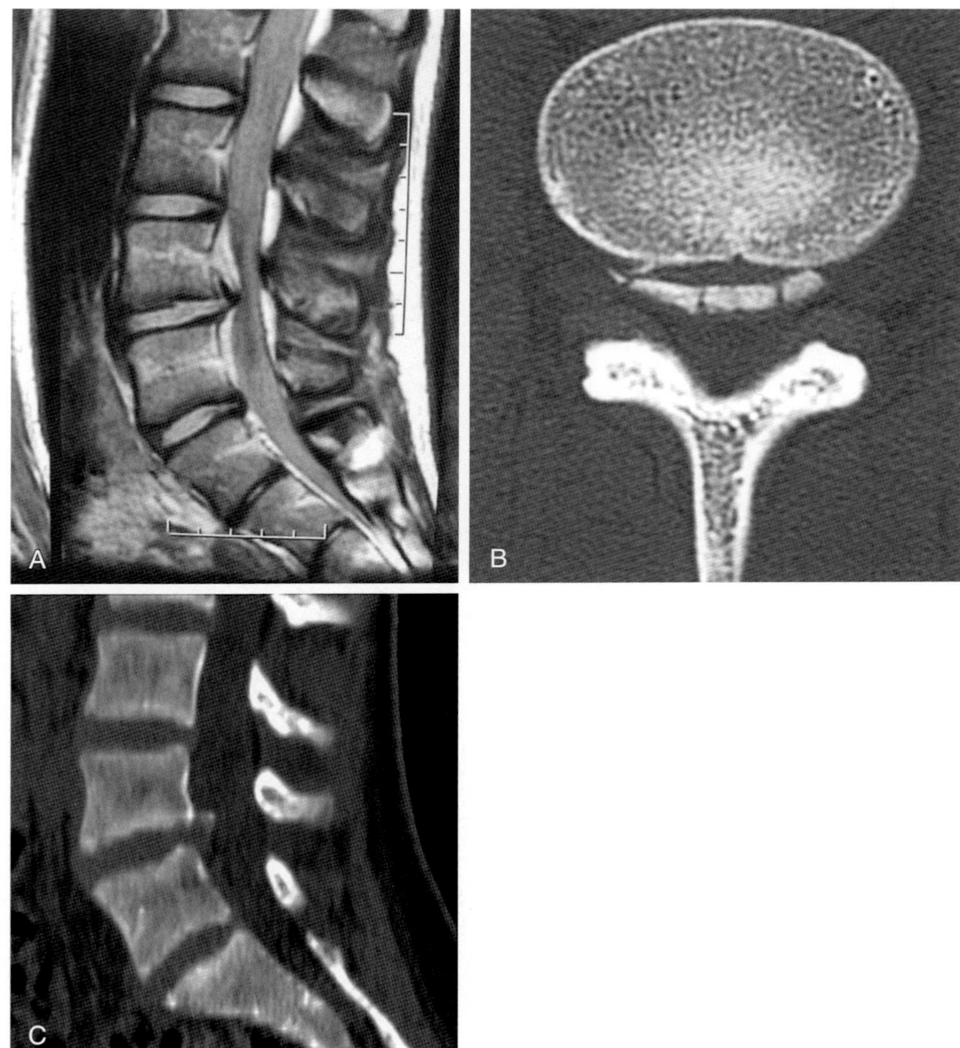

FIGURE 138-11 Magnetic resonance imaging (**A**) gives the appearance of a disk herniation, but a computed tomography scan (**B** and **C**) clearly shows that it is in fact an apophyseal ring fracture. *(Courtesy Children's Orthopedic Center, Los Angeles, CA.)*

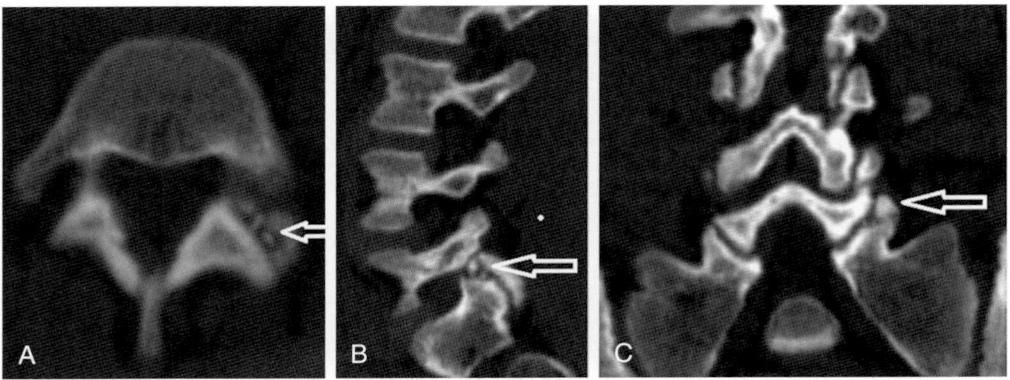

FIGURE 138-12 Magnetic resonance imaging scan (**A**) and A computed tomography scans (**B** and **C**) depicting a sacral facet fracture (*arrows*). *(Courtesy Children's Orthopedic Center, Los Angeles, CA.)*

Suggested Readings

Citation: Jackson RS, Banit DM, Rhyne AL, et al: Upper cervical spine injuries. *J Am Acad Orthop Surg* 10:271–280, 2002.
Level of Evidence: III
Summary: The authors describe the unique anatomy of the upper cervical spine, mechanisms of injury, and injury patterns and review nonoperative and operative treatment of these injuries.

Citation: Bull MJ: Clinical report: Health supervision for children with Down syndrome. *Pediatrics* 128:393–406, 2011.
Level of Evidence: V
Summary: This article includes guidelines from the American Academy of Pediatrics on caring for patients with Down syndrome and managing associated conditions.

Citation: Tokunaga S, Ishii Y, Alzawa T, et al: Remodeling capacity of malunited odontoid process fractures in kyphotic angulation in infancy. *Spine* 36:E1515–E1518, 2011.
Level of Evidence: III
Summary: The authors performed a retrospective study of odontoid fractures that occurred in children younger than 3 years of age with a minimum of 20-year follow-up; they compared these patients with 127 patients who did not have a history of cervical spine trauma. At final follow-up, patients who had sustained odontoid fractures did not demonstrate a difference in odontoid process tilt angle compared with control subjects.

Citation: Sankar WN, Wills BP, Dormans JP, et al: Os Odontoideum revisited: The case for a multifactorial etiology. *Spine* 31:979–984, 2006.
Level of Evidence: IV
Summary: The authors reviewed 519 cervical spine radiographs for cases of os odontoideum. A history of trauma was reported in only 8 of 16 cases, supporting the theory that two separate etiologies may exist for the os odontoideum: posttraumatic and congenital.

Citation: Grinsell MM, Showalter S, Gordon KA, et al: Single kidney and sports participation: perception versus reality. *Pediatrics* 118(3):1019–1027, 2006.
Level of Evidence: III/V
Summary: The authors report a combination of a survey of 135 American Society of Pediatric Nephrology members (level of evidence: V) and a review of literature on sports-related kidney injuries (38 articles; level of evidence: III). Although only one article reported one injury to a single kidney that was managed conservatively without sequelae, 62% of respondents said they would not allow sports participation by patients with a single kidney.

Citation: Launay F, Leet AI, Sponseller PD: Pediatric spinal cord injury without radiographic abnormality. *Clin Orthop Rel Res* 433:166–170, 2005.
Level of Evidence: III
Summary: The authors provide a metaanalysis of 392 published cases of spinal cord injuries without radiographic abnormalities and evaluation of the mechanism of injury, risk factors, treatment, and prognosis.

Citation: Weinstein SL, Zavala DC, Ponseti IV: Idiopathic scoliosis: Long-term follow-up and prognosis in untreated patients. *J Bone Joint Surg Am* 63A:702–712, 1981.
Level of Evidence: III
Summary: The authors provide a classic article on the prognosis of persons with idiopathic scoliosis that is untreated with an average follow-up of 39 years.

Citation: Fabricant PD, Admoni SH, Green DW, et al: Return to athletic activity after posterior spinal fusion for adolescent idiopathic scoliosis: analysis of independent predictors. *J Pediatr Orthop* 32(3):259–265, 2012.
Level of Evidence: II
Summary: The authors performed a retrospective cohort study of patients with adolescent idiopathic scoliosis in which 60% returned to sports at an equal or higher level of physical activity after surgery. A distal level of fusion, Lenke classification, and postoperative SRS-22 scores were each independent predictors of rate of return to the preoperative level of activity.

Citation: Hu S, Tribus CB, Diab M, et al: Spondylolisthesis and spondylolysis. *J Bone Joint Surg Am* 90A:656–671, 2008.
Level of Evidence: Instructional Course Lecture
Summary: The authors provide a review on nonoperative and operative management and prognosis of patients with spondylolisthesis and spondylolysis.

Citation: Higashino K, Sairyo K, Katoh S, et al: Long term outcomes of lumbar posterior apophyseal end plate lesions in children and adolescents. *J Bone Joint Surg Am* 94A:e74, 2012.
Level of Evidence: III
Summary: This study demonstrated a favorable outcome for pediatric patients with posterior endplate lesions in both operatively and nonoperatively managed cases with a mean follow-up of 14 years.

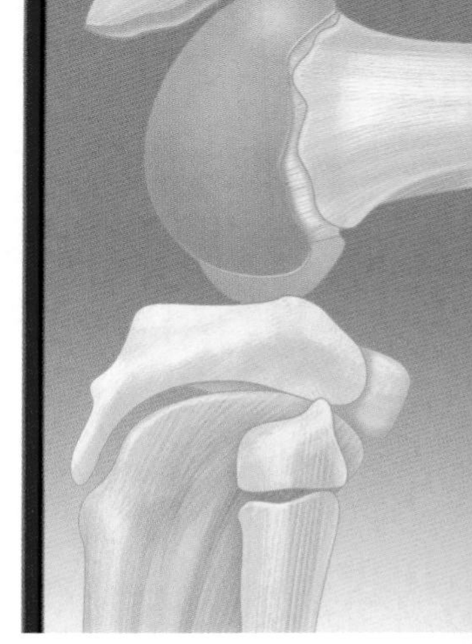

Appendix

Sports Medicine Terminology

DEAN C. TAYLOR • ROBERT A. ARCIERO •
DONALD T. KIRKENDALL • WILLIAM E. GARRETT JR

This appendix defines commonly used sports medicine terms and presents a basis for standardized orthopaedic sports medicine terminology. The language must be understandable for patients, health care providers, the media, orthopaedic surgeons, and sports medicine specialists. If we want to communicate our ideas to others, then we need to do so in a comprehensible way. If the language we use is ambiguous, confusing, contradictory, inconsistent, or filled with nonexistent words (as it often is), then our communication is ineffective, misleading, and potentially problematic.

The bases for the presentation of the material are not our own opinions or pet peeves. We have solicited suggestions from experts (editors of major orthopaedic journals and established medical editors) to assist in improving the language of sports medicine. We have attempted to synthesize the collective wisdom of sports medicine organizations to help develop consensus when possible. We hope that this appendix can serve as a starting point for standardizing sports medicine terminology and lead to further refinement of our unique language.

The use of consistent and proper terms helps research findings to be more accessible and understandable to the audience. But more importantly, misuse of the language can affect patient care. Physicians in the same group using different definitions of terms could compromise patient care when treating a common patient. This problem could also extend to supporting health care personnel such as nurses, nurse practitioners, physician assistants, physical therapists, athletic trainers, and others.

This appendix is divided into two segments—commonly accepted sports medicine terminology and some special topics, along with sports medicine classification systems. We point out common misuses of terminology. In situations in which there are good arguments for consensus, we recommend acceptance of the terminology or the classifications. If usage is conflicting, we point out the strengths, the weaknesses, or the limitations of the terminology or classification.

Sports Medicine Terminology

Sports medicine terminology is a highly descriptive mix of athletic, lay, and medical language. It is filled with athletic terms such as "jumper's knee," "tennis elbow," "skier's thumb," and "footballer's ankle," as well as common terms such as "shoulder separation" and "hip pointer." The language is colorful and has developed over time as prominent athletes, media personnel, trainers, and physicians have added their own terms, or misuse of terms, to the mix. This rich and vivid language can also be confusing because many terms are used improperly or have developed different meanings over time. For example, the media routinely confuse strain and sprain. Or how does a dislocation differ from a frank dislocation? What is a nonfrank dislocation, what is the "line" to be crossed when identifying a dislocation as "frank," and do all physicians understand where this line is? How about stomach versus abdomen? Do patients place their hands on their stomach or their abdomen? Unless they have an incision to reach into, it is probably their abdomen. Where is the line separating the lower abdomen from the groin? These examples may seem to be nonsensical, but misuse of such terms leads to confusion and miscommunication. For example, medical professionals are aware that humans have upper and lower extremities, not arms and legs (the upper extremity includes the arm and the forearm, and the lower extremity includes the thigh and leg).

Some definitions of commonly used sports medicine terms are listed in Table A-1. Some of these terms can be misleading. It may be difficult to eliminate these terms from our sports medicine language, but eliminating them is necessary if we are to improve our ability to communicate consistently. For example, how can one explain to a medical student that an athlete with tenderness of the proximal patellar tendon has a localized degenerative process, not an inflammatory process, when the terminology we use to describe the condition is "patellar tendinitis"? Maffulli and associates[1] have discussed this common incorrect usage of the term *tendinitis*. The Magellan Orthopaedic Society, the alumni society for the international sports medicine traveling fellowships, considered this terminology problem while attempting to develop an international consensus on the description of tendon problems. The Society decided that most overuse tendon problems are associated with noninflammatory degenerative-type changes in the tendon, which histologically should be called tendinosis. Inflammation around a tendon is more commonly tenosynovitis, such as in De Quervain or Achilles tenosynovitis. Because tendinitis, tenosynovitis, and tendinosis are all histologic diagnoses, however, these terms should not be used for the clinical diagnosis of an overuse tendon problem. Rather, the term *tendinopathy* is a better descriptor for the clinical diagnosis (see Table A-1). This distinction may seem insignificant to some people, but when terminology interferes with

TABLE A-1

DEFINITIONS OF COMMONLY USED SPORTS MEDICINE TERMS

Term	Definition
Abrasion	A worn-away area of skin
Arm	The part of the upper extremity between the shoulder and the elbow (sometimes used incorrectly in place of "forearm")
Arthritis	Inflammation of a joint (commonly used to describe arthrosis)
Arthrosis	Degeneration of a joint
Bursitis	Inflammation of a bursa
Cartilage	The tissue covering the articular surface of bones
Chondromalacia	Softening of articular cartilage (frequently used incorrectly for patellofemoral pain before operative inspection of the patellar articular cartilage)
Cramp	A painful spasmodic muscle contraction
Dislocation	Displacement of the bones of a joint from their normal position; usually implies loss of articulation of the joint surfaces that are normally in apposition
Forearm	The part of the upper extremity between the elbow and the wrist
Instability	A condition of increased joint motion due to ligament injury; a symptom
Laceration	An open wound, commonly referred to as a "cut"
Laxity	Looseness or slackness, usually when describing the character of a ligament; may be used when describing a normal or an abnormal ligament; a sign
Leg	The part of the lower extremity between the knee and the ankle (sometimes used incorrectly in place of "thigh")
Lower extremity	Thigh + leg + ankle + foot
Meniscus	Within the knee, a crescent or crescent-shaped tissue of fibrous cartilage
Operation	An act performed by a surgeon; a surgical procedure
Radiograph (or roentgenogram)	The image produced by passing x-rays through the body onto specially sensitized film
Sprain	Injury to a ligament as a result of an excessive load (sometimes used incorrectly to describe a muscle-tendon unit injury)
Strain	Injury to a muscle-tendon unit as a result of an excessive contractile or stretching load (sometimes used incorrectly to describe a ligament injury)
Subluxation	A partial dislocation
Surgery	The branch of medicine that treats injuries, diseases, and deformities by manual or operative methods, or conceptually, the work performed by a surgeon (often used incorrectly in place of "operation")
Tendinitis	Inflammation of a tendon
Tendinopathy	Disease process of a tendon
Tendinosis	Degeneration of a tendon
Tenosynovitis	Inflammation of a tendon sheath
Thigh	The part of the lower extremity between the hip and knee
Upper extremity	Arm + forearm + wrist + hand
X-ray (or roentgen ray)	The actual electromagnetic radiation used to make radiographs (commonly used as a synonym for radiograph)

accuracy when teaching students, residents, and patients, it is a real problem because our language loses clarity.

Another problem is the use of terms or phrases in the wrong context. Frequently, the term "strain"—an injury to a muscle—is incorrectly used to describe a "sprain"—an injury to a ligament—and vice versa. "Incidence" and "prevalence" are other terms that are sometimes incorrectly interchanged.

Two examples of the meanings of inappropriately used words being accepted and ingrained in our use are "arthritis" and "x-ray." *Arthritis* is often used incorrectly to describe a degenerative joint; the term *arthrosis* may be the accurate term. *X-ray* is commonly used instead of the accurate term *radiograph* to refer to the image made by radiography. We use these terms so frequently on a day-to-day basis that the incorrect meanings have become accepted. This acceptance then becomes a problem when we are communicating with newcomers to the sports medicine language and in formal writing and presentations. The correct terminology is defined in Table A-1.

Surgery is another word that is frequently used incorrectly in place of "operation," as in "The knee surgery we performed on the patient yesterday was a success." Surgery is defined as a field of medicine or the concept of the work performed by a surgeon, not an actual surgical procedure. An operation is the act performed by the surgeon. "The knee operation we performed…" is the correct usage.

Many times, commonly used terminology has evolved because a certain term may be easier to use than more accurate language. These terms are not incorrect but can be misleading. For example, it may be difficult to explain to a patient how tennis elbow can develop in someone who does not play tennis. In these cases, it is important to know the synonyms. The common usage is unlikely to disappear, but it is necessary to know the accurate terminology to improve understanding and for formal writing or presentation. Some examples of common terms and their associated precise synonyms and definitions are listed in Table A-2.[2]

TABLE A-2

COMMONLY USED SPORTS MEDICINE TERMS

Common Term	Precise Term
Break	Fracture
Bruise	Contusion/ecchymosis
Burner/stinger	Brachial plexus traction injury
Dead arm	Condition of transient episodes of upper extremity loss of function associated with recurrent, transient anterior subluxation (Rowe[2])
High ankle sprain	Syndesmosis ankle sprain
Hip pointer	Iliac crest contusion or abdominal muscle strain at iliac crest insertion
Jumper's knee	Patellar tendinopathy
Muscle pull	Muscle strain
Shin splints	Nonspecific term for leg pain; usually implies a condition of overuse; specific conditions (stress reaction, stress fracture, tendinopathy, exertional compartment syndrome, and the like) should be used as a diagnosis
Shoulder separation	Acromioclavicular sprain
Skier's/gamekeeper's thumb	Ulnar collateral ligament sprain of the thumb metacarpophalangeal joint
Tennis elbow	Lateral epicondylar tendinopathy

Other words that are used in a questionable context include the "-logy" words, such as pathology, morphology, and symptomatology. The -logy suffix comes from the Greek *logos*, meaning work or reason, and refers to the science or study of the subject designated by the stem to which it is affixed.[3] Thus the traditional meaning of the word "pathology" is the science or study of disease processes. "Morphology" refers to the science of the forms and structure of organisms,[3] and "symptomatology" refers to the science of disease symptoms.

Common usage has led to other definitions for these -logy words. A secondary meaning of pathology has become "the structural and functional manifestations of disease"[3]; for morphology, "the form and structure of a particular organism, organ or part"[8]; and for symptomatology, "the combined symptoms of a disease."[3] For example, orthopaedists frequently refer to intraarticular pathology when describing abnormalities in a joint or the appearance of a meniscal tear. These forms of common usage have become accepted in presentations and verbal communication but are not accepted by some journal editors. In addition, our communication will be easier if we can keep our language as simple as possible. Therefore we would recommend using the -logy words in their more traditional meanings. The common form of pathology could be replaced with words such as "injury," "lesion," "finding," or "damage." Similarly, "shape," "appearance," "structure," or "form" can replace morphology, and "symptoms" can be used instead of symptomatology. "Methods" should be used consistently, not "methodology," when referring to "the methods we used in our study."

"Suffer" is a word that is commonly used inappropriately, as in "the patient suffered a tibia fracture." This usage is more common in the lay media but is still present in medical writing and presentations. Inasmuch as the extent of suffering associated with injuries is often unknown and difficult to quantify, it is better to use the word "sustain" to denote an injury, as in "the patient sustained a tibia fracture."

Some nouns in sports medicine are now being used as verbs. Examples include scope or arthroscope ("we arthroscoped his knee"), biopsy ("we biopsied the lesion"), and radiograph or x-ray, as described previously ("we x-rayed his leg"). These usages are common in sports medicine but are not acceptable. The use of nouns as new verbs should be avoided in formal presentations or writing.

We can offer numerous other similar instances. Consider gender versus sex. Inanimate objects have gender in languages such as Spanish, French, and others, whereas sex is biologic. The more proper term for males and females is "sex," but many editors will ask that the word "gender" be used.

We also use many nonexistent words in sports medicine. This practice can make us look unintelligent and lead to poor communication, especially with persons for whom English may be a second language. At best, these terms sometimes become so ingrained in usage that they are adopted as accepted words. Some of the nonexistent words are listed in Table A-3.

Several common terms are incorrectly used in the plural form. For example, the phrase, "The data is shown in Figure 1," should be stated as, "The data are shown in Figure 1." Table A-4 provides some commonly misused plural forms of singular words.

Some terms remain controversial, and no consensus on usage exists. For example, the patellar ligament or the ligamentum patella fits the strict definition of a ligament in that it connects two bones, the patella and the tibia; however, as an extension of the quadriceps muscle group, it functionally acts as a tendon, the connection between a muscle and a bone, and can also be called the patellar tendon. Both usages are accepted and understood, but no consensus exists among orthopaedic journals with regard to which term to use. We use "patellar tendon" because the patella is a large sesamoid, and the collagen that extends distally from the patella acts as a tendon to extend the knee when the quadriceps muscle group contracts. Similarly, the flexor hallucis longus tendon extends distally from the plantar sesamoid bones to the head of the first metatarsal.

Sports Medicine Classification Systems

We create classification systems to improve our ability to communicate both clinically and in research. We also use the

TABLE A-3

NONEXISTENT WORDS COMMONLY USED IN SPORTS MEDICINE

Nonexistent Word	Correct Word
Allograph	Allograft
Crepitance	Crepitus/crepitation
Patulent	Patulous
Sublux	Suluxate or subluxation

TABLE A-4

COMMONLY MISUSED PLURAL FORMS OF SINGULAR WORDS

Singular	Plural
Bacterium	Bacteria
Basis	Bases
Criterion	Criteria
Curriculum	Curricula
Datum	Data
Fungus	Fungi
Maximum	Maxima
Medium	Media
Patella	Patellae
Septum	Septa
Sequela	Sequelae

classifications to help decide courses of action when presented with a clinical problem.

A few classification systems are widely accepted, make sense, and contribute to the understanding of a process. The Rockwood classification of acromioclavicular joint sprains is an example of a classification that is well accepted in North America.[4] The Seddon classification of nerve injuries (neurapraxia, axonotmesis, and neurotmesis) is also well accepted because the terms describe the extent of injury and are easy to understand and remember.[5]

Most of our classification systems, however, are plagued by the existence of other competing classification systems, by lack of acceptance, or by varied interpretation of the grading. These problems create a significant communication dilemma. When multiple classification systems are in place, using them is equivalent to a situation in which everyone is speaking different languages and no one knows which languages the others are speaking. For example, according to the Hughston classification,[6] a grade II medial collateral ligament knee sprain has no medial joint space opening with valgus stress at 30 degrees of flexion, but according to the Fetto and Marshall classification,[7] a grade II injury is "unstable … with a firm end point if chronic and soft if acute." When different classifications are used, understanding is impaired.

A system that is not widely accepted can be used to communicate only with those who understand and use the system. For example, if an English-speaking physician is trying to describe a Lauge-Hanson supination-eversion type IV ankle fracture to another English-speaking physician who does not know the Lauge-Hanson classification, communication will be as effective as if one of them were speaking a foreign language. When our goal is to expand education and understanding, it is not effective to have a language with limited acceptance.

Perhaps the worst situation is when a classification system has different interpretations so that one person may have a completely different idea of what another person is intending to communicate. This situation is common in communications about articular cartilage lesions. These lesions are usually graded I to IV based on the Outerbridge classification of chondromalacia patellae[8]; however, several modifications of the Outerbridge classification have been proposed, and these modified grading schemes are now applied to articular cartilage lesions throughout the knee and in other joints. As a result, in a lecture on cartilage injury, a grade II lesion may mean many different things to an audience, rendering the use of all the classifications ineffective.

The existence of confusion regarding classification systems is well recognized. Results of a 1997 questionnaire sent to Herodicus Society members showed that 97% of respondents believed that there was confusion in grading of knee ligament injuries (personal communication, Richard J. Hawkins, MD). However, even though the Society's members recognized that there was no agreement regarding the grading of injuries, 82% still used some type of classification. Although we need classification systems to communicate, many of the ones we have now are inadequate.

General Concerns

Lack of Consensus Regarding Grading and Measurement

Most classification systems in orthopaedic surgery and sports medicine have three grades—I/II/III, 1/2/3, or 1+/2+/3+. (What the "+" means in grading is unclear, but it has become a common part of the sports medicine language. One might think "1+" is greater than a "1" but not quite a "2." If so, then what is a "3+"?). The three-level method of grading is simple and easily understood. It generally provides information about the magnitude of injury or measurement. In medicine, these classifications are widely recognized to represent adjectives such as mild/moderate/severe, small/medium/large, or little/moderate/big. Therefore use of general grading scales usually leads to understanding, although it is often inexact. Communication could be greatly improved if descriptive words instead of numbers were used for the purpose of classification. In the story of Goldilocks, it is much better to talk about a papa bear, a momma bear, and a baby bear instead of a type III, type II, and type I bear. Similarly, it is clearer to describe a nerve injury as neurapraxia, axonotmesis, or neurotmesis instead of type I, II, or III.

In efforts to make the classification systems more exact, authors have applied quantitative values to the gradations. Differences of opinion have led to different classification systems based on differing magnitudes of the measurements used to define the classification grades. As a result, we find several different classifications in place and are unable to compare one study with another.

Because of the existence of many different classification systems, it might be reasonable to eliminate grading systems and instead quantify measurements precisely. The problem with this concept is that our measurements are so imprecise that comparisons between different examiners have little agreement. The members of the International Knee Documentation Committee clearly illustrated this point. When examining patients with different knee conditions, the International Knee Documentation Committee members differed appreciably in their measurements of translation on the Lachman test and grading of the pivot shift and reverse pivot shift tests.[9] Additionally, wide variability existed among examiners in how instability tests were performed.[10,11] Using different methods for making the same measurement affects the results, thus contributing to the general lack of agreement regarding the measurement values.

We have a significant problem in sports medicine if even the experts, such as the International Knee Documentation

Committee members, cannot agree on what is measured, how to measure it, or the results of the measurement. Partly for this reason, when the Anterior Cruciate Ligament (ACL) Study Group examined the problem of knee classifications in 2000, the members agreed that when examining a knee, providing a general description of the findings was better than providing exact measurements in millimeters. The group decided that better agreement could be reached with regard to the assessment of whether an ACL was torn and whether a collateral ligament injury was mild, moderate, or severe (grade I, II, or III) than with measurements of displacement during a physical examination in millimeters (personal communication, Richard J. Hawkins, MD). We agree that physical examinations can determine if an injury exists and can generally approximate the extent of injury.

Whenever possible, injuries, findings, and examination results for individual cases should be described in common language, and if measurements are reasonably accurate, they can be included in this description. Going back to the example of the three bears, it is much clearer to say that we were chased by an 8-foot (2.4-meter) male bear than by a type III bear, even if the bear in question was only 7 feet 6 inches (2.25 meters tall). More to the point, an articular cartilage lesion is better described as a 2 × 2 cm half-thickness lesion than as a type II or III lesion (depending on the classification system used) of the femoral condyle.

To provide some understanding of the language, the following subsections outline and clarify the qualities and deficiencies of the classification systems that have been created to (1) describe anatomic changes associated with pathologic conditions, (2) define physical examination findings, and (3) grade the extent of an injury.

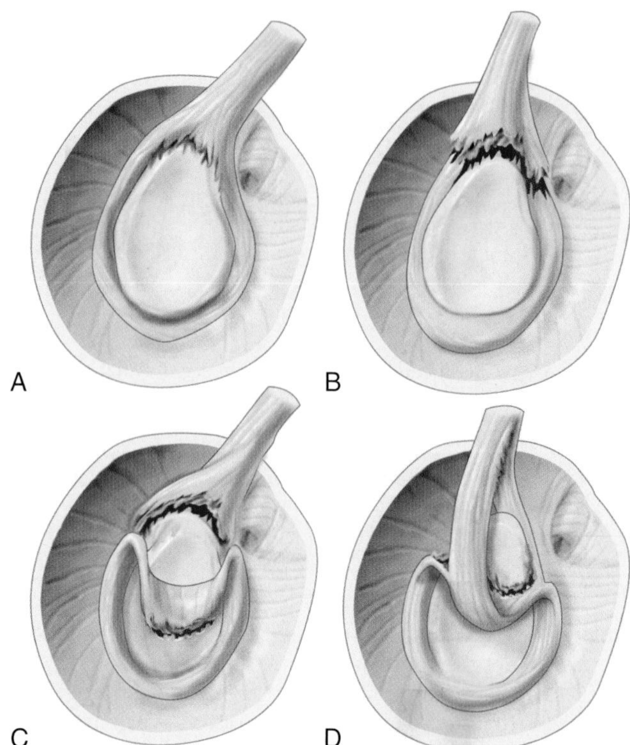

FIGURE A-1 Classification of superior labrum injuries. **A,** Type I, fraying and degeneration of the superior labrum. **B,** Type II, detachment of the superior labrum and the biceps anchor from the superior glenoid. **C,** Type III, bucket-handle tear of the superior labrum, with the peripheral labrum and the biceps anchor remaining intact. **D,** Type IV, bucket-handle tear of the superior labrum with extension of the tear into the biceps tendon. *(From Snyder SJ, Karzel RP, Del Pizzo W, et al: SLAP lesions of the shoulder.* Arthroscopy *6:274–279, 1990.)*

Classifications

Anatomic Changes Associated with Pathologic Conditions

Anatomic changes due to injury or disease that are seen repetitively intraoperatively or on imaging studies are often classified for research purposes or to assist in treatment. The following classifications are examples of these grading schemes.

Superior Labral Injuries

With the development of shoulder arthroscopy has come the realization that a severe injury to the superior glenoid labrum can be a source of symptoms. Snyder and colleagues[12] coined the term “superior labrum anterior to posterior” (SLAP), which has become associated with superior labral injuries. This term is so firmly ingrained in shoulder terminology that it is often used without clarifying the severity of the injury, the precise diagnosis, and a description of loss of function, and hence the acronym may be confusing for persons just learning about shoulder injuries. Snyder and colleagues[12] also described the classification of superior labral injuries (Fig. A-1).

Acromion Shape

Bigliani and coworkers[13] described various shapes of the acromion that are associated with impingement syndrome of the shoulder (Fig. A-2). These shapes are usually defined on a suprascapular outlet view radiograph. Obtaining a good outlet view can be difficult, and the shape of the acromion can vary depending on the angle of the x-ray beam. Therefore, as in any classification system, variability can exist in the measurements.

Radiographic Changes of the Knee

In 1948, Fairbank[14] outlined radiographic changes associated with previous meniscectomy (Table A-5).[15] These radiographic findings have come to be known as Fairbank's changes and are telltale signs of arthrosis that can follow partial or complete meniscectomy. Fairbank's changes are now commonly used to describe any radiographic evidence of arthrosis of the knee.

Articular Cartilage Lesions

In 1961, Outerbridge[8] published his classification of articular cartilage lesions associated with chondromalacia patellae. This classification has subsequently been used to classify articular cartilage lesions in general throughout the knee and in other joints. Furthermore, the Outerbridge classification has been modified on the basis of arthroscopic findings. The grading criteria of the Outerbridge classification have been modified and misquoted in various articles on cartilage injury. Others have attempted to use grading scales based on lesion depth,[16] shape,[17] and a combination of measures.[18,19] Noyes and

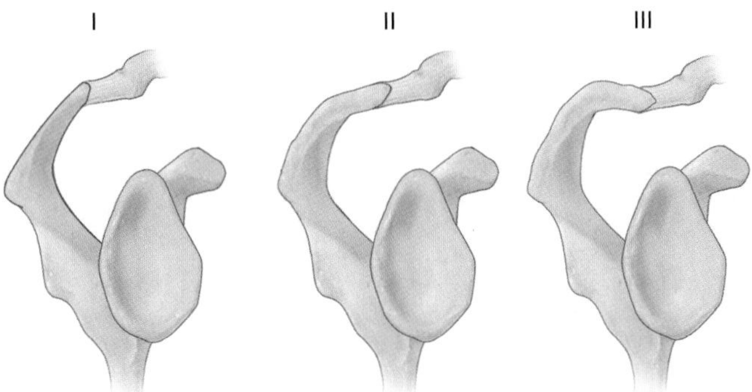

FIGURE A-2 Classification of acromion shapes. *I,* A flat acromion from posterior to anterior. *II,* The anterior acromion has an inferior curve relative to the remainder of the acromion slope. *III,* The anterior acromion has an acute angle, or "hooked" shape, relative to the remainder of the acromion slope. *(From O'Brien SS, Allen AA, Fealy S, et al: Developmental anatomy of the shoulder and anatomy of the glenohumeral joint. In Rockwood CA, Matsen FA, editors:* The shoulder, *ed 2, Philadelphia, 1998, WB Saunders.)*

Stabler[19] have reviewed many of the classification systems in their article describing their system.

Unless a clear definition exists of the classification system being used to describe a lesion, confusion will ensue. We propose that for simplicity's sake and for general understanding, the appearance of individual cartilage lesions be described by size, depth, and location; for example, a 1.5 × 2.0 cm partial-thickness lesion of the medial femoral condyle. When classifying a series of lesions in a research study, it is important that the classification be clearly defined. We suggest the Outerbridge classification for general research use when grading cartilage lesions because it is the original scale for cartilage injury, is widely accepted, and remains the best-known grading scale. The only modification we make is changing the cutoff between grades II and III from 0.5 inch to 1 cm because of the conversion to the metric system after the publication of the original article (Table A-6). In research, if the Outerbridge classification is not used, the classification that is used should be well described and defined.

TABLE A-5

FAIRBANK'S CHANGES

Term	Definition
Marginal ridge	Ridge or osteophyte formation at the margin of the outer aspect of the femoral condyle
Femoral condyle flattening	Flattening of the femoral condyle's normally concave curvature as visualized on an anteroposterior radiograph
Joint space narrowing	Narrowing of the space between the femoral condyle and the tibial plateau; usually best defined on an anteroposterior radiograph with the patient bearing weight; an anteroposterior radiograph taken with the patient bearing weight and the knee flexed 45 degrees is often helpful in demonstrating joint space narrowing and has come to be known as the Rosenberg view[15]

TABLE A-6

MODIFIED OUTERBRIDGE CLASSIFICATION OF ARTICULAR CARTILAGE LESIONS

Grade	Description
I	Cartilage softening and swelling
II	Fragmentation and fissuring, ≤1-cm diameter area
III	Fragmentation and fissuring, >1-cm diameter area
IV	Erosion of cartilage to bone

The International Cartilage Society has recently developed a rating scale to assess articular cartilage lesions. Although the use of this scale is increasing, interrater and intrarater reliability data are lacking.

Classification of Physical Examination Findings

Physical examination findings are frequently classified into different gradations, especially in the evaluation of ligaments and the translational or rotational changes that may result from injury. Noyes and colleagues[20] have provided clear definitions for much of the terminology that is used to document examination findings. Quantitative physical examination measurements should be described as translations or rotations and not as the amount of "laxity" in a particular ligament. Laxity implies the general slackness present in a structure and should not be used when discussing measurements. "Instability" refers to the presence of abnormal displacements between the two opposing bones of a joint as a result of traumatic injury. Like the term "laxity," "instability" should be used in a general sense. It is better to state that anterior translation is present on Lachman's examination than to say that 2+ laxity or 2+ instability of the ACL is present. Additionally, the history of traumatic injury to a joint and symptomatic excessive translations differentiates instability from laxity. In this sense, the term "multidirectional instability of the shoulder" sometimes is used incorrectly to imply generalized shoulder laxity in the absence of trauma.

In 1968, the Committee on the Medical Aspects of Sports of the American Medical Association (AMA) published *Standard Nomenclature of Athletic Injuries.*[21] Many physical examination grading scales and injury classifications used today follow the AMA guidelines. The grading for ligament testing is shown in Table A-7. Using this system, an 8-mm posterior drawer test would be graded as 2+, or grade II. Often the "+" is used to clarify that one is referring to a measurement grade and not a grade of injury, which is discussed in the next section.

This grading system for evaluation of ligaments can also be used to quantify joint space opening to rotational stress, such as valgus stress to assess a medial collateral ligament (MCL) injury of the knee or the elbow. In this case, 7 mm would be considered a 2+, or grade II, opening to valgus stress.

The following sections outline some commonly used physical examination grading scales.

TABLE A-7

GENERAL GRADING OF TRANSLATION/JOINT OPENING FOR LIGAMENT TESTING

Measurement	Grade
1-5 mm	1+ or grade I
>5 mm and <10 mm	2+ or grade II
≥10 mm	3+ or grade II

Shoulder Instability Examination (Translation)

Scapulothoracic, acromioclavicular, and glenohumeral motion combined provide the shoulder with tremendous mobility in positioning the hand, both in daily activities and in sports that involve throwing. Any attempt to quantify glenohumeral translation when evaluating a shoulder for instability is difficult because of these multiple articulations. The load and shift test[22] and the drawer test[23] are common methods that attempt to quantify the amount of glenohumeral translation. The presence of different classifications for the load shift test has resulted in confusion and difficulty in comparing studies in the shoulder literature. Additionally, different examiners conduct the test differently. Despite these problems, grading of the load and shift or drawer tests is useful to provide a general idea of the anterior and posterior translation of the humerus relative to the glenoid. For uniformity, we recommend use of the American Shoulder and Elbow Surgeons (ASES) grading scale for glenohumeral translation (Table A-8).[24] The ASES grading scale can also be applied to inferior translation of the humerus when evaluating the sulcus sign. The grading results are reported for each shoulder in isolation and not in comparison with the contralateral shoulder.

In 1990, Hawkins and Bokor[25] proposed a four-level grading of glenohumeral translation (Fig. A-3). In 1998, they subsequently modified this grading scale[24] (Table A-9), and this grading scale was then used as part of the ASES evaluation. Subsequently, McFarland et al.[26] and Bahk et al.[27] have described great interrater and intrarater variability when using the ASES grading scale. One of the reasons for this variability is that grading by tactile appreciation of translation short of subluxation (as in the original grading scale) is easier to identify than millimeters of translation (as used in the ASES scale).[24] In fact, a 0.3 greater reliability occurs if the grading of translation is based on whether the humeral head translates over either the anterior or posterior glenoid rim.[27] McFarland

TABLE A-8

THE AMERICAN SHOULDER AND ELBOW SURGEONS GRADING FOR THE LOAD SHIFT TEST

Grade	Humeral Head Translation	Degree of Translation
0	No translation	None
I	Slight up the glenoid face	Mild (0 to 1-cm translation)
II	Translation to the glenoid rim, but not over	Moderate (1- to 2-cm translation)
III	Translation over rim	Severe (>2-cm translation)

TABLE A-9

RECOMMENDED GRADING SCALE FOR ANTERIOR AND POSTERIOR SHOULDER TRANSLATIONS

Grade	Humeral Head Translation
1	Humeral head translation up to but not over the glenoid rim
2	Humeral head translation over the glenoid rim with spontaneous reduction
3	Humeral head translation over the glenoid rim without spontaneous reduction ("locked out")

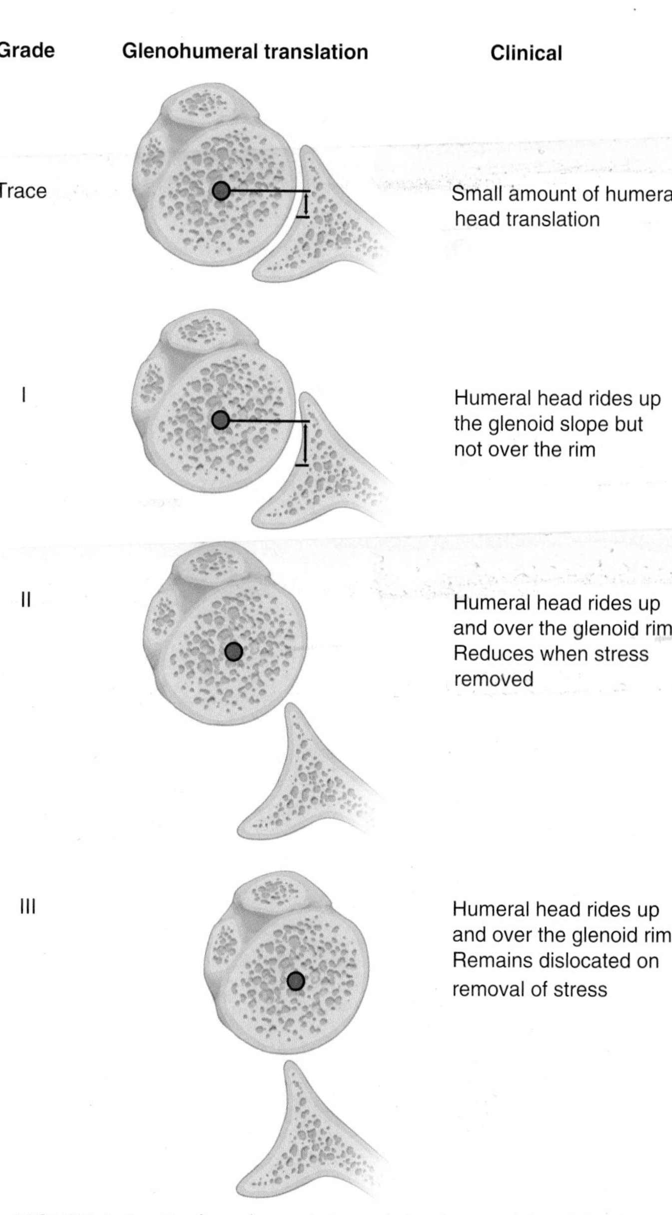

FIGURE A-3 Grades of translation of the humeral head in the glenoid fossa during the load and shift test. *(From Hawkins RJ, Bokor DJ: Clinical evaluation of shoulder problems. In Rockwood CA Jr, Matsen FA 3rd, editors:* The shoulder, vol 1, *Philadelphia, 1990, WB Saunders.)*

TABLE A-10

PIVOT SHIFT TEST

Grade	Description
I	Mild (also known as pivot glide), slight subluxation upon testing, but no "jump" or "shift"
II	Moderate; an obvious jump or clunk occurs with reduction of the tibia
III	Severe; a marked clunk is observed; the tibia may remain subluxated unless a reduction maneuver is used

also suggested that the lowest grades (trace and 1 in the first edition of the book or 0 and 1 in the second edition) be combined. When grades 0 (or trace) and 1 are combined, the intrarater and interrater reliability are improved.[26] Therefore we recommend using the classification system of Hawkins and Bokor as modified by McFarland et al.[26] for reporting glenohumeral translation (see Table A-9).

Inferior translation has been measured most commonly with use of an inferior traction force applied to the upper extremity as described in the sulcus sign by Neer and Foster.[28] As Bahk et al.[29] point out, the sulcus sign usually is graded as I (<1 cm translation), II (1.0 to 2.0 cm), or III (>2.0 cm). An alternative for describing the sulcus sign when measuring the amount of inferior translation is to simply use centimeters, which may be a more accurate method of communication.

Anterior Cruciate Ligament

The diagnosis of an ACL injury is largely based on two physical examination techniques—the Lachman test and the pivot shift test. The Lachman test can be based on manual examination, an instrumented examination, or radiographic analysis. The measurement in millimeters is usually the difference between the measurements in the injured knee and in the normal contralateral knee. Different grades have been described. We recommend the use of a three-grade scale based on grading described by the AMA (see Table A-7).[21]

Additionally, the end point is graded as A—a firm end point, or B—a soft, or not a well-defined, end point. Compared with the normal knee, a knee with 8 mm of increased anterior translation with a soft end point would be a grade IIB on the Lachman test.

Numerous descriptions and different grading schemes have been applied to the pivot shift test. Because of varying degrees of the pivot shift phenomenon, we have used a grading system (Table A-10) based on the classification of Bach and associates.[27] The one deficiency of this grading scheme is that a 2+ pivot shift encompasses a wide range of findings; however, this system allows the examiner to assign different grades based on the magnitude of abnormal examination findings.

Posterior Cruciate Ligament

The primary test for evaluating the posterior cruciate ligament is the posterior drawer test. Traditionally, the posterior drawer test has been graded similarly to other ligament tests (see Table A-7). Posterior tibial translation so that the anterior tibia is flush with the femoral condyles has generally been considered to be 10 mm of posterior translation, or the dividing point between a 2+ or 3+ posterior drawer findings. Obviously, patient size varies, and thus the flush position does not always equate to 10 mm of posterior translation. To improve the understanding of posterior drawer measurement, the "thumb sign" has been introduced. The examiner performs the thumb sign test by sliding his or her thumbs off the femoral condyles onto the tibial plateau. The test is graded as anterior, flush, or posterior depending on the position of the anterior tibial plateau relative to the femoral condyles. The consensus of the ACL Study Group was that the thumb sign was a better assessment than millimeters of posterior tibial translation in documenting the posterior drawer findings.

Collateral Ligaments of the Knee

The integrity of the knee collateral ligaments is assessed by applying a valgus (MCL) or varus (fibular collateral ligament) rotational stress to the knee positioned in 30 degrees of flexion. The amount of opening in millimeters of the medial or the lateral joint space is measured and is compared with the normal contralateral knee or is considered an isolated examination. The amount of opening is classified with use of the AMA grading scale (Table A-11) or by documenting the measurement in millimeters. Based on the ACL Study Group consensus, using the 1+, 2+, and 3+ grades may be the best way to communicate, especially because measuring joint space opening is not reproducible to within 1 or 2 mm.

Classification Systems Used to Describe Sports Injuries

General

Ligament

Ligament injuries are generally graded on three levels based on the AMA guidelines (see Table A-11).[21] This classification can be confusing because three grades also are used for measuring translation on the physical examination, as discussed in the previous section. Some authors use these translational changes to classify the extent of injury. This usage results in conflicting classifications and confusion, because they are not the same. For example, a grade I MCL injury of the knee will have no increased medial knee opening to valgus stress, but a grade II injury may have 1+ or 2+ medial joint opening to valgus stress. Additionally, some authors use their own grading

TABLE A-11

AMERICAN MEDICAL ASSOCIATION LIGAMENT INJURY CLASSIFICATION

Grade	Description
I	Mild, minor tearing of ligament fibers and no demonstrable increase in translation on examination
II	Moderate, partial tear of the ligament without complete disruption, with a slight to moderate increased translation upon examination
III	Severe, complete tear of the ligament, with a marked increase in translation upon examination

TABLE A-12

CLASSIFICATION OF MUSCLE STRAIN INJURIES

Injury Type	Swelling/ Ecchymosis	Defect
Interstitial strain	Absent	Absent
Intramuscular strain	Present	Absent
Partial rupture	Present	Present, incomplete
Complete rupture	Present	Present, complete loss of continuity

scales for ligament injuries. The lack of uniformity is the biggest communication problem in grading the severity of ligament injuries.

Muscle Strains

Currently, no good classification exists for muscle strain injuries. Unlike ligament injuries, partial disruption of a muscle-tendon unit is difficult to assess with mechanical testing; use of a scale similar to the ligament injury classification is therefore not exact. The physical examination findings that can be assessed in a strain are tenderness, muscle strength, swelling, ecchymosis, and the presence of a defect in the muscle-tendon unit. Based on these findings, muscle strain injuries can be classified as interstitial strains, intramuscular strains, partial ruptures, or complete ruptures (Table A-12). Interstitial injury without disruption of blood vessels or muscle fibers is the mildest form of strain. Mild to moderate tenderness and mild strength loss may be present, but the patient has no swelling ecchymosis or defect with an interstitial strain. Intramuscular injuries are the next-highest level of severity in muscle strains. In intramuscular strains, there is enough tensile force to cause limited muscle fiber and capillary disruption. The injury is usually localized adjacent to a muscle-tendon junction, where, because of the fiber disruption, swelling and possibly ecchymosis are seen. Tenderness and weakness may be moderate to severe, but a defect is not palpable at the injury site.

Persons with partial muscle ruptures have a palpable defect, and tenderness, weakness, and swelling may be more severe than in intramuscular strains. Persons with complete muscle ruptures have a disruption of all muscle fibers and a total loss of function of the muscle that is injured. Complete ruptures are uncommon injuries.

Nerve Injuries

Based on his extensive experience treating peripheral nerve injuries during World War II, Seddon[5] classified nerve injuries as neurapraxia, axonotmesis, or neurotmesis. Neurapraxia is defined as a "failure of conduction in a nerve in the absence of structural changes, due to blunt injury, compression or ischemia; return of function normally ensues."[3] Axonotmesis is a "nerve injury characterized by disruption of the axon and myelin sheath but with preservation of the connective tissue fragments, resulting in degeneration of the axon distal to the injury site; regeneration of the axon is spontaneous and of good quality."[3] Neurotmesis is a "partial or complete severance of a nerve, with disruption of the axon and its myelin sheath and the connective tissue elements; regeneration does not occur."[3]

Sunderland[30] classified nerve injuries into five types (see Fig. A-4). Types I and II are neurapraxia and axonotmesis, respectively. Types III to V represent increasing severity of nerve injury to complete transection.

Both classifications are used and well known. Seddon's classification probably has the greatest acceptance among all orthopaedists because of its descriptive nature and because it is simple and easy to understand. Sunderland's classification may be better accepted among hand surgeons and neurosurgeons because it provides additional clarification that can be helpful in deciding between treatment alternatives.

Specific Injury Classifications

Acromioclavicular Joint Injuries

Rockwood[4] has presented a classification for acromioclavicular joint injuries that is well accepted and commonly used. This classification is shown in Table A-13.

Medial Collateral Ligament

Several grading schemes exist for MCL injuries, and as a result, confusion ensues when trying to compare studies of these injuries. Many investigators use the AMA nomenclature for damage to the ligament as a basis for injury classification. Other researchers use the instability classification of 1+, 2+, and 3+ for grades I, II, and III. Hughston[6] clearly outlines how study results can vary because of differences in

TABLE A-13

CLASSIFICATION OF ACROMIOCLAVICULAR JOINT SPRAINS

Type	Description
I	AC ligament sprain only; interstitial without evidence of injury to the AC joint on radiographs
II	AC ligament disruption without injury to the CC ligaments; widening of the AC space on radiographs with minimal increase in the CC distance
III	Disruption of the AC and CC ligaments; increase in the CC distance on radiographs
IV	Ligaments injured as in type III with posterior translation of the lateral clavicle relative to the acromion and displacement of the clavicle into or through the trapezius muscle; posterior translation of the clavicle is seen on the axillary lateral radiograph
V	Ligaments injured as in type III with detachment of the deltoid and the trapezius from the lateral clavicle; a marked increase in the CC separation, with CC space 100% to 300% of normal
VI	Ligaments injured as in type III with inferior translation of the lateral clavicle; the clavicle is inferior to the acromion and coracoid on radiographs

AC, Acromioclavicular; *CC,* coracoclavicular.

Data from Rockwood CA: Fractures and dislocations of the shoulder: part II, subluxations and dislocations about the shoulder. In Rockwood CA, Green DP, editors: *Fractures in adults,* ed 2, Philadelphia, 1984, JB Lippincott.

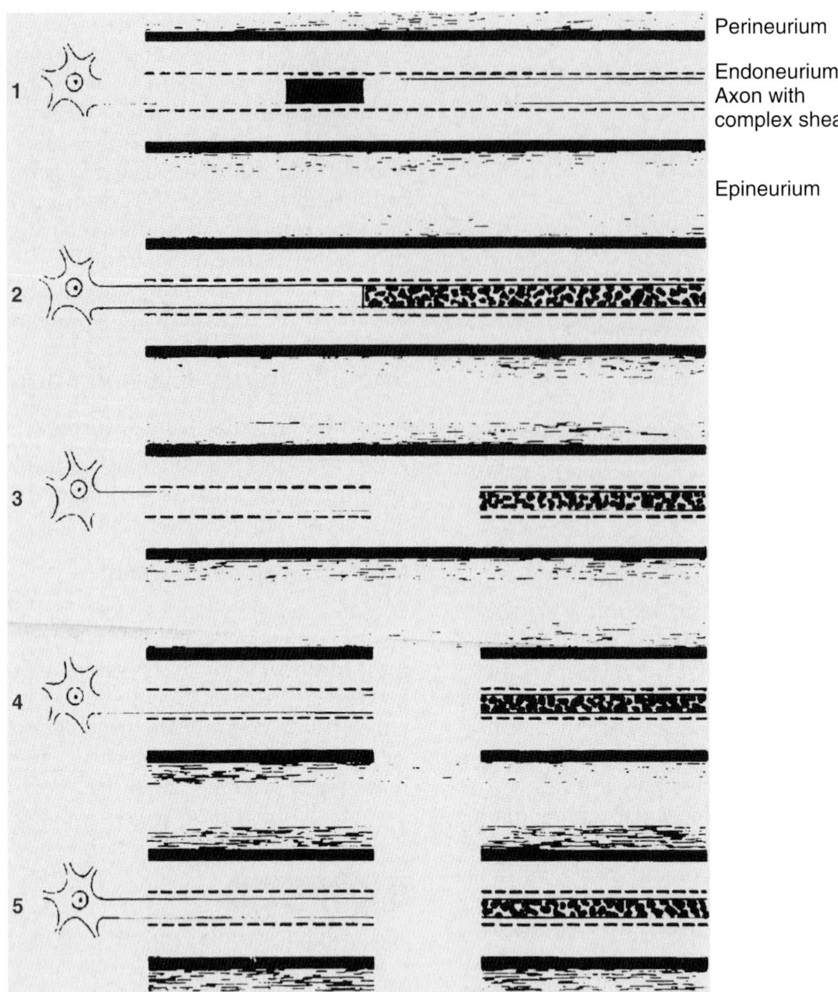

FIGURE A-4 The five degrees of nerve injury based on the Sunderland classification of peripheral nerve injuries. *1,* Neurapraxia is equivalent to conduction block. *2,* Axonotmesis is equivalent to intact endoneurium resulting in wallerian degeneration. *3,* Loss of nerve fiber continuity; the perineurium and epineurium are intact. *4,* Loss of nerve fascicle continuity; only the epineurium is intact. *5,* Complete nerve transection. *(From Sunderland S:* Nerve Injuries and Their Repair: A Critical Appraisal, *Edinburgh, 1991, Churchill Livingstone.)*

classification systems used. He compared several studies with his own work and found that each study had a different definition for a grade III MCL sprain. Hughston's classification is similar to that of the AMA; however, his interpretation is that only grade III injuries can have medial opening to valgus stress. Hughston further subdivides grade III injuries by the extent of the medial opening—1+, 2+, or 3+. According to the interpretation of other investigators, grade II may have increased opening of the medial joint space consistent with a partial tear (1+ or 2+ opening).

As Hughston[6] demonstrated, our understanding of the best way to treat MCL injuries is impaired by the use of various classifications. We recommend use of the AMA system because of its simplicity and the overall awareness of the classification. Based on physical examination findings, grade I (interstitial) injuries have no increased medial opening to valgus stress, grade II (partial injuries) have 1+ or 2+ opening, and grade III (complete tears) have 3+ opening. We recommend that authors clearly define their classifications, and readers should understand that many classifications exist so that the data are properly presented and interpreted.

Fibular Collateral Ligament

The grading of fibular collateral ligament injuries usually follows the standard I, II, and III scheme for ligament injuries. Instability is usually graded on the basis of the amount of lateral joint-line opening to varus stress with the knee in 30 degrees of flexion. Again, some authors use the instability grading as injury grading, which results in confusion and the inability to compare studies. We recommend use of the AMA guidelines for ligament injury, as described for MCL injuries.

Anterior and Posterior Cruciate Ligaments

It is unusual to classify ACL or posterior cruciate ligament injuries using the AMA nomenclature because identifying grade I injuries is difficult. ACL and posterior cruciate ligament injuries therefore are usually considered to be either partial or complete. Additionally, the method of treatment of cruciate ligament injuries is dependent on the presence or the absence of injuries to other knee ligaments. ACL and posterior cruciate ligament injuries therefore are usually classified as "isolated" injuries, with no other ligamentous injury evident on examination, or as "combined" injuries, if evidence exists of injury to the ACL and one of the collateral ligaments.

Ankle Sprains

Ankle sprains are usually separated into medial, lateral, and syndesmosis types. Grading of ankle sprains using the AMA classification can be difficult because often more than one ligament is involved. As a result, a "mild, moderate, or severe" grading scheme is usually used to document the severity of injury. The West Point Ankle Grading System[31] (Table A-14) provides guidelines for grade I, II, and III injuries.

Concussive Injury

Although brain injury is not an orthopaedic issue, recognizing and reporting these injuries is an important aspect of caring for athletes involved in contact and collision sports. Few injuries are as polarizing or are more confusing than a concussion injury. The earlier comments on the grading of injury are magnified here because of the lack of agreement on the definition of injury and the lack of standardization of terms.

Two primary concerns exist with regard to a concussive head injury: first, recognizing that an injury has occurred, and second, when to allow a player to return to play (which is beyond the scope of this appendix). Recognition of the injury is a function of the definition of the injury. The Concussion in Sport group offers this lengthy definition: "(1) Concussion may be caused by a direct blow to the head, face, neck, or elsewhere on the body with an 'impulsive' force transmitted to the head. (2) Concussion typically results in the rapid onset of short-lived impairment of neurological function that resolves spontaneously. (3) Concussion may result in neuropathological changes, but the acute clinical symptoms largely reflect a functional disturbance rather than structural injury. (4) Concussion results in a graded set of clinical syndromes that may or may not involve loss of consciousness. Resolution of the clinical and cognitive symptoms typically follows a sequential course. (5) Concussion is typically associated with grossly normal structural neuroimaging studies."[32]

After recognizing that an injury has occurred, many health care professionals will attempt to grade the severity of injury. Table A-15 shows three popular grading schemes (out of well over a dozen recognized scales). With most grading scales, each higher grade suggests a more serious injury to a specific location, such as in grading ligament injuries. In general, the higher the grade of injury, the more challenging the prognosis. As the aforementioned definition states, this injury is functional, not structural, and the presence or length of loss of consciousness is not prognostic of outcome. Thus using loss of consciousness or memory loss or other features as criteria for injury severity is problematic.

Many physicians who deal with concussive injury prefer not to use a grading system. They prefer simply to describe the injury as "concussion with less than 1 minute loss of consciousness" or "concussion with retrograde amnesia" because the qualifier is suggestive of where the functional

TABLE A-14

WEST POINT ANKLE GRADING SYSTEM

Criteria	Grade I	Grade II	Grade III
Evidence of instability	None	None or slight	Definite
Reaction to manual ligament stress testing	Mild to moderate discomfort	Moderate to intense discomfort	No pain or intense discomfort
Localization of Tenderness			
Lateral sprains	Mild to moderate over ATaFL only	Moderate to intense over ATaFL+ CFL	Intense over ATaFL + CFL+ PTaFL
Medial sprains	Deltoid only	Deltoid	Deltoid
Syndesmosis sprains	Distal syndesmosis only	Distal syndesmosis and proximally ≤4 cm	Distal syndesmosis and proximally >4 cm
Suspected disorder	Stretch to ligaments involved without macroscopic disruption	Partial tear/partial macroscopic disruption to ligaments involved	Complete tear of ligaments involved
Weight-bearing capability	Full or partial without significant pain	Difficult or impossible without supportive device (i.e., brace, tape, cane)	Impossible
Edema/ecchymosis	Well localized	± Localized	Diffuse
Syndesmosis sprains	Slight	Significant	Significant
Special Tests			
Squeeze or external rotation stress tests	Positive	Positive	Signs and symptoms of grade II sprain but will have mortise widening radiographically
Radiograph	No mortise widening	No mortise widening	
Edema	Minimal edema superior and anterior to lateral malleolus	Moderate edema superior and anterior to lateral malleolus	

ATaFL, Anterior talofibular ligament; *CFL,* calcaneal fibular ligament; *PTaFL,* posterior talofibular ligament.
Modified from Gerber JP, Williams GN, Scoville CR et al: Persistent disability associated with ankle sprains: a prospective examination of an athletic population. *Foot Ankle Int* 19:655, 1998.

TABLE A-15

CONCUSSION GRADING SCALES

Grade	Cantu	Colorado	AAN
1 (Mild)	No LOC PTA <30 min	No LOC Confusion No amnesia	No LOC Symptoms <15 min
2 (Moderate)	LOC <5 min or PTA >30 min	No LOC Confusion Amnesia	No LOC Symptoms >15 min
3 (Severe)	LOC >5 min or PTA >24 h	LOC	Any LOC Brief vs. prolonged

AAN, American Academy of Neurology; *LOC*, loss of consciousness; *PTA*, posttraumatic amnesia.

deficit is focused in the brain. Many grading scales are available, and no clear consensus exists on which scale is best. Assigning a grade to a concussion injury can be very confusing to patients and health care colleagues alike. Until a definitive grading scale is defined and validated, grading of concussion injury probably should be avoided.

Basic Statistical Terms

The language of statistics can be as confusing to orthopaedic surgeons as the language of medicine is to the lay public. However, in a profession in which advances are a result of research, proper understanding of some statistical terms is important because it affects decisions about the quality of research and whether results are meaningful to any particular physician's practice.

Provision of a statistics course is far beyond the scope of this appendix; however, we discuss basic statistical terms that are used on a regular basis and require an understanding for communication between professionals and patients alike.

Researchers communicate their results in three forms: as text, tables, or figures (notice there is no "and" in that statement). Text explains the data, tables present data in a small space, and figures augment through visual images the text table, and data. Statistics are most commonly encountered when reading a journal article or a chapter in a book or while listening to a research presentation. Statistics provide objectivity to research results and their interpretation, which makes them a key component of any discussion of research. Having a passing understanding of some basic statistical concepts is critical to being a wise consumer of research.

Reliability and Validity

The fundamental definition of reliability is the degree of consistency with which an instrument or rater measures a variable.[33] Within this definition are multiple levels of reliability. For example, one of the most common types of reliability is test-retest reliability (or intrarater reliability). A test is said to be reliable if measurements taken today and tomorrow by the same rater are similar. Another aspect of reliability is objectivity. Do two (or more) raters obtain the same results when administering a test? For example, do two different surgeons rate a manual muscle or range of motion or other clinical test the same? This aspect of reliability is sometimes called *interrater reliability*. Other aspects of reliability are internal consistency and split-half reliability, which are critical for development of a questionnaire.

The definition of validity is multifaceted. The most commonly applied definition is the degree to which an instrument measures what it is supposed to measure. In research, studies are designed to allow reasonable interpretations of the data based on controls (interval validity), definitions (construct validity), analysis (statistical validity), and generalizations (external validity).[33] Researchers generally need the assistance of a statistician to help with the design and analysis of a project to ensure that all the nuances of the research process are satisfied.

Samples and Populations

Research (especially clinical research) attempts to make some generalization about a population, and thus the population needs to be defined at the outset of a project. A population is the entire set of cases or units the study attempts to generalize, and a sample is a subset of the population under study.[33] Selecting the sample from a defined population requires special procedures to ensure a representative group of cases.

Dependent and Independent Variables

Almost all research projects include a variable of interest and a variable modified to affect the variable of interest. The dependent variable is assumed to depend on or be caused by another variable. The independent variable is the variable presumed to cause or determine a dependent variable—the variable manipulated or controlled by the researcher.[33] For example, an article is about outcomes after patellar ligament versus hamstring grafts for ACL rupture. The independent variable is graft (hamstrings vs. patellar ligament) and the dependent variable is outcome.

Power

Power is the ability of a statistical procedure to find a significant difference that really exists.[33] In planning a project, the researchers need to consider what difference is important, the inherent variability in the measurements, and the planned level of significance. When all this is known, the appropriate number of cases to detect the desired difference can be determined. This determination is probably the most commonly requested service of a statistician in the planning stages of a project.

Clinical Versus Statistical Significance

An article shows that there is a 0.8-degree difference in range of motion between two groups and that this difference is statistically significant. The question the reader might ask is whether this difference is of any practical significance and whether the researcher's methods are sensitive enough to detect such a small difference. One way that clinical significance is reported is through the use of confidence intervals, which allow the clinician to more easily determine if the detected difference is sufficient enough to warrant a change in practice. Part of the issue is the use of the word "significant." To avoid confusion in medicine and research, the use of the word "significant" should be reserved for statistical reporting and not be used as a synonym for "important," "critical," "distinctive," or other similar terms.

Proper use of the term "significant" does not provide much help in evaluating the magnitude of a difference, that is, the practical significance. For that, one can use effect size to assign a measure of the strength of a relationship or difference between two variables by complementing inferential statistics and the resulting *P* value. Although a number of methods may be used to arrive at the calculated effect size (the choice is dictated by the research question), when comparing differences between two groups, most methods are variations on the difference between means divided by some statement of pooled variability. The resulting effect is compared with tabled benchmarks. The classifications are most commonly small, medium, or large, but some researchers expand on this classification by adding extremes such as very small and very large effects. Thus including effect size (the method and benchmarks would be noted in an article's methods) in the example that opened this section might yield a statement such as, "Although the 0.8-degree difference in range of motion between the two groups was significant ($P = .03$), the intervention resulted in a very small effect." Although the calculations can look deceptively simple, it is best to consult a statistician to evaluate the research question, choose the appropriate statistic, and apply the proper benchmark.

Epidemiology Terms

Epidemiology is a special class of statistics that deals with the incidence, distribution, and control of disease in a population. Whether one is aware of it or not, the basic concepts are a common feature of dealing with colleagues and patients. Many basic epidemiologic statistics are based on the simple 2 × 2 table (Table A-16) that asks, in this case, if a diagnostic procedure actually does find the existence of a clinical condition.

Sensitivity Versus Specificity

Sensitivity and specificity are generally used to describe the utility of a test. Sensitivity is the fraction of true positives detected by a test (in Table A-16, that would be a/a + c). Specificity is the fraction of true negatives detected by a test (as d/b + d). For example, assume that a test has a sensitivity of around 70% and a specificity of 95%. This means that about 70% of people with the condition will have a positive test (the remaining 30% will have a false negative test) and 95% of people without the condition will have a negative test (the remaining 5% will have a false-positive test).

TABLE A-16

THE BASIC 2 × 2 TABLE

	Disease Present? Yes	**Disease Present? No**
Test positive? Yes	a	b
Test positive? No	c	d

Relative Risk and Odds Ratio

Relative risk (routinely abbreviated as RR) estimates the degree of an association between exposure to a condition and the likelihood of developing the condition in the exposed group relative to those not exposed.[34] In general, the RR is computed for prospective, randomized clinical trials or cohort studies. For example, change the rows in Table A-16 to exposure to some risk and the columns to the outcome. RR is calculated as [a/(a + b)] / [c/(c + d)]. Consider prior ankle injury as a risk of subsequent injury. Records are reviewed for injury history in a sample of athletes and then they are followed up over the course of some predefined duration. Exposure would be prior ankle sprain (yes/no) and the outcome would be a new sprain (yes/no). At the end of the study, if the calculated relative risk were 4.5, this would mean an athlete with a prior ankle sprain is 4.5 times as likely to sustain another sprain as a player with no prior ankle sprain. A relative risk of 1.0 means the rate of disease in the exposed and unexposed groups is similar. An RR greater than 1.0 is a positive association (a prior ankle sprain is associated with a subsequent ankle sprain) and an RR less than 1.0 is a negative association (greater flexibility is associated with fewer strain injuries). The odds ratio is a special case of relative risk and is usually used in retrospective or case-controlled studies.[33]

Prevalence Versus Incidence

Prevalence is the proportion of persons in a population with the particular condition at a specific point in time (e.g., as of today, how many residents of a nursing home have osteoporosis?). Incidence is the number of new cases that develop in a population during a defined time interval (e.g., how many new cases of osteoporosis are diagnosed in this nursing home during a 3-year period?)[33]

For a complete list of references, go to expertconsult.com.

Index

Page numbers followed by "f" indicate figures, "t" indicate tables, and "b" indicate boxes.

B

C

D

E

G

H

J

K

M

N

P

Q

T

U